JANUARY 1980 VOLUME 29 NUMBER 1

diabetes

E JOURNAL OF
E AMERICAN
BETES
SOCIATION

ORIGINAL CONTRIBUTIONS

Effects of glucose on insulin release and on intermediary metabolism of isolated perifused pancreatic islets from fed and fasted rats MICHAEL TRUS, HOWARD WARNER, AND FRANZ MATSCHINSKY 1

Morphologic study of cultured pancreatic fetal islets during maturation of the insulin stimulus-secretion mechanism RONALD W. DUDEK, NORBERT FREINKEL, NANCY JO LEWIS, CLAES HELLERSTRÖM, AND ROBERT C. JOHNSON 15

The glucose intolerance of acute pancreatitis: hormonal response to arginine SOLOMON S. SOLOMON, WILLIAM C. DUCKWORTH, PANDURANGA JALLEPALLI, MARY ALICE BOBAL, AND RAMAMURTHI IYER 22

Insulin degradation by mononuclear cells ALVIN C. POWERS, SOLOMON S. SOLOMON, AND WILLIAM C. DUCKWORTH 27

Effects of sodium DL-lactate on insulin secretion in anesthetized dogs G. FEDERSPIL, M. ZACCARIA, S. PEDRAZZOLI, E. ZAGO, C. DEPALO, AND C. SCANDELLARI 33

One month of sustained release of insulin from a polymer implant HALIMENA M. CREQUE, ROBERT LANGER, AND JUDAH FOLKMAN 37

Ten-year follow-up of subjects with impaired glucose tolerance: prevention of diabetes by tolbutamide and diet regulation GUNNAR SARTOR, BENGT SCHERSTÉN, SVEN CARLSTRÖM, ARNE MELANDER, ÅKE NORDÉN, AND GUNNAR PERSSON 41

Kinetic modeling of insulin binding to receptors and degradation in vivo in the rabbit MONES BERMAN, ELIZABETH A. McGUIRE, JESSE ROTH, AND ANTHONY J. ZELEZNIK 51

Diabetic neuropathy in the mutant mouse [C57BL/ks(db/db)]: a morphometric study DAVID M. ROBERTSON AND ANDERS A. F. SIMA 60

The histocompatibility (HLA) antigen distribution in diabetes in southern African blacks (Xhosa) BRIAN R. BRIGGS, W. P. U. JACKSON, ERNETTE D. DUTOIT, AND MARTIN C. BOTHA 68

Somatostatin concentration responds to arginine in portal plasma: effects of fasting, streptozotocin diabetes, and insulin administration in diabetic rats TSUTOMU KAZUMI, MASAFUMI UTSUMI, GEN YOSHINO, KAZUHIDE ISHIHARA, YOSHIKAZU HIROSE, HIROYUKI MAKIMURA, AND SHIGEAKI BABA 71

RAPID PUBLICATIONS

Stimulation of adenylate cyclase by Ca^{2+} and calmodulin in rat islets of Langerhans: explanation for the glucose-induced increase in cyclic AMP levels GEOFFREY W. G. SHARP, DAYNA E. WIEDENKELLER, DENISE KAELIN, EBERHARD G. SIEGEL, AND CLAES B. WOLLHEIM 74

Overnight basal insulin requirements in fasting insulin-dependent diabetics WILLIAM L. CLARKE, MOREY W. HAYMOND, AND JULIO V. SANTIAGO 78

The effect of aprotinin on the absorption of subcutaneously injected regular insulin in normal subjects MICHAEL BERGER, HANS J. CÜPPERS, PHILIPPE A. HALBAN, AND ROBIN E. OFFORD 81

Disparate effects of enkephalin and morphine upon insulin and glucagon secretion by islet cell cultures R. A. KANTER, J. W. ENSINCK, AND W. Y. FUJIMOTO 84

DIAEAZ 29(1) 1–86 (1980)
ISSN 0012-1797

Upjohn

Diabetes management and the problem of water retention

In the management of maturity-onset diabetes when diet alone fails, an oral agent should offer effective blood-glucose control, convenient once-a-day dosage, and potency. Tolinase® (tolazamide tablets, USP) offers all these and in addition does not cause fluid retention.

FEBRUARY 1980 VOLUME 29 NUMBER 2

diabetes

E JOURNAL OF
E AMERICAN
ABETES
SSOCIATION

ORIGINAL CONTRIBUTIONS

Prevention of hypophosphatemia by phosphate infusion during treatment of diabetic ketoacidosis and hyperosmolar coma ULRICH KELLER AND WILLI BERGER 87

Erythrocyte insulin receptors in non-insulin-dependent diabetes mellitus ROBERTO DePIRRO, ANGELO FUSCO, RENATO LAURO, IVANO TESTA, FABRIZIO FERRETI, AND CARLO DeMARTINIS 96

Development of adipose tissue in newborns of gestational-diabetic and insulin-dependent diabetic mothers G. ENZI, E. M. INELMEN, F. CARETTA, F. VILLANI, V. ZANARDO, AND F. DeBIASI 100

Insulin recoverable from tissues JOHN ENG AND ROSALYN S. YALOW 105

Hypothesis: the frequencies of juvenile diabetes in American blacks and Caucasians are consistent with dominant inheritance MICHAEL J. MACDONALD 110

Response: racial differences in juvenile-type diabetes are consistent with more than one mode of inheritance JEROME I. ROTTER AND SUSAN E. HODGE 115

Diabetes and cell growth—lack of differences in growth characteristics of fibroblasts from diabetic and nondiabetic Pima Indians BARBARA V. HOWARD, ROSE M. FIELDS, DAVID M. MOTT, PETER J. SAVAGE, M. NAGULESPARAN, AND PETER H. BENNETT 119

Stimulation of counterregulatory hormonal responses in diabetic man by a fall in glucose concentration RALPH A. DeFRONZO, ROSA HENDLER, AND NIELS CHRISTENSEN 125

Short-term regulation of insulin receptor affinity in man J. R. INSEL, O. G. KOLTERMAN, M. SAEKOW, AND J. M. OLEFSKY 132

Inhibition of gastric inhibitory polypeptide (GIP) release by insulin and glucose in juvenile diabetes W. CREUTZFELDT, M. TALAULICAR, R. EBERT, AND B. WILLMS 140

Streptozotocin-induced diabetes in athymic and conventional BALB/c mice G. BEATTIE, R. LANNOM, J. LIPSICK, N. O. KAPLAN, AND A. G. OSLER 146

Defective regulation of Cl^- permeability in islets of diabetic mice [C57BL/KsJ(db/db)] OVE BERGLUND AND JANOVE SEHLIN 151

RAPID PUBLICATIONS

Transformation of glicentin-containing L-cells into glucagon-containing cells by enzymatic digestion MARIELLA RAVAZZOLA AND LELIO ORCI 156

Direct evidence for downregulation of insulin receptors by physiologic hyperinsulinemia in man VIJAY R. SOMAN AND RALPH A. DeFRONZO 159

Influence of the age of erythrocytes on their insulin receptors JOHN ENG, LILLY LEE, AND ROSALYN S. YALOW 164

ORGANIZATION SECTION 167

FUTURE MEETINGS 168

DIAEZ 29(2)87–168 (1980)
ISSN 0012-1797

The merits of a simple

Compliance: the key to metabolic control

Metabolic control in maturity-onset diabetes requires adherence to a complex regimen.

This regimen often includes drastic changes in diet, substantial weight reduction, an exercise program, routine monitoring, and the daily use of medication.

Factors such as a language barrier, or lack of understanding of the disease, can lead to noncompliance—often the major impediment to successful management.

Therefore, the simpler the regimen, the greater the likelihood of compliance ... and the better the chances of metabolic control.

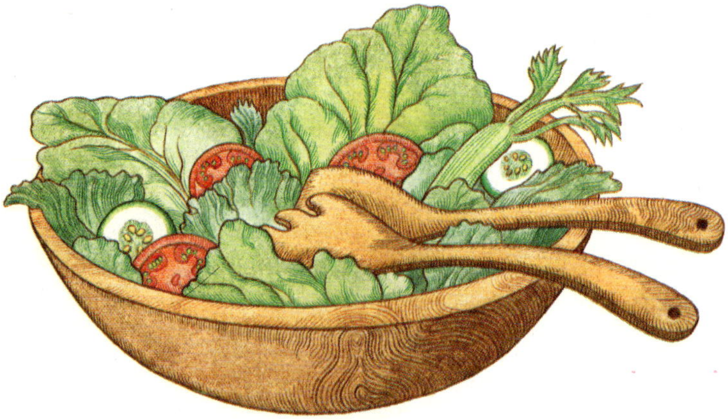

Diet: the essential element

Diabetic patients must follow strict rules regarding diet to achieve better blood sugar control and substantial weight loss.

These rules are often difficult to comply with.

More flexible approaches to diet—as reflected in the food "exchange" system and the restriction of total calories rather than carbohydrates—permit greater flexibility in meal plans and therefore enhance patient compliance.

Carbohydrates—which represent almost one-half the diabetic's diet—can be supplied by high-fiber foods.

These may satisfy hunger while reducing caloric intake and thus improve dietary compliance.

And data indicate that in some patients plasma glucose as well as lipid levels may be reduced by an increase in dietary fiber.

Monitoring: a new measure of control ... HbA_{1c}

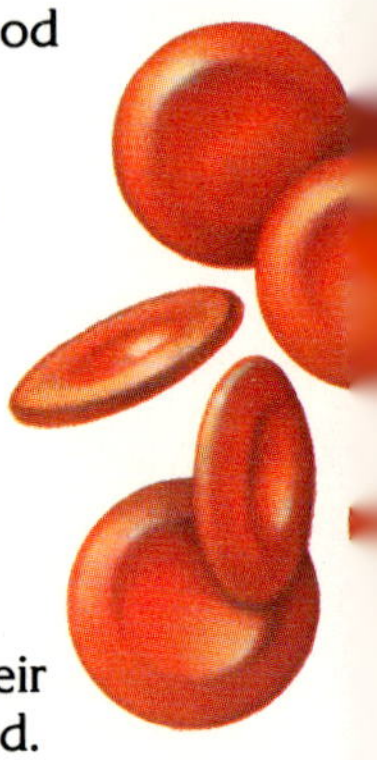

The measurement of hemoglobin A_{1c} (glycosylated hemoglobin) is one of the most important recent developments in the monitoring of blood glucose.

The concentration of HbA_{1c} is a measure of the ambient level of blood glucose that has interacted with hemoglobin over several weeks.

When blood glucose values are elevated above 150 mg/100 ml for any substantial period of time, HbA_{1c} levels begin to rise.

Glycosylated hemoglobin accumulates in the red cells during their 120-day life span and can be measured.

Hence, HbA_{1c} concentration reflects the time-averaged exposure of red cells to glucose.

While random postprandial blood glucose determination indicates the patient's glucose control at a given time, HbA_{1c} represents a reading of blood glucose for long-term evaluation of average blood glucose levels.

Thus, HbA_{1c} levels help the physician determine patient compliance.

Both HbA_{1c} levels and postprandial levels should be considered before making adjustments in the therapeutic regimen.

Exercise: more effective glucose utilization

Recent literature confirms the importance of exercise—from simple calisthenics to strenuous activities such as jogging—in the control of diabetes.

With a routine exercise program, insulin sensitivity may be improved and glucose utilization enhanced.

A specific exercise program should be developed with each individual patient.

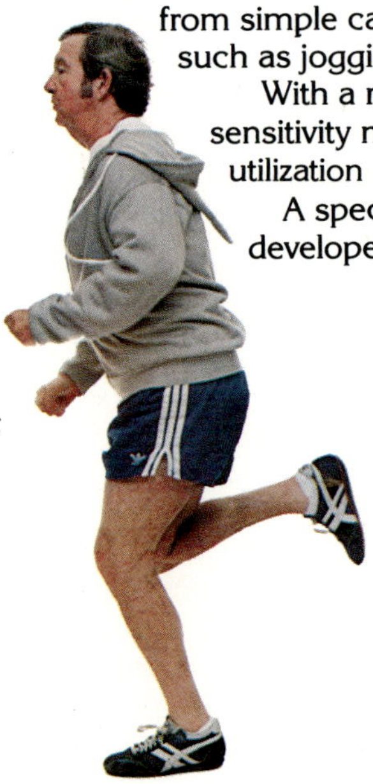

MARCH 1980 VOLUME 29 NUMBER 3

diabetes

E JOURNAL OF
E AMERICAN
BETES
SOCIATION

ORIGINAL CONTRIBUTIONS

Insulin resistance in obesity as analyzed by the response of glucose kinetics to glucagon infusion MLADEN VRANIC, SOICHIRO MORITA, AND GEORGE STEINER **169**

Ketonuria in pregnancy—with special reference to calorie-restricted food intake in obese diabetics E. J. COETZEE, W. P. U. JACKSON, AND P. A. BERMAN **177**

Reduced perikaryal volume of lower motor and primary sensory neurons in early experimental diabetes P. SIDENIUS AND J. JAKOBSEN **182**

A decreased response of cyclic adenosine monophosphate concentrations to glucagon in liver slices from streptozotocin-induced diabetic rats KAMEJIRO YAMASHITA, SOMO YAMASHITA, HIROKO YASUDA, YUJI OKA, AND ETSURO OGATA **188**

Mode of action of clonidine upon islet function: dissociated effects upon the time course and magnitude of insulin release V. LECLERCQ-MEYER, A. HERCHUELZ, I. VALVERDE, E. COUTURIER, J. MARCHAND, AND W. J. MALAISSE **193**

Glucocorticoid-induced recovery from streptozotocin diabetes in the adult rat MICHEL ROUDIER, BERNARD PORTHA, AND LUC PICON **201**

Continuous subcutaneous infusion of insulin in the management of diabetes mellitus M. C. CHAMPION, G. A. A. SHEPHERD, N. W. RODGER, AND J. DUPRE **206**

Inhibition of alloxan action in isolated pancreatic islets by superoxide dismutase, catalase, and a metal chelator L. J. FISCHER AND S. A. HAMBURGER **213**

Impaired glycogen synthase activating system in human diabetic polymorphonuclear leukocytes DAVID E. GOLDSTEIN AND RANDALL T. CURNOW **217**

Decreased insulin binding and degradation associated with depressed intracellular ATP content BORIS DRAZNIN, CLIVE C. SOLOMONS, CAROL A. EMLER, DON S. SCHALCH, AND KARL E. SUSSMAN **221**

Abnormal sciatic nerve *myo*-inositol metabolism in the streptozotocin-diabetic rat: effect of insulin treatment REX S. CLEMENTS, JR. AND CECIL R. STOCKARD **227**

Effects of exogenous fatty acid concentration on glucagon-induced changes in hepatic fatty acid metabolism J. DENIS McGARRY AND DANIEL W. FOSTER **236**

RAPID PUBLICATION

Nonaggregating insulin solutions for long-term glucose control in experimental and human diabetes A. MICHAEL ALBISSER, WILLIAM LOUGHEED, KUSIEL PERLMAN, AND ANDREJ BAHORIC **241**

ORGANIZATION SECTION **244**

FUTURE MEETINGS **245**

DIAEAZ 29(3) 169–245 (1980)
ISSN 0012-1797

The merits of a simpl

Compliance: the key to metabolic control

Metabolic control in maturity-onset diabetes requires adherence to a complex regimen.

This regimen often includes drastic changes in diet, substantial weight reduction, an exercise program, routine monitoring, and the daily use of medication.

Factors such as a language barrier, or lack of understanding of the disease, can lead to noncompliance—often the major impediment to successful management.

Therefore, the simpler the regimen, the greater the likelihood of compliance ... and the better the chances of metabolic control.

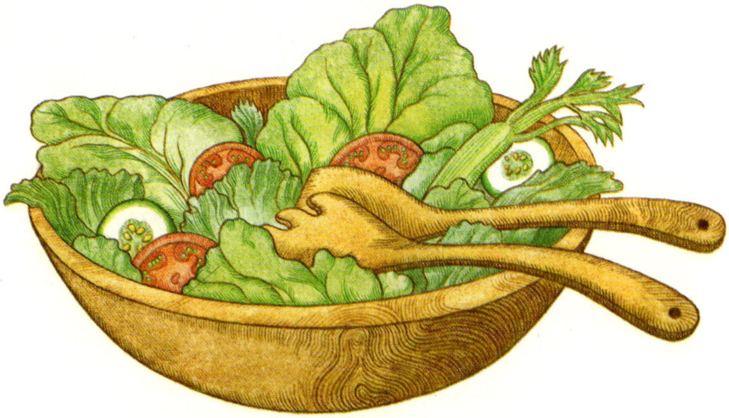

Diet: the essential element

Diabetic patients must follow strict rules regarding diet to achieve better blood sugar control and substantial weight loss.

These rules are often difficult to comply with.

More flexible approaches to diet—as reflected in the food "exchange" system and the restriction of total calories rather than carbohydrates—permit greater flexibility in meal plans and therefore enhance patient compliance.

Carbohydrates—which represent almost one-half the diabetic's diet—can be supplied by high-fiber foods.

These may satisfy hunger while reducing caloric intake and thus improve dietary compliance.

And data indicate that in some patients plasma glucose as well as lipid levels may be reduced by an increase in dietary fiber.

Monitoring: a new measure of control ... HbA_{1c}

The measurement of hemoglobin A_{1c} (glycosylated hemoglobin) is one of the most important recent developments in the monitoring of blood glucose.

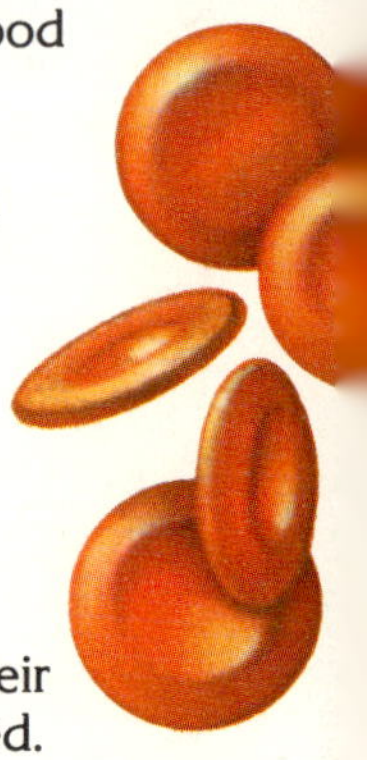

The concentration of HbA_{1c} is a measure of the ambient level of blood glucose that has interacted with hemoglobin over several weeks.

When blood glucose values are elevated above 150 mg/100 ml for any substantial period of time, HbA_{1c} levels begin to rise.

Glycosylated hemoglobin accumulates in the red cells during their 120-day life span and can be measured.

Hence, HbA_{1c} concentration reflects the time-averaged exposure of red cells to glucose.

While random postprandial blood glucose determination indicates the patient's glucose control at a given time, HbA_{1c} represents a reading of blood glucose for long-term evaluation of average blood glucose levels.

Thus, HbA_{1c} levels help the physician determine patient compliance.

Both HbA_{1c} levels and postprandial levels should be considered before making adjustments in the therapeutic regimen.

Exercise: more effective glucose utilization

Recent literature confirms the importance of exercise from simple calisthenics to strenuous activities such as jogging—in the control of diabetes.

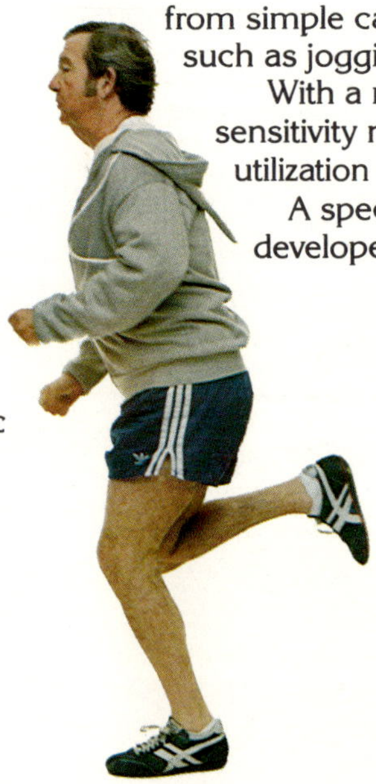

With a routine exercise program, insulin sensitivity may be improved and glucose utilization enhanced.

A specific exercise program should be developed with each individual patient.

APRIL 1980 VOLUME 29 NUMBER 4

diabetes

OURNAL OF
AMERICAN
BETES
SOCIATION

HLA-DRw antigens in Mexican-American and black-American diabetic patients ADINA ZEIDLER, JIMMY LOON, S. DOUGLAS FRASIER, DINESH KUMAR, ROBERT PENNY, AND PAUL TERASAKI 247

Metabolic activity of diabetic monocytes MITSUO KITAHARA, HARMON J. EYRE, ROBERT E. LYNCH, MARVIN L. RALLISON, AND HARRY R. HILL 251

Impaired responses of catecholamines, growth hormone, and cortisol to graded exercise in diabetic autonomic neuropathy JANNIK HILSTED, HENRIK GALBO, AND NIELS JUEL CHRISTENSEN 257

Beta-cell electrical activity in response to high glucose concentration PAUL M. BEIGELMAN AND BERNARD RIBALET 263

Effects of acute variation of fetal glycemia on glycogen storage and on glycogen synthase and phosphorylase activities in the liver of the rat fetus M. GILBERT AND J. BOURBON 266

HbA_1 in subjects with abnormal glucose tolerance but normal fasting plasma glucose GEREMIA BOLLI, PIETRO COMPAGNUCCI, MARIA G. CARTECHINI, FAUSTO SANTEUSANIO, CARLO CIROTTO, LUCIANO SCIONTI, AND PAOLO BRUNETTI 272

Effect of insulin, glucose, and 2-deoxy-glucose infusion into the third cerebral ventricle of conscious dogs on plasma insulin, glucose, and free fatty acids G. J. TABORSKY, JR. AND R. N. BERGMAN 278

Altered responsiveness to cortisol, epinephrine, and glucagon in insulin-infused juvenile-onset diabetics: a mechanism for diabetic instability HARRY SHAMOON, ROSA HENDLER, AND ROBERT S. SHERWIN 284

Effects of insulin and pancreatic polypeptide on gastric somatostatin release TSUTOMU CHIBA, TOMOHIKO TAMINATO, SEIZO KADOWAKI, HIROMI ABE, KAZUO CHIHARA, SHIGERU MATSUKURA, YASUO GOTO, YUTAKA SEINO, AND TAKUO FUJITA 292

Glycosylation of plasma protein and its relation to glycosylated hemoglobin in diabetes D. K. YUE, K. MORRIS, S. McLENNAN, AND J. R. TURTLE 296

Hagfish insulin: the discrepancy between binding affinity and biologic activity STEFAN O. EMDIN, OLE SONNE, AND JØRGEN GLIEMANN 301

Pancreatic islets: a tissue rich in serotonin JANICE L. BIRD, EUGENE E. WRIGHT, AND JEROME M. FELDMAN 304

Impaired granulocyte adherence in mildly diabetic patients: effects of tolazamide treatment J. D. BAGDADE AND E. WALTERS 309

Glucose and insulin responses to oral glucose in overt non-insulin-dependent diabetics with and without the islet cell antibody R. S. GRAY, W. J. IRVINE, E. H. D. CAMERON, AND L. J. P. DUNCAN 312

Complement-mediated cytotoxic effects on pancreatic islets with sera from diabetic patients HARRY G. RITTENHOUSE, DALE L. OXENDER, SUMER PEK, AND DIANE AR 317

Starvation-induced changes of somatostatin, glucagon, and insulin secretion from the isolated perfused rat pancreas SUSUMU SEINO, HIDEO SAKURAI, YUTAKA SEINO, KINSUKE TSUDA, KEIICHIRO TANIGAWA, HIDESHI KUZUYA, YASUO GOTO, AND HIROO IMURA 323

RAPID PUBLICATIONS

Diurnal episodic pattern of insulin secretion in the dog WALTER P. VANHELDER, ANNA SIREK, OTAKAR V. SIREK, KENNETH H. NORWICH, ZDENKA POLICOVA, AND TOMAS VANHELDER 326

Phenformin increases insulin binding to human cultured breast cancer cells D. COHEN, V. PEZZINO, R. VIGNERI, R. AVOLA, R. D'AGATA, AND P. POLOSA 329

ORGANIZATION SECTION 332

AZ 29(4)247–334(1980)
0012-1797

For the stable, maturity-onset
diabetic patient when diet alone has failed.

An effective choice to help control blood sugar

- ☐ Single or multiple dosing
- ☐ Two tablet strengths
- ☐ Documented bioavailability
- ☐ Severe hypoglycemia uncommon, but may occur*
- ☐ Twenty years of clinical use

Orinase®

tolbutamide, USP, Upjohn

0.25 and 0.5 Gm tablets

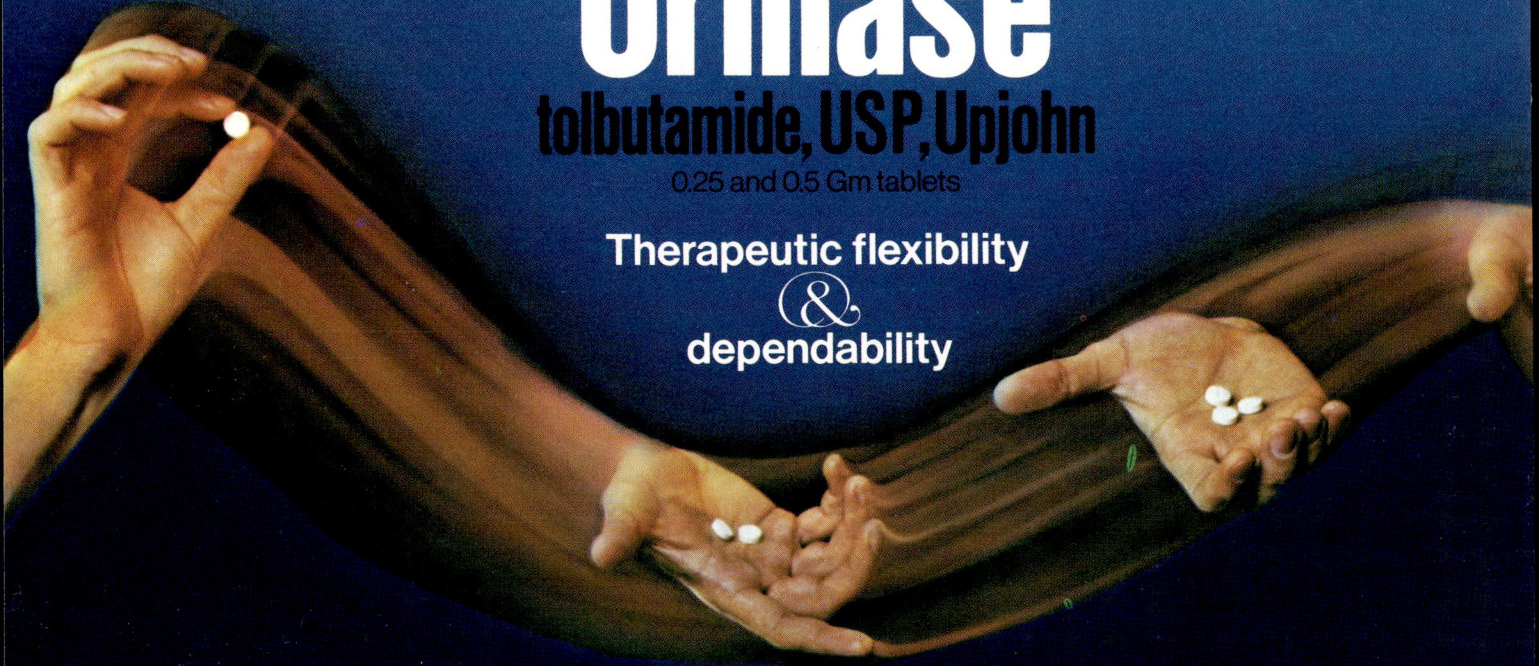

Therapeutic flexibility & dependability

Contraindications:
Orinase (tolbutamide) alone is not effective in juvenile or growth-onset diabetes nor in unstable brittle diabetes where insulin therapy is required.

Orinase tablets should not be used in diabetes complicated by acidosis, ketosis, or coma, or when a history of repeated bouts of acidosis or coma is obtained, in the presence of other acute complications such as fever, severe trauma, or infections, nor in patients with severe renal insufficiency. Insulin is indicated in these circumstances.

Pregnancy Warning: The safety and usefulness of *Orinase* during pregnancy has not been established. Animal studies have demonstrated feticidal and teratogenic effects. *Orinase* is not recommended for the pregnant diabetic, and should be used cautiously in women of childbearing age.

Precautions: Diagnostic and therapeutic measures necessary for optimal control with insulin are also necessary with *Orinase*. The patient on *Orinase* must be fully instructed about the nature, complications, and necessary personal measures needed to maintain control of the disease.

Caution: Very close observation, and careful adjustment of dose are necessary when: insulin is withdrawn during the trial period in order to avoid ketosis, acidosis, and coma; thiazide diuretics are administered, since they may aggravate the diabetic state and increase tolbutamide requirement, temporary loss of control, or even secondary failure; treating patients with impaired hepatic and/or renal function and debilitated, malnourished, or semistarved patients to avoid severe hypoglycemia; and treating patients with severe trauma, infection, or surgical procedures where temporary return to insulin or addition of insulin may be necessary. Beta-blocking agents reduce response to tolbutamide.

Patients must be under continuous medical supervision, and during the initial test period should communicate with the physician daily, and during the first month report at least once weekly for physical examination and definitive evaluation. After a month, examinations are recommended monthly or as indicated. Ketonuria, increased glycosuria, unsatisfactory lowering or persistent elevation of blood sugar, or poor clinical response indicate nonresponsiveness to *Orinase*. *Orinase* does not obviate the need for maintaining standard diet regulation. In treating mild asymptomatic diabetic patients with abnormal glucose tolerance, glucose tolerance tests should be obtained at 3-6 month intervals. *Orinase* is not an oral insulin or a substitute for insulin and must not be used as sole therapy *in juvenile diabetes or in diabetes complicated by acidosis or coma where insulin is indispensable.

Adverse Reactions: Severe hypoglycemia, though uncommon, may occur and may mimic acute neurologic disorders such as cerebral thrombosis. Certain factors such as hepatic and renal disease, malnutrition, advanced age, alcohol ingestion, and adrenal and pituitary insufficiency may predispose to hypoglycemia. Certain drugs such as insulin, sulfonamides, oxyphenbutazone, salicylates, probenecid, monamine oxidase inhibitors, phenylbutazone, bishydroxycoumarin, and phenyramidol may prolong or enhance the action of *Orinase* (tolbutamide) and increase risk of hypoglycemia. *Orinase* long-term therapy has been reported to reduce RAI uptake without producing clinical hypothyroidism or thyroid enlargement. High doses are mildly goitrogenic in animals. Photosensitivity reactions, disulfiram-like reactions after alcohol ingestion, and false positive tests for urine albumin have been reported.

Although usually not serious, gastrointestinal disturbances (nausea, epigastric fullness, and heartburn) and headache appear to be dose related and frequently disappear with reduction of dose or administration with meals. Allergic skin reactions (pruritus, erythema, urticaria, and morbilliform or maculopapular eruptions) are transient, usually not serious, and frequently disappear with continued administration. *Orinase* should be discontinued if skin reactions persist. Reports indicate that long-term use of *Orinase* has no appreciable effect on body weight.

Orinase appears to be remarkably free from gross clinical toxicity. Crystalluria or other renal abnormalities have not been observed, incidence of liver dysfunction is remarkably low, and jaundice has been rare and cleared readily on discontinuation of drug (carcinoma of the pancreas or other biliary obstruction should be ruled out in persistent jaundice).

Leukopenia, agranulocytosis, thrombocytopenia, hemolytic anemia, aplastic anemia, pancytopenia, and hepatic porphyria and porphyria cutanea tarda have been reported.

How Supplied: *250 mg Tablets* — bottle of 100, *0.5 Gram Tablets* — bottles of 50, 100, 200, 500 or 1000, Unit-Dose packages of 100, and Unit-of-Use packages of 30.

For additional product information, see your Upjohn representative or consult the package insert.

MED B-7-S

Upjohn

MAY 1980 VOLUME 29 NUMBER 5

diabetes

JOURNAL OF
E AMERICAN
BETES
SOCIATION

ORIGINAL CONTRIBUTIONS

Potentiation of insulin secretion to nonglucose stimuli in normal man by tolbutamide MICHAEL A. PFEIFER, JEFFREY B. HALTER, RON GRAF, AND DANIEL PORTE, JR. 335

Effects of intraportal islet transplantation on the transplanted tissue and the recipient pancreas. I. Functional studies E. R. TRIMBLE, C. KARAKASH, F. MALAISSE-LAGAE, I. VASSUTINE, L. ORCI, AND A. E. RENOLD 341

Clearance rates of metabolizable and nonmetabolizable sugars in insulin-infused dogs and in exercising dogs B. ISSEKUTZ, JR. 348

Effect of adrenergic agents on the secretion of gastrointestinal immunoreactive glucagon in depancreatized dogs TOSHIHIDE YOSHIDA AND MOTOHARU KONDO 355

Duodenal contribution to pancreaticoduodenal vein islet hormones during stimulation of the canine pancreas with calcium K. HERMANSEN 361

Effects of therapy on the nature and quantity of fuels oxidized during diabetic ketoacidosis O. E. OWEN, V. E. TRAPP, G. A. REICHARD, JR., M. A. MOZZOLI, R. SMITH, AND G. BODEN 365

A comparison of basal and insulin-stimulated glucose transport in rat adipocyte plasma membranes CARL LUDVIGSEN AND LEONARD JARETT 373

Effects of indomethacin on acute insulin release in man ERIC TOPOL AND ROBERT G. BRODOWS 379

Induction of hyperglycemia with insulin antibodies to B-chain determinants JOHN M. KELSO, IRENE Y. TAMAI, MICHAEL D. ROTH, IGNACIO VALDES, AND EDWARD R. ARQUILLA 383

Integrated concentration of growth hormone in juvenile-onset diabetes JOHN T. HAYFORD, MARK M. DANNEY, JAMES A. HENDRIX, AND ROBERT G. THOMPSON 391

REVIEW

Insulin action and the regulation of hexose transport MICHAEL P. CZECH 399

RAPID PUBLICATIONS

Pirogliride: an oral hypoglycemic drug which accelerates glucose usage and insulin secretion by islets of Langerhans WALTER S. ZAWALICH, VICTORIA A. WEILL, AND FRANZ M. MATSCHINSKY 410

Nonenzymatically glycosylated serum protein: spurious elevation due to free glucose in serum ALLAN LAURENCE KENNEDY, THOMAS D. MEHL, AND THOMAS J. MERIMEE 413

ORGANIZATION SECTION 416

DIAEAZ 29(5)335–416 (1980
ISSN 0012-1797

For the stable, maturity-onset diabetic patient when diet alone has failed.

An effective choice to help control blood sugar

- ☐ Single or multiple dosing
- ☐ Two tablet strengths
- ☐ Documented bioavailability
- ☐ Severe hypoglycemia uncommon, but may occur*
- ☐ Twenty years of clinical use

Orinase®

tolbutamide, USP, Upjohn

0.25 and 0.5 Gm tablets

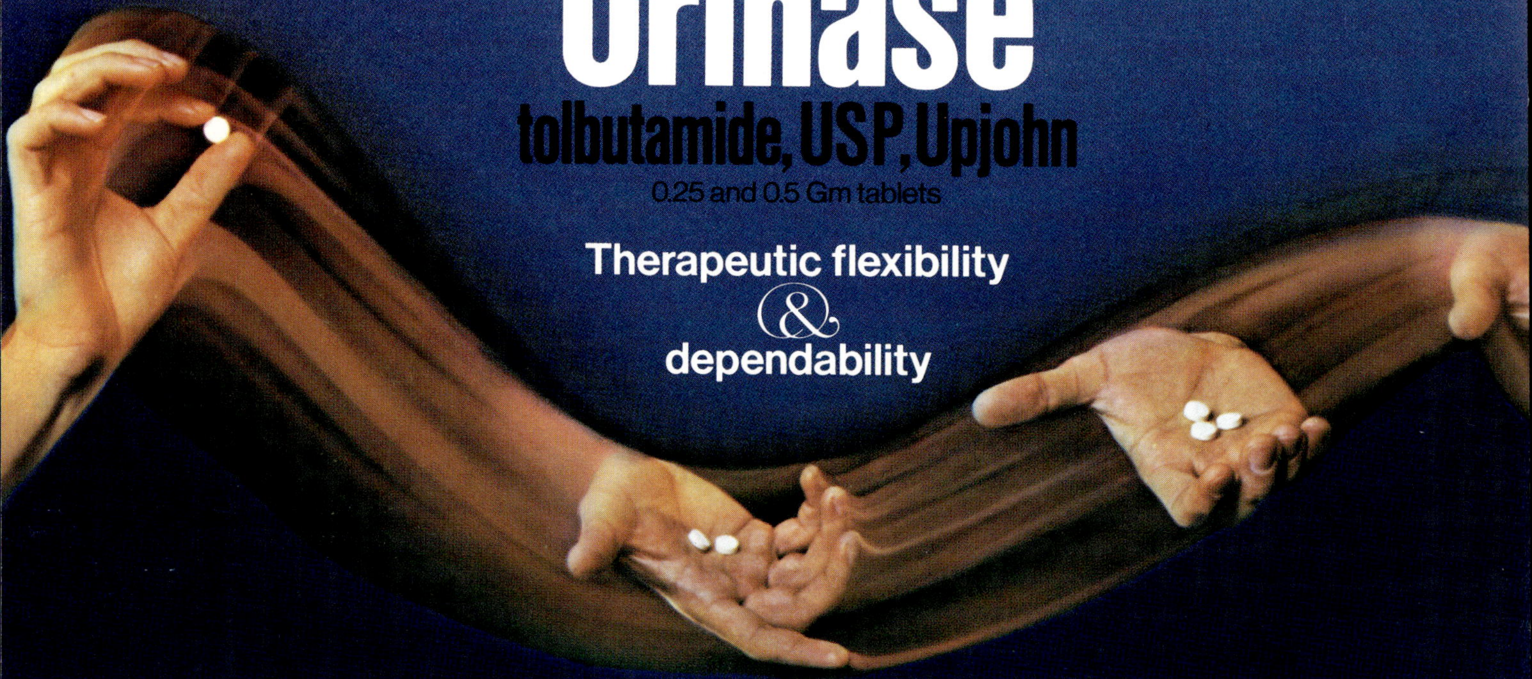

Therapeutic flexibility & dependability

Contraindications:
Orinase (tolbutamide) alone is not effective in juvenile or growth-onset diabetes nor in unstable brittle diabetes where insulin therapy is required.

Orinase tablets should not be used in diabetes complicated by acidosis, ketosis, or coma, or when a history of repeated bouts of acidosis or coma is obtained, in the presence of other acute complications such as fever, severe trauma, or infections, nor in patients with severe renal insufficiency. Insulin is indicated in these circumstances.

Pregnancy Warning: The safety and usefulness of *Orinase* during pregnancy has not been established. Animal studies have demonstrated feticidal and teratogenic effects. *Orinase* is not recommended for the pregnant diabetic, and should be used cautiously in women of childbearing age.

Precautions: Diagnostic and therapeutic measures necessary for optimal control with insulin are also necessary with *Orinase*. The patient on *Orinase* must be fully instructed about the nature, complications, and necessary personal measures needed to maintain control of the disease.

Caution: Very close observation, and careful adjustment of dose are necessary when: insulin is withdrawn during the trial period in order to avoid ketosis, acidosis, and coma; thiazide diuretics are administered, since they may aggravate the diabetic state and increase tolbutamide requirement, temporary loss of control, or even secondary failure; treating patients with impaired hepatic and/or renal function and debilitated, malnourished, or semistarved patients to avoid severe hypoglycemia; and treating patients with severe trauma, infection, or surgical procedures where temporary return to insulin or addition of insulin may be necessary. Beta-blocking agents reduce response to tolbutamide.

Patients must be under continuous medical supervision, and during the initial test period should communicate with the physician daily, and during the first month report at least once weekly for physical examination and definitive evaluation. After a month, examinations are recommended monthly or as indicated. Ketonuria, increased glycosuria, unsatisfactory lowering or persistent elevation of blood sugar, or poor clinical response indicate nonresponsiveness to *Orinase*. *Orinase* does not obviate the need for maintaining standard diet regulation. In treating mild asymptomatic diabetic patients with abnormal glucose tolerance, glucose tolerance tests should be obtained at 3-6 month intervals. *Orinase* is not an oral insulin or a substitute for insulin and must not be used as sole therapy in juvenile diabetes or in diabetes complicated by acidosis or coma where insulin is indispensable.

*****Adverse Reactions:** Severe hypoglycemia, though uncommon, may occur and may mimic acute neurologic disorders such as cerebral thrombosis. Certain factors such as hepatic and renal disease, malnutrition, advanced age, alcohol ingestion, and adrenal and pituitary insufficiency may predispose to hypoglycemia. Certain drugs such as insulin, sulfonamides, oxyphenbutazone, salicylates, probenecid, monamine oxidase inhibitors, phenylbutazone, bishydroxycoumarin, and phenyramidol may prolong or enhance the action of *Orinase* (tolbutamide) and increase risk of hypoglycemia. *Orinase* long-term therapy has been reported to reduce RAI uptake without producing clinical hypothyroidism or thyroid enlargement. High doses are mildly goitrogenic in animals. Photosensitivity reactions, disulfiram-like reactions after alcohol ingestion, and false positive tests for urine albumin have been reported.

Although usually not serious, gastrointestinal disturbances (nausea, epigastric fullness, and heartburn) and headache appear to be dose related and frequently disappear with reduction of dose or administration with meals. Allergic skin reactions (pruritus, erythema, urticaria, and morbilliform or maculopapular eruptions) are transient, usually not serious, and frequently disappear with continued administration. *Orinase* should be discontinued if skin reactions persist. Reports indicate that long-term use of *Orinase* has no appreciable effect on body weight.

Orinase appears to be remarkably free from gross clinical toxicity. Crystalluria or other renal abnormalities have not been observed, incidence of liver dysfunction is remarkably low, and jaundice has been rare and cleared readily on discontinuation of drug (carcinoma of the pancreas or other biliary obstruction should be ruled out in persistent jaundice).

Leukopenia, agranulocytosis, thrombocytopenia, hemolytic anemia, aplastic anemia, pancytopenia, and hepatic porphyria and porphyria cutanea tarda have been reported.

How Supplied: *250 mg Tablets* – bottle of 100. *0.5 Gram Tablets* – bottles of 50, 100, 200, 500 or 1000, Unit-Dose packages of 100, and Unit-of-Use packages of 30.

For additional product information, see your Upjohn representative or consult the package insert.

Upjohn

MED B-7-S

JUNE 1980 VOLUME 29 NUMBER 6

diabetes

JOURNAL OF
E AMERICAN
ABETES
SOCIATION

ORIGINAL CONTRIBUTIONS

Increased glycosylation of serum albumin in diabetes mellitus R. DOLHOFER AND O. H. WIELAND 417

Properdin factor B(Bf) allele Bf^{F1} specifies an HLA-B18 diabetogenic haplotype JOHN DORNAN, PATRICIA ALLAN, ELKE P. NOEL, BODIL LARSEN, AND NADIR R. FARID 423

Low plasma levels of pancreatic polypeptide in obesity VÉRONIQUE LASSMANN, PHILIPPE VAGUE, BERNARD VIALETTES, AND MARIE-CHRISTINE SIMON 428

The stimulus-secretion coupling of amino acid-induced insulin release: metabolic and cationic effects of leucine WILLY J. MALAISSE, JOHN C. HUTTON, ANGELO R. CARPINELLI, ANDRÉ HERCHUELZ, AND ABDULLAH SENER 431

Immunohistochemical localization of aldose reductase. I. Enzyme purification and antibody preparation—localization in peripheral nerve, artery, and testis MARK A. LUDVIGSON AND ROBERT L. SORENSON 438

Immunohistochemical localization of aldose reductase. II. Rat eye and kidney MARK A. LUDVIGSON AND ROBERT L. SORENSON 450

Acute changes in brain tryptophan and serotonin after carbohydrate or protein ingestion by diabetic rats ELIZABETH A. CRANDALL AND JOHN D. FERNSTROM 460

Critical factors in the chromatographic measurement of glycohemoglobin (HbA_1) M. SIMON AND J. EISSLER 467

Lysosomal degradation of receptor-bound ^{125}I-labeled insulin by rat adipocytes: its characterization and dissociation from the short-term biologic effects of insulin GLENN T. HAMMONS AND LEONARD JARETT 475

LILLY LECTURE 1979

Role of insulin in the regulation of protein synthesis LEONARD S. JEFFERSON 487

RAPID PUBLICATION

Monolayer cultures of adult pancreatic islet cells on osmotically disrupted fibroblasts P. MEDA, E. L. HOOGHE-PETERS, AND L. ORCI 497

ORGANIZATION SECTION XV

DIAEAZ 29(6)417-500(1980)
ISSN 0012-1797

For the stable, maturity-onset diabetic patient when diet alone has failed.

An effective choice to help control blood sugar

- ☐ Single or multiple dosing
- ☐ Two tablet strengths
- ☐ Documented bioavailability
- ☐ Severe hypoglycemia uncommon, but may occur*
- ☐ Twenty years of clinical use

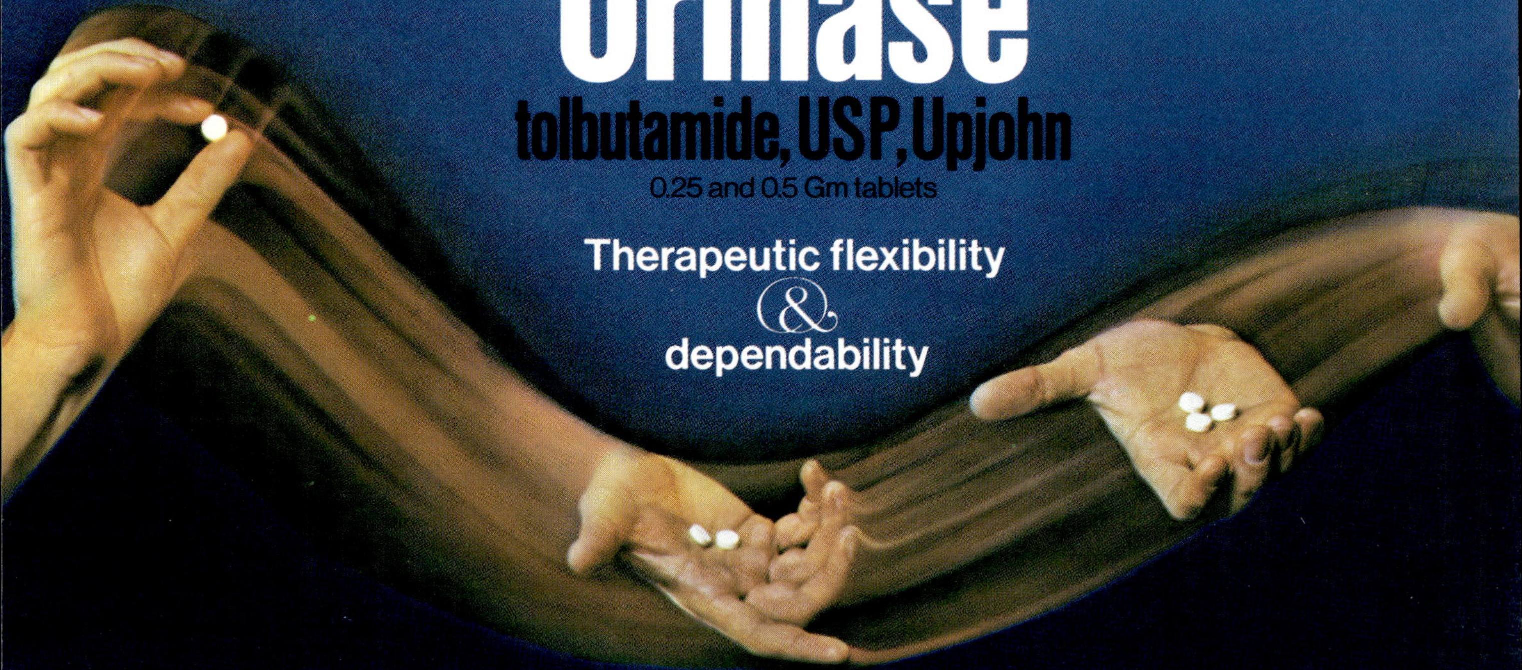

Orinase®

tolbutamide, USP, Upjohn

0.25 and 0.5 Gm tablets

Therapeutic flexibility & dependability

Contraindications:
Orinase (tolbutamide) alone is not effective in juvenile or growth-onset diabetes nor in unstable brittle diabetes where insulin therapy is required.

Orinase tablets should not be used in diabetes complicated by acidosis, ketosis, or coma, or when a history of repeated bouts of acidosis or coma is obtained, in the presence of other acute complications such as fever, severe trauma, or infections, nor in patients with severe renal insufficiency. Insulin is indicated in these circumstances.

Pregnancy Warning: The safety and usefulness of *Orinase* during pregnancy has not been established. Animal studies have demonstrated feticidal and teratogenic effects. *Orinase* is not recommended for the pregnant diabetic, and should be used cautiously in women of childbearing age.

Precautions: Diagnostic and therapeutic measures necessary for optimal control with insulin are also necessary with *Orinase*. The patient on *Orinase* must be fully instructed about the nature, complications, and necessary personal measures needed to maintain control of the disease.

Caution: Very close observation, and careful adjustment of dose are necessary when: insulin is withdrawn during the trial period in order to avoid ketosis, acidosis, and coma; thiazide diuretics are administered, since they may aggravate the diabetic state and increase tolbutamide requirement, temporary loss of control, or even secondary failure; treating patients with impaired hepatic and/or renal function and debilitated, malnourished, or semistarved patients to avoid severe hypoglycemia; and treating patients with severe trauma, infection, or surgical procedures where temporary return to insulin or addition of insulin may be necessary. Beta-blocking agents reduce response to tolbutamide.

Patients must be under continuous medical supervision, and during the initial test period should communicate with the physician daily, and during the first month report at least once weekly for physical examination and definitive evaluation. After a month, examinations are recommended monthly or as indicated. Ketonuria, increased glycosuria, unsatisfactory lowering or persistent elevation of blood sugar, or poor clinical response indicate nonresponsiveness to *Orinase*. *Orinase* does not obviate the need for maintaining standard diet regulation. In treating mild asymptomatic diabetic patients with abnormal glucose tolerance, glucose tolerance tests should be obtained at 3-6 month intervals. *Orinase* is not an oral insulin or a substitute for insulin and must not be used as sole therapy in juvenile diabetes or in diabetes complicated by acidosis or coma where insulin is indispensable.

Adverse Reactions: Severe hypoglycemia, though uncommon, may occur and may mimic acute neurologic disorders such as cerebral thrombosis. Certain factors such as hepatic and renal disease, malnutrition, advanced age, alcohol ingestion, and adrenal and pituitary insufficiency may predispose to hypoglycemia. Certain drugs such as insulin, sulfonamides, oxyphenbutazone, salicylates, probenecid, monamine oxidase inhibitors, phenylbutazone, bishydroxycoumarin, and phenyramidol may prolong or enhance the action of *Orinase* (tolbutamide) and increase risk of hypoglycemia. *Orinase* long-term therapy has been reported to reduce RAI uptake without producing clinical hypothyroidism or thyroid enlargement. High doses are mildly goitrogenic in animals. Photosensitivity reactions, disulfiram-like reactions after alcohol ingestion, and false positive tests for urine albumin have been reported.

Although usually not serious, gastrointestinal disturbances (nausea, epigastric fullness, and heartburn) and headache appear to be dose related and frequently disappear with reduction of dose or administration with meals. Allergic skin reactions (pruritus, erythema, urticaria, and morbilliform or maculopapular eruptions) are transient, usually not serious, and frequently disappear with continued administration. *Orinase* should be discontinued if skin reactions persist. Reports indicate that long-term use of *Orinase* has no appreciable effect on body weight.

Orinase appears to be remarkably free from gross clinical toxicity. Crystalluria or other renal abnormalities have not been observed, incidence of liver dysfunction is remarkably low, and jaundice has been rare and cleared readily on discontinuation of drug (carcinoma of the pancreas or other biliary obstruction should be ruled out in persistent jaundice).

Leukopenia, agranulocytosis, thrombocytopenia, hemolytic anemia, aplastic anemia, pancytopenia, and hepatic porphyria and porphyria cutanea tarda have been reported.

How Supplied: *250 mg Tablets* – bottle of 100. *0.5 Gram Tablets* – bottles of 50, 100, 200, 500 or 1000, Unit-Dose packages of 100, and Unit-of-Use packages of 30.

For additional product information, see your Upjohn representative or consult the package insert.

MED B-7-5 **Upjohn**

Effects of Glucose on Insulin Release and on Intermediary Metabolism of Isolated Perifused Pancreatic Islets from Fed and Fasted Rats

MICHAEL TRUS, HOWARD WARNER, AND FRANZ MATSCHINSKY

SUMMARY

We examined the relationship between glucose-induced insulin release and the intermediary metabolism of islets from fed and fasted rats. Isolated islets were perifused and insulin release measured in the effluent. At various times after switching islets from 2.4 to 8.6 or 14.5 mM glucose or from 2.4 to 14.5 and back to 2.4 mM glucose, islets were quickly frozen, freeze dried, and subsequently analyzed for tissue content of glucose-6-P, fructose-1,6-P_2 plus triose-P, P_i, ATP, ADP, 5′-AMP, NADH, NADPH, total NAD, and total NADP using enzymatic fluorometric procedures. When islets from fed rats were exposed to high glucose, there were concomitant increases of insulin release and islet content of glucose-6-P, fructose-1,6-P_2 plus triose-P, NADH, and NADPH. During stimulation P_i and 5′-AMP content fell markedly. The total adenine nucleotide content remained constant. Similar secretory and metabolic changes occurred when 1.5 mM P_i was added to the perifusion fluid. When glucose-stimulated islets were switched back to low glucose for 10 min, all substances but fructose-1,6-P_2 plus triose-P, 5′-AMP, NADPH, and possibly ATP returned to the prestimulatory level. Starvation of rats for 3 days blocked the secretory response to 8.6 mM glucose. Fructose-1,6-P_2 plus triose-P rose but it did not attain the level existing in islets from fed rats. The ratios (ATP)/(5′-AMP) and (ATP)/(P_i)(ADP) increased to the values observed in glucose-stimulated islets of fed rats.

The metabolic changes in islets from fed rats exposed to high glucose are consistent with an activation of glycolysis occurring concomitantly with stimulated rates of insulin release. This occurs despite the decrease of important activators of glycolysis—P_i and 5′-AMP. The enhanced glycolysis possibly results from P-fructokinase activation by increased fructose-6-P levels. Activation of glycolysis with 8.6 mM glucose was not as pronounced in islets from starved rats. Despite the different secretory response of islets from fed and fasted rats, the changes of phosphorylation state in the islets, in particular, P_i and 5′-AMP levels, were similar. **DIABETES *29*:1–14, January 1980.**

An understanding of the regulatory characteristics of glucose metabolism in pancreatic islet tissue would help to explain the glycolytic events that occur during the activation of insulin release by glucose and other stimulants. Knowledge of this aspect of islet biochemistry is still fragmentary.[1–3] The known enzymatic properties found in islets implicate the glycolytic events in stimulus secretion coupling. Glucose transport across the outer cell membrane is rapid,[4,5] so that intracellular glucose levels rapidly adjust to extracellular levels. Kinetic evidence exists for the presence of both hexokinase and glucokinase in islets,[4,6,7] thus indicating that glucose phosphorylation is related to glucose levels over a large physiologic range. Similar properties of glucose metabolism are found in liver,[8–10] where glucose is primarily shunted into glycogen synthesis.[9,11] Islets, however, do not store large amounts of glycogen.[1] Most glucose use occurs by means of glycolysis[12] and the rate of glycolysis is related to the level of extracellular glucose over a wide range of physiologic concentrations.[13] Presumably, these characteristics of islet cell metabolism serve to relate glucose levels to some important cell function other than glycogen synthesis. One possible function is insulin release, which could be mediated by a glycolytic event or a combination of events.

From the Department of Pharmacology, Washington University School of Medicine, St. Louis, Missouri 63110.
Dr. Matschinsky's present address is Department of Biochemistry and Biophysics, University of Pennsylvania School of Medicine, Philadelphia, Pennsylvania 19104.
Received for publication 14 May and in revised form 23 August 1979.

The present work describes the relationships observed among the kinetic changes of glucose-induced insulin release, levels of various glycolytic intermediates, pyridine nucleotides, adenine nucleotides, and inorganic phosphate in isolated, perifused rat islets. The changes in levels of glucose-6-P and fructose diphosphate serve as a useful indicator of changes in glycolytic flux.[14,15] Changes of reduced pyridine nucleotide content might indicate alterations of the cellular redox state.[16] ATP, ADP, 5′-AMP, and P_i are important regulators of glycolysis.[14,15] Some of these intermediates and cofactors have been implicated to have a role in the stimulus secretion–coupling process.[2,17–19] Measurements were made before and after the initiation of glucose stimulation of islets and after switching stimulated islets back to low glucose. Adaptive characteristics of the metabolic response were studied by starvation of rats, which interferes with glucose-induced insulin release. It is hoped that these studies help to clarify the relationship of intermediary metabolism and its regulation to the fuel-induced hormone release process.

EXPERIMENTAL PROCEDURE*

Reagents. The sources, specific activities, and preparations of enzymes used for the fluorometric assays are shown in Table 1. Collagenase from *Clostridium histolyticum* was used for the islet isolation procedure. The enzyme was obtained from Worthington and it had a specific activity of 150–180 U/mg. Crystalline bovine serum albumin for preparing the perifusion fluid was from Armour (Reheis Co. subsidiary). It had no detectable insulin contamination at the concentrations used. Rabbit muscle glycogen was obtained from Boehringer. It was prepared for use in the P_i and 5′-AMP assays by dialysis as described previously.[20] α-D-glucose was obtained from Mallinckrodt. It was added to the perifusion fluid with sufficient time before perifusion to allow the α and β anomers to equilibrate. Note that, although the level of glucose in control perifusion fluid was prepared from analytic grade glucose as 2.8 mM on the basis of weight, the level indicated by enzymatic assay of the perifusion effluent was 2.36 mM. In perifusion fluid prepared as 16.7 mM glucose, enzymatic assay indicated a level of 14.5 mM. Analysis of subsequent preparations of glucose from Koch Light indicated glucose levels the same as that prepared on the basis of weight.

Hanks' solution was used for the islet isolation procedure. It contained NaCl, 137 mM; KCl, 5.4 mM; $CaCl_2$, 1.2 mM; $MgSO_4$, 0.81 mM; Na_2HPO_4, 0.34 mM; KH_2PO_4, 0.44 mM; and glucose, 2.4 mM. The pH was titrated to 7.4 by addition of a 7% $NaHCO_3$ solution. Hanks' solution was stored at 4°C between use. The glucose was added immediately before the islet isolation procedure.

The basic perifusion fluid consisted of NaCl, 115 mM; KCl, 5 mM; $MgCl_2$, 1.0 mM; $NaHCO_3$, 24 mM; $CaCl_2$, 2.2 mM; BSA, 0.3%; and inulin, 10 mM (fructose equivalents). Inulin was added as a marker to quantitate the extracellular space of islet tissue. This precautionary measure proved unnecessary in the present study and inulin measurements were not done. For perifusion experiments in the presence of P_i, KH_2PO_4 (1.5 mM) was added to the basic perifusion fluid.

Treatment of animals and isolation of islets. Male Holtzman rats weighing 250–450 g were used. Rats were either given free access to water and Purina rat chow or starved with only water present 3 days before the islets were isolated.

For each experiment at 50–80 min before perifusion began, one rat was anesthetized with Nembutal (sodium pentobarbital, Abbott), 50 mg/kg injected intraperitoneally. The islet isolation procedure has been described previously.[21] Pancreatic parenchymal tissue was disrupted by slow injection of about 20 ml of Hanks' solution into the common bile duct. After distention of the pancreas, it was removed. Most animals died at this point, although some died earlier in the procedure. Pancreatic tissue was digested with 20–25 mg of collagenase. After collagenase treatment, islets were transferred from Hanks' solution to a plastic 5 ml beaker containing perifusion fluid at 22–25°C. The yield was 50–120 islets from a single rat pancreas. The average dry weight of single islets from fed rats, measured with a quartz fiber balance,[22] was about 0.8 μg. The DNA content, determined by a fluorometric assay,[23] was 44 ng/μg dry weight.

Perifusion[24] and tissue-sampling protocols. Islets were transferred with a 1 ml syringe to a nylon filter placed on the filter support of a plastic perifusion chamber (Millipore Corp.). The nylon filter (Tetko, Inc.) had a pore size of 20 μm and a diameter of 1.2 cm. It was prepared for use by heating at 100°C in 8% $NaHCO_3$ for 30 min and then rinsing with distilled water. The time required from removal of the pancreas to the beginning of perifusion was 40–60 min. Perifusion was driven with a peristaltic pump (Harvard Corp.) at a flow rate of 1.8–2.2 ml/min. The chamber containing islets was placed between the pump and the reservoir end on the tubing. In a typical experiment, two chambers, usually a control and an experimental chamber, each containing 25–60 islets from the same rat, were perifused simultaneously. The dead space between the reservoir of fluid and the chamber containing islets was roughly 0.5 ml, which is equivalent to 15 s in this system. The dead space between the islets and the effluent end was about 2 ml, or, 1 min. When perifusions were switched from 2.4 to 14.5 mM glucose, increased glucose started to appear in the effluent 1 min after the switch. Because of the dead space and the time needed for sampling (see below), the metabolic changes depicted in Figures 3 through 9 are displaced about 45 s to the left of the corresponding insulin release rates.

In order to study the metabolic state of freshly isolated islets at room temperature (22–25°C), groups of islets were placed on a nylon filter, briefly rinsed with perifusion fluid containing 2.4 mM glucose, and then quick frozen. To observe the immediate effect of perifusion at 37°C, there were also groups of islets perifused for 3 min with 2.4 mM glucose before freezing. In all other experiments, islets were perifused with 2.4 mM glucose for 30 min. At 30 min, some of the perifusions were switched to fluid reservoirs containing 8.6 or 14.5 mM glucose; a sham switch was made for controls. Finally, there were perifusions in which the high glucose stimulus was switched off.

Frequent, 1 min samples of effluent were collected throughout the perifusions. These samples were stored at

* These abbreviations are used: AMP_2, 2-amino-2-methyl propanol; BSA, bovine serum albumin; DH, dehydrogenase; DTT, dithiothreitol; EDTA, ethylenediaminetetraacetate; ME, B-mercaptoethanol; and tris, tris(hydroxymethyl)aminomethane.

TABLE 1
Enzyme preparations used for metabolite and cofactor assays

Enzyme	Biologic source (manufacturer)	Specific activity	Preparation
Alcohol DH	Yeast (Boehringer)	300 U/mg	Use stock suspension in 3.2 M $(NH_4)_2SO_4$ (30 mg/ml).
Aldolase	Rabbit muscle (Boehringer)	9 U/mg	Centrifuge at 2500 rpm in Sorvall GLC-1 for 30 min at 4°C. Remove supernatant and resuspend in reag A (1.0 mg/ml).
Catalase	Beef liver (Boehringer)	65,000 U/mg	Use stock suspension in 0.01% alkylbenzyldimethylammonium chloride (20 mg/ml).
Glucose-6-P DH	L. mesenteroides (Sigma)	235 U/mg	Suspend in reag A (5 mg/ml).
Glucose-6-P DH	Yeast (Boehringer)	140 U/mg	Centrifuge at 2500 rpm in Sorvall GLC-1 for 30 min at 4°C. Remove supernatant and resuspend in reag A (5 mg/ml).
Glutamate DH	Beef liver (Boehringer)	90 U/mg	Centrifuge at 2500 rpm in Sorvall GLC-1 for 30 min at 4°C. Remove supernatant. Resuspend in reag A (20 mg/ml).
Glyceraldehyde-P DH	Yeast (Boehringer)	100 U/mg	Centrifuge at 2500 rpm in Sorvall GLC-1 for 30 min at 4°C. Remove supernatant and resuspend in Imidazole HCl, 100 mM, pH 7 (10 mg/ml).
Hexokinase	Yeast (Boehringer)	140 U/mg	Use stock suspension in 3.2 N $(NH_4)_2SO_4$ (10 mg/ml)
Lactate DH	Beef heart (Worthington)	204 U/mg	Use stock suspension (33.2 mg/ml).
Malic enzyme	Chicken liver (Sigma)	13.5 U/mg	Use stock suspension in 2.9 M $(NH_4)_2SO_4$, 10 mM KH_2PO_4, 3 mM EDTA, 10 mM $MnCl_2$, 5 mM ME (0.74 mg/ml).
Malic DH	Pig heart (Boehringer)	1200 U/mg	Use stock suspension in 3.2 M $(NH_4)_2SO_4$ (5 mg/ml).
Phosphorylase a (for 5′-AMP assay)	Rabbit muscle (Sigma)	12.4 U/mg	Add 5 mg to 1 ml of reag C. Incubate 20 min at 37°C (5 mg/ml).
Phosphorylase a (for P_i assay)	Rabbit muscle (Sigma)	12.4 U/mg	Add 62 mg to 1 ml water. Dialyze against 1 liter of reag B (62 mg/ml).
Phosphoglucomutase (for 5′-AMP assay)	Rabbit muscle (Boehringer)	200 U/mg	Centrifuge at 10,000 rpm in Sorvall RC 2-B for 30 min at 2°C. Remove supernatant and resuspend in reag A (10 mg/ml).
Phosphoglucomutase (for P_i assay)	Rabbit muscle (Boehringer)	200 U/mg	Centrifuge at 2500 rpm in Sorvall GLC-1 for 30 min at 4°C. Remove supernatant and resuspend in 3.3 M $(NH_4)_2SO_4$ (10 mg/ml).
6-P-gluconate DH	Yeast (Boehringer)	12 U/mg	Dilute stock suspension in 3.2 M $(NH_4)_2SO_4$ 1:12 with reag A (0.83 mg/ml).
Pyruvate kinase	Rabbit muscle (Boehringer)	200 U/mg	Use stock suspension in 3.2 M $(NH_4)_2SO_4$ (10 mg/ml).
Triose-P isomerase	Rabbit muscle (Boehringer)	5000 U/mg	Centrifuge at 2500 rpm in Sorvall GLC-1 for 30 min at 4°C. Remove supernatant and resuspend in reag A (2 mg/ml).

Number in parentheses indicates the approximate concentration of enzyme prepared.
Reag A—Tris HCl, 20 mM, pH 8.2; BSA, 0.02%. Reag B—Imidazole HCl, 20 mM, pH 7; EDTA, 1 mM; 5′-AMP, 10 μM; DTT, 500 μM.
Reag C—Imidazole-HCl, 20 mM, pH 7; B-mercaptoethanol, 5 mM; BSA, 0.02%.

−20°C until assayed for insulin and sometimes for glucose.

After the indicated times of perifusion, the chambers were opened and the filters with islets removed. The filters were quickly blotted on Whatman filter paper and immersed in liquid Freon-12 cooled to its freezing point with liquid N_2. It took 10 to 15 s to remove and freeze islets. The filters were then transferred to 25 ml glass vials cooled with solid CO_2. The vials were stored at −70°C.

Preparation of islet tissue for assay.[22] To lyophilize the islet tissue on filters, they were transferred at −20°C to 1-ml beakers and placed in a vacuum bottle. Islet tissue was kept at this temperature for a maximum of 45 min. Lyophilization was carried out for a minimum of 2 days at −40°C with a vacuum of less than 1 μm. The vacuum bottle was transferred to room temperature for the final 1.0 to 1.5 h of lyophilization. Afterwards, samples were stored in a vacuum at −20°C.

In order to obtain islet specimens for assay, the vacuum bottle containing islet specimens was transferred to room temperature, 18–20°C, at least 45 min before releasing the vacuum. The bottle was opened and the filters containing islet tissue removed. The opening of the vacuum tube and all subsequent manipulations were carried out in a room with a temperature of 18–20°C and a relative humidity of 50%. Islet specimens were obtained by scraping an islet from the surface of the filter with a microdissection knife. In some instances, portions of an islet were sampled using the dissecting knife. The specimens were transferred to a tissue holder and weighed with a quartz fiber balance. The weights ranged from 25 to 1500 ng. After weighing, the samples were transferred to an oil well rack [25] for assay.

Analytic procedures. To measure tissue content of cofactors and metabolities, fluorometric assays were employed with enzymatic cycling and oil well techniques to obtain the sensitivity required.[22,25,26] Tables 2 and 3 indicate the analytic conditions for each of these assays. The malate or 6-P-gluconate formed during cycling was measured using malic enzyme or 6-P-gluconate DH as described previously.[22,26]

Alkali-enhanced fluorescence was used after the indicator step to measure NADH and NADPH in islet specimens weighing less than 50 ng in order to achieve adequate sensitivity.[22] After completion of the cycling step, the droplet was transferred to 100 μl of the indicator reagent for malate or 6-P-gluconate. Incubation with the indicator reagent was for 35 (6-P-gluconate) or 60 (malate) min. Excess $NADP^+$ in the indicator reagent then was destroyed by adding 100 μl of phosphate buffer (250 mM Na_3PO_4 plus 250 mM K_2HPO_4), pH 11.5. Incubation was at 60°C for 20 min. Final fluorescence was developed by adding 1 ml of 7 N NaOH plus 0.03% H_2O_2 and heating at 60°C for 15 min. After cooling the tubes to room temperature, fluorescence was measured.

For the assays of total NAD and total NADP, the extraction with the first step reagent was short because of the lability of oxidized pyridine nucleotides in dilute alkali.[27,28] In order to assay many samples, it was necessary to add the first step reagent to a group of five islet samples. Two minutes later, the cycling reagent was added to these samples. The sequence was then repeated. Standards were prepared in the dilute alkali immediately before cycling. The standards consisted of the oxidized form of the pyridine nucleotide for the

TABLE 2
Analytic conditions prior to the cycling step*

Substance measured	First step	Second step (reagent)	Second step (volume)
Glucose-6-P	0.049 μl 0.015 N HCl, 20 min at 80°C	Tris·HCl, 200 mM, pH 8.2; DTT, 0.25 mM; BSA, 0.19%; $NADP^+$, 27 μM; glucose-6-P DH, 0.55 μg/ml	0.049 μl
Fructose-1,6-P_2 plus triose-P	0.058 μl 0.025 N HCl, 20 min at 70°C	Imidazole·HCl, 0.4 M, pH 7.5; ME, 4 mM; EDTA, 2 mM; NaH_2AsO_4, 2 mM; BSA, 0.5%; NAD^+, 50 μM; aldolase, 5 μg/ml; triose-P isomerase, 1 μg/ml; glyceraldehyde-P DH, 75 μg/ml	0.058 μl
P_i	0.16 μl 0.1 N NaOH, 15 min at 60°C	Imidazole·HCl, 54 mM, pH 6.9; glycogen, 5.7 mM; EDTA, 1 mM; 5′-AMP, 11 μM; DTT, 0.55 mM; magnesium acetate, 0.55 mM; glucose-1,6-P_2, 1.1 μM; BSA, 0.04%; $NADP^+$, 60 μM; glucose-6-P DH, 1.1 μg/ml; phosphoglucomutase, 4 μg/ml; phosphorylase a, 50 μg/ml	3 μl
ATP	0.32 μl 0.1 N NaOH, 15 min at 60°C	Tris·HCl, 112 mM, pH 8.2; $MgCl_2$, 2.3 mM; DTT, 570 μM; glucose, 340 μM; $NADP^+$, 85 μM; BSA 0.35%; hexokinase, 2.3 μg/ml; glucose-6-P DH, 0.58 μg/ml	3 μl
ADP	0.1 μl 0.1 N NaOH plus 6 mM H_2O_2, 20 min at 60°C	Imidazole·HCl, 56 mM, pH 6.9; NaOH, 56 mM; ascorbic acid, 56 mM; KCl, 83 mM; $MgCl_2$, 2.3 mM; BSA, 0.023%; P-enolpyruvate, 23 μM; NADH, 11 μM; catalase, 11 μg/ml; pyruvate kinase, 5.5 μg/ml; lactate DH, 7.5 μg/ml	1 μl
5′-AMP	0.52 μl† 32 mM Imidazole 32 mM NaOH 58 mM $HClO_4$	Imidazole·HCl, 49 mM, pH 6.7; Na_2HPO_4, 0.44 mM; glycogen, 1.2 mM (glucose eq.); BSA, 0.1%; glucose-1,6-P_2, 0.49 μM; ME, 2.5 mM; magnesium acetate, 2 mM; ME, 2.5 mM; magnesium acetate, 2 mM; glucose-6-P DH, 1 μg/ml; phosphoglucomutase, 3 μg/ml; phosphorylase a, 3 μg/ml	0.51 μl‡
NADH	0.16 μl 0.02 N NaOH plus 0.5 mM cysteine, 15 min at 70°C	See Table 3	
Total NAD	0.44 μl 0.02 N NaOH plus 0.5 mM cysteine, 2 min at 20–22°C	See Table 3	
NADPH	0.16 μl 0.02 N NaOH plus 0.5 mM cysteine, 15 min at 70°C	See Table 3	
Total NADP	0.16 μl 0.02 N NaOH plus 0.5 mM cysteine, 2 min at 20–22°C	See Table 3	

* All steps were carried out under oil. The incubation period for all assays was 30–60 min at 22–26°C.

† This was carried out in two steps. First, 0.13 μl of 0.3 N $HClO_4$ was added to the islet specimens. Next, 0.10 μ of the supernatant was transferred to 0.42 μl of a solution containing 0.04 N NaOH and 0.04 N imidazole. The final pH of the neutralized extract was about 7.

‡ This reagent was added in two steps. To the neutralized extract was added 0.32 μl of a reagent containing imidazole·acetate, 160 mM, pH 6.7; ME, 8.1 mM; magnesium acetate, 6.4 mM; glucose-1,6-P_2, 1.6 μM; BSA, 0.32%; glucose-6-P DH, 3.2 μg/ml; phosphoglucomutase, 9.6 μg/ml; phosphorylase a, 9.6 μg/ml. The phosphorylase reaction was started by adding 0.19 μl of 1.43 mM Na_2HPO_4 plus 3.3 mM glycogen at 10-s intervals to the oil wells.

TABLE 3
Preparation and conditions for cycling step

Substance measured*	Preparation for cycling	Cycling conditions†	Incubation conditions‡	Range of sensitivity (10^{-14} mol)
Glucose-6-P (NADPH)	0.049 μl 0.4 N NaOH, 20 min at 75°C	Glucose-6-P DH, 30 μg/ml; glutamate DH, 400 μg/ml; 22,000 cycles/h	1.5 h, 37°C in 1.7 μl	1.5–10
Fructose-1,6-P_2 plus triose-P (NADH)	0.058 μl 0.45 N NaOH, 20 min at 70°C	Alcohol DH, 330 μg/ml; malic DH, 31 μg/ml; 6,500 cycles/h	2 h, 26°C in 1.7 μl	1.8–8.1
P_i (NADPH)	2 μl 0.3 N NaOH, 25 min at 60°C§	Glucose-6-P DH, 1.25 μg/ml; glutamate DH, 2.5 μg/ml; 370 cycles/h	2 h, 37°C in 52 μl	330–3300
ATP (NADPH)	2 μl 0.45 N NaOH, 25 min at 70°C‖	Glucose-6-P DH, 1.25 μg/ml; glutamate DH, 2.5 μg/ml; 250 cycles/h	2 h, 37°C in 54 μl	150–1200
ADP (NAD^+)	0.1 μl 2.5 N HCl¶	Alcohol DH, 16 μg/ml; malic DH, 1.33 μg/ml; 900 cycles/h	1.4 h, 25°C in 51 μl	200–400
5′-AMP (Glucose-6-P)**	(1) 5 μl 50 mM AMP_2 HCl, pH 8.7; 125 μM $NADP^+$; 30 min at 22–25°C (2) 1.5 μl 0.55 N NaOH, 25 min at 75°C	Glucose-6-P DH, 2.5 μg/ml; glutamate DH, 5 μg/ml; 500 cycles/h	2 h, 37°C in 52 μl	17–130
NADH (NADH)	See Table 2	Alcohol DH, 300 μg/ml; malic DH, 31 μg/ml; 12,000 cycles/h	1.25 h, 25°C in 3 μl	1.4–16.7 0.8–5.0††
Total NAD (NAD^+ and NADH)	See Table 2	Alcohol DH, 48 μg/ml; malic DH, 4 μg/ml; 2000 cycles/h	1.4 h, 25°C in 5 μl	7.0–16
NADPH (NADPH)	See Table 2	Glucose-6-P DH, 20 μg/ml; glutamate DH, 400 μg/ml; 15,000 cycles/h	1.5 h, 37°C in 3 μl	1.8–9.5 0.8–5.8††
Total NADP ($NADP^+$ and NADPH)	See Table 2	Glucose-6-P DH, 5 μg/ml; glutamate DH, 200 μg/ml; 17,000 cycles/h	1.5 h, 37°C in 2 μl	1.5–17

* The product of the second step reaction (Table 2) is given in parentheses.

† Cycling rates are only approximate.

‡ Incubations in volumes of 5 μl or less were carried out in oil wells; the rest were carried out in test tubes (10 × 75 mm). Cycling in oil wells was terminated by addition of NaOH, 100 mM base excess to the oil wells followed by heating at 80°C for 15 min. For all other assays but ADP, cycling was terminated by 2 min of incubation in a 100° bath.

§ A 2 μl aliquot was transferred to the cycling reagent.

‖ A 4 μl aliquot was transferred to the cycling reagent.

¶ The cycling procedure was begun by addition of a 0.94 μl aliquot to cycling reagent in tubes in an ice bath. Cycling was stopped in the same time sequence that it was started by adding 50 μl of 0.26 N NaOH to the tubes in an ice bath and then heating for 2 min in a 100°C bath.

** Preparation occurred in two steps. The first reagent was added to the oil wells at 10 s intervals. After incubation with this reagent, the second step was carried out. A 1.6 μl aliquot was then transferred to the cycling reagent.

†† Alkali-enhanced fluorescence was used to increase sensitivity.

assays of total NADP and total NAD. Cycling was stopped with alkali addition in the same time sequence that it was started.

There was a danger of NADH and NADPH loss from lyophilized islets during storage and repeated handling.[22,28] Therefore, these assays (NADH first) were the first ones done on the islet tissue after lyophilization. These were followed by the assays for P_i, total NAD, total NADP, 5′-AMP, ATP, ADP, glucose-6-P, and fructose-1,6-P_2 plus triose-P. There was not much tissue remaining for the assay for glucose-6-P or fructose-1,6-P_2 plus triose-P. As a consequence, for some experimental conditions, only one or two perifusions were analyzed.

Glucose assays of the perifusion effluent were done by a direct fluorometric procedure.[22]

Insulin in the effluent was measured with a radioimmunoassay procedure using rat insulin standards.[29,30]

RESULTS

Analytic considerations. The analytic capacities of the fluorometric assays used to measure metabolic and cofactor levels in islets are summarized in Table 4. The lower limit of sensitivity of these assays, as a rule of thumb, was considered as the level equal to from 20% to 50% of the overall blank. Recovery for the assays was tested by adding known amounts of standards in the first step reagent to tissue. There was no effect on any assay of adding glucose to the first step reagent at levels comparable to those expected from islet tissue. This test was necessary, since glucose was present in varying amounts in the islet specimens assayed.

TABLE 4
Standard deviations and overall blanks of assays

Substance measured	Standard deviations, % Assays with standards	Assays with tissues	Overall blank 10^{-14} mol	% recovery
Glucose-6-P	5.6 (7)	37 (28)	1.7 (7)	98
Fructose-1,6-P_2 plus triose-P	5.4 (8)	29 (15)	1.7 (7)	95
P_i	5.5 (11)	13 (22)	370 (9)	113
ATP	2.0 (5)	10 (15)	170 (6)	110
ADP	7.3 (10)	13 (20)	180 (10)	107
5′-AMP	17 (13)	27 (34)	19 (13)	116
NADH	3.5 (15)	22 (20)	1.7 (14)	104
Total NAD	5.0 (4)	12 (16)	7.1 (4)	99
NADPH	3.2 (18)	27 (15)	1.7 (16)	not tested
Total NADP	4.8 (5)	15 (16)	1.6 (5)	not tested

The number of analyses considered in calculating the standard deviations and blanks is given in parentheses. The overall blank is the equivalent of total fluorescence obtained in the absence of standard or tissue. Recovery was calculated as (total measured/total expected) × 100. Total measured is the amount of metabolite or cofactor measured in tissue with known amount of standard added. Total expected is the sum measured in standard alone and in tissue alone.

Comments made below concern specific problems and tests made with regard to these assays.

In the first step reagent for the ATP assay, no significant hydrolysis of ATP occurred in the presence or absence of islet tissue. This was tested by quantitating the ADP level of the reagents.

In the ADP assay, a substantial tissue blank was present when dilute alkali alone was used as a first step reagent. The tissue blank, determined in the absence of pyruvate kinase, was 16% of the total substance measured in tissue when pyruvate kinase was present. The lactate DH preparation used did not have pyruvate kinase activity and the tissue blank, probably pyruvate, was eliminated by addition of H_2O_2 to the first step reagent, a measure practiced previously.[31] Since H_2O_2 could oxidize NADH during step 2, catalase was added to the second step reagent.

For assaying NADPH or total NADP, it was necessary to use the cycling enzyme, glucose-6-P DH, from yeast. The enzyme from *Leuconostoc mesenteroides* cycled NAD at 11% of the rate for NADP.[32] Since NAD predominated in islet tissue, this would contribute to erroneously high values for total NADP or NADPH. The yeast enzyme did not result in any detectable cycling of NAD.

NADH levels for a given experimental condition were constant over a large range of specimen sizes analyzed, 0.05–1.0 μg. In samples larger than 1 μg, there was an indication of lower NADH levels. Since most samples in this study were less than 0.6 μg, the effect of weight on NADH levels was neglected. In contrast to NADH, the levels of observed NADPH were greatly affected by sample size (Figure 1) in the range analyzed. A similar weight dependency of NADPH levels was noted for islets exposed to 8.6 or 14.5 mM glucose. This tissue dependency was unexpected from previous experience and became apparent only after completion of the analysis of reduced pyridine nucleotides. There were two possibilities: Large islets could have lower NADPH levels than small islets; alternatively, sample size could affect the analysis. Large islets were sliced into fragments. Assay of each fragment separately indicated higher levels of NADPH than were present in other large islets from the same group. Therefore, the weight dependency of NADPH was due to the effect of sample size on the analysis. It appeared that islet specimens below 50 ng had NADPH levels independent of sample weight. The average NADPH levels in these small samples, 50 ng or less, perifused for 50 min with 2.4 mM glucose was 85.3 ± 4.7 (N = 13) μmol/kg dry wt. The average value of NADPH in islet specimens, 50 ng or less, which were perifused with 2.4 mM glucose for 30 min and then stimulated with 14.5 mM glucose for 20 min, was 116 ± 4.3 (N = 14) μmol/kg dry wt. Altogether, these results suggest that the present NADPH levels are underestimated by about 50%. The weight averages of islet speci-

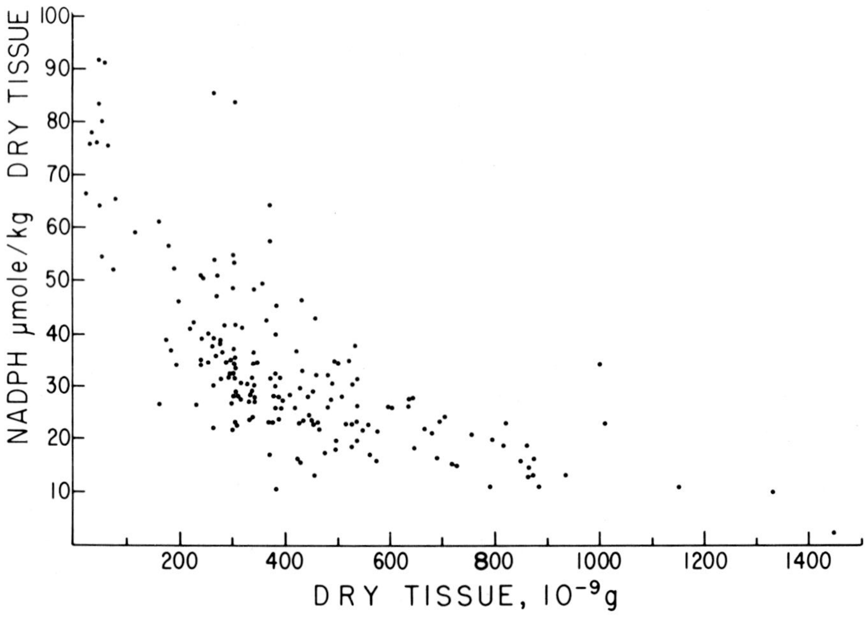

FIGURE 1. NADPH levels in islet specimens of different weights. Each point represents a value obtained from one islet sample. The data for this figure were obtained from islets perifused with 2.4 mM glucose for from 30 to 60 min.

mens analyzed for NADPH did not vary much among the experimental conditions described in this study. Thus, the relative changes of NADPH observed in islets exposed to different glucose levels are likely to be of significance. It is possible that NADPH loss occurs in large specimens when the dilute alkali, used to make the tissue extract, penetrates too slowly. Use of a stronger alkali in making the initial tissue extract might solve the problem.

To determine if loss of reduced pyridine nucleotide occurred in freeze-dried islet tissue during the time required for microdissecting, weighing, and loading,[22,28] islets were sampled at different times in a day and kept in the dissection room atmosphere at 18–20°C and 50% humidity until assayed. No significant loss of NADH occurred for at least 490 min before the first step reagent was added to tissue. There was no apparent loss of NADPH during 300 min of air exposure. For the remaining studies of reduced pyridine nucleotides, the maximum time of air exposure of lyophilized islet tissue was 120 min for NADH assays and 150 min for NADPH assays.

Metabolite and cofactor levels of freshly isolated islets kept at 25°C and islets briefly perifused at 37°C (Table 5). These experiments were done to assess the effects of the islet isolation procedure, which includes collagenase treatment, on islet viability. The levels of ATP, ADP, 5′-AMP, and P_i in freshly isolated islets were similar to those found in vivo for many other tissues.[33] This suggests that the islets survive collagenase treatment without an energy deficit. The levels of glucose-6-P are lower than those previously reported, which were 100–400 μmol/kg dry tissue for rat islets.[31,34–36] Glucose-6-P content doubled after perifusion for 3 min at 37°C. The levels of fructose-1,6-P_2 plus triose-P remained unchanged. P_i levels increased about twofold after perifusion. If one assumes an islet water content of 3.2 L/kg dry tissue,[37] then islet P_i levels can be expressed as 4.8 and 9.3 mmol/kg wet wt before and after brief perifusion. ATP fell 30% and ADP increased 30% after islets were perifused. The rise of 5′-AMP was 131% after perifusion at the higher temperature. Total adenine nucleotides decreased 14% after perifusion. Brief perifusion at 37°C also resulted in a 30% loss of NADH content. There were no obvious differences in the levels of total NAD, NADPH, and total NADP in the two groups of islets. The changes of ATP, ADP, 5′-AMP, and P_i during brief perifusion at 37°C should stimulate glycolysis and respiration.[14,15] The decrease of NADH observed is consistent with enhanced respiration. These changes might have resulted from the temperature rise from 25° to 37°C. Basal insulin release rates at these two temperatures were not measured.

TABLE 5
Metabolite and cofactor levels in pancreatic islets immediately after isolation and after perifusion for 3 min

Metabolite or cofactor	Islets immediately after isolation	Islets after 3 min of perifusion	P
Glucose-6-P	20.9 ± 2.3 (5)	40.2 ± 3.2 (4)	0.002
Fructose-1,6-P_2 plus triose-P	53.2 ± 3.6 (3)	52.9 ± 8.5 (4)	NS
P_i	15.4 ± 0.86 (6)	29.7 ± 1.3 (6)	0.001
ATP	17.4 ± 0.75 (6)	12.2 ± 1.3 (5)	0.008
ADP	4.22 ± 0.44 (5)	5.62 ± 0.36 (5)	0.04
5′-AMP	493 ± 42 (6)	1141 ± 233 (6)	0.022
NADH	123 ± 7.5 (6)	83.7 ± 10 (6)	0.011
Total NAD	1.14 ± 0.27 (4)	1.54 ± 0.035 (4)	—
	1.55 ± 0.81 (4)	1.40 ± 0.13 (4)	
	1.41 ± 0.08 (4)		
NADPH	32.9 ± 3.6 (12)	27.7 ± 1.0 (15)	NS
Total NADP	148 ± 10 (4)	158 ± 9.4 (4)	—
	154 ± 18 (4)	142 ± 29 (3)	

Data in the left column were obtained from islets after isolation at room temperature (20–25°C) in the presence of 2.4 mM glucose. Before freezing, the islets were transferred with a syringe to a nylon filter on a Millipore chamber filter support. After washing the islets with an aliquot of perifusion fluid containing 2.4 mM glucose, the filter was removed, plunged into liquid Freon and lyophilized. The middle column shows values obtained from islets perifused at 37°C for 3 min with 2.4 mM glucose. Dimensions of P_i ATP, ADP, and total NAD are mmol/kg dry wt. Glucose-6-P, fructose-1,6-P_2 plus triose-P, NADH, 5′-AMP, NADPH, and total NADP are expressed as μmol/kg dry tissue. Standard errors are included. The number of perifusion experiments assayed is given in parentheses. The right column indicates the statistical significance of differences in cofactor and metabolite levels of the two groups of islets. NS denotes a P value greater than 0.15. Values of total NAD and total NADP are mean ± SE of individual observations of a single perifusion experiment. Here, (N) refers to number of islet samples analyzed.

Secretory and metabolic changes during and after stimulation with 14.5 mM glucose. Switching from 2.4 to 14.5 mM glucose caused a rapid increase of glucose in the effluent beginning at 1 min and reaching a maximum 3 min after the switch (not shown). A similar transition time was noted when perifusions were switched back to 2.4 mM glucose.

When islets were switched from 2.4 to 14.5 mM glucose, there was biphasic release of insulin (Figure 2). After 2 min, insulin release had doubled. The first peak occurred at 5 min; there was a sevenfold increase at this time. A 14% decrease at 8 min marked the end of the first phase of release. After 9 min of exposure to high glucose, the insulin-secretory rate increased continually with time.

Stimulation of islets with 14.5 mM glucose induced a monophasic rise of glucose-6-P (Figure 2). A 110% increase occurred within 2 min. At 20 min the increase was threefold. Unlike the rate of insulin release, the level of glucose-6-P did not continue to increase further after 20 min. When stimulated islets were switched back to basal glucose, a 38% decrease occurred within 3 min. Glucose-6-P returned to basal levels 10 min after the switch to low glucose.

Within 2 min after glucose stimulation began, a 73% increase of fructose-1,6-P_2 plus triose-P occurred (Figure 2). The increase continued throughout the stimulatory period. When islets were switched back to basal glucose, fructose-1,6-P_2 plus triose-P was lower at 3 and 10 min, but at 10 min it was still twice the prestimulatory level.

There was a loss of P_i content in islets stimulated with 14.5 mM glucose (Figure 3). The loss was first observed at 5 min and ceased by 10 min. The loss of P_i at 10 min was 14 mmol/kg dry wt, or, about 46%. P_i increased again by 6 mmol/kg dry wt in islets switched back from 14.5 to 2.4 mM glucose for 10 min, but it reached only 68% of the level seen in islets treated only with 2.4 mM glucose.

ATP increased 10%–15% after 10–30 min of exposure to high sugar (Figure 3). There was a marginal fall of ATP when islets were switched from stimulatory to basal glucose.

ADP levels decreased 30% after 20 min of stimulation (Figure 3). After switching back to low glucose for 3 min, ADP rose to prestimulatory levels.

A marked loss of 5′-AMP content occurred during stimulation with 14.5 mM glucose (Figure 3). The loss at 2 min was about 40% and at 5 min, 70%. There were no further decreases after 5 min. After switching islets back to basal glucose, 5′-AMP rose again but it reached only 75% of the

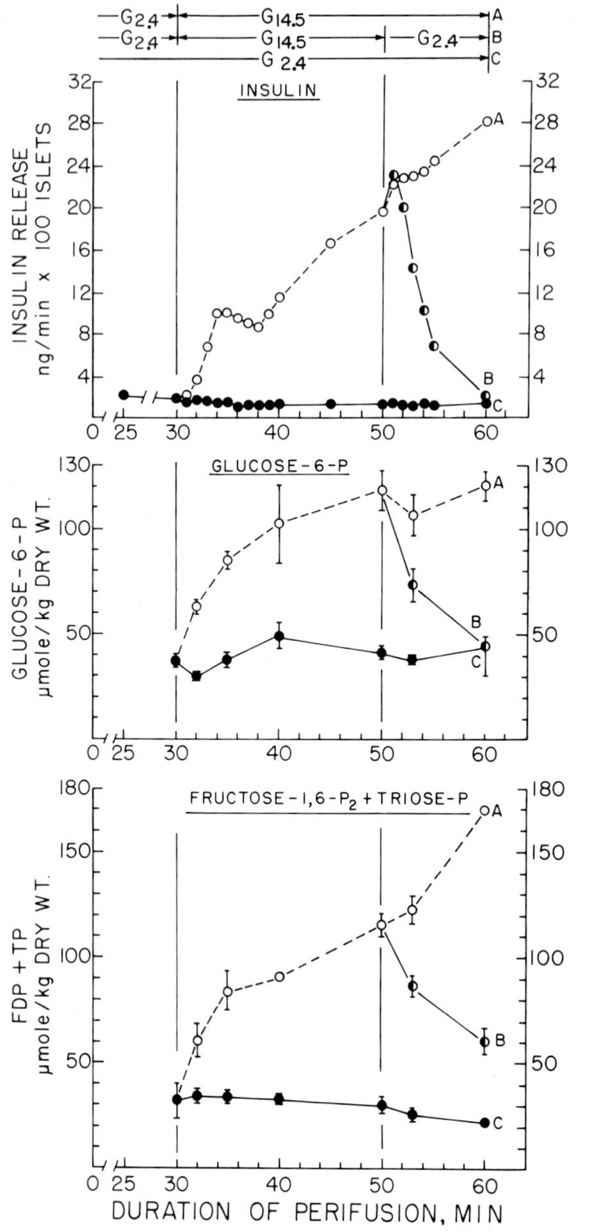

FIGURE 2. Insulin release and glucose metabolites in isolated perifused islets. The upper panel depicts the hormone release elicited by 2.4 or 14.5 mM glucose. The lower panels show the corresponding profiles of glucose-6-P and fructose-1,6-P$_2$ plus triose-P. Broken lines denote data from stimulated islets and solid lines, controls. For each perifusion condition, two to eight perifusions were analyzed for islet content of glucose-6-P and fructose-1,6-P$_2$ plus triose-P. Standard errors are given where graphically feasible. A statistical treatment is given in Table 6.

Only two perifusions were analyzed for fructose-1,6-P$_2$ plus triose-P after stimulation with 14.5 mM glucose for 10 and 30 min. The means ± SE of four individual observations of each of these perifusion experiments are as follows: at 10 min of stimulation, 104 ± 14 and 76.2 ± 5.9 and at 30 min, 149 ± 24 and 189 ± 23 μmol/kg dry wt.

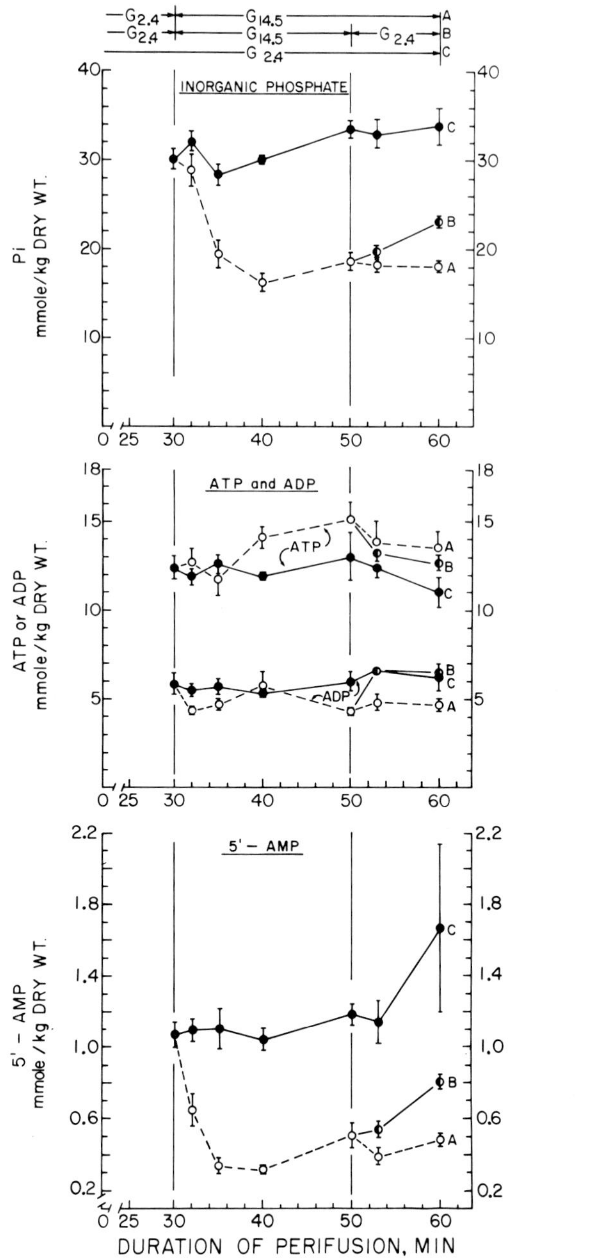

FIGURE 3. P$_i$, ATP, ADP, and 5′-AMP levels in isolated perifused islets. In the panel depicting P$_i$ levels, each point indicates the mean of 5 to 20 perifusion experiments. The panel for ATP and ADP levels shows the mean of three to five perifusions for each point. For 5′-AMP, the mean of 5 to 22 experiments is depicted. Standard errors are included. A statistical treatment of these data is given in Table 6.

prestimulatory level. Total adenine nucleotides—(ATP) + (ADP) + (5′-AMP)—did not change at any time of stimulation or perifusion with 2.4 mM glucose.

NADH levels increased in glucose-stimulated islets (Figures 4 and 7). The increase of NADH at 2 min of stimulation was 35%. After islets were switched back to basal glucose, NADH decreased within 10 min to prestimulatory levels. The changes of NADH were due to a change in the redox state—NADH/NAD$^+$—since total NAD was constant (not shown). The average total NAD content of islets exposed to 2.4 or 14.5 mM glucose for different times was 1.4 ± 0.02 (N=45) mmol/kg dry wt.

There was an increase of NADPH with stimulation (Figures 4 and 7); the increase was 125% at 10 min. A switch of stimulated islets back to basal glucose resulted in a 30% loss of NADPH, but the level was still higher than that found in islets not stimulated with 14.5 mM glucose. There was no effect on total NADP content of switching islets to high or low glucose. The average total NADP content of islets ex-

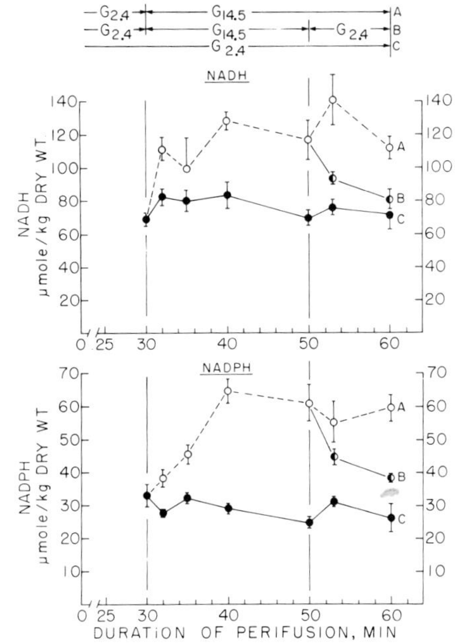

FIGURE 4. NADH and NADPH levels in isolated perifused islets. Each point indicates the mean of 5 to 26 perifusion experiments. The SE is included and a statistical treatment of these data is given in Table 6.

posed to 2.4 or 14.5 mM glucose for different times was 140 ± 3 (N= 30) μmol/kg dry wt.

The kinetics of the level changes of intermediates and cofactors differed (Figures 2–4): 5′-AMP and NADH levels attained their maximal alteration most rapidly, within 2–5 min, whereas glucose-6-P and NADPH achieved a steady state level only after 10–20 min of glucose stimulation. Fructose diphosphate plus triose-P did not seem to reach a steady state level throughout the 30-min period of stimulation.

A statistical treatment of the data shown in Figures 2 through 4 is given in Table 6.

Effect of adding 1.5 mM P_i to the perifusion fluid (Table 7). These experiments were done to determine if the P_i loss observed in glucose-stimulated islets also occurred when the islets were perifused in the presence of a P_i level similar to that of extracellular fluid. P_i added to the perifusion fluid did not change the response of most cofactors and metabolites to glucose stimulation. P_i content of islets in the presence of 2.4 mM glucose was 23% higher than that observed when islets were perifused without added P_i. After 10 min of stimulation with 14.5 mM glucose, there was a decrement of islet P_i of 18 mmol/kg dry wt, or, 46%. Thus, the decreased P_i content from glucose-stimulated islets could be of physiologic significance.

Effects of 2.4 and 8.6 mM glucose on islets from fed or fasted rats. When islets from fed rats were stimulated with 8.6 mM glucose, increased insulin first appeared in the effluent 3 min after the switch (Figure 5). The release induced by 8.6 mM glucose was biphasic. The rates of release induced by 8.6 mM glucose were about half of those obtained with 14.5 mM glucose. Starvation for 3 days completely abolished the insulin-secretory response of islets to 8.6 mM glucose.

Stimulation with 8.6 mM glucose of islets from fed rats resulted in a rise of glucose-6-P content, obvious at 2 min (Figure 5). The increase of glucose-6-P content after 20 min of stimulation was 96% or about 68% of the level attained with 14.5 mM glucose. Islets from starved rats exhibited a slow, marginal rise of glucose-6-P.

Perifusion with 8.6 mM glucose also induced a rise of fructose-1,6-P_2 plus triose-P in islets from fed or starved rats (Figure 5). Note that the increase at 2 min, about 60%, was the same in islets from fed or fasted rats. At later periods of treatment with 8.6 mM glucose, fructose-1,6-P_2 plus triose-P continued to increase only in islets from fed rats.

Islets from fed rats had decreased P_i levels after stimulation with 8.6 mM glucose (Figure 6). The P_i decrement at 20 min was 12.5 mmol/kg dry wt or 37%, only slightly less than the loss observed with 14.5 mM glucose. The loss of P_i with 8.6 mM glucose was rapid; no further loss occurred after 5 min. In the presence of 2.4 mM glucose, P_i in islets from

TABLE 6
Statistical treatment of data presented in Figures 4 through 6

Perifusion time (min)	Glucose-6-P	Fructose-1,6-P_2 plus triose-P	P_i	ATP	ADP	5′-AMP	NADH	NADPH
A vs. C comparison								
32	0.001	0.04	NS	NS	0.015	0.001	0.003	0.004
35	0.001	0.003	0.001	NS	0.14	0.001	NS	0.002
40	0.04	—	0.001	0.015	NS	0.001	0.001	0.001
50	0.001	0.001	0.001	NS	0.017	0.001	0.001	0.001
53	0.001	—	0.001	NS	NS	0.001	0.003	0.005
60	—	—	0.001	0.11	NS	0.04	0.005	0.001
A vs. B comparison								
53	0.04	0.001	NS	NS	0.006	0.045	0.01	NS
60	0.001	0.001	0.001	NS	NS	0.001	0.004	0.001
B vs. C comparison								
53	0.005	0.001	0.001	NS	NS	0.001	0.01	0.001
60	—	—	0.001	NS	NS	0.095	NS	0.02

This table indicates the P values obtained from Student's *t* test[38] for comparison of means among the experimental conditions A, B, and C, which are described in Figures 4 through 6: NS denotes a P value greater than 0.15. No P values were calculated for comparison of groups where the number of degrees of freedom was 3 or less. Since a large number of comparisons of means were made, caution should be used in evaluating P values such as 0.04 and 0.045 that are normally considered significant.

TABLE 7
Insulin release and metabolite and cofactor levels in islets stimulated with glucose in the presence of 1.5 mM P_i

Substance measured	$G_{2.4}$	$G_{14.5}$	P
Insulin release	1.28 ± 0.15 (6)	8.15 ± 1.2 (6)	0.001
Glucose-6-P	49.5 ± 8.8 (5)	83.5 ± 12 (3)	0.064
Fructose-1,6-P_2 plus triose-P	32.9 ± 7.8 (5)	79.8 ± 3.5 (3)	0.002
P_i	39.2 ± 0.46 (6)	21.2 ± 0.31 (6)	0.001
ATP	11.9 ± 0.43 (5)	14.0 ± 0.59 (3)	0.029
ADP	5.69 ± 0.26 (5)	4.46 ± 0.20 (4)	0.075
5'-AMP	935 ± 67 (6)	360 ± 25 (5)	0.001
NADH	66.0 ± 5.1 (6)	107 ± 11 (6)	0.072
Total NAD	1.51 ± 0.026 (4)	1.49 ± 0.048 (4)	—
	1.63 ± 0.063 (4)	1.47 ± 0.11 (4)	—
NADPH	35.6 ± 3.2 (6)	60.7 ± 7.0 (6)	0.009
Total NADP	111 ± 3.1 (4)	117 ± 14 (4)	—
	146 ± 18 (4)	147 ± 34 (3)	—

The left column shows data from islets perifused with 2.4 mM glucose for 40 min. Data in the right column were obtained from islets perifused with 2.4 mM glucose for 30 min and then switched to medium containing 14.5 mM glucose for 10 min. Insulin release is expressed in terms of ng/min per 100 islets and was measured at 40–41 min. Other dimensions are as indicated in Table 5. Standard errors are included. The number of perifusion experiments assayed is given in parentheses. Each value for total NAD and total NADP is the mean ± SE of individual observations of a single perifusion experiment.

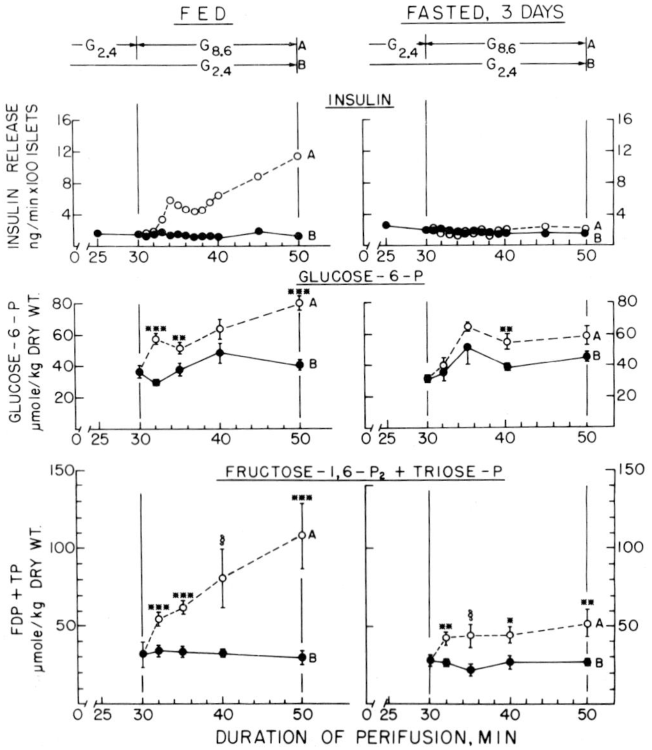

FIGURE 5. Effects of starvation on insulin release and islet content of glucose-6-P and fructose-1,6-P_2 plus triose-P. The left panels depict the hormone release and content of glucose-6-P and fructose-1,6-P_2 in islets from fed rats. The right panels show the corresponding profiles obtained from rats starved for 3 days. Solid lines denote data from islets perifused with 2.4 mM glucose. Broken lines indicate data from islets perifused with 8.6 mM glucose. Standard errors are given where graphically feasible. Asterisks denote statistical significance of differences between controls and experimentals (*0.1 > P > 0.05, **0.05 > P > 0.01, ***P < 0.01).

§Only two perifusion experiments were analyzed to obtain this point; a P value was not calculated.

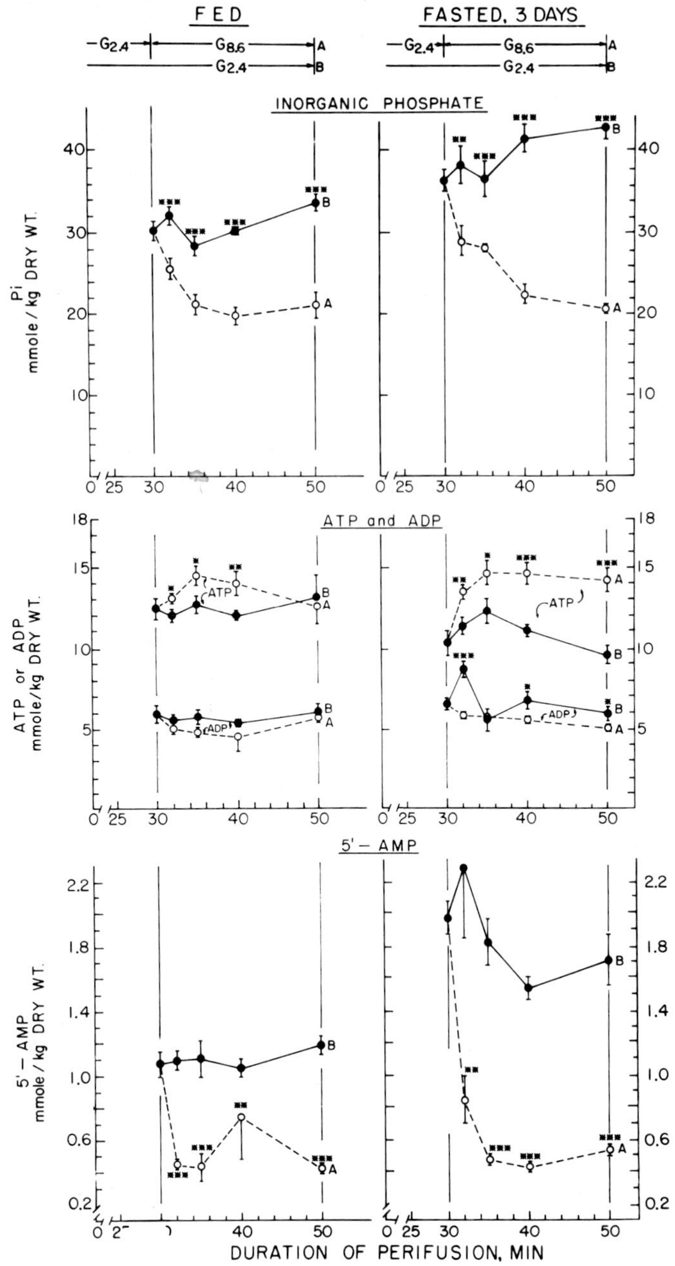

FIGURE 6. Effects of starvation on levels of P_i, ATP, ADP, and 5'-AMP in islets perifused with 2.4 or 8.6 mM glucose. The meaning of symbols is given in legend to Figure 5. Each point is the mean ± SE of three to five experiments.

starved rats were an average of 27% higher than in islets from fed rats. Starvation did not prevent the loss of P_i observed in islets switched to 8.6 mM glucose.

ATP in islets from fed rats increased 14% at 5 and 10 min during perifusion with 8.6 mM glucose (Figure 6). Increases of ATP were not as pronounced at 10 and 20 min of stimulation. Exposure to 8.6 mM glucose resulted in a more obvious and sustained increase in the ATP content of islets from starved rats.

ADP levels did not change in a consistent manner in islets from fed or starved rats. There was a tendency for islets exposed to 8.6 mM glucose to have lower values.

During perifusion with 2.4 mM glucose, the levels of 5'-AMP were an average of 70% higher in islets from starved rats when compared with islets from fed rats (Figure 6). After treatment with 8.6 mM glucose, there was a loss of 5′-AMP content in islets from both fed and starved rats, resulting in similar levels for the two groups of islets. In islets from fed rats, 5′-AMP levels were similar after exposure to 8.6 or 14.5 mM glucose.

The total adenine nucleotide contents of islets from fed or fasted rats were indistinguishable and did not appear to change after exposure to 8.6 mM glucose.

Stimulation with 8.6 mM glucose of islets from fed rats elicited a slow rise of NADH content, which reached statistical significance only at 20 min (Figure 7). The rise of NADH was marginal in islets from starved rats.

NADPH content appeared to rise during perifusion with 8.6 mM glucose of islets from fed or fasted rats (Figure 7). The rise of NADPH in islets from starved rats was apparent only at 10 and 20 min of exposure to 8.6 mM glucose.

DISCUSSION

Metabolic changes in islets during glucose stimulation of insulin release. The results of this study make possible a general evaluation of the relationships in islets among insulin release, glycolysis, and the cellular redox and phosphorylation state. The interpretation of metabolite and cofactor changes observed here in glucose-stimulated islets is guided by previous observations with static incubations indicating an increase of glycolytic flux during exposure to high glucose.[13,39,40] It is reasonable to assume that increased glycolysis occurs also in the present dynamic system when islets are switched from 2.4 to 8.6 or 14.5 mM glucose. The elevations of glucose-6-P, fructose-1,6-P_2 plus triose-P, and NADH are consistent with this interpretation. The behavior of ATP, ADP, 5′-AMP, and P_i during glucose stimulation indicates that activation of glycolysis is probably not a consequence of lower levels of high energy intermediates resulting from the increased energy demand of hormone secretion. Fructose-6-P, considering its behavior in other tissues, probably increases with increasing glucose-6-P levels.[41,42] It is presumably responsible for the increase of glycolysis at the phosphofructokinase step.[15] A similar conclusion has been made with observations of islets of the perfused pancreas, although not as many substances were measured.[43] Previous evidence indicates that islet content of glucose-6-P and fructose-1,6-P_2 plus triose-P are related to glucose levels over a physiologic range. This has been observed with islets from rats[34,36] and normal mice[34,39,44] incubated in batches. With the obese hyperglycemic mouse, the relationship has been observed in batch-incubated islets,[40] perifused islets,[45] and islets in vivo.[4] A recent study of islets in the perfused rat pancreas is in general agreement[43] and also indicates a rise of NADH[46] when insulin release is induced by glucose. The change of redox state accompanying elevated glucose is also suggested by the measurement of NAD(P)H specific fluorescence, which increases in isolated perifused islets of rats and of normal or obese hyperglycemic mice.[47] There are ambiguities associated with the interpretation of tissue surface fluorescence measurements, however.[48] The state of binding of NADPH and NADH can affect the fluorescence of these compounds.[49] Furthermore, it is not possible to assess changes of NAD^+ and $NADP^+$ with fluorescence measurement. Few reports include direct measurement of both oxidized and reduced forms of pyridine nucleotides in islets.[50–52] In one study, both oxidized and reduced forms of pyridine nucleotides were measured in batch-incubated rat islets.[52] Islets exposed to 11.1 mM glucose had a 2.7-fold higher $NADH/NAD^+$ compared with islets incubated in the absence of glucose. In the presence of 27.8 mM glucose, however, islet content of NADH, NAD^+, and $NADH/NAD^+$ was slightly lower than that in islets exposed to 11.1 mM glucose. It is difficult to interpret these results. The different levels of pyridine nucleotides in islets incubated with 0 or 11.1 mM glucose could result from a possible fuel deficit or other metabolic defect in islets incubated in the absence of glucose. The results might not reflect the normal characteristics of glucose metabolism of islets in vivo, which are always exposed to a physiologic level of glucose.

A report of adenine nucleotide levels in batch-incubated rat islets[52] indicates no difference of ATP levels in islets exposed to 11.1 or 16.7 mM glucose. Islets exposed to 11.1 mM glucose had 1.4-fold higher levels of ATP than islets incubated in the absence of glucose. ADP levels also were similar in islets exposed to 11.1 or 16.7 mM glucose but were 50% higher in islets incubated in the absence of glucose. 5′-AMP levels were 1.7, 1.04, and 0.73 pmol/islet in islets exposed to 0, 11.1, and 16.7 mM glucose, respectively. As mentioned above, these results could reflect a fuel deficit in islets incubated in the absence of glucose and might not be related to physiologic aspects of islet glucose metabolism. In batch-incubated mouse islets,[53] ATP levels increase almost twofold with increasing glucose levels in the range of 0 to 5 mM. There is a 12% further increase when glucose is increased from 5 to 20 mM. When perifused islets of the obese hyperglycemic mouse are switched from 3 to 17 mM glucose, a biphasic rise of ATP occurs.[45] In studies with rats, either in vivo[35] or using the isolated perfused pancreas,[31] there seems to be, at most, only a marginal effect of different physiologic levels of glucose on islet ATP or ADP content. These results and those of the present study suggest that the effect of physiologic glucose levels on ATP levels of viable islets is minimal.

FIGURE 7. Effects of starvation on islet content of NADH and NADPH. The meaning of symbols is given in legend to Figure 5. Each point represents the mean ±SE of from 5 to 21 perifusion experiments.

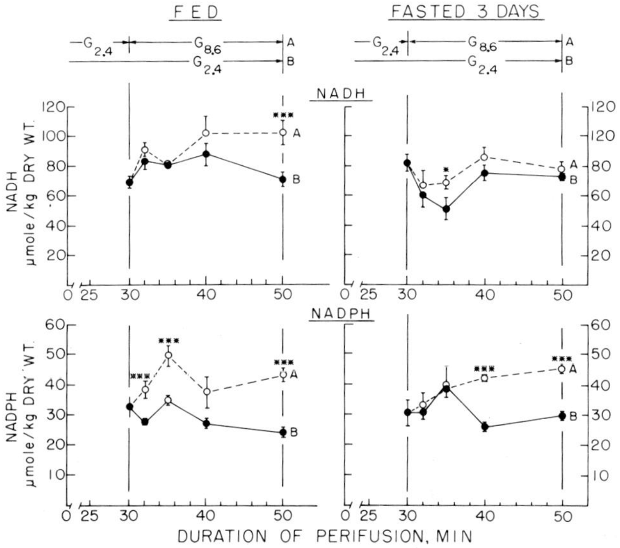

A threefold increase of ATP and ADP release into the effluent was observed when perifused rat islets were switched from 1.67 to 16.7 mM glucose.[19] The ATP and ADP lost into the effluent during the initial 30 min of stimulation was about 6.3 pmol/islet. In the present study, no change of total adenine nucleotide content occurred to coincide with this loss. Although 5′-AMP content decreased, the loss was an order of magnitude less. Only an unexpected high rate of de novo synthesis of adenine nucleotides could account for the discrepancy. Another explanation, however, consistent with the present data, is that no significant loss of adenine nucleotides occurs either by extrusion from the cell or by deamination. The decrease of 5′-AMP levels would result from phosphorylation to form ADP and ATP. Since the decrease of 5′-AMP content is small compared with ATP and ADP levels, the change in the latter two substances would not be easily detected. This conclusion is supported by changes of ^{32}P-labeling patterns in rat islets after glucose stimulation.[54,55] Increases in labeled ATP content and reductions in labeled ADP, 5′-AMP, and P_i content have been reported after 5 and 10 min[54] or 7 and 14 min of stimulation with glucose in perifused collagenase-isolated islets.

Glucose stimulation of isolated perifused islets labeled with $^{32}P_i$ results in release of radioactive phosphate into the effluent[18] in a manner parallel to the loss of P_i content observed in the present work. The present results for total tissue P_i confirm earlier observations under similar conditions.[56] The earlier report indicates that labeled and unlabeled tissue P_i content decreases to a similar extent after 30 min glucose stimulation of perifused islets. Since the specific activity of P_i within the islet does not change during glucose stimulation, the loss of P_i content is not primarily caused by increased incorporation into an organic cellular store. The net decrement of tissue $^{32}P_i$ can account for all the radioactive P_i lost during the phosphate efflux.[56] This indicates that the labeled phosphate efflux originates primarily from a labile pool of tissue P_i and not from labeled ATP, ADP, or 5′-AMP. Moreover, no release of P-labeled ATP, ADP, or 5′-AMP is seen in the effluent. In the present study, the similar decrement of P_i content of islets switched to 8.6 or 14.5 mM glucose is expected in view of the dose response characteristics of glucose-stimulated phosphate efflux from islets.[57] The biologic significance of this phosphate efflux is unknown. It has been postulated as an early event in stimulus secretion coupling.[18]

Effects of starvation and the implication of glycolysis in stimulus secretion coupling. Starvation was used to interfere with glucose stimulation of insulin release.[58-60] The effect of starvation does not seem to be due to a loss of insulin content from the islets.[59] It has been held that starvation interferes with the production of a metabolic signal needed for stimulus secretion coupling.[7] This metabolic signal presumably results from the enhancement of glycolysis and glucose oxidation when islets are exposed to increased levels of glucose. One report indicates that glucokinase and phosphofructokinase in rat islets are decreased to 36% and 49% of the control values, respectively, after a 2-day fast.[7] Thus, the impaired formation of a hypothetical metabolic signal during fasting could have resulted from adaptive changes of these enzymes. Other work indicates that glycolytic events occurring after glucose phosphorylation do not seem to be responsible for the effect of starvation on glucose-induced insulin release.[60] Starvation of rats for 1 day results in a threefold reduction of insulin release elicited by 8 mM glucose with no apparent effect on glucose use as measured by the isotopic exchange of two or five tritiated glucose with water.

In the present study, the profiles of glucose-6-P, fructose-1,6-P_2 plus triose-P, and NADH, considered together with the previous flux measurements, indicate some activation of glycolysis when islets of starved rats are switched from 2.4 to 8.6 mM glucose. This occurs despite the complete interference of stimulated rates of insulin release by 3 days' starvation. The glucose-induced changes of glucose-6-P, fructose-1,6-P_2 plus triose-P, and NADH content seem to be less pronounced in islets from starved rats than in islets from fed rats. This is especially apparent with the fructose-1,6-P^2 plus triose-P profile. There is also some attenuation of glucose use in islets of rats starved 3 days compared with islets of fed rats. The effect of starvation on insulin release is much more dramatic.[60]

The reduced secretory responsiveness of islets from starved rats does not seem to be caused by loss of the response of 5′-AMP and P_i to increased glucose. If the P_i efflux from glucose-stimulated islets is an early event in stimulus secretion coupling, starvation must interfere with events that occur later in this sequence. This is corroborated by a study of $^{32}P_i$-labeled islets from fed and 2-day-fasted rats.[61] When the perifused islets were switched from 2.8 to 8.3 mM glucose, the P_i efflux was preserved in islets of fasted rats. Nevertheless, there is some indication that starvation affects the dose response relationship betwen glucose levels and the P_i efflux.[61]

The results of the present work generally seem to agree with those of a previous study using mouse islets incubated in batches for 30 min.[44] Starvation of the mice for 2 days did not alter islet content of glucose-6-P in vitro in the presence of 16.7 mM glucose, although fructose-1,6-P_2 plus triose-P content was 25% lower. Starvation also resulted in higher levels of ATP in islets exposed to 16.7 mM glucose compared with islets from fed mice. When perifused islets from 17- or 18-h-starved obese hyperglycemic mice were switched from 3 to 17 mM glucose, the rise of glucose-6-P was similar to but that of fructose-1,6-P_2 plus triose-P was lower than in islets from fed animals.[45] These results are consistent with a block at phosphofructokinase. With the obese hyperglycemic mouse, there was no change of ATP in islets from starved animals when switched from 3 to 17 mM glucose. In the present work, the rise of ATP and other changes of the phosphate potential during glucose stimulation were more pronounced in islets from starved rats.

The procedures used in this study offer some advantages over earlier comparable endeavors. Comparisons of the tissue concentrations of metabolites and cofactors among reports are hindered by the common practice of expressing data on an islet rather than on a weight or DNA basis. Many of the previous experiments, with islets from both fed and fasted animals, were done with islets incubated in batches. In this system, temporal resolution of secretory and metabolic changes is difficult. The response could be complicated by the accumulation of products of metabolism, for example, lactate and hormones secreted, such as insulin, glucagon, and somatostatin. Although the islet perifusion system is better, it is probably not ideal, since circulation does not occur primarily through the islet capillary and diffusion of solutes into the islet might be rate limiting. The outer portion of the islet is initially exposed to higher concentrations of glucose, and stimulated insulin release there could alter secretory and metabolic events in the core of the islet. Nevertheless, the perifused islet is a dynamic system, which allows for a modicum of temporal resolution. Islet responses can be studied in the absence of neural[62] and, possibly, other influences that occur in vivo. The prior removal of exocrine tissue by collagenase treatment makes it relatively easy to measure a large number of metabolites and cofactors in islets under a variety of secretory conditions.

Conclusions. The results demonstrate that application of the sensitive fluorometric microanalytic techniques to isolated perifused islets can provide useful information on the physiologic and metabolic responses of pancreatic islet cells. The study provides basic information on the phosphorylation state and the oxidation reduction state changes of islet tissue from fed and fasted rats caused by glucose. The results suggest a close relationship between insulin release and glycolytic changes in islets. This might suggest to some that glucose stimulation of insulin release is mediated by events associated with enhanced glucose metabolism. A corollary would be that the impaired glucose-induced insulin release following starvation results from changes in the normal pattern of glucose metabolism. Other interpretations of the data are possible, however. For instance, there seems to be some dissociation of glucose metabolism from insulin release in islets of starved animals. The metabolic effects of glucose could reflect merely one aspect of a dual action on islet cells. Such processes as glucose recognition at a specific site on the cell membrane, transport, or phosphorylation would be able to rapidly relate in a direct manner the level of extracellular glucose to the rate of hormone release. If the initial recognition of glucose requires one of these events, its activation should be related to glucose levels in a manner similar to the dose response curve for insulin release. Such an event might account for the adaptive nature of glucose-induced insulin release. Changes of islet responsiveness to glucose during development, pregnancy, or starvation and refeeding might result from alterations in the level or function of this so-called glucoreceptor.

ACKNOWLEDGMENTS

This study was supported by United States Public Health Service grant AM-22122, by Diabetes and Endocrinology Centers grant AM-17094, and by United States Public Health Service neuropharmacology training grant 5-T01-NS-05221.

The figures were drawn by Ann Fuller Dillon, and the manuscript was typed by Gloria M. Jourdon.

REFERENCES

1 Matschinsky, F. M.: Enzymes, metabolites and cofactors involved in intermediary metabolism of islets of Langerhans. *In* Handbook of Physiology. Section 7, Endocrinology. Steiner, D. F., and Freinkel, N., eds. Baltimore, Williams and Wilkins, 1972, pp. 199–214.

2 Malaisse, W. J., Levy, J., Sener, A., and Herchuelz, A.: The stimulus secretion coupling of glucose induced insulin release. XXII. Qualitative and quantitative aspects of glycolysis in isolated islets, Acta Diabetol. Lat. *XIII*:202–15, 1976.

3 Lambert, A. E.: The regulation of insulin secretion. Rev. Physiol. Biochem. Pharmacol. *75*:97–159, 1976.

4 Matschinsky, F. M., and Ellerman, J.: Metabolism of glucose in islets of Langerhans. J. Biol. Chem. *243*:2730–36, 1968.

5 Hellman, B., Sehlin, J., and Taljedal, I.-B.: Evidence for mediated transport of glucose in mammalian pancreatic B-cells. Biochim. Biophys. Acta *241*:147–54, 1971.

6 Ashcroft, S. J. H., and Randle, P. J.: Enzymes of glucose metabolism in islets of Langerhans. Biochem. J. *119*:5–15, 1970.

7 Malaisse, W. J., Sener, A., and Levy, J.: The stimulus secretion coupling of glucose induced insulin release: fasting induced adaption of key glycolytic enzymes in isolated islets. J. Biol. Chem. *251*:1731–37, 1976.

8 Cahill, G. F., Ashmore, J., Earle, A. S., and Zottu, S.: Glucose penetration into liver. Am. J. Physiol. *192*:491–96, 1958.

9 Cahill, G. F., Ashmore, J., Renold, A. E., and Hastings, A. B.: Blood glucose and the liver. Am. J. Med. *26*:264–82, 1959.

10 Weinhouse, S.: Regulation of glucokinase in liver. Curr. Top. Cell. Regul. *11*:1–50, 1976.

11 Stalmans, W.: The role of the liver in the homeostasis of blood glucose. Curr. Top. Cell Regul. *11*:51–97, 1976.

12 Ashcroft, S. J. H., Weerassinghe, L. C. C., Bassett, J. M., and Randle, P. J.: The pentose cycle and insulin release in mouse pancreatic islets. Biochem. J. *126*:525–32, 1972.

13 Zawalich, W. S., and Matschinsky, F. M.: Sequential analysis of the releasing and fuel functions of glucose in isolated perifused pancreatic islets. Endocrinology *100*:1–8. 1977.

14 Krebs, H. A.: The Pasteur effect and the relation between respiration and fermentation. Essays Biochem. *8*:1–33, 1972.

15 Passonneau, J. V., and Lowry, O. H.: The role of phosphofructokinase in metabolic regulation. Adv. Enzyme Regul. *2*:265–74, 1964.

16 Chance, B., Williamson, J. R., Jamieson, D., and Schoener, B.: Properties and kinetics of reduced pyridine nucleotide fluorescence of the isolated and *in vivo* rat heart. Biochem. Z. *341*:357–77, 1965.

17 Watkins, D. F., Cooperstein, S. J. and Lazarow, A.: Stimulation of insulin secretion by pyridine nucleotides. Endocrinology *88*:1380–84, 1971.

18 Freinkel, N., Younsi, C. E., Bonnar, J., and Dawson, R. M. C.: Rapid transient efflux of phosphate ions as an early action of insulin secretagogues. J. Clin. Invest. *54*:1179–88, 1974.

19 Leitner, J. W., Sussman, K. E., Vatter, A. E., and Schneider, F. H.: Adenine nucleotides in the secretory granule fraction of rat islets. Endocrinology *96*:662–77, 1975.

20 Shultz, D. W., Passonneau, J. V., and Lowry, O. H.: An enzymic method for the measurement of inorganic phosphate. Anal. Biochem. *19*:300–14, 1967.

21 Lacy, P. E., and Kostianovsky, M.: Method for the isolation of intact islets of Langerhans from the rat pancreas. Diabetes *16*:35–39, 1967.

22 Lowry, O. H., and Passonneau, J. V.: A Flexible System of Enzymatic Analysis. New York and London, Academic Press, 1972.

23 Kissane, J. M. and Robins, E.: The fluorometric measurement of deoxyribonucleic acid in animal tissues with special reference to the central nervous system. J. Biol. Chem. *233*:184–88, 1958.

24 Lacy, P. E., Young, D. A., and Fink, C. J.: Studies on insulin secretion *in vitro* from isolated islets of the rat pancreas. Endocrinology *83*:1155–61, 1968.

25 Matschinsky, F. M., Passonneau, J. V., and Lowry, O. H.: Quantitative histochemical analysis of glycolytic intermediates and cofactors with an oil well technique. J. Histochem. Cytochem. *16*:29–39, 1968.

26 Kato, T., Berger, S. J., Carter, J. A., and Lowry, O. H.: An enzymatic cycling method for nicotinamide-adenine dinucleotide with malic and alcohol dehydrogenases. Anal. Biochem. *53*:86–97, 1973.

27 Burch, H. B., Bradley, M. E., and Lowry, O. H.: The measurement of triphosphopyridine nucleotide and reduced triphosphopyridine nucleotide and the role of hemoglobin in producing erroneous triphosphopyridine nucleotide values. J. Biol. Chem. *242*:4546–54, 1967.

28 Matschinsky, F. M.: Quantitative histochemistry of nicotinamide adenine nucleotides in retina of monkey and rabbit. J. Neurochem. *15*:643–57, 1968.

29 Yalow, R. S., and Berson, S. A.: Immunoassay of endogenous plasma insulin in man. J. Clin. Invest. *39*:1157–75, 1960.

30 Morgan, C. R., and Lazarow, A.: Immunoassay of insulin: two antibody system; plasma insulin levels of normal, subdiabetic and diabetic rats. Diabetes *12*:115–26, 1963.

31 Matschinsky, F. M., Landgraf, R., Ellerman, J. E., and Kotler-Brajtburg, J.: Glucoreceptor mechanisms in islets of Langerhans. Diabetes *21* (Suppl. 2):555–69, 1972.

32 Chi, Maggie M.-Y., Lowry, C. V., and Lowry, O. H.: An improved enzymatic cycle for nicotinamide-adenine dinucleotide phosphate. Anal. Biochem. *89*:119–29, 1978.

33 Williamson, D. H., and Brosnan, J. T.: Concentrations of metabolites in animal tissues. *In* Methods of Enzymatic Analysis. Bergmeyer, H. V., Ed. New York, Academic Press, 1974, pp. 2293–2300.

34 Ashcroft, S. J. H., Capito, K., and Hedeskov, C. J.: Time course studies of glucose induced changes in glucose-6-phosphate and fructose-1,6-diphosphate content of mouse and rat pancreatic islets. Diabetologia *9*:299–302, 1973.

35 Matschinsky, F. M., Ellerman, J. E., Krzanowski, J., Jr., Kotler-Brajtburg, J., Landgraf, R., and Fertel, R.: The dual function of glucose in islets of Langerhans. J. Biol. Chem. *246*:1007–11, 1971.

36 Montague, W., and Taylor, K. W.: Islet cell metabolism during insulin

release; effects of glucose, citrate, octanoate, tolbutamide, glucagon and theophylline. Biochem. J. *115*:257–62, 1969.

[37] Pace, C. S., Ellerman, J., Hover, B. A., and Matschinsky, F. M.: Multiple metabolic functions of glucose in rat pancreatic islets. Diabetes *24*:476–88, 1976.

[38] Snedecor, G. W., and Cochran, W. G.: Statistical Methods, 6th edit. Ames, Iowa State University Press, 1967.

[39] Ashcroft, S. J. H., and Randle, P. J.: Glucose metabolism in mouse pancreatic islets. Biochem. J. *118*:143–54, 1970.

[40] Hellman, B., Idahl, L. A., Sehlin, J., and Taljedal, I.-B.: Influence of anoxia on glucose metabolism in pancreatic islets: lack of correlation between fructose-1,6-diphosphate and apparent glycolytic flux. Diabetologia *11*:495–500, 1975.

[41] Lowry, O. H., Passonneau, J. V., Hasselberger, F. X., and Schulz, D.: Effect of ischemia on known substrates and cofactors of the glycolytic pathway in brain. J. Biol. Chem. *239*:18–30, 1964.

[42] Lowry, O. H., and Passonneau, J. V.: The relationships between substrates and enzymes of glycolysis in brain. J. Biol Chem. *239*:31–42, 1964.

[43] Trus, M. T., Hintz, C. S., Weinstein, J. B., Williams, A. D., Pagliara, A. S., and Matschinsky, F. M.: A comparison of the effects of glucose and acetylcholine on insulin release and intermediary metabolism in rat pancreatic islets. J. Biol. Chem. *254*:3921–29, 1979.

[44] Hedeskov, C. J., and Capito, K: The effect of starvation on insulin secretion and glucose metabolism in mouse pancreatic islets. Biochem. J. *140*:423–33, 1974.

[45] Idahl, L. A.: Dynamics of the pancreatic B-cell response to glucose. Diabetologia *9*:403–12, 1973.

[46] Trus, M. D., Hintz, C. S., Weinstein, J. B., Williams, A. D., Pagliara, A. S., and Matschinsky, F. M.: Effects of glucose and acetylcholine on islet tissue NADH and insulin release. Life Sci. *22*:809–16, 1978.

[47] Panten, U., Christians, J. V., Kriegstein, E., Poser, W., and Hasselblatt, A.: Effect of carbohydrates upon fluorescence of reduced pyridine nucleotides from perifused isolated pancreatic islets. Diabetologia *9*:477–82, 1973.

[48] Matschinsky, F. M., Hintz, C. S., Reichlmeier, K., Quistorff, B., and Chance, B.: The intralobular distribution of oxidized and reduced pyridine nucleotides in the liver of normal and diabetic rats. *In* Microenvironments and Metabolic Compartmentation. Eastabrook and Srere, Eds. New York and London, Academic Press, 1978.

[49] Galeotti, T., van Rossum, G. D. V., Mayer, D. H., and Chance, B.: On the fluorescence of NAD(P)H in whole-cell preparations of tumors and normal tissues. Eur. J. Biochem. *17*:485–96, 1970.

[50] Montague, W., and Taylor, K. W.: The role of the pentose phosphate pathway in insulin secretion. *In* The Structure and Metabolism of the Pancreatic Islets, Vol. 16. Falkmer, S., Hellman, B., and Taljedal, I.-B., Eds. Oxford, Pergamon Press, 1970, pp. 263–73.

[51] Ammon, H. P. T.: Effect of glucose and methylene blue (MB) on NADP, NADPH and insulin secretion of isolated pancreatic rat islets. Arch. Pharm. (Weinheim) *272* (Suppl.): RI Abstr., 1973.

[52] Malaisse, W. J., Hutton, J. C., Kawazu, S., and Sener, A.: The stimulus secretion coupling of glucose-induced insulin release. Metabolic effects of menadione in isolated islets. Eur. J. Biochem. *87*:121–30, 1978.

[53] Ashcroft, S. J. H., Weerasinghe, L. C. C., and Randle, P. J.: Interrelationship of islet metabolism, adenosine triphosphate content and insulin release. Biochem. J. *132*:223–31, 1973.

[54] Asplund, K., and Freinkel, N.: Phosphate metabolism and glucose-initiated efflux of phosphate ions in islets of fetal pancreas. Diabetes *27*:611–19, 1978.

[55] Pierce, M., Freinkel, N., Dawson, R. M. C., Asplund, K., and Bukowiecki, L.: ^{32}P-labeling patterns in rat pancreatic islets: tissue source of the radiophosphate released after glucose stimulation. Endocrinology *103*:971–77, 1978.

[56] Bukowiecki, L., Trus, M., Matschinsky, F., and Freinkel, N.: Alterations in pancreatic islet phosphate content during secretory stimulation with glucose. Biochim. Biophys. Acta *583*:370–77, 1979.

[57] Pierce, M., Bukowiecki, L., Asplund, K., and Freinkel, N.: Orthophosphate efflux from pancreatic islets: graded response to glucose stimulation. Horm. Metab. Res. *8*:358–61, 1976.

[58] Cahill, G. F., Jr., Herrera, M. G., Morgan, A. P., Soeldner, J. S., Steinke, J., Levy, P. L., Reichard, G. A., Jr., and Kipnis, D. M.: Hormone-fuel interrelationships during fasting. J. Clin. Invest. *45*:1751–69, 1966.

[59] Grey, N. J., Goldring, S., and Kipnis, D. M.: The effect of fasting, diet and actinomycin on insulin secretion in the rat. J. Clin. Invest. *49*:881–89, 1970.

[60] Zawalich, W. S., and Matschinsky, F. M.: Starvation diabetes in the rat: onset, recovery and specificity of reduced responsiveness of pancreatic B-cells. Endocrinology *104*:1344–51, 1979.

[61] Asplund, K., and Freinkel, N.: Effect of fasting on ^{32}P translocation in pre-labeled pancreatic islets. Acta Endocrinol. (Copenh) *88*:545–55, 1978.

[62] Woods, S. C., and Porte, D., Jr.: Neural control of the endocrine pancreas. Physiol. Rev. *54*:596–619, 1974.

Morphologic Study of Cultured Pancreatic Fetal Islets During Maturation of the Insulin Stimulus-secretion Mechanism

RONALD W. DUDEK, NORBERT FREINKEL, NANCY JO LEWIS, CLAES HELLERSTRÖM, AND ROBERT C. JOHNSON

SUMMARY

We recently described a tissue culture system in which 21.5-day-old fetal rat islets underwent an in vitro maturation of insulin stimulus-secretion coupling over a period of 7 days. During the same period, the acinar part of the explanted fragments degenerated and the islets became isolated, seeming to increase in mass. In the present study, we have utilized these characteristic morphologic changes in an attempt to evaluate the extent that apparent islet growth reflects multiplication of preformed beta cells or the neogenesis of these cells from ductular or acinar cells. In the first days of culture, continuity between islets and ducts could be demonstrated, and the islets appeared to "bud" from the ducts. During this time, only insulin- and glucagon-positive cells could be demonstrated immunocytochemically, and the ^{3}H-thymidine incorporation index of the beta cells (expressed as the percentage of beta cells labeled during 24 h of exposure to ^{3}H-thymidine and 3 h of "chase") in the "budding" islets was 28.7 ± 2.6. After 7 days in culture, i.e., after maturation of the insulin stimulus-secretion mechanism, the islets were no longer associated with ductular epithelium. At this stage, insulin-, glucagon-, and occasional somatostatin-positive islet cells could be demonstrated, and the ^{3}H-thymidine incorporation index of the beta cells was significantly decreased to 16.7 ± 2.8. These observations are taken to support previous suggestions of a possible neogenesis of beta cells from duct epithelium in the rat. This tissue culture technique appears well suited for further detailed studies of this neogenesis. DIABETES 29:15–21, January 1980.

To elucidate the molecular mechanisms involved in the maturation of the stimulus-secretion coupling in pancreatic islet beta cells this laboratory recently developed a tissue culture technique for the enrichment of large numbers of fetal rat islets.[1] The inherent properties of this technique are the characteristic morphologic changes, shown by the explanted pancreatic fragments, involving a marked degeneration of acinar cells and an apparent growth of islets. Within 1 wk of culture, the explants thus become transformed into numerous isolated islets, loosely attached to a monolayer of fibroblastoid cells. This process would indeed provide a unique possibility to study, under the strictly controlled conditions of tissue culture, the important question whether, in the perinatal period, beta cells arise solely by multiplication of preformed beta cells or if neogenesis from duct or acinar cells also occurs. In the present study, we followed, by light microscopy, the morphologic events that take place during culture of the fetal rat pancreas, with particular regard to the relationship between islets and ductular epithelium. In addition, we performed autoradiographic studies of the DNA replication in cultured cells with the aid of ^{3}H-labeled thymidine.

MATERIALS AND METHODS

Animals. Primiparous pregnant rats, mated at 41–57 days of age, were obtained from Charles River Laboratories (Boston, Massachusetts) at least 1 wk before the experiment. The time of mating was assessed with an accuracy of ± 12 h and was considered day 0 of pregnancy. In this strain, the length of gestation is 22–22.5 days, and all experiments with fetal rats were performed on day 21.5 of pregnancy. All animals were allowed free access to Purina rat chow and drinking water until they were killed.

Tissue culture. Tissue culture of the fetal pancreas was performed as previously described in detail.[1] Pancreases were partially digested with collagenase and cultured in RPMI-1640 containing 11.1 mM glucose, 10% heat-inactivated fetal bovine serum (Gibco, Grand Island, New York), 20 mM HN-2-hydroxyethylpiperazine-N′-2-ethanesulfonic acid buffer (HEPES), and antibiotics (penicillin 100 U/ml and streptomycin 0.1 mg/ml). The complete growth medium was changed daily.

From the Center for Endocrinology, Metabolism and Nutrition, and the Departments of Medicine, Anatomy, and Biochemistry, Northwestern University Medical School, Chicago, Illinois 60611.
Received for publication 20 August 1979.

Light microscope immunocytochemistry. Tissue was prepared for light microscopy immediately after partial digestion with collagenase and 60 min of stirring,[1] and after 48, 120, and 192 h of tissue culture. Tissue attached to the bottom of the culture dish was gently blown free with a sterilized Pasteur pipette. The culture medium, with suspended tissue, was then transferred to a test tube and pelleted by centrifugation. After washing with serum-free growth medium, the tissue was fixed in Bouin's for 2–3 h at room temperature, subsequently washed 3 times with distilled water, and enclosed in a fibrin clot to facilitate handling.[2] Tissue in the fibrin clot was dehydrated through a graded series of alcohols, three changes of xylene, and finally embedded in paraffin. Four-micron-thick serial sections were cut and mounted on glass slides.

Guinea pig antiserum to bovine insulin (GP-AIS) was supplied by the Department of Anatomy, University of Minnesota. Rabbit antiserum to glucagon (F-AGS) was a generous gift of Dr. Robert McEvoy (Mount Sinai Hospital, New York). Rabbit antiserum to synthetic somatostatin (R-ASRIF) was a gift from Dr. Robert Elde (Department of Anatomy, University of Minnesota). Sheep anti-rabbit immunoglobulin G (S-AR$_\gamma$G), capable of recognizing and binding both guinea pig and rabbit immunoglobulins, was purchased from Antibodies, Inc. (Davis, California). The soluble horseradish peroxidase-rabbit anti-peroxidase (PAP) complex was purchased from Cappel Laboratories Inc. (Downington, Pennsylvania). Normal sheep serum (NSS) was purchased from Grand Island Biological Co. All antisera were diluted with 0.05 M Tris-buffered saline (TBS), pH 7.6, containing 1% NSS.

The immunocytochemical localization of pancreatic islet cell hormones was accomplished by employing the unlabeled antibody enzyme method described by Sternberger et al.[3] The staining procedure for localization of a single antigen (hormone) consisted of exposing deparaffinized tissue sections to the following sequence of antisera: 1:1000 dilution of either GP-AIS, R-AGS, or R-ASRIF for 24 h at 4°C and then S-AR$_\gamma$G for 30 min at room temperature. Between each step in the staining sequence, the slides were rinsed with 0.05 M Tris buffer, pH 7.6. The localization of specific binding of antibody to antigen was accomplished by demonstrating the peroxidase activity of the PAP complex by incubating tissue sections in 0.05 M Tris buffer, pH 7.6, solution containing 0.03% 3-3 diamino-benzidene (Sigma) and 0.05% hydrogen peroxide. Immunocytochemical staining was identified by the deposition of a brown-colored reaction product. Slides were counterstained with Harris hematoxylin for 30 s.

Two types of control procedures were used to substantiate specific immunocytochemical staining. The first specificity control consisted of substituting normal sheep serum for the primary antisera (GP-AIS, R-AGS, R-ASRIF). The second specificity control used primary antisera, which was absorbed with an excess of purified antigen. In each case, immunocytochemical staining of the controls was negative.

Radioautography. Tissue was taken at 24, 96, and 168 h after the start of the culture and replated onto a new culture dish containing 1 μCi of ^{3}H-thymidine (New England Nuclear, Boston, Massachusetts, specific activity 6.7 Ci/mmol) per milliliter of tissue culture medium. The islets were then pulse labeled for exactly 24 h. After the pulse period, the islets were rinsed 3 times with nonradioactive medium, replated onto a new culture dish, and incubated for 3 additional h of "chase." Control islets were processed exactly as above except that the initial culture media contained 1 μCi/ml of ^{3}H-thymidine with 25 mM hydroxyurea to inhibit DNA synthesis. Islets were then histologically processed according to the following protocols.

1. The islets were harvested and fixed in Bouin's for 2 h. They were then embedded in paraffin and immunocytochemically stained for the presence of insulin, as described earlier. After staining, the slides were dried overnight at room temperature and coated, in the dark, with NTB-3 Kodak photographic emulsion. The emulsion-coated slides were dried and placed in slide boxes containing Drierite. The emulsion was exposed to the radioactive emission for 2 days at 4°C and then developed in Kodak D-19 for 2 min. Development was stopped in distilled water and the emulsion fixed in Kodak Ektaflo fixer for 6 min. The slides were then washed under running tap water for 1 h and counterstained with Harris' hematoxylin.

2. The islets were harvested and fixed, in the dark, with 3% glutaraldehyde and 2% osmium tetroxide containing 5% sucrose and 0.05% $CaCl_2$ in 0.1 M cacodylate buffer, pH 7.2 at 4°C. Islets were dehydrated through a graded series of alcohols, propylene oxide, and then embedded in Epon-Araldite. One-micron-thick plastic sections were cut with glass knives and mounted on glass slides. The plastic sections were then either directly stained with Richardson's stain or coated with Kodak NTB-3 emulsion. After exposure, development, and fixation of the photographic emulsion, the tissue was stained through the emulsion with Richardson's stain for 30 s at 40°C.

Quantitation of radioautographs. To assess the frequency of beta cells with labeled nuclei, slides were viewed with a 100× objective under oil immersion. To aid in the counting of the cells, a 100-square grid disc was installed in a 10× eyepiece. Only those cells in which both immunocytochemical staining in the cytoplasm and radioautographic labeling in the nucleus could be observed in the same plane of section were considered as beta cells that had entered the S-phase during the 24-h-labeling period. The ^{3}H-thymidine incorporation index was expressed as the number of labeled beta cell nuclei per 100 beta cells.

Counting background radiation. The average nuclear diameter of the islet cells was determined by means of the smaller grid in the center square of the micrometer grid. Using this diameter as the unit area for counting background radiation, 10 random spots in the slide (not occupied by any tissue) were selected, and the number of silver grains were counted per unit area. A nucleus was considered labeled only when it contained three or more silver grains above the average background radiation.

Microscopy. In this study and others conducted in our laboratory, the identification (in culture) of isolated islets has been facilitated by the use of a Wild M5A darkfield stereomicroscope (Wild Heerbrugg, Ltd., Heerbrugg, Switzerland). Because of the heterogeneity of tissue fragments in the culture system, the need to specifically identify islet tissue for biochemical and morphologic studies was essential. Using the Wild M5A darkfield stereomicroscope, islets were easily delineated as round, grayish structures with a bright beaded halo at the perimeter, whereas nonislet tissue, even if rounded, appeared white and opaque.

Islet perifusion and insulin assay. After 24, 96, and 168 h of culture, islets were gently blown free from the culture dish and washed 3 times with Krebs-Ringer bicarbonate buffer (KRB) modified to contain 0.5 mM HPO_4^{2-}, 1.7 mM Ca^{2+}, 5.5 mM glucose, and 0.5 mg/ml fatty acid–free albumin, pH 7.4. The islets were then perifused with apparatus and techniques as previously described.[4] After 30 min of stabilizing perifusion with KRB containing 2.8 mM glucose, fresh perifusion medium was introduced containing either 2.8 or 16.8 mM glucose. Total release of immunoreactive insulin into the nonrecirculating perifusion medium during the subsequent 15 min was collected and quantified.[4] The 15-min interval was selected in view of the evidence that acute release of insulin may be the most sensitive index of secretory responsiveness to glucose stimulation in fetal rat islets.[5,6]

RESULTS

Light microscope examination of the immunocytochemically stained sections showed that, in the freshly collagenase-treated 21.5-day-old fetal pancreas, islets remained intact but were still surrounded by a significant amount of acinar tissue (Figure 1a). Within the islets, only insulin- and glucagon-positive cells could be immunocytochemically identified at this time (Figures 1b and 1c). No somatostatin reactive components could be detected.

After 48 h in culture, insulin-positive and glucagon-positive cells appeared to "bud" from large heterogeneous structures containing degenerating acinar cells, healthy-looking ductular epithelium, and fibroblasts (Figures 2a and 2b). In all cases, some cellular continuity between the "budding islets" and ductular epithelium within the large heterogeneous structures could be demonstrated (Figure 3a). In some cases, as many as three islets budding from one large heterogeneous structure were observed. Radioautographs showed ^{3}H-thymidine-labeled cells in budding islet tissue as well as within ductular epithelium and fibroblasts (Figure 3b). Although no strict quantitative estimate was obtained, it was clearly apparent that the majority of islet tissue in culture at this point in time was in the form of budding islets, although some free-floating islets were present—as visualized in darkfield illumination.

The explanted tissue appeared to enter a transition period after 120 h in culture. It was apparent that the number of free-floating isolated islets markedly increased, whereas the number of budding islets declined. Morphologic evidence also suggested that budding islets broke free from the large heterogeneous structures and became free-floating isolated islets (Figure 4). At this time, only insulin- and glucagon-positive cells could be identified in either the budding or free-floating islets. After 192 h in culture, the vast majority of fetal islets were isolated—either free-floating or lightly attached to the bottom of the culture dish. At this time, insulin-, glucagon- and somatostatin-positive cells could be recognized within the islets (Figures 5a,5b,5c).

The ^{3}H-thymidine incorporation index of the fetal beta cells after various culture periods is given in Table 1. The highest labeling index was found at 48 h of culture, when most islets were still attached to ductular epithelium. After 120 h, the labeling frequency showed a slight, but insignificant, decrease and appeared similar in the budding islets as in the free islets. However, after 192 h in culture, when

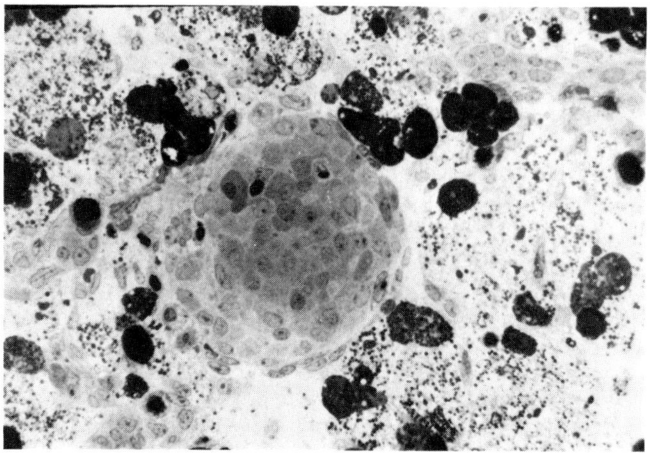

FIGURE 1. 21.5-day-old fetal pancreas after partial digestion with collagenase and 60 min of washing with HBSS as described in text. (a). One-micron-thick plastic section stained with Richardson's. Fetal islet appears intact while surrounded by acinar tissue in various states of degradation. (×500)

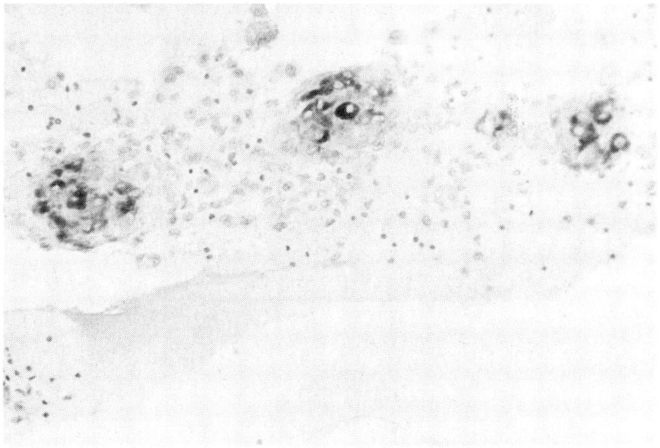

FIGURE 1(b). Paraffin section immunocytochemically stained with anti-insulin serum demonstrating the presence of insulin. (×320)

FIGURE 1(c). Paraffin section immunocytochemically stained with anti-glucagon serum demonstrating the presence of glucagon. (×320)

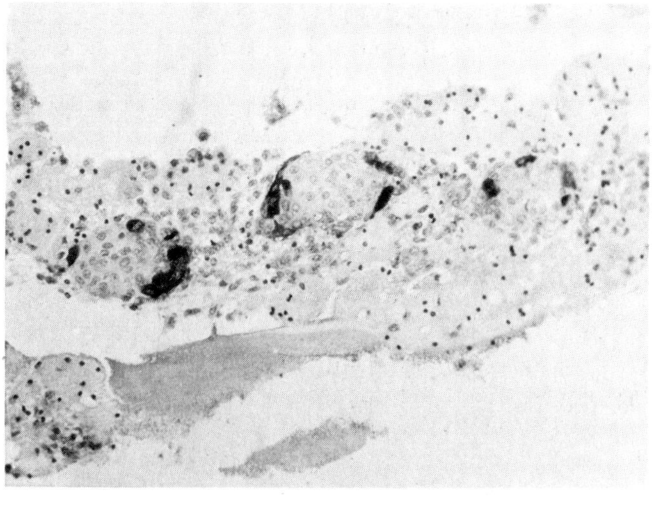

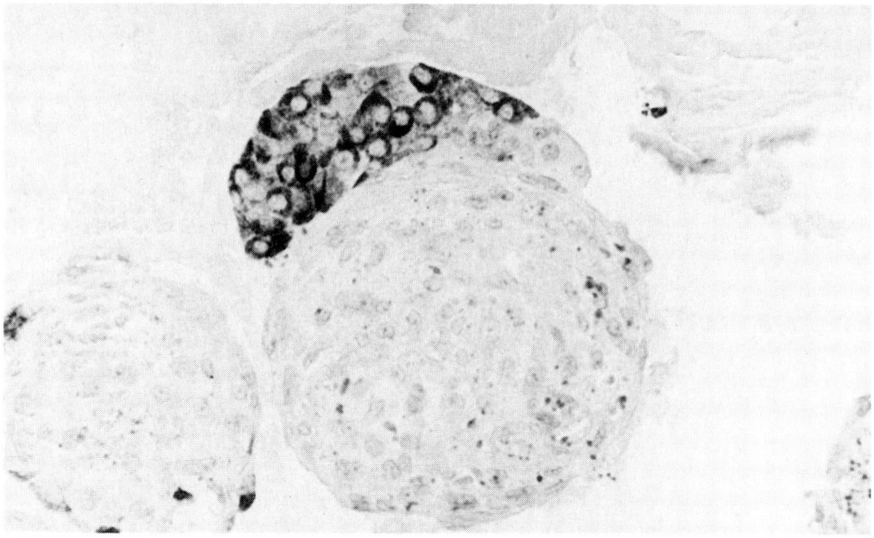

2(a)

FIGURE 2. 21.5-day-old fetal pancreas after 48 h of culture. (a). Paraffin section immunocytochemically stained demonstrating insulin-positive beta cells as a "bud" or "cap" attached to a larger heterogeneous structure. (×480)

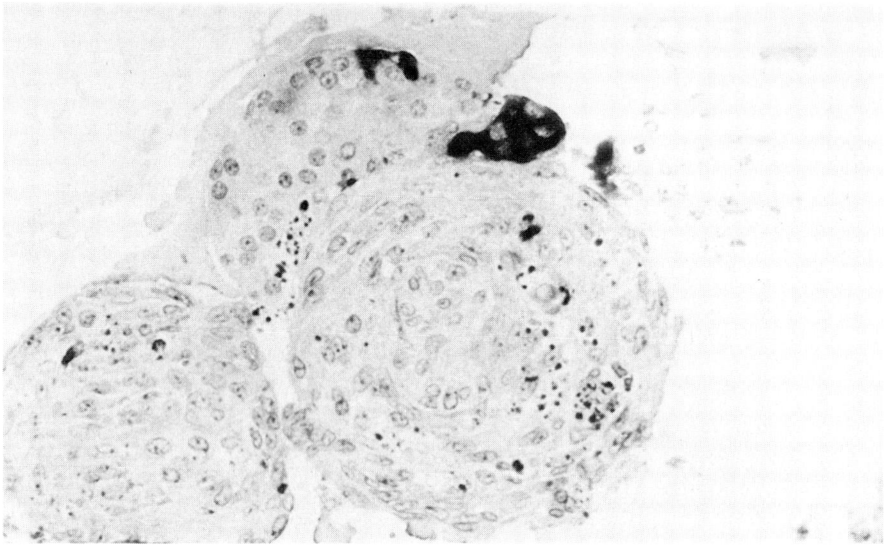

2(b)

FIGURE 2(b) Paraffin section immunocytochemically stained demonstrating glucagon-positive alpha cells also in the "bud" and preferentially located at the periphery. (×480)

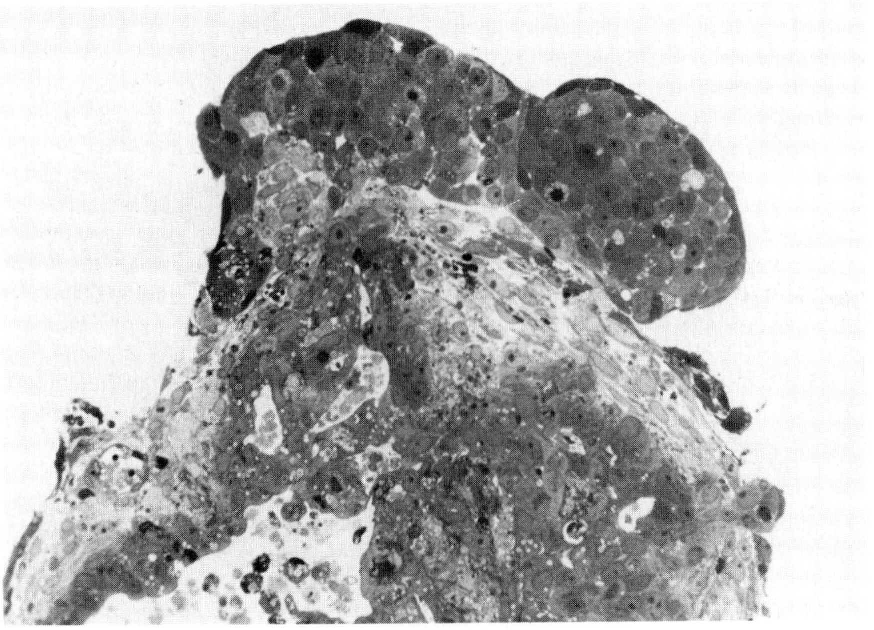

3(a)

FIGURE 3. 21.5-day-old fetal pancreas after 48 h of culture. (a). One-micron plastic section stained with Richardson's demonstrating cellular continuity between the "budding islet" and the large heterogeneous structure. The latter contains ductular epithelium and thin, flat cells that may be fibroblasts, degenerating acinar cells, and/or pluripotential precursor cells. (×500)

3(b)

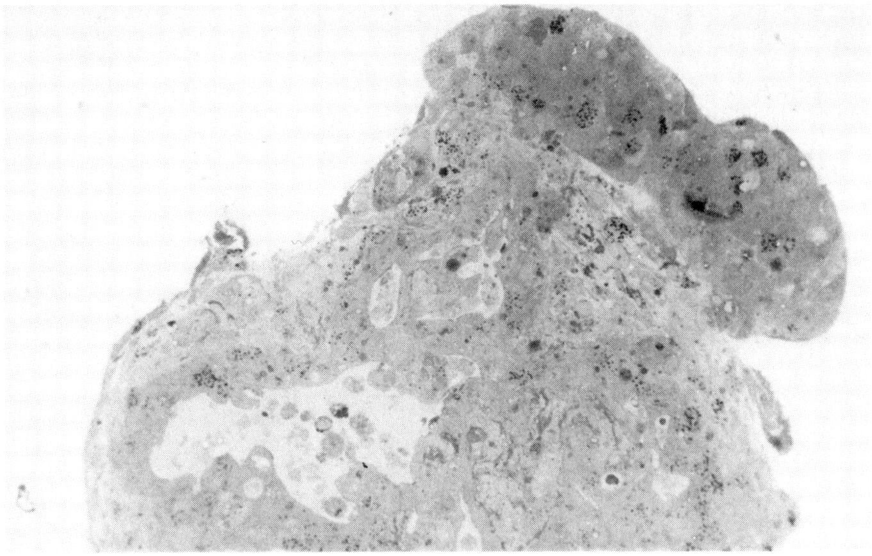

FIGURE 3(b). Radioautograph of 1-μm-thick plastic section demonstrating labeling with ^{3}H-thymidine in the nuclei of cells in the budding islet, ductular epithelium, and the thin, flat cells. (×500)

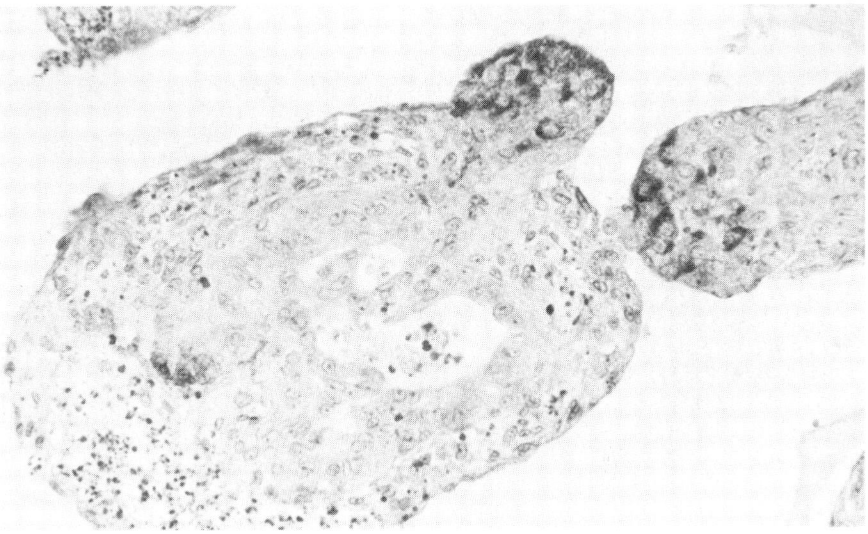

FIGURE 4. 21.5-day-old fetal pancreas after 120 h of culture. Paraffin section, immunocytochemically stained, demonstrating a smaller budding islet with insulin-positive beta cells and another larger budding islet breaking away from the large heterogeneous structure. (×480)

budding islets were no longer present, the labeling index had significantly decreased. Control islets incubated with ^{3}H-thymidine, in the presence of hydroxyurea, showed a negligible labeling irrespective of the time in culture.

Values for insulin release by cultured islets during 15 min of nonrecirculating perifusion are summarized in Table 2. Mean values for basal release of insulin per islet in the presence of 2.8 mM glucose tended to rise as culture was extended from 24 to 96 and 168 h. At each time point, stimulation with 16.8 mM glucose elicited significant acute enhancements of insulin release above basal values. However, the increases were relatively small with islets that had been cultured for only 24 or 96 h, whereas much greater stimulation was observed after 168 h of tissue culture (Table 2).

DISCUSSION

This laboratory had previously reported[1] an in vitro technique in which tissue culture of minced and mildly collagenase-digested fetal rat pancreas led to the enrichment of a large number of isolated islets. It was furthermore documented that the maturation of insulin-secretory responsiveness is related to the glucose concentration in the growth medium. Thus, fetal islets cultured for 192 h in RPMI 1640 containing 11.1 mM glucose showed a marked and significant insulin release in response to glucose stimulation during 60 min of incubation in batch-type systems. When the culture period was confined to 24 h in RPMI 1640 with 11.1 mM glucose, there was, however, an insignificant insulin response to glucose. Corresponding observations were made in the present study, although a statistically significant glucose stimulation of the insulin release was already observed after 24 h of culture. This presumably was due to the greater sensitivity that is achieved during shorter observations with the use of the perifusion system. The data nevertheless reemphasize the gradual maturation of the stimulus-secretion coupling that takes place during culture of fetal beta cells.

The present data furthermore suggest that, during culture, there was de novo formation of beta cells, as judged by ^{3}H-thymidine incorporation index at various time periods. These results, together with the observation of cellular conti-

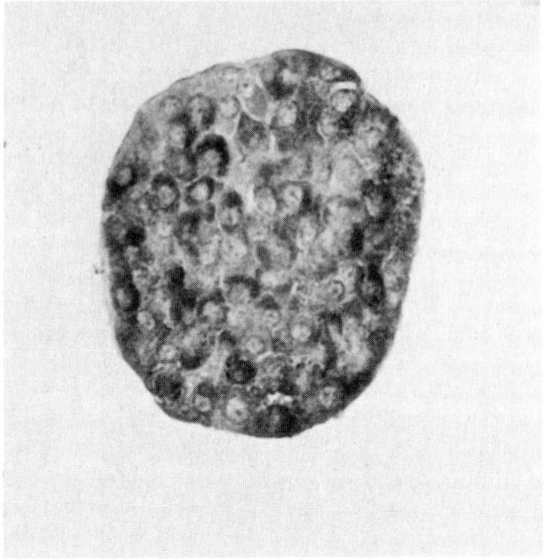

5(a)

FIGURE 5. 21.5-day-old fetal pancreas after 192 h of culture. (a). Paraffin section immunocytochemically stained with anti-insulin serum. The islet is completely isolated from any surrounding tissue and consists principally of insulin-positive beta cells. (×560)

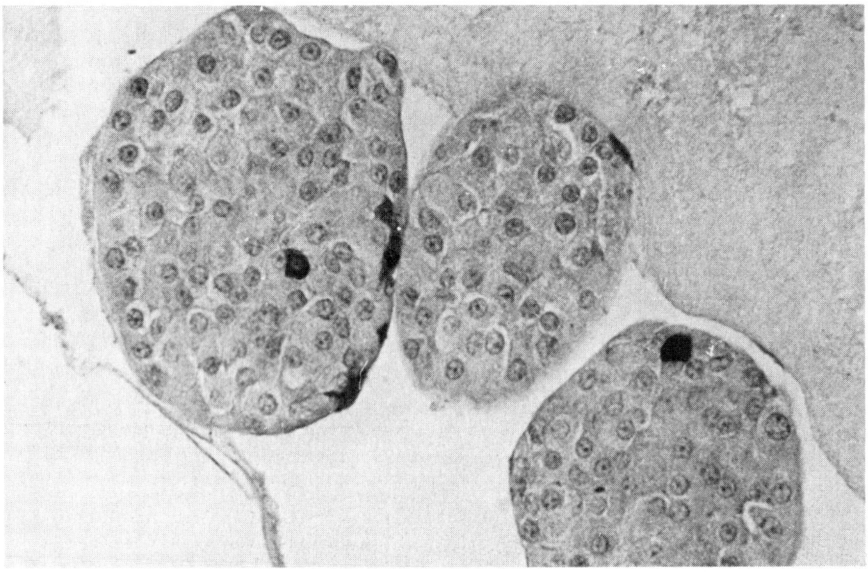

5(b)

FIGURE 5(b). Paraffin section immunocytochemically stained with anti-glucagon serum demonstrating relatively few glucagon-positive alpha cells. (×560)

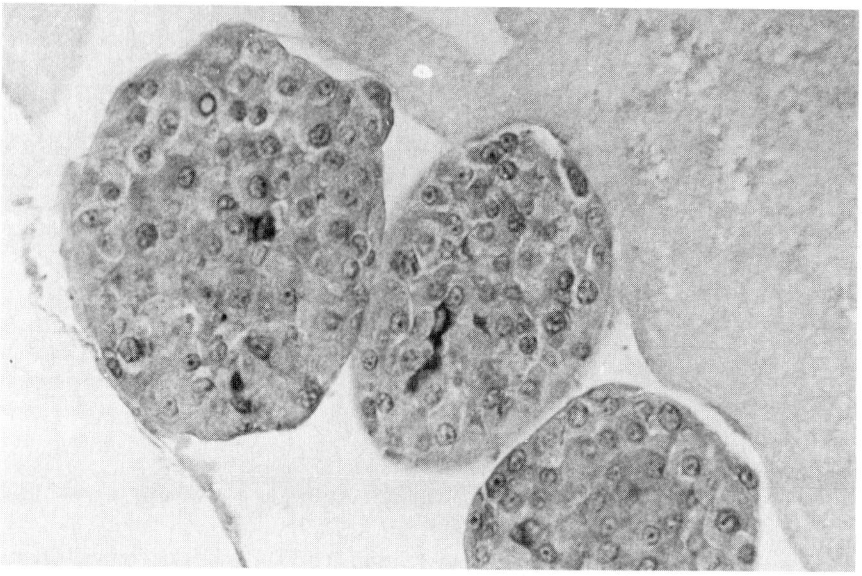

5(c)

FIGURE 5(c). Paraffin section, immunocytochemically stained with anti-somatostatin serum, demonstrating a few delta cells within the islets. (×560)

TABLE 1
^{3}H-Thymidine incorporation index of beta cells*

Hours in culture	Budding islets†	Free islets†	Hydroxyurea treated
48 + 3	28.7 ± 2.7[a] (3)	—	2.8 ± .06 (3)
120 + 3	23.9 ± 1.4[b] (6)	22.1 ± 1.8[c] (6)	4.8 ± 0.9 (6)
192 + 3	—	16.7 ± 1.7[d] (3)	4.1 ± 0.2 (3)

* Islets were pulse labeled in the presence of ^{3}H-thymidine for the final 24 h of culture and then "chased" in nonradioactive media for 3 additional h, as described in the text. Values for the ^{3}H-thymidine incorporation index (i.e., number of labeled beta cell nuclei per 100 beta cells) have been presented as mean ± SEM; parentheses denote the number of cultures examined.

† Statistical analysis by Student's *t* test disclosed: a vs d, $P < 0.05$; b vs d, $P < 0.05$; a vs b, b vs c, c vs d, not significant.

TABLE 2
Insulin release by fetal islets cultured for various time periods*

	μU/islet/15 min	
Hours in culture	2.8 mM glucose†	16.8 mM glucose†
24	1.05 ± 0.1[a] (3)	2.50 ± 0.4[b] (4)
96	1.62 ± 0.5[c] (4)	5.72 ± 0.9[d] (7)
168	2.31 ± 0.5[e] (4)	21.0 ± 1.1[f] (13)

* Mean ± SEM values for the total release of immunoreactive insulin into the perifusion medium during 15 min of nonrecirculating perifusion with KRB containing 2.8 or 16.8 mM glucose are presented. Parentheses denote the number of cultures perifused.

† Statistical analysis by Student's *t* test disclosed: a vs c, c vs e, not significant; a vs e, $P < 0.05$; a vs b, $P < 0.05$; c vs d, $P < 0.02$; e vs f, $P < 0.001$; b vs d, $P < 0.02$; b vs f, $P < 0.001$; d vs f, $P < 0.001$.

nuity between budding islets and ductular epithelium, support the idea that beta cell neogenesis is somehow related to duct epithelium. This postulate is reinforced by the observation of islet tissue breaking off from the large heterogeneous structures, the similarity of ^{3}H-thymidine incorporation index in budding islets, and free-floating isolated islets after 120 h in culture (i.e., when both budding and free-floating islets are present). In addition, there was a significant difference in the ^{3}H-thymidine incorporation index between budding islets after 48 or 120 h in culture and the isolated islets after 192 h in culture. This increased propensity for ^{3}H-thymidine incorporation in budding islets after 48 and 120 h in culture may be due, at least in part, to a possible precursor relationship of ductular epithelium to budding islets.

In summary, the present culture technique seems to offer better possibilities for a detailed study of the perinatal growth of the beta cells than have hitherto been available. Islets budding from ductular epithelium have been described before, but thus far, only after pancreatic exocrine atrophy caused by duct ligation in adult animals.[7–9] In these experiments, autoradiography revealed a much greater regeneration of both islet and duct epithelium in the atrophic pancreas than in the normal pancreas.[10] It cannot be excluded that the in vitro atrophy of the acinar part, which is a characteristic of the present culture method, enables the fetal beta cells to replicate at an even higher rate than normally occurs in vivo. Electron microscope studies are underway to see if some of these cells are in the process of transforming from duct epithelial cells to granule-containing beta cells. Needless to say, a demonstration of beta cell neogenesis from duct cells in vitro will have important implications with regard to delineating the factors that promote this process.

ACKNOWLEDGMENTS

This investigation was supported by research grants AM 10699 and MRP HD 11021 and training grants AM 05071 and AM 07169 from the National Institutes of Health, Bethesda, Maryland; a research grant from the Kroc Foundation; and by Fellowship AM 05873 from the National Institutes of Health to Dr. Dudek. Dr. C. Hellerström was a Visiting Scientist in the Center for Endocrinology, Metabolism and Nutrition, Northwestern University Medical School, in 1977 and his work was supported in part by grants from the Swedish Diabetes Association, Stiftelsen Expressens Prenatalforskningsfond, and the Swedish Medical Research Council (12X-109).

REFERENCES

[1] Hellerström, C., Lewis, N. J., Borg, H., Johnson, R., and Freinkel, N.: Method for large-scale isolation of pancreatic islets by tissue culture of fetal rat pancreas. Diabetes *28*:769–77, 1979.

[2] Furtado, J. S.: The fibrin clot: a medium for supporting loose cells and delicate structures during processing for microscopy. Stain Technol. *45*:19–20, 1970.

[3] Sternberger, L. A., Hardy, P. H., Cuculis, J. J., and Meyer, H. G.: The unlabeled antibody method of immunohistochemistry. J. Histochem. Cytochem.*18*:315–27, 1970.

[4] Freinkel, N., El Younsi, C., Bonnar, J., and Dawson, R. M. C.: Rapid transient efflux of phosphate ions from pancreatic islets as an early action of insulin secretagogues. J. Clin. Invest. *54*:1179–89, 1974.

[5] Burr, I. M., Kanazawa, Y., Marliss, E. B., and Lambert, A. E.: Biphasic insulin release from perifused cultured fetal rat pancreas. Diabetes *20*:592–97, 1971.

[6] Asplund, K., and Freinkel, N.: Phosphate metabolism and glucose-initiated efflux of phosphate ions in islets of fetal pancreas. Diabetes *27*:611–19, 1978.

[7] Hultquist, G. T., and Jonsson, L. E.: Ligation of the pancreatic duct in rats. Acta Soc. Med. Ups. *70*:82–88, 1965.

[8] Edström, C., and Falkmer, S.: Pancreatic morphology and blood glucose levels in rats at various intervals after duct ligation. Virchows Arch. [Pathol. Anat.] *345*:134–53, 1968.

[9] Boquist, L., and Edström, C.: Ultrastructure of pancreatic acinar and islet parenchyma in rats at various intervals after duct ligation. Virchows Arch. [Pathol. Anat.] *349*:69–79, 1970.

[10] Hultquist, G., Karlsson, U., and Hallner, A. C.: The regenerative capacity of the pancreas in duct ligated rats. Exp. Pathol. *17*:44–52, 1979.

The Glucose Intolerance of Acute Pancreatitis
Hormonal Response to Arginine

SOLOMON S. SOLOMON, WILLIAM C. DUCKWORTH, PANDURANGA JALLEPALLI, MARY ALICE BOBAL, AND RAMAMURTHI IYER

SUMMARY

Patients with acute pancreatitis were studied by arginine infusion at 48–72 h, 7–10 days, and 18–21 days after onset of their illness. Plasma glucose, insulin, and glucagon values were determined. Acute pancreatitis was characterized by fasting hyperglycemia and hyperglucagonemia, associated with relative hypoinsulinemia. Arginine stimulation early in the disease (48–72 h) demonstrated hyperglycemia and hyperglucagonemia, which normalized by 18–21 days. Both phases of the normal biphasic insulin response to arginine were decreased during the initial arginine infusion. By 18–21 days, although the first phase was completely normal, the second phase of insulin secretion remained depressed.

Acute pancreatitis is associated with damage to both the endocrine and exocrine pancreas. Glucose intolerance seen with this disease appears to be the result of hyperglucagonemia and relative hypoinsulinemia. Although the healing process at 3 wk is associated with return of plasma glucose and glucagon concentrations to normal, the impaired second phase insulin secretion persists. DIABETES 29:22-26, January 1980.

Clinicians have long observed the presence of transient hyperglycemia in patients with acute pancreatitis[1–3] and the development of diabetes mellitus in patients with chronic pancreatitis.[1,3–5] In chronic pancreatitis the carbohydrate intolerance is most frequently attributed to hormonal deficiency, with absolute decreases in both insulin and glucagon secretion as the pancreatic insufficiency progresses.[2,4–6] In contrast, the pathogenesis and progression (or resolution) of the hyperglycemia associated with acute pancreatitis and the nature of the alterations in insulin and glucagon secretion are less clear.[2] In the initial phase of acute pancreatitis (first 24 h), hyperglycemia is almost invariably present and is accompanied by hyperglucagonemia.[2,7] The increase in glucagon levels is much greater than that caused by stress alone.[7] Insulin levels have also been reported to be elevated during the first 24 h of acute pancreatitis,[2,8] but, in another study, insulin levels were considered low relative to the blood glucose.[7]

Because the changing patterns of pancreatic endocrine function have not been adequately described past the first 24 h of acute pancreatitis, we examined basal and stimulated insulin and glucagon secretion in a group of patients with acute pancreatitis. Following are the results of this study, in which repeated arginine infusions were given for 21 days after the acute episode.

MATERIALS AND METHODS

Patients. Twelve patients who had a diagnosis of acute pancreatitis received arginine infusions to study the effects of the disease on pancreatic endocrine function. The diagnosis was established by finding consistent clinical features—elevated serum and urine amylase and/or lipase and an appropriate history. Nine patients had no prior history, two had a history of one episode, and one had had two previous episodes of acute pancreatitis. No evidence of chronic pancreatitis[1,3,9] was present by clinical, laboratory, or x-ray findings. No patient had previously been diagnosed to have diabetes mellitus or glucose intolerance. The patients ranged in age from 24 to 61 yr, were all within 15% of their ideal body weight, and were male veterans (Tables 1 and 2). The population studied was compared with an age-, weight-, sex-, and race-matched population without pancreatitis, hospitalized for unrelated problems, who had the same degree of ambulation as the pancreatitis population. All patients were taking or had just discontinued intravenous therapy and were receiving only narcotics for pain. All drugs were discontinued during the study. Arginine infusions were given at three times after admission: 48–72 h

From the Research and Medical services of the VA Medical Center and University of Tennessee Center for the Health Sciences, Memphis, Tennessee 38104.
Address reprint requests to Solomon S. Solomon, M. D., Research Service, VA Medical Center, 1030 Jefferson Avenue, Memphis, Tennessee 38104.
Received for publication 8 June and in revised form 11 September 1979.

TABLE 1
Clinical findings in 12 patients with acute pancreatitis

Subject	Age (yr)	Height	Weight (lb)	History of alcoholism	Previous attack of pancreatitis	Evidence of chronic pancreatitis, gallstones, x-ray, malabsorption	Other diseases and medication
L.C.	44	5′11″	163	+	1	−	0
W.J.	40	6′	170	+	0	−	Diet controlled AODM; Maalox PRN
C.A.	28	5′6″	142	+	0	−	0
J.C.	38	6′	153	+	0	−	0
M.L.	28	6′3″	180	+	0	−	Maalox for ? ulcer
W.C.	55	5′9″	165	+	2	−	0
P.F.	57	5′7″	152	+	0	−	0
F.M.	50	5′11″	141	+	0	−	0
M.C.	61	5′9″	166	−	0	−	Thorazine (schizophrenia); motrin (arthritis)
W.B.	24	6′	200	−	0	−	0
R.S.	47	5′11″	158	+	0	−	0
T.R.	50	6′1″	150	−	1	−	Maalox, Valium, Tylenol
Ave $\bar{X}$	43.5	5′9″	162	+			

(ARG-I), 7–10 days (ARG-II), and 18–21 days (ARG-III). Twenty-two individual patient studies in 12 subjects were conducted. Six patients from ARG-I were restudied in ARG-II. Four patients in ARG-II were restudied in ARG-III. Additional fasting plasma samples for determination of glucose, insulin, and glucagon were obtained from other patients recovering from an episode of acute pancreatitis. A total of 53 fasting samples was obtained from 26 patients at varying times after admission for acute pancreatitis.

All studies were conducted under the auspices of the Human Studies Committee of the VA Hospital and the University of Tennessee Center for the Health Sciences. Informed consent was obtained from all patients and from volunteer control subjects.

Studies. All studies were conducted in the morning after an overnight fast. Fasting blood samples (N = 53) were taken for 21 days from the time of admission and the plasma was analyzed for glucose, insulin, and glucagon.

The patients chosen for investigation received an arginine infusion, amounting to 11.7 mg/kg body wt/min, i.v., in normal saline, for 40 min. Blood samples were taken at 0, 2, 5, 10, 20, 30, 40, 50, 60, 75, and 90 min and again analyzed for glucose, insulin, and glucagon. Arginine infusions were done three times, at 48 h, 7–10 days, and 18–21 days.

Laboratory methods. Plasma glucose was determined by the glucose oxidase method.[10] Plasma insulin and glucagon were determined by previously described radioimmunoassay procedures, employing 30K glucagon antiserum for glucagon determinations.[11–13] Statistical analyses were done by standard Student's *t* test.[14]

RESULTS

Data shown in Table 1 establish a clinical profile of patients studied who had the diagnosis of acute pancreatitis. Data shown in Table 2 establish baseline laboratory findings in these patients. These patients have decreased serum proteins, elevated serum and urinary amylase, and elevated alkaline phosphatase, SGOT, LDH, and CPK. With the history

TABLE 2
Laboratory findings in 12 patients with acute pancreatitis*

Subject	Ca (mg/dl)	P (mg/dl)	Proteins (g/dl)	Amylase (U/dl)	Urinary amylase (U/dl)	Alk PO_4 (mU/ml)	Direct bilirubin (mg/dl)	SGOT (IU/ml)	LDH (IU/L)	CPK (IU/L)	CHOL (mg/dl)	TG (mg/dl)
L.C.	9.2	2.3		960	1296	73	0.7	22	279	109	261	77
W.J.	9.9	2.9	6.0	264	1535	123	0.8	14	294	67	189	191
C.A.	9.2	3.6	6.3	690	1540	60	0.7	43	437	608	177	51
J.C.	10.4	0.8		240	2720	189	—	91	381	226	198	112
M.L.	9.7	3.0	6.7	91	270	—	—	13	255	280	—	—
W.C.	9.2	2.3		88	375	85	1.0	96	334	38	190	156
P.F.	—	—		400	—	—	—	—	—	—	—	—
F.M.	8.8	2.1		336	2240	123	0.8	89	240	—	133	72
M.C.	11.2	2.1		371	1720	107	0.4	15	130	74	154	86
W.B.	8.4	3.4		320	1200	84	1.1	30	—	—	146	100
R.S.	10.1	4.3		272	4336	114	—	48	235	178	234	72
T.R.	8.7	—		272	112	—	—	—	—	—	116	65
N	11	10	3	12	11	9	7	10	9	8	10	10
$\bar{X}$	9.5	2.7	6.3	358	1577	106	0.8	46	287	207	180	98
Normal	8.4–10.7	2.5–4.5	6.4–7.9	80–150	90–560	30–110	0.2–1.0	0–20	130–290	0–50	310	160

* Unless indicated otherwise, values are for serum.

and clinical findings, these laboratory data are diagnostic of acute pancreatitis.

Fasting plasma glucose, insulin, and glucagon values were obtained from a group of pancreatitis patients at various times after an acute attack (data not shown). Patients studied shortly after the acute episode have fasting hyperglycemia, hyperglucagonemia, and relative hypoinsulinemia. With time, the glucose and glucagon values gradually decreased, returning to normal by about 2 wk.

In order to evaluate the ability of the pancreas to respond to a stimulus, arginine infusions were performed at 48–72 h, 7–10 days, and 18–21 days after admission for acute pancreatitis. Plasma glucose, insulin, and glucagon levels were measured during each of these infusions. Figure 1 shows the glucose values. Acute pancreatitis results in hyperglycemia. All glucose values obtained during the first arginine infusion were significantly greater than control. In contrast to control subjects, the average glucose values of the pancreatitis patients did not increase in response to arginine, but this apparent lack of response was caused by the more erratic pattern seen in pancreatitis patients. If the maximal change from basal glucose (fasting) to peak glucose is determined for each patient regardless of time of occurrence, then the response for pancreatitis patients and controls is similar (Table 3).

By 7–10 days after admission (ARG-II), glucose values had decreased but fasting levels remained significantly elevated over controls, as did values at the early times of the arginine infusion (Figure 1). By 18–21 days, all values were within the normal range. Table 4 shows the total area under the glucose curve for the three arginine infusions, demonstrating the progressive decrease in plasma glucose response to arginine with time.

In response to an arginine infusion, insulin is secreted in a biphasic manner in normal subjects (Figure 2). In pancreatitis patients 48–72 h after admission, first phase insulin secretion was significantly decreased and very little second phase secretion could be identified. All insulin values during the arginine infusion (ARG-I) were significantly less than control (Figure 2). If the maximal change for each patient is calculated, the average increase during the first 5 min of the arginine infusion (peak 1) was 34 ± 5 μU/ml for control and 15 ± 3 μU/ml for pancreatitis patients ($P < 0.005$) (Table 3). For peak 2 (highest value after 5 min) the control value was 59 ± 7 μU/ml and for pancreatitis patients, 11 ± 3 μU/ml ($P < 0.001$).

By 7–10 days, the first phase insulin secretion was completely restored, but the second phase remained impaired (Figure 2 and Table 3). Even at 18–21 days after the acute episode, second phase insulin secretion remained significantly decreased compared with control.

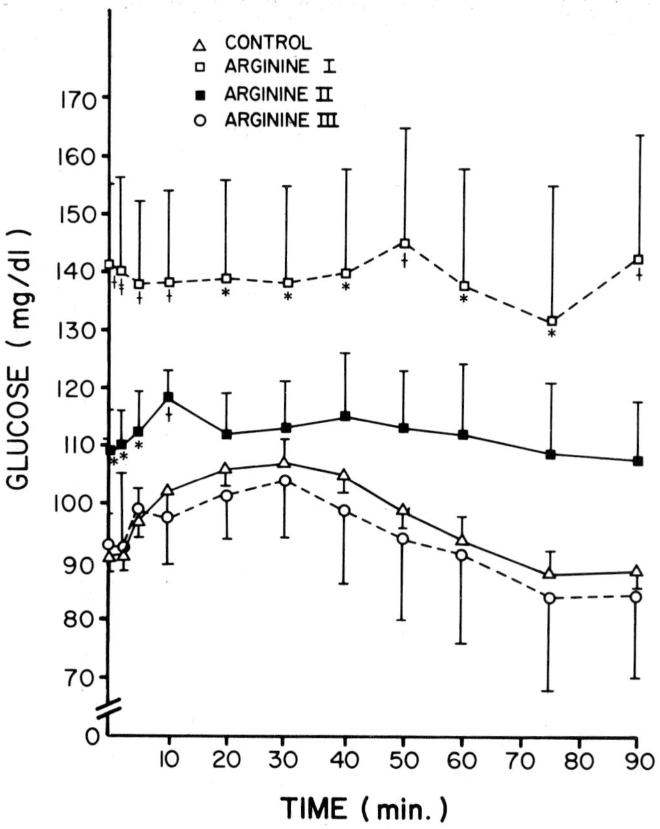

FIGURE 1. Studies of three arginine infusions in 12 patients with acute pancreatitis. Control values are shown (N = 9). Arginine (ARG) infusions were performed at 48–72 h (ARG-I, N = 7), at 7–10 days (ARG-II, N = 11), and at 18–21 days (ARG-III, N = 4). Plasma samples were analyzed for glucose (mg/dl). Values are shown as average ± SEM. Statistical significance for each point compared with control: *P < 0.05; †P < 0.01; and ‡P < 0.001.

Glucagon levels were strikingly elevated in patients with acute pancreatitis. During the first arginine infusion, all glucagon levels were significantly increased in patients with acute pancreatitis (Figure 3). The net change (basal to peak), however, although greater in patients with pancreatitis than in controls, was not statistically significant because of a wide variation in individual responses (Table 3).

TABLE 3
Plasma glucose, insulin, and glucagon after three arginine (ARG) infusions

		Glucose (mg/dl)			Insulin (μU/ml)					Glucagon (pg/ml)		
	N	B	P	P − B	B	P_1	P_2	$P_1 - B$	$P_2 - B$	B	P	P − B
Control	9	91 ± 3	107 ± 4	17 ± 2	12 ± 1	46 ± 6	71 ± 7	34 ± 5	59 ± 7	171 ± 26	588 ± 117	410 ± 115
ARG-I	7	141 ± 14	154 ± 19	13 ± 8	15 ± 1	30 ± 2	25 ± 3	15 ± 3	11 ± 3	648 ± 177	1394 ± 325	710 ± 333
		0.001	0.001	NS	NS	0.01	0.001	0.005	0.001	0.001	0.01	NS
ARG-II	11	110 ± 7	126 ± 9	16 ± 5	17 ± 3	50 ± 7	44 ± 7	34 ± 5	28 ± 7	301 ± 39	678 ± 89	378 ± 74
		0.025	0.05	NS	NS	NS	0.005	NS	0.001	0.01	NS	NS
ARG-III	4	93 ± 7	107 ± 9	14 ± 5	16 ± 1	48 ± 13	43 ± 12	32 ± 14	26 ± 13	196 ± 44	610 ± 126	414 ± 106
		NS	NS	NS	0.025	NS	0.025	NS	0.01	NS	NS	NS

B = basal; P = peak; P_1 = first peak, 0–5 min; P_2 = second peak, after 5 min; and (P − B) = net difference. Values shown are average ± SEM. N = number of patients studied. P values are shown against controls in each case.

TABLE 4
Integrated area under curve for glucose, insulin, and glucagon after three arginine infusions

	Control (N = 9)	ARG-I (N = 7)		ARG-II (N = 11)		ARG-III (N = 4)	
Glucose	8,713 ±301	12,456 ±1,674	0.01	9,763 ±1,262	NS	8,438 ±1,017	NS
Insulin	3,481 ±379	1,655 ±201	0.001	2,578 ±322	NS	2,781 ±450	NS
Glucagon	34,684 ±4,180	94,498 ±14,293	0.001	41,510 ±3,740	NS	42,229 ±9,478	NS

Values shown are average ± SEM. N = number of patients studied. P values are shown against controls in each case. Integrated areas for glucose, mg/dl/90 min; insulin, μU/ml/90 min; and glucagon, pg/ml/90 min.

By 7–10 days, although fasting plasma glucagon levels remained significantly elevated, most of the stimulated values were within the normal range (Figure 3 and Table 3), and the total area under the curve was not significantly different from that of control (Table 4). By 21 days, all values had returned to normal.

DISCUSSION

These data demonstrate that patients with acute pancreatitis, examined within 48–72 h after onset of their illness, have fasting hyperglycemia, hyperglucagonemia, and relative hypoinsulinemia. With recovery from the acute episode, these changes gradually reverse, reaching normal by about 15 days. In other studies, hyperglycemia and hyperglucagonemia have been demonstrated during the acute phase (first 24 h) of pancreatitis,[2,7] but the time required for restoration of normal fasting levels has not previously been well defined.

We have also examined the response of the endocrine pancreas to stimulation at various times after an episode of acute pancreatitis. Elevated glucagon levels are characteristic of acute pancreatitis, and all glucagon values obtained during an arginine infusion 72 h after the acute episode were significantly greater than control values. The change in glucagon levels (basal to peak) in response to arginine was greater in patients with pancreatitis, but, because of marked variability in individual responses, this did not achieve statistical significance. In any case, certainly, the ability of the pancreas to respond to the glucagon secretagogue was not decreased. This is consistent with earlier reports.[2,7,8] With time, glucagon levels and responses gradually returned to normal, and, by 21 days, all aspects of glucagon secretion were normal.

The mechanism for the marked hyperglucagonemia in acute pancreatitis remains unclear. The prolonged duration of the elevation, the normal or excessive response to a stimulus, and the lack of comparable insulin increases would all suggest that the hyperglucagonemia does not result merely from release of stored hormone from damaged or destroyed

FIGURE 2. Studies of three arginine infusions in 12 patients with acute pancreatitis. Control values and arginine (ARG) infusions were performed as indicated in the legend to Figure 1. Plasma samples were analyzed for insulin (μU/ml). Values are shown as average ± SEM.

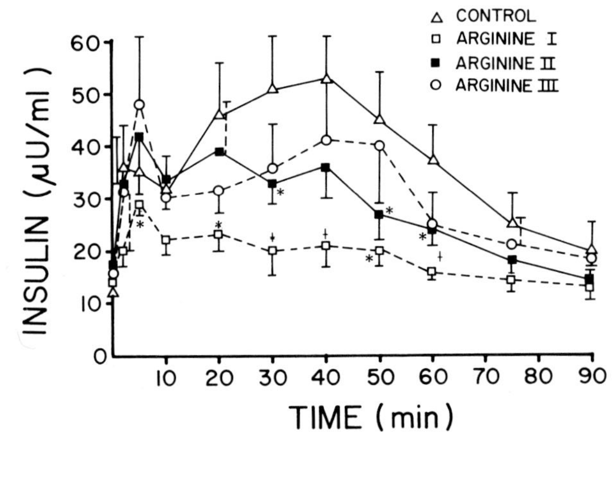

FIGURE 3. Studies of three arginine infusions in 12 patients with acute pancreatitis. Control values and arginine (ARG) infusions were performed as indicated in the legend to Figure 1. Plasma samples were analyzed for glucagon (pg/ml). Values are shown as average ± SEM.

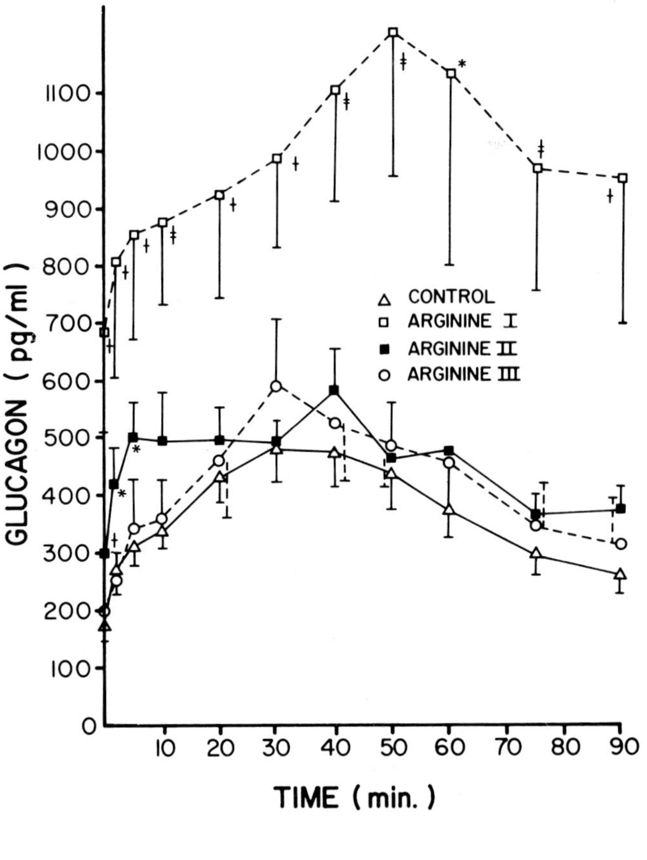

alpha cells. In addition, the nature of the glucagon secreted is not yet clarified, so that abnormal or "big" glucagon, which has a slower clearance rate, remains a real possibility in pancreatitis.

Insulin responses to arginine were clearly abnormal early after the illness and also at subsequent times. At 48–72 h after the patients were admitted for acute pancreatitis, the fasting insulin levels were in the normal range but were low for the level of blood glucose. After arginine stimulation, both first and second phase insulin secretion was decreased. By 7–10 days after the patients were admitted, the first phase was restored to normal but the second phase was significantly decreased; even at 21 days, when all glucose and glucagon responses had returned to normal, second phase insulin secretion remained impaired. Further sequential studies of patients with persistent defects in second phase secretion are needed in order to see if this could prove useful as a test for continuing damage or recovery in pancreatitis.

In an earlier study, Donowitz et al.[2] found hyperinsulinemia and an exaggerated response to alanine in patients with acute pancreatitis examined within 24 h after admission. Differences between the present studies and those of Donowitz et al. may in part be a result of the use of different provocative stimuli, i.e., arginine vs. alanine, or to the timing of the test. It is possible that the insulin stores in the pancreas are sufficient to produce a normal or even excessive response to a stimulus early after the acute insult, but, by 48–72 h, insulin stores are so depleted that the response becomes subnormal.[17] Damage to the beta cells by pancreatitis could result in impairment of the biosynthetic process and decreased insulin production, resulting in inadequate stores of hormone.

Of considerable interest is the persistent defect in second phase insulin secretion after acute pancreatitis. Although the occurrence of a biphasic insulin response to an infusion of glucose or arginine (in the presence of glucose) has been well established, the mechanism(s) responsible for this has not. Although several theories have been advanced, the most widely held one, perhaps, is that insulin is stored in two compartments—a rapidly releasable and a slowly releasable pool.[15] The relative importance of these two pools for the maintenance of glucose tolerance is not known, but the rapidly releasable component is most often found to be abnormal in diabetes.[16] The finding that acute pancreatitis affects the second phase response more than the first phase is of considerable interest, but the explanation for this is not readily apparent. It could be caused by a defect in the release process or to a deficiency of hormone stored in the second phase pool. Thus, the demonstration that patients recovering from acute pancreatitis have a selective abnormality in second phase secretion may facilitate studies of the importance of this aspect of insulin secretion.

ACKNOWLEDGMENTS

The authors are indebted to Louise Holliday for technical assistance and to Dr. A. E. Kitabchi for review of the manuscript prior to submission. The authors are also grateful to the house staff of the Department of Medicine, University of Tennessee, and the nursing staff of the VA Medical Center for sharing access to and care of patients.

The work was supported by grants from the Veterans Administration, NIH grant AM18022, CRC grant RR-00211, Juvenile Diabetes Foundation, and Memphis Mid-South Diabetes Association.

Dr. Duckworth is the recipient of a career development award of the NIH, AM00187.

REFERENCES

[1] Ohlsen, P.: Endocrine and exocrine pancreatic function in pancreatitis. Acta Med. Scand. [Suppl.] *484*:7–99, 1968.

[2] Dunowitz, M., Hendler, R., Spiro, H. M. et al.: Glucagon secretion in acute and chronic pancreatitis. Ann. Intern. Med. *83*:778–81, 1975.

[3] Marks, I. N., and Banks, S.: The aetiology, clinical features and diagnosis of pancreatitis in the South Western Cape; a review of 243 cases. S. Afr. Med. J. *37*:1039–53, 1963.

[4] Jaffee, B. J., Jackson, W. P. U., Banks, S. et al.: Insulin reserve in patients with chronic pancreatitis. Lancet *2*:890–92, 1968.

[5] Johansen, K., and Ornsholt, J.: Frequency of diabetes after acute pancreatitis. Metabolism *21*:291–96, 1972.

[6] Banks, S., Keller, P., Jackson, W. P. U. et al.: Serum-insulin response to glucose in "pancreatic diabetes". Postgrad. Med. J. *44*:214–17, 1968.

[7] Drew, S. I., Jaffe, B., Vinik, A. et al.: The first 24 hours of acute pancreatitis. Am. J. Med. *64*:795–803, 1978.

[8] Day, J. L., Knight, M., and Condon, J. R.: The role of pancreatic glucagon in the pathogenesis of acute pancreatitis. Clin. Sci. *43*:597–603, 1972.

[9] Carey, L. C.: Acute and chronic pancreatitis. Surg. Clin. North Am. *55*:325–39, 1975.

[10] Tietz, N. W.: Fundamentals of Clinical Chemistry. Philadelphia, W. B. Saunders Co., 1970.

[11] Morgan, C. R., and Lazarow, A.: Immunoassay of insulin: two antibody system. Plasma insulin levels of normal, sub-diabetic and diabetic rats. Diabetes *13*:114–26, 1963.

[12] Duckworth, W. C., Solomon, S. S., and Kitabchi, A. E.: Effect of chronic sulfonylurea therapy on plasma proinsulin levels. J. Clin. Endocrinol. Metab. *35*:585–81, 1972.

[13] Unger, R. H.: *In* Handbook of Physiology Section 7. Greep, R. O., and Astwood, E. B., Eds. Vol. 1. Steiner, D. F., and Freinkel, N., Eds. Washington, D. C., Am. Physiol. Soc., 1972, p. 529.

[14] Waugh, A. E.: Elements of Statistical Methods, 3rd edit. New York, McGraw-Hill, 1952.

[15] Grodsky, G. M., Landahl, H., Curry, D. et al.: In-vitro studies suggesting a two compartment model for insulin secretion. *In* Second Wenner-Genn Symposium on the Structure and Metabolism of the Pancreatic Islets. Falkner, S., Hellman, B., and Täljedal, I. B., Eds. London, Pergamon Press, 1970, pp. 409–20.

[16] Robertson, R. P., and Porte, D., Jr.: The glucose receptor: a defective mechanism in diabetes mellitus distinct from the beta-adrenergic receptor. J. Clin. Invest. *52*:870–76, 1973.

[17] Pi-Sunyer, X., Byrne, J. J., and Freinkel, N.: Effects of acute experimental pancreatitis on insulin metabolism in the dog: application of a new equilibrium infusion technic. Diabetes *17*:437–43, 1968.

Insulin Degradation by Mononuclear Cells

ALVIN C. POWERS, SOLOMON S. SOLOMON, AND WILLIAM C. DUCKWORTH

SUMMARY

Mononuclear cells from peripheral blood possess insulin receptors that are altered in number or binding affinity in certain metabolic diseases as obesity. The monocyte, and not the lymphocyte, is the cell with the capacity to specifically bind insulin. Furthermore, this binding appears to mirror the receptor status on such insulin target tissues as liver, muscle, and fat. Since liver, muscle, and fat also degrade insulin, mononuclear cells from the blood of normal volunteers were examined for insulin-degrading activity. Intact cells were incubated with ^{125}I-insulin and the amount of degraded insulin was measured by the trichloroacetic acid–precipitation technique. Insulin-degrading activity increased when the number of cells and the time of incubation were increased. Total insulin binding behaved in a similar fashion. Very little degradation was seen at 4° or 15°. The K_m for insulin-degrading activity was 7.03 × 10^{-8} M. Homogenized mononuclear cells degraded two to five times more insulin than did intact cells and also demonstrated cell concentration, time, and temperature dependence for degradation. The K_m of degradation for homogenized mononuclear cells was 2.2 × 10^{-8} M. Subcellular fractionation revealed significant degrading activity in the 100,000 × *g* supernatant, but little activity in the 100,000 × *g* pellet. A purified lymphocyte preparation did not bind insulin and contained little insulin-degrading activity.

DIABETES *29*:27–32, January 1980.

Insulin-sensitive tissues, such as muscle,[1] liver,[2] fat,[3] and kidney,[4] have been shown not only to possess membrane receptors that specifically bind insulin but also to contain systems that degrade insulin. Studies have demonstrated insulin-degrading activity in isolated hepatocytes,[2,5] adipocytes,[3] in muscle fibers and homogenates,[1] in kidney and liver plasma membranes,[6,7] and in other subcellular fractions.[4,8] Kahn and Baird have suggested that, following the initial binding of insulin to a specific membrane receptor, the insulin was both altered and compartmentalized.[4] This parallels work by Ascoli and Puett, who proposed that human choriogonadotrophin binding to a specific membrane receptor is followed by an internalization of this receptor-ligand complex.[9] The work of Schlessinger and co-workers demonstrated an internalization of fluorescently labeled insulin following the incubation of insulin and fibroblasts.[10]

Mononuclear cells from peripheral blood possess insulin receptors[11,12] that are altered in number or binding affinity in certain metabolic diseases as obesity.[13,14] The monocyte and not the lymphocyte is the cell with the capacity to specifically bind insulin.[15] Furthermore, this binding appears to mirror receptor status in such insulin-sensitive tissues as liver and fat.[12] Since liver, muscle, and fat all degrade insulin, we have examined human mononuclear cells for insulin-degrading activity. Herein, we demonstrate that both intact and homogenized mononuclear cells and their subcellular fractions actively degrade insulin. The insulin-degrading mechanism is characterized and the effects of time and temperature examined.

MATERIALS AND METHODS

Materials. Bovine serum albumin (BSA) was obtained from Miles Laboratories and HN-2-hydroxyethylpiperazine-N-2-ethanesulfonic acid (HEPES) from Calbiochem. Pork crystalline zinc insulin, from Dr. R. Chance of Lilly Research Laboratories, was prepared as a stock solution and diluted in 0.1M HEPES-1% BSA buffer, pH 7.4, to the desired insulin concentrations. ^{125}I-insulin was obtained from Immuno Nuclear Corporation at an activity of 150–200 μCi/μg and further purified by chromatography on DEAE cellulose column and the appropriate peaks were diluted in HEPES-BSA buffer.

Isolation of mononuclear cells. Blood from normal, fasted human volunteers was placed in heparinized containers and diluted 1.1 with phosphate-buffered saline (PBS), pH

From the Department of Medicine, Veterans Administration Medical Center, and the University of Tennessee Center for the Health Sciences, Memphis, Tennessee 38104.
Received for publication 8 June and in revised form 17 September 1979.

7.4. The mononuclear cells were isolated by the method of Boyum.[16] Ficoll-Hypaque was added to the PBS-diluted blood and centrifuged at 500 × *g* for 40 min at room temperature in an International Equipment centrifuge. The mononuclear cell layer was removed and suspended in a 0.1M HEPES-1% BSA buffer, pH 7.4. The number of mononuclear cells was quantitated with a hemacytometer. Cell viability was assessed by trypan blue exclusion and found to be consistently greater than 95%. As estimated by a nonspecific esterase stain,[17] monocytes comprised from 15 to 20% of the mononuclear preparation.

Insulin degradation by intact mononuclear cells. A suspension of 25 × 10^6 mononuclear cells was added to ^{125}I-insulin at a concentration of 5 × 10^{-11} M (0.3 ng/ml) and diluted to a total volume of 500 μl by the addition of HEPES-BSA buffer, pH 8.0. This mixture was incubated for 30 min at pH 8.0 and 37°C. Experiments were performed that varied in the number of mononuclear cells, the length of incubation, and the temperature of incubation. To one incubation medium, no ^{125}I-insulin was added. This medium was incubated under the customary conditions and then placed in a Beckman microfuge and spun at 13,000 × *g* for 5 min. The resulting cell pellet was discarded, and the supernatant was combined with ^{125}I-insulin and incubated for 30 min at pH 8.0 and 37°C. An aliquot of this supernatant was then analyzed for degrading activity as outlined below. After incubation with labeled insulin, 200-μl aliquots were removed from the remaining incubation mixtures and placed in plastic microfuge tubes containing 150 μl of HEPES-BSA buffer, pH 8.0, at 4°C. A cell pellet was obtained by centrifuging the mixture at 13,000 × *g* for 5 min at 4°C in a Beckman microfuge. The resulting supernatant was combined with trichloroacetic acid (TCA) at a final concentration of 5% TCA. Binding and degradation were determined as described previously.[18,19] Nonspecific binding averaged about 20% of the total binding, in agreement with previous studies.[13,20]

Preparation of homogenized mononuclear cells and subcellular fractions. Mononuclear cell homogenates were prepared from a suspension of cells obtained by the Ficoll-Hypaque method outlined above. After suspension in a 0.35M sucrose solution, the cells were homogenized in a hand-powered, glass on glass, Pyrex homogenizer and then partitioned into an incubation mixture at a concentration of 5 × 10^6 cells. The mixture was brought to a final volume of 500 μl with the addition of HEPES-BSA buffer, pH 7.4, and incubated for 30 min at pH 7.4 and 37°C. Aliquots of 200 μl were removed immediately after incubation to a solution containing a final concentration of 5% trichloroacetic acid.[18,19]

Subcellular fractions were obtained as follows. Mononuclear cells were diluted in 0.1 mM $NaHCO_3$ and homogenized. This homogenate was centrifuged at 500 × *g* for 30 min. The supernatant produced was recentrifuged at 30,000 × *g* for 30 min at 4°C in a Beckman model L5-65 ultracentrifuge. The resulting supernatant was centrifuged at 100,000 × *g* for 30 min at 4°C. The three pellets and the 100,000 × *g* supernatant were incubated with labeled insulin at pH 7.4 and 37°C. Aliquots were analyzed for degraded insulin by the TCA method.

K_m determinations. The intact mononuclear cell preparations, the mononuclear homogenates, and the subcellular fractions were incubated under identical conditions with labeled insulin and varying amounts of unlabeled insulin. The K_m of the insulin-degrading mechanism was calculated by the customary Lineweaver-Burke plot and linear regression analysis.

Lymphocyte and monocyte preparations. Lymphocyte and monocyte preparations were obtained from Dr. Arnold Postlethwaite (Veterans Administration Medical Center, Memphis, Tennessee). Mononuclear cells were prepared from whole blood by the method of Boyum[16] and separated according to cell size by countercurrent centrifugation. These were 95% pure lymphocytes and 60% pure monocytes, by staining with nonspecific esterase.

Assay of binding and degradation by lymphocytes and monocytes. Binding of ^{125}I-insulin was determined as reported previously.[13] A lymphocyte preparation with 20 ×10^6 cells was incubated with 10^{-11} M ^{125}I-insulin (0.3 ng/ml) for 90 min at pH 8.0 and 22°C. After incubation, a 200μl aliquot was spun in a Beckman microfuge. The supernatant and the pellet were quantitated for radioactivity and the net percent insulin bound to the lymphocytes was calculated from the radioactivity in the cell pellet over the total radioactivity in the cell pellet and the supernatant.

A lymphocyte preparation and a monocyte suspension were homogenized in a 0.35M sucrose solution as outlined above. The lymphocyte homogenate and the monocyte homogenate were incubated for 60 min at pH 7.4 and 37°C. The percent insulin degraded was derived as previously mentioned.

Degradation by a 95% pure intact lymphocyte preparation and a 60% pure intact monocyte preparation (the remaining cells being large lymphocytes) was measured as outlined above.

RESULTS

Insulin degradation by intact mononuclear cells. Figure 1 is a diagram of the relation between the amount of insulin degraded and the number of mononuclear cells placed in the incubation medium. Total binding of insulin also exhibited a similar response to increasing cell concentration. It should be noted that the total binding is not corrected for nonspecific binding. As a control, mononuclear cells were incubated without labeled insulin under identical circumstances and then removed by centrifugation. The resulting supernatant did not degrade insulin.

FIGURE 1. Insulin degradation and binding at varying cell concentrations (expressed as by 10^6 cells in each 500 μl). Mononuclear cells were incubated with ^{125}I-insulin for 30 min at pH 8.0 and 37°C in 0.1 M HEPES-1% BSA buffer. The percent insulin degraded was measured by TCA precipitation. The incubation mixture did not degrade insulin after removal of the mononuclear cells.

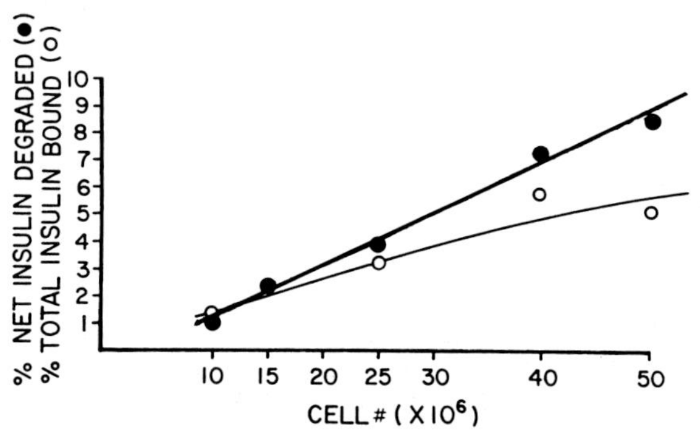

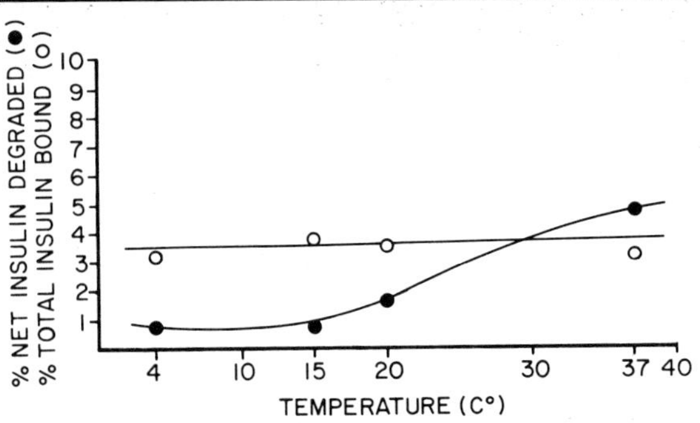

FIGURE 2. Insulin degradation and binding at varying incubation temperatures (°C). A volume of 500 μl, containing 25 $\times$ 10^6 mononuclear cells and ^{125}I-insulin, was incubated for 30 min at pH 8.0 and 4°C, 15°C, 20°C, and 37°C. The percent insulin degraded was measured by TCA precipitation. The incubation mixture did not degrade insulin after removal of the mononuclear cells.

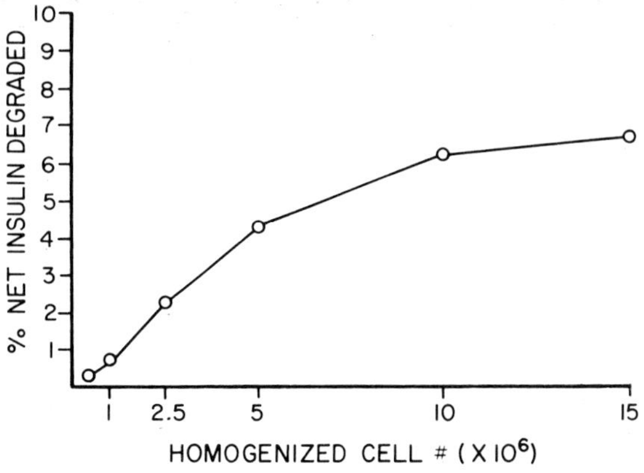

FIGURE 4. Insulin degradation by homogenized mononuclear cells at varying cell concentrations (expressed as by 10^6 homogenized cells in each 500 μl). Homogenized mononuclear cells were incubated with ^{125}I-insulin for 30 min as pH 7.4 and 37°C in 0.1M HEPES-BSA buffer. The percent insulin degraded was measured by TCA precipitation.

When insulin degradation was plotted against the temperature of incubation, the resultant curve is shown in Figure 2. Total insulin binding changed little over the temperature range examined. After removal of the mononuclear cells, the incubation mixture did not degrade insulin.

As shown in Figure 3, increasing the time of incubation produced an appropriate increase in the amount of insulin degraded. Unlike the studies shown in Figures 1 and 2, however, the incubation medium possessed insulin-degrading activity after removal of the cells. The amount of degrading activity in the cell-free medium depended on the length of incubation and represents the major percentage of degrading activity measured. Incubation of mononuclear cells and labeled insulin for 30 min produced an average of 5.46% of the insulin degraded, while the media following removal of the cells degraded 4.27% of the insulin at the end of a 30-min incubation. This activity in the media represents either continuous leakage from the cells or degrading activity that is only loosely attached to the cell surface. Various adjustments in the experimental protocol, as balanced salt buffers and preincubation of the cells before adding the labeled insulin, failed to prevent this extracellular degradation. Total insulin binding increased with longer periods of incubation and appeared to reach a maximum at 60 min.

Insulin degradation by homogenized mononuclear cells. Homogenized mononuclear cells degraded approximately fivefold more insulin than did intact cells (Table 1). This degradation is related both to the number of cells in each homogenate and the length of incubation, as shown in Figures 4 and 5, respectively. Figure 6 indicates the relationship between degradation and the temperature of incubation by homogenized mononuclear cells.

K_m determination. Using a Lineweaver-Burke plot and linear regression analysis, the K_m for the insulin-degrading mechanism was determined. For intact cells, the K_m was 7.03 $\times 10^{-8}$ M; for homogenized mononuclear cells, the K_m was 2.2 $\times 10^{-8}$. The incubation medium possessed insulin-degrading activity after the removal of cells. Table 2 contains a comparison of the kinetic constants of degradation for intact and homogenized cells.

FIGURE 3. Insulin degradation and binding at increasing lengths of incubation (minutes). A volume of 500 μl, containing 25 $\times$ 10^6 mononuclear cells and ^{125}I-insulin, was incubated at pH 8.0 and 37°C for increasing periods of time. The percent insulin degraded was measured by TCA precipitation. The incubation mixture after the removal of the mononuclear cells degraded a significant amount of insulin.

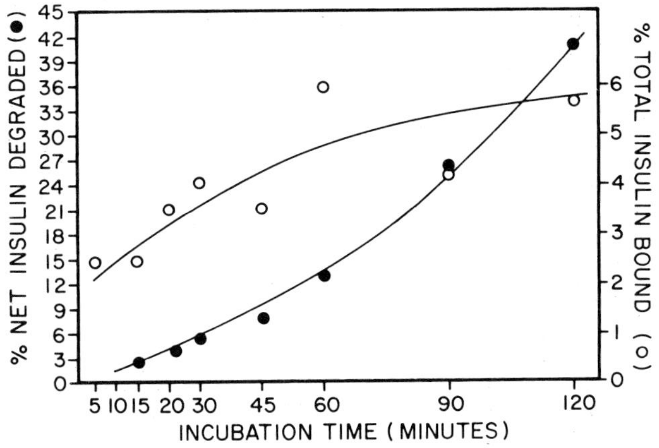

FIGURE 5. Insulin degradation by homogenized mononuclear cells at increasing lengths of incubation (minutes) shown along the x axis. A volume of 500 μl, containing 5 $\times$ 10^6 homogenized mononuclear cells and labeled insulin, was incubated at pH 7.4 and 37°C for increasing periods of time. The percent insulin degraded was measured by TCA precipitation.

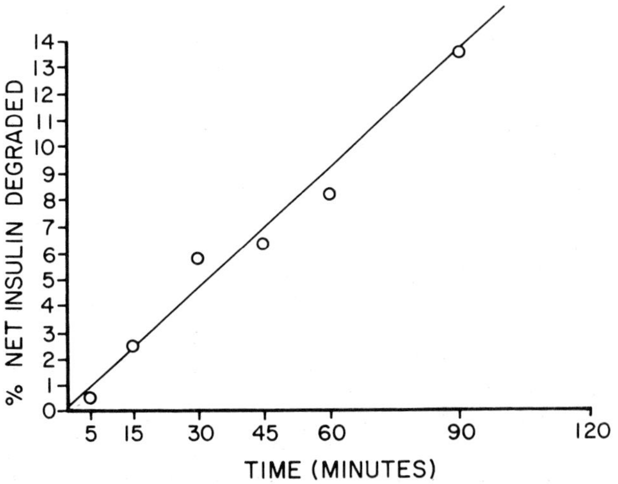

TABLE 1
Insulin degradation by intact and homogenized mononuclear cells

Intact cells	Insulin binding	Insulin degraded (moles)	Total degrading activity
Total mononuclear cells (25 × 10⁶ cells)	Yes	5.46×10^{-13}	100%
Intact lymphocytes (20–21.25 × 10⁶ cells*)	None detected	None detected	0%
Intact monocytes (3.75–4.0 × 10⁶ cells*)	Not assessed	$2.5–3.3 \times 10^{-13}$	46–61%
Total mononuclear cells (5 × 10⁶ cells)		5.73×10^{-13}	100%
Homogenized lymphocytes (4.0–4.25 × 10⁶ cells*)		$1.78–1.89 \times 10^{-13}$	31–33%
Homogenized monocytes (0.75–1.0 × 10⁶ cells*)		$1.34–1.79 \times 10^{-13}$	23–31%

* This represents the approximate number of these cells in the mononuclear cell preparation. All incubations were at 37° for 30 min.

Insulin degradation by mononuclear subcellular fractions. Table 3 illustrates the amount of insulin-degrading activity present in a 500 × *g*, a 30,000 × *g*, and a 100,000 × *g* pellet and in the 100,000 × *g* supernatant. Most of the activity resided within the cytosol fraction. Only small amounts of activity were found in the 500 × *g*, the 30,000 × *g*, and the 100,000 × *g* pellet. The cells were homogenized in 0.1 mM $NaHCO_3$, and this released considerably more degrading activity than did homogenizing the cells in a 0.35 M sucrose solution.

The K_m constant of the cytosol-associated insulin-degrading system was 1.97×10^{-7} M (R = 0.985), as determined by a Lineweaver-Burke plot and linear regression analysis.

Insulin binding and degradation by lymphocytes and monocytes. A 95% pure lymphocyte preparation exhibited no ability to specifically bind insulin.

An intact lymphocyte preparation of 95% purity possessed no significant insulin-degrading activity; an intact monocyte preparation of 60% purity, with no significant degrading activity in the media, degraded 1.96×10^{-13} mol of insulin in 30 min (5×10^6 cells). Homogenized lymphocytes of 95% purity degraded 2.31×10^{-13} mol of insulin in 30 min (5×10^6 cells), while a homogenized monocyte preparation of 60% purity degraded 5.4×10^{-13} mol of insulin in 30 min (5×10^6 cells). Large lymphocytes constituted the remaining percentage of cells in the monocyte preparation (Table 1).

DISCUSSION

The relation of insulin binding by membrane receptors and insulin degradation is uncertain, but studies have suggested that receptor interaction is a necessary prerequisite for insulin degradation.[2,21] Gliemann and Sonne have concluded that degradation of receptor-bound insulin does occur.[22] Terris and Steiner have shown that inhibition of insulin binding by the addition of unlabeled insulin or by treatment with trypsin produces an equal degree of depression of insulin degradation.[2] Following the incubation of intact hepatocytes and iodinated insulin, the demonstration of an unalterable lag phase preceding the appearance of degradation products supports the concept of a mandatory transport of the bound insulin to a membrane-associated or intracellular site.[2] This is consistent with the recent work of Kahn and Baird, in which insulin was both altered and compartmentalized after being bound to adipocytes.[3] The form and location of the internalized insulin is unknown. Schlessinger et al. have visualized the sequence of insulin binding, receptor aggregation, and intracellular uptake of the insulin label, and this series of reactions depends on time, temperature, and energy.[10]

In this study, intact mononuclear cells were shown to actively degrade insulin in a time-, temperature-, and cell concentration–dependent manner. As shown in Figures 1 and 3, both total insulin bound and insulin degraded increased with length of incubation and enlargement of the cell concentration. Insulin degradation displayed a temperature-dependent relationship. However, total insulin binding (specific insulin bound plus insulin nonspecifically bound) appeared unrelated to the temperature of incubation. This is in agreement with previously reported insulin receptor activity in kidney and liver membranes[6] and mononuclear cells,[23] in which insulin binding was of comparable magnitude—regardless of incubation temperature—for incubations of less than 45 min. With greater lengths of incubation, differences in insulin binding with varying temperatures of incubation have been reported.[6,23] Maximum insulin-degradative activity occurred at 37°C, with only minor amounts of

FIGURE 6. Insulin degradation by homogenized mononuclear cells at varying incubation temperatures (°C). A volume of 500 μl, containing 5 × 10⁶ homogenized mononuclear cells and ¹²⁵I-insulin, was incubated for 30 min at pH 7.4 and 4°C, 15°C, 20°C, and 37°C. The percent insulin degraded was measured by TCA precipitation.

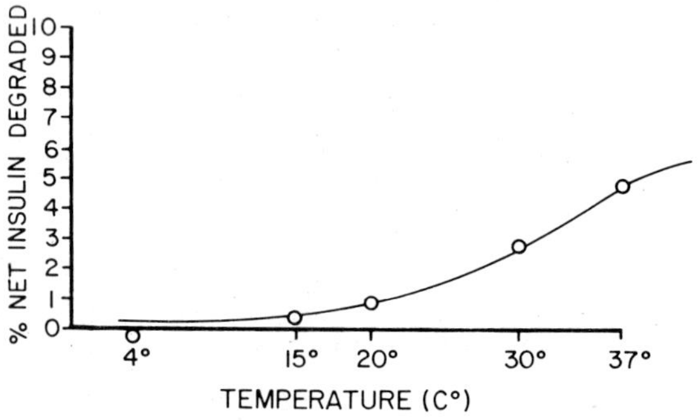

TABLE 2
Kinetic constants for insulin degradation by intact and homogenized mononuclear cells

		× 10⁻¹⁰ mol	
	K_m (× 10⁻⁸ M)	V_{max} (5 × 10⁶ cells, 30 min, 37°C)	*R*
Intact cells	7.03	5.66	0.9809
Homogenized cells	2.2	11.93	0.9890

TABLE 3
Subcellular fractionation of insulin-degrading activity*

	< 10^{-9} mol of insulin degraded	% of total degrading activity
Complete mononuclear homogenate	20.2	100
500 × g pellet	0.96	4.8
30,000 × g pellet	0.74	3.7
100,000 × g pellet	0.56	2.8
100,000 × g supernatant	15.6	77.2

* Activity for equivalent of 5 × 10^6 cells, at 37°C, for 30 min.

degraded products found with incubation temperatures of 4°C and 15°C, and an intermediate quantity of degradation at 22°C. Similar temperature relationships are seen in liver membranes,[6,7] kidney membranes,[6] isolated hepatocytes,[5,7] and fat cell membranes.[8]

After incubation, the intact mononuclear cells were removed by centrifugation and the remaining media were examined for degrading activity. During the studies on optimum cell concentration and temperature of incubation, the incubation media minus the mononuclear cells did not degrade insulin. However, the data obtained for varying lengths of incubation represent degradation by intact mononuclear cells and by degrading activity in the media. In twenty separate attempts, the incubation media's degradation accounted for the major portion of the degradation measured. We were unable to alter the experimental protocol to rid our experimental system of this cell-independent-degrading activity. Since samples of the cell-free suspension at various points in the isolation of the mononuclear cells contained degrading activity, it was felt that this media activity represents cell trauma and rupture by the experimental procedure. Gross cell viability, as assessed by trypan blue exclusion, was always greater than 95%, however.

Homogenized mononuclear cells degrade two- to fivefold more insulin than do intact cells. Hammond and Jarett have demonstrated a fourfold difference in degradative activity in homogenized and intact fat cells.[8] The mononuclear cell homogenates exhibited similar relationships to length and temperature of incubation as intact cells.

The K_m for intact mononuclear cells, as determined by a Lineweaver-Burke plot and linear regression analysis, was 7.03 × 10^{-8} M. Olefsky has reported a K_m of 5 × 10^{-7} M for insulin degradation by hepatocytes,[7] Le Cam et al. a value of 2.7 × 10^{-7} M for hepatocytes,[5] and Duckworth a value of 2.2 × 10^{-7} M for kidney membranes[6] and 2.2 × 10^{-8} M for insulin protease isolated from muscle.[1]

As shown in Table 3, most of the insulin-degrading activity following subcellular fractionation resides in the 100,000 × g fraction. This is consistent with several previous subcellular fractionation studies,[4,5,24] all of which located the major portion of insulin-degrading activity in the cytosol fraction. The K_m of degradation by the cytosol fraction is 1.97 × 10^{-7} M and this is comparable to the K_m for the total mononuclear cell homogenate and the K_m determinations from other investigators.[1,5–7] However, there is almost a 10-fold difference in homogenate and cytosolic K_m. It is possible the homogenate contains materials that interact with the enzyme in some way to alter the kinetic properties of the enzyme. Other tissues, specifically liver and kidney, do contain activators and inhibitors of insulin protease. In general, caution must always be taken in interpreting kinetic values in crude preparations.

Our present study indicates that intact lymphocytes of 95% purity possess insignificant insulin-binding and -degrading capability. The inability of circulating lymphocytes to bind insulin is well known,[11,12,23,25] although PHA-stimulated lymphocytes do contain receptors.[26] In contrast, isolated monocytes of 60% purity (the remainder of the cells being large lymphocytes) degraded 1.96 × 10^{-13} mol of insulin for each 5 × 10^6 cells in 30 min. The total mononuclear cell suspensions, composed of from 15 to 20% monocytes with the remainder being lymphocytes, degraded 5.46 × 10^{-13} mol for each 25 × 10^6 cells in 30 min. Therefore, it appears that the monocyte accounts for the major degradative activity demonstrated in intact mononuclear cell suspensions (Table 1).

Mononuclear cells from peripheral blood degrade insulin in a time- and temperature-dependent fashion. The major insulin-degrading activity in intact mononuclear cell preparations resides in the monocyte, since intact lymphocytes exhibit little ability to bind or degrade insulin. Homogenized mononuclear cells, which degrade two- to fivefold more insulin than do intact cells and lymphocytes, are responsible for only slightly more of this degradation than are monocytes—despite their fivefold greater representation in the homogenate. Homogenized monocytes degrade approximately fourfold more insulin than a like number of homogenized lymphocytes. The cytosol is the site for the major portions of this activity. The location and the K_m of insulin degradation for mononuclear cells closely resemble the characteristics of insulin protease and insulin degradation in such insulin-responsive tissues as liver, muscle, and fat. Mononuclear cell preparations may prove useful in the study of the insulin-degrading mechanism.

ACKNOWLEDGMENTS
This work was supported in part by funds from the Veterans Administration and by a Research Career Development Award AM00187 (to WCD) from the National Institutes of Health.

REFERENCES

1 Duckworth, W. C., Heinemann, M., and Kitabchi, A. E.: Purification of insulin specific protease by affinity chromatography. Proc. Natl. Acad. Sci. USA 69:3698–3702, 1972.

2 Terris, S., and Steiner, D. F.: Binding and degradation of ¹²⁵I-insulin by rat hepatocytes. J. Biol. Chem. *250*:8389–98, 1975.

3 Kahn, R. C., and Baird, K.: The fate of insulin bound to adipocytes. J. Biol. Chem. *253*:4900–06, 1976.

4 Duckworth, W. C.: Insulin and glucagon degradation by the kidney. Biochim. Biophys. Acta *437*:518–30, 1976.

5 Le Cam, A., Freychet, P., and Lenoir, P.: Degradation of insulin by isolated rat liver cells. Diabetes *24*:566–73, 1975.

6 Duckworth, W. C.: Insulin and glucagon degradation by kidney cell membranes. Endocrinology *102*:1766–74, 1978.

7 Olefsky, J. M., Johnson, J., Liu, F., Edwards, P., and Baur, S.: Comparison of ¹²⁵I-insulin binding and degradation to isolated rat hepatocytes and liver membranes. Diabetes *24*:801–10, 1975.

8 Hammond, J. M., and Jarett, L.: Insulin degradation by isolated fat cells and their subcellular fractions. Diabetes *24*:1011–19, 1975.

9 Ascoli, M., and Puett, D.: Degradation of receptor bound human choriogonadotrophin by murine leydig tumor cells. J. Biol. Chem. *253*:4892–99, 1978.

10 Schlessinger, J., Shecter, Y., Willingham, M. C., and Pastan, I.: Di-

rect visualization of binding, aggregation, and internalization of insulin and epidermal growth factor on living fibroblastic cells. Proc. Natl. Acad. Sci. USA *75*:2659–63, 1978.

[11] Beck-Nielsen, H., Pedersen, O., Kragballe, K., and Sorensen, N. S.: The monocyte as model for the study of insulin receptors in man. Diabetologia *13*:563–69, 1977.

[12] Gavin, J. R., III, Roth, J., Jen, P., and Freychet, P.: Insulin receptors in human circulating cells and fibroblasts. Proc. Natl. Acad. Sci. USA *69*:747–51, 1972.

[13] Bar, R. S., Gordon, P., Roth, J., Kahn, C. R., and De Meyts, P. O.: Fluctuations in the affinity and concentration of insulin receptors of circulating monocytes of obese patients. J. Clin. Invest. *58*:1123–35, 1976.

[14] Olefsky, J. M.: Decreased insulin binding to adipocytes and circulating monocytes in obesity. J. Clin. Invest. *57*:1165–72, 1976.

[15] Schwartz, R. H., Branco, A. R., Hardwerger, B. S., and Kahn, R. C.: Demonstration that monocytes rather than lymphocytes are the insulin binding cells in preparations of human peripheral blood mononuclear leukocytes: implications for studies of insulin resistance in man. Proc. Natl. Acad. Sci. USA *72*:474–78, 1975.

[16] Boyum, A.: A one stage procedure for the isolation of granulocytes and lymphocytes from human blood. Scand. J. Clin. Lab. Invest. *58*:1123–35, 1976.

[17] Yam, L. T., Li, C. V., and Crosby, W. H.: Cytochemical identification of monocytes and granulocytes. Am. J. Clin. Pathol. *55*:283–90, 1971.

[18] Duckworth, W. C.: Insulin degradation by liver cell membranes. Endocrinology *104*:1758–64, 1979.

[19] Duckworth, W. C., and Kitabchi, A. E.: Insulin and glucagon degradation by the same enzyme. Diabetes *23*:536–43, 1974.

[20] Olefsky, J. M., and Reaven, G. M.: Insulin binding in diabetes. Diabetes *26*:680–88, 1977.

[21] Gammeltoft, S., Kristensen, L. O., and Sestaft, L.: Insulin receptors in isolated rat hepatocytes. J. Biol. Chem. *253*:8406–13, 1978.

[22] Gliemann, J., and Sonne, O.: Binding and receptor-mediated degradation of insulin in adipocytes. J. Biol. Chem. *253*:7857–63, 1978.

[23] Pedersen, O., and Beck-Neilsen, H.: A study of insulin receptors in human mononuclear leucocytes. Acta Endocrinol. *83*:556–64, 1976.

[24] Freychet, P., Kahn, R., Roth, J., and Neville, D. M.: Insulin interactions with liver plasma membranes. Independence of binding of the hormone and its degradation. J. Biol. Chem. *247*:3953–61, 1972.

[25] DeFronzo, R. A., Soman, V., Sherwin, R. W., Hendler, R., and Felig, P.: Insulin binding to monocytes and insulin action in obesity starvation. J. Clin. Invest. *62*:204–13, 1978.

[26] Helderman, J. H., and Strom, T. B.: Emergence of insulin receptors upon alloimmune T cells in the rat. J. Clin. Invest. *59*:338–44, 1977.

Effects of Sodium DL-Lactate on Insulin Secretion in Anesthetized Dogs

G. FEDERSPIL, M. ZACCARIA, S. PEDRAZZOLI, E. ZAGO, C. DEPALO, AND C. SCANDELLARI

SUMMARY

The effect of sodium DL-lactate administration on insulin release in anesthetized dogs has been studied. Eleven mongrel dogs were infused with sodium DL-lactate for 20 min at the rate of 20 mg/kg · min. Lactate infusion produced simultaneous increases in blood glucose and plasma insulin levels in the pancreaticoduodenal vein. To determine whether lactate stimulated insulin secretion directly, sodium DL-lactate was rapidly injected into the pancreatic artery of six dogs; this pulse induced a significant increase in insulin release from pancreatic B-cells, even in the absence of a measurable change in blood glucose. Diazoxide, when infused in six dogs, blocked lactate-induced insulin secretion. These findings indicate that lactate, as do other circulating energy fuels, may play a role in the physiologic control of insulin secretion.

DIABETES 29:33–36, January 1980.

Insulin secretion is stimulated by glucose and other metabolic substrates, such as free fatty acids (FFA), triglycerides, ketone bodies, and amino acids.[1–4] Blood concentration of these metabolic substrates varies in some physiologic conditions, including food intake, starvation, psychological stress, and prolonged physical activity.

During muscular exercise the blood lactate level increases and, at present, it is not well understood whether in vivo this metabolite constitutes a signal for pancreatic insulin release.

The present research was undertaken to verify whether lactate, when administered in paraphysiologic amounts to anesthetized dogs, modifies pancreatic insulin secretion. Our results show that sodium DL-lactate can stimulate insulin secretion directly.

MATERIALS AND METHODS

Experimental procedure. Seventeen overnight-fasting mongrel dogs weighing 16 ± 2 kg were used. All dogs were anesthetized with Nembutal and secured in a supine position until the end of the experiment. After anesthesia a right subcostal laparotomy was performed and the pancreaticoduodenal vein (PDV) was isolated. Two cannulas, connected by a T-fitting, were inserted into the pancreaticoduodenal vein. During the experiments, pancreaticoduodenal venous effluent was drained off at intervals and blood samples were drawn by free flow from the lateral branch of the tap. Blood flow was estimated by direct measurement in a graduated heparinized vessel.

Insulin production (IP) was calculated according to the formula:

$$IP\ (mU/min) = I_{PDV} \times BF \times (1 - Ht)/1000$$

where I_{PDV} is insulin concentration in PDV, BF is the blood flow, and Ht is the hematocrit of perfusing blood. Ten minutes was allowed between cannulation of the vein and the beginning of the experiment itself to avoid irregularities of blood flow.

Three types of experiments were carried out. In the first experiment sodium DL-lactate was infused in the femoral vein of 11 dogs at the rate of 20 mg/kg · min for 20 min. Blood samples were drawn at 20–10–0 min before, 5–10–15–20 min during, and 5–10–20 min after the end of infusion. In the second experiment, six dogs received an injection directly into the pancreatic artery, with pulses of 400 mg sodium DL-lactate over 2 min, to evaluate its direct insulin secretory capacity. In the third experiment, diazoxide was infused in eight dogs over a 60-min period at the rate of 5 mg/min. From the 20th to 40th minute an infusion of sodium DL-lactate (20 mg/kg · min) was added.

Analytical procedure. In all samples, blood glucose, plasma insulin, and blood lactate were measured. Blood glucose was determined by the glucose-oxidase method,[5]

From the Institute of Semeiotic Medicine and Surgical Clinic, University of Padua, Padova, Italy.
This research was supported by CNR grant 76-01321-04-115-1187.
These data have been presented in a preliminary form (International Diabetes Federation, Bruxelles, 1973) (EASD Annual Meeting 1975).
Address reprint requests to G. Federspil, M.D., Istituto di Semeiotica Medica, Via Ospedale 105, 35100 Padova, Italy.
Received for publication 3 February 1978 and in revised form 13 July 1979.

plasma insulin was measured by the method of Herbert et al.,[6] and blood lactate was determined using lactate dehydrogenase (Boehringer-Mannheim). In all experiments sodium DL-lactate (British Drug Houses Ltd, B.D.H. Laboratory Chemicals Division) was used.

Statistical analysis. The Student's paired *t* test was used to examine the significance of changes during sodium DL-lactate or sodium DL-lactate plus diazoxide infusion compared with 20-min values. The same test was used to compare values of insulin production at time 0 with values at 2 and 5 min after acute sodium DL-lactate injection into the pancreatic artery.

RESULTS

Infusion of sodium DL-lactate. As shown in Figure 1, sodium DL-lactate infusion progressively increased the mean blood lactate concentration from 19 to 56 mg/dl. At the end of the infusion, blood lactate decreased slowly. Twenty minutes after lactate infusion, blood glucose rose slightly but significantly. Insulin production, which appeared stable during the control period, increased progressively and significantly during lactate administration and began to drop after the infusion stopped. Insulin concentration in the femoral vein rose slightly but significantly during lactate administration and decreased progressively from the 45th min.

Injection of sodium DL-lactate into the pancreatic artery. As shown in Figure 2, rapid injection of 400 mg sodium DL-lactate increased lactate concentration in the pancreatic venous effluent (from 14.9 ± 2.7 to 30.5 ± 4.7 mg/dl by the second minute; $P < 0.01$). Rapid administration of lactate did not modify either blood glucose level or pancreatic blood flow.

The sodium DL-lactate pulse elicited a rapid and significant increase of the plasma insulin concentration in PDV (from 205 ± 24 to 395 ± 78 μU/ml at the second minute; $P < 0.05$). As a result, insulin production was increased significantly ($P < 0.05$) by the sodium DL-lactate injection (Figure 2).

Infusion of sodium DL-lactate during diazoxide administration. As shown in Figure 3, diazoxide administration did not modify the blood lactate level; however, blood glucose concentration increased 20 min after the start of the infusion. The blood glucose level was not further modified following sodium DL-lactate administration. Basal insulin secretion was inhibited by diazoxide (pancreaticoduodenal

FIGURE 1. Effect of infusion of sodium DL-lactate (20 mg/kg · min) into the femoral vein on peripheral blood lactate, blood glucose, plasma insulin, and pancreatic insulin production. Results are expressed as mean ± SEM; n indicates the number of experiments.

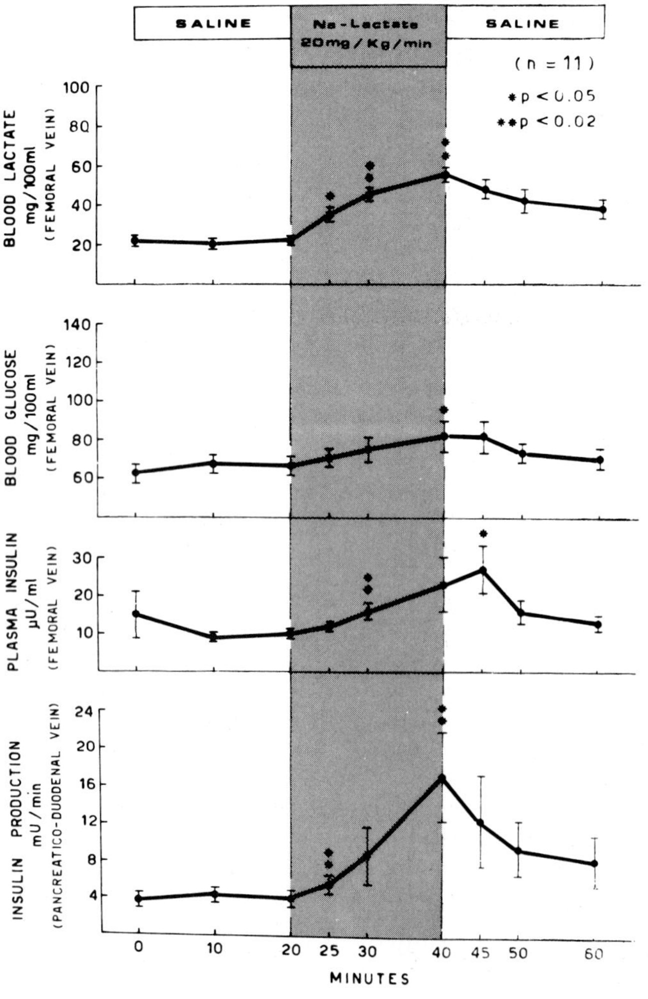

FIGURE 2. Effect of injection of sodium DL-lactate (▨) (400 mg over 2 min) into the superior pancreaticoduodenal artery on pancreatic venous lactate, glucose, and insulin production. Results are expressed as mean ± SEM; n indicates the number of experiments.

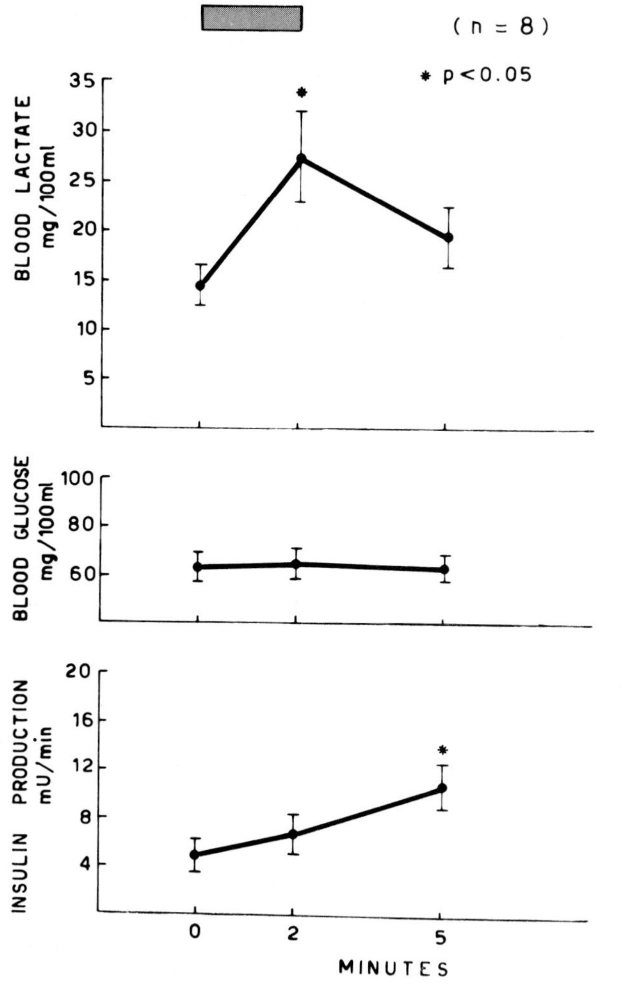

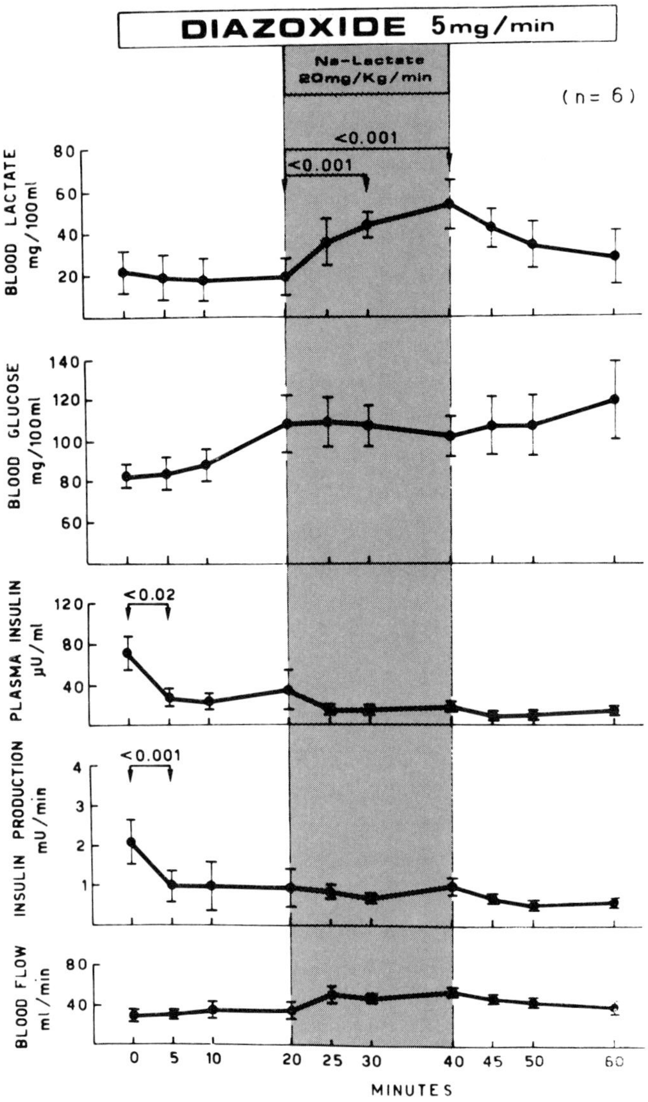

FIGURE 3. Effect of infusion of sodium DL-lactate (20 mg/kg · min) into the femoral vein during diazoxide administration (5 mg/min) on femoral blood lactate, blood glucose, and pancreatic insulin production. Results are expressed as mean ± SEM; n indicates the number of experiments.

insulin production: from 2.13 ± 0.56 to 0.85 ± 0.14 mU/min). The sodium DL-lactate infusion, during diazoxide administration, increased the blood lactate level in the same way as in dogs treated with sodium DL-lactate alone. However, sodium DL-lactate did not change insulin secretion during diazoxide administration.

DISCUSSION

Infusion of 20 mg/kg · min of sodium DL-lactate increases blood lactate to levels similar to those obtained during exhaustive muscular exercise.[7–9] Our results show that such a lactate infusion increases insulin concentration in the superior pancreaticoduodenal vein of anesthetized dogs and that the rise of insulin concentration corresponds to an increased insulin release from pancreatic B-cells.

Sodium DL-lactate increases the blood glucose level slightly but significantly. This effect raises the question of whether lactate-induced insulin secretion is mediated by hyperglycemia. To ascertain whether lactate stimulates pancreatic B-cells directly, this substance was injected into the pancreatic artery. Acute sodium DL-lactate administration causes a prompt rise of insulin concentration in PDV and an increase of the pancreatic insulin release, although there are no measurable changes in blood glucose.

These results, therefore, show a direct effect of sodium DL-lactate on pancreatic B-cells and suggest that the increase of insulin secretion, which was observed during lactate infusion, is independent of the small blood glucose increase. The stimulatory effect of sodium DL-lactate on insulin secretion is supported also by the experiments of Loubatières-Mariani et al.,[10] who report that sodium DL-lactate increases insulin release from the isolated and perfused rat pancreas.

The mechanism responsible for lactate-stimulated insulin secretion remains to be fully determined. Lactate is a product of glycolysis. Malaisse[11] has shown that, in isolated islets, various sugars increase lactate output according to their relative insulinotropic capacity. Therefore, it is reasonable to assume that lactate itself may be an intracellular trigger for insulin secretion, although it may provoke B-cell secretory response through another intermediate.

To further investigate the effect of blood lactate on insulin secretion, we used diazoxide, which has a direct inhibitory effect on pancreatic B-cells,[12] and have shown that this drug blocks lactate-stimulated insulin secretion. Since diazoxide inhibits glucose- and tolbutamide-stimulated insulin secretion, but does not affect glucagon- and 3′,5′-AMP-induced insulin release,[13,14] our findings support the idea that lactate does not stimulate the 3′,5′-AMP system; however, it may act through a mechanism similar to that stimulated by glucose.

Physiologic experiments[15] have shown that, during glucose infusion, diazoxide modifies the labile insulin pool in pancreatic B-cells and inhibits transfer of insulin to the distal labile compartment; therefore, it is possible that lactate may act on the labile compartment of insulin.

The possible physiologic significance of these findings deserves some comment. It is well known that hyperlactacidemia occurs in such pathologic conditions as diabetes mellitus.[16,17] Moreover, an increase of blood lactate concentration to levels similar to those obtained with our infusion, in addition to a decrease of plasma insulin, has been shown during prolonged muscular exercise.[7,9,18] Thus, the present findings suggest that blood lactate concentration may contribute to the control of pancreatic B-cell secretion in physiologic as well as in spontaneous pathologic conditions. Lactate action on insulin secretion during muscular exercise looks similar to that of FFA: in fact it has been shown that plasma FFA stimulate insulin release[1,2] and also rise during muscular exercise.[18] It therefore seems reasonable to suppose that the increase of blood lactate and of plasma FFA concentrations during muscular exercise may act together in preventing an excessive plasma insulin fall.

In conclusion, the present observations support the concept that the release of insulin from pancreatic B-cells is regulated by an interaction between many circulating energy fuels, i.e., glucose, FFA, ketone bodies, and lactate, and that these fuels are therefore not only metabolic intermediates, but also signals for endocrine pancreatic function.

REFERENCES

[1] Crespin, S. R., Greenough, W. B., and Steinberg, D.: Stimulation of insulin secretion by long chain free fatty acids. A direct pancreatic effect. J. Clin. Invest. *52*:1979–84, 1973.

[2] Balasse, E. O.: Interactions of insulin, ketone bodies and free fatty acids in the regulation of peripheral utilization of substrates. *In* Diabetes. Malaisse, W. J., and Pirart, J., Eds. Amsterdam, Excerpta Medica, 1974, pp. 231–40.

[3] Greenberger, H. J., Tzagournis, M., and Graves, T. M.: Stimulation of insulin secretion in man by medium chain triglycerides. Metabolism *17*:796–801, 1968.

[4] Floyd, J., Fajans, S., Conn, J., Knopf, R., and Rull, J. A.: Stimulation of insulin secretion by amino acids. J. Clin. Invest. *45*:1487–1502, 1966.

[5] Hugget, A., and Nixon, D.: Use of glucose-peroxidase in determination of blood and urinary glucose. Lancet *2*:368–70, 1957.

[6] Herbert, A., Lau, K., Gottleib, C., and Bleicher, B.: Coated charcoal immunoassay of insulin. J. Clin. Endocrinol. Metab. *25*:1375–84, 1965.

[7] Keul, J., and Keppler, D.: The substrate supply of the human skeletal muscle at rest, during and after work. Experientia *23*:974–79, 1967.

[8] Jrka, Z., and Dolezel, J.: Changes in cholesterol serum levels after spiroergometric examination in children. *In* Biochemistry of Exercise. Poortmans, J., Ed. Basel, S. Karger, 1969, pp. 152–55.

[9] Paul, P.: Uptake and oxidation of substrates in the intact animal during exercise. *In* Muscle Metabolism during Exercise. Pernaow, B., and Saltin, B., Eds. New York, Plenum Press, 1971, pp. 225–47.

[10] Loubatières-Mariani, M. M., Blayac, J. P., Alric, R., Valette, G., and Loubatières, A.: Effets du DL-lactate de sodium sur les sécrétions d'insuline et du glucagon. Etude sur le pancréas isolé at perfusé de rat. Compt. Rend. Soc. Biol. (Paris), 168:1038–44, 1974.

[11] Malaisse, W. J.: The possible link between glycolysis and insulin release in isolated islets. *In* Diabetes Research Today. Meeting of the Minkowsky Prize-Winners'. Stuttgart, F. K. Schattauer Verlag, 1976, pp. 191–206.

[12] Basabe, J. C., Lopez, N. L., Viktora, J. K., and Wolff, F. W.: Insulin secretion studied in the perfused rat pancreas. I. Effect of tolbutamide, leucine and arginine; their interaction with diazoxide and relation to glucose. Diabetes *20*:449–56, 1971.

[13] Brech, J., Kaess, H., Schlierf, G., and Rohs, M.: Effects of diazoxide on the glucagon-induced secretion of insulin. Klin. Wochenschr. *46*:449–50, 1968.

[14] Basabe, J. C., Lopez, N. L., Viktora, J. K., and Wolff, F. W.: II. Effect of glucose, glucagon, 3′,5′adenosine monophosphate, theophylline, imidazole and phenoxybenzamine; their interaction with diazoxide. Diabetes *20*:457–66, 1971.

[15] Levin, S. R., Charles, M., O'Connor, M., and Grodsky, G.: Use of diphenylhydantoin and diazoxide to investigate insulin secretory mechanisms. Am. J. Physiol. *229*:49–54, 1975.

[16] Alberti, K. G., Dornhorst, A., and Rowe, A.: Metabolic rhythms in normal and diabetic man. Isr. J. Med. Sci. *11*:571–80, 1975.

[17] Kanter, Y., Gerson, J. R., and Bessman, A. N.: 2-3-diphosphoglycerate, nucleotide phosphate, and organic and inorganic phosphate levels during the early phases of diabetic ketoacidosis. Diabetes *26*:429–33, 1977.

[18] Federspil, G., Lefèbvre, P., and Luyckx, A.: Effets d'un exercise musculaire continu (nage forcée) sur la glycémie et le taux plasmatique des acides gras libres, de l'insuline et de la corticostérone chez le rat. Arch. Int. Physiol. Biochem. *77*:778–86, 1969.

One Month of Sustained Release of Insulin from a Polymer Implant

HALIMENA M. CREQUE, ROBERT LANGER, AND JUDAH FOLKMAN

SUMMARY

Rats made diabetic with streptozotocin received a single subcutaneous implant of an insulin polymer pellet that released insulin continuously at approximately 2 U/day. Continuous normoglycemia was achieved for up to 1 mo. Mean glucose level for treated animals was 113 mg/dl as compared with 398 mg/dl for untreated diabetic controls. Diurnal blood glucose values for treated animals ranged from 71 to 116 mg/dl. Polyuria and glycosuria were corrected by the presence of the insulin + polymer. Treated animals gained weight normally and reached a mean weight of 350 g, whereas untreated control animals lost weight, to a mean of 150 g. When insulin + polymer preparations were periodically implanted and removed at 7-day intervals, normoglycemia was only associated with the presence of implants. DIABETES 29:37–40, January 1980.

In a previous report,[1] we demonstrated that a variety of macromolecules could be continuously released in a biologically active form from pellets of vinyl acetate-ethylene copolymer. We now show that diabetic rats can be made normoglycemic for 1 mo after a single subcutaneous implant of such a polymer that releases insulin in a sustained manner.

MATERIALS AND METHODS

Animals. Twenty-three male cesarean-delivered rats (21 days old) (Charles River Breeding Laboratories), weighing from 150 to 250 g, were made diabetic with streptozotocin and were distributed into four experimental groups: (1) 15 animals received single insulin + polymer implants; (2) 1 animal received an insulin + polymer that was repeatedly implanted and removed every 7 days; (3) 2 untreated control animals received no polymers; (4) 2 untreated control animals received empty polymers. Animals received water and rat chow ad libitum. Body weights were measured every 8–10 days.

From the Department of Surgery, Children's Hospital Medical Center and Harvard Medical School, Boston, Massachusetts, and the Department of Nutrition and Food Science, Massachusetts Institute of Technology, Cambridge, Massachusetts 02139.

Address reprint requests to Judah Folkman, M.D., Children's Hospital Medical Center, 300 Longwood Avenue, Boston, Massachusetts 02115.

Received for publication 1 August 1979.

Induction of diabetes mellitus and determination of blood glucose levels. Each animal received an intravenous injection of 75 mg/kg of streptozotocin, suspended in 0.4 ml of 0.005 M citric acid at pH 4.5. The rats were left untreated for 6 days and were then entered into the experimental design. During the 6-day period, glucose determinations were made at days 1, 3, and 6 to insure a consistently high blood glucose value.

To measure glucose levels, 200 μl of blood was withdrawn from the tail (samples were generally taken in the morning or early afternoon, except for the diurnal study) and centrifuged at 15,000 × *g*. Twenty-microliter samples of plasma were analyzed on a YSI glucose analyzer. Glucose levels were determined about every 3 days.

Preparation and implantation of sterile polymer implants. A number of preliminary experiments were conducted to determine a polymer design that would release about 2 U of insulin a day in vitro. The insulin released in vitro was monitored spectrophotometrically at 220 nm. Insulin + polymer preparations were incubated in physiologic saline in glass tubes coated with Siliclad. The spectrophotometric measurements were corroborated by both an insulin radioimmunoassay[2] and injections of released insulin into diabetic rats. In both cases, it was found that all the released insulin was active.

The polymer implants were made using a modification[3] of our previously described procedure.[1] First, 100 mg of bovine pancreatic insulin (Sigma or Calbiochem, 25 IU/mg) was mixed with 0.4 cc of 10% (w/v) vinyl acetate-ethylene copolymer (Eluax 40, Dupont) in methylene chloride. The resulting suspension was vortexed and poured into circular glass molds, which were supercooled over dry ice. Molds containing insulin + polymer were then refrigerated overnight at −20°C. To evaporate methylene chloride, the molds were then placed under vacuum (600 mm Hg) for 24 h. The resulting discs (1.3 cm by 1 mm) were incubated in lactated Ringer's solution (Abbott) for 24 h and then implanted subcutaneously in the lower abdomen. Implant sites were closed with Michel's wound clamps.

Variation in diurnal serum glucose, urine glucose, and urine volume. Blood and urine samples from two treated animals and one control were analyzed with the YSI glucose analyzer every 2–5 h for 31 h. Urine was collected by housing the animals in metabolic cages.

RESULTS

Glucose analysis. At 24 h after the administration of streptozotocin, glucose levels were elevated to 374–412 mg/dl. Within the first 24 h after implantation of insulin + polymer, glucose levels fell from 374–412 mg/dl to 87–127 mg/dl and remained stable for 26 days. During the 29-day experiment, the mean glucose level for all treated animals was 113 ± 29 mg/dl. The mean glucose level for controls was 398 ± 22 mg/dl. On the 27th day of the test, 27% of the treated animals had glucose levels between 252 and 295 mg/dl compared with the original values of between 382 and 411 mg/dl before treatment. On the 29th day, all animals were hyperglycemic (Figure 1). In contrast, all diabetic control animals displayed a mean value of 398 ± 22 mg/dl throughout the experiment.

Diurnal glucose measurements and urine analysis. Figure 2 illustrates the variation in blood glucose concentrations on the 16th day of treatment for two experimental animals and one control. During the 31 h of monitoring, glucose levels for treated animals ranged from 71 to 116 mg/dl, with a mean daily concentration of 95 ± 13 mg/dl. Mean glucose concentration for the control was 338 ± 61 mg/dl. Values ranged from 297 to 470 mg/dl.

Treated animals voided a total of 38 and 44 ml of urine in 31 h. Glucose was not detected in the urine of treated animals. In contrast, the untreated control voided 183 ml of urine during the 31 h and urine glucose concentrations exceeded 500 mg/dl.

FIGURE 1. Implantation of single insulin-containing polymers into diabetic rats. Control animals were diabetic rats receiving empty polymers or no polymers.

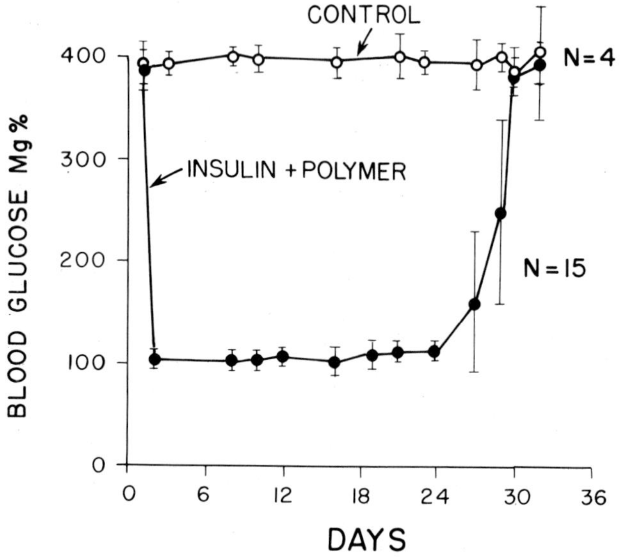

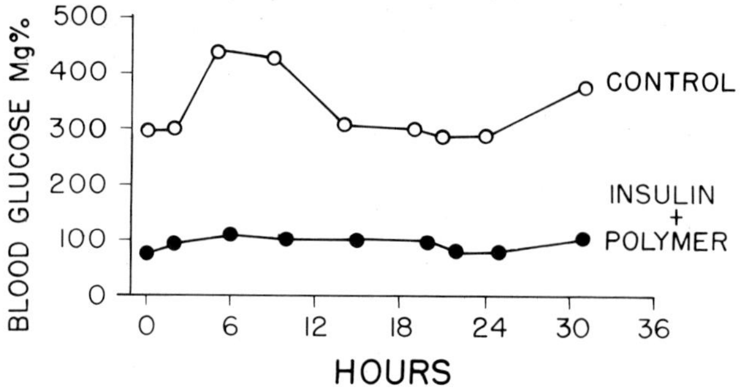

FIGURE 2. Determinations of blood glucose, made every few hours around the clock, for two treated animals and one control animal.

Periodic implantation and removal of the polymer. When a diabetic animal was treated with the insulin + polymer for 7 days, glucose levels ranged between 87 and 106 mg/dl. After the implant was removed, values rose to 378–440 mg/dl. After reimplantation, glucose fell to between 105 and 119 mg/dl (Figure 3).

Polymer activity. After 31 days, all insulin + polymer preparations appeared to have stopped releasing insulin. They were removed, washed in saline, and implanted in untreated diabetic animals. No effect on hyperglycemia was observed. When a new, unexpended insulin + polymer was placed in a diabetic animal previously treated for 31 days, glucose levels were again lowered to 103 mg/dl.

Growth and development. Figure 4 shows the change in body weight for all experimental animals. The weight gain of controls was depressed as a result of the disease. Treated animals gained weight at the normal rate of approximately 40 g/wk. Some became slightly obese, to over 400 g. The mean body weight for treated animals at 28 days was 350 ± 55 g. By contrast, untreated controls lost weight or maintained their starting weight. By the end of the experiment, they averaged 105 ± 23 g.

DISCUSSION

These experiments show that a small subcutaneous implant of vinyl acetate-ethylene copolymer can release insulin in biologically active form for 29 days. Each implant released about 2 U of insulin a day throughout the 1-mo period. Diabetic rats carrying the implanted insulin + polymer main-

FIGURE 3. An experiment in which a diabetic rat was used as its own control. Without the insulin + polymer, blood glucose levels were about 400 mg/dl. Implantation and reimplantation of the same polymer caused glucose levels to be nearly 100 mg/dl.

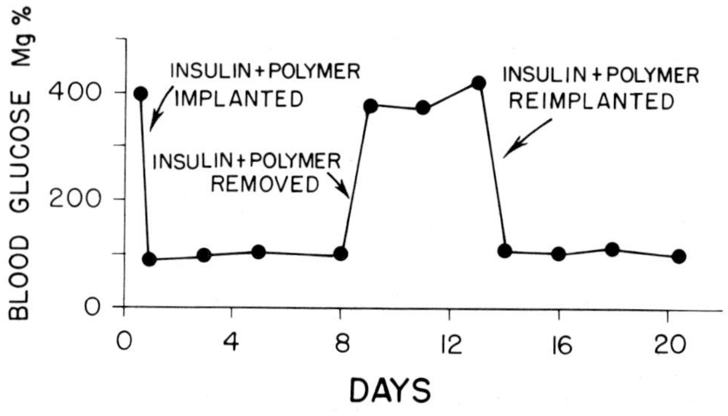

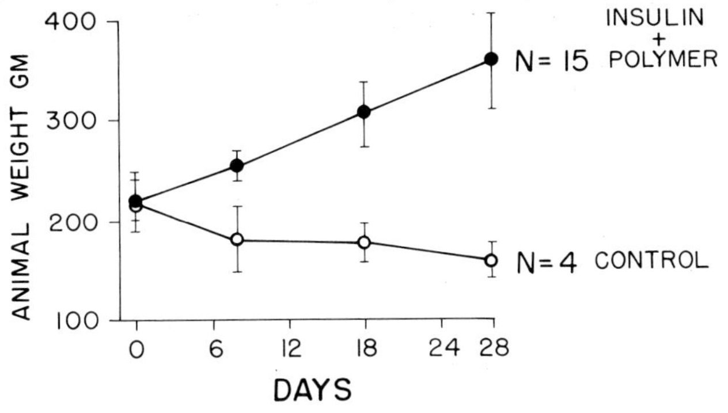

FIGURE 4. Weight determinations of control and treated animals.

tained normoglycemia and gained weight normally. This indicates that the rats adjusted their dietary intake to match insulin levels in their blood.

Blood glucose levels in the treated animals were not erratic, as shown by the glucose determinations made every 2–5 h (Figure 2). The polymer implants all stopped releasing insulin at the same time. This release time span was a function of such design factors as percent loading and particle size of the insulin + polymer configuration, as well as the external coating of the polymer.[1,3] In fact, the polymer design in the present study was not effectively optimized. Our calculations show that only about 3% of the insulin incorporated into the polymer escaped at the level of 2 U a day. The insulin was apparently not denatured, because we have taken insulin released from polymers in vitro at day 25, subjected it to both an insulin radioimmunoassay and injection into diabetic rats, and found that nearly 100% of the insulin released, as determined by protein measurement, was biologically active. Current experiments in our laboratory show that such simple adjustments as increasing the particle size of lyophilized proteins before incorporation into the polymers or increasing the drug loading can alter release rates by as much as 50 times.[3] In the case of insulin, particle size appears to be a critical factor, because the commercial insulin powder we used is less than 50 μm in diameter (which is much smaller than most protein powders) and release is slow, with much of the drug retained, unless extremely high loadings are employed. Future experimentation in our laboratory will be directed toward achieving an insulin-releasing system that more optimally utilizes the drug and releases insulin for far longer periods of time. Nevertheless, the present experiments are the first to demonstrate that even one month of sustained release of insulin can be accomplished.

No rats in this study spontaneously recovered from their diabetes. To further strengthen the experiments, diabetic rats were used as their own controls. Periodic implantation and removal of an insulin + polymer in the same animal correlated with normoglycemia or hyperglycemia. When an expended polymer was removed from a diabetic rat and implanted into a previously untreated diabetic rat, there was still no effect from the polymer. This indicated that the shutdown of insulin release was intrinsic to the polymer itself and not due to fibrous encapsulation or to a foreign body reaction around it. Furthermore, when a fresh insulin + polymer pellet was implanted into the first rat (i.e., the previously treated rat), glucose levels returned to normal. This indicated that the shutdown of insulin release from the expended polymer was unrelated to any type of "resistance" to insulin by the host animal.

The only previous report in which insulin released from long-term implants was studied was by Davis,[4] who used polyacrylamide as a vehicle. He measured weights of diabetic animals receiving such implants for 2–3 wk, but blood glucose was not measured. Also, polyacrylamide implants are inflammatory[1] and acrylamide monomers have been shown to be toxic to both animals and humans.[5] The ethylene-vinyl acetate copolymer used in our study causes no detectable tissue reaction.[1]

Several other novel approaches for maintaining normoglycemia in diabetic animals and patients have been investigated recently; these include pancreatic islet cell transplants, infusion pumps, servomechanisms, and glucose-sensing artificial pancreases.[6–13] The sustained release of low levels of insulin from a single polymer implant offers another potential therapeutic approach or adjunct. One could speculate that, with further development, these insulin + polymer implants might be used clinically in conjunction with dietary control or as an insulin depot linked to a regulatory feedback control with a glucose sensor.[14,15] It is also conceivable that insulin + polymers could maintain a constantly low level of insulin and that additional insulin release could be triggered by some external force, such as temperature. While any future clinical applications of these implants remain to be seen, their immediate practical use may be as a means of studying the kinetics of dietary intake and blood glucose level when insulin input is continuous.

ACKNOWLEDGMENTS

We are grateful to Dr. Kenneth Gabbay for helpful advice and for reviewing the manuscript and for the use of the Beckman YSI glucose analyzer. We also thank Dr. Antoine Augustin, Dr. Joseph Vacanti, and Dr. Julian Kadish for their help and advice, and Mary Jo Canavan for her secretarial assistance.

This study was supported by a grant from the Alza Corporation and by a gift to Harvard University from the Monsanto Company.

REFERENCES

[1] Langer, R., and Folkman, J.: Polymers for the sustained release of proteins and other macromolecules. Nature *263*:797–800, 1976.

[2] Soeldner, J. S., and Slone, D.: Critical variables in the radioimmunoassay of serum insulin using the double antibody technic. Diabetes *14*: 771–79, 1965.

[3] Rhine, W. D., Hsieh, D. S. T., and Langer, R.: Kinetics of polymeric delivery systems for proteins and other macromolecules. Polymer Preprints *20*:596–99, 1979.

[4] Davis, B. K.: Control of diabetes with polyacrylamide implants containing insulin. Experientia *28*:348, 1972.

[5] McCollister, D. D.: Toxicology of acrylamide. Toxicol. Appl. Pharmacol. *6*:172–81, 1964.

[6] Renner, R., Hepp, K. D., Mehnert, H., Franetzki, M., Reese, H., and Geisen, K.: Continuous insulin therapy with a portable miniaturized infusion system. Diabetologia *13*:427, 1977.

[7] Gonet, A. E., and Renold, A. E.: Homografting of fetal rat pancreas. Diabetologia *1*:91–95, 1965.

[8] Gates, R. J., and Lazarus, N. R.: Reversal of streptozotocin-induced diabetes in rats by intraperitoneal implants of encapsulated neonatal rabbit pancreatic tissue. Lancet *2*(8051):1257–59, 1977.

[9] Tze, W. J., Wong, F. C., Chen, L. M., and O'Young, S.: Implantable artificial endocrine pancreas unit used to restore normoglycemia in the diabetic rat. Nature *264*:466–67, 1977.

[10] Pickup, J. C., Keen, H., Parsons, J. A., and Alberti, K.: Continuous

subcutaneous insulin infusion: an approach to achieving normal glycaemia. Br. Med. J. *1*:204–07, 1978.

[11] Genuth, S., and Martin, P.: Control of hyperglycemia in adult diabetics by pulsed insulin delivery. Diabetes *26*:571–81, 1977.

[12] Slama, G., Hautecouverture, M., Assan, R., and Tchobroutsky, G.: One to five days of continuous intravenous infusion on seven diabetic patients. Diabetes *23*:732–38, 1974.

[13] Slama, G., Klein, J. C., Merouani, A., and Frantz, A.: Artificial pancreas for renal transplantation in a diabetic. Lancet *1*(8065):665, 1978.

[14] Soeldner, J. S., Chang, K. W., Aisenberg, S., Hiebert, J., and Egdahl, R.: Diabetes Mellitus, vol. 14, chap. 20. Fogarty Int. Center Ser. Prev. Med., DHEW, (NIH), 1976, pp. 267–77.

[15] Cahill, G. F., Soeldner, J. S., and Harris, G. W.: Practical developments in diabetes research. Diabetes *21*:703–12, 1972.

Ten-year Follow-up of Subjects with Impaired Glucose Tolerance
Prevention of Diabetes by Tolbutamide and Diet Regulation

GUNNAR SARTOR, BENGT SCHERSTÉN, SVEN CARLSTRÖM, ARNE MELANDER, ÅKE NORDÉN, AND GUNNAR PERSSON

SUMMARY

In a diabetes detection survey carried out between 1962 and 1965, 2477 (1.1%) of 228,883 subjects had Clinistix-positive glucosuria after a carbohydrate-rich luncheon meal. Of these 2477, 578 displayed impaired tolerance to oral glucose without having manifest diabetes. From this group, 267 men were divided into five groups and subjected to the following treatments and controls: (a) diet regulation and 0.5 g tolbutamide t.i.d. (N = 49), annual oral glucose tolerance test (OGTT); (b) diet regulation and one placebo tablet t.i.d. (N = 48), annual OGTT; (c) diet regulation only (N = 50), annual OGTT; (d) no treatment (N = 61), annual OGTT; and (e) no treatment, OGTT at follow-up (N = 59 at follow-up). In addition, a control group was included comprised of men with normal OGTT (N = 52). At follow-up, 29% of those without diet regulation and medication (group e; N = 59) had developed diabetes. Of those on diet regulation, but without active medication (group b plus group c, N = 98), 13% had diabetes. No individual maintaining tolbutamide and diet regulation (N = 23) had progressed to diabetes. In this group, 80% of those later examined (N = 11) had serum tolbutamide concentrations in the therapeutic range. No individual with initially normal OGTT developed diabetes or impaired OGTT.

The findings suggest that normal oral glucose tolerance signifies little risk of progress to impaired glucose tolerance and manifest diabetes, whereas impaired glucose tolerance is associated with a high risk of progression to diabetes. In addition, it seems possible that treatment with diet regulation, in combination with tolbutamide, may prevent or postpone progression from impaired glucose tolerance to manifest diabetes. DIABETES 29:41–49, January 1980.

Since the 1940s, several diabetes surveys[1–3] have been carried out with the intention to detect the disease at an early stage and, by the institution of various therapeutic measures, postpone or prevent the late complications of the disease. For such purposes, a diabetes detection campaign was started in 1962[4] in Malmöhus County in southern Sweden. As defined in a separate study,[5] impaired tolerance to oral glucose was found in a number of subjects. These individuals were assumed to be in an early phase of diabetes, and it was decided, therefore, to examine whether impaired glucose tolerance carries a significant risk of development into overt diabetes, and if diet regulation and sulfonylurea medication could prevent or postpone such development. The present report is comprised of follow-up data from 1974 to 1976 as to the effects of tolbutamide and diet regulation on glucose tolerance and progression to diabetes.

MATERIALS AND METHODS

Population. From 1962 to 1965, a diabetes detection survey[4–6] was conducted in Malmöhus County in southern Sweden. The screening was based on Clinistix testing of urine collected 2 h after a carbohydrate-rich luncheon meal. The survey covered 82% of the population over 16 yr of age. Of the 228,833 participants, 2477 (1.08%) had glucosuria (Figure 1). In 2180 of these, a 3-hr oral glucose tolerance test (OGTT) was performed. All subjects were asked to include bread in each meal for 3 consecutive days preceding the OGTT.

Oral glucose tolerance test (OGTT). An oral glucose dose of 30 g/m² body surface was given as a 10% solution between 8 a.m. and 9 a.m. after overnight fasting. Samples of capillary blood for glucose determination were taken before and 15, 30, 45, 60, 75, 90, 120, 150, and 180 min after glucose administration. During the test, the subjects rested in half-recumbent position, except for the movements necessary to deliver urine samples at 60 and 120 min.

Diagnostic criteria. Diagnostic criteria for evaluation of the OGTT were established from a subset of the population collected at random among those without a history of diabetes, as earlier described.[5] All 10 blood glucose values of the

From the Departments of Internal Medicine (Lund University Hospital) and Clinical Pharmacology (Malmö General Hospital), University of Lund; and the Department of Community Care Sciences, Dalby, Sweden.
Received for publication 9 July 1979.

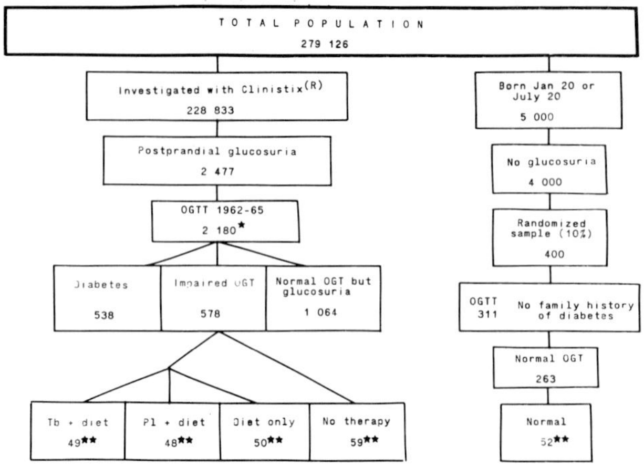

FIGURE 1. Flow chart of a diabetes prevention study. x: OGT = oral glucose tolerance, OGTT = oral glucose tolerance test. xx = males only. Tb = tolbutamide, Pl = placebo.

OGTT above the mean plus three standard deviations (SD) were taken to indicate diabetes, and all 10 blood glucose values below the mean plus 2 SD were considered to represent the normal state. Impaired glucose tolerance was defined as the condition when neither the criteria for diabetes nor those for normality were fulfilled. Table 1 gives the standards for normal oral glucose tolerance and diabetes.

Blood pressure, heart rate, body weight, and height. Systolic and diastolic blood pressure (phase 5) was measured after the OGTT, when the subject had been in the recumbent position for at least 10 min. A mercury manometer with standard cuff (rubber balloon 12 × 35 cm) was used. Heart rate was calculated as number of beats per min by auscultation during 30 s at the time of blood pressure measurement. Body weight and height were measured in a standardized way according to the Expert Committee of Medical Assessment of Nutritional Status.[7]

Blood glucose. Throughout the study, capillary blood was used for blood glucose determination. Samples were taken during fasting and 15, 30, 45, 60, 75, 90, 120, 150, and 180 min after glucose ingestion. The blood glucose concentrations were determined by the glucose oxidase method of Marks,[8] as modified by Scherstén.[9] Analyses were always made on the day of blood sampling.

Plasma insulin. Venous blood samples were obtained through an indwelling antebrachial polyethylene catheter. Plasma was separated by centrifugation and was frozen and stored at −20°C until assessed for insulin content. Plasma insulin concentrations were measured by a commercial solid phase radioimmunoassay[10] (Phadebas Insulin Test, Pharmacia, Uppsala, Sweden).

Plasma insulin was determined only at follow-up. Determinations were made on samples obtained before and during the OGTT, at the same time intervals as for blood glucose determinations.

Serum lipids. Serum cholesterol and serum triglyceride concentrations were determined on venous blood samples obtained before the OGTT, when the patients were in the fasting state. Standard enzymatic methods were used.[11,12]

Serum tolbutamide. The serum concentrations of unmetabolized tolbutamide were measured by gas chromatography.[13] As such measurements were not part of the original plan, determinations could be carried out only in 11 of the 23 subjects maintaining tolbutamide medication throughout the study. The samples were obtained during 1977.

Statistical methods. The statistical significance of differences was calculated by paired or nonpaired Student's t tests or by chi-square tests. The levels of significance are given as $P < 0.05$, $P < 0.01$, and $P < 0.001$.

Impaired glucose tolerance: randomization and information. By consecutive randomization procedure, the 578 subjects with impaired glucose tolerance were divided into five groups:

(a) 0.5 g tolbutamide t.i.d. plus diet regulation, annual OGTT.*
(b) one placebo tablet t.i.d. plus diet regulation, annual OGTT.*
(c) diet regulation only, annual OGTT.*
(d) no regulations, annual OGTT.*
(e) no regulations, 1–2 OGTT in the 1960s, 1 OGTT at follow-up, 1974–1976.

Randomization followed the schedule a-e-b-e-c-e-d-e-e-e.

Subjects in groups a–c were informed that they were at

* At least annual OGTT in the 1960s, then at longer intervals until follow-up, 1974–1976.

TABLE 1
Blood glucose concentrations at OGTT, mean + 2 SD and 3 SD, in a random sample of 121 men used to define the criteria of normal oral glucose tolerance, impaired glucose tolerance, and diabetes (see text and ref. 5 for further information)

		Blood glucose (mM)									
Age group (yr)		0	15	30	45	60	75 (min)	90	120	150	180
	M	4.3	7.3	8.9	8.1	7.1	6.1	5.6	4.8	4.0	3.9
≤39*	M + 2 SD	4.9	9.1	11.3	11.3	10.3	8.9	8.0	7.2	5.0	4.9
	M + 3 SD	5.2	10.0	12.5	12.9	11.9	10.3	9.2	8.4	5.5	5.4
	M	4.4	8.1	9.7	9.6	8.8	7.2	6.1	4.8	3.9	3.8
40–59†	M + 2 SD	5.4	10.1	12.7	13.2	12.8	11.6	10.3	7.8	5.7	5.0
	M + 3 SD	5.9	11.1	14.2	15.0	14.8	13.8	12.4	9.3	6.6	5.6
	M	4.5	8.0	9.8	10.0	9.5	8.2	7.5	5.7	4.3	3.8
≥60‡	M + 2 SD	5.5	10.6	13.2	13.4	13.7	12.2	11.3	8.9	6.5	5.0
	M + 3 SD	6.0	11.9	14.9	15.1	15.8	14.2	13.2	10.5	7.6	5.6

*N = 49, †N = 41, and ‡N = 31; M = mean.

TABLE 2
Age and blood glucose concentrations at OGTT, mean ± SEM, at start of study in men with impaired and men with normal glucose tolerance

			Blood glucose (mM)									
Group	N	Age (yr)	0	15	30	45	60 (min)	75	90	120	150	180
Tolbutamide plus diet	49	54 ± 2	4.7 ± 0.1	8.1 ± 0.2	10.7 ± 0.2	11.7 ± 0.2	11.6 ± 0.2	10.3 ± 0.2	9.3 ± 0.2	6.9 ± 0.2	4.9 ± 0.2	4.0 ± 0.2
Placebo plus diet	48	55 ± 2	4.9 ± 0.1	8.3 ± 0.2	10.6 ± 0.2	11.7 ± 0.3	11.5 ± 0.3	10.2 ± 0.3	9.4 ± 0.3	7.2 ± 0.3	5.0 ± 0.2	4.2 ± 0.2
Diet	50	55 ± 2	4.9 ± 0.1	8.4 ± 0.2	11.0 ± 0.2	12.1 ± 0.3	11.8 ± 0.2	10.3 ± 0.2	9.2 ± 0.2	6.6 ± 0.2	4.6 ± 0.2	3.9 ± 0.1
No therapy	59	48 ± 1	5.0 ± 0.1	8.3 ± 0.2	10.5 ± 0.2	11.3 ± 0.3	11.2 ± 0.3	10.2 ± 0.3	9.5 ± 0.3	7.5 ± 0.3	5.7 ± 0.2	4.8 ± 0.2
Normal	52	50 ± 2	4.4 ± 0.1	7.3 ± 0.1	8.8 ± 0.1	8.5 ± 0.2	7.5 ± 0.2	6.2 ± 0.2	5.6 ± 0.2	4.7 ± 0.2	3.9 ± 0.1	3.9 ± 0.1

risk of developing diabetes, that they should limit their intake of carbohydrates and lipids, and that (when overweight) they should reduce their total energy intake.

After the randomization, there were no differences between groups a, b, and c as to age, blood glucose, blood pressure, heart rate, or body weight (Tables 2 and 3).

Subjects in groups d and e were informed that the OGTT had given a normal result and that no therapy was necessary.

At follow-up in 1974, a retrospective sample of 59 men was drawn from group e. They are presented below as the "untreated group." The untreated group was younger than the group given tolbutamide plus diet regulation ($P < 0.05$), than the group given placebo plus diet regulation ($P < 0.001$), and than that given diet regulation only ($P < 0.01$). In the untreated group, the mean OGTT blood glucose level was higher than that in group c at 120 min ($P < 0.05$), than that in groups a ($P < 0.05$), b ($P < 0.05$), and c ($P < 0.001$) at 150 min, and than that in groups a ($P < 0.01$), b ($P < 0.05$), and c ($P < 0.001$) at 180 min. Blood pressure, heart rate, and body weight did not differ (Tables 2 and 3).

Subjects belonging to group d were not examined at this follow-up. A family history of diabetes at the start of the study was found in 22% of the subjects in group a. The corresponding figures were 25%, 20%, and 31% in groups b, c, and e, respectively. There were no significant differences between the groups (chi-square test).

Normal glucose tolerance. From the subset of the population with normal OGTT at the start of the study, and having no family history of diabetes,[5] 52 men were selected at random at the time of follow-up. They are presented as the "normal group."

The normal group was younger than group b ($P < 0.05$). The mean systolic blood pressure was lower than that of group c ($P < 0.01$) and group e ($P < 0.05$). The heart rate was lower than that of groups b, c, and e ($P < 0.05$). Normal group body weight was lower than that of group a ($P < 0.01$) (Tables 2 and 3).

Follow-up. Groups a, b, and c underwent yearly OGTT during the 1960s and then at longer intervals until follow-up in 1974–1976. A similar schedule was held for group d. Group e underwent OGTT twice during the 1960s and again at follow-up.

Standardization of OGTT conditions. The subjects were instructed to include bread with every meal during the 3 days preceding the OGTT. Eating and drinking was not allowed from 10 p.m. on the day before the study. No smoking or medication was allowed on the day of examination.

Adherence to treatment. Adherence to medication was assessed by direct questioning during each visit and by a retrospective analysis of the rate of tablet issue from the local pharmacy, which distributed the tablets independently. After the follow-up had been performed, a method became available for the determination of serum tolbutamide.[13] Therefore, a special check on adherence to tolbutamide medication was performed in 1977 by measurements of the steady state concentrations of tolbutamide in serum.

Distribution of tablets. Tolbutamide and placebo tablets

TABLE 3
Blood pressure, heart rate, and body weight, mean ± SEM, at start of study in men with impaired and men with normal glucose tolerance

		Blood pressure			
Group	N	Systolic (mm Hg)	Diastolic (mm Hg)	Heart rate (beats/min)	Body weight (kg)
Tolbutamide plus diet	49	149 ± 3	90 ± 2	76 ± 2	82 ± 2
Placebo plus diet	48	148 ± 3	88 ± 2	76 ± 2	78 ± 1
Diet	50	153 ± 3	90 ± 1	77 ± 2	77 ± 2
No therapy	59	151 ± 3	91 ± 1	76 ± 2	78 ± 2
Normal	52	143 ± 3	88 ± 1	71 ± 2	75 ± 1

TABLE 4
Follow-up 1974–1976 of 206 men with impaired and 52 men with normal glucose tolerance

Group at start of study		Diagnosis at follow-up: Diabetes		No diabetes			
					Alive		
		Alive	Deceased	Deceased	Examined	Dropout	Total
Tolbutamide plus diet	Tolbutamide continued	0	0	3	20	0	23
	Tolbutamide discontinued	2	3	3	15	3	26
Placebo plus diet	Placebo continued	1	3	5	17	0	26
	Placebo discontinued	1	1	5	7	8	22
Diet		5	2	6	27	10	50
No therapy		15	2	4	36	2	59
Total		24	11	26	122	23	206
Normal		0	0	7	39	6	52

were originally given by double-blind technique. The code was broken in 1972 to allow for studies of cardiovascular conditions in the population examined.[14]

Reclassification. At follow-up, group a (tolbutamide plus diet regulations) was divided into two subgroups: one subgroup had continued with tolbutamide plus diet regulation for the entire period of study, while another discontinued tolbutamide but had continued diet regulation. At follow-up, nondiabetic subjects from group b (placebo plus diet regulation, placebo discontinued but diet regulation continued) and group c (diet regulation only) were considered as one group. This new group was labeled the "dietary group." The reclassification seemed justified, as the code was already broken and as the effect of the placebo was judged to be negligible during long-term observation.

Attenders at follow-up. For those who did not develop diabetes during the study period, and who were examined by OGTT at follow-up (Table 4), the average time elapsed from start of study to follow-up was: group a (i.e., continuation of tolbutamide plus dietary regulation) 9.9 (9.1–10.8) yr; group having discontinued tolbutamide but having continued dietary regulation 9.9 (9.4–11.0) yr; dietary group (i.e., dietary regulation with or without placebo) 10.1 (9.3–11.8) yr; untreated group 11.3 (9.3–13.6) yr; and normal group 10.1 (8.5–11.3) yr.

Nonattenders at follow-up. Diabetics. During the study, 35 subjects developed diabetes (Table 4). The diagnosis was verified by fasting capillary whole blood glucose of 10.0 mM or more in 13 subjects, or between 7.8 and 9.9 mM on more than one occasion in 10 subjects. Another six subjects had obvious diabetic symptoms (overt diabetes) and were treated by their own physicians with insulin (N = 3) or oral antidiabetic drugs (N = 3). In two subjects, the diagnosis of diabetes was based on their death certificates. Four

TABLE 5
Morbidity in diabetes*

Group		N	Diabetes at follow-up N	%	Level of significance
Tolbutamide plus diet	Tolbutamide continued	23	0	0	
	Tolbutamide discontinued	26	5	19	
Placebo plus diet	Placebo continued	26	4	15	$P < 0.01$
	Placebo discontinued	22	2	9	$P < 0.05$
Diet		50	7	14	
No therapy		59	17	29	
Total		206	35	17	$P < 0.01$
Normal		52	0	0	

*Statistical method: chi-square tests.

TABLE 6
Characteristics at start of study of those later developing diabetes compared with those not developing diabetes

Group	N	Age (yr)	Body wt (kg)	Blood pressure: Systolic (mm Hg)	Blood pressure: Diastolic (mm Hg)	Blood glucose at OGTT (mM): 0 (min)	60	75	90	120	150	180
Not developing diabetes	171	52 ± 1	78 ± 1	150 ± 2	89 ± 1	4.8 ± 0.1	11.4 ± 0.1	10.0 ± 0.1	9.1 ± 0.1	6.9 ± 0.1	4.9 ± 0.1	4.1 ± 0.1
Developing diabetes	35	55 ± 2	83 ± 2*	154 ± 4	94 ± 1†	5.3 ± 0.1‡	12.2 ± 0.4*	11.3 ± 0.4‡	10.5 ± 0.4‡	8.0 ± 0.4†	5.9 ± 0.3‡	4.9 ± 0.2†

Values given as mean ± SEM.
Statistical method: nonpaired Student's *t* test.
Significance of the difference: * $P < 0.05$; † $P < 0.01$; ‡ $P < 0.001$. Values greater than $P < 0.05$ are omitted.

subjects had a fasting blood glucose of 6.6–7.0 mM. At OGTT all had a 2-h blood glucose level above 10.4 mM. In addition, at least four of the six values between 0 and 2 h were above 10.4 mM.

Deceased. Thirty-seven subjects with impaired glucose tolerance and seven with normal glucose tolerance at the start of the study died before follow-up (Table 4). Cause of death was obtained by hospital files, autopsy protocols, and death certificates. Autopsies had been performed in less than half of the deceased subjects.

Dropouts. For various reasons (moving from the area, unwillingness to participate, disability), 29 subjects were not examined by OGTT at follow-up. Their health situation was judged from a questionnaire, answered by 18 out of 21 dropouts from the treatment groups, by the two dropouts from the untreated group, and by five of six dropouts from the normal group. None who answered the questionnaire had diabetes. The vital register indicated that those who did not answer the questionnaire were alive. There was no overt difference in initial clinical or laboratory results between the 29 dropouts and those remaining in the study.

RESULTS

Morbidity in diabetes. Diabetes developed in 35 of the 206 subjects (17%) with initially impaired glucose tolerance, while none of the 52 subjects with initially normal glucose tolerance developed either impaired glucose tolerance or diabetes ($P < 0.01$) (Table 5). Among the subjects with impaired glucose tolerance, the incidence of diabetes was lower in those given dietary regulations (with or without placebo, plus those who had discontinued tolbutamide; 18 of 124 subjects = 15%) than in those left untreated (17 of 59 subjects = 29%; $P < 0.05$). It was further reduced, to nil, in the group treated with diet regulation in combination with tolbutamide (0 of 23 subjects = 0%; $P < 0.01$ versus the untreated group). The cumulative frequency distribution of the incidence of diabetes in treated and untreated subjects is demonstrated in Figure 2. The difference in the incidence of diabetes was apparently not the effect of an age difference at diabetes onset in untreated [60.2 ± 2.6 (SEM) yr] and treated groups [63.4 ± 3.1 (SEM) yr].

At entrance, those who subsequently developed diabetes had higher mean values of fasting blood glucose ($P < 0.001$), as well as blood glucose at 60–180 min during OGTT, than those who did not develop diabetes (N =171) ($P < 0.05$–$P < 0.001$) (Table 6). In addition, they had a higher mean diastolic blood pressure ($P < 0.01$) and were more obese ($P < 0.05$).

Total mortality. Among subjects with initially impaired glucose tolerance, the mortality was 31% in those who subsequently developed diabetes, while it was only 15% in those who remained nondiabetic ($P < 0.05$) (Table 7). There was no obvious difference in death rates between different treatment groups (Table 4). Among those who died, the mean ages at the start of the study (range 61.4 – 66.6 yr) and at death (range 66.4 – 73.1 yr) did not differ between diabetics and nondiabetics.

Those who died after having developed diabetes were, at entrance, older ($P < 0.001$) than those still alive at follow-up

FIGURE 2. Cumulative diabetes morbidity (%) within the different groups. Total number of subjects in each group indicated within brackets. •——• No therapy (N = 59). *——* Diet, diet plus placebo continued or discontinued; diet and tolbutamide discontinued (N = 124). ▲——▲ Tolbutamide plus diet (N =23).

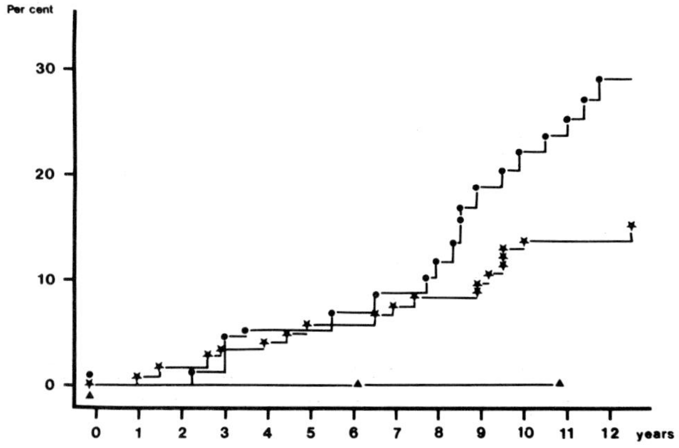

TABLE 7
Mortality*

Group	N	Deceased N	Deceased %	Level of significance	
Impaired glucose tolerance					
Nondiabetic	171	26	15	P < 0,05 (Nondiabetic vs Diabetic)	NS (Impaired vs Normal)
Diabetic	35	11	31	NS (Diabetic vs Normal)	
Normal glucose tolerance	52	7	13		

* Statistical method: chi-square tests.

TABLE 8
Characteristics at start of study of those later deceased compared with those alive at follow-up

Group	N	Age (yr)	Blood pressure Systolic (mm Hg)	Blood pressure Diastolic (mm Hg)	Blood glucose at OGTT (mM) 0 (min)	60	75	90	120	150	180
Impaired glucose tolerance											
Alive	169	50 ± 1	148 ± 1	89 ± 1	4.9 ± 0.1	11.2 ± 0.2	10.0 ± 0.1	9.1 ± 0.1	6.8 ± 0.1	4.9 ± 0.1	4.1 ± 0.1
Nondiabetic deceased	26	67 ± 2††	165 ± 5‡	94 ± 3*	4.8 ± 0.1	12.3 ± 0.3*	11.2 ± 0.4‡	10.4 ± 0.5‡	8.1 ± 0.5‡	5.9 ± 0.5‡	4.8 ± 0.4*
Diabetic deceased	11	66 ± 2††	161 ± 6*	99 ± 3‡	5.2 ± 0.2	12.7 ± 0.6*	11.7 ± 0.6‡	11.2 ± 0.6††	8.5 ± 0.5‡	5.9 ± 0.4*	5.0 ± 0.3*
Normal glucose tolerance											
Alive	45	48 ± 2	140 ± 2	87 ± 1	4.3 ± 0.1	7.3 ± 0.2	6.0 ± 0.2	5.4 ± 0.2	4.6 ± 0.2	3.9 ± 0.1	3.9 ± 0.1
Deceased	7	61 ± 2**	162 ± 9**	91 ± 5	4.5 ± 0.2	9.2 ± 0.6**	7.8 ± 0.7**	6.6 ± 0.5†	4.9 ± 0.4	3.8 ± 0.2	3.8 ± 0.1

Values given as mean ± SEM.
Statistical method: nonpaired Student's *t* test.
* and †: Significance of the difference of those alive in the impaired glucose tolerance group (N = 169) and in the normal glucose tolerance group (N = 45), respectively.
*,† P < 0.05; ‡,** P < 0.01; ††,P < 0.001. Values greater than P < 0.05 are omitted.

(N = 169) (Table 8). At entrance, the former had higher mean blood glucose values at 60–180 min during OGTT (P < 0.05–P < 0.01) and higher mean systolic (P < 0.05) and diastolic blood pressures (P < 0.01) (Table 8). The same was true for those who subsequently died but had remained nondiabetic, as compared with those still alive at follow-up (Table 8).

Glucose tolerance. Oral glucose tolerance improved in all groups with initially impaired glucose tolerance (P < 0.05–P < 0.001) but most markedly in those given some kind of treatment. The glucose tolerance remained unchanged in the normal group (Table 9 and Figure 3).

Plasma insulin values. At follow-up, plasma insulin levels (both fasting and during OGTT) tended to be higher in those

TABLE 9
Age, blood glucose concentrations at OGTT, blood pressure, heart rate, and body weight (mean ± SEM) in men with impaired and men with normal glucose tolerance at start and at follow-up of study

Group	Time of OGTT	N	Age (yr)	Blood glucose (mM) 0 (min)	30	60	90	120	180	Blood pressure Systolic (mm Hg)	Blood pressure Diastolic (mm Hg)	Heart rate (beats/min)	Body wt (kg)
Tolbutamide	1962–5	20	52 ± 2	4.8 ± 0.1	10.8 ± 0.3	11.8 ± 0.3	8.9 ± 0.4	6.3 ± 0.3	3.8 ± 0.1	146 ± 3	89 ± 2	73 ± 2	80 ± 3
plus diet	1974–6		62 ± 2	4.6 ± 0.1	9.3 ± 0.2‡	9.6 ± 0.3‡	7.6 ± 0.5†	5.9 ± 0.4	3.8 ± 0.2	142 ± 4	84 ± 2*	61 ± 1†	79 ± 3
Discontinued tolbutamide	1962–5	15	46 ± 2	4.5 ± 0.2	10.7 ± 0.3	11.0 ± 0.3	8.9 ± 0.2	6.9 ± 0.3	3.7 ± 0.2	140 ± 5	86 ± 2	79 ± 4	83 ± 2
continued diet	1974–6		56 ± 2	4.6 ± 0.2	10.0 ± 0.3	10.0 ± 0.5	7.2 ± 0.5†	5.4 ± 0.5†	3.6 ± 0.2	143 ± 4	90 ± 2	59 ± 3*	85 ± 3
Diet with or without placebo	1962–5	51	52 ± 2	4.8 ± 0.1	10.9 ± 0.2	11.3 ± 0.2	8.8 ± 0.2	6.3 ± 0.2	3.7 ± 0.1	148 ± 3	87 ± 1	79 ± 2	77 ± 2
(dietary group)	1974–6		62 ± 2	4.4 ± 0.1‡	9.2 ± 0.2‡	9.3 ± 0.2‡	7.2 ± 0.3‡	5.7 ± 0.3†	3.5 ± 0.1	148 ± 3	90 ± 2	66 ± 2‡	77 ± 2
No therapy	1962–5	36	44 ± 2	5.0 ± 0.1	10.5 ± 0.3	10.7 ± 0.4	8.9 ± 0.4	6.9 ± 0.3	4.6 ± 0.2	147 ± 3	89 ± 2	76 ± 2	77 ± 2
	1974–6		55 ± 2	4.8 ± 0.1	9.7 ± 0.2†	9.7 ± 0.3*	7.8 ± 0.4*	6.5 ± 0.4	4.1 ± 0.2	147 ± 4	91 ± 2	67 ± 2*	78 ± 2
Normal	1962–5	39	48 ± 2	4.4 ± 0.1	8.6 ± 0.1	7.3 ± 0.2	5.4 ± 0.2	4.6 ± 0.2	3.8 ± 0.1	139 ± 2	87 ± 1	68 ± 2	73 ± 1
	1974–6		57 ± 2	4.4 ± 0.1	8.4 ± 0.2	7.1 ± 0.3	5.3 ± 0.2	4.6 ± 0.2	3.6 ± 0.1*	140 ± 3	88 ± 2	61 ± 1*	75 ± 1*

Statistical method: paired Student's *t* test.
* Significance of the difference within each of the five groups at start and at follow-up of study,
* P < 0.05; † P < 0.01; ‡ P < 0.001. Values greater than P < 0.05 are omitted.

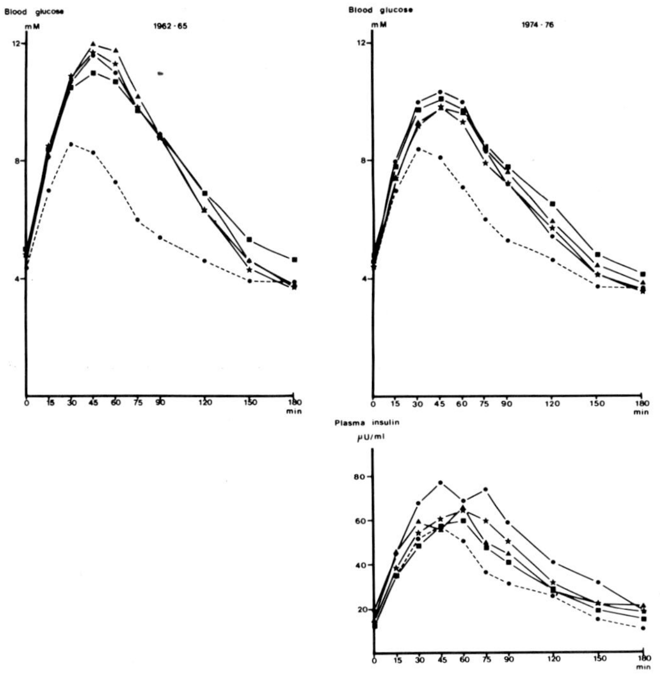

FIGURE 3. Mean concentrations of blood glucose (at OGTT 1962–65 and 1974–76) and plasma immunoreactive insulin (at OGTT 1974–76) in normal subjects and in the different subgroups of subjects with initially impaired glucose tolerance. •---• Normal, N = 39 (glucose), N = 28 (insulin). ■——■ No therapy, N = 36 (glucose), N = 26 (insulin). ▲——▲ Tolbutamide plus diet, N = 20. •——• Diet, tolbutamide discontinued, N = 15. *——* Diet, diet plus placebo continued or discontinued, N = 51.

with initially impaired glucose tolerance than in the normal group, but the levels showed no overt difference between the various groups with initially impaired glucose tolerance (Table 10 and Figure 3). The group that continued tolbutamide medication had a mean time of "peak insulin appearance" most similar to that in the normal group. However, a significantly earlier time of peak insulin appearance was found only when the normal group was compared with the dietary group ($P < 0.001$). The mean (±SEM) time of peak insulin appearance for the different groups were: normals, 46.1 (±3.2) min; tolbutamide continued, 50.3 (±5.2) min; tolbutamide discontinued, 56.0 (±4.5) min; diet 61.2 (±2.4) min; and untreated, 56.0 (±3.9) min.

Blood pressure and heart rate. Systolic blood pressure was unaltered, but diastolic blood pressure was reduced ($P < 0.05$) in the tolbutamide-treated group (Table 9). The heart rate was reduced in all groups ($P < 0.05$–$P < 0.001$), and no difference was recorded with respect to consumption of antihypertensive drugs or drugs that affect heart rate.

Body weight and serum lipids. Body weight remained unaltered in the groups with initially impaired glucose tolerance, but was increased in the normal group ($P < 0.05$) (Table 9). Mean serum cholesterol was lower in the tolbutamide-treated group and the dietary group than in the untreated group ($P < 0.05$) (Table 10). Mean serum triglycerides were lower in the tolbutamide-treated group and the dietary group than in the group having discontinued tolbutamide ($P < 0.05$) and in the untreated group ($P < 0.01$) (Table 10).

Medication compliance. One year after the follow-up had been concluded, the steady state concentrations of tolbutamide in serum were measured in those (N = 11) of the tolbutamide-treated subjects (N = 23) who could be reached and who agreed to blood sampling. Nine of the 11 subjects had measurable concentrations, ranging from 56 to 222 μM (15–60 μg/ml), while two had nonmeasurable concentrations.

DISCUSSION

In the present study, almost one-third of the subjects with initially impaired glucose tolerance developed diabetes when left untreated and uninformed. In contrast, no subject with initially normal glucose tolerance developed either impaired glucose tolerance or diabetes. It should be mentioned in this context that the Swedish Board of Social Health and Welfare estimates the prevalence rate of diabetes to be 1.5% in Sweden, but gives no figure for the incidence of diabetes. In the region studied, the prevalence rate is 1.6% and the incidence (all ages) is 0.14%. These figures may explain why no case of diabetes appeared in the normal group (N = 52) during the study time of 10 yr. In addition, all cases with a family history of diabetes had been excluded initially from the normal group. The shortest time from entrance to follow-up was 8.5 yr in subjects with normal glucose tolerance and 9.1 yr in subjects with impaired glucose tolerance. The subjects at the greatest risk to develop diabetes seemed to be those initially characterized by the most pronounced OGTT abnormalities and having the highest body weights. Development of diabetes could not be associated with the use of diabetogenic drugs such as thiazides or glucocorticoids.

TABLE 10
Plasma insulin concentrations at OGTT and serum lipids (mean ± SEM) in men with impaired and men with normal glucose tolerance

Group	N	Plasma insulin (μU/ml) 0 (min)	30	45	60	120	180	Serum lipids: Cholesterol (mM)	Triglycerides (mM)
Tolbutamide plus diet	20	15 ± 2	60 ± 7	56 ± 7	66 ± 10	28 ± 5	21 ± 4	5.4 ± 0.2	0.72 ± 0.1
Discontinued tolbutamide, continued diet	15	20 ± 3	68 ± 11	78 ± 15	69 ± 12	41 ± 9	19 ± 4	5.6 ± 0.3	1.28 ± 0.2
Diet with or without placebo (dietary group)	51	14 ± 1	55 ± 5	61 ± 4	65 ± 5	32 ± 4	18 ± 2	5.6 ± 0.1	0.91 ± 0.06
No therapy	26	13 ± 2	49 ± 5	58 ± 6	60 ± 7	29 ± 4	15 ± 2	6.1 ± 0.2*	1.17 ± 0.09†
Normal	28	13 ± 2	52 ± 4	57 ± 6	51 ± 5	26 ± 4	11 ± 2	6.3 ± 0.2*	1.02 ± 0.09†

* N = 36.
† N = 39.

In contrast to the high frequency of development of diabetes in untreated subjects with impaired glucose tolerance, only 13% progressed to diabetes when maintaining dietary regulation. The most striking outcome, however, was that in the group given tolbutamide in combination with dietary regulation; indeed, none of the subjects developed diabetes.

Direct comparisons with other studies on the prevention of diabetes are difficult, as the selection of subjects, time of follow-up, and type of therapy have been different. In three prospective studies[15–18] with randomized design, sulfonylurea therapy did not appear to affect diabetes morbidity. There is no obvious explanation of this discrepancy; however, the dosage of tolbutamide was 50% higher in the present study than in the Bedford study[15] and in the study by Feldman.[16] Stowers[17,18] used chlorpropamide instead of tolbutamide, and the dosage, moreover, was lower than conventional (100 mg). It should be added, in this context, that chlorpropamide seems to have less efficacy than tolbutamide at equimolar serum concentrations.[19,20] Furthermore, recent studies have shown that there is a great interindividual variation in the steady state concentrations of tolbutamide and chlorpropamide and that several patients are at risk of attaining suboptimal concentrations at conventional dosage.[19] Reasonably, this risk should be increased with the low doses of tolbutamide (1.0 g) and chlorpropamide (100 mg) used in the Bedford, Feldman, and Stowers-Logie studies. Measurements of the serum concentrations of sulfonylurea were not carried out in the studies referred to. In the present study such determinations were performed, although only in 11 of the 23 cases claiming that they were maintaining tolbutamide medication as prescribed. Nine of these 11 subjects had serum tolbutamide concentrations similar to the mean of a tolbutamide-treated diabetes population, i.e., 104 μM.[19] Accordingly, it seems probable that the majority of the tolbutamide-treated group was exposed to effective concentrations of the drug.

Another important factor is the compliance with drug therapy. There is reason to assume that the compliance with sulfonylurea therapy in patients with manifest diabetes is far from complete,[19,21–23] and it is not likely that compliance is any better when sulfonylurea is given to subjects without overt diabetic symptoms. Neither of the previously cited studies[15–17] gives information as to the compliance with sulfonylurea medication. In the present study, half the subjects spontaneously admitted that they had ceased tolbutamide medication prematurely, and this may also suggest that some of those allegedly remaining on the drug were not taking it appropriately. Indeed, among those claiming that they were still taking the drug as prescribed, 2 of 11 had nonmeasurable concentrations of tolbutamide in serum, suggesting compliance failure.

While this study was in progress, the possibility of a relationship between moderate hyperglycemia and increased cardiovascular morbidity and mortality was brought up.[24–26] In the present study, a higher mortality was found among those who subsequently developed diabetes than in those who did not. Irrespective of whether they had developed diabetes or not, those who died during the study differed from the survivors by having higher mean age, higher mean blood pressure, and higher mean blood glucose levels, both fasting and during OGTT, at the time of entrance into the study.

Following the UGDP study, there has been an intense debate as to whether sulfonylurea therapy increases cardiovascular mortality.[27–30] The cardiovascular morbidity in the present material was assessed in a separate study,[14] based on interviews, plethysmography, and ECG during exercise. It was found that cardiovascular morbidity was higher in subjects with impaired glucose tolerance than in those with normal glucose tolerance. However, cardiovascular morbidity was less frequent in those subjects with impaired glucose tolerance who had been taking tolbutamide. The current experience on the influence of tolbutamide on body weight, glucose tolerance, and plasma insulin can hardly explain the difference in cardiovascular morbidity. Rather, changes in diastolic blood pressure and serum lipoproteins (below) may help to explain the difference. It should be mentioned that risk factors present at the start of the study, such as obesity and hypertension, were equally distributed among the groups. Another major risk factor, smoking, was incompletely registered and its influence could not be evaluated.

The significance of plasma insulin levels and the influence of treatment thereon is difficult to evaluate, as plasma insulin was not determined in the initial phase of the study. Comparison of the peak insulin appearances suggested a difference between those with impaired glucose tolerance and normal subjects. In addition, treatment with tolbutamide seemed to reduce this difference.

There is reason to assume that the blood glucose-lowering effects of sulfonylurea, at least in part, may be due to extrapancreatic mechanisms,[20,23,31] and long-term studies[32–36] have failed to show an association between the sulfonylurea influence on plasma insulin, on the one hand, and blood glucose on the other. In the present study, the combination of tolbutamide and diet regulation tended to yield the most pronounced reduction of blood glucose. However, the evaluation of the blood glucose–reducing effect was obscured by the surprising finding that blood glucose levels were diminished in all groups with impaired glucose tolerance, irrespective of treatment and despite the fact that subjects were more than 10 yr older at follow-up and that no weight reduction had occurred. The reduced blood glucose was probably not due to unknown changes in laboratory routines. Blood glucose levels remained unchanged in the normal group that was studied concurrently, according to the same procedures and in the same laboratory as were the subjects with impaired glucose tolerance.

Treatment with tolbutamide and diet regulation in combination could be associated with a reduction in diastolic blood pressure. In agreement with earlier data,[37–39] moreover, the tolbutamide-treated group displayed reduced concentrations of serum lipids. These findings stress the need for further studies on tolbutamide effects on specific plasma lipoproteins in diabetics, with special reference to cardiovascular morbidity.[40]

In this long-term study, about 50% of those on medication with tolbutamide or placebo ceased tablet intake before follow-up. It appears that this lack of adherence to medication was not dependent on any side effects but, rather, due to the discontinuation of annual check-ups with OGTT. This emphasizes the importance of extensive information and frequent check-ups when a symptomless disorder is being treated.

In conclusion, it appears that impaired glucose tolerance carries a great risk of development toward manifest diabetes, whereas normal glucose tolerance signifies little risk of such development. In addition, it seems possible that diet regulation in combination with tolbutamide, at adequate dosage, may prevent or postpone progression from impaired glucose tolerance to manifest diabetes. Thus, this study stresses the necessity to identify such subjects and suggests active treatment of them. For practical purposes, this requires the development of a simple screening method for detecting subjects at risk.

ACKNOWLEDGMENTS

This work was supported by the County Council of Malmöhus County, by grants 19X-3784 and O4X-5657 from the Swedish Medical Research Council, and by a grant from the Swedish Board of Health and Social Welfare (the Dalby project). Boehringer-Mannheim GmbH, Mannheim, Federal Republic of Germany, supplied tolbutamide (Artosin) and placebo tablets.

REFERENCES

[1] Scherstén, B.: Untersuchung über die Diabetesfrequenz in einem Schwedischen Bezirk von 145.000 Einwohnern. 4e Congrès de la Fédération internationale du Diabète, Genève, 1961, pp. 249–52.

[2] Wilkerson, H. L. C., and Krall, L. P.: Diabetes in a New England town. JAMA *135*:209–15, 1947.

[3] Jorde, R.: The Diabetic Survey in Bergen, Norway, 1956. Bergen, Norwegian Universities Press, 1962.

[4] Brandt, L., Nordén, Å., Scherstén, B., and Tryding, N.: A diabetes detection campaign in southern Sweden. Results of 69,000 examinations. Acta Med. Scand. *176*:555–61, 1964.

[5] Lundquist, I., Nordén, Å., and Scherstén, B.: Studies in subjects with positive postprandial Clinistix test. I. Serum insulin-like activity and free cortisol in newly discovered diabetics. Acta Med. Scand. *187*:163–68, 1970.

[6] Carlström, S., Lundquist, A., Lundquist, I., Nordén, Å., Scherstén, B., and Wollmark, G.: Studies in subjects with positive postprandial Clinistix test. III. Special studies and follow-up of cases with borderline glucose tolerance. Acta Med. Scand. *189*:415–22, 1971.

[7] Expert Committee of Medical Assessment of Nutritional Status. Technical Report Series 258, 1963.

[8] Marks, V.: An improved glucose-oxidase method for determining blood, C.S.F. and urine glucose levels. Clin. Chim. Acta *4*:395–400, 1959.

[9] Scherstén, B.: Clinical evaluation of a rapid enzyme strip method (Dextrostix) for blood glucose estimation. Acta Med. Scand. *178*:583–90, 1965.

[10] Wide, L., Axén, R., and Porath, J.: Radioimmunosorbent assay for proteins. Chemical couplings of antibodies to insoluble dextran. Immunochemistry *4*:381–86, 1967.

[11] Roeschlau, P., Bernt, E., and Gruber, W.: Enzymatische Bestimmungen des gesamt-Cholesterins in Serum. J. Klin. Chem. Klin. Biochem. *12*:226, 1974.

[12] Wahlefeld, A. W.: Triglyceride determination after enzymatic hydrolysis. *In* Method of Enzymatic Analysis, 2nd Eng. edit. Weinheim, Verlag Chemie, and New York, Academic Press, 1974.

[13] Prescott, L. F., and Redman, D. R.: Gas-liquid chromatographic estimation of tolbutamide and chlorpropamide in plasma. J. Pharm. Pharmacol. *24*:713–16, 1972.

[14] Persson, G.: Cardiovascular complications in diabetics and subjects with reduced glucose tolerance. Acta Med. Scand. (Suppl.) 605, 1977.

[15] Keen, H.; Jarrett R. J., and Fuller, J. H.: Tolbutamide and arterial disease in borderline diabetics. *In* Proceedings, VIII Congress of the International Diabetes Federation. Malaisse, W. J., and Pirart, J., Eds. Amsterdam, Excerpta Medica, 1973, pp. 588–602.

[16] Feldman, R., Crawford, D., Elashoff, R., and Glass, A.: Progress report on the prophylactic use of oral hypoglycemic drugs in asymptomatic diabetes: neurovascular studies. Adv. Metab. Dis. *2* (Suppl. 2):557–67, 1973.

[17] Stowers, J.: Treatment of chemical diabetes with chlorpropamide and the associated mortality. Adv. Metab. Dis. 2 (Suppl. 2):549–55, 1973.

[18] Logie, A. W., Stowers, J. M., and Dingwall-Fordyce, I.: Longitudinal study of untreated chemical diabetes. Br. Med. J. *4*:630–32, 1974.

[19] Melander, A., Sartor, G., Wåhlin-Boll, E., Scherstén, B., and Bitzén, P. O.: Serum tolbutamide and chlorpropamide concentrations in patients with diabetes mellitus. Br. Med. J. *1*:142–44, 1978.

[20] Sartor, G., Melander, A., Scherstén, B., and Wåhlin-Boll, E.: Influence of food and of age on the single dose kinetics and effects of tolbutamide and chlorpropamide. Eur. J. Clin. Pharmocol. In press.

[21] Eshelman, F. N.: Drug compliance in diabetics. Br. Med. J. *1*:581, 1978.

[22] Melander, A.: Drug compliance in diabetics. Br. Med. J. *1*:990, 1978.

[23] Sartor, G., Melander, A., Scherstén, B., and Wåhlin-Boll, E.: Serum glibenclamide in diabetic patients, and influence of food on the kinetics and effects of glibenclamide. Diabetologia. In press.

[24] Epstein, F. K.: Hyperglycemia. A risk factor in coronary heart disease. Circulation *36*:609–19, 1967.

[25] Keen, H., and Jarrett, R. J.: Modern concepts in the diagnosis of diabetes. *In* The Management of Stable Adult Diabetes. Weller, C., Ed. Springfield, Ill., Charles C Thomas, 1969, p. 3.

[26] Wahlberg, F.: Intravenous glucose tolerance in myocardial infarction, angina pectoris and intermittent claudication. Acta Med. Scand. (Suppl.) *453*:37–73, 1966.

[27] University Group Diabetes Program: A study of the effects of hypoglycemic agents on vascular complications in patient with adult-onset diabetes. Diabetes *19* (Suppl. 2):1970.

[28] Bradley, R. F., Dolger, H., Forsham, P. H., and Seltzer, H.: Settling the UGDP controversy. JAMA *232*:813–17, 1975.

[29] O'Sullivan, J. B., and D'Agostino, R. B.: Decisive factors in the tolbutamide controversy. JAMA *238*:825–29, 1975.

[30] Marigo, S.: The UGDP report after four years. Acta Diabetol. Lat. *XI*:357–422, 1974.

[31] Feldman, J. M., and Lebovitz, H. E.: Appraisal of the extrapancreatic actions of sulfonylureas. Arch. Intern. Med. *123*:314–22, 1969.

[32] Reaven, G., and Dray, J.: Effect of chlorpropamide on serum glucose and immunoreactive insulin concentrations in patients with maturity-onset diabetes mellitus. Diabetes *16*:487–92, 1967.

[33] Boshell, B. R., Fox, O. J., Roddam, R. F., and Hill, P. S.: *In* Tolbutamide. . . After Ten Years. Amsterdam, Excerpta Medica Foundation, 1967, pp. 286–97.

[34] Turtle, J. R.: Glucose and insulin secretory response patterns following diet and tolazamide therapy in diabetes. Br. Med. J. *3*:606–10, 1970.

[35] Barnes, A. J., Garbien, K. J. T., Crowley, M. F., and Bloom, A.: Effect of short and long term chlorpropamide treatment on insulin release and blood-glucose. Lancet *2*:69–72, 1974.

[36] Tan, M. H., Grahma, C. A., Bradley, R. F., Gleason, R. E., and Soeldner, J. S.: The effects of long-term therapy with oral hypoglycemic agents on the oral glucose tolerance test dynamics in male chemical diabetics. Diabetes *26*:561–70, 1977.

[37] Shipp, J. C., and Munroe, J. F.: Effects of sulfonylurea components on hyperlipemia and hypercholesteremia in patients with minimal impairment of glucose tolerance. Diabetes *11*:69–73, 1962.

[38] Holman, R. R., and Turner, R. C.: Basal normoglycemia attained with chlorpropamide in mild diabetes. Metabolism *27*:539–47, 1978.

[39] Simpson, R. W., Mann, J. J. Hockaday, J. M., Turner, R. C., and Jelfs, R.: Lipid abnormalities in untreated maturity-onset diabetics and the effect of treatment. Diabetologia *16*:101–06, 1979.

[40] Reckless, J. P. D., Betteridge, D. J., Wu, P., Payne, B., and Galton, D. J.: High density and low density lipoproteins and prevalence of vascular disease in diabetes mellitus. Br. Med. J. *1*:883–86, 1978.

Kinetic Modeling of Insulin Binding to Receptors and Degradation In Vivo in the Rabbit

MONES BERMAN, ELIZABETH A. McGUIRE, JESSE ROTH, AND ANTHONY J. ZELEZNIK

SUMMARY

In vivo metabolism of insulin, with emphasis on the distribution, binding, and degradation from receptor and nonreceptor sites, has been studied in rabbits by analyzing the kinetics of antibody-bindable, TCA-precipitable, and TCA-soluble components in plasma. Tracer amounts of ^{125}I- and ^{131}I-labeled high affinity (pork) and low affinity (guinea pig) insulins were injected simultaneously into rabbits in the basal state or after a large bolus of unlabeled pork insulin. In one series of experiments, a bolus of unlabeled pork insulin was given from 5 to 30 min after the tracers. Based on the kinetic curves derived in these experiments, a model is developed for insulin metabolic pathways in vivo. A number of features are contained in the model. First, some of the kinetics are caused by distribution spaces in the body and some by specific binding sites, presumably receptors. Two equilibration phases between plasma insulin and receptors can be detected. The first and major one occurs within about one minute. The second one takes about 15 or 20 min. Partial degradation of the insulin molecule can be detected rapidly by the kinetics and is associated with the rapid (1 min) receptor phase. About 27% of the labeled insulin molecules are partially degraded via this pathway. There is, also, irreversible loss of insulin from the receptors without significant return of label to plasma during the experiment. This loss could be a result of internalization of insulin by the cells. About 48% of the insulin injected follows this pathway. The remaining degradation of insulin (~24%) takes place at other sites in the body. The results of the kinetic analysis also suggest that there are two populations of receptors. The high affinity population has an equilibrium dissociation constant equal to about 9×10^{-9} M, a value comparable to that observed in vitro (~5×10^{-9} M). The low affinity population has an equilibrium dissociation constant about 100 times greater than that of the high affinity population; its capacity, however, is about 30 times greater. It is, further, concluded that the TCA-soluble degradation products observed in plasma could *not* be accounted for by the partial and irreversible degradation pathways identified in the insulin model. They could be accounted for, however, by a 5%–15% subpopulation of injected labeled TCA-precipitable molecules that decay monoexponentially from plasma. DIABETES *29*:50–59, January 1980.

From the Laboratory of Theoretical Biology, Division of Cancer Biology and Diagnosis, National Cancer Institute, and Diabetes Branch, NIAMDD, National Institutes of Health, Bethesda, Maryland.
Address reprint requests to Mones Berman, Ph.D., Laboratory of Theoretical Biology, NCI, 9000 Rockville Pike, Bethesda, Maryland 20205.
Received for publication 14 June 1979.

Extensive quantitative studies have been done for more than two decades on the fate of labeled and unlabeled insulin in vivo.[1–5] However, the role of the receptor and its binding of hormone was rarely, if ever, considered explicitly in these studies.

Methods to study directly the binding of ligands to cell surface receptors, introduced for the study of ACTH and angiotensin, have been used widely for the study of insulin binding to its receptors. These studies have been restricted almost entirely to in vitro systems using receptors on isolated cells or subcellular particles.

Zeleznik and Roth, in a recent paper,[6] introduced a method to study the interaction of insulin with its specific receptors in the whole animal in vivo. It was shown that such radioiodinated insulins as pork insulin and chicken insulin, which have a high affinity for receptors (and high biologic activity), distribute in vivo into a larger apparent volume than do insulins like guinea pig insulin or pork proinsulin, which have low affinities for receptors (and reduced biologic activity). It was concluded that the increased "space" reflected binding of the high affinity hormone to receptors and that these results paralleled previous findings of receptor experiments in vitro.[7] The analysis of the data, however, was mostly qualitative.

Since a variety of protocols and perturbations was carried out in the kinetic studies of Zeleznik and Roth,[6] we decided to analyze the data in the context of a formal mathematical model in order to extract more information from the data and to gain a better insight into the kinetics of insulin. The initial

TABLE 1
List of experiments

Series	Rabbits	Cold pork insulin load: Amount	Cold pork insulin load: Time admin. (min)	High* affinity insulin	Low* affinity insulin	Measurements: TCA Precip-itable	Measurements: TCA Sol-uble	Measurements: Anti-body precip-itable
Ia	1	None	—	^{131}I-P	^{125}I-GP	x		
(tracer)	6B	"	—	^{125}I-P	^{131}I-GP	x		
Ib	2	"	—	"	"	x	x	
(tracer)	3	"	—	"	"	x	x	
	6A	"	—	"	"	x	x	
II	7	3 mg	−2	^{125}I-P	^{131}I-GP	x		
(preload)	8	"	"	"	"	x		
	9	300 μg	"	"	"	x		
	10	"	"	"	"	x		
	11	30 μg	"	"	"	x		
	12	"	"	"	"	x		
III	5W	3 mg	+5	^{125}I-CH	^{131}I-GP	x		
(washout)	7W	"	+7	"	"	x		
	15W	"	+15	"	"	x		
	30W	"	+30	"	"	x		
IV	2X	None	—	^{125}I-P	^{131}I-PRO	x	x	x
(tracer)	3X	"	—	^{131}I-P	^{125}I-PRO	x	x	x
	4X	"	—	"	"	x	x	x

* P stands for pork, GP for guinea pig, CH for chicken insulin, and PRO for pork proinsulin.

modeling results led to additional experiments which were then used to validate and further refine the model.* It was, indeed, possible to identify and quantify several mechanisms and features in the kinetics of radioiodinated insulins that were not previously appreciated. However, some anomalies in the results remain to be resolved.

METHODS

The laboratory methods and materials are described in detail in a previous publication.[6] Briefly, after a 16 h fast, rabbits were injected simultaneously with a high and a low affinity insulin, one labeled with ^{125}I and the other with ^{131}I. In most cases, pork insulin served as the high affinity insulin, but in several experiments, chicken insulin was used instead. In the initial studies, guinea pig insulin was used as the low affinity insulin, but in the most recent experiment, proinsulin was substituted. In all studies, potassium iodide (1 mg/kg) was given intravenously before the tracers were injected.

Four series of experiments were carried out, as summarized in Table 1. In the first series, labeled insulin in tracer amounts was administered to the rabbits in the basal state. In the second series, the tracers were injected after preloading with varying amounts of cold, high affinity insulin (30, 300, and 3000 μg of pork insulin) and 2 min before injecting the tracers. The highest preloading dose was shown to saturate receptor sites.[6] In the third series, washout experiments were carried out by giving 3000 μg of unlabeled high affinity (pork) insulin at 5, 7, 15, or 30 min after the tracers were injected. In these three series of experiments, plasma TCA-precipitable activity (measured using 5% trichloroacetic acid) was followed for 60 min after the injection of the tracer. The fourth series of experiments was similar to the first series with the additional measurement of the amount of plasma radioactivity bindable by anti-insulin antibody. In six rabbits (series Ib and series IV) the amount of tracer in the plasma TCA-soluble fraction was measured also. The integrity of the labeled insulin was measured by its precipitability in 5% TCA or by its binding to an excess of anti-insulin antibody.

The model evolved in several stages. First, the tracer studies (series I) were analyzed using the TCA-precipitable (series Ia and Ib) and TCA-soluble data (series Ib). The washout experiments (series III) were analyzed next. New tracer experiments (series IV) were then carried out and the kinetic structure of the proposed model was finalized. All the data, including those from series II, were then reanalyzed using the proposed model.

The modeling and data analysis were carried out with the SAAM computer program[8,9] using simulation and least squares data-fitting techniques previously described.[10–12]

MODEL DEVELOPMENT

A typical set of plasma TCA-precipitable data for high and low affinity insulins is shown in Figure 1. These data are from a tracer experiment without any preloading with cold insulin (series I). The underlying assumption (AI) in the modeling is that the kinetics of the high and low affinity insulins differ only in their affinities for the insulin receptor and are identical with respect to other total body distributions. The strongest support for this derives from the preloading experiments (series II), in which at high levels of cold insulin the plasma curve for high affinity insulin became nearly superimposable on that for the low affinity insulin (data shown in Figure 3 of ref. 6). Since low affinity insulin does not

* A preliminary report of the model was published in abstract form in the Program of the 37th Annual Meeting of the American Diabetes Association, held in St. Louis, Missouri. (Berman, M., McGuire, E. A., and Zeleznik, A. J.: Kinetic model for *in vivo* distribution and receptor binding of insulin in the rabbit. DIABETES *26*:387, 1977.)

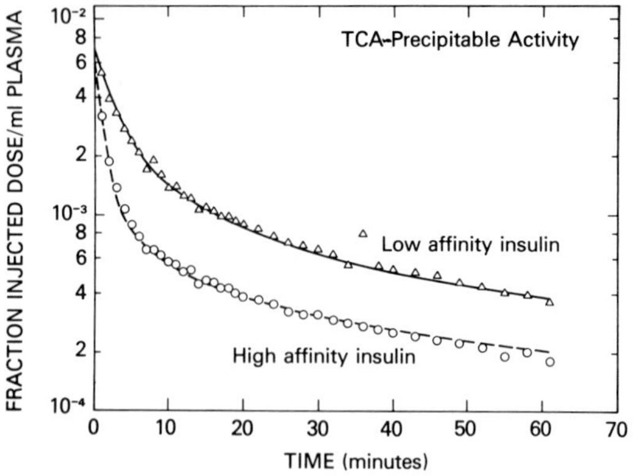

FIGURE 1. Plasma TCA-precipitable low affinity (guinea pig) and high affinity (pork) tracer insulin. The symbols indicate data, the curves being the corresponding fits derived by the final model.

bind avidly to insulin receptors, its kinetics are assumed to reflect predominantly body distributions.

Low affinity insulin data—initial model. The low affinity guinea pig insulin data could be fitted to a sum of at least three exponentials, and, hence, a simple three compartment model was initially proposed (Figure 2). The series arrangement for the compartments is arbitrary, and so is the degradation site (compartment 1).

TCA-soluble data—heterogeneity of label. In three rabbits (2, 3, and 6A), TCA-soluble plasma radioactivities for both high and low affinity insulins were also measured (Figure 3). Three features are recognizable in these curves. First, there is a rapid, initial decay that closely parallels the TCA-precipitable curve. It was assumed (A2), therefore, that this was caused by residual TCA-precipitable activity in the supernatant (it averaged about 5% of the TCA-precipitable activity). Second, there is a distinct delay of several minutes before the curve begins to build up. It was necessary to introduce a delay component in the conversion from the TCA-precipitable to the TCA-soluble material to account for this. The third feature is the build-up and relatively flat, final phase of the curve. Both the high and low affinity TCA-soluble curves for two of the three rabbits whose data were available at this point in the modeling effort (and the curves for three rabbits studied later in series IV) showed this flat, final phase. The data for the third rabbit (6A) showed a continual build-up over the 60 min of the experiment, especially for the low affinity TCA-soluble material. It seemed reasonable to propose that (1) the soluble material was an insulin degradation product and (2) one or more of the compartments in the model (Figure 4) would serve as its precursor. This, however, was not the case. No combination of outputs from the various compartments could be made to satisfy the TCA-soluble data. It was observed, however, that one of the *exponentials* (the intermediate one)—used originally to fit the TCA-precipitable data—served very well as a sole precursor. This observation was found to hold very well for five of the six sets of data in the three rabbits for which data were available, i.e., for both the low and the high affinity insulins. This strongly suggested that initially there were two distinct moieties in the plasma for each of the labeled insulins, only one of which served as the precursor for the TCA-soluble data. The model was therefore restructured as two independent subsystems (Figure 5)—an exchangeable two compartment subsystem (compartments 1 and 8) for the TCA-precipitable material and a single compartment subsystem (compartment 2), accounting for the one exponential (intermediate) of the plasma TCA-precipitable curve that served as the precursor for the nonprecipitable TCA material. Based on the magnitude of the intermediate exponential

FIGURE 2. Compartmental model initially proposed for the low affinity (guinea pig) insulin. Circles represent compartments, and arrows are transition pathways. The triangle represents site of sampling. *IC = 1 represents a unit bolus injection into plasma. The numbering of the compartments is only for identification purposes and is arbitrary.

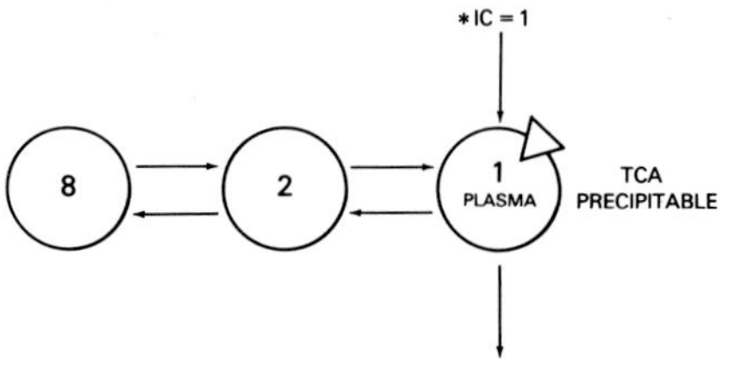

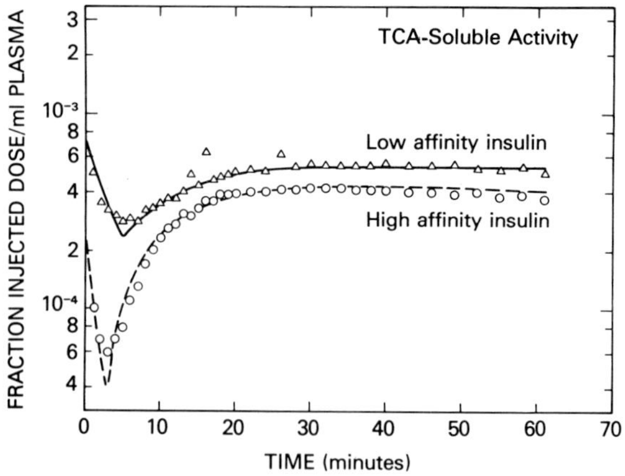

FIGURE 3. Plasma TCA-soluble low affinity (guinea pig) and high affinity (pork) tracer insulin. Symbols indicate observed data. The curves were generated by the final model.

FIGURE 4. Model employed for testing possible sites of degradation to account for the TCA-soluble material. The notation is the same as for Figure 2. Rectangle 15 represents a delay component to account for the observed lag in the appearance of labeled TCA-soluble material in plasma.

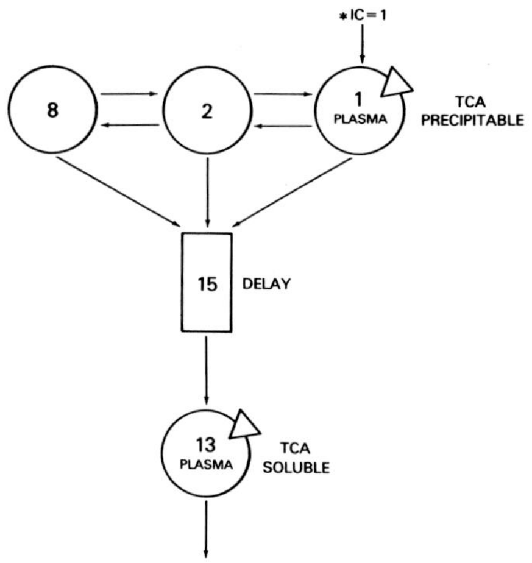

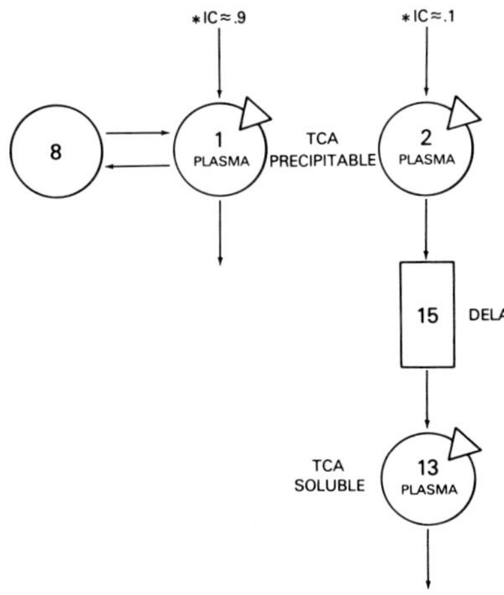

FIGURE 5. Low affinity insulin model to account for TCA-soluble material in plasma. Two labeled moieties of insulin are necessary. About 10% of the injected insulin is required to account for the plasma TCA-soluble fraction.

component, about 10% (range, 5–15%) of the injected material was necessary to account for the TCA-soluble material. With this value and the observed concentration of the TCA-soluble label in plasma, the estimated space of distribution of the TCA-soluble material was, approximately, plasma space. Hence, in the subsequent modeling, plasma was assumed (A3) to be the space of distribution of the TCA-soluble material. Fits of the data using this model are represented by the lines in Figure 3.

High affinity insulin data—initial model. Since it was assumed (AI) that high affinity insulin behaves like low affinity insulin except for a high affinity insulin receptor compartment, the model shown in Figure 6 was proposed. In this model, compartments 1 and 8 are the same as for the low affinity insulins while the additional compartment, compartment 3, represents the receptors. The subsystem generating the TCA-soluble material (compartments 2, 13, and 15) is structurally the same as that in the low affinity insulin model, although it required somewhat different values for its rate constants. This model yielded good fits for the rabbits studied in the tracer experiments (series I), except for the low affinity study of rabbit 6A in which all the losses from the TCA-

FIGURE 6. High affinity insulin model to account for both TCA-soluble and TCA-precipitable material. $L_{3,1}$ is the rate constant for the binding of insulin to a receptor. The model is the same as in Figure 5, except for the addition of the receptor compartment, compartment 3.

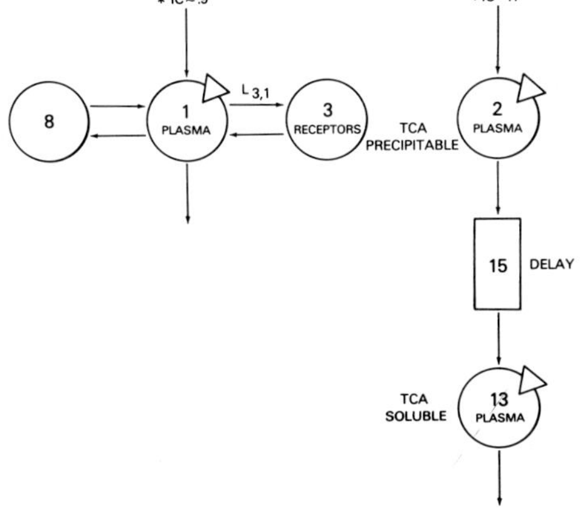

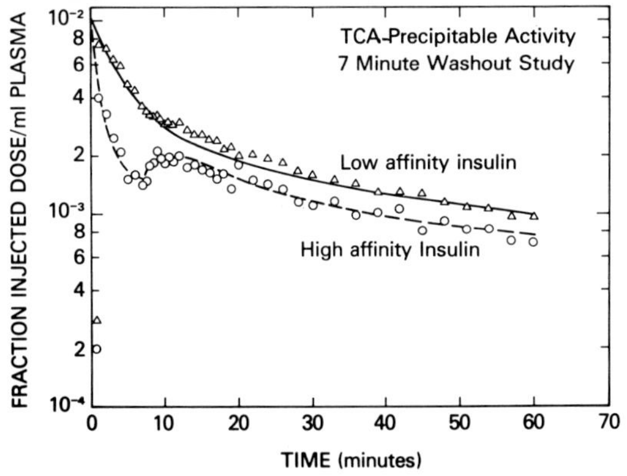

FIGURE 7. Washout experiments for high affinity (chicken) and low affinity (guinea pig) insulins. Cold pork insulin (3 mg) was given 7 min after the labeled insulins were injected.

precipitable compartments were required to account for a continuously rising plasma-soluble activity.

Washout experiments—receptor subsystem. We next tested the model against the data from the washout experiments (series III). In these experiments, a large dose (3000 μg) of high affinity (pork) insulin was given 5, 7, 15, or 30 min after injection of the tracers. The response for a 7-minute washout is shown in Figure 7. Since the washout experiments showed a relatively minor perturbation in the plasma low affinity insulin curves, it seemed reasonable to assume that the effects of the loading were predominantly on the receptor part of the model. Hence, only the high affinity insulin washout curves were initially used in testing the model further.

Problem of fitting the washout data. In simulating the washout experiments, it was assumed (A4) that the only effect of a large dose of unlabeled high affinity insulin is the immediate saturation of the receptors and, hence, the blockage of further binding of tracer insulin to them ($L_{3,1} = 0$, Figure 6). However, when this assumption was incorporated into the model and the washout experiments simulated, the observed curves could not be reproduced. The simulated plasma responses following the pulses of unlabeled insulin were larger than observed, especially for loads given at the later times. It was apparent that some of the receptor insulin was not readily available for washout. The addition of a loss pathway from compartment 3 did not remove the inconsistency. A second receptor compartment, in exchange with the first one, was introduced, therefore (compartment 12, Figure 8), to divert some of the receptor insulin to a state that

FIGURE 8. Intermediate four-compartment TCA-precipitable insulin model. The difference between high and low affinity insulin kinetics is fully accounted for by a change in the value of parameter $L_{3,1}$ only. This model has two receptor states. The data could have been fitted equally well by an irreversible loss pathway from compartment 12 instead of compartment 3.

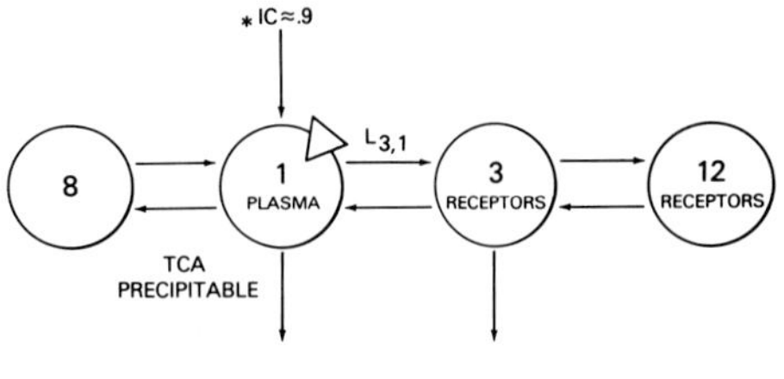

was less readily available for washout. This model, with the addition of a direct loss pathway from the receptors ($L_{0,3}$ or $L_{0,12}$), was found adequate to fit each of the washout curves. However, in comparing the derived parameter values for the four washout experiments, it was found that the rate constant $L_{12,3}$ had to assume an increasingly higher value the later the washout occurred. This, of course, should not be the case, since the same parameter value should fit all experiments.

Partial degradation of hormone. It was then proposed that some of the receptor-bound insulin returning to plasma was partially degraded, so that it remained TCA precipitable but could no longer bind to the receptors. A hint that this may indeed have occurred is provided by the data in the previous paper[6] (cf. Figure 6 and Table 2) where it can be seen that antibody-bindable activity disappears from plasma more rapidly than TCA-precipitable activity. To account for the kinetics of partially degraded insulin, a subsystem was added to the model with the assumption (A5) that the partially degraded insulin follows the nonreceptor kinetics of insulin (Figure 9). This modification added only one additional independent parameter to the model ($L_{7,3}$), the partial degradation path of insulin at the receptors. The addition of this degradation path was sufficient to satisfy all the washout data with a common set of parameter values. However, an additional irreversible degradation pathway from the receptor compartment was still required. Although the irreversible loss could occur from either compartment 12 or compartment 3, we chose compartment 12, because, as already discussed, the TCA-soluble data was not compatible with the appearance of TCA-soluble degradation products during the 60 min of these studies.

To validate directly the two TCA-precipitable moieties (antibody bindable and nonbindable) and to improve on the estimates for the parameter values, additional experiments were carried out (series IV). In these experiments, proinsulin was used as the low affinity insulin and antibody-bindable activity was determined.

Antibody-bindable data—final model. The antibody-bindable data for low affinity insulin (Figure 10) suggest that there is little degraded proinsulin in plasma over the first 10–15 min, but there is considerable degradation thereafter. This pattern cannot be explained by the degradation pathway from receptor compartments 3 and 12, since they contain too little proinsulin. In addition, the delay of several minutes was too long to be consistent with a loss from compartment 8. It was therefore proposed that partial degradation of the antibody-bindable proinsulin occurred in a deeper compartment in the body. Compartment 23 (Figure 11) was then added as a further refinement, with an equivalent compartment 17 for the TCA-precipitable antibody-soluble subsystem, and a partial degradation pathway $L_{17,23}$ was introduced. The irreversible loss pathway was also shifted to the deeper compartment ($L_{0,23}$), since little, if any, of the degradation products was seen in the plasma TCA-soluble fraction during the experiment. This subsystem was used for both the high and low affinity insulins. The rapid drop in plasma antibody-bindable high affinity insulin activity (Figure 10) supported the need for a receptor-mediated partial degradation pathway, $L_{7,3}$.

The model developed from the high affinity insulin data was reapplied to the low affinity insulin data with the refinement that some binding of low affinity insulins to the receptors took place. The extent of binding was set in the ratios of 0.05:1:3 for guinea pig, pork, and chicken insulins, respectively, as determined in previous experiments in vitro.[13]

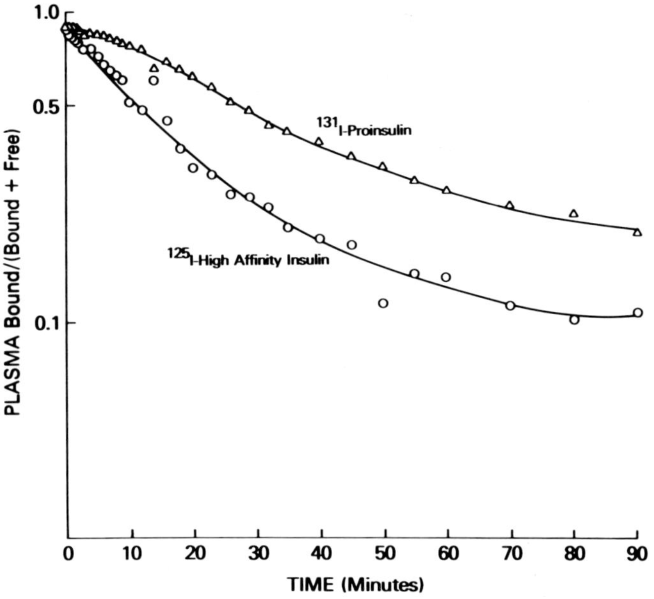

FIGURE 10. Ratios of antibody-bindable to total radioactivities in plasma for high affinity pork insulin and for low affinity pork proinsulin. Symbols represent data, and the curves are generated by the model.

FIGURE 9. Modified model to account for the partial degradation of insulin molecules on receptors (compartment 3), resulting in a TCA-precipitable moiety that no longer binds to receptors (compartments 7 and 10) or to anti-insulin antibody.

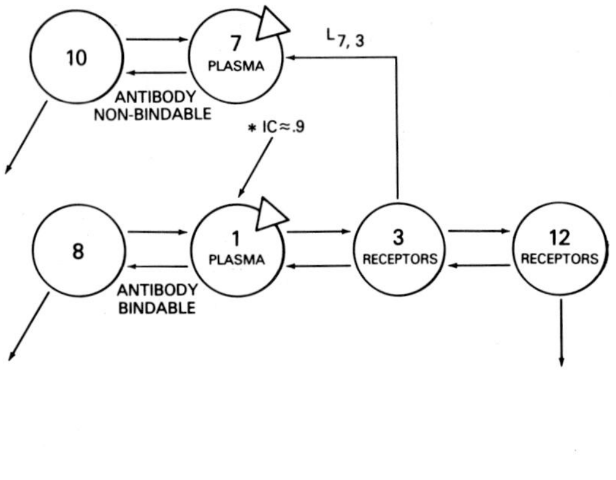

RESULTS

The final model for high and low affinity insulins, including parameter values, is shown in Figure 11. The values given are a composite for the entire population of rabbits. The steady state values are all relative and are based on a unit input rate of insulin into plasma. Hence, the irreversible losses from the system and subsystems, calculated in the steady state, represent directly the fractions of the input that are lost or degraded via these pathways, and the compartmental steady state masses are numerically equal to residence times.[12]

Pathways of insulin degradation. For high affinity insulin, about 75% of the 'good' insulin entering plasma is either partially degraded or lost irreversibly via the receptors and the

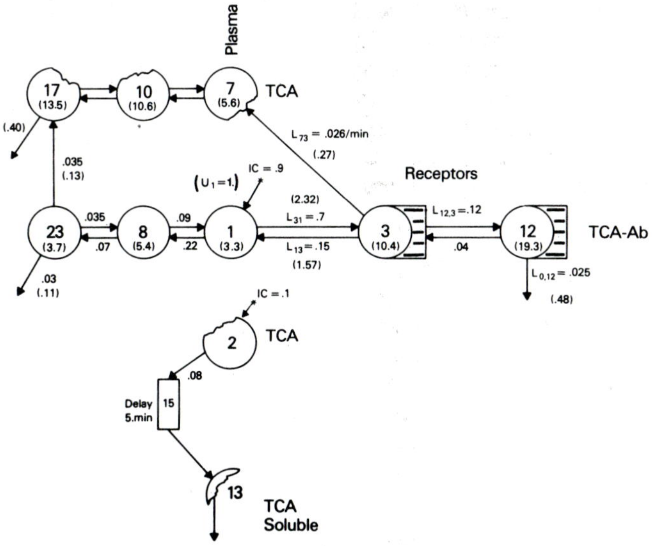

FIGURE 11. Final insulin model for both high and low affinity insulins. The only difference lies in parameter $L_{3,1}$, which has a value of 0.7 min^{-1} for pork insulin and 0.035 min^{-1} for guinea pig insulin. Compartments 2, 15, and 13 account for the plasma TCA-soluble data and are slightly different for the two insulins. Compartment 13 is a TCA-soluble product derived from compartment 2, which is a TCA-precipitable labeled moiety in the injectate that does not bind to the receptors. Compartments 1, 8, and 23 represent total body nonreceptor antibody-bindable insulin, and compartments 3 and 12 represent insulin bound to receptors (hatched areas). Compartments 7, 10, and 17 represent partially degraded insulin, which is TCA precipitable but not antibody bindable. The values given along the arrows are estimates for the population rate constants expressed as the fraction per minute. The values in parentheses inside compartments represent the residence time (in minutes) of insulin molecules in these compartments when first introduced into the system by way of compartment 1 (plasma). They also represent steady state insulin masses in these compartments for a unit infusion rate into plasma (represented by $U_1 = 1$). The values given in parentheses along the arrows represent the fractions of insulin molecules entering plasma that go by way of these pathways as well as steady state flow rates per unit input rate into plasma. For example, 27% of the insulin entering plasma is partially degraded from the receptors by way of pathway $L_{7,3}$ and 48% is irreversibly lost from the receptors via $L_{0,12}$.

rest is lost by way of other (nonreceptor) pathways. About one-third of the insulin lost via receptor-associated processes returns to plasma as TCA-precipitable material (via $L_{7,3}$), and about two-thirds are lost by an, as yet, undefined path (via $L_{0,12}$). On the other hand, only about 13% of the low affinity insulin entering plasma is degraded by way of the receptors (not shown). It is of special note that, for high affinity insulin, 2.32 molecules attach to the receptors per molecule entering the plasma (as compared with 0.41 molecules for low affinity insulin), indicating a considerable degree of reutilization of the molecule despite its degradation at the receptor compartment. On a single pass, about two-thirds of the molecules binding to receptors return to plasma as intact insulin and about one third is degraded.

Receptor compartments and apparent volumes of distribution. A plasma equivalent volume (PEV) is defined as the volume a substance would occupy if its mass (M) were distributed at a concentration equal to that in the plasma (c_p): $PEV = M/c_p$. The PEV of antibody-bindable insulin, from the model, is $V_1(M_1 + M_8 + M_{23} + M_3 + M_{12})/M_1$, where V_1 is plasma volume. Expressed as percent body weight (%BW), assuming a plasma volume of 4%BW, the total PEV is 50%BW for high affinity and 17%BW for low affinity insulin. The PEV for the nonreceptor spaces is 15%BW for both insulins. Hence, the receptors account for about two-thirds of the total high affinity insulin space.

The PEV for TCA-precipitable insulin is a somewhat artificial quantity, since one does not usually measure insulin fragments, except, of course, when insulin is labeled and the amount of TCA-precipitable label is measured, as was the case in the Zeleznik-Roth experiments. A total TCA-precipitable PEV can be calculated directly from the model, as, $PEV = V_1(M_1 + M_8 + M_{23} + M_3 + M_{12} + M_7 + M_{10} + M_{17})/(M_1 + M_7)$. For high affinity insulin, this space is about 32%BW (compared with 50%BW for the antibody-bindable label) and, for low affinity insulin, the space is about 20%BW (compared with 17%BW for the antibody-bindable label).

The calculated values for PEVs are given in Table 2. For comparison, the results for two other methods of calculation —the input-output (I/O) analysis[14] and the intercept

TABLE 2
Calculated parameter values for insulin system using various computational methods

	Proposed model		Input-output* (Tracer curve)		Intercept†	
	High affinity	Low affinity	High affinity	Low affinity	High affinity	Low affinity
Ab-B FCR min^{-1}	0.300	0.085	0.300	0.085		
TCA-P FCR min^{-1}	0.112	0.064	0.112	0.064		
Ab-B $\bar{t}_{sys}$ (min)	42.4	49.5	23.0	30.1		
TCA-P $\bar{t}_{sys}$ (min)	71.9	80.0	65.9	53.6		
Ab-B PEV (%BW)	50.9	16.8	26.9	10.2	96.8	19.1
TCA-P PEV (%BW)	32.3	20.3	30.0	13.7	48.8	24.3

* The input-output analysis is based on the assumption that all inputs enter plasma and all irreversible losses are from plasma.[14]

† The intercept method is based on extrapolation to $t = 0$ of the final exponential in the plasma concentration curve for a unit injection. The plasma equivalent volume (PEV) is set equal to $1/I(0)$, where $I(0)$ is the value of the intercept.

Plasma volume (V_p) is assumed to be 4% of body weight.

Ab-B: Antibody-bindable material.

TCA-P: TCA-precipitable material.

FCR: Fractional catabolic rate. For a unit tracer input into plasma, its value is:

$$FCR = \frac{1}{V_p \int_0^\infty C_p^*(t)dt},$$

where C_p^* is plasma concentration of tracer. For tracee, its value is: $FCR = U_p/M_p$, where U_p is input rate of tracee into plasma and M_p is plasma tracee mass.

$\bar{t}_{sys}$: Mean residence time of injected particles in the system. For a unit tracer input into plasma, using the input-output method of analysis, $\bar{t}_{sys} = (\Sigma A_i\alpha_i^2)/(\Sigma A_i\alpha_i)$, where A_i and α_i are parameters in fitting the plasma curve, f_p, to a sum of exponents: $f_p = \Sigma A_i e^{-\alpha_i t}$. For our model, $\bar{t}_{sys} = M_T/U_p$, where M_T is total tracee mass and U_p is plasma tracee input rate.

PEV: Plasma equivalent volume. Its value is derived from the relation, $PEV = FCR_p \cdot \bar{t}_{sys} \cdot V_p$.

%BW: Percent body weight.

method[15]—are also given. In addition, the table contains values for the fractional catabolic rates (FCR)* and mean residence times of insulin particles in the system using the various methods of calculation. As can be seen, the FCR value for low affinity insulin is considerably smaller than for high affinity insulin, which means that the low affinity insulin generates a higher concentration in plasma than the high affinity insulin per unit input. This tends to counteract, to some extent, the effect of the measured differences in affinities by making more low affinity insulin available for binding to the receptors. The mean residence time for insulin in the entire system, † $\bar{t}_{sys}$, is poorly estimated by the input-output method of analysis when compared with our model.

DISCUSSION

In their interpretation of the high and low affinity insulin data, Zeleznik and Roth[6] proposed that the increase in plasma equivalent space for the high affinity insulin reflects binding to receptors. Our more detailed kinetic analysis is based on a similar proposition, namely, that some of the kinetics are common to both insulins and that the difference is accounted for by the difference in affinities for the receptor subsystem. Basically, our results support the conclusions of Zeleznik and Roth, but there are important qualitative and quantitative differences. In addition, interesting new structure and insights as to the binding of insulin to specific receptors and its degradation in vivo emerged from the modeling. Finally, the modeling led to additional experiments designed to test the validity of assumptions introduced and conclusions drawn during the modeling. Experiments for further validation of the model are also indicated.

To appreciate the new findings, a brief review of our knowledge derived from the in vitro systems appears to be in order. In vitro receptor studies have shown that the initial interaction of insulin and other peptide hormones (H) with their target cells is a reversible binding to specific receptors (R) on the cell surface to form hormone-receptor complexes (HR), i.e., $H + R \leftrightarrows HR$. In the case of insulin and other hormones, receptors are not restricted to cells that are well established as targets for the hormone, but are found on many, if not most, cell types. The specific receptors are found not only on the plasma membrane of the cell but also on such intracellular membranous structures as Golgi, rough endoplasmic reticulum, and, possibly, the nuclear envelope. While the role of these intracellular receptors is not yet known, there is agreement that binding to the cell surface receptors is the essential initial step in hormone action.

At 37°C, the initial reversible binding of hormones to receptors is followed quickly by time-dependent and temperature-dependent processes, which result in the loss of reversibility, and by degradation of the hormone.[16] Autoradiographic studies indicate that these processes include translocation of the hormone to submembranous regions of the cell, including lysosomes.[17,18] Using fluorescent probes, it can be shown that these processes promote aggregation of receptor-bound hormones on the cell surface followed by internalization and association with cytoskeletal elements.[19] What role each of these events plays in hormone action is not yet known.

The physiologic mechanisms of hormone degradation are less well known. Although hormone degradation in vitro is often detected in the extracellular medium (owing to the enzymes released from cells), insulin is not degraded in plasma. Rather, insulin degradation in vivo is regarded as a cellular process that takes place through both receptor-mediated and receptor-independent pathways,[20–22] although the relative role of these two pathways is not known. Proponents of the receptor-mediated pathways suggest that insulin binds to its receptor, which leads to transfer of the hormone, after a delay of several minutes, to a degradation site.[20] Thus, there appears to be agreement, supported by studies of the components of the system, that the receptor has no degrading action but acts only to expedite the delivery of bioactive hormone to a degradative site.

The receptor subsystem. In our model of the kinetics of insulin in vivo, the insulin-specific subsystem is thought to reflect receptors and is characterized by two states, which are designated compartments 3 and 12. The rate constant $L_{3,1}$ is the probability per unit time for an insulin molecule in plasma to bind to a receptor. This probability depends on the accessibility of insulin molecules in plasma to the receptors and is *directly proportional* to the number of free receptors available. Calculated in the steady state, the amount of insulin retained on the receptors, $M_3 + M_{12}$, is also proportional to the number of free receptors present, but depends on the dissociation, transfer, and degradation rate constants ($L_{1,3}$, $L_{12,3}$, $L_{0,12}$, $L_{3,12}$, $L_{7,3}$), as well. Hence, $L_{3,1}$ is a more direct measure of the free receptor population. The initial decay slopes of the high and low affinity plasma insulin tracer curves reflect the information on the rate of association, $L_{3,1}$, of insulin to the receptors.

In the proposed model, compartment 3 is the initial receptor-binding state, and compartment 12, in exchange with it, represents some alteration which makes the insulin in that state less rapidly exchangeable with plasma. The initial equilibration time between plasma insulin and the receptors (compartment 3) is short, on the order of one minute. The partial degradation process for high affinity insulin is also rapid, as can be seen from the almost immediate drop of the fraction of antibody-bindable high affinity insulin in plasma (Figure 10). This suggests that the partial degradation process takes place either directly on the receptors or in close proximity to them.

There is growing evidence that the insulin-receptor complex forms aggregates and is internalized.[17–19] The exchange kinetics between compartments 3 and 12 require about the same time (15–20 min) as aggregation. By this interpretation, the irreversible degradation pathway from compartment 12 ($L_{0,12}$) corresponds to internalization. Carpentier et al. have reported that 30%–40% of the ^{125}I-in-

* FCR is usually defined with respect to plasma, as, the fraction of plasma material that is irreversibly lost per unit time via all pathways. It can also be expressed as the reciprocal of the plasma residence time, $\bar{t}_p$ (or plasma mass per unit input rate of material into plasma): $FCR = \frac{1}{\bar{t}_p} = \frac{1}{M_p^{(1)}}$, where $M_p^{(1)}$ is the calculated mass of all plasma compartments for a unit insulin input into plasma. It can be shown[12] that, for a plasma insulin tracer curve, $f_p^*(t)$, derived after a unit injection of tracer, $FCR = \frac{1}{\int_0^\infty f_p^*(t)dt}$.

† The residence time in the entire system for particles entering the system at some given sites equals the generated mass (ΣM_i) in the system per unit input rate of particles. For a tracer introduced into plasma, it is given by

$$\bar{t}_{sys} = \frac{\int_0^\infty t f_p^*(t)dt}{\int_0^\infty f_p^*(t)dt},$$ where $f_p^*(t)$ is the plasma tracer activity.[14]

sulin bound to rat hepatocytes is internalized.[18] This value compares favorably with the value of 48%, found to be that portion of the total loss which occurs by way of $L_{0,12}$.

Compartment 12 was introduced to satisfy the washout experiments. Its series arrangement with compartment 3, although compatible with a possible aggregation scheme, is not unique. From the kinetic point of view, the data are equally compatible with a compartment 12 in direct exchange with plasma and in parallel with compartment 3. In such an arrangement, compartment 12 would constitute a second population of receptors having a different affinity constant, or, it could represent receptors in less well perfused tissues (e.g., muscle). In previous insulin-glucose studies by Sherwin et al.[4] and by Insel et al.,[23] it was pointed out that glucose utilization was controlled by a slowly turning over insulin compartment (compartment 3 in their model), whereas endogenous glucose production responded within minutes to changes in insulin. If one considers that compartment 3, the rapidly exchanging receptor compartment in our model, is mostly in liver, it could explain the rapid effect on glucose production. The slow response of glucose utilization would then have to be associated with the deeper insulin compartment (e.g., compartment 12).

Number of insulin receptors and effective affinity in vivo. When the rabbits were preloaded with various amounts of unlabeled high affinity insulin (30–3000 μg), the only change found necessary and sufficient to explain the loading effects was a change in the value of $L_{3,1}$, the rate constant for association of plasma insulin to receptors. A relation can be established between the values of $L_{3,1}$, the size of the receptor populations, R_0, and the equilibrium dissociation constant, K_d, between insulin and the receptors.

Let R_0 be the total receptor concentration in a solution, and let R be the concentration of the free receptors. Let S be the concentration of insulin and K_d the dissociation equilibrium constant for insulin and receptors. Hence,

$$K_d \equiv \frac{k_{13}}{k_{31}} = \frac{S \quad R}{(R_0 - R)}, \qquad (1)$$

where k_{31} and k_{13} are the association and dissociation rate constants. Solving for R,

$$R = \frac{K_d R_0}{K_d + S} \qquad (2)$$

The parameters in vivo, L_{31} and L_{13}, can be related to the idealized solution parameters as follows: $L_{31} = k_{31}R$ and $L_{13} = k_{13}$.

Combining these relations with Eqs. (1) and (2), we get:

$$\frac{L_{13}}{L_{31}} = \frac{1}{R_0} S + \frac{K_d}{R_0} \qquad (3)$$

Hence, a plot of $L_{1,3}/L_{3,1}$ against S yields a straight line with a slope $1/R_0$ and an intercept K_d/R_0. Using the $L_{1,3}$ and $L_{3,1}$ values derived in the preloading experiments (series II), one obtains $R_0 = 1 \times 10^{-6}$ M and $K_d = 0.75 \times 10^{-6}$ M (Figure 12) over most of the range. However, if one uses the first two sets of data, namely, the basal state (0.1×10^{-9} M) and the 30 μg preload, one obtains [using Eq. (3)] a value of $K_d = 9 \times 10^{-9}$ M and $R_0 = 36 \times 10^{-9}$ M. Thus, there seem to be two populations of receptors. The value of $K_d = 9 \times 10^{-9}$ M, derived for low concentrations, is quite comparable to that reported for studies in vitro ($\sim 5 \times 10^{-9}$ M). The value $K_d = 0.75 \times 10^{-6}$ M, derived for high concentrations of insulin, is about 100 times greater than that for low concentrations. The concentration of receptors having low affinity ($R_0 = 1 \times 10^{-6}$ M) is about 20–30 times greater than the concentration of high affinity receptors ($R_0 = 0.036 \times 10^{-6}$ M). At basal insulin levels (0.1 nM), the low affinity receptors have an occupancy [from Eq. (2), occupancy equals $(R_0 - R)/R_0 = 1/1 + (K/S)$] about 100 times lower than that of the high affinity receptors (0.01% vs 1%).

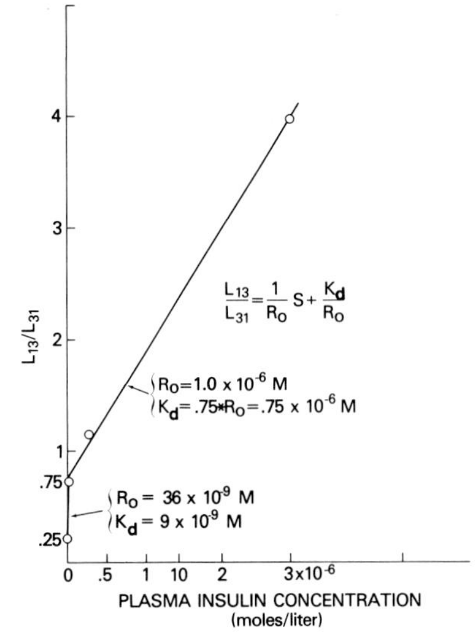

FIGURE 12. Plot of the ratio $L_{1,3}/L_{3,1}$ versus plasma insulin concentration in the preloading experiments (see text).

There was no apparent pattern of change in the value of the dissociation rate constant, $L_{1,3}$, in the preloading experiments. Nor was there a need to change $L_{1,3}$ in the washout experiments. There is some suggestion, however, that $L_{12,3}$ may decrease with loading. This means that no negative cooperativity on the dissociation rate constant, $L_{1,3}$, seemed necessary in the range covered by these studies. On the other hand, if $L_{12,3}$ tends to saturate at high doses of insulin, the over-all apparent rate of release of insulin from the receptors will increase with load, and this could be interpreted as negative cooperativity.

Nonreceptor subsystem. The nonreceptor insulin subsystem for both high and low affinity insulins has a PEV of about 15%BW, somewhat smaller than the extracellular space (~20%BW). The fact that one does not see significant degradation products in the form of TCA-soluble material from this subsystem over the 60 min of these studies argues that either degradation takes place in the deep compartment (compartment 23) or the irreversible losses are actually reversible exchanges with compartments that turn over more slowly. Direct support for *partial* degradation from compartment 23 ($L_{17,23}$) comes from the combined antibody-bindable and TCA-precipitable data (series IV) for proinsulin. There was a considerable delay (Figure 10) before the fraction of antibody-bindable proinsulin in the plasma started to drop, as opposed to the fraction of antibody-bindable insulin, which dropped almost immediately. It is not clear now whether the partial degradation path, $L_{17,23}$, is unique to proinsulin or applies also to insulin. Studies to clarify this are underway.

It is quite possible that the nonreceptor subsystem is not fully a passive domain. In the washout experiments (Figure 7), there is some indication that guinea pig insulin washes out to a greater extent than is predicted by the model on the basis of the relative affinities in vitro obtained from the literature. This could mean that the affinity of insulin receptors for guinea pig insulin relative to the affinity for chicken insulin is higher in the rabbit than the values in vitro. Alternatively, there may be another class of receptors that also cross reacts with pork insulin but has a higher affinity for guinea pig insulin relative to chicken insulin than the insulin receptors measured in vitro. These possibilities are presently under investigation.

Heterogeneity of the injected labeled insulin. Efforts to fit the TCA-soluble activity in plasma as iodide or iodotyrosine by-products arising from the degradation of insulin in one or more of the exchangeable insulin compartments failed, and they led to the conclusion that the measured plasma TCA-precipitable (and antibody-bindable) material is inhomogeneous. It was subsequently observed that a 5% to 15% TCA-precipitable subpopulation in the injectate could fully account for the TCA-soluble fraction in plasma, provided it did not diffuse into extraplasma spaces. This is not a particularly attractive assumption, in view of the fact that in vitro experiments do show iodide and iodotyrosine degradation products, and these do exchange with the extravascular, extracellular spaces. Some arguments can be made for heterogeneity of the injected labeled insulin (e.g., 80% labeling in the A14 position and 20% in A19, or partially degraded insulin molecules). An argument against iodide (or iodinated tyrosine) as a major degradation product can also be made, since its space of distribution is at least five or eight times greater than that of plasma,[24,25] and 10% labeled iodide in plasma would correspond to 50% to 80% of the injected label in the extracellular spaces. This, however, is somewhat inconsistent with the predicted amounts of labeled insulin remaining in the various compartments of the model. Obviously, this problem is not resolved, and experiments are necessary to identify more fully the nature of the labeled components in plasma.

Plasma equivalent distribution volumes (PEVs) and FCR. One question raised by the model concerns the significance of a PEV. By definition, a PEV is a hypothetic volume that a substance would occupy if it were distributed at a concentration equal to that of plasma. By this definition, a different volume is calculated for plasma antibody-bindable material than for TCA-precipitable material, as shown in Table 2. Using our model, TCA-precipitable material has a PEV of 32.3%BW for pork insulin and 20.3%BW for guinea pig insulin, or, a ratio of about 1.5. This compares with the ratio of about 2.1 approximated by Zeleznik and Roth. On the other hand, using antibody-bindable material, the PEV is 50.9%BW for the high affinity insulin and 16.8%BW for the low affinity insulin, or, a ratio of 3. The model indicates that TCA-precipitable material in plasma includes partially degraded insulin, which can no longer bind to receptors. Therefore, studies using this technique to quantitate receptors in vivo in various physiologic states should measure antibody-bindable activity in plasma. A better indicator of the insulin receptor population, however, is the initial decay phase of the plasma curves. This is nearly the same for the TCA-precipitable and antibody-bindable data.

An initial distribution volume (IDV) for insulin is sometimes calculated and is shown to vary as a result of various clinical perturbations.[5] Our model suggests that the calculation of an IDV is highly dependent on the early plasma data. Since initial equilibration with receptors takes place within about one minute in the rabbit, failure to recognize this phase of the kinetic curve would lead to the inclusion of receptors bound as well as plasma insulin in the calculation of the plasma equivalent space of IDV. This also means that the time it takes to inject insulin could affect the calculated value of the IDV.

There is considerable variation in the literature as to values of FCRs (fractional catabolic rates) and distribution spaces for insulin.[1-5] It is obvious from the results shown in Table 2 that these parameters are dependent on a number of factors: mode of perturbation (tracer vs nontracer), method of assay (TCA vs antibody bindable), affinities of insulin for its receptors, and duration of the experiment. Not until a full model of insulin kinetics is worked out and the various exchange and degradation pathways are defined will it be possible to reconcile completely the various results.

SUMMARY OF MODEL ASSUMPTIONS

A1. High and low affinity insulins follow identical kinetics with respect to total body distributions and degradation and differ only in their affinities for insulin receptors.

A2. Measured TCA-soluble material in plasma contains a small fraction of TCA-precipitable material.

A3. TCA-soluble material, measured during the course of these experiments (60 min), is restricted to plasma space.

A4. Large insulin load acutely blocks tracer uptake ($L_{3,1}$) by receptors, with no other effects on the system.

A5. Insulin molecules, partially degraded in association with the receptors (TCA precipitable but not antibody bindable), cannot rebind to the insulin receptors, but do follow the kinetics of the total body distribution subsystem for insulin.

REFERENCES

1 Berson, S. A., Yalow, R. S., and Volk, B. W.: In vivo and in vitro metabolism of insulin-I[131] and glucagon-I[131] in normal and cortisone-treated rabbits. J. Lab. Clin. Med. *49*:331–42, 1957.

2 Silvers, A., Swenson, R. S., Farquhar, J. W., and Reaven, G. M.: Derivation of three compartment model describing disappearance of plasma insulin-^{131}I in man. J. Clin. Invest. *48*:1461–69, 1969.

3 Genuth, S. M.: Metabolic clearance of insulin in man. Diabetes *21*:1003–12, 1972.

4 Sherwin, R. S., Kramer, K. J., Tobin, J. D., Insel, P. A., Liljenquist, J. E., Berman, M., and Andres, R.: A model of the kinetics of insulin in man. J. Clin. Invest. *53*:1481–92, 1974.

5 Navalesi, R., Pilo, A., and Ferrannini, E.: Kinetic analysis of plasma insulin disappearance in nonketotic diabetic patients and in normal subjects. J. Clin. Invest. *61*:197–208, 1978.

6 Zeleznik, A. J., and Roth, J.: Demonstration of the insulin receptor in vivo in rabbits and its possible role as a reservoir for the plasma hormone. J. Clin. Invest. *61*:1363–74, 1978.

7 Freychet, P., Roth, J., and Neville, D. M., Jr.: Insulin receptors in the liver. Specific binding of ^{125}I-insulin to the plasma membrane and its relation to insulin bioactivity. Proc. Natl. Acad. Sci. USA *68*:1833–37, 1971.

8 Berman, M., Weiss, M. F., and Shahn, E.: Some formal approaches to the analysis of kinetic data in terms of linear compartmental systems. Biophys. J. *2*:289–316, 1962.

9 Berman, M., and Weiss, M. F.: SAAM Manual. DHEW, (NIH)78-180. Washington, D.C., U.S. Government Printing Office, 1978, p. 196.

[10] Berman, M.: The formulation and testing of models. Ann. NY Acad. Sci. *108*:182–94, 1963.

[11] Berman, M.: A postulate to aid in model building. J. Theor. Biol. *4*:229–36, 1963.

[12] Berman, M.: Kinetic analysis of lipoprotein turnover data. *In* Progress in Biochemical Pharmacology. Eisenberg, S., Ed. Basel, S. Karger AG, 1979, pp. 67–108.

[13] Simon, J., Freychet, P., and Rosselin, G.: Chicken insulin: radioimmunological characterization and enhanced activity in rat fat cells and liver plasma membranes. Endocrinology *95*:1439–49, 1974.

[14] Rescigno, A., and Gurpide, E.: Estimation of average times of residence, recycle and interconversion of blood-borne compounds using tracer methods. J. Clin. Endocrinol. Metab. *36*:263–76, 1973.

[15] Shipley, R. A., and Clark, R. E.: Tracer Methods for In Vivo Kinetics, Theory and Applications. New York and London, Academic Press, 1972, p. 19.

[16] Kahn, C. R., and Baird, K. L.: The fate of insulin bound to adipocytes: evidence for compartmentalization and processing. Diabetes *26*:354, 1977 (abstract).

[17] Bergeron, J. J. M., Levine, G., Sikstrom, R., Nadler, N. J., Kopriwa, B., and Posner, B. I.: Localization of liver insulin receptors by radioautography. J. Cell Biol. *75*:182a, 1977 (abstract).

[18] Carpentier, J-L., Gorden, P., Freychet, P., LeCam, A., and Orci, L.: Lysosomal association of internalized ^{125}I-insulin in isolated rat hepatocytes. J. Clin. Invest. *63*:1249–61, 1979.

[19] Schlessinger, J., Shechter, Y., Willingham, M. C., and Pastan, I.: Direct visualization of binding, aggregation, and internalization of insulin and epidermal growth factor on living fibroblastic cells. Proc. Natl. Acad. Sci. USA *75*:2659–63, 1978.

[20] Terris, S., and Steiner, D. F.: Binding and degradation of ^{125}I-insulin by rat hepatocytes. J. Biol. Chem. *250*:8389–98, 1975.

[21] Terris, S., and Steiner, D. F.: Retention and degradation of ^{125}I-insulin by perfused livers from diabetic rats. J. Clin. Invest. *57*:885–96, 1976.

[22] Gliemann, J., and Sonne, O.: The mechanism of action of polypeptide hormones with special reference to insulin's action on glucose transport. Clin. Endocrinol. (Oxf) *7*:405–15, 1977.

[23] Insel, P. A., Liljenquist, J. E., Tobin, J. D., Sherwin, R. S., Watkins, P., Andres, R., and Berman, M.: Insulin control of glucose metabolism in man: a new kinetic analysis. J. Clin. Invest. *55*:1057–66, 1975.

[24] Berman, M.: Iodine kinetics. *In* Methods of Investigative and Diagnostic Endocrinology. Amsterdam, North-Holland Publishing Company, 1972, pp. 172–203.

[25] Belshaw, B. E., Barandes, M., Becker, D. V., and Berman, M.: A model of iodine kinetics in the dog. Endocrinology *95*:1078–93, 1974.

Diabetic Neuropathy in the Mutant Mouse [C57BL/ks(db/db)]

A Morphometric Study

DAVID M. ROBERTSON AND ANDERS A. F. SIMA

SUMMARY

Detailed studies of peripheral nerves were undertaken in the mutant diabetic mouse of the [C57BL/ks(db/db)] strain using electrophysiologic and morphometric techniques.

Electrophysiologic studies showed severely impaired motor nerve conduction velocity (MNCV), which developed promptly during the early phase of the diabetic syndrome. Morphometric changes occurred first after 20 wk of diabetes in both myelinated and unmyelinated fibers. There were both loss and shrinkage of myelinated fibers, most pronounced in the sural nerve and the ventral root. Changes appeared late in the dorsal root and in the peroneal and vagus nerves. Unmyelinated fibers showed both shrinkage and loss of axons, presumably involving sympathetic and afferent somatic fibers.

Teased fiber studies and calculations of axon-myelin ratios confirmed our earlier suggestion[18] that the neuropathy is primarily axonal in nature.

The temporal discrepancy between functional and structural impairments in the present model strongly suggests a metabolic cause of the early neuropathy. This was further supported by the positive effect of insulin treatment on MNCV during the early phase of diabetes, whereas, during the late phase, treatment failed to show any effect.

DIABETES 29:60–67, January 1980.

Previous reports on the pathology of experimental diabetic neuropathy have yielded conflicting results concerning structural and morphometric changes.[5–7,10,14,15] Early reports on chemically induced diabetes in rats claimed that segmental demyelination was the cardinal morphologic change,[5,10,13] but these results have not been confirmed by recent investigations.[6,7,14]

From the Department of Pathology, Queen's University, and Kingston General Hospital, Kingston, Ontario, Canada.

Received for publication 20 February 1979 and in revised form 13 September 1979.

Sharma and Thomas[14] were unable to demonstrate morphometric changes in streptozotocin- and alloxan-diabetic rats which had survived for 1 yr. Disproportionate atrophy of axons compared with myelin sheaths has, however, recently been demonstrated in peroneal nerves of streptozotocin-diabetic rats.[6]

Common to all reports on chemically induced and spontaneous experimental diabetes is the finding of reduced motor nerve conduction velocity, which occurs almost simultaneously with the elevation of blood glucose.[2,11,13,14]

The discrepancy between morphologic and functional changes led to the suggestion that the reduced nerve conduction velocity occurring in experimental diabetes is most likely due to metabolic alterations rather than morphologic changes.[4,22]

In a preliminary report,[18] we demonstrated decreased diameters of myelinated fibers of peripheral nerves and structural changes suggestive of a primary axonopathy of old diabetic mice.

In the present report these observations have been extended to include morphometric studies of motor, sensory, and autonomic peripheral nerves, including both myelinated and unmyelinated fibers in several age groups. Blood glucose levels and motor nerve conduction velocity were measured at regular intervals. In addition, a preliminary trial of the effects of insulin treatment on motor nerve conduction velocity was undertaken.

MATERIALS AND METHODS

ANIMALS

The experimental animals were of the mutant diabetic mouse strain [C57BL/ks(db/db)] (Jackson Laboratories, Bar Harbor, Maine), which is characterized by an autosomal recessive gene (db). The homozygote (db/db) mouse, which shows full penetrance of the diabetic syndrome, was used as the experimental animal. The heterozygote (db/m) nonpenetrant genotype was used as the control animal. The animals were genotyped by the Jackson Laboratory before delivery. All experimental and control animals used were females, to minimize interindividual differences.

The homozygote (db/db) develops gross obesity at 5–6 wk, followed by hyperglycemia, polyuria, and glycosuria.[19,21]

Animals investigated at the age of 4 wk were obtained as weanlings at 24 days of age. The diabetic mice in this age group were identified at the age of 7 wk according to the phenotypic characteristics of obesity and fasting blood glucose elevation above two standard deviations (SD) of the control value. The mean value of the control animals was 77.4 ± 21.5 mg% and of the diabetics, 156.4 ± 44.4 mg%, at this age.

CLINICAL MONITORING

Blood glucose. Blood glucose levels were determined in the morning (8 a.m.–9 a.m.), after 16 h of fasting, using an Ames Colimeter. Blood glucose was measured every 4–7 days in animals up to 8 wk of age and at monthly intervals in older animals.

Motor nerve conduction velocity (MNCV). MNCV was measured at weekly intervals in animals younger than 8 wk. In older animals, MNCV was measured on a monthly basis. The measurements were performed using light methoxyflurane anesthesia and a constant warm room temperature (22–23°C). In most instances, measurements were completed within 2–3 min of induction of anesthesia so that body temperature was unaffected. The nerve was not exposed during measurement. Two stimulation points were used on the left hind leg, the sciatic nerve at the sciatic notch and tibial nerve posterior to the ankle. Recordings were obtained from the muscle of the first interosseous space. Supramaximal stimuli (6V) were delivered at a frequency of 8/s from a Grass SD9 stimulator. The action potentials of the interosseous muscle were recorded from an oscilloscope. The MNCV was calculated by dividing the distance between the two stimulation points (18–21 mm) by the difference of the two latencies.

Treatment trial. Six diabetic animals were treated with subcutaneous Lente insulin (Connaught Laboratories Ltd., Toronto, Canada) at 13 wk of age for a period of 17 days. Since the mice are largely nocturnal feeders, the amount of insulin was titrated according to the postprandial blood glucose measured early in the morning. Insulin was subcutaneously given at 11 p.m. to control the late nocturnal blood glucose peak. The amount of insulin required was between 2 and 12 U. In treated mice, the morning blood glucose was kept below 150 mg%. Eight control animals were subcutaneously injected with physiologic saline and studied in the same fashion.

A second period of treatment was undertaken, starting at the age of 23 wk and lasting for 3 wk. Six previously untreated diabetic mice and nine control animals were used, and the treatment procedure was the same as that described above.

Longitudinal growth. As an indication of longitudinal growth, the lengths of femur and tibia were measured with the aid of a vernier caliper. Eight diabetic and eight control animals were measured at 25 wk of age and seven diabetic and nine controls at 33 wk of age.

MORPHOMETRIC METHODS

Morphometric investigations were performed at 4, 8, 15, 25, and 33 wk of age. In 4-wk-old prediabetic mice the sural and peroneal nerves of the right hind leg were excised under methoxyflurane anesthesia and immersed in cacodylate-buffered paraformaldehyde-glutaraldehyde fixative for 4 h. These animals were then kept alive to 7 wk of age to determine which developed diabetes. The nerves from five animals that developed diabetes and from five that did not were investigated.

In each of the other age groups, five diabetic (db/db) and five nondiabetic (db/m) mice were anesthetized with methoxyflurane and perfused with cacodylate-buffered paraformaldehyde-glutaraldehyde fixative through the left heart. From the right side, dorsal and ventral roots of the fifth lumbar segment, the sural and peroneal nerves were obtained. From the left side, the phrenic nerve and the ventral vagus nerve cranially to the diaphragm were taken. All specimens were taken from a defined level along the course of the respective nerve. All nerves were postfixed in 1% cacodylate-buffered osmium tetroxide, dehydrated, and embedded in Epon.

Caliber spectra of myelinated fibers. Measurements of myelinated fiber size and number were performed blindly from photographs of semithin toluidine-blue–stained sections at a final magnification of 1000×, with the aid of a Zeiss particle size analyzer. Myelinated fibers were measured in the ventral and dorsal roots, the sural, peroneal, phrenic, and ventral vagus nerves.

Caliber spectra of unmyelinated fibers. Randomly chosen areas from the sural, peroneal, and ventral vagus nerves were photographed and the measurement of fibers was performed from electron micrographs with a final magnification of 5000×. The criteria used for examining unmyelinated fibers were in accordance with those outlined by Ochoa.[12]

Fascicular areas, fiber number per fascicle, and fiber densities. The area of the cross-sectioned nerve fascicle was calculated by planimetry from photographs with a final magnification of 150×. All myelinated fibers were counted in each fascicle. The number of unmyelinated fibers per fascicle was calculated by multiplying the number of measured fibers by the factor fascicular area/measured area. The fiber densities for both myelinated and unmyelinated fibers were calculated by dividing the number of measured fibers by the measured areas.

Teased fibers. Specimens from the sural and peroneal nerves, proximal to those used for caliber spectra, measuring up to 4 mm in length, were stained overnight in osmium tetroxide. Single fibers were obtained by teasing in 30% glycerol in water. The fiber caliber and the internodal length were measured using an ocular scale. The types of qualitative changes were classified according to Dyck et al.[1] Nerves from mice 8, 25, and 33 wk of age were investigated.

Relationship between axonal area and number of myelin lamellae. Randomly selected myelinated fibers from the sural and peroneal nerves were studied. Micrographs with a final magnification of 12,500× were used to measure the axonal area with the aid of a planimeter. The number of myelin lamellae was counted from micrographs with a final magnification of 55,000×. Only fibers cut perpendicularly, as judged by circular appearances of microtubules, were measured. The area was plotted against the number of myelin lamellae. This method was applied to three diabetic and three control animals, of each 25- and 33-wk age groups. A

TABLE 1
Length of femur and tibia

Age	Bone	Diabetic mice	Control mice	P value
25 wk	Femur	15.0 ± 0.3 (N = 8)	15.2 ± 0.6 (N = 8)	P > 0.1
	Tibia	19.2 ± 0.6 (N = 8)	19.2 ± 0.9 (N = 8)	P > 0.1
33 wk	Femur	15.3 ± 0.5 (N = 7)	15.3 ± 0.4 (N = 9)	P > 0.1
	Tibia	20.1 ± 0.7 (N = 7)	20.2 ± 0.7 (N = 9)	P > 0.1

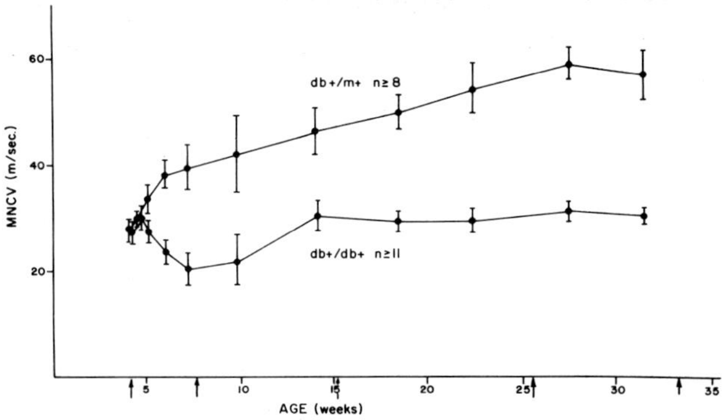

FIGURE 2. Mean ±SD of MNCV in diabetic and control mice. Arrows indicate points at which morphometry was performed.

minimum of 70 observations were made on each nerve of each age group.

STATISTICAL METHODS

For the statistical evaluation of the caliber measurements, an approximate analysis using analysis of variance on the logarithms of the fiber counts was used.

The data of fascicular areas, fiber numbers, and densities were subjected to paired Student's t tests. The slopes for the linear relationships between fiber diameter and internodal length and between the number of myelin lamellae and axonal area were also subjected to paired Student's t tests.

RESULTS

CLINICAL OBSERVATIONS

Growth. With the development of the diabetic syndrome at the age of 5 wk, the diabetic mice became progressively obese and at 3 mo were about 2.5 times the weight of the age-matched controls.

The lengths of femur and tibia measured in 25- and 33-wk-old animals (Table 1) showed no difference between diabetic and control mice.

Blood glucose. The mean fasting blood glucose values are shown in Figure 1. The diabetic mice exhibited a marked increase in blood glucose after the age of 5 wk, which continued to increase over the observation period to a highest mean value of 325 mg% at the age of 33 wk. The control animals showed a mean value of 78.9 ±14.2 mg% throughout the observation period.

MNCV. The results of MNCV measurements are illustrated in Figure 2. The control animals showed a progressive increase in MNCV up to the age of 27 wk. In animals younger than 5 wk, there was no difference between control and presumptive diabetic mice. From the age of 7 wk onward, the diabetic mice showed MNCV values that were significantly lower than those of age-matched control mice. The diabetic mice revealed an absolute decrease in MNCV. At 15 wk of age, the diabetic mice had reached prediabetic values of MNCV and remained at these values until the end of the observation period.

Treatment trial. The results of MNCV recordings during periods of insulin treatment are shown in Figure 3. During the early treatment period, commencing at 13 wk of age, the diabetic mice showed a marked and highly significant increase in MNCV, which, however, did not reach normal control values and which fell promptly to previous levels on cessation of therapy. With treatment at 23 wk, there was no significant change in MNCV in response to insulin administration.

MORPHOMETRIC RESULTS

Myelinated fibers. In prediabetic animals, only the sural and the peroneal nerves were investigated. No difference was demonstrated between the animals that subsequently developed diabetes and the control animals.

FIGURE 1. Mean ±SD of fasting blood glucose in diabetic and control animals.

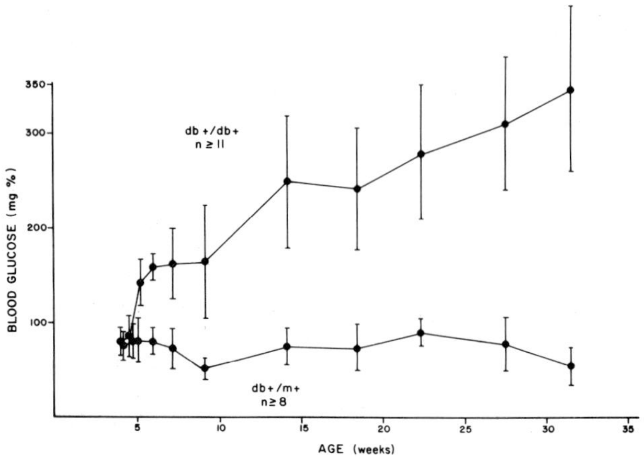

FIGURE 3. Mean ±SD of MNCV during insulin treatment. Shaded areas indicate periods of insulin treatment.

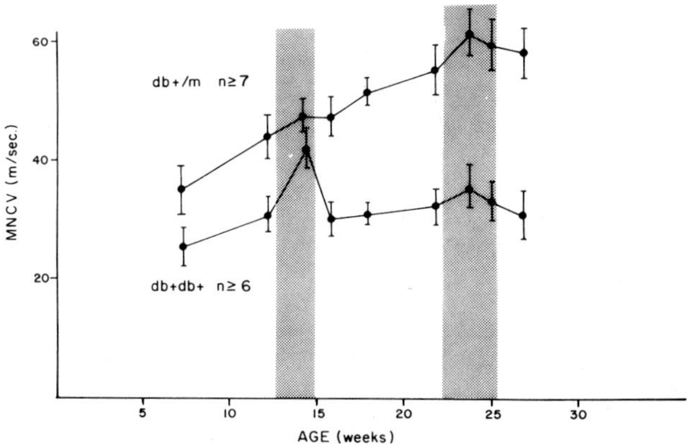

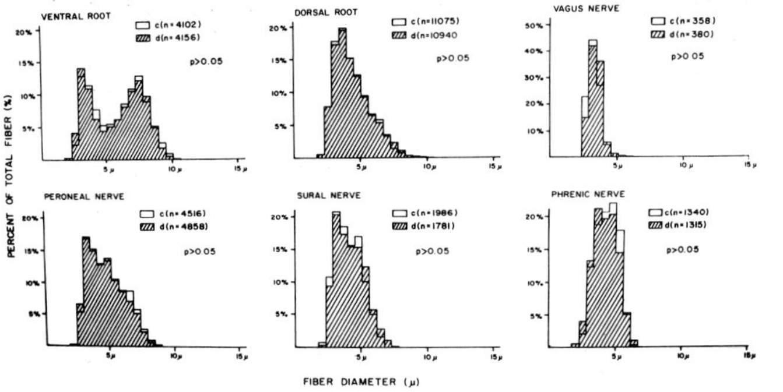

FIGURE 4. Caliber spectra of myelinated fibers in 8-wk-old diabetic (shaded bars) and control mice (open bars).

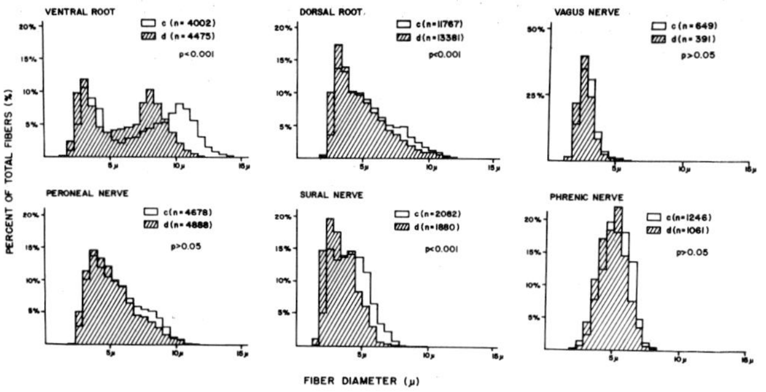

FIGURE 6. Caliber spectra of myelinated fibers in 33-wk-old diabetic (shaded bars) and control mice (open bars).

During the early period of diabetes, no significant differences were observed in any of the nerves (Figure 4). In 15-wk-old animals, a nonsignificant shift of the fiber distribution toward smaller diameters was noted in the ventral root, sural, phrenic, and ventral vagus nerves.

In 25-wk-old mice, 20 wk after the onset of diabetes, the ventral root and the sural nerve showed significant shifts of the fiber distribution toward smaller diameters (Figure 5). In the oldest age group investigated, 32 wk (Figure 6), the shift in fiber distribution toward smaller diameters is highly significant in the ventral root, the sural nerve, and the dorsal root. The peroneal, phrenic, and vagus nerves showed nonsignificant shifts.

Caliber spectra of unmyelinated fibers. Unmyelinated fibers were measured in the peroneal, the sural, and the ventral vagus nerves. In prediabetic animals, no differences were obtained between presumptive diabetic and control animals. No significant differences were found between diabetic and control mice 8 wk of age. However, the diabetic animals exhibited a small proportion of very large unmyelinated fibers measuring up to 1.6 μm. The fiber sizes were not found in control animals.

In 15-wk-old diabetic mice, the peroneal and the sural nerves showed a bimodal distribution of unmyelinated fibers. The shift of fibers to smaller diameters was, however, not significant (Figure 7). Diabetic mice, 25 wk of age, showed highly significant shifts of unmyelinated fibers toward smaller diameters in the peroneal, the sural, and the ventral vagus nerves. This was also the case in 33-wk-old diabetic mice (Figure 8).

FIGURE 5. Caliber spectra of myelinated fibers in 25-wk-old diabetic (shaded bars) and control mice (open bars).

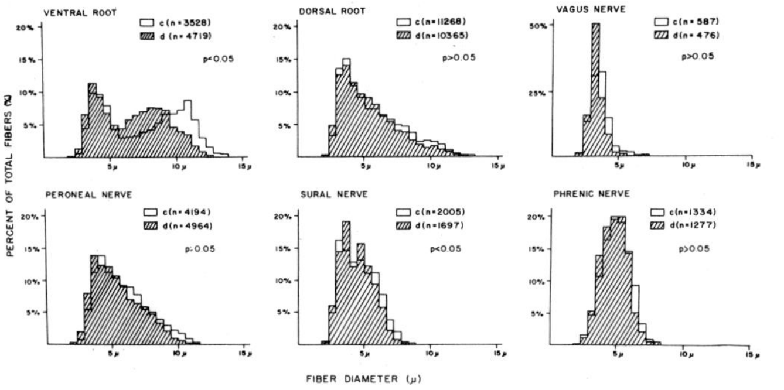

Fiber numbers, fascicular areas, and fiber densities. These parameters were measured in 25- and 33-wk-old mice (Tables 2 and 3). The number of myelinated fibers in 25-wk-old diabetic mice was not significantly altered except in the sural nerve, in which the number of myelinated nerves was significantly reduced. The number of unmyelinated fibers was reduced in the vagus nerve.

The fascicular areas of the ventral and dorsal roots of the sural and the vagus nerves were reduced to a significant degree in diabetic animals 25 wk of age. When myelinated fiber densities were calculated, they were found to be significantly increased in all nerves except for the peroneal and phrenic (Table 2). The densities of unmyelinated fibers were increased in all three nerves examined (Table 2). In 33-wk-old mice (Table 3), the number of myelinated fibers was significantly reduced, not only in the sural nerve, but also in the ventral root and the ventral vagus nerve. Unmyelinated fibers were absolutely reduced in both the sural and the vagus nerves. The nerve fascicular areas were significantly smaller in all nerves but the phrenic. Myelinated fiber densities were significantly increased in all nerves except for the peroneal and phrenic. The densities of unmyelinated fibers were significantly increased in all three nerves.

Teased fibers. Teased fibers were examined in the sural and peroneal nerves in 8-, 25-, and 33-wk-old mice, to determine the relationship between fiber diameter and internodal length. The regression lines were calculated. Statistical comparison between the slopes revealed no significant difference in the sural and the peroneal nerves of 8-wk-old mice (Table 4). In 25-wk-old mice, the peroneal nerves of the diabetic mice were not significantly different from those of control mice, whereas the sural nerve showed significantly thinner fiber diameters for a given internodal length. In 33-wk-old diabetic mice, the peroneal nerves were also significantly different from those of control mice. The differences between the sural nerves in each group were highly significant.

FIGURE 7. Caliber spectra of unmyelinated fibers in 15-wk-old diabetic (shaded bars) and control mice (open bars).

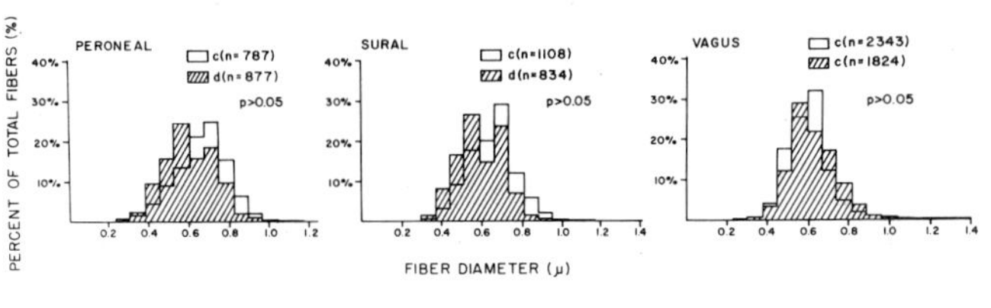

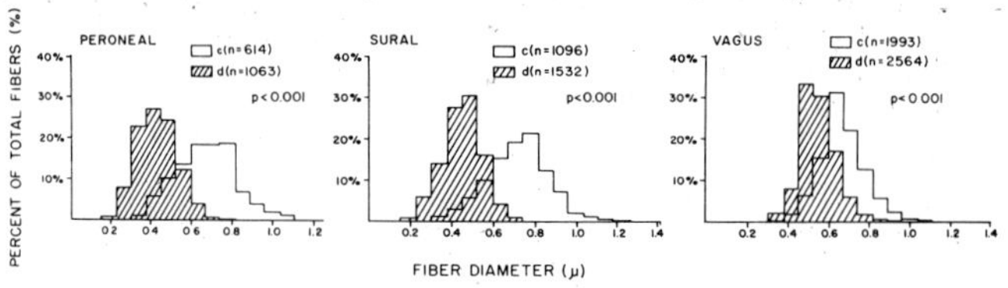

FIGURE 8. Caliber spectra of unmyelinated fibers in 33-wk-old diabetic (shaded bars) and control mice (open bars).

Qualitative classification of teased fibers (Table 5) according to Dyck et al.,[1] showed a large proportion of B and C fibers in sural nerves of diabetic mice 8, 25, and 33 wk old. The incidence of the same changes in the peroneal nerve was less, but was increased compared with control mice at 25 and 33 wk.

Relationship between axonal area and number of myelin lamellae. The relationship between the thickness of the myelin sheath and axonal area was obtained in 25- and 33-wk-old mice. The sural nerves of diabetic mice showed, in both age groups, significantly smaller axonal sizes in proportion to the number of myelin lamellae. The same was true for the peroneal nerves of diabetic mice, although the differences between diabetic and control nerves were not as marked as in the sural nerves. The regression lines for 25-wk-old mice are given in Figure 9, and the regression coefficients for both ages are compared in Table 6.

DISCUSSION

The present study has demonstrated a reduction in MNCV in early diabetes. Not only did the MNCV fail to increase with the normal maturation of the peripheral motor nerve, but it showed an absolute decrease. The decrease in MNCV occurred almost simultaneously with the elevation of blood glucose levels in 5-wk-old diabetic mice, long before any morphometric changes were detectable. These MNCV changes are similar to those previously reported for chemically induced diabetes in rats.[2,11,13,14]

Myelinated fibers first showed significant morphometric changes in 25-wk-old diabetic mice, 20 wk after the onset of diabetes. Morphometric changes in myelinated fibers were first discernible in the sural nerve and the ventral root and consisted of a shift of fibers toward smaller diameters. In 33-wk-old diabetic mice, this shift became more pronounced, and, in addition, the dorsal root showed a significant shift of myelinated fibers toward thinner diameter. The peroneal, phrenic, and ventral vagus nerves failed to demonstrate significant reduction in myelinated fiber size.

The temporal discrepancy between the occurrence of functional and morphometric deficits strongly indicates that the neuropathy is primarily metabolic in origin. This concept is further supported by the findings in the preliminary insulin treatment trial. This revealed a partial functional recovery during the early phase of the diabetic syndrome, whereas no recovery could be demonstrated during the late phase. Similar findings have been reported by Eliasson[2] and Greene et al.,[4] for chemically induced diabetes in rats.

Peripheral nerves were not obtained for morphometric analysis from treated animals. It would be most interesting to subject diabetic mice to prolonged insulin therapy to study its effect on morphometric and morphologic changes.

Although the vagus nerve failed to show a significant shift in fiber size distribution of myelinated fibers, it showed a significant reduction in the number of fibers, indicating the involvement of presynaptic parasympathetic fibers.

This study has, for the first time, demonstrated morphometric changes in the unmyelinated fiber populations of somatic and autonomic nerves in experimental diabetes. Although the changes of unmyelinated fibers in the sural, peroneal, and ventral vagus nerves reached significant levels first in 25-wk-old diabetic mice, it is interesting to follow the early changes. Diabetic mice 8 wk of age revealed a small population of unusually large fibers not found in the

TABLE 2
Fiber number: fascicular areas and fiber densities in 25-wk-old mice

Nerve	Fiber number (P-values)		Fascicula area (mm^2) (P-values)	Fiber density (N/mm^2) (P-values)	
	Myelinated	Unmyelinated		Myelinated	Unmyelinated
Ventral root C [5]	882 ± 84		0.0769 ± 0.0056	11666 ± 749	
Ventral root D [5]	814 ± 28		0.063 ± 0.0073	16217 ± 1902	
	(P > 0.05)		(P < 0.05)	(P < 0.01)	
Dorsal root C [5]	2296 ± 102		0.0980 ± 0.0058	22716 ± 1161	
Dorsal root D [5]	2377 ± 400		0.0778 ± 0.0090	31048 ± 3522	
	(P > 0.05)		(P < 0.0025)	(P < 0.01)	
Peroneal C [4]	943 ± 16	2513 ± 540	0.0476 ± 0.0069	19832 ± 3048	49925 ± 5441
Peroneal D [4]	992 ± 123	2347 ± 434	0.0456 ± 0.0062	24027 ± 2870	63502 ± 8444
	(P > 0.05)	(P > 0.05)	(P > 0.05)	(P > 0.05)	(P < 0.01)
Sural C [4]	401 ± 11	890 ± 61	0.0156 ± 0.022	24801 ± 3304	59051 ± 5426
Sural D [4]	339 ± 40	876 ± 90	0.0107 ± 0.0014	35326 ± 6974	78627 ± 15383
	(P < 0.01)	(P > 0.05)	(P < 0.01)	(P < 0.05)	(P < 0.05)
Vagus C [5]	103 ± 15	4392 ± 376	0.0090 ± 0.0007	11110 ± 1179	423618 ± 14101
Vagus D [5]	95 ± 26	3072 ± 472	0.0072 ± 0.0011	14262 ± 1468	484902 ± 16300
	(P > 0.05)	(P < 0.01)	(P < 0.025)	(P < 0.025)	(P < 0.0005)
Phrenic C [5]	266 ± 44		0.0102 ± 0012	25073 ± 3378	
	255 ± 23		0.0092 ± 0.0016	28232 ± 59566	
	(P > 0.05)		(P > 0.05)	(P > 0.05)	

C = control mice, D = diabetic mice; number of animals in brackets.

TABLE 3
Fiber numbers: fascicular areas and fiber densities in 33-wk-old mice

Nerve	Fiber number		Fascicular area (mm²) (P-values)	Fiber density (N/mm²) (P-values)	
	Myelinated	Unmyelinated		Myelinated	Unmyelinated
Ventral root C [5]	869 ± 44		0.0730 ± 0.0211	11095 ± 1178	
Ventral root D [5]	800 ± 53		0.0560 ± 0.0163	17500 ± 1115	
	(P < 0.025)		(P < 0.035)	(P < 0.001)	
Dorsal root C [5]	2476 ± 191		0.0924 ± 0.0084	26547 ± 2411	
Dorsal root D [5]	2353 ± 174		0.0767 ± 0.0055	29964 ± 2648	
	(P > 0.05)		(P < 0.005)	(P < 0.025)	
Peroneal C [5]	935 ± 41	2932 ± 324	0.0468 ± 0.0091	20632 ± 3213	63817 ± 4647
Peroneal D [5]	926 ± 38	2370 ± 417	0.0404 ± 0.0080	23444 ± 4291	73673 ± 3495
	(P > 0.05)	(P > 0.05)	(P < 0.01)	(P > 0.05)	(P < 0.05)
Sural C [5]	421 ± 29	934 ± 132	0.0153 ± 0.0031	27296 ± 2596	67788 ± 6823
Sural D [5]	351 ± 24	693 ± 93	0.0094 ± 0.0017	38875 ± 1658	84216 ± 10652
	(P < 0.0025)	(P < 0.025)	(P > 0.005)	(P < 0.001)	(P < 0.001)
Vagus C [5]	127 ± 22	3211 ± 318	0.0083 ± 0.0014	11941 ± 4511	402044 ± 34186
Vagus D [5]	78 ± 13	2489 ± 304	0.0060 ± 0.0011	15116 ± 1331	485408 ± 28661
	(P < 0.0025)	(P < 0.0025)	(P < 0.0025)	(P < 0.05)	(P < 0.01)
Phrenic C [5]	265 ± 13		0.0104 ± 0.0012	24122 ± 4447	
Phrenic D [5]	238 ± 39		0.0092 ± 0.0018	27868 ± 4300	
	(P > 0.05)		(P > 0.05)	(P > 0.05)	

C = control mice, D = diabetic mice; number of animals in brackets.

TABLE 4
Regression coefficients for the relationship between fiber diameter and internodal length

Age (wk)	Sural			Peroneal		
	Control		Diabetic	Control		Diabetic
8 wk	0.050 ± 0.008		0.0569 ± 0.0011	0.0410 ± 0.0010		0.0420 ± 0.0012
		P > 0.05			P > 0.05	
25 wk	0.0580 ± 0.0012		0.0700 ± 0.0014	0.0260 ± 0.0017		0.0290 ± 0.0010
		P < 0.001			P > 0.05	
33 wk	0.0460 ± 0.0015		0.0340 ± 0.0016	0.0324 ± 0.0037		0.0607 ± 0.0076
		P < 0.001			P < 0.05	

TABLE 5
Distribution of teased myelinated fibers

Nerve and number of fibers*	Age (wk)	Type of myelinated fibers†								
		A	B	C	D	E	F	G	H	I
Sural C [300]	8	289	3	7		1	1			
Sural D [300]	8	266	14	15		1	4			
Peroneal C [300]	8	289	6	4			1			
Peroneal D [300]	8	285	6	6			3			
Sural C [300]	25	278	8	11		1	2			
Sural D [300]	25	217	32	40	3		8			
Peroneal C [300]	25	280	8	8		1	3			
Peroneal D [300]	25	249	23	19	2		7			
Sural C [300]	33	277	11	9	2					
Sural D [300]	33	153	42	66	28	5	4			
Peroneal C [300]	33	287	6	3		1	3			
Peroneal D [300]	33	247	28	17	4		4			

Teased myelinated fibers evaluated according to the classification by Dyck et al.[1]
* C = control mice; D = diabetic mice.
† A = Normal appearance; B = wrinkling and folding of myelin; C = para- and internodal segmental demyelination, thinnest myelin thicknesss > 50% of thickest myelin thickness; D = para- and internodal segmental demyelination, thinnest myelin thickness < 50% of thickest myelin thickness; E = linear rows of myelin ovoids; F = intercalated nodes; G = excessive variability of myelin thickness "sausage formations"; H = myelin ovoids contiguous in two or more internodes; I = segmental demyelination with distal myelin ovoids.

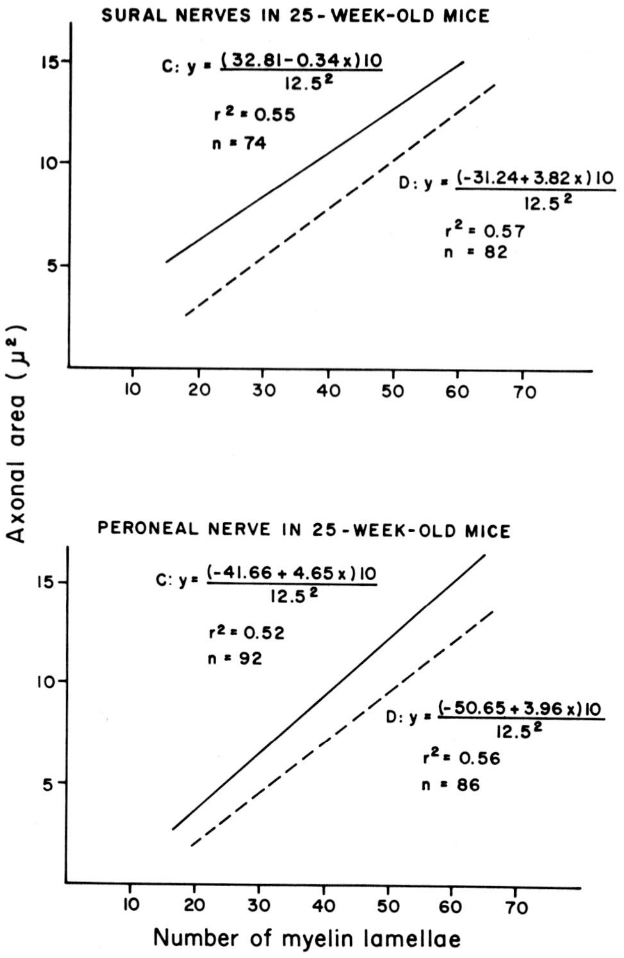

FIGURE 9. The relationship between axonal area and number of myelin lamellae in the sural and peroneal nerves of 25-wk-old diabetic (dotted lines) and control mice.

control animals. These were shown by us[20] to consist of greatly distended axons containing electron dense irregular organelle debris. At the age of 15 wk, the unmyelinated fiber spectra showed a bimodal configuration, which may indicate a new population of small regenerating fibers.

The unmyelinated fibers in the sural and peroneal nerves are both somatic afferent and sympathetic in type. The involvement of these fibers, therefore, probably reflects sympathetic fiber damage. This hypothesis is consistent with the suppressed activity of sympathetic nerves in db/db mice, as demonstrated by Giachetti.[3] The present findings, therefore, are consistent with the involvement of both sympathetic and parasympathetic fibers in this model of diabetic neuropathy.

The calculation of fascicular areas and the number of myelinated and unmyelinated fibers is interesting in view of the findings of Jakobsen.[6] This author found increased fascicular areas of the peroneal nerves in rats with early streptozotocin diabetes. Contrary to his results, we found decreased fascicular areas. However, the fascicular areas were decreased only in nerves that were otherwise involved by the neuropathy, with fiber-caliber shifts and decreased number of fibers. For example, the phrenic nerve, which did not show any of these changes, also failed to show decreased fascicular area. It is therefore unlikely that this shrinkage of the nerve fascicles is due to fixation artifacts. It should be noted, however, that these changes were observed in mice with longstanding diabetes (20–28 wk), and these parameters were not investigated in early diabetes. Therefore, these results do not necessarily contradict those of Jakobsen, who investigated diabetic rats 4 wk after diabetes was induced with streptozotocin.

Seneviratne[15] found an increased permeability of the perineurium and the endoneurial vessels to bovine albumin in alloxan diabetic rats, which, in an elegant way, could explain endoneurial edema. However, these findings were not confirmed in our studies of streptozotocin-diabetic rats or the present diabetic model.[19]

In the present model, we believe that the decreased fascicular area is, at least in part, due to reduction in number of both myelinated and unmyelinated fibers and to the shrinkage of single nerve fibers.

It has been suggested that the reduced fiber diameter in diabetic rats could be due to the impaired growth of these rats after the induction of diabetes,[6] since it has been shown that stunted growth causes reduced fiber growth, with a proportional reduction in nerve conduction velocity.[16,17] This possibility was ruled out in the present study, since we failed to demonstrate any difference in longitudinal limb growth between diabetic and control mice.

In a preliminary report,[19] quantitative and qualitative findings were suggestive of a primary axonal degeneration. In order to obtain objective morphometric evidence for this suggestion, axonal areas were measured and plotted against the number of myelin lamellae. Both the sural and the peroneal nerve showed disproportionally small axons for a given myelin thickness in diabetic mice 25 and 33 wk of age, the changes being more severe in the sural nerve. These findings thus indicate an axonal dwindling and are in agreement with those made by Jakobsen.[6,7] These findings are also in keeping with an increased ratio between internodal length and fiber diameter in teased fiber preparations, also more pronounced in the sural nerve. In addition, teased fibers showed substantial wrinkling in the sural nerve. These changes were also noted in the peroneal nerve, to a

TABLE 6
Regression coefficients for the relationship between axonal area and number of myelin lamellae

	Sural			Peroneal		
Age (wk)	Control		Diabetic	Control		Diabetic
25 wk	3.42 ± 0.04		3.82 ± 0.11	4.65 ± 0.46		3.96 ± 0.27
		$P < 0.001$			$P < 0.05$	
33 wk	6.29 ± 0.10		3.47 ± 0.17	4.45 ± 0.17		4.21 ± 0.13
		$P < 0.001$			$P < 0.05$	

lesser extent, and are interpreted as being secondary to the axonal dwindling. The more advanced changes in the sural nerve have been ultrastructurally illustrated in a previous report.[20] These morphometric procedures, which are more sensitive to subtle changes of the nerve fiber than, for instance, caliber spectra, indicate that the peroneal nerve is involved in the neuropathic process, although the changes tend to occur at a later stage than in the sural nerve. However, whether these changes in the peroneal nerve involve motor fibers cannot be ascertained, since this nerve also contains a small proportion of sensory fibers. The caliber spectra of the central root, however, clearly shows involvement of motor fibers at a proximal level.

In conclusion, this study has shown that the early onset of MNCV deficit is not due to visible morphologic damage, but is, rather, metabolic in nature. This concept is supported by the partial reversibility of MNCV deficit during insulin treatment.

Long-term studies of morphometric parameters have shown degeneration of axons in somatic sensory, motor, and autonomic fibers of progressive severity during the time studied. At no stage was there significant evidence of primary demyelination.

ACKNOWLEDGMENT

This work was supported by grant MA 5857 from the Medical Research Council of Canada.

REFERENCES

[1] Dyck, P. J., Johnson, W. J., Lambert, E. H., and O'Brien, P. C.: Segmental demyelination secondary to axonal degeneration in uremic neuropathy. Mayo Clin. Proc. *46*:400–31, 1971.

[2] Eliasson, S. G.: Nerve conduction studies in experimental diabetes. J. Clin. Invest. *43*:2352–59, 1964.

[3] Giachetti, A.: The functional state of sympathetic nerves in spontaneously diabetic mice. Diabetes *27*:345–52, 1978.

[4] Greene, D. A., DeJesus, P. V., and Winegrad, A. I.: Effects of insulin and dietary myoinositol on impaired peripheral motor nerve conduction velocity in acute streptozotocin diabetes. J. Clin. Invest. *55*:1326–36, 1975.

[5] Hildebrand, J., Joffray, A., Graff, G., and Coers, C.: Neuromuscular changes with alloxan hyperglycemia. Electrophysiological, biochemical and histological study in rats. Arch. Neurol. *18*:633–41, 1968.

[6] Jakobsen, J.: Axonal dwindling in early experimental diabetes. I. A study of cross sectioned nerves. Diabetologia *12*:547–53, 1976.

[7] Jakobsen, J.: Axonal dwindling in early experimental diabetes. II. A study of isolated nerve fibers. Diabetologia *12*:547–53, 1976.

[8] Jakobsen, J., Malmgren, L., and Olsson, Y.: Permeability of the blood-nerve barrier in the streptozotocin diabetic rat. Exp. Neurol. *60*:277–85, 1978.

[9] Like, A. A., and Chick, W. L.: Studies in diabetic mutant mouse: I. Light microscopy and radio-autography of pancreatic islets. Diabetologia *6*:207–16, 1970.

[10] Lovelace, R. E.: Experimental neuropathy in rats made diabetic with alloxan. Electroencephalogr. Clin. Neurophysiol. *26*:393, 1968.

[11] Miyoshi, T., and Goto, I.: Serial in vivo determinations of nerve conduction velocity in rat tails. Physiological and pathological changes. Electroencephalogr. Clin. Neurophysiol. *35*:125–31, 1973.

[12] Ochoa, J.: Recognition of unmyelinated fiber disease: Morphologic criteria. Muscle Nerve *1*:375–87, 1978.

[13] Preston, F. M.: Peripheral neuropathy in the alloxan diabetic rat. J. Physiol. (Lond.) *189*:49–50, 1967.

[14] Sharma, A. K., and Thomas, P. K.: Peripheral nerve structure and function in experimental diabetes. J. Neurol. Sci. *23*:1–15, 1974.

[15] Seneviratne, K. N.: Permeability of blood nerve barriers in the diabetic rat. J. Neurol. Neurosurg. Psychol. *35*:156–62, 1972.

[16] Sima, A.: Studies on fiber size in developing sciatic nerve and spinal roots in normal, undernourished, and rehabilitated rats. Acta Physiol. Scand. *91*(Suppl.):406, 1974.

[17] Sima, A., and Jankowska, E.: Sensory nerve conduction velocity as correlated to fiber size in experimental undernutrition in the rat. Neuropathol. Appl. Neurobiol. *1*:31–37, 1975.

[18] Sima, A. A. F., and Robertson, D. A.: Peripheral neuropathy in mutant diabetic mouse [C57BL/Ks(db/db)]. Acta Neuropathol. (Berl.) *41*:85–89, 1978.

[19] Sima, A. A. F., and Robertson, D. M.: The perineurial and blood-nerve barriers in experimental diabetes. Acta Neuropathol. (Berl.) *44*:189–96, 1978.

[20] Sima, A. A. F., and Robertson, D. M.: Peripheral neuropathy in the diabetic mutant mouse [C57BL/Ks(db/db)]. An ultrastructural study. Lab. Invest. *40*:627, 1979.

[21] Staats, J.: Diabetes in the mouse due to two mutant genes—a bibliography. Diabetologia *11*:325–27, 1975.

[22] Winegrad, A. I., and Greene, D. A.: Diabetic polyneuropathy: The importance of insulin deficiency, hyperglycemia and alterations in myoinositol metabolism in its pathogenesis. N. Engl. J. Med. *295*:1416–21, 1976.

The Histocompatibility (HLA) Antigen Distribution in Diabetes in Southern African Blacks (Xhosa)

BRIAN R. BRIGGS, W. P. U. JACKSON, ERNETTE D. DuTOIT, AND MARTIN C. BOTHA

SUMMARY

The frequency distributions of HLA antigens in 25 juvenile-onset diabetics (JOD) and 56 maturity-onset diabetics (MOD) belonging to a southern African black tribe (Xhosa) were compared with those of 153 nondiabetic Xhosa blacks. Unlike the findings in white JODs, there was no increase of B8 or B15 nor a reduced frequency of B7 but an apparently, significantly increased frequency of Bw35 and A2 in both Xhosa JODs and Xhosa MODs, respectively.

This is the first ethnic group in which an HLA antigen marker has been found for MOD. Furthermore, these findings suggest that diabetes, both JOD and MOD, in white people is a different genetic disease from the diabetes among the Xhosa tribe.

DIABETES *29*:68–71, January 1980.

The associations of HLA antigens with juvenile-onset diabetes (JOD) have been reported in various populations. In Caucasians the associations with HLA-B8 and HLA-B15 are now well known.[1–5] In Japanese JODs, however, a significant positive association has been found to occur with HLA-Bw54[6] and not with B15 or B8 (though it should be noted that B8 is extremely rare among Japanese).

The HLA antigen frequency distribution in southern African blacks is distinctive and differs from that found in southern African whites, who are similar to European Caucasians. Certain antigens (e.g., HLA-A11) are absent, and other antigens (e.g., Aw43) are confined to some southern African populations, including the Xhosa. With the regard to specificities relevant to Caucasian JODs, B8 and B15 are both less common.[7] Hence, we decided to investigate the situation among JODs and MODs in the Xhosa population.

MATERIALS AND METHODS

The Xhosa chiefdom or tribe accounts for about 26% of the Negro population of southern Africa (1970 census). This chiefdom constitutes a large branch of the Nguni linguistic division of the Bantu-speaking Negroes.

The clinical criteria used to select for JOD were patients who were insulin dependent and in whom the age of onset of diabetes had been below 30 yr. None of these patients were obese, about 50% had been in ketoacidosis at some stage, and all were grossly symptomatic before treatment. Only two JOD patients had a family history of diabetes: In both cases the affected members were paternal, but it was not possible to ascertain into which category the diabetes fell. It was also ensured that the patients were unrelated and were members of the Xhosa tribe, having no admixture of other southern African genes. The infrequency of JOD in southern African blacks and the small numbers living in the Cape Peninsula caused our sample to be limited to 25 patients. As a control group, 153 unrelated healthy Xhosa individuals were randomly selected from the same geographic area, i.e., the Cape Peninsula.

A further group of 56 adult Xhosa maturity-onset diabetics were also typed. About 50% of these were obese. All were clearly diabetic, with some random blood glucose levels over 200 mg/dl. None became insulin dependent or ketoacidotic. In all, the age of onset was over 30 yr. In the MOD group, family histories were usually negative. Seven patients were able to give a history of siblings being affected, but again the category was difficult to ascertain. Only two gave doubtful histories of paternal involvement. In neither group were data on fasting C-peptide levels or anti-islet cell antibodies available.

Serologic tests. HLA typing was performed using the microlymphocytotoxicity test of Terasaki et al.[8]

Patients and controls were tissue typed for the following HLA antigens: A1, A2, A3, A9, A10, A11, A28, A29, A19, Aw23, Aw24, A25, A26, Aw30, Aw31, Aw32, Aw33, Aw34, Aw36, and Aw43 of the A locus series and B5, B7, B8, B12, B13, B14, B18, B27, B15, Bw16, B17, Bw21, Bw22, Bw35,

From the Department of Medicine, University of Cape Town (Dr. Jackson), and the Provincial Blood Grouping Laboratory, Observatory, Cape, South Africa.

Address reprint requests to Dr. Brian R. Briggs, Provincial Blood Grouping Laboratory, Private Bag 4, Observatory, 7935, Cape, South Africa.

Received for publication 2 July 1979.

B37, Bw38, Bw39, B40, Bw41, Bw47, and Bw42 of the B locus series.

The sera used were highly selected, sources being the authors' own laboratory and interchange with other laboratories. A minimum of three sera was used for the identification of each antigen. In those few cases where the antigen assignment was ambiguous, the individuals concerned were retyped using specially selected sera.

Statistical evaluation of the results. Since the sample was not large, and since it has proved almost impossible to increase the sample, due cognizance of the sample size was taken into account. This consideration has been discussed fully elsewhere.[9,10]

Thus, for each antigen given that (a) patients carry and (b) patients lack and that (c) controls possess and (d) lack, where (a), (b), (c), and (d) are the entries of the appropriate 2 × 2 table, the formula given by Haldane[9] was used:

$$\text{the relative risk, } X = \frac{(2a + 1)(2d + 1)}{(2b + 1)(2c + 1)}$$

The natural logarithm y = ln x, with a variance given by

$$V = \frac{1}{a + 1} + \frac{1}{b + 1} + \frac{1}{c + 1} + \frac{1}{d + 1}$$

and weight, w = 1/V, were computed.

The significance of the divergence of Y from zero was measured by $\chi^2 = wy^2$ for one degree of freedom.

In addition, Fisher's test was used to determine the exact probability (P) of finding differences as extreme or more extreme than those observed between the antigen frequencies in patients and controls by chance alone, if there is no true difference.

RESULTS

In the tables, only those results in which a P value of less than 0.1 was obtained are shown.

The HLA antigen frequencies in the control population were similar to those found previously in healthy unrelated Xhosa,[7] and the JOD results are shown in Table 1. The MOD results are similarly shown in Table 2.

Bw35 was found to be increased in the JOD patient group (P = 0.009), while Bw42 was found to be decreased (P = 0.019).

Among the maturity-onset diabetics (MODs), A2 showed an increased frequency compared with controls, the P value of the difference for A2 being 0.006. In addition, B12 (P = 0.041) was found to be marginally increased while Bw41, a low frequency antigen, was increased, with a P value of 0.034. Bw35, while not significantly increased, was found to be more frequent than in the control group. A29 was decreased (P = 0.038).

When, however, as suggested by Grumet et al.,[11] the P values were corrected by multiplying by the number of antigens tested for, all the deviations became nonsignificant.

TABLE 1
HLA antigen frequencies in juvenile-onset diabetes in the Xhosa

HLA antigen	Patients (N = 25) % positive	Controls (N = 153) % positive	Relative risk (x)	P value
A2	36	23	1.92	0.074
B7	28	17	1.95	0.092
Bw35	20	4	6.09	0.009
Bw42	0	16	0.10	0.019

TABLE 2
HLA antigen frequencies in maturity-onset diabetes in the Xhosa

HLA antigen	Patients (N = 56) % positive	Controls (N = 153) % positive	Relative risk (x)	P value
A2	41	23	2.34	0.006
A3	14	8	1.98	0.096
A29	7	17	0.41	0.038
B8	21	14	1.73	0.081
B12	25	14	1.99	0.041
B17	46	39	1.38	0.086
Bw35	11	4	2.92	0.068
Bw41	9	2	4.59	0.034
Bw42	9	16	0.56	0.095

DISCUSSION

The questions are whether juvenile-onset diabetes follows the same pattern of HLA frequencies in the Xhosa as in other populations and whether maturity-onset diabetes shows any relation to the HLA system.

Clinically, there are no clear differences in type of JOD or MOD in black Xhosa people compared with white, except in the low frequency of JOD and of a positive family history of diabetes among the Xhosa people.

From our results, it would appear that (1) the frequencies of B8 and B15 are not increased in JOD in the Xhosa, (2) the frequency of B7 is not reduced as has been found among white JODs,[3] and (3) the frequencies of Bw35 and A2 may be markedly increased in the JOD and MOD Xhosa people, respectively. It is possible that Bw35 is also increased in MODs.

Although no relation has previously been reported in other races between MOD and the HLA system, we suggest that the increased frequency of A2 in Xhosa is too great to be dismissed summarily.

Our results, therefore, suggest that the marker HLA antigens for JOD among the Xhosa people are quite different from those in white people and that maturity-onset diabetes among Xhosa may also be related to the HLA system.

ACKNOWLEDGMENTS

This work was supported in part by the Medical Research Council grant to the Endocrine/Diabetic Research Group.

REFERENCES

1 Singal, D. P., and Blajchman, M. A.: Histocompatibility (HLA) antigens, lymphocytotoxic antibodies and tissue antibodies in patients with diabetes mellitus. Diabetes *22*:429–32, 1973.

2 Nerup, J., Platz, P., Anderson, O. O., Christy, M., Lyngse, J., Poulsen, J. E., Ryder, L. P., Nielsen, L. S., Thomsen, M., and Svejgaard, A.: HLA antigens and diabetes mellitus. Lancet *2*:864–66, 1974.

3 Cudworth, A. G., and Woodrow, J. C.: HLA system and diabetes mellitus. Diabetes *24*:345–49, 1975.

[4] Cudworth, A. G., and Woodrow, J. C.: Evidence for HLA linked genes in "juvenile diabetes mellitus". Br. Med. J. *3*:133–35, 1975.

[5] Cudworth, A. G., and Woodrow, J. C.: Genetic susceptibility in diabetes mellitus: analysis of the HLA association. Br. Med. J. *2*:846–48, 1976.

[6] Okomoto, K., Juji, T., Ishiba, S., Maruyama, H., Tohyama, H. and Kosaka, K.: HLA-Bw54 (Bw22-J, J-1) antigen in juvenile onset diabetes mellitus in Japan. Tissue Antigens *11*:418–22, 1978.

[7] Botha, M. C., Campbell, E., Briggs, B. R., and Du Toit, E. D.: Differences in serological definition and frequency of some HL-A antigens among southern African populations. *In* Histocompatibility Testing. Copenhagen, Munksgaard, 1975, pp. 151–72.

[8] Terasaki, P. I., McClelland, J., Min Sik Park, and McCurdy, B.: Microdroplet lymphocyte cytotoxicity test. *In* Manual of Tissue Typing Techniques. Ray, J. G., Hare, D. B., Pedersen, P. D., and Kayhoe, D. E., Eds. Bethesda, NIH, 1974, pp. 66–72.

[9] Haldane, J. B. S.: The estimation and significance of the logarithm of a ratio of frequencies. Ann. Hum. Genet. *20*:309–11, 1955.

[10] Svejgaard, A., Jersild, C., Staub Nielsen, L., and Bodmer, W. F.: HL-A antigens and disease: statistical and genetical considerations. Tissue Antigens *4*:95–195, 1974.

[11] Grumet, F. C., Coukell, A., Bodmer, J. G., Bodmer, W. F., and McDevitt, H. O.: Histocompatibility (HL-A) antigens associated with systemic lupus erythematosis. N. Engl. J. Med. *285*:193–96, 1971.

[12] Botha, M. C., Briggs, B. R., Du Toit, E. D., Campbell, E., Taljaard, D., and Jackson, W. P. U.: Associations between HLA-A and B loci and maturity onset diabetes in southern African populations. Tissue Antigens *10*:201, 1977.

Somatostatin Concentration Responds to Arginine in Portal Plasma

Effects of Fasting, Streptozotocin Diabetes, and Insulin Administration in Diabetic Rats

TSUTOMU KAZUMI, MASAFUMI UTSUMI, GEN YOSHINO, KAZUHIDE ISHIHARA, YOSHIKAZU HIROSE, HIROYUKI MAKIMURA, AND SHIGEAKI BABA

SUMMARY

Changes of somatostatin concentration in response to a single i.v. injection of arginine (400 mg/kg body weight) were examined in extracted portal plasma of normal and diabetic rats in the fully fed state and after 24 h of fasting, as well as in diabetic rats treated with insulin for one week. In both normal and diabetic animals fasted for 24 h, the basal level of somatostatin declined but the magnitude of the arginine-induced elevation of somatostatin was not affected, suggesting a physiologic role of the tetradecapeptide in nutrient homeostasis.

When compared with intact rats, diabetic animals were shown to have increased levels of somatostatin before and after arginine administration, both of which were attenuated by insulin replacement therapy. These findings suggest that alterations of D cell function in streptozotocin diabetes may be related to either insulin deficiency or its metabolic consequences.
DIABETES 29:71–73, January 1980.

Increases in somatostatin-containing D cells[1] and in the somatostatin content of the pancreatic islets and the stomach[2] have been found in rats with insulin-deficient diabetes. Recent studies[3,4] revealed that circulating levels of somatostatin were elevated in dogs with alloxan diabetes of long duration. On the other hand, it is well known that fasting results in changes of pancreatic hormone secretion.[5] Therefore, the present studies were undertaken to determine changes of somatostatin levels in response to arginine in portal plasma of normal and streptozotocin-diabetic rats in the fed and fasted state. In addition, effects of insulin treatment on somatostatin concentration were also examined in diabetic rats.

From the Second Department of Internal Medicine, Kobe University School of Medicine, Kobe, Japan.
Address requests for reprints to Professor Shigeaki Baba, Second Department of Internal Medicine, Kobe University School of Medicine, Kusunoki-cho, Ikuta-ku, Kobe 650, Japan.
Received for publication 23 July 1979.

MATERIALS AND METHODS

Male Wistar rats (310–390 g) were used throughout the study. Diabetes was induced by a single i.v. injection of streptozotocin (Upjohn, Kalamazoo, Michigan), 40mg/kg body weight, after overnight fasting. (The diabetogenic activity of streptozotocin is enhanced in older rats.[6]) Four days after injection, rats developed hyperglycemia in excess of 400 mg/dl in the fed state, though they did not develop ketosis. They had free access to water and were fed ad libitum on rat chow pellets, except during periods of fasting.

Two weeks after streptozotocin treatment, rats in the fully fed state and after being fasted for 24 h were laparotomized under pentobarbital anesthesia. Blood (2 ml each) was taken from the portal vein by syringes containing 1.25 mg of EDTA and 1000 KIU of Trasylol in each milliliter of whole blood, before and after a single injection of L-arginine (Taisho Seiyaku, Osaka, Japan), 400 mg/kg body weight in a 20% solution, into the jugular vein. Blood was withdrawn 2 min after arginine injection, as preliminary studies in intact rats revealed that an identical arginine load resulted in a prompt and significant rise of somatostatin in portal plasma, which peaked at 2 min and was followed by a decline thereafter towards baseline levels. Normal rats were subjected to arginine-loading tests in the same manner. In another group of diabetic rats, 4–6 U of NPH insulin was injected subcutaneously at 6 p.m. for four consecutive days beginning 7 days after streptozotocin treatment, after which 3–4 U was administered for an additional 3 days. Identical arginine loading was performed in these animals in the fed state 15 h after the last insulin injection. Diabetic rats given saline served as controls. All experiments were performed between 9 and 11 a.m.

Blood was centrifuged immediately after each sampling. Plasma (0.5 ml each) was extracted by sonification in 4 vol of acid-acetone for somatostatin determinations as previously reported.[7] Plasma and its extracts were kept at −20°C until assayed.

Glucose and insulin were measured by the glucose-oxidase method using commercially available kits (Green Cross Corporation, Osaka, Japan) and by radioimmunoassay (RIA[8]), with rat insulin used as a standard, respectively. Somatostatin was determined by a double antibody RIA.[7]

Data are expressed as mean ± SEM and statistical analysis was performed by the nonpaired Student's *t* test.

RESULTS

Figure 1 shows the effects of arginine on glucose, insulin, and somatostatin in portal plasma of normal and diabetic rats in the fully fed state and after 24 h of being fasted. Streptozotocin administration produced diabetes characterized by hyperglycemia associated with hypoinsulinemia. Somatostatin levels in diabetic rats were significantly elevated when compared with those of normal animals in both the fasted (235 ± 23 vs. 151 ± 12 pg/ml, $P < 0.005$) and fed state (401 ± 43 vs. 201 ± 10 pg/ml, $P < 0.001$). Somatostatin (151 ± 12 vs. 201 ± 10 pg/ml, $P < 0.02$) as well as glucose (113 ± 4 vs. 153 ± 4 mg/dl, $P < 0.001$) and insulin (3.85 ± 0.35 vs. 6.83 ± 0.79 ng/ml, $P < 0.005$) were significantly lower in normal, fasted rats as compared with fed controls. In diabetic animals as in normal rats, fasting resulted in a marked decrease in both glucose (459 ± 15 vs. 175 ± 12 mg/dl, $P < 0.001$) and somatostatin levels (401 ± 43 vs. 235 ± 23 pg/ml, $P < 0.005$), although there was no significant change in insulin values.

Arginine injection resulted in a significant elevation of insulin and somatostatin levels in all animals used in this study. Normal rats, regardless of the nutrient state, showed 1.3-fold increases of somatostatin in response to arginine. However, the mean somatostatin level in portal plasma of diabetic animals rose from 401 ± 43 to 726 ± 103 pg/ml in the fed state and from 235 ± 23 to 395 ± 30 pg/ml in the fasted state. Thus, arginine administration produced an approximately twofold elevation of somatostatin in diabetic rats. Arginine loading resulted in threefold increases of insulin in diabetics. By contrast, intact rats showed 4.5-fold and 3.7-fold elevations of insulin in the fed (from 6.83 ± 0.79 to 30.99 ± 4.17 ng/ml) and fasted state (from 3.85 ± 0.35 to 14.16 ± 1.56 ng/ml), respectively.

Plasma glucose was significantly lower in the insulin-treated rats, which showed steady weight gain, than in saline-treated diabetic animals, though insulin-treated rats continued to show moderate hyperglycemia (Figure 2). Mean somatostatin levels before and after arginine injection were markedly lower in the insulin-treated group than in the saline-treated group (157 ± 16 vs. 338 ± 31 pg/ml at 0 min, $P < 0.01$; 280 ± 32 vs. 737 ± 63 pg/ml at 2 min, $P < 0.001$). They returned to the levels found in normal rats in the fed state (see Figure 1). Arginine administration resulted in a 1.8-fold elevation of somatostatin in the insulin-treated group, whereas it produced a 2.2-fold elevation of the tetradecapeptide in saline-treated diabetic rats.

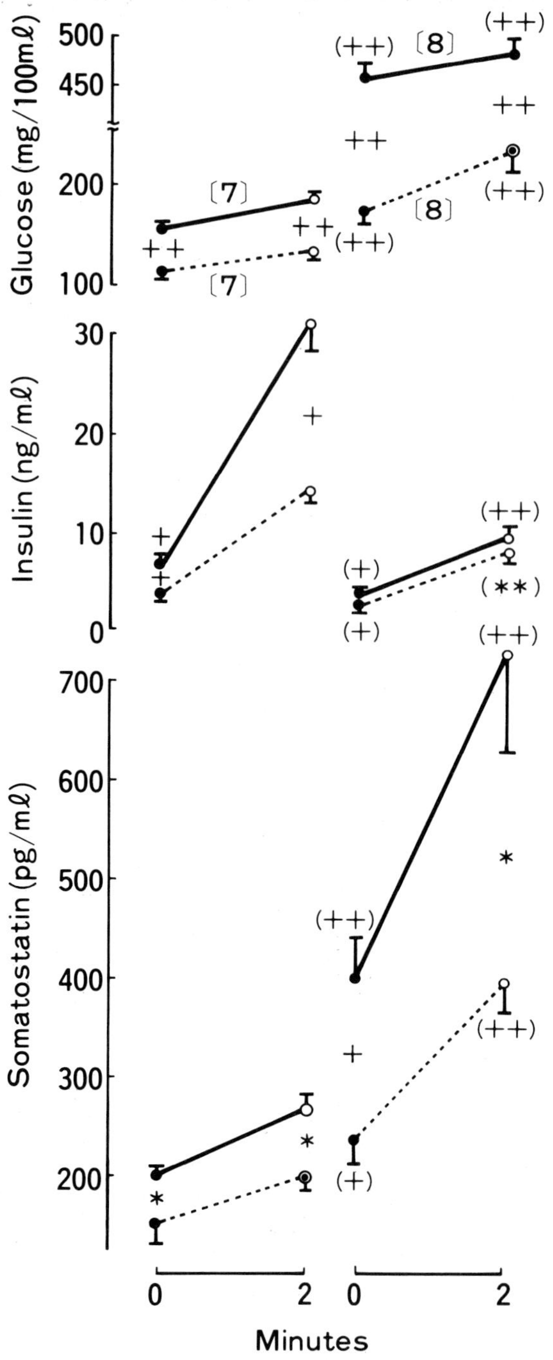

FIGURE 1. Effects of a single i.v. injection of arginine, 400 mg/kg body weight, on portal plasma glucose, insulin, and somatostatin in normal (left panel) and diabetic rats (right panel) in the fully fed state (solid lines) and after 24 h of fasting (dotted lines). The number of animals is in square brackets. Mean data ± SEM. Significance of difference between fasted and fed states: *$P < 0.05$, **$P < 0.01$, +$P < 0.005$, ++$P < 0.001$. Symbols in parentheses indicate differences between normal and diabetic rats in the fed and fasted states, respectively, at each corresponding time period. ⊙ and ○ indicate significant differences vs. zero values ($P < 0.05$ or 0.01, and $P < 0.005$ or less, respectively).

DISCUSSION

The present study demonstrates that rats with streptozotocin diabetes of 2-wk duration have increased levels of somatostatin in portal plasma. A similar result was obtained from the in vitro study[9] using perfused pancreases from alloxan-diabetic rats that had had the disease for a short time. Furthermore, in the present study, insulin replacement therapy for one week significantly lowered the increased levels of tetradecapeptide before and after arginine administration. A recent study[10] in streptozotocin-diabetic rats revealed that insulin therapy lowered the increased pancreatic somatostatin content but did not affect that of the stomach and colon. These findings suggest that alterations in islet D-cell function may be related to either insulin deficiency or its metabolic consequences and that the reduced portal so-

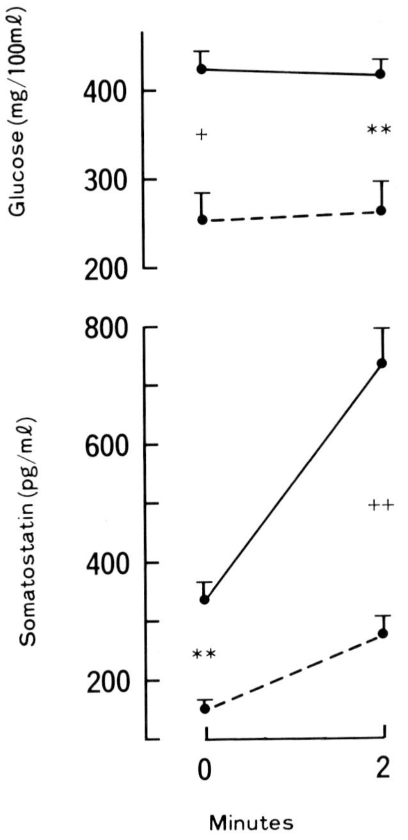

FIGURE 2. Effects of insulin replacement therapy for 1 wk on arginine-induced elevation of somatostatin in portal plasma of streptozotocin-diabetic rats. Dotted and solid lines represent data from insulin-treated (N = 7) and saline-treated (N = 7) diabetic rats, respectively. Mean ± SEM. For significance of difference between the two groups, see legend for Figure 1.

matostatin response to insulin therapy found in the present study is of pancreatic origin.

These results in intact rats confirm the previous finding[11] that fasting results in a decrease in portal somatostatin, which appears to reflect its release from the pancreas and gastrointestinal tract. These two studies are not consistent with the recent study[12] using perifused rat islets, which indicated that fasting produced a high secretory activity of D cells. The reason for the discrepancy between in vivo and in vitro results is unclear but may be a result of the different experimental designs employed. Though the effect of arginine on somatostatin's release from the rat stomach is obscure to us, an elevation of portal somatostatin in response to arginine appears to be consistent with the observations[13,14] that arginine can stimulate somatostatin's release from the rat pancreas.

REFERENCES

1 Orci, L., Baetens, D., Rufener, C., Amherdt, M., Ravazzola, M., Studer, P., Malaisse-Lagae, F., and Unger, R. H.: Hypertrophy and hyperplasia of somatostatin-containing D cells in diabetes. Proc. Natl. Acad. Sci. USA *73*: 1338–42, 1976.

2 Patel, Y. C., Cameron, D. P., Bankier, A., Malaisse-Lagae, F., Ravazzola, M., Studer, P., and Orci, L.: Changes in somatostatin concentration in pancreas and other tissues of streptozotocin diabetic rats. Endocrinology *103*:917–23, 1978.

3 Schusdziarra, V., Rouiller, D., Harris, V., Conlon, J. M., and Unger, R. H.: The response of somatostatin-like immunoreactivity to nutrients in normal and alloxan diabetic dogs. Endocrinology *103*:2264–73, 1978.

4 Schusdziarra, V., Dobbs, R. E., and Unger, R. H.: Immunoreactive somatostatin levels in plasma of normal and alloxan diabetic dogs. FEBS Lett. *81*:69–72, 1977.

5 Buchanan, K. D., Vance, J. E., and Williams, R. H.: Effect of starvation on insulin and glucagon release from isolated islets of Langerhans of the rat. Metabolism *18*:155–62, 1969.

6 Masiello, P., Depaoli, A., and Bergamini, E.: Age-dependent changes in the sensitivity of the rat to a diabetogenic agent (streptozotocin). Endocrinology *96*:787–89, 1975.

7 Utsumi, M., Makimura, H., Ishihara, K., Morita, S., and Baba, S.: Determination of immunoreactive somatostatin in rat plasma and responses to arginine, glucose and glucagon infusion. Diabetologia *17*:1–5, 1979.

8 Morgan, C. R., and Lazarow, A.: Immunoassay of insulin: two antibody system. Plasma insulin levels of normal and diabetic rats. Diabetes *12*:115–16, 1963.

9 Hara, M., Patton, G., and Gerich, J.: Increased somatostatin release from pancreases of alloxan diabetic rats perfused in vitro. Life Sci. *24*:625–28, 1979.

10 Berelowitz, M., Shapiro, B., Pimstone, B., and Kronheim, S.: Growth hormone release inhibitory hormone-like immunoreactivity in pancreas and gut in streptozotocin diabetes in the rat and response to insulin administration. Clin. Endocrinol. *10*:195–98, 1979.

11 Shapiro, B., Berelowitz, M., Pimstone, B. L., Kronheim, S., and Sheppard, M.: Tissue and serum somatostatin-like immunoreactivity in fed, 15-h-fasted, and 72-h-fasted rats. Diabetes *28*:182–84, 1979.

12 Schauder, P., McIntosh, C., Arends, J., and Frerichs, H.: Effect of fasting on the release of insulin and somatostatin from perifused islets of Langerhans. Diabetes *28*:204–07, 1979.

13 Patton, G. S., Ipp, E., Dobbs, R. E., Orci, L., Vale, W., and Unger, R. H.: Response of pancreatic immunoreactive somatostatin to arginine. Life Sci. *19*:1957–60, 1976.

14 Efendić, S., Nylen, A., Roovete, A., and Uvnäs-Wallenstein, K.: Effects of glucose and arginine on the release of immunoreactive somatostatin from the isolated perfused rat pancreas. FEBS Lett. *92*:33–35, 1978.

Rapid Publications

Stimulation of Adenylate Cyclase by Ca^{2+} and Calmodulin in Rat Islets of Langerhans

Explanation for the Glucose-induced Increase in Cyclic AMP Levels

GEOFFREY W. G. SHARP, DAYNA E. WIEDENKELLER, DENISE KAELIN, EBERHARD G. SIEGEL, AND CLAES B. WOLLHEIM

SUMMARY

The effect of Ca^{2+} and calmodulin has been studied on adenylate cyclase activity in homogenates of rat islets of Langerhans. EGTA had a stimulatory effect on the enzyme in accord with the known inhibitory effect of Ca^{2+}. In contrast, the addition of Ca^{2+} together with calmodulin is stimulatory and demonstrates the existence of a Ca^{2+}-dependent adenylate cyclase in islets of Langerhans. It is suggested that the glucose-induced increase in cyclic AMP concentrations in intact islets is a secondary consequence of the glucose-induced increase in cytosol free-Ca^{2+} concentrations which, with calmodulin, causes an increase in the activity of adenylate cyclase. DIABETES 29:74–77, January 1980.

Cyclic AMP has been shown to have a marked potentiating effect on the ability of glucose to stimulate insulin release from islets of Langerhans.[1] In addition, intracellular concentrations of cyclic AMP in islets can be modestly increased by stimulatory levels of glucose.[2,3] These two effects, and a variety of studies that demonstrate a strong correlation between the glucose-induced increase in cyclic AMP and the rate of insulin release,[4–8] suggest a role for cyclic AMP in the mechanism of glucose-stimulated insulin release. However, agents such as theophylline can cause a greater increase in intracellular cyclic AMP concentration than glucose and have only minor effects on insulin release at nonstimulatory glucose concentrations. For this and other reasons, a straightforward association of glucose causing stimulation of insulin release by raising cyclic AMP levels is unlikely. It seems more likely that the glucose-induced rise in cyclic AMP has a self-potentiating effect on the glucose-stimulated insulin release.[2]

From the Department of Physiology, Tufts University Schools of Medicine, Dental Medicine, and Veterinary Medicine, Boston, Massachusetts 02111, and the Institut de Biochimie Clinique, University of Geneva, Geneva, Switzerland.

Address reprint requests to Geoffrey W.G. Sharp, Department of Physiology, Tufts University School of Medicine, Boston, Massachusetts 02111.

Received for publication 2 October 1979.

The mechanism by which glucose increases intracellular cyclic AMP is not understood. Only one report[9] out of eight published reports[1] claims that glucose does stimulate adenylate cyclase in broken cell preparations of islets. Repeated studies in this laboratory have also failed to detect a stimulatory effect (unpublished work). An explanation involving inhibition of cyclic nucleotide phosphodiesterase activity seems unlikely as no such effect has been demonstrated.[10–13]

In seeking an explanation for the effect of glucose to elevate cyclic AMP levels, the possibility was considered that raised intracellular Ca^{2+} concentrations in response to glucose could be responsible for the stimulation of adenylate cyclase. The effect of glucose to raise cyclic AMP levels, like that of insulin release, depends on the presence of extracellular calcium,[14–16] but calcium, by itself, is inhibitory to adenylate cyclase in islets.[1] The possibility that a factor important for the regulation of adenylate cyclase in the intact cell is missing when the enzyme is studied in the broken cell situation was suggested by the fact that calmodulin, a calcium-dependent regulator protein, activates adenylate cyclase in the brain.[17–19] Thus we have studied the possibility that calcium, in the presence of calmodulin, might stimulate adenylate cyclase in islets of Langerhans and thereby afford an explanation for the glucose-induced rise in cyclic AMP levels.

METHODS

Pancreatic islets were isolated from male Wistar rats by the collagenase digestion technique of Lacy and Kostianovsky.[20] Adenylate cyclase activity was measured by the method of Salomon et al.[21] and protein by the method of Lowry et al.[22] Islets were assayed for adenylate cyclase activity under two sets of conditions: (1) Approximately 1500 islets were sonicated in 500 μl of a buffer solution (A) containing 75 mM Tris-HCl (pH 7.5) and 5 mM $MgCl_2$. Twenty microliters of this sonicate was then mixed with 20 μl of the appropriate reaction mixture and 10 μl of test agents or control solution. (2) Approximately 2000 islets were homogenized in a ground glass hand homogenizer in 1 ml of 10 mM

TABLE 1
The effects of fluoride, calcium, calmodulin, and the combination of calcium and calmodulin on adenylate cyclase activity of rat islets in the presence of 200 μM EGTA (expressed as pmol · cyclic AMP · mg^{-1} · min^{-1})

Basal	F^- (10 mM)	Cal (6.6 μM)	Ca^{2+} (150 μM)	Cal + Ca^{2+}	Δ	SEM	P	% change	N
1.93	8.22				6.29	1.04	<0.001	326	10
1.93		2.19			0.26	0.14	<0.1		10
1.93			1.87		−0.06	0.16	<0.8		10
1.93				2.57	0.64	0.15	<0.01	33	10

imidazole buffer (pH 7.5) containing 1 mM EDTA. The homogenate was centrifuged for 15 min at 3600 rpm in a Beckman JS-4.0 rotor at 4°C. The supernatant was discarded and the pellet resuspended in 600 μl of a buffer solution (B) containing 125 mM glycylglycine, 10 mM imidazole, 12.5 mM $MgCl_2$, 2.5 mM dithiothreitol, and 0.5 mM EGTA at pH 7.5. Twenty microliters of this suspension was then mixed with 20 μl of the appropriate reaction mixture and 10 μl of water or test agents for assay. The final assay mixture contained, in addition to the islet suspensions, α-^{32}P-ATP, 0.1 mM; cyclic AMP, 0.1 mM; and an ATP regenerating system of phosphoenolpyruvate, myokinase, and pyruvate kinase. Protein concentration was approximately 20 μg per assay and activity was measured over 20 min at 37°C. Under these conditions the reaction rate is linear for at least 30 min. Blanks were always close to background levels of radioactivity. Statistics were performed using Student's *t* test.

RESULTS

In the first group of studies, removal of Ca^{2+} by the addition of 500 μM EGTA had a stimulatory effect on adenylate cyclase activity. The basal activity in the absence of EGTA (buffer solution A) was 1.00 ± 0.24 pmol · mg^{-1} · min^{-1} and increased to 1.49 ± 0.24 in the presence of EGTA ($\Delta = 0.49 \pm 0.12$, $P < 0.01$, $N = 8$). Assuming that each islet has a calcium content of 11 pmol,[23] the concentration of Ca^{2+} in the assay could be as high as 13 μM. Simple addition of calmodulin to the sonicate had no effect on the activity of adenylate cyclase; in these experiments basal activity was 0.94 ± 0.27 pmol · mg^{-1} · min^{-1}, and in the presence of calmodulin the activity was 0.88 ± 0.23 ($\Delta = -0.06 \pm 0.10$, $P < 0.6$, $N = 7$). Because of the possible inhibitory effects of Ca^{2+} and the lack of response to calmodulin, the second group of experiments was performed with a buffer containing EGTA (buffer solution B) in the presence or absence of Ca^{2+}. These conditions were similar to those used by Brostrom et al.[17,18] in their studies on calmodulin stimulation of adenylate cyclase in brain tissue. The results are presented in Table 1. Calmodulin alone (6.6 μM) caused a small but nonsignificant increase in activity. Ca^{2+} (150 μM), in the presence of 200 μM EGTA, did not affect the activity of the enzyme, whereas the combination of calmodulin and 150 μM Ca^{2+} caused a reproducible and highly significant 33% increase in adenylate cyclase activity. NaF (10 mM) caused, as expected, a marked stimulation of adenylate cyclase.

Further studies were performed with higher concentrations of free Ca^{2+} by carrying out experiments in the 200 μM EGTA buffer, but increasing the Ca^{2+} concentration to 200 and 250 μM. These results are shown in Table 2. No significant effects were detected, although the activity decreased from 1.76 to 1.34 pmol · mg^{-1} · min^{-1} with 250 μM Ca^{2+}.

DISCUSSION

Calmodulin is a ubiquitous protein involved in a variety of calcium-dependent control mechanisms. With Ca^{2+} it has been shown to stimulate adenylate cyclase,[17–19] cyclic nucleotide phosphodiesterase,[24–26] Ca^{2+}-dependent ATPase,[27] NAD-kinase,[28] myosin light chain kinase,[29] glycogen synthase phosphorylation,[30] and membrane protein phosphorylation.[31] The results presented here demonstrate the existence of a Ca^{2+}-dependent adenylate cyclase in rat islets of Langerhans which is dependent on calmodulin for its expression. Ca^{2+} alone is inhibitory to adenylate cyclase, as has been demonstrated directly (results not shown) and as can be deduced from the stimulatory effect of EGTA. Calmodulin alone was without effect. This is similar to the result obtained with brain tissue, and presumably reflects the need for careful control of free Ca^{2+} to strike a balance between the Ca^{2+} concentration that interacts with calmodu-

TABLE 2
The effects of calmodulin in the presence of 200 μM EGTA and two different concentrations of Ca^{2+} (200 and 250 μM) (expressed as pmol · cyclic AMP · mg^{-1} · min^{-1})

Basal	Cal (6.6 μM)	Ca^{2+} (200 μM)	Cal + Ca^{2+}	Δ	SEM	P	N
1.76	2.05			0.29	0.21	<0.3	5
1.76		1.74		−0.02	0.42	>0.9	5
1.76			1.85	0.09	0.23	<0.8	5
		Ca^{2+} (250 μM)					
1.76	2.05			0.29	0.21	<0.3	5
1.76		1.34		−0.42	0.37	<0.4	5
1.76			1.78	0.02	0.23	>0.9	5

lin and stimulates adenylate cyclase and the concentration that directly inhibits adenylate cyclase. That the Ca^{2+} concentration has to be maintained between critical constraints can be seen from the results presented. In the presence of EGTA-Ca^{2+} buffer, comprising 200 μM EGTA and 150 μM Ca^{2+}, calmodulin caused a significant stimulation of adenylate cyclase. With 200 μM Ca^{2+} no effect was observed. With 250 μM Ca^{2+} there was a tendency toward inhibition by Ca^{2+}.

This demonstration of a Ca^{2+}-calmodulin-dependent adenylate cyclase in islets of Langerhans could provide an explanation for the glucose-induced rise in cyclic AMP levels. Given that glucose stimulates insulin release by a mechanism that involves increased cytosol Ca^{2+} concentrations, the increased Ca^{2+} could, with calmodulin, cause a secondary rise in adenylate cyclase activity and an increase in the cyclic AMP content. This proposed mechanism is in accord with the following observations: (1) the Ca^{2+}-dependency of the effect,[14,15] (2) the similar anomeric specificity of glucose-induced insulin release and elevation of cyclic AMP,[5-8] (3) the increase in cyclic AMP which has been observed during treatment of islets with ionophore A23187 in the presence of Ca^{2+},[32] and (4) the reduced insulin release and reduced cyclic AMP responses to glucose under fasting conditions,[33,34] in neonatal rats,[5] and in islets from diabetic animals.[35-37] Furthermore, as glucose causes only a small increase in cyclic AMP levels in intact islets, the relatively small (30%) increase in adenylate cyclase activity seen with Ca^{2+} and calmodulin would be appropriate for such a response. It suggests that, of the total adenylate cyclase in the islet, only a small portion is calmodulin-sensitive. The presence of calmodulin-sensitive and -insensitive adenylate cyclases in tissues has already been demonstrated.[38] It should be noted that as rat islets of Langerhans are composed of approximately 80% β-cells, the conclusions on the mechanism of the glucose-induced increase in cyclic AMP levels depend on the absence of a large effect of calcium and calmodulin on the remaining 20% non-β-cells. Further studies on the role of calmodulin with respect to Ca^{2+}-dependent adenylate cyclase and the control of insulin release are in progress.

ACKNOWLEDGMENTS

The authors are grateful to Dr. Claude B. Klee for a generous gift of calmodulin derived from brain tissue and to Dr. Paul Leavis for his help and advice.

This investigation was supported by U.S. Public Health Service grant 5 ROI AM 18460 from the NIAMDD.

Note added in proof. Two papers dealing with the roles of calmodulin in islets of Langerhans were published recently.[39,40]

REFERENCES

1 Sharp, G.W.G.: The adenylate cyclase-cyclic AMP system in islets of Langerhans and its role in the control of insulin release. Diabetologia *16*:287–96, 1979.

2 Charles, M. A., Fanska, R., Schmid, F. G., Forsham, P. H., and Grodsky, G. M.: Adenosine 3′,5′-monophosphate in pancreatic islets: Glucose-induced insulin release. Science *179*:569–71, 1973.

3 Grill, V., and Cerasi, E.: Activation by glucose of adenyl cyclase in pancreatic islets of the rat. FEBS Lett. *33*:311–14, 1973.

4 Grill, V., and Cerasi, E.: Stimulation by D-glucose of cyclic adenosine 3′,5′-monophosphate accumulation and insulin release in isolated pancreatic islets of the rat. J. Biol. Chem. *249*:4196–201, 1979.

5 Grill, V., Asplund, K., Hellerstrom, C., and Cerasi, E.: Decreased cyclic AMP and insulin response to glucose in isolated islets of neonatal rats. Diabetes *24*:746–52, 1975.

6 Grill, V., and Cerasi, E.: Glucose-induced cyclic AMP accumulation in rat islets of Langerhans: Preferential effect of the alpha anomer. FEBS Lett. *54*:80–83, 1975.

7 Niki, A., Niki, H., Miwa, I., and Okuda, J.: Insulin secretion of anomers of D-glucose. Science *186*:150–51, 1974.

8 Grodsky, G. M., Fanska, R., West, L., and Manning, M.: Anomeric specificity of glucose-stimulated insulin release: Evidence for a glucoreceptor? Science *186*:536–38, 1974.

9 Capito, K., and Hedeskov, C. J.: Effects of glucose metabolites and calcium ions on adenylate cyclase activity in homogenates of mouse pancreatic islets. Biochem. J. *162*:569–73, 1977.

10 Sams, D. J., and Montague, W.: The role of adenosine 3′,5′-monophosphate in the regulation of insulin release. Properties of islet cell adenosine 3′,5′-monophosphate phosphodiesterase. Biochem. J. *129*:945–52, 1972.

11 Ashcroft, S. J. H., Randle, P. J., and Täljedal, I.-B.: Cyclic nucleotide phosphodiesterase activity in normal mouse pancreatic islets. FEBS Lett. *20*:263–66, 1972.

12 Bowen, W., and Lazarus, N. R.: Glucose mediated insulin release: 3′,5′-cyclic AMP phosphodiesterase. Diabetes *22*:738–43, 1973.

13 Schubart, U. K., Udem, L., Baum, S. G., and Rosen, O. M.: Characterization of cyclic 3′,5′-nucleotide phosphodiesterase activity in an islet cell tumor of the Syrian hamster. Mol. Cell. Endocrinol. *1*:227–47, 1974.

14 Charles, M. A., Lawecki, J., Pictet, R., and Grodsky, G. M.: Insulin secretion: inter-relationships of glucose, cyclic adenosine 3′,5′-monophosphate and calcium. J. Biol. Chem. *250*:6134–40, 1975.

15 Zawalich, W. S., Karl, R. C., Ferrendelli, J. A., and Matschinsky, F. M.: Factors governing glucose-induced elevation of cyclic adenosine 3′,5′-monophosphate in pancreatic islets. Diabetologia *11*:231–35, 1975.

16 Katada, T., and Ui, M.: Islet-activating protein. Enhanced insulin secretion and cyclic AMP accumulation in pancreatic islets due to activation of native calcium ionophores. J. Biol. Chem. *254*:469–79, 1979.

17 Brostrom, C. O., Huang, Y.-C., Breckenridge, B. McL., and Wolff, D. J.: Identification of a calcium-binding protein as a calcium-dependent regulator of brain adenylate cyclase. Proc. Natl. Acad. Sci. USA *72*:64–68, 1975.

18 Brostrom, C. O., Brostrom, M. A., and Wolff, D. J.: Calcium-dependent adenylate cyclase from rat cerebral cortex: Reversible activation by sodium fluoride. J. Biol. Chem. *252*:5677–85, 1977.

19 Brostrom, M. A., Brostrom, C. O., and Wolff, D. J.: Calcium-dependent adenylate cyclase from rat cerebral cortex: Activation by guanine nucleotides. Arch. Biochem. Biophys. *191*:341–50, 1978.

20 Lacy, P., and Kostianovsky, M.: Method for the isolation of intact islets of Langerhans from the rat pancreas. Diabetes *16*:35–39, 1967.

21 Salomon, Y., Londos, C., and Rodbell, M.: A highly sensitive adenylate cyclase assay. Anal. Biochem. *58*:541–48, 1974.

22 Lowry, O. H., Rosebrough, N. S., Farr, A. L., and Randall, R. J.: Protein measurement with the Folin-phenol reagent. J. Biol. Chem. *193*:265–75, 1951.

23 Kikuchi, M., Wollheim, C. B., Cuendet, G. S., Renold, A. E., and Sharp, G. W. G.: Studies on the dual effects of glucose on $^{45}Ca^{++}$ efflux from isolated rat islets. Endocrinology *102*:1339–49, 1978.

24 Cheung, W. Y.: Cyclic 3′,5′-nucleotide phosphodiesterase. Evidence for and properties of a protein activator. J. Biol. Chem. *246*:2859–69, 1970.

25 Wolff, D. J., and Brostrom, C. O.: Calcium-binding phosphoprotein from pig brain: Identification as a calcium-dependent regulator of brain cyclic nucleotide-phosphodiesterase. Arch. Biochem. Biophys. *163*:349–58, 1974.

26 Brostrom, C. O., and Wolff, D. J.: Calcium-dependent cyclic nucleotide phosphodiesterase from glial tumor cells. Arch. Biochem. Biophys. *165*:715–27, 1974.

27 Luthra, M. G., Hildenbrandt, G. R., and Hanahan, D. J.: Studies on the soluble activator of Ca^{++}-Mg^{++} ATPase found in various mammalian erythrocytes. Biochim. Biophys. Acta *419*:164–79, 1976.

28 Anderson, J. M., and Cormier, M. J.: Calcium-dependent regulator of NAD kinase in higher plants. Biochem. Biophys. Res. Commun. *84*:595–602, 1978.

29 Yazawa, M., Kuwayama, H., and Yagi, K.: Modulator protein as a Ca^{2+}-dependent activator of rabbit skeletal myosin light-chain kinase. Purification and characterization. J. Biochem. (Tokyo) *84*:1253–58, 1978.

30 Srivastava, A. K., Waisman, D. M., Brostrom, C. O., and Soderling, T. R.: Stimulation of glycogen synthase phosphorylation by calcium-dependent regulator protein. J. Biol. Chem. *254*:583–86, 1979.

31 Schulman, H., and Greengard, P.: Ca^{2+}-dependent protein phosphorylation system in membranes from various tissues, and its activation by calcium dependent regulator. Proc. Natl. Acad. Sci. USA *75*:5432–36, 1978.

32 Karl, R. C., Zawalich, W. S., Ferrendelli, J. A., and Matschinsky, F. M.: The role of Ca^{2+} and cyclic adenosine 3′,5′-monophosphate in insulin released induced in vitro by the divalent cation ionophore A23187. J. Biol. Chem. *250*:4574–79, 1975.

33 Wolters, G. H. J., Konijnendijk, W., and Bouman, P. R.: Effects of fasting on insulin secretion, islet glucose metabolism, and the cyclic adenosine

3′,5′-monophosphate content of rat pancreatic islets in vitro. Diabetes *26*:530–37, 1977.

[34] Rabinovitch, A., Grill, V., Renold, A. E., and Cerasi, E.: Insulin release and cyclic AMP accumulation in response to glucose in pancreatic islets of fed and starved rats. J. Clin. Invest. *58*:1209–16, 1976.

[35] Rabinovitch, A., Renold, A. E., and Cerasi, E.: Decreased cyclic AMP and insulin responses to glucose in pancreatic islets of diabetic Chinese hamsters. Diabetologia *12*:581–87, 1976.

[36] Rabinovitch, A., Gutzeit, A., Grill, V., Kikuchi, M., Renold, A. E., and Cerasi, E.: Defective insulin secretion in the spiny mouse (*Acomys cahirinus*), possible value in the study of the pathophysiology of diabetes. Isr. J. Med. Sci. *11*:730–37, 1975.

[37] Boquist, L., Hellman, B., Lernmark, Å., and Täljedal, I.-B.: Content of adenosine 3′,5′-cyclic monophosphate in the pancreatic islets of mice with a hereditary defect of insulin secretion. Biochem. Biophys. Res. Commun. *60*:1391–96, 1974.

[38] Westcott, K. R., La Porte, D. C., and Storm, D. R.: Resolution of adenylate cyclase sensitive and insensitive to Ca^{2+} and calcium-dependent regulatory protein (CDR) by CDR-Sepharose affinity chromatography. Proc. Natl. Acad. Sci. USA *76*:204–08, 1979.

[39] Valverde, I., Vandermeers, A., Anjaneyulu, R., and Malaisse, W. J.: Calmodulin activation of adenylate cyclase in pancreatic islets. Science *206*:225–27, 1979.

[40] Sugden, M. C., Christie, M. R., and Ashcroft, S. J. H.: Presence and possible role of calcium-dependent regulator (calmodulin) in rat islets of Langerhans. FEBS Lett. *105*:95–100, 1979.

Overnight Basal Insulin Requirements in Fasting Insulin-dependent Diabetics

WILLIAM L. CLARKE, MOREY W. HAYMOND, AND JULIO V. SANTIAGO

SUMMARY

Overnight basal insulin requirements to maintain eugycemia were determined in six insulin-requiring diabetic subjects using a feedback-controlled (closed loop) insulin infusion system. Mean hourly insulin infusion rates, required to maintain plasma glucose concentrations at approximately 100 mg/dl, were remarkably stable from 2400 h to 0600 h; however, a twofold to threefold increase in insulin requirements was observed in each subject between 0600 h and 0900 h. This increase in amount of basal insulin required was not associated with increases in plasma glucagon or growth hormone concentrations, but occurred simultaneously with normal diurnal increases in plasma cortisol. These findings suggest that normal diurnal increases in plasma cortisol, independent of the content of the morning meal, contribute to the increased amount of morning insulin required in diabetic subjects. Programs designed for optimal open loop insulin delivery may benefit from modifications designed to coincide with this increase in amount of basal insulin required in the early morning. DIABETES *29*:78–80, January 1980.

The development of closed-loop and open-loop devices for improved metabolic control in diabetes has focused interest on the insulin delivery rate required to normalize blood glucose concentrations in insulin-dependent diabetics. During the course of studies designed to determine the amount of insulin required to maintain euglycemia overnight with a feedback-controlled (closed loop) insulin infusion system, we have observed a striking increase in inulin requirements in diabetic subjects between 0600 h and 0900 h. This diurnal variability in basal insulin requirements is synchronous with the diurnal increase in plasma cortisol seen in these diabetic subjects.

From the Department of Pediatrics, Divisions of Endocrinology and of Diabetes, University of Virginia Medical Center, Charlottesville, Va.; the Edward Mallinckrodt Department of Pediatrics and the Department of Medicine, Washington University School of Medicine; and the Division of Metabolism and Endocrinology, St. Louis Children's Hospital, St. Louis, Missouri.

Address reprint requests to William L. Clarke, M.D., Department of Pediatrics, Box 386, University of Virginia Medical Center, Charlottesville, Virginia 22908.

Received for publication 17 September 1979.

METHODS

Six insulin-requiring diabetic subjects (ages 12–36 yr), each within 10% of ideal body weight (Metropolitan Life Insurance Tables), were studied on the Clinical Research Units at the University of Virginia and at Washington University. Informed consent was obtained from each subject and his parents where applicable. Each subject had presented in diabetic ketoacidosis at the time of original diagnosis and had required subcutaneous insulin therapy for at least 1 yr before the study.

Control of each subject's plasma glucose concentrations was initiated with a bedside, closed-loop, insulin delivery system (Biostator, Miles Laboratories) before breakfast or after the evening meal. Four subjects were studied on the day of admission, while two were studied 4 days after admission. The characteristics of the Biostator and its use in diabetic subjects have been reported previously.[1,2] Postprandial hyperglycemia was corrected within 6 h of Biostator control, and plasma glucose concentrations were maintained at approximately 100 mg/dl from 2400 h to 0900 h. All patients slept from 2400 h to 0900 h. Mean hourly basal insulin requirements, defined as the amount of insulin required to maintain euglycemia after the plasma glucose concentrations had been lowered to 100 mg/dl for at least 1 h, were calculated from the printout of the minute-by-minute insulin delivery by the Biostator. Blood samples were obtained at 2400 h and at 0600 h for determination of cortisol, glucagon, and growth hormone concentrations. Plasma cortisol was measured in a competitive protein-binding assay,[3] while plasma glucagon[4] and growth hormone[5] were measured by radioimmunoassay.

Statistical analyses were performed utilizing a paired *t* test, and all data are expressed as mean ± 1 SE.

RESULTS

Mean plasma glucose concentrations were maintained at 96 ± 1 mg/dl from 2400 h to 0900 h (Table 1). No patient

TABLE 1
Mean hourly plasma glucose concentrations (mg/dl) and mean plasma glucose concentrations (mg/dl ± SE) from 2400 h to 0600 h and from 0600 h to 0900 h in six insulin-requiring diabetic subjects

Patient no.:	1	2	3	4	5	6	X̄	SEM	
2400–0100	103	72	106	84	112	95			
0100–0200	107	74	95	78	102	117			
0200–0300	101	66	118	74	105	124			
0300–0400	91	72	98	76	104	102			
0400–0500	100	78	94	84	101	112			
0500–0600	98	74	98	86	101	106			
X̄, 2400–0600	100 ± 2	73 ± 2	102 ± 4	80 ± 2	104 ± 2	109 ± 4	95	2.0	
0600–0700	98	84	88	94	96	111			
0700–0800	96	85	99	102	113	115			NS
0800–0900	99	84	102	96	102	—			
X̄, 0600–0900	98 ± 1	84 ± 0.3	96 ± 4	97 ± 2	104 ± 5	112 ± 2	96	1.0	

exhibited a mean hourly plasma glucose concentration of less than 66 mg/dl or greater than 124 mg/dl, and neither of these extremes occurred within 3 h of 0600 h. Mean hourly basal insulin requirements were low and constant (12 ± 0.5 mU/kg/h) in each individual from 2400 h to 0600 h, but increased significantly to 23 ± 2 mU/kg/h ($P < 0.025$) between 0600 h and 0900 h (Table 2). The increase in individual insulin requirements ranged from 38 to 1300%. No consistent correlation was observed between the degree of nocturnal decrease in plasma glucose and the subsequent rise in insulin requirements after 0600 h. Infusions of dextrose were not required to correct for overinsulinization at any time. Plasma glucagon concentrations averaged 163 ± 22 pg/ml by 0600 h ($P < 0.01$), while plasma growth hormone concentrations fell from 10.3 ± 6 ng/ml at 2400 h to 1.6 ± 0.5 ng/ml at 0600 h (Table 3). Mean plasma cortisol concentrations increased from 2.4 ± 0.5 μg/ml at 2400 h to 13.2 ± 1.4 μg/ml ($P < 0.001$) at 0600 h.

DISCUSSION

In previous studies using feedback-controlled (closed loop) insulin delivery systems, it was demonstrated that significantly greater amounts of insulin are required intravenously to normalize blood glucose concentrations after breakfast than after either lunch or dinner.[2,6,7] This finding has been corroborated in recent studies utilizing nonfeedback-controlled preprogrammed (open loop) insulin delivery systems, which infuse insulin either intravenously or subcutaneously.[8,9] The increased amount of insulin required by diabetics during breakfast occurs even when subsequent meals contain a larger caloric content. In normal subjects, it has been demonstrated that endogenous insulin release is greater after breakfast than after either lunch or dinner.[10,12]

In the present study, the basal insulin required to maintain euglycemia remain remarkably constant from 2400 h to 0600 h under closed loop glucose control. At 0600 h, a significant increase in insulin requirements is detected. This increase in insulin requirements occurs at a time when plasma glucagon and growth hormone concentrations are low, but plasma cortisol concentrations are significantly elevated. Although it could be postulated that the changes in insulin requirements observed in our patients within a single 24 h period are transient, parallel studies in four insulin-requiring diabetic patients on 3–10 consecutive days utilizing an open-loop (preprogrammable) insulin delivery system have uncovered a 68 ± 9% rise in plasma glucose concentration from 0600 h to 0800 h when insulin was delivered at a constant rate (0.2 to 1.3 U/h) from 2400 h to 0800 h.

Previous studies in our laboratories[13,14] have demonstrated that overnight-fasted normal children and adults, as well as nondiabetic obese adults, maintain stable plasma glucose, insulin, glucagon, and growth hormone concentrations despite significant increases in early morning plasma cortisol concentrations. However, Shanoon et al.[15] have recently reported that infusions of cortisol (5 mg/m²/h), designed to mimic physiologic cortisol increments into normal and insulin-treated euglycemic diabetic subjects, resulted in significant elevations in blood glucose concentrations only in the diabetic subjects. They suggest that diabetic patients are exquisitely sensitive to cortisol and that normal

TABLE 2
Hourly insulin infusion rates (mU/kg/h) and mean insulin infusion rates (mU/kg/h ± SE) from 2400 h to 0600 h and from 0600 h to 0900 h in six insulin-requiring diabetic subjects

Patient no.:	1	2	3	4	5	6	X̄	SEM	
2400–0100	24	3	5	8	22	4			
0100–0200	23	1	2	16	17	15			
0200–0300	31	1	2	13	25	7			
0300–0400	23	2	3	4	19	7			
0400–0500	28	1	4	6	20	16			
0500–0600	25	2	6	10	19	9			
X̄, 2400–0600	26 ± 1	2 ± 0.3	4 ± 1	10 ± 2	20 ± 1	10 ± 2	12	0.5	
0600–0700	25	16	16	12	24	12			
0700–0800	49	29	24	15	18	16			P < 0.025
0800–0900	34	27	14	16	36	—			
X̄, 0600–0900	36 ± 7	24 ± 4	18 ± 3	14 ± 1	26 ± 5	14 ± 2	23	2.0	

TABLE 3
Plasma cortisol (μg/ml), glucagon (pg/ml), and growth hormone (ng/ml) concentrations, obtained at 2400 h and 0600 h, in six insulin-requiring diabetic subjects

Patient no.:	1	2	3	4	5	6	$\bar{X}$	SEM	
				Cortisol (μg/ml)					
2400 h	1.0	1.0	1.8	3.0	3.8	3.9	2.4	0.5	$P < 0.001$
0600 h	14.4	12.9	13.9	7.6	12.2	18.5	13.2	1.4	
				Glucagon (pg/ml)					
2400 h	187	84	93	173	114	228	163	22	$P < 0.01$
0600 h	140	50	79	106	89	180	107	19	
				Growth Hormone (ng/ml)					
2400 h	2.1	1.1	8.0	40.0	8.6	1.9	10.3	6.0	NS
0600 h	2.1	0.8	3.7	1.7	0.9	0.7	1.6	0.5	

elevations in plasma cortisol may be responsible, in part, for glucose instability in insulin-treated diabetic patients.

Our findings suggest that overnight-fasted insulin-requiring diabetic subjects are sensitive to normal diurnal rises in plasma cortisol and that a twofold to threefold increase in early morning basal insulin requirements is necessary to maintain euglycemia in these individuals. It would appear that normal diurnal elevations in plasma cortisol, independent of the content of the morning meal, contribute to the increased morning insulin requirements observed in diabetic subjects. These observations indicate that programs for optimal open-loop insulin delivery may benefit from modifications designed to coincide with the increased basal insulin requirements that occur in diabetic subjects in the early morning hours.

ACKNOWLEDGMENTS
This work was supported, in part, by NIH grants 1P60AM22125, 5SO7RR05431-17, RR-00847, AM20579, RR-00036, AM01921, and 1F32AM05544 and by a grant from the St. Louis Chapter of the American Diabetes Association.

REFERENCES

[1] Clarke, W., and Santiago, J.: The characteristics of a new glucose sensor for use in an artificial pancreatic beta cell. Artif. Organs *1*:78, 1977.
[2] Clarke, W., Thomas, L., and Santiago, J.: Clinical evaluation and preliminary studies on the use of an artificial pancreatic beta cell in juvenile diabetes mellitus. J. Pediatr. *91*:590, 1977.
[3] Beitins, I., Shaw, M., Kowarski, A., and Migeon, C.: Comparison of competitive protein binding radioassay of cortisol to double isotope dilution and Porter-Silber methods. Steroids *15*:765, 1975.
[4] Leichter, S., Pagliara, A., Grieder, M., Pohl, S., Rosai, J., and Kipnis, D.: Uncontrolled diabetes mellitus and hyperglucagonemia associated with an islet cell carcinoma. Am. J. Med. *48*:285, 1975.
[5] Schalch, D., and Parker, M.: A sensitive double antibody immunoassay for human growth hormone in plasma. Nature *203*:1141, 1964.
[6] Santiago, J., Clarke, W., and Arias, F.: Studies with a pancreatic beta cell simulator in the third trimester of pregnancies complicated by diabetes. Am. J. Obstet. Gynecol. *132*:455, 1978.
[7] Santiago, J., Clemens, A., Clarke, W., and Kipnis, D.: Closed-loop and open-loop devices for blood glucose control in normal and diabetic subjects. Diabetes *28*:71, 1979.
[8] Genuth, S., and Martin, P.: Control of hyperglycemia in adult diabetics by pulsed insulin delivery. Diabetes *23*:397, 1974.
[9] Tamborlane, W., Sherwin, R., Genel, M., and Felig, P.: Reduction to normal of plasma glucose in juvenile diabetes by subcutaneous administration of insulin with a portable infusion pump. N. Engl. J. Med. *300*:573, 1979.
[10] Tasaka, Y., Sekine, M., Wakatsuki, M. et al.: Levels of pancreatic glucagon, insulin and glucose during twenty-four hours of the day in normal subjects. Horm. Metab. Res. *7*:205, 1975.
[11] Hansen, A., and Johansen, K.: Diurnal patterns of blood glucose, serum free fatty acids, insulin, glucagon and growth hormone in normals and juvenile diabetics. Diabetologia *6*:27, 1970.
[12] Genuth, S.: Plasma insulin and glucose profiles in normal, obese, and diabetic persons. Ann. Intern. Med. *79*:812, 1973.
[13] Santiago, J., Haymond, M., Karl, I., Clarke, W., Pagliara, A., and Kipnis, D.: Comparative substrate and hormone response to fasting in normal adults and children. Presented at the 56th Annual Meeting of the Endocrine Society, Atlanta, Ga., June 1974.
[14] Santiago, J., Haymond, M., Clarke, W., and Pagliara, A.: Glucagon, insulin and glucose responses to physiologic testing in normal and massively obese adults. Metabolism *25*:1115, 1977.
[15] Shanoon, H., Hendler, R., and Sherwin, R.: Hypersensitivity to cortisol (C) and epinephrine (E) in normoglycemic insulin-treated diabetics: a mechanism for diabetic instability. Diabetes *28* (Program):353, 1979 (abstract 36).

The Effect of Aprotinin on the Absorption of Subcutaneously Injected Regular Insulin in Normal Subjects

MICHAEL BERGER, HANS J. CÜPPERS, PHILIPPE A. HALBAN, AND ROBIN E. OFFORD

SUMMARY

The effect of aprotinin on the absorption of regular insulin was assessed in normal man. Ten units of Actrapid insulin were subcutaneously injected together with 1.4 mg aprotinin (i.e., 0.5 ml of Trasylol) or an equivalent volume of physiologic saline (controls) into the thighs of overnight-fasted normal subjects. Aprotinin caused an increase in the rate of insulin entry into the circulation; the absolute amount of insulin that was detected in the circulation during the course of the experiment was also higher. In addition, the onset of the hypoglycemic action of exogenous insulin was significantly accelerated when insulin was administered together with aprotinin. These data suggest that aprotinin increases the absorption rate of subcutaneously injected insulin from its depot into the circulation, possibly by an inhibition of the local degradation of exogenous insulin at the injection site. DIABETES *29*:81–83, January 1980.

We have recently reported that a considerable proportion of subcutaneously injected insulin is degraded at the site of injection, i.e., before it even reaches the circulation.[1] In addition, we have demonstrated that the degradative activity of rat adipose tissue in vitro is at least partially specific to insulin and that the degradation of insulin by adipose tissue slices in vitro can be inhibited by the bovine pancreatic protease inhibitor aprotinin.[2] This study indicates that the absorption into the circulation of subcutaneously injected insulin in normal man is accelerated when the hormone is administered together with aprotinin.

From the Department of Medicine E, Düsseldorf University, Düsseldorf, West Germany; the Institut de Biochimie Clinique, University of Geneva, Geneva, Switzerland; and the Laboratory of Molecular Biophysics, Department of Zoology, Oxford University, Oxford, England.
Address reprint requests to Michael Berger, M.D., Department of Medicine E, University Düsseldorf, Moorenstrasse 5, 4 Düsseldorf, West Germany.
Received for publication 1 October 1979.

MATERIALS AND METHODS

The experiments were carried out in accord with the Helsinki Declaration of 1975 in four male volunteers of normal body weight (mean weight 73 kg, range 67–78 kg; mean height 178 cm, range 170–186 cm), mean age 24 yr (range 21–27 yr), and free of acute or chronic illnesses, who had never been injected with insulin or aprotinin before. The individuals reported to the laboratory on two consecutive mornings after an overnight fast. Throughout the experiments they rested in a supine position. A Teflon catheter was inserted into an antecubital vein, kept patent with 0.9% saline, and was used to draw venous blood samples at indicated time intervals (Figure 1). At time zero, 10 U of Actrapid insulin (Novo Industri, Copenhagen, Denmark) was subcutaneously injected into the thigh. Immediately before administration, insulin was mixed within the injection syringe with 0.5 ml 0.9% saline or with 0.5 ml aprotinin solution (Trasylol, Bayer AG, Leverkusen, West Germany), obtained in ampules of isotonic saline solution at 20,000 kallikrein inhibitor units (KIU) per ml, equivalent to 10,000 KIU. Separate sets of experiments showed that the rate of entry of 10 U exogenous insulin into the circulation was independent of the concentration of the injected solution over the range from 40 to 12 U insulin/ml. In two subjects insulin mixed with saline was injected on the first experimental day; in the two remaining subjects the insulin-Trasylol mixture was injected first.

Except for one individual presenting some minor symptoms of hypoglycemia during both experimental conditions at 1 h following the insulin administration, no untoward side effects of the test procedure became apparent.

In control experiments, the effect of aprotinin (10,000 KIU Trasylol) subcutaneously injected together with 0.25 ml 0.9% saline was examined in four healthy volunteers, matched for age, sex, height, and weight.

Blood glucose and serum insulin were measured as previously reported;[3] serum C-peptide levels were determined according to Kaneko et al.[4] using a commercially available kit system (Byk-Mallinckrodt, 6057 Dietzenbach, West Germany).

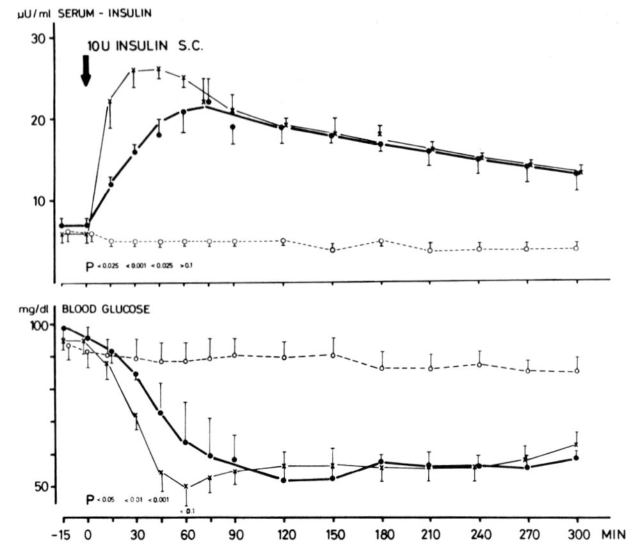

FIGURE 1. Effect of aprotinin on the increase of serum insulin and the fall of blood glucose levels after the subcutaneous injection of 10 U Actrapid insulin in four normal men. Means ±SEM are given. P values indicate statistical significance of differences for the time points indicated by paired comparison. (—×—): 0.5 ml aprotinin Trasylol, equivalent to 10,000 KIU, was added to 10 U of Actrapid insulin. (—•—): 0.5 ml 0.9% saline was added to 10 U of Actrapid insulin. (--O--): the results of control experiments are given, in which 0.5 ml aprotinin Trasylol, equivalent to 10,000 KIU, was subcutaneously injected together with 0.25 ml 0.9% saline in four matched control subjects.

RESULTS

The addition of aprotinin to subcutaneously injected insulin accelerated the rise of circulating insulin and induced significantly higher serum insulin levels at 15, 30, and 45 min after the administration of the hormone (Figure 1). In addition, the maximal serum insulin concentration reached during the experimental procedure was significantly higher when insulin was injected together with aprotinin, compared with the control injections (28 ± 2 SD versus 22 ± 2 SD μU/ml, $P < 0.01$ on paired comparison). As a consequence, the onset of the hypoglycemic action of the subcutaneously injected regular insulin was accelerated by the protease inhibitor; during the first hour following the insulin injection, blood glucose levels were significantly lower when insulin had been injected together with aprotinin, compared with the control experiments (Figure 1). Under both sets of experimental conditions, there was a continuous fall of circulating C-peptide levels, indicating the expected suppression of endogenous insulin secretion. No additional effect of aprotinin on the course of C-peptide levels was observed (Table 1).

In control experiments, any effect of aprotinin on blood glucose or serum insulin levels was ruled out (Figure 1).

DISCUSSION

This study demonstrates that the early rise of circulating insulin levels, following the subcutaneous injection of regular insulin in normal man, is accelerated and increased when the hormone is injected together with 10,000 KIU aprotinin, a bovine pancreatic protease inhibitor. This effect of aprotinin is corroborated by a significant amplification of the early hypoglycemic effect of subcutaneously injected insulin. On the other hand, there was no apparent effect of aprotinin on the suppression of endogenous insulin secretion, induced presumably via the rapid fall of glycemia, under the experimental conditions. Thus, it is assumed that the aprotinin-induced rise of circulating insulin levels in the first hour after the subcutaneous injection of regular insulin is due to an acceleration of insulin absorption into the circulation. This assumption is in agreement with the view that the early phase of the rise of exogenous insulin concentration in the circulation is primarily determined by the rate of absorption of insulin from its subcutaneous depot.[5–9] The molecular mechanisms involved in the absorption of subcutaneously injected insulin into the bloodstream remain to be elucidated. Aprotinin, however, could influence this process in a variety of possible ways, such as alterations of the local circulation or simply by working as an insulin carrier.

On the basis of our recent observations,[1,2] it might also be suggested that aprotinin increases the absorption rate of subcutaneously injected insulin, and amplifies its biological effect by inhibition of the local degradation of exogenous insulin at the injection site. If aprotinin were to likewise increase the biological effectiveness of subcutaneously injected insulin in diabetic patients, this observation should not be without therapeutic implications.

ACKNOWLEDGMENTS

The authors thank M. Schütte for her excellent technical assistance.

This study has been supported in part by the German Research Association, grant G 2 (Diabetology Düsseldorf), and the Medical Research Council of the United Kingdom.

REFERENCES

[1] Berger, M., Halban, P. A., Girardier, L., Seydoux, J., Offord, R. E., and Renold, A. E.: Absorption kinetics of subcutaneously injected insulin. Evidence for degradation at the injection site. Diabetologia *17*:97–99, 1979.

TABLE 1
Effect of insulin, 10 U Actrapid, subcutaneously injected together with aprotinin, 10,000 KIU Trasylol or an equivalent volume of 0.9% saline, on circulating C-peptide levels in four healthy men (means ± SEM).

	Time (min)														
	−15	0	15	30	45	60	75	90	120	150	180	210	240	270	300
Controls (ng/ml) (insulin injected together with saline)	1.74 ± 0.10	1.73 ± 0.09	1.58 ± 0.01	1.43 ± 0.08	1.14 ± 0.06	0.94 ± 0.11	0.91 ± 0.07	0.86 ± 0.06	0.68 ± 0.05	0.57 ± 0.04	0.58 ± 0.05	0.51 ± 0.06	0.45 ± 0.05	0.43 ± 0.07	0.43 ± 0.06
Aprotinin experiments (ng/ml) (insulin injected together with Trasylol)	1.66 ± 0.08	1.65 ± 0.08	1.58 ± 0.02	1.28 ± 0.09	1.11 ± 0.15	0.89 ± 0.09	0.77 ± 0.08	0.74 ± 0.04	0.58 ± 0.04	0.59 ± 0.04	0.52 ± 0.02	0.51 ± 0.03	0.50 ± 0.03	0.48 ± 0.02	0.46 ± 0.03

[2] Offord, R. E., Philippe, J., Davies, J. G., Halban, P. A., and Berger, M.: The inhibition of degradation of insulin by ophthalmic acid and a bovine pancreatic protease inhibitor. Biochem. J. *182*:249–51, 1979.

[3] Berger, M., Berchtold, P., Cüppers, H. J., Drost, H., Kley, H. K., Müller, W. A., Wiegelmann, W., Zimmerman-Telschow, H., Gries, F. A., Krüskemper, H. L., and Zimmermann, H.: Metabolic and hormonal effects of muscular exercise in juvenile type diabetics. Diabetologia *13*:355–65, 1977.

[4] Kaneko, T., Oda, H., and Munemura, M.: Radioimmunoassay of human proinsulin C-peptide using synthetic human connecting peptide. Endocrinol. Jpn. *21*:141–45, 1974.

[5] Galloway, J., Root, M. A., Rathmacher, R. P., and Carmichael, R. H.: A comparison of acid regular and neutral regular insulin. Diabetes *22*:471–79, 1973.

[6] Teorell, T.: Kinetics of distribution of substances administered to the body. Arch. Int. Pharmacodyn. *37*:205–25, 1957.

[7] Schou, J.: Absorption of drugs from subcutaneous connective tissue. Pharmacol. Rev. *13*:441–64, 1961.

[8] Berger, M., Halban, P. A., Müller, W. A., Offord, R. E., Renold, A. E., and Vranic, M.: Mobilization of subcutaneously injected tritiated insulin in rats: effects of muscular exercise. Diabetologia *15*:133–40, 1978.

[9] Schlichtkrull, J.: The absorption of insulin. Acta Paediatr. Scand. Suppl. *270*:97–102, 1978.

Disparate Effects of Enkephalin and Morphine upon Insulin and Glucagon Secretion by Islet Cell Cultures

R. A. KANTER, J. W. ENSINCK, AND W. Y. FUJIMOTO

SUMMARY

Insulin and glucagon release from monolayer pancreatic islet cell cultures were inhibited in a dose-response fashion by various enkephalins. Morphine, however, stimulated insulin and glucagon release. Both effects were blocked by naloxone, while naloxone alone had no effect. In isolated and denervated islet cells, opiates directly influence secretion from islet cells. DIABETES 29:84–86, January 1980.

Endogenous opiates (endorphins and enkephalins) are widely distributed in the nervous system and gastrointestinal tract of animals, including man. They have been shown to affect rates of neuronal transmission and the secretion of several pituitary hormones (ADH, prolactin, growth hormone, and gonadotrophins).[1–3] By immunocytochemical techniques, endorphin-like substances have been demonstrated in the A-cells of the islets of Langerhans of the rat,[4] and morphine and B-endorphin have been reported to enhance insulin and glucagon release from the isolated perfused dog pancreas.[5]

Since islets are richly enervated by sympathetic, parasympathetic, and peptidergic systems, opiates might alter islet secretion indirectly by modulating these neuronal influences or directly by interacting with receptors on the islet secretory cells. We have used pancreatic islet cell monolayer cultures, an isolated and denervated islet cell system, to determine if opiates have a direct effect on islet cells and if all opiates act in a similar fashion.

MATERIALS AND METHODS

Pancreatic monolayer cultures were established according to previously described techniques.[6–8] These cultures have been shown by immunocytochemistry to contain cells that stain for insulin, glucagon, somatostatin (SRIF), gastric inhibitory polypeptide, secretin, gastrin, and pancreatic polypeptide.[9–15] Experiments were performed on the fourth day of culture. Experimental incubation medium was Eagle's minimal essential medium supplemented with nonessential amino acids, Earle's salts, and 0.5% (v/v) heat-inactivated fetal bovine serum. All dishes were preincubated for 2 h in 5.5 mM glucose. This was followed by a 1-h incubation during which secretagogues plus varying concentrations of opiate were added to experimental cultures and compared with control cultures with segretagogues alone. Insulin and glucagon were measured in the incubation media by radioimmunoassay.[16,17] Statistical analysis was performed using Newman-Keul's multiple comparison procedure.[18]

The naturally occurring peptides leucine- and methionine-enkephalin, D-ala²-leucine-, and D-phe⁴-leucine-enkephalin analogues were generously provided by Dr. Richard J. Miller of the University of Chicago.

RESULTS

With glucose 16.5 mM, the naturally occurring opiates leucine-enkephalin (LEK) and methionine-enkephalin (MEK) produced, over a concentration range of 0.02 to 2.0 μM, a dose-related suppression of both insulin and glucagon release (Figure 1). D-ala²-leucine-enkephalin (DLE) is an enkephalin analogue that has been reported to resist metabolic degradation.[1] Over the same concentration range, DLE produced a similar suppression of insulin and glucagon release (Figure 1). This suggests that the natural peptides are not significantly degraded in our system. D-phe⁴-leucine-enkephalin is an analogue that has been shown to be less potent in classic opiate bioassays.[1] It required a 10-fold greater concentration than MEK, LEK, or DLE to achieve a similar suppression of insulin and glucagon release.

Enkephalins also reversed insulin and glucagon release stimulated by other secretagogues. The effects of 10 mM arginine and 5 mM theophylline were both significantly diminished by the addition of enkephalin (2.0 μM) to 74% and 83%, respectively, of control insulin levels, and 50% and 45%, respectively, of control glucagon levels.

From the Division of Metabolism and Endocrinology, Department of Medicine, RG 20, University of Washington, Seattle, Washington.
Address reprint requests to John W. Ensinck, M.D., Department of Medicine, Division of Metabolism and Endocrinology, RG 20, University of Washington, Seattle, Washington 98195.
Received for publication 1 October 1979.

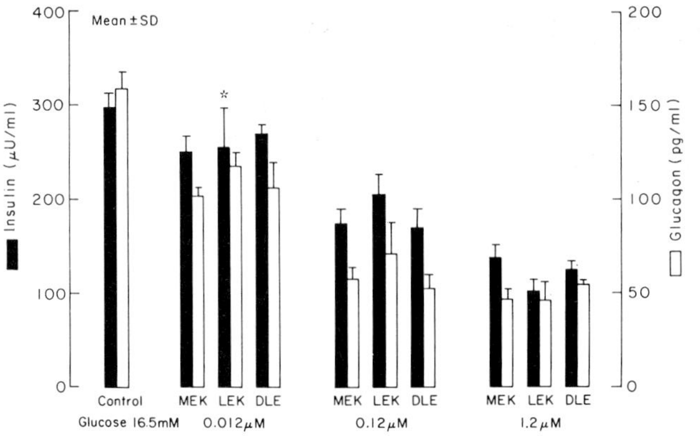

FIGURE 1. The mean (± SD) of insulin and glucagon responses in neonatal rat pancreatic monolayer cultures after 1-h incubation. Control: 16.5 mM glucose alone. Experimental: 16.5 mM glucose plus varying concentrations of methionine-enkephalin (MEK), leucine-enkephalin (LEK), and D-ala²-leucine-enkephalin (DLE). N = 4; when compared with control, *P < 0.05 and for all other experimental values P < 0.01.

Morphine sulfate, an opiate of plant origin, had an effect opposite to that of enkephalin. Morphine (20 μM) significantly enhanced insulin and glucagon secretion (Figure 2). Under similar conditions (5.5 mM glucose plus 10 mM arginine), enkephalin (1.2 μM) inhibited insulin and glucagon levels by 36% and 50%, respectively.

The effects of both enkephalins and morphine were reversed by the opiate antagonist naloxone (20 μM). Naloxone alone did not influence hormonal secretion.

DISCUSSION

In a system free of neuronal input, opiates were found to influence insulin and glucagon secretion. This would suggest that opiates have a direct effect on islet cells and, therefore, may have a role in glucose homeostasis.

FIGURE 2. The mean (± SD) of insulin and glucagon responses in neonatal rat pancreatic monolayer cultures after 1-h incubation. Control: glucose (5.5 mM) and arginine (10 mM). Experimental: glucose (5.5 mM), arginine (10 mM), and morphine sulfate (2.0–20 mM). N = 4, *P < 0.01.

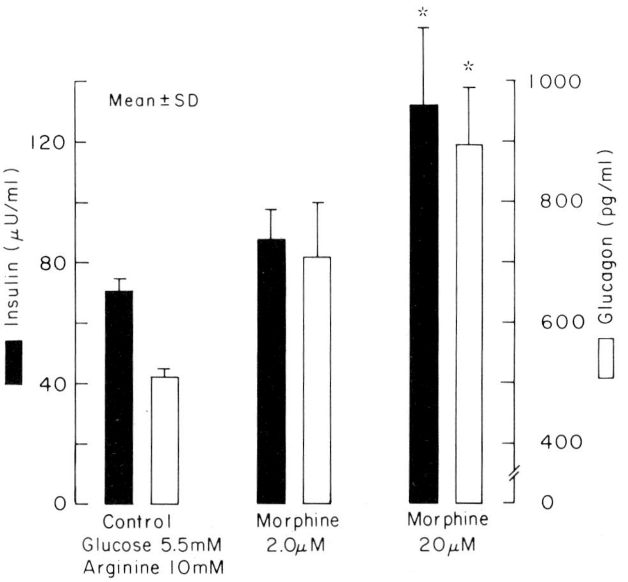

Stubbs et al.[19] found no significant change in insulin, glucagon, or glucose levels with intravenous infusion of a long-acting enkephalin in humans. However, serum growth hormone, prolactin, TSH, and cortisol were significantly altered in those subjects. Thus, although widespread effects of enkephalins were observed, specific effects on insulin and glucagon secretion may have been obscured. Our findings in an isolated system are in agreement with Ipp et al.,[5] who found morphine enhanced stimulated insulin and glucagon secretion in the perfused dog pancreas.

Although opiates perturb the secretion of several pituitary hormones in vivo, they have no effect on their release from isolated pituitary glands.[3] The site of opiate action is the hypothalamus, where they influence the activity of neurosecretory cells that secrete releasing hormones into the hypophyseal portal system. By altering releasing hormone concentrations, opiates secondarily modify pituitary hormone release. This modulating role is analogous to the postulated function of opiates in the spinal cord, where they alter afferent impulse conduction by interacting with presynaptic neurons. By increasing presynaptic membrane potentials, the threshold for conduction is increased and the rate of firing is decreased.[20] The influence of opiates on insulin and glucagon secretion in an isolated and denervated system implies a different mechanism of opiate action: direct effect on islet secretory cells.

Ipp et al.[5] found that both morphine and β-endorphin decreased SRIF secretion in the isolated perfused dog pancreas. Since a fall in SRIF levels is compatible with greater secretion of insulin and glucagon, they raised the possibility that the effects on secretion from A- and D-cells may be mediated through suppression of SRIF release. Because pancreatic monolayers also contain SRIF cells, it is conceivable that enkephalins and morphine also act on D-cells in the cultured islet system.

Recently, at least two different classes of opiate receptors have been identified in rat brain.[21] The μ-receptor is more specific for morphine and other narcotics while the δ-receptor binds enkephalin with much greater affinity. Furthermore, Martin et al.[22] have shown that activation of different opiate receptors may result in opposite physiologic responses. Whether the disparate effects of morphine and enkephalin on insulin and glucagon secretion in rat monolayer islet cultures are due to interaction with different classes of opiate receptors remains to be determined.

A physiologic role of opiates in glucose homeostasis is as yet speculative. Due to their well-documented metabolic instability, enkephalins are unlikely to function as circulating hormones. β-endorphin has been measured in the circulation.[23] But even after stimulation with metyrapone, it is present only in femtomole amounts. Ipp et al.[5] found that micromolar concentrations of β-endorphin were necessary to alter insulin and glucagon secretion in the perfused dog pancreas.

It is conceivable that endogenous opiates reach the islets by neural pathways and modify insulin and glucagon secretion either by directly interacting with A- and B-cells or by influencing SRIF secretion from D-cells, which in turn perturbs adjacent cells.

The finding, in animals, of met-enkephalin in nerve terminals of other endocrine glands (adrenal medulla) is consistent with our hypothesis.[24] In addition, a nonpeptide opiate with chemical properties similar to morphine was found in the nervous system of animals.[25] This makes the postulated presence of "morphine-specific" receptors more physiologically reasonable.

In conclusion, despite the uncertain nature of the exact mechanism of action, our results suggest that opiates have a direct effect on the hormone-producing cells of the islets of Langerhans.

ACKNOWLEDGMENTS

This work has been supported by USPHS grants AM02456, AM15312, AM16008, and AM17047. We wish to acknowledge the excellent technical assistance of Jeanette Teague and Claudine Nist in the performance of these studies and Myrna Anderson for typing the manuscript.

REFERENCES

[1] Miller, R., Chang, K. J., Cuatrecasas, P., Wilkinson, S., Lowe, L., Beddell, C., and Fotlenfant, R.: Distribution and pharmacology of enkephalins and related peptides. *In* Centrally Acting Peptides. Hughes, J., Ed. Baltimore, University Park Press, 1978, pp. 195–213.

[2] Polak, J. M., Bloom, S. R., Sullivan, S. N., Facer, P., and Pearse, A. G. E.: Enkephalin-like immunoreactivity in the human gastrointestinal tract. Lancet *1*:972–73, 1977.

[3] Meites, J., Bruni, J. F., Van Vugt, D. A., and Smith, A. F.: Relation of endogenous opiate peptides and morphine to neuroendocrine functions. Life Sci. *24*:1325–36, 1979.

[4] Grube, D., Voight, K. H., and Weber, E.: Pancreatic glucagon cells contain endorphin-like immunoreactivity. Histochemistry *59*:75–79, 1978.

[5] Ipp, E., Dobbs, R., and Unger, R. H.: Morphine and beta-endorphine influence the secretion of the endocrine pancreas. Nature *276*:190–91, 1978.

[6] Lambert, A. E., Blondel, B., Kanazawa, Y., Orci, L., and Renold, A. E.: Monolayer cell culture of neonatal rat pancreas: light microscopy and evidence for immunoreactive insulin synthesis and release. Endocrinology *90*:239–48, 1972.

[7] Fujimoto, W. Y., Ensinck, J. W., and Williams, R. H.: Somatostatin inhibits insulin and glucagon release by monolayer cell cultures of rat endocrine pancreas. Life Sci. *15*:1999–2004, 1974.

[8] Fujimoto, W. Y., Williams, R. H., and Ensinck, J. W.: Gastric inhibitory polypeptide, cholecystokinin, and secretin effects on insulin and glucagon secretion by islet cell culture. Proc. Soc. Exp. Biol. Med. *160*:349–53, 1979.

[9] Orci, L., Like, A. A., Amherdt, M., Blondel, B., Kanazawa, Y., Marliss, E. B., Lambert, A. E., Wollheim, C. B., and Renold, A. E.: Monolayer cell culture of neonatal rat pancreas: an ultrastructural and biochemical study of functioning endocrine cells. J. Ultrastruct. Res. *43*:270–97, 1973.

[10] Rufener, C., Amherdt, M., DuBois, M. P., and Orci, L.: Ultrastructural immunocytochemical localization of somatostatin in rat pancreatic monolayer culture. J. Histochem. Cytochem. *23*:866–69, 1975.

[11] Smith, P. H., Merchant, F. W., Johnson, D. G., Fujimoto, W. Y., and Williams, R. H.: Immunocytochemical localization of a gastric inhibitory polypeptide-like material within A cells of the endocrine pancreas. Am. J. Anat. *149*:585–90, 1977.

[12] Fujimoto, W. Y., Ensinck, J. W., Merchant, F. W., Williams, R. H., Smith, P. H., and Johnson, D. G.: Stimulation by gastric-inhibitory polypeptide of insulin and glucagon secretion by rat islet culture. Proc. Soc. Exp. Biol. Med. *157*:89–93, 1978.

[13] Braaten, J. T., Greider, M. H., McGuigan, J. E., and Mintz, D. H.: Gastrin in the perinatal rat pancreas and gastric antrum: immuno fluorescent localization of pancreatic gastrin cells and gastrin secretion in monolayer cell culture. Endocrinology *99*:684–91, 1976.

[14] Rufener, C., Amherdt, M., Baltens, D., Yanaihara, N., and Orci, L.: Immunofluorescent localization of secretin in pancreatic monolayer culture. Histochemistry *47*:171–73, 1976.

[15] Rufener, C., Baetens, O., and Orci, L.: Localization of bovine pancreatic polypeptide (BPP)-like immunoreactivity in rat pancreatic monolayer culture. Experientia *32*:919–20, 1976.

[16] Zaharko, D. S., and Beck, L. V.: Studies of a simplified plasma insulin immunoassay using cellulose powder. Diabetes *17*:445–57, 1968.

[17] Ensinck, J. W., Shepard, C., Dudl, R. J., and William, R. H.: Use of benzamidine as a proteolytic inhibitor in the radioimmunoassay of glucagon in plasma. J. Clin. Endocrinol. Metab. *35*:463–67, 1972.

[18] Zar, Z. H.: Biostatistical Analysis. Englewood Cliffs, N.J., Prentice-Hall, 1974, pp. 151–55.

[19] Stubbs, W. A., Jones, A., Edwards, C. R. W., Delitala, G., Jeffcoate, W. J., and Ratter, S. J.: Hormonal and metabolic responses to an enkephalin analogue in normal man. Lancet *2*:1225, 1978.

[20] Chang, K. W., and Cuatrecasas, P.: Multiple opiate receptors. Enkephalins and morphine bind to receptors of different specificity. J. Biol. Chem. *254*: 2610, 1979.

[21] Jessell, T. M., and Iversen, L. L.: Opiate analgesics inhibit substance P release from rat trigeminal nucleus. Nature *268*:549–51, 1977.

[22] Martin, W. R., Eades, C. G., Thompson, J. A., Huppler, R. E., and Gilbert, P. E.: The effects of morphine and nalorphine-like drugs in the non dependent and morphine dependent chronic spinal dog. J. Pharm. Exp. Ther. *197*:517–32, 1976.

[23] Wardlan, S. L., and Franz, A. G.: Measurement of B-endorphin in human plasma. J. Clin. Endocrinol. Metab. *48*:176–80, 1979.

[24] Schultzberg, M., Lundberg, J. M., Hokfelt, T., Terenius, L., Brandt, J., Eide, R. P., and Goldstein, M.: Enkephalin-like immunoreactivity in glands cells and nerve terminals of the adrenal medulla. Neuroscience *3*:1169–86, 1978.

[25] Blume, A. J., Shorr, J., Finberg, J. P. M., and Spector, S.: Binding of the endogenous non-peptide morphine-like compound to opiate receptors. Proc. Natl. Acad. Sci. USA *74*:4927–31, 1977.

Prevention of Hypophosphatemia by Phosphate Infusion During Treatment of Diabetic Ketoacidosis and Hyperosmolar Coma

ULRICH KELLER AND WILLIE BERGER

SUMMARY

To assess the effect of phosphate replacement therapy on the course of diabetic coma, 24 patients with severe diabetic ketoacidosis and 16 patients with nonketotic hyperosmolar coma were randomly assigned either to standardized conventional treatment alone or combined with phosphate infusions. Insulin and fluid therapy produced a rapid fall of plasma phosphorus; almost all patients not receiving phosphate infusions developed marked hypophosphatemia within 12 h. Hypophosphatemia was prevented by administration of 62 ± 5 mmol (range 35–140) sodium phosphate. Initial red blood cell 2,3-diphosphoglycerate (2,3-DPG) concentrations were markedly decreased in ketoacidotic patients. The recovery of 2,3-DPG upon institution of therapy was accelerated when phosphate replacement infusions were given. The increase in 2,3-DPG during the first 48 h was 56% greater ($P < 0.02$) when phosphate was administered, but later the difference between the two treatment groups disappeared. Nonketotic hyperosmolar coma patients revealed normal 2,3-DPG concentrations on admission, and a similar decline of plasma phosphorus occurred, as in ketoacidosis, during treatment. 2,3-DPG levels remained unaffected by phosphate therapy. While plasma calcium levels declined during the initial 48 h in both groups, transient postinfusion hyperphosphatemia was noted in 7 of 17 patients. A favorable effect of phosphate therapy on the clinical course of diabetic ketoacidosis or hyperosmolar coma could not be demonstrated.
DIABETES 29: 87–95, February 1980.

The occurrence of excessive urinary phosphorus excretion in patients with uncontrolled diabetes mellitus has been recognized for more than 100 yr.[1] Severe phosphorus depletion ensued when insulin was withdrawn from diabetic subjects,[2] and marked hypophosphatemia occurred soon after insulin therapy was instituted.

Treatment of phosphorus depletion usually remained neglected until phosphate replacement therapy was reported to be accompanied by an improvement of the mental state and by a statistically significant decrease in fatality rates.[3] Thus, earlier recommendations for treatment of diabetic coma included the administration of phosphate-containing infusions.[4–6] However, a clinical benefit of phosphate therapy was not observed in other studies.[7,8] The opinion regarding the importance of phosphate replacement is divided in more recent reports. Some authors deny the necessity of phosphate therapy[9–11] while others recommend it.[12,13]

The observation of decreased concentrations of red blood cell 2,3-diphosphoglycerate (2,3-DPG) in diabetic ketoacidosis[14–16] and the potential deleterious effects of lowered 2,3-DPG levels on hemoglobin oxygen affinity[17] have refocused attention on the importance of phosphate replacement therapy. Phosphate infusions might accelerate the recovery of 2,3-DPG-levels,[15–18] thereby decreasing hemoglobin-oxygen affinity and improving tissue oxygenation. Hypophosphatemia has recently been recognized to be associated with various clinical ill-effects, and correction by phosphate administration has been advocated.[19]

The present study was performed to evaluate the effect of phosphate replacement therapy on phosphate economy and on 2,3-DPG concentrations, and to assess its clinical significance.

METHODS

Twenty-four patients with severe diabetic ketoacidosis and 16 patients with nonketotic hyperosmolar coma were studied. Ketotic patients were selected when all the following conditions were fulfilled: positive plasma ketone test using Acetest tablets at a dilution of more than 1:2, pH of less than 7.25, and plasma glucose exceeding 400 mg/dl on admission. Cases with nonketotic hyperosmolar coma were included when initial plasma glucose was more than 550

From the Department of Internal Medicine, University Hospital, CH-4031 Basel, Switzerland.
Accepted for publication 14 August 1979.

mg/dl and calculated osmolality exceeded 340 mosmol/kg. Plasma osmolality was calculated as follows:

$$\text{mosmol/kg} = (\text{Na} + \text{K})(\text{mval/L}) \times 2 + \frac{\text{glucose (mg/dl)}}{18} + \frac{\text{urea (mg/dl)}}{6}$$

The disturbance of consciousness was graded as follows: patients in grade 1 were awake and fully responsive; grade 2 indicated obtundance, somnolence, or disorientation; grade 3 indicated stupor with motor reactions to pain but without appropriate verbal responses; and patients in grade 4 were in deep coma without reactions to external stimuli. Consciousness on admission was impaired in all cases except for one patient with severe ketoacidosis. The patients were treated by the house staff on the Medical Intensive Care Unit according to a set schedule. Treatment with fluids, sodium, and potassium chloride was performed as outlined in Table 1 and as described previously.[20,21] Insulin was administered by constant infusion at 4 U/h. The rate was increased to 8 U/h in the rare event that the blood glucose level failed to decline within 4 h. All infusions were administered through a central venous catheter. The rate of fluid therapy was guided by the central venous pressure (CVP). The patients were randomly assigned on admission either to phosphate therapy or to conventional treatment alone (controls). Phosphate was administered by separate infusions containing isotonic-buffered solutions of sodium phosphate (65 mmol/L). Ketotic patients received between 40 and 130 mmol phosphate (Table 3); the first infusion was 65 mmol given over 8 h, except in oliguric patients who received lower amounts as indicated. The dose of phosphate was chosen on the basis of previous experience;[3] the infusion was repeated when hypophosphatemia persisted. Nonketotic patients were treated with 33 mmol phosphate infused over 8 h (Table 5), and the same dose was repeated when hypophosphatemia persisted.

This group of patients purposely received lower amounts of phosphate, since data on phosphate requirements in nonketotic patients were not available. The phosphate infusions were started as soon as diuresis was noted to be present. In most patients bladder catheterization was necessary. Phosphate infusions were started on the average after 8 h and were terminated by 36 h. A bland diet was allowed in fully conscious patients after the second day of treatment.

The first blood samples were drawn on the emergency ward before any therapy was started. Thereafter, blood samples were collected at 1, 2, 4, 6, 12, 24, 48, 72, and 96 h after instituting insulin and fluid therapy. Data of all individual sampling points were obtained in 15 ketotic and in 12 non-

TABLE 1
Treatment of diabetic coma

A. Initial therapy
1. Insulin
   a. Actrapid 16 U i.m.
   b. Continuous infusion of 4 U/h (prepare by adding 50 U Actrapid to 500 ml NaCl 0.9%, discard initial 50 ml)
      If blood glucose fails to decline after 4 h, increase to 8 U/h
      Monitor blood glucose, electrolytes, and blood gases q2h
2. Fluids

Serum-Na (mval/L)	Composition	CVP (cm H_2O)	Amount* (L)	Rate
>165	Glucose 2.5%	<3	1.0	First 8 h (per 1 h)
145–165	NaCl 0.45%	3–8	0.5–1.0	
<145	NaCl 0.9%	8–12	0.5	After 8 h (per 5 h)
		>12	0.25	

* Maximal amount: 10% of body weight per 12 h.

3. Potassium

Serum-K^+	Amount (mval)* pH < 7.1	Amount (mval)* pH > 7.1	Rate
<3.0†	30	20	First 8 h (per 1 h)
3.0–3.9	20	15	
4.0–4.9	15	10	
5.0–5.9	10	5	After 8 h (per 5 h)
>6.0	—	—	

* If patient is oliguric, give K^+ only in case of hypokalemia.
† If hypokalemia is severe, double the K^+ infusion rate (monitor plasma-K^+ q1h).

4. Bicarbonate (only used if pH < 7.1)
   Amount: 0.1 × base excess × BW (kg) = mval Na-bicarbonate/2h

B. If blood glucose has declined to below 300 mg/dl,
infuse 1000 ml glucose 5% over 5 h (if CVP > 10 cm: 500 ml)

Add: Actrapid:

Blood glucose	<200	200–300
Actrapid (U)	10	20–30

Potassium:

Serum K^+	<3.5	3.5–4.9	5–6
Potassium (mval)	80	40	20

ketotic patients. pH was determined initially on arterial blood samples and later in central venous blood. Plasma was obtained by immediate centrifugation, and plasma glucose was measured by an enzymatic method.[22] Plasma inorganic phosphorus was measured using a spectrophotometric method.[23] Calcium was determined on a Technicon Multiple Channel Analyzer, and sodium and potassium by flame photometry. A portion of the blood samples was frozen and stored at −20°C for later determination of 2,3-DPG[24] and of hemoglobin concentration. The normal range of 2,3-DPG in our laboratory, as determined in normal volunteers, is 14.4 ± 2.4 μmol/g Hb (mean ± 2 SD, N = 16).

Student's *t* test was employed for statistical analysis. The data are expressed as means ±SEM unless stated otherwise.

RESULTS

Clinical and biochemical data of patients with ketoacidosis (Tables 2 and 3). Patients' ages ranged from 16 to 85 yr; males and females were equally distributed. The majority of cases were insulin-dependent diabetics. Ketoacidosis developed in 46% of the cases in association with infections. Mean blood glucose concentrations on admission and arterial pH were not statistically different between phosphate-treated patients and controls. Acidosis was usually corrected within the first few hours of therapy, and the pH values were normal after 24 h in both groups of patients.

Plasma phosphorus levels were elevated in 17 of the 24 patients before the institution of therapy, but in 2 cases the initial phosphorus concentrations were below the normal range (<2.5 mg/dl). The degree of hyperphosphatemia was not related to the severity of acidosis or to the impairment of renal function, as suggested by the lack of correlation with urea levels (data not shown). Mean plasma phosphorous concentrations were below normal after 48 h in patients not receiving phosphate compared with phosphate-treated cases (2.2 and 3.6 mg/dl, respectively, $P < 0.02$). Mean plasma calcium levels fell by 1.0 and 0.9 mg/dl in phosphate-treated subjects and in controls, respectively, during the first 48 h. One patient (no. 13) developed hypocalcemia (5.4 mg/dl) after phosphate administration. The decline of calcium was associated with a significant decrease of hemoglobin concentration, which was similar in either group; the mean hemoglobin concentration decreased within 48 h from 15.1 ± 0.5 to 11.1 ± 0.5 and from 15.8 ± 0.5 to 12.0 ± 0.4 g/dl in controls and phosphate-treated patients, respectively. 2,3-DPG levels were markedly lowered in patients with ketoacidosis; the correlation between pH and 2,3-DPG was significant ($r = 0.83$, $P < 0.001$). Cases 4 and 5 as well as 19 and 20 refer to consecutive episodes in two patients. It was noted that in the consecutive episodes 2,3-DPG levels were remarkably similar.

No significant correlation was found between phosphorus and 2,3-DPG concentrations on admission.

Clinical and biochemical data of patients with nonketotic hyperosmolar coma (Tables 4 and 5). The mean age of patients with nonketotic diabetic coma was considerably higher than that of ketotic patients. Nonketotic coma was not observed below age 50. The condition occurred predominantly in females; only one-fifth were males. All patients had maturity-onset diabetes. Diabetes mellitus was unknown before admission in more than 50% of the cases; thus, fre-

TABLE 2
Clinical and biochemical data of patients with ketoacidosis without phosphate therapy

Case	Age, sex	Prior therapy	Associated conditions	Blood glucose (mg/dl)	pH 0 h*	pH 24 h	Plasma phosphorus (mg/dl) 0 h*	Plasma phosphorus (mg/dl) 48 h	Calcium (mg/dl) 0 h*	Calcium (mg/dl) 48 h	2,3-DPG (μmol/g Hb)	Consciousness (grade) 0 h*	Consciousness (grade) 48 h	Complication
1	52 M	Insulin	Spondylitis	820	7.00	7.40	7.0	1.5	10.0	8.4	6.8	2	1	Septicemia following
2	28 M	Insulin	Omission of insulin	685	6.96	7.41	3.3	2.0						recovery
3	85 M	Insulin	Urinary tract infection	670	7.20	7.49	5.3	3.4	8.7	8.6	6.3	2	1	
4	25 F	Insulin	Pharyngitis	770	6.90	7.30	6.5	3.7	—	—	10.0	2	1	
5	26 F	Insulin	None detected	640	7.00	—	7.0	2.9	8.8	—	5.5	3	1	
6	70 M	D.M. unknown	Saddle embolus aorta	1650	7.24	7.42	7.8	—	—	—	6.0	3	1	
									—	—	12.6	3	—	Died after 18 h in
7	75 F	Oral agents	Change of therapy	1030	6.98	7.41	—	—						circulatory shock
			(previously insulin)						10.6	6.2	3.4	2	1	
8	69 M	D.M. unknown	Transient ischem. attack	1020	6.93	7.48	6.1	1.2	8.6	7.8	3.3	3	2	Cholecystitis
9	46 F	D.M. unknown	Urinary tract infection	1500	7.11	7.40	6.8	2.5	—	—	7.7	4	1	
10	43 F	D.M. unknown	Fever of undeterm. origin	940	6.92	7.30	9.7	1.2	—	—	6.1	2	1	Bronchitis
11	33 M	Insulin	None detected	574	6.98	7.31	9.2	2.4	9.8	8.4	5.5	3	1	
12	39 F	Insulin	None detected	952	6.92	7.40	10.0	1.7	—	—	—	3	1	
Mean	49			938	7.00	7.39	7.2	2.2	9.4	8.3	6.6	2.6	1.1	
± SEM	6			97	0.03	0.02	0.6	0.3	0.3	0.1	0.8	0.2	0.1	

* Admission.

TABLE 3
Clinical and biochemical data of patients with ketoacidosis treated with phosphate infusions

Case	Age, sex	Prior therapy	Associated condition	Blood glucose (mg/dl)	pH 0 h*	pH 24 h	Plasma phosphorus (mg/dl) 0 h*	Plasma phosphorus (mg/dl) 48 h	Calcium (mg/dl) 0 h*	Calcium (mg/dl) 48 h	2,3-DPG (μmol/g Hb)	P therapy (mmol)	Consciousness (grade) 0 h*	Consciousness (grade) 48 h	Complication
13	63 M	Insulin	Mesenterial and cerebral infarction	1000	7.08	—	10.0	6.9	7.8	5.4	5.9	40	4	—	Died after 48 h
14	21 M	Insulin	None detected	427	6.96	7.36	6.8	4.1	6.9	8.0	2.9	65	2	1	
15	75 F	Insulin	Fever, unknown origin	796	6.87	—	6.0	2.8	10.6	9.2	—	65	3	1	
16	83 M	Insulin	None detected	790	7.12	7.40	4.7	5.4	8.5	8.1	9.4	75	2	1	
17	18 F	Insulin	Vulvitis	556	6.99	7.33	1.5	3.6	9.8	8.8	3.1	130	4	1	
18	38 F	Insulin	Pneumonia	1190	6.72	7.36	8.2	3.2	7.3	7.0	3.1	65	2	1	Respiratory failure
19	34 M	Insulin	Pneumonia	950	6.89	7.43	3.1	2.0	—	—	1.5	65	4	1	
20	36 M	Insulin	None detected	926	6.90	7.39	8.0	—	8.7	8.0	2.3	65	3	1	
21	33 F	Insulin	Vulvitis	446	7.10	7.42	3.9	2.6	7.7	7.1	5.4	65	1	1	
22	16 M	Oral agents	Pharyngitis	1500	7.15	7.36	2.6	4.0	—	—	8.3	65	4	1	
23	81 M	Oral agents	Skull fracture	1000	7.22	7.45	2.2	3.0	9.5	8.4	8.0	65	3	1	Bronchopneumonia after 48 h
24	41 M	Insulin	Osteomyelitis	750	6.80	7.36	8.6	2.3	10.2	8.3	3.0	65	2	1	
Mean	45			863	6.98	7.39	5.5	3.6	8.70	7.83	4.8	69	2.8	1	
± SEM	7			88	0.04	0.01	0.8	0.4	0.40	0.34	0.8	6	0.3	0	

* Admission.

TABLE 4
Clinical and biochemical data of patients with nonketotic coma treated without phosphate infusions

Case	Age, sex	Prior therapy	Associated condition	Blood glucose (mg/dl)	pH 0 h*	Plasma phosphorus (mg/dl) 0 h*	Plasma phosphorus (mg/dl) 48 h	Calcium (mg/dl) 0 h*	Calcium (mg/dl) 48 h	2,3-DPG (μmol/g Hb)	Consciousness (grade) 0 h*	Consciousness (grade) 48 h	Complication
25	77 F	D.M. unknown	None detected	1580	7.30	5.1	2.0	8.9	7.3	8.5	2	1	Urinary tract infection after 3 days
26	62 F	Insulin	Omission of insulin	920	7.39	4.6	2.3	8.1	6.9	15.8	3	2	Urinary tract infection
27	75 F	D.M. unknown	Urinary tract infection	2350	7.31	6.1	2.0	8.0	7.9	11.0	2	1	Decubitus, pyelonephritis
28	77 M	D.M. unknown	Cerebral infarction	1211	7.29	8.9	2.0	—	—	—	2	1	Pneumonia after 2 days
29	51 F	D.M. unknown	Septicemia	2500	7.20	3.4	1.7	9.5	8.8	10.6	4	2	Large ovarian tumor detected
30	74 F	Oral agents	None detected	1040	7.30	6.3	1.8	9.6	7.2	10.7	2	1	Urinary tract infection
31	67 M	None	Cerebral infarction	1360	7.30	8.4	1.7	—	—	17.5	4	3	Died after 6 days of acute myocardial infarction
32	70 F	D.M. unknown	Erysipela	1170	7.44	4.4	2.8	10.9	6.8	19.0	2	1	
33	65 F	Oral agents	Heart failure	1250	7.40	4.8	1.6	8.4	—	16.8	4	2	
34	76 F	Oral agents	Mesenterial infarction	900	7.34	4.3	—	7.5	—	18.6	4	—	Died after 12 h of mesenterial infarction and acute cerebral infarction
Mean	69			1428	7.33	5.6	2.0	8.9	7.5	14.3	2.9	1.6	
± SEM	3			178	0.02	0.6	0.1	0.4	0.3	1.3	0.3	0.2	

* Admission.

TABLE 5
Clinical and biochemical data of patients with nonketotic coma treated with phosphate infusions

Case	Age, sex	Prior therapy	Associated condition	Blood glucose (mg/dl)	pH	Plasma phosphorus (mg/dl) 0 h*	48 h	Calcium 0 h*	48 h	2,3 DPG (μmol/g Hb)	P therapy (mmol)	Consciousness (grade) 0 h*	48 h	Complication
35	73 F	Insulin	Erysipela	570	7.40	3.0	3.1	9.5	6.9	10.6	33	2	1	Septicemia
36	71 M	D.M. unknown	Pneumonia	940	7.45	4.6	4.2	7.9	8.2	20.8	52	3	1	Urinary tract infection after 3 days
37	69 F	D.M. unknown	Gangrene, sepsis	2175	7.33	4.9	1.6	9.2	7.1	17.5	65	3	2	Died after 6 days of cerebral infarction and pneumonia
38	75 F	Oral agents	Urinary tract infection	660	7.37	5.9	2.2	9.2	7.8	16.8	33	2	1	
39	75 F	D.M. unknown	Pharyngitis	1160	7.32	7.4	2.0	9.5	7.2	17.7	33	3	1	
40	50 F	D.M. unknown	Vulvitis	1450	7.27	6.7	2.3	10.6	8.5	11.7	65	2	1	
Mean	69			1159	7.36	5.4	2.6	9.3	7.6	15.9	47	2.5	1.2	
± SEM	4			242	0.03	0.7	0.4	0.4	0.3	1.6	6	0.2	0.2	

* Admission.

quently the coma was the first manifestation of the disease. As expected, mean blood glucose on admission was significantly higher in nonketotic hyperosmolar coma than in ketoacidosis ($P < 0.005$). pH was normal in most cases. Case no. 29 revealed metabolic acidosis without ketoacidosis. The cause of the acidosis remained unclear; it resolved following fluid administration. Initial inorganic phosphorus concentrations were elevated in 14 of the 16 patients. Thus, nonketotic patients presented with a similar incidence of hyperphosphatemia as ketotic patients. Hypophosphatemia persisted without phosphate replacement at 48 h. Phosphate-treated nonketotic patients had lower mean phosphorus levels at 48 h than ketotic patients, which was probably caused by the lower amounts of phosphate infused. Plasma calcium concentrations fell during the initial 48 h of therapy to a similar degree as in ketotic patients and regardless of phosphate therapy.

In contrast to ketoacidosis, nonketotic hyperosmolar coma was not associated with decreased 2,3-DPG levels, the mean concentrations on admission being in the normal range.

Effects of phosphate replacement therapy on plasma phosphorus and red cell 2,3-DPG concentrations in ketotic patients. Figure 1 illustrates the course of the mean plasma phosphorus and red blood cell 2,3-DPG concentrations in nine phosphate-treated patients and in six controls during the initial 96 h. Plasma phosphorus declined precipitously after beginning insulin therapy. In control patients, phosphorus concentrations reached 24% of the initial

FIGURE 1. Plasma phosphorus and change of red blood cell 2,3-DPG concentrations following institution of therapy in patients with ketoacidotic coma (means ± SEM). Straight line indicates patients treated without phosphate infusions (N = 6) and the broken line patients treated with phosphate infusions (N = 9). An average of 71 ± 7 mmol sodium phosphate was administered between 2 and 36 h following institution of therapy.

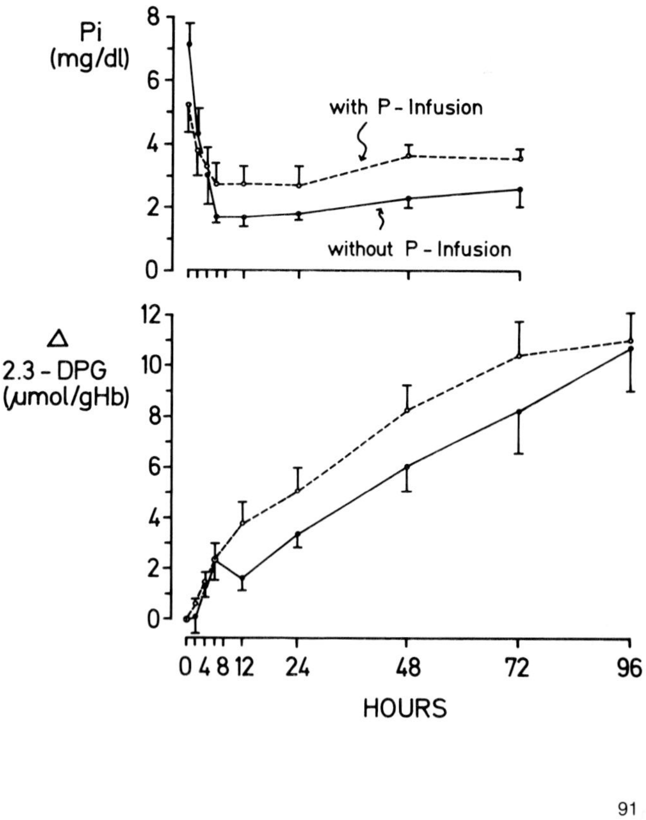

values after 6 h. Plasma phosphorus levels of less than 2.0 mg/dl were noted in two-thirds of these patients.

Administration of phosphate infusions maintained the plasma phosphorus concentrations in the normal range, and the development of persistent hypophosphatemia was prevented. Plasma phosphorus levels were significantly higher after 24 h ($P < 0.05$) and after 48 h ($P < 0.02$) when phosphate was administered. Seventy-two hours after onset of therapy, mean phosphorus levels reached the lower limit of normal (2.6 ± 0.6 mg/dl) in untreated patients, at which time plasma phosphorus was 3.6 ± 0.3 mg/dl in phosphate-treated patients ($P > 0.05 < 0.1$).

Transient postinfusion hyperphosphatemia (5.0–6.0 mg/dl) was noted in 4 of the 12 phosphate-treated patients. Red blood cell 2,3-DPG levels rose gradually during the initial 96 h of observation. Administration of phosphate infusions was associated with a faster increase in 2,3-DPG levels. Between 0 and 48 h, 2,3-DPG had risen by 5.9 ± 0.6 μmol/g Hb in 10 patients receiving phosphate infusions (56% difference, $P < 0.02$). At 72 and 96 h the difference between treated and untreated patients had lost the level of significance. The increase in 2,3-DPG in case no. 19 was particularly remarkable, because 2,3-DPG rose within 4 days from 1.5 to 17.3 μmol/g Hb during phosphate infusions.

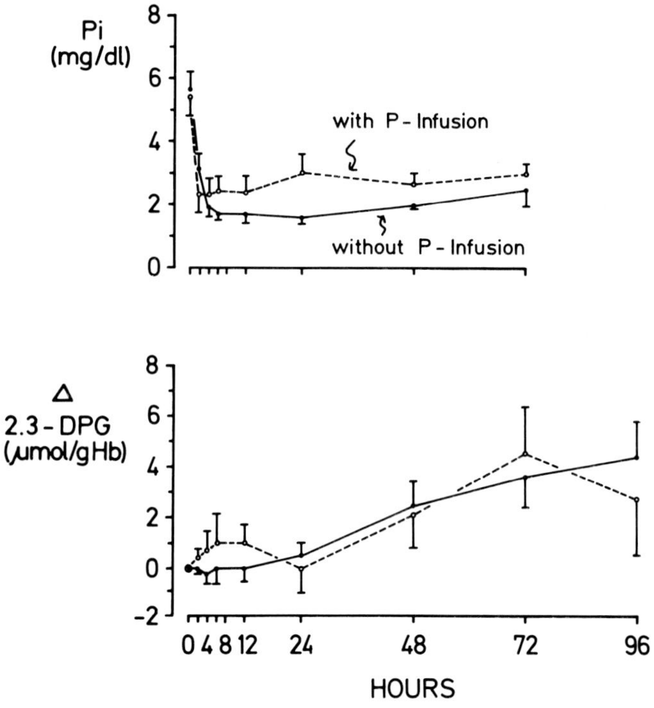

FIGURE 2. Plasma phosphorus and red blood cell 2,3-DPG concentrations in patients with nonketotic hyperosmolar coma. Data represent means ± SEM of five and seven patients treated with and without phosphate infusions, respectively. Phosphate (47 ± 6 mmol) was administered between 4 and 36 h.

Effects of phosphate replacement therapy on plasma phosphorus and red cell 2,3-DPG concentrations in nonketotic patients (Figure 2). Plasma phosphorus concentrations declined again within the first hours of insulin therapy. Marked hypophosphatemia persisted in patients not treated with phosphate infusions until 48 h, while later a gradual rise of plasma phosphorus to normal values occurred.

Phosphate replacement infusions resulted in normalization of plasma phosphorus concentrations in the majority of patients. At 24 h phosphorus levels were significantly higher than in controls ($P < 0.025$). The plasma phosphorus concentrations in phosphate-treated nonketotic patients were slightly lower than those in ketotic patients, possibly because of the lower amount of phosphate infused (mean dose 48 versus 71 mmol phosphate). Transient hyperphosphatemia was observed in three patients after termination of the phosphate infusion.

2,3-DPG levels increased slightly after instituting therapy in both groups of patients with and without phosphate replacement. After 48 h, 2,3-DPG had risen by 2.1 ± 1.5 and 2.5 ± 1.1 μmol/g Hb in phosphate-treated patients and in controls, respectively.

Urinary phosphate excretion (Table 6). Urinary phosphate excretion was measured in five patients receiving phosphate replacement and in three patients treated without phosphate infusions. During the first 24 h after instituting therapy, considerable amounts of phosphate were lost in the urine. Without phosphate therapy, phosphate excretion gradually declined, and after 72 h only minimal amounts of phosphate were excreted.

In contrast, phosphate-treated patients exhibited continuing urinary phosphate losses persisting for 72 h, although phosphate therapy was only administered up to 36 h. The balance between phosphate input and output indicated that during the initial 72 h, urinary phosphate losses amounted to 95% of the phosphate infused. Phosphate administration appeared to increase phosphate excretion, as suggested by comparison of the results of the two groups of patients. Phosphate infusion enhanced phosphate excretion by an average of 26.5 mmol (one-third of the administered dose).

Blood glucose concentrations (Figure 3). Blood glucose levels decreased rapidly in ketotic and in nonketotic patients when insulin and fluid therapy was started. Blood glu-

TABLE 6
Phosphate excretion in patients treated with and without phosphate infusions

	Hours following institution of insulin therapy				
	0–12	12–24	24–48	48–72	72–96
With P therapy (N = 5)					
Phosphate administered (mmol)	75 ± 16				
Phosphate excreted (mmol)	19.1 ± 4.2	15.5 ± 8.3	19.0 ± 4.4	17.9 ± 2.0	1.0 ± 0.3
Without P therapy (N = 3)					
Phosphate excreted (mmol)	22.1 ± 9.2	8.3 ± 1.5	7.0 ± 2.4	7.6 ± 3.9	0.9 ± 0.1

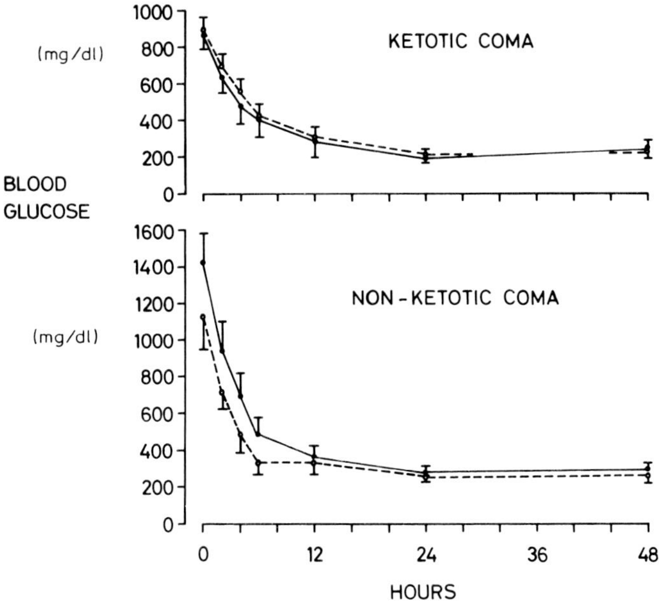

FIGURE 3. Blood glucose concentrations during the initial 48 h of treatment. Upper panel: data obtained from 11 ketotic patients treated with (●- - -●) and 11 patients treated without (●——●) phosphate infusions. Lower panel: 6 and 10 nonketotic patients treated with (●- - -●) and without (●——●) phosphate infusions, respectively.

cose fell below 300 mg/dl on the average after 10 ± 3 h in ketotic patients, and somewhat later, after 12.5 ± 3 h, in nonketotic patients who presented with higher initial values. The rate of fall of blood glucose was similar in patients with and without phosphate therapy.

Effects of phosphate therapy on the clinical course and on mortality rates. As noted in Tables 2 and 3, consciousness was restored after 24 h in virtually all ketotic patients irrespective of phosphate replacement. The time required for the patients to regain full consciousness was 18 ± 4 h in controls and 24 ± 6 h in phosphate-treated patients, which represented no statistically significant difference. Associated conditions such as infections were frequently present on admission (Tables 2–5). Infections occurred with a similar incidence in ketotic and in nonketotic patients; infections were noted in 7 of 22 controls and in 13 of 18 phosphate-treated cases. An effect of phosphate therapy on the course of complications could not be demonstrated. Discharge from the hospital following recovery from diabetic coma was possible after a duration of 14 ± 4 days and 29 ± 5 days in ketotic and nonketotic cases, respectively, and after 23 ± 3 days in phosphate-treated patients compared with 22 ± 4 days in controls. Two patients with ketotic coma and three with nonketotic coma died of complications related to diabetic coma. This represented 8% and 16% of the cases, respectively.

Two of the five fatalities occurred in phosphate-treated patients. In each instance the lethal course was due to thromboembolic complications. In four of the five patients who eventually died, the complication was already present on admission; in the fifth (case no. 37) cerebral infarction occurred on day 6.

Treatment with insulin, potassium, and fluids in the first 24 h (Table 7). Administration of insulin at rates between 4 and 8 U/h resulted in similar amounts of insulin being in-

TABLE 7
Treatment with insulin, potassium, and fluids in the first 24 h (means ± SEM)

	N	Insulin (U/24 h)	Potassium (mval/24 h)	Fluids (L/24 h)
Ketotic coma				
Without P therapy	12	160 ± 35	206 ± 30	8.8 ± 1.0
With P therapy	12	136 ± 13	252 ± 29	8.3 ± 0.8
Nonketotic coma				
Without P therapy	10	128 ± 24	221 ± 42	8.5 ± 0.8
With P therapy	6	166 ± 30	244 ± 32	9.4 ± 1.2

fused in ketotic and in nonketotic patients. In cases no. 9 and 36, the insulin infusion rate had to be increased to 16 U/h because blood glucose failed to decline with the lower rates. Thereafter, the glucose values gradually decreased.

Potassium requirements were similar in ketotic and in nonketotic patients, and fluid balance was achieved by the administration of approximately 8 L of fluids in the first 24 h in either group of patients. The amounts of insulin, fluids, and potassium administered were not significantly different in patients with and without phosphate replacement.

DISCUSSION

The present study, in agreement with previous reports, demonstrates that plasma phosphorus levels in diabetic ketoacidosis decline within a few hours following institution of insulin treatment,[3,5] whereas blood cell 2,3-DPG concentrations are markedly lowered before therapy[26,27] and are slowly restored after several days of treatment.[15,25] Prevention of hypophosphatemia by phosphate infusions results in a more rapid increase in 2,3-DPG concentrations in ketoacidosis, whereas in nonketotic patients initial 2,3-DPG levels are not decreased and remain uninfluenced by phosphate therapy.

The significance of red blood cell 2,3-DPG in regulating hemoglobin oxygen affinity has been elucidated in recent years.[17] Earlier studies suggested that these organic phosphate compounds of blood served as an intracellular storage pool of inorganic phosphorus.[14,27] Their concentration would be lowered as a result of diabetic acidosis and phosphorus depletion, whereas their resynthesis would produce hypophosphatemia during treatment with insulin.

However, red blood cell 2,3-DPG concentrations in our nonacidotic patients were not significantly lowered, while hypophosphatemia eventually developed with a similar incidence as in acidotic patients. This indicates that the phosphorus shifts into organic phosphates of blood cells play a minor role in the fall of plasma phosphorus levels after treatment. Moreover, the similar occurrence of hypophosphatemia in acidotic as in nonacidotic patients suggests that phosphate depletion in diabetic coma is not related to the presence of acidosis but is more likely a consequence of insulin lack and its attendant glucosuria.[29] Following treatment with insulin, phosphorus levels fall, largely due to the insulin-induced shifts of plasma phosphorus from the extracellular space into tissues.[30] The tendency to develop hypophosphatemia in the early phase of treatment was augmented by continuing urinary phosphate losses. As noted in Table 6, we found an average phosphate excretion of 30 mmol during the initial 24 h in untreated patients, which later gradually decreased to very low excretion rates. Furthermore, the observation that hypophosphatemia did not occur in oliguric patients supports the contention that phosphorus losses in the urine were important. Phosphate excretion was probably enhanced by fluid therapy, since phosphate excretion has been reported to be increased following expansion of the extracellular volume in man.[31]

In contrast to plasma phosphorus levels, 2,3-DPG concentrations on admission were markedly influenced by the presence of acidosis. 2,3-DPG concentrations during ketoacidosis were significantly lowered, whereas in nonacidotic patients they remained within the normal range. In spite of the diminished 2,3-DPG concentrations, hemoglobin-oxygen affinity has been reported to be normal in diabetic acidosis before insulin therapy,[16,17] because of the opposing effects of decreased 2,3-DPG levels and acidosis on hemoglobin oxygen dissociation.[32] The fact that 2,3-DPG concentrations in our patients only gradually increased to normal within 4–5 days following insulin therapy while acidosis was corrected within a few hours might have resulted in increased hemoglobin-oxygen affinity and, thus, in impaired oxygen delivery to the tissues. A rationale for administering phosphate infusions was to attempt an accelerated increase in 2,3-DPG, since inorganic phosphorus plays a regulatory role in 2,3-DPG synthesis.[33] Indeed, phosphate infusions have been reported to increase 2,3-DPG concentrations in patients with hypophosphatemia associated with parenteral nutrition[34] and in a few cases of diabetic coma.[18]

The data of the present study demonstrated that phosphate replacement therapy resulted in a slight but significant acceleration of the recovery of 2,3-DPG concentrations in acidotic patients. In contrast to an earlier case report,[16] however, normalization of 2,3-DPG did not occur within a few hours. In view of the known correlation of 2,3-DPG concentration and the position of the hemoglobin oxygen dissociation curve,[16] the estimated effect of phosphate therapy on the hemoglobin dissociation curve can be calculated. In the phosphate-treated patients the increase in 2,3-DPG within 48 h exceeded that observed in controls by 3.3 μmol/g Hb; this difference of 2,3-DPG concentration would increase p_{50} of the hemoglobin dissociation curve by 2.3 mm Hg.* Although the effect is small, the associated decrease in hemoglobin-oxygen affinity might be beneficial in certain patients by improving tissue oxygenation. Furthermore, if restoration of other intracellular phosphates parallels that of 2,3-DPG,[34] phosphate therapy might at least have a transient accelerating effect on the resynthesis of other organic phosphates such as adenine nucleotides, as has been shown in liver and kidney of phosphate-depleted rats.[35]

A clinical benefit of phosphate replacement therapy was not evident in the patients in this study: an effect on the blood glucose response to insulin, an accelerated recovery of the mental state, and a lower mortality rate[3] could not be demonstrated. However, it remains possible that in a larger number of patients a clinical benefit could be detected. We were unable to note clinically signs that have been reported to be associated with hypophosphatemia such as impaired myocardial performance,[36] depressed ventilation,[37] or delayed recovery from infections.[38] This observation and the apparent clinical ineffectiveness of phosphate replacement might be related to the short duration of hypophosphatemia in diabetic coma as opposed to the clinical manifestations of prolonged hypophosphatemia reported in the studies mentioned above.

The present results demonstrate that administration of approximately 70 mmol of phosphate increased plasma phosphorus levels to the low normal range. The amount of phosphate infused was similar to that employed by Franks et al.[3] The urinary loss of phosphorus during the first days of treatment was about 30 mmol, which compares well with the previously reported 26 mmol excreted before insulin treatment.[2] Phosphate excretion was augmented when phosphate infusions were given; therefore, the amount excreted within the first 3 days almost equaled the amount infused.

Potassium and phosphorus concentrations decline in parallel after administration of insulin;[5,27] thus, the use of potassium phosphate solutions in the therapy of diabetic coma has been recommended.[6] However, potassium replacement may be necessary before diuresis is established,[39] whereas in view of the present findings phosphate infusions should be withheld in the absence of adequate urine output. Therefore, potassium should be administered independent of phosphate.

If phosphate infusions are given, we consider it mandatory to monitor plasma phosphorus and calcium levels to guide the effectiveness of the replacement therapy and to avoid the development of hyperphosphatemia or hypocalcemia, although these conditions occurred only transiently in a minority of our patients.

The mortality rate in the present series of patients was lower than in our past report,[20] but still a considerable number of patients died due to complications of diabetic coma. The majority of fatalities was due to thromboembolic complications that had already developed during the period of dehydration and had exerted deleterious effects before any therapy was begun.

The data of the present study demonstrate that phosphate therapy does not improve the course of patients with diabetic coma. However, the possibility remains that it might have a favorable effect in a certain patient, particularly if hypophosphatemia is severe and persistent. Nonetheless, the results indicate that phosphate replacement is not a necessary measure in the standard treatment of diabetic coma.

ACKNOWLEDGMENTS

We are obliged to Dr. R. Ritz, head of the Intensive Care Unit, and to the nursing staff of the Kantonsspital Basel for their collaboration. The technical help of U. Büchler and Mr. Rajacic and the secretarial assistance of L. Eidenbenz are gratefully acknowledged. We thank Prof. W. Stauffacher for critical review of the manuscript.

REFERENCES

1 Neubauer, C.: Ueber die Erdphosphate des Harns. J. F. Prakt. Chem. *67*:65–97, 1856.

2 Atchley, D. W., Loeb, R. F., Richards, D. W., Jr., Benedict, E. M., and Driscoll, M. E.: On diabetic acidosis. A detailed study of electrolyte balances following the withdrawal and reestablishment of insulin therapy. J. Clin. Invest. *12*:297–326, 1933.

3 Franks, M., Berris, R. F., Kaplan, N. O., and Myers, G. B.: Metabolic studies in diabetic acidosis. Arch. Intern. Med. *81*:42–55, 1948.

* P_{50} indicates the pO_2 level at which 50% of the hemoglobin is saturated.

[4] Nabarro, J. D. N., Spencer, A. G., and Stowers, J. M.: Treatment of diabetic ketosis. Lancet *1*:983–88, 1952.

[5] Butler, A. M., Talbot, N. B., Burnett, C. H., Stanbury, J. B., and MacLachlan, E. A.: Metabolic studies in diabetic coma. Trans. Assoc. Am. Physicians *60*:102–09, 1947.

[6] Daughaday, W. H.: The nature and correction of diabetic ketoacidosis. Diabetes *7*:230–35, 1958.

[7] Martin, H. E., Smith , K., and Wilson, M. L.: The fluid and electrolyte therapy of severe diabetic acidosis and ketosis. Am. J. Med. *24*:376–89, 1958.

[8] Harwood, R.: Diabetic acidosis. Results of treatment in 67 consecutive cases. N. Engl. J. Med. *245*:1–8, 1951.

[9] Bradley, R. F.: Diabetic ketoacidosis and coma. *In* Joslin's Diabetes Mellitus. Marble, A., White, P., Bradley, R. F., and Krall, L. P., Eds. Philadelphia, Lea & Febiger, 1971, pp. 361–66.

[10] Gibby, O. M., Veale, K. E. A., Hayes, T. M., Jones, J. G., and Wardrop, C. A. J.: Oxygen availability from the blood and the effect of phosphate replacement on erythrocyte 2.3-diphosphoglycerate and haemoglobin-oxygen affinity in diabetic ketoacidosis. Diabetologia *15*:381–85, 1978.

[11] Alberti, K. G. M. M.: Severe diabetic ketoacidosis. Med. Clin. North Am. *62*:799–814, 1978.

[12] Sperling, M. A.: Diabetic ketoacidosis in childhood. Pediatr. Clin. North Am. *26*:152–59, 1979.

[13] Kreisberg, R. A.: Diabetic ketoacidosis. New concepts and trends in pathogenesis and treatment. Ann. Intern. Med. *88*:681–95, 1978.

[14] Guest, G. M., and Rapoport, S.: Progress in pediatrics. Role of acid-soluble phosphorus compounds in red blood cells. Am. J. Dis. Child. *58*:1072–89, 1939.

[15] Alberti, K. G. M. M., Darley, J. H., Emerson, P. M., and Hockaday, T. D. R.: 2,3-Diphosphoglycerate and tissue oxygenation in uncontrolled diabetes mellitus. Lancet *2*:391–95, 1972.

[16] Ditzel, J.: Effect of plasma inorganic phosphate on tissue oxygenation during recovery from diabetic ketoacidosis. Adv. Exp. Med. Biol. *37A*:163–72, 1973.

[17] Bellingham, A. J., Detter, J. C., and Lenfant, C.: The role of hemoglobin affinity for oxygen and red-cell 2,3-diphosphoglycerate in the management of diabetic ketoacidosis. Trans. Assoc. Am. Physicians *83*:113–20, 1970.

[18] Ditzel, J., and Anderson, H.: Importance of plasma inorganic phosphate in the treatment of diabetic ketoacidosis. Diabetes *22* (Suppl. 1):293, 1973.

[19] Knochel, J. P.: The pathophysiology and clinical characteristics of severe hypophosphatemia. Arch. Intern. Med. *137*:203–20, 1977.

[20] Keller, U., Berger, W., Ritz, R., and Truog, P.: Course and prognosis of 86 episodes of diabetic coma. A five year experience with a uniform schedule of treatment. Diabetologia *11*:93–100, 1975.

[21] Berger, W.: Diagnose und Behandlung diabetischer Notfall-situationene in der Praxis und im Spital. Schweiz. Med. Wochenschr. *102*:1008–16, 1972.

[22] Scholer, A., and Pianezzi, A.: Micromethod for the determination of glucose with glucose dehydrogenase in the AutoAnalyzer. J. Clin. Chem. Clin. Biochem. *14*:189–95, 1976.

[23] Fiske, Ch., and Subbarow, Y.: The colorimetric determination of phosphorus. J. Biol. Chem. *66*:375–400, 1925.

[24] Keitt, A. S.: Reduced nicotinamide adenine dinucleotide-linked analysis of 2,3-diphosphoglyceric acid; spectrophotometric and fluorometric procedures. J. Lab. Clin. Med. *77*:470–75, 1971.

[25] Ditzel, J., and Standl, E.: The oxygen transport system of red blood cells during diabetic ketoacidosis and recovery. Diabetologia *11*:255–60, 1975.

[26] Kanter, Y., Gerson, J. R., and Bessman, A. N.: 2,3-Diphosphoglycerate, nucleotide phosphate, and organic and inorganic phosphate levels during the early phases of diabetic ketoacidosis. Diabetes *26*:429–33, 1977.

[27] Guest, G. M.: Organic phosphates of the blood and mineral metabolism in diabetic acidosis. Am. J. Dis. Child *64*:401–12, 1942.

[28] Danowski, T. S., Hald, P. M., and Peters, J. P.: Sodium, potassium and phosphates in the cells and serum of blood in diabetic acidosis. Am. J. Physiol. *149*:667–77, 1947.

[29] Levitan, B. A.: Effect in normal man of hyperglycemia and glucosuria on excretion and reabsorption of phosphate. J. Appl. Physiol. *4*:224–26, 1951.

[30] Forsham, P. H., and Thorn, G. W.: Changes of organic serum phosphorus during the intravenous glucose tolerance test as an adjunct to the diagnosis of early diabetes mellitus. Proc. Am. Diabetes Assoc. *9*:101–22, 1950.

[31] Steele, T. H.: Increased urinary phosphate excretion following volume expansion in normal man. Metabolism *19*:129–39, 1970.

[32] Bellingham, A. J., Detter, J. C., and Lenfant, C.: Regulatory mechanisms of hemoglobin oxygen affinity in acidosis and alkalosis. J. Clin. Invest. *50*:700–06, 1971.

[33] Schrier, St. L.: ATP synthesis in human erythrocyte membranes. Biochim. Biophys. Acta *135*:591–98, 1967.

[34] Lichtman, M. A., Miller, D. R., Cohen, J., and Waterhouse, Ch.: Reduced red cell glycolysis, 2,3-diphosphoglycerate and adenosine triphosphate concentration, and increased hemoglobin-oxygen affinity caused by hypophosphatemia. Ann. Intern. Med. *74*:562–68, 1971.

[35] Morris, R. C., Nigon, K., and Reed, E. B.: Evidence that the severity of depletion of inorganic phosphate determines the severity of the disturbance of adenine nucleotide metabolism in the liver and renal cortex of the fructose-loaded rat. J. Clin. Invest. *61*:209–20, 1978.

[36] O'Connor, L. R., Wheeler, W. S., and Bethune, J. E.: Effect of hypophosphatemia on myocardial performance in man. N. Engl. J. Med. *297*:901–03, 1977.

[37] Newman, J. H., Neff, T. A., and Ziporin, P.: Acute respiratory failure associated with hypophosphatemia N. Engl. J. Med. *296*:1101–03, 1977.

[38] Craddock, P. R., Yawata, Y., Van Santen, L., Gilberstadt, S., Silvis, S., and Jacob, H. S.: Acquired phagocyte dysfunction. A complication of the hypophosphatemia of parenteral hyperalimentation. N. Engl. J. Med. *290*:1403–07, 1974.

[39] Soler, N. G., Dixon, K., Bennet, M. A., Fitzgerald, M. G., and Malins, J. M.: Potassium balance during treatment of diabetic ketoacidosis. Lancet *2*:665–67, 1972.

Erythrocyte Insulin Receptors in Non-insulin-dependent Diabetes Mellitus

ROBERTO DEPIRRO, ANGELO FUSCO, RENATO LAURO, IVANO TESTA, FABRIZIO FERRETI, AND CARLO DEMARTINIS

SUMMARY

Insulin binding was studied on circulating erythrocytes isolated from 12 normal and 12 untreated, adult, nonobese, nonketotic, non-insulin-dependent diabetic subjects. Insulin binding in normal subjects was higher than in diabetics ($P < 0.01$); binding variation was caused mainly by a reduction in insulin receptor concentration. Insulin binding was inversely correlated with fasting serum insulin levels ($R = 0.49$; $P < 0.01$). The close agreement between the present data and previous data on other cell populations suggests that isolated erythrocytes may be a useful tool in clinical investigations on the human insulin receptor.
DIABETES *29*:96–99, February 1980.

Now that insulin receptors have been identified on the monocyte cell membrane,[1,2] it is no longer necessary to take biopsy specimens when doing human studies.[3–11] A major drawback in the use of the monocyte method, however, is the large quantity of blood (100 ml or more) required for each receptor study, because of the low monocyte concentration in white blood cells.

It has recently been shown that insulin receptors are also present on circulating erythrocytes,[12,13] and their binding characteristics are almost identical to those of the monocyte system. Since a sufficient number of erythrocytes are easily isolated from 15 ml of blood, it was suggested that they may provide an ideal model for clinical evaluation of insulin receptors.[12] Nevertheless, before replacing the monocyte model, the insulin receptor present on the erythrocyte should be evaluated in some of the conditions previously studied on other cell membranes.

In the present investigation the insulin receptor on erythrocytes in normal subjects is compared with that in subjects with non-insulin-dependent diabetes mellitus.

MATERIAL AND METHODS

Subjects. 12 male volunteers with normal glucose tolerance and 12 nonketotic, non-insulin-dependent diabetic male patients who had fasting blood glucose concentrations >140 mg $\cdot$ dl^{-1} on at least three occasions were studied. All subjects were of normal body weight (Geigy table, 7th edit.), and none presented with any disease other than diabetes. None was taking any drug known to affect carbohydrate or insulin metabolism. No females were included in the study, because there is a wide variation in insulin receptors during the menstrual cycle.[4,14]

Buffer used for binding studies consisted of Hepes (50 mM), Tris (50 mM), $MgCl_2$ (10 mM), EDTA (2 mM), dextrose (10 mM), $CaCl_2$ (10 mM), NaCl (50 mM), KCl (5 mM), and bovine serum albumin (0.1%; pH 8 at 15°C).[12,13]

Preparation of cells. Blood (15 ml) was collected from an antecubital vein in tubes containing 4 ml 3.8% sodium citrate. Each sample was diluted with isotonic saline to a final volume of 30 ml and then transferred on a Ficoll-Angiographin gradient for cell fractionation according to the method of Boyum.[15] Saline, lymphomonocytes, Ficoll-Angiographin, granulocytes, and the upper layer of the erythrocyte phase were aspirated after centrifugation ($600 \times g$ at 4°C for 30 min). The cell pellet was resuspended with 20 ml isotonic saline and the above procedure repeated. The new eythrocyte pellet was washed first with 20 ml isotonic saline and then with 20 ml buffer. The last pellet was suspended with buffer at the final cell concentration; contamination by mononuclear cells was minimal. Cell concentration was determined using an automatic Coulter counter (Royco 920-A, California) and by hematocrit.

Binding studies were performed as previously described.[12,13] Erythrocytes ($2.5 \times 10^9 \times$ ml^{-1}) were incubated at 15°C with ^{125}I-insulin (34 pmol/L, 110–130 μCi/μg, Sorin, Italy), with or without varying amounts of native insulin (Organon, Holland), in a total volume of 0.5 ml. After 210 min of incubation, duplicate 200-μl samples were placed in 1.5-ml

Medica, Università degli Studi di Ancona, Ancona, Italy.
Address reprint requests to Roberto De Pirro, M.D., Policlinico Umberto 1°, Università degli Studi di Roma, Viale del Policlinico, 00100 Roma, Italy.
Received for publication 15 May and in revised form 11 July 1979.

TABLE 1
Clinical and metabolic characteristics of the study group*

	No.	Age (yr)	Wt (kg)	Ht (cm)	Fasting blood glucose (mg · dl⁻¹)	Fasting serum insulin (μU/ml)	Specific cell† binding fraction (2.5 × 10⁹ eryth./ml)
Normals	12	48 ± 10	72 ± 11	169 ± 10	85 ± 5	10.4 ± 1.7	6.39 ± 0.50
Diabetics	12	49 ± 11	69 ± 10	165 ± 9	208 ± 30	14.5 ± 2.0	5.39 ± 0.56

* Mean ± SD.
† Insulin specifically bound/total insulin (× 10^{-2}) at the tracer concentration of 34 pmol/L.

tubes containing 0.8 ml ice-cold buffer and 200 μl di-n-butyl phthalate (density=1.044). Cell-bound and free insulin were separated by centrifugation in a Microfuge B (Beckman Instruments, Fullerton, California) for 2.5 min. TCA precipitation or rebinding of supernatants with freshly prepared cells showed that ^{125}I-insulin degradation was less than 3%. Nonspecific binding was defined as the amount of labeled insulin that remained bound in the presence of 17 μmol/L of native insulin. Nonspecific binding was about 16% of total binding (~1% of total radioactivity).

Analytic procedures. Plasma glucose was determined by the glucose-oxidase method using a Beckman glucose analyzer.[16] Serum immunoreactive insulin was measured with the method described by Herbert et al.;[17] the coefficient of interassay variation was 8.1% and that of intra-assay was 7.8%.

Statistical analysis. Analysis of variance was employed to compare results from normal and diabetic subjects. Spearman's coefficient of rank was applied in correlation studies.

RESULTS

Clinical characteristics and results are briefly reported in Table 1. The specific cell-binding fraction in normal subjects (6.39 ± 0.05) is higher than in diabetics (5.39 ± 0.56)($P < 0.01$;df = 1.22;F = 18.57). In the presence of a single class of binding sites exhibiting negative cooperativity, the decrease in binding is caused mainly by a decreased receptor concentration (R_0) rather than by a change in receptor affinity ($\bar{K}_e$), even if a change in receptor affinity cannot be excluded (Figure 1). On the other hand, if the so-called "apparently higher affinity binding sites" are taken into account, it can be seen that changes are due only to variations in receptor concentration (Figure 2).

A significant inverse relationship ($R = 0.49$, $P < 0.01$) was found between fasting serum insulin concentration and the insulin-specific cell-binding fraction (Figure 3).

DISCUSSION

Insulin binding on erythrocytes from non-insulin-dependent diabetics is significantly lower than it is in normal subjects. According to the negative cooperativity model,[18] the decrease in binding is caused mainly by a lower concentration of insulin receptors rather than by a change in receptor affinity; on the other hand, a change in receptor affinity cannot be excluded, since average affinity profiles do not entirely overlap (Figure 1,inset). In this regard, it is well known that the slope of the profiles is considerably influenced by the R_0

FIGURE 1. Scatchard plot[39] of mean values from competition-inhibition studies in 12 normal subjects (■——■) and 12 non-insulin-dependent diabetic subjects (●——●) in fasting conditions. Bound and free ratio of ^{125}I-insulin (B/F) is plotted as a function of the insulin bound. Extrapolation of the curve to the horizontal axis is used to obtain the total receptor concentration (R_0) (Inset[18]) Average affinity ($\bar{K}$) is plotted as a function of the occupancy of insulin receptors at that concentration of insulin (B/R_0). Theoretically, $\bar{K}_e$ represents the highest affinity reached at zero occupancy of the insulin receptor. In practice, $\bar{K}_e$ has been taken to be equal to $\bar{K}$ at an insulin concentration of 0.2 ng/ml (34 pmol/L).

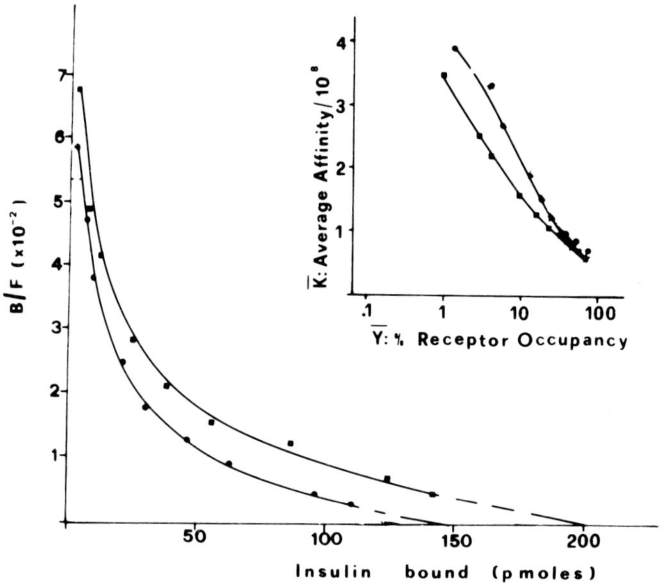

FIGURE 2. Scatchard plots, given in figure 1, on a larger scale. Straight lines represent so-called "apparently higher affinity binding sites".

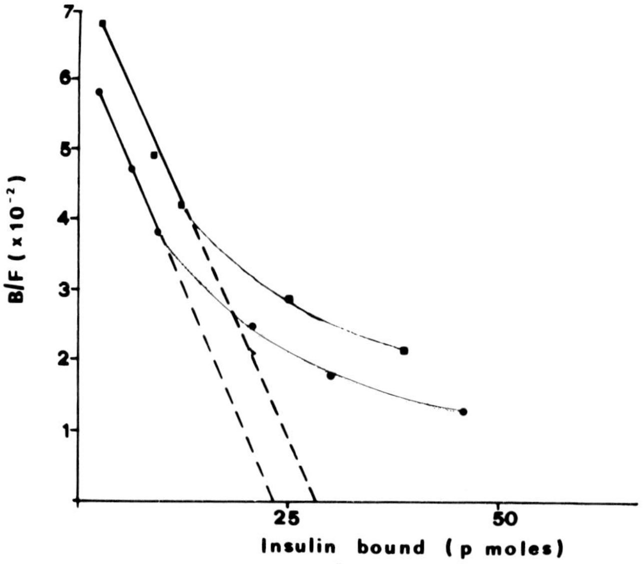

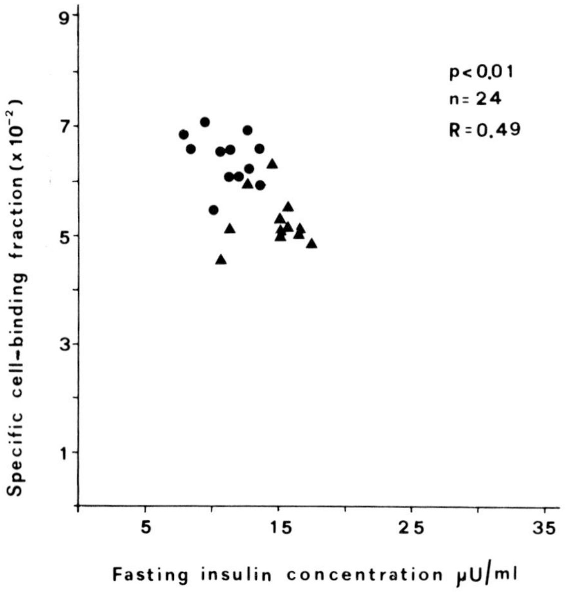

FIGURE 3. Relationship between specific cell-binding fraction (per 2.5 × 10⁹ erythrocytes/ml) and fasting serum insulin level in 12 normal subjects (●) and 12 non-insulin-dependent diabetic subjects (▲).

value, which is an extrapolation and is grossly evaluated.[19,20]

The question of negative cooperativity[21] versus the presence of two or more classes of binding sites,[22] or a single class of sites not exhibiting negative cooperativity,[23] is still under debate; therefore, at present, the so-called "apparently higher affinity binding sites" should also be taken into consideration. According to this model the decrease in binding is caused only by a reduction of insulin receptors. The present data are in agreement with results obtained on other tissues.[8,10,11,24–30]

Subsequent to the hypothesis advanced by Gavin et al.[31] that the insulin receptor may be subject to negative feedback regulation by the height of ambient insulin concentration (downregulation), significant negative correlations between insulin binding and fasting insulin levels have been found in certain hyperinsulinemic states.[3,9,32–34] In the present study, a negative correlation was found between insulin binding and fasting serum insulin levels, suggesting that insulin might also regulate the erythrocyte insulin receptor. On the other hand, the ability of insulin to modulate its receptor is based primarily on studies in vitro, and situations in which insulin receptor variations do not appear to be related to insulinemia have been described.[4–7,35,36] The relationship found might, thus, be an epiphenomenon of a more important, controlling influence.

These data suggest that changes exist in the erythrocyte insulin receptor associated with or occurring with diabetes mellitus in a similar form to those described for other cell populations. Therefore, even if excessive amounts of cells have to be employed (because of the low number of receptor sites per cell), sufficient information about the insulin receptor may be obtained from erythrocytes.

The close parallelism between findings on monocytes[8,10,11] and those on erythrocytes seems to support the possibility that the erythrocyte model might replace the monocyte model in future clinical studies; this would undoubtedly have certain advantages. In fact, about 15 ml of blood is used for each erythrocyte receptor determination versus 80–100 ml for monocytes. Moreover, erythrocytes can easily be separated as a pure preparation, while monocyte samples are composed of a mixed cell population of lymphocytes, monocytes, and granulocytes.[1,2,5] The biologic role of insulin receptors present on monocytes and erythrocytes has not yet been elucidated, and, even if it has been suggested that monocyte insulin reflect a similar situation to that occurring on the cell membrane of other tissues,[33] it has not yet been shown that insulin binding on different cells is regulated by the same factors. In this respect, it must be borne in mind that the erythrocyte has certain peculiarities distinguishing it from other cells (lack of nucleus and lack of internalization of cell surface proteins). Thus, if it is assumed that the nucleus plays a role in insulin action and that cells internalize insulin as a consequence of insulin receptor interaction,[37,38] some differences might also exist between erythrocytes and other cells.

In conclusion, the present report demonstrates that, in agreement with previous studies on other cell populations, non-insulin-dependent diabetes mellitus is associated with a loss of insulin receptors on the erythrocyte membrane, thus suggesting that erythrocytes might be used in clinical studies instead of monocytes. In this respect, it is interesting to note that the monocyte and the erythrocyte insulin receptors from three obese subjects (~200% of ideal body weight) have shown the same behavior during a 5-day-fasting period (data not reported) and that patients with impaired glucose tolerance in basal conditions have a reduced number of erythrocyte insulin receptors in comparison with normals.[40] Nevertheless, before replacing the monocyte model, further comparative studies are required.

ACKNOWLEDGMENTS

We are indebted to Dr. G. Tamburrano for serum insulin analysis and to D. Minelli for skillful technical assistance.

This work was supported, in part, by a grant from ISIS, sezione scientifica.

REFERENCES

1 Schwartz, R. H., Bianco, A. R., Handwerger, B. S., and Kahn, C. R.: Demonstration that monocytes rather than lymphocytes are the insulin-binding cells in preparation of human peripheral blood mononuclear leukocytes preparation: implication for studies of insulin-resistance states in man. Proc. Natl. Acad. Sci. USA. *72*:474–78, 1975.

2 Beck-Nielsen, H., Pedersen, O., Kragballe, K., and Sørensen N. S.: The monocyte as a model for the study of insulin receptors in man. Diabetologia *13*:563–69, 1977.

3 Bar, R. S., Gordon, P., Roth, J., and Kahn, C. R.: Fluctuations in the affinity and concentration of the insulin receptors on circulating monocytes of obese patients. J. Clin. Invest. *58*:1123–35, 1976.

4 De Pirro, R., Fusco, A., Bertoli, A., Greco, A. V., and Lauro, R.: Insulin receptors during the menstrual cycle in normal women. J. Clin. Endocrinol. Metab. *47*:1387–89, 1978.

5 De Pirro, R., Bertoli, A., Greco, A. V., Gelli, A. S., and Lauro, R.: The effect of food intake on insulin receptor in man. Acta Endocrinol. (Copen) *90*:473–80, 1979.

6 De Pirro, R., Tamburrano, G., Fusco, A., Natoli, C., and Lauro, R.: Insulin receptor during arginine infusion test in man. Diabetologia *15*:227, 1978. Abstract.

7 Muggeo, M., Bar, R. S., and Roth, J.: Change in affinity of insulin receptors following oral glucose in normal adults. J. Clin. Endocrinol. Metab. *44*:1206–09, 1977.

8 Beck-Nielsen, H.: The pathogenic role of an insulin-receptor defect in diabetes mellitus of the obese. Diabetes *27*:1175–81, 1978.

9 Beck-Nielsen, H. Pedersen, O., Bagger, J. P., and Sorensen, N. S.: The insulin receptor in normal and obese persons. Acta Endocrinol. (Copen) *83*:565–75, 1976.

[10] Olefsky, J. M., and Reaven, G. M.: Insulin binding to monocytes and total mononuclear leukocytes from normal and diabetic patients. J. Clin. Endocrinol. Metab. *43*:232–34, 1976.

[11] Olefsky, J. M., and Reaven, G. M.: Insulin binding in diabetes. Diabetes *26*:680–88, 1977.

[12] Gambhir, K. K., Archer, J. A., and Bradley, C. J.: Characteristics of human erythrocyte insulin receptors. Diabetes *27*:701–08, 1978.

[13] Lauro, R., Greco, A. V., Bertoli, A., Fusco, A., Spallone, L., Magnatta, R., and De Pirro, R.: A study on insulin receptors of human erythrocytes. LAB, J. Res. Lab. Med. *6*:297–308, 1979.

[14] De Pirro, R., Bertoli, A., Greco, A. V., Fusco, A., and Lauro, R.: Differences in erythrocyte insulin receptor between man and woman. Acta Endocrinol. (Copen) (Suppl.) *225*:310, 1979. Abstr.

[15] Boyum, A.: Separation of leukocytes from blood and bone marrow. Scand. J. Clin. Lab. Invest. *21* (Suppl. 97):77–89, 1968.

[16] Hugget, A. St. G., and Nixon, D. A.: Use of glucose oxidase, peroxidase and o-dianisidine in determination of blood and urinary glucose. Lancet *2*:368–70, 1957.

[17] Herbert, V., Lan, K. S., Gottlieb, C. W., and Bleicher, S.: Coated charcoal immunoassay of insulin. J. Clin. Endocrinol. Metab. *25*:1375–84, 1965.

[18] De Meyts, P., and Roth, J.: Cooperativity in ligand binding: a new graphic analysis. Biochem. Biophys. Res. Commun. *66*:1118–26, 1975.

[19] Muggeo, M., Bar, R. S., Roth, J., Kahn, C. R., and Gorden, P.: The insulin resistance in acromegaly: evidence for two alterations in the insulin receptor on circulating monocytes. J. Clin. Endocrinol. Metab. *48*:17–25, 1979.

[20] Beck-Nielsen, H., and Pedersen, O.: Diurnal variation in insulin binding to human monocytes. J. Clin. Endocrinol. Metab. *47*:385–90, 1978.

[21] Pollet, R. J., Standaert, M. L., and Haase, B. A.: Insulin binding to the human lymphocyte receptor. Evaluation of the negative cooperativity model. J. Biol. Chem. *252*:5828–34, 1977.

[22] Krupp, M. N., and Livingstone, J. N.: Insulin binding to solubilized material from fat cell membranes: evidence for two binding species. Proc. Natl. Acad. Sci. USA *75*:2593–97, 1978.

[23] Maturo, J. M., III, and Hollemberg, M. D.: Insulin receptor: interaction with nonreceptor glycoprotein from liver cell membranes. Proc. Natl. Acad. Sci. USA *75*:3070–74, 1978.

[24] Kern, P., Picard, J., Caron, M., and Veissiere, D.: Decreased binding of insulin to liver plasma membrane receptors in hereditary diabetic mice. Biochim. Biophys. Acta *389*:281–89, 1975.

[25] Harrison, L. C., Billington, T., Clark, S., Nichols, R., East, I., and Martin, F.: Decreased binding of insulin by receptors on placenta membranes from diabetic mothers. J. Clin. Endocrinol. Metab. *44*:206–09, 1977.

[26] Freychet, P., and Forgue, E.: Insulin receptors in the heart muscle: impairment of insulin binding to the plasma membrane in the obese hyperglycemic mouse. Diabetes *23* (Suppl. 1):354, 1974. Abstr.

[27] Freychet, P., Laudat, M. H., Laudat, P., Rosselin, G., Kahn, C. R., Gorden, P., and Roth, J.: Impairment of the insulin binding to the fat cell membrane in the obese hyperglycemic mouse. FEBS Lett. *25*:339–42, 1972.

[28] Soll, A. H., Goldfine, I. D., Roth, J., and Kahn, C. R.: Thymic lymphocytes in obese (ob/ob) mice: a mirror of the insulin receptor defect in liver and fat. J. Biol. Chem. *249*:4127–31, 1974.

[29] Dahms, W. T., Atkinson, R. L., and Bray, G. A.: Insulin resistance and the binding of insulin to adipocytes. Clin. Res. *24*:116A, 1976. Abstract.

[30] Goldstein, S., Blecher, M., Binder, R., Perrino, P. V., and Recant, L.: Hormone receptors: binding of glucagon and insulin to human circulating mononuclear cells in diabetes mellitus. Endocr. Res. Commun. *2*:367–76, 1975.

[31] Gavin, J. R., III, Roth, J., Neville, D. M., Jr., De Meyts, P., and Buell, D. N.: Insulin-dependent regulation of insulin receptor concentrations: a direct demonstration in cell culture, Proc. Natl. Acad. Sci. USA *71*:84–88, 1974.

[32] Olefsky, J. M.: Decreased insulin binding to adipocytes and circulating monocytes from obese persons. J. Clin. Invest. *57*:1165–72, 1976.

[33] Olefsky, J. M.: The insulin receptor: its role in insulin resistance of obesity and diabetes. Diabetes *25*:1154–64, 1976.

[34] Harrison, L. C., Martin, F. I., and Melick, R.: Insulin receptor binding in isolated fat cells and insulin sensitivity in obesity. J. Clin. Invest. *58*:1435–41, 1976.

[35] Bennet, G. V., and Cuatrecasas, P.: Insulin receptor of fat cells in insulin-resistant metabolic states. Science *176*:805–06, 1972.

[36] Kahn, C. R., Goldfine, I. D., Neville, D. M., Jr., and De Meyts, P.: Alterations in insulin binding induced by changes in vivo in the levels of glucocorticoids and growth hormone. Endocrinology *103*:1054–66, 1978.

[37] Goldfine, I. D., and Smith, G. J.: Binding of insulin to isolated nuclei. Proc. Natl. Acad. Sci. USA *73*:1427–31, 1976.

[38] Goldfine, I. D., Jones, A. L., Hradek, G. T., Wong, K. Y., and Mooney, J. S.: Entry of insulin into human cultured lymphocytes: electron microscope autoradiographic analysis. Science *202*:760–63, 1978.

[39] Scatchard, G.: The attraction of proteins for small molecules and ions. Ann. N.Y. Acad. Sci. *51*:660–72, 1949.

[40] De Pirro, R., Fusco, A., Lauro, R., Testa I., Ferretti, F., and De Martinis, C.: Erythrocyte insulin receptor in patients with impaired glucose tolerance. Submitted for publication.

Development of Adipose Tissue in Newborns of Gestational-diabetic and Insulin-dependent Diabetic Mothers

G. ENZI, E. M. INELMEN, F. CARETTA, F. VILLANI, V. ZANARDO, AND F. DEBIASI

SUMMARY

Some parameters of adipose tissue development have been studied in normal, full-term infants of gestational-diabetic mothers (GDM) and insulin-dependent diabetic mothers (IDDM). Values of skinfold thickness, body fat mass, and fat cell weight in full-term newborns of GDM and IDDM are greater than in infants of nondiabetic mothers. Fat mass enlargement in newborns of diabetic mothers seems to be caused almost exclusively by an increase in the triglyceride content of the single adipocytes. Results of determinations of fat cell weight are in fact significantly higher in newborns of GDM and IDDM and correlate closely with skinfold thickness and body fat mass: No differences resulted in the approximate estimate of fat cell number. Neither maternal weight gain during pregnancy nor pregravidic overweight seem to be directly related to the expansion of adipose tissue observed in newborns of diabetic mothers. Maternal blood glucose levels and neonatal IRI levels in cord blood significantly correlated with fat cell weight. Maternal FFA levels are not related to parameters of adipose tissue development in newborns of normal, GD, and IDD mothers.

In conclusion, enlargement of body fat mass in full-term infants of GDM and IDDM is dependent on glucose availability and, thus, on the insulin-induced enhancement of triglyceride synthesis and storage in single adipocytes. Free fatty acids do not seem to play an important role in regulating the triglyceride content of fat cells in newborns of gestational-diabetic or insulin-dependent diabetic mothers.

DIABETES 29:100–104, February 1980.

Fetal macrosomia is frequently observed in newborns of gestational-diabetic mothers (GDM) and insulin-dependent diabetic mothers (IDDM). Excessive fetal size is partially related to an enlargement in body fat mass.[1–4] However, the factors that provoke fat mass expansion in newborns of diabetic mothers have not been defined. It has been hypothesized that increased glucose availability to the fetus and enhanced insulin release by the fetal pancreas could cause fat mass enlargement in newborns of diabetic mothers.[5]

An increase in fat cell size in newborns of diabetic mothers[4] and a correlation between blood glucose area after an oral glucose tolerance test (OGTT) and fat cell size in newborns of presumably healthy, casually selected mothers have been reported.[6] Moreover, chronic exposure to elevated levels of insulin in utero could induce hypercellularity of adipose tissue. In vitro observations[7] confirm the mitogenic activity of insulin on adipose tissue cultures, while increased cellularity of the retroperitoneal fat pad in offspring of alloxan-diabetic rats has been described in vivo.[8]

The aim of this work was to study some developmental aspects of adipose tissue in connection with hormonal or metabolic factors in newborns of GDM and IDDM.

PATIENTS AND METHODS

Seventeen GDM, class A of White's classification[9] (abnormal GTT that reverted to normal postpartum), eight IDDM, two class B (overt diabetes, onset after age 20, duration of less than 10 yr), and six class C (overt diabetes, onset before age 20, duration of from 10 to 20 yr) and their respective infants born at term of clinically normal pregnancies were evaluated. A reference group of 17 normal mothers was also considered.

Maternal pregravidic body weight, overweight, weight gain during pregnancy, and tricipital, subscapular, and crural skinfold thickness (Harpenden caliper) were recorded. Overweight was calculated as percent difference between actual body weight and theoretic ideal body weight.[10]

GDM were instructed to follow a low carbohydrate diet (1200 cal each day: proteins = 72 g; carbohydrates = 120

From the departments of Internal Medicine, Division of Gerontology and Metabolic Diseases (G. E., E.M.I., F.C., and F.D.), and of Pediatrics (V.Z.), University of Padua, and the Antidiabetic Center (F.V.), City Hospital, Padua, Italy. Address reprint requests to Dr. Giuliano Enzi, Department of Internal Medicine, Via Giustiniani 2, 35100 Padova, Italy.
Received for publication 14 May and in revised form 26 September 1979.

g; lipids = 45 g). IDD mothers followed a 1500-cal diet (proteins = 93 g; carbohydrates = 160 g; lipids = 60 g). Insulin was administered three times daily with total doses of 30 to 65 U each day. Insulin requirement during the last 3 mo of gestation progressively increased in five patients.

Normal and GD mothers underwent a 100-g standard oral glucose tolerance test (OGTT) at the 35th wk of pregnancy for determination of blood glucose (BG) and plasma immunoreactive insulin (IRI). Venous blood samples were collected at 0, 30, 60, 90, 120, and 180 min of the test. Glucose tolerance and insulin release were then expressed as BG or IRI areas during the test. Repeated venous blood samples were collected in all the patients during the last 4 wk of gestation for fasting BG, plasma free fatty acid (FFA),[11] IRI,[12] and placental lactogen (HPL)[13] determinations. The mean of at least three determinations of each parameter was considered the basal value for each patient.

At the 21st, 24th, 27th, 30th, 33rd, and 36th wk of gestation, IDD mothers were hospitalized for 24 h. At each hospitalization, venous blood samples were collected at 0800 h (fasting state), 1100 h (after breakfast), 1500 h (after lunch), and at 1800 h (before dinner) for BG and plasma IRI, FFA, glycerol, and β-hydroxybutyrate (β-OHB)[14] determinations. Six nondiabetic pregnant women were similarly studied at the 33rd wk of pregnancy.

Body weight at birth, body length in supine position, and skinfold thickness at the subscapular, subcostal, tricipital, and crural regions were recorded in the newborn infants. A cord blood sample was also collected for blood glucose and plasma FFA and IRI determinations.

After receiving written parental consent, we performed a percutaneous microbiopsy of subcutaneous adipose tissue (butterfly needle, gauge 19), under local anesthesia with Nupercainal, in the gluteal region within 10 h of birth. The diameter of 100 adipocytes was determined on frozen-cut samples of tissue.[15] Mean fat cell volume and weight were calculated using Goldrik's formula.[16] Body fat mass was calculated from anthropometric measurements.[17] An approximate estimate of fat cell number was calculated for each infant from the ratio between fat mass weight and fat cell weight.

RESULTS

GDM group. As reported in Table 1, the GDM showed greater mean values of body weight, overweight, and body weight gain than did the controls. BG and IRI areas during OGTT were significantly higher than in controls. Fasting plasma FFA and HPL values were not significantly different in the GDM and controls.

The newborns of GDM (Table 2) presented greater, though statistically not significantly different, mean values of body weight, body length, and body fat mass.

Statistically significant differences were observed in the sum of skinfold thickness (23.0 ± 1.4 mm vs. 17.8 ± 0.7 mm; $P < 0.05$), in fat cell weight (0.37 ± 0.06 μg vs. 0.19 ± 0.02 μg; $P < 0.01$), and in percent values of fat mass (17.4 ± 1.7% vs. 12.2 ± 0.5%; $P < 0.05$) in the newborns of GDM group. IRI values in newborns of the GDM were higher, though not significantly different, than those in controls.

IDDM group. As reported in Table 1, the IDDM showed significantly greater mean values of gravidic weight gain (15.0 ± 1.7 vs. 8.4 ± 0.8 kg; $P < 0.01$) and plasma HPL values (9.9 ± 0.7 μg/ml vs. 4.6 ± 1.4 μg; $P < 0.01$) than did the controls. No statistically significant differences were found in the other parameters considered. Body fat mass (BFM) (718 ± 51 g vs. 386 ± 22 g; $P < 0.001$), sum of skinfold thickness (30.8 ± 1.7 mm vs. 17.8 ± 0.7 mm; $P < 0.001$), fat cell weight (FCW) (0.44 ± 0.02 μg vs. 0.19 ± 0.02 μg; $P < 0.001$), and body fat mass as percent of total body weight (20.3 ± 1.1% vs. 12.2 ± 0.5%; $P < 0.001$) (Table 2) were significantly higher in the newborns of these mothers. Mean IRI values in cord blood were markedly higher, though the difference was not statistically significant, in these newborns as compared with controls (Table 2).

Diurnal substrate variations in IDD mothers. The fluctuations in diurnal blood glucose and in plasma glycerol and β-OHB levels in the IDDM, observed from the 21st to the 36th wk of pregnancy, are reported in Figure 1. An improvement in the control of diabetes was observed late in pregnancy (35th wk). Diurnal FFA and glycerol variations did not exceed those in the normal pregnant women, thus confirming good control of lipid mobilization in the IDDM (Figure 1). Mean plasma β-OHB values at times 1100 h and 1800 h did not exceed the range of variations of the normal mothers at the corresponding times. Markedly higher fasting β-OHB values in IDDM were observed only at the 30th and 33rd wk of gestation.

The evaluation of the relationship between the hormonal and metabolic parameters in the mothers globally considered and parameters of adipose tissue development in newborns shows a significant correlation between maternal fasting blood glucose and neonatal BFM and FCW (Figure 2). A significant correlation was also found between IRI levels in

TABLE 1
Anthropometric, metabolic, and hormonal parameters in gestational-diabetic mothers (GDM), insulin-dependent diabetic mothers (IDDM), and normal mothers (mean ± SEM)

	Age (yr)	Pregravidic body weight (kg)	Pregravidic overweight (%)	Body weight gain (kg)	OGTT BG area	OGTT IRI area	Fasting FFA (μeq/L)	HPL (μg/ml)
Controls	28.4	59.2	12.5	8.4	297	116	291	4.6
(N = 17)	±1.4	±2.7	±5.0	±0.8	±10	±5.6	±30	+1.4
GDM	31.7	66.3	20.5	12.4*	420‡	209‡	337	9.9
(N = 17)	±1.9	±2.6	±3.6	±1.5	±22	±17.6	±38	±3.4
IDDM	25.9	58.1	10.5	15.0†	—	—	319	9.9†
(N = 8)	±1.5	±2.9	±6.9	±1.7			±35	±0.7

Statistical analysis was carried out using the Student's *t* test: * $P < 0.05$; † $P < 0.01$; ‡ $P < 0.001$.

TABLE 2
Adipose tissue development in newborns of gestational-diabetic mothers (GDM), insulin-dependent diabetic mothers (IDDM), and normal mothers (mean ± SEM)

	Gestational age (wk)	Body weight (kg)	Body length (cm)	Σ of S.T. (mm)	Body fat mass (g)	Body fat mass (% of BW)	Fat cell weight (μg)	Fat cell number (×10⁹)	Blood glucose (mg/dl)	Plasma IRI (μU/ml)
Controls	39.2	3.103	48.9	17.8	386	12.2	0.19	2.29	58	7.0
(N = 17)	±0.5	±0.10	±0.6	±0.7	±22	±0.5	±0.02	±0.2	±5	±3.1
GDM	38.0	3.508	50.9	23.0*	553	17.1*	0.37†	2.65	79	15.7
(N = 17)	±0.5	±0.20	±0.8	±1.4	±49	±1.7	±0.06	±0.6	±10	±3.3
IDDM	37.7	3.518	48.9	30.8‡	718‡	20.3‡	0.44‡	2.16	67	25.1
(N = 8)	±0.4	±0.18	±0.8	±1.7	±51	±1.1	±0.02	±0.2	±12	±9.1

Statistical analysis was carried out using the Student's *t* test: * $P < 0.05$; † $P < 0.01$; ‡ $P < 0.001$.

cord blood and neonatal body weight, FCW, and BFM (Figure 3). Considering each group separately, significant correlations between IRI levels in cord blood and BFM ($r = 0.822$; $P < 0.001$) or FCW ($r = 0.859$; $P < 0.001$) were found in the newborns of GDM.

No correlations were found between maternal pregravidic overweight, or weight gain during pregnancy and parameters of adipose tissue development in newborns, as well as between maternal plasma FFA levels and neonatal BFM and FCW.

In the newborns globally considered, a singificant correlation resulted between fat cell weight and body fat mass (Figure 4) or sum of skinfold thickness ($r = 0.604$; $P < 0.001$).

FIGURE 1. Diurnal profile of blood glucose, plasma FFA, β-hydroxybutyrate (βOHB), and glycerol levels (mean ± SEM) in insulin-dependent diabetic pregnant women studied at different weeks of gestation. Dashed areas represent the range of variations observed in six nondiabetic pregnant women studied at the 33rd wk of gestation.

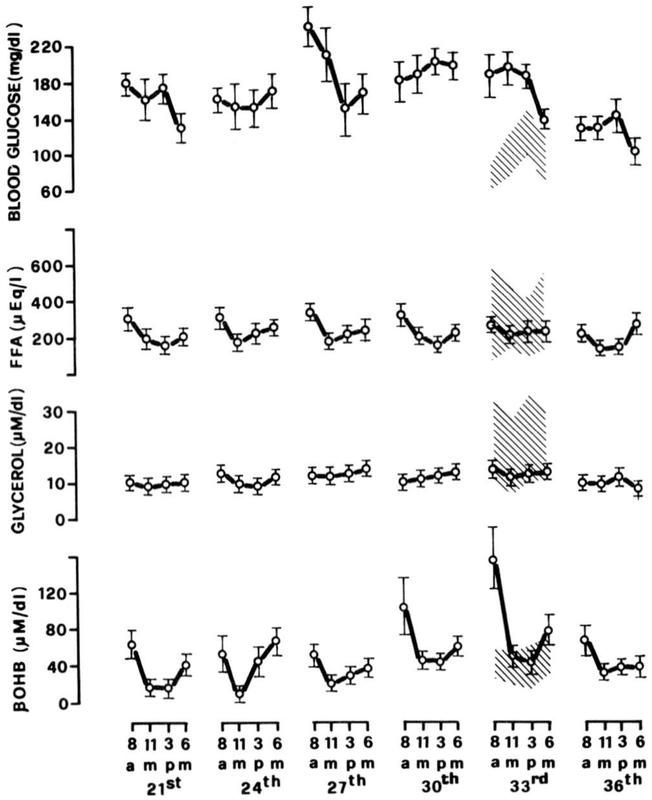

FIGURE 2. Relationship between maternal fasting blood glucose levels and parameters of adipose tissue development in newborns (○ = normal mothers; ● = GDM; △ = IDDM).

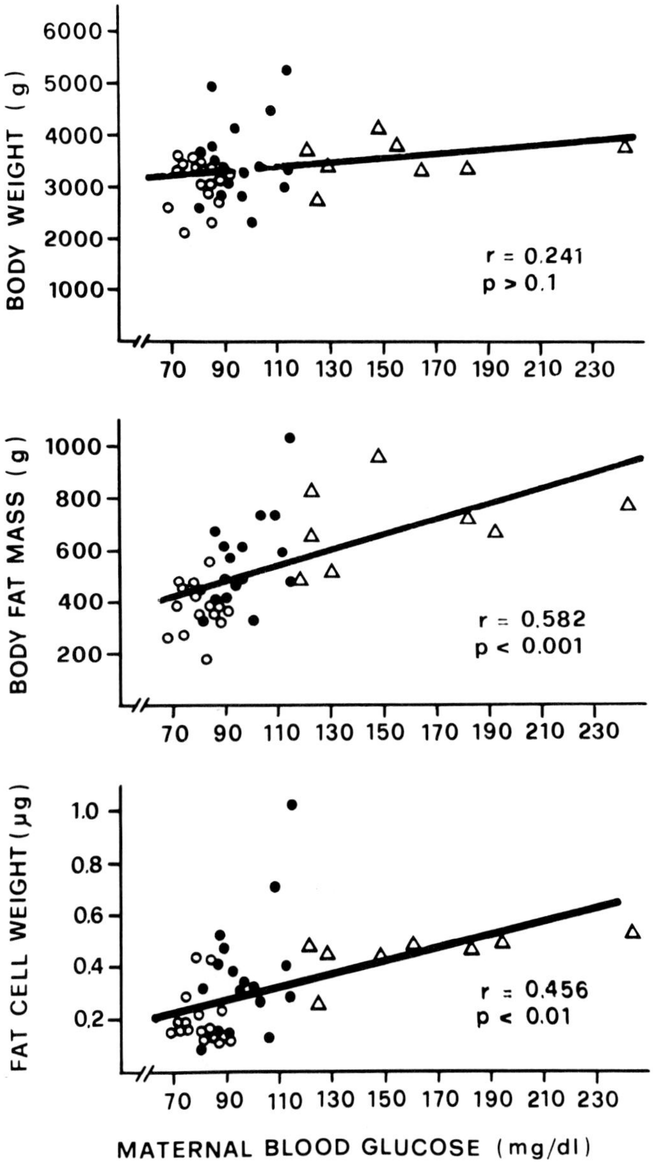

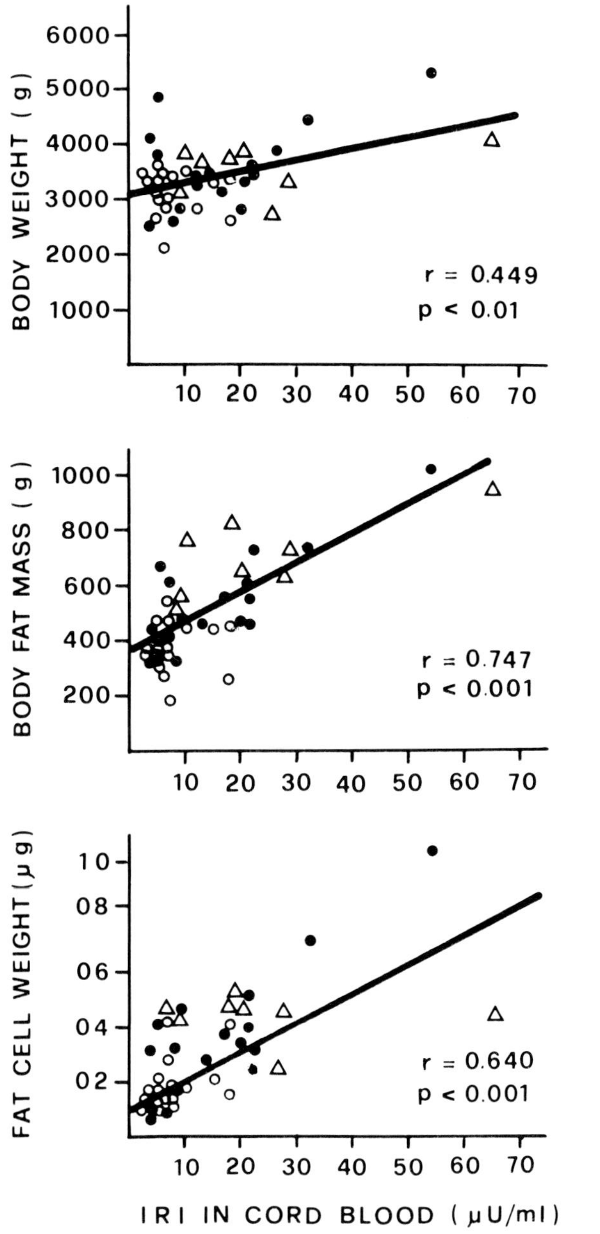

FIGURE 3. Relationships between immunoreactive insulin (IRI) levels in cord blood and parameters of adipose tissue development in newborns of normal and diabetic mothers (○ = normal mothers; ● = GDM; △ = IDDM).

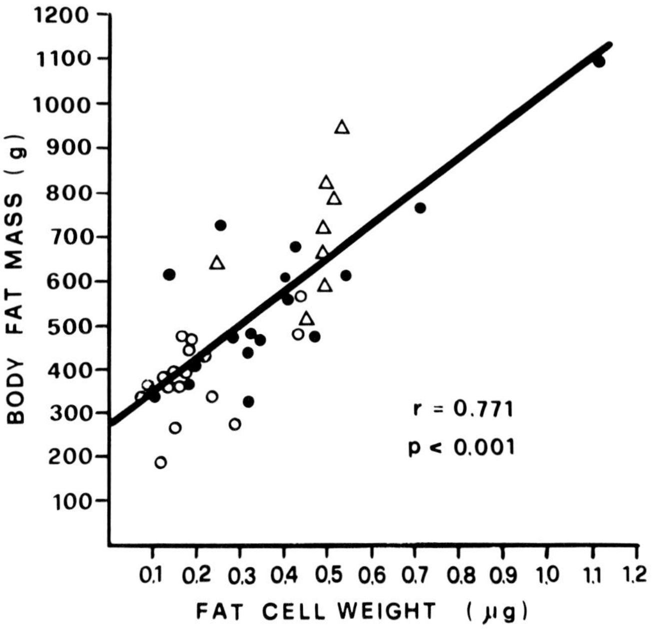

FIGURE 4. Relationships between fat cell weight and body fat mass in newborns of normal and diabetic mothers (○ = newborns of normal mothers; ● = newborns of GDM; △ = newborns of IDDM).

DISCUSSION

An enlargement in BFM was observed in full-term newborns of GDM and IDDM as compared with that observed in the controls. The difference is more evident when BFM is expressed as percent values of total body weight. Other authors have previously demonstrated that body fat mass and skinfold thickness are increased in infants of diabetic mothers.[4] In the present study, it has been shown that the expansion of body fat mass correlates with fat cell size. Estimation of fat cell number does not suggest an increase in this parameter in infants of diabetic mothers, and, to the extent that such measurements (obtained from a single biopsy site) are truly representative of adipose depots throughout the body, the data would suggest that fat cell hypertrophy, rather than an increase in fat cell number, is the primary change that characterizes the adiposity in infants of diabetic mothers.

Several factors may be responsible for fat cell hypertrophy in newborns of diabetic mothers. The GDM presented significantly higher pregravidic body weight and overweight than did controls, and several were overtly obese. It has been reported that newborn infants or obese mothers have a greater body weight at birth[18,19] even independently from a reduced glucose tolerance of the mother.[20] In newborns of diabetic mothers, however, no correlation was found between maternal pregravidic body weight or overweight and neonatal skinfold thickness, body fat mass, and fat cell weight. This seems to exclude a relationship between maternal obesity and neonatal fat mass enlargement.

In a previous study dealing with full-term newborns of presumably healthy mothers,[6] a significant correlation was found between maternal weight gain during pregnancy and the expansion of adipose tissue in newborns. In the present work, a significantly higher body weight gain was observed in the IDDM than in the controls. Nevertheless, no correlation resulted between maternal weight gain during pregnancy and parameters of adipose tissue development in newborns. Neither weight gain during pregnancy nor pregravidic overweight seem to be related to the increased development of adipose tissue observed in the offspring of diabetic mothers.

HPL has been defined as the true "growth hormone" for the fetus.[21] Both GDM and IDDM show a tendency towards higher plasma HPL levels. In normal conditions, maternal HPL values closely correlate with neonatal BFM and fat cell size.[6] It has been suggested that, by reducing carbohydrate tolerance in the mother,[22-25] HPL augments the amount of glucose available to the fetus and, thus, enhances triglyceride synthesis and storage in adipose tissue. In the present study, no correlations emerged between maternal HPL values and parameters of adipose tissue development in newborns. These observations, and the finding of significantly higher HPL values in insulin-treated diabetic women (in which the diabetic condition precedes the pregnancy), may suggest that hyperglycemia could be the cause and not the consequence of an elevation in plasma HPL levels in IDDM.

Maternal circulating free fatty acids could be a source for triglyceride synthesis in fetal adipose tissue. FFA availability to the fetus is regulated, at least in part, by maternal plasma FFA levels.[26–29] However, from studies in vitro, Dancis et al.[28] calculated a fatty acid transfer rate that was too slow to account for relevant fat storage by the fetus during the last trimester. On the other hand, when the FFA concentration increases up to normal in the maternal blood, a positive uptake of FFA occurs in the fetus.[27,30] It has been suggested that elevated levels of circulating FFA, caused by uncontrolled lipid mobilization in IDDM, could be responsible for fetal macrosomia.[31] In a previous study in infants of presumably normal mothers, no relationship was observed between maternal FFA levels and parameters of adipose tissue development in newborns.[6]

In the present investigation, fasting FFA levels in the IDDM were not significantly different from those in controls, while the diurnal profile of plasma glycerol and FFA excluded an abnormal lipid mobilization late in pregnancy. No correlation was demonstrated between FFA levels in IDDM and adipose tissue development in newborns.

Plasma IRI levels in cord blood are higher in newborns of GD and IDD mothers and closely correlate with parameters of adipose tissue development (that is, skinfold thickness, body fat mass, and fat cell weight). Cord blood IRI values in neonates of insulin-treated diabetic women may be in part artifactually elevated, owing to the presence of insulin-binding antibodies crossing the placenta. Nevertheless, a good correlation between IRI levels in cord blood and BFM and FCW was confirmed in the group, separately considered, of newborns from gestational-diabetic mothers who did not receive insulin treatment. Therefore, the putative enhancement of insulin production by the fetal pancreas and the greater amount of glucose made available by the mother may be important factors regulating triglyceride synthesis and storage in adipose tissue in newborns of diabetic mothers.

In conclusion, no evidence has been found suggesting fat cell multiplication in full-term infants of GDM and IDDM, while the hypertrophic mechanism seems to account almost entirely for fat mass enlargement. Fat cell hypertrophy depends on increased insulin production by the fetal pancreas, which, in turn, is secondary to a larger glucose availability in utero. In newborns of insulin-treated IDDM, FFAs do not represent a further substrate for the enhanced triglyceride synthesis and storage in adipose tissue.

ACKNOWLEDGMENTS

This work was supported by the National Research Council (CNR, Rome, Italy) grant 77.01332.4.

REFERENCES

[1] Osler, M.: Body water of newborn infants of diabetic mothers. Acta Endocrinol. (Copenh) *34*:261–76, 1960.

[2] Malins, G. M., and Fitzgerald, M. G.: Childbearing prior to recognition of diabetes. Recollected birth weights and stillbirth rate in babies born to parents who developed diabetes. Diabetes *14*:175–78, 1965.

[3] Oakley, N. W., Beard, R. W., and Turner, R. C.: Effect of sustained maternal hyperglycemia on the fetus in normal and diabetic pregnancies. Br. Med. J. *1*:466–69, 1972.

[4] Whitelaw, A.: Subcutaneous fat in newborn infants of diabetic mother: an indication of quality of diabetic control. Lancet *1*:15–18, 1977.

[5] Pedersen, J.: Weight and length at birth of infants of diabetic mothers. Acta Endocrinol. (Copenh) *16*:330–42, 1954.

[6] Enzi, G., Inelman, E. M., Caretta, F., Rubaltelli, F., Grella, P., and Baritussio, A.: Adipose tissue development "in utero". Relationships between some nutritional and hormonal factors and body fat mass enlargement in newborns. *In* Diabetes, Obesity and Hyperlipoproteinemias. Crepaldi, G., Lefèbvre, P., and Alberti, K. G. M. M., Eds. London, Academic Press, 1978, pp. 143–47.

[7] Kazdova, L., Fabry, P., and Vrana, A.: Effect of small doses of insulin in vivo on the proliferation and cellularity of adipose tissue. Diabetologia *10*:77–83, 1974.

[8] Björntorp, P., Enzi, G., Karlsson, K., Krotkiewski, M., Sjöström, L., and Smith, U.: The effect of maternal diabetes on adipose tissue cellularity in man and rat. Diabetologia *10*:205–09, 1974.

[9] White, P.: Classification of obstetric diabetes. Am. J. Obstet. Gynecol. *130*:228–30, 1978.

[10] Duncombe, W. G.: The colorimetric micro-determination of non-esterified fatty acids in plasma. Clin. Chim. Acta *9*:122–25, 1964.

[11] Metropolitan Life Insurance Company: Frequency of overweight and underweight. Stat. Bull. *41*:4, 1960.

[12] Yalow, R. S., and Berson, S. A.: Immunoassay of endogenous plasma insulin in man. J. Clin. Invest. *39*:1157–75, 1960.

[13] Pennisi, F., and Vancheri, L.: Il dosaggio radioimmunologico di ormoni in gravidanza. *In* Semeiotica della gravidanza a rischio. Destro, F., Ed. Rome, Verucci Press, 1977, pp. 322–31.

[14] Olsen, C.: An enzymatic fluorimetric micromethod for the determination of acetoacetate, β-hydroxybutyrate, pyruvate and lactate. Clin. Chim. Acta *33*:293–300, 1971.

[15] Sjöström, L., Björntorp, P., and Vrana, J.: Microscopic fat cell size measurement on frozen-cut adipose tissue in comparison with automatic determination of osmium fixed fat cells. J. Lipid Res. *12*:521–30, 1971.

[16] Goldrick, R. B.: Morphological changes in the adipocyte during fat deposition and mobilization. Am. J. Physiol. *212*:777–82, 1967.

[17] Dauncey, M. J., Gandy, G., and Gairner, D.: Assessment of total body fat in infancy from skinfold thickness measurements. Arch. Dis. Child. *52*:233–27, 1977.

[18] Whitelaw, A. G. L.: Influence of maternal obesity on subcutaneous fat in the newborn. Br. Med. J. *1*:985–86, 1976.

[19] Love, E. J., and Kinch, R. A.: Factors influencing the birth weight in normal pregnancy. Am. J. Obstet. Gynecol. *91*:342–49, 1965.

[20] Enzi, G., Inelmen, E. M., Caretta, F., Zanardo, V., and Baritussio, A.: Adipose tissue development in newborn of obese mothers. *In* Obesity and Diabetes. Vague, J., and Vague, Ph., Eds. Amsterdam, Excerpta Medica Found., 1979, ICS *xv*, pp. 763–67.

[21] Grumbach, M. M., Kaplan, J. L., Sciarra, J. J., and Burr, I. M.: Chorionic growth hormone prolactin (CGP): secretion, disposition, biologic activity in man and postulated functions as the "growth hormone" of the second half of pregnancy. Ann. N.Y. Acad. Sci. *148*:501–31, 1968.

[22] Kalkhoff, R., Schalch, D. S., Walker, L., Beck, P., Kipnis, D. M., and Daughaday, W. H.: Diabetogenic factors associated with pregnancy. Trans. Assoc. Am. Physicians *77*:270–73, 1964.

[23] Beck, P., and Daughaday, W. H.: Human placental lactogen: studies of its acute metabolic effects and disposition in normal man. J. Clin. Invest. *46*:103–10, 1967.

[24] Samaan, N., Yen, S. S. C., Gonzalez, D., and Pearson, O. H.: Metabolic effects of placental lactogen (HPL) in man. J. Clin. Endocrinol. Metab. *28*:485–91, 1968.

[25] Malaisse, W. J., Malaisse-Lagae, F., Picard, C., and Flament-Durand, J.: Effects of pregnancy and chorionic growth hormone upon insulin secretion. Endocrinology *84*:41–44, 1969.

[26] Szabo, A. J., Grimaldi, R. D., and Jung, W. F.: Palmitate transport across perfused human placenta. Metabolism *18*:406–15, 1960.

[27] Sheath, J., Grimwade, J., Waldron, K., Bikley, M., Taft, P., and Wood, C.: Arteriovenous non-esterified fatty acids and glycerol differences in the umbilical cord at term and their relationships to fetal metabolism. Am. J. Obstet. Gynecol. *113*:358–62, 1972.

[28] Dancis, J., Jansen, V., Kayden, M. J., Schneider, M., and Levitz, M.: Transfer across perfused human placenta. II. Free fatty acids. Pediatr. Res. *7*:192–97, 1973.

[29] Dancis, J., Jansen, V., Kayden, H. J., Björnson, L., and Levitz, M.: Transfer across the perfused human placenta: III. Effect of chain length on transfer of free fatty acids. Pediatr. Res. *8*:796–99, 1974.

[30] Rubaltelli, F., Enzi, G., De Biasi, F., Bondio, M., and Rondinelli, M.: Effect of lipid loading on the fetal uptake of free fatty acids, glycerol and β-hydroxybutyrate. Biol. Neonate *33*:320–26, 1978.

[31] Szabo, A. J., and Szabo, O.: Placental free fatty acid transfer and fetal adipose tissue development. An explanation of fetal adiposity in infants of diabetic mothers. Lancet *2*:498–99, 1974.

Insulin Recoverable from Tissues

JOHN ENG AND ROSALYN S. YALOW

SUMMARY

In this report we describe the insulin concentrations in plasma and in brain, kidney, liver, heart, and other tissues of rabbits and dogs as well as of rats and mice of different strains. In the larger animals, insulin concentrations in the brain never exceeded plasma levels. In rats, brain concentration averaged no more than twice plasma levels, compared with the 25-fold tissue:plasma ratio reported by others. Since there is no reason to believe that the biosynthetic mechanisms are different in the brains of large and small mammals, our results suggest that the insulin found in the brain is due in part to that in vascular spaces and perhaps also to that crossing the blood-brain barrier, diffusing through the brain and then concentrating on brain receptor sites. In our preliminary abstract we reported that kidney and liver concentrations in rabbits and dogs exceeded plasma levels but noted no pattern of relationship between tissue and plasma concentrations. However, we have observed that when hyperinsulinism persists, as in a dexamethasone-treated dog or hyperphagic, obese rodents, the insulin content of some organs, particularly the kidney, does reflect plasma levels. In rats and mice, the insulin concentrations in kidney extracts appear to increase linearly with plasma levels. Liver and heart insulin concentrations initially appear to increase with plasma but then plateau, suggesting a saturable mechanism. We believe that insulin extractable from tissues reflects binding of insulin to receptors and that the total content of insulin receptors in a tissue may be the sum of unoccupied receptor sites, as measured in receptor assays, and the sites occupied by insulin extractable from the tissue.
DIABETES 29:105–109, February 1980.

It is now generally appreciated that several peptides such as substance P,[1] somatostatin,[2,3] vasoactive intestinal peptide,[4] and cholecystokinin[5] or its COOH-terminal fragments[5–7] are common to and synthesized in the brain and digestive system. The recent report by Havrankova et al.[8] that insulin concentrations in acid-ethanol extracts of rat brain averaged 25 times higher than plasma levels, coupled with their suggestion that this peptide, known to be synthesized in the pancreas, might also be synthesized by cells in the central nervous system stimulated our investigations of the insulin content of the brains of larger animals as well as the possibility of insulin production in other body tissues. In this report we describe the insulin concentrations in brain, kidney, liver, heart, and other tissues of rabbit and dog as well as of rats and mice of different strains.

MATERIALS AND METHODS

Tissue extraction. New Zealand white rabbits, mixed-breed dogs, C57BL/6J ob/ob and C57BL/KsJ db/db mice and their nonobese littermates (Jackson Memorial Labs, Bar Harbor, Maine), Sprague-Dawley rats, and Zucker rats (Fab Labs, New City, New York) were fed ad lib. and blood samples obtained before they were killed. One dog was treated with dexamethasone, producing an elevated plasma insulin.

Rabbits and dogs were bled from ear or leg veins and then killed by intravenous injection of lethal doses of sodium pentobarbital. Blood was taken from tail vein or heart puncture in rats and mice after anesthesia with intraperitoneal sodium pentobarbital (5 mg/100 g). Animal tissues were quickly removed, placed on dry ice, and later stored at −20°C before extraction. During tissue removal, contamination by pancreatic tissue was carefully avoided.

Tissues were extracted with a Teflon grinder in 10 vol of 0.18 N HCl-75% ethanol (acid-ethanol). The suspension was centrifuged at 2000 × *g* for 30 min at 4°C and the supernatants were removed and stored at −10°C before radioimmunoassay.

From the Solomon A. Berson Research Laboratory, Veterans Administration Medical Center, Bronx, New York.
Address reprint requests to John Eng, Solomon A. Berson Research Laboratory, Veterans Administration Medical Center, Bronx, New York 10468.
Received for publication 7 August 1979.

Radioimmunoassay (RIA). RIA was performed using a guinea pig anti-porcine insulin serum prepared in our laboratory and porcine monoiodoinsulin (380 $\mu Ci^{125}I/\mu g$) obtained after purification on starch gel electrophoresis according to methods generally used in our laboratory.[9-12] The standard diluent for the assay contained 0.25 g human serum albumin (HSA)/dl 0.02 M barbital buffer (pH 8.6). Standards were prepared with pork (gift from Novo Laboratories, courtesy of Dr. J. Schlichtkrull), dog (gift from Dr. I. Arthur Mirsky), and rat and mouse insulins (gift from Novo Laboratories, courtesy of Dr. L. Heding). Extracts of a rabbit pancreas were assayed over a 100-fold concentration range. Insulin concentrations reported here are in terms of the appropriate animal insulin standard. The assay volume was 2.5 ml and plasma and tissue extracts were added in volume between 5 and 250 μl. When acid-ethanol extracts were assayed, an equal volume of 0.18 N NaOH was added for neutralization to diluent pH. Standard curves contained volumes of acid-ethanol and NaOH corresponding to volume of tissue extracts. For some studies neutralized tissue extracts were freed of insulin by absorption to talc and then used for preparation of standard curves. Since the Sephadex gel chromatography elution buffer was the same as standard diluent, eluates in volumes up to 1 ml were used directly in the assay. Separation of bound from free ^{125}I-insulin was effected by addition of 0.2 ml of 100 mg charcoal/ml 0.02 M barbital buffer.

Validation procedures. Nonspecific interference in the immune reaction by substances in tissue extracts and damage to the ^{125}I-peptide can result in diminished binding of tracer to antibody and be falsely interpreted as resulting from the presence of hormone. The integrity of the tracer was monitored in two ways. ^{125}I-insulin was incubated with tissue extracts under simulated assay conditions, and the Sephadex gel filtration patterns of radioactivity after incubation were unchanged from those before incubation. In addition, when an excess of anti-insulin antibody was added in a double-antibody assay system, the radioactivity precipitated by antiserum to guinea pig gamma globulin was the same in tubes with the unknown samples as in standard tubes.

The nature of the immunoreactive material in tissue extracts was examined using Sephadex G50 gel chromatography. Because undiluted acid-alcohol causes marked gel shrinkage and distortion, tissue extracts were either diluted in up to 10 vol of standard diluent or first concentrated to one-tenth of original volume before addition of standard diluent. The extracts were applied to Sephadex G50 fine columns (1 × 50 cm) and eluted with standard diluent. The columns were calibrated with ^{125}I-albumin, ^{125}I-insulin, and $Na^{125}I$. Immunoreactive insulin content of the successive 1-ml eluates was determined by RIA.

RESULTS

The antiserum used for these studies was about 15-fold more sensitive than that used by Havrankova et al.[8] In our RIA 10 pg pork insulin/ml incubation mixture reduced to about one-half the initial B/F ratio (~1) (Figure 1). Dog and pork insulins react identically and a dilution curve of rabbit pancreas is superposable on the standard curve. However, rat insulin reacts more poorly in this system and a dilution of this insulin is not superposable on the pork insulin curve (Figure 1). Rat and mouse insulins react identically. The sensitivity of our RIA makes it possible to assay plasma and

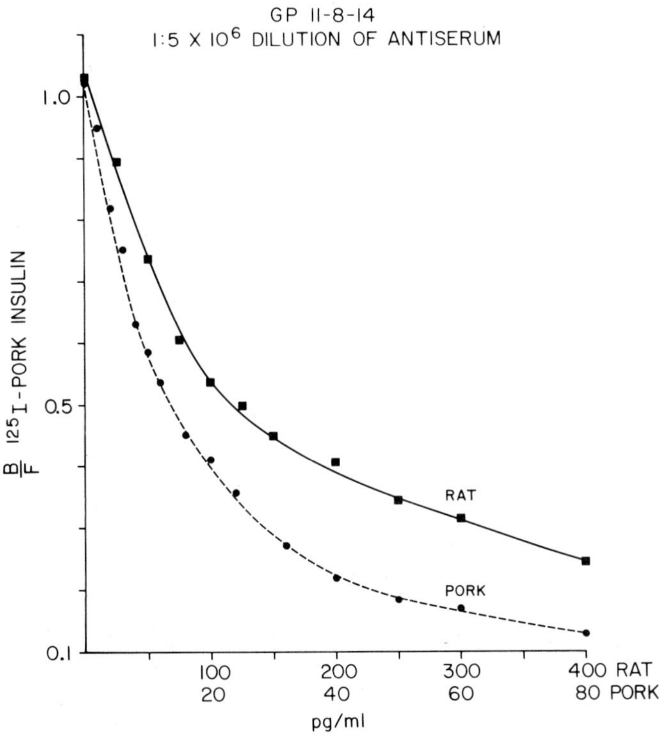

FIGURE 1. Standard curves for the insulin assay. Dog and pork insulins react identically in this assay and dilutions of rabbit pancreatic extracts are superposable on the pork standard curve. Mouse and rat insulins react identically.

tissue extracts directly without prior purification and concentration.

Extracts of various portions of the brains and other tissue of rabbits and dogs were compared with plasma levels (Table 1). For these studies the acid-ethanol extracts (0.1 g wet tissue/ml) were assayed directly at a dilution of 1:10 or greater in the final incubation mixture. The minimum detectable concentration of insulin in dog or rabbit tissues would therefore be ~0.2 ng/g. The apparent concentration in the brains of these animals was at or near this minimal level (Table 1). The plasma levels ranged from 0.5 to 3.5 ng/ml. In no case did the insulin concentration in the brain exceed the plasma level. However, insulin concentrations in several peripheral tissues did exceed that in plasma. In the few animals studied, there appeared to be no particular pattern in the relationship between plasma and tissue concentrations except that kidney concentrations were usually the highest.

TABLE 1
Concentration of insulin in plasma (ng/ml) and tissue (ng/g)

	Rabbit 1	Rabbit 2	Dog 1	Dog 2	Dog (dexamethasone-treated)
Plasma	0.9	1.2	1.8	0.5	3.5
Cortex	0.7	0.5	0.2	0.5	0.4
Hypothalamus	0.7	0.8	0.2		
Cerebellum	0.4	0.5	0.2		
Brain stem	0.5	0.6	0.5		
Heart	1.5	3.6	1.0	0.6	1.5
Liver	3.1	5.7	2.0	0.6	1.0
Kidney	5.0	4.5	6.5	3.0	25.0
Muscle	0.7	2.3	1.0	1.3	1.1

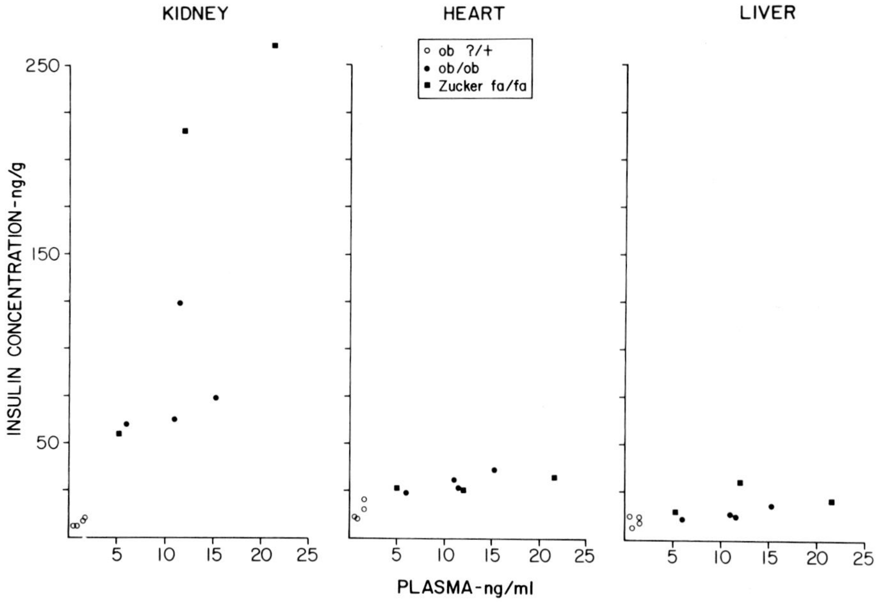

FIGURE 2. Concentrations of insulin in extracts of kidney (left), heart (middle), and liver (right) plotted as a function of the plasma concentrations. Obese rodents are shown in solid symbols and nonobese littermates in open symbols. All obese rodents were hyperinsulinemic. There appears to be a linear relationship between the insulin concentration in the kidney and that in plasma.

The highest kidney concentration was found in a dexamethasone-treated dog with sustained hyperinsulinism (Table 1).

Since our antiserum is less sensitive for the detection of rat and mouse insulins, the minimum detectable level is about 2 ng/g rat or mouse tissue. Extracts of the whole brains of four normal rats averaged just at the limit of detectability, i.e., 2.0 ± 0.2 ng/g (SEM) compared with plasma levels of 1.1 ± 0.5 ng/ml (SEM). The brain concentrations seem to exceed plasma levels but are considerably below those found by Havrankova et al.[8] Shown in Figure 2 are the relative concentrations of insulin in the plasma and kidney, heart, and liver extracts of ob/ob mice and their lean littermates and of Zucker (fa/fa) rats. In each of these organs increased plasma insulin levels are associated with an increase in tissue levels. However, the rate of increase is organ dependent. The kidney generally has the highest insulin concentration, the levels increasing almost linearly with plasma level (Figure 2, left). The concentrations in heart and liver appear to rise and then plateau with increasing plasma concentration (Figure 2, middle and right). All hyperinsulinemic mice of the ob/ob or db/db strains have

FIGURE 3. Insulin concentrations in extracts of kidney of db/db mice, ob/ob mice, and of their nonobese littermates.

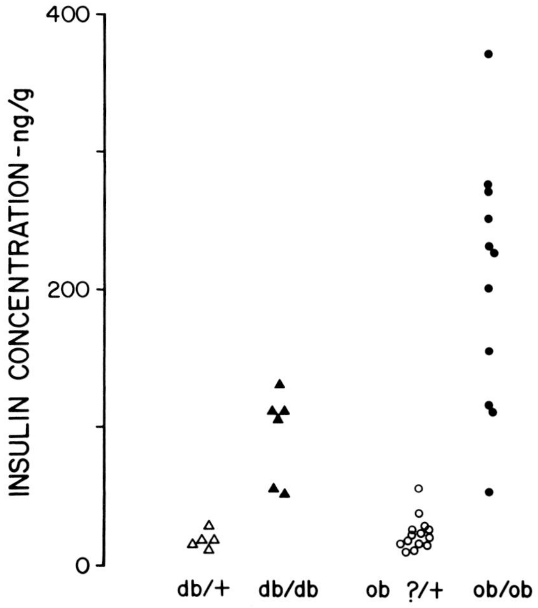

FIGURE 4. Sephadex G50 gel filtration patterns of immunoreactive insulin in plasma and in extracts of heart, liver, and kidney of a Zucker (fa/fa) rat. The major peak of immunoreactivity coelutes with authentic insulin.

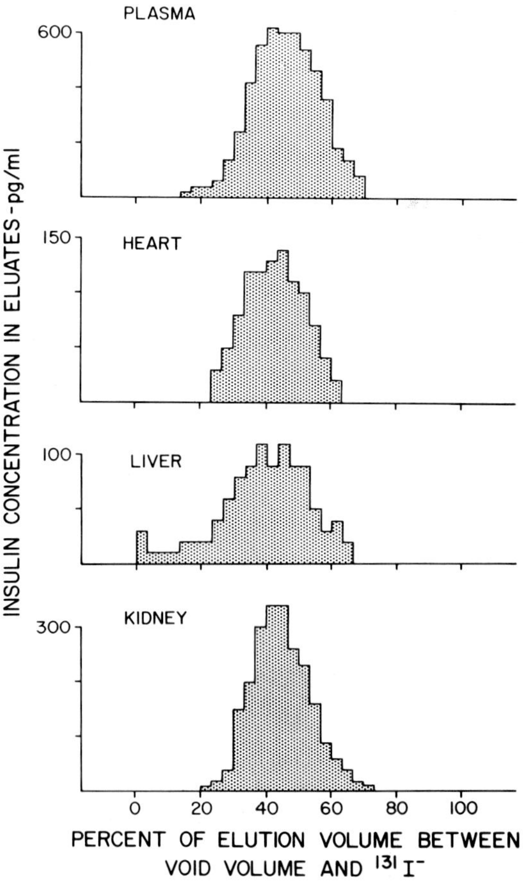

marked elevations of kidney insulin compared with that of their lean littermates (Figure 3).

That the immunoreactivities extracted from the kidney, heart, and liver of the Zucker (fa/fa) rat are authentic insulin is evident from the Sephadex G50 gel filtration patterns (Figure 4). We have not detected immunoreactivity in the proinsulin region in Sephadex gel eluates of rat plasma or tissue extracts. The failure to detect rat proinsulin may be due to poor cross-reactivity of proinsulin with the antiserum employed.

DISCUSSION

Our observations fail to confirm the report of Havrankova et al.[8] that on the average insulin is concentrated in the rat brain to levels 25 times higher than in plasma. In fact, in a subsequent report by the same group,[13] the brain:plasma ratio in control rats was 4, a ratio much closer to the one in this report (ratio = 1.8) than the value they previously reported.[8] The decrease in their ratio was due to a marked decrease in brain insulin in the control rats in the second study[13] (6 ± 1 ng/g) compared with the levels previously measured[8] (22 ± 8 ng/g). The authors[8,13] did not account for the striking decrease in brain content in rats of the same strain and sex, with the only evident difference being that the second group weighed slightly less (200–250 g) than the first group (250–300 g). In animals with larger brains such as the rabbit and dog, the insulin levels are certainly below that of plasma. Since there is no reason to believe that the biosynthetic mechanisms are different in the brains of large and small mammals, our results would suggest that insulin found in the brain is due in part to that in vascular spaces and perhaps also to that crossing the blood-brain barrier, diffusing through the brain (which occurs to a greater extent in small-brained animals), and then concentrating on brain receptor sites.

In our preliminary abstract describing the content of insulin in the tissues of dog and rabbit, [14] we could find no pattern of relationship between tissue and plasma hormone levels. However, when hyperinsulinism persists as in hyperphagic, obese rodents, the insulin content of some organs does reflect plasma levels. These results are strikingly different from those of Rosenzweig et al.,[15] who also found that insulin is present in many tissues in concentrations higher than plasma, but who concluded that the insulin concentrations in these tissues vary little or not at all with extreme fluctuations in plasma insulin.

It is difficult to account for the differences between our laboratories. Part of the discrepancies may be due to the marked differences in sensitivities of the different antisera. With the sensitivity of the antiserum we employed, it was not necessary to concentrate insulin from tissue extracts before assay. We employed mouse or rat insulin as standard and dilution curves of tissue extracts of the hyperinsulinemic rats and mice were superposable along the standard curve. In the studies of Havrankova et al.,[8] dilution curves of the brain and hypothalamic extracts were not superposable on the pork insulin curve used as standard. This does of course introduce some error into the assay. However, neither the limited sensitivity nor the lack of superposability could explain the failure of this group to find marked elevations of insulin in the kidneys of hyperinsulinemic animals. Although there is some increase in liver insulin concentration with increase in plasma level, the difference is not large and might easily be missed. Our studies are consistent with the earlier work of Elgee et al.,[16] who reported that in rats 5 min after intravenous administration of ^{131}I-insulin, the kidney:blood ratio averaged more than 10:1 whereas the liver:blood ratio was only about 2:1. These authors[16] also demonstrated from autoradiographs of the kidney that the hormone is concentrated in the proximal convoluted tubules. Since in the absence of insulin, massive glycogen accumulation occurs in the terminal straight portion of the proximal convoluted tubules,[17,18] it is possible that the presence of insulin on receptor sites in this region is required to prevent glycogen deposition or to hasten its disappearance.

The difference in insulin concentration for kidney and other organs is perhaps best explained in terms of receptor site content. At physiologic concentrations of insulin the kidney appears to have a nonsaturable mechanism for retaining or sequestering the insulin that is filtered through it. In contrast, the insulin concentrations of the heart and liver plateau with increase in plasma level, indicating that in these organs the receptor sites are readily saturable. Our findings are consistent with those of Sodoyez-Goffaux et al.,[19] who concluded from studies with ^{125}I-insulin that its binding to fetal rat liver was saturable but that binding to kidney was not. In similar studies on binding of labeled insulin to tissue sites Zeleznik and Roth,[20] after observing that large doses of unlabeled insulin do not affect uptake of radioactivity by the kidney, concluded that such binding was "predominantly not related to the specific insulin receptor." However, an equally tenable interpretation of their observations is that the receptor sites in this organ are not readily saturable. Such an interpretation would be consistent with our studies. Since, according to the studies of Elgee et al.,[16] insulin concentration in the kidney appears to be found primarily in the proximal convoluted tubules, the concentration of insulin and, by inference, of receptor sites in this region is likely to exceed that in any other tissue site.

ACKNOWLEDGMENTS

This work was supported by the Medical Research Program of the Veterans Administration.

REFERENCES

1 Leeman, S. E., Mroz, E. A., and Carraway, R. E.: Substance P and neurotensin. *In* Peptides in Neurobiology. Gainer, H., Ed. New York, Plenum Press, 1977, pp. 99–144.

2 Brownstein, M., Ariumra, A., Sato, H., Schally, A. V., and Kizer, J. S.: The regional distribution of somatostatin in the rat brain. Endocrinology *96*:1456–61, 1975.

3 Hokfelt, T., Efendic, S., Hellerstrom, C., Johnson, O., Luft, R., and Arimura, A.: Cellular localization of somatostatin in endocrine-like cells and neurons of the rat with special reference to the A-cells of the pancreatic islets and to the hypothalamus. Acta Endocrinol. *80* (Suppl. 200):141, 1975.

4 Bryant, M. G., Polak, S. M., Modlin, B., Bloom, S. R., Albuguerque, R. H., and Pearse, A. G. E.: Possible dual role for vasoactive intestinal peptide as gastrointestinal hormone and neurotransmitter substance. Lancet *1*:991–93, 1976.

5 Muller, J. E., Straus, E., and Yalow, R. S.: Cholecystokinin and its C-terminal octapeptide in the pig brain. Proc. Natl. Acad. Sci. USA *74*:3035–37, 1977.

6 Dockray, G. J.: Immunochemical evidence of cholecystokinin-like peptides in the brain. Nature *264*:568–70, 1976.

7 Dockray, G. J., Gregory, R. A., and Hutchinson, J. B.: Isolation structure and biological activity of two cholecystokinin octapeptides from sheep brain. Nature *274*:711–13, 1978.

8 Havrankova, J., Schmechel, D., Roth, J., and Brownstein, M.: Identification of insulin in rat brain. Proc. Natl. Acad. Sci. USA *75*:5737–41, 1978.

9 Yalow, R. S., and Berson, S. A.: Assay of plasma insulin in human subjects by immunological methods. Nature *184*:1648–49, 1959.

[10] Yalow, R. S., and Berson, S. A.: Immunoassay of endogenous plasma insulin in man. J. Clin. Invest. *39*:1157–75, 1960.

[11] Berson, S. A., and Yalow, R. S.: General radioimmunoassay. *In* Methods in Investigative and Diagnostic Endocrinology, Part I, General Methodology. Berson, S. A., and Yalow, R. S., Eds. Amsterdam, North-Holland Publishing Co., 1973, Chap. 4, Sec. 2.1, pp. 84–120.

[12] Yalow, R. S., and Berson, S. A.: Radioimmunoassay of insulin. *In* Methods in Investigative and Diagnostic Endocrinology, Part III, Non-Pituitary Hormones. Berson, S. A., and Yalow, R. S., Eds. Amsterdam, North-Holland Publishing Co., 1973, Chap. 3, Sec. 3.2, pp. 864–70.

[13] Havrankova, J., Roth, J., and Brownstein, M. J.: Concentrations of insulin and of insulin receptors in the brain are independent of peripheral insulin levels. J. Clin. Invest. *64*:636–42, 1979.

[14] Eng, J., and Yalow, R. S.: Insulin recoverable from tissues. Endocrinology (Suppl. A-384):168, 1979.

[15] Rosenzweig, J. L., Havrankova, J., Lesniak, M. A., Brownstein, M. J., and Roth, J.: Insulin at high concentrations in a broad range of extrapancreatic tissues of rodent and man. Diabetes *28*:346A, 1979. Abstract.

[16] Elgee, N. J., Williams, H., and Lee, N. D.: Distribution and degradation studies with insulin-I^{131}. J. Clin. Invest. *33*:1252–60, 1954.

[17] Ritchie, S., and Waugh, D.: The pathology of Armanni-Ebstein diabetic nephropathy. Am. J. Pathol. *35*:1035–57, 1957.

[18] Warren, S.: Glycogen deposits in diabetes mellitus. Am. J. Med. Sci. *179*:482–88, 1930.

[19] Sodoyez-Goffaux, F. R., Sodoyez, J. C., and De Vos, C. J.: Insulin secretion and metabolism during the perinatal period in the rat. J. Clin. Invest. *63*:1095–1102, 1979.

[20] Zeleznik, A. J., and Roth, J.: Demonstration of the insulin receptor in vivo in rabbits and its possible role as a reservoir for the plasma hormone. J. Clin. Invest. *61*:1363–74, 1978.

Hypothesis:

The Frequencies of Juvenile Diabetes in American Blacks and Caucasians Are Consistent with Dominant Inheritance

MICHAEL J. MACDONALD

SUMMARY

A test is described that can be used to distinguish whether a trait (in this case juvenile diabetes) is inherited in an autosomal dominant or a recessive manner. The frequencies of the trait are compared in two populations in which there has been a unidirectional influx of genes from the gene pool of one of the populations into that of the other. Before the racial admixture, the trait should be primarily a characteristic of the first population. If the trait is dominant, its frequency in the second population will be equal to the number of individuals carrying at least one gene causing the trait and thus directly proportional to the overall percentage of its genes received from the first population. If the trait is recessive, its frequency in the second population, relative to that in the first, will be far lower than the overall percentage of its genes received from the first population, because the rate of homozygotes is equal to the square of the gene frequency. The American Caucasian and black populations fulfill the criteria for the test. Racial admixture between the two groups has been entirely from the Caucasian to the black population, and juvenile diabetes was very likely nonexistent in black people before their arrival in North America. About 20% of the American black gene pool is composed of Caucasian genes and the frequency of juvenile diabetes in the American black population is 20%–30% that in American Caucasians. Because juvenile diabetes in American blacks is associated with the same HLA genes as in Caucasians, and these genes are also about 20%–30% as common in American blacks as in Caucasians, the occurrence of juvenile diabetes in American blacks is very likely due to Caucasian genes. If susceptibility to juvenile diabetes is inherited in a recessive manner, its frequency in black Americans should be about $(1/5)^2$ or 1/25 the frequency in Caucasians. However, since the ratio of the frequency of juvenile diabetes in American blacks to that in Caucasians is roughly equal to, or certainly not lower than, the fraction of Caucasian genes in the American black gene pool, the data fit the criterion for dominant better than for recessive inheritance. Because population data are used in the test, factors that confound genetic studies in families, such as incomplete penetrance and recombination should not confound this test.

DIABETES 29:110–114, February 1980.

Because the causation of insulin-dependent, juvenile-onset diabetes probably involves environmental as well as hereditary factors,[1–5] it has not been easy to determine its mode(s) of inheritance. In addition, there might be genetic heterogeneity within the syndrome.[6–8] Recently, it was discovered that juvenile diabetes is associated with the HLA complex on chromosome number 6.[9] Several investigators have attempted to use this association to determine whether the susceptibility to juvenile diabetes is inherited in an autosomal recessive or dominant manner by measuring the percentages of pairs of diabetic siblings who shared HLA haplotypes (0, 1, or 2 haplotypes) in families in which more than one offspring was a juvenile diabetic. In all the studies it was found that the frequency of pairs of diabetic siblings with two identical haplotypes was 50%–60%, which was higher than expected by chance.[10–14] (If juvenile diabetes is not linked to the HLA complex, about 25% of the pairs would have shared two haplotypes). Although this result demonstrated that genes associated with juvenile diabetes are indeed linked to genes in the HLA complex, it did not yield clear interpretations about the inheritance of diabetes. If the genes associated with juvenile diabetes are tightly linked to the HLA complex, 100% of the pairs of diabetic siblings should have shared two haplotypes if juvenile diabetes is recessive; if it is dominant, 50% of the pairs should have shared two haplotypes. (See Appendix I.) These proportions do not depend on the penetrance of the genes giving susceptibility to diabetes since, in the cases studied, penetrance was essentially complete, i.e., the subjects studied

From the Department of Pediatrics and Institute for Enzyme Research, University of Wisconsin, Madison.
Address reprint requests to Michael J. MacDonald, M.D., Institute for Enzyme Research, 1710 University Avenue, Madison, Wisconsin 53706.
Received for publication 10 August 1979.

obviously had the genes giving susceptibility to juvenile diabetes. If the genes causing susceptibility to juvenile diabetes are not closely linked to the HLA complex, such that there was recombination between these genes and the HLA complex, the proportion of sibling pairs sharing two haplotypes would have been lower than 100% if diabetes is recessive and lower than 50% if it is dominant. (To determine how much lower, the amount of recombination and the mode of inheritance must be known.) If diabetes is recessive, a high rate of homozygous but unaffected parents could also explain a lower than expected percentage of shared haplotypes, but as noted by Spielman et al.,[14] this explanation is not very plausible. The interpretation involving the fewest assumptions is, of course, that the studies of HLA haplotypes in pairs of diabetic siblings indicate that the inheritance of susceptibility to juvenile diabetes is dominant. However, due to our current lack of knowledge of the genetics of diabetes, other more complex interpretations of these HLA data cannot be excluded.[6]

Besides studies of families, population data can be used to distinguish whether a trait is autosomal dominant or recessive. In the test discussed here the frequency of the trait is compared in two populations in which there has been a unidirectional influx of genes from the gene pool of one of the populations into that of the other. If the disorder was almost nonexistent in the second population before the influx of genes, the test is more rigorous. If the trait is autosomal dominant, its frequency in the second population will be equal to the number of individuals carrying at least one gene causing the trait and thus directly proportional to the overall number of genes received from the first population. If the trait is inherited in an autosomal recessive manner, its frequency in the second population, relative to that in the first, will be far lower than the overall percentage of its genes received from the first population, since the rate of homozygotes is equal to the square of the gene frequency as predicted by the Hardy-Weinberg law. If the trait depends on the simultaneous presence of two or more genes, even if they are dominant, or if the trait is quasicontinuous (multifactorial with a threshold), this would in most cases mimic recessive inheritance by the criterion employed here.* That is, the frequency of the trait will be equal to the product of the frequencies of the individual genes and also far lower in the second population than in the first.

The American Caucasian and black populations fulfill the criteria for this test. Racial admixture between the two groups has been entirely from the Caucasian to the black population and juvenile diabetes was very likely nonexistent in black people before their arrival in North America. The data indicate that most cases of juvenile diabetes are inherited in a dominant manner. The information important to this argument follows:

1. Idiopathic juvenile-onset, insulin-dependent diabetes is extremely rare in blacks in western Africa,[15–21] where 99% of the American black slaves originated,[22] as it is in all populations in which there has been no admixture of genes from Caucasians.[23,24] When insulin-dependent diabetes is found in western Africa, it is often associated with pancreatitis with pancreatic calcifications visible on x-rays,[20,21] characteristics not associated with juvenile diabetes in Caucasians.

2. More than 15 studies of blood groups show that an average of 20% of the genome of black Americans is composed of genes received through racial admixture during the last three and one-half centuries (for a review, see ref. 22).

3. In surveys in which the rates in both ethnic groups were determined concomitantly, the frequency of insulin-dependent, juvenile-onset diabetes among black Americans was no lower than 20%–30% of the frequency of juvenile-onset diabetes among white Americans,[25–29] and estimates ranged as high as 50%.[28,29]

4. The HLA genes DW3 and DW4, which are the ones most strongly associated with juvenile diabetes in Caucasians, are also increased among American black juvenile diabetics. About 50%–60% of Caucasian juvenile diabetics are DW3 and about 40%–50% are DW4.[30,31] About 75% of black juvenile diabetics are DW3 and about 40% are DW4.[32,33] In the general Caucasian population about 20%–30% are DW3 or DW4[30,31] and 7%–14% of the general black American population are DW3 or DW4.[32,33] The frequencies of the HLA genes A1, A2, B8, B15, and CW3 that are in linkage disequilibrium with either DW3 or DW4 in Caucasians[34] have also been found to be increased in black juvenile diabetics,[32,35] but to a lesser extent than DW3 or DW4, as is the case in white juvenile diabetics.[9,13,30,36]

5. The frequencies of the HLA genes A1, A2, B8, B15, DW3, and DW4 in nondiabetic blacks in the United States are about 20%–30% of those in nondiabetic Caucasians.[30,32,37,38] Therefore, these antigens may be in part, or predominately, of Caucasian origin.

The case-finding procedures used in the studies in which almost no juvenile-onset diabetics were found among blacks in western Africa[14–20] seem adequate. There is virtually no juvenile-onset diabetes among blacks in western Africa, but juvenile-onset diabetes occurs among blacks in the United States, whose gene pool has been diluted significantly with Caucasian genes. These findings suggest that the occurrence of juvenile-onset diabetes among black Americans is the result of the admixture of Caucasian genes, which cause a susceptibility to the disease. The associations of juvenile diabetes in blacks with HLA genes that are also associated with the disorder in Caucasians (and that may well be of Caucasian origin) are good evidence that the genetic components of juvenile-onset diabetes in the two ethnic groups are similar.

According to the studies referred to above and the experience of physicians who see juvenile diabetics in areas of the United States where there are large concentrations of blacks, the ratio of the frequency of juvenile-onset diabetes in American blacks to the frequency in American whites is roughly equal to, or certainly not lower than, the fraction of Caucasian genes in the American black gene pool, i.e., about one-fifth to one-third. If susceptibility to juvenile-onset diabetes is inherited in an autosomal recessive manner, the frequency of the disorder in black Americans should be far lower than this, i.e., about $(1/5)^2$ or 1/25 the frequency in whites.

Recent estimates of the frequency of juvenile-onset diabetes in American Caucasian children range from about 1/600 to 1/1,500.[27–29,39] Choosing the average value of about

* This statement is true for most patterns of inheritance except in uncommon types of epistasis, e.g., such that two or more genes are required for the expression of juvenile diabetes and the black genome contained all these genes except one that was a Caucasian gene.

1/900 for the calculations, then if susceptibility to juvenile diabetes is autosomal recessive, the gene frequency in Caucasians is equal to $\sqrt{1/900} = 1/30$. Assuming that 1/5 of the black American gene pool is composed of Caucasian genes, the frequency of the gene causing diabetes in blacks should be $1/30 \times 1/5 = 1/150$ and the frequency of juvenile-onset diabetics in blacks should be equal to $(1/150)^2$ or about 1 in 22,500 (or 900/22,500 that in whites).

If juvenile-onset diabetes is inherited as an autosomal dominant disorder, the frequency of Caucasians who have a gene that causes the disorder is equal to the frequency of the disorder, and the frequency of the disorder in blacks will be merely one-fifth that in Caucasians or about 1/4,500.

Figure 1 shows the expected frequencies in American blacks of traits inherited from Caucasians should the traits be due to a gene at a single locus and inherited in autosomal dominant or recessive manners. The single point in the figure represents the lowest estimate of juvenile diabetes in American blacks and shows that the frequencies of juvenile diabetes in blacks and Caucasians fit the criterion predicted for dominant far better than that for recessive inheritance.

Contrasting the frequency of juvenile diabetes in blacks with that of cystic fibrosis, a disorder known to be autosomal recessive,[40] supports the idea that juvenile diabetes is not inherited in an autosomal recessive manner. Cystic fibrosis is far less common among American blacks than among American whites. Even though the reporting of cases of cystic fibrosis in blacks has been increasing, it still appears to be 10 to 30 times less frequent among American blacks than among whites.[41,42]

Since the concordance for juvenile diabetes in monozygotic twins is 50% or lower,[2] the gene that causes juvenile diabetes must be incompletely penetrant and therefore environmental factors must play a role in the causation of juvenile diabetes. In the calculations shown above, taking incomplete penetrance into consideration would increase the calculated gene frequencies to the same extent in blacks and whites, but it would not alter the calculated frequencies of the disorder in blacks or whites in either the model for recessive or dominant inheritance. In calculating the frequencies of the disorders, a penetrance factor would be canceled out. For example, if the penetrance was 50%, the calculated frequency of individuals possessing a susceptible genotype would be doubled, but only one-half would have the disorder. If penetrance, for example because of a higher rate of contact with a specific environmental agent that leads to juvenile diabetes, is much higher in the American black than in the American Caucasian population, recessive inheritance might simulate dominant inheritance in the proposed model. Whether this situation might exist is simply unknown at present. The similar frequencies of specific HLA types associated with juvenile diabetics in the two ethnic groups suggest that the amount of genetic influence on the expression of the disorder in both groups is similar. The majority of cases of diabetes in American black children and adolescents are clinically identical to those in whites, with ketosis and an insulin requirement.[26]

Nerup et al.[30] and Rotter and Rimoin[7] have suggested that there is some evidence for heterogeneity within juvenile diabetes on the basis of different clinical pictures associated with antigens B8 and B15 in Caucasian juvenile diabetes. They find in juvenile diabetics an association of HLA gene B8 with coexistent autoimmune phenomena, such as Hashimoto's thyroiditis or Addison's disease, and antibodies to various endocrine organs, including pancreatic islets. They find another association between HLA B15 in cases of juvenile diabetes not associated with autoimmune phenomena. B8 and B15 are less strongly associated with juvenile diabetes than are DW3 and DW4. It is likely that B8 and B15 are associated with diabetes because, in Caucasians, they are in linkage disequilibrium with DW3 and DW4, respectively.[34,36,43] Even if juvenile diabetes associated with DW3 is considered as a separate disorder from juvenile diabetes associated with DW4, the frequency of cases associated with either antigen in blacks is too high to indicate recessive inheritance.[32,33,43] It should be noted, however, that although many geneticists believe that there could be heterogeneity in the causation of juvenile diabetes, many also regard heterogeneity as currently unproven. Arguments have been advanced that there is no convincing evidence for more than one juvenile diabetes susceptibility allele associated with the HLA complex and that a single susceptibility allele could be associated with both Dw3 and Dw4.[44,45]

To summarize, population data indicate that the gene(s) giving susceptibility to juvenile diabetes is (are) dominantly inherited, so 50% of first degree relatives of juvenile diabetics should be genetically susceptible. The low frequencies (5–15%) of affected first degree relatives of juvenile diabetics[46,47] can be accounted for by incomplete penetrance, possibly caused by lack of contact with, or acquired resistance to, the putative environmental factors that cause juvenile diabetes in genetically susceptible individuals. This concept, even though based on current information,

FIGURE 1. Expected frequencies of traits in American blacks inherited from Caucasians should the inheritance be autosomal recessive or dominant. To calculate the expected frequencies of traits in blacks, the frequency of genes of Caucasian origin in the gene pool of American blacks was taken as 20%.[22] The single point represents the frequency of juvenile diabetes in Caucasians (averaged from values given in refs. 27–29 and 39) and the lowest estimate found for the frequency of juvenile diabetes in American blacks, 0.28 that in whites (taken from ref. 26).

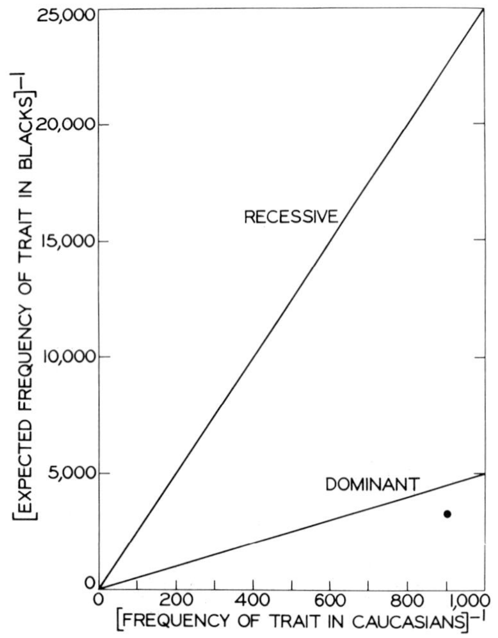

is at best an hypothesis. Whether it will eventually be elevated to the status of theory will depend on the outcome of studies with better markers for juvenile diabetes.

ACKNOWLEDGMENTS

The author is indebted to Professors James F. Crow, Carter Denniston, and Martin Curie-Cohen for critically reviewing this manuscript. The author is thankful for a Research Career Development Award from the Juvenile Diabetes Foundation.

APPENDIX I

If the gene for juvenile diabetes is closely linked to the HLA locus, the expectations for HLA types among affected sibs is as shown below. D or d designates the diabetes gene, according to whether it is dominant or recessive; + indicates the normal allele; and w, x, y, and z designate HLA haplotypes.

	Dominant	Recessive	
Parents	$\frac{D\ w}{+\ x} \times \frac{+\ y}{+\ z}$	$\frac{d\ w}{+\ x} \times \frac{d\ y}{+\ z}$	$\frac{d\ w}{+\ x} \times \frac{d\ w}{+\ z}$
Diabetic offspring	$\frac{D\ w}{+\ y}$ $\frac{D\ w}{+\ z}$	$\frac{d\ w}{d\ y}$	$\frac{d\ w}{d\ w}$

If the trait is dominant, half the offspring will have identical HLA types; if recessive, all will have identical HLA types. These proportions will be reduced if there are recombinants, which will be rare if the loci are closely linked. The number of HLA haplotypes is large enough so that almost always all four haplotypes in the two parents will be different. The pattern on the extreme right shows a case in which the parents have one identical haplotype. Note that these expected proportions do not depend on the penetrance of the diabetes gene.

REFERENCES

[1] Pyke, D. A.: The genetics of diabetes. Postgrad. Med. J. *46*:604–06, 1970.

[2] Tattersall, R. B., and Pyke, D. A.: Diabetes in identical twins. Lancet *2*:1120, 1972.

[3] Fajans, S. S.: Diabetes mellitus. *In* The Year in Metabolism 1975–76. Freinkel, N., Ed. New York, Plenum Press, 1976, pp. 45–71.

[4] Ganda, O. P., and Soeldner, S. S.: Genetic, acquired and related factors in the etiology of diabetes mellitus. Arch. Intern. Med. *137*:461–69, 1977.

[5] Barbosa, J., Chern, M., and Greenberg, L.: Segregation analysis of juvenile-onset insulin-dependent diabetes in 136 families. Diabetes *27*:458, 1978. Abstract.

[6] Neel, J. V.: The genetics of juvenile-onset type diabetes mellitus. N. Engl. J. Med. *297*:1062–63, 1977.

[7] Rotter, J. I., and Rimoin, D. L.: Heterogeneity in diabetes mellitus—update, 1978. Evidence for further genetic heterogeneity within juvenile-onset insulin-dependent diabetes mellitus. Diabetes *27*:599–608, 1978.

[8] Fajans, S. S., Cloutier, M. C., and Crowther, R. L.: Clinical and etiologic heterogeneity of idiopathic diabetes mellitus. Diabetes *27*:1112–25, 1978.

[9] Nerup, J., Platz, P., Ortved-Anderson, O., Christy, M., Lyngsoe, J., Poulsen, J. E., Ryder, L. P., Staub-Nielsen, L., Thomsen, M., and Svejgaard, A.: HLA antigens and diabetes mellitus. Lancet *2*:864–66, 1974.

[10] Cudworth, A. G., and Woodrow, J. C.: Evidence for HLA-linked genes in "juvenile" diabetes mellitus. Br. Med. J. *3*:133–35, 1975.

[11] Barbosa, J., King, R., Noreen, H., and Junis, E. J.: The histocompatibility system in juvenile, insulin-dependent diabetic multiplex kindreds. J. Clin. Invest. *60*:989–98, 1977.

[12] Rubinstein, P., Suciu-Foca, N., and Nicholson, J. F.: Genetics of juvenile diabetes mellitus. A recessive gene closely linked to HLA D and with 50 percent penetrance. N. Engl. J. Med. *297*:1036–40, 1977.

[13] Cudworth, A. G.: Type I diabetes mellitus. Diabetologia *14*:281–91, 1978.

[14] Spielman, R. S., Baker, L., and Zmyewski, C.: Genetics of juvenile diabetes: dosage of susceptibility genes. Diabetes *27*:459, 1978. Abstract.

[15] Dodu, S. R.: The incidence of diabetes in Accra (Ghana). A study of 4,000 patients. West Afr. Med. J. *7*:129–34, 1958.

[16] Dodu, S. R., and deHeer, N.: A diabetes case-finding survey in Ho, Ghana. Ghana Med. J. *3*:75–80, 1964.

[17] Dodu, S. R., and Harthorn, M. H.: Diabetes in Accra. Ghana Med. J. *5*:2–7, 1966.

[18] Sankale, M., and Wade, F.: Le diabete sucre in milieu hospitalier dakarois (a propos de 260 cas). Bull. Soc. Med. Afr. Noire Lang. Fr. *11*:730–39, 1966.

[19] Sankale, M., Sow, A. M., and Signate, S.: Aspects du diabete sucre chez le Noir African au Senegal. Afr. J. Med. Sci. *1*:17–31, 1970.

[20] Kinnear, T. W.: The pattern of diabetes mellitus in a Nigerian teaching hospital. East Afr. Med. J. *40*:288–94, 1963.

[21] Osuntokun, B. O., Akinkugbe, F. M., Francis, T. I., Reddy, S., Osuntokun, O., and Taylor, G. O. L.: Diabetes mellitus in Nigerians. A study of 932 patients. West Afr. Med. J. *20*:295–312, 1971.

[22] Reed, T. E.: Caucasian genes in American Negroes. Science *165*:762–68, 1969.

[23] Pyke, D. A.: The geography of diabetes. Postgrad. Med. J. *45*(Suppl.):796–801, 1969.

[24] Chao, P.-Y.: The prevalence of diabetes mellitus among the Chinese. Diabetes *21*:353, 1972. Abstract.

[25] MacDonald, M. J.: Characteristics of diabetes mellitus in American Negro children. Washington University School of Medicine Senior Research Report, 1970, pp. 11–12.

[26] MacDonald, M. J.: Lower frequency of diabetes among hospitalized Negro than white children: Theoretical implications. Acta Genet. Med. Gemellol (Rome) *24*:119–26, 1975.

[27] Sultz, H. A., Schlesinger, E. R., and Mosher, W. W.: The Erie County survey of long-term childhood illness II. Incidence and prevalence. Am. J. Public Health *58*:491–98, 1968.

[28] Sultz, H. A., Schlesinger, E. R., Mosher, W. E., and Feldman, J. G.: Childhood diabetes mellitus. *In* Long Term Childhood Illness. Pittsburgh, University of Pittsburgh Press, 1972, pp. 223–48.

[29] Gorwitz, K., Howen, G. G., and Thompson, T.: Prevalence of diabetes in Michigan school-age children. Diabetes *25*:122–27, 1976.

[30] Nerup, J., Platz, P., Ortved-Andersen, O., Christy, M., Egelberg, J., Lyngsoe, J., Poulsen, J. E., Ryder, L. P., Thomsen, M., and Svejgaard, A.: HLA, autoimmunity and insulin-dependent diabetes mellitus. *In* The Genetics of Diabetes Mellitus. Creutzfeld, W., Köbberling, J., and Neel, J. V. Berlin, Springer-Verlag, 1976, pp. 106–14.

[31] Möller, E., Persson, B., and Sterky, G.: HLA phenotypes and diabetic retinopathy. Diabetologia *14*:155–58, 1978.

[32] Duquesnoy, R. J., MacDonald, M. J., Mullins, P., Hackbarth, S. A., Traisman, H. S., and Levitsky, L. L.: Increased frequency of HLA-DW3 in North American black patients with juvenile onset diabetes. Tissue Antigens *13*:369–72, 1979.

[33] Mullins, P., Collins, J., MacDonald, M. J., and Duquesnoy, R. J.: Unusual MLC responses of black patients with juvenile onset diabetes. Transplantation Proc. In press.

[34] Svejgaard, A., Hauge, M., Jersild, C., Platz, D., Ryder, L. P., Staub-Nielsen, L., and Thomsen, M.: The HLA System. Basel, S. Karger, 1975, pp. 25–28.

[35] Patel, R., Ansari, A., and Covarrubias, C. L.-P.: Leukocyte antigens and disease: III. Association of HLA-B8 and HLA-BW15 with insulin-dependent diabetes in three different population groups. Metabolism *26*:487–92, 1977.

[36] Solow, H., Hidalgo, R., and Singal, D. P.: Juvenile-onset diabetes: HLA-A, -B, -C and DR alloantigens. Diabetes *28*:1–4, 1979.

[37] Payne, R., Feldman, M., Cann, H., and Bodner, J. G.: A comparison of HLA data of the North American black with African black and North American Caucasoid population. Tissue Antigens *9*:135–47, 1977.

[38] Nerup, J., Cathelineau, G., and Seignalet, J.: HLA and endocrine disease. *In* HLA and Disease. Dausset, J., and Svejgaard, A., Eds. Copenhagen, Munksgaard, 1977, pp. 149–67.

[39] U.S. Public Health Service: Diabetes Source Book. Washington, D.C., U.S. Government Printing Office, 1969 (PHS publication No. 1168), pp. 8–11.

[40] Crow, J. F.: Problems of ascertainment in the analysis of family data. *In* Genetics and the Epidemiology of Chronic Diseases. Neel, J. V., Shaw, M. W., and Schull, W. J., Eds. Washington, D.C., U.S. Government Printing Office, 1965 (PHS publication No. 1163).

[41] Kulczycki, L. L., and Schauf, V.: Cystic fibrosis in blacks in Washington, D.C. Am. J. Dis. Child. *127*:64–67, 1974.

[42] Schaap, T., and Cohen, M. M.: A proposed model for the inheritance of cystic fibrosis. *In* Cystic Fibrosis: Projections into the Future. Mangos, J. A., and Talamo, R. C., Eds. New York, Stratton International, 1976, pp. 291–303.

[43] Rodey, G. E., White, N., Frazer, T. E., Duquesnoy, R. S., and Santiago, S. V.: HLA associations with juvenile onset diabetes in American blacks—evidence for the primary nature of D locus associations with diabetes. Diabetes *28*:395, 1979. Abstract.

[44] Bengsch, N., and Köbberling, J.: No evidence for two HLA-associated genes. 10th Congress of the International Diabetes Federation. Waldhäusl, N., and Alberti, K. G., Ed. Amsterdam, Excerpta Medica, 1979, p. 19. (Abstract)

[45] Watson, B., Sachs, J., Jaraquamada, D., and Festenstein, H.: Type I diabetes and the D-locus. 10th Congress of the International Diabetes Federation. Waldhäusl, W., and Alberti, K. G., Ed. Amsterdam, Excerpta Medica, 1979, pp. 249–250. (Abstract)

[46] MacDonald, M. J.: Equal incidence of adult-onset diabetes among ancestors of juvenile diabetics and nondiabetics. Diabetologia *10*:767–73, 1974.

[47] Köbberling, J.: Genetic heterogeneities within idiopathic diabetes. *In* The Genetics of Diabetes Mellitus. Creutzfeldt, W., Köbberling, J., and Neel, J. V., Eds. Berlin, Springer-Verlag, 1976, pp. 79–87.

Response:

Racial Differences in Juvenile-type Diabetes Are Consistent with More Than One Mode of Inheritance

JEROME I. ROTTER AND SUSAN E. HODGE

SUMMARY

The ratio of the prevalences of insulin-dependent type (juvenile) diabetes (IDDM) in blacks and Caucasians is examined. It has been argued that this ratio is of the same order as the estimated proportion of Caucasian genes in the American black population. It has been further argued that this observation, together with an assumption of equal penetrances in the two races, is consistent with autosomal dominant inheritance for IDDM. The present paper shows that the ratio is equally compatible with a three-allele model which, moreover, incorporates observed immunogenetic heterogeneity within IDDM. This three-allele heterogeneity model exhibits some features of both dominant and recessive inheritance. The model predicts that, compared with Caucasians, there will be less pancreatic autoimmunity in the black IDDM population and lower recurrence risks to relatives of black diabetics. These predictions can be tested in future studies. **DIABETES 29:115–118, February 1980.**

There currently exists a lively debate regarding the mode of inheritance of insulin-dependent type (juvenile) diabetes (IDDM).[1] Susceptibility to IDDM has been variously proposed to be inherited in autosomal dominant or recessive fashion, based on population studies of HLA antigens and family studies of HLA haplotypes.[2–5] Recently, MacDonald,[6] making ingenious use of cross-racial data, has argued that the U.S. black-Caucasian differences in the frequency of IDDM are of the same order as the estimated admixture of Caucasian genes in the American black population. This observation, together with the assumption that the penetrances are equal in the two groups, would imply that the susceptibility to IDDM is transmitted in an autosomal dominant as opposed to autosomal recessive manner.

For the most part these models ignore the increasingly documented heterogeneity within IDDM.[1,7,8] Other genetic models, besides simple autosomal dominant or recessive ones, must be developed to take this heterogeneity into account. In particular, we have recently developed a three allele model for a diabetic susceptibility locus, tightly linked to the HLA complex, which incorporates the immunogenetic heterogeneity observed within IDDM.[9,10] This paper will demonstrate that the racial differences which MacDonald describes can also be explained by this heterogeneity model.

MODEL AND METHODS

The model was developed to take into account two sets of observations in the diabetic literature that indicate heterogeneity within the insulin-dependent diabetic phenotype. These include (1) the increased relative risk for individuals who have two *different* associated HLA alleles (e.g., B8/B15 or Dw3/Dw4) as compared with those with only one such allele (B8/x or B15/x, where x is any nondiabetogenic HLA allele) or those with two *identical* such alleles (B8/B8 or B15/B15)[1,2,7,8,11–17] and (2) differential immunologic associations with these different HLA alleles, i.e., persistent islet cell antibodies associated with HLA B8/Dw3 and antibody response to exogenous insulin associated with HLA B15.[1,7,8,14,18–27] Neither observation can be explained by simple autosomal or recessive inheritance of IDDM susceptibility.

The three allele model[9,10] makes the following assumptions. (1) There exists a diabetes susceptibility locus "S," which is tightly linked to the HLA locus (recombination fraction within 1–2%). (2) This S locus has two diabetogenic alleles, S_1 and S_2, which are in linkage disequilibrium (and thus in association) with B8 and B15, respectively. All other alleles (assumed nondiabetogenic) at the S locus are subsumed under the name "little s." (3) Different allelic combinations at the S locus are at risk for different forms of IDDM,

From the Division of Medical Genetics, Departments of Medicine and Pediatrics, Harbor-UCLA Medical Center, Torrance, California and the Mental Retardation Research Center, Neuropsychiatric Institute, 760 Westwood Plaza UCLA, Los Angeles, California.
Address reprint requests to Jerome I. Rotter, Division of Medical Genetics, Departments of Medicine and Pediatrics, Harbor-UCLA Medical Center, Torrance, California 90509.
Received for publication 8 October 1979.

TABLE 1
Forms of IDDM resulting from different allelic combinations at the postulated S locus

S genotype class number	Description	Disease form	Associated alleles	Characteristics
1	S_1S_1 or S_1s	1	B8	Autoimmunity to the pancreas
2	S_2S_2 or S_2s	2	B15	Antibody response to exogeneous
3	S_1S_2	3	Both of above	Both of above
4	ss	No disease	—	—

TABLE 2
Input for calculations

	Frequency of alleles			Penetrances		
	S_1	S_2	s	ϕ_1 (Form 1)	ϕ_2 (Form 2)	ϕ_3 (Form 3)
Blacks	0.0222	0.0012	0.9766	0.001	0.107	0.436
Caucasians	0.111	0.006	0.833	0.001	0.107	0.436

The Caucasian gene frequencies and penetrances are given for comparison. These were obtained as described under METHODS.[9,10] In blacks, the gene frequencies are reduced by a factor of 5, and the penetrances are kept the same.

as shown in Table 1. Persons who have the S_1 allele, in either single or double dose, but without the S_2 allele, are found in association with the B8 allele of the HLA complex. They are subject to what is denoted as "Form 1" of the disease, the autoimmune form. The penetrance ϕ_1 is defined as the probability that a person with this genotype will in fact become diabetic. As seen in Table 1, similar descriptions apply to Forms 2 and 3. This "little s-little s" genotype is assumed not to be at risk.

The underlying mathematical structure of this model involves seven parameters. The model was fitted to eight observations from the literature—the population prevalence,[3,28] 3 HLA relative risks,[2,7,11,12,13,29] the concordance rates in monozygotic twins and sibs,[30–36] and the number of HLA haplotypes shared in common by pairs of affected sibs.[3,23,37,38] All these observations were made on Caucasian diabetics. One solution set which provided a particularly good fit to the observations gave gene frequencies of 0.111, 0.006, and 0.883 for S_1, S_2, and little s, respectively, and penetrances $\phi_1 = 0.001$, $\phi_2 = 0.107$, and $\phi_3 = 0.436$, as shown in Table 2. Table 3 shows the corresponding population prevalence and the predicted relative proportions of the three forms among all juvenile diabetics in the Caucasian population, a prediction consistent with various reported immunologic studies. The model also predicts, due to the higher penetrance of Form 3, that the distribution of the forms of the disease differs among affected individuals and families with multiple members affected, as shown in Table 4.

To apply this model to the black-Caucasian differences, we reduced the gene frequencies to one-fifth that in Caucasians, the gene admixture ratio that MacDonald[6] utilizes, while keeping the penetrances constant (Table 2). Predicted population and familial parameters were then calculated for the U.S. black population.

RESULTS

The predicted black-Caucasian differences are shown in Tables 3 and 4. First, this model predicts the population prevalence of IDDM in the U.S. black population to be about one-sixth that of the Caucasian population. This is well within the estimates that MacDonald reports.[6] Second, the predicted proportions of the three forms are different in the black and Caucasian populations. The combined Form 3 in the black diabetic population is predicted to be one-fourth that among Caucasian diabetics (7% compared with 30%). The proportion of insulin-dependent diabetics with an autoimmune component to their disorder would be half that in the Caucasian population (21% compared with 41%). Third, the familial distribution would be markedly different in the two racial groups. Whereas among Caucasians, some 37% of pairs are predicted in which both siblings have Form 2, this increases to 77% among the black population. In contrast, pairs in which one or both siblings have Form 3 would be reduced by a factor of 3, 63% to 22% (columns 5 and 6 of Table 4). Fourth, if the risks for diabetes to the sib or twin of an insulin-dependent diabetic are 8% and 20%, respectively, in the Caucasian population, this risk is predicted to fall to a corresponding 5.4% and 11.6% in the black population.

DISCUSSION

The mathematical modeling of IDDM performed in this paper demonstrates that other genetic models, besides simple autosomal recessive or dominant, are consistent with the observed population and family data. These simpler models have failed to take into account the now well-documented immunogenetic heterogeneity within IDDM—specifically, the differential immunologic features of B8/Dw3 and B15 diabetics and the increased risk of the B8/B15 compound heterozygote.[1,7,8,14,25] The mathematical model presented is the first to take this heterogeneity into account

TABLE 3
Population frequencies

	Population prevalence	Proportion of each form (%)		
		Form 1	Form 2	Form 3
Blacks	0.000318	14	79	7
Caucasians	0.001927	11	59	30

TABLE 4
Family distribution

	Affected sib pairs (%)							
	Both Form 1	Form 1, Form 2	Form 1, Form 3	Both Form 2	Form 2, Form 3	Both Form 3	Prevalence in sibs (%)	Prevalence in twins (%)
Blacks	0.1	0.0	0.1	77.5	7.1	15.1	5.4	11.6
Caucasians	0.1	0.1	0.2	37.0	17.8	44.8	8.0	20.0

by including all these observations in a single genetic model and deriving the population and genetic implications of their existence.

There are several predictions and conclusions from this modeling process. First, it demonstrates that other models, besides dominant and recessive, can account for the population and HLA observations as well as the racial differences. Second, in a sense this model has both dominant and recessive features. Since only one diabetogenic allele is required for susceptibility, genetic transmission mimics dominant inheritance on a population basis. However, the familial forms often involve two alleles, especially in the Caucasian group, and therefore can mimic recessive inheritance within families. Third, the model predicts that there will be less pancreatic autoimmunity in the black insulin-dependent diabetic population and that the risk to relatives will be less than that in the Caucasian population because of the greatly reduced proportion of the compound Form 3.

It should be pointed out that this is a modeling process, and it still remains to be determined whether it will prove fruitful for IDDM. The model incorporates certain assumptions that have been enumerated previously.[9,10] In addition, for this cross-racial analysis we assumed, as did MacDonald,[6] that the penetrance of the diabetic susceptibility gene does not vary between the black and Caucasian populations. This assumption remains to be validated.

If this model proves accurate, it will have direct implications for the recurrence risk to relatives in the two racial groups. Since Form 3 is the most penetrant, its relative reduction in the black population would imply that the recurrence risk for diabetes within families would be reduced compared with that among Caucasians. The strength of the model lies in its incorporation of both the described heterogeneity of the disorder and the increased compound relative risk, something which other genetic models of IDDM susceptibility have failed to do. It is consistent with currently reported data and makes predictions about racial and family differences that can be immediately tested in appropriately designed clinical genetic and epidemiologic investigations.

ACKNOWLEDGMENTS

Supported in part by NIAMDD Clinical Investigator Award AM 00523 to Jerome I. Rotter, a grant from the Kroc Foundation, and USPHS Fellowship Award HD 07032 (to Susan E. Hodge) and HD 05616.

REFERENCES

[1] Rotter, J. I., and Rimoin, D. L.: Diabetes mellitus: the search for genetic markers. Diabetes Care *12*:215–26, 1979.

[2] Svejgaard, A., Platz, P., Ryder, L. P., Staub Nielsen, L., and Thomsen, M.: HLA and disease associations: a survey. Transplantation Rev. *22*:3–34, 1975.

[3] Spielman, R. S., Baker, L., and Zmijewski, C. M.: Inheritance of susceptibility to juvenile onset diabetes. *In* Genetic Analysis of Common Diseases: Applications to Predictive Factors in Coronary Heart Disease. Sing, C. F., and Skolnick, M. H., Eds. New York, Alan R. Liss, 1979, pp. 567–585.

[4] Thomson, G., and Bodmer, W.: The genetic analysis of HLA and disease associations. *In* HLA and Disease. Dausset, J., and Svejgaard, A., Eds. Copenhagen, Munksgaard, 1977, pp. 84–93.

[5] Rubinstein, P., Suciu-Foca, N., and Nicholson, F.: Genetics of juvenile diabetes mellitus, a recessive gene closely linked to HLA and with 50 percent penetrance. N. Engl. J. Med. *297*:1036–40, 1977.

[6] MacDonald, M. J.: Hypothesis: the frequencies of juvenile diabetes in American Blacks and Caucasians are consistent with dominant inheritance of juvenile diabetes. Diabetes *29*:110–114, 1980.

[7] Rotter, J. I., and Rimoin, D. L.: Heterogeneity in diabetes mellitus—update 1978, evidence for further genetic heterogeneity within juvenile onset insulin dependent diabetes mellitus. Diabetes *27*:599–608, 1978.

[8] Rotter, J. I.: Genetic heterogeneity within diabetes mellitus, a review. *In* Genetic Analysis of Common Diseases: Applications to Predictive Diseases in Coronary Heart Disease, Sing, C. F., and Skolnick, M. H., Eds. New York, Alan R. Liss, 1979, pp. 135–155.

[9] Hodge, S. E., Rotter, J. I., and Lange, K. L.: A three allele model for heterogeneity within insulin dependent diabetes. November, 1979. Presented at the Plenary Session, American Society of Human Genetics, October 3, 1979 (abstract). Am. J. Hum. Genet. *31*:135A, 1979.

[10] Hodge, S. E., Rotter, J. I., and Lange, K. L.: A three allele model for heterogeneity of juvenile onset insulin dependent diabetes. Ann. Hum. Genet. In press.

[11] Cudworth, A. G., and Woodrow, J. C.: Genetic susceptibility in diabetes mellitus: analysis of the HLA association. Br. Med. J. *2*:846–48, 1976.

[12] Barta, L., and Simon, S.: Role of HLA-B8 and Bw15 antigens in diabetic children. N. Engl. J. Med. *296*:397, 1977.

[13] Svejgaard, A., and Ryder, L. P.: Associations between HLA and disease, notes on methodology and a report from the HLA and disease registry. *In* HLA and Disease. Dausset, J., and Svejgaard, A., Eds. Copenhagen, Munksgaard, 1977, pp. 46–71.

[14] Cudworth, A. G., and Festenstein, H.: HLA genetic heterogeneity in diabetes mellitus. Br. Med. Bull. *34*:285–90, 1978.

[15] Farid, N. R., Barnard, J. P., Pepper, B., Noel, E. P., Kelly, F., Davis, A. J., Hoberika, C., and Marshall, W. H.: The association of HLA with juvenile diabetes in Newfoundland. Tissue Antigens *2*:215–22, 1978.

[16] Christy, M., Green, A., Christau, B., Kromann, H., Nerup, J., Platz, R., Thomsen, M., Ryder, L. P., and Svejgaard, A.: Studies of the HLA-system and insulin-dependent diabetes mellitus. Diabetes Care *2*:209–14, 1979.

[17] Farid, J. R., Sampson, L., Noel, P., Barnard, J. M., Davis, A. J., and Hillman, D. A.: HLA-D-related (DRW) antigens in juvenile diabetes mellitus. Diabetes *28*:552–57, 1979.

[18] Nerup, J., Platz, P., Ortved Anderson, O., Christy, M., Egeberg, J., Lyngsoe, J., Poulsen, J. E., Ryder, L. P., Thomsen, M., and Svejgaard, A.: HLA autoimmunity and insulin-dependent diabetes mellitus. *In* The Genetics of Diabetes Mellitus. Creutzfeldt, W., Kobberling, J., and Neel, J. V., Eds. Berlin, Springer-Verlag, 1976, pp. 106–14.

[19] Morris, P. J., Vaughn, H., Irvine, W. J., McCallum, F. J., Gray, R. S., Campbell, C. J., Duncan, L. J. P., and Farquhar, J. W.: HLA and pancreatic islet cell antibodies in diabetes. Lancet *2*:652–53, 1976.

[20] Bertrams, J., Jansen, F. K., Gruneklee, D., Reis, H. F., Drost, H., Beyer, J., Gries, F. A., and Kuwert, E.: HLA antigens and immunoresponsiveness to insulin in insulin dependent diabetes mellitus. Tissue Antigens *8*:13–19, 1976.

[21] Irvine, W. J., McCallum, C. J., Campbell, C. J., Duncan, L. J. P., Farquhar, W., Vaughan, H., and Morris, P. J.: Pancreatic islet-cell antibodies in diabetes mellitus correlated with the duration and type of diabetes, coexistent autoimmune disease and HLA type. Diabetes *26*:138–47, 1977.

[22] Ludwig, H., Schernthaner, G., and Mayr, W. R.: Inselzellantikorper beim juvenilea diabetes mellitus. Dtsch. Med. Wochenschr. *102*:1221–26, 1977.

[23] Cudworth, A. G.: Type I diabetes mellitus. Diabetologia *14*:281–91, 1978.

[24] Irvine, W. J., Mario, U. D., Feck, C. M., Gray, R. S., Ting, A., Morris, P. J., and Duncan, L. J. P.: Autoimmunity and HLA antigens in insulin dependent (type I) diabetes. J. Clin. Lab. Immunol. *1*:107–10, 1978.

[25] Irvine, W. J., Mario, U. D., Feek, G. M., Ting, A., Morris, P. J., Gray, R.

S., and Duncan, L. J. P.: Insulin antibodies in relation to islet cell antibodies and HLA antigens in insulin dependent (type I) diabetes. J. Clin. Lab. Immunol. *1*:111–14, 1978.

[26] Schernthaner, G., Ludwig, H., and Mayr, W. R.: Immunoglobulin G-insulin antibodies and immune region-associated alloantigens in insulin-dependent diabetes mellitus. J. Clin. Endocrinol. Metab. *48*:403–07, 1979.

[27] Ludwig, H., Schernthaner, G., and Mayr, W. R.: Ia type alloantigens and hormonal autoimmune responsiveness in insulin-dependent diabetes mellitus. Metabolism *28*:797–800, 1979.

[28] Palumbo, P. J., and Labarthe, D. R.: The incidence of diabetes mellitus in Rochester, Minnesota, 1945–1969. Adv. Metab. Disord. *9*:13–28, 1978.

[29] Cudworth, A. G., and Woodrow, J. C.: HLA system and diabetes mellitus. Diabetes *24*:345–49, 1975.

[30] Gottlieb, M. S., and Root, H. F.: Diabetes mellitus in twins. Diabetes *17*:693–704, 1968.

[31] Pyke, D. A., and Nelson, P. G.: Diabetes mellitus in identical twins. *In* The Genetics of Diabetes Mellitus. Creutzfeldt, W., Kobberling, J., and Neel, J. V., Eds. Berlin, Springer-Verlag, 1976, pp. 194–202.

[32] Cahill, G. F., Jr.: Current concepts of diabetic complications with emphasis on hereditary factors: a brief review. *In* Genetic Analysis of Common Diseases: Applications to Predictive Factors in Coronary Heart Disease. Sing, C. F., and Skolnick, M. H., Eds. New York, Alan R. Liss, 1979, pp. 113–125.

[33] Harris, H.: The familial distribution of diabetes mellitus: a study of the relatives of 1241 diabetic propositi. Ann. Eugenics *15*:95–110, 1950.

[34] Simpson, N.: Multifactorial inheritance: a possible hypothesis for diabetes. Diabetes *13*:462–71, 1964.

[35] Kobberling, J.: Genetic heterogeneities within idiopathic diabetes. *In* The Genetics of Diabetes Mellitus. Creutzfeldt, W., Kobberling, J., and Neel, J. V., Eds. Berlin, Springer-Verlag, 1976, pp. 79–87.

[36] Degnbol, B., and Green, A.: Diabetes mellitus among first- and second-degree relatives of early onset diabetics. Ann. Hum. Genet. *42*:25–47, 1978.

[37] Cudworth, A. G., and Woodrow, J. C.: Evidence for HLA-linked genes in "juvenile" diabetes mellitus. Br. Med. J. *3*:133–35, 1975.

[38] Barbosa, J., King, R., Noreen, H., and Yunis, E. J.: The histocompatibility (HLA) system in juvenile insulin-dependent diabetic multiplex kindreds. J. Clin. Invest. *60*:989–98, 1977.

Diabetes and Cell Growth—Lack of Differences in Growth Characteristics of Fibroblasts from Diabetic and Nondiabetic Pima Indians

BARBARA V. HOWARD, ROSE M. FIELDS, DAVID M. MOTT, PETER J. SAVAGE, M. NAGULESPARAN, AND PETER H. BENNETT

SUMMARY

Skin biopsies were obtained from diabetic and nondiabetic Pima Indians and nondiabetic Caucasian controls to compare fibroblast growth characteristics. The Pima population were used because they have a high prevalence of well-characterized diabetes mellitus, and extensive clinical and demographic data are available for selection of subjects. Cultures were derived from 19 subjects between the ages of 20 and 42 yr. Seven were from Pimas with severe diabetes who had two diabetic parents and relatively early age of onset. Six were from Pima nondiabetics who had two nondiabetic parents. Six control cultures were established from Caucasian nondiabetics with no family history of diabetes. Cell density at confluence, plating efficiency, thymidine incorporation, and population doubling rates were monitored as a function of cell population doublings until the senescence of each culture. Fibroblast cultures from the Pima diabetics did not differ from those of the Pima nondiabetics in replicative life span or any of the measured culture parameters. When cultures from the Pimas were compared with those of the Caucasian controls, however, they had decreased cell density at confluence, slower population doubling times, decreased thymidine incorporation, shorter replicative life spans, and lower plating efficiency. The data suggest that altered growth properties of cultures from diabetics may not be a requisite of diabetic status; they may reflect a genetic background that accompanies the expression of diabetes. DIABETES 29:119–124, February 1980.

Human diploid fibroblastic cells in culture have a finite population life span, which has been found in most cases to be inversely proportional to the donor's age.[1–5] Furthermore, this loss of division potential is often correlated with other growth characteristics such as cell density at confluence,[5] plating efficiency,[2] and proliferative activity.[6] Diabetes mellitus in man has been associated with accelerated aging, and epidemiologically a strong positive correlation exists between aging and the incidence of diabetes.[7,8] For this reason, diabetic cells have been studied in culture. Several laboratories have demonstrated altered growth properties in fibroblasts cultured from diabetics, including decreased replicative life span,[3,9,10] decreased plating efficiency,[2,11] lower saturation density at confluence,[9,12] and longer population doubling times.[9,11,12]

The interpretation of the findings in diabetic cells is subject, however, to the variable of genetic heterogeneity, both in the source of control donors and in the selection of diabetics, since diabetes is a genetically heterogeneous disease.[13] Rosenbloom and Rosenbloom[14] have recently failed to demonstrate growth differences in cultured fibroblasts from two insulin-dependent diabetics compared with matched controls, and Golstein et al.[9] have shown that cultures from prediabetics exhibit altered growth parameters compared with those from controls having no family history of diabetes.

The Pima Indians are a genetically isolated group[15] with a high prevalence of non-insulin-dependent diabetes mellitus, which appears to be a more homogeneous disease in this population.[16] The availability of extensive demographic and clinical data on the individuals in this population makes them an ideal group for selection of diabetic and nondiabetic individuals for comparative studies of their fibroblasts. This report presents data on several growth parameters of fibroblastic lines derived from Pima Indian diabetics and nondiabetics and from nondiabetic Caucasian controls of similar ages.

MATERIALS AND METHODS

Skin biopsies were obtained with informed consent from 13 Pima Indians and 6 Caucasian controls between the ages of 20 and 42 yr (Table 1). Criteria for classification of diabetics and nondiabetics in the Pimas were based on previous

From the Phoenix Clinical Research Section and the Human Diabetes Center, National Institute of Arthritis, Metabolism, and Digestive Diseases, National Institutes of Health, Phoenix, Arizona.
Address reprint requests to Dr. Barbara V. Howard, NIAMDD, 4212 N. 16th Street, Phoenix, Arizona 85016.
Received for publication 20 August 1979.

TABLE 1
Characteristics of biopsy donors

	Age/sex	Relative weight* (kg/m²)	Age of onset	Glucose levels fasting/2 h (mg/dl)	Diabetic status of Father	Diabetic status of Mother
Pima diabetic†						
E.J.	37/M	26.8	27	221/364	+	+
F.E.	26/F	31.3	16	239/356	+	+
C.L.	25/M	22.2	20	231/506	+	+
P.B.	37/M	21.2	20	170/329	+	+
M.L.	24/F	34.0	20	103/225	+	+
G.S.‡	42/F	31.3	22	265/383	−	+
P.J.‡	23/M	29.4	21	152/270	+	+
Pima nondiabetic						
P.T.	28/F	44.2		106/143	−	−
K.D.	41/F	29.0		95/157	−	−
C.C.	20/M	26.8		89/103	−	−
C.T.	22/F	42.9		92/140	−	−
B.S.	41/M	29.4		100/156	−	−
R.W.‡	23/M	39.2		99/127	−	−
Caucasian nondiabetic						
G.M.‡	26/F	NA§		NA§		
A.W.	22/M	22.5		96/		
D.M.	37/M	21.9		95/		
G.J.	25/F	21.1		81/		
J.K.	40/F	24.0		69/		
L.B.	35/M	25.0		87/		

* Percent desirable weight is equal to kg/m² × 4.39 for males and kg/m² × 4.76 for females.
† All diabetics were of the non-insulin-dependent type. P.B., G.S., and M.L. had been treated with insulin.
‡ Biopsies from these individuals were processed and the cell line stored frozen at the Institute for Medical Genetics, Camden, New Jersey (culture numbers GM2416, GM2440, GM3234, and GM945, respectively). Cultures were then sent to the Phoenix Clinical Research Section for measurements of cell growth characteristics.
§ Not available.

studies of plasma glucose levels and their relation to complications in this population.[17] The Pima diabetics had symptomatic non-insulin-dependent diabetes with no evidence of ketoacidosis. They were selected as having severe glucose intolerance and relatively early age of onset. In addition, both parents of all but one patient were diabetic, as documented by glucose levels greater than 200 mg/dl 2 h following a 100-g oral carbohydrate load. The nondiabetic Indians had no symptoms of diabetes and 2-h glucose levels less than 160 mg/dl; both parents had normal oral glucose tolerance. Caucasian controls had normal fasting glucose levels and neither symptoms nor family history of diabetes.

Cell cultures were established from 3-mm full-thickness punch biopsies obtained from the medial aspect of the forearm after cleansing with PhisoHex and ethanol and administration of a local anesthetic (Xylocaine). The skin specimen was placed in Eagle's Minimal Essential Medium (MEM) supplemented with penicillin (50 μU/ml) and streptomycin (50 μg/ml) and processed within 1 h. For explantation the pieces were minced into 16–20 pieces with a fine scissors, and 5–7 fragments were transferred into each of three 25-cm² polystyrene culture vessels (Corning Glass Works, Corning, New York). The pieces were allowed to adhere to the vessel bottom for 3–5 min and then carefully covered with 2–3 ml of MEM supplemented with 20% fetal bovine serum and penicillin and streptomycin. After overnight equilibration in 5% CO_2 in air, the vessels were sealed and incubated at 37°C. Medium was replaced weekly with 7–10 ml volumes, and cultures were scored for numbers of pieces resulting in fibroblast outgrowth. Cultures were subcultivated after 4–5 wk using a solution of 0.05% trypsin, 0.02% sodium EDTA in calcium, and magnesium-free Dulbecco's phosphate-buffered saline (DPBS). The primary confluent monolayer was designated as 1 cell population doubling (CPD).

Cultures were grown in MEM supplemented with nonessential amino acids, glutamine (4.6 mM), penicillin, streptomycin, 10% fetal bovine serum, and HEPES buffer (10 mM). Two batches of fetal bovine serum with apparently equal growth promoting abilities were used for the entire study. Cells were screened periodically for mycoplasma using the Flow Laboratories Testing Service (Rockville, Maryland), and only mycoplasma-free cultures were used for these studies.

Cells were subcultivated weekly using an inoculum of 7.5×10^5 cells in 75-cm² polystyrene culture vessels containing 40 ml growth medium. Cell attachment, or settling efficiency, under these conditions after 24 h was found to be 80%–90% and did not appear to differ significantly among donors. Confluent density was determined as the number of cells/flask after 1 wk, and CPD were calculated directly by dividing this number by the number of cells inoculated. No correction for settling efficiency was made since it was high and did not differ between groups. All cell counts were performed using a hemocytometer. When cell size was determined, the trypsinized cell suspension was photographed and the cell diameters of the photographed cells were measured. The cell culture was declared "senescent" when the weekly cultivation did not result in at least one CPD.

Plating efficiency was determined at biweekly intervals by plating 200 cells in 25-cm² polystyrene culture flasks containing 5 ml growth medium supplemented with 20% fetal bovine serum and 4.6 mM glutamine.[18] These were incubated, after overnight pH equilibration, in the closed vessel for 2 wk. Flasks were then rinsed with DPBS, fixed for 30 s with methanol/acetic acid (3/1), and stained with Giemsa (Buffered Blood Staining Solution, Baker, Phillipsburg, New Jersey). Colonies were counted using a dissecting microscope.

Growth curves were determined between CPD 10 and 15 for each culture at least twice by inoculating replicate 25-cm² vessels containing 12 ml medium with 7.5×10^4 cells. Duplicate vessels were harvested and counted at 1- or 2-day intervals. Population doubling times were determined during the period of logarithmic growth (1–3 days after inoculation).

For determination of thymidine incorporation, 2×10^5 cells were added to 25-cm² petri dishes containing two 11 × 22-mm cover slips.[19] Forty-eight hours later, [methyl-^{3}H] thymidine (0.5 μCi/ml, 21 Ci/mmol) was added to each culture. After 24 h, the cover slips were removed, rinsed in DPBS, placed in 15% and then 5% trichloroacetic acid for 1 min each, and then rinsed with alcohol. Radioactivity was quantified by placing the cover slips in vials containing a 2:1 mixture of LSC-complete (Yorktown Research, S Hackensack, New Jersey) and Triton X-100.

RESULTS

Initial outgrowth rates were quantified by observing the number of pieces adhering to the culture vessels and the percentage of pieces resulting in fibroblast outgrowth. These did not differ among the three groups (85% for Pima diabetics, 77% for Pima normals, and 82% for Caucasians). Moreover, the time between explantation and the first trypsinization was 4–5 wk in all three groups.

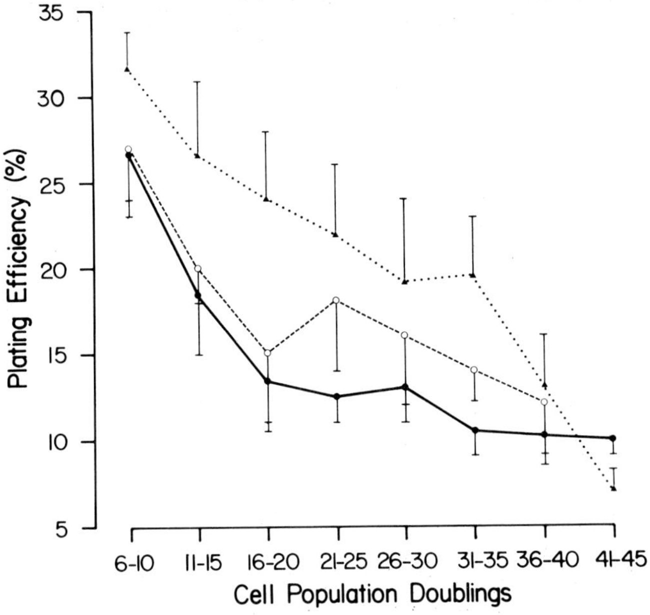

FIGURE 2. Plating efficiency as a function of cell population doublings. Legend corresponds to that of Figure 1. Differences in plating efficiency between Caucasians and Pimas are significant at $P < 0.05$ only for CPD 16–20.

Cell density at confluence (Figure 1), plating efficiency (Figure 2), and thymidine incorporation (Figure 3) were measured throughout the in vitro life span of all lines and tabulated in intervals of 5 CPD. Significance between means was assessed using the Student's *t* test procedure. All three culture parameters were found to decrease with increasing CPD. There were no significant differences between the diabetic and nondiabetic Pima cells in these parameters. Significant differences were observed, however, between both Pima types and the Caucasian controls. Cell density at confluence and thymidine incorporation were higher in the Caucasian lines until the later passage levels. There was much more variability in the determination of plating efficiency;

FIGURE 1. Cell number at confluency as a function of cell population doublings (CPD) in cultures from Pima diabetics (●), Pima nondiabetics (○), and Caucasian nondiabetics (▲). Values represent the mean and standard error of all determinations in increments of 5 CPD. Confluent density for Caucasians is significantly different from Pimas at $P < 0.05$ or smaller for all points up to CPD 21–25.

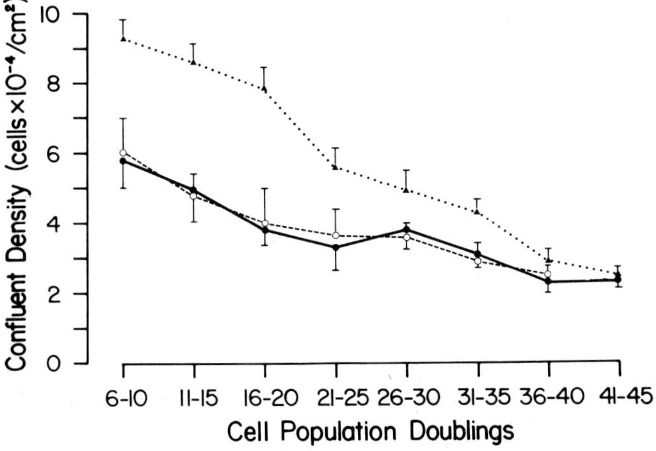

FIGURE 3. Thymidine incorporation as a function of cell population doublings. Legend corresponds to that of Figure 1. Values are dpm/cover slip, which contained approximately 21,000 cells. Values for Caucasians are significantly different from Pimas at $P < 0.05$ or smaller for points up to CPD 16–20.

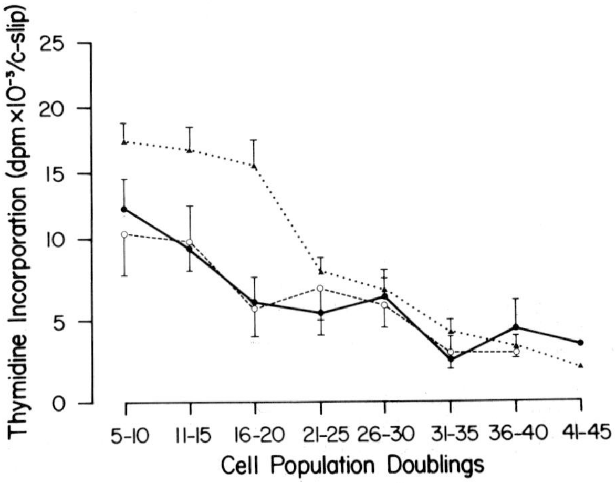

TABLE 2
Size of Pima and Caucasian fibroblasts

Cell	N	CPD	Diameter (μm)
Caucasian	8	13 ± 1*	16.1 ± 0.48*
Pima	14	15 ± 1	18.2 ± 0.47

* Mean ± SEM. Cell diameters were measured from photographs of trypsinized, suspended cells.

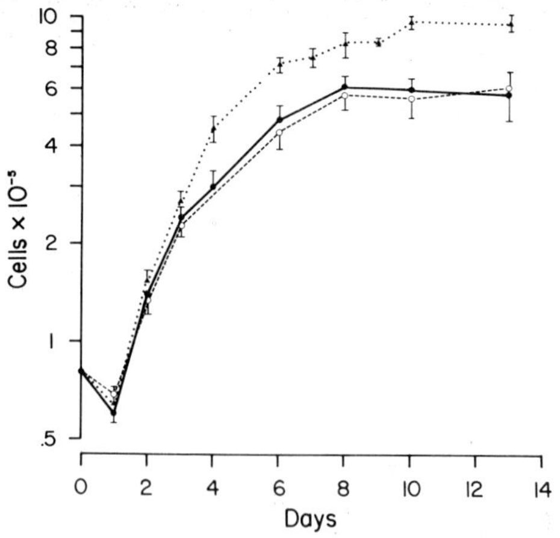

FIGURE 4. Cell population growth curves of cultures from Pima diabetics (●), Pima nondiabetics (○), and Caucasian nondiabetics (▲). Population doubling rates were estimated from the slope between days 1 and 3 and are summarized in Table 3. Caucasian cell number is significantly different from Pimas at P < 0.05 or smaller for days 4–14.

both Pima diabetic and nondiabetic lines appeared to have lower plating efficiencies than the Caucasian lines, but the differences were not significant. Settling efficiency, that is, the proportion of cells surviving 18 h after the routine weekly subcultivation, was determined for several of the lines studied. These ranged from 80% to 90%, and there did not appear to be significant differences between the three types of cells. Cell size was measured for a sample of the cell lines below CPD 20 (Table 2), and the diameter of Pima cells was larger than that of Caucasians (P < 0.01).

Growth curves were determined for early passage cultures of each cell line (Figure 4). Growth rates were similar for the diabetic and nondiabetic cells. The Caucasian lines, however, had lower population doubling times and also reached a higher confluent density.

The relationships between cell growth characteristics and the age of the donor were assessed by simple correlation analysis. All Pima cells were combined for this analysis (Table 3). No significant correlations were found between age of the donor and any of the measured growth parameters. In addition there were no significant correlations when all of the cell lines were combined (N = 19, data not shown). Since there were no significant correlations between the growth parameters and age, and since all the cultures were derived from individuals in a relatively narrow age range (20–42 yr), culture parameters were summarized without adjustment for age (Table 4). Culture parameters up to CPD 15 were averaged for all three groups, and differences between the groups were assessed using the Student's *t* test procedure. There were no significant differences between the diabetic and nondiabetic Pima fibroblasts in any of the culture characteristics or in the final CPD achieved. In all cases, cultures from the Pimas differed from those from the Caucasian control group. The Pimas had significantly higher cell density at confluence, higher thymidine incorporation, shorter population doubling times, and longer replicative life spans. Plating efficiency also appeared to be greater in the Caucasian cultures, but this difference was not significant because of the large variability.

DISCUSSION

The present data on culture parameters of Pima cells indicate that no significant differences in confluent cell density, plating efficiency, population doubling times, and thymidine incorporation were specifically associated with cells from diabetic individuals. Extensive epidemiologic and clinical studies of diabetes in the Pima population have indicated that it is a relatively homogenous, non-insulin-dependent or ketosis-resistant type.[16,20] Thus, our data suggest that the hyperglycemia of this form of diabetes is not a determinant of altered cell growth properties in vitro. In contrast, differences were observed in all culture parameters between the cultures from Pima donors and those from the Caucasian control group. Although this small group cannot be representative of the Caucasian race, it suggests that there may be differences between cultured cells from individuals of differing racial backgrounds. If so, then differences in growth characteristics previously described in cells from diabetics[2,3,9–12] may reflect other aspects of the genetic background of diabetic individuals.

The results of any study of cultures derived from skin biopsies are influenced by many experimental variables; by far the most difficult to control are in the period before the first subcultivation. Although every attempt was made to standardize the site and depth of biopsy, explant conditions, and time, these are all difficult to control. There is no evidence, however, that difference in these variables could

TABLE 3
Correlation coefficients between donor age and culture parameters

		Density at confluency	Population doubling time	Plating efficiency	Thymidine incorporation	Replicative life span
Pima	r*	−0.40	0.22	−0.023	−0.42	−0.063
(N = 12)	P	0.20	0.49	0.94	0.18	0.85
Caucasian	r	−0.11	0.070	−0.15	−0.59	−0.22
(N = 7)	P	0.81	0.88	0.75	0.16	0.64

* r values are simple correlation coefficients.

TABLE 4
Comparison of Pima and Caucasian cell cultures (culture parameters up to CPD = 15)

	Cell density (cells × 10^{-4}/cm^2)	Population doubling rate (days)	Plating efficiency (%)	Thymidine incorporation (dpm)	Replicative life span (CPD)
Pima nondiabetic (N = 6)	5.4 ± 1.0*	1.9 ± 0.21	24 ± 5.0	12.4 ± 2.3	29 ± 3.9
Pima diabetic (N = 7)	5.5 ± 0.63	1.7 ± 0.11	11.6 ± 1.8	11.6 ± 1.8	31 ± 3.8
P†	NS	NS	NS	NS	NS
Pima (N = 13)	5.4 ± 0.53	1.8 ± 0.11	22 ± 2.5	11.9 ± 1.7	30 ± 2.6
Caucasian (N = 6)	8.8 ± 0.73	1.3 ± 0.07	29 ± 3.2	16.6 ± 1.3	38 ± 2.2
P†	0.001	0.005	0.15	0.05	0.05

* Mean ± SEM.
† Values for P were obtained treating the inferences as independent events; P values might be higher since the various growth characteristics are correlated.

account for the large differences in cell culture parameters observed between the Caucasian and Pima cells.

The most consistent differences observed between the cells of Pima and Caucasian origin were in cell density at confluence. The Pima cells were found to be larger, but it is difficult to relate spherical size to the adherent cell configuration. Although cell size has been shown to increase at advanced stages of replicative life span,[21–23] it has not been found by other investigators to be the major determinant of the decreased confluent density associated with in vitro culture age.[24]

Although the cell culture parameters such as confluent density, plating efficiency, thymidine incorporation, and growth rate correlated significantly with each other (data not shown), no significant correlation was observed between any of these and the age of the donor. This was in part due to the very narrow age range of the biopsies, since previous studies had established these correlations in individuals ranging from 10 to 80 yr of age.[3,5,9] It should also be noted that culture senescence was determined by relatively strict criteria, which would minimize any possible differences due to age that might occur between the culture lines.

In summary, the results of the present study suggest that the non-insulin-dependent type of diabetes did not lead to differences in cellular growth properties in vitro. In contrast, differences in in vitro cell growth behavior were observed between cells derived from differing racial groups. Both the determinants of cell growth properties in vitro and their relationship to in vivo functions are not well understood. Since cell density at confluence was the most striking difference observed between the cells from the two populations, it is possible that genetic differences in cell surface characteristics influence cellular in vitro growth behavior. Alternatively, the different proliferative capacities may be a reflection of differences in the cellularity of the dermis itself;[25] this could be related to the differences in weight between the Pima and Caucasian groups (Table 1). The present data are of interest in relationship to the data of Goldstein et al.,[9] who showed differences between cultures from individuals with a family history of diabetes (prediabetics) and cultures from those individuals with neither evidence nor family history of diabetes. They postulated that they have identified a group with altered fibroblast growth potential and the propensity for diabetes. Since the entire Pima population appears to have a propensity for obesity and hyperinsulinemia,[17] it is possible that in vitro cell growth behavior is a reflection of a genetic background, as in the ob/ob and db/db mouse,[26] upon which the diabetes gene is superimposed and/or favored in expression. This hypothesis will require further investigation using larger sample sizes and individuals from other genetic backgrounds.

ACKNOWLEDGMENTS
The authors wish to acknowledge the excellent technical assistance of Michael Davis and Karen Stone. We also wish to thank the Institute for Medical Research, Camden, New Jersey. This work was supported in part by NIH contract #N01-AM-6-0219.

REFERENCES

1 Hayflick, L.: The limited in vitro lifetime of human diploid cell strains. Exp. Cell Res. *37*:614–36, 1965.

2 Goldstein, S., Littlefield, J. W., and Soeldner, J. S.: Diabetes mellitus and aging: diminished plating efficiency of cultured human fibroblasts. Proc. Natl. Acad. Sci. USA *65*:155–60, 1969.

3 Martin, G. M., Sprague, C. A., and Epstein, C. J.: Replicative life-span of cultivated human cells. Lab. Invest. *23*:86–92, 1970.

4 LeGuilly, Y., Simon, M., Lenoir, P., and Bourel, M.: Long term culture of adult liver cells: morphological changes related to in vitro senescence and effect of donor's age on growth potential. Gerontologia *19*:303–13, 1973.

5 Schneider, E. L., and Mitsui, Y.: The relationship between in vitro cellular aging and in vivo human age. Proc. Natl. Acad. Sci. USA *73*:3584–88, 1976.

6 Cristofalo, V. J., and Sharf, B. B.: Cellular senescense and DNA synthesis. Exp. Cell Res. *76*:419–27, 1973.

7 Andres, R., Pozefsky, T., Sverdloff, S., and Tobin, J. D.: Effect of aging on carbohydrate metabolism in early diabetes. *In* Advances in Metabolic Disorders, Suppl. 1. Camerini-Davalos, R. A., and Cole, H. S., Eds. New York, Academic Press, 1970, pp. 349–55.

8 Knowler, W. C., Bennett, P. H., Hamman, R. F., and Miller, M.: Diabetes incidence and prevalence in Pima Indians: a 19-fold greater incidence than in Rochester, Minnesota. Am. J. Epidemiol. *108*:497–505, 1978.

9 Goldstein, S., Moerman, E. J., Soeldner, J. S., Gleason, R. E., and Barnett, D. M.: Diabetes mellitus and genetic prediabetes. Decreased replicative capacity of cultured skin fibroblasts. J. Clin. Invest. *63*:358–70, 1979.

10 Vracko, R., and Benditt, E. P.: Restricted replicative life-span of diabetic fibroblasts in vitro: its relation to microangiopathy. Fed. Proc. *34*:68–70, 1975.

11 Archer, J., and Kaye, R.: Cultured skin fibroblasts and juvenile diabetes: senescence and collagen synthesis. Diabetes *26* (Suppl. 1):36, 1977.

12 Rowe, D. W., Starman, B. J., Fujimoto, W. Y., and Williams, R. H.: Abnormalities in proliferation and protein synthesis in skin fibroblast cultures from patients with diabetes mellitus. Diabetes *26*:284–90, 1977.

[13] Rotter, J. I., and Rimoin, D. L.: Heterogeneity in diabetes mellitus—update 1978. Evidence for further genetic heterogeneity within juvenile-onset insulin-dependent diabetes mellitus. Diabetes *27*:599–605, 1978.

[14] Rosenbloom, A. L., and Rosenbloom, E. K.: Insulin-dependent childhood diabetes. Normal viability of cultured fibroblasts. Diabetes *27*:338–41, 1978.

[15] Matson, G. A., Burch, T. A., and Polesky, H. F.: Distribution of hereditary factors in the blood of Indians of the Gila River, Arizona. Am. J. Phys. Anthropol. *29*:311–38, 1968.

[16] Savage, P. J., Bennett, P. H., Senter, R. G., and Miller, M.: High prevalence of diabetes in young Pima Indians: evidence of phenotypic variation in a genetically isolated population. Diabetes *28*:937–42, 1979.

[17] Rushforth, N. B., Miller, M., and Bennett, P. H.: Fasting and two hour post-load glucose levels for the diagnosis of diabetes. The relationship between glucose levels and complications of diabetes in the Pima Indians. Diabetologia *16*:373–79, 1979.

[18] Ham, R. G., Hammond, S. L., and Miller, L. L.: Critical adjustment of cysteine and glutamine concentrations for improved clonal growth of WI-38 cells. In Vitro *13*:1–9, 1977.

[19] Cristofalo, V. J.: The effect of hydrocortisone on DNA synthesis and cell division during aging in vitro. *In* Cell Impairment in Aging and Development. Holekova, E., and Cristofalo, V. J., Eds. New York, Plenum Press, 1975, pp. 7–22.

[20] Bennett, P. H., Rushforth, N. B., Miller, M., and LeCompte, P.: Epidemiological studies of diabetes in the Pima Indians. Recent Prog. Horm. Res. *32*:333–76, 1976.

[21] Cristofalo, V. J., and Kritchevsky, D.: Cell size and nucleic acid content in the diploid human cell line WI-38 during aging. Med. Exp. *19*:313–20, 1969.

[22] Bowman, P. D., Meek, R. L., and Danell, C. W.: Aging of human fibroblasts in vitro I. Correlations between DNA synthetic ability and cell size. Exp. Cell Res. *93*:184–90, 1975.

[23] Mitsui, Y., and Schneider, E. L.: Relationship between cell replication and volume in senescent human diploid fibroblasts. Mech. Aging Dev. *5*:45–56, 1976.

[24] Greenberg, S. B., Grove, G. L., and Cristofalo, V. J.: Cell size in aging monolayer cultures. In Vitro *5*:297–300, 1977.

[25] Harper, R. A., and Grove, G.: Human skin fibroblasts derived from papillary and reticular dermis: differences in growth potential in vitro. Science *204*:526–27, 1979.

[26] Coleman, D. L.: Obese and diabetes: two mutant genes causing diabetes-obesity syndromes in mice. Diabetologia *14*:141–48, 1978.

Stimulation of Counterregulatory Hormonal Responses in Diabetic Man by a Fall in Glucose Concentration

RALPH A. DEFRONZO, ROSA HENDLER, AND NIELS CHRISTENSEN

SUMMARY

The effect of a falling plasma glucose concentration, from one hyperglycemic to another lower, yet still hyperglycemic, level, on the release of counterregulatory hormones was examined in nine diabetic subjects. The fasting plasma glucose concentration (201 ± 22 mg/dl) was lowered at the rate of 2.3 ± 0.3 mg/min with an exogenous insulin infusion and maintained between 100 and 110 mg/dl for an additional 60 min employing the glucose clamp technique. During the phase of rapidly falling glucose concentration, or shortly thereafter while the plasma glucose was being maintained at or above 100 mg/dl, eight of nine diabetics released growth hormone, five of nine released cortisol, six of nine released epinephrine, and five of nine released norepinephrine. No subject demonstrated any increase in plasma glucagon. One subject experienced a frank hypoglycemic reaction when her plasma glucose concentration had decreased to 149 mg/dl. In contrast, control subjects did not demonstrate the release of any counterregulatory hormones despite a similar rate of decline in plasma glucose concentration. These results indicate that diabetic subjects with fasting hyperglycemia have an upward resetting of the glucostat at which counterregulatory hormones are released and provide direct support for the clinical observation of hypoglycemic reactions in some diabetics with "normal" or high plasma glucose concentrations. DIABETES 29:125–131, February 1980.

Previous studies by DeFronzo et al. have demonstrated that a rapidly falling blood glucose concentration in normal subjects does not result in the release of counterregulatory hormones as long as the glucose concentration remains above fasting values.[1] Not until absolute levels of hypoglycemia (decrease in glucose concentration = 20–40 mg/dl below basal) were achieved was any increase in plasma cortisol, growth hormone, glucagon, or catecholamines observed. However, these results may not be applicable to diabetic subjects with long-standing hyperglycemia, in whom a different level at which counterregulatory hormones are released may occur. Such an upward resetting of the glucostat at which counterregulation occurs may explain the development of hypoglycemic symptoms in the absence of absolute hypoglycemia.[2] To examine this possibility we infused insulin into diabetic subjects with fasting hyperglycemia to induce a rapid decline in blood glucose concentration. The glucose concentration was allowed to drop to 100 mg/dl, at which it was maintained employing the glucose clamp technique.[3]

From the Department of Internal Medicine, Yale University School of Medicine, New Haven, Connecticut, and the Department of Internal Medicine and Endocrinology, Herlev Hospital, Denmark.

Address reprint requests to Dr. Ralph A. DeFronzo, Department of Internal Medicine, Yale University School of Medicine, New Haven, Connecticut 06510.

Received for publication 15 June 1979 and in revised form 22 October 1979.

METHODS

SUBJECTS

Five non-insulin-dependent and four insulin-dependent diabetics of long-standing duration (greater than 5 yr) and five control subjects were studied. The diabetics ranged in age from 22 to 61 yr (mean = 47 ± 6 yr) and all were within 17% of ideal body weight (mean = 105 ± 3) as determined by Metropolitan Life Insurance Tables, 1959. There were four males and five females. Other than insulin, the last dose of which was taken 24 h before study, none of the diabetics were consuming any medications. There was no clinical evidence of diabetic neuropathy as determined by history and clinical examination. The control group consisted of four males and one female ranging in age from 22 to 49 yr and in obesity index from 1.00 to 1.11. None had a family history of diabetes mellitus, none were taking any medications, and all had a normal oral glucose tolerance test. During the 3 days before study, all subjects consumed at least 200 g of carbohydrate per day. All studies were carried out in the postabsorptive state at 8:00 a.m. following a 12-h overnight fast. The purpose and potential risks of the study were carefully explained to all subjects and written voluntary consent was obtained before their participation.

STUDY PROTOCOL

Before each study a polyethylene catheter was inserted into an antecubital vein for the administration of insulin and glucose. A second catheter was inserted into a hand vein for blood sampling and the hand was then inserted into a heated chamber to insure arterialization of venous blood.[4] After a 40-min control period during which two to four samples were collected for analysis of glucose, insulin, cortisol, growth hormone, glucagon, and catecholamines, subjects received one of two types of studies.

Study 1. In five diabetic subjects (two insulin dependent and 3 non-insulin dependent) the plasma glucose concentration was acutely raised and maintained at 125 mg/dl above the basal level for 60 min with a variable intravenous glucose infusion.[3] After 60 min of sustained hyperglycemia, a prime-continuous insulin infusion (1 mU/kg · min) was begun[3] and the glucose infusion was stopped. The plasma glucose concentration was allowed to decrease to 100 mg/dl, at which level it was clamped for an additional 60 min with a variable intravenous infusion of glucose.[3] The insulin infusion was continued until the end of the study. Plasma cortisol, growth hormone, insulin, and glucagon were determined at 10–15-min intervals throughout the study. Plasma catecholamines were determined at 15–30-min intervals. Five control subjects were similarly studied.

Study 2. In four diabetic subjects (two insulin dependent and two non-insulin dependent) the prime-continuous insulin infusion (1 mU/kg · min) was started immediately after the control period and maintained until the end of the study. No glucose was infused until the plasma glucose concentration had decreased to 100 mg/dl. At this time the glucose infusion was begun and the plasma glucose concentration was maintained at 100 mg/dl for an additional 60–80 min. Plasma samples were obtained as previously described.

Since we have previously shown that intravenous injection of insulin may result in a decrease in plasma volume, which could increase adrenergic venous system activity,[5] all blood losses were replaced quantitatively with normal saline and above this an additional 750 ml of normal saline was administered during the study period. Subjects also received between 200 and 400 ml of a 20% glucose solution to maintain the plasma glucose concentration at the desired level. Blood pressure and pulse were monitored at 15–30-min intervals and, except for one subject who experienced a hypoglycemic reaction, no changes from baseline were observed.

ANALYTICAL METHODS

Plasma glucose concentration was determined using the glucose oxidase method (Glucostat, Beckman Instruments Corp., Fullerton, California). Methods for the determination of plasma immunoreactive glucagon (with Unger antibody

Figure 1. Time course of change in plasma glucose, glucagon, cortisol, and growth hormone concentrations after sustained hyperglycemia in diabetic subjects.

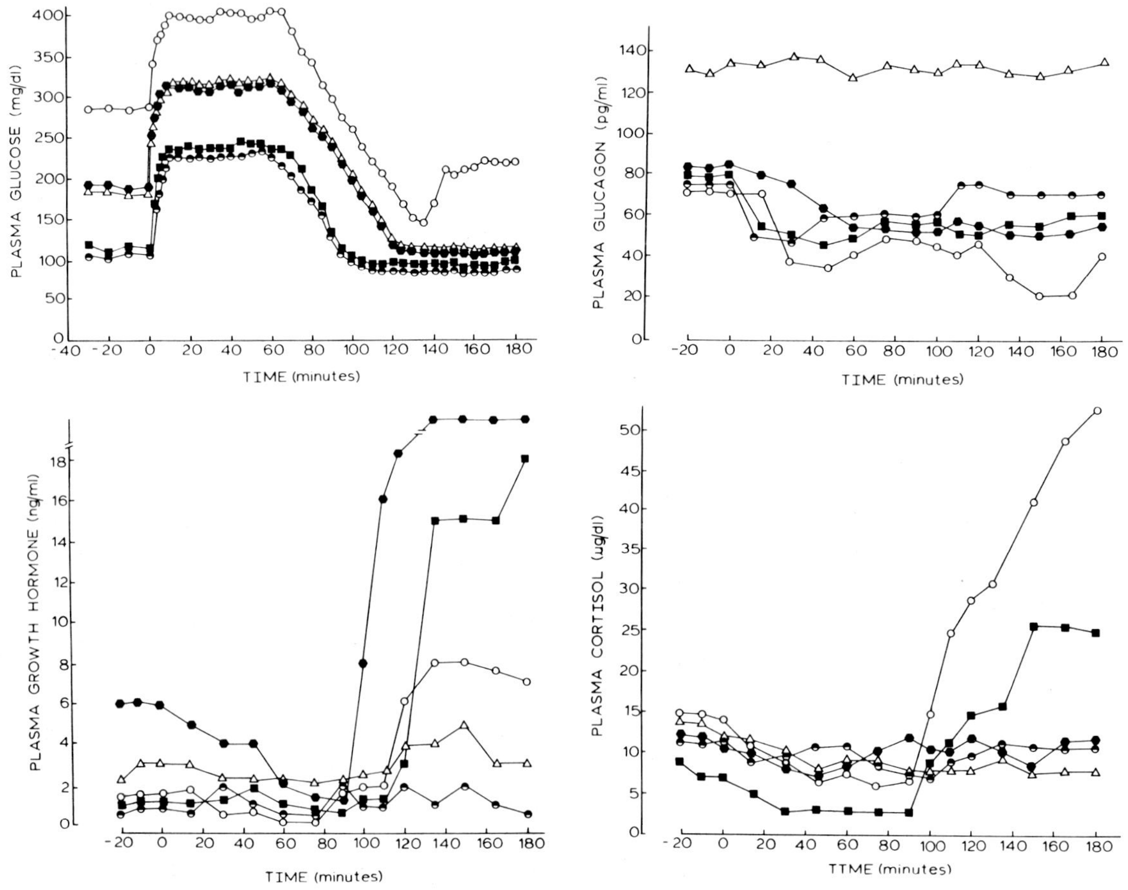

30K) and insulin,[6] growth hormone and cortisol,[1] and catecholamines[7] have previously been described. All results are expressed as mean ±SEM.

RESULTS

FALLING GLUCOSE PRECEDED BY HYPERGLYCEMIA IN DIABETICS

Glucose. The mean fasting plasma glucose concentration in the nine diabetics was 201 ± 22 mg/dl. In five diabetics (Figure 1) the plasma glucose concentration was raised and maintained by 126 ± 3 mg/dl above basal levels for the first 60 min with a coefficient of variation of 1.8 ± 0.4%. Following discontinuation of the glucose infusion, the plasma glucose concentration fell rapidly by 2.8 ± 0.2 mg/min, and in all but one subject the plasma glucose concentration had declined to 100 mg/dl by 120 min. This one subject (open circles) experienced a hypoglycemic reaction (tachycardia, sweating, anxiety, tremor, headache, blurred vision, faintness) when the plasma glucose concentration reached 149 mg/dl, which was associated with an increase in plasma glucose concentration to 170 mg/dl within 10 min. The glucose infusion was restarted at this point and the plasma glucose concentration was maintained at 215 ± 2 mg/dl until the end of the study. In the other four subjects the plasma glucose concentration was maintained at 102 ± 2 mg/dl (range = 98–109 mg/dl) for the last 60 min of study.

Insulin. In the three maturity-onset diabetics who had not received prior insulin therapy, the fasting plasma insulin concentration was 14 ± 1 μU/ml. During the period of sustained hyperglycemia (0–60 min) the plasma insulin concentration averaged 50 ± 9 μU/ml. For the 60–180-min time period, during which exogenous insulin was infused at the rate of 1 mU/kg · min, the mean plasma insulin concentration increased to 204 ± 9 μU/ml.

Glucagon. Basal glucagon levels averaged 87 ± 10 pg/ml (Figure 1). During the period of sustained hyperglycemia, four of five subjects demonstrated a decline in plasma glucagon concentration to a mean of 67 ± 16 pg/ml ($P < 0.05$). During the rapidly falling phase of plasma glucose, glucagon remained suppressed and continued so until the end of the study.

Growth hormone. Basal growth hormone concentration was 2.3 ± 0.9 ng/ml and fell slightly to 1.4 ± 0.5 ng/ml during the period of sustained hyperglycemia (Figure 1). During the phase of rapidly falling glucose concentration, two subjects (hexagons, open circles) released growth hormone and during the last hour of study, when the plasma glucose concentration was maintained at 100 mg/dl, two additional subjects (squares, open triangles) released growth hormone. Thus, four of five diabetic subjects demonstrated an increase in growth hormone in the absence of hypoglycemia.

Cortisol. Basal plasma cortisol, 12 ± 1 mg/dl, fell slightly to 8 ± 1 mg/dl following hyperglycemia (Figure 1). During the phase of rapidly falling glucose concentration, two subjects (open circles, squares) demonstrated an increase in plasma cortisol levels. No changes were observed in the other three.

Catecholamines. Baseline plasma epinephrine and norepinephrine concentrations were 0.03 ± 0.01 and 0.09 ± 0.01 ng/dl, respectively (Figure 2). During the phase of rapidly falling glucose concentration, two subjects released epinephrine (open circles and half-closed circles) and two released norepinephrine (hexagons, half-closed circles). During the last 60 min, when the plasma glucose concentration was maintained at 100 mg/dl, one subject released epinephrine (squares) and one norepinephrine (triangles). Thus, three of five subjects released epinephrine and norepinephrine in the absence of hypoglycemia.

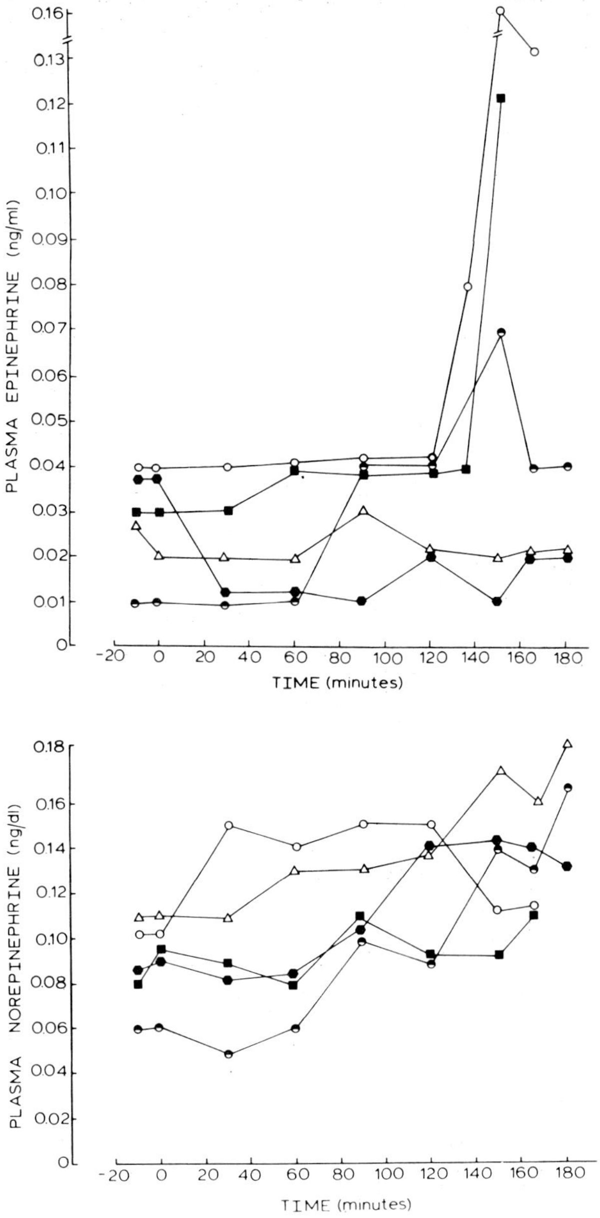

FIGURE 2. Time course of change in plasma epinephrine and norepinephrine concentrations after sustained hyperglycemia in diabetic subjects.

FALLING GLUCOSE WITHOUT PRECEDING HYPERGLYCEMIA IN DIABETICS

Glucose. In four diabetic subjects (Figure 3) the exogenous insulin infusion was begun immediately after the basal

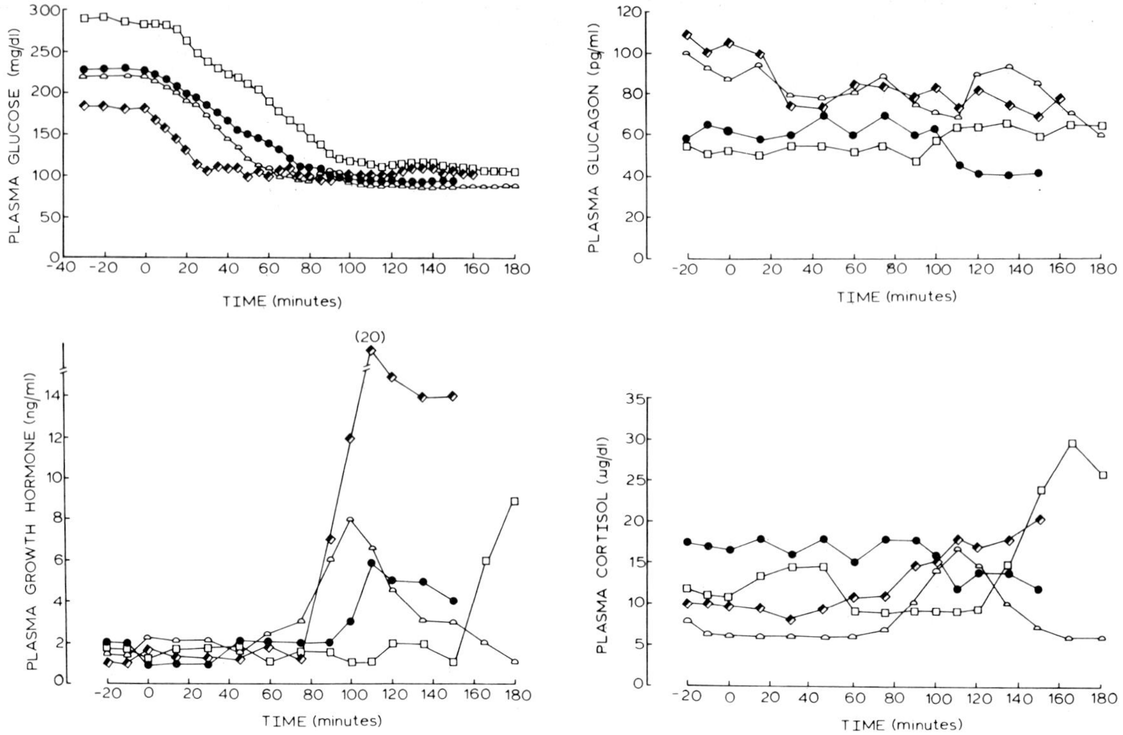

Figure 3. Time course of change in plasma glucose, glucagon, cortisol, and growth hormone concentrations after insulin infusion to diabetic subjects.

period without any preceding period of hyperglycemia. The rate of decline of plasma glucose concentration averaged 1.6 ± 0.1 mg/min during the rapidly falling phase and the plasma glucose concentration declined to 100 mg/dl within 40–100 min in all subjects. The glucose infusion was begun at this point and the plasma glucose concentration was maintained at 102 ± 2 mg/dl (range = 98–112 mg/dl) for an additional 60–100 min.

Insulin. In the two maturity-onset diabetics who had not received prior insulin therapy, the fasting plasma insulin concentration averaged 13 μU/ml. During the phase of rapidly falling glucose concentration and thereafter, the insulin concentration averaged 123 μU/ml.

Glucagon. Fasting plasma glucagon concentration was 79 ± 13 pg/ml and either remained unchanged or fell slightly during the study period (Figure 3).

Growth hormone. Mean fasting plasma growth hormone was 1.4 ± 0.1 ng/ml (Figure 3). During the phase of rapidly falling glucose concentration, no subject released growth hormone. However, all four subjects released growth hormone while the glucose concentration was being maintained at 100 mg/dl.

Cortisol. Basal plasma cortisol was 11 ± 2 mg/dl (Figure 3). Plasma cortisol remained unchanged during the period of rapidly falling glucose concentration, but increased in three of four subjects while the plasma glucose was being held constant at 100 mg/dl.

Catecholamines. Fasting plasma epinephrine and norepinephrine levels averaged 0.04 ± 0.01 and 0.14 ± 0.02 ng/ml, respectively (Figure 4). During the phase of rapidly falling glucose concentration, one subject (open squares) released epinephrine and in two others (closed circles and half circles) epinephrine was released shortly after the glucose concentration reached 100 mg/dl. Small increases in plasma norepinephrine were observed in two subjects (closed circles and half-closed diamonds).

FALLING GLUCOSE IN CONTROLS (FIGURE 5)

The mean fasting glucose concentration in the five control subjects was 91 ± 1 mg/dl. Following the 60-min period of sustained hyperglycemia (mean glucose = 218 ± 1 mg/dl), the plasma glucose concentration fell at the rate of 4.0 ± 0.3 mg/min and returned to basal levels within 35 min. The plasma glucose concentration was maintained at or above basal levels (range = 95–109 mg/dl) for an additional 60–80 min. One subject released growth hormone during the rapid falling of plasma glucose concentration (solid circles) and one subject (solid triangles) released growth hormone after the plasma glucose concentration had been lowered to 100 mg/dl. In a third subject (solid squares) growth hormone was released during the hyperglycemic plateau but eventually was suppressed and remained suppressed. No other counterregulatory hormones were released either during or after the period of rapidly declining plasma glucose concentration.

DISCUSSION

The response of the four counterregulatory hormones–glucagon, growth hormone, cortisol, catecholamines—after a fall in blood glucose concentration from hyperglycemic levels has not been systematically examined in diabetic subjects. Although clinical studies in diabetics have suggested that hypoglycemic symptoms can occur in response to a falling blood glucose concentration even before abso-

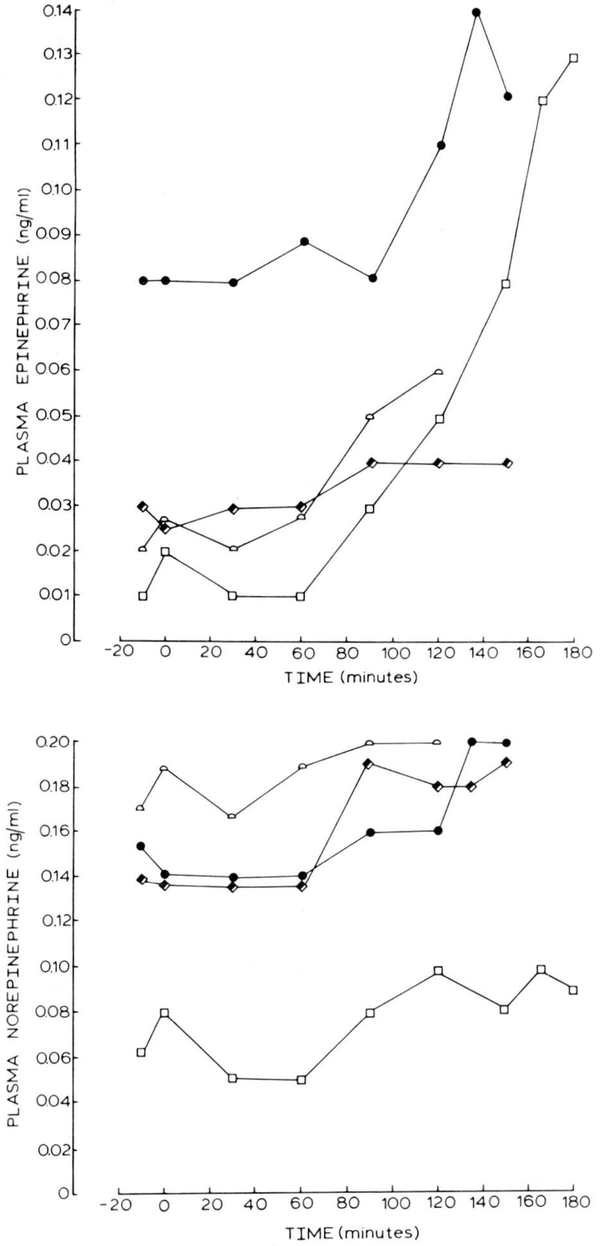

FIGURE 4. Time course of change in plasma epinephrine and norepinephrine concentrations after insulin infusion to diabetic subjects.

lute hypoglycemia is achieved,[2,8] previous studies from our laboratory in normal subjects failed to document an increase in any counterregulatory hormones during this period. A similar lack of response to a falling glucose concentration was also observed in the control group in the present study. However, in diabetic subjects with long-standing hyperglycemia an upward resetting of the glucostat may occur at which counterregulatory hormones are released.

In the present study we acutely decreased the plasma glucose concentration from hyperglycemic levels (214–400 mg/dl) in nine diabetic subjects. The plasma glucose concentration was measured at 5-min intervals throughout the study and at no time did the glucose concentration fall below 98 mg/dl. Thus, absolute hypoglycemia was avoided in all subjects. Nonetheless, the release of cortisol (five of nine subjects), growth hormone (eight of nine), epinephrine (six of nine), and norepinephrine (five of nine) was commonly observed. Only glucagon failed to show any consistent increase. This pattern of release of counterregulatory hormones was similar in both insulin-dependent and non-insulin-dependent diabetics and occurred whether or not the phase of rapidly falling glucose concentration was preceded by a period of hyperglycemia or not.

Two previous studies[1,9] have examined the plasma growth hormone response during a fall in blood glucose from one hyperglycemic to yet another hyperglycemic level in normal subjects. In one study[1] no release of growth hormone was observed during the rapidly falling phase of plasma glucose concentration while in the other[9] sporadic increases were reported. In the present study only two of five control subjects released growth hormone in response to a rapidly falling plasma glucose concentration. In contrast, eight of nine diabetic subjects demonstrated an increase in plasma growth hormone either during the period of rapidly falling glucose concentration or while the plasma glucose was being maintained at or above 100 mg/dl. Similarly, plasma cortisol increased in five of nine diabetic subjects whereas no increase was observed in normal subjects as long as the glucose concentration did not decrease below fasting levels. Previous studies in normal subjects employing insulin-induced hypoglycemia have shown that growth hormone[1,10–19] and cortisol[1,10,15,16,19,21] are not consistently released until the blood glucose concentration has decreased to 30–40 mg/dl below basal levels.

Plasma epinephrine and norepinephrine levels increased in six of nine and five of nine diabetic subjects, respectively, in response to a falling glucose concentration, despite plasma glucose concentrations ≥ 98 mg/dl. A consistent increase in both epinephrine[18,19] and norepinephrine[5,18,19,22,23] has been reported in both normal[1,18,19,20,23] and diabetic[5,19,23] subjects after insulin-induced hypoglycemia. In previous studies[5,23] we have demonstrated an increase in plasma norepinephrine levels in diabetic subjects after intravenous insulin despite the absence of hypoglycemia. The release of norepinephrine correlated closely with the decrease in plasma volume, which averaged 265 ml, and a rise in pulse rate, suggesting that the stimulation of norepinephrine was a compensatory response to a plasma volume-lowering effect of insulin. Recently, Parving et al.[24] have questioned the premise that insulin causes a decrease in plasma volume. To avoid any possible contribution of an insulin-mediated decrease in plasma volume to the rise in circulating plasma catecholamine levels, subjects received an excess of 750 ml of normal saline in addition to 200–400 ml of water (given as 20% glucose to maintain the plasma glucose concentration constant) during the study period. No changes in either pulse rate or blood pressure were observed. Thus, it is unlikely that the increase in norepinephrine observed in the present study was secondary to an insulin-mediated decrease in the circulating plasma volume. An increase in plasma epinephrine levels was also observed in six of nine diabetic subjects. In three, epinephrine was released during the rapidly falling phase of plasma glucose concentration and in three others it was released while the plasma glucose concentration was being maintained at or above 100 mg/dl. To our knowledge this represents the first docu-

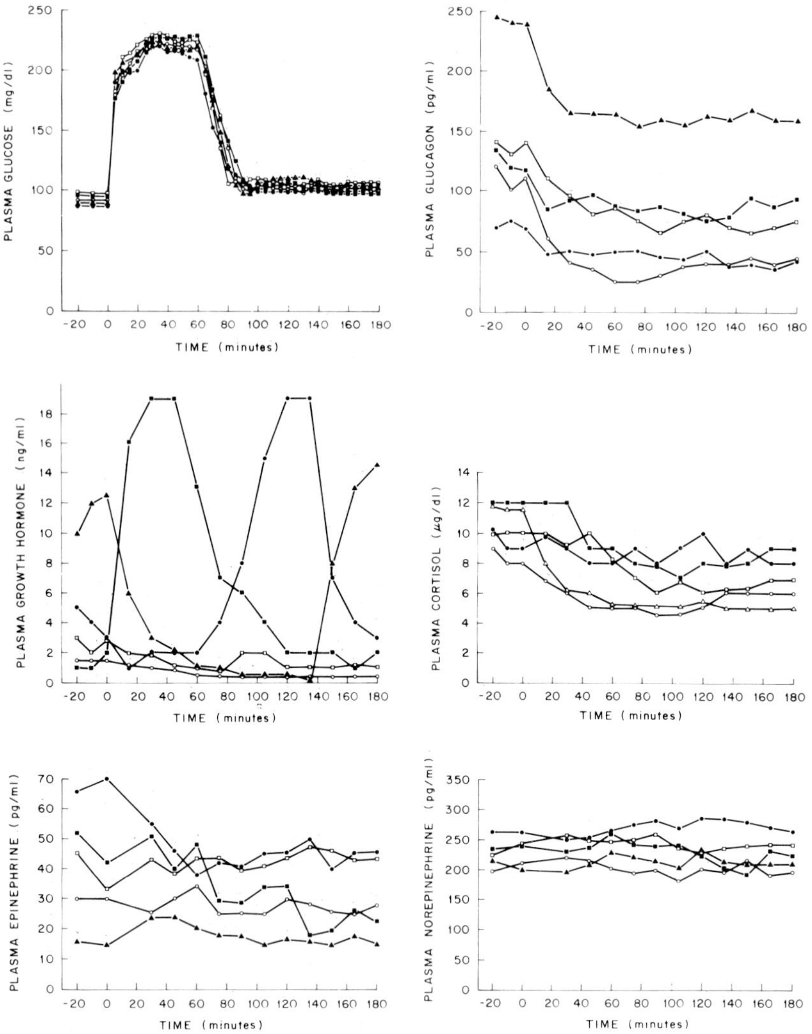

FIGURE 5. Time course of change in plasma glucose, glucagon, cortisol, growth hormone, epinephrine, and norepinephrine concentrations after sustained hyperglycemia in control subjects.

mentation of catecholamine release in response to a falling blood glucose concentration in the absence of overt hypoglycemia (plasma glucose concentration $\leq$100 mg/dl). It should be noted, however, that the rise in plasma epinephrine is significantly less than that observed during insulin-induced hypoglycemia (blood glucose concentration = 20 −40 mg/dl below basal levels).[18,23]

In contrast to the stimulatory effect of a falling glucose concentration on growth hormone, cortisol, and catecholamines, no increase in plasma glucagon concentration was observed in any of the diabetic subjects. Since the controls also failed to demonstrate a rise in plasma glucagon levels, our results cannot be interpreted to indicate that a defect in alpha-cell function exists in diabetic subjects. However, it should be noted that previous studies have demonstrated defective glucagon release in response to a fall in plasma glucose concentration below fasting levels.[25]

The present results clearly establish that in both insulin-dependent and non-insulin dependent diabetics with fasting hyperglycemia, there is an upward resetting of the glucostat, which regulates the release of counterregulatory hormones. Our results also give credence to the clinical observation that diabetic subjects may experience hypoglycemic symptoms in the absence of frank hypoglycemia. Thus, one diabetic (open circles) experienced a typical hypoglycemic reaction with a plasma glucose concentration of 149 mg/dl and this was temporally correlated with the release of epinephrine. Despite this hypoglycemic reaction, no increase in plasma glucagon was observed. The release of cortisol, growth hormone, and norepinephrine significantly preceded the onset of hypoglycemic symptoms.

In summary, a rapidly falling blood glucose concentration from one hyperglycemic to a lower, yet, still, hyperglycemic level is capable of stimulating the release of counterregulatory hormones and resulting in a hypoglycemic reaction.

ACKNOWLEDGMENTS

The authors would like to thank Joan Vieira for secretarial assistance in preparation of this manuscript and Lois Michiwiec for her help in performing the studies.

This work was supported in part by grants from the Danish Medical Research Council, the National Institutes of Health (AM24092), the Juvenile Diabetes Foundation (78R294), and the American Diabetes Association.

REFERENCES

[1] DeFronzo, R. A., Andres, R., Bledsoe, T. A., Boden, G., Faloona, G. A., and Tobin, J. D.: A test of the hypothesis that the rate of fall in glucose

concentration triggers counterregulatory hormonal responses in man. Diabetes *26*:445–52, 1977.

[2] Schade, D. S., and Eaton, R. P.: Dose response to insulin in man: differential effects on glucose and ketone body regulation. J. Clin. Endocrinol. Metab. *44*:1038–53, 1977.

[3] DeFronzo, R. A., Tobin, J. D., and Andres, R.: The glucose clamp technique. A method for quantifying insulin secretion and resistance. Am. J. Physiol. *237*:E214–23, 1979.

[4] McGuire, E. A. H., Helderman, J. H., Tobin, J. D., Andres, R., and Berman, M.: Effects of arterial versus venous sampling. An analysis of glucose kinetics in man. J. Appl. Physiol. *41*:565–73, 1976.

[5] Gundersen, H. J. G., and Christensen, N. J.: Intravenous insulin causing loss of intravascular water and albumin and increased adrenergic nervous activity in diabetics. Diabetes *26*:551–57, 1977.

[6] Wise, J. K., Hendler, R., and Felig, P.: Influence of glucocorticoids on glucagon secretion and plasma aminoacid concentrations in man. J. Clin. Invest. *52*:2774–82, 1973.

[7] Christensen, N. J.: Plasma noradrenaline and adrenaline in patients with thyrotoxicosis and myxoedema. Clin. Sci. *45*:163–71, 1973.

[8] Harries, M., and Prout, B. J.: Relative hypoglycemia. Lancet *2*:317–19, 1970.

[9] Roth, J., Glick, S. M., Yalow, R. S., and Berson, S. A.: Secretion of human growth hormone: physiologic and experimental modification. Metab. Clin. Exp. *12*577–79, 1963.

[10] Gerich, J. E., Schneider V., Dippe, S. E., Langlois, M., Noacco, C., Karam, J. H., and Forsham, P. H.: Characterization of the glucagon response to hypoglycemia in man. J. Clin. Endocrinol. Metab. *38*:77–82, 1974.

[11] Roth, J., Glick, S. M., Yalow, R. S., and Berson, S. A.: The influence of blood glucose on the plasma concentration of growth hormone. Diabetes *13*:355–61, 1964.

[12] Glick, S. M.: Hypoglycemic threshold for human growth hormone release. J. Clin. Endocrinol. Metab. *30*:619–23, 1970.

[13] Sonksen, P. H., Tompkins, C. V., Srivastava, M. D., and Nabarro, J. D. N.: Growth hormone and cortisol responses to insulin infusion in patients with diabetes mellitus. Lancet *2*:155–60, 1972.

[14] Fatourechi, V., Molnar, G. D., Service, F. J., Ackerman, E., Rosevear, J. W., Moxness, K. E., and Taylor, W. F.: Growth hormone and glucose interrelationships in diabetes: studies with insulin infusion during continuous blood glucose analysis. J. Clin. Endocrinol. Metab. *29*319–27, 1969.

[15] Greenwood, F. C., Landon, J., and Stamp, T. C. B.: The plasma sugar, free fatty acid, cortisol, and growth hormone response to insulin. I. In control subjects. J. Clin. Invest. *45*:429–36, 1966.

[16] Nakagawa, K., Horiuchi, Y., and Mashimo, K.: Further studies on the relation between growth hormone and corticotrophin secretion in insulin-induced hypoglycemia. J. Clin. Endocrinol. Metabl. *32*:188–91, 1971.

[17] Koh, C. S., Kohn, J., Catt, K. J., and Burger, E. G.: Lack of relation between plasma growth hormone levels and small decrements in blood sugar. Lancet *1*:13–14, 1968.

[18] Garber, A. J., Cryer, P. E., Santiago, J. V., Haymond, M. W., Pagliara, A. S., and Kipnis, D. M.: The role of adrenergic mechanisms in the substrate and hormonal response to insulin-induced hypoglycemia in man. J. Clin. Invest. *58*:7–14, 1976.

[19] Clarke, W. L., Santiago, J. V., and Cryer, P. E.: Catecholamine and growth hormone release with physiologic decrements in the plasma glucose concentration in normal and diabetic man. Clin. Res. *25*:561A, 1977.

[20] Plonk, J. W., Bivens, C. H., and Feldman, J. M.: Inhibition of hypoglycemia-induced cortisol secretion by the serotonin antagonist cyproheptadine. J. Clin. Endocrinol. Metab. *38*:836–40, 1974.

[21] Donald, R. A.: Plasma immunoreactive corticotrophin and cortisol response to insulin hypoglycemia in normal subjects and patients with pituitary disease. J. Clin. Endocrinol. Metab. *32*:225–31, 1971.

[22] Christensen, N. J., Alberti, K. G. M. M., and Brandsborg, O.: Plasma catecholamines and blood substrate concentrations: studies in insulin induced hypoglycemia and after adrenaline infusions. Eur. J. Clin. Invest. *5*:415–23, 1975.

[23] Christensen, J. N.: Plasma epinephrine and norepinephrine in untreated diabetics during fasting and after insulin administration. Diabetes *23*:1–8, 1974.

[24] Parving, H. H., Noer, I., Deckert, T., and Lassen, N. A.: Intravenous insulin has no effect on transcapillary escape rate of albumin and on plasma volume in short-term juvenile diabetics. Diabetes *28*:282–86, 1979.

[25] Gerich, J. E., Langlois, M., Noacco, C., Karam, J. H., and Forsham, P. H.: Lack of glucagon response to hypoglycemia in diabetes: evidence for an intrinsic pancreatic alpha cell defect. Science *182*:171–73, 1973.

Short-term Regulation of Insulin Receptor Affinity in Man

J. R. INSEL, O. G. KOLTERMAN, M. SAEKOW, AND J. M. OLEFSKY

SUMMARY

We have studied the short term regulation of insulin receptors by serially measuring insulin binding to erythrocytes during 5 h of infusions of glucose and insulin. Two infusion protocols were employed: (1) Hyperinsulinemic study. Subjects were infused with insulin (80 mU/min) to induce sustained hyperinsulinemia, while euglycemia was approximated by infusion of glucose (8 mg/kg/min). (2) Hyperglycemic study. Subjects were infused with glucose (7 mg/kg/min) and a small amount of insulin (10 mU/min), while endogenous insulin secretion was inhibited with epinephrine and propranolol. Insulin binding to erythrocyte insulin receptors was measured serially during both of these infusion protocols for 5 h. The results demonstrated no change in insulin binding during the first 3 h of either infusion. However, by 5 h of either infusion, a striking 36% decrease in insulin binding, from 6.3 ± 0.5% to 4.0 ± 0.6%, was observed. Scatchard analysis and average affinity analysis of the binding data demonstrated that this decrease in insulin binding was entirely caused by a decrease in receptor affinity. Insulin binding to circulating monocytes was also measured, and comparable effects were observed. When cells were removed from the in vivo environment at 3 h and were incubated in vitro for a subsequent 2 h, decreased insulin binding developed during the incubation. Thus, this short term regulation of insulin receptor affinity occurred in vivo or in vitro, and cells that were programmed during the first 3 h of the infusion study could develop a decrease in insulin receptor affinity in vitro in the absence of plasma factors. DIABETES *29*:132–139, February 1980.

Insulin binding to receptors is the first event in insulin action, and this step represents a major control point for insulin's effects in vivo.[1] Insulin binding to receptors is not a fixed biologic process but is subject to modulation by alterations in either receptor number or affinity.[2,3] In particular, there are numerous reports documenting changes in the number of insulin receptors under a variety of experimental conditions.[2–4] However, changes in insulin receptor number appear to take several days to develop in man[5–7] and do not provide an adaptive mechanism for short term (within 24 to 48 h) regulation of insulin binding. Several situations have been reported in which acute (up to 48 h) alterations in insulin binding occur, and these effects are secondary to modulation of receptor affinity.[5–9] Recently, we have reported that short term (5 day) high carbohydrate feeding in man lead to a decrease in the binding affinity of adipocyte insulin receptors, whereas long term high carbohydrate ingestion leads to a reduction in adipocyte insulin receptor number.[7] Thus, the short term adaptive response of the insulin receptor appears to be mediated through changes in receptor affinity whereas the long term response requires a change in receptor number. To further explore the mechanisms whereby receptor affinity can be regulated, we have serially assessed the ability of insulin to bind to human erythrocytes during 5 h of glucose and insulin infusions.

MATERIALS AND METHODS

Materials. Porcine monocomponent insulin was generously supplied by Dr. Ronald Chance of Eli Lilly and Co. (Indianapolis, Ind.). [^{125}I]Na was purchased from New England Nuclear (Boston, Mass.), bovine serum albumin (BSA fraction V) from Armour and Co. (Chicago, Ill.), and collagenase from Worthington Biochemical Corp. (Freehold, N.J.).

Subjects. The study group consisted of nine nonobese normal subjects (two men and seven women), whose ages ranged from 26 to 58 yr. The subjects' relative weights ranged from 0.75 to 1.20, with a mean of 0.95. After informed consent was obtained from them, subjects were admitted to

From the Departments of Medicine, University of Colorado Medical Center and the Veterans' Administration Hospital, Denver, Colorado 80262.
Address reprint requests to: Dr. Jerrold M. Olefsky, University of Colorado Health Science Center, Department of Medicine; B151, 4200 East Ninth Avenue, Denver, Colorado 80262.
Received for publication 4 September 1979.

the University of Colorado Clinical Research Center. No patient had a history of recent weight change or a history of illness known to affect glucose metabolism. All oral glucose tolerance tests were normal.

Diet. The subjects consumed a weight-maintaining liquid diet consisting of 45% carbohydrate, 40% fat, and 15% protein. The daily intake of 35 kcal/kg/day was divided into portions of 1/5, 2/5, and 2/5 served at 8 a.m., 12 noon, and 6 p.m. Daily weights were monitored for all subjects and were constant throughout the study. Each subject was allowed to stabilize on the diet for at least 48 h before any study.

Protocol. After 12 h of an overnight fast, blood samples were obtained for measurements of plasma glucose, plasma insulin, and insulin binding to erythrocytes. Each subject was then given an intravenous injection of 5 mg of propranolol, followed in 5 min by an infusion of glucose (7 or 8 mg/kg/min), epinephrine (6 μg/min), propranolol (0.08 mg/min), and insulin. The insulin was infused at either 10 or 80 mU/min. The solution was infused continuously for 5 h via a Harvard infusion pump (Millis, Mass.) into an antecubital vein. Blood samples were obtained at 3 h and 5 h for determination of plasma glucose, insulin, growth hormone, cortisol, and insulin binding to erythrocytes. These samples were drawn from the opposite arm through a needle kept patent by a slow saline infusion.

Under these experimental conditions, endogenous insulin secretion is suppressed by the epinephrine and propranolol, and steady state plasma glucose and insulin levels are reached by 90 min.[10] During one of the two infusion protocols—termed the hyperglycemic infusion—insulin was infused at 10 mU/min to maintain a steady state insulin concentration at, or near, basal levels while it allowed hyperglycemia to occur in response to the glucose infusion (7 mg/kg/min). During the other infusion protocol—termed the hyperinsulinemic infusion—insulin was given at 80 mU/min to achieve hyperinsulinemia while it maintained plasma glucose near basal levels via the administration of glucose (8 mg/kg/min). Studies were performed at least 2 days apart; both infusion protocols were carried out in five of the nine subjects, while only one protocol was given in the other subjects.

CELL PREPARATION AND INSULIN BINDING STUDIES

Erythrocytes. Insulin binding to erythrocytes was measured according to a modification of the method of Gambhir et al.[11–13] Whole blood (10 ml) was drawn into heparinized tubes and centrifuged for 10 min (400 *g* at 20°). The resulting cell pellet was diluted 1:1 with phosphate-buffered saline and the red cells were fractionated on a Ficoll-Hypaque gradient. After isolating the resultant red cell pellet, the latter two steps were repeated and the cell pellet was diluted 1:2 with a buffer containing 50 mM Hepes, 50 mM Tris, 50 mM sodium chloride, 10 mM CaCl, 10 mM $MgCl_2$, 5 mM KCl, 10 mM glucose, 2 mM EDTA, and 1%BSA, pH 8.0, 15°. The erythrocyte suspension was centrifuged and the pellet was resuspended in 1% BSA buffer to yield a final cell concentration of 4.4×10^9/ml. Cell viability was always >98%, as determined by exclusion of trypan blue. Cell counts were performed with a hemacytometer.

Insulin-binding studies. [^{125}I]insulin was prepared with a specific activity of between 100 and 150 μCi/μg by the modification of Freychet et al.[14] of the method of Hunter and Greenwood.[15] Insulin binding to receptors was assessed by incubating cells with [^{125}I]insulin (3.3×10^{-11} M) and by increasing the concentrations of unlabeled insulin at 15°C for 2.5 h in a total volume of 0.5 ml. At the end of the incubation, duplicate 200 μl aliquots were added to prechilled plastic tubes containing 100 μl of dibutyl phthalate and 100 μl of the 1% BSA buffer. The microfuge tubes were centrifuged for 120 s in a Beckman Microfuge, and the radioactivity in the cell pellets was determined. Nonspecific binding was defined as the amount of cell-associated [^{125}I]insulin in the presence of a large excess, 10^5 ng/ml, of unlabeled insulin. All data were corrected for this factor and represent specific insulin binding. The amount of insulin specifically bound was normalized to a cell concentration of 3.5×10^9/ml.

Monocytes. Isolated monocytes were prepared and insulin-binding studies were performed according to previously described methods.[4,16,17]

Analytic procedures. Blood to measure glucose and insulin was drawn into test tubes containing EDTA, the plasma quickly separated, and aliquots stored at −20°C until insulin determinations were done. Plasma glucose was measured by the glucose oxidase method in a glucose analyzer (Beckman Instruments, Fullerton, Calif.). Plasma insulin was measured by a two antibody radioimmunoassay according to the method of Desbuquois and Aurbach.[18] Glucose and insulin values are reported as the mean (±SE).

Statistical Analysis. All P values were obtained by use of the paired Student's *t* test.

RESULTS

Insulin binding to erythrocytes in the basal state. At a tracer concentration (3.3×10^{-11} M), the mean (±SE) percent [^{125}I]insulin specifically bound for every 3.3×10^9 erythrocytes was 6.1 ± 0.4% for the entire study group. Interassay variation was 8% and nonspecific binding averaged 15% of total binding.

Plasma glucose and insulin levels during the infusion studies. Two separate 5 h infusion protocols were employed. The first infusion was designed to produce hyperinsulinemia and maintain euglycemia; it will be called the hyperinsulinemic infusion, hereafter. This was accomplished by suppressing endogenous insulin secretion with epinephrine and propranolol so that the resultant steady state plasma insulin levels were essentially a reflection of the infused exogenous insulin (80 mU/min). Euglycemia was approximated by administering glucose at 8 mg/kg/min. Many samples (5–11) were obtained during the final 2 h of the infusion, and steady state levels were clearly achieved in all subjects. The coefficients of variation of all values obtained from 180 to 300 min for each of the six individual studies were 7, 4, 5, 3, 4, and 8 for glucose levels and 8, 4, 4, 4, 7, and 14 for insulin levels. The mean (±SE) glucose values (mg/100 ml) during the steady state were 90 ± 18 at 180 min, 91 ± 18 at 240 min, 85 ± 17 at 280 min, 92 ± 22 at 290 min, 86 ± 17 at 295 min, and 85 ± 16 at 300 min. The mean (±SE) insulin values (μU/ml) during the steady state were 118 ± 12 at 180 min, 108 ± 15 at 280 min, 100 ± 15 at 285 min, 108 ± 15 at 290 min, 110 ± 14 at 295 min, and 107 ± 13 at 300 min. The basal glucose value was 90 ± 3 mg/100 ml. Thus, substantial hyperinsulinemia was achieved in the face of euglycemia. The second infusion protocol was designed to produce hyperglycemia and to maintain insulin near basal values; it is termed the hyperglycemic infusion. During this protocol, endogenous insulin secretion was suppressed by epinephrine and propranolol, and a small amount of exogenous insulin was infused (10 mU/min) to maintain basal levels. Hyperglycemia was produced by infusing glucose at 7 mg/kg/min. Steady state values were clearly achieved in all subjects, and the coefficient of variation of all values obtained from 180 to 300 min for each of the nine individual studies were 9, 6, 5, 1, 2, 2, 1, 3, and 1 for glucose levels and 15, 9, 6, 14, 7, 14, 6, 7, and 10 for insulin levels. The mean (±SE) glucose values (mg/100 ml) during the steady state were 256 ± 25 at 180 min, 233 ± 31 at 280 min, 228 ± 30 at 285 min, 231 ± 31 at 290 min, 232 ± 29 at 295 min, and 228 ± 28 at 300 min. The mean (±SE) insulin values (μU/ml) during the steady state were 30 ± 7 at 180 min, 28 ± 5 at 280 min, 27 ± 5 at 285 min, 27 ± 5 at 290 min, 30 ± 7 at 295 min, and 31 ± 9 at 300 min. The basal insulin value was 7 ± 2 μU/ml. Thus, substantial hyperglycemia was achieved with a minimal elevation of the insulin level. Three of the eight subjects who received this infusion had 3 h and 5 insulin levels of less than 15 μU/ml. The mean (±SE) basal and steady state glucose and insulin values during both infusion protocols are presented in Figure 1.

Insulin-binding studies in vivo. Cells were prepared for insulin binding studies before and at both 3 h and 5 h of each infusion protocol; the results are presented in Table 1. As

FIGURE 1. Mean ± SE plasma glucose and insulin values at 3 h and 5 h of either the hyperinsulinemic infusion (middle panels) or the hyperglycemic infusion (right hand panels). Basal glucose and insulin values are given in the left hand panels: Since the mean fasting plasma glucose and insulin levels were the same for each group, the data have been combined.

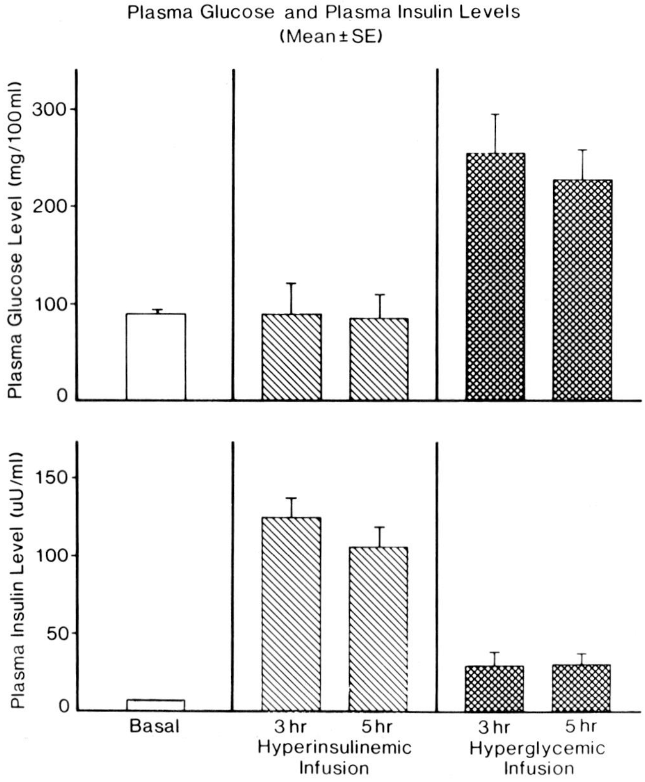

TABLE 1
Percent red cell insulin binding at tracer concentrations (3.5×10^9 erythrocytes)

Subject	Basal	3 Hours	5 Hours
Hyperinsulinemic Study			
1	8.93	8.67	4.77
2	6.24	5.73	3.83
3	6.62	7.19	6.11
4	5.62	5.00	4.09
5	5.49	5.62	2.54
6	4.80	4.23	2.92
Mean ± SE	6.3 ± 0.6	6.1 ± 0.6	4.0 ± 0.5
		NS	P < 0.005
Hyperglycemic Study			
1	8.91	9.06	3.81
2	5.06	5.23	2.00
3	7.61	7.13	7.30
4	5.65	5.93	4.42
5	4.90	4.31	2.34
7	6.48	5.17	2.05
8	6.59	6.50	5.61
9	6.00	5.83	5.37
Mean ± SE	6.4 ± 0.5	6.2 ± 0.5	4.1 ± 0.7
		NS	P < 0.005

can be seen, no change in insulin binding to erythrocytes occurred after 3 h of either infusion. On the other hand, a highly significant 36% decrease in the ability of cells to specifically bind tracer concentrations of insulin was observed at 5 h. The magnitude of this change was similar with both infusion protocols as was the level of insulin binding under basal conditions.

To see if this decrease in insulin binding was due to a change in receptor number or affinity, the complete competition curves were analyzed. The data in Figure 2 demonstrate that, after 5 h of either infusion, insulin binding is decreased at the lower insulin concentrations, but the curves converge at the higher insulin levels. This pattern suggests a change in receptor affinity rather than a change in receptor number, and this point is made clearer by analyzing the Scatchard plots[19] of these data. With this method of analysis, the x-intercept represents the number of insulin receptor sites per cell and, as Figure 3 demonstrates, these intercepts are the same for all groups. Calculations reveal that there are ~30 receptor sites per cell under all conditions. Therefore, the decrease in insulin binding induced by either infusion must be the result of a decrease in receptor affinity, and this is confirmed by plotting the data on an average affinity graph (Figure 4), as described by De Meyts and Roth.[20] The average affinity ($\bar{K}$) is decreased by 38% at levels of receptor occupancy less than 50%, supporting the concept that 5 h of either infusion leads to a decrease in receptor affinity with no change in receptor number.

In seven of the eight subjects who received the hyperglycemic infusion and in five of the six subjects who received the hyperinsulinemic infusion, a clear-cut decrease was observed in insulin binding caused by reduced receptor affinity. One subject (no. 3), who received both infusions, did not exhibit any change in the binding curves.

To be certain these changes were not limited to erythrocyte insulin receptors, insulin binding to isolated monocytes

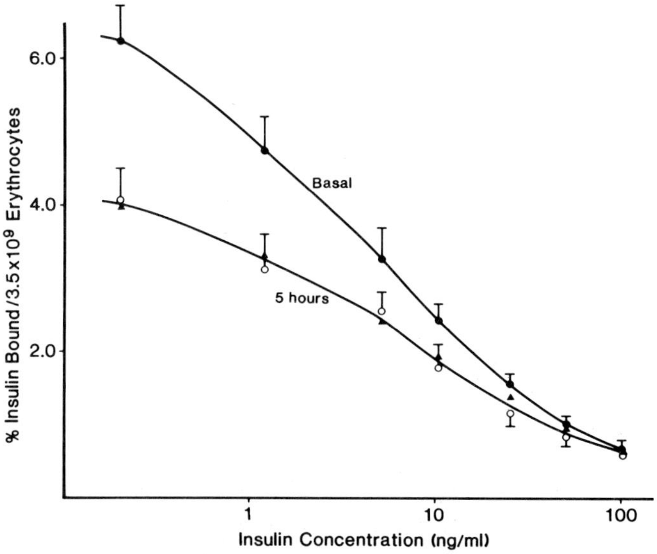

FIGURE 2. Ability of erythrocytes obtained in the basal state (●——●) and after 5 h of either the hyperglycemic (○——○) or hyperinsulinemic (▲——▲) infusion to specifically bind insulin. Cells were incubated for 150 min at 15° with 25 pM (0.15 ng/ml) [^{125}I]insulin plus unlabeled insulin to give the indicated total insulin concentrations. All data are corrected for nonspecific binding by subtracting the amount of radioactivity remaining bound at an insulin concentration of 2 × 10^5 ng/ml from the amount of radioactivity in the cell pellet at all other insulin concentrations. Data represent the mean of 15 studies in the basal group, six studies in the hyperinsulinemic group, and eight studies in the hyperglycemic group. Since the basal values before either the hyperglycemic or hyperinsulinemic infusion were the same, these results have been combined.

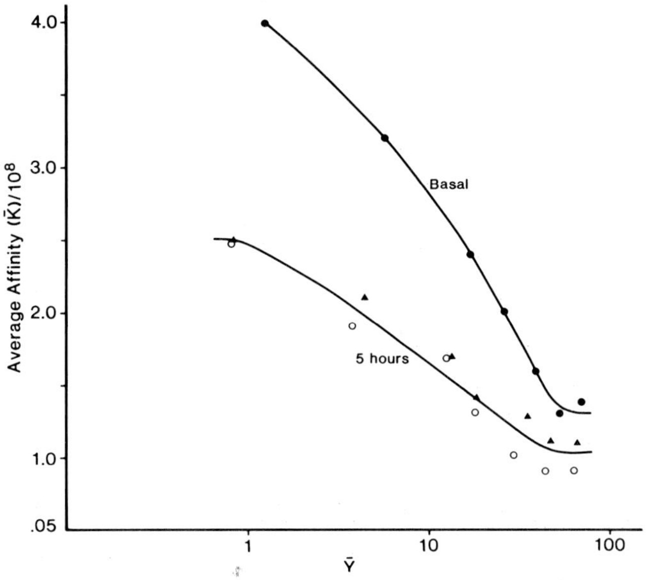

FIGURE 4. Average affinity profile plot of insulin-binding data from Figure 3. Calculations were performed according to the method of De Meyts and Roth.[21] The average affinity ($\bar{K}$) = [(B/F)/R_0-B)] × 10^8 and is plotted as a function of fractional receptor occupancy ($\bar{Y}$) $\bar{Y}$ = the fraction of the total number of available receptors that is occupied, and it is computed by dividing the amount bound (B) by R_0 (the total receptor concentration as calculated from the ascissal intercept of the Scatchard plot). $\bar{Y}$ is expressed as percentage and $\bar{K}$ is expressed as $M^{-1} \times 10^{-8}$.

was determined in one subject during a hyperinsulinemic infusion: The results are presented in Figure 5. After 5 h of the infusion, insulin binding to monocytes was decreased by 37%, and the shapes of these curves are identical to those seen in Figure 2. Scatchard and average affinity analysis demonstrate a decrease in receptor affinity only (data not shown). The basal insulin and glucose values were 7 μU/ml and 82 mg/100 ml, respectively, and were 82 μU/ml and 79 mg/100 ml at 5 h of the infusion. Erythrocyte insulin binding decreased 39% during the hyperinsulinemic infusion in this same subject. Thus, the effects were comparable in both cell types.

To determine if the epinephrine and propranolol in the infusion mixture were responsible for any of the receptor alterations, two subjects who had already demonstrated a decrease in insulin binding in response to the hyperglycemic infusion were given epinephrine (6 μg/min) and propranolol (0.08 mg/min) in normal saline, and insulin binding to erythrocytes was measured at 0 and 5 h of this infusion. A small amount of exogenous insulin (10 mU/min) was administered to prevent a fall in basal insulin values. In these studies, basal glucose and insulin levels were 90 mg/100 ml

FIGURE 3. Scatchard plots of the insulin-binding data of Figure 2. The ratio of the bound to free insulin (B/F) is plotted on the ordinate, and bound insulin is on the abscissa. Symbols are the same as in Figure 2.

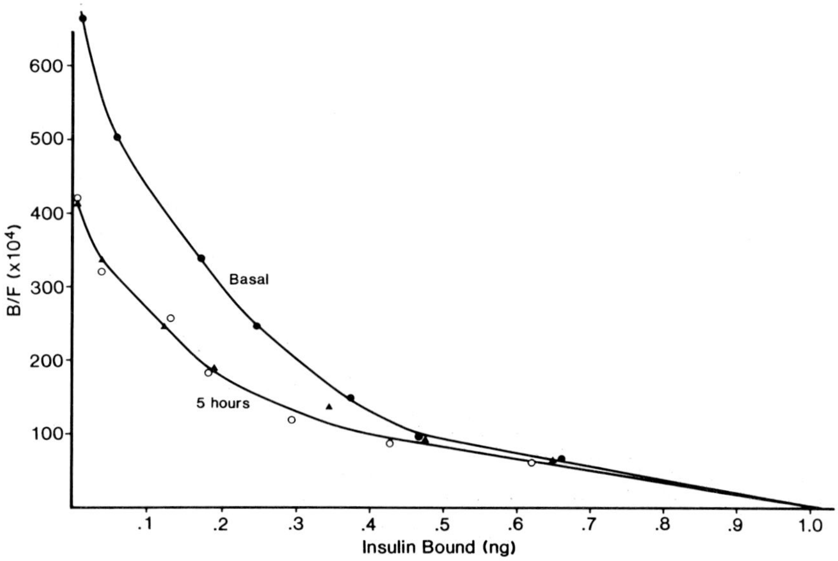

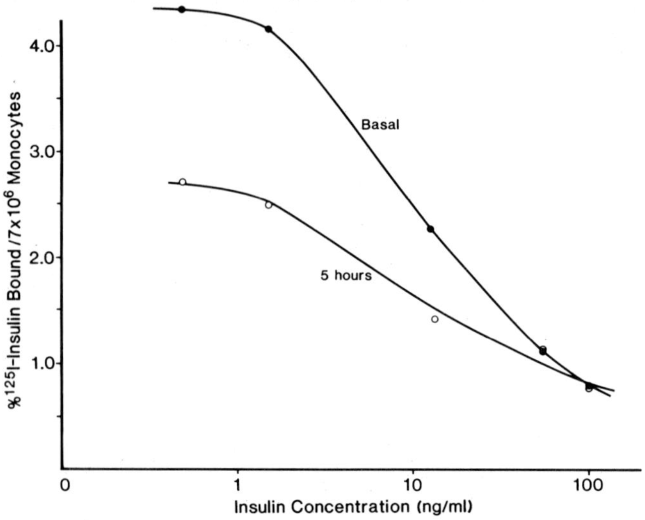

FIGURE 5. Comparison of [^{125}I]insulin binding to isolated, circulating monocytes prepared in the basal state and after 5 h of a hyperglycemic infusion in one patient. Data are corrected for nonspecific binding and are normalized to a monocyte concentration of 7 × 10^6 cells/ml.

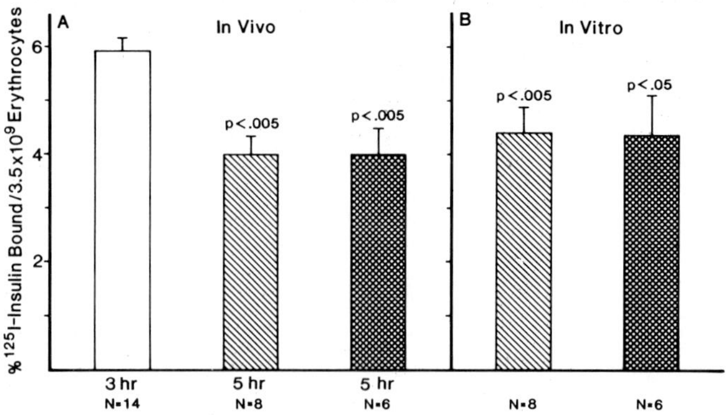

FIGURE 7. Decreased insulin binding to erythrocytes after 5 h of in vivo infusion (A) or 3 h of in vivo infusion followed by 2 h of in vitro incubation (B). Insulin binding to erythrocytes was measured after 3 h of either the hyperglycemic or hyperinsulinemic infusion protocol. At this point, blood was drawn and incubated in vitro for 2 h as whole blood at 4°, and the infusion was continued for another 2 h. Insulin binding was then determined after the 2 h of incubation. Binding was also assessed using cells obtained at 5 h of the infusion study. Insulin binding decreased to a comparable degree during the 2 h in vivo (A) and in vitro (B) with either the hyperglycemic (lined) or hyperinsulinemic (crosshatched) infusion. All data are corrected for nonspecific binding and represent the mean ± SE.

and 10 μU/ml, respectively, and were 85 mg/100 ml and 16 μU/ml at 5 h. As Figure 6 demonstrates, the infusion of epinephrine and propranolol in saline for 5 h had no effect on erythrocyte insulin binding.

Insulin-binding studies in vitro. Thus far, the data show that, after 5 h of either the hyperglycemic or hyperinsulinemic infusion, insulin receptor affinity decreases in vivo. Next, it was of interest to determine whether similar changes could occur in vitro. As seen in Table 1, no change in insulin binding was seen using cells prepared immediately after 3 h of infusion. On the other hand, when blood was obtained at 3 h and was incubated as whole blood in vitro at 4° for 2 h, a striking decline was observed in the amount of insulin that bound to subsequently prepared erythrocytes (Figure 7). As can be seen in Figure 7, the decrease in insulin binding that developed during the 2 h of in vitro incubation was identical to the decline in insulin binding that occurred in vivo between the third and fifth hours of the infusions. Analysis of the complete binding curves demonstrated that this decrease in insulin binding was due to a decrease in receptor affinity, comparable to the in vivo results (Figures 2–4).

FIGURE 6. Ability of erythrocytes to bind insulin before (●) and after (○) 5 h of infusion of epinephrine (6 μg/min), propranolol (0.08 mg/ml), and insulin (10 mU/min). All data are corrected for nonspecific binding and represent the mean of two studies.

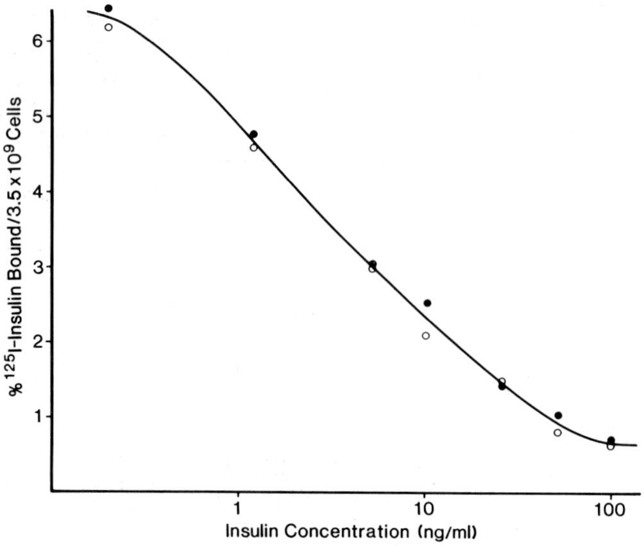

To determine whether this in vitro change in insulin binding was dependent on a plasma factor present during the incubation, blood was obtained at 3 h of the hyperglycemic infusion, plasma was removed from the cell pellet, and the cells were incubated in vitro with buffer at 4° (N = 4). Insulin binding to the erythrocytes prepared at the end of 2 h of incubation in buffer decreased the same as was seen when the in vitro incubation was performed in whole blood (Table 2). Comparable changes occurred when the in vitro incubation was carried out at 22° or 37°. Furthermore, no changes in insulin binding could be induced when cells prepared in the basal state were incubated for 5 h with plasma obtained at the end of 5 h of infusion previously performed in the same subject. Lastly, in vitro changes in insulin binding were not induced when cells prepared in the basal state were incubated for 5 h with 20 mM glucose. Thus, it appears that the signal which triggers the change in receptor affinity is generated during the first 3 h of the infusion and can be subsequently expressed either in vitro or in vivo.

To better characterize the time course of the changes in

TABLE 2
Insulin binding to erythrocytes after in vitro incubation

	% [^{125}I] insulin bound
Cells studied at 3 h of infusion	5.6
Cells obtained at 3 h, incubated in whole blood for 2 h	3.8
Cells obtained at 3 h, incubated in buffer for 2 h	3.7

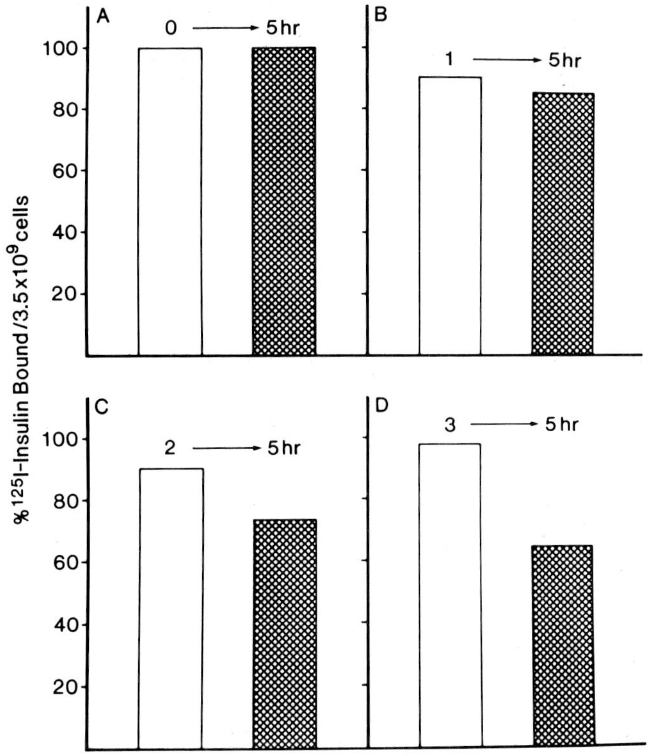

FIGURE 8. Time course of the development of the in vivo decrease in insulin binding to erythrocytes. Cells were obtained at 0 h (A), 1 h (B), 2 h (C), and 3 h (D) of the infusion study and were incubated in vitro at 4° for 5 h, 4h, 3 h, and 2 h, respectively. At this point, cells were prepared and insulin binding was determined. Thus, the total time from the start of the infusion study was 5 h in all cases.

insulin binding seen in Figure 7, erythrocytes were prepared hourly during 5 h of hyperglycemic infusions in two subjects. As can be seen in panel A of Figure 8, cells obtained during the basal state and incubated in vitro for 5 h, failed to show any change in insulin binding. The same is true for cells obtained at 1 h of the infusion and incubated in vitro for 4 h (panel B). When cells were obtained at 2 h of the infusion and incubated in vitro for 3 h (panel C), an 18% decrease in insulin binding was noted. Although a change occurred under these conditions, it was less than the full effect (35% decrease in insulin binding) observed when cells were prepared at 3 h and incubated for 2 h (panel D). Thus, 2 h to 3 h of exposure to the in vivo infusion conditions appears critical to the activation and subsequent expression of the binding changes.

Counterregulatory hormone levels. Table 3 presents the mean (± SE) levels of cortisol and growth hormone at 0 and 5 h of each type of infusion study. Cortisol levels decline slightly during the infusion, and this might be expected on the basis of either normal diurnal variation or the suppressive effects of glucose metabolism. No consistent change in growth hormone levels were observed.

TABLE 3
Serum cortisol and growth hormone levels during the infusion studies
(Mean ± SE)

	Hyperinsulinemic infusion		Hyperglycemic infusion	
	0	5 Hours	0	5 Hours
Growth hormone (ng/ml)	2.1 ± 0.7	1.4 ± 0.2	1.7 ± 0.5	2.7 ± 1.0
Cortisol (μg%)	17.7 ± 2.1	17.3 ± 2.5	19.2 ± 2.6	12.6 ± 0.9

DISCUSSION

Many conditions have been reported in which the binding of insulin to its receptor is altered.[2,3] Although a number of studies have corroborated the concept that insulin may control its receptors—hyperinsulinemia leading to a decrease in receptors, and hypoinsulinemia leading to an increase in receptors[2-4]—the existing evidence suggests that this process may take several days in man.[6,7] Given the short term dynamics and crucial homeostatic importance of the insulin–insulin receptor–glucose metabolism sequence, it seemed reasonable to suspect that a short term regulatory mechanism for alteration in insulin binding might also exist. In support of this hypothesis, there have been recent reports of acute insulin receptor affinity changes associated with fasting,[5,6,8,21] exercise,[22] and oral glucose ingestion.[9] In the present study, we have demonstrated that an acute phase change in insulin binding occurs in response to 5 h of either a hyperglycemic or hyperinsulinemic intravenous infusion.

The feasibility of investigating rapid changes in insulin binding is contingent on access to a readily available tissue source for serial studies. The erythrocyte provides an ideal tool for such purposes, since sufficient numbers of cells can be prepared from 10 ml of whole blood to perform a complete competition study. Although a physiologic role for insulin receptors in these cells has not been described, these receptors are highly specific for insulin, with binding characteristics comparable to insulin receptors of other tissues.[11,12]

Using this approach, we have found that in vivo exposure to either hyperinsulinemia and euglycemia or hyperglycemia and a minimal change of basal insulin levels leads to a striking decrease in insulin binding. Both Scatchard[19] and average affinity analysis[20] demonstrate that this decrease in insulin binding is caused by a decrease in receptor affinity. The time course of these in vivo changes was such that, when cells were prepared after 3 h of either infusion, no alterations in insulin binding were observed; however, after 5 h of infusion, this effect was fully evident. We do not know whether other changes would have occurred had the infusions been carried out for a longer time. The data in Figure 5 show that these events were not limited to erythrocytes, since identical results were obtained when isolated monocytes were studied, consistent with the possibility that these effects are expressed in other tissues.

The results also show that identical changes can occur in vitro if the cells are removed from the in vivo setting. Thus, when cells were obtained after 3 h of either infusion and then incubated in vitro for an additional 2 h, the same change in receptor affinity that would have occurred between the third and fifth hours in vivo could be demonstrated. This is an intriguing observation which indicates that some process is activated which programs the cell to develop the observed changes in receptor affinity in a time-dependent fashion, independent of maintenance of the in vivo environment. When the temporal sequence of these events was studied more carefully, we found that cells obtained at 2 h of the infusion were partially programmed to develop the decrease in insulin binding, whereas after only 1 h of infusion no changes developed in vitro. Whether this implies incremental activation of these processes in all cells or a gradual recruitment of cells into the fully programmed state is unclear. It should be noted that the apparent time sequence of these events is only semiquantitative, since the time required to prepare cells and to measure insulin binding is not considered. However, this latter interval is the same under all conditions.

Whatever the nature of this triggering process, it is most probable that this signal is intrinsic to the cell itself. Thus, when erythrocytes obtained at 3 h of infusion were incubated in vitro in buffer, the decrease in receptor affinity could still develop fully. This suggests that this process is unrelated to plasma factors, at least after 3 h of in vivo exposure. Furthermore, when cells were obtained at basal conditions and were incubated for 5 h with plasma obtained at the end of 5 h of infusion in the same subject (on the previous day) or buffer containing 20mM glucose, no change in insulin binding was noted. Although a highly labile plasma factor could be missed with this approach, this finding is still most consistent with the idea of an intrinsic cellular signal. On balance, the results support the hypothesis that a signal(s) is generated during the first 2 or 3 h of the infusion, which, by that time, is intrinsic to the cells; after 2 or 3 h of a latent period, this signal then leads to a decrease in receptor affinity. Since erythrocytes lack nuclei, do not internalize insulin,[23] and contain sparse intracellular metabolic processes, it is difficult to conceive of a mechanism whereby changes in receptor number occur. However, the alterations we observed were in receptor affinity and are most likely mediated through some direct plasma membrane perturbation in response to the infusion or perhaps via some aspect of the glycolytic pathway.

Clearly the mechanisms underlying this regulatory process remain to be elucidated. Although the magnitude of the prevailing plasma insulin level has been previously shown to have a major influence on insulin receptor number, this effect takes a relatively long time in man,[5–7] and our data suggest that the plasma insulin concentration is not the primary factor producing these acute phase changes. First, comparable changes in receptor affinity were seen with both infusion protocols despite marked differences in insulin levels. Secondly, in the hyperglycemic protocol, plasma insulin levels increased only modestly and not in all subjects. When these subjects are divided into those whose plasma insulin levels during the infusion were ≤ 15 μU/ml (N = 3) and those whose insulin levels were >15 μU/ml (N = 5), the decrease in maximal insulin binding was 43% in the former group and 32% in the latter group. Lastly, during the epinephrine, propranolol, and insulin (10 mU/min) infusions (Figure 6), which did not lead to changes in receptor affinity, the plasma insulin level at 5 h was 16 μU/ml. This is greater than the plasma insulin level at 5 h in the three subjects with the greatest change in receptor affinity during the hyperglycemic infusion. Although these arguments do not eliminate the possibility that the modest increase in plasma insulin levels during the hyperglycemic infusion are critical to the observed changes in receptor affinity, we believe that, on balance, the results make this formulation unlikely. However, further studies will be necessary to completely evaluate this issue.

The evidence also indicates that hyperglycemia per se is not critical to the development of the receptor changes. During the hyperinsulinemic infusions, euglycemia was approximated, and yet the receptor changes were identical to those produced by the hyperglycemic infusion. Furthermore, control studies indicated that 5 h of infusion of epinephrine and propranolol in saline led to no alteration in insulin binding, demonstrating that the epinephrine and propranolol did not induce the observed effects. Lastly, in the hyperinsulinemic infusions, the decrease in insulin binding was not simply a result of the occupancy of receptors in vivo, with subsequent masking of receptors during the in vitro assay, since addition of a large amount of insulin (100 ng/ml) to whole blood did not affect the subsequent determination of insulin binding (data not shown). The reason for this is that the multiple dilutions and washings involved in cell preparation are sufficient to allow all previously bound insulin to dissociate from the cells.

Since plasma glucose or insulin levels per se do not appear to be the primary mediators of these acute phase changes in insulin binding, other factors need to be considered. As one example, growth hormone levels increase in fasting, exercise, and acromegaly, and all these conditions have been associated with an increase in insulin receptor affinity.[5,6,8,22,24] Conversely, carbohydrate loading leads to a decrease in receptor affinity[7,25] and is associated with lower growth hormone levels. These in vivo associations are consistent with the possibility that growth hormone may influence insulin receptor affinity. However, a direct effect of growth hormone on insulin binding has not been demonstrated in vitro,[26] and the data in Table 2 show no consistent change in the level of this hormone during the infusion studies. Obviously, the plasma levels of a variety of other hormones and substrates also change in these conditions, but data to implicate such factors are not yet available. Another possibility is that the signal responsible for these changes in receptor affinity is an intracellular product of cellular metabolism. In this event, since erythrocytes use only a few metabolic pathways, some product of glucose catabolism may be operative. With this formulation, however, it should be noted that insulin has not been shown to exert physiologic effects on erythrocyte metabolism.

The relationship between these acute phase changes in receptor affinity and total glucose homeostasis is unclear. Beck-Nielson and Pedersen have reported a diurnal variation in insulin binding to monocytes, with a decrease during the day associated with food ingestion,[27] although others have not confirmed this observation.[28] Additionally, sustained high carbohydrate feedings will lead to depressed insulin receptor affinity.[7] It is possible that some aspect of the fed state may lead to a fall in receptor affinity, whereas fasting has the opposite effect. The data of Muggeo et al.[9] are a possible exception to this line of reasoning. These workers found an increase in binding affinity after an oral glucose load. However, this effect was only noted 5 h after an oral glucose tolerance test; at this time the body is shifting from the fed to the fasted state and is recovering from the normal insulin-induced hypoglycemia that commonly occurs between 3 h and 5 h of this procedure.

Since insulin binding falls at 5 h of the infusion, one might expect to see some manifestation of decreased insulin sensitivity at this time. Inspection of the steady state plasma glucose levels at 3 h and 5 h of the infusions gives no support to this prediction. If anything, glucose levels are somewhat lower at 5 h compared with at 3 h (Figure 2), suggesting a possible increase in overall insulin effectiveness. Several situations exist in which insulin binding and insulin action can be dissociated (e.g., fasting[8,29] and high carbohydrate feedings[6,25]), and the net effect of any given perturbation on insulin action is a result of changes in postreceptor events as well as changes in insulin binding. In this regard, high carbohydrate ingestion leads to increased insulin effectiveness, and the enhanced activity of such postreceptor steps as the glucose transport system and intracellular metabolism have been demonstrated.[25,30] It is possible that 5 h of glucose plus insulin infusions can lead to some augmentation of these processes.

In summary, we have demonstrated that 5 h of either hyperinsulinemia or hyperglycemia will lead to decreased insulin receptor affinity. This decrease in receptor affinity will develop in vivo or in vitro, and, once a cell is programmed to develop these changes, this will be expressed in the absence of any plasma factors. The exact nature of the signal that mediates these effects remains to be elucidated.

ACKNOWLEDGMENTS

This work was supported in part by funds from the Medical Research Service of Veterans Administration and by grant AM 25242 from the National Institute of Arthritis, Metabolism, and Digestive Diseases of the National Institutes of Health.

Dr. Kolterman was an Associate Investigator with the Veterans' Administration during the course of these studies.

REFERENCES

[1] Roth, J.: Peptide hormone binding to receptors: a review of direct studies in vitro. Metabolism *22*:1059–73, 1973.

[2] Roth, J., Kahn, C. R., Lesniak, M. A., Gorden, P., De Meyts, P., Megyesi, K., Neville, D. M., Jr., Gain, J. R., III, Soll, A. H., Freychet, P., Goldfine, I. D., Bar, R. S., and Archer, J. A.: Receptors for insulin, NSILA-s, and growth hormone: applications to disease states in man. Recent Prog. Horm. Res. *31*:95–126, 1976.

[3] Olefsky, J. M.: The insulin receptor: its role in insulin resistance in obesity and diabetes. (Review.) Diabetes *25*:1154–64, 1976.

[4] Gavin, J. R., III, Roth, J., Neville, D. M., Jr., De Meyts, P., and Buell, D. W.: Insulin-dependent regulation of insulin receptor concentrations: a direct demonstration in cell culture. Proc. Natl. Acad. Sci. USA *71*:84–88, 1974.

[5] Bar, R. S., Gorden, P., Roth, J., Kahn, C. R., and De Meyts, P.: Fluctuations in the affinity and concentration of insulin receptors on circulating monocytes of obese patients: effects of starvation, refeeding, and dieting. J. Clin. Invest. *58*:1123–35, 1976.

[6] Kolterman, O. G., Saekow, M., and Olefsky, J. M.: The effects of acute and chronic starvation on insulin binding to isolated human adipocytes. J. Clin. Endocrinol. Metab. *48*:836–42, 1979.

[7] Kolterman, O. G., Greenfield, M., Reaven, G. M., Saekow, M., and Olefsky, J. M.: Effect of a high carbohydrate diet on insulin binding to adipocytes and in vivo insulin action in man. Diabetes *28*:731–36, 1979.

[8] Olefsky, J. M.: Effect of fasting on insulin binding, glucose transport, and glucose oxidation in isolated rat adipocytes: relationship between insulin receptors and insulin action. J. Clin. Invest. *38*:1450–60, 1976.

[9] Muggeo, M., Bar, R. S., and Roth, J.: Changes in affinity of insulin receptors following oral glucose in normal adults. J. Clin. Endocrinol. Metab. *44*:1206–09, 1977.

[10] Shen, S. W., Reaven, G. M., and Farquhar, J. W.: Comparison of impedance to insulin-mediated glucose uptake in normal subjects and in subjects with latent diabetes. J. Clin. Invest. *49*:2151–60, 1970.

[11] Gambhir, K. K., Archer, J. A., and Canter, L.: Insulin radioreceptor assay for human erythrocytes. Clin. Chem. *23*:1590–95, 1977.

[12] Gambhir, K. K., Archer, J. A., and Bradley, C. J.: Characteristics of human erythrocyte insulin receptors. Diabetes *27*:701–08, 1978.

[13] Wachslight-Rodbard, H., Gross, H. A., Rodbard, D., Ebert, M. H., and Roth, J.: Increased insulin binding to erythrocytes in anorexia nervosa. N. Engl. J. Med. *300*:882–87, 1979.

[14] Freychet, P. J., Roth, J., and Neville, D. M., Jr.: Monoiodoinsulin: demonstration of its biological activity and binding to fat cells and liver membranes. Biochem. Biophys. Res. Commun. *43*:400–08, 1971.

[15] Hunter, W. M., and Greenwood, F. C.: Preparation of iodine-131 labeled human growth hormone of high specific activity. Nature (Lond.) *194*:495–96, 1962.

[16] Olefsky, J. M., and Reaven, G.: The human lymphocyte: a model for the study of insulin-receptor interaction. J. Clin. Endocrinol. Metab. *38*:554–60, 1974.

[17] Gavin, J. R., III, Gorden, P., Roth, J., Archer, J. A., and Buell, D. N.: Characteristics of the human lymphocyte insulin receptor. J. Biol. Chem. *248*:2202–07, 1973.

[18] Desbuquois, B., and Aurbach, G. D.: Use of polyethylene glycol to separate free and antibody-bound peptide hormones in radioimmunoassays. J. Clin. Endocrinol. Metab. *33*:732–38, 1971.

[19] Scatchard, G.: The attraction of proteins for small molecules and ions. Ann. N.Y. Acad. Sci. *51*:660–72, 1949.

[20] De Meyts, P., and Roth, J.: Cooperativity in ligand binding: a new graphic analysis. Biochem. Biophys. Res. Commun. *66*:1118–26, 1975.

[21] Kasuga, M., Akanuma, Y., Iwamoto, Y., and Kosaka, K.: Effects of fasting and refeeding on insulin receptors and glucose metabolism in rat adipocytes. Endocrinology *100*:1384–90, 1977.

[22] Soman, R. V., Koivisto, V. A., Grantham, P., and Felig, P.: Increased insulin binding to monocytes after acute exercise in normal man. J. Clin. Endocrinol. Metab. *47*:216–19, 1978.

[23] Marshall, S., and Olefsky, J. M.: Effects of lysosomotropic agents on insulin interactions with adipocytes: evidence for a lysosomal pathway for insulin processing and degradation. J. Biol. Chem. In press, 1979.

[24] Muggeo, M., Bar, R. S., Roth, J., Kahn, C. R., and Gorden, P.: The insulin resistance of acromegaly: evidence for two alterations in the insulin receptor on circulating monocytes. J. Clin. Endocrinol. Metab. *48*:17–25, 1979.

[25] Olefsky, J. M., and Saekow, M.: The effects of dietary carbohydrate content on insulin binding and glucose metabolism by isolated rat adipocytes. Endocrinology *103*:2252–63, 1978.

[26] Olefsky, J. M., and Kobayashi, M.: Mechanisms of the fasting-induced increase in insulin binding to rat adipocytes. J. Clin. Invest. *61*:329–38, 1978.

[27] Beck-Nielsen, H., and Pedersen, O.: Diurnal variations in insulin binding to human monocytes. J. Clin. Endocrinol. Metab. *47*:385–90, 1978.

[28] De Pirro, R., Bertoli, A., Greco, A. V., Gelli, A. S., and Lauro, R.: The effect of food intake on insulin receptor in man. Acta Endocrinol. (Copenh.) In press, 1979.

[29] De Fronzo, R. A., Soman, V., Sherwin, R., Hendler, R., and Felig, P.: Insulin binding to monocytes and insulin action in human obesity: starvation and refeeding. J. Clin. Invest. *62*:204–13, 1978.

[30] Ip, C., Tepperman, H. M., Holohan, P., and Tepperman, J.: Insulin binding and insulin response to adipocytes from rats adapted to fat feeding. J. Lipid Res. *17*:588–99, 1976.

Inhibition of Gastric Inhibitory Polypeptide (GIP) Release by Insulin and Glucose in Juvenile Diabetes

W. CREUTZFELDT, M. TALAULICAR, R. EBERT, AND B. WILLMS

SUMMARY

The effect of glucose and insulin on fat- and glucose-induced gastric inhibitory polypeptide (GIP) release has been studied in insulin-dependent juvenile-type diabetics. Blood glucose and serum immunoreactive GIP (IR-GIP) were measured after an oral load of 100 g glucose or 100 g fat was given and during an infusion of one of the following: saline, glucose, glucose plus insulin, or insulin. The infusion of insulin alone (in the presence of elevated glucose levels) or together with glucose significantly suppressed the IR-GIP rise after fat ingestion, but it did not alter the GIP response to oral glucose. Intravenous infusion of glucose had a slight but significant inhibitory effect on fat-stimulated increase of IR-GIP, which cannot be related to endogenous insulin release in these insulin-deficient diabetics. It is suggested that an insulin-mediated increase of glucose utilization in the GIP cell interferes only with increased GIP secretion stimulated by the utilization of fatty acids but not of glucose. This could explain the existence of a negative feedback control between insulin and GIP secretion for fat but not for glucose-induced GIP release. DIABETES 29:140–145, February 1980.

Gastric inhibitory polypeptide (GIP)[1] is a potent insulin releaser in the presence of hyperglycemia.[2–4] GIP is released by ingestion of glucose,[1,5,6] fat,[1,6,7] or amino acids.[8] The GIP response to fat ingestion is diminished during an intravenous (i.v.)[6,9,10] or oral[11] glucose load or exogenous insulin injection.[1] Therefore, a feedback regulation between GIP and insulin has been postulated. However, the effects of glucose and insulin cannot be differentiated in normal subjects, since glucose results in an increased secretion of endogenous insulin. Furthermore, it has not been decided whether this feedback control is operating during ingestion of all nutrients or only during fat-induced GIP release. Therefore, the effect of glucose and exogenous insulin on GIP secretion stimulated by an oral load of glucose or triglyceride was studied in insulin-dependent juvenile-type diabetics who did not secrete endogenous insulin. Some of the results have been published in abstract form.[12]

From the Division of Gastroenterology and Metabolism, Department of Medicine, University of Göttingen, and the Fachklinik für Diabetes und Stoffwechselkrankheiten, Bad Lauterberg im Harz, FRG.

Address reprint requests to Dr. Werner Creutzfeldt, Medizinische Universitätsklinik, Robert-Koch-Straße 40, D-3400 Göttingen, FRG.

Received for publication 26 June and in revised form 4 October 1979.

MATERIALS AND METHODS

SUBJECTS

The studies were performed in 40 insulin-dependent diabetics. Some subjects participated in more than one experiment. Informed consent was obtained from all test persons. The clinical characteristics of each group are given in Table 1. The subjects fulfilled the following criteria: good control of diabetes, onset of diabetes before 30 yr of age, insulin treatment for 5 yr or longer, body weight within 10% of the ideal according to the Metropolitan Life Insurance Co. tables,[13] good general health, no clinical or laboratory evidence of abnormal liver or renal function; and no drug treatment except insulin, which was given as an intermediate-acting form before breakfast and before supper. The complete insulin deficiency of the test subjects was confirmed by estimating the C-peptide levels in serum samples drawn before and at 60 and 120 min after i.v. or oral glucose load. Significant levels of C-peptide could not be detected in these patients.

TEST PROCEDURE

All tests were done in the morning after an overnight fast. The evening before, insulin was withheld and only half the amount of carbohydrates for supper and bedtime snack was given. After 3 days, each subject served as his own control. The tests were given in random sequence. After 45 min of rest in the supine position, an indwelling cannula was inserted into an antecubital vein and the catheter was kept patent by slow infusion of saline.

Blood samples were drawn at −30, −15, 0, 15, 30, 45, 60,

TABLE 1
The clinical data of the 40 juvenile diabetics studied

Protocol	N	Sex: Men	Sex: Women	Age (mean ± SEM)	% Ideal body wt (mean ± SEM)	Insulin (U/24 h) (mean ± SEM)
Oral glucose load without and with i.v. insulin infusion	16	11	5	37 ± 3	100 ± 1	52 ± 4
Oral triglyceride load and i.v. glucose infusion without and with i.v. insulin infusion	14	10	4	33 ± 2	99 ± 1	55 ± 4
Oral triglyceride load without and with i.v. glucose infusion	8	4	4	32 ± 3	97 ± 2	57 ± 5
Oral triglyceride load without and with i.v. insulin infusion	7	4	3	31 ± 3	99 ± 1	47 ± 3

90, 120, 150, 180, 210, and 240 min, except for protocol 1, where blood sampling was continued for only 180 min. The samples were immediately placed on ice and centrifuged at 4°C. Five aliquots of each serum sample were frozen and stored at −20°C until assayed.

Oral glucose load was given as 400 ml Dextro O.G.T. (Boehringer Mannheim GmbH), containing 17 g glucose, 13 g maltose, 11 g maltotriose, and 53 g oligosaccharides, corresponding to 100 g rapidly absorbable glucose, within 2 min.

Oral triglyceride load was given as 150 ml of a suspension of corn oil (Lipomul, Upjohn Co., Kalamazoo), corresponding to 100 g triglyceride, within 5 min.

Insulin was given as pork regular insulin (Insulin Novo Actrapid MC, Novo Industrie GmbH, Mainz) by i.v. bolus (0.2 IU/kg body wt) and was followed by continuous i.v. infusion (0.033 IU/kg body wt/h) dissolved in human albumin solution (1 g/100 ml saline 0.154 mol/L) using an automatic perfusion pump (Perfusor, B. Braun Melsungen AG) immediately after ingestion of glucose or fat.

Intravenous glucose (1 mol/L) was given as constant infusion at a rate of 0.7 g glucose/kg body wt/h immediately after ingestion of fat.

Protocols. (1) Oral glucose load without and with i.v. insulin infusion—insulin was administered for 180 min. (2) Oral triglyceride load and intravenous glucose infusion without and with i.v. insulin infusion—insulin was administered for 90 min. (3) Oral triglyceride load without and with i.v. infusion of glucose. (4) Oral triglyceride load without and with i.v. insulin infusion for 90 min.

LABORATORY ANALYSIS

Blood glucose was immediately measured in duplicate by the hexokinase method.[14] Serum IR-GIP was determined within 4 wk after the test by the radioimmunoassay method of Kuzio et al.,[15] modified[11] to improve the sensitivity of the assay. The GIP antiserum used in this study (Gö 5/77/11) did not cross-react with glucagon, VIP, secretin, CCK, gut glucagon I, gastrin, insulin, motilin, or pancreatic polypeptide. Pork GIP was used as standard. The antiserum Gö 5/77/11 stems from a later bleeding of the same rabbit as antiserum Gö 5/76/9, which has been described in detail elsewhere.[27] It measures the same molecular species on gel chromatography of serum as does antiserum VAN 8: the values were about 10% lower than with antiserum VAN 8. The titer of antiserum Gö 5/77/11 was higher than that of Gö 5/76/9. At a final dilution of 1:70,000, about 40% of ^{125}I-GIP was bound. The lower limit of sensitivity varied from 3–5 pg. Since final serum dilution in our assays was 1:10, the actual sensitivity for practical determination varied from 30–50 pg/ml of serum. The interassay variance was 15% to 18% and the intra-assay variance, 6% to 9%.

C-peptide was estimated using a commercial kit produced by Novo Industrie, Copenhagen.[28]

STATISTICAL ANALYSIS

The values are given as means ±SEM. Results were analyzed using Student's *t* test for paired values. Integrated responses for blood glucose and serum IR-GIP were calculated from summation of the products of the mean concentration during each time period and the number of minutes in the time period minus the product of the fasting value and the total number of minutes after a test.[16]

RESULTS

Fasting levels. The fasting blood glucose and serum IR-GIP levels were markedly elevated because all test persons had not received their evening insulin injection on the preceding day. The mean concentration of blood glucose was 291 ± 15 mg/dl and of serum IR-GIP, 611 ± 39 pg/ml (normal controls, 169 ± 20 pg/ml; N = 27). The fasting levels in the four experimental groups did not differ from each other.

Oral glucose load without and with i.v. insulin infusion (Figure 1 and Table 2). After oral glucose, mean blood glucose concentrations increased slowly, reaching a plateau at 90 min and their maximum at 150 min (509 ± 31 mg/dl) and persisting at this level to the end of the test. Serum IR-GIP rose sharply, nearly reaching maximum levels already at 30 min and the peak at 90 min (1742 ± 127 pg/ml). Thereafter, a slight decrease was observed until 180 min (1141 ± 105 pg/ml).

When insulin was infused after the glucose ingestion, blood glucose levels did not rise. However, the increase of the mean levels of serum IR-GIP was similar to that obtained with oral glucose alone. Significant differences were only found at 15 and 180 min, and the integrated IR-GIP response was not significantly different without and with insulin (Table 2).

Oral triglyceride load and i.v. glucose infusion without and with i.v. insulin infusion (Figure 2, Table 2). In the first experiment, the blood glucose concentration rose sharply when glucose was infused, to a peak value of 598 ± 39 mg/dl at 90 min; afterwards, it decreased, to 377 ± 29

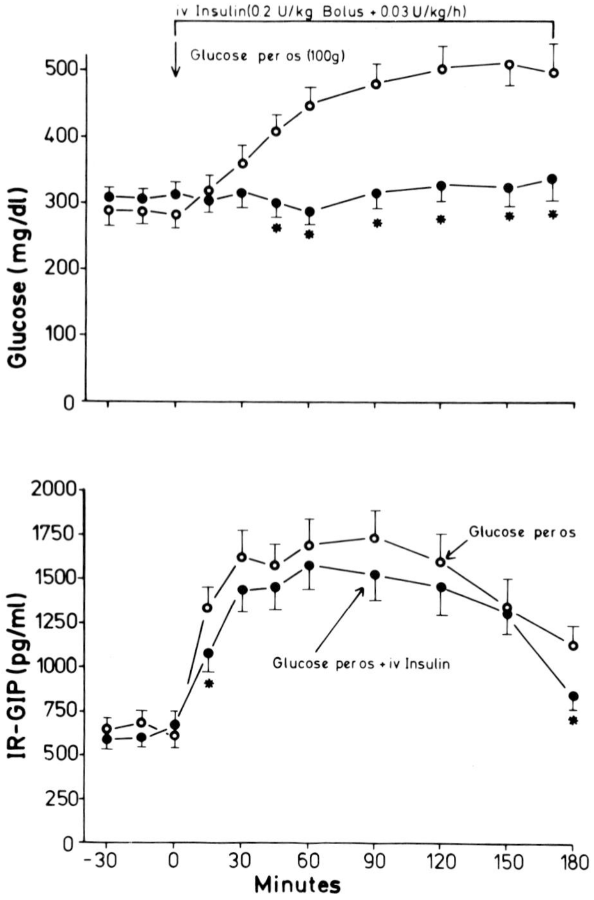

FIGURE 1. Blood glucose and serum IR-GIP levels (mean ± SEM) after oral glucose load without (○) and with (●) i.v. insulin infusion in 16 normal weight subjects with insulin-dependent juvenile-type diabetes. Significant differences are indicated as * = P < 0.02 and less.

mg/dl at 240 min. The serum IR-GIP concentration increased steadily to a peak value of 1588 ± 177 pg/ml at 90 min; then the levels declined gradually—at 210 min, a mean concentration of 926 ± 71 pg/ml was found.

The infusion of insulin resulted in a significantly smaller increase of blood glucose; a small rise at 15 min (384 ± 24 mg/dl) persisted through 90 min; then, the mean values decreased, to 210 ± 25 mg/dl at 240 min. Also the increase of the serum IR-GIP levels was significantly smaller after the insulin infusion. Mean serum IR-GIP values rose to 926 ± 71 pg/ml at 15 min and stayed at this level until 30 min after the end of the insulin infusion. Then a significant increase of IR-GIP occurred in contrast to the decrease at the same time in the study without insulin infusion. This late serum IR-GIP peak attained higher levels than the initial response without insulin. Despite this late rebound-like IR-GIP increase, the 180-min integrated IR-GIP response to oral fat was significantly smaller in the experiment with the combined i.v. infusion of glucose plus insulin than with the infusion of glucose alone (Table 2).

Oral triglyceride load without and with i.v. infusion of glucose (Figure 3, Table 2). Fat ingestion alone did not change blood glucose levels. Mean serum IR-GIP levels reached a peak value of 1935 ± 148 pg/ml at 90 min and

TABLE 2
Integrated response (180 min) of serum levels of IR-GIP and blood glucose (mean ± SEM) to the ingestion of 100 g glucose or 100 g triglyceride with and without an i.v. infusion of glucose and/or insulin

Protocol	N	Serum IR-GIP (ng/ml · 180 min)	Blood glucose (g/dl · 180 min)
1.1—oral glucose load	16	146.5 ± 12.7	29.4 ± 1.3
1.2—oral glucose load with i.v. infusion of insulin		127.2 ± 9.4	1.3 ± 0.1*
2.1—oral triglyceride load and i.v. infusion of glucose	14	150.8 ± 6.9	39.1 ± 2.0
2.2—oral triglyceride load and i.v. infusion of glucose plus insulin		104.1 ± 8.0†	7.8 ± 0.4*
3.1—oral triglyceride load	8	188.6 ± 15.9‡	−4.1 ± 0.3
3.2—oral triglyceride load with i.v. infusion of glucose		164.1 ± 15.5	32.9 ± 1.9*
4.1—oral triglyceride load	7	215.2 ± 16.3§	−3.5 ± 0.4
4.2—oral triglyceride load with i.v. infusion of insulin		95.5 ± 7.8*	−22.6 ± 1.8*

Significant differences: * P < 0.005 or less compared with the respective control experiment; † P < 0.02 compared with the respective control experiment; ‡ P < 0.02 compared with protocol 2.1; § P < 0.001 compared with protocol 2.1.

then slowly decreased to a value of 1367 ± 145 pg/ml at 240 min.

Glucose infusion resulted in an immediate increase of the mean blood glucose concentration and remained between 420 and 500 mg/dl until the end of the infusion. Thereafter, blood glucose decreased to 328 ± 30 mg/dl at 240 min. The mean levels of serum IR-GIP were similar to those obtained with oral triglycerides alone, all values being slightly lower under oral fat and i.v. glucose. However, significant differences were found only at 15, 180, and 210 min, and the integrated 180-min IR-GIP response was not significantly different (Table 2).

Oral triglyceride load without and with i.v. insulin infusion (Figure 4, Table 2). Ingestion of triglycerides alone did not alter blood glucose and resulted in a rapid increase of mean serum IR-GIP levels, reaching a near-maximum at 90 min (2018 ± 204 pg/ml) and a peak value of 2129 ± 278 pg/ml at 180 min. Then it fell slowly to a value of 1768 ± 94 pg/ml at 240 min.

Insulin infusion resulted in a decrease of the blood glucose concentration during the infusion time, without producing hypoglycemia in any patient. At 90 min after termination of the insulin infusion, the blood glucose concentration increased again to a mean value of 173 ± 16 mg/dl at 240 min. The IR-GIP response was significantly lower during the insulin infusion compared with that after fat alone, amounting to only 1006 ± 84 pg/ml at 90 min, i.e., at the end of the insulin infusion. Thereafter, the serum IR-GIP levels started

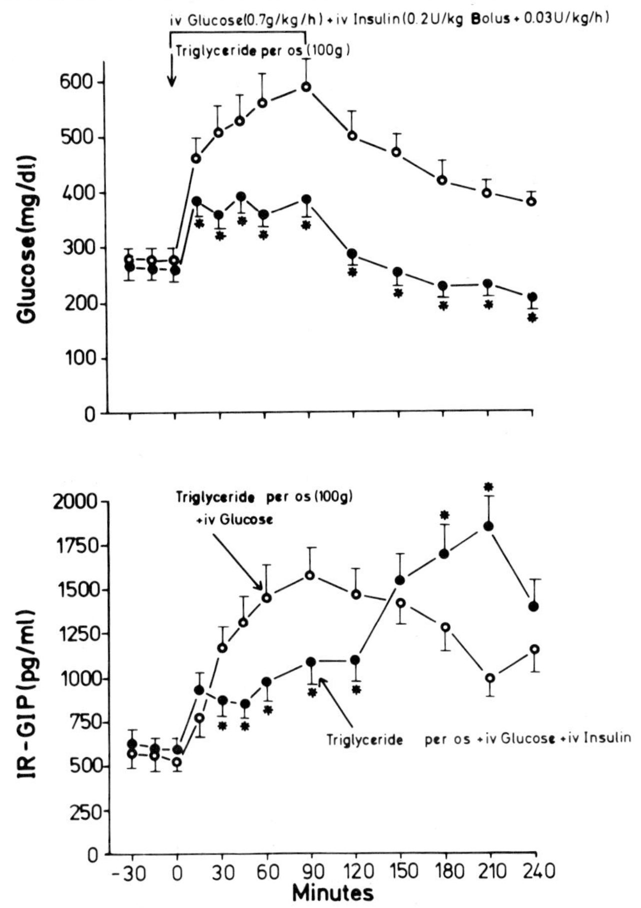

FIGURE 2. Blood glucose and serum IR-GIP levels (mean ± SEM) after oral triglyceride load and i.v. glucose infusion without (○) and with (●) i.v. insulin infusion in 14 normal weight subjects with insulin-dependent juvenile-type diabetes. Significant differences are indicated as * = P < 0.02 and less.

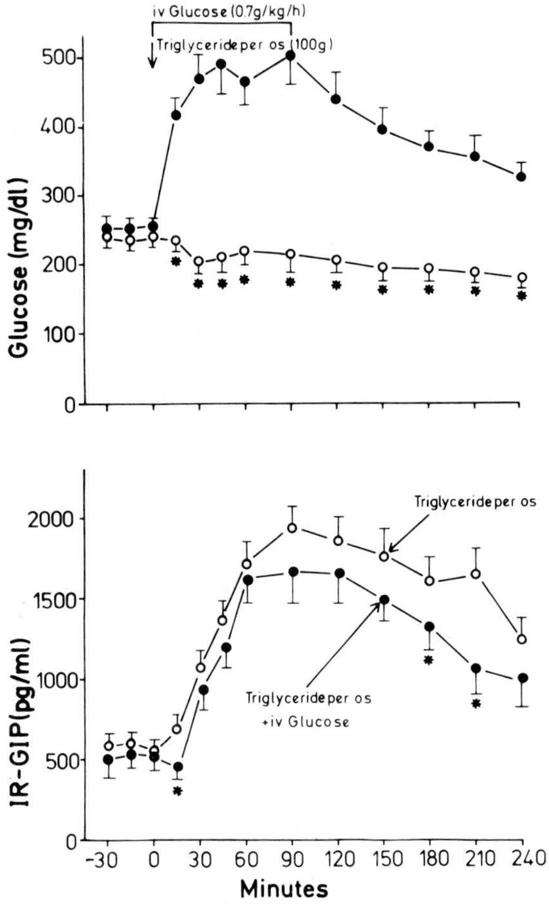

FIGURE 3. Blood glucose and serum IR-GIP levels (mean ± SEM) after oral triglyceride load without (○) and with (●) i.v. infusion of glucose in eight normal weight subjects with insulin-dependent juvenile-type diabetes. Significant differences are indicated as * = P < 0.02 and less.

to rise and were not significantly different with and without insulin at 210 and 240 min. At this time the glucose levels started to rise again.

The integrated 180-min IR-GIP response to fat ingestion was significantly smaller in the experiment with insulin infusion than without it (Table 2).

DISCUSSION

Fasting GIP levels. The fasting serum levels of IR-GIP found in the present study are higher than those obtained in this laboratory in well controlled juvenile diabetics. Elevated serum IR-GIP concentrations have been described in untreated, ketotic, juvenile diabetics; these levels normalized after insulin treatment.[17,18] Botha et al.[19] reported a rise of basal levels of GIP when insulin was withheld and a significant lowering of them by insulin treatment in four subjects with chronic pancreatitis and insulin-dependent diabetes. Therefore, the elevated fasting IR-GIP levels may be the result of withholding the intermediate-acting insulin dose the evening before the test in all subjects, resulting in elevated, fasting blood glucose levels. This suggests that the basal values of GIP are related to the serum insulin or blood glucose levels.

Inhibition of fat-induced GIP secretion by insulin. In these experiments is demonstrated the inhibition of fat-stimulated GIP secretion by exogenous insulin in the presence of moderate hyperglycemia in juvenile diabetics.

A negative feedback control of fat-stimulated GIP in normal subjects has been suggested by Brown et al.[1] These authors demonstrated in a few subjects that insulin, given as a bolus together with an i.v. glucose infusion, diminishes the GIP response to the ingestion of triglycerides. Significantly lower GIP levels following fat ingestion during i.v. glucose infusion[6,9,10] or simultaneous oral glucose administration[11] have been observed than with fat ingestion alone. In these latter experiments, either the increase of insulin levels after i.v. or oral glucose load or the elevated blood glucose concentration itself could have been responsible for the diminished response of the GIP-producing cells to oral fat. The observation of a decreased IR-GIP response to fat during an insulin infusion, leading to increased glucose utilization, as documented by lowering of the elevated blood glucose levels in a situation of complete lack of endogenous insulin, shows that an insulin (not a glucose) effect inhibits fat-stimulated GIP secretion. This effect is present only briefly after cessation of the insulin infusion. Thereafter the IR-GIP levels start to rise in a rebound-like fashion (Figures 2 and 4).

Lack of a suppressive effect of insulin on glucose-induced GIP secretion. A significant attenuation of the response to an oral glucose load by exogenous insulin did not

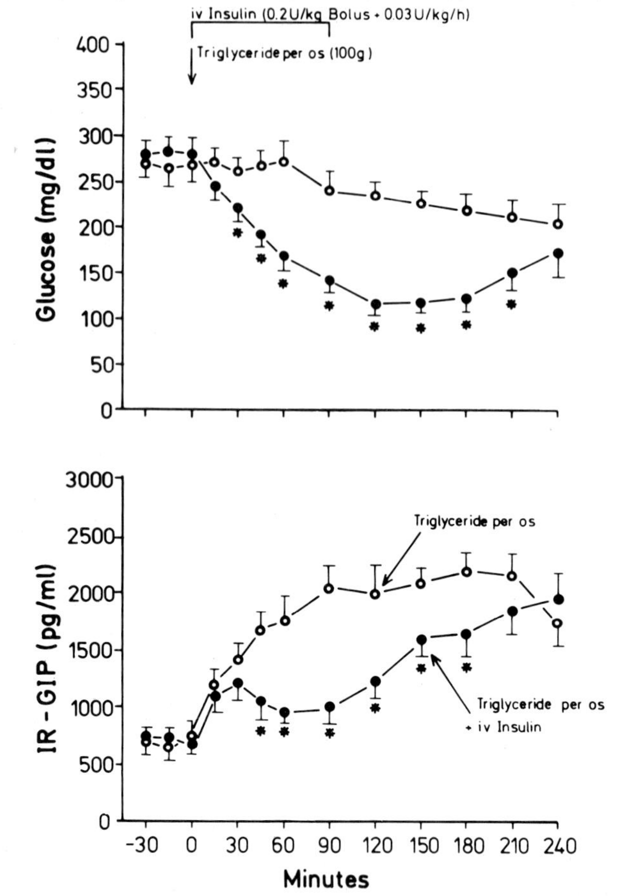

FIGURE 4. Blood glucose and serum IR-GIP levels (mean ± SEM) after oral triglyceride load without (○) and with (●) i.v. insulin infusion in seven normal weight subjects with insulin-dependent juvenile-type diabetes. Significant differences are indicated as * = P < 0.02 and less.

occur in this study, although the insulin dose was effective, as indicated by suppression of the blood glucose increase. Contradictory findings have been reported regarding the question. Andersen et al.[20] examined the effect of oral glucose administration on GIP secretion in normal subjects using the glucose clamp technique. The lowest GIP responses were found during marked hyperglycemia and moderate endogenous hyperinsulinemia; the highest responses occurred in the presence of marked exogenous hyperinsulinemia and moderate hyperglycemia. Thus, hyperinsulinemia did not inhibit glucose-induced GIP secretion. In contrast to these observations in man, Sirinek et al.[21] described a marked blunting of the GIP response to intraduodenal glucose during i.v. insulin infusion in dogs prepared with a Mann-Bollman fistula. Possibly, species differences are responsible for this.

Mechanism of insulin-mediated inhibition of GIP release. One explanation for the different insulin effect on glucose- or fat-induced GIP release could be the possibility that different molecular forms of GIP are released after glucose or fat ingestion.[1] Subsequently, only the secretion of a high molecular weight GIP, released by fat, might be inhibited by insulin. This possibility can be ruled out, because it has been demonstrated that the IR-GIP components secreted after fat and glucose ingestion are identical.[22]

It has been postulated previously that the GIP-producing cells of the gut are equipped with insulin receptors.[11] To explain the different insulin effect on fat- or glucose-induced GIP release, one has to assume that the insulin-induced increase in glucose utilization in the GIP cells interferes only with the GIP release stimulated by the entry and utilization of fatty acids but not of glucose.

Considering GIP as one of the strongest incretin candidates, a feedback loop between GIP and insulin would protect the organism against the hyperinsulinemia following food ingestion.[23] Teleologically, such a safeguard against GIP-mediated insulin hypoglycemia would be important at a time when normoglycemia is present, i.e., after fat but not after glucose ingestion.

Influence of hyperglycemia on fat-induced GIP secretion. Juvenile diabetics, treated for longer than 5 yr with insulin, lack significant amounts of endogenous insulin.[24,25] Therefore, the effect of hyperglycemia, as such, can be studied in these subjects. In one experiment (protocol 3 of Table 2), the marked hyperglycemia produced by i.v. glucose infusion in eight juvenile diabetics lowered the GIP response to fat ingestion (Figure 3). However, the difference of the integrated GIP responses did not attain significance. The capacity of marked hyperglycemia to alter the fat-induced GIP release became obvious if the other experimental groups were evaluated (Table 2): the IR-GIP response to fat ingestion was significantly higher in the two experiments without simultaneous i.v. glucose infusion (protocol 3.1 and 4.1) than with glucose, if compared with a larger group of patients (N = 14, protocol 2.1). This suggests that hyperglycemia, even in the absence of insulin, has a slight suppressive effect on fat-induced GIP release. Conceivably, the metabolic events initiated by fatty acids in the GIP cell do not respond to insulin, as such, but rather to the increased glucose utilization induced by insulin. Since glucose is metabolized by insulin-sensitive tissues to some degree, also in the absence of insulin, provided the glucose levels are markedly elevated,[26] an inhibitory effect of i.v. glucose infusion on fat-induced GIP release could be expected.

ACKNOWLEDGMENTS

We want to thank K. Illmer and U. Kleinschmidt for their expert technical assistance. This work was supported by the Deutsche Forschungsgemeinschaft, Bonn-Bad Godesberg, grant Cr 20/12.

REFERENCES

[1] Brown, J. C., Dryburgh, J. R., Ross, S. A., and Dupré, J.: Identification and actions of gastric inhibitory polypeptide. Recent Prog. Horm. Res. *31*:487–532, 1975.

[2] Dupré, J., Ross, S. A., Watson, D., and Brown, J. C.: Stimulation of insulin secretion by gastric inhibitory polypeptide in man. J. Clin. Endocrinol. Metab. *37*:826–28, 1973.

[3] Pederson, R. A., Schubert, H. E., and Brown, J. C.: Gastric inhibitory polypeptide. Its physiologic release and insulinotropic action in the dog. Diabetes *24*:1050–56, 1975.

[4] Pederson, R. A., and Brown, J. C.: The insulinotropic action of gastric inhibitory polypeptide in the perfused isolated rat pancreas. Endocrinology *99*:780–85, 1976.

[5] Cataland, S., Crockett, S. E., Brown, J. C., and Mazzaferri, E. L.: Gastric inhibitory polypeptide (GIP) stimulation by oral glucose in man. J. Clin. Endocrinol. Metab. *39*:223–28, 1974.

[6] Cleator, J. G. M., and Gourlay, R. H.: Release of immunoreactive gastric inhibitory polypeptide (IR-GIP) by oral ingestion of food substances. Am. J. Surg. *130*:128–35, 1975.

[7] Falko, J. M., Crockett, S. E., Cataland, S., and Mazzaferri, E. L.: Gastric inhibitory polypeptide (GIP) stimulated by fat ingestion in man. J. Clin. Endocrinol. Metab. *41*:260–65, 1975.

[8] Thomas, F. B., Mazzaferri, E., Crockett, S. E., Mekhjiam, H. S., Gruemer, H. D., and Cataland, S.: Stimulation of secretion of gastric inhibitory polypeptide and insulin by intraduodenal amino acid perfusion. Gastroenterology *70*:523–27, 1976.

[9] Crockett, S. E., Cataland, S., Falko, J. M., and Mazzaferri, E. L.: The insulinotropic effect of endogenous gastric inhibotory polypeptide in normal subjects. J. Clin. Endocrinol. Metab. *42*:1098–1103, 1976.

[10] Ebert, R., Frerichs, H., and Creutzfeldt, W.: Impaired feedback control of fat induced gastric inhibitory polypeptide (GIP) secretion by insulin in obesity and glucose intolerance. Eur. J. Clin. Invest. *9*:129–35, 1979.

[11] Creutzfeldt, W., Ebert, R., Willms, B., Frerichs, H., and Brown, J. C.: Gastric inhibitory polypeptide (GIP) and insulin in obesity: increased responses to stimulation and defective feedback control of serum levels. Diabetologia *14*:15–24, 1978.

[12] Ebert, R., Creutzfeldt, W., Talaulicar, M., and Willms, B.: Inhibition of fat, but not glucose induced release of gastric inhibitory polypeptide (GIP), by insulin or glucose. Diabetologia *15*:229, 1978. Abstract.

[13] Wissenschaftliche Tabellen. Documenta Geigy, 7th edit. Stuttgart, Thieme, 1975, p. 701.

[14] Schmidt, F. H.: Die enzymatische Bestimmung von Glucose und Fructose nebeneinander. Klin. Wochenschr. *39*:1244–47, 1961.

[15] Kuzio, M., Dryburgh, J. R., Malloy, K. M., and Brown, J. C.: Radioimmunoassay for gastric inhibitory polypeptide. Gastroenterology *66*:357–64, 1974.

[16] Stern, D. H., and Walsh, J. H.: Gastrin release in postoperative ulcer patients: evidence for release of duodenal gastrin. Gastroenterology *64*:363–69, 1973.

[17] Creutzfeldt, W., and Ebert, R.: Release of gastric inhibitory polypeptide (GIP) to a test meal under normal and pathological conditions in man. *In* Diabetes. Proc. IDF, New Delhi, 1976. Bajaj, J. S., Ed. Amsterdam, Excerpta Medica, 1977, pp. 63–75.

[18] Ebert, R., and Creutzfeldt, W.: Aspects of GIP pathology. *In* Gut Hormones. Bloom, S. R., Ed. Edinburgh-London-New York, Churchill Livingstone, 1978, pp. 294–300.

[19] Botha, J. L., Vinik, A. I., and Child, P. T.: Gastric inhibitory polypeptide in acquired pancreatic diabetes: effects of insulin treatment. J. Clin. Endocrinol. Metab. *47*:543–49, 1978.

[20] Andersen, D. K., Elahi, D., Brown, J. C., Tobin, J. D., and Andres, R.: Oral glucose augmentation of insulin secretion. Interactions of gastric inhibitory polypeptide with ambient glucose and insulin levels. J. Clin. Invest. *62*:152–61, 1978.

[21] Sirinek, K. R., Pace, W. G., Crockett, S. E., O'Dorisio, T. M., Mazzaferri, E. L., and Cataland, S.: Insulin-induced attenuation of glucose-stimulated gastric inhibitory polypeptide secretion. Am. J. Surg. *135*:151–55, 1978.

[22] Finke, U., Ebert, R., and Creutzfeldt, W.: Different forms of immunoreactive gastric inhibitory polypeptide (IR-GIP) in human serum and intestinal mucosa. Diabetologia *15*:232, 1978. Abstract.

[23] Creutzfeldt, W.: The incretin concept today. Diabetologia *16*:75–85, 1979.

[24] Heding, L. G.: Insulin, C-peptide, and proinsulin in nondiabetics and insulin-treated diabetics. Characterization of the proinsulin in insulin-treated diabetes. Diabetes *27* (Suppl. 1):178–83, 1978.

[25] Madsbad, S., Faber, O. K., Binder, C., McNair, P., Christiansen, C., and Transbøl, I.: Prevalence of residual beta-cell function in insulin-dependent diabetics in relation to age at onset and duration of diabetes. Diabetes *27* (Suppl. 1): 262–64, 1978.

[26] Levine, R., and Goldstein, M. S.: On the mechanism of action of insulin. Recent Prog. Horm. Res. *11*:343–75, 1955.

[27] Ebert, R., Illmer, K., and Creutzfeldt, W.: Release of gastric inhibitory polypeptide (GIP) by intraduodenal acidification in rats and humans and abolishment of the incretin effect of acid by GIP-antiserum in rats. Gastroenterology *76*:515–23, 1979.

[28] Heding, L. G.: Radioimmunological determination of human C-peptide in serum. Diabetologia *11*:541–48, 1975.

Streptozotocin-induced Diabetes in Athymic and Conventional BALB/c MICE

G. BEATTIE, R. LANNOM, J. LIPSICK, N. O. KAPLAN, AND A. G. OSLER

SUMMARY

Spleen cells from conventional BALB/c or athymic mice with streptozotocin (SZ)-induced hyperglycemia failed to raise blood sugar levels when injected into athymic or thymus-sufficient recipients. Passive transfer efforts were unsuccessful despite variations in donor-recipient pairs with respect to age, thymic function, or time after sensitization of donor mice. Athymic mice develop hyperglycemia following SZ but fail to mount an inflammatory lymphocyte infiltration. In contrast, the heterozygotes show a marked cellular response, which seems to follow the onset of hyperglycemia. The injection of spleen cells from thymus-sufficient mice to athymic recipients confers immunologic competence on the latter as tested by antibody formation to sheep erythrocytes.
DIABETES 29:146–150, February 1980.

Recently accumulated evidence tends to support the concept of an immunologic component in the pathogenesis of juvenile-onset-type diabetes mellitus (reviewed in ref. 1). Among the pertinent findings in affected patients are the presence of islet-specific immunoglobulins,[2] cytotoxic lymphocytes for cultured insulinoma cells,[3] an increased association of this disease with several HLA types,[4] and the frequency with which this diabetic state is observed in other endocrinopathies that are immunologically mediated.[5,6] Moreover, the induction of diabetes with streptozotocin (SZ) has also been attributed, in part, to immune processes.[7] Important evidence in this regard has been offered by Buschard and co-workers.[8,9] In these studies the hyperglycemic state was produced in athymic or thymus-sufficient mice that received lymphocytes from human diabetics or from SZ-treated mice. The potential significance of these reports prompted attempts in this laboratory to reproduce these results in order to use this animal model for studies of the mechanism(s) involved in the passive transfer of the diabetic state.

From the Departments of Chemistry and Medicine, University of California, San Diego, La Jolla, California 92093.
Received for publication 21 August 1979.

MATERIALS AND METHODS

Mice. Conventional BALB/c mice were purchased from Leonell Strong Foundation (San Diego, California). BALB/c homozygous athymic nu/nu mice originally obtained from Bomholtsgaard (Ry, Denmark) were bred under pathogen-free conditions in the Athymic Mouse Research Center of this laboratory. Mice of both sexes were used. However, in any one experiment either only males or females were used.

Streptozotocin. SZ [2-deoxy-2(3-methyl-3-nitrosoureido)-D-glucopyranose] was obtained through the courtesy of Upjohn (Kalamazoo, Michigan). The drug was dissolved in 0.15 M NaCl adjusted to pH = 4.5 with 0.1 N citric acid and administered intraperitoneally (i.p.) immediately after solubilizing in five daily doses of 60–80 mg/kg. The results of several preliminary experiments clearly indicated that the following minimum dosage schedules yielded consistently reproducible results: male mice (nu/nu or nu/+) 60–70 mg SZ/kg/day; female mice (nu/nu or nu/+) 70–80 mg SZ/kg/day.

Blood glucose determinations. Blood (20 μl) was collected in heparinized capillary tubes from the tail vein and glucose levels estimated as follows. Two aliquots of the heparinized blood (10 μl each) were added to 2.0 ml of distilled water, thus maintaining stable glucose values for at least 2 h at room temperature (R.T.).[10] The diluted blood was deproteinized by rapid mixing with 100 μl of 5% $ZnSO_4$, and 100 μl of 0.3 N NaOH was then added. The contents were mixed and incubated for 5 min before centrifugation for 5 min at 1200 *g*. The following enzyme mixture (100 μl) was then added to 1.0 ml of the supernatant: 1.0 μM each of ATP and NAD plus 3.0 mM $MgSO_4$ plus 50 mM Tris buffer, pH = 7.5; glucose 6-phosphate dehydrogenase (leuconostoc) 1–2 U/ml and hexokinase 0.7 U/ml.

The NADH formed after 15 min at R.T. was estimated at 340 nm and the glucose content of the supernate was calculated with the aid of a standardized calibration curve prepared with glucose. The linear calibration curve thus obtained was prepared for each assay and found to be reproducible to within 10% and linear up to 500 mg/dl. The leuconostoc enzyme was obtained as a gift from Hyland Corporation (Costa Mesa, California) and the hexokinase was purchased from Sigma (St. Louis, Missouri).

This assay for glucose yielded better reproducibility than the methods using glucose oxidase or orthotoluidine. In addition, removal of the proteins from the test samples in the present assay minimized interference from hemoglobin.

Histological studies. For light microscopy, the pancreata of male and female mice were fixed in 10% neutralized formalin and paraffin sections were prepared and stained with hematoxylin and eosin. The immunoperoxidase technique of Sternberger et al.[11] was used to identify beta cells within the pancreatic islets. Formalin-fixed sections were incubated with guinea pig antiserum to bovine insulin (Miles-Yeda lot. no GP-14), diluted 50-fold for 90 min at 22°C. The secondary and tertiary antisera (goat anti-rabbit gamma globulin, cross-reactive with guinea pig IgG, at 1/40 dilution, peroxidase–anti-peroxidase at a dilution of 1/400, Cappel Labs) were each added to the slides and incubated for 30 min at 22°C. Insulin-specific staining was visualized by flooding the slides with 0.02% of 3,3′-diaminobenzidine (Sigma Chemical Co., St. Louis, Missouri) in 0.05 M Tris buffer at pH = 7.6. The slides were kept in the dark for 10 min before adding hydrogen peroxide. The appearance of brown, insulin-containing islets was monitored by light microscopy. To control the specificity of the staining procedure, normal guinea pig serum and guinea pig anti-insulin serum absorbed with insulin replaced the primary anti-bovine insulin preparation.

RESULTS

Before initiating the passive transfer experiments, it was necessary to determine whether the homozygous athymic mice responded to hyperglycemia induction by SZ in a manner comparable to their heterozygous (nu/+) counterparts. Groups of 10 nu/nu and nu/+ BALB/c mice were injected with SZ as indicated above. These mice, as well as 10 controls injected with citrate-NaCl, were bled 15 days after beginning the treatment with SZ. The following nonfasting, mean blood glucose values were obtained: control nu/nu mice, 149 mg/dl ± 15; SZ-treated nu/nu mice, 261 mg/dl ± 44; control nu/+ mice, 118 mg/dl ± 6; SZ-treated nu/+ mice, 225 mg/dl ± 49.

There was no significant difference in the response of the athymic mice compared with the heterozygotes. The results of a typical passive transfer experiment involving 10 donors from each of the above groups are given in Table 1.

The donor spleen cells for the SZ-treated animals were obtained from a group of 10 nu/+ mice whose blood glucose values all exceeded 250 mg/dl. The cells were pooled and checked for viability by trypan blue exclusion (viable cells, 95%). The 10 control mice received an equivalent number of viable spleen cells from donors injected with the citrate-NaCl used as diluent for the SZ.

In view of the failure to observe any hyperglycemia in these recipient mice and in those of replicated experiments, several variables were altered in subsequent passive transfer trials. These included the following:

1. Spleen cell transfers from (a) conventional BALB/c to conventional BALB/c; (b) conventional BALB/c to nu/nu mice; (c) nu/+ to nu/nu; and (d) nu/nu to nu/nu.
2. Athymic recipients of ages 3, 6, 8, and 12 wk were used in different experiments.
3. Donor nu/+ or conventional BALB/c mice were killed on days 7, 9, 10, 12, 13, 14, 16, 17, 19, 20, and 30 after the initial SZ injection and their spleen cells used for passive transfer.
4. Blood glucose values were measured in fasting (14 h) or nonfasting mice.
5. Number of spleen cells transferred ranged from 10^7 to 10×10^7.

In none of these experiments did we succeed in the passive transfer of hyperglycemia.

Since the success of these experiments apparently involved viable and functional T lymphocytes in the spleen cells used for passive transfer, we sought to determine whether these criteria were met. Repeated assays for functional viability clearly indicated that living T-cells were indeed present in recipient mice for at least 2 wk after transfer. This assay simply determined that nu/nu mice, recipients of conventional BALB/c or nu/+ spleen cells, unlike their untreated controls, were able to mount an immune response to the T-dependent antigens in sheep erythrocytes.[12] For this purpose, 1×10^8 SRBC were injected i.p. into the recipient nu/nu mice. Blood taken 6 days after antigen challenge in the recipients showed a variable but unequivocal hemagglutinin response in all nu/nu recipients of nu/+ or BALB/c spleen cells without regard to SZ treatment of the donors. Positive responses were also observed in nu/+ mice, but none in nu/nu animals that were not spleen cell recipients or were recipients of nu/nu spleen cells.

The results of the histological studies can be summarized as follows: The pancreata of the heterozygous mice showed a moderate infiltration of lymphocytes around the islet cells within 10 days after the initial injection of SZ and became more intense with time (Figures 1–4). By day 35 after the

TABLE 1
Fasting blood glucose levels in 3-wk-old nu/nu mice recipients of 1×10^8 spleen cells from SZ-treated nu/+ mice

nu/+ donor mice treated with	No.	Day after spleen cell injection			
		4	7	12	19
SZ	10	118.6 ± 7.6	126.6 ± 13.3	131 ± 13.4	127.5 ± 7.3
Citrate NaCl (pH = 4.5)	5	103.4 ± 17.7	109.6 ± 9.7	135 ± 3.7	127.7 ± 11.1

The mean fasting blood glucose level in 47 untreated mice was 111 ± 30.6.
The blood glucose values are expressed as mg/dl ± 1 SD.

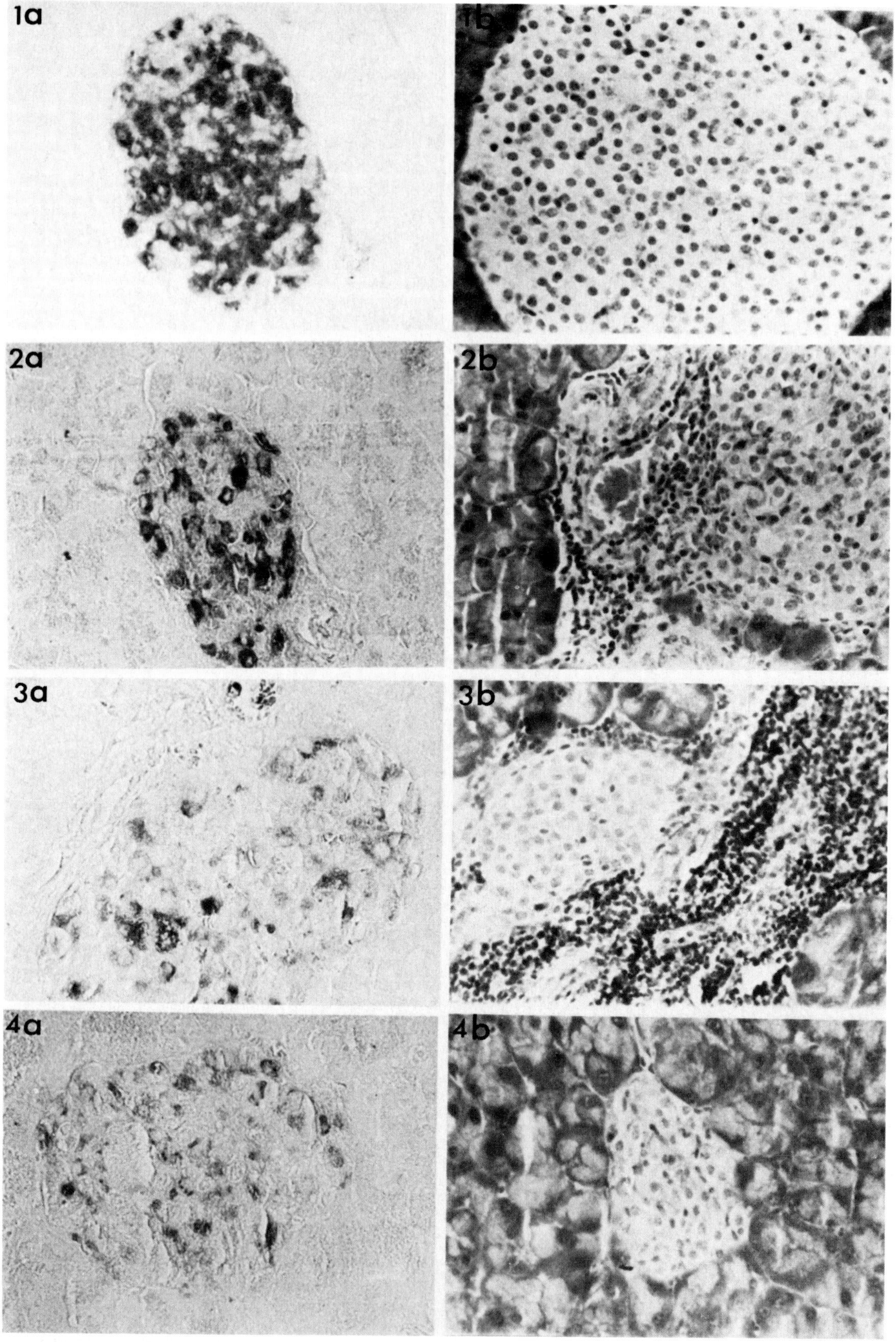

FIGURES 1-8. Histological samples from heterozygote (Figures 1–4) and nude mice (Figures 5–8). Specific immunoperoxidase staining of insulin in beta cells (1a–8a)and hematoxylin and eosin staining of islet cells of pancreas (1b–8b) are shown. Day 0—normal islet of heterozygote (1a,b) and nude (5a,b). Blood glucose 121 mg/dl in heterozygote and 131 mg/dl in nude. Day 10 following first SZ injection (Figures 2 and 6). Moderate infiltration of lymphocytes around the islet cells in heterozygote (2b) but none in nude (6b). Loss of specific insulin staining in both heterozygote

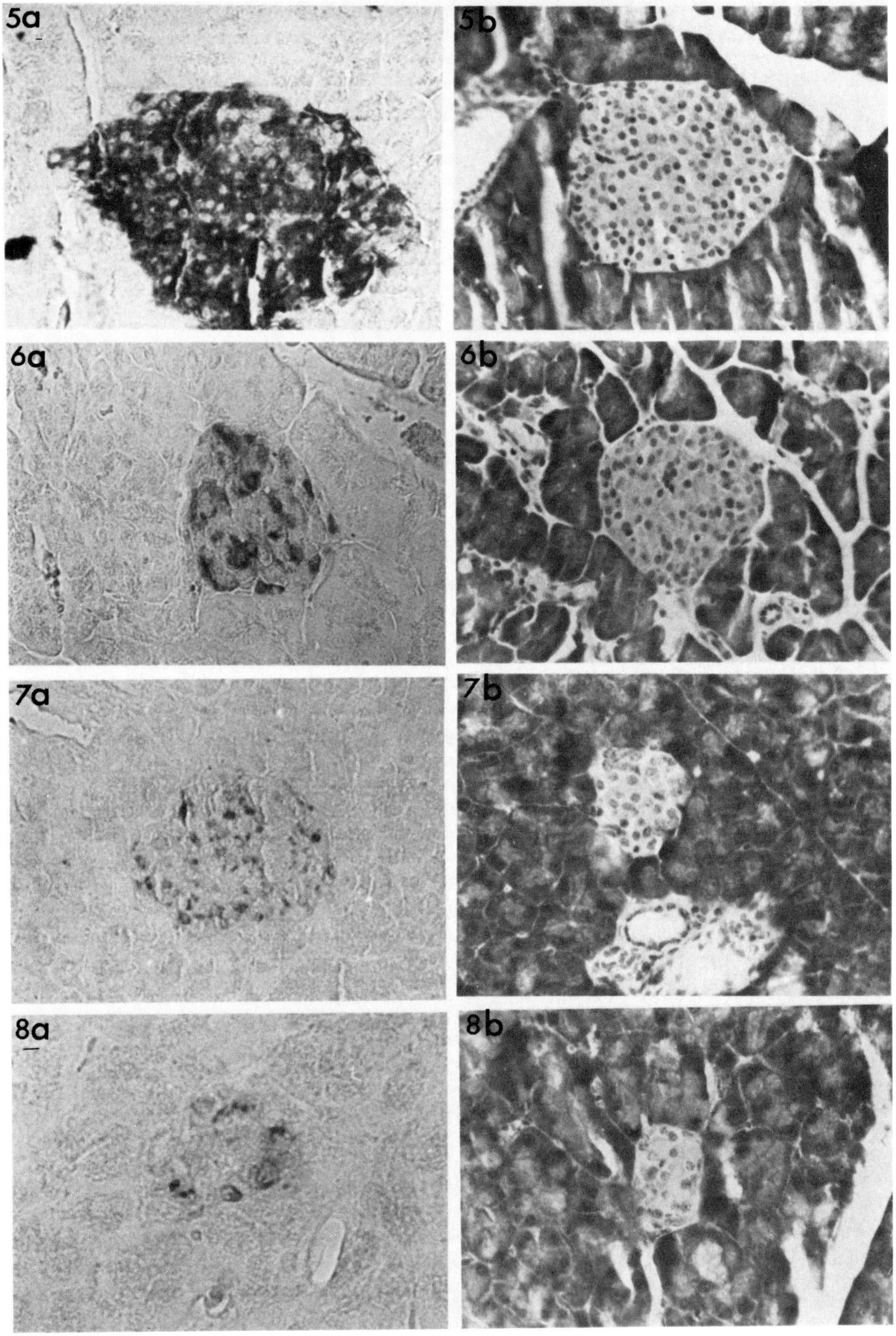

and nude (2a, 6a). Blood glucose 395 mg/dl in heterozygote and 312 mg/dl in nude. Day 17—heavy infiltration of lymphocytes (Figures 3 and 7) around the islets in heterozygote (3b) but still none in the nude (7b). Further decrease in insulin-specific staining in both heterozygote and nude (3a, 7a). Blood glucose 423 mg/dl in heterozygote and 431 mg/dl in nude. Day 35 (Figures 4 and 8) infiltration has receded from heterozygote (4a). Islets of both heterozygote and nude distorted with marked loss of insulin-specific staining (4a,b, 8a,b). Blood glucose >500 mg/dl in heterozygote and nude.

first SZ injection, the islets were markedly diminished in size, their characteristic architecture was distorted, and their content of insulin-containing cells greatly reduced as judged by the immunoperoxidase staining.

The tissues of the athymic mice revealed no lymphocytic invasion during the entire period of observation (Figures 5–8). It is noteworthy, however, that despite the lack of an inflammatory response, the islets appeared, in all apparent respects, similar to those of the heterozygous mice, i.e., there was disruption of the normal topography with concomitant loss of insulin-stained cells. The gradual injury to the beta cells over a period of 35 days after the initial injection of SZ correlated with a gradual rise in blood sugar from 120 to >500 mg/dl in both heterozygous and athymic mice.

DISCUSSION

The negative results obtained in all passive transfer experiments described above are obviously at variance with early reports of passive transfer of SZ-induced diabetes from mouse to mouse.[8] We had hoped that success in these efforts would provide unambiguous evidence for an immunologic role for the hyperglycemic state in this animal model and permit further mechanistic studies. It must also be noted that our attempts at human to mouse transfer were similarly unsuccessful.[13] The recent report that the injection of dead lymphocytes from SZ-induced diabetic mice leads to insulitis and abnormal glucose tolerance in recipient mice[14] suggests the need to consider alternative facets of the mechanism underlying previously successful findings. The possibility of viral transfer merits serious consideration, particularly in view of the reports that SZ-induced insulitis may be associated with the presence of virus particles in mouse pancreatic islet tissues.[7,15] It should be noted that our strain of BALB/c mice require more SZ than those used by Buschard et al.[9] and Like and Rossini[7] to sustain hyperglycemia in all mice. This observation is in agreement with Rossini et al.'s[16] study of variations in strain susceptibility. We also confirmed their finding that male mice are more susceptible to SZ-induced hyperglycemia than are females. At lower doses some, but not all, our experimental mice became hyperglycemic and the dosages we used insured consistently reproducible results. Levels of the α anomer of SZ (the more active form) in our SZ preparations may be lower than that of other investigators, necessitating higher dosages.

Also, electron microscopic observation of damaged beta cells in our mice failed to reveal any signs of induction of type C viruses, as described by Like and Rossini.[7]

The histological studies provide data for an interesting comparison between the responses of the nude and heterozygous mice to injections of SZ. Within 10 days after the first administration of SZ, the islets of the heterozygous animals showed a well-established lymphocytic infiltration, which became more marked with time. By day 35 the islets lost their normal structure as well as their content of insulin-containing cells. The lymphocytic infiltration did not develop in the nude mice, but the destruction of islet cells was of the same intensity as in their heterozygous counterparts. These findings indicate that under the influence of SZ, islet cell damage can proceed in the absence of an inflammatory cell response. Moreover, the hyperglycemia due to SZ is apparent as early as 8 days after the first injection, much before the lymphocytic invasion is most marked. The toxicity of SZ is therefore primary and precedes the cellular immune response. Since several workers have detected an immune response to islet cells in patients with juvenile-onset-type diabetes, it might be anticipated that the peri-islet lymphocytes would be capable of inducing hyperglycemia in recipient, congenic animals. This has not been the case in our studies as noted above. In attempting to reconcile our findings with those of the Danish investigators, we can only surmise that passive transfer of hyperglycemia requires some stimulus in addition to the sensitized lymphocytes. Its identification is obviously of material importance in furthering our understanding of the pathogenesis of the diabetic syndrome.

Our results also suggest that cancer chemotherapeutic drugs such as SZ may act solely by cytotoxic mechanisms without involvement of the immune system.

ACKNOWLEDGMENTS

This work was supported in part by grants from the National Institutes of Health PHS [CA-11683-09, CA-23052-01, GM-07198-05 (J.L.) and AI-15798-01 (A.G.O.)] and the American Cancer Society (BC-60). We thank Sheryl Slimmer and Beverly Kelly for excellent technical assistance.

REFERENCES

[1] Doniach, D., and Buttazzo, G. F.: Autoimmunity and the endocrine pancreas. Pathobiol. Annu. 7:327–46, 1977.

[2] Lendrum, R., Walker, J. G., and Gamble, D. R.: Islet-cell antibodies in juvenile diabetes mellitus of recent onset. Lancet 1:880, 1975.

[3] Huang, S. W., and MacLaren, N. K.: Insulin dependent diabetes: a disease of autoaggression. Science 192:64–66, 1976.

[4] Cudworth, A. G., and Woodrow, J. C.: Genetic susceptibility in diabetes mellitus. Analysis of the HLA associations. Br. Med. J. 2:846, 1976.

[5] Landing, B. H., Pettit, R. N., Wiens, R. L., Knowles, H., and Guest, G. M.: Antithyroid antibody and chronic thyroiditis in diabetes. J. Clin. Endocrinal. Metab. 23:119, 1963.

[6] MacCuish, A. C.: Autoimmunity and diabetes mellitus. Br. J. Clin. Pract. 30:131–35, 1976.

[7] Like, A. A., and Rossini, A. A.: Streptozotocin-induced pancreatic insulitis: new model of diabetes mellitus. Science 193:415–17, 1976.

[8] Buschard, K., and Rygaard, J.: Passive transfer of streptozotocin induced diabetes mellitus with spleen cells. Acta Pathol. Microbiol. Scand [C] 85:469–72, 1977.

[9] Buschard, K., Madsbad, S., and Rygaard, J.: Passive transfer of diabetes mellitus from man to mouse. Lancet 1:908–10, 1978.

[10] Meites, S.: Ultramicro glucose (enzymatic). Standard Methods of Clin. Chem. 5:113–20, 1965.

[11] Sternberger, L. A., Hardy, P. H., Jr., Cuculis, J. J., and Meyer, H. G.: The unlabeled antibody method of immunohistochemistry. Preparation and properties of soluble antigen-antibody complex (horseradish peroxidase-antiperoxidase) and its use in identification of spirochetes. J. Histochem. Cytochem. *18*:315, 1970.

[12] Kindred, B., and Weiler, E.: The response to SRBC by nude mice injected with lymphoid cells other than thymus cell. J. Immunol. 109:382–87, 1972.

[13] Lipsick, J., Beattie, G., Osler, A. G., and Kaplan, N. O.: Passive transfer of lymphocytes from diabetic man to athymic mouse. Lancet *1*:1290–91, 1979.

[14] Kiesel, V., Kolb, H., and Freytag, G.: Streptozotocin-induced diabetes—a transmissible disease. Presented at 14th Annual Meeting of the European Assoc. for the Study of Diabetes, Zagreb, 1978, Vol. 9, pp. 23–30.

[15] Rayfield, E. J., and Seto, Y.: Viruses and the pathogenesis of diabetes mellitus. Diabetes *27*:1126–40, 1978.

[16] Personal communication.

Defective Regulation of Cl^- Permeability in Islets of Diabetic Mice [C57BL/KsJ(db/db)]

OVE BERGLUND AND JANOVE SEHLIN

SUMMARY

Efflux of $^{36}Cl^-$ from prelabeled, collagenase-isolated islets of noninbred ob/ob mice, inbred diabetic [C57BL/KsJ(db/db)] mice, and nondiabetic [C57BL/KsJ(+/+)] mice was studied by nonrecirculating perifusion. Islets of both ob/ob mice and nondiabetic KsJ mice showed similar rates of basal $^{36}Cl^-$ efflux, D-glucose stimulation of the $^{36}Cl^-$ efflux, and net uptake of $^{36}Cl^-$ at apparent isotope equilibrium. The $^{36}Cl^-$ efflux in islets from both young and old KsJ-db/db mice was almost insensitive to the D-glucose concentration. The basal rate of $^{36}Cl^-$ efflux in islets from young and old db/db mice was increased, indicating an abnormally high Cl^- permeability. It is suggested that the defective regulation of the membrane potential in B-cells from [C57BL/KsJ(db/db)] mice may at least partly be caused by a db-mediated defect in the regulation of Cl^- permeability.

DIABETES 29:151–155, February 1980.

Mice with the genetic background C57BL/KsJ and the gene db in homozygous form develop a spontaneous diabetes with deficient insulin release.[1] The B-cells of diabetic KsJ-db/db mice exhibit persistent depolarization with irregular spike activity,[2] suggesting impairment of the transmembrane ionic movements. Studies of islet $^{86}Rb^+$ fluxes indicated that the glucose sensitivity of K^+ permeability found in islets of normal mice was absent in the diabetic ones.[3] This unresponsiveness was found in both young (7 wk) and older diabetic animals, although the young animals still exhibited glucose-stimulated insulin release.[1] It was therefore suggested that disturbed regulation of the K^+ permeability may be an early step in the development of B-cell dysfunction in diabetes.[3] In the present work we have studied $^{36}Cl^-$ fluxes in islets from diabetic and nondiabetic mice, because Cl^- fluxes may be important for the regulation of normal insulin release. Experiments using well-functioning islets from ob/ob mice suggested a metabolism-dependent inward transport of Cl^- against the electrochemical gradient and a glucose-stimulated passive exit.[4] It was suggested that the resulting net efflux of Cl^- may participate in the depolarization of the B-cells, which is connected with secretion. We have now tested whether the abnormal regulation of B-cell electrical activity and the deterioration of insulin release in [C57BL/KsJ(db/db)] islets might at least partly be due to impairment of the Cl^- fluxes in the B-cells.

From the Department of Histology, University of Umeå, S-901 87 Umeå 6, Sweden.
Address reprint requests to Dr. Ove Berglund, Department of Histology, University of Umeå, S-901 87 Umeå, Sweden.
Received for publication 19 June 1979 and in revised form 8 October 1979.

MATERIALS AND METHODS

Chemicals. $Na^{36}Cl$ was obtained from the Radiochemical Centre, Amersham, Bucks., England. Aquasol was from NEN Chemicals GmbH, Frankfurt/Main, Germany; Hyamine from Packard Instrument Co., Inc., Downers Grove, Illinois; Bovine serum albumin, fraction V, from Miles Laboratories Inc., Elkhart, Indiana; collagenase (CLS type IV) from Worthington Biochemical Corp., Freehold, New Jersey; 2-(N-hydroxyethylpiperazine-N′-yl)ethane-sulphonic acid (Hepes) from Sigma Chemical Co., St. Louis, Missouri; D-glucose from BDH Chemicals Ltd., Poole, England; and inorganic salts from E. Merck AG., Darmstadt, Germany. Water was deionized, charcoal-treated, and filtered through a Millipore cartridge before being used.

Animals. Inbred diabetic [C57BL/KsJ(db/db)] mice and normal [C57BL/KsJ(+/+)] mice from a local colony were used. Six young diabetic animals (two males and four females) were taken at the age of 7 ± 1 wk (range), whereas seven older diabetic animals (four males and three females) were selected when they had shown a significant loss of body weight for the preceding 4 wk (weighing at 2-wk intervals). These animals had a mean age of 48 ± 11 wk (range). Young controls had a mean age of 7 ± 2 wk (range for four males and six females). In each experiment islets from two young control animals were pooled. Older controls were 43 ± 5 wk (range for three males and three females). In some experiments 6-mo-old, noninbred obese-hyperglycemic mice (Umeå-ob/ob) of both sexes were used. All animals were fasted for about 18 h before being killed.

Experimental. Pancreatic islets were isolated by collagenase digestion of the pancreas. They were then subjected to a preliminary incubation for 30 min at 37°C in basal medium. The basal medium had the same composition as Krebs-Ringer bicarbonate medium[5] except that the bicarbonate was replaced by 20 mM 2-(N-hydroxyethylpiperazine-N′-yl)ethane-sulphonic acid (Hepes), the gas phase was ambient air, and 0.5% (W/V) bovine serum albumin and 3 mM D-glucose were added. The Cl^- concentration was 139.8 mM. After the preliminary incubation, the islets were labeled for 60 min at 37°C in 200 μl basal medium supplemented with $^{36}Cl^-$ (4.4 GBq/mol). After labeling they were rapidly washed in 10 ml nonradioactive basal medium and transferred to the small chamber (30 μl) in a perifusion apparatus, placed in an incubator maintained at 37°C. One minute after removing the islets from the labeling medium, perifusion was started by pumping (Peristaltic Pump P-3, Pharmacia Fine Chemicals AB, Uppsala, Sweden) nonradioactive basal medium at a flow rate of 1.2 ml/min through the chamber. Fractions of the effluent were collected every 30 s. Change of perifusion medium from one reservoir to the other was made without interrupting the perifusion. Control experiments showed that the time required for the new medium to reach the islets was 140 s. Correction for this lag period has been made in the figures and tables.

In one experiment the perifusion chamber was loaded with $^{36}Cl^-$ (61,570 cpm) without islets. Figure 1 shows efflux of $^{36}Cl^-$ from the islet-free chamber compared with the efflux from chambers loaded with prelabeled islets. The washout of label from the islet-free chamber was rapid; after the first 30 s only 3.1%, and after 2.5 min, less than 0.2% of the initial radioactivity remained. In the islet-containing chambers about 36% of the initial radioactivity remained after 2.5 min. Data on $^{36}Cl^-$ efflux from prelabeled islets after the initial 2.5 min should therefore not be significantly affected by washout of extracellular label, even if this constituted a marked fraction of the total label initially placed in the chamber.

Samples (5 μl) from each radioactive medium were used as external standards for calculation of the specific radioactivity in each experiment. Islets were collected directly after the perifusion was stopped. They were then freeze-dried overnight (−40°C, 0.1 Pa) and weighed on a quartz-fiber balance. Radioactivity in the effluent fractions, the external standards, and the islets was measured in a liquid-scintillation spectrometer using Aquasol as scintillant.

FIGURE 1. Time dependence of $^{36}Cl^-$ efflux from ob/ob islets and the islet-free perifusion chamber. The islets (10–15) were prelabeled for 60 min in basal medium with $^{36}Cl^-$. They were then placed in a small chamber and perifused with nonradioactive basal medium. Mean values for five separate but identical experiments are given (●). In one experiment the islet-free perifusion chamber was labeled by pipetting $^{36}Cl^-$ (61,570 cpm) directly into the chamber and perifusing with water (○). Results are expressed in percent of the initial content of labeled Cl^- in the chamber at start of perifusion and are plotted in a semilogarithmic graph.

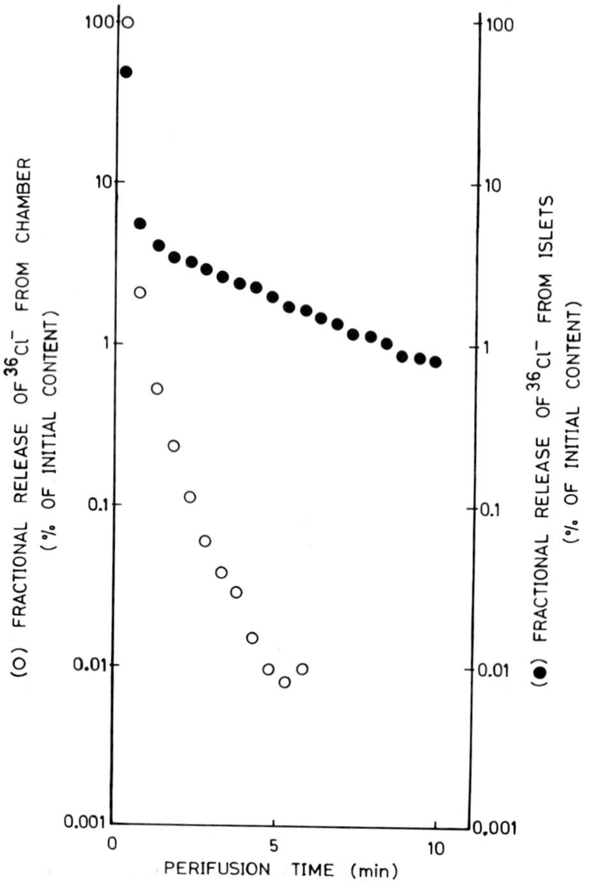

RESULTS

Transmembrane $^{36}Cl^-$ fluxes in islets from ob/ob mice have been described.[4] Those results were obtained by measuring labeled Cl^- retained by the islets after various treatments in static incubations. Figure 1 shows $^{36}Cl^-$ efflux from prelabeled collagenase-isolated ob/ob islets, as measured by perifusing them with nonradioactive basal medium. The $^{36}Cl^-$ efflux approached a first-order function with a rate constant of -0.18 ± 0.03 min^{-1} (N = 5). The rapid efflux during the first minutes probably represented the washout of extracellular label. Figure 2 (left panel) indicates that the rate of

FIGURE 2. The left panel shows effects of changing medium from one reservoir to another when both contain identical basal media. Islets (10–15 in each experiment) from ob/ob mice were prelabeled for 60 min in basal medium with $^{36}Cl^-$. They were then perifused with nonradioactive basal medium for 5 min, at which time the medium was changed to a second reservoir with identical medium. Mean values ± SEM (bars) for three separate but identical experiments are given in a semilogarithmic graph. The right panel shows effects of 20 mM D-glucose on $^{36}Cl^-$ efflux from ob/ob islets. The islets were prelabeled and perifused as in the left panel except that after 5 min, the basal medium was changed to a new medium containing 20 mM D-glucose. Mean values ± SEM (bars) for six separate but identical experiments are given.

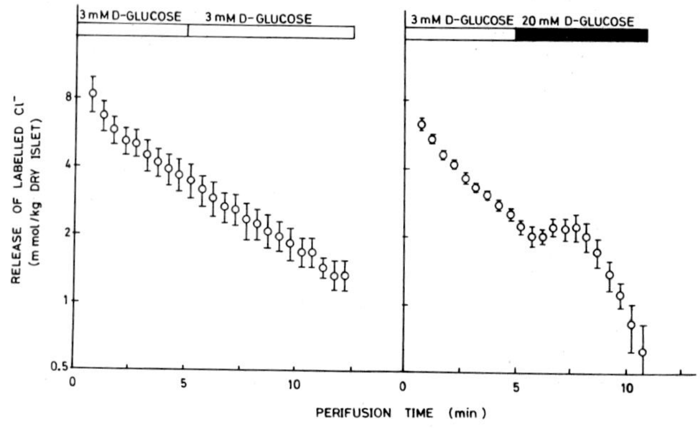

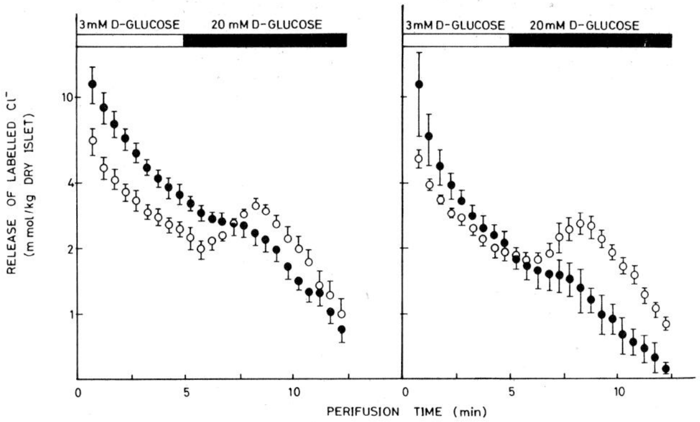

FIGURE 3. Effects of 20 mM D-glucose on $^{36}Cl^-$ efflux from islets of diabetic [C57Bl/KsJ(db/db)] mice and nondiabetic [C57BL/KsJ(+/+)] mice. The islets (50–100 from diabetic mice or 80–140 from nondiabetics) were prelabeled and perifused as in Figure 2. The left panel shows the experiments with young (7 wk) animals and the right with old (>37 wk) animals. In each panel experiments with diabetic mice (●) and nondiabetic mice (○) are plotted together in a semilogarithmic graph. Mean values ± SEM (bars) for six (young diabetics), five (young controls), seven (old diabetics), and six (old controls) separate but identical experiments are given.

$^{36}Cl^-$ efflux from ob/ob islets was not affected by switching between reservoirs containing media of identical composition. The rate constant for efflux with the first medium was -0.16 ± 0.01 min^{-1} and for the second medium -0.13 ± 0.01 min^{-1} (P-value for equality > 0.3). These rate constants comform well with those of −0.12 to −0.14 min^{-1} obtained by static incubations in the same type of medium.[4]

Previous experiments showed that D-glucose increased the rate of $^{36}Cl^-$ efflux from prelabeled hand-dissected ob/ob islets.[4] Figure 2 (right panel) extends this observation to perifused collagenase-isolated ob/ob islets. Shortly after changing medium from 3 to 20 mM D-glucose, a peak of labeled Cl^- in the perifusate appeared, after which a new first-order function with a higher rate constant was approached. Nondiabetic animals with the genetic background C57BL/KsJ showed kinetics and D-glucose sensitivity of islet $^{36}Cl^-$ efflux very similar to those of the ob/ob islets (Figure 3 and Table 1). There was no marked difference between young (7 wk) and older (43 wk) nondiabetic mice.

TABLE 2
Net uptake of labeled Cl^-

Gene type	Age group	Islet content of labeled Cl^- (mmol/kg dry islet)
+/+	Young	88.2 ± 7.1 (5)
db/db	Young	121.2 ± 9.3 (6)*
+/+	Old	79.5 ± 4.0 (6)
db/db	Old	77.6 ± 9.5 (7)
ob/ob		86.9 ± 4.3 (6)

Net uptake of labeled Cl^- in islets from diabetic (db/db) or nondiabetic (+/+) mice was calculated from data in Figures 2 (right panel) and 3. The sum of the islet content of label after perifusion, the pooled label released during min 3–12.5, and the extrapolated release during min −1 to 2.5 was calculated for each experiment. Mean values ± SEM are given for the number of identical but separate experiments given in parentheses.
* $P < 0.025$ for difference between +/+ and db/db (two-tailed Student's *t* test).

In contrast to the results obtained with ob/ob islets and islets from nondiabetic KsJ mice, the $^{36}Cl^-$ efflux from KsJ-db/db islets was only slightly modified by elevating the D-glucose concentration from 3 to 20 mM (Figure 3 and Table 1). D-glucose had no significant effect on the rate constants and only small peaks of radioactivity in the effluent were obtained. Table 1 and Figure 3 also indicate that the rate of basal $^{36}Cl^-$ efflux was higher in islets from diabetic mice as compared with the controls. This was demonstrated by a significantly higher fractional efflux and higher mean values of the rate constants for $^{36}Cl^-$ efflux at 3 mM D-glucose.

From the data in Figures 2 (right panel) and 3 and the radioactivity remaining in the islets after perifusion, the islet cell content of labeled Cl^- after 60 min of labeling (apparent isotope equilibrium[4]) was computed (Table 2). With an intracellular water space of 1.2 L/kg dry islet weight,[6,7] the estimated intracellular concentration of Cl^- was 73.5 mM for islets from young controls, 101.1 mM for young diabetics, 66.3 mM for old controls, 64.6 mM for old diabetics, and 72.3 mM for ob/ob mice. These values correspond well with those previously reported for ob/ob islets.[4] Mice homozygous for the db gene showed no reduction of their content of

TABLE 1
Effect of D-glucose on islet efflux of labeled Cl^-

Gene type	Age group	Characteristics of $^{36}Cl^-$ efflux: Rate constants (min^{-1}): min 3–5 (3 mM glucose)	min 9–12.5 (20 mM glucose)	Effect of glucose	Fractional efflux during min −1 to 5 (3 mM glucose)
+/+	Young	−0.14 ± 0.02	−0.32 ± 0.04	−0.17 ± 0.04†	0.51 ± 0.02
db/db	Young	−0.22 ± 0.03	−0.26 ± 0.03	−0.04 ± 0.05	0.68 ± 0.03‡
+/+	Old	−0.17 ± 0.02	−0.28 ± 0.03	−0.11 ± 0.04*	0.46 ± 0.02
db/db	Old	−0.22 ± 0.03	−0.20 ± 0.03	+0.03 ± 0.06	0.64 ± 0.03§

Effects of D-glucose on $^{36}Cl^-$ efflux from islets of diabetic (db/db) or nondiabetic (+/+) mice. The values were calculated from the data in Figure 3. Rate constants for basal efflux (3 mM D-glucose) were computed for each experiment from the first-order function obtained during min 3–5; rate constants at 20 mM D-glucose were derived from the values on efflux during min 9–12.5. The fractional efflux at 3 mM D-glucose was calculated by extrapolation from the first-order functions obtained for min 3–5. The data represent the fractions of the initial cellular $^{36}Cl^-$, which was released during min −1 to 5. Mean values ± SEM for the number of experiments given in the legend to Figure 3. * $P < 0.05$, † $P < 0.02$ for effect of D-glucose, ‡ $P < 0.005$ (between 0.68 and 0.51), § $P < 0.005$ (between 0.64 and 0.46), two-tailed Student's *t* test.

labeled Cl^- as compared with the controls. On the contrary, islets from 7-wk-old diabetic mice accumulated more $^{36}Cl^-$ than those from the age-matched controls.

DISCUSSION

Previous work with hand-dissected ob/ob mouse islets suggested that Cl^- is nonpassively transported into the B-cells and that D-glucose, by increasing the membrane permeability to Cl^-, may induce an electrogenic efflux of this anion.[4,8] These basic observations are confirmed here using nonrecirculating perifusion of collagenase-isolated islets from ob/ob mice and nondiabetic [C57BL/KsJ(+/+)] mice. Basal rates of $^{36}Cl^-$ efflux and the D-glucose sensitivity of this efflux were very similar for the two types of mice. The estimated intracellular concentration of Cl^- was 65–74 mM, corresponding to a $[Cl^-]_{in}/[Cl^-]_{out}$ ratio of 0.46–0.53. This conforms well with the previously reported values for ob/ob islets.[4] If the intracellular activity coefficient for Cl^- is not markedly different from the extracellular activity coefficient, such a distribution ratio is much too high to fit a passive distribution. According to the Nernst equation, a Cl^- distribution ratio of 0.46–0.53 corresponds to an equilibrium potential (E_{Cl}) of about −17 to −21 mV, which is much lower than the apparent resting membrane potential (E_m) in mouse B-cells.[9,10] The results thus support the idea of a nonpassive influx of Cl^- into the B-cells against its electrochemical gradient. This mechanism seems not to be depressed by inheritance of the db gene, since islets from diabetic KsJ-db/db mice had at least the same capacity as normal islets to keep a high intracellular $^{36}Cl^-$ concentration in spite of the higher rate of basal $^{36}Cl^-$ efflux. In fact, islets from young, only mildly diabetic animals showed even a higher equilibrium concentration of $^{36}Cl^-$ than islets from age-matched controls. This suggests that the inward transport of Cl^- in KsJ-db/db islets may be accelerated.

Inheritance of the db gene in homozygous form on the C57BL/KsJ background seems to induce two major effects on the islet $^{36}Cl^-$ efflux. The basal rate is elevated and the D-glucose-induced acceleration of the efflux is greatly reduced. These differences are probably not due to a marked change of islet cellular composition, because the proportion of B-cells in [C57BL/KsJ (db/db)] islets is only slightly lower than that in islets from the nondiabetic mice.[11] The results may rather demonstrate an inherited basic anomaly of the B-cells of diabetic mice. Since the rate of $^{36}Cl^-$ efflux probably reflects the B-cell permeability to Cl^-,[4] the results suggest, more specifically, that B-cells of the diabetic mice have both an abnormally high basal Cl^- permeability and a disturbed D-glucose control of this permeability. This was seen already in the young, mildly diabetic mice, which may indicate that it represents an early step in the development of diabetes mellitus. The results also support the previous notion that D-glucose-induced Cl^- efflux is not merely the result of insulin release,[4] since this D-glucose effect was almost abolished in islets from young diabetic mice, whereas such islets retain the major part of their insulin-releasing capacity in response to D-glucose.[1]

B-cells of [C57BL/KsJ(db/db)] mice are characterized by an increased rate of basal insulin release and a reduced D-glucose-stimulated release.[1] Microelectrode impalements demonstrate that these cells are constantly depolarized with an irregular spike activity, which is not dependent on D-glucose concentration.[2] It appears likely that the disturbed electric pattern is due to impairment of ionic mechanisms in the B-cells, and that it may partly be explained by an abnormal regulation of the B-cell Cl^- permeability. If, as suggested by the present and previous[4,8] data, Cl^- is nonpassively distributed across the B-cell plasma membrane, the membrane potential may at least partly depend on the Cl^- permeability in such a way that increase of this permeability participates in depolarization of the B-cell membrane. The reduced membrane potential in KsJ-db/db B-cells may, therefore, be partly due to the elevated basal Cl^- permeability indicated in the present results. The low membrane potential may in turn be responsible for the increased basal insulin release, as has been suggested.[2] It also appears likely that a relationship may exist between the unresponsiveness to D-glucose of the membrane potential and the Cl^- permeability. However, the details of such a relationship are not clear at the moment.

We have previously shown that the D-glucose-induced decrease of Rb^+ (K^+-analogue) permeability is virtually abolished in the islets of diabetic mice.[3] Since decrease of K^+ permeability may participate in the depolarization of the B-cells,[12] the idea was forwarded that a defective control of K^+ permeability might explain the abnormal regulation of the membrane potential.[3] Recent data[13] show, furthermore, that KsJ-db/db islets display a decreased rate of basal $^{86}Rb^+$ efflux, which may be partly responsible for the constant depolarization of their B-cells. It thus appears that the operation of two ionic mechanisms (Cl^- and K^+), in which both may have electrogenic properties and participate in the electrical activity of the B-cells, is disturbed by the inheritance of the db gene in homozygous form. With the present state of knowledge, one cannot exclude the possibility that the increased basal B-cell Cl^- permeability might be secondary to depolarization induced by decreased permeability to K^+. On the other hand, it cannot be ruled out that K^+ permeability is voltage dependent and is affected by depolarization due to an increase in Cl^- permeability. However, even if Cl^- and K^+ permeabilities are regulated separately, the co-appearance of the defects might be explained by a defect step in the stimulus-secretion coupling before the ion permeability regulation.

ACKNOWLEDGMENTS

This work was supported by the Swedish Medical Research Council (12x-04756), the Swedish Diabetes Association, the Magnus Bergvall Foundation, the Clas Groschinsky Memorial Foundation, and the Kempe Memorial Foundation.

REFERENCES

1 Berglund, O., Frankel, B. J., and Hellman, B.: Development of the insulin secretory defect in the genetically diabetic (*db/db*) mouse. Acta Endocrinol. (Kbh.) *87*:543–51, 1978.

2 Meissner, H. P., and Schmidt, H.: The electrical activity of pancreatic B-cells of diabetic mice. FEBS Lett. *67*:371–74, 1976.

3 Berglund, O., Sehlin, J., and Täljedal, I.-B.: $^{86}Rb^+$ fluxes and K^+-stimulated nitrophenyl phosphatase activity in the pancreatic islets of genetically diabetic mice (C57BL/KsJ-*db/db*). Diabetologia *15*:191–95, 1978.

4 Sehlin, J.: Interrelationship between chloride fluxes in pancreatic islets and insulin release. Am. J. Physiol. *235*:E501–E508, 1978.

5 DeLuca, H. F., and Cohen, P. P.: Suspending media for animal tissues. *In* Manometric Techniques. Umbreit, W. W., Burris, R. H., and Stauffer, J. F., Eds. Minneapolis, Burgess Publishing Co., 1964, 4th ed., pp. 131–33.

[6] Hellman, B., Sehlin, J., and Täljedal. I.-B.: Transport of α-aminoisobutyric acid in mammalian pancreatic B-cells. Diabetologia *7*:256–65, 1971.

[7] Hellman, B., Sehlin, J., and Täljedal, I.-B.: Evidence for mediated transport of glucose in mammalian pancreatic B-cells. Biochim. Biophys. Acta *241*:147–54, 1971.

[8] Sehlin, J.: Univalent ions in islet cell function. Horm. Metab. Res. In press.

[9] Matthews, E. K., and Sakamoto, Y.: Electrical characteristics of pancreatic islet cells. J. Physiol. (Lond.) *246*:421–37, 1975.

[10] Meissner, H. P.: Electrical characteristics of the beta-cells in pancreatic islets. J. Physiol. (Paris) *72*:757–67, 1976.

[11] Boquist, L., Hellman, B., Lernmark, Å., and Täljedal, I.-B.: Influence of the mutation "diabetes" on insulin release and islet morphology in mice of different genetic backgrounds. J. Cell Biol. *62*:77–89, 1974.

[12] Sehlin, J., and Täljedal, I.-B.: Glucose-induced decrease in Rb^+ permeability in pancreatic B-cells. Nature *253*:635–36, 1975.

[13] Berglund, O., Sehlin, J., and Täljedal, I.-B.: Defective ion transport in diabetic mouse islet cells, Acta Physiol. Scand. *106*:489–90, 1979.

Rapid Publications

Transformation of Glicentin-containing L-Cells into Glucagon-containing Cells by Enzymatic Digestion

MARIELLA RAVAZZOLA AND LELIO ORCI

SUMMARY

Exposure of sections of ileal mucosa to enzymatic digestion with trypsin and carboxypeptidase B reveals a population of immunofluorescent cells after incubation with a specific C-terminally directed antiglucagon serum. These cells, unreactive before enzyme treatment, were identified as L-cells by their immunoreactivity to antiglicentin serum and to cross-reacting (N-terminal) antiglucagon sera. The presence in the L-cells of antigenic sites characteristic of the glucagon-containing cells (A-cells) emphasizes the close relationships between these two cell types, and it further supports the hypothesis of glicentin as a glucagon precursor. DIABETES *29*:156–158, February 1980.

Recently, the immunocytochemistry of the pancreatic and gastric A-cell and of the intestinal L-cell has been extensively investigated in our laboratory.[1–5] Three types of antisera were used: specific (C-terminal) and nonspecific (N-terminal) antiglucagon sera and the R64 antiglicentin serum. This latter, which does not bind glucagon, was raised against the purified gut GLI of 100 amino acids called glicentin.[3,4] Glicentin contains the full amino acid composition and the entire sequence of glucagon[6,7] and, except for the inversion of two amino acids, the same C-terminal peptide as the proglucagon fragment of Tager and Steiner.[8]

With these antisera, it was demonstrated that the A-cell of the endocrine pancreas and of the oxyntic mucosa contains the immunoreactive sites that bind C- and N-terminally directed antiglucagon sera and the glicentin immunoreactive site, whereas the L-cell of the postduodenal mucosa reacts solely with N-terminal antiglucagon and with the antiglicentin sera.[4,5] These immunocytochemical and biochemical studies lead to the following hypothesis: (1) glicentin might be a precursor of glucagon biosynthesis; (2) the A-cells and L-cells differ in the degree to which they shorten a common primary gene product. In the A-cell, the biosynthetic pathway of glucagon would expose the 23–29 immunodeterminant, whereas in the L-cell this sequence would be masked by maintaining the C-terminal prolongation present in the proglucagon fragment. In support of this hypothesis, Tager and Markese[9] have been able to show recently that enzymatic digestion of two large glucagon-like substances isolated from rabbit intestine resulted in tryptic peptides immunologically and electrophoretically indistinguishable from those of glucagon. In this work, we performed similar enzymatic treatment on sections of ileal mucosa, and we provide morphologic evidence that such treatment leads to the unmasking of a C-terminal glucagon immunodeterminant in the L-cells.

From the Institute of Histology and Embryology, University of Geneva Medical School, 1211 Geneva 4, Switzerland.
Received for publication 8 November 1979.

MATERIALS AND METHODS

Segments of dog ileum were fixed in Bouin's fluid, washed overnight in tap water, dehydrated in alcohol, and embedded in paraffin. Fragments of the same tissue were fixed in 4% phosphate-buffered glutaraldehyde, dehydrated, and embedded in Epon 812 without osmification.

The indirect immunofluorescence method of Coons et al.[10] was applied to rehydrated sections of paraffin-embedded ileum and to semithin sections (1 μm thick) pretreated to remove resin.[11]

The following antisera were used: rabbit antiglicentin serum (R64 provided by Dr. A. J. Moody, Novo, Copenhagen), rabbit antiglucagon serum 05Y, which reacts with intestinal L-cells and is considered a cross-reactive antiglucagon serum, and the specific rabbit antiglucagon serum 15K, which only reacts with pancreatic and gastric A-cells.[1] (05Y and 15K antisera were gifts of Dr. R. H. Unger, Dallas, Texas.) Sections were incubated for 2 h at room temperature in a moist chamber with the primary antiserum, repeatedly washed with PBS, and incubated for an additional hour with sheep antirabbit IgG serum coupled to FITC. The sections were then stained with 0.01% Evans blue and were observed in a Leitz Orthoplan fluorescence microscope equipped with a Pleomopak illuminator.

Enzymatic digestion. The enzymatic treatment was performed after rehydration of paraffin-embedded tissue or after resin removal of Epon-embedded sections. The following schedule was used: first, a solution of 0.06% trypsin in 0.5 M Tris buffer was applied to the sections, and they were left at room temperature for 30 min. After rinsing with the same buffer, carboxypeptidase B (20 μg/ml in PBS) was applied for 30 min. The sections were then washed with Tris buffer, transferred to PBS, and finally processed for indirect immunofluorescence.

Controls of the specificity were carried out by absorbing each antiserum with glicentin, glucagon, or the related peptides VIP, GIP, and secretin (100 μg/ml of undiluted antiserum). The antigen-antibody mixture was left for 1 h at room temperature or overnight at 4°C before being applied to the sections.

RESULTS

Sections of paraffin- or Epon-embedded ileal mucosa, incubated with antiglicentin serum or with nonspecific N-terminally directed antiglucagon sera, showed the same population of cells stained by the two antisera. No immunoreactive cells were detected by the specific (C-terminally directed) antiglucagon serum (Figure 1A). If exposure to the specific antiglucagon serum was preceded by enzymatic treatment with trypsin and carboxypeptidase B, however, numerous cells in the glands and in the villi appeared brightly fluorescent (Figure 1B). These glucagon-immunoreactive cells could be easily identified as L-cells on the consecutive semithin section exposed to the antiglicentin serum without enzymatic treatment (compare Figures 1B and 1C). No fluorescent cells were found when the specific antiglucagon serum was preabsorbed with glucagon, whereas glicentin, VIP, GIP, and secretin did not quench the immunofluorescence. Treatment with enzymes did not appreciably alter immunofluorescence after exposure to antiglicentin or N-terminal antiglucagon sera.

DISCUSSION

The data presented in this paper clearly demonstrate that the intestinal L-cell contains antigenic sites that bind a specific antiglucagon serum. In this respect the L-cell does not differ from the glucagon-containing cell (A-cell) of the endocrine pancreas and the oxyntic mucosa, since each cell type contains the immunodeterminants of antiglicentin and of N-terminally and C-terminally directed antiglucagon sera. However, the L-cell does differ from the A-cell in that the C-terminal sequence of glucagon is usually not available for the corresponding antibody. For this reason, the L-cell cannot be identified by specific antiglucagon sera under conditions that allow the same cell to be easily detected by nonspecific antiglucagon sera and by the antiglicentin serum.[4,5]

This is reflected biochemically by the fact that the family of glucagon-like peptides extracted from the intestine, including glicentin, easily reacts with nonspecific antiglucagon sera but not with specific antiglucagon sera.[1,3,9,12] After limited enzymatic digestion, these peptides have been reported to yield tryptic fragments indistinguishable from the 18–29 sequence of glucagon.[7,9]

These findings perfectly correlate with the present morphologic demonstration that a similar enzymatic digestion on fixed tissue provokes the unmasking of antigenic sites

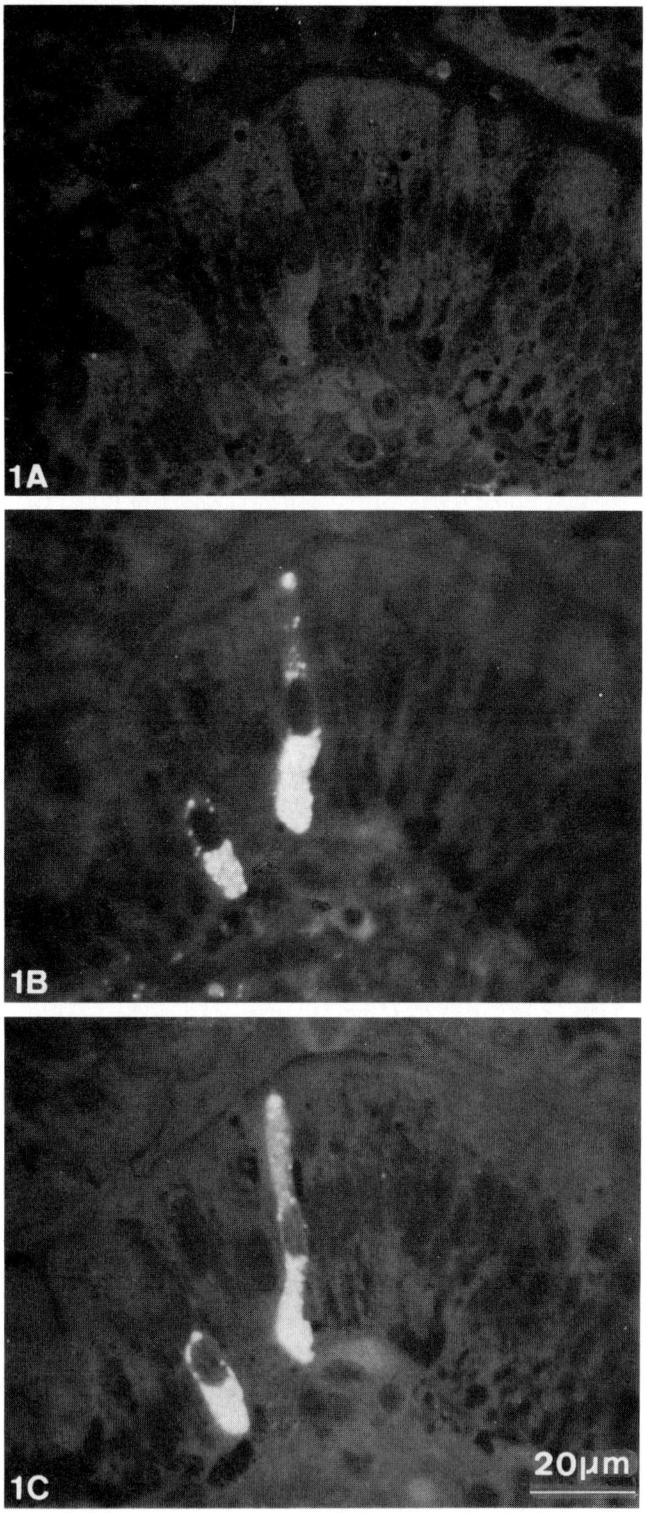

FIGURE 1. Consecutive semithin sections of dog ileum mucosa showing that glucagon C-terminal immunodeterminant is present in the L-cells and can be revealed by enzymatic digestion.

(A) Section not exposed to trypsin and carboxypeptidase B and incubated with specific antiglucagon serum: no fluorescent cells are revealed.

(B) Section exposed to trypsin and carboxypeptidase B and incubated with specific antiglucagon serum: immunofluorescent cells are present.

(C) Section not exposed to trypsin and carboxypeptidase B and incubated with antiglicentin serum: glicentin immunoreactive cells are the same as those positive to glucagon shown in B.

reacting with a specific antiglucagon serum in the same cell that contains glicentin[4,5] or gut GLIs.[13-16]

From this work, it can be concluded that the L-cell shares the same antigenic sites with the glucagon-containing cell (A-cell) and that, in the L-cell, the C-terminal sequence of glucagon is usually concealed but can be exposed by enzymatic digestion. The possible physiologic importance of this finding remains to be established.

ACKNOWLEDGMENTS

This work was supported by the Swiss National Science Foundation (3.120.77).

The skillful assistance of A. M. Lucini, I. Bernard, and M. Sidler is gratefully acknowledged.

REFERENCES

[1] Baetens, D., Rufener, C., Srikant, B. C., Dobbs, R., Unger, R., and Orci, L.: Identification of glucagon-producing cells (A-cells) in dog gastric mucosa. J. Cell Biol. *69*:455–64, 1976.

[2] Moody, A. J., Frandsen, E. K., Jacobsen, H., Sundby, F., and Orci, L.: The structural and immunologic relationship between gut GLIs and glucagon. Metabolism *25* (Suppl. 1):1336–38, 1976.

[3] Moody, A. J., Jacobsen, H., Sundby, F., Frandsen, E. K., Baetens, D., and Orci, L.: Heterogeneity of gut glucagon-like immunoreactivity (GLI). *In* Glucagon: Its Role in Physiology and Clinical Medicine. Foà, P. P., Bajaj, J. S., and Foà, N. L., Eds. Berlin, Springer Verlag, 1977, pp. 129–35.

[4] Ravazzola, M., Siperstein, A., Moody, A. J., Sundby, F., Jacobsen, H., and Orci, L.: Glicentin immunoreactive cells: their relationship with glucagon producing cells. Endocrinology *105*:499–508, 1979.

[5] Ravazzola, M., Siperstein, A., Moody, A. J., Sundby, F., Jacobsen, H., and Orci, L.: Glicentin. A precursor of glucagon? Life Sci. *25*:287–90, 1979.

[6] Jacobsen, H., Demandt, A., Moody, A. J., and Sundby, F.: Sequence analysis of porcine gut GLI-1. Biochim. Biophys. Acta *493*:452–59, 1977.

[7] Holst, J. J., and Hagerup, M.: Evidence that the glicentin molecule contains the entire glucagon sequence. 10th Congr. IDF, Vienna, 1979. Amsterdam, Excerpta Medica. Abstract.

[8] Tager, H. S., and Steiner, D. F.: Isolation of a glucagon-containing peptide: primary structure of a possible fragment of proglucagon. Proc. Natl. Acad. Sci. USA *70*:2321–25, 1973.

[9] Tager, H. S., and Markese, J.: Intestinal and pancreatic glucagon-like peptides. Evidence for higher molecular weight forms. J. Biol. Chem. *254*:2229–33, 1979.

[10] Coons, A. H., Leduc, E. H., and Connolly, J. M.: Studies on antibody production. I. A method for the histochemical demonstration of specific antibody and its application to a study of the hyperimmune rabbit. J. Exp. Med. *102*:49–63, 1955.

[11] Maxwell, M. H.: Two rapid and simple methods used for the removal of resin from 1.0 μm thick epoxy sections. J. Microsc. *112*:253–55, 1978.

[12] Heding, L. G., Frandsen, E. K., and Jacobsen, H.: Structure-function relationship: immunologic. Matabolism *25* (Suppl. 1). 1327–29, 1976.

[13] Polak, J. M., Bloom, S., Coulling, I., and Pearse, A. G. E.: Immunofluorescent localization of enteroglucagon cells in the gastrointestinal tract of the dog. Gut *12*:311–18, 1971.

[14] Larsson, L.-I., Holst, J., Håkanson, R., and Sundler, F.: Distribution and properties of glucagon immunoreactivity in the digestive tract of various mammals: an immunohistochemical and immunochemical study. Histochemistry *44*:281–90, 1975.

[15] Grimelius, L., Capella, C., Buffa, R., Polak, J. M., Pearse, A. G. E., and Solcia, E.: Cytochemical and ultrastructural differentiation of enteroglucagon and pancreatic type glucagon cells of the gastrointestinal tract. Virchows Arch. (Cell Pathol.) *20*:217–28, 1976.

[16] Ito, S., and Kobayashi, S.: Immunocytochemical demonstration of glucagon- and GLI-containing cells in the canine gut and pancreas. Arch. Histol. Jpn. *39*:193–202, 1976.

Direct Evidence for Downregulation of Insulin Receptors by Physiologic Hyperinsulinemia in Man

VIJAY R. SOMAN AND RALPH A. DEFRONZO

SUMMARY

To directly examine whether physiologic hyperinsulinemia regulates insulin receptors in normal man, we studied the effect of insulin infusion (employing the euglycemic insulin clamp technique) on ^{125}I-insulin binding to monocytes. In Study I (9 subjects), when the steady-state plasma insulin concentration was raised to approximately 100 μU/ml, insulin binding to monocytes remained unchanged at 1 h, but decreased significantly by 3 h (20%, $P < 0.01$) and fell further by 5 h (37%, $P < 0.001$) following the insulin infusion. In Study II (5 subjects) increments in plasma insulin concentration to 31 μU/ml resulted in no change in insulin binding at 3 h ($P > 0.5$) but resulted in a significant decrease at 5 h (25%, $P < 0.01$). The plasma glucose concentration was maintained at basal levels in both infusion protocols. The decrease in insulin binding in both studies was due to a decrease in insulin receptor concentration. No significant change in receptor affinity was observed. In a control study (5 subjects) 5 h of saline infusion had no effect on insulin binding to monocytes.

We conclude that in normal humans, increments in the plasma insulin concentration in the physiologic range downregulates the number of insulin receptors in a dose- and time-dependent manner. DIABETES 29:159–163, February 1980.

Recent studies have shown that receptors for various polypeptide hormones are regulated by the ambient hormone concentration.[1–6] While growth hormone,[2] glucagon,[3,4] and TRH[5] have been shown to downregulate their receptors, prolactin[6] is known to induce its own receptor. These observations have important implications in the modulation of hormone action at the cellular level. With respect to the insulin receptor, Gavin et al.[1] were the first to demonstrate that in vitro exposure (5–16 h) of IM–9 lymphocytes in culture to supraphysiologic, but not physiologic, concentrations of insulin resulted in a decrease in the number of insulin receptors. In vivo studies in animals indicate that chronic (14 days) hyperinsulinemia in healthy rats leads to a decrease in insulin binding to adipocytes.[7] Whether physiologic hyperinsulinemia in humans can regulate insulin receptors has not been examined previously. Indirect evidence for such a possibility has been provided by studies from several laboratories, demonstrating an inverse correlation between insulin binding to monocytes and fasting plasma insulin levels under various conditions.[8–13] However, this inverse relationship between insulin binding and insulin concentration does not establish causality and has not been a universal observation.[14,15] Consequently the present study, employing the insulin clamp technique,[11] was undertaken to directly examine in humans the effect of physiologic hyperinsulinemia on insulin binding to monocytes. This technique, by maintaining the glucose concentration constant at the basal level, allows one to assess the effect of insulin on its receptor independent of changes in plasma glucose concentration, and avoids the release of counterregulatory hormones which might of themselves affect insulin binding.[16] Our findings indicate that in healthy humans, short-term physiologic hyperinsulinemia leads to a decrease in insulin binding to monocytes.

From the Department of Internal Medicine, Yale University School of Medicine, New Haven, Connecticut.
Address reprint requests to Vijay R. Soman, Department of Internal Medicine, Yale University School of Medicine, 333 Cedar Street, New Haven, Connecticut 06510.
Received for publication 19 October 1979.

MATERIALS AND METHODS

Subjects and experimental protocol. Nineteen healthy adults (14 males, 5 females, age 30 ± 3 yr) were studied. All subjects were within 10% of their ideal body weight (Metropolitan Life Insurance Tables, 1959) and were consuming a weight-maintaining diet containing at least 200 g of carbohydrate per day for 3 days before the initiation of the study. None of the subjects were consuming any medication. The purpose, nature, and the potential risks of the study were explained to all subjects before obtaining their voluntary consent to participate in the study.

All studies were performed in the postabsorptive state at 8

a.m. after a 12-h overnight fast. Blood samples were obtained for the determination of fasting plasma glucose and insulin levels and for insulin binding to monocytes before the initiation of glucose and insulin infusions (euglycemic insulin clamp technique). The details of the insulin clamp technique have been described previously.[11,17] In Study I (9 subjects) insulin was infused at a rate of 1 mU/kg · min and blood samples were obtained for insulin binding studies at 1 h (N = 4), 3 h (N = 8), and 5 h (N = 5) following insulin infusion. The second study (II) consisted of a separate group of 5 subjects who received an insulin infusion at a rate of 0.25 mU/kg · min. Insulin binding to monocytes was determined at 3 h and 5 h in all 5 subjects. In an additional group of five subjects, insulin binding to monocytes was determined before and after a 5-h saline infusion alone.

Analyses. Plasma glucose was measured by the glucose oxidase method and plasma insulin levels were determined by radioimmunoassay.[18] ^{125}I-insulin binding to monocytes was determined by the previously described techniques.[11,14] In the binding assay, mononuclear cells (3–5 × 10^7 cells/ml) were incubated in tubes containing 0.2 ng/ml of ^{125}I-monoiodoinsulin with and without unlabeled porcine insulin in Hepes buffer, pH 8.0 at 22°C for 3 h. The percentage of monocytes remained unaltered by glucose and insulin infusion (Study I: 16.5 ± 1.5% basal, 16.4 ± 2.0% at 3 h, and 18.0 ± 1.9% at 5 h; Study II: 16.5 ± 1.2% basal, 17.6 ± 1.2% at 3 h, and 15.9 ± 2.0% at 5 h).

Calculations. During insulin clamp studies, the glucose infusion rate and the steady-state plasma glucose and insulin concentrations were determined by calculating the mean of the values observed between various time intervals as shown in Table 1. Insulin binding data were analyzed by the Scatchard analysis[19] and by the average affinity profile plot method of DeMeyts and Roth.[20] Statistical analyses were done by the paired Student's *t* test.[21] All data are presented as mean ± SEM.

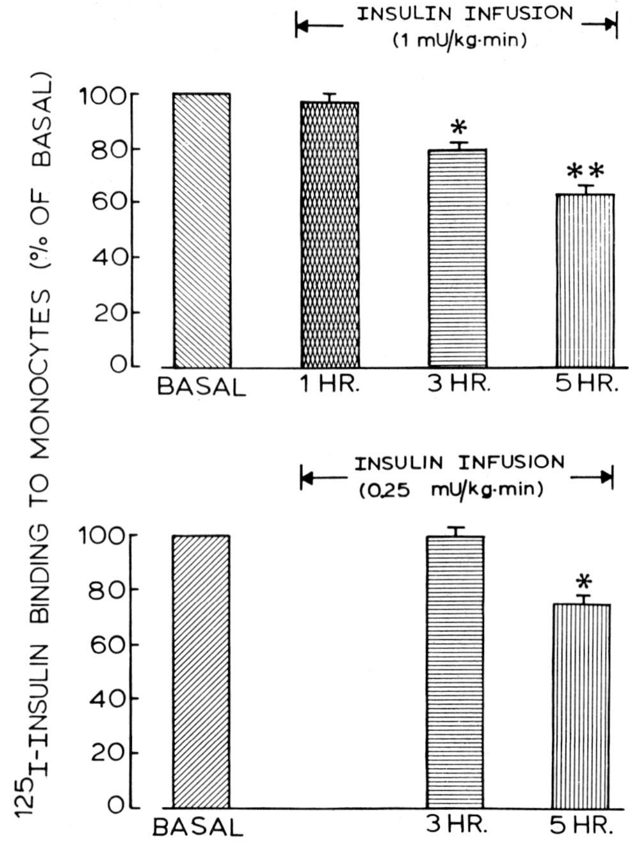

FIGURE 1. Effect of insulin infusion (by euglycemic insulin clamp technique) on ^{125}I-insulin binding to monocytes in 9 healthy subjects. *P < 0.01, **P < 0.001.

RESULTS

Study I. During the 1-mU/kg · min insulin clamp study (Table 1) the steady-state plasma insulin concentration was maintained at 102 ± 6 μU/ml. This represented a mean increase of 89 μU/ml above basal levels. The plasma glucose concentration was maintained close to the basal level with little variation throughout the study period. The glucose infusion rate required to maintain euglycemia during the insulin clamp study rose rapidly during the first hour of study and

TABLE 1
Plasma glucose and insulin levels and glucose infusion rates during euglycemic insulin clamp studies*

	Fasting plasma glucose (mg/dl)	Steady-state plasma glucose** (mg/dl)	C. V. of plasma glucose† (%)	Fasting plasma insulin (μU/ml)	Steady-state plasma insulin** (μU/ml)	C. V. of plasma insulin‡ (%)	Glucose infusion rate during insulin clamp (mg/kg/min) Time (min) 20–60	60–120	120–180	180–240	240–300
Study I (Insulin infusion rate: 1 mU/kg/min) (N = 9)	90 ± 2	91 ± 2	3.4 ± 0.1	13 ± 2	102 ± 6	8.5 ± 0.8	6.0 ± 0.8	7.5 ± 0.7	8.4 ± 0.6	8.9 ± 0.8§	9.3 ± 0.8§
Study II (Insulin infusion rate: 0.25 mU/kg/min) (N = 5)	92 ± 2	91 ± 2	2.3 ± 0.2	16 ± 2	31 ± 2	1.3 ± 0.2	2.6 ± 0.5	3.2 ± 0.4	3.5 ± 0.4	4.2 ± 0.5	4.6 ± 0.6

* Data are shown as mean ± SEM.
† Coefficient of variation of steady-state plasma glucose during insulin clamp.
‡ Coefficient of variation of steady-state plasma insulin during insulin clamp.
§ Represents data in 5 subjects.
** Represents mean concentrations between 20 min to the end of insulin clamp.

then tended to plateau. During the last 3 h of study the increase in glucose metabolism was small, averaging 5% per hour.

The total specific binding of ^{125}I-insulin to monocytes (determined at the tracer concentration of insulin) remained unaltered at 1 h after the initiation of insulin infusion (Figure 1 and Table 2). However at 3h, insulin binding fell an average of 20% ($P < 0.01$), and at 5 h it declined further to levels which were 37% ($P < 0.001$) below those observed during the basal preinfusion period (Figure 1 and Table 2). The competition curves of insulin binding to monocytes are shown in Figure 2 (upper panel). At 5 h after the insulin infusion, insulin binding was significantly lower at all insulin concentrations up to 100 ng/ml as compared with the preinfusion study (Figure 2, upper panel). Scatchard analysis of these data revealed that the Scatchard plots were curvilinear and parallel (Figure 2, lower panel). The calculated insulin receptor concentration was about 33% lower at 5 h following insulin infusion (9200 ± 750 sites/monocyte) as compared with the basal period (13,500 ± 1050 sites/monocytes, $P < 0.005$). The average affinity profile plots revealed that both the highest ($\bar{K}e$ 0.39 ± 0.04 nM^{-1} basal and 0.38 ± 0.05 nM^{-1} after infusion, $P > 0.5$) and the lowest ($\bar{K}f$ 0.06 ± 0.01 nM^{-1} before and 0.05 ± 0.01 nM^{-1} after infusion; $P > 0.5$) insulin binding affinity was not significantly altered during the 5 h infusion period. Similarly, at 3 h during insulin clamp, insulin binding affinity was unchanged (not shown), whereas the insulin receptor concentration decreased by 22% (10,480 ± 490 sites/monocyte, $P < 0.01$).

Study II. When insulin was infused at the rate of 0.25 mU/kg · min, the mean steady-state plasma insulin concentration was 31 ± 2 μU/ml (Table 1). This represented an increase of only 15 μU/ml above basal levels. Again, the steady-state plasma glucose concentration was maintained at the basal fasting level throughout the study period.

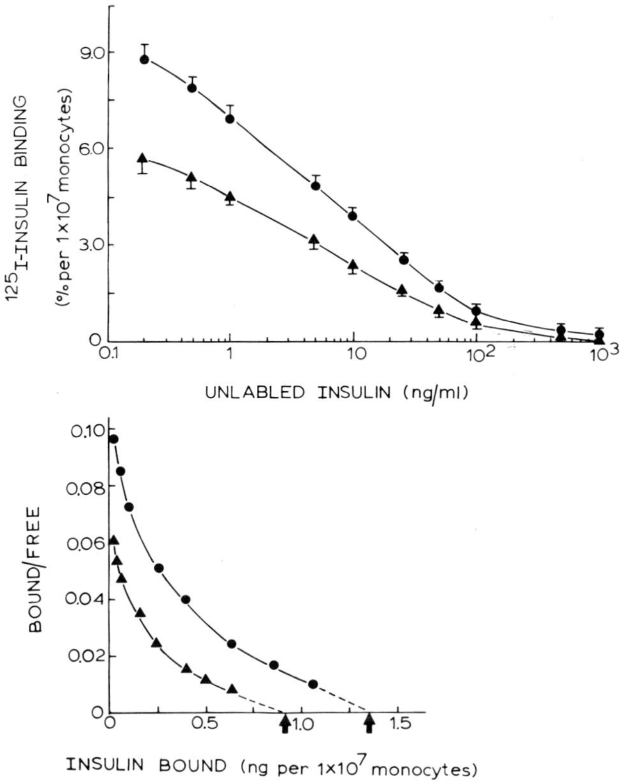

FIGURE 2. Upper panel: Competition curves of ^{125}I-insulin binding to monocytes before (●, N = 9) and 5 h after (▲, N = 5) insulin infusion in healthy subjects. Insulin was infused at a rate of 1 mU/kg/min by the euglycemic insulin clamp technique. Data are corrected for nonspecific binding. Lower panel: Scatchard analysis of insulin binding to monocytes. The Scatchard plots were obtained by analysis of the individual competition curves shown in the upper panel for each of the subjects before (●, N = 9) and 5 h after (▲, N = 5) insulin infusion. The mean values are shown. The intercepts at the abscissa represent the total insulin binding capacity in each group.

As shown in Figure 1 and Table 2, the total specific binding of ^{125}I-insulin to monocytes was unaltered at 3 h after the initiation of insulin infusion, but it fell significantly by 25% ($P < 0.01$) following 5 h of sustained hyperinsulinemia. The decrease in insulin binding observed at 5 h of insulin infusion was demonstrable at all insulin concentrations examined (Figure 3, upper panel). Scatchard analysis (Figure 3, lower panel) of the insulin binding data showed that at 5 h, the number of binding sites/monocyte (9100 ± 680) were 28% lower as compared with the preinfusion, basal period (12,850 ± 760, $P < 0.01$). However, the insulin binding affinity, as revealed by the average affinity profile plots, remained unaltered following insulin infusion ($\bar{K}e$ 0.35 ± 0.05 nM^{-1} before and 0.36 ± 0.04 nM^{-1} at 5 h after infusion, $P > 0.5$).

In five control subjects receiving saline infusion (5 h), ^{125}I-insulin binding to monocytes was similar before (7.5 ± 0.5%) and after saline infusion (7.7 ± 0.6%, P = NS).

Among the fourteen subjects receiving insulin clamp, we observed an inverse correlation between fasting plasma in-

TABLE 2
Effect of insulin infusion (euglycemic insulin clamp technique) on ^{125}I-insulin binding to monocytes

		Postinfusion		
	Basal	1 h	3 h	5 h
Study I		Specific binding of insulin* (%)		
(Insulin infusion rate: 1 mU/kg/min)				
Subjects				
1	10.2	9.9	8.3	—
2	7.0	7.2	5.9	—
3	8.9	8.4	7.0	—
4	8.4	8.6	—	—
5	11.0	—	9.2	7.0
6	7.6	—	6.1	5.2
7	10.8	—	8.0	6.4
8	8.2	—	6.5	5.8
9	7.2	—	5.5	4.0
Study II				
(Insulin infusion rate: 0.25 mU/kg/min)				
Subjects				
1	6.8	—	6.2	4.8
2	7.0	—	7.1	5.1
3	9.6	—	9.4	7.0
4	7.8	—	8.3	6.2
5	6.6	—	6.4	5.1

* Represents the total specific binding of ^{125}I-insulin to monocytes determined at the tracer concentration (0.2 ng/ml) of insulin.

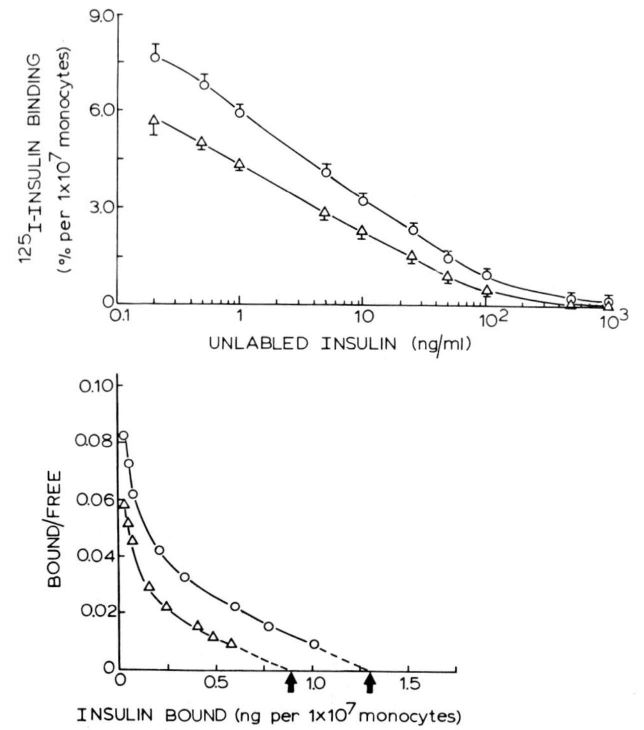

FIGURE 3. Upper Panel: Competition curves of ^{125}I-insulin binding to monocytes before (o, N = 5) and 5 h after (△, N = 5) insulin infusion in healthy subjects. Insulin was infused at a rate of 0.25 mU/kg/min by the euglycemic insulin clamp technique. Data are corrected for nonspecific binding. Lower panel: Scatchard analysis of insulin binding to monocytes. The Scatchard plots were obtained by analysis of the individual competition curves shown in the upper panel for each of the subjects before (o, N = 5) and 5 h after (△, N = 5) insulin infusion. The mean values are shown. The intercepts at the abscissa represent the total insulin binding capacity in each group.

sulin levels and insulin receptor concentration ($r = -0.62$, $P < 0.01$).

DISCUSSION

The current data provide direct evidence for in vivo downregulation of insulin receptors by physiologic hyperinsulinemia in normal man. The decrease in insulin binding to monocytes was found to be dependent upon the degree and duration of hyperinsulinemia. When the plasma insulin concentration was increased by 89 μU/ml above basal (Study I), a significant decrease in insulin binding was observed at 3 h, which averaged 20 ± 2% ($P < 0.01$). At 5 h insulin binding declined further (37 ± 3%, Figure 1). During Study II, when the plasma insulin concentration was raised by as little as 15 μU/ml above basal, the decrease in insulin binding did not become significant until 5 h (Figure 1), and the magnitude (25 ± 2%) was significantly lower ($P < 0.05$) than observed with the higher insulin infusion dose (Study I). The analyses of insulin binding data revealed that the decrease in insulin binding in both insulin clamp studies was due entirely to a decrease in insulin receptor concentration without any change in the receptor affinity (Figures 2 and 3). These data are thus consistent with previous studies demonstrating that homologous regulation of polypeptide hormones generally involves alterations in hormone receptor concentration rather than changes in receptor affinity.[1–7]

The steady-state plasma insulin levels achieved in the present study are well within the physiologic range. In Study I plasma insulin concentration increased to a mean of 102 μU/ml, a level which is commonly observed following the ingestion of oral glucose. The low dose insulin clamp (Study II) resulted in a mean steady-state plasma insulin concentration of only 31 μU/ml, which is in the same range of fasting insulin levels observed in obesity[8,9,11] and acromegaly.[12]

It has been proposed that the decrease in insulin receptor concentration in these insulin resistant states[8–11] may be secondary to the elevated fasting insulin levels characteristic of these conditions. This hypothesis has been based on the finding that decreased insulin binding in these patients is inversely correlated with the fasting plasma insulin concentration.[8–13] However, this observation does not necessarily indicate causality. The current data thus provide direct support for the thesis that the fasting hyperinsulinemia in these insulin-resistant states may, at least in part, be responsible for the decrease in insulin receptor concentration. Although the monocyte is not a conventional target organ for insulin action, previous data have shown that monocytes mirror the changes in insulin receptors in target tissues in both man[22] and animals.[23] Therefore, to the extent that insulin binding to monocytes reflects muscle, adipose, and liver cells, it would appear that physiologic hyperinsulinemia can downregulate insulin receptor concentration in insulin-sensitive target organs.

We considered the possibility that the decrease in insulin binding may have been secondary to insulin bound to monocyte membranes as a direct result of the insulin infusion. This seems unlikely for the following reasons. 1) During the insulin binding assay, multiple washing steps are performed and insulin is known to almost completely dissociate from its membrane receptor under these conditions.[23] 2) We failed to observe any decrease in insulin binding at 1 h following insulin infusion, the time required to achieve steady-state binding equilibrium at 37°C. 3) If insulin had bound to the membrane, one would expect an alteration in the shape of the competition curve of insulin binding. This would be most evident at low insulin concentrations, reflecting a change in insulin receptor affinity. No change in affinity was observed in the present study. Since no change in insulin binding was seen in control studies, when saline was infused, it is unlikely that the decrease in binding was the result of diurnal variation.

An obvious question raised by our findings is the possible functional consequence of the downregulation of insulin receptors induced by hyperinsulinemia. In this regard, it is noteworthy that the insulin sensitivity, as reflected by the insulin-mediated glucose uptake (Table I), did not decrease at 5 h of insulin infusion in Study I. In fact, there was a small (10%) but significant ($P < 0.05$) increase in insulin-mediated glucose uptake between the third and fifth hours of insulin infusion. It should be pointed out, however, that insulin-mediated glucose uptake, as measured by the insulin clamp technique, reflects an effect of insulin on overall cellular glucose metabolism—a function of post-receptor as well as receptor-mediated events. Thus, it is possible that the decrease in insulin binding was compensated for by an increased efficiency of post-receptor events. Whether more prolonged hyperinsulinemia will result in a decrease in insulin sensitivity remains to be established. In any event, the present findings indicate that in normal human subjects, increments in plasma insulin concentration well within the physiologic range are capable of downregulating the number of insulin receptors.

ACKNOWLEDGMENT

Dr. Soman is the recipient of a Clinical Investigator Award (AM-00356) from the National Institutes of Health, Bethesda, Maryland.

REFERENCES

[1] Gavin, J. R., III, Roth, J., Neville, D. M., Jr., DeMeyts, P., and Buell, D. N.: Insulin-dependent regulation of insulin receptor concentrations: A direct demonstration in cell culture. Proc. Natl. Acad. Sci. U.S.A. *71*:84–88, 1974.

[2] Lesniak, M. A., and Roth, J.: Regulation of receptor concentration by homologous hormone. Effect of human growth hormone on its receptor in IM-9 lymphocytes. J. Biol. Chem. *251*:3720–29, 1976.

[3] Soman, V., and Felig, P.: Regulation of the glucagon receptor by physiological hyperglucagonemia. Nature (London) *272*:829–32, 1978.

[4] Srikant, C. B., Freeman, D., McCorkle, K., and Unger, R. H.: Binding and biologic activity of glucagon in liver cell membranes of chronically hyperglucagonemic rats. J. Biol. Chem. *252*:7434–36, 1977.

[5] Hinkle, P. M., and Tashijian, A. M., Jr.: Thyrotropin-releasing hormone regulates the number of its own receptors in GM_3 strain of pituitary cells in culture. Biochemistry *14*:3845–51, 1975.

[6] Manni, A., Chambers, M. J., and Pearson, O. H.: Prolactin induces its own receptor in rat liver. Endocrinology *103*:2168–71, 1978.

[7] Kobayaski, M., and Olefsky, J. M.: Effect of experimental hyperinsulinemia on insulin binding and glucose transport in isolated rat adipocytes. Am. J. Physiol. *235*(1):E53–E62, 1978.

[8] Soll, A. M., Kahn, C. R., Neville, D. M., Jr., and Roth, J.: Insulin receptor deficiency in genetic and acquired obesity. J. Clin. Invest. *56*:769–80, 1975.

[9] Bar, R. S., Gorden, P., Roth, J., Kahn, C. R., and DeMeyts, P.: Fluctuations in the affinity and concentration of insulin receptors on circulating monocytes of obese subjects. J. Clin. Invest. *58*:1123–35, 1976.

[10] Olefsky, J. M., and Reaven, G. M.: Insulin binding in diabetes: relationships with plasma insulin levels and insulin sensitivity. Diabetes *26*:680–88, 1977.

[11] DeFronzo, R. A., Soman, V., Sherwin, R. S., Hendler, R., and Felig, P.: Insulin binding to monocytes and insulin action in human obesity, starvation and refeeding. J. Clin. Invest. *62*:204–13, 1978.

[12] Muggeo, M., Bar, R. S., Roth, J., Kahn, C. R., and Gorden, P.: The insulin resistance of acromegaly: Evidence for two alterations in the insulin receptor on circulating monocytes. J. Clin. Endocrinol. Metab. *48*:17–25, 1979.

[13] DeFronzo, R. A., Deibert, D., Hendler, R., Felig, P., and Soman, V.: Insulin sensitivity and insulin binding to monocytes in maturity-onset diabetes. J. Clin. Invest. *63*:939–46, 1979.

[14] Soman, V., Tamborlane, W., DeFronzo, R., Genel, M., and Felig, P.: Insulin binding and insulin sensitivity in isolated growth hormone deficiency. New Eng. J. Med. *299*:1025–30, 1978.

[15] Soman, V., Coustan, D., and Felig, P.: Dissociation between insulin binding to monocytes and insulin sensitivity in normal pregnancy. Program of 61st Annual Meeting of the Endocrine Society, p. 118, 1979.

[16] Kahn, C. R., Goldfine, I. D., Neville, D. M., Jr., and DeMeyts, P.: Alterations in insulin binding induced by changes in vivo in the levels of glucocorticoids and growth hormone. Endocrinology *103*:1054–66, 1978.

[17] Sherwin, R. S., Karmer, K. J., Tobin, J. D., Insel, P. A., Liljenquist, J. E., Berman, M., and Andres, R.: A model of the kinetics of insulin in man. J. Clin. Invest. *53*:1481–92, 1974.

[18] Wise, J. K., Hendler, R., and Felig, P.: Influence of glucocorticoids on glucagon secretion and plasma amino acid concentrations in man. J. Clin. Invest. *52*:2774–82, 1973.

[19] Scatchard, G.: The attractions of proteins for small molecules and ions. Ann. N.Y. Acad. Sci. *51*:660–72, 1949.

[20] DeMeyts, P., and Roth, J.: Cooperativity in ligand binding: A new graphic analysis. Biochem. Biophys. Res. Commun. *66*:1118–26, 1975.

[21] Snedecor, G. W., and Cochran, W. G.: Statistical Methods. Ames, Iowa State University Press, 6 ed., 1967.

[22] Olefsky, J. M.: Decreased insulin binding to adipocytes and circulating monocytes in obesity. J. Clin. Invest. *57*:1165–72, 1976.

[23] Roth, J., Kahn, C. R., Lesniak, M., Gorden, P., DeMeyts, P., Megyesi, K., Neville, D. M., Jr., Gavin, J. R., III, Soll, A. H., Freychet, P., Goldfine, I. D., Bar, R. S., and Archer, J. A.: Receptors for insulin, NSILA-S and growth hormone: applications to disease states in man. Recent Prog. Horm. Res. *31*:95–139, 1976.

Influence of the Age of Erythrocytes on Their Insulin Receptors

JOHN ENG, LILLY LEE, AND ROSALYN S. YALOW

SUMMARY

Specific binding of ^{125}I-insulin to erythrocyte receptors increased linearly with reticulocyte count in routine blood specimens from hospitalized patients. Specific binding as high as 30–35% is observed in patients with reticulocyte counts in the range of 20–25% compared with 9.0 ± 0.5% specific binding in healthy control subjects with normal reticulocyte counts. It is concluded that care must be exercised in interpreting elevations of specific ^{125}I-insulin binding to erythrocyte receptors as due to specific disease processes without considering how the disease itself may alter mean erythrocyte age at the time of sampling. **DIABETES 29:164–166, February 1980.**

There have been a number of recent studies describing changes in insulin binding to human erythrocyte receptors in disease states, including diabetes[1] and anorexia nervosa.[2] In view of a report by Thomopoulos et al.[3] that rabbit reticulocytes have 10-fold greater insulin binding sites than mature rabbit red blood cells, we thought it important to determine the influence of the age of human erythrocytes on insulin binding. The reticulocyte count is one index of erythrocyte age. In this report we determined the variation in insulin binding to erythrocytes in the blood of normal subjects and of hospitalized patients with normal or elevated reticulocyte counts.

MATERIALS AND METHODS

Blood for insulin binding study was obtained from specimens sent to the hematology laboratory for reticulocyte counts or from normal volunteers. Plasma from the bloods was saved for insulin assay. Monoiodinated ^{125}I-insulin was prepared as previously published.[4] Erythrocytes were prepared according to the procedure described by Gambhir et al.[5] with the following modifications. At each step of preparation, white blood cells were carefully aspirated while avoiding excessive removal of the upper layer of erythrocytes. On completion of preparation, erythrocytes were suspended to a concentration of 4.4×10^9 cells/ml and a reticulocyte count was done. Loss of reticulocytes during the preparation procedure ranged from 10 to 50%. Leukocyte contamination was less than 10^5/ml. ^{125}I-insulin binding to erythrocytes was determined by incubating 0.3 ml of the cell suspension with 50 pg of ^{125}I-insulin and varying concentrations of unlabeled insulin in a final volume of 0.5 ml. After overnight incubation at 4°C, 0.2 ml portions were placed into chilled test tubes and washed with 2.5 ml cold normal saline. The tubes were quickly vortexed and centrifuged at $2000 \times g$ at 4°C for 5 min, after which the supernatant was aspirated and the cell pellet counted. ^{125}I-insulin binding in the presence of 10^5 ng/ml of unlabeled insulin was taken to be nonspecific binding and accounted for 2–4% of total radioactivity added. In one experiment, a portion of an erythrocyte suspension was taken for assay of insulin binding and the remainder of the suspension was centrifuged at $400 \times g$ for 20 min. The top and bottom quarter portions of the sedimented cells were resuspended and also assayed for insulin binding. In all cases the percentage is expressed in terms of ^{125}I-insulin binding to 2.64×10^9 erythrocytes/ml incubation volume.

RESULTS

A plot of erythrocyte insulin binding as a function of reticulocyte count for each patient studied is shown in Figure 1. The high correlation is obvious, and regression analysis of the data gives a correlation coefficient of 0.87. Individual competitive binding curves were analyzed for most of the blood samples, and in all cases the half-maximal binding of labeled insulin to erythrocytes occurred in the presence of 4–5 ng/ml unlabeled insulin. The Scatchard plots were essentially parallel. Taken together, these data suggest that the differences in binding are due, at least in part, to a greater

From the Solomon A. Berson Research Laboratory, Veterans Administration Hospital, Bronx, New York and the Department of Clinical Sciences, Albert Einstein College of Medicine at the Montefiore Hospital and Medical Center, Bronx, New York.

Address reprint requests to Rosalyn S. Yalow, Solomon A. Berson Research Laboratory, VA Hospital, Bronx, New York 10468.

Received for publication 17 December 1979.

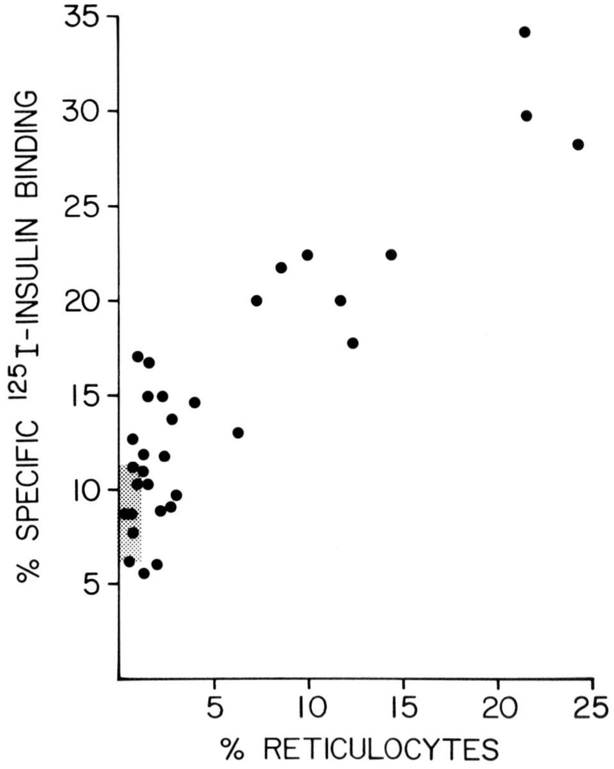

FIGURE 1. Specific ^{125}I-insulin binding (%) to erythrocyte receptors as a function of reticulocyte count in blood from hospitalized patients sent to the routine hematology laboratory. The shaded area represents the range for normal, healthy laboratory personnel.

number of binding sites on human reticulocytes than on mature erythrocytes.

The illnesses which produced the reticulocytosis were blood loss, hemolysis from various causes, and pernicious anemia during cyanocobalamin therapy. Although erythrocyte mean cell volumes tended to be higher than normal in bloods with elevated reticulocyte counts, quite often the mean cell volumes were normal—especially when hemolysis was the cause of reticulocytosis. Specific ^{125}I-insulin binding to erythrocytes from nine normal laboratory controls ranged from 6.2 to 11.6% with an average of 9.0 ± 0.5%. Insulin binding was not related to plasma insulin levels in the bloods studied.

A patient with pernicious anemia was followed during the course of treatment with cyanocobalamin (Table 1). It is evident that insulin binding to his erythrocytes remained elevated despite a decrease in the percentage of reticulocytes from 21.4% at 6 days to 2.1% at 20 days. These data suggest that early mature erythrocytes, like reticulocytes, also have an increased number of insulin receptors per cell.

Since erythrocytes are thought to form an age-related gradient on centrifugation, with younger cells sedimenting on top and older cells on the bottom,[6] we determined the insulin binding to various centrifuged erythrocyte fractions. Insulin binding to an erythrocyte preparation with a modestly elevated reticulocyte count was compared with suspensions of erythrocytes taken from the top and bottom quarters of the same preparation after it had been centrifuged at 400 × *g* for 20 min (Table 2). The data suggest that even a relatively low centrifugal force can separate erythrocytes into at least two populations of cells. The top portion contains erythrocytes with a larger cell size and higher insulin binding. Erythrocytes from the bottom portion have smaller cell size and lower insulin binding.

TABLE 1
Percent specific ^{125}I-insulin bound to red cells in a treated pernicious anemia patient

B_{12} therapy, day:	6	10	20
Mean cell volume (μm^3)	123.0	115.0	110.0
Reticulocytes (%)	21.4	15.0	2.1
Specific ^{125}I-insulin bound (%)	28.6	26.5	29.9

TABLE 2
Percent specific ^{125}I-insulin bound to red cells before and after centrifugation

	Initial mixture	Top ¼	Bottom ¼
Mean cell volume (μm^3)	93.0	109.0	82.0
Reticulocytes (%)	2.7	7.8	0.1
Specific ^{125}I-insulin bound (%)	10.3	16.9	7.6

DISCUSSION

These data demonstrate that, in man, not only reticulocytes but also early mature erythrocytes have more insulin binding sites per cell than older erythrocytes. As a result in some hospitalized patients, even those whose reticulocytes appeared to be in the normal range, manifest erythrocyte insulin binding increased above the levels found in healthy control subjects. (This was most evident in the case of the cyanocobalamin-treated pernicious anemia patient whose insulin binding, even after the reticulocyte count had returned to 2%, remained elevated to three times the mean value for normals.) Since a variety of disease states may alter erythrocyte survival, the mean circulating erythrocyte age in patients with these diseases may be significantly less than in normal subjects. Thus, in the absence of a simple method capable of measuring differences in mean cell age between erythrocytes from normal and disease populations, we must rely on a clinical history to determine if the mean cell age of the patient is likely to be younger than that of the control group. Care must therefore be exercised in interpreting elevations of insulin binding to erythrocytes, as due to specific disease processes, without considering how the disease itself may affect mean erythrocyte age at the time of the sampling.

ACKNOWLEDGMENT

This work was supported by the Medical Research Program of the Veterans Administration.

REFERENCES

[1] Robinson, T. J., Archer, J. A., Gambhir, K. K., Hollis, V. W., Jr., Carter, L., and Bradley, C.: Erythrocytes: A new cell type for the evaluation of insulin receptor defects in diabetic humans. Science *205*:200–02, 1979.

[2] Wachslicht-Rodbard, H., Gross, H. A., Rodbard, D., Ebert, M. H., and

Roth, J.: Increased insulin binding to erythrocytes in anorexia nervosa. N. Engl. J. Med. *300*:882–87, 1979.

[3] Thomopoulos, P., Berthellier, M., and Laudat, M.-H.: Loss of insulin receptors on maturation of reticulocytes. Biochem. Biophys. Res. Commun. *85*:1460–65, 1978.

[4] Schneider, B. S., Straus, E., and Yalow, R. S.: Some considerations in the preparation of radioiodoinsulin for radioimmunoassay and receptor assay. Diabetes *25*:260–67, 1976.

[5] Gambhir, K. K., Archer, J. A., and Carter, L.: Insulin radioreceptor assay for human erythrocytes. Clin. Chem. *23*:1590–95, 1977.

[6] O'Connell, D. J., Caruso, C. J., and Sass, M. D.: Separation of erythrocytes of different ages. Clin. Chem. *11*:771–81, 1965.

Insulin Resistance in Obesity as Analyzed by the Response of Glucose Kinetics to Glucagon Infusion

MLADEN VRANIC, SOICHIRO MORITA, AND GEORGE STEINER

SUMMARY

A new approach has been developed to examine insulin sensitivity and resistance in vivo in man. In it, tracer methods are used, which permit the assessment of nonsteady state glucose kinetics by a method that is noninvasive and does not use pharmacologic agents. Graded doses of glucagon, infused intravenously, are used to drive glucose out of steady state and to stimulate the release of insulin into the portal circulation. By relating the changes in the rates of glucose production, utilization, and fractional disappearance to immunoreactive glucagon and insulin, it is possible to assess the body's sensitivity to physiologic levels of these two hormones.

The utility of this approach was examined in obesity, a known human model of insulin resistance. The data demonstrated that glucose production in the obese subjects responded normally to glucagon. They also showed that insulin was much less effective in promoting glucose utilization in the obese persons than it was in the normal ones. In the obese subjects who were studied, the pancreatic B-cells were shown to be normally responsive to the stimulatory effects of either glucose or glucagon. Hence, they did not release sufficient insulin to overcome the insulin resistance, and these obese individuals had impaired glucose tolerance. Thus, it is suggested that, in the presence of insulin resistance, the responsiveness of B-cells will determine whether the glucose tolerance will be normal or abnormal in obese persons. This approach can now be used to explore glucose homeostasis in other conditions associated with glucose intolerance, the metabolic basis of which is undefined.
DIABETES 29:169–176, March 1980.

From the Departments of Physiology and of Medicine, University of Toronto, Ontario, Canada. Present address of Dr. Morita is Department of Internal Medicine, Kobe University School of Medicine, Kusunoki-cho, Ikuta, Kobe, Japan.

Address reprint requests to Mladen Vranic, M.D., D.Sc., Department of Physiology, University of Toronto, Medical Sciences Building, Toronto, Ontario, Canada M5S 1A8.

Received for publication 8 June and in revised form 5 October 1979.

In these studies, we examined the effects of insulin and glucagon on glucose turnover in lean and obese subjects. Glucoregulation was studied under both steady state and nonsteady state conditions. This was done because we felt that any alteration in glucoregulatory processes would be more pronounced and, therefore, easier to detect when glucose homeostasis was perturbed. To drive glucose out of steady state, we infused stepwise-incremental doses of glucagon. This hormone is known to stimulate in vivo hepatic glucose production[1] and to promote insulin release from the pancreatic B-cell.[2] The latter effect was also desirable for the study, because it allowed us to examine the glucoregulatory consequences of insulin delivered into the portal, rather than peripheral, circulation. To examine nonsteady state glucose kinetics, the method of primed infusion of radioactive glucose[3] was used. This method was previously validated in dogs[4,5] and applied to man.[6–8]

The obese subjects were studied because they provided a model known to be resistant to insulin and, hence, could be easily contrasted with normal subjects. Insulin sensitivity has been assessed in vivo by a variety of methods. One approach has been to measure the plasma insulin/glucose ratio under different conditions.[9] However, the meaning of this ratio is uncertain, as it is the product of a feedback loop, which includes not only the effect of glucose on insulin release, but also the effect of insulin on glucose metabolism, both its production and utilization. Another approach has been to use measurements of trans-splanchnic glucose balance.[10] This is essentially applicable only to steady state conditions. A third approach has been to clamp the levels of glucose and insulin and, then, to examine their interrelations.[11] Since this approach may be complicated by the influence of release of pancreatic insulin, others have stabilized endogenous insulin reaction by the combined infusion of glucose, insulin, epinephrine, and a beta-adrenergic–blocking drug.[12] Not only were there uncertainties about the many effects of these drugs, but this third approach is also limited by its requirement for steady glucose concentration and, in man, for peripheral insulin administration.

In the present study, we used tracer techniques to measure nonsteady and steady state glucose kinetics under the influence of varying concentrations of glucagon and insulin. While an infusion of glucose, combined with tracer, could provide similar information about the peripheral response to insulin, the present approach was chosen because it permitted us to examine not only the response to insulin, but also the response to glucagon and the interaction of these two hormones, which are so important in regulating glucose homeostasis. Insulin gained access to the body by its physiologic route. We have shown how the glucoregulatory effect of these hormones differs in lean and obese persons and have suggested that this approach may be used to analyze the bases of other types of abnormalities in glucose homeostasis.

MATERIALS AND METHODS

Subjects. Two groups of volunteers were studied. All had given written informed consent before participating in the study. The control group consisted of five individuals of normal weight; the second group consisted of five grossly obese individuals. The characteristics of all volunteers are summarized in Table 1. Volunteers were of both sexes. The controls were somewhat younger: however, the ages of the groups' members overlapped, and there was no relationship between any of the parameters measured and the ages of the subjects. All subjects were selected to be healthy and to have normal, fasting plasma glucose and lipid concentrations. None had liver, kidney, or thyroid disease. The normal (lean) control group members were 102 ± 4% of ideal body weight[13] and had a body mass index of 20.9 ± 0.8. The body mass, or Quetelet, index is obtained by dividing the weight, in kilograms, by the height, in meters squared; it has been shown by Keys et al.[14] to be the anthropometric index that gives the best correlation with body fatness, as determined by body density measurements. The obese groups were 199 ± 11% of ideal weight and had a body mass index of 40.0 ± 2.2.

All individuals were studied in the Clinical Investigation Unit of the Toronto General Hospital. They were placed on a weight-maintaining diet that contained 250 g of carbohydrate. The fat and protein contents of the diet constituted between 30 and 35% and 12 and 15% of the total calories, respectively. After 3 days on the diet, they underwent an oral glucose tolerance test—1.75 g glucose/kg ideal body weight—according to the procedure described by Fajans and Conn.[15] During the glucose tolerance test, samples were taken for assay of plasma glucose, serum insulin, and plasma glucagon levels. Each individual has been classified, in Table 1, as normal or abnormal by the criteria of Fajans and Conn for plasma glucose levels.[15] In addition, the glucose concentrations were scored according to the USPHS-Wilkerson System[16] or summed, as in the University Group Diabetes Program.[17] It should be noted that the glucose load given by the Fajans and Conn procedure is more than the 100 g given in the USPHS procedure or the 50 g given by the University Group Diabetes Program. All controls and two of the five obese subjects had normal glucose tolerance tests by all three criteria. After a further 3 days, on the same diet as before the glucose tolerance tests, all the participants underwent the glucose turnover study.

Glucose turnover protocols and methods. After the dietary preparation noted above, all participants underwent a protocol designed to permit the determination of glucose concentration and turnover—before, during, and after an infusion of stepwise-graded increments of glucagon. Each person was fasting from 12 h before the study until its end. All materials were administered, and blood was taken via separate, indwelling venous cannulae. These were placed 45 min before the study started and, when not in use, were kept patent with a slow saline infusion. The subjects remained recumbent and quietly relaxed throughout the study.

TABLE 1
Anthropometric data and immunoreactive insulin (IRI), glucagon (IRG), and glucose tolerance in five normal and five obese subjects

			Anthropometric data				Fasting values			Glucose tolerance test criteria†		
Subject	Sex	Age	Ht (cm)	Wt (kg)	Relative wt (% ideal)	BMI*	Plasma glucose (mg/dl)	Basal IRI (μU/ml)	Basal IRG (pg/ml)	Conn, Fajans	Wilkerson score	Sum of glucoses
Normal												
J.H.	M	26	175	66	100	21.6	70	18	120	N	0	301
J.P.	M	33	174	68	100	22.5	82	17	174	N	0	426
L.J.	F	24	163	51	100	19.2	83	18	120	N	0	330
M.N.	F	30	163	59	115	22.2	72	8	108	N	0	304
E.C.	F	30	158	47	94	18.8	77	15	102	N	0	323
Mean ± SE		29 ± 2			102 ± 4	20.9 ± 0.8	77 ± 2.6	15.2 ± 1.9	125 ± 13			336 ± 23
Obese												
M.G.	M	29	180	140	209	43.2	97	26	117	Abn	2	527
L.M.	F	55	152	80	170	34.6	105	15	80	N	0	336
D.D.	F	40	170	133	229	46.0	108	42	159	Abn	2	653
P.S.	F	48	173	105	178	35.1	89	10	77	N	0	394
M.G.	F	25	159	104	208	41.1	67	25	80	Abn	2	619
Mean ± SE		39 ± 6			199 ± 11	40.0 ± 2.2	93 ± 7.3	23.6 ± 5.4	103 ± 16			511 ± 58

* Body mass (Quetelet) index = wt(kg) ÷ [ht(m)]².

† The glucose tolerance test was conducted using the glucose load defined by Fajans and Conn.[15] It was considered normal (N) or abnormal (Abn) according to their criteria. It was also rated by the criteria of Wilkerson[16] and of the University Group Diabetes Program,[17] although both of these had used lower glucose loads.

Glucose turnover was determined by the primed-infusion procedure, the details of which have been described for dogs[18] and man.[7] Glucose-1-^{14}C (New England Nuclear, Montreal, P.Q.), tested to be sterile and pyrogen free, was used. The priming dose contained an amount of glucose-1-^{14}C equal to the amount infused in 120 min. The total infusion, designed to be at a rate of 0.107 Ci/min, was continued for 265 min. The precise dose infused was determined in each experiment from the calibrated pump rate and the actual specific activity measured in an aliquot of the infusate. The methods used to assay glucose concentrations and specific activities, the procedures used to correct for recycling of ^{14}C, and the calculation of glucose kinetics were exactly as previously described.[7,18]

During the first 100 min of the turnover study, samples were drawn to determine both basal concentrations of insulin and glucagon and basal glucose kinetics. An infusion of glucagon (Eli Lilly Co., Indianapolis, Ind.) was then started. With the aid of a calibrated Sage pump, it could be given in gradually increasing doses. From 100 to 110 min, the glucagon infusion rate was 5.7 ng/kg-min; from 110 to 125 min, 9.3 ng/kg/min; from 125 to 145 min, 12.9 ng/kg/min; from 145 to 170 min, 10.3 ng/kg/min; from 170 to 190 min, 25.7 ng/kg/min. This schedule of doses was based on previous experience with dogs[19] and was aimed at producing, for some period of time, plasma glucagon levels within a range extending from basal levels to high levels seen in poorly controlled diabetes or in patients with severe stress.[2] The glucose-1-^{14}C infusion was continued for a further 45 min after the glucagon infusion was stopped (235–280 min).

Plasma glucagon levels and serum insulin levels were measured by previously described methods.[20,21] Antiserum 30K, supplied by Dr. R. Unger, was used for the glucagon assay.

RESULTS

Oral glucose tolerance test. Neither the obese nor the normal individuals had fasting hyperglycemia (Figure 1 and Table 1). After an oral glucose load, the glucose concentrations were higher in the obese subjects. The fasting serum IRI values were not significantly different from normal in the obese group. However, as with the glucose levels, the obese subjects displayed significantly higher IRI concentration at 60, 90, and 180 min after an oral glucose load. The responses of our patients to an oral glucose load were similar to those frequently observed by others.[22]

The fasting plasma IRG levels in the obese group were not significantly different from the normal (Table 1). The IRG levels did not decrease significantly in normal subjects after an oral glucose load (Figure 2). This is consistent with the frequent experience that a glucose load does not always suppress IRG levels. However, in the obese subjects, after the glucose load, IRG fell by as much as 35%. At 90, 120, and 180 min the IRG levels were significantly less than the basal levels.

Glucose administration and glucose kinetics. Glucose turnover was measured before, during, and after the infusion of progressively increasing doses of glucagon (Figure 3, panels c and f). The decision to use stepwise increments in glucagon was made because it has been shown in dogs[1,19] and in man[23–25] that, within both physiologic and pharmacologic ranges, the effect of glucagon on glucose production is transient, and we wished to sustain the increased rate of glucose production. The mean fasting plasma glucose level in the normal group was 80 mg/dl and in the obese, it was 90 mg/dl (Figure 3,a and d). The mean basal rate of glucose turnover was 80 mg/m²/min in the lean group and 75 mg/m²/min in the obese one (Figure 3,b and e). These differences were not significant.

In the normal subjects, the glucose concentration increased as soon as the glucagon infusion was started (100 min). It plateaued at 160 min, despite continued infusion of greater amounts of glucagon. The rise of glucose during the first 60 min of glucagon infusion occurred because the rate of glucose production (Ra) exceeded the rate of glucose utilization (Rd) (Figure 3b). Both rates then became equal and therefore the glucose concentration plateaued. Only by using turnover techniques was it possible to analyze the basis of these two steady states and the mechanisms responsible for the change from one to the other. After the glu-

FIGURE 1. Oral glucose tolerance test (1.75 g glucose/kg ideal body weight) in five normal and five grossly obese individuals. Left panel depicts the plasma glucose concentrations and the right panel, the serum concentrations of immunoreactive insulin (IRI). Concentrations of glucose and IRI were higher in the obese at 60, 90, and 180 min (P < 0.05).

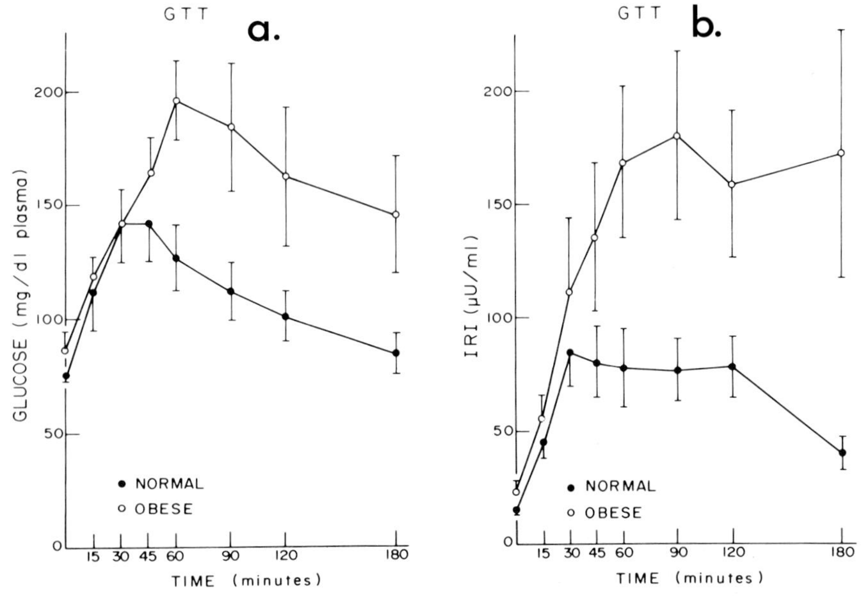

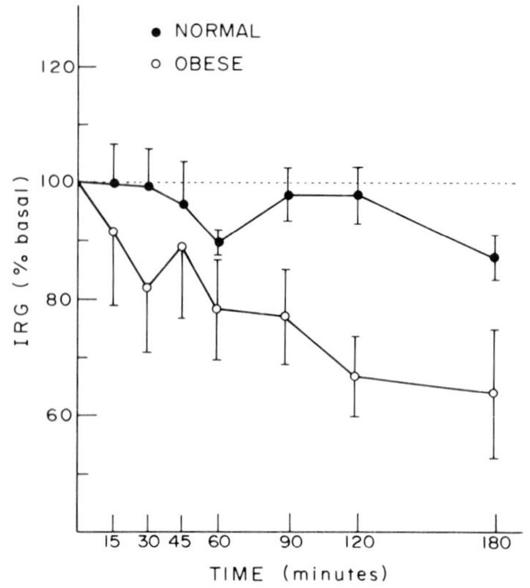

FIGURE 2. Plasma concentrations of immunoreactive glucagon (IRG) in five normal and five grossly obese individuals after an oral glucose tolerance test. Basal IRG was 125 ± 13 pg/ml in the lean subjects and 103 ± 16 pg/ml in the obese. A significant suppression of IRG was noted in the obese at 90, 120, and 180 min ($P < 0.05$) but not in the lean.

cagon infusion was stopped, the plasma glucose concentration decreased. This occurred because the decrease in Ra was greater than the decrease in Rd.

The glucose concentrations also rose during the glucagon infusion in the obese group. However, the rise was more rapid than it was in the lean group (Figure 3,a and d). Furthermore, in contrast with the lean subjects, the glucose concentrations in the obese did not plateau during the glucagon infusion. This occurred because, throughout the glucagon infusion in the obese group, glucose production always exceeded glucose utilization (Figure 3e). After stopping the glucagon infusion, there was a prompt fall in plasma glucose concentration, because Ra fell below Rd. In both groups, this difference between Ra and Rd could reflect a rapid response of hepatic glucose production to the decrease in glucagon and a less rapid response of glucose utilization to the decrease in insulin.

FIGURE 3. The effect of a graded glucagon infusion (panels c and f) on concentration, production, and utilization of glucose in five normal (left panel) and five grossly obese subjects (right panel). At 160 min, plasma glucose reached a steady state, whereas glucose concentrations in the obese subjects were steadily increasing throughout the glucagon infusion period. Glucose concentrations were significantly higher in the obese than in the lean subjects from 180 to 230 min ($P < 0.05$–0.01).

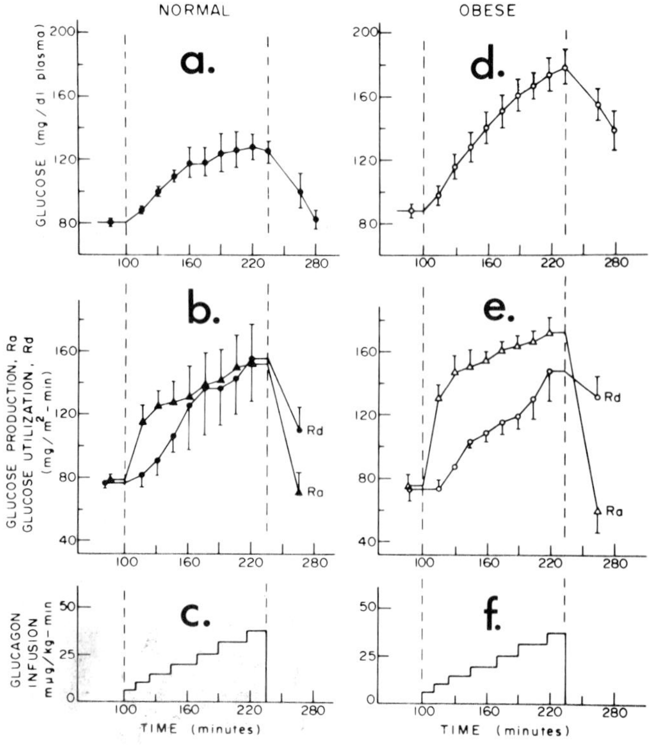

Glucagon administration and IRI. There were no significant differences in mean fasting IRG between the normal (110 pg/ml) and the obese (125 pg/ml) groups. The IRG levels rose in both groups during the infusion. By the end of the infusion period, the mean IRG was 900 pg/ml in the normal group and 1200 pg/ml in the obese group (Figure 4,b and e). The higher IRG in the obese group reflects the fact that the glucagon infusion in all individuals was the same in relation to their body weight. This presumably resulted in a higher rate of infusion per unit of extracellular fluid volume in the obese. The peak IRG values correspond to the high IRG concentrations reported in poorly controlled diabetes or in patients with severe stress.[2] The mean fasting insulin

FIGURE 4. Concentrations of serum immunoreactive insulin (IRI) and plasma immunoreactive glucagon (IRG) before, during, and after a graded infusion of glucagon.

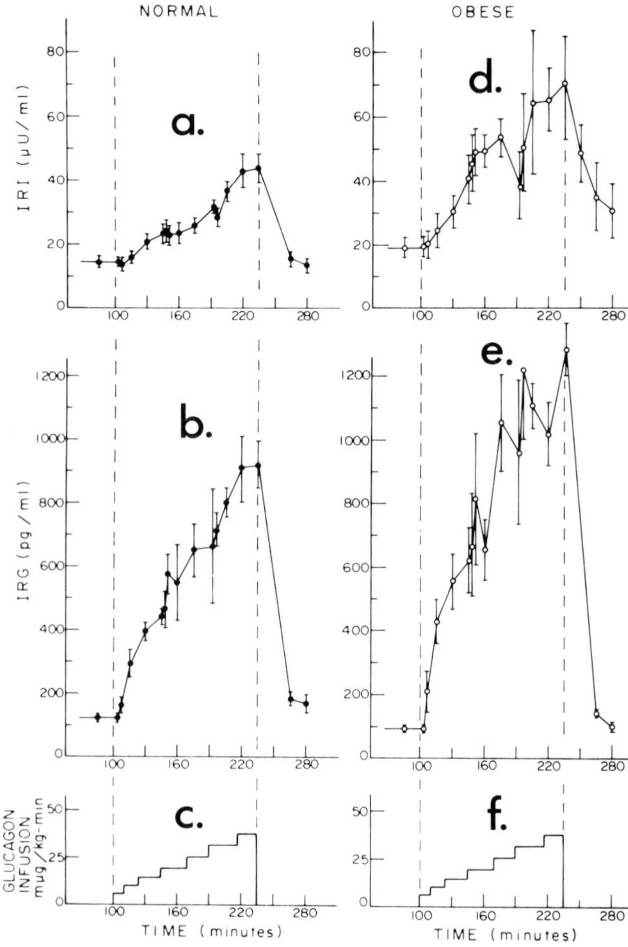

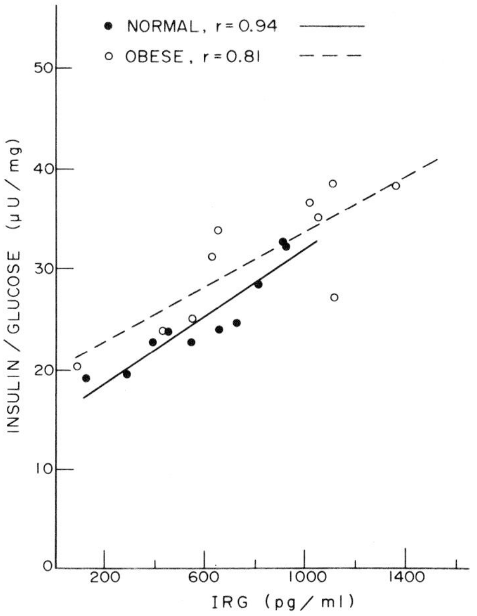

FIGURE 5. Correlation between mean plasma concentration of immunoreactive glucagon (IRG) and the mean insulin-glucose ratio from 80 to 235 min. Highly significant correlations were found in both the normal and the obese subjects, and the correlation was the same for both groups of individuals.

levels in the obese group (20 μU/ml) were similar to those in the normal one (15 μU/ml) (Figure 4,a and d). Although not significant, this small difference was similar to that observed for the fasting insulin levels before the glucose tolerance tests (see Table 1). During the infusion of glucagon, the serum IRI rose progressively to a peak of 40 μU/ml in the lean group and to 70 μU/ml in the obese one.

Correlation of insulin and glucagon. We next examined the relationship between glucagon and insulin in the normal and in the obese groups. In exploring the effect of glucagon on pancreatic B-cells, insulin concentrations were normalized for the prevailing glucose concentration and were expressed as the IRI/glucose ratio. The IRI/glucose ratio was directly related to IRG concentration (Figure 5). This reflected the stimulatory effect of glucagon on the pancreatic B-cell.[2] Since it was shown that, after an intravenous glucose injection, the relationship between glucose and insulin is linear,[26] the rise in IRI during the glucagon infusion was not merely an effect of glucagon on plasma glucose. As the correlation between IRG and IRI/glucose was the same, the sensitivity of the B-cell to glucagon was similar in both groups.

Correlation of glucose kinetics with glucagon and with insulin. To examine the correlation of glucose production and IRG, we used data from the first 30 min of the glucagon infusion only (Figure 6). We chose this interval for two reasons: first, because the effect of a given concentration of glucagon on glucose production declines with time,[1,19,23–25] and second, because during this interval the glucagon and insulin concentrations were within the physiologic range and were similar in both populations (Figure 4, from 100 to 130 min). Glucose production and glucagon were positively correlated, and the correlation was the same for both normal and obese subjects (Figure 6,a and b).

As shown in Figure 7, glucose utilization was positively correlated to the IRI in both normal and obese subjects. However, the regression line for the obese group was shifted to the right and its slope was much less steep than that for the normal group, indicating that insulin had less effect on glucose utilization in the obese than in the normal subjects (statistical comparison of the two slopes revealed a highly significant difference, $t = 3.33$, $P < 0.01$).

The rate of glucose utilization is governed by the concentration of both glucose and insulin. To examine the effect of insulin itself on glucose utilization, the correlation between IRI and the fractional disappearance rate of glucose (k = Rd divided by the glucose mass) was also determined (Figure 8). In dogs receiving similar glucagon infusions but with plasma insulin fixed at different constant levels,[4] or in dogs infused with glucose and having both insulin and glucagon levels fixed,[27] the fractional glucose disappearance rate was independent of glucose concentration. However, the fractional disappearance of glucose was directly, and predictably, related to plasma insulin levels.[28] Davis et al. have now shown that a similar situation exists in man.[29]

In our studies (Figure 8), at basal insulin concentrations, the fractional disappearance of glucose was much greater

FIGURE 6. Correlation between the concentration of immunoreactive glucagon (IRG) and the rate of glucose production in lean (panel a) and obese (panel b) individuals. In both groups, the correlations were significant and the correlation was the same for both groups of individuals. All individual data were plotted before and during the first 30 min of glucagon infusion.

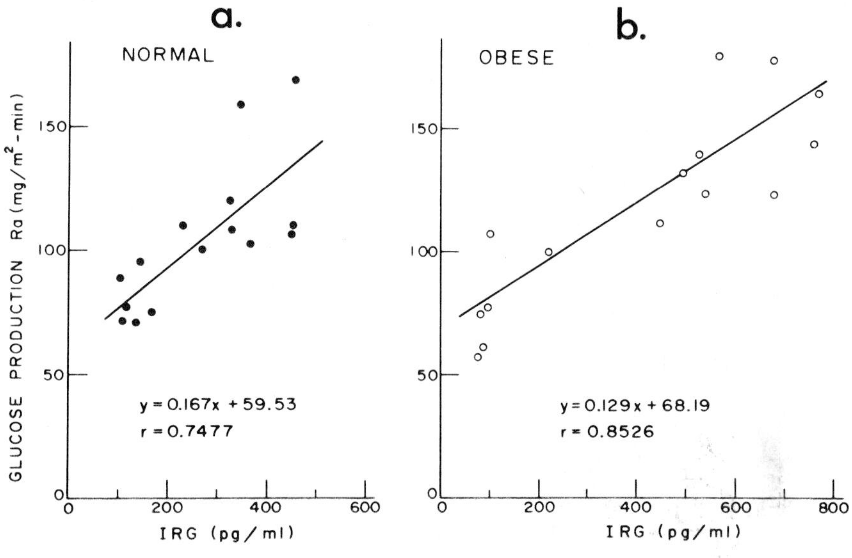

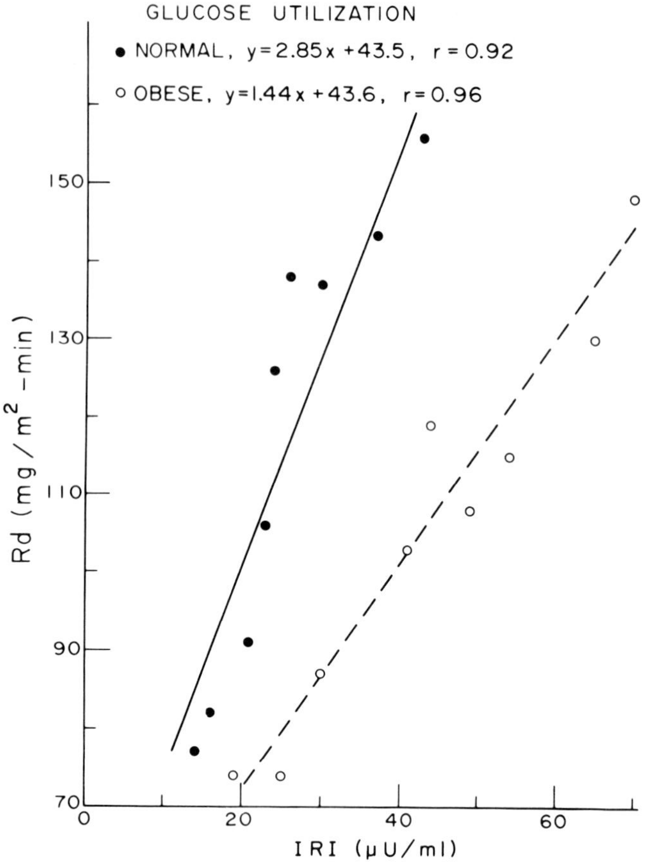

FIGURE 7. Correlation between the mean concentrations of immunoreactive insulin (IRI) and the mean rate of glucose utilization (Rd) in lean and obese subjects at from 80 to 220 min of the experiment.

in the lean than it was in the obese group. With higher concentrations of insulin, K rose significantly in the lean but not in the obese group. Thus the obese were resistant to the effect of all observed levels of insulin on the fractional glucose disappearance. Such a conclusion could already have been inferred from the data in Figures 3 and 4. There it can be seen that, despite a greater increment in IRI, any given increment in glucose concentration resulted in a smaller increment in the absolute rate of glucose utilization (Rd) in the obese than in the lean group.

FIGURE 8. Correlation between mean concentrations of immunoreactive insulin (IRI) and mean fractional disappearance rate of glucose (k) at from 80 to 220 min of the experiment. A highly significant correlation was found in the lean, but no correlation was observed in the obese subjects. [fractional disappearance rate of glucose (min⁻¹) = rate of glucose utilization (mg/min) divided by glucose mass (mg)].

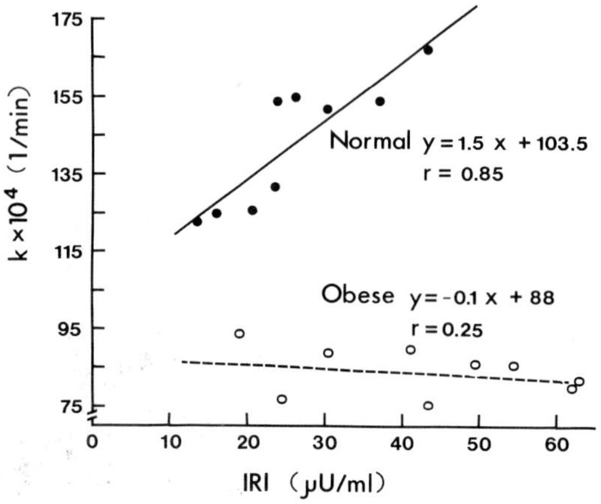

DISCUSSION

A variety of in vivo methods has suggested that the obese individual is resistant to the effect of insulin on glucose metabolism.[9–11,30–32] Each contains a number of assumptions and, therefore, has inherent limitations. We have applied tracer methods to the examination of glucose kinetics in normal and in obese persons; the latter group was chosen as a model of insulin resistance.

Tracer methods were used to quantitate both glucose production and utilization, as they required neither invasive nor pharmacologic manipulations. The studies were conducted under nonsteady state conditions to obtain a sensitive assessment of the effects of insulin and glucagon on the processes of glucoregulation. A graded infusion of glucagon was used to stimulate glucose production and B-cell insulin release. The plasma levels of glucagon started from basal and ranged up to the near maximal concentrations seen in the portal circulation.[2] This approach also permitted us to examine the effects of insulin release into the portal bed in response to a physiologic stimulus.

The lean and the obese groups both had similar basal glucose turnover rates, expressed in relation to body surface area. When glucagon was infused, glucose production rose promptly. Because of the previously described transient effect of glucagon,[1] the glucagon infusion was increased incrementally and glucose production did not decline. This is analogous to such physiologic situations as strenuous exercise of limited duration.[18]

During the glucagon infusion, glucose production rose promptly in both groups. Glucose utilization followed more slowly; it finally equaled glucose production in the lean subjects but not in the obese ones. As noted earlier, only the data from the first 30 min of the glucagon infusion were used to examine the relationship of glucagon to Ra. This was the time at which the liver was highly responsive to increments in glucagon and at which we would have expected the greatest likelihood of any difference to show up. Previously, it had been shown that insulin, even at higher concentrations, did not influence the response of glucose production to glucagon infusions lasting up to 1 h.[19] The positive correlation between IRG and glucose production was the same in both populations. Since glucose production had not plateaued, even at the highest levels examined in Figure 6, this portion of the study did not reach maximally effective concentrations of glucagon. Therefore, one interpretation of these data would be that both populations were equally sensitive to glucagon. However, if the behavior of the human liver is not like that previously characterized in the dog,[19] one would not rule out the possibility that obesity might be associated with altered hepatic sensitivity to glucagon.

Glucose disappearance rose in both groups during the glucagon infusion. This could have resulted from an increase in the concentration of either insulin, or glucose, or both. Therefore, it became necessary to examine the effect of glucagon on human B-cell function in vivo. We noted (Figure 4) that plasma insulin increased during the course of the glucagon infusion and that this increase was greater in the obese group than in the lean one. This could have been a result of the higher levels of either glucagon, or plasma glucose, or both. The relationship between this insulin/glucose ratio and the plasma level of glucagon suggested that, in both groups, the B-cells were similarly responsive to glucagon.

The insulin level and the rate of glucose utilization were positively correlated in both lean and obese subjects (Figure 7). The line relating insulin to glucose utilization was steeper in the lean group than in the obese one. At basal insulin concentrations, the rate of glucose utilization in the lean subjects appeared to be higher than in the obese ones. This was observed even though the basal glucose concentrations in both groups were similar. Glucose utilization is influenced by both glucose concentration and insulin's effectiveness on insulin-sensitive tissues.[18] As the basal glucose concentrations were similar, the data in Figure 7 suggested that insulin was indeed less effective in promoting glucose utilization in the obese subjects than it was in the lean ones. This difference in sensitivity also could have accounted for the difference in the slopes of the lines relating glucose utilization (Rd) to IRI.

To explore the effectiveness of insulin divorced from the influence of glucose concentration, we examined the relationship between the fractional disappearance of glucose and the plasma insulin concentrations. A significant positive correlation was found in the lean subjects but no correlation was observed in the obese ones. This is another demonstration of the insulin sensitivity in the lean group and of the insulin resistance in the obese group.

These studies of glucose turnover permitted us to examine some factors that might have led to differences in glucose tolerance of the lean and the obese subjects whom we studied. Theoretically these could have included the following. First, the pancreatic B-cells of the obese subjects might have responded inadequately to the glucose load. Second, their pancreatic A cells' release of glucagon might not have been suppressed. Third, hepatic glucose production may not have been adequately suppressed in the obese group. Finally, as suggested by a number of studies,[9-11,30-32] insulin's ability to promote glucose utilization might have been markedly decreased in the obese subjects. Perley and Kipnis[30] challenged the lean and obese subjects with glucose and examined the glucose concentration patterns and insulin responses. They found that certain obese subjects were able to maintain normal glucose tolerance by releasing much more insulin than did the lean ones. In other words, this subgroup of carbohydrate-tolerant obese individuals had markedly hyper-responsive B-cells. Other obese individuals had insulin responses to glucose that, although higher than those of the lean nondiabetic, were lower than those of the obese nondiabetic. This subgroup of obese subjects was carbohydrate intolerant. Hence, an obese individual is likely to become carbohydrate intolerant if his B cells are not sufficiently hyper-responsive.

The B-cells of the obese subjects in the present study responded normally to glucagon. During the glucose tolerance test, their insulin levels were higher than those of the lean subjects. However, there was little difference between the two groups in the relationship between insulin and glucose concentrations. This suggested that the B-cells in our population of obese subjects were normally, but not excessively, responsive to a glucose or glucagon challenge.

Carbohydrate intolerance in the obese subjects did not appear to have resulted from a failure to suppress A-cell function. In fact, glucagon concentrations during the glucose tolerance test were suppressed to a greater extent in the obese subjects than they were in the lean, which could improve rather than impair glucose tolerance. This could have resulted from either the greater hyperglycemia or the greater hyperinsulinemia seen in the obese subjects or from both. In addition, an altered responsiveness of liver to glucagon could not be demonstrated. Thus, the glucose intolerance of the obese group could not have resulted from an excessive rate of glucagon-stimulated glucose production.

Therefore, it appeared that carbohydrate intolerance was not a consequence of either pancreatic A-cell's or B-cell's failure to respond normally to hyperglycemia. Rather, it resulted from an abnormal hormonal effect on glucose kinetics. These studies were not designed to assess the effect of insulin on glucose production; however, they did demonstrate that the obese individual was markedly resistant to the effect of insulin on glucose utilization. This was presumably the main reason for the glucose intolerance of the obese group. It is probable that, had the B-cells of these obese subjects been hyper-responsive rather than normally responsive to a glucose challenge, they would have secreted enough insulin to overcome this resistance. This group would then have had normal glucose tolerance. This was the case in one of the groups of obese individuals studied by Perley and Kipnis.[30]

In these studies, we have shown that the combination of glucagon infusion and measurements of nonsteady state glucose kinetics is a useful tool to study glucoregulation. Obesity has been used as a model of an insulin resistance state to explore the applicability of this approach to the examination of the basis of carbohydrate intolerance. This method could now be extended to the study of other less well defined states of carbohydrate intolerance.

ACKNOWLEDGMENTS
We are grateful to N. Kovacevic, J. Wilkins, and the nursing and dietary staff of the Clinical Investigation Unit at the Toronto General Hospital for their excellent assistance. The work was supported by the Medical Research Council of Canada. Dr. Morita was a postdoctoral fellow supported by an Ontario provincial health grant.

REFERENCES

1 Cherrington, A., and Vranic, M.: Role of glucagon and insulin in the control of glucose turnover. Metabolism *20*:625–28, 1971.

2 Unger, R. H., and Orci, L.: Physiology and pathophysiology of glucagon. Physiol. Rev. *56*:778–826, 1976.

3 De Bodo, R. C., Steele, R., Altszuler, N., Dunn, A., and Bishop, J.: On the hormonal regulation of carbohydrate metabolism: studies with C^{14} glucose. Recent Prog. Horm. Res. *19*:445–88, 1963.

4 Radziuk, J., Norwich, K., and Vranic, M.: Measurement and validation of non-steady turnover rates with application to the insulin and glucose system. *In* Tracer Methodology and Glucose Turnover Symposium. Fed. Proc. *33*:1855–64, 1974.

5 Radziuk, J., Norwich, K. H., and Vranic, J.: Experimental validation of measurements of glucose turnover in nonsteady state. Am. J. Physiol. *234*:E84–93, 1978.

6 Steiner, G., Morita, S., and Vranic, M.: Tolerance of the grossly obese to physiologic amounts of glucagon. Diabetes *23* (Suppl. 1):383, 1974 (abstract).

7 Steiner, G., Wilson, D., and Vranic, M.: Studies of glucose turnover and renal function in an unusual case of hereditary fructose intolerance. Am. J. Med. *62*:150–53, 1977.

8 Garber, A. J., Cryer, P. E., Santiago. J. V., Haymond, M. W., Pagliara,

A. S., and Kipnis, D. M.: The role of adrenergic mechanisms in the substrate and hormonal response to insulin-induced hypoglycemia in man. J. Clin. Invest. *58*:7–15, 1976.

[9] Seltzer, H. S., Allen, E. W., Herron, A. L., Jr., and Brennan, M. T.: Insulin secretion in response to glycemic stimulus: relation of delayed initial release to carbohydrate intolerance in mild diabetes mellitus J. Clin. Invest. *46*:323–35, 1967.

[10] Felig, P., and Wahren, J.: The liver as site of insulin and glucagon action in normal, diabetic and obese humans. Isr. J. Med. Sci. *11*:528–39, 1975.

[11] DeFronzo, R. A., Soman, V., Sherwin, R. S., Hendler, R., and Felig, P.: Insulin binding to monocytes and insulin action in human obesity, starvation and refeeding. J. Clin. Invest. *62*:204–13, 1978.

[12] Ginsberg, H., Kimmerling, G., Olefsky, J., and Reaven, G. M.: Demonstration of insulin resistance in untreated adult onset diabetic subjects with fasting hyperglycemia. J. Clin. Invest. *55*:454–61, 1975.

[13] Metropolitan Life Insurance Company: New weight standards for men and women. Stat. Bull. Metropol. Life Ins. Co. *40*:1–10, 1959.

[14] Keys, A., Fidanza, F., Kawanen, M. J., Kimura, N., and Taylor, H. J.: Indices of relative weight and obesity. J. Chronic Dis. *25*:329–43, 1972.

[15] Fajans, S., and Conn, J. W.: The early recognition of diabetes mellitus. Ann. N.Y. Acad. Sci. *82*:208–18, 1959.

[16] Remein, Q. R., and Wilkerson, H. L. C.: The efficiency of screening tests for diabetes. J. Chronic Dis. *13*:6–21, 1961.

[17] Klimt, C. R., Knatterud, G. L., Meinert, C. L., and Prout, T. E.: The University Group Diabetes Program: a study of the effect of hypoglycemic agents on vascular complications in patients with adult-onset diabetes. I. Design, methods and baseline characteristics. II. Mortality results. Diabetes *19* (Suppl. 2):474–830, 1970.

[18] Vranic, M., Kawamori, R., Pek, S., Kovacevic, N., and Wrenshall, G. A.: The essentiality of insulin and the role of glucagon in regulating glucose turnover during strenuous exercise. J. Clin. Invest. *57*:245–55, 1976.

[19] Cherrington, A., and Vranic, M.: Effect of interaction between insulin and glucagon on glucose turnover and FFA concentration in normal and depancreatized dogs. Metabolism *23*:729–44, 1974.

[20] Hales, G. N., and Randle, P. J.: Immunoassay of insulin with insulin antibody precipitate. Biochem. J. *88*:137–46, 1968.

[21] Faloona, G. R., and Unger, R. H.: Glucagon. *In* Methods of Hormone Immunoassays. Jaffe, B. M., and Berman, H. R., eds. New York, Academic Press, 1974, pp. 317–30.

[22] Bagdade, J. D., Bierman, E. L., and Porte, D., Jr.: The significance of basal insulin levels in the evaluation of the insulin response to glucose in diabetic and non-diabetic subjects. J. Clin. Invest. *46*:1549–57, 1967.

[23] Felig, P., Wahren, J., Sherwin, R., and Hendler, R.: Insulin, glucagon and somatostatin in normal physiology and diabetes mellitus. Diabetes *25*:1091–99, 1976.

[24] Bomboy, J., Lewis, S., Lacy, W., Sinclair-Smith, B., and Liljenquist, J.: Transient stimulatory effect of sustained hyperglucagonemia on splanchnic glucose production in normal and diabetic man. Diabetes *26*:177–84, 1977.

[25] Rizza, R. A., and Gerich, J. E.: Persistent effect of sustained hyperglucagonemia on glucose production in man. J. Clin. Endocrinol. Metab. *48*:352–55, 1979.

[26] Soeldner, J. S., Gleason, R. E., Rojas, L., Kahn, C. B., and Marble, A.: Serum insulin and blood glucose relationships in genetic prediabetic males with normal glucose tolerance. *In* Diabetes, Osterman, J., and Milner, R. D. G., eds. Amsterdam, Excerpta Medica Foundation, ICS *172*:505–14, 1969.

[27] Cherrington, A. D., Williams, P. E., and Harris, M. S.: Relationship between the plasma glucose level and glucose utilization in the conscious dog. Metabolism *27*:787–91, 1978.

[28] Vranic, M., Radzuik, J., and Cherrington, A.: The role of glucagon and insulin in the glucoregulatory system as assessed by tracer methods. *In* Regulation and Control in Physiological Systems. Iberall, A. S., and Guyton, A. C., eds. International Federation of Autonomic Control. Pittsburgh, Instrument Society of America, 1973, pp. 487–90.

[29] Davis, B. M., Bernstein, R., Kolterman, O., Olefsky, J. M., and Reaven, G. M.: Defect in glucose removal in nonketotic diabetic patients with fasting hyperglycemia. Diabetes *28*:32–34, 1979.

[30] Perley, M., and Kipnis, D. M.: Plasma insulin responses to glucose and tolbutamide of normal weight and obese diabetic and nondiabetic subjects. Diabetes *15*:867–74, 1966.

[31] Rabinowitz, D., and Zierler, K. L.: Forearm metabolism in obesity and in response to intra-arterial insulin. J. Clin. Invest. *41*:2173–81, 1962.

[32] Olefsky, J. M., Reaven, G. M., and Farquhar, J. W.: Effects of weight reduction on obesity: studies of carbohydrate and lipid metabolism. J. Clin. Invest. *53*:64–76, 1974.

Ketonuria in Pregnancy—With Special Reference to Calorie-restricted Food Intake in Obese Diabetics

E. J. COETZEE, W. P. U. JACKSON, AND P. A. BERMAN

SUMMARY

Early morning ketonuria, as judged by Ketostix testing, occurred in 19% of urine samples from insulin-independent diabetic pregnant women eating 1000 calorie diets, in 14% from diabetics on higher calorie diets, and in 7% of urines from nondiabetic pregnant women. Ketostix test was never found to be positive in blood, even when it was 2+ in urine samples, and acetoacetate levels were always below 1 mmol/L.

Enzymatic estimations of acetoacetate (AA) and beta-hydroxybutyrate (BB) in urine and plasma samples revealed (1) no significant differences in range or mean between the groups receiving different restricted diets or full diets, the highest value observed for plasma AA being 0.34 mmol/L; (2) that Ketostix became positive at a concentration of AA above 1 mmol/L and that such a value in urine corresponded to plasma levels of between 0.06 and 0.1 mmol/L, i.e., double the normal; and (3) a 50–100-fold increase in urine AA when blood levels exceeded 0.08 mmol/L.

Neonates born to diabetic mothers with ketonuria had no fetal distress or asphyxia neonatorum. The lowest Apgar score at 5 min was 8; 80% of neonates had a score of 10. Hence, positive Ketostix tests in urine samples do not indicate toxic levels in the blood, and a 1000 calorie diet for obese pregnant diabetics appears to be safe as regards neonatal outcome. DIABETES *29*:177–181, March, 1980.

It is well known that diabetic ketoacidosis in a pregnant woman seriously endangers the life of the fetus. In this condition, the maternal serum concentrations of the ketone bodies acetoacetate (AA) and beta-hydroxybutyrate (BB) are 100–200 times greater than normal, i.e., about 10–20 mmol/L.[1] The resultant depression of cerebral function cannot be accounted for by the acidosis or the BB alone,[2] though AA at levels of 10 mmol/L may depress cerebral oxygen utilization.[3]

The majority of pregnant diabetics managed at Groote Schuur Hospital have mild metabolic disturbances and are of the non-insulin-dependent, adult-onset type, whether their diabetes was previously known or arose during gestation.[4] Some cases are of long duration, some have fasting blood glucose levels of about 200 mg/dl, and the overall late fetal loss is about 25% for untreated mothers.[5] More than half of these patients are obese (more than 20% above standard body weight, based on Kemsley's tables[6]) and their raised blood glucose levels can be controlled by a 1000-calorie reducing diet.[4] The question may be asked whether such calorie restriction could produce significant ketosis and endanger fetal well-being, especially in view of a report suggesting that ketonuria during pregnancy is associated with a lower IQ in young children.[7]

We have accordingly attempted to (A) compare the frequency of ketonuria in various diet groups; (B) assess the blood ketone levels in various diet groups, with and without ketonuria; (C) relate urine and blood ketone levels; and (D) relate fetal outcome to ketonuria.

SUBJECTS AND METHODS

1. The frequency of positive Ketostix tests made by nurses on fasting (early morning) urine specimens was analyzed in the case of all 146 patients in one of the maternity wards of Groote Schuur Hospital over a 3-mo period.

2. Plasma Ketostix readings were taken in the ward in 45 instances after urine Ketostix tests had been found positive.

3. The subjects in this separate study were 69 pregnant non-insulin-dependent diabetics and nondiabetics admitted to one of the maternity wards during the past 18 mo. All subjects had normal blood urea concentrations. The obese subjects were given a 1000-calorie diet, and nonobese diabetics between 1400 and 1800 calories, depending upon various factors (1600 calories is the average intake of our hospital's nonobese pregnant population on a free diet). Blood concentrations of AA and BB were measured often on

From the Departments of Obstetrics and Gynaecology, Medicine and Chemical Pathology, Groote Schuur Hospital and University of Cape Town, Observatory, South Africa.
Address reprint requests to Dr. E. J. Coetzee, Department of Obstetrics and Gynaecology, University of Cape Town Medical School, Rep. of South Africa.
Received for publication 22 June and in revised form 4 October 1979.

TABLE 1
Positive Ketostix on fasting urine in pregnant women during a 3-mo period

	Diabetic Non-insulin-dependent			
	On 1000 calories	On ± 1600 calories	J.O.D.	Nondiabetic
Number of patients	18	17	4	107
Number of patients showing positive tests	11	7	4	25
Total number of tests	250	243	66	501
Tests positive	48	34	5	33
Per cent positive	19	14	8	7

several occasions in the same patient, and they were correlated with simultaneous urine Ketostix tests. Approximately three-quarters of tests were performed on patients in the third trimester in each group and one-quarter during the second trimester. The fetal morbidity was recorded with particular attention to fetal distress, Apgar scores, and asphyxia neonatorum.

4. Laboratory estimations of AA and BB were made on blood and urine specimens from patients, after an overnight fast, often on several occasions. Similar studies were made on normal volunteers from the department of chemical pathology, after different periods of fasting, in order to observe a definite rise in blood ketone levels in normal subjects.

Blood and urine samples for ketone body measurements were taken directly into tubes containing perchlorate and were stored at 4°C; estimations were performed the same day or at the latest on the next day. Measurement was by enzymatic NAD-linked assays, using purified beta-hydroxybutyrate dehydrogenase made from Rhodopseudomonas spheroides, obtained from Boehringer-Mannheim.[8] The end-point determination uses the extinction coefficient of NADH to calculate the concentrations. Weighed-out standards of acetoacetate and beta-hydroxybutyrate were used as recovery controls. For acetoacetate, these varied between 80 and 85%, and for beta-hydroxybutyrate, between 85 and 95%.

RESULTS

1. In the 3-mo survey of all early morning urine tests in 18 patients on 1000-calorie intake, ketonuria (by Ketostix) was recorded in 11 patients in 48 tests out of a total of 250 (19%); among 17 diabetic patients on higher calorie intakes, the test was positive in seven patients, in 14% of a total of 243 tests; among four insulin-dependent diabetics, it was positive at times in all four patients, in 8% of 66 tests; and, among 107 nondiabetic patients, it was positive in 25 subjects, in 7% of 501 tests (Table 1).

2. After 2+ ketones had been found in a patient's urine by nurses' Ketostix testing, the *plasma* Ketostix was immediately studied in 45 instances. It was never positive (i.e., the plasma AA level was always below 1 mmol/L, as confirmed by our figures below, which showed that the highest plasma AA measured in these pregnant patients was 0.34 mmol/L).

3. Normal nonpregnant levels (after fasting overnight) were established as: blood AA, 0–0.05 mmol/L, and blood BB, 0–0.15 mmol/L (these values are similar to those quoted by other authors[9]).

Of 36 obese patients seen during the past 18 mo taking 1000 calorie diets, whose blood was drawn for ketone estimations in the fasting state, 14 showed positive Ketostix reactions in their urines at the time of the first blood estimation. The mean AA and BB values of the whole group and of those who were urine-Ketostix-negative and positive are shown in Table 2. Data are also shown for 23 patients on higher calorie intakes, of whom 7 had ketonuria, and for 10 nondiabetic pregnant women, of whom 2 had ketonuria. There was no statistically significant difference between the values obtained in diabetics and in nondiabetics.

The 22 obese patients (on 1000-calorie diets) who did *not* have ketonuria at the time of measuring the blood ketone concentrations had a mean age of 32.9 yr, a mean height of 158 cm, a mean weight at 30 wk of 89.0 kg (range, 69–109), and a mean weight at term of 90.6 kg. Twenty-one of these have been delivered at the time of writing. The mean gestational age of these neonates was 38 wk (range, 34–40 wk) and their mean birth weight was 3389 g (range, 2300–4640 g). The lowest Apgar score at 5 min was 8, and 81% of the neonates had scores of 10. One infant was recorded as needing intubation and assisted respiration, but had fully recovered by 5 min.

The 14 obese mothers in whom ketonuria was recorded had a mean age of 32.1 yr, a mean height of 160 cm, a mean weight at 30 wk of 92.7 kg (range, 71–139) and at term of 92.4 kg. The mothers produced 13 neonates with a mean gestational age of 38 wk (range, 36–40 wk) and a mean birth weight of 3463 g (range, 2850–5300 g). The lowest 5 min Apgar score was 8 and 69% had a score of 10. As-

TABLE 2
Fasting plasma ketone levels in pregnant women (Mean values, with standard deviations, in mmol/L)

	Diabetic		Nondiabetic free diet
	on 1000 calories	on ± 1600 calories	
Total patients	36	23	10
Acetoacetate	0.084 (±0.06)	0.058 (±0.04)	0.068 (±0.05)
β-hydroxybutyrate	0.22 (±0.18)	0.23 (±0.21)	0.17 (±0.21)
Patients with negative Ketostix	22	16	8
Acetoacetate	0.062 (±0.03)	0.04 (±0.02)	0.05 (±0.02)
β-hydroxybutyrate	0.13 (±0.12)	0.19 (±0.20)	0.10 (±0.05)
Patients with positive Ketostix	14	7	2
Acetoacetate	0.116 (±0.08)	0.102 (±0.02)	0.149
β-hydroxybutyrate	0.36 (±0.18)	0.34 (±0.17)	0.46

phyxia neonatorum and fetal distress were not recorded. One mother aborted.

Among the 23 patients of normal weight who were receiving less restrictive diets, there were 16 patients who had *no* ketonuria recorded. Their mean age was 36.5 yr, mean height was 155.4 cm, mean weight at 30 wk 69.4 kg (range, 53–75 kg), and at term 70.3 kg. Of the 16 neonates (one twin) already delivered, the mean gestational age was 37.6 wk (range, 35–39 wk) and the mean birth weight (excluding the twins) was 3109 g (2200–4260 g). Asphyxia neonatorum was observed in two neonates, fetal distress in one, and two infants had 5 min Apgar scores of 5.

The mean age of the seven patients of normal weight in whom ketonuria was recorded was 27.4 yr, mean height was 161 cm, mean weight gain at 30 wk was 69.0 kg (range, 58–88 kg), and at term 70.6 kg. Seven neonates (one twin) have been delivered from this group. The mean gestational age was 36.8 wk (34–38 wk) and the mean birth weight (twins excluded) was 2908 g (range, 2070–3310 g). All the infants had 5-min Apgar scores of 10.

4. From the relationship between blood and urine AA and BB estimations and Ketostix readings on urine in both pregnant and nonpregnant subjects (Tables 2 and 3 and Figures 1 and 2), the following generalizations appear:

(A) Ketostix indicates the presence of AA in urine by the nitroprusside reaction at levels greater than 1 mmol/L (i.e., a level that develops when the blood AA level is twice normal). When the blood concentration of the total ketone bodies (AA and BB) reached 1 mmol/L, urine Ketostix tests were positive in 100% of cases (Figure 1).

(B) A massive progressive increase in urine levels of AA

TABLE 3
Blood and urine acetoacetate and β-ohbutyrate in fasting state

Blood acetoacetate (mmol/L)	Urine acetoacetate (mmol/L)	Blood β-ohbutyrate (mmol/L)	Urine β-ohbutyrate (mmol/L)	Blood BB/AA ratio
Pregnant women				
0.012	0.08	0.070	0.26	5.8
0.016	0.02	0.099	0.10	6.2
0.022	0.03	0.080	0.19	3.9
0.035*	0.14	0.128	0.21	3.7
0.038	0.05	0.084	0.21	2.2
0.046	0.05	0.088	0.16	1.9
0.049	0.04	0.153	0.12	3.1
0.053	0.03	0.139	0.06	2.6
0.059	0.05	0.139	0.17	2.4
0.066	0.02	0.121	0.17	1.8
0.067	0.05	0.168	0.10	2.5
0.068	5.30†	0.420	5.50	6.2
0.078	0.02	0.178	0.14	2.3
0.079	0.02	0.202	0.05	2.6
0.081	0.07	0.112	0.20	1.4
0.098*	1.98	0.151	1.45	1.5
0.114	11.60 †	0.530	7.92	4.6
0.123	1.06 †	0.459	1.02	3.7
0.134	4.19 †	0.420	3.38	3.1
0.171	4.24 †	0.542	4.76	3.2
0.176	4.12 †	0.616	2.43	3.5
0.235	6.96 †	0.840	3.83	3.6
0.263	4.08 †	0.944	3.51	3.6
Normal control subjects, fasting up to 62 h				
0.016	0.02	0.033	0.04	2.1
0.018	0.02	0.062	0.03	3.4
0.019	0.02	0.025	0.01	1.3
0.024	0.02	0.097	0.05	4.0
0.032	0.04	0.026	0.07	0.8
0.071	3.35 †	0.416	1.75	5.9
0.078	0.04	0.183	0.08	2.3
0.078	2.20 †	0.310	1.36	4.0
0.086	6.65 †	0.558	4.40	6.5
0.095	0.03	0.278	0.09	2.9
0.102	1.33 †	0.465	0.68	4.6
0.106	0.04	0.258	0.05	2.4
0.106	0.53	0.275	0.31	2.6
0.136	6.29 †	0.455	2.61	3.3
0.122	11.30 †	0.710	20.60	3.9
0.197	3.54 †	0.719	1.78	3.6
0.251	2.73 †	0.713	1.86	2.8
0.416	7.75 †	1.280	9.08	3.1

* Nondiabetic.
† Ketostix.

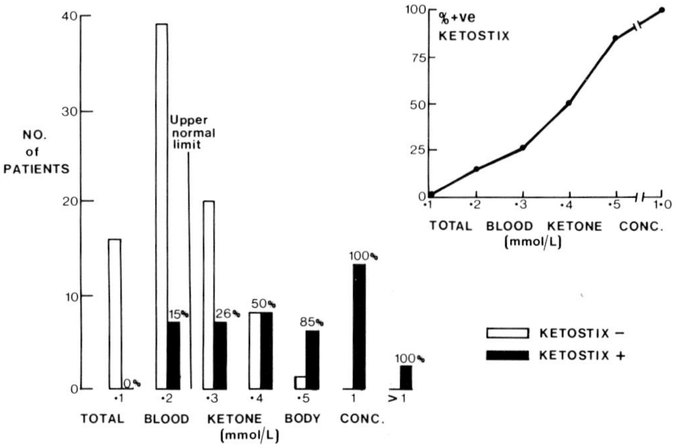

FIGURE 1. Frequency of ketonuria with increasing total blood ketone levels in pregnant patients. Total blood ketone concentration indicates the sum of acetoacetate and beta-hydroxybutyrate concentrations. Note that all subjects have positive Ketostix test in urine before blood level of ketones reaches 1 mmol/L.

FIGURE 2. Correlation of blood and urine acetoacetate concentrations. The values shown here are taken from Table 3. Note marked increase in urinary AA at a blood level between 0.05 and 0.1. All urine AA levels are below 0.2 or above 1.0.

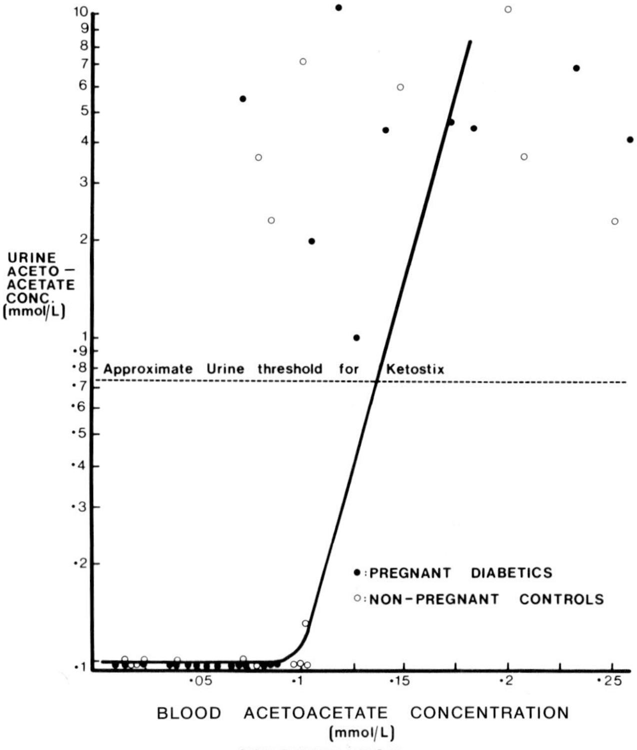

occurs when blood levels reach 0.06–0.1 mmol/L. The increase in urine AA may reach 50–100-fold with a rise of AA in the blood of only twofold (Figure 2). The same trend occurs with BB (Table 3). Thus, the blood level at which AA starts to rise steeply in the urine lies between 0.06 and 0.1 mmol/L, but never far from the limit of the normal range for blood. Further, there appears to be little or no correlation between urine and blood AA concentrations above this level (Figure 2).

(C) There was no apparent difference between pregnant diabetic women, pregnant nondiabetic women, and normal controls as regards the renal handling of ketone bodies.

DISCUSSION

The oft-quoted study of reduced intelligence relating to ketonuria during pregnancy was based on reports from many different hospitals of nurses' single urine tests made on patients on the day of delivery.[7] No measurements of serum ketone levels or of blood sugar measurements were made. It seemed difficult to imagine that such records could produce valid conclusions. It seems more difficult now that it is apparent that the urine ketone levels bear little relation to blood levels once the acetoacetate values reach values as low as 0.1 mmol/L, which is about double the normal and 100 times less than is needed to depress cerebral oxygen utilization.[3]

Although ketonuria, as judged by positive Ketostix tests in the early morning urines, was found in 19% of tests on the diabetics on reducing diets, this was only slightly more frequent than in diabetics allowed their usual higher calorie intake (14%), while as many as 7% of the tests on nondiabetics taking completely free diets were positive. Since simultaneous plasma Ketostix tests were never positive, it would appear that the corresponding blood levels of AA never exceeded 1 mmol/L. In fact, in all our blood ketone tests, the highest blood level discovered in nearly 200 estimations was 0.34 mmol/L, with a corresponding BB level of 0.39. The highest BB was 0.94 mmol/L and this patient also had the highest total keto-acids, i.e., 1.2 mmol/L. No measurable change in base excess or pH would therefore be found, and this must surely be a nontoxic level. (Huckabee[10] demonstrated that a change of 5 mmol/L is needed to alter the acid-base balance.)

Diabetic patients on 1000 calories had minimally higher mean blood AA levels (0.08 mmol/L) than pregnant nondiabetics on uncontrolled diets (0.07 mmol/L) and than diabetics on higher restricted calorie intakes (0.06 mmol/L, Table 2). These differences were small and were all slightly above the normal nonpregnant range (below 0.05 mmol/L).

Thus, ketonuria in these circumstances does not herald ketoacidosis.[11] Small changes in blood ketones may be associated with massive ketonuria and strongly positive urine Ketostix tests, the blood levels being well below those associated with ketoacidosis.[12] Yet, in true diabetic ketoacidosis, with blood AA levels 100 fold above normal (i.e., 5 mmol/L), the Ketostix test on urine gives the same positive result.

Judging by the weight changes between 30 wk of gestation and term, it is evident that not all patients on "1000 calorie" diets really complied with this. The obese mothers who showed ketonuria actually lost a mean of 0.3 kg, while those in whom ketonuria was not recorded gained 1.6 kg. On restricted but higher calorie diets, those with ketonuria recorded gained 1.6 kg, those in whom ketonuria was not recorded gained 0.9 kg. Mean weight gain in nondiabetics on unrestricted diet was 2.9 kg over the same period of time. While it is evident that 1000 calorie diets are more likely to be associated with Ketostix-positive ketonuria than are more liberal intakes, we question the significance of this observation.

At blood concentrations of AA and BB below a certain level (i.e., about 0.08 mmol/L for AA and about 0.4 mmol/L for BB) the urinary losses are slight (below 0.1 mmol/L for AA and below 1 mmol/L for BB). When these "thresholds" are exceeded, there is a sudden, manyfold increase in urinary excretion (Figure 2). Thus a massive increase in urinary AA is seen at blood levels varying between 0.06 and 0.1—in all cases close to the upper limit of normal (0.05 mmol/L).

The observation that, after an overnight fast, blood ketone body concentrations are about threefold higher in pregnant women than in nonpregnant women has been published already.[13] Since ketone bodies can be used by the brain (including fetal brain) as natural fuel,[14] and there is evidence that the synthesis of essential cerebral lipids occurs from these substances,[15] it is inconceivable that the blood levels reached during calorie-restricted diets could cause harm. Kraus and Stumpf[16] calculated that ketone bodies account for 13% of the total cerebral oxygen consumption at 2 and 4 wk of neonatal life and thought that this percentage would be even higher in the first week of life. Nevertheless, our policy in patients who show repeated positive Ketostix tests on fasting urine is to add or increase a late-night carbohydrate-containing snack.

The obese mothers in group 2, Ketostix-positive and Ketostix-negative, delivered infants with a mean birth weight of 3463 and 3389 g, respectively, while the mothers with normal weight delivered infants with a mean birth weight of 2908 and 3109 g, respectively, in the case of Ketostix-positive and Ketostix-negative groups. Heavier mothers, therefore, still had heavier children than normal weight mothers, despite the calorie restriction, and there was no difference between the Ketostix-positive and Ketostix-negative groups as judged by birth weights. There was no fetal distress, asphyxia neonatorum, or low 5-min Apgar scores in the neonates of the Ketostix-positive group or in those mothers who had had plasma ketone levels above the normal range. All these untoward events occurred in neonates of Ketostix-negative mothers, who thus appeared to do less well than neonates of mothers who showed ketonuria! We presume this is a random event, but at least it indicates an absence of damage connected with Ketostix-positive ketonuria.

Recently Naeye[17] has suggested that low IQ values and psychomotor impairment may be a result of amniotic fluid infection syndrome rather than of ketosis, as noninfected infants of ketotic gestations had normal IQ values and no excess of neurologic abnormalities at 4 and 7 yr of age.

We therefore believe, on the above evidence, that 1000 calories is a safe intake during pregnancy in obese persons, more desirable from the patient's point of view, and that occasional positive Ketostix tests can be disregarded.

ACKNOWLEDGMENTS

This work was supported by a grant from the Medical Research Council of South Africa to the Endocrine/Diabetic Research Group and forms part of the program of this unit.

We wish to thank Professor W. Gevers of the Medical Biochemistry Department, University of Cape Town, for helpful criticism concerning this paper.

We acknowledge grants from Messrs. Hoechst, S. A., Boehringer-Mannheim, Rona Laboratories, and Propan Ethicals (Pty) Ltd.

We are grateful for the excellent service of the Neonatal Unit. We also thank H. A. Coetzee, A. Mason, and Sr. J. Allan for such splendid assistance.

REFERENCES

[1] Oakley, W. S., Pyke, D. A., and Taylor, K. W.: *In* Clinical Diabetes and Its Biochemical Basis. Oxford, Blackwell, 1968, p. 430.

[2] Daughaday, W. H.: Diabetic acidosis. *In* Diabetes, chap. 37. Williams, R. H., Ed. New York, Paul Hoeber, 1960, pp. 515–48.

[3] Kety, S. S., Polis, B. D., Nadler, C. S., and Schmidt, C. F.: The blood flow and oxygen consumption of the human brain in diabetic acidosis and coma. J. Clin. Invest. *37*:500–10, 1948.

[4] Coetzee, E. J., and Jackson, W. P. U.: Diabetes newly diagnosed during pregnancy. A 4 year experience at Groote Schuur Hospital. S. Afr. Med. J. *56*:467–75, 1979.

[5] Coetzee, E. J., and Jackson, W. P. U.: Metformin in management of pregnant insulin-independent diabetics. Diabetologia *16*:241–45, 1979.

[6] Kemsley, W. F. F.: Body weight at different ages and heights. Ann. Hum. Genet. *16*:316–34, 1952.

[7] Churchill, J. A., Berendes, H. W., and Nemore, J.: Neuropsychological deficits in children of diabetic mothers. Am. J. Obstet. Gynecol. *105*:257–68, 1969.

[8] Bergmeyer, H. U., and Gawehn, K.: *In* Methods of Enzymatic Analysis, second edit. New York, Academic Press, 1974, pp. 1836–43.

[9] Wieland, O.: Ketogenesis and its regulation. Adv. Metab. Disord. *3*:1–47, 1968.

[10] Huckabee, W. E.: Abnormal resting blood lactate. Am. J. Med. *30*:837–39, 1961.

[11] Watkins, P. J., Fitzgerald, M. G., and Malind, J. M.: Inter-relationships of blood sugar and ketones in insulin-treated diabetes. Br. Med. J. *4*:648–51, 1969.

[12] Watkins, P. J., and Fitzgerald, M. G.: An evaluation of Ketostix strips. Diabetes *17*:398–401, 1968.

[13] Felig, P., and Lynch, V.: Starvation in human pregnancy: hypoglycemia, hypoinsulinemia and hyperketonemia. Science *170*:990–92, 1970.

[14] Hawkins, R. A., Williamson, D. H., and Krebs, H. A.: Ketone body utilization by adult and suckling rat brain in vivo. Biochem. J. *122*:13–18, 1971.

[15] Patel, M. S., Johnson, C. A., Rajan, R., and Owen, O. E.: The metabolism of ketone bodies in developing human brain: development of ketone body utilizing enzymes and ketone bodies as precursors for lipid synthesis. J. Neurochem. *25*:905, 1975.

[16] Kraus, H., and Stumpf, B.: Interrelationship of glucose and ketone body metabolism in brain during early infancy. Regulatory role of pyruvate dehydrogenase. *In* Biochemical and Clinical Aspects of Ketone Body Metabolism. Söling, H-D, and Seufert, C-D., Eds. Stuttgart, George Thieme Publishers, 1978, pp. 233–41.

[17] Naeye, R. L.: The outcome of diabetic pregnancies: a prospective study. *In* Pregnancy Metabolism, Diabetes and the Fetus; Ciba Foundation Symposium 63. Amsterdam, Oxford, New York, Excerpta Medica, 1979, pp. 227–41.

Reduced Perikaryal Volume of Lower Motor and Primary Sensory Neurons in Early Experimental Diabetes

P. SIDENIUS AND J. JAKOBSEN

SUMMARY

The volume of nerve cell bodies of the anterior horn of the fifth lumbar segment and of the fifth lumbar dorsal root ganglion were measured by stereological methods in rats with 4-wk duration of streptozotocin diabetes and in age-matched controls. The perikaryal volume of motor and sensory neurons was reduced by 18% in diabetic rats and a shift between the number of A- and B-cells was observed in the dorsal root ganglion.

The findings are in accordance with our earlier observation of reduced axonal size of myelinated fibers in the common peroneal nerve. Furthermore, the data lead us to suppose that the nervous system abnormalities in early diabetes are not exclusively restricted to the peripheral nerves. DIABETES 29:182–186, March 1980.

Abnormalities of peripheral nerve function are present very early in juvenile diabetes mellitus. At the time of diagnosis, slowing of the never conduction and preservation of peripheral nerve function for a longer period during ischemia have been demonstrated.[1–3] Both abnormalities are present in rats after a few weeks duration of streptozotocin diabetes.[4,5]

In our laboratory the streptozotocin-diabetic rat has been used as a model in structural and physiological studies of early peripheral nerve changes. In previous studies we have found that the fibers of peripheral nerves are thinner than normal, mostly due to a thinning of the axon.[5–7] We have recently shown a distinct change of the axonal transport of glycoproteins, consisting of a decrease of the retrograde flux.[8,9]

We have also pursued the morphometric studies by examining the size of the cell bodies associated with the motor and sensory fibers of peripheral nerves.

The present paper reports the results of a morphometric study of the anterior horn cells and the spinal ganglion cells of the fifth lumbar segment in streptozotocin-diabetic rats.

MATERIALS AND METHODS

Male Wistar rats, 24 wk of age and weighing between 350 and 450 g, were allocated for a diabetic group and a control group. The animals were raised on a standard rat chow and had free access to the diet during the experiment. Diabetes was induced by intravenous injection of 40 mg streptozotocin per kg body wt. Blood samples were taken from a tail vein and glucose was measured by Dextrostix and an Ames Reflectance Meter. Only rats having a blood glucose value above 250 mg/dl on the day following streptozotocin injection were included in the study. The diabetic state was estimated 2 and 4 wk later by measuring 24-h urine output as well as blood glucose.

After a 4-wk experimental period, a group of 12 diabetic rats and 12 controls were selected at random for the morphological study. For tissue preparation, osmolarity of fixatives and buffer solutions were controlled by freezing-point determination and maintained constant. Fixation was carried out by whole body perfusion with 0.5 L of a buffered paraformaldehyde-glutaraldehyde solution delivered during 10 min at 150 mm Hg. The spinal cord and the fifth lumbar ganglia were removed and immersed in the paraformaldehyde-glutaraldehyde fixative overnight. The fifth segment of the lumbar enlargement of the spinal cord was then cut into four 0.6–1.0-mm-thick transverse sections. To visualize white and gray matter, the sections were stained with 2% osmium tetroxide for 10 min. The anterolateral quadrant of both anterior horns was cut out from each of the four transverse sections. Subsequently, the small cubes of anterior horns and ganglia were postfixed in osmium tetroxide for 4 h, rinsed in the corresponding buffer, dehydrated in graded acetone, and embedded in Vestopal.

One animal was excluded from the diabetic group because tissues were obtained from less than three of the four

From the Second University Clinic of Internal Medicine and Institute of Pathology, Kommunehospitalet, DK-8000 Aarhus C, Denmark.
Address reprint requests to J. Jakobsen, Institute of Anatomy, Universitetsparken, DK-8000 Aarhus C, Denmark.
Received for publication 2 July 1979.

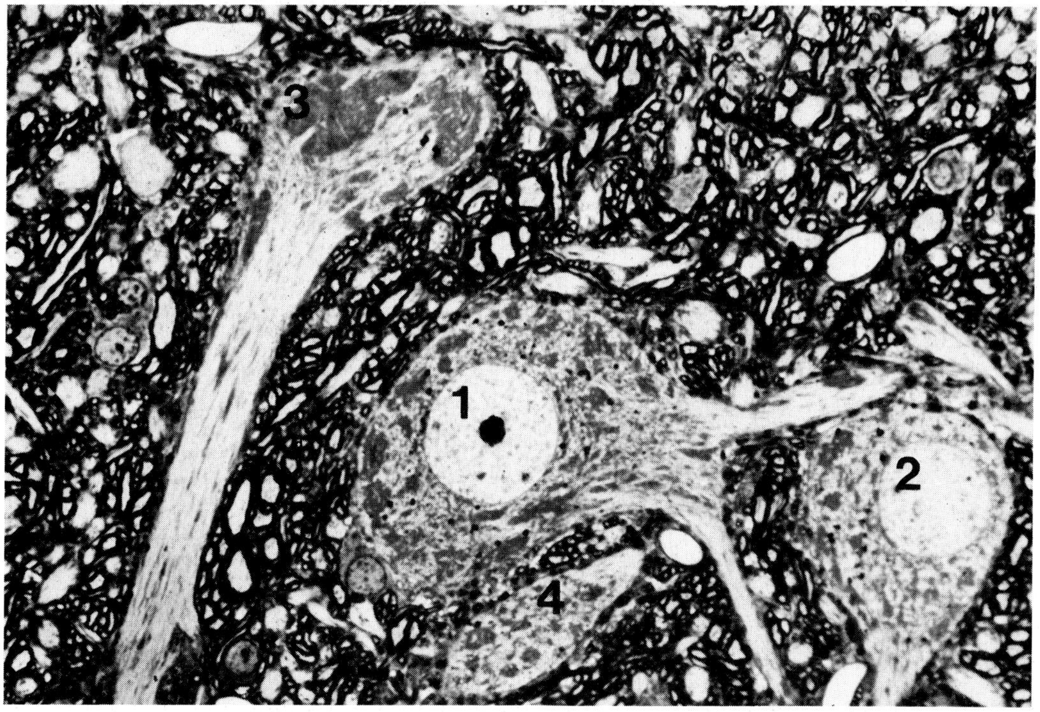

FIGURE 1. Micrograph of four nerve cell profiles of the anterior horn of the fifth lumbar segment in a normal rat (semithin toluidine-stained section at magnification ×880). One profile contains nucleus as well as nucleolus (1), another is without nucleolus (2), and two profiles lack nuclei (3 and 4). All the various profiles were included for the measurement. For determination of perikaryal size, axon and dendrites were excluded by drawing a line in continuation with the outer limits of the cell body across the outrunners.

0.6–1.0-mm-thick transverse sections of the fifth lumbar segment of the spinal cord.

Morphometry of anterior horn cells. Semithin sections (0.1–0.2 μm) of the randomly oriented cubes of anterior horn cells were cut on an LKB Ultrotome, stained with toluidine blue, and photographed at a final magnification of ×830. The anterolateral group, which almost exclusively consists of alpha motor neurons, was outlined and all nerve cell profiles within the group (also those devoid of nuclei) were included for the measurements. The tissues were also well preserved at the electronmicroscopic level. In Figure 1 a group of anterior horn cells are shown. The perikaryon was defined as nerve cell cytoplasm not including axon and dendrites. The selection of tissues, the outlining of cell groups and cell bodies, and all measurements were performed by the authors who were unaware of the identity of the specimens.

The size of the nerve cells was obtained according to stereological techniques.[10] The nuclei of anterior horn cells approximate spheres. The mean nuclear volume, therefore, can be estimated from diameter measurements.* For all individual nuclear profiles the two largest diameters at right angle to each other were measured in halves of millimeter and averaged. From the mean profile radius ($\bar{r}$) of each animal, the mean nuclear volume was calculated from the formula $\bar{V}_N = 4/3\pi \cdot [\sqrt{(3/2)} \cdot \bar{r}]^3$.[10] Since every nerve cell has one and only one nucleus, the mean perikaryal volume can be obtained from the mean volume of the nuclei multiplied by the ratio between the perikaryal and nuclear volumes: ($\bar{V}_P = \bar{V}_N \cdot P_P/P_N$). The fractional volumes of nuclei and perikaryons were estimated with a point-counting technique using grids with point densities of one point per 13 and 115 μm^2, respectively.

To obtain information about the amounts of nucleoli and Nissl substance (granular endoplasmic reticulum), their volume fractions were also estimated by point counting using grids with densities of one point per 2 and 210 μm^2. The mean nucleolar volume was calculated as the mean nucleus volume multiplied by the volume ratio between nucleoli and nuclei:

$$\bar{V}_{(nucleoli)} = \bar{V}_{(nuclei)} \cdot [P_{(nucleoli)}/P_{(nuclei)}].$$

The mean volume of the Nissl substance was similarly estimated using the perikaryon as the reference volume.

Morphometry of dorsal root ganglion cells. From each animal, a single semithin section of the randomly oriented ganglia including more than 50 nerve cell profiles was projected onto a screen at a final magnification of ×333. Light A-cells with granular cytoplasm and dark B-cells with a more homogeneous cytoplasm were identified, and counting and calculation procedures were performed separately for each of these cell populations. In Figure 2 a group of dorsal root ganglion cells is shown. In two diabetic animals and one control, less than 50 nerve cells per section were found; these animals were excluded. Diameters of nuclei were measured in halves of millimeter, and volumes of nuclei and perikayrons were estimated with point densities of one point per 80 and 720 μm^2, respectively, as described above.

The number of myelinated nerve fibers in the mixed common peroneal nerve is unchanged in rats with a similar degree and duration of diabetes as those used in the present experiment.[6] It is therefore assumed that the number of nerve cells in the fifth lumbar dorsal root ganglion is unchanged in the diabetic rats of the present study. Based on this assumption, the mean cell volume of A- and B-cells

* Abbreviations used in the formulas are: $\bar{V}$, mean volume; P, number of test points; and N, number. The subscripts refer to the structure in question.

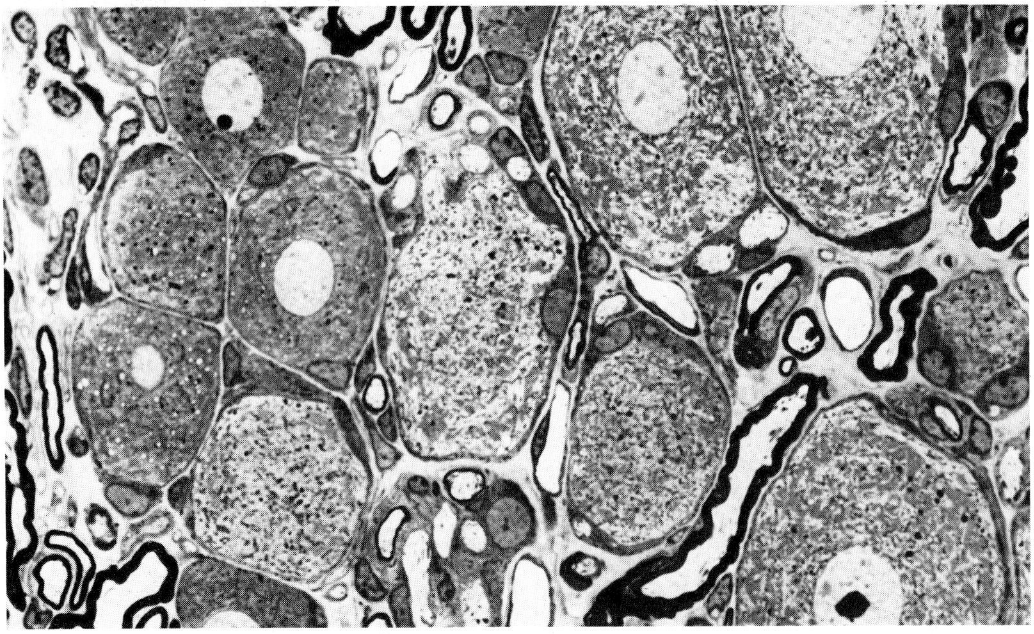

FIGURE 2. Micrograph of a group of nerve cell profiles of the fifth lumbar dorsal root ganglion (semithin toluidine-stained section at magnification ×880). Profiles were divided into light granular A-cells and dark B-cells with a more homogeneous cytoplasm.

taken together can be calculated. The ratio between the number of A- and B-cells can be obtained from the equation $P_A/P_B = (N_A \cdot \bar{V}_A)/(N_B \cdot \bar{V}_B)$, in accordance with the assumption $N_A + N_B$ is held constant. From these two equations the percentage of A- and B-cells can be calculated. Subsequently, the mean cell volume for all ganglion cells equals $(N_A\% \cdot \bar{V}_A + N_B\% \cdot \bar{V}_B) \cdot 0.01$.

RESULTS

The diabetic rats all lost weight (mean loss 63 g, range 25–115 g), whereas the mean body weight was increased in the control group (17 g, range 5–30 g). Blood glucose values varied between 72 and 88 mg/dl in 10 controls (mean = 81). In the diabetic rats the values varied between 280 and 420 mg/dl (mean = 356) 24 h after the injection of streptozotocin and between 310 and 520 mg/dl (mean = 404) at the end of the experiment. The mean 24-h urine output in the diabetic group was 145 ml (range 100–180) and 135 ml (range 90–190) 14 and 28 days, respectively, after the induction of diabetes.

No qualitative histologic signs of nerve cell degeneration or of cell loss were observed.

For the calculation of perikaryal volume it was assumed that the nuclei approximate spheres. The ratio between the two largest diameters at right angle to each other was calculated for each animal. In the control group the value for anterior horn cells was 0.90 ± 0.02 (mean ± SD) and in the diabetic group 0.90 ± 0.02. For the A-cells of the dorsal root ganglions, the ratios were 0.85 ± 0.04 in controls and 0.84 ± 0.04 in the diabetic rats, and the corresponding values for the B-cells were 0.87 ± 0.03 and 0.87 ± 0.02. No differences were observed of the variance of the diameter ratios between the two groups.

In Figure 3 the distribution of profile diameters of the motor nuclei are shown for the control and diabetic groups. There are no statistical differences between the two groups and the distributions approximate those of spheres all of identical volume cut by random sections. The same is true for the distributions of the nuclei diameters of A- and B-cells of the dorsal root ganglion.

Anterior horn cells. In Table 1 the mean volumes of nucleoli, nuclei, and perikaryons are shown for the ventrolateral group of anterior horn cells of the fifth lumbar segment in the control group and in the diabetic group. The perikaryal volume was reduced by 18% in the diabetic group whereas the reductions in nucleus and nucleolus volume were statistically insignificant.

In Figure 4 the individual values of the perikaryal volumes are shown for each animal of both groups.

The absolute amount of Nissl substance was 12,720 ± 3190 μm^3 in the control group and 10,780 ± 2490 μm^3 in the diabetic group, the difference being statistically

FIGURE 3. Size-frequency histograms of nuclear diameters of anterior horn cell profiles of the fifth lumbar segment in the group of diabetic rats (solid line) and in the group of controls (dashed line). Values are means ± SEM.

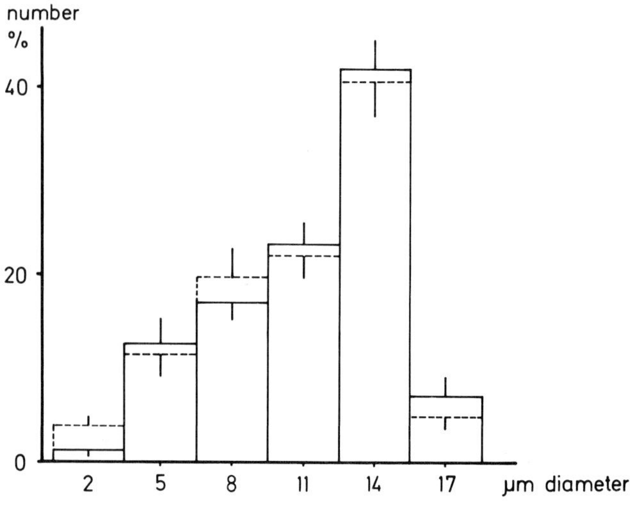

TABLE 1
Volumes of nucleoli, nuclei, and perikaryons of anterior horn cells of the fifth lumbar segment and of the fifth lumbar dorsal root ganglion cells in diabetic rats and in controls (values are means ± SD)

Cell type		Nucleolus (μm^3)			Nucleus (μm^3)			Perikaryon ($\times 10^3$ μm^3)		
		Control	Diabetes	2P	Control	Diabetes	2P	Control	Diabetes	2P
Anterior horn cell		103 ± 38 (N = 12)	87 ± 32 (N = 11)	NS	2548 ± 580	2227 ± 289	NS	33.28 ± 6.93	27.45 ± 5.09	0.033
Dorsal root ganglion	A-cell	106 ± 36 (N = 11)	88 ± 39 (N = 10)	NS	1840 ± 250	1815 ± 460	NS	51.31 ± 14.10	45.32 ± 12.06	NS
	B-cell	41 ± 9	34 ± 13	NS	855 ± 102	792 ± 108	NS	10.10 ± 1.46	10.34 ± 3.19	NS

insignificant. The amount of cytoplasm free of Nissl substance was, however, statistically reduced from 20,560 ± 4130 μm^3 in controls to 16,704 ± 2970 μm^3 in diabetics (2P = 0.019).

Dorsal root ganglion cells. In Table 1 the mean volumes of nucleoli, nuclei, and perikaryons are shown for A- and B-cells of the fifth lumbar dorsal root ganglion in both groups of rats. None of the differences between the two groups were statistically significant.

However, the mean perikaryal volume of A- and B-cells taken together was reduced by 18% in diabetic rats as compared with controls. In Figure 4 the mean values for individual rats are shown. In the diabetic group the mean perikaryal volume was 18,520 ± 3230 μm^2 compared with 22,680 ± 3460 μm^2 in the control group, the 2P value being 0.011. The explanation for this apparent discrepancy is that the number of the large A-cells is decreased in the diabetic rats and that the number of the smaller B-cells is correspondingly increased. In Figure 5 the relative number of A-cells is shown for each rat of both groups. The number of A-cells was 23.9 ± 5.5% in the diabetic group and 31.7 ± 8.0% in controls. The difference was statistically significant, the 2P value being 0.018.

DISCUSSION

The present experiment has demonstrated that the perikaryons of rat sciatic nerve have reduced volume after 4 wk of streptozotocin diabetes; perikaryal size and axon size presumably are directly related.[11] The present finding, therefore, is in accordance with our previous observation of reduced axon caliber in rats with a similar degree and duration of diabetes. Furthermore, the magnitude of the reduction is similar for the perikaryal volume and the axon volume, namely 18% and 14–20%, respectively.[5,6]

It has been doubted whether myelinated nerve fiber caliber is reduced in streptozotocin-diabetic rats. Sharma and Thomas[12] and Sharma et al.[13] have claimed that peripheral nerve structure is normal in streptozotocin-diabetic rats. However, close analysis of the results reported in these two papers clearly indicate a smaller myelinated nerve fiber caliber in the diabetic rats. Recently, Sima and Robertson[14] observed a similar difference in myelinated nerve fiber caliber in a preliminary report on the obese hyperglycemic db/db mouse.

Commenting on an earlier report from this laboratory, Thomas and Sharma[15] suggested that the axon caliber is reduced in our rats because of weight loss and retarded skeletal growth. This explanation, however, is unlikely for the following reasons. We have shown that rats with a weight loss comparable to that of the diabetic animals have normal caliber.[6] Moreover, we have found that nerve fiber internodal length is normal despite reduced caliber and that tibial

FIGURE 4. Mean perikaryal volume of anterior horn cells of the fifth lumbar segment and of the fifth lumbar dorsal root ganglion cells (A- and B-cells taken together) for individual diabetic rats (○) and controls (●).

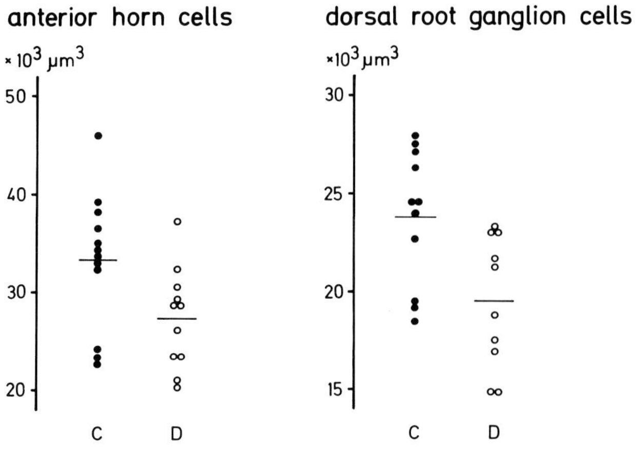

FIGURE 5. Relative number (%) of A-cells in the fifth lumbar dorsal root ganglion for individual diabetic rats (○) and controls (●).

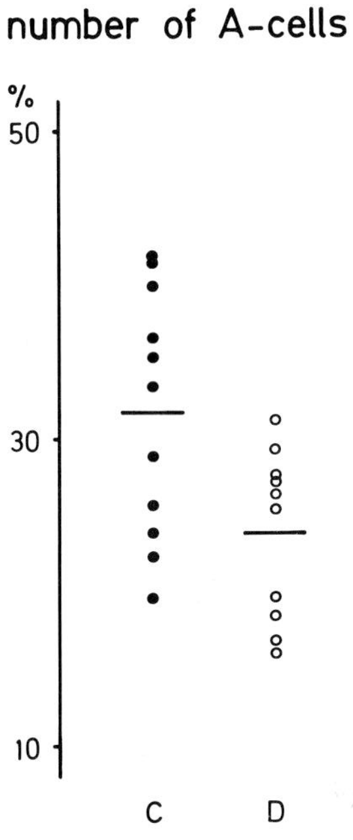

length is identical in diabetic rats and controls.[5,7] We have also shown that the difference in fiber caliber can be prevented by insulin treatment.[5] These results indicate that the reduction of axon caliber is caused by metabolic derangement of the diabetic rats, not by general poor condition of the animals, and it is reasonable to assume that the same is true of the reduced perikaryal volume demonstrated in the present paper. Furthermore, our results rule out the possibility that the abnormalities observed are due to a toxic effect of streptozotocin.

Reduced perikaryal volume as found in the present study may be generated in at least two different ways. It might arise because of shrinkage of nerve cell bodies or because of inhibition of normal increase of the perikaryal volume during the experimental period. At present it seems most likely that both mechanisms are involved. In our previous experiments, increase of axon caliber was demonstrated in the control rats during the 4-wk experimental period whereas the axon caliber remained statistically unchanged in diabetic rats. The axon-myelin ratio, however, was decreased, indicating that axonal shrinkage also occurs. Inhibition of the normal increase in cell body volume as well as in shrinkage, therefore, is suggested to explain the present observation.

The classification on light microscopic criteria of the A- and B-cells in the spinal root ganglion is widely held to reflect different cell populations subserving different modalities. Studies on the ultrastructure and biochemistry of the ganglion cells have resulted in further subdivisions.[16–18] The most prominent differences have been the intracellular architecture, especially the amounts of neurofilament and transmitter enzyme, and the localization of potential transmitter substances. Although these differences have been interpreted as expressions of mutually exclusive cell populations, it is possible to envisage these differences as expressions of different stages in a biochemical series of events in one and the same kind of cell.

In regenerating nerves an increased amount of neurofilaments and decreased acetylcholinesterase activity have been demonstrated.[19,20] These changes follow an increased retrograde, axonal transport of proteins.[21,22] Recently we have demonstrated a decreased flux of retrogradely transported glycoproteins in axons of diabetic rats.[8,9] The present changed ratio of A-cells to B-cells, as well as the decreased amount of cytoplasm free of Nissl substance, may imply a decrease in the amount of structural proteins, e.g., neurofilaments and neurotubuli. It is possible that the structural and biochemical changes found in this and other studies are responses to the changes in retrograde transport.[21–23]

Recently an abstract by Felten[24] has appeared, in which it is stated that there is a significant loss of alpha motor neurons in the anterior horn throughout the spinal cord in rats with 16-wk duration of streptozotocin diabetes. The neuronal loss was found to be associated with an altered dendritic field of the remaining alpha motor neurons and denervation of trunk and proximal limb musculature, and it was also observed in alloxan diabetic rats and genetically diabetic (db/db) mice.

There are no histologic studies on the nerve cells of peripheral nerves from short-term diabetic patients. In reports on the spinal cord from patients dying after many years of diabetes, loss of anterior horn cells and dorsal root ganglion cells has been documented.[25–27]

Our report has demonstrated that motor and sensory neurons are involved in the peripheral nerve abnormalities present in rats after a few weeks of streptozotocin diabetes. It appears that the nervous system abnormalities in the streptozotocin-diabetic model are not limited to the peripheral nerves only, but also involve the central nervous system.

ACKNOWLEDGMENTS

The skillful assistance of Helle Danvad Jensen, Karin Wiedemann, and Uffe Dalsgaard Hansen is gratefully acknowledged. The study was supported by the Danish Medical Research Council (512–15466) and Novo.

REFERENCES

[1] Gregersen, G.: Diabetic neuropathy: influcence of age, sex, metabolic control, and duration of diabetes on motor conduction velocity. Neurology (Minneap.) *17*:972–80, 1967.

[2] Fraser, D. M., Campbell, I. W., Ewing, D. J., Murray, A., Neilson, J. M. M., and Clarke, B. F.: Peripheral and autonomic nerve function in newly diagnosed diabetes mellitus. Diabetes *26*:546–50, 1977.

[3] Terkildsen, A. B., and Christensen, N. J.: Reversible nervous abnormalities in juvenile diabetics with recently diagnosed diabetes. Diabetologia *7*:113–17, 1971.

[4] Jakobsen, J.: Early peripheral nerve abnormalities in diabetes: an animal model. Horm. Metab. Res., 1979. In press.

[5] Jakobsen, J.: Early and preventable changes of peripheral nerve structure and function in insulin-deficient diabetic rats. J. Neurol. Neurosurg. Psychiatr. *42*:509–18, 1979.

[6] Jakobsen, J.: Axonal dwindling in early experimental diabetes. I. A study of cross sectioned nerves. Diabetologia *12*:539–46, 1976.

[7] Jakobsen, J.: Axonal dwindling in early experimental diabetes. II. A study of isolated nerve fibres. Diabetologia *12*:547–53, 1976.

[8] Sidenius, P., and Jakobsen, J.: Axonal transport in early experimental diabetes. Brain Res. *173*:315–30, 1979.

[9] Jakobsen, J., and Sidenius, P.: Decreased axonal flux of retrogradely transported glycoproteins in early experimental diabetes. J. Neurochem. *33*:1055–60, 1979.

[10] Underwood, E. E.: Quantitative Stereology. Reading, Mass., Addison-Wesley, 1970, pp. 23–47, 80–147.

[11] Wässle, H., Levick, W. R., Kirk, D. L., and Cleland, B. G.: Axonal conduction velocity and perikaryal size. Exp. Neurol. *49*:246–51, 1975.

[12] Sharma, A. K., and Thomas, P. K.: Peripheral nerve structure and function in experimental diabetes. J. Neurol. Sci. *23*:1–15, 1974.

[13] Sharma, A. K., Thomas, P. K., and De Molina, A. F.: Peripheral nerve fiber size in experimental diabetes. Diabetes *26*:689–92, 1977.

[14] Sima, A. A. F., and Robertson, D. M.: Peripheral neuropathy in mutant diabetic mouse [C57BL/Ks(db/db)]. Acta Neuropathol. [Berl.] *41*:85–89, 1978.

[15] Thomas, P. K., and Sharma, A. K.: Neuropathy in experimental diabetes. Br. Med. J. *2*:478, 1976.

[16] Andres, K. H.: Untersuchung über den Feinbau von Spinalganglien. Z. Zellforsch. *55*:1–48, 1961.

[17] Duce, I. R., and Keen, P.: An ultrastructural classification of the neuronal cell bodies of the rat dorsal root ganglion using zinc iodide-osmium impregnation. Cell Tissue Res. *185*:263–77, 1977.

[18] Ambrose, W. W., and McNeill, M. E.: Graphic representation of the distribution of acetylcholinesterase in cat dorsal root ganglion neurons. Histochem. J. *10*:711–20, 1978.

[19] Aldskogius, H.: Fine structural changes in nerve cell bodies of the adult rabbit dorsal motor vagal nucleus during axon reaction. Neuropathol. Appl. Neurobiol. *4*:323–41, 1978.

[20] Koenig, H. L.: Relations entre la distribution de l'activité acétylcholinestérasique et celle de l'ergastoplasme dans les neurones du ganglion ciliaire du poulet. Arch. Anat. Microsc. Morphol. Exp. *54*:937–64, 1965.

[21] Bisby, M. A., and Bulger, V. T.: Reversal of axonal transport at a nerve crush. J. Neurochem. *29*:313–20, 1977.

[22] Bulger, V. T., and Bisby, M. A.: Reversal of axonal transport in regenerating nerves. J. Neurochem. *31*:1411–18, 1978.

[23] Kristensson, K., and Olsson, Y.: Diffusion pathways and retrograde axonal transport of protein tracers in peripheral nerves. Prog. Neurobiol. *1*:87–109, 1973.

[24] Felten, D. L.: Spinal cord alterations in streptozotocin-induced dia-

betes. Anat. Rec. *193*:741–42, 1979.
[25] Greenbaum, D., Richardson, P. C., Salmon, M. V., and Urich, H.: Pathological observations on six cases of diabetic neuropathy. Brain *87*:201–14, 1964.
[26] Reske-Nielsen, E., and Lundbæk, K.: Pathological changes in the central and peripheral nervous system of young long-term diabetics. II. The spinal cord and peripheral nerves. Diabetologia *4*:34–43, 1968.
[27] Olsson, Y., Säve-Söderbergh, J., Sourander, P., and Angervall, L.: A patho-anatomical study of the central and peripheral nervous system in diabetes of early onset and long duration. Pathol. Europ. *3*:62–79, 1968.

A Decreased Response of Cyclic Adenosine Monophosphate Concentrations to Glucagon in Liver Slices from Streptozotocin-induced Diabetic Rats

KAMEJIRO YAMASHITA, SOMO YAMASHITA, HIROKO YASUDA, YUJI OKA, AND ETSURO OGATA

SUMMARY

Responses to glucagon from the adenylate cyclase–cyclic adenosine monophosphate (cAMP) system in liver slices from control and streptozotocin-induced diabetic rats were compared. Tissue cAMP levels were similar in the basal state but responded poorly to glucagon (20 pg/ml–2 μg/ml) in diabetic rats. Insulin treatment of diabetic rats in vivo led to a reversal of the glucagon stimulation towards the values in the control rats. The basal and glucagon-stimulated activities of adenylate cyclase in crude membrane fractions were similar in both groups.

Plasma immunoreactive glucagon levels in diabetic rats were approximately three times higher than those in normal rats.

Liver slices obtained from normal rats, which were injected with glucagon (0.2 mg, i.m.) 45 min previously, also showed an impaired responsiveness to glucagon of tissue cAMP levels, while no significant difference in adenylate cyclase activity was observed between the normal and glucagon-treated rats.

These results suggest that the responsiveness of liver slices from the streptozotocin-induced diabetic rat has been modified by the preceding hyperglucagonemia. The reason for the observed differences between slices and crude membranes is not known.
DIABETES 29:188–192, March 1980.

Diabetes has been described as a bihormonal disease caused not only by insulin deficiency but also by glucagon excess.[1] From this point of view, it is conceivable that deteriorations in hepatic metabolism in diabetes are attributable to abnormal plasma levels of either hormone or both.

Recently it has been demonstrated that several hormones, including insulin and catecholamines, regulate the concentration and function of their own receptors in target cells.[2,3] For example, hyperinsulinemia due to a variety of causes is accompanied by a decrease in the specific insulin-binding capacity of target cells. Regarding glucagon, Soman and Felig reported that the hyperglucagonemia, lasting 5 h, in rats resulted in a 45% decrease in glucagon binding and a comparable decrease in the glucagon-stimulated adenylate cyclase activity of a membrane fraction from the liver.[4] However, preceding and subsequent reports of theirs and of others were or were not in harmony with this conclusion.[5–7] It is possible that the disparity in conclusions may come from a difference in the tissue preparations employed in the experiments.

The present study was undertaken to determine if responses to glucagon of the hepatic adenylate cyclase–cyclic AMP (cAMP) system were altered in streptozotocin-induced–diabetic rats and whether the alteration resulted from the preceding hyperglucagonemia. For this purpose the responses of liver slices and those of liver membrane preparations were compared.

Evidence is presented in this communication that the preceding hyperglucagonemia may cause a diminished response of the adenylate cyclase–cAMP system in the slices but not in the membrane fractions.

MATERIALS AND METHODS

Wistar rats, weighing between 200 and 250 g, were used. Diabetes was induced by a single injection of streptozotocin (SZ) (60 mg/kg of body weight) into the tail vein. Control rats received the vehicle. SZ was dissolved immediately before use in a citric acid buffer (50 mM) adjusted to pH 4.5, and 0.3 ml of solution was injected. On days 7–14 after SZ injection, plasma glucose was measured, and only those rats with fasting plasma glucose of 200 mg/dl or higher were used in the study. Several rats in the diabetic group were injected subcutaneously with 0.5 U of Lente insulin per day for four days, and those rats with fasting plasma glucose of 120 mg/dl or lower were used as insulin-treated diabetic rats. In another set of experiments the normal

From the Department of Medicine, University of Tsukuba, the Department of Medicine, University of Tokyo, and the Division of Endocrinology, National Cancer Institute, Japan.
Address reprint requests to Kamejiro Yamashita, M.D., Department of Medicine, University of Tsukuba, Niihari-gun, Ibaraki-ken, 300-31, Japan.
Received for publication 8 January and in revised form 22 October 1979.

animals received 200 μg of glucagon i.m. 45 min before sacrifice, with the control receiving the appropriate vehicle (saline). The rats had free access to standard rat chow and tap water. The experiments were started at between 10 and 11 a.m. The animals were anesthetized with pentobarbital (50 mg/kg, i.p.), and the abdominal wall was opened. Two milliliters of blood was withdrawn from the abdominal aorta with a heparinized syringe; 20 μl of the blood sample was used for glucose determination. An aliquot of the plasma was stored for immunoreactive insulin (IRI) assay. For glucagon assay, 50 μl of Trasylol (250 U) was added immediately to 1 ml of the blood (before separation of the plasma).

After being perfused with 20–40 ml of cold normal saline from the portal vein, the liver was removed and sliced. Thirty to 40 mg of the slices was incubated at 37°C in test tubes containing 1 ml of Krebs-Ringer bicarbonate buffer, glucose (1 mg/ml), theophylline (10^{-2}M), bovine albumin (1 mg/ml), and appropriate substances to be tested. In all incubations the gas phase was 95% O_2 and 5% CO_2. The slices were preincubated for 10 min without test substances, and then the incubation was performed as indicated in the legends of the figures. After incubation, the tissue was extracted with 0.5 ml of hot 50 mM sodium acetate. After centrifugation, the cAMP content in the supernate was determined by radioimmunoassay[8] using the Yamasa kit.

Liver homogenates were prepared in 0.25 M sucrose and filtered through four layers of gauze. The 8000 *g* pellet of the filtrate was used as a crude membrane fraction.

Adenylate cyclase activity in the liver crude membrane fraction was assayed according to the procedure described previously.[9] In short, incubation of 10–30 μg of membrane protein was performed at 37°C in 200 μl of a medium consisting of 2.5 mM ATP, 5 mM $MgCl_2$, 1 mM EDTA, 30 mM Tris-HCl buffer (pH 7.6), and an ATP-regenerating system (10 mM phosphenolpyruvate and 5 μg of pyruvate kinase). The reaction was terminated by boiling for 3 min. After centrifugation, the supernate was assayed for cAMP by the above-mentioned method. Glucagon was added in the concentrations indicated in the figures. The rate of cAMP production was used as an index of the enzyme activity.

The specific activity of a plasma membrane marker enzyme, 5′-nucleotidase, and a microsomal marker enzyme, glucose-6-phosphatase, was measured by the method described by Aronson and Touster.[10] Protein content was estimated by the method of Lowry et al.[11]

Plasma glucose was measured by a glucose oxidase method.[12] IRI was assayed with the two antibody method by use of a kit provided by Daiichi Isotope Co., and immunoreactive glucagon was assayed with the two antibody method employing antiserum 30 K.[13] Glucagon was a generous gift from Kodama Co. SZ was purchased from Upjohn Co., Kalamazoo, Michigan.

RESULTS

As summarized in Table 1, plasma glucose and glucagon levels were higher and insulin levels were much lower in the diabetic than in the control rats.

Figure 1 indicates that glucagon (200 pg/ml to 2 μg/ml) significantly stimulated cAMP levels in a dose-dependent fashion during 3 min of incubation in slices from control rats. The stimulation by glucagon of cAMP levels in liver slices was much lower than that obtained in perfusion experiments,[14] but it was consistent with the results obtained by others in slice experiments.[15] In contrast, no significant stimulation was observed in slices from diabetic rats by glucagon at concentrations lower than 200 ng/ml. The stimulation of cAMP levels by 2 μg/ml glucagon in liver slices from the diabetic rats was markedly lower than that from the normal rats. Basal levels (obtained without glucagon) were the same between the two groups.

In liver slices from the control rats, the peak tissue cAMP response to glucagon was obtained at 3 min of incubation (Figure 2). Thereafter, the cAMP levels declined, reaching the basal by 10 min. The response was significantly lower in slices from diabetic than in the control rats at 3 and 5 min of incubation. Insulin treatment (0.5 U of Lente insulin subcutaneously for 4 days) led to a reversal of the glucagon stimulation towards the values in the control group.

TABLE 1
Plasma glucagon, insulin, and glucose levels in normal and streptozotocin-induced diabetic rats

	Glucagon (pg/ml)	Insulin (μU/ml)	Glucose (mg/100 ml)
Normal rats (N = 10)	115 ± 8.6	13.7 ± 2.1	104 ± 5.0
Diabetic rats (N = 8)	296 ± 38.3	2.3 ± 1.2	381 ± 44.7

Data are presented as means ± SE.

FIGURE 1. Effect of various concentrations of glucagon on cAMP levels in liver slices from control and SZ-induced diabetic rats.

After preincubation for 10 min, the slices were incubated in triplicate for 3 min in the medium containing various concentrations of glucagon, as described under MATERIALS AND METHODS. The basal levels (obtained in the absence of glucagon) of tissue cAMP in the control and the diabetic rats were 0.22 ± 0.03 and 0.20 ± 0.04 (mean ± SE of five experiments in each group) nmol/g tissue, respectively, and the difference between them was not significant statistically. In each experiment the basal levels were compared, the difference being not significant statistically. The values (mean ± SE, N = 5) in the figure are expressed as percentage of the basal of the respective group. The differences of values between the respective counterparts are significant (P < 0.05 by Student's *t* test) from 200 pg/ml to 2μg/ml of glucagon concentrations. (●——● Normal, N = 5; ○------- ○ diabetic, N = 5.)

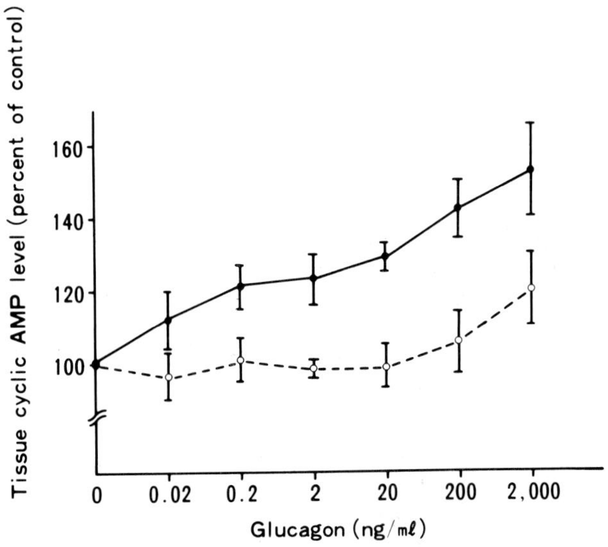

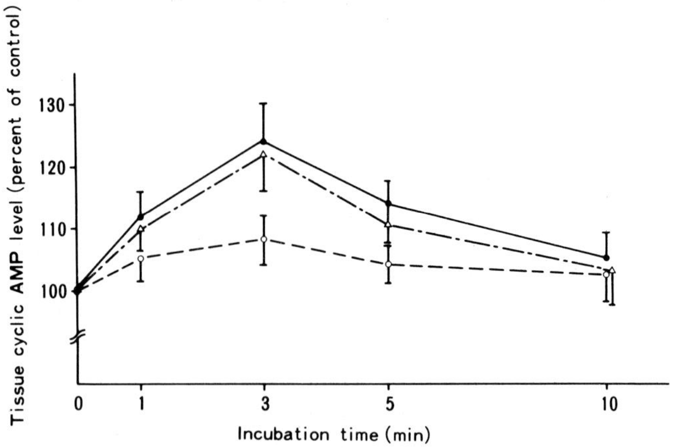

FIGURE 2. Time course of glucagon stimulation of cAMP levels in liver slices from control, SZ-induced diabetic, and insulin-treated diabetic rats.

Slices were incubated for various times in the medium containing glucagon (200 pg/ml). The values in the figure are expressed as percent of the basal. The other details are as in Figure 1. The cAMP responses of the diabetic rats at 3 and 5 min are significantly lower than the respective counterparts of control rats and insulin-treated diabetic rats ($P < 0.05$). (●——● Normal, N = 10; ○-------○ diabetic, N = 8; △— — — — —△ insulin-treated diabetic, N = 8.)

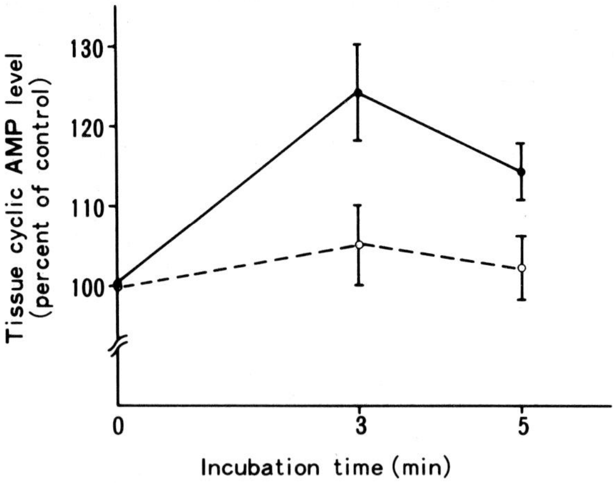

FIGURE 3. Time course of glucagon stimulation of cAMP levels in liver slices from control and glucagon-pretreated rats.

Normal rats were injected with 200 μg of glucagon or the vehicle (saline) i.m. 45 min before sacrifice. The other procedures were as described under MATERIALS AND METHODS. The slices were incubated in the medium containing 200 pg/ml glucagon.

The basal levels of tissue cAMP in the control and the glucagon-pretreated rats were 0.24 ± 0.04 and 0.25 ± 0.06 nmol/g tissue, respectively (N = 4 in each group), and the difference was not significant statistically. The values in the figure are expressed as in Figure 1. The values of the glucagon-pretreated rats are significantly lower than those of the respective control rats at 3 and 5 min of incubation ($P < 0.05$). (●———● Control, ○------○ glucagon-pretreated.)

Although the cAMP levels stimulated by norepinephrine (100 μM) were much lower than those by glucagon, the hormone-induced change was statistically significant (data not shown). Similar small but significant stimulation by norepinephrine was reported in liver perfusion experiments.[14] The rate of stimulation was identical in both the normal and the diabetic rats.

To examine adenylate cyclase activity in the membrane fraction, we prepared the crude membrane fraction as described in METHODS. The purity of the preparation was checked by assaying 5′-nucleotidase and glucose-6-phosphatase activities. As previously reported,[16] liver homogenates and membrane fractions from diabetic rats had significantly decreased 5′-nucleotidase activity when compared with controls (normal liver: homogenates 0.34 ± 0.05 μmol/mg protein/10 min, crude membranes 0.67 ± 0.06; diabetic liver: homogenates 0.20 ± 0.03, crude membranes 0.41 ± 0.06; values are mean ± SEM of four different experiments in each group), whereas glucose-6-phosphatase activity was increased in diabetic rats (normal liver: homogenates 0.71 ± 0.06 μmol/mg protein/10 min, crude membranes 1.24 ± 0.15; diabetic liver: homogenates 1.16 ± 0.21, crude membranes 2.32 ± 0.35). Comparison of these data indicates that the membrane fraction was concentrated by approximately twofold in both the control and the diabetic sample and that both preparations were accompanied by similar contamination with microsomal fractions. The adenylate cyclase activity in the crude membrane fraction prepared from either the normal or the diabetic livers was increased in a similar fashion by increasing concentrations of glucagon (20 pg/ml to 2 μg/ml) (data not shown). These results contrast sharply with those obtained in the slice experiments (Figure 1).

The effect of glucagon administration in vivo on the hepatic cAMP response to glucagon in vitro was next examined in normal rats (Figure 3). The basal tissue cAMP levels were the same for control and glucagon-pretreated animals. However, the response to glucagon in the tissue from the glucagon-pretreated animals was significantly lower than that in the control animals. The cAMP response to norepinephrine in slices and the adenylate cyclase activity in the crude membrane fractions were similar between the two groups of animals (data not shown).

Glucose (1.5 g/kg body weight) was injected i.p. 45 min before sacrifice to induce similar hyperglycemia (higher than 200 mg glucose/100 ml) to that produced by glucagon or SZ treatment, and the liver tissue cAMP response to glucagon was examined. The responsiveness was not altered by this maneuver (data not shown).

DISCUSSION

The present study demonstrates that SZ-diabetic rats exhibit hyperglycemia, hypoinsulinemia, and hyperglucagonemia. These results are consistent with the previous report.[16] Furthermore, we have demonstrated that responses to glucagon of the adenylate cyclase–cAMP system in liver slices from these diabetic rats are significantly lower than those in liver slices from normal rats and that insulin treatment of diabetic rats leads to a reversal of the responsiveness towards the values of the control rats. These phenomena were observed when physiologic or supraphysiologic quantities of glucagon were employed in the stimulation of the cAMP system.

Several, conflicting observations have been reported regarding the binding and biologic activity of glucagon in liver preparations from SZ-diabetic rats.[7,16] Srikant et al. reported that the concentration of specific glucagon-binding sites was significantly reduced in SZ-diabetic rats.[7] In isolated hepatocytes, Bhathena et al. demonstrated that specific glucagon binding was decreased in diabetic rats compared with controls and that hepatocyte cAMP response to glucagon was almost abolished in diabetic rats.[17] When adenylate cyclase activity was examined in membrane fractions, Pilkis et al.[18] and Srikant et al.[7] observed that glucagon-stimulated adenylate cyclase activities were not different in SZ-diabetic rats and control rats.

In contrast, Soman and Felig reported that the specific binding of ^{125}I-glucagon to liver plasma membranes was approximately twofold higher in the diabetic as compared with the control rats.[16] They suggested that it was due to an increase in the number of binding sites rather than to a change in the binding affinity. Simultaneously, they reported that both the basal and glucagon-stimulated adenylate cyclase activities in the SZ-treated rats were twofold higher than in controls. Similar results were reported in membrane fractions by Hepp.[19] It is difficult to reconcile these diverse conclusions, but one likely explanation is that they are due to the difference in the experimental settings, particularly to that in liver preparations. To minimize inclusion of possible artifacts in the present study, we relied on a simple tissue slice system, and the results indicate, as in the case of those in the isolated cell experiments,[17] that tissue cAMP response to glucagon was diminished in diabetic rats. In our hands, also, the crude liver membrane preparation (intentionally prepared without drastic manipulations) did not exhibit the differences in the responsiveness to glucagon between diabetic, glucagon-treated, and control rats. Therefore, the results of membrane experiments including ours were much different from those obtained in intact cells. Similar dissociation between the glucagon-responsive hepatic adenylate cyclase activity and the hepatic cAMP response to glucagon was reported in hyperglucagonemic rats previously.[19] It seems likely that such factors as phosphodiesterase activity contribute to regulation of the tissue cAMP levels in diabetic livers, since phosphodiesterase activity in homogenates is still present, even after the addition of 10 mM theophylline. The reduced responsiveness to glucagon in vitro in liver slices from glucagon-injected rats has been shown, although the level and time course of hyperglucagonemia may be different from those in diabetic states. The present results are consistent with the report of DeRubertis and Craven.[21] Similar line of results was also reported by Soman and Felig in the rats pre-infused with glucagon for 5 h.[4] In addition, our results indicate that hyperglycemia per se did not reproduce the state of diabetic rats. These data support the thesis that impairment of the liver cAMP response to glucagon in diabetic rats is caused by preceding hyperglucagonemia. Similar reduction in hepatic cAMP responses to glucagon has been described in cultured fetal hepatocytes after preceding exposure to glucagon.[20]

Since Exton et al.[14] and Hepp[19] reported the activation of adenylate cyclase by norepinephrine, we also examined the effect of norepinephrine on tissue cAMP levels. In contrast with the glucagon stimulation, no difference in the norepinephrine stimulation of tissue cAMP levels was observed between diabetic and normal livers and between glucagon-pretreated and control rats (data not shown). The abovementioned phenomenon (the reduced responsiveness to glucagon in vitro in liver slices from the diabetic and glucagon-injected rats) may be explainable as a hormone-specific desensitization or refractoriness induced by endogenous overproduction or an exogenous administration of the α-cell hormone. Similar phenomena have been reported in terms of other peptide hormones and catecholamines.[22–24]

The pathophysiologic significance of hyperglucagonemia and of altered glucagon responses in diabetic states has not been elucidated. However, it seems that the hyperglycemia maintained in the diabetic rats is an expression of a persistent, though less efficient, action of glucagon on hepatic glucose production. In conclusion, the present data support the concept that regulation by glucagon of hepatic metabolism is impaired in diabetic livers.

ACKNOWLEDGMENTS

The authors thank Dr. James B. Field for his help in preparing the manuscript.

REFERENCES

1 Unger, R. H.: Diabetes and the alpha cell. Diabetes *25*:136–51, 1976.

2 Gavin, J. R., Roth, J., Neville, D. M., Jr., DeMeyts, P., and Buell, D. N.: Insulin-dependent regulation of insulin receptors' interactions: a direct demonstration in cell culture. Proc. Natl. Acad. Sci. USA *71*:84–88, 1974.

3 Mukherjee, C., and Lefkowitz, R. J.: Desensitization of β-adrenergic receptors by β-adrenergic agonist in a cell-free system: resensitization by guanosine 5'-(β, γ-imino) triphosphate and other purine nucleotides. Proc. Natl. Acad. Sci. USA *73*:1494–98, 1976.

4 Soman, V., and Felig, P.: Regulation of the glucagon receptor by physiological hyperglucagonaemia. Nature *272*:829–32, 1978.

5 Fouchereau-Peron, M., Rancon, F., Freychet, P., and Rosselin, G.: Effect of feeding and fasting on the early steps of glucagon action in isolated rat liver cells. Endocrinology *98*:755–60, 1976.

6 Soman, V., and Felig, P.: Glucagon and insulin binding to liver membranes in a partially nephrectomized uremic rat model. J. Clin. Invest. *60*:224–32, 1977.

7 Srikant, C. B., Freeman, D., McCorkle, K., and Unger, R. H.: Binding and biologic activity of glucagon in liver cell membranes of chronically hyperglucagonemic rats. J. Biol. Chem. *252*:7434–36, 1977.

8 Steiner, A. L., Pagliara, A. S., Chase, L. R., and Kipnis, D. M.: Radioimmunoassay for cyclic nucleotides. II. Adenosine 3', 5'-monophosphate and guanosine 3',5'-monophosphate in mammalian tissues and body fluids. J. Biol. Chem. *247*:1114–20, 1972.

9 Oka, H., Kaneko, T., Yamashita, K., Suzuki, S., and Oda, T.: The glucagon and fluoride sensitive adenyl cyclase in plasma membrane of rat liver. Endocrinol. Jpn. *20*:263–70, 1973.

10 Aronson, N. N., Jr., and Touster, O.: Isolation of rat liver plasma membrane fragments in isotonic sucrose. *In* Methods in Enzymology, vol. 31. Fleischer, S., and Packer, L. Eds. New York, Academic Press, 1974, p. 90.

11 Lowry, O. H., Rosenbrough, N. J., Farr, A. L., and Randall, R. J.: Protein measurement with the Folin phenol reagent. J. Biol. Chem. *193*:265–75, 1951.

12 Huggett, A. S. G., and Dixon, D. A.: Use of glucose oxidase, peroxidase and O-dianisidine in determination of blood and urinary glucose. Lancet *2*:368–70, 1957.

13 Aguilar-Parada, E., Eisentraut, A. M., and Unger, R. H.: Effects of starvation on plasma pancreatic glucagon in normal man. Diabetes *18*:717–23, 1969.

14 Exton, J. H., Robison, G. A., Sutherland, E. W., and Park, C. R.: Studies on the role of adenosine 3', 5'-monophosphate in the hepatic actions of glucagon and catecholamines. J. Biol. Chem. *246*:6166–77, 1971.

15 Leichter, S. B., and Poffenbarger, P. L.: The effects of nonsuppressible insulin-like protein (NSILP) on cyclic nucleotide metabolism in rat liver. Biochem. Biophys. Res. Commun. *84*:403–10, 1978.

16 Soman, V., and Felig, P.: Glucagon binding and adenylate cyclase activity in liver membranes from untreated and insulin-treated diabetic rats. J. Clin. Invest. *61*:552–60, 1978.

17 Bhathena, S. J., Voyles, N. R., Smith, S., and Recant, L.: Decreased glucagon receptors in diabetic rat hepatocytes. Evidence for regulation of glucagon receptors by hyperglucagonemia. J. Clin. Invest. *61*:1488–97, 1978.

18 Pilkis, S. J., Exton, J. H., Johnson, R. A., and Park, C. R.: Effects of glucagon on cyclic AMP and carbohydrate metabolism in livers from diabetic rats. Biochim. Biophys. Acta *343*:250–67, 1974.

19 Hepp, K. D.: Adenylate cyclase and insulin action. Eur. J. Biochem. *31*:266–76, 1972.

20 Plas, C., and Nunez, J.: Glycogenolytic response to glucagon of cultured fetal hepatocytes; refractoriness following prior exposure to glucagon. J. Biol. Chem. *250*:5304–11, 1975.

21 DeRubertis, F. R., and Craven, P.: Reduced sensitivity of the hepatic adenylate cyclase-cyclic AMP system to glucagon during sustained hormonal stimulation. J. Clin. Invest. *57*:435–43, 1976.

[22] Shuman, S. J., Zor, U., Chayoth, R., and Field, J. B.: Exposure of thyroid slices to thyroid-stimulating hormone induces refractoriness of the cyclic AMP system to subsequent hormone stimulation. J. Clin. Invest. *57*:1132–41, 1976.

[23] Mickey, J., Tate, R., and Lefkowitz, R. J.: Subsensitivity of adenylate cyclase and decreased β-adrenergic receptor binding after chronic exposure to (−)-isoproterenol in vitro. J. Biol. Chem. *250*:5727–29, 1975.

[24] Aiyoshi, Y., Yamashita, K., Yamashita, S., and Ogata, E.: Effects of norepinephrine on cyclic nucleotide levels in dog thyroid slices. Endocrinology *102*:1527–33, 1978.

Mode of Action of Clonidine Upon Islet Function

Dissociated Effects Upon the Time Course and Magnitude of Insulin Release

V. LECLERCQ-MEYER, A. HERCHUELZ, I. VALVERDE, E. COUTURIER, J. MARCHAND, AND W. J. MALAISSE

SUMMARY

Clonidine (0.08 to 80.0 ng/ml) caused a dose-related inhibition of glucose-stimulated insulin release, but failed to affect glucose oxidation, glucose-stimulated ^{45}Ca net uptake, and adenylate cyclase activity in isolated rat islets. Phentolamine antagonized the effect of clonidine upon insulin release. Despite profound inhibition of insulin secretion, the drug failed to affect the time course for the changes evoked by glucose in either ^{45}Ca fractional outflow rate from perifused islets or insulin release from the isolated perfused pancreas. The latter changes were multiphasic, revealing an initial secretory peak, a period of low secretory activity, and a second secretory elevation before establishing a period characterized by a steadily and slowly increasing insulin output. In the clonidine-treated islets, the secretory rate was not significantly different from the basal value during the period after the initial secretory response. Thus, despite continuous stimulation with glucose, insulin release appears as a discontinuous phenomenon, even when little insulin is secreted during the initial phase of stimulation.
DIABETES 29:193–200, March 1980.

Clonidine, an α-adrenergic agonist, inhibits glucose-induced insulin release.[1] In the present work, we have first explored the influence of the drug upon several parameters of islet function to assess its possible mode of action in the B-cell. The data suggested that clonidine does not affect the process of glucose identification by the pancreatic B-cell. The drug was then used to compare the time course of ^{45}calcium efflux and insulin release from the endocrine pancreas under normal conditions and when insulin secretion is severely depressed. The results obtained indicate that the magnitude of insulin release is not an essential determinant of the phasic pattern of functional events in the endocrine pancreas.

From the Laboratory of Experimental Medicine, Brussels University, Brussels, Belgium.
Address reprint requests to W. J. Malaisse, Laboratoire de Médecine Expérimentale, 115, Boulevard de Waterloo, B-1000 Brussels (Belgium).
Received for publication 8 May and in revised form 5 September 1979.

MATERIALS AND METHODS

Experiments with intact isolated islets. Isolated islets were prepared[2] from the pancreases of fed female albino rats of the Wistar strain (body weight, 150–200 g). The methods used to measure insulin release,[3] glucose oxidation,[4] and ^{45}Ca net uptake[5] in static incubations and to monitor ^{45}Ca efflux and insulin release from perifused islets[6] are described in detail elsewhere.

Measurement of adenylate cyclase activity in islet homogenates. Groups of 200–400 islets each were homogenized in Tris-HCl buffer (25 mM, pH 7.6) containing $MgCl_2$ (5.0 mM), EGTA (1.5 mM), and dithiothreitol (3.0 mM) in a ratio of 100 islets/0.2 ml of buffer. Cell debris and intact cells were removed by a 1-min centrifugation at 100 *g*. The reaction mixture (75 μl) contained (final concentration) Tris-HCl (25 mM, pH 7.6), $MgCl_2$ (5.0 mM), EGTA (0.3 mM), 3-isobutyl-1-methylxanthine (0.5 mM), dithiothreitol (0.6 mM), bovine albumin (0.5 mg/ml; fraction V, Sigma Chemicals, St. Louis, Mo.), [α-^{32}P]ATP (13 μM; 20 μCi/ml), an ATP-regenerating system consisting of creatine phosphate (20 mM) and creatine kinase (0.8 mg/ml), and 15 μl of the islet homogenate (4.6 ± 0.1 μg of protein/15 μl). The enzymatic reaction was initiated by addition of the islet homogenate and was terminated by adding 0.5 ml of a 2% sodium dodecyl-sulfate solution containing 1 mM ATP and 0.5 mM cyclic (8-^{3}H)AMP.[7] The separation of cyclic AMP from ATP was achieved by the procedure of Salomon et al.[8] with the use of Dowex 50W-X4 and neutral alumina columns.

Most measurements were performed after 20 min of incubation at 37°C. Control experiments indicated that both the basal and NaF-stimulated formation of cyclic AMP was proportional to the time of incubation (Figure 1, panel A) and amount of islet protein. The temperature dependency of the reaction (Arrhenius' plot) yielded an apparent energy activation of 8.0 and 18.4 kcal/mol in the absence and presence of NaF, respectively (Figure 1, panel B).

All data were corrected for the blank values found in the

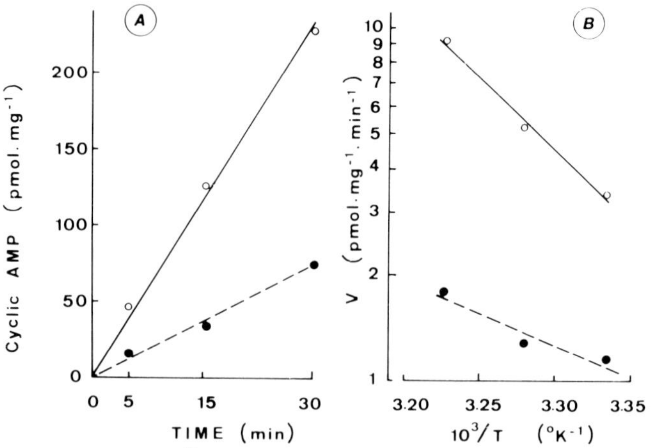

FIGURE 1. Kinetics of cyclic AMP formation (panel A) and Arrhenius' plot for the activity of adenylate cyclase (panel B) in islet homogenates incubated in the absence (closed circles) or presence (open circles) of NaF (10.0 mM). The data in each panel were collected in separate experiments. Each point represents the mean of three or more individual determinations.

absence of homogenate, which averaged 20.6 ± 1.5% (n = 11) of the basal activity. Protein was determined by the method of Lowry et al.[9] using bovine albumin as the standard. Results were expressed as picomoles of cyclic AMP formed per minute and per milligram of islet protein.

Insulin released by the isolated perfused pancreas. Fed female albino rats were used (mean body weight ± SEM: 366 ± 11 g, n = 8). The perfusion technique has been detailed previously.[10] The animals were anesthetized with sodium pentobarbital (42 mg/kg, i.p.), and the whole pancreas, excluding the duodenum, was perfused through the celiac and mesenteric arteries via a cannula inserted into the aorta. The rats were given heparin (125 U, i.v.) before cannulation. The perfusion medium contained the following salts, in millimoles per liter: NaCl, 118.5; KCl, 4.7; KH_2PO_4, 1.2; $MgSO_4$, 1.2; $NaHCO_3$, 25.0; and $CaCl_2$, 2.0. It was supplemented with dextran (40 g/L, T70, Pharmacia, Uppsala, Sweden) and bovine albumin (5 g/L, fraction V, Sigma Chemicals, St. Louis, Mo.). The medium was equilibrated against oxygen and carbon dioxide (95:5, v/v), with a resulting pH of 7.4, and entered the pancreas with a temperature of 37.5°C. The measured flow rate was similar in the control (1.99 ± 0.02 ml/min, n = 4) and in the clonidine experiments (1.95 ± 0.02 ml/min; n = 4). The perfusate contained a low amount of glucose (60 mg/dl), and the increase in the concentration of glucose (up to 200 mg/dl) was induced through a sidearm syringe working at a flow rate of 0.075 ml/min. The increase in osmolarity induced by glucose was corrected by an appropriate decrease in the amount of NaCl during the infusion period. Samples of the effluent were collected at 18-s intervals in chilled tubes containing 600 KIU Trasylol (generously donated by Drs. G. Wald and A. Pirart, Bayer, Brussels, Belgium) and were frozen at −25°C until time of assay. Insulin was estimated on 0.2-ml or 0.05-ml aliquots using the radioimmunoassay previously described,[11] in which the standard was rat insulin (lot R170, a gift from Dr. J. Schlichtkrull, Novo, Bagsvaerd, Denmark). All samples in each experiment were assayed in the same run and were referred to the same standard curve. The eight experiments reported in the present study were assayed in a total of three separate runs. The data illustrated in Table 1 indicate the variability attributable to the assay procedure at increasing rates of insulin secretion. Glucose was titrated in the pancreatic effluent with the glucose oxidase method using a first generation Technicon analyzer. Clonidine was administered at doses varying from 0.05 to 1 μg/ml of the perfusate. These dosages induced increases in the perfusion pressure that were not, however, statistically significant, owing to the limited number of experiments. The mean pressure recorded at the beginning of the samplings was 31 ± 5 mm Hg (n = 4) in the control experiments and 52 ± 16 mm Hg (n = 4) in the clonidine experiments.

Presentation of results. All results are expressed as mean values (± SEM) together with the number of individual determinations (n). The statistical significance of differences between control and experimental values was assessed by use of the Student's *t* test.

TABLE 1
Variability of the measurements for insulin release by the endocrine pancreas over short collection intervals (18 s)

Vol	Range	Mean	$\sqrt{(\Sigma\Delta^2/2n)}$	CV (%)	n
200 λ	<20	2.25	0.63	27.8	50
50 λ	<20	8.08	3.18	39.4	50
50 λ	20–200	93.8	7.2	7.6	47
50 λ	200–500	295.8	17.7	6.0	50
50 λ	>500	1,182	456	38.6	20

The Table indicates, from left to right, the volume of effluent used in each assay (flow rate: 0.6 ml/18 s), the range and mean value of readings in each class (expressed as μU/min), the estimate of within-assay variability based on the difference (Δ) between duplicate measurements, the corresponding coefficient of variation (CV), and the number of samples examined (n), each of which was assayed in duplicate.

RESULTS

Effects of clonidine upon metabolic and functional events in isolated islets. Clonidine inhibited glucose-induced insulin release in isolated islets in a dose-related fashion (Table 2). A clonidine concentration of 0.08 ng/ml was sufficient to cause a significant fall ($P < 0.005$) in glucose-stimulated insulin secretion. A close-to-basal rate of release was seen in the presence of clonidine, 80.0 ng/ml. The concentrations of clonidine used in further experiments were usually close to the latter value. Phentolamine, an alpha-adrenergic–blocking agent, markedly reduced but failed to abolish the inhibitory effect of clonidine upon insulin release (Table 2, last line).

Clonidine failed to affect the oxidation of glucose and the glucose-stimulated net uptake of ^{45}calcium by the islets (Table 2). The drug also failed to affect the basal or NaF-stimulated activity of adenylate cyclase in islet homogenates (Table 3).

Effect of clonidine upon ^{45}calcium efflux from prelabeled islets. In good agreement with the data obtained in the static experiments (Table 2), the insulinotropic action of glucose was virtually abolished in perifused islets exposed to clonidine (50 ng/ml). When glucose was removed from the perifusate during continuous exposure to clonidine, a paradoxic off-response occurred in the form of a transient increase in insulin output (Figure 2, lower panel).

Despite obliteration of insulin release, the administration

TABLE 2
Effect of clonidine upon insulin output, ^{45}Ca uptake, and glucose oxidation in isolated islets

Glucose (mg/dl)	Clonidine (ng/ml)	Phentolamine (μg/ml)	Insulin output (μU/90 min per islet)	^{45}Ca net uptake (pmol/90 min per islet)	[U-^{14}C] glucose oxidation (pmol/120 min per islet)
—	—	—	38.3 ± 10.8 (24)		
300	—	—	319.0 ± 11.2 (36)	6.1 ± 0.4 (12)	45.3 ± 2.8 (12)
300	0.08	—	245.9 ± 20.1 (13)		
300	0.8	—	151.8 ± 13.7 (13)		
300	8.0	—	69.2 ± 11.5 (12)	6.9 ± 0.4 (12)	
300	80.0	—	43.8 ± 7.9 (11)	6.2 ± 0.3 (12)	45.1 ± 3.4 (12)
300	8.0	50.0	221.4 ± 11.5 (13)		

Mean values (±SEM) are shown together with the number of individual determinations (in parentheses).

of glucose to the clonidine-treated islets provoked both the initial fall and later increase in ^{45}calcium fractional outflow rate (FOR) normally seen in the present system (Figure 2, upper panel). Before the introduction of glucose, the ^{45}Ca FOR tended to be lower in the presence of clonidine (FOR at the 44th min, 0.62 ± 0.06%/min) than in its absence (FOR at the 44th min, 0.90 ± 0.12%/min; $P < 0.08$). When glucose, but not clonidine, was removed from the perifusate, a modest and transient increase in ^{45}Ca efflux was occasionally observed. Within 4 min or less of glucose deprivation, the ^{45}Ca FOR decreased (Figure 2, upper panel). It eventually stabilized (from the 76th min onwards) at values that are significantly lower (paired difference in ^{45}Ca FOR, −0.204 ± 0.058; $P < 0.05$) than those recorded at the end of period of exposure to glucose (i.e., at the 69th min).

A closer examination of the individual data revealed that, in both control and clonidine-treated islets, a multiphasic pattern of changes in ^{45}calcium efflux was observed in response to glucose (Table 4). These changes consisted not only of the already mentioned initial fall and secondary rise in ^{45}Ca FOR; in addition, the latter phenomenon could itself be dissected into two successive peaks. In the clonidine-treated islets, there was an almost perfect synchrony of behavior in the four individual experiments. The lowest value during the initial fall was always reached at the 47th min. Thereafter, the ^{45}Ca FOR increased and reached its maximal value in all cases at the 50th min. A fall was then again observed at the 53rd or 54th min. This was followed by a second rise in ^{45}Ca efflux, peaking at the 57th min. The ^{45}Ca FOR eventually fell again, the values recorded from the 59th to 61st min being already significantly lower than those seen at the 57th min. In the control islets not exposed to clonidine, exactly the same pattern of changes was observed: initial fall, first peak, second peak, and eventual equilibration. The magnitude of each excursion was not vastly different in the control and clonidine-treated islets, respectively (Table 4). There was a trend, however, (1) for the two peaks in ^{45}Ca FOR to occur somewhat earlier in the control than in the clonidine-treated islets, (2) for a better synchrony of each event in the latter islets, and (3) for the ascending excursions in ^{45}Ca FOR to be less marked in the clonidine-treated islets, such ascensions averaging 79.6 ± 6.1% ($n = 8$) of their appropriate mean control values.

TABLE 3
Effect of clonidine upon adenylate cyclase activity in islet homogenates

NaF (mM)	Clonidine (μg/ml)	Adenylate cyclase activity (pmol cyclic AMP · min^{-1} · mg^{-1})
—	—	1.915 ± 0.137 (6)
—	10–20	1.928 ± 0.056 (6)
10.0	—	7.907 ± 0.174 (6)
10.0	10–20	8.073 ± 0.198 (6)

Mean values (±SEM) are shown together with the number of individual determinations (in parentheses).

FIGURE 2. Effect of a rise and fall in glucose concentration (G_0: no glucose; G_{300}: glucose, 300 mg/dl) at the time shown by the vertical dotted lines upon ^{45}Ca FOR (upper panel) and insulin release (lower panel) by prelabeled isolated islets exposed throughout perifusion to clonidine (50 ng/ml; closed circles and solid lines). Control data for ^{45}Ca FOR, obtained in the absence of clonidine, are shown by the open circles and dotted line. Mean values (±SEM) refer to four individual experiments in each case. The abscissas represent the time (minutes) from the onset of perifusion.

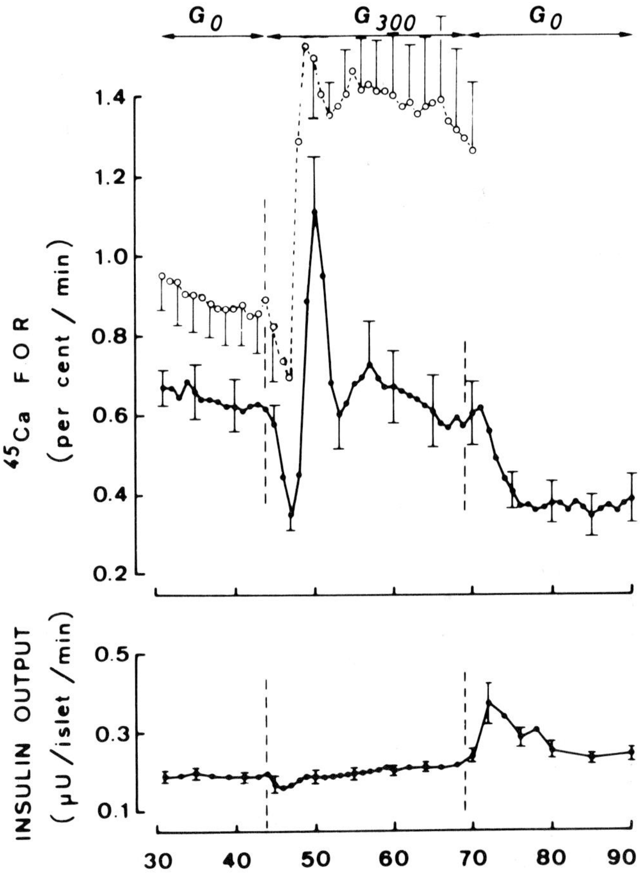

TABLE 4
Time course of glucose-induced changes in ^{45}Ca fractional outflow rate (FOR)

Control islets

Time (min)	Paired difference in ^{45}Ca FOR (per thousand/min)	(P)
44-44-44-44 → 46-46-47-47	−1.94 ± 0.23	<0.005
46-46-47-47 → 48-49-49-50	+9.66 ± 1.66	<0.020
48-49-49-50 → 50-50-53-52	−3.66 ± 1.11	<0.050
50-50-53-52 → 53-55-55-55	+1.82 ± 0.44	<0.030
53-55-55-55 → Mean 59th to 61st	−0.85 ± 0.39	N.S.

Clonidine-treated islets

Time (min)	Paired difference in ^{45}Ca FOR (per thousand/min)	(P)
44-44-44-44 → 47-47-47-47	−2.67 ± 0.17	<0.001
47-47-47-47 → 50-50-50-50	+7.66 ± 1.09	<0.010
50-50-50-50 → 53-53-53-54	−5.30 ± 0.44	<0.005
53-53-53-54 → 57-57-57-57	+1.46 ± 0.13	<0.005
57-57-57-57 → Mean 59th to 61st	−0.63 ± 0.09	<0.010

In each experiment, the difference in ^{45}calcium fractional outflow rate (FOR, expressed as per thousand/min) was established between the individual times indicated in the first and fourth columns. The mean values (±SEM; n = 4) for such paired differences are given with their statistical significance. The 44th min corresponds to the last sample collected during the control period, i.e., before raising the glucose concentration from zero to 300 mg/dl. Data collected between the 59th and 61st min inclusive were pooled, since the FOR of ^{45}calcium remained fairly constant over this three-minute period.

Effects of clonidine upon insulin released by the isolated perfused pancreas. Figure 3 is an illustration of the mean values for the concentration of glucose and insulin in the effluent from pancreases first exposed to a low (60 mg/dl) and then to a high (200 mg/dl) glucose concentration in the absence or presence of clonidine. In the control experiments, a typical biphasic response was observed, which was virtually abolished by clonidine.

In the control experiments, an increase in insulin output was first detected in sample 12, i.e., within 36 s after the moment when an increase in the glucose concentration of the effluent might have first occurred (Table 5). The highest secretory rate (mean value, 2534 μU/min; range, 993–5698 μU/min) was reached in samples 15 (two cases), 16 (one case), or 18 (one case) and was three orders of magnitude higher than the prestimulatory value (about 3 μU/min). In the same samples, the concentration of glucose averaged no more than 131.5 ± 12.2 mg/dl. In two of four experiments (B and D), the early response to glucose displayed a double peak in samples 15 and 18, respectively (Figure 4). A rapid fall in secretory rate always occurred between samples 18 and 22, at a time when the glucose concentration of the effluent was still steadily increasing from 157.0 ± 3.6 to 180.3 ± 3.4 mg/dl. After the initial secretory response, the lowest rates of insulin release were enregistered in samples 23 to 26 inclusive (Table 6). Thereafter, i.e., in sample 27 and subsequent samples, a reascension in insulin output occurred in all cases. The existence of a second secretory peak was obvious in only one experiment—D. However, in all cases, a second fall in secretory rate was noticed after the aforementioned reascension in insulin output. Thus, in each individual experiment, the three to six consecutively lowest values, seen in samples 40 to 46, were significantly lower than both the three consecutively highest values seen in samples 32 to 37 and the three last values in samples 55 to 57 (Table 6). As judged by linear regression, the secretory rate steadily increased during the late period (samples 46 to 57 inclusive), with a mean increment of +8.9 ± 0.8 μU/min for each sample. When the regression line corresponding to such a late increase was extrapolated to earlier times, and, when the values so obtained were subtracted from the observed insulin output, an apparently peak-shaped secretory component could be isolated for the 5-min period elapsing between samples 29 and 46 (see inset of Figure 3).

Although clonidine (see Table 6 for dosage) inhibited glucose-induced insulin release (Figure 3), the drug failed to totally suppress the insulinotropic action of the sugar (Figure 4 and Table 6). Both an early (samples 13 to 21) and a late (samples 27 to 57) secretory responses to glucose were still present, yielding mean secretion rates significantly higher than the basal value (Table 6). In the period separating the early from the late response (samples 22 to 26 inclusive), however, the mean insulin output was not significantly different from its prestimulatory value (Table 6). There was a strict temporal similarity in the secretory response to glucose in control and clonidine-treated pancreases, respectively, despite the fact that the secretory rate was 30 to 100 times higher in the former than in the latter case (Table 6). For instance, the early secretory response to glucose always started with samples 12 or 13 and terminated with samples 21 or 22 (Table 1, Figure 4); in the clonidine-treated islets, this early response always appeared as a double peak (Figure 4). Likewise, the later secretory response to glucose in the clonidine-treated pancreases started at exactly the same time (sample 27) when the reascension in insulin output was first seen in the control experiments. During the first minute of this late secretory response in the clonidine-treated pancreases, an apparently rhythmic pattern of release was observed in both individual (Figure 4) or pooled (Figure 5) experimental data.

DISCUSSION

Mode of action of clonidine in the B-cell. Clonidine, an alpha-adrenergic agonist,[12] is one of the most powerful inhibitors of insulin release so far investigated, as little as 0.08 ng/ml (0.3 nM) being sufficient to decrease glucose-stimulated insulin release. Clonidine failed to affect glucose oxidation and adenylate cyclase activity in the islets. These findings suggest that the drug does not interfere directly with either the process of glucose identification by the B-cell, a process tightly linked with the metabolism of the

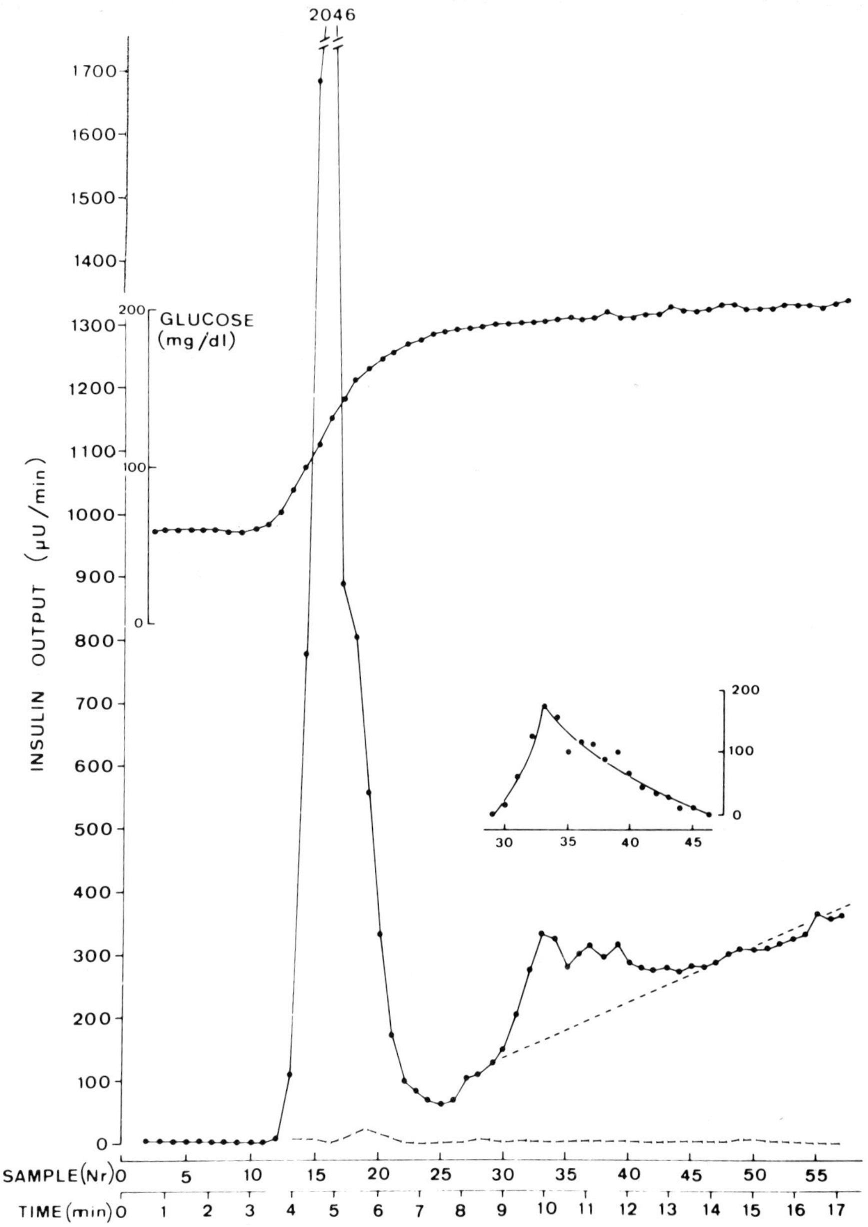

FIGURE 3. Time course for the mean increase in glucose concentration and insulin output in isolated perfused pancreases. Samples 2 to 57 were collected over successive periods of 18 s each. The output of insulin is shown as closed circles (control experiments) or dashes (clonidine-treated pancreases). The dotted line corresponds to the regression line for insulin release calculated for samples 46 to 57 inclusive. The inset illustrates the difference in secretory rate between mean experimental values and those obtained by extrapolation of the regression line.

sugar,[13] or with the synthesis of cyclic AMP at the level of adenylate cyclase. An indirect effect of clonidine upon cyclic AMP formation cannot be ruled out by the present data. Clonidine failed to affect glucose-stimulated ^{45}calcium net uptake. The situation found in the presence of clonidine is reminiscent of that encountered with epinephrine, which, at low concentrations (less than 10^{-6} M), also fails to abolish glucose-stimulated ^{45}calcium net uptake (Mahy and Malaisse, unpublished observation) and the glucose-induced increase in ^{45}calcium efflux.[14] Higher concentrations of epi-

TABLE 5
Glucose concentration and insulin output during the first minute of stimulation

Sample no.	Time (s)	Glucose (mg/dl)	Insulin output (μU/min)	
			Control	Clonidine
9	−36 to −18	59.0 ± 0.7 (8)	3.8 ± 0.3 (4)	1.7 ± 0.3 (4)
10	−18 to zero	60.2 ± 1.4 (8)	2.8 ± 0.3 (4)	2.2 ± 0.4 (4)
11	zero to +18	64.1 ± 1.9 (8)	3.4 ± 0.4 (4)	2.0 ± 0.3 (4)
12	+18 to +36	71.8 ± 2.9 (8)	7.8 ± 1.0 (4)	2.6 ± 0.6 (4)
13	+36 to +54	86.3 ± 3.1 (8)	109.0 ± 36.5 (4)	9.2 ± 2.6 (4)

Mean values for glucose concentration in the effluent and insulin output are given together with the number of individual determinations (in parentheses). The zero time is arbitrarily taken as the end of the last period during which the glucose concentration remained within the prestimulatory range.

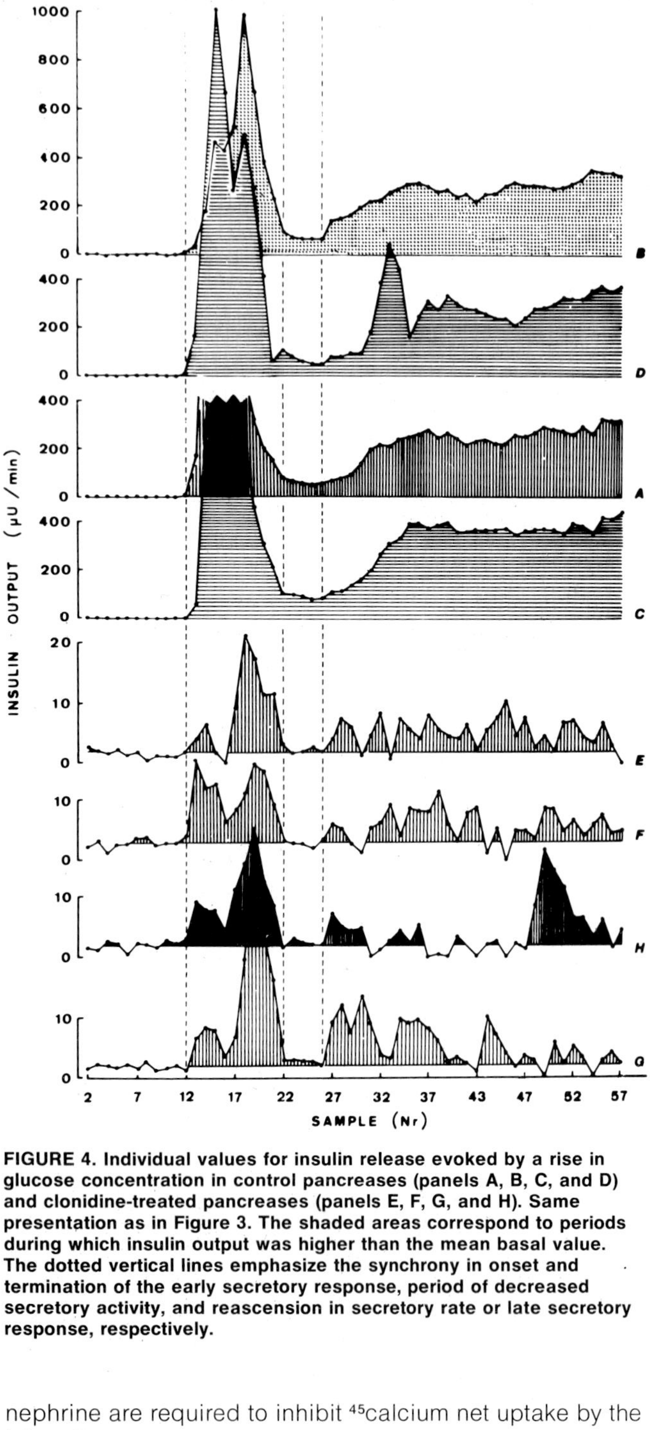

FIGURE 4. Individual values for insulin release evoked by a rise in glucose concentration in control pancreases (panels A, B, C, and D) and clonidine-treated pancreases (panels E, F, G, and H). Same presentation as in Figure 3. The shaded areas correspond to periods during which insulin output was higher than the mean basal value. The dotted vertical lines emphasize the synchrony in onset and termination of the early secretory response, period of decreased secretory activity, and reascension in secretory rate or late secretory response, respectively.

nephrine are required to inhibit ^{45}calcium net uptake by the islets.[15]

A possible explanation for these findings is that α-adrenergic agonists, rather than altering the inflow of calcium into islet cells, reduce the concentration of cytosolic calcium by causing the sequestration of this cation in subcellular organelles.[16] This is supported by the present finding that clonidine tended to decrease both the basal fractional outflow rate of ^{45}calcium and the augmentation of such a rate seen in response to glucose after an initial fall in ^{45}calcium efflux. Part of the basal release of ^{45}calcium and the major fraction of the glucose-induced secondary rise in effluent radioactivity apparently correspond to a process of calcium-calcium exchange,[17] which may indeed depend on the ability of influent calcium to displace calcium of high specific activity from intracellular organelles.

Timing of ^{45}calcium efflux from perifused islets. It is known from previous work[18–20] that glucose exerts a dual effect upon ^{45}calcium efflux, namely, a rapid decrease in ^{45}calcium fractional outflow rate followed, a few minutes later, by a marked and sustained increase in effluent radioactivity. The initial fall was recently attributed to inhibition of Na-Ca counter transport,[21] and the secondary rise to stimulation of a process of Ca-Ca exchange.[17,20,22,23] At normal extracellular calcium concentration, the latter process masks the underlying and sustained inhibition of Na-Ca counter transport.[21] The data illustrated in Figure 2 emphasize the view, already expressed on several occasions,[20,23,24] that the glucose-induced secondary rise in ^{45}calcium is not merely linked with exocytosis of the secretory granules, as initially proposed.[18]

The present study reveals that this secondary rise can itself be dissected in two successive peaks before establishment of a steady-state situation characterized by a slow and progressive fall in ^{45}calcium fractional outflow rate. In the absence of clonidine, the existence of successive peaks coincides with the phasic pattern of insulin release.[20] These peaks in effluent radioactivity are thought to reflect increases in the rate of ^{40}calcium influx in the prelabeled islet cells.[17] It is conceivable, therefore, that the phasic pattern of insulin release is, in part at least, attributable to a phasic regulation of calcium movements in the islet cells.

The early secretory response. The findings illustrated in Figures 3 and 4 indicate that the rate of insulin release during the initial secretory peak is at least 4 to 14 times higher than the values recorded during the second phase, up to the 15th min of stimulation with glucose. This difference could be accounted for by the fact that, at some moment during the early response, most B-cells within each islet and most islets within the same pancreas are simultaneously in an active phase of release, whereas this may never be the case during the later phase of secretory response.

The early peak was initiated at a time when the effluent glucose concentration was raised to no more than 70 or 80 mg/dl, a value often considered as below the threshold concentration for stimulation of insulin release by the sugar. The concentration of glucose in the immediate vicinity of the B-cell was not measured, however. The secretory activity of the B-cell is not solely regulated by the incremental change in glucose concentration: during the 3rd and 4th min of stimulation by glucose, a dramatic fall in insulin output occurred, despite a persistent and steady increase in the glucose concentration. Some other factor(s) inherent to the functional organization of the endocrine pancreas must be responsible for the peak-shaped pattern of the initial secretory response. Incidentally, this early response displayed an apparently double peak in some of the control and all the clonidine-treated pancreases (Figure 4). This could reflect a discrepancy between two populations of B-cells or islets in the same pancreas. A heterogeneous anatomic distribution of islets rich in either pancreatic polypeptide- or somatostatin- and glucagon-producing cells was recently identified in different species, including the rat.[25] These hormones may play a role in intraislets' regulatory processes.[26]

The silent phase. During the fifth minute of exposure to the high concentration of glucose, the release of insulin

TABLE 6
Time course of glucose-induced insulin release

Expt	2–9 (8)	10–11 (2)	12 (1)	14–19 (6)	23–26 (4)	27–30 (4)	32–37 (3)[a]	40–46 (3–6)[b]	55–57 (3)
A	3.5 ± 0.4	2.6 ± 0.6	6.2	941 ± 241	62 ± 3	100 ± 16	267 ± 9	232 ± 4	333 ± 3
B	2.9 ± 0.3	3.9 ± 0.7	8.3	548 ± 110	70 ± 2	167 ± 11	295 ± 5	244 ± 10	342 ± 5
C	2.6 ± 0.6	2.5 ± 0.0	6.4	2009 ± 820	89 ± 3	129 ± 12	387 ± 7	357 ± 4	424 ± 7
D	3.9 ± 0.2	3.4 ± 0.1	10.3	1022 ± 116	64 ± 8	92 ± 4	462 ± 46	240 ± 11	370 ± 8
Mean	3.3 ± 0.2	3.1 ± 0.3	7.8 ± 1.0	1131 ± 232	71 ± 4	122 ± 9	353 ± 25	265 ± 13	365 ± 12
Expt	2–9 (8)	10–12 (3)	13 (1)	14–20 (7)	22–26 (5)	27–57 (31)			
E	1.8 ± 0.3	1.6 ± 0.3	4.2	9.3 ± 2.8	2.4 ± 0.3	5.1 ± 0.4			
F	2.7 ± 0.3	3.3 ± 0.4	16.5	11.6 ± 1.3	2.9 ± 0.3	5.7 ± 0.5			
G	2.0 ± 0.2	1.6 ± 0.2	6.8	15.3 ± 4.5	2.7 ± 0.2	5.4 ± 0.7			
H	1.7 ± 0.2	2.7 ± 0.3	9.3	11.8 ± 2.4	2.3 ± 0.3	4.3 ± 0.8			
Mean	2.0 ± 0.1	2.3 ± 0.3	9.2 ± 2.6	12.0 ± 1.5	2.6 ± 0.1	5.1 ± 0.3			

Insulin-secretory rates (expressed as μU/min per pancreas) were measured over successive periods of 18 s each in pancreas first perfused for 40 min at a low glucose concentration (60 mg/dl; samples 2 to 10 inclusive) and then exposed to a high glucose concentration (200 mg/dl; samples 11 to 57) for the ensuing 17 min. Control experiments (A to D) are illustrated in the upper part of the Table. At the top of each column are mentioned the rank number of the first and last samples in each period together with the total number of samples in the same period (in parentheses). In (a), the three consecutively highest values in this period corresponded to samples 35 to 37 in three cases (A, B, C) and 32 to 34 in the last case (D). In (b), the three to six consecutively lowest values in this period corresponded to samples 40 to 42 (or 40 to 45) in three cases (A, B, C) and 43 to 46 in the last case (D). The lower part of the Table refers to experiments performed in the presence of clonidine, which was administered either throughout the experiment (E: 0.08 μg/ml; F and G: 0.05 μg/ml) or only for 10 min (20th to 30th min) before stimulation with glucose (from the 40th min onwards) at a 1.0-μg/ml concentration (H).

occurred at a steady low rate. In the control experiments, this rate was higher than the prestimulatory value, while in the clonidine-treated pancreases, the rate of secretion measured in five consecutive samples was not significantly different from the prestimulatory value. The latter finding indicates that a virtually complete arrest of secretory activity may be seen in the period in-between the early and late phases of insulin release. This finding is reminiscent of the silent bioelectric phase recorded in single islet cells in-between the first and second bursts of spikes,[27] and it demonstrates that the secretory, like the bioelectric activity, indeed, both represent discontinuous processes. With this idea in mind, the fact that the release of insulin during the silent phase failed to reach a basal value in the control experiments may well be attributable, in part at least, to heterogeneity in the precise timing of secretory events in different

FIGURE 5. Mean values (± SEM) for insulin release evoked by a rise in glucose concentration in pancreases treated with clonidine (same presentation as in Figure 3; n = 4).

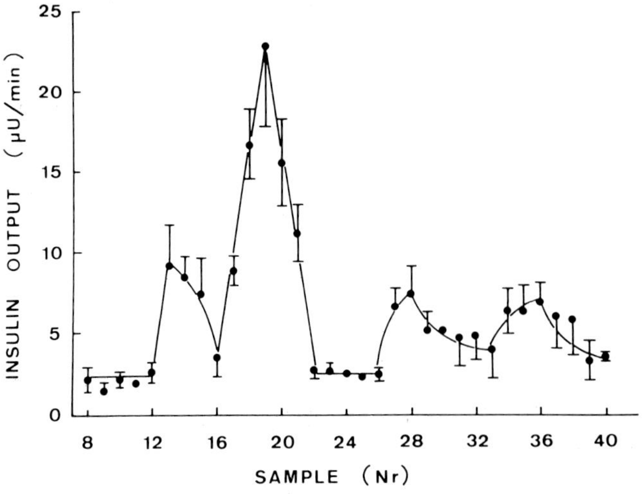

islets within the same pancreas and different B-cells within the same islet.

Several explanations have already been proposed to account for the phasic pattern of insulin release, such as the functional segregation of secretory granules[28] or a feedback effect of insulin on its own rate of secretion.[29] Although we do not wish to rule out the existence of such phenomena, it is unlikely that they are solely responsible for the precise timing of the secretory response to glucose. Indeed, exactly the same timing was observed in the absence or presence of clonidine, despite the caricatural difference in (1) the secretory rate and, hence, (2) potential depletion of a readily releasable pool of secretory granules, and (3) potential feedback effect of insulin upon its own rate of secretion. Since clonidine apparently interferes with insulin release at a level distal to the site of glucose identification and failed to affect the chronology of the secretory response, the pacemaker for the rhythmic nature of insulin release could conceivably be located at an early step of the secretory sequence, e.g., at the level of these metabolic events that help the B-cell to identify glucose.[13]

The late secretory response. The progressive build-up in secretory rate seen during the latest phase of the secretory response, i.e., beyond the 10th min of stimulation, probably reflects a true increase in the activity of each secretory unit. However, before such a phenomenon occurs, the second phase of the secretory response to glucose was characterized by (1) a rapid increase in secretory rate above the level seen in the silent period and, somewhat later, (2) a modest but significant second fall in secretory rate. This oscillatory phenomenon could reflect a synchronous onset of the second phase of secretory activity in different functional units (initial reascension in secretory rate) followed sometime later by the disappearance of such a synchrony (second fall in secretory rate). This tentative explanation is supported by the findings collected in the clonidine-treated pancreases, in which a rhythmic secretory pattern was indeed observed immediately after the silent period but faded out thereafter (Figure 5).

In conclusion, the present findings are compatible with the view that insulin release may occur according to a rhythmic pattern[30,31] and suggest that such a biorhythm is not regulated by the absolute rate of insulin secretion.

ACKNOWLEDGMENTS

This work was supported in part by grants from the Belgian Foundation for Scientific Medical Research. We thank C. Demesmaeker for secretarial help.

REFERENCES

[1] Metz, S. A., Halter, J. B., and Robertson, R. P.: Induction of defective insulin secretion and impaired glucose tolerance by clonidine. Diabetes *27*:554–62, 1978.

[2] Lacy, P. E., and Kostianovsky, M.: Method for the isolation of intact islets of Langerhans from the rat pancreas. Diabetes *16*:35–42, 1967.

[3] Malaisse, W. J., Brisson, G., and Malaisse-Lagae, F.: The stimulus-secretion coupling of glucose-induced insulin release. I. Interaction of epinephrine and alkaline earth cations. J. Lab. Clin. Med. *76*:895–902, 1970.

[4] Malaisse, W. J., Sener, A., and Mahy, M.: The stimulus-secretion coupling of glucose-induced insulin release. XVIII. Sorbitol metabolism in isolated islets. Eur. J. Biochem. *47*:365–70, 1974.

[5] Malaisse-Lagae, F., and Malaisse, W. J.: Stimulus-secretion coupling of glucose-induced insulin release. III. Uptake of ^{45}calcium by isolated islets of Langerhans. Endocrinology *88*:72–80, 1971.

[6] Herchuelz, A., and Malaisse, W. J.: The dual regulation of calcium efflux from pancreatic islets. Horm. Metab. Res., in press, 1980.

[7] Robberecht, P., Deschodt-Lanckman, M., Morgat, J.-L., and Christophe, J.: The interaction of caerulein with the rat pancreas. 3. Structural requirements for in vitro binding of caerulein-like peptides and its relationship to increased calcium outflux, adenylate cyclase activation, and secretion. Eur. J. Biochem. *91*:39–48, 1978.

[8] Salomon, Y., Londos, C., and Rodbell, M.: A highly sensitive adenylate cyclase assay. Anal. Biochem. *58*:541–48, 1974.

[9] Lowry, O. H., Rosebrough, N. J., Farr, A. L., and Randall, R. J.: Protein measurement with the Folin phenol reagent. J. Biol. Chem. *193*:265–75, 1951.

[10] Leclercq-Meyer, V., Marchand, J., Leclercq, R., and Malaisse, W. J.: Glucagon and insulin release by the in vitro perfused rat pancreas. Influence of the colloid composition of the perfusate. Diabete Metab. *2*:57–65, 1976.

[11] Leclercq-Meyer, V., Marchand, J., Rebolledo, O., Malaisse, W. J., and Leclercq, R.: A combined radioimmunoassay for glucagon and insulin. Diabetologia *11*:419–25, 1975.

[12] Van Zwieten, P. A.: The central action of antihypertensive drugs, mediated via central α-receptors. J. Pharm. Pharmacol. *25*:89–95, 1973.

[13] Malaisse, W. J.: The possible link between glycolysis and insulin release in isolated islets. *In* Diabetes Research Today. Lindenlaub, F., Ed. Stuttgart-New York, F. K. Schattauer Verlag, 1976, pp. 191–206.

[14] Wollheim, C. B., Kikuchi, M., Renold, A. E., and Sharp, G. W. G.: Somatostatin- and epinephrine-induced modifications on $^{45}Ca^{++}$ fluxes and insulin release in rat pancreatic islets maintained in tissue culture. J. Clin. Invest. *60*:1165–73, 1977.

[15] Malaisse-Lagae, F., Mahy, M., and Malaisse, W. J.: Effect of epinephrine upon ^{45}Ca uptake by isolated islets of Langerhans. Horm. Metab. Res. *1*:319–20, 1969.

[16] Brisson, G. R., and Malaisse, W. J.: The stimulus-secretion coupling of glucose-induced insulin release. XI. Effects of theophylline and epinephrine on ^{45}Ca efflux from perifused islets. Metabolism *22*:455–65, 1973.

[17] Herchuelz, A., Couturier, E., and Malaisse, W. J.: Regulation of calcium fluxes in pancreatic islets. III. Glucose-induced calcium-calcium exchange. Am. J. Physiol., in press.

[18] Malaisse, W. J., Brisson, G. R., and Baird, L. E.: Stimulus-secretion coupling of glucose-induced insulin release. X. Effect of glucose on ^{45}Ca efflux from perifused islets. Am. J. Physiol. *224*:389–94, 1973.

[19] Bukowiecki, L., and Freinkel, N.: Relationship between efflux of ionic calcium and phosphorus during excitations of pancreatic islets with glucose. Biochim. Biophys. Acta *436*:190–98, 1976.

[20] Herchuelz, A., and Malaisse, W. J.: Regulation of calcium fluxes in pancreatic islets. I. Dissociation between calcium and insulin release. J. Physiol. (Lond) *283*:409–24, 1978.

[21] Herchuelz, A., Sener, A., and Malaisse, W. J.: Regulation of calcium fluxes in rat pancreatic islets. IV. Calcium extrusion by sodium-calcium counter transport. Submitted for publication.

[22] Frankel, B. J., Imagawa, W. T., O'Connor, M. D. L., Lundquist, I., Kromhout, J. A., Fanska, R. E., and Grodsky, G. M.: Glucose-stimulated ^{45}calcium efflux from isolated rat pancreatic islets. J. Clin. Invest. *62*:525–31, 1978.

[23] Kukuchi, M., Wollheim, C. B., Cuendet, G. S., Renold, A. E., and Sharp, G. W. G.: Studies on the dual effects of glucose on $^{45}Ca^{++}$ efflux from isolated rat islets. Endocrinology *102*:1339–49, 1978.

[24] Gylfe, E., and Hellman, B.: Calcium and pancreatic B-cell function. 2. Mobilisation of glucose-sensitive ^{45}Ca from perifused islets rich in B-cells. Biochim. Biophys. Acta *538*:249–57, 1978.

[25] Orci, L., Baetens, D., Ravazzola, M., Stefan, Y., and Malaisse-Lagae, F.: Pancreatic polypeptide and glucagon: non-random distribution in pancreatic islets. Life Sci. *19*:1811–16, 1976.

[26] Unger, R. H.: Diabetes and the alpha cell. Diabetes *25*:136–51, 1976.

[27] Meissner, H. P., and Atwater, I. J.: The kinetics of electrical activity of beta-cells in response to a "square wave" stimulation with glucose or glibenclamide. Horm. Metab. Res. *8*:11–16, 1976.

[28] Grodsky, G. M.: A threshold distribution hypothesis for packet storage of insulin and its mathematical modeling. J. Clin. Invest. *51*:2047–59, 1972.

[29] Pace, C., Matschinsky, F. M., Lacy, P. E., and Conant, S.: Electrophysiological evidence for the autoregulation of B-cell secretion by insulin. Biochim. Biophys. Acta *497*:408–14, 1977.

[30] Beigelman, P. M., Thomas, L. J., Slavin, T. B., Shu, M. J., and Bessman, S. P.: Insulin from individual isolated islets of Langerhans. 1. Response to glucose. Biochem. Med. *8*:392–402, 1973.

[31] Garcia-Hermida, O., and Gomez-Acebo, J.: A different pattern of insulin release in the perifused islets of the rabbit. Biochem. Biophys. Res. Commun. *57*:209–15, 1974.

Glucocorticoid-induced Recovery from Streptozotocin Diabetes in the Adult Rat

MICHEL ROUDIER, BERNARD PORTHA, AND LUC PICON

SUMMARY

The effect of a large dose of cortisol (5 mg/kg), injected 24h and 3h before or 3h and 24h after streptozotocin (SZ), on the course of SZ-induced diabetes has been studied in the rat. Glucose tolerance tests, performed 1 or 2, 8, and 30 days after the SZ injection (35 mg/kg), gave the same results in cortisol-treated rats regardless of the time of cortisol injection [before SZ (C.SZ) or after it (SZ.C)]. During the first test, elevated plasma glucose, decreased glucose tolerance, and decreased glucose-induced insulin secretion were present in SZ, C.SZ, and SZ.C rats. During the second and the third tests, glucose tolerance and insulin secretion were significantly improved in both groups of cortisol-treated rats. On the contrary, rats receiving only SZ showed a worsening of the diabetic state. It should be noted that cortisol-induced recovery of diabetes was not obtained with larger doses of SZ (50 mg/kg).

These findings indicate that an improvement of diabetes can be obtained by cortisol treatment after the onset of chemically induced diabetes. Whether this effect is obtained through an effect on pancreatic regeneration and/or through the anti-inflammatory properties of glucocorticoids is unknown at the present time. DIABETES *29*:201–205, March 1980.

It has recently been proposed that the diabetogenic effect of streptozotocin in the rat is reduced by pretreatment with cortisol.[1] Unlike several agents known to modify the diabetogenic activity of streptozotocin,[2–7] cortisol did not improve the diabetic state during the first day, but the diabetes became milder in cortisol-treated rats, with glycemia returning to normal values in the fed state after one week.[1] It was important to know the long-term efficiency of this cortisol treatment and to determine the relationship between (1) the cortisol dose and the degree of recovery from diabetes and (2) the severity of diabetes and the degree of recovery.

From the Laboratoire de Physiologie du Développement, Laboratoire associé au CNRS no. 307. Tour 23-33, Université Paris 7, 2 Place Jussieu, 75221-Paris Cedex 05, France.
Received for publication 26 July and in revised form 11 October 1979.

MATERIAL AND METHODS

Female rats of the Sherman strain, weighing about 150 g, were fed ad libitum with commercial, pelleted food containing 47% carbohydrates, 8% lipids, and 20% proteins (U.A.R. France). Streptozotocin (SZ) (lot 60 140 U 9899) (Upjohn Laboratories) was dissolved in citrate buffer (pH 4.5) and immediately injected intravenously under slight ether anesthesia at the doses of 20, 35, and 50 mg per kg body weight. The concentration of SZ in the buffer varied according to the doses, and the volume of citrate buffer injected was always 100 μl/100 g body weight. Cortisol acetate (2.5, 5, 10, or 25 mg/kg), methylprednisolone acetate (5 mg/kg), and dexamethasone acetate (5 mg/kg), as a 100 μl/100 g b.w. solution, was injected subcutaneously 24h and 3h before the injection of SZ (C.SZ rats) or 3h and 24h after it (SZ.C rats).

Intravenous glucose tolerance tests (IVGTT) (0.5 g glucose/kg b.w.) were performed under pentobarbital anesthesia (4 mg/100 g b.w., i.p.) 1, 8, and 30 days after the SZ injection for the C.SZ rats or 2, 8, and 30 days for the SZ.C rats. Blood was withdrawn from the tail vein in the fed state. Blood samples (300 μl) were immediately centrifuged at 4°C; plasma was stored at −20°C until assayed. After dissection, the pancreas was weighed and homogenized for 1 min by ultrasonic disintegration at 4°C (sonifier Branson B12, Heat Systems-Ultrasonics, Plainview, N.Y.) in acid alcohol solution (75% ethanol, 1.5% v/v 12 mol/L, HCl, 23.5% distilled water). After one night at −20°C, the extracts were centrifuged and the supernatant was kept at −20°C until assayed.

Plasma glucose was determined using a glucose analyzer (Beckman Inc., Palo Alto, Calif.). Pancreatic and plasma immunoreactive insulin (IRI) was estimated using purified rat insulin as standard (R 171, Novo, Copenhagen, Denmark), antibody to human insulin,[8] and porcine monoiodinated ^{125}I-insulin.[9] The method allows the determination of 6 μU/ml (0.25 ng/ml) with a coefficient of variation within

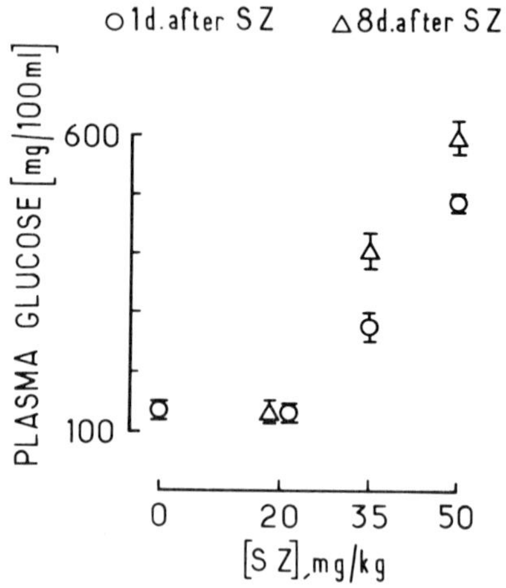

FIGURE 1. Streptozotocin dose response curve. Plasma glucose in the fed state was determined 1 day (○) and 8 days (△) after i.v. streptozotocin injection. Each point is the mean ±SEM of 5 to 10 rats.

and between assays of 10%. Silicate was used to separate free from bound hormone.[10] Results are given as mean ±SEM. Statistical analysis was performed using Student's unpaired *t* test.

RESULTS

Effect of the dose of streptozotocin on plasma glucose. A relationship exists between the dose of streptozotocin and plasma glucose values in fed rats (Figure 1). With 20 mg/kg, plasma glucose was not modified 1 day and 8 days after streptozotocin and was not different from the control values. With 35 mg/kg, plasma glucose was significantly increased on the first day, was still higher on the eighth day, and remained high on the 30th day (356 ± 88 mg/100 ml). With 50 mg/kg, plasma glucose values were higher than with 35 mg/kg. We checked (Table 1) that the citrate buffer injection per se had no effect on glucose tolerance. As a consequence, all the SZ-treated groups were compared with the nontreated group.

Effect of a pretreatment with cortisol (two injections of 25 mg/kg) on the course of diabetes induced by 50 or 35 mg/kg of streptozotocin. With the higher dose of streptozotocin, no protective effect of the cortisol was observed; plasma glucose values were the same in C.SZ and SZ rats on the first day (496 ± 10 versus 480 ± 11 mg/100 ml) and on the eighth day (595 ± 16 versus 598 ± 64 mg/100 ml).

With the lower dose of streptozotocin (35 mg/kg), pretreatment with cortisol improved the glucose tolerance on the eighth day (Table 1). However, this treatment resulted in a worsening of the diabetic state on the first day. So, in an effort to obtain an improvement of the glucose tolerance on the eighth day without increased hyperglycemia on the first day, we checked the effect of smaller doses of cortisol.

Effect of different doses of cortisol in rats injected with 35 mg/kg of streptozotocin. Table 1 indicates that, after a pretreatment with 5 mg/kg of cortisol, the glucose tolerance was better than with any other dose of cortisol both on the first and on the eighth day after streptozotocin injection. So, this dose of cortisol was chosen for further experiments. Methylprednisolone (2 × 5 mg/kg) had an effect similar to that of cortisol (2 × 10 mg/kg); with dexamethasone (2 × 5 mg/kg), the glucose tolerance test was normal on the eighth day, but hyperglycemia was important on the first day.

Comparison of the effect of cortisol (5 mg/kg) given before or after streptozotocin on the course of the diabetes. On the eighth day after streptozotocin treatment (Figure 2), diabetes was improved in SZ.C rats and C.SZ rats when compared with the SZ rats. During the IVGTT, plasma glucose values in C.SZ or SZ.C rats were not significantly different from each other and were significantly different from values of SZ rats. Plasma IRI was lower in SZ rats (15 ± 3 μU/ml) than in C.SZ rats (39 ± 9 μU/ml, $P < 0.05$) and in SZ.C rats (35 ± 9 μU/ml, $P < 0.05$).

On the 30th day (Figure 2) as compared with the 8th day, there was no improvement in SZ rats: the basal plasma glucose value was high, glucose tolerance was similar, and insulin secretion was not significantly increased by i.v. glucose. In SZ.C and C.SZ rats, the basal plasma glucose value and the glucose tolerance did not differ from those in

TABLE 1
Plasma glucose (PG) values (mg/100 ml) during an IVGTT (0.5 g/kg) performed 1 or 8 days after streptozotocin (SZ) injection (35 mg/kg) in nontreated rats, in rats receiving citrate buffer only, in SZ rats, and in SZ rats pretreated with glucocorticoids.

	1 day after SZ Minutes after glucose load				8 days after SZ Minutes after glucose load			
Treatment	0	5	15	90	0	5	15	90
None	142 ± 4	263 ± 10	207 ± 8	116 ± 3	142 ± 4	263 ± 10	207 ± 8	116 ± 3
Citrate buffer	135 ± 3	246 ± 9	202 ± 13	124 ± 4	130 ± 2	260 ± 12	199 ± 12	120 ± 4
SZ	276 ± 26	399 ± 26	362 ± 25	288 ± 39	401 ± 40	488 ± 25	478 ± 28	447 ± 60
Cortisol + SZ								
25 mg/kg	373 ± 60	495 ± 58	485 ± 68	352 ± 81	186 ± 20	278 ± 47	328 ± 41	292 ± 60
10	264 ± 50	382 ± 41	376 ± 47	301 ± 47	253 ± 43	346 ± 36	292 ± 34	212 ± 42
5	201 ± 28	324 ± 33	308 ± 34	175 ± 23	173 ± 10	258 ± 15	248 ± 15	171 ± 28
2.5	228 ± 42	342 ± 37	316 ± 37	190 ± 42	265 ± 52	318 ± 49	323 ± 44	251 ± 40
Dexamethasone + SZ								
5 mg/kg	444 ± 41	501 ± 40	531 ± 38	529 ± 23	140 ± 12	251 ± 12	199 ± 7	96 ± 13
Methylprednisolone + SZ								
5 mg/kg	328 ± 43	416 ± 35	394 ± 36	337 ± 41	248 ± 47	363 ± 50	299 ± 46	218 ± 43

Values are the mean ± SEM. Number of rats was between 8 and 10. On the first day, all the PG values of pretreated rats are significantly higher than values in controls ($P < 0.05$). Only dexamethasone-pretreated rats have PG values higher than values in SZ rats ($P < 0.05$). On the eighth day, all glucocorticoid-pretreated rats have lower PG values as compared with SZ rats ($P < 0.05$).

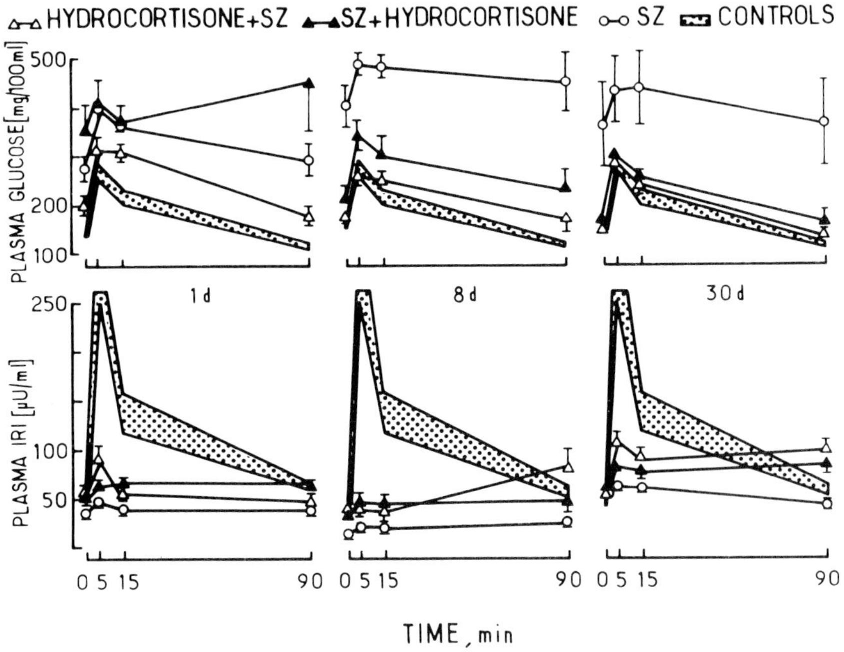

FIGURE 2. Normalization of glucose tolerance after cortisol pre (C.SZ) or post (SZ.C) treatment (2 × 5 mg/kg) of streptozotocin-diabetic rats (SZ). Glucose tolerance (0.5 g/kg, i.v.) and plasma insulin response were determined 1 (or 2), 8, and 30 days after streptozotocin injection in SZ rats (○), in C.SZ rats (△), and in SZ.C rats (▲).
Each point is the mean ± SEM of 5 to 10 animals in each group. The same animals were studied sequentially; the dotted shadow refers to five control rats.

the controls. Although basal plasma IRI was almost the same in all groups of rats (control rats: 46 ± 5 μU/ml, C.SZ rats: 53 ± 5, SZ.C rats: 57 ± 5, SZ rats: 56 ± 5), plasma IRI 5 min after injection of glucose was significantly higher in C.SZ (107 ± 11 μU/ml) and SZ.C rats (81 ± 7 μU/ml) than in SZ rats (56 ± 5 μU/ml). However, even in cortisol-treated rats, insulin secretion at this time remained severely impaired as compared with the controls (292 ± 42 μU/ml). On the contrary, 90 min after glucose injection, plasma IRI was increased in cortisol-treated rats as compared with the controls (C.SZ rats: 101 ± 6 μU/ml, SZ.C rats: 83 ± 10 μU/ml, control rats: 57 ± 6 μU/ml, $P < 0.05$). To relate the value of plasma IRI and glycemia, the plasma IRI/glucose ratio during the IVGTT was calculated in each group of rats (Figure 3). In control rats, there was an early increase of the ratio in contrast to the cortisol-treated rats and the SZ rats. In cortisol-treated rats, an increase of the ratio took place at the later time of IVGTT. In the SZ rats, the IRI/glucose ratio remained low.

The pancreatic IRI was measured in control, C.SZ, and SZ.C rats killed on day 1 or 2, 8, and 30 after SZ injections (Table 2). In the SZ rats, the pancreatic IRI was 14% of the control value on day 8, and it was 20% of the control value on day 30. In C.SZ and SZ.C rats, pancreatic IRI was also decreased (24% and 28% of the control values on day 8, respectively) but was significantly higher than in SZ rats. Moreover there was an increase of the pancreatic IRI between the 8th and the 30th day by 94% in C.SZ and by 42% in SZ.C rats.

DISCUSSION

In rats, a relationship between the dose of streptozotocin and the level of plasma glucose has been observed.[11] Ganda et al.[7] obtained the maximum diabetogenic effect in their rats given 60 mg/kg. Our results confirm the lack of spontaneous recovery from the streptozotocin-induced diabetes in adult rats[12] in contrast to the findings in neonatal rats.[13] A pharmacologic dose of cortisol has been found to have a protective effect only against a moderate dose of streptozotocin (35 mg/kg). Although we did not find any improvement of diabetes induced with a dose of 50 mg/kg, Katada and Ui[1] have reported such an improvement. However, in their study, diabetes induced with higher doses of streptozotocin did not improve with the cortisol pretreatment; thus, differences in diabetogenic activity of various batches of streptozotocin could explain this discrepancy. Their contents of α or β anomers are not always the same, and α anomer has been proved to be more diabetogenic.[14] Well-

FIGURE 3. Plasma $\frac{\text{insulin } (\mu\text{U/ml})}{\text{glucose (mg/100 ml)}}$ ratio during IVGTT performed 30 days after streptozotocin (SZ) injection (35 mg/kg) in rats treated with SZ only (○), in rats pretreated (△) or post-treated (▲) with cortisol, and in control rats (□).
Values are taken from Figure 2 and are the means ± SEM of 5 to 10 animals in each group.
* $P < 0.05$, * * $P < 0.01$, * * * $P < 0.001$ as compared with SZ rats.
+ $P < 0.05$, + + $P < 0.01$, + + + $P < 0.001$ as compared with control rats.

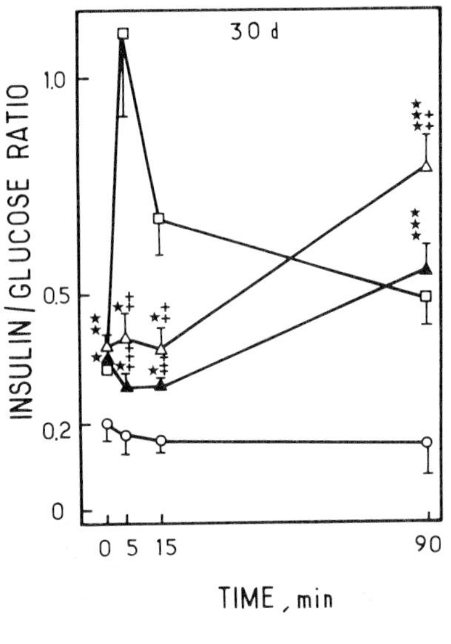

TABLE 2
Pancreatic insulin values 1 (or 2), 8, and 30 days after streptozotocin (SZ) injection in rats treated with SZ only, pretreated (C.SZ), or post-treated (SZ.C) with cortisol

		Pancreatic insulin (mU/mg) Days after SZ			
		1	2	8	30
Controls	2.59 ± 0.45 (5)				
SZ		0.88 ± 0.15 (6)		0.36 ± 0.05 (9)	0.54 ± 0.23 (5)
C.SZ		0.91 ± 0.23 (6)		0.63 ± 0.07* (8)	1.22 ± 0.20* (7)†
SZ.C			0.66 ± 0.24 (5)	0.72 ± 0.08* (7)	1.02 ± 0.08* (6)†

Values are the means ± SEM. The number of observations is shown in parentheses.
* The difference from the corresponding value of SZ rats is significant ($P < 0.05$).
† The difference from the corresponding value on day 8 in the same group is significant ($P < 0.05$).

mann and Volk[15] found lower blood glucose values and a persistence of identifiable, but poorly granulated, β cells on the seventh day after streptozotocin (65 mg/kg) after 6 wk of pretreatment with cortisol, but the mortality in cortisol-pretreated rats was greater than in rats receiving streptozotocin alone. Pretreatment with cortisol has also been found to improve alloxan diabetes in rabbit[16] and guinea pig.[17] The ineffectiveness of cortisol on diabetes induced by a high dose of streptozotocin indicates that the mechanism of the protective effect of corticosteroids against streptozotocin differs from that of protective agents like glucose and its analogues,[7,13] which have an effect even against high doses of streptozotocin and are said to compete with the glucose moiety of the streptozotocin molecule, thus preventing its interaction with the β cells. These agents must be injected before streptozotocin. The protective effect of cortisol injected before streptozotocin is not caused by the hyperglycemia, since at the time of the injection of streptozotocin (3 h after the last injection of cortisol), we observed decreased plasma glucose values (86 ± 5 mg/100 ml in cortisol-treated as compared with 142 ± 4 mg/100 ml in controls, $n = 10$, $P < 0.001$), probably because of insulin secretion induced by cortisol.

Houssay et al.[18] found that 6 mo of cortisol treatment in subtotally pancreatectomized rats resulted in a diminution of the percentage of rats becoming diabetic; the insulin secretion and the glucose tolerance were, however, not studied and the course of diabetes after interruption of cortisol treatment was not checked. In our study, we find that basal plasma glucose and glucose tolerance are much improved on the 30th day after cortisol treatment, but glucose-induced insulin secretion is only moderately increased with a particularly prolonged increase of the plasma IRI/glucose ratio. In cortisol-treated rats, the pancreatic insulin content is increased on the 30th day; however, we do not know whether the number of β cells is larger in C.SZ or SZ.C than in SZ rats.

It has been found, in vivo, that corticoid treatment results in an increased β cell number in rodents and subhuman primates;[19] on the contrary, in vitro, corticosteroids decrease the replication of β cells in pancreatic monolayer cultures.[20] Cortisol could act by another mechanism; Rossini et al.[21] have reported that, in some strains of mice injected with multiple subdiabetogenic doses of streptozotocin, there is insulitis, progressive β cell destruction, and diabetes. Immunosuppressive treatment has been used successfully in this model.[22] In streptozotocin-injected rats, one may speculate that cortisol could also be effective, owing to its anti-inflammatory or immunosuppressive properties. As a matter of fact, this possibility is presently without supporting data in the rat, since the SZ-induced insulitis model has been observed only in mice. Nevertheless, whatever the mechanism of action, the ability of cortisol, injected *after* the action of a diabetogenic agent, to improve the course of the subsequent diabetes deserves further analysis in view of the possible clinical implications in recent human diabetes.

ACKNOWLEDGMENTS
Streptozotocin was kindly provided by Dr. J. P. Paturaud (Upjohn France, Paris). We wish to thank Dr. G. Rosselin (INSERM-U55) for the gift of iodinated insulin.

The technical assistance of Jean-Claude Cros is gratefully acknowledged.

This study was supported in part by the Université Paris VII and the Institut National de la Santé et de la Recherche Médicale (INSERM) (contrat de recherche libre no. 76 1 022 4).

REFERENCES
[1] Katada, T., and Ui, M.: Spontaneous recovery from streptozotocin induced diabetes in rats pretreated with pertussis vaccine or hydrocortisone. Diabetologia *13*:521–25, 1977.
[2] Schein, P., Cooney, D., and Vernon, L.: The use of nicotinamide to modify the toxicity of streptozotocin diabetes without loss of antitumor activity. Cancer Res. *27*:2324–32, 1967.
[3] Dulin, W. E., and Wyse, B. M.: Studies on the ability of compounds to block the diabetogenic activity of streptozotocin. Diabetes *18*:459–66, 1969.
[4] Iwatsuka, H., Shino, A., and Taketomi, S.: Streptozotocin resistance of the genetically diabetic KK mouse. Diabetes *23*:856–57, 1974.
[5] Anderson, T., Schein, P. S., McMenamin, M. G., and Cooney, D. A.: Streptozotocin diabetes. Correlation with extent of depression of pancreatic islet nicotinamide adenine dinucleotide. J. Clin. Invest. *54*:672–77, 1974.
[6] Culbert, S., Sharp, R., Rogers, M., Felts, P., and Burr, I. M.: Diazoxide modification of streptozotocin-induced diabetes in rats. Diabetes *23*:282–86, 1974.
[7] Ganda, O. P., Rossini, A. A., and Like, A. A.: Studies on streptozotocin diabetes. Diabetes *25*:595–603, 1976.
[8] Rosselin, G., and Dolais, J.: Application de la méthode radioimmunologique au dosage de l'insuline humaine et au dosage de l'hormone folliculo-stimulante (H.F.S.H.). Monogr. Annu. Soc. Fr. Biol. Clin. *1*:189–217, 1967.
[9] Freychet, P., Roth, J., and Neville, D. M.: Monoiodo-insulin: demon-

stration of its biological activity and binding to fat cells and liver membranes. Biochem. Biophys. Res. Commun. *43*:400–08, 1971.

[10] Rosselin, G., Assan, R., Yalow, R. S., and Berson, S. A.: Separation of antibody-bound and unbound peptide hormones labelled with iodine 131 by talcum powder and precipitated silica. Nature *212*:355–57, 1966.

[11] Junod, A., Lambert, A. E., Stauffacher, W., and Renold, A. E.: Diabetogenic action of streptozotocin: relationship of dose to metabolic response. J. Clin. Invest. *48*:2129–39, 1969.

[12] Steiner, H., Oelz, O., Zahn, G., and Froesch, E. R.: Studies on islet regeneration, hyperplasia and intrainsular interrelations in long-lasting streptozotocin diabetes in rats. Diabetologia *6*:558–64, 1970.

[13] Portha, B., Levacher, C., Picon, L., and Rosselin, G.: Diabetogenic effect of streptozotocin in the rat during the perinatal period. Diabetes *23*:889–95, 1974.

[14] Rossini, A. A. Like, A. A., Dulin, W. E., and Cahill, G. F., Jr.: Pancreatic beta cell toxicity by streptozotocin anomers. Diabetes *26*:1120–24, 1977.

[15] Wellmann, K. F., and Volk, B. W.: Modification of streptozotocin-induced diabetes in rats by pretreatment with cortisone. Diabetologia *13*:331–37, 1977.

[16] Lazarus, S. S., and Volk, B. W.: Studies on a latent diabetic state in cortisone-alloxan treated rabbits. Diabetes *13*:54–59, 1964.

[17] Wellmann, K. F., and Volk, B. W.: Fine structure of pancreas in cortisone treated guinea-pigs and rabbits. Arch. Pathol. Lab. Med. *100*:334–38, 1976.

[18] Houssay, B. A., Rodriguez, R. R., and Cardeza, A. F.: Prevention of experimental diabetes with adrenal steroids. Endocrinology *54*:550–52, 1954.

[19] Like, A. A., and Chick, W. L.: Pancreatic beta cell replication induced by glucocorticoids in subhuman primates. Am. J. Pathol. *75*:329–48, 1974.

[20] Chick, W. L.: Beta-cell replication in rat pancreatic monolayer cultures. Diabetes *22*:687–93, 1973.

[21] Rossini, A. A., Appel, M. C., Williams, R. M., and Like, A. A.: Genetic influence of the streptozotocin-induced insulitis and hyperglycemia. Diabetes *26*:916–20, 1977.

[22] Rossini, A. A., Williams, R. M., Appel, M. C., and Like, A. A.: Complete protection from low-dose streptozotocin-induced diabetes in mice. Nature *276*:182–84, 1978.

Continuous Subcutaneous Infusion of Insulin in the Management of Diabetes Mellitus

M. C. CHAMPION, G. A. A. SHEPHERD, N. W. RODGER, AND J. DUPRE

SUMMARY

Control of glycemia by means of continuous subcutaneous infusion of insulin (CSII) was examined in insulin-dependent diabetes mellitus (IDDM). A battery-powered portable infusion pump was employed to deliver insulin at a constant basal rate designed to maintain plasma glucose within the normal range in the postabsorptive state, and empirically determined supplementary infusions of insulin were delivered before meals by the same system with the objective of maintaining excursions of plasma glucose within the normal range during absorption of a meal. The effects of CSII were compared with those of optimized conventional treatment using twice daily injections of mixed intermediate-acting and crystalline insulins in the same groups of volunteers in short term (1 wk) studies in hospital and in longer term (1 to 7 mo) studies with unrestricted activity under normal conditions after leaving hospital. The control of glycemia obtained with CSII in hospital was closely approximated by optimized conventional treatment under these conditions. In studies in hospital, continued infusion of insulin by the CSII program at basal rates with omission of meals and with vigorous exercise did not result in hypoglycemia. Abrupt cessation of CSII for 12 h overnight resulted in moderate ketoacidosis, which was rapidly corrected on resumption of insulin infusion. After the subjects were discharged from hospital, their mean postabsorptive plasma glucose concentrations and mean excursions of plasma glucose after ingestion of meals were maintained within normal limits with CSII but not with optimized conventional therapy. The control of glycemia with CSII was associated with significant reduction of daily dose of insulin by comparison with conventional treatment. During CSII, plasma free immunoreactive insulin (IRI) concentrations were in the normal range in the postabsorptive state. The supplementary doses of insulin before meals with the CSII program were shown to be essential for control of glycemia and were associated with dose-related increments of plasma free IRI, which were detectable within 15 min of delivery, rose to peaks at between 60 and 90 min, and declined to baseline at between 3 and 4 h. It is concluded that the management of IDDM by CSII is effective and safe and provides normalization of mean diurnal plasma glucose concentration through prolonged unrestricted activities under everyday conditions. The treatment can be maintained by the unaided subject and permits the undertaking of long term studies of its effects on the complications of diabetes mellitus. DIABETES *29*:206–212, March 1980.

Subcutaneous infusion of insulin has been proposed as a means of controlling glycemia in insulin-dependent diabetes mellitus.[1–4] The technique employs a continuous infusion of insulin at basal rates, designed to hold the plasma concentrations of glucose in the normal range in the overnight-fasted state and immediately before meals (referred to as the postabsorptive state), with empirically determined supplementary infusions given before meals. In studies cited above, this method was shown to be capable of maintaining the concentrations of glucose and other metabolites in the blood within or near the normal range when subjects were in hospital. It has also been claimed that treatment by continuous subcutaneous infusion of insulin (CSII) can be continued effectively after the subjects are discharged from hospital for periods of at least 3 mo,[2–5] but the regulation of glycemia under these conditions has not been documented. In the present study, we have compared the control of glycemia by conventional and CSII techniques in the same subjects in hospital. Under these conditions, we assessed the risk of hypoglycemia with omission of meals and vigorous exercise during CSII, and we examined the hazards of simulated failure of the insulin delivery system. We then compared the control of glycemia by conventional and CSII techniques in a further paired study through 1 to 7 mo of normal activity after volunteers left hospital. We also examined the timing and dosage of the

From University Hospital and St. Joseph's Hospital, London, Ontario, Canada.
Received for publication 13 August 1979.

supplementary infusions of insulin necessary to control the excursions of plasma glucose concentration after meals during CSII, while monitoring the concentrations of free immunoreactive insulin (FIRI) in the plasma.

SUBJECTS, MATERIALS, AND METHODS

The subjects were 12 volunteers who had insulin-dependent ketosis-prone diabetes mellitus; they are characterized in Table 1. Nine of the 12 subjects showed clinical evidence of either retinopathy, nephropathy, or neuropathy.

The study was carried out in two stages. The first stage was designed to provide a comparison of optimized conventional treatment with treatment by CSII under in-hospital conditions and to examine possible hazards of the infusion technique. To compare the treatments, five subjects were admitted to the Clinical Investigation Unit for two periods of 7 days each. During one of these admissions, depot injection treatment was optimized by administration of mixed intermediate-acting and regular (crystalline) insulins before breakfast and before the main evening meal. After 5 days' adjustment of dosage, the treatment was continued for a further 48 h while the plasma glucose was measured before each main meal, at bedtime, and 1½ h after starting each meal. Glycosuria was monitored by estimating glucose in consecutive 24-h collections. The same five subjects were readmitted within the next 2 to 4 wk for a trial of the effects of CSII. After a similar period of 5 days' adjustment of insulin dosage, the effects were again studied during a further period of 48 h. In this first stage of the study, mixed beef-pork insulins were employed.

To assess the risk of hypoglycemia during CSII and while fasting, nine diabetic volunteers received infusions of insulin at the optimized rates overnight and omitted breakfast before undertaking 30 min of exercise on a bicycle ergometer. The exercise was interrupted for 2 min at the midtime point to permit blood sampling, and the work load was adjusted so that 75% maximum exertion was required, as indicated by attainment of age-adjusted target heart rates. After exercise the subjects rested fasting until 1200 h. To assess the possible hazards of a failure to deliver insulin, the previously optimized subcutaneous infusions were discontinued abruptly in four subjects at 2000 h, and the plasma concentrations of glucose, ketoacids, and hydrogen and bicarbonate ions were monitored overnight.

The second stage of the study was designed to compare CSII with the conventional technique in everyday conditions after subjects were discharged from hospital. Depot treatment and CSII were optimized for each volunteer in hospital, as described above. After volunteers left hospital, the control of blood glucose was assessed for periods of 1 to 5 mo on conventional treatment under everyday conditions, and for periods of 1 to 6 mo of treatment by CSII under the same conditions. These assessments were carried out in varied order. To facilitate the assay of serum FIRI concentrations, pure pork crystalline insulin was employed with the infusion technique in this stage of the study.

TABLE 1

The age, duration of diabetes, and body weight of the 12 subjects who took part in the studies: A, stage 1 in hospital; and B, stage 2 after leaving hospital. The daily insulin dose on optimized depot therapy and CSII, the duration of studies of control of glycemia by the two techniques in stage 2, the number of days on which plasma postabsorptive glucose concentration was monitored in each subject, the mean of these concentrations in each subject, and the mean 24 h urine glucose output, where estimated, are set out for each individual

Subject	Age (yr)	Duration diabetes (yr)	% Ideal body weight	Daily insulin dose (U/day)		Weeks studied		Days monitored		Mean postabsorptive plasma glucose (mg/dl)		24-Hour urine glucose output (g/day)	
				Depot	CSII	Depot	CSII	Depot	CSII	Depot	CSII	Depot	CSII
(A) G.D.	45	1	92	31	20	1	1						
T.L.	23	18	102	73	42	1	1						
C.K.	36	18	105	43	33	1	1	(see text and Figure 1)					
K.J.	26	9	111	43	34	1	1						
K.S.	49	34	102	57	44	1	1						
Mean (N = 5)	36 ±5.1	16 ±7.1	100 ±3.7	49 ±7.1	35 ±4.2								
(B) K.S.*	49	34	102	57	48	16	28	8	8	106	98	2.62	0.34
D.G.	48	39	98	35	21	20	28	8	8	95	94	3.73	0.21
P.O.	39	26	100	33	20	4	12	7	7	255	87	—	—
V.L.	34	4	130	40	45	4	10	3	4	211	107	55	0.33
D.K.	16	2	107	43	23	4	11	3	5	268	117	—	—
G.M.	33	3	92	52	41	4	4	6	6	87	99	0.17	0.22
L.M.	28	6	98	39	33	4	4	4	4	135	95	4.53	0.59
N.P.	51	26	102	80	60	4	4	3	4	137	114	—	—
Mean (N = 8)	37	18	103	47.4	36.4					162	101	13.3	0.34
± SEM	4.2	5.4	4	5.5	5.1					26	3.6	10	0.09
Total days						420	707	42	46				

* K.S. took part in both stages of the study.

Technique of subcutaneous insulin infusion. The first stage study (in hospital) was carried out following the technique described by Pickup et al., employing the Muirhead Mill-Hill battery-powered infusion pump modified to deliver insulin at an increase rate (eightfold), initiated by the subject for 17 or 34 min before meals.[1] In subsequent studies, it was found more convenient and effective to employ the Muirhead infusion pump model 1001-HM. This instrument delivers infusate at a rate of 60 μl/h with the 6 ml syringe employed. The infusion rate can be increased manually with an extension of the driveshaft, which delivers 50 μl on each half revolution, registered by a palpable and audible click. The pump (dimensions, 12 cm × 5 cm × 2 cm; weight, 300 g) was worn on a light harness, and the infusate was delivered via either a "butterfly" needle or a fine nylon catheter inserted through a larger plastic cannula, which was withdrawn, bisected, and removed. One technique was selected by each volunteer: some preferred to manage the infusion entirely themselves, reloading the syringe once a day and changing the "butterfly" needle once every 1 to 3 days, while others preferred the catheter, which could be left in place for up to 3 wk but had to be replaced by a nurse or physician. Except where otherwise indicated, the pre-meal supplement of insulin was delivered as a series of clicks (one a second) 15 min before each meal, including snacks, and the supplementary dose was adjusted with the objective of preventing plasma glucose concentration from rising above 150 mg/dl (see RESULTS).

During optimization of dosage of insulin with CSII or with conventional treatment, the objectives were to maintain plasma glucose within the limits of excursions defined in other studies in subjects with normal glucose tolerance[6] and to avoid symptomatic hypoglycemia.

Laboratory techniques. Plasma and urine glucose concentrations were estimated by a glucose oxidase technique using the Beckman glucose analyzer. For purposes of management of treatment and for documentation, subjects were instructed in the use of the Ames reflectance meter and Dextrostix reagent strip for measurement of capillary blood glucose concentrations. Plasma FIRI concentration was assayed following precipitation of antibody-bound insulin with polyethylene glycol after equilibration of plasma at 37° for at least 2 h.[7] Ketoacids in the blood were assayed in the laboratory of Dr. N. Toews, McMaster Medical Centre, by a modified enzymatic technique.[8]

RESULTS

No local complication was encountered with the subcutaneous infusion technique. Occasionally the infusion line was accidentally withdrawn: the subject could easily replace a "butterfly" needle, and those using the catheter without a needle were supplied with "butterflies" to deal with this problem. In the course of the experiences with this technique that are documented in this report, two episodes of intercurrent infection were encountered: one subject developed a paronychia, requiring incision of the finger under local anesthetic, and another suffered an influenza-like febrile illness for several days. Both subjects became hyperglycemic while using the previously established continuous infusion insulin dosage, but the delivery of extra doses of insulin in the form of clicks, on the advice of one of us, served to control the glycemia. The supplementary doses of insulin regularly employed before meals varied from subject to subject and ranged from 4 to 12 clicks before main meals and 0 to 3 clicks before snacks. After determination of the infusion dose regimen during the early optimization period, no systematic trend in the amount of doses needed to control glycemia was apparent in the course of longer term management.

Stage 1. Comparisons of conventional and infusion techniques in hospital. After optimization of treatment as described, the mean plasma glucose concentrations were similar with the two techniques at the times indicated in Figure 1, except before breakfast after overnight subcutaneous infusion, when the mean plasma glucose concentration was significantly below that determined concurrently in normal subjects (55 ± 12 mg/dl cf. 77 ± 3.1 mg/dl, $P < 0.01$). Under these conditions the subjects were free of symptoms of hypoglycemia. The mean 24 h outputs of glucose in the urine were low by conventional criteria and were similar with both techniques (Figure 1). These studies confirm the reports that excellent control of the blood glucose can be achieved by CSII and show that this can be closely approximated by conventional treatment, with insulin given at least twice a day in hospital.

In the course of optimization of insulin dosage with CSII, a reduction of the total daily dose occurred in each subject. The mean reduction, expressed as a percentage of the optimized conventional depot requirement, was statistically significant, in spite of the attainment of comparable or superior control of glycemia with CSII (30% ± 3.4 SEM, $P < 0.01$).

To study the effects of fasting with continued administration of insulin, the overnight (basal) infusion was continued with omission of breakfast through to 1200 h in nine diabetic subjects. In the course of this 15-h fast, at 0900 h, the subjects undertook 30 min of vigorous exercise on a bicycle ergometer and then rested until lunchtime. As shown in Table 1, there was no fall in mean plasma glucose concentration with continued administration of insulin before, during, or after exercise. No subject developed symptomatic hypoglycemia during this procedure.

To examine the effects of abrupt cessation of delivery of insulin, the previously optimized infusions were discontin-

FIGURE 1. Mean plasma glucose concentrations (mg/dl ± SEM) on two consecutive days after optimization of treatment by depot injection or CSII in five volunteers with IDDM. The mean 24 h urine glucose outputs (g/day ± SEM) are shown below the figure.

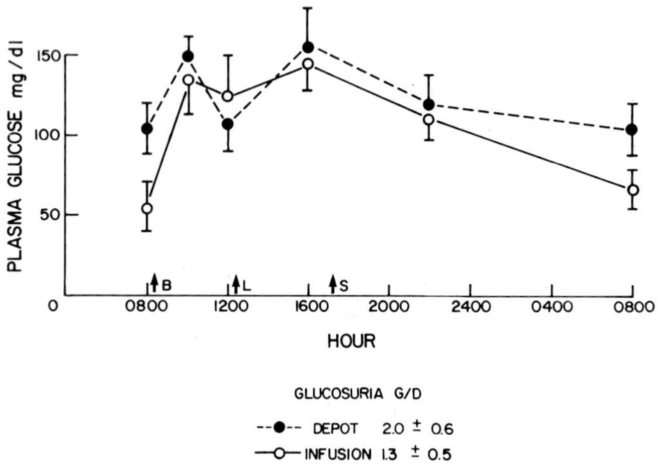

ued at 2000 h in four diabetic subjects (K.S., P.O., V.L., and D.K. in Table 1), and blood samples were drawn at intervals through the next 12 h. As seen in Figure 2, the mean plasma glucose concentration had returned to normal after the evening meal, and it then rose overnight to reach a mean level of 215 mg/dl (range, 160–420 mg/dl) at 0800 h the next morning. All subjects showed heavy glycosuria and ketonuria by conventional urine testing. The concentrations of ketoacids in the blood also rose progressively through the night. There was a mean reduction in plasma bicarbonate concentration of 6 mEq/L, and a slight fall in venous plasma pH in each subject, during the same interval. One of the four subjects developed nausea 12 h after termination of insulin infusion and was given a supplementary subcutaneous infusion of 5 U of insulin when the pump was reactivated. The other three subjects resumed the basal infusion rate, and by noon all four were asymptomatic. Normoglycemia was achieved in all four on continuation of the infusion during the afternoon.

Stage 2. Comparison of conventional and subcutaneous infusion treatments under everyday conditions. In the light of the results obtained in hospital, it was decided to undertake a comparison of conventional and CSII techniques under everyday conditions after volunteers left the Unit. The treatment by each technique was optimized during a brief admission to the Unit, as described above. An appropriately diluted solution of pork insulin in saline was prepared by injection of U-100 insulin into 20 ml bacteriostatic saline in a multidose vial by the subject. The volunteers measured capillary blood glucose concentration at least twice a day (before breakfast and at bedtime) and frequently made additional determinations. One of us was always available by radio call, and alterations of insulin dose and other problems were dealt with at visits to hospital or by telephone call.

Table 1 indicates the clinical characteristics and mean individual results of the eight volunteers who took part in this stage of the study. The comparison of the effects of the two treatments is based on observations of plasma glucose concentrations before breakfast, lunch, and the main evening meal, determined when subjects attended the laboratory. In addition, the capillary blood glucose concentration, determined by each subject at bedtime on these days, was corrected empirically to the equivalent glucose value. As shown in Figure 3, with CSII, the mean plasma glucose concentration before meals and at bedtime was held close to 100 mg/dl, whereas the mean values during injection were significantly higher at each time. These values for postabsorptive plasma glucose concentrations represent the means of all observations, with closely similar numbers of sets for each subject in the course of each treatment regimen, but with greater numbers of observations from subjects studied through longer periods of time. The results in Table 1 indicate that the significance of this difference was not dependent on the great number of observations in longer term subjects, since the means of averaged individual values for postabsorptive plasma glucose concentrations determined on hospital-visit days during the two treatments were also significantly different, in the same sense. The representative nature of these determinations on hospital-visit days is supported by the closely similar values for self-determined capillary blood glucose concentrations recorded on other days. The latter values were determined a.c. breakfast and a.c. supper. In the course of conventional treatment, the means of averaged individual values for capillary blood glucose concentrations at these times were 156 ± 16 mg/dl compared with 165 ± 16 mg/dl for venous plasma glucose on hospital-days. The corresponding values in the course of CSII were 97 ± 4.5 mg/dl for capillary blood glucose concentration on non-hospital-days, and 93 ± 5.2 mg/dl for venous plasma glucose concentration on

FIGURE 2. Means ± SEM of plasma glucose and ketoacid concentrations (K-A: A-A, acetoacetic acid; B-OHB, beta-hydroxybutyric acid), after abrupt cessation of infusion of insulin at 2000 h and through the next 12 h, in four volunteers with IDDM in the course of CSII. Below the figure are shown the mean values for venous plasma pH and bicarbonate (mEq/L) at the beginning and end of the study period.

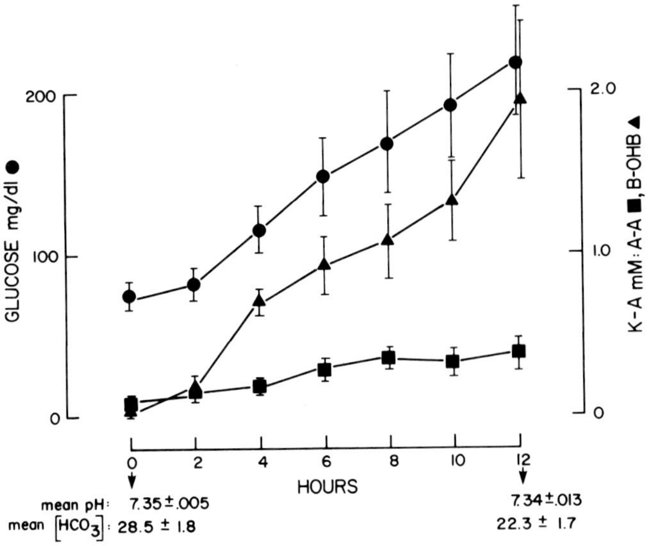

FIGURE 3. Plasma glucose concentrations before breakfast, lunch, main evening meal, and at bedtime in eight volunteers with IDDM in the course of studies of glycemia outside hospital during treatment by depot injection of CSII. Each value represents the mean ± SEM of all estimates made at the given times. The durations of studies and number of sets of estimates in each subject are shown in Table 2. The values at HS are based on self-determined capillary blood glucose concentrations, which were corrected to equivalent plasma concentrations. Below the figure are shown mean urine glucose output per 24 h and daily insulin dose for the two regimens.

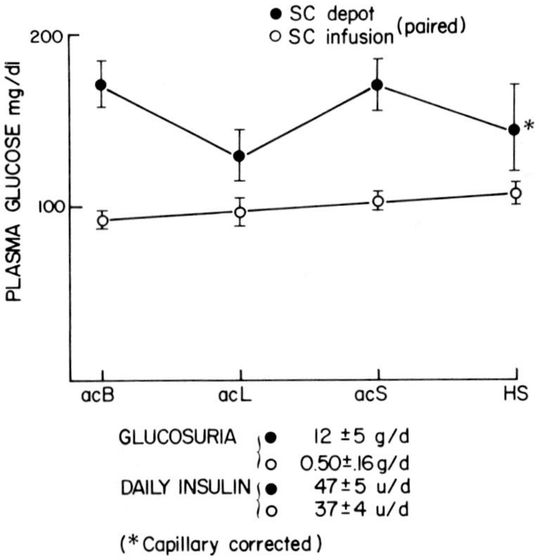

TABLE 2
Plasma glucose concentration during 16 h of a fast in nine subjects undergoing continuous subcutaneous insulin infusion at basal rates. Subjects undertook 30 min of vigorous exercise between 1300 and 1330 h (see text)

Time	0800	0900	0915	0930	0945	1000	1100	1200
			EXERCISE					
Hours of fasting	1200	1300	1315	1330	1345	1400	1500	1600
Plasma glucose, mg/dl	73	75	81	85	89	94	93	96*
± SEM	15	16	13	12	12	13	18	22

* The values at noon (1200 h) were self-determined capillary blood glucose concentrations corrected to equivalent plasma concentrations (see METHODS).

hospital-days. Five subjects also furnished 24-h collections of urine at, approximately, 2-wk intervals of each regimen, and as shown in Table 1 the mean of averaged individual values was significantly lower during CSII.

Meal tolerance tests during continuous subcutaneous insulin infusion. To assess the control of glycemia after ingestion of food during CSII, the volunteers attended the Investigation Unit at intervals to eat a variety of test meals.

In one of these studies, six volunteers attended the Unit for meals matching breakfast, lunch, or supper, according to the individual diet, and took the empirically determined pre-meal supplements of insulin, according to the usual program. Blood samples were drawn at the intervals shown in Figure 4. Each subject attended for the same meal at the same time on two occasions: on one occasion the insulin supplement was given according to the routine adopted, i.e., at 15 min before the meal, and on the other occasion the same supplement was taken immediately before the meal (Figure 4). The mean plasma glucose concentration was in the normal postabsorptive range immediately before the meal and was held below 120 mg/dl through the next 3 h on both occasions. Although the mean plasma glucose concentration was lower when the insulin supplement was given 15 min before the meal, the difference was not significant. When the insulin supplement was given 15 min before the meal, the mean plasma glucose concentration fell significantly in terms of paired differences in the interval between the taking of the supplement and conclusion of the meal. This effect of the insulin supplement was not apparent when it was given immediately before the meal. The mean plasma FIRI concentration rose within 15 min of delivery of the supplement and returned to baseline between 2 and 3 h after the meal.

To assess the dependence of control of glycemia after ingestion of food on the dose of insulin given as the pre-meal supplement during CSII, seven subjects took part in a further study, in which they attended on three occasions to eat a standard meal containing 75 g of carbohydrate. Each subject attended at the same time of day for each meal and took the meal with continued basal infusion of insulin but with no supplement, or with the usual pre-meal supplement, or with a pre-meal supplement amounting to twice the usual dose for that subject. It can be seen from Figure 5 that mean plasma FIRI remained constant when no supplement was given and plasma glucose concentration rose from normal pre-meal values to a mean peak exceeding 300 mg/dl at 3 h after the meal. When the empirically determined usual supplement was taken, the mean plasma glucose concentration was held below 160 mg/dl, and when twice the usual supplement was taken by each subject, the mean plasma glucose concentration was held below 110 mg/dl through the period of study. The mean plasma FIRI again rose by 15 min after delivery of the supplements. With the high dose of insulin, plasma FIRI reached a higher peak mean level at a later time. The mean plasma glucose again fell in the interval between delivery of the supplement and conclusion of the meal, but this was significant (in terms of paired concentration differences) only with the higher dosage.

FIGURE 4. Means ± SEM of free IRI and glucose concentrations in six volunteers with IDDM in course of treatment with CSII who ingested a meal corresponding to lunch or supper, according to the individualized diet, and took the pre-meal insulin supplement empirically determined for each subject. On one occasion the supplement was taken 15 min before the meal (——) and on the other occasion the supplement was taken immediately before starting the meal (------). Time 0 is 15 min before the meal.

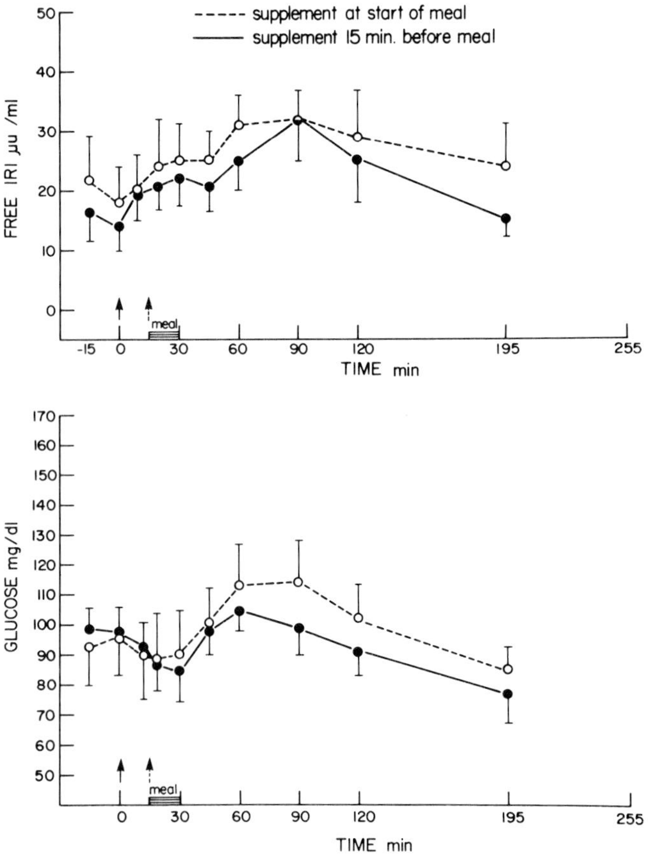

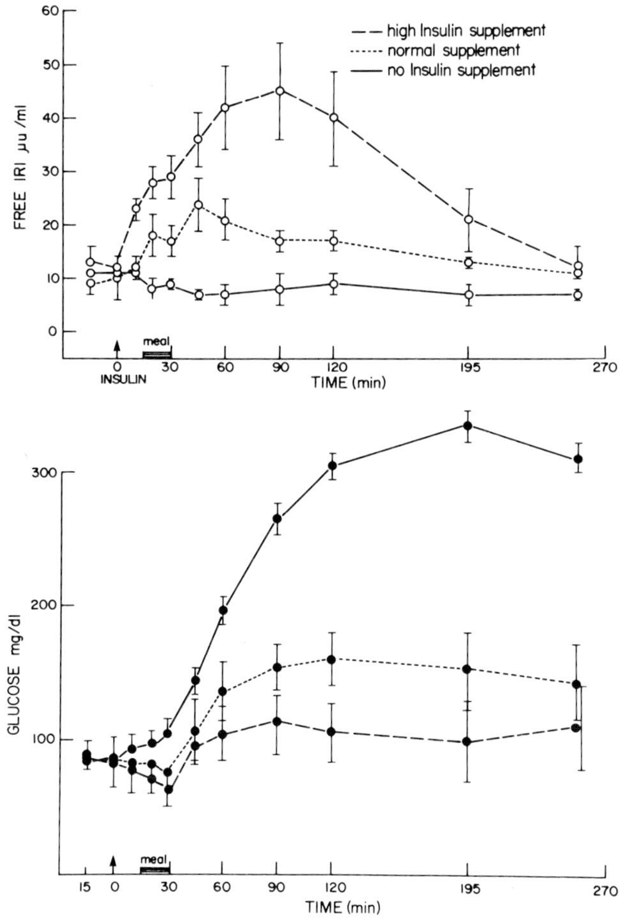

FIGURE 5. Means ± SEM of plasma free-IRI and glucose concentrations in seven subjects who ingested a standard 75 g carbohydrate meal in the course of CSII on three separate occasions. On one occasion, subjects took the meal with no insulin supplement, but with continued subcutaneous infusion of insulin at basal rates (——). On another occasion they took the insulin supplement usually employed 15 min before starting the meal (......), and on a third occasion they took twice the supplement 15 min before the meal (------). The meals were taken in varied order. Time 0 is the time the insulin supplement was taken.

DISCUSSION

The studies with CSII in hospital confirm that excellent control of plasma glucose concentration can be achieved with this technique under these conditions, and they show also that similar results can be obtained with optimized intermittent depot injection of insulin. The possible hazards of the infusion technique, in terms of the risk of hypoglycemia, and the risks associated with the failure to deliver insulin, appear to be small under the conditions of this study. Continued infusion of insulin at basal rates during prolonged fasting, accompanied by vigorous exercise, did not result in depression of plasma glucose. The interruption of infusion of insulin under experimental conditions for 12 h in four subjects resulted in development of glycosuria and ketonuria, but the acidosis was mild and readily reversed on resumption of infusion. This study was carried out overnight in the belief that the longest period of unnoticed failure of insulin delivery that would be likely to occur under everyday conditions would be through part, or the whole, of this interval. It is important to note that individual variation of responses in this situation may be considerable and, also, the potential dangers of this accident are common to all continuous delivery systems that administer insulin.

With the procedure employed, the program of CSII could be roughly predicted on the basis of the dose of insulin used with optimized conventional treatment. The basal rate needed to maintain plasma glucose concentration within the normal range in the fasting or postabsorptive state amounted to 30%, approximately, of the total daily depot injection dose, and the supplements given before meals amounted cumulatively to a further 35% to 55% of the depot injection dose. With these guidelines and subsequent adjustments of basal infusion rates and pre-meal supplement volumes, the mean daily dose of insulin required for comparable or superior control of glycemia by CSII was established within 3–7 days and was significantly less than that employed with the optimized depot technique. The mean reductions of 30% in the stage 1 study, when beef-pork insulins were employed with both techniques, and of 22% in the later study, when pork insulin was administered by the continuous infusion technique, were rapidly apparent during the optimization period. Thus, the maintained fall in insulin requirement is not likely to be a result of reduced neutralization of insulin by antibodies, and it may depend on more appropriate timing of delivery of insulin in relation to meals with this program and, perhaps, on factors affecting the bioavailability of insulin given in this way. The fact that subjects in this study consistently achieved equivalent or improved control of glycemia with reduced doses of insulin during CSII, whereas many of those in other studies using similar techniques received increased daily doses of insulin after initiation of the infusion technique,[1,3] may be accounted for by the optimization of depot injection therapy in all our subjects before initiation of CSII.

With respect to the comparisons of the effects of the infusion technique and those of conventional depot injection technique, it is, clearly, quite difficult to design a trial that would satisfy the most rigid criteria. It is suggested that the procedure employed represents an acceptable compromise, in that depot injection therapy, according to a demanding but practicable regimen, was optimized under the same conditions as those employed for CSII, and comparisons of the effectiveness of the treatments were made under similar in-hospital and everyday conditions. In stage 1 of this study, the only difference between the results of the two techniques was the low mean fasting plasma glucose after breakfast in the subjects treated by infusion (range, 45 to 70 mg/dl, approximately), and this clearly resulted from the use of unnecessarily high basal infusion rates in these subjects, since overnight fasting plasma glucose concentrations in the normal range (80–100 mg/dl, approximately) were later achieved under the same conditions, as well as in outpatients, as a result of reduction of basal infusion rates.

The results of the study done after discharge of the volunteers from hospital demonstrate superior control of glycemia with CSII. The mean plasma glucose concentrations before meals and at bedtime were lower with the infusion technique and were maintained with less variation. The observations on glycosuria were less numerous but confirmed the superior control of glycemia attained by the infusion technique. Detailed observations of excursions of plasma glucose after ingestion of meals in the course of depot treatment were not made in this study. The results of the study of plasma glucose after ingestion of test meals, corresponding to those usually taken by subjects undergoing CSII with the usual supplementary doses of insulin, show control of glycemia within the limits established under everyday conditions in studies of diurnal plasma glucose concentrations in subjects who had normal glucose tolerance.[6] To compare estimated mean diurnal plasma glucose concentrations in our subjects during CSII with values determined in subjects with normal glucose tolerance,[6] we can interpolate the mean plasma glucose concentrations after normal meals (three a day) and snacks (two a day) into the observed mean curve for postabsorptive plasma glucose concentration. The mean value for a plasma glucose concentration estimated in this way in the eight subjects during CSII outside hospital was 107 mg/dl, and it can be compared with the value of 109 mg/dl derived from the observations in normal subjects cited above. The studies with the standard 75 g carbohydrate meal showed that control of glycemia depended on the administration of the pre-meal supplementary infusion of insulin in a dose-related fashion, and thus it could probably not be matched by any regimen that did not require administration of rapidly acting insulin before each meal. Even though this meal exceeded the largest normally taken by some of the diabetic subjects, the mean peak plasma glucose concentration attained after the usual supplementary dose of insulin was 152 ± 18 mg/dl, similar to that of four normal subjects who took the same standard meal (the authors, 172 ± 7.6 mg/dl).

The studies of immunoreactive insulin in the plasma showed that the concentration of FIRI increased within 15 min of delivery of supplementary doses of insulin during CSII. The peak mean increments were achieved at 60 to 90 min after delivery, and individual peaks tended to be greater and later after administration of higher doses. The control of glycemia was clearly related to the dose of insulin and blood concentrations of FIRI. In some studies with the so-called artificial pancreas, requiring administration of insulin by peripheral intravenous infusion at rates dependent on continuous monitoring of blood glucose concentration, normalization of plasma glucose levels has been achieved only in association with supranormal concentrations of FIRI in the plasma, in the postabsorptive state, as well as in the course of absorption of a meal,[9] and it was suggested that the apparent need for supraphysiologic doses of insulin administered by the systemic route depends on greater effectiveness of insulin reaching the liver by the portal route under physiologic conditions. However, other studies with a different program for peripheral intravenous infusion of insulin, initiated before the rise of blood glucose after a meal, have shown normalization of plasma glucose concentrations when plasma FIRI concentrations were closer to the normal range.[10] Thus, even with continuous administration of insulin, the blood levels of the free hormone necessary for control of glycemia vary widely with the programs employed. It is also important to recognize that the biologic significance of apparent FIRI, determined by the antibody-precipitation-extraction procedures used in these studies, is uncertain and may not be equivalent to that of plasma IRI in the absence of insulin antibodies. However, it is notable that the time courses of changes in free IRI in the present study were not obviously different from those of IRI in subjects without insulin antibodies in a recent study employing CSII.[11] Further studies of the pharmacology of insulin administered by the systemic route in diabetic subjects with and without antibodies to insulin, with particular attention to the timing of supplementary dosage, are necessary for interpretation of the observations presently available.

In spite of the fact that the infusion system used in this study could be made more convenient by further miniaturization and by simplification of the technique for prolonged cannulation, treatment by CSII proved to be remarkably acceptable to the subjects. The program is simple and the apparatus easily managed by the unaided subjects, who found the flexibility of timing of meals particularly advantageous. On the basis of their experience, a growing number of volunteers have opted to continue the treatment through a long term trial. While much remains to be learned of the range of applications of the technique and the details of its effects on metabolism, it is now possible to plan studies of the effects of control of mean glycemia within the normal range on the complications of the disease in insulin-dependent diabetes mellitus.

ACKNOWLEDGMENTS

This study was carried out with the aid of a grant from the Physician's Services Incorporated Foundation, Ontario.

REFERENCES

[1] Pickup, J. C., Keen, H., Parsons, J. A., and Alberti, K. G. M. M.: Continuous subcutaneous insulin infusion: an approach to achieving normoglycemia. Br. Med. J. *1*:204, 1978.

[2] Shepherd, G. A. A., Champion, M. C., Rodger, N. W., and Dupre, J.: Blood glucose during subcutaneous insulin infusion in the treatment of diabetes mellitus. Clin. Res. *26*:865A, 1978. Abstract.

[3] Tamborlane, W. V., Sherwin, R. S., Genel, M., and Felig, P.: Administration of insulin to juvenile diabetics via portable pump. N. Engl. J. Med. *300*:573, 1979.

[4] Pickup, J. C., Keen, H., Parsons, J. A., Alberti, K. G. M. M., and Rowe, A. S.: Continuous subcutaneous insulin infusion: improved blood glucose and intermediary metabolite control in diabetics. Lancet *1*:1255, 1979.

[5] Tamborlane, W. V., Sherwin, R. S., Genel, M., and Felig, P.: Restoration of normal lipid and amino acid metabolism in diabetic patients treated with a portable insulin infusion pump. Lancet *1*:1258, 1979.

[6] Genuth, S. M.: Plasma insulin and glucose profiles in normal, obese and diabetic persons. Ann. Intern. Med. *79*:812, 1973.

[7] Kuzuya, H., Blix, P. M., Horwitz, D. L., Steiner, D. F., and Rubenstein, A. H.: Determination of free and total insulin and C-peptide in insulin-treated diabetics. Diabetes *26*:22, 1977.

[8] Williamson, D. H., Lund, P., and Krebs, H. A.: The redox-state of free-nicotinamide-adenine dinucleotide in the cytoplasm and mitochondria of rat liver. Biochem. J. *103*:514, 1967.

[9] Marliss, E. B., Nakhooda, A. F., and Hanna, A. K.: Insulin, glucagon and amino acid profiles during glycemic control by the closed-loop artificial endocrine pancreas (AEP). Diabetes *28*:377, 1979. Abstract.

[10] Horwitz, D. L., Granger, J. F., Nattrass, M., Martin, M. J., and Ash, S. L.: Combined preprogrammed and feedback-controlled insulin administration with an artificial beta cell. Diabetes *28*:376, 1979. Abstract.

[11] Slama, G., Buu, K. N. P., Tchobroutsky, G., Delage, A., and Desplanque, N.: Plasma insulin and C-peptide levels during continuous subcutaneous insulin infusion. Diabetes Care *2*:251, 1979.

Inhibition of Alloxan Action in Isolated Pancreatic Islets by Superoxide Dismutase, Catalase, and a Metal Chelator

L. J. FISCHER AND S. A. HAMBURGER

SUMMARY

The possible participation of superoxide anions, hydrogen peroxide, and hydroxyl radicals in the action of alloxan was investigated using isolated rat pancreatic islets. Exposure of islets for 5 min to alloxan (0.15 or 0.2 mg/ml) inhibited subsequent glucose-stimulated insulin release. The presence of superoxide dismutase (1000 U/ml), catalase (50 μg/ml), or a metal chelator diethylenetriaminepentacetic acid (1 mM) markedly attenuated this effect of alloxan. Use of these agents afforded complete protection from the lower concentration of alloxan and partial protection from the higher concentration of the toxic compound. Inactivation of the enzymes or addition of excess iron to the chelating agent before its use with alloxan eliminated the protective action of these agents. The results are consistent with the proposal that hydroxyl radicals, generated via reactions that involve superoxide anions, hydrogen peroxide, and iron, mediate the deleterious effect of alloxan in pancreatic islets. DIABETES *29*:213–216, March 1980.

It has been suggested that the diabetogenic action of alloxan includes the production of highly reactive oxygen-containing radicals, which are cytotoxic to the insulin-producing B cells of the pancreas.[1] Such oxygen-containing species as superoxide anion, hydrogen peroxide, and hydroxyl radical have been detected in oxygenated solutions containing alloxan and its reduced form, dialuric acid.[2] Any or all of these species may produce cell damage. Hydroxyl radical, the most reactive species, probably arises from reactions that involve superoxide anions, hydrogen peroxide, and iron.[3] Hydroxyl radical has been implicated in the diabetogenic effect of alloxan, because animals pretreated with such radical scavengers as n-butanol and dimethylurea are protected from alloxan-induced permanent hyperglycemia.[1,4] Other results do not support the hydroxyl radical mechanism for alloxan. For example, the radical scavenger n-butanol was shown to protect animals in vivo by an indirect mechanism[5] and was not effective against alloxan action in vitro.[6]

Exposure of isolated pancreatic islets to alloxan for short periods (e.g., 5 min) is known to reduce subsequent glucose-stimulated insulin release.[7] This action has been widely used as an in vitro model for alloxan action on the pancreatic B cell. In an attempt to investigate in a more direct manner the possible role of reactive oxygen-containing radicals in alloxan cytotoxicity, we have tested the ability of superoxide dismutase (SOD), catalase, and a chelator of iron, diethylenetriaminepentacetic acid (DETAPAC), to protect isolated rat pancreatic islets from the inhibitory effects of alloxan on glucose-stimulated insulin release. Addition of these agents in vitro to pancreatic islets before addition of alloxan should reduce the amount of hydroxyl radicals present in the solution bathing the islets, provided the radicals are produced according to the scheme shown in Figure 1. This report shows that pretreatment of pancreatic islets with the agents interfered with the action of alloxan and, thereby, provides more definitive evidence than that currently available to implicate hydroxyl radicals in the alloxan-induced damage to insulin-secreting cells.

MATERIALS AND METHODS

Animals and chemicals. Male Wistar rats (Lab Supply, Indianapolis, Indiana), weighing between 200 and 250 g, were used for the isolation of pancreatic islets. Superoxide dismutase (SOD), purchased from Biotics Research, Houston, Texas, had a specific activity of about 30,000 U/mg. Catalase (3000 U/mg) and alloxan monohydrate were from Sigma Chemical, St. Louis, Missouri. Diethylenetriaminepentacetic acid (DETAPAC) was purchased from Aldrich Chemical, Milwaukee, Wisconsin, and Trasylol was from FBA Pharmaceuticals, New York.

Experimental procedure. All experiments were performed with islets of Langerhans isolated by collagenase digestion

From the Department of Pharmacology, College of Medicine, University of Iowa, Iowa City, Iowa 52242.
Address reprint requests to L. J. Fischer, Ph.D., Department of Pharmacology, Basic Sciences Building, University of Iowa, Iowa City, Iowa 52242.
Received for publication 12 July 1979.

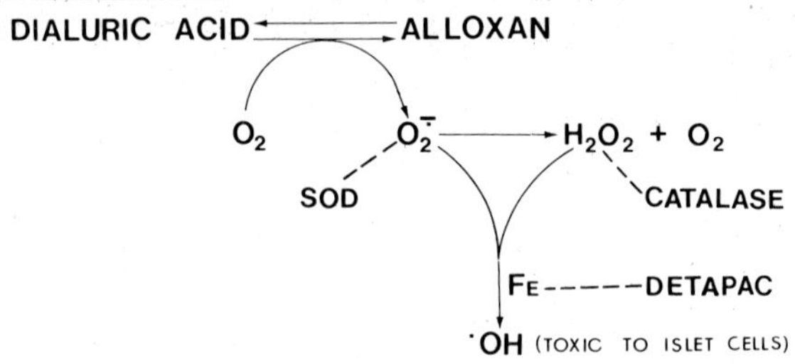

FIGURE 1. Proposed scheme for alloxan-generated hydroxyl free radicals (˙OH) and inhibition of this process by various agents (broken lines indicate site of action of inhibitors). Dialuric acid, when reoxidized to alloxan, produces superoxide anions (O_2^{-}) that dismute to form hydrogen peroxide (H_2O_2).[1] In a series of reactions, these products and iron interact to form the reactive and potentially toxic ˙OH free radical.[3] Superoxide dismutase (SOD) and catalase should reduce formation of ˙OH by reducing amounts of O_2^{-} and H_2O_2, respectively. An iron chelator (DETAPAC) should sequester the metal component of the system, thereby reducing ˙OH radical formation.

of the pancreas.[8] Islets were placed into a reservoir containing oxygenated (95% O_2 and 5% CO_2) Krebs-Ringer bicarbonate (KRB) buffer with 2 mg/ml bovine serum albumin (BSA). Groups of 20 islets, collected in a 0.1-ml volume from the islet reservoir, were added to 13 × 100-mm, siliconized glass tubes. Immediately, 0.8 ml of KRB buffer with 2 mg/ml BSA and containing low glucose (0.75 mg/ml) was added to the tubes so that a final volume of 1 ml contained 0.6 mg/ml glucose. The tubes were placed in a 37°C shaking, water bath, and 0.05 ml of a solution containing SOD, catalase, DETAPAC, or 0.05 ml of KRB buffer (control) was added. The concentrations of the agents used in the experiments (see figures) were the highest concentrations that, by themselves, would not alter subsequent glucose-stimulated insulin release. Pretreatment of islets in oxygenated buffer for 10 min with the agents was followed by addition of 0.05 ml of a freshly prepared alloxan solution or a similar volume of KRB buffer (control). The agents used for pretreatment were present during alloxan exposure. A 5-min alloxan exposure period was used in a manner identical to that used by others to study the effects of alloxan on subsequent glucose-stimulated insulin release.[6,9] After the alloxan exposure period, the tubes were centrifuged at 1000 rpm for 2 min to settle the islets and the supernatant was aspirated and discarded. KRB buffer (1 ml with 2 mg/ml BSA), containing either low glucose (0.6 mg/ml) or high glucose (3.0 mg/ml), was added to the appropriate tubes. The addition of an inhibitor of insulin degradation (Trasylol, 1000 U/0.05 ml) to all tubes was followed by immediate flushing of the tubes with oxygen and capping to prevent loss of the gas phase. The tubes were placed in a shaking water bath at 37°C for 45 min and then removed for centrifugation to pellet the tissue (2000 rpm for 2 min). The supernatant was diluted with an equal volume of 1N acetic acid and frozen until assayed for immunoreactive insulin (IRI) using the method of Makulu et al.[10] Rat insulin (Novo, Copenhagen) was used as the standard and guinea-pig antiserum to porcine insulin (P. Wright) was the antibody source. Results were expressed as nanograms of rat insulin released per islet over the 45-min test period. Values for basal insulin release (low glucose control), determined in each experiment, were subtracted from the values obtained for islets exposed to high glucose. Basal insulin release was always below 1 ng/islet/45 min. Mean values for glucose-stimulated insulin release were compared by an analysis of variance followed by Dunnett's procedure or the least significant difference test.[11]

In certain experiments the agents used in pretreatment of islets were inactivated before their use. For SOD and catalase, this was accomplished by heating solutions of the enzymes at 100°C for 1 hr. The iron chelator (DETAPAC) was inactivated by adding a 10-fold molar excess of $FeSO_4$ to a solution containing DETAPAC and allowing it to remain at room temperature for 20 min before its use with isolated islets.

RESULTS

Exposure of isolated pancreatic islets to alloxan for 5 min significantly inhibited subsequent glucose-stimulated insulin release. Addition to SOD (1000 U/ml) to islets before their alloxan exposure protected the insulin-secreting cells from the effects of alloxan (Figure 2). The lower concentration of alloxan (0.15 mg/ml) produced a 62% inhibition of glucose-stimulated insulin release, but, in the presence of SOD, normal insulin release could be obtained. A higher concentration of alloxan (0.2 mg/ml) almost completely abolished glucose-stimulated insulin release and pretreatment with SOD permitted release to return to 60% of the nontreated control value. Heat-inactivated SOD was unable to protect islet cells from the effects of alloxan, indicating that the protection was due to enzymatic activity. Pretreatment of islets with SOD in the absence of alloxan had no effect on subsequent glucose-stimulated insulin release.

The ability of catalase to antagonize the effects of alloxan was studied in a separate series of experiments and the results are shown in Figure 3. Catalase pretreatment was able to almost completely antagonize the effects of the lower concentration of alloxan. The protective effect of catalase was apparent, but not complete, when the higher concentration of alloxan was used. The protective action of catalase was not evident when the enzyme had been inactivated by heat. Catalase alone had no effect on glucose-stimulated insulin release.

Pretreatment with the iron chelator DETAPAC was also

FIGURE 2. Effect of superoxide dismutase (SOD) on alloxan-induced inhibition of glucose-stimulated insulin release from isolated pancreatic islets. Islets were pretreated with SOD (indicated by +) and then exposed to various concentrations of alloxan for 5 min. After removal of alloxan and SOD, glucose-stimulated insulin release was measured. The symbol △ indicates the enzyme was inactivated by heat; * indicates a significant ($P < 0.05$) difference from control. The number of experiments is indicated at the bottom of each bar.

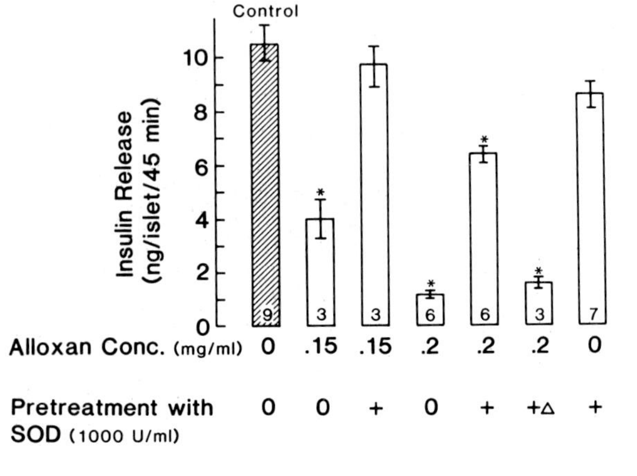

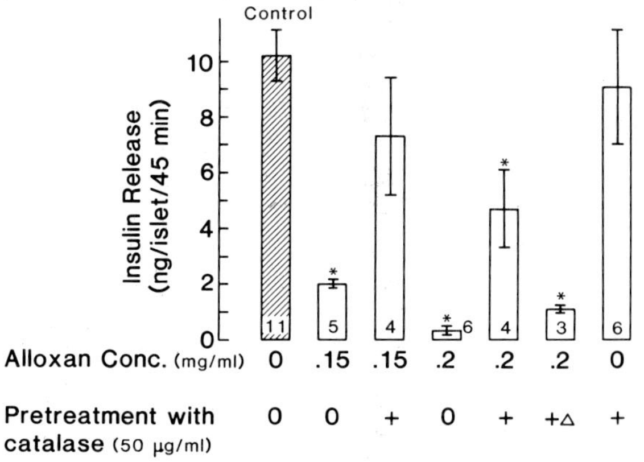

FIGURE 3. Effect of catalase on alloxan-induced inhibition of glucose-stimulated insulin release from isolated pancreatic islets. Format, same as in Figure 2.

able to protect islets from the action of alloxan (Figure 4). Similar to SOD and catalase, DETAPAC completely antagonized the insulin-inhibitory effect of 0.15 mg/ml of alloxan and showed partial antagonism at the higher concentration of the cytotoxic compound. DETAPAC protection was abolished when the compound was allowed to chelate in an excess of iron before its use with alloxan. This result is consistent with a protective role for DETAPAC, owing to its chelation of metal. In preliminary experiments, exposure of isolated islets to iron alone (10 mM) had no effect on subsequent glucose-stimulated insulin release. DETAPAC pretreatment alone also had no effect on glucose-stimulated insulin release (Figure 4).

DISCUSSION

The data presented here are consistent with the involvement of hydroxyl radicals in the effects of alloxan on isolated pancreatic islets. Utilizing agents that should reduce the amounts of key components needed for the production of highly reactive hydroxyl, free radicals, it was possible to reduce or eliminate the ability of alloxan exposure to damage the insulin release mechanism. This is the first evidence obtained from isolated pancreatic islets to implicate hydroxyl radicals in the mechanism of alloxan action.

FIGURE 4. Effect of DETAPAC on alloxan-induced inhibition of glucose-stimulated insulin release. Format, same as in Figure 2, except that +FE indicates that DETAPAC was allowed to chelate an excess of iron before its use as a pretreatment.

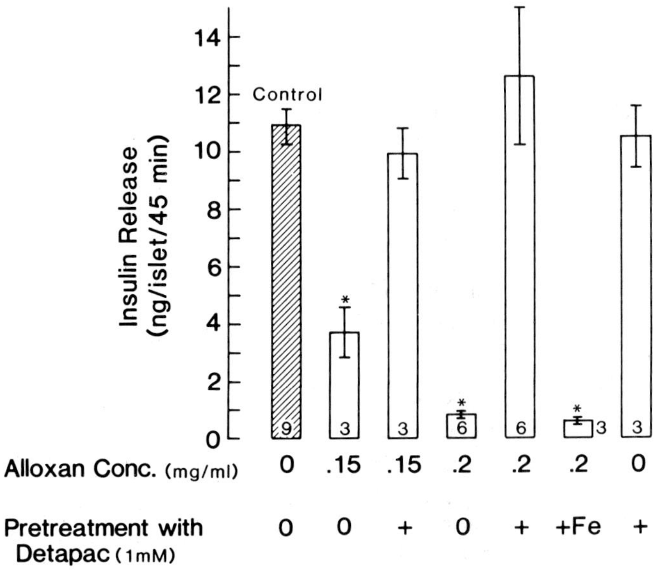

Because SOD inhibits alloxan action on islet cells, the involvement of superoxide anions is evident, but superoxide does not appear to be the ultimate toxic substance. Superoxide anions dismute to form hydrogen peroxide, and, because catalase also antagonizes the alloxan effect, peroxide appears to be involved. It has been reported that a series of reactions involving superoxide anions, hydrogen peroxide, and iron will generate hydroxyl, free radicals.[3,12] DETAPAC has been reported to chelate iron and prevent the generation of hydroxyl radicals in systems similar to those used in the present study.[13] The ability of the iron chelator to inhibit the action of alloxan, when considered with the inhibitory actions of SOD and catalase, provides evidence that hydroxyl free radicals mediate the deleterious action of alloxan on pancreatic islets.

Inactivation of SOD and catalase eliminated the ability of these enzymes to protect from alloxan, and this supports their presumed action to reduce superoxide anions and hydrogen peroxide, respectively. However, protection by all the agents used here could occur if they reduced, in some way, the autooxidation of dialuric acid, thereby preventing the formation of superoxide anions. This possibility was examined by measuring autooxidation in solutions of alloxan and ascorbic acid according to published methods.[12] Autooxidation, as measured by rate of oxygen consumption, occurred at rates that were essentially unaltered by the presence of SOD, catalase, or DETAPAC (data not shown). These results indicated that alloxan and dialuric acid were not altered by the protective agents in a manner that would prevent their participation in the autooxidative process presumed to be needed for the production of free radicals.

If hydroxyl radicals mediate alloxan action, it should be possible to observe a similar action after exposure of pancreatic islets to another known generator of oxygen-containing free radicals. Dihydroxyfumarate produces superoxide anions[14] and hydroxyl radicals,[15,16] and exposure of islets to this substance for 5 min will inhibit subsequent glucose-stimulated insulin release.[17] This effect of dihydroxyfumarate, like that reported here for alloxan, was inhibited by SOD, catalase, and DETAPAC.[17] These similarities in the actions of dihydroxyfumarate and alloxan provide additional support that the latter compound acts on pancreatic islets through the generation of hydroxyl free radicals.

Certain compounds (e.g., n-butanol and thiourea) are known to chemically react with hydroxyl radicals and have been used in vivo as potential scavengers of these free radicals.[1] It may be possible to protect isolated pancreatic islets from the effects of alloxan by utilizing hydroxyl radical scavengers. In experiments similar to those described here, n-butanol (40 mM) and thiourea (40 mM) were unable to protect isolated islets from the effects of alloxan (data not shown). Others have been unsuccessful in attempts to protect isolated islets from alloxan using n-butanol.[6] It may be difficult to protect cells from the effects of hydroxyl radicals by using scavengers of these extremely reactive substances. Hydroxyl radicals, after their formation, should immediately react with adjacent cellular components unless they reacted preferentially with scavengers present in high concentrations. Scavengers possessing a high affinity for radicals and a low toxicity to islets have yet to be found. An inability to protect or an incomplete protection of isolated islets from alloxan by hydroxyl radical scavengers should not, in our opinion, be considered adequate evidence to rule out the participation of hydroxyl radicals.

It is not clear whether the alloxan-induced generation of superoxide anions and hydroxyl radicals takes place extracellularly or within the B cells. It seems likely that the enzymes, SOD and catalase, and, possibly, the metal chelator, DETAPAC, will not freely enter cells, but we have no evidence to rule out the possibility of an intracellular action for one or more of these inhibitors of alloxan action. It should be emphasized that the present results do not exclude the possibility that alloxan, in addition to participating in the generation of hydroxyl free radicals, may have other actions that damage insulin-producing cells. The interaction of alloxan with membrane components, possibly near a glucose receptor, can still be considered.[18] Clearly, additional studies will be needed for a full understanding of the role that free radicals play in the action of alloxan.

ADDENDUM

While this manuscript was in press K. Grankvist et al. reported that superoxide dismutase, catalase, and some radical scavengers attenuated the ability of alloxan to produce an inhibition of rubidium uptake in isolated pancreatic islets and to cause cell death (dye exclusion) in isolated endocrine cells (Biochem. J. *182*:17, 1979).

ACKNOWLEDGMENTS

This work was supported by USPHS grant GM-12675. The helpful comments of Dr. A. P. Autor during the course of this study are gratefully acknowledged.

REFERENCES

[1] Heikkila, R. E., Winston, B., and Cohen, G.: Alloxan-induced diabetes—evidence for hydroxyl radical as a cytotoxic intermediate. Biochem. Pharmacol. *25*:1085–92, 1976.

[2] Cohen, G., and Heikkila, R. E.: The generation of hydrogen peroxide, superoxide radical, and hydroxyl radical by 6-hydroxydopamine, dialuric acid and related cytotoxic agents. J. Biol. Chem. *249*:2447–52, 1974.

[3] Czapski, G., and Ilan, Y. A.: On the generation of the hydroxylation agent from superoxide radical. Can the Haber-Weiss reaction be the source of ˙OH radicals. Photochem. Photobiol. *28*:651–53, 1978.

[4] Heikkila, R. E., and Cabbat, F. S.: Protection against alloxan-induced diabetes in mice by hydroxyl radical scavenger dimethylurea. Eur. J. Pharmacol. *52*:57–60, 1978.

[5] Schauberger, C. W., Thies, R. L., and Fischer, L. J.: Mechanism of protection from alloxan diabetes provided by n-butanol. J. Pharmacol. Exp. Ther. *201*:450–55, 1977.

[6] McDaniel, M. L., Roth, C. E., Bry, C. A., Fink, C. J., Swanson, J. A., and Lacy, P. L.: Effect of ethanol and n-butanol on alloxan inhibition of glucose-induced insulin release in isolated pancreatic islets. Biochem. Pharmacol. *27*:1749–51, 1978.

[7] Tomita, T., Lacy, P. E., Matschinsky, F. M., and McDaniel, M. L.: Effect of alloxan on insulin secretion in isolated rat islets perfused in vitro. Diabetes *23*:517–24, 1974.

[8] Lacy, P. E., and Kostianovsky, M.: Method for the isolation of intact islets of Langerhans from the rat pancreas. Diabetes *16*:35–39, 1967.

[9] Niki, A., Niki, H., Miwa, I., and Lin, B. J.: Interaction on alloxan and anomers of D-glucose on glucose-induced insulin secretion and biosynthesis in vitro. Diabetes *25*:574–79, 1976.

[10] Makulu, D. R., Vichick, D., and Wright, P. H.: Insulin immunoassay by back titration using alcohol precipitation of insulin-antibody complexes. Diabetes *18*:660–69, 1969.

[11] Steel, R. G. D., and Torrie, J. H.: Principles and Procedures of Statistics. New York, McGraw-Hill, 1960.

[12] Borg, D. C., Schaich, K. M., Elmore, J. J., and Bell, J. A.: Cytotoxic reactions of free radical species of oxygen. Photochem. Photobiol. *28*:887–907, 1978.

[13] Buettner, G. R., Oberley, L. W., and Chan-Leuthauser, S.: The effect of iron on the distribution of superoxide and hydroxyl radicals as seen by spin trapping and on the superoxide dismutase assay. Photochem. Photobiol. *28*:693–95, 1978.

[14] Halliwell, B.: Generation of peroxide, superoxide and hydroxyl radicals during the oxidation of dihydroxyfumaric acid by peroxidase. Biochem. J. *163*:441–48, 1977.

[15] Autor, A. P., McLennan, G., and Fox, A. W.: Oxygen free radicals generated by dihydroxyfumarate and ionizing radiation: cytotoxic effect on isolated pulmonary macrophages. *In* Molecular Mechanisms of Environmental Toxicity. Bhatnagar, R. S., Ed. Ann Arbor, Michigan, Ann Arbor Science, 1979, In press.

[16] Autor, A. P., and Kapke, G.: Cytotoxicity of autooxidixing dihydroxyfumarate on isolated rat pulmonary macrophages. In preparation.

[17] Fischer, L. J., and Hamburger, S.: Inhibition of insulin secretion from isolated pancreatic islets treated with dihydroxyfumarate. Fed. Proc. *38*:528, 1979.

[18] Weaver, D. C., McDaniel, M. L., Naber, S. P., Barry, C. D., and Lacy, P. E.: Alloxan stimulation and inhibition of insulin release from isolated rat islets of Langerhans. Diabetes *27*:1205–14, 1978.

Impaired Glycogen Synthase Activating System in Human Diabetic Polymorphonuclear Leukocytes

DAVID E. GOLDSTEIN AND RANDALL T. CURNOW

SUMMARY

The effects of diabetes mellitus on glycogen synthase and its activating system (synthase phosphatase) were studied using human polymorphonuclear leukocytes (PMN). PMN were obtained from control subjects and diabetic patients by a gradient sedimentation technique. Enzyme activities of synthase-*I* and total synthase were not statistically different in diabetic and control cells. For measurement of endogenous synthase phosphatase, cells were sonicated in 50 mM Tris buffer (pH 7.5) and incubated at 30°C. Conversion of endogenous synthase-*D* to -*I* was linear for 20 min and maximal by 30 min. The rate of conversion of synthase-*D* to -*I* and the maximum percent synthase-*I* attained were decreased in homogenates of diabetic cells. There was no correlation between the plasma glucose concentration and the rate of conversion of synthase-*D* to -*I*. Synthase phosphatase activities were also measured using a purified synthase-*D* substrate. Under these experimental conditions, glycogen synthase phosphatase activities did not differ in control and diabetic cells. These results are consistent with a diabetes-induced defect in conversion of endogenous synthase-*D* to -*I* at the level of the synthase enzyme rather than at that of the activating phosphatase. DIABETES 29:217–220, March 1980.

Although diabetes mellitus has been shown to cause alterations in glycogen metabolism in experimental animals,[1–5] few studies have been carried out using human tissue. In this paper, the effects of diabetes mellitus on glycogen synthase and its activating enzyme in human polymorphonuclear leukocytes are described.

From the Division of Clinical Pharmacology, Departments of Internal Medicine and Pharmacology, University of Virginia School of Medicine, Charlottesville 22903, and the Department of Child Health, University of Missouri-Columbia School of Medicine, Columbia, Missouri 65212.
Received for publication 27 July and in revised form 10 October 1979.
Address reprint requests to David E. Goldstein, M.D., Department of Child Health, University of Missouri-Columbia School of Medicine, Columbia, Missouri 65212.

Glycogen synthase is the rate-limiting enzyme catalyzing glycogen synthesis.[6] The enzyme has been characterized in a variety of tissues, where it has been shown to exist in active and inactive forms interconvertible by phosphorylation-dephosphorylation reactions. The dephospho-*I* form of synthase is active in vivo, while the phospho-*D* form is thought to be completely inactive under physiologic conditions. The *D* to *I* conversion is catalyzed by synthase-*D* phosphatase.[7]

The present results show that the rate of the conversion of synthase-*D* to -*I* in homogenates of human polymorphonuclear leukocytes is decreased in diabetes.

METHODS

Polymorphonuclear leukocytes (PMN) were obtained by Ficoll-Hypaque separation,[8] followed by dextran sedimentation and hypotonic lysis of the residual erythrocytes. Cells were suspended in phosphate-buffered saline (PBS), pH 7.4, were 99% viable, as determined by trypan-blue exclusion, and consisted of essentially pure PMN (95–99%), as determined by Wright's stain differential counts. Blood specimens (50–100 ml) were obtained from eight diabetic patients and 18 nondiabetic control subjects at 8 a.m. after an overnight fast. Patients were selected at random from the diabetic outpatient clinic. Informed consent was obtained from all diabetic patients and control subjects. Plasma glucose concentrations were determined by the glucose oxidase method using a Beckman glucose analyzer. Diabetic patients ranged in age from 13 to 72 yr (mean = 35 yr).

Of the eight diabetic patients, seven were receiving daily insulin injections and one was being treated with diet alone. None was ketotic at the time of blood sampling. Fasting plasma glucose concentrations ranged from 135 to 526 mg/dl (mean ± SD = 314 ± 138). Control subjects ranged in age from 18 to 66 yr (mean = 33 yr) and gave no history of chronic illness or glucose intolerance (Table 1).

For measurement of conversion of endogenous synthase-*D* to -*I*, cells suspended in PBS were centrifuged at 1200 *g* for 15 min. The cell pellet was resuspended in 50 mM Tris/HCl (pH 7.5) at a concentration of 10^8 PMN per milliliter,

TABLE 1
Clinical characteristics of diabetic patients and control subjects and their endogenous polymorphonuclear leukocyte synthase phosphatase activities

Diabetic patients			Fasting plasma glucose	Insulin dose	Synthase phosphatase activity
No.	Sex	Age (yr)	(mg/dl)	(U/day)	(Δ % synthase-*I*, 0–15 min)
1	F	28	350	35	14.6
2	M	14	163	28	15.9
3	F	13	135	18	42.4
4	M	53	526	55	25.7
5	F	36	360	30	16.9
6	M	28	298	25	35.5
7	F	39	461	0§	21
8	M	72	222	26	24.8
					24.60 ± 3.5‡
Control subjects					
9–22 10 M 4 M		33 (18–66)*	76 (66–80)*	—	40.35 ± 5.12†

* Mean and range, respectively.
† Mean ± SEM.
‡ $P < 0.002$ as compared with control subjects.
§ Treated with diet alone.

sonicated, and incubated at 30°C. At intervals, 100 μl aliquots were removed and placed in chilled tubes, containing 5 μl 1 M KF and 10 μl 100 mM EDTA, and were assayed immediately for glycogen synthase-*I* and total synthase (*I* + *D* forms) activities. In some experiments, cells were disrupted by freeze-thawing or by resuspension of the pellet in buffer containing 1% Triton X-100. However, these techniques caused complete and irreversible loss of synthase-*I* activity without altering synthase-*D* activity. In other experiments, cells were sonicated and then centrifuged at 12,000 *g* at 4°C for 15 min. The supernatant was filtered through a column of Sephadex G-25, which had been equilibrated with the sonication buffer, and the eluent was used for incubation experiments. Gel filtration did not alter appreciably the conversion of synthase-*D* to -*I* in either diabetic or control cells. Gel filtration through Sephadex G-25 after incubations, but before enzyme assays, did not alter measurements of enzyme activities in control or diabetic cells. Thus, gel filtration was not performed routinely before incubations or enzyme assays. For measurement of leukocyte synthase phosphatase activities using an exogenous synthase substrate, synthase-*D* was purified from dog muscle by the method of Takeda et al.[9] except that the Sepharose 4B column chromatography and α-amylase digestion steps were omitted. The enzyme preparation contained glycogen (1.1 mg/ml final concentration), which greatly enhanced the stability of the enzyme. The synthase activity in this preparation was 5.8 U/ml prep and contained 2.7 mg protein per milliliter (1 U = 1 μmol of glucose converted to glycogen per minute per milligram protein in the presence of 10 mM glucose 6-phosphate). Residual synthase-*I* activity represented approximately 3% of total synthase activity. For this assay, the cell pellet was resuspended in 50 mM Tris/HCl (pH 7.8), 5mM EDTA, 10 mM MgCl, 2 mM phenylmethylsulfonyl fluoride (PMSF) at a concentration of 2 × 10^8 cells per milliliter. Cells were then sonicated and incubated with the purified synthase-*D* preparation. Each incubation tube contained 50 μl cell homogenate and 25 μl synthase-*D*, which had been diluted 1:3 in 2 mg/ml BSA, 50 mM Tris/HCl (pH 7.8), 5 mM EDTA, and 3.5 μl 8% column-treated rabbit muscle glycogen. The reaction was terminated by the addition of 700 μl ice-cold 200 mM KF, and each tube was assayed immediately for synthase activity. The conversion of exogenous synthase-*D* to -*I* was linear for approximately 30 min. The addition of 0.1-1% glycogen to the incubation mixture did not alter appreciably the rate of *D* to *I* conversion. Conversion of endogenous synthase-*D* to -*I* represented less than 10% of the total *D* to *I* conversion and was subtracted from the results.

Glycogen synthase activity was determined by the filter paper method of Thomas et al.,[10] measuring the incorporation of radioactive glucose into glycogen. To assay synthase, 25 μl of leukocyte homogenate was added to 50 μl of an assay mixture containing 50 mM Tris/HCl (pH 7.8), 5 mM EDTA, 6.7 mM UDP-^{14}C-glucose, and 10 mg/ml column-treated rabbit muscle glycogen. After 10 min of incubation at 30°C, a 60 μl aliquot was removed, spotted immediately on a square of filter paper, and processed by the method of Thomas et al.[10] Under these assay conditions, the activity of leukocyte phosphorylase, the enzyme catalyzing glycogen degradation, is low.[11,12] For measurement of synthase-*I* activity, 10 mM Na_2SO_4 was added to the assay mixture.[13] Total synthase activity was measured in the presence of 6.7 mM glucose 6-phosphate, which is saturating at 4 mM UDP glucose. Enzyme activities of total glycogen synthase (synthase) and synthase in the *I*-form (synthase-*I*) are expressed as units (micromoles of glucose incorporated into glycogen per min per 10^8 cells). Synthase-*I* activities are also expressed as percent of total synthase. Phosphatase activity is expressed in units, where 1 U = △ GS-*I* U/min/10^6 PMN.

All reagents were of the highest purity available. (U-^{14}C)

UDP-glucose was obtained from New England Nuclear. Differences between mean values for each variable measured were analyzed for significance by the Student *t* test for paired and, where appropriate, unpaired observations. Correlation coefficients between selected parameters were calculated using standard methods.

RESULTS AND DISCUSSION

Table 2 shows basal activities of synthase-*I* and total synthase in homogenates of polymorphonuclear leukocytes from diabetic patients and control subjects. These enzyme activities were not statistically different in diabetic and control cells. Figure 1 shows the time course of synthase activation in homogenates of diabetic and control cells. Total synthase activities did not change during incubations. Conversion of endogenous synthase-*D* to -*I* was linear for approximately 20 min and was maximal by 30 min in homogenates from both diabetic and control cells. Both the rate of the conversion of synthase-*D* to -*I* (Table 1) and the maximal percent synthase-*I* attained were significantly decreased in homogenates of diabetic polymorphonuclear leukocytes ($P < 0.02$ and < 0.01, respectively). There was no correlation between the plasma glucose concentration and the rate of conversion of synthase-*D* to -*I*.

Insulin has been shown to promote the activation of glycogen synthase in many tissues.[14] It has been reported that conversion of synthase-*D* to -*I* in liver extracts from diabetic rats is decreased with restoration of conversion to normal following treatment with insulin in vivo.[1,2] Studies of glycogen synthase and its activation in human polymorphonuclear leukocytes have yielded conflicting results. Insulin has not been shown to have direct effects on synthase in intact human polymorphonuclear leukocytes.[15,16] It was reported initially that glycogen synthase in human polymorphonuclear leukocytes was exclusively in the *D*-form and that conversion of synthase-*D* to -*I* could not be demonstrated.[17] It was also reported that polymorphonuclear leukocytes from diabetic human beings showed slightly decreased total synthase (measured as the *D*-form only) as compared with controls, but in contrast to controls, conversion of synthase-*D* to -*I* was demonstrable.[18] The rate of conversion was found to be increased in some of the diabetic patients after insulin treatment in vivo.

In accord with the present findings, more recent studies have demonstrated both the presence of synthase-*I* and conversion of synthase-*D* to -*I* in homogenates of polymorphonuclear leukocytes from nondiabetic human beings.[16,19]

From the present results, the mechanism of the impaired conversion of synthase-*D* to -*I* is consistent with a diabetes-induced abnormality of either the synthase substrate or possibly the synthase-activating phosphatase. To further define the defect, the activation of a purified synthase-*D* substrate by homogenates of diabetic and control polymorphonuclear leukocytes was compared (Table 3). Under the present experimental conditions using an exogenous synthase-*D* substrate, glycogen synthase phosphatase activities in control and diabetic polymorphonuclear leukocytes did not differ. These results are consistent with a diabetes-induced defect in conversion of endogenous synthase-*D* to -*I* at the level of the synthase enzyme rather than at that of the activating phosphatase. Thus, diabetes mellitus could decrease synthase activation in human polymorphonuclear leukocytes by making the synthase enzyme a less favorable substrate for its activating phosphatase. However, there are both specific and nonspecific phosphatases present in many tissues, and it is possible that activation of the exoge-

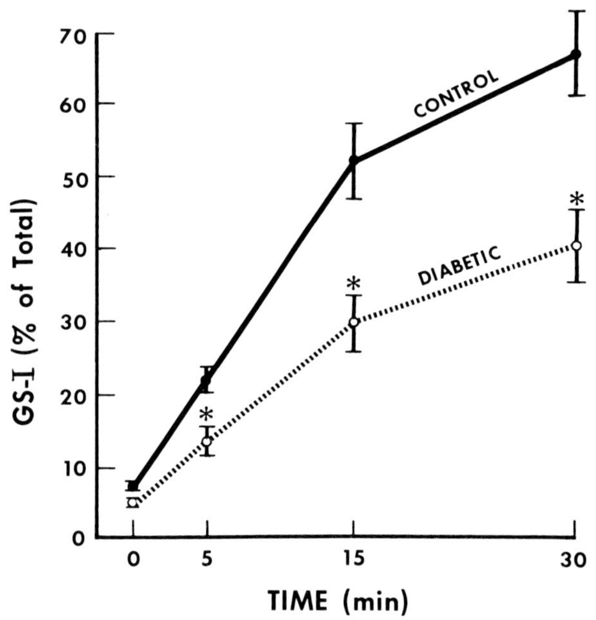

FIGURE 1. Homogenates from human polymorphonuclear leukocytes were prepared as described under METHODS. Homogenates were incubated at 30°C, and aliquots were removed at intervals for assays of synthase-*I* and total synthase activities. Conversion of synthase-*D* to -*I* was maximal by 30 min in homogenates from both diabetic and control cells. Points and vertical bars represent means ± SE, respectively, of values from 8 diabetic patients and 18 control subjects. Asterisks show $P < 0.01$ as compared with control subjects.

TABLE 2
Glycogen synthase activity in polymorphonuclear leukocytes from diabetic patients and control subjects

	Synthase-*I* (% of total)	Total synthase
Control	7.74 ± 0.51	78.20 ± 4.72
Diabetic	5.35 ± 0.66	74.52 ± 4.14
P	NS	NS

Homogenates from human PMN leukocytes were prepared as described under METHODS. Values are means ± SE of leukocyte synthase activities from 8 diabetic patients and 18 control subjects and are expressed as units (nanomoles of glucose incorporated into glycogen per minute) per 10^8 leukocytes.

TABLE 3
Glycogen synthase phosphatase activity in diabetic and control polymorphonuclear leukocytes using a purified synthase-*D* substrate

Controls	9.63 ± 0.97	P = NS
Diabetics	8.56 ± 1.62	

Purified dog muscle synthase-*D* and homogenates from human PMN leukocytes were prepared as described under METHODS. Values are means ± SE of leukocyte synthase phosphatase activities from nine diabetic patients and nine control subjects and are expressed as miliunits synthase-*I* formed from the purified synthase-*D* substrate/min/10^6 PMN leukocytes.

nous synthase under the present assay conditions was catalyzed by a nonspecific leukocyte phosphatase.[20] Thus, it is possible that the specific synthase-activating phosphatase is subtly altered by diabetes such that its activity is decreased in respect to its specific synthase substrate.

Additional studies will be required to clearly define the mechanisms and physiologic significance of the present findings.

ACKNOWLEDGMENTS

The work was supported by grants AM 447 and AM 1702 (University of Virginia Diabetes Research and Training Center) from the USPHS.

REFERENCES

[1] Gold, A. H.: The effect of diabetes and insulin on liver glycogen synthetase activation. J. Biol. Chem. *245*:903–05, 1970.

[2] Nichols, W. K., and Goldberg, N. D.: The relationship between insulin and apparent glucocorticoid-promoted activation of hepatic glycogen synthetase. Biochim. Biophys. Acta *279*:245–59, 1972.

[3] Tan, A. J., and Nuttall, F. Q.: Characteristics of the dephosphorylated form of phosphorylase purified from rat liver and measurement of its activity in crude liver preparations. Biochim. Biophys. Acta *410*:45–60, 1975.

[4] Khandelwal, R. L., Zinman, S. M., and Zebrowski, E. J.: The effect of streptozotocin-induced diabetes and of insulin supplementation on glycogen metabolism in rat liver. Biochem. J. *168*:541–48, 1977.

[5] Hornbrook, K. R.: Synthesis of liver glycogen in starved alloxan-diabetic rats. Diabetes *19*:916–23, 1970.

[6] Hizukuri, S., and Larner, J.: Studies on UDPG: α-1, 4-glucan α-4 glucosyl transferase. VII. Conversion of the enzyme from glucose-6-phosphate dependent to independent form in liver. Biochemistry *3*:1783–88, 1963.

[7] Hers, H. G., Stalmans, W., DeWulf, H., LaLous, M., and Hue, L.: The control of glycogen metabolism in the liver. *In* Metabolic Interconversion of Enzymes. Fischer, E. H., Ed. Berlin, Springer, 1973, pp. 89–98.

[8] Boyum, A.: Separation of leukocytes from blood and bone marrow. Scand. J. Clin. Lab. Invest. *21*:97, 1968.

[9] Takeda, Y., Brewer, H. B., and Larner, J.: Structural studies on rabbit muscle glycogen synthase. 1. Subunit composition. J. Biol. Chem. *250*:8943–50, 1975.

[10] Thomas, J. A., Schlender, K. K., and Larner, J.: A rapid filter paper assay for UDP glucose-glycogen glycosyltransferase, including an improved biosynthesis of UDP-^{14}C-glucose. Anal. Biochem. *25*:486–99, 1968.

[11] Wang, P., and Esmann, V.: A new assay of phosphorylase based on the filter paper technique. Anal. Biochem. *47*:495–500, 1972.

[12] Newman, J. D., and Armstrong, J. McD.: On the activities of phosphorylase and glycogen synthase in the liver of the rat. Biochim. Biophys. Acta *544*:225–33, 1978.

[13] DeWulf, H., and Hers, H. G.: The role of glucose, glycogen and glucocorticoids in the regulation of liver glycogen synthesis. Eur. J. Biochem. *6*:558–64, 1968.

[14] Curnow, R. T., Rayfield, E. J., George, D. T., Zenser, T. V., and DeRubertis, F.: Control of hepatic glycogen metabolism in the rhesus monkey: effect of glucose, insulin and glycogen administration. Am. J. Physiol. *228*:80–87, 1975.

[15] Esmann, V.: Effect of insulin on human leucocytes. Diabetes *12*:545–49, 1963.

[16] Wang, D., Plesner, L., and Esmann, V.: The effect of glucose and glucose analogues on the conversion of glycogen synthetase from phosphorylated to dephosphorylated form in human polymorphonuclear leukocytes. Eur. J. Biochem. *27*:297–300, 1972.

[17] Rosell-Perez, M., and Esmann, V.: UDPG-glucan-glucosyl-transferase in human polymorphonuclear leukocytes. Acta Chem. Scand. *19*:679, 1965.

[18] Esmann, V., Hedeskov, C. J., and Rosell-Perez, M.: UDP-glucose-glucan-glycosyl-transferase activity of polymorphonuclear leukocytes from diabetic subjects. Diabetologia *4*:181–87, 1968.

[19] Nahas, N., and Gutman, A.: In vitro activation of leukocyte glycogen synthase. Biochem. Biophys. Res. Commun. *52*:21–26, 1973.

[20] Curnow, R. T., and Larner, J.: Biochemical Actions of Hormones, vol. 6. New York, Academic Press, 1979, pp. 77–119.

Decreased Insulin Binding and Degradation Associated with Depressed Intracellular ATP Content

BORIS DRAZNIN, CLIVE C. SOLOMONS, CAROL A. EMLER, DON S. SCHALCH, AND KARL E. SUSSMAN

SUMMARY

The effect of metabolic inhibitors, 2,4-dinitrophenol (DNP) and NaF, on insulin binding and degradation has been studied in cultured Buffalo rat liver (BRL) cells. In control studies, 1.8 fmol of ^{125}I-insulin binds to 1.2 × 10^{6} cells, possessing approximately 40,000 receptor sites per cell with binding affinity of 5.52 × 10^{-8}M. When the cells were preincubated with increasing concentrations of either DNP or NaF, a dose- and time-dependent decrease in both insulin binding and degradation was observed. The total amount of ^{125}I-insulin bound to BRL cells preincubated with metabolic inhibitors was reduced to 1.2 fmol per 1.2 × 10^{6} cells. The point of ½ B max was achieved in the presence of 50 ng/ml of native insulin, 1.7 times that of the control level. The number of receptor sites was unaffected by either DNP or NaF, but an average affinity profile revealed a decrease in the affinity of the ATP-depleted cells for insulin (K_D: 7.31 × 10^{-8} M and 7.06 × 10^{-8} M in DNP- and NaF-treated cells, respectively). The decrease in insulin binding and degradation following the exposure of the BRL cells to the metabolic inhibitors was associated with a 20% reduction in intracellular ATP and adenylate energy charge. DNP and NaF did not affect the equilibrium constant for the myokinase catalyzed reaction and the intracellular concentration of hypoxanthine was stable, confirming the integrity of the cells during the experiments.

It is suggested that ATP levels must remain intact to maintain normal insulin receptor affinity. Furthermore, the rate of insulin degradation by ATP-depleted cells is slower than that of intact cells. It is conceivable that the depression of insulin degradation by partially ATP-depleted cells results from either diminished binding or decreased endocytosis and lysosomal activity, all of which appear to be energy dependent.

DIABETES *29*:221–226, March 1980.

The action of insulin is mediated via specific interactions with its plasma membrane receptors. Detailed information has been accumulated concerning the binding of insulin to the cell surface and much is also known about the effects of insulin on intermediary metabolism in target tissues. In contrast, relatively little is known about the influence of cellular metabolic events that might modulate or control insulin binding to its receptor sites.

Acute changes in the affinity of insulin receptors following oral[1] and intravenous[2] glucose challenges in normal volunteers have recently been described. These studies indicated that major changes in receptor affinity occur rather rapidly (within 2–5 h), while changes in receptor concentration probably occur in the range of hours to days. The molecular mechanisms that mediate the effect of glucose on insulin receptor affinity have not yet been elucidated. Insulin,[3–6] cyclic AMP,[7] H^+,[8] B-OH butyrate,[9] and antibodies to the insulin receptors[10] have all been suggested to be mediators and/or modulators of some changes in either insulin receptor affinity or concentration.

Recent studies have revealed that high energy phosphate bonds appear to be involved not only in the step linking insulin binding to accelerated glucose transport,[11] but possibly also in the binding process itself.[12,13] In addition, receptor-mediated lysosomal insulin degradation[14–16] may be inhibited by ATP depletion.[17] The focus of the present investigation is to examine the possible role and importance of high energy phosphate compounds in either controlling or modulating insulin binding and degradation by liver cells. The model selected for study was the cultured Buffalo rat liver (BRL) cell.

MATERIALS AND METHODS

Materials. All tissue culture media and sera were obtained from Grand Island Biological Co. (GIBCO, Grand Island,

From the Departments of Medicine and Orthopedics of the University of Colorado Health Science Center and the Veterans Administration Medical Center, Denver, Colorado.

Address reprint requests to Dr. Boris Draznin, Division of Endocrinology, UCHSC, Box B151, 4200 East 9th Avenue, Denver, Colorado 80262.

Received for publication 4 September 1979 and in revised form 22 October 1979.

New York). Porcine monocomponent insulin was generously supplied by Dr. Ronald Chance of Eli Lilly and Company (Indianapolis, Indiana). Na (^{125}I) was purchased from New England Nuclear (Boston, Massachusetts); bovine serum albumin (fraction V) from Armour Pharmaceutical Co. (Phoenix, Arizona); and 2,4-dinitrophenol (DNP) and NaF from Sigma (St. Louis, Missouri).

Cell culture technique. BRL cells were cultured in Petri dishes (35 × 10 mm) in Ham's F-12 medium containing 5% fetal calf serum under an atmosphere of 95% air/5% CO_2 at 37°C in a humidified incubator. The medium was changed 2–3 times per week and cells were subcultured every 10–14 days. For all studies, serum-free Ham's F-12 medium was introduced at least 24 h before each experiment.

Iodination of insulin. ^{125}I-labeled insulin (specific activity = 100–200 μCi/μg) was prepared according to the Freychet et al.[18] modification of the method of Hunter and Greenwood,[19] as previously described.[20]

Binding studies. Except where noted, binding experiments were performed directly in Petri dishes (35 × 10 mm) to minimize the proteolytic activity released by cells broken during scraping. Monolayer cultures of BRL cells, covered with 1 ml of Ham's F-12 serum free medium containing 1% BSA, were incubated for varying times with mixtures of ^{125}I-insulin (0.4 ng/ml) and unlabeled insulin at 22°C. At termination of the incubation the media were aspirated. The cells were washed three times with ice-cold phosphate-buffered solution (PBS), then dissolved with 1 ml of 1 N NaOH, transferred to scintillation vials, and the radioactivity counted. Cells from identical dishes were separated by trypsin digestion and counted in a hemocytometer or dissolved in 0.1 N NaOH for protein determinations.[21] The cell density was 1.2 ± 0.5 × 10^6 cells per dish (mean ± SEM), which corresponded to 250 ± 28 μg of protein. The viability of BRL cells in monolayer culture was greater than 90% at all time points of incubation, as judged by trypan blue exclusion.

Nonspecific binding. For these studies, nonspecific binding is defined as the amount of ^{125}I-labeled insulin remaining in the cell layer in the presence of a large excess (100 μg/ml) of unlabeled insulin. All values were corrected for nonspecific binding, which ranged between 10 and 20% of the total radioactivity attached to liver cells.

Insulin degradation. Degradation of insulin was determined by examining the ability of the free ^{125}I-insulin remaining in the incubation medium to precipitate with 10% trichloroacetic acid. The validity of this method has been previously evaluated and justified.[20]

ATP depletion studies. In addition to experiments in which insulin binding and degradation by intact BRL cells were assessed, the cells were preincubated with either DNP (0.2, 0.5, or 1 mM) or NaF (1, 5, or 10 mM) for 30, 60, and 120 min before the 60-min incubation with ^{125}I-insulin. Insulin binding to the cells pre-exposed to these metabolic inhibitors was studied as described above. In selected experiments, cellular ATP, ADP, AMP, and hypoxanthine levels were determined by high performance liquid chromatography.[22]

Statistical analysis. The nonpaired Student's *t* test was employed for comparison between experimental groups.

RESULTS

Control experiments. Figure 1 depicts the time course of ^{125}I-insulin binding and degradation by cultured BRL cells at 22°C. It can be seen that the binding reaction reaches an equilibrium by 60 min, which is maintained for at least an additional 60 min of incubation. The rate of insulin degradation ranged between 10 and 15% per hour of incubation. Specific insulin binding under these conditions averaged 1.8 fmol per 1.2 × 10^6 cells, which is three- to fivefold lower than insulin binding to freshly isolated hepatocytes[23–25] and to cloned neonatal rat hepatocytes.[26] However, insulin binding to cultured BRL cells appears to be twice that obtained with Zajdela rat ascites hepatoma cells.[27] On the basis of these initial studies to establish steady state conditions, all subsequent experiments were carried out for 60 min at room temperature.

The binding of ^{125}I-insulin to BRL cells was competitively inhibited by native insulin with 50% inhibition (½ B max) occurring at 30 ng/ml (Figure 2A). The Scatchard analysis of these data is depicted on Figure 2B. The Scatchard plot, by far the most common method of the graphical analysis of binding data, is based on several assumptions. We believe that in the system studied, these numerous assumptions (i.e., identical behavior of labeled and unlabeled hormone, homogeneity and univalency of the ligand, reversibility and equilibrium of the binding reaction, and perfect separation of bound and free hormone) have been fulfilled to justify the

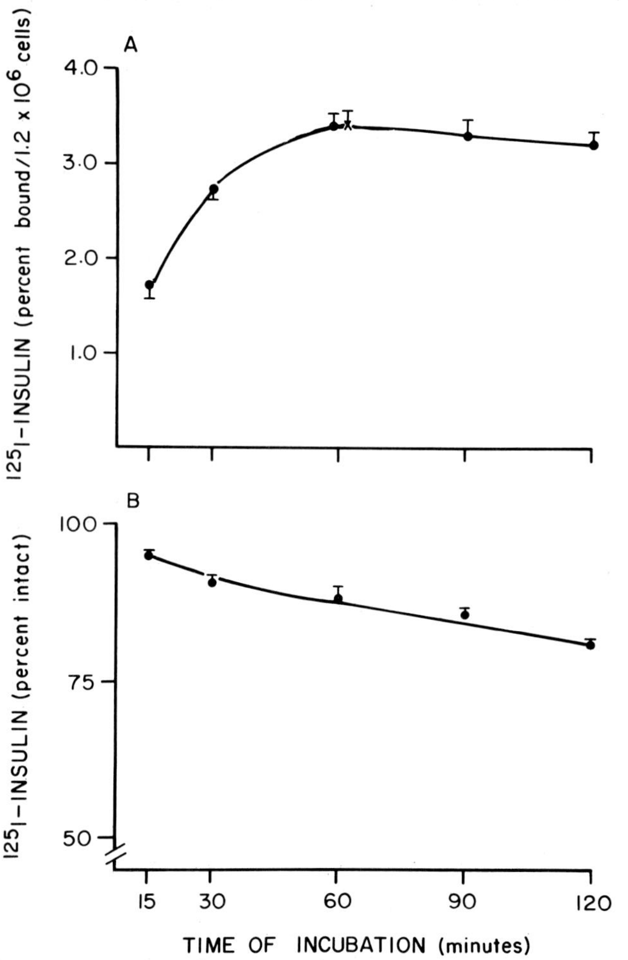

FIGURE 1. Time-dependent ^{125}I-insulin binding (A) and degradation (B) by cultured BRL cells at 22°C. The data represent mean ± SEM of six experiments.

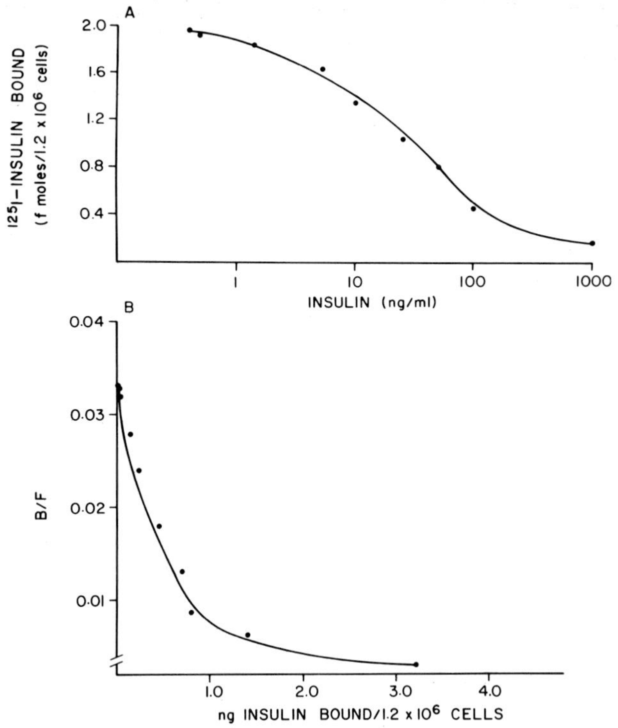

FIGURE 2. Insulin binding to BRL cells. Cells were incubated for 60 min at 22°C with 0.4 ng/ml ^{125}I-insulin and increasing concentrations of unlabeled insulin (A). Scatchard plot (B) is calculated from the insulin binding data (A). The data represent mean values from two separate experiments (four dishes per point).

validity of the analysis employed. We have specifically checked the effect of the metabolic inhibitors on the reversibility and equilibrium of the binding reaction, and neither process was altered by exposure of the cells to energy depletors. In the steady state, the binding affinity of insulin to these cells (KD:5.52 $\times$ 10^{-8}M) was found to be considerably lower than that observed in isolated hepatocytes.[14,23] The number of binding sites, however, was about one-fifth (30,000–50,000 sites/cell) that seen in intact fresh liver cells[23–26] but higher than that reported for ascites hepatoma cells.[27] The abscissa intercept (Ro) was calculated from the linear equation of the low affinity portion of the Scatchard plot and represents gross evaluation of the number of binding sites.

Effect of metabolic inhibitors. When the cells were preincubated with increasing concentrations of either DNP or NaF, a dose- and time-dependent decrease in insulin binding was observed (Figures 3A and 4A). The amount of cell-associated radioactivity was significantly reduced after 30 min of exposure of the cells to either metabolic inhibitor. The preincubation of the cells with metabolic inhibitors was necessary to demonstrate their effect on insulin binding. Although the results of the experiments reported herein were obtained at 22°C, a similar decrease in insulin binding was seen when the cells were preincubated with metabolic inhibitors at 37°C.

The degradation of insulin was significantly prevented by both DNP and NaF (Figures 3B and 4B). These findings are consistent with previous data relative to receptor-mediated degradation of insulin,[14–16] wherein both insulin internaliza-

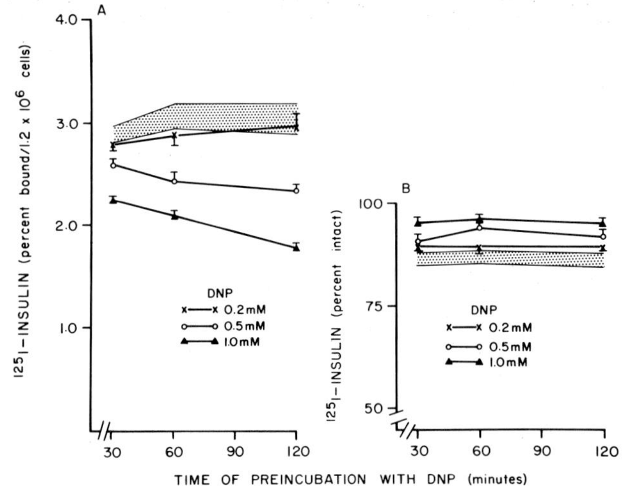

FIGURE 3. Effect of DNP on insulin binding (A) and degradation (B) by BRL cells. Cells were preincubated with 0.2 mM, 0.5 mM, and 1 mM DNP for 30, 60, and 120 min. Insulin binding to these cells was then performed as described in MATERIALS AND METHODS. The data represent mean ± SEM of six experiments. Insulin binding and degradation by BRL cells not exposed to DNP shown by shadow area.

tion and its lysosomal handling are energy dependent and preceded by initial insulin binding.[18,29,30] The DNP of NaF-induced inhibition of insulin degradation by BRL cells was also dose dependent.

In two selected experiments, BRL cells were preincubated with DNP and NaF, and intracellular purine nucleotide content assessed at the end of the binding reaction (Table 1). Both DNP (0.5 mM) and NaF (5 mM) significantly reduced intracellular ATP content, as well as insulin binding to BRL cells, after 60 min of preincubation ($P < 0.05$). The equilibrium constant for the reaction catalyzed by myokinase (2 ADP $\rightarrow$ ATP + AMP),[31,32] however, was unchanged under the present experimental conditions, reflecting stability of the total purine nucleotide pool. Adenylate

FIGURE 4. Effect of NaF on insulin binding (A) and degradation (B) by BRL cells. Cells were preincubated with 1 mM, 5 mM, and 10 mM of NaF for 30, 60, and 120 min. Insulin binding to these cells was then performed as described in MATERIALS AND METHODS. The data represent mean ± SEM of six experiments. Insulin binding and degradation by BRL cells not exposed to NaF shown by shadow area.

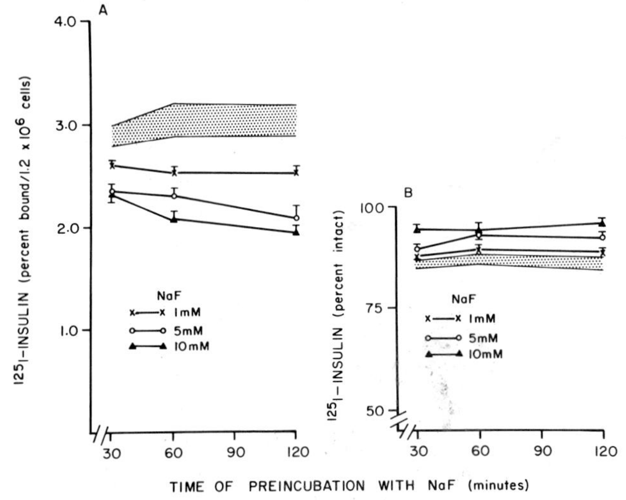

TABLE 1
Effect of DNP and NaF on insulin binding and cellular content of purine nucleotides in cultured BRL cells

	^{125}I-insulin* (percent bound/1.2 × 10^6 cells)	ATP‡	ADP‡	AMP‡	Hypoxanthine‡	K myokinase	Adenylate energy charge
Control	3.47 ± 0.07	35.0	13.0	26.9	4.5	0.18	0.55
		36.8	13.7	25.8	3.9	0.19	0.57
DNP (0.5 mM)	2.15 ± 0.08†	20.8	10.0	28.7	4.2	0.16	0.43
		21.2	9.3	21.8	3.7	0.19	0.49
NaF (5 mM)	2.11 ± 0.11†	20.2	8.8	22.8	5.9	0.17	0.47
		19.0	9.0	24.6	4.6	0.17	0.44

* Mean ± SEM for four experimental dishes; † $P < 0.05$ versus control; and ‡ 10^{-10} M/mg protein. K myokinase = $(ADP)^2/(ATP)(AMP)$. Adenylate energy charge = (ATP + ½ ADP)/(ATP + ADP + AMP).

energy charge represents a linear measure of the metabolic energy stored as component nucleotides and was calculated from the equation[33] (ATP + ½ ADP)/(ATP + ADP + AMP). As can be seen from Table 1, the incubation of BRL cells with either DNP or NaF resulted in a 20% reduction in the adenylate energy charge. The absence of ATP in the extracellular fluid and the stable concentration of intracellular hypoxanthine suggest sustained integrity and viability of BRL cells in these experiments. Moreover, the effect of energy inhibitors on insulin binding was completely reversible, confirming the viability of the cells under experimental conditions.

Figure 5A demonstrates that the total amount of ^{125}I-insulin bound to BRL cells preincubated with metabolic inhibitors was reduced to 1.2 fmol per 1.2 × 10^6 cells and the point of ½ B max was achieved in the presence of 50 ng/ml of native insulin, a value 1.7 times that of the control level. The Scatchard analysis of these data (Figure 5B) revealed that the number of receptor sites was unchanged following the exposure to metabolic inhibitors, but an average affinity profile[34] (Figure 5C) demonstrated a decreased affinity of ATP-depleted cells for insulin (KD:7.31 × 10^{-8} M and 7.06 × 10^{-8} M in DNP- and NaF-treated cells, respectively).

FIGURE 5. Insulin binding to ATP-depleted BRL cells. Control cells and cells exposed to DNP (0.5 mM) and NaF (5 mM) for 60 min were incubated with ^{125}I-insulin (0.4 ng/ml) and increasing concentrations of unlabeled insulin (A). Scatchard plots (B) and average affinity profiles (C) were calculated from these experiments. The data represent mean values from two experiments (four dishes per point).

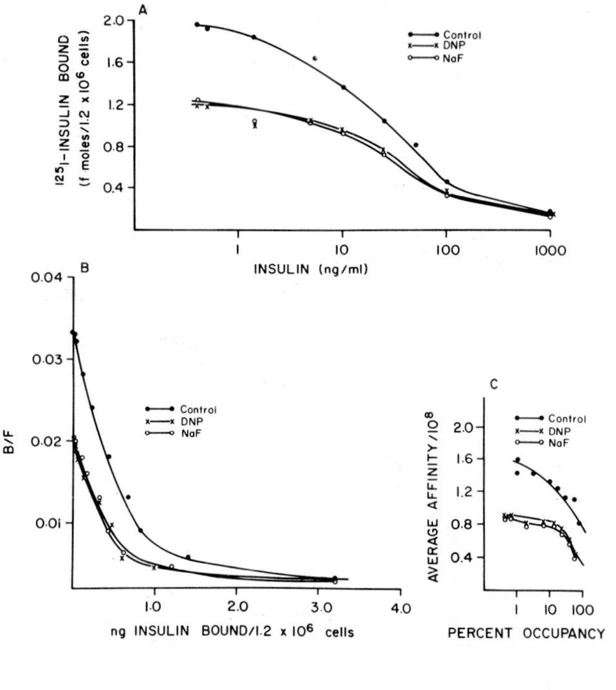

DISCUSSION

The thrust of the present investigation was to establish the possible role and need of high energy phosphate compounds for insulin binding to liver cells. Insulin binding to cultured BRL cells was examined. These cells are derived from the livers of normal 5-wk-old female Buffalo rats[35] that have been maintained for several years in continuous culture, and presumably are fully adapted to tissue culture conditions. The assumption that these cells represent hepatic parenchymal cells is based on their retention of some liver-specific functions,[35] although they do not exhibit the broad range of functions demonstrated in primary cultures.[36,37] Various studies have demonstrated that many of the altered properties of transformed cells involve modifications in cell surface functions.[38,39] These membrane alterations may be responsible for the diminished insulin binding to cultured, transformed liver cells as compared with freshly isolated hepatocytes.[27,40] Thus, BRL cells possess a decreased number of specific insulin receptor sites (40,000 sites/cell) compared with normal cells.[27] Furthermore, the affinity of BRL binding sites for insulin is lower than that found in freshly isolated hepatocytes.[14,23,25] Unlike many other clones of cultured cells, BRL cells are able to grow and replicate in serum-free medium—suggesting the possible acquired independence of their intermediary metabolism from conventional hormonal regulation. Decreased insulin binding capacity and receptor affinity may well represent another facet of this adaptation.

The magnitude and rate of insulin degradation was not rapid when these studies were performed directly in the Petri dish. This is consistent with insulin degradation being mediated via a pathway that involves insulin's binding to its receptor.[14–16,29,30] In contrast, when the cells were harvested into an incubation tube by either trypsin digestion (0.05% trypsin in 0.9% NaCl with 0.1 M Na_2PO_4) or by physical removal from the dish, the degradation of insulin was markedly accelerated. A suspension of BRL cells inactivated approximately 40% of extracellular insulin within 30 min. It is conceivable that in the experimental settings in which the

BRL cells were manipulated or treated with trypsin, some degree of cellular destruction occurred with release of intracellular enzymes capable of degrading insulin more rapidly. It is rational to assume that with the destruction of a small number of cells, significant changes in insulin degradation might occur.

Kono et al.[12] and Yu and Gould[13,41] have shown an association between the inhibitory effect of DNP on insulin-stimulated sugar transport and insulin binding to rat adipocytes and muscle. Several other reports, however, have failed to demonstrate an effect of metabolic inhibitors on insulin binding.[11,17,42,43] BRL cells recently have been shown to use glucose as a primary source for ATP production.[37] Therefore, the generation of ATP by these cells could be easily prevented by interference with either glycolysis or oxidative phosphorylation. Glycolysis is effectively inhibited by NaF, whereas oxidative phosphorylation is uncoupled by 2,4-dinitrophenol. The results of the present studies demonstrated a 30–40% decrease in insulin binding in partially ATP-depleted BRL cells and suggest at least a permissive effect of ATP on insulin binding to its receptor. The use of cultured cells for binding studies has the potential drawback that perturbations in energy metabolism can lead to major changes in cell morphology, particularly in plasma membrane topology. However, in the present study such a possibility appears remote for the following reasons. First, although the examination of the cell morphology was limited to light microscopy, no apparent morphological changes were found during the experimental period. Second, to maintain cell viability only partial ATP depletion was produced. Third, the complete reversibility of the decreased binding and the depressed ATP levels was achieved within 30 min after removal of the metabolic inhibitors, suggesting the lack of significant permanent structural changes in cell membrane.

Terris and Steiner[14] previously demonstrated a highly significant correlation between insulin binding to isolated hepatocytes and its degradation velocity. They have, therefore, concluded that binding of insulin to the plasma membrane receptor is the initial and rate-limiting step in regulating insulin degradation by intact cells. Our observations of both decreased insulin binding and degradation by ATP-depleted BRL cells are consistent with the thesis that receptor-mediated "delivery" of insulin to lysosomes is crucial for its subsequent degradation.[14–16,29,30]

Scatchard analysis of binding experiments in which ^{125}I-insulin was incubated with BRL cells (pre-exposed for 60 min to either DNP or NaF) revealed a further decline in affinity of these cells for insulin without any change in receptor number. These findings are compatible with a suggestion that changes in receptor affinity occur faster than those in receptor concentration.[1] DeMeyts and Roth[34] have recently introduced a new graphic analysis of binding experiments, which is now known as an "average affinity profile." According to this analysis, plotting $\bar{K}$ as a function of fractional occupancy (B/Ro) could reveal several situations wherein the function of the binding site is altered. The average affinity profile calculated from the present experiments (Figure 5C) clearly demonstrates a significantly diminished affinity of ATP-depleted BRL cells for insulin. The affinity profiles of the cells exposed to either DNP or NaF could be interpreted as "decreased K_e" (affinity of empty sites) or partially "locked in K_f" (affinity of fully occupied sites) pattern.[34] ATP dependence of receptor affinity seems to be a generalized regulatory phenomenon. Thus, the activation and stabilization of the glucocorticoid receptors in cytosol preparations from both mouse fibroblasts and thymocytes have been recently shown to be ATP dependent.[44,45]

There are several pitfalls and limitations in interpreting the studies involving metabolic inhibitors. The assumption that the inhibitors are specific in terms of their locus of action may not be altogether true. Notwithstanding these limitations, however, one can draw the following tentative conclusions: (1) BRL cells partially depleted of ATP by either DNP or NaF have decreased ability to bind insulin; (2) this decrease in insulin binding reflects the changes in receptor affinity without alteration in receptor number; and (3) a permissive effect of ATP on insulin binding and energy-dependent modulation of receptor affinity are strongly suggested. Furthermore, the state of ATP depletion appears to depress the rate of insulin degradation. It is not clear whether the depression of insulin degradation is a result of diminished binding or due to decreased endocytosis and/or lysosomal degradation, all of which may be inhibited in the state of ATP depletion.

ACKNOWLEDGMENTS

The iodination of insulin was performed in Dr. J. M. Olefsky's laboratory. The work was supported by grants from the American Diabetes Association, the Colorado Affiliate of the American Diabetes Association, NIH grant AM 18617, the Rocky Mountain Chapter of the Western Orthopedic Association, and the Medical Research Service of the Veterans Administration Medical Center (MRIS #8227), Denver, Colorado. The authors wish to thank Drs. J. M. Olefsky and O. G. Kolterman for their helpful comments.

We are indebted to Evelyn Fitzgerald for her excellent secretarial assistance.

REFERENCES

1 Muggeo, M., Bar, R. S., and Roth, J.: Change in affinity of insulin receptors following oral glucose in normal adults. J. Clin. Endocrinol. Metab. *44*:1206–09, 1977.

2 Kolterman, O. G., Insel, J. R., Saekow, M., and Olefsky, J. M.: Short-term regulation of insulin receptors in man. Clin. Res. *27*:86A, 1979.

3 Olefsky, J. M.: The insulin receptor: its role in insulin resistance of obesity and diabetes. Diabetes *25*:1154–65, 1976.

4 Gavin, J. R., III, Roth, J., Neville, D. M., Jr., DeMeyts, P., and Buell, D. N.: Insulin-dependent regulation of insulin receptor concentrations. A direct demonstration of cell culture. Proc. Natl. Acad. Sci. USA *71*:84–88, 1974.

5 Davidson, M. B., and Kaplan, S. A.: Increased insulin binding by hepatic plasma membranes from diabetic rats. Normalization by insulin therapy. J. Clin. Invest. *59*:22–30, 1977.

6 Kobayashi, M., and Olefsky, J. M.: Effect of experimental hyperinsulinemia on insulin binding and glucose transport in isolated rat adipocytes. Am. J. Physiol. *234*:E53–62, 1978.

7 Thomopoulos, P., Kosmakos, F. C., Pastan, I., and Lovelace, E.: Cyclic AMP increases the concentration of insulin receptors in cultured fibroblasts and lymphocytes. Biochem. Biophys. Res. Commun. *75*:246–52, 1977.

8 Cuatrecasas, P.: Properties of the insulin receptor of isolated fat cell membrane. J. Biol. Chem. *246*:2756–74, 1971.

9 Merimee, T. J., Pulkkinen, A. J., and Lofton, S.: Increased insulin binding by lymphocyte receptors induced by β-OH butyrate. J. Clin. Endocrinol. Metab. *43*:1190–92, 1976.

10 Flier, J. S., Kahn, C. R., Roth, J., and Bar, R. S.: Antibodies that impair insulin receptor binding in an unusual diabetic syndrome with severe insulin resistance. Science *190*:63–65, 1975.

11 Chandramouli, V., Milligan, M., and Carter, J. R., Jr.: Insulin stimulation of glucose transport in adipose cells. An energy dependent process. Biochemistry *16*:1151–57, 1977.

12 Kono, T., Robinson, F. W., Sarver, J. A., Vega, F. V., and Pointer, R. H.: Action of insulin in fat cells. J. Biol. Chem. *252*:2226–33, 1977.

[13] Yu, K. T., and Gould, M. K.: Effect of prolonged anaerobiosis on ^{125}I-insulin binding to rat soleus muscle: permissive effect of ATP. Am. J. Physiol. *235*:E606–13, 1978.

[14] Terris, S., and Steiner, D. F.: Binding and degradation of ^{125}I-insulin by rat hepatocytes. J. Biol. Chem. *250*:8389–98, 1975.

[15] Gorden, P., Carpentier, J. L., Freychet, P., LeCam, A., and Orci, L.: Intracellular translocation of iodine-125-labeled insulin: direct demonstration in isolated hepatocytes. Science *200*:782–85, 1978.

[16] Gliemann, J., and Sonne, O.: Binding and receptor-mediated degradation of insulin in adipocytes. J. Biol. Chem. *253*:7857–63, 1978.

[17] Marshall, S., and Olefsky, J. M.: Effects of lysosomotropic agents on insulin interactions with adipocytes: evidence for a lysosomal pathway for insulin processing and degradation. J. Biol. Chem. *254*:10153–60, 1979.

[18] Freychet, P., Roth, J., and Neville, D. M., Jr.: Moniodoinsulin: demonstration of its biological activity and binding to fat calls and liver membranes. Biochem. Biophys. Res. Commun. *43*:400–08, 1971.

[19] Hunter, W. M., and Greenwood, F. C.: Preparation of iodine-131 labeled human growth hormone of high specific activity. Nature (London) *194*:495–96, 1962.

[20] Olefsky, J. M., and Reaven, G. M.: The human lymphocyte: a model for the study of insulin-receptor interaction. J. Clin. Endocrinol. Metab. *38*:554–60, 1974.

[21] Lowry, D. H., Rosenborough, W. J., Farr, A. L., and Randall, R. J.: Protein determination with the Folin Phenol reagent. J. Biol. Chem. *193*:265, 1951.

[22] Solomons, C. C., and McDermott, N.: Use of high performance liquid chromatography and thin layer chromatography in the rapid detection of human cellular toxicity of environment substance. 12th Annual Conference on Trace Substances in Environmental Health. Hemphill, D., Ed. University of Missouri, Columbia, Missouri, 1978, pp. 447–54.

[23] Olefsky, J. M., Johnson, J., Liu, F., Edwards, P., and Baur, S.: Comparison of ^{125}I-insulin binding and degradation to isolated rat hepatocytes and liver membrane. Diabetes *24*801–10, 1975.

[24] Broer, J., Freychet, P., and Rosselin, G.: Insulin and glucagon receptor interactions in the genetically obese Zucker rat: studies of hormone binding and glucagon-stimulated cyclic AMP levels in isolated hepatocytes. Endocrinology *101*:236–49, 1977.

[25] Blackard, W. G., Guzelian, P. S., and Small, M. E.: Down regulation of insulin receptors in primary cultures of adult rat hepatocytes in monolayer. Endocrinology *103*:548–53, 1978.

[26] Petersen, B., Beckner, S., and Blecher, M.: Hormone receptors. 7. Characteristics of insulin receptors in a new line of cloned neonatal rat hepatocytes. Biochem. Biophys. Acta *542*:470–85, 1978.

[27] Capeau, J., Picard, J., and Caron, M.: Insulin receptors in Zajdela rat ascites hepatoma cells and their sensitivity to certain enzymes and lectins. Cancer Res. *38*:3930–37, 1978.

[28] DeMeyts, P.: Insulin and growth hormone receptors in human cultured lymphocytes and peripheral blood monocytes. *In* Methods in Receptor Research. Blecker, M., Ed. New York, Marcel Dekker, 1976, pp. 301–83.

[29] Carpentier, J.-L., Gorden, P., Barazzone, P., Freychet, P., LeCam, A., and Orci, L.: Intracellular localization of ^{125}I-labeled insulin in hepatocytes from intact rat liver. Proc. Natl. Acad. Sci. USA *76*:2803–07, 1979.

[30] Carpentier, J.-L., Gorden, P., Freychet, P., LeCam, A., and Orci, L.: Lysosomal association of internalyzed ^{125}I-insulin in isolated rat hepatocytes. J. Clin. Invest. *63*:1249–60, 1979.

[31] Kalckar, H. M.: The role of myokinase in transphosphorylations. II. The enzymatic action of myokinase on adenine nucleotides. J. Biol. Chem. *148*:127–37, 1943.

[32] Lehninger, A. L.: Biochemistry. New York, Worth Publishers, Inc., 1970, p. 308.

[33] Atkinson, D. E.: Cellular Energy Metabolism and its Regulation. New York, Academic Press, 1977, p. 90.

[34] DeMeyts, P., and Roth, J.: Cooperative ligand binding: a new graphic analysis. Biochem. Biophy. Res. Commun. *66*:1118–26, 1975.

[35] Coon, H. C.: Clonal culture of differentiated rat liver cell. J. Cell Biol. *39*:29A, 1968.

[36] Bissell, D. M.: Study of hepatocyte function in cell culture. Prog. Liver Dis. *5*:69–82, 1976.

[37] Bissell, D. M., Levine, G. A., and Bissell, N. J.: Glucose metabolism by adult hepatocytes in primary culture and by cell lines from rat liver. Am. J. Physiol. *234*:C122–30, 1978.

[38] Hynes, R. O.: Cell surface proteins and malignant transformation. Biochem. Biophys. Acta *458*:73–107, 1976.

[39] Nicolson, G. L.: Trans-membrane control of the receptors of normal and tumor cells. II. Surface changes associated with transformation and malignancy. Biochem. Biophys. Acta *458*:1–72, 1976.

[40] Pezzino, V., Vigneri, R., Siperstein, M. D., and Goldfine, I. D.: Insulin and glucagon receptors in Morris hepatomas of varying growth rates. Cancer Res. *39*:1443–46, 1979.

[41] Yu, K. T., and Gould, M. K.: Insulin-stimulated sugar transport and ^{125}I-insulin binding by rat soleus muscle: permissive effect of ATP. Biochem. Biophys. Res. Commun. *77*:203–10, 1977.

[42] Terris, S., Hoffman, C., and Steiner, D. F.: Mode of uptake and degradation of ^{125}I-insulin by isolated hepatocytes and H4 hepatoma cell. Can. J. Biochem. *57*:459–68, 1979.

[43] Olefsky, J. M., Kobayashi, M., and Ghang, H.: Interactions between insulin and its receptors after the initial binding event: functional heterogeneity and relationship to insulin degradation. Diabetes *28*:460–71, 1979.

[44] Sando, J. J., LaForest, A. C., and Pratt, W. B.: ATP-dependent activation of L cell glucocorticoid receptors to the steroid binding form. J. Biol. Chem. *254*:4772–78, 1979.

[45] Sando, J. J., Hammond, N. D., Stratford, C. A., and Pratt, W. B.: Activation of thymocyte glucocorticoid receptors to the steroid binding form. J. Biol. Chem. *254*:4779–89, 1979.

Abnormal Sciatic Nerve *Myo*-inositol Metabolism in the Streptozotocin-diabetic Rat

Effect of Insulin Treatment

REX S. CLEMENTS, JR., AND CECIL R. STOCKARD

SUMMARY

The metabolism of *myo*-inositol and its phospholipids has been studied in the sciatic nerves of control, two weeks' streptozotocin-diabetic, and insulin-treated diabetic rats. The concentrations of glucose, fructose, and sorbitol were increased and the concentration of *myo*-inositol was decreased in the sciatic nerves of the diabetic animals; these abnormalities were only partially corrected by insulin therapy that was adequate to obviate hyperglycemia. Whereas the space of distribution of 2-^{3}H-*myo*-inositol was found to exceed the total water space of the nerves of control animals, the 2-^{3}H-*myo*-inositol space approximated the water space in the nerves of diabetic animals and was only slightly increased after insulin therapy. During the first 2 h after the intraperitoneal injection of 2-^{3}H-*myo*-inositol, the recovery of radioactivity in nerve lipids was decreased by 69% in the untreated diabetics and by 77% in the insulin-treated diabetics. Analysis of the individual phosphoinositides revealed a proportional increase in the radioactivity recovered with phosphatidylinositol and a decrease in the recovery with triphosphatidylinositol in the diabetic nerves.

CDP-diglyceride:inositol transferase activity was decreased by 44% in homogenates of sciatic nerves from untreated diabetic rats, but it was normal in nerve homogenates from insulin-treated diabetics. The pattern of incorporation of radioactivity into phospholipids after 1 h of incubation of nerve homogenates with 2-^{3}H-*myo*-inositol was similar to that observed in vivo. The fractional recovery of radioactivity with phosphatidylinositol was increased, whereas the recovery of label as triphosphatidylinositol was decreased by 11% in the presence of homogenates of sciatic nerves from diabetic rats.

These observations indicate that 2 wk of acute streptozotocin diabetes results in a decrease in the sciatic nerve content and space of distribution of *myo*-inositol and suggests that nerve *myo*-inositol transport may be defective in the diabetic animal. The observed abnormalities in the amount and pattern of incorporation of 2-^{3}H-*myo*-inositol into diabetic nerve phospholipids could be explained, in part, by decreased activities of CDP-diglyceride:inositol transferase and phosphatidylinositol 4-phosphate kinase activities in the diabetic nerves. However, the fact that the incorporation of 2-^{3}H-*myo*-inositol into phospholipids was decreased in the nerves of insulin-treated–diabetic animals despite a normal CDP-diglyceride:inositol transferase activity suggests that defective *myo*-inositol transport may also contribute to the abnormal neural phosphoinositide metabolism in this model. The possibility that these abnormalities are related to the development of the structural and functional changes associated with diabetic neuropathy requires further investigation. **DIABETES *29*:227–235, March 1980.**

During the past decade, considerable evidence has accumulated to suggest that the metabolism of *myo*-inositol and its phospholipid derivatives may play an important role in peripheral nerve function.[1–14] Under normal circumstances, the concentration of free *myo*-inositol within the rat sciatic nerve is approximately thirty times higher than that of the plasma.[7–9,15,16] Neither the mechanisms responsible for the maintenance of this gradient nor the relative contribution of the axons, the Schwann cells, the epineurial space, and the endoneurial space to the total free *myo*-inositol content of nerve homogenates are known. Similarly, the significance of this gradient with regard to peripheral nerve function is unclear. However, since the turnover of *myo*-inositol–containing phospholipids has been found to increase after nerve impulse and synaptic transmission,[1–6,10,11] it is possible that the metabolism of phosphoinositides may participate in the cationic fluxes that accompany neural excitation.[2,4–6,10,11] Furthermore, since the enzyme responsible for the synthesis

From the Metabolic Research Laboratory, Veterans' Administration Medical Center, and the Department of Medicine and the Diabetes Research and Training Center of the University of Alabama School of Medicine, Birmingham.
Address reprint requests to Rex S. Clements, Jr., M. D., Veterans' Administration Medical Center, 700 South 19th Street, Birmingham, AL 35233.
Received for publication 27 April and in revised form 22 October 1979.

of phosphatidylinositol (CDP-diglyceride:inositol transferase, E.C. 2.7.8.11) has been found (in other tissues) to have a high K_m for *myo*-inositol,[17,18] it is reasonable to speculate that the high concentration of *myo*-inositol within the nerve may serve to facilitate the synthesis of this phospholipid and to permit its rapid replenishment after neural stimulation. This speculation is bolstered by the observations that CDP-diglyceride:inositol transferase activity is present in the axoplasm of the giant squid axon[19] and newly synthesized phosphatidylinositol appears (by radioautographic techniques) to be laid down in the axolemma of the mouse sciatic nerve.[20] If the metabolism of *myo*-inositol and the phosphoinositides does, in fact, play a role in nerve function, then one would anticipate that any abnormality in the metabolism of these compounds should result in dysfunction of the peripheral nerves.

The induction of acute experimental diabetes in the rat is known to cause a prompt decrease in sciatic motor nerve conduction velocity[7,8,21,22] as well as a decrease in the concentration of *myo*-inositol within this nerve.[7-9,15,16] Both these abnormalities can be obviated by careful insulin treatment.[7,22] In addition, oral *myo*-inositol supplementation, sufficient to normalize the peripheral nerve *myo*-inositol content, has been found by some[7] but not all investigators[23] to improve the sciatic motor nerve conduction velocity in the diabetic rat. The possibility that the decrease in nerve *myo*-inositol content resulting from exposure of this tissue to hyperglycemia may cause impairment of nerve phosphoinositide synthesis is suggested by the recent observations that the peripheral nerve phosphatidylinositol content is decreased in rats with acute (but not chronic) experimental diabetes,[9] the CDP-diglyceride:inositol transferase activity is decreased in homogenates of streptozotocin-diabetic rat nerves,[13] and the total acidic phospholipid content (phosphatidylinositol and phosphatidylserine content) of the peripheral nerve is decreased in human beings with diabetes mellitus.[24]

Since virtually nothing is known concerning the neural uptake of *myo*-inositol and its subsequent incorporation into the phosphoinositides, we have studied these phenomena in normal rat sciatic nerves using radioisotopic techniques. In addition, we have examined the influence of acute experimental diabetes (both with and without careful insulin treatment) on the recovery of water-soluble and lipid-bound radioactivity from the sciatic nerve after the intraperitoneal injection of 2-^{3}H-*myo*-inositol as well as on the CDP-diglyceride:inositol transferase activity in sciatic nerve homogenates. This report describes the abnormalities in these phenomena that we observed in the diabetic rat nerve as well as the effect of careful insulin treatment on these alterations.

MATERIALS AND METHODS

Animal models. Male Sprague-Dawley rats, whose ages were between 7 and 8 wk, were employed for all experiments. The animals were maintained in wire-bottomed cages and were fed Wayne Lab-Blox ad libitum throughout the 2-wk study. Three groups of animals were studied—controls, untreated streptozotocin diabetics, and insulin-treated streptozotocin diabetics. Experimental diabetes was induced in overnight-fasted rats by the intraperitoneal injection of streptozotocin (SZ) (65 mg/kg body wt, Sigma Chemical, St. Louis, Mo.) freshly dissolved in approximately 0.4 ml of a 0.85% sodium chloride solution in 0.05 M citric acid (pH 4.2). Those animals whose tail vein blood glucose concentration was in excess of 300 mg/dl on the third morning after SZ injection were considered to be diabetic. One group of diabetic animals was untreated for 14 days after the SZ was administered, and the other group was treated with insulin as described below.

The insulin treatment regimen was similar to that employed by Greene et al.[7] On the evening of the third day, the insulin-treated animals were given a subcutaneous injection of 10 U of Lente insulin for every 100 g body wt. Subsequently, twice daily injections of Lente insulin were administered at 9 a.m. and 5 p.m., and the individual doses were titrated against the morning and evening tail vein blood glucose concentrations. After day 5, the total amount of insulin administered per day averaged approximately 9 U for each animal. The final dose of insulin was given on the evening of the thirteenth day, and the animals were studied on the morning of the fourteenth day after SZ was administered. To avoid the risk of hypoglycemia in the insulin-treated diabetic animals, all study groups had free access to food until the time of study.

Analysis of blood and sciatic nerve *myo*-inositol specific activity and nerve phospholipid-bound radioactivity after intraperitoneal 2-^{3}H-*myo*-inositol injection. Animals from each of the three experimental groups were studied before, at 30 min (only the controls and the untreated diabetics), and at four 1-h intervals after the intraperitoneal injection of 50 μCi of 2-^{3}H-*myo*-inositol (New England Nuclear, Boston, Mass., specific activity 12.5 Ci/mmol) dissolved in 0.5 ml of a sodium chloride solution (0.85%). Samples of tail vein blood (0.1 ml) were collected in heparinized capillary tubes, added to 1.9 ml of distilled water containing 1 μg of α-methylmannose (Sigma), and deproteinized by the sequential addition of 1.0 ml portions of barium hydroxide (0.3 N) and zinc sulfate (5%). Blood glucose concentration was determined by an hexokinase-glucose-6-phosphate dehydrogenase enzymatic assay of duplicate 0.1 ml aliquots of the clear supernatant.[25] Duplicate 0.4 ml aliquots of the supernatant were lyophilized in scintillation vials for the subsequent analysis of radioactivity by liquid scintillation spectrometry.[26] The remainder of the supernatant (approximately 2.0 ml) was lyophilized for gas-liquid chromatographic analysis of *myo*-inositol content as previously described.[26]

At hourly intervals after the intraperitoneal injection of 2-^{3}H-*myo*-inositol, animals were anesthetized by the intraperitoneal injection of Nembutal (36 mg/kg body wt). One sciatic nerve was exposed from the sciatic notch to the popliteal fossa by blunt dissection and then removed and placed in 0.85% sodium chloride at 4°C (the contralateral nerve was removed later). The nerves were bisected, and the proximal portions (approximately 10 mg) were blotted on filter paper and weighed before homogenization in a glass vessel containing 2.0 ml of distilled water, 1.0 mg of zinc sulfate (5%), and 10 μg of α-methylmannose. The resultant suspension was rehomogenized after the addition of barium hydroxide (1.0 ml, 0.3 N) and centrifuged. The water-soluble radioactivity present in the nerve homogenates was determined in duplicate 0.4 ml aliquots treated as previously described for the blood samples. The remainder of the supernatant was lyophilized for analysis of glucose, fructose, sorbitol, and *myo*-inositol content by gas-liquid chromatography of their trimethylsilyl ethers.[27]

The distal portions of the nerves (approximately 15 mg) were blotted on filter paper, weighed, and homogenized in 3.0 ml of 0.1 N HCl in methanol in glass vessels. After the addition of 6.0 ml of chloroform, the solution was mixed, decanted into a glass-stoppered tube, and maintained overnight at 4°C. Subsequently, the chloroform-methanol solution was extracted with four 2.0 ml washes of 1 M $MgCl_2$.[28] The resultant chloroform layer was dried under nitrogen at room temperature. The residue was dissolved in 1.0 ml of chloroform, and a 0.5 ml portion was placed in a liquid scintillation vial, dried under a stream of nitrogen, dissolved in 5 ml of a solution of toluene-Triton X-100 (2:1, vol/vol) containing 11 g/L of PPO and 0.1 g/L of POPOP, and counted in a liquid scintillation spectrometer. The remaining 0.5 ml of chloroform was dried under nitrogen, taken up in 0.05 ml of a solution of chloroform, methanol, and 4.3 N ammonium hydroxide (90:65:20, vol/vol/vol), and spotted on thin-layer chromatography plates, which were developed as previously described.[28,29] The localization of mono-, di-, and triphosphatidylinositol standards was made by exposure of the plates to iodine vapor, the corresponding areas from the channels containing nerve extract being removed with a spatula and counted, as described previously.[28]

Assay of nerve CDP-diglyceride:inositol transferase. For analysis of the activity of CDP-diglyceride:inositol transferase, sciatic nerves were removed from animals that had not received injections of radioactive *myo*-inositol and then weighed and homogenized in 2.0 ml of 0.25 M sucrose in glass vessels. The homogenates were centrifuged at 550 *g* for 5 min, and the supernatant was utilized for enzyme assay and protein determination.[30] The assay system employed was a slight modification of the method of Takenawa and Egawa.[18] To 0.9 ml of homogenate was added 0.1 ml of a solution of asolectin (16 mg/ml, Associated Concentrates, Woodside, L.I., N.Y.), containing 6% sodium cholate (Sigma), and 0.01 ml of β-mercaptoethanol (4 M, Sigma). After mixing, triplicate 0.05 ml aliquots, containing between 20 and 120 μg of nerve protein, were added to test tubes containing 0.05 ml of 0.4 mM CDP-dipalmitate (Serdary Research Laboratories, London, Ontario, Canada) in 0.6% sodium cholate. After gentle mixing, 0.1 ml of glycyl-glycine buffer (0.1 M, pH 8.4) containing 0.5 M $MgCl_2$ and 10 mM 2-^{3}H-*myo*-inositol (1.0 μCi/μmol) was added. For each assay, control tubes (one without CDP-dipalmitate and one without enzyme) were run in parallel. After mixing, the tubes were incubated for 60 min at 37°C in a water bath. To each tube was added 1.0 ml of HCl (0.1 N) in methanol, followed by 2.0 ml of chloroform and 0.7 ml of $MgCl_2$ (1 M). The tubes were mixed and centrifuged, and the upper phase was discarded. This washing procedure was repeated three times, and the resultant chloroform layer was taken to dryness in scintillation vials for the determination of lipid-soluble radioactivity as previously described. The incorporation of radioactivity into lipid in the absence of CDP-dipalmitate was subtracted from the mean value of that observed in its presence, and this difference was considered to be due to CDP-diglyceride:inositol transferase activity. Nonspecific exchange activity was estimated by the difference between the rate of incorporation of 2-^{3}H-*myo*-inositol into lipid in the presence of enzyme without added CDP-dipalmitate and that observed in the absence of enzyme. The distribution of radioactivity in the phosphoinositides at the end of the assay was determined by the thin-layer chromatography technique previously described.[29]

Statistical methods. All results are expressed as means ± SEM. Statistical differences between means were determined by Student's *t* test.

RESULTS

Effect of insulin treatment on the blood glucose concentrations of streptozotocin-diabetic rats. The mean blood glucose concentrations observed in the insulin-treated diabetic rats are given in Table 1. With the exception of the value observed on the morning of day 13, after insulin treatment had been initiated, all mean blood glucose concentrations were within (or below) the range observed in the morning samples from the control animals (122.9 ± 8.4, n = 26). After the eleventh day, the fluctuations in blood glucose increased in amplitude; eight animals died of presumed hypoglycemia (overall mortality rate = 30.8%). These values for blood glucose, as well as for mortality, are in excellent agreement with the data of Greene et al.[7] and suggest that this model is adequate for the study of the effect of insulin treatment on peripheral nerve metabolism in the streptozotocin-diabetic rat.

Characteristics of the animal models. As indicated in Table 2, the mean body weight of the untreated diabetic animals was less than that of the controls at the time of study. In contrast, since the insulin-treated diabetic animals gained weight during the course of the study, their mean weight was slightly greater than that of the controls and the untreated diabetics. As anticipated, on the morning of study the blood glucose was elevated in the untreated diabetic rats and was normal in the insulin-treated animals. The blood *myo*-inositol concentrations were similar in all groups at the outset (Table 2) and did not change during the course of the experiment.

TABLE 1
Tail vein blood glucose concentrations of diabetic rats treated twice daily with subcutaneous injections of Lente insulin

Blood glucose (mg/dl)	Days after streptozotocin administration											
	3	4	5	6	7	8	9	10	11	12	13	14
Morning (8 a.m.)	409.1 ±12.1	157.0 ±23.3	117.7 ±15.5	136.6 ±14.4	108.0 ±16.9	161.5 ±21.5	141.2 ±22.8	152.3 ±21.3	119.4 ±16.3	164.0 ±19.6	183.6 ±23.3	139.4 ±24.0
Evening (4 p.m.)	379.4 ±14.4	120.9 ±18.1	90.5 ±12.5	73.8 ±6.0	63.1 ±4.7	84.4 ±10.1	79.8 ±14.0	69.9 ±9.5	92.5 ±19.8	117.3 ±19.3	79.2 ±14.0	— —
N	26	26	26	26	26	26	26	26	26	25	25	18

TABLE 2
Characteristics of the control, streptozotocin-diabetic, and insulin-treated streptozotocin-diabetic rats on the morning of study

Study group	Body weight (g)	Blood glucose (mM)	Blood *myo*-inositol (μM)	Nerve carbohydrate content (mmol/kg wet wt)			
				Glucose	Fructose	Sorbitol	*Myo*-inositol
Controls (N = 26)	287.3 ±11.8	6.8 ±0.5	99.9 ±13.5	1.96 ±0.45	0.63 ±0.15	0.26 ±0.10	2.78 ±0.24
Diabetics (N = 20)	278.4 ±8.7	22.9 ±0.7‡	82.4 ±7.9	7.21 ±0.69‡	1.13 ±0.15*	0.74 ±0.15*	2.02 ±0.15†
Insulin-treated diabetics (N = 18)	291.8 ±8.4	7.7 ±1.3§	79.5 ±7.6	3.19 ±0.39*§	0.50 ±0.14‖	0.30 ±0.10‖	2.24 ±0.17

* P vs controls < 0.05, † P vs controls < 0.01, ‡ P vs controls < 0.001, § P vs untreated diabetics < 0.001, ‖ P vs untreated diabetics < 0.025.

Nerve carbohydrate content. The mean values for the various carbohydrates measured in homogenates of nerves obtained from the various study groups are also given in Table 2. The expected increase in the glucose, sorbitol, and fructose content as well as the decrease in *myo*-inositol content was observed in the nerves of untreated diabetic rats. Amelioration of these abnormalities was observed in the nerves of insulin-treated animals, and the mean values for both fructose and sorbitol were normalized. However, neither the nerve glucose nor the nerve *myo*-inositol concentrations were restored to normal values. This suggests that the insulin treatment regimen may not have been as effective in the correction of the fluctuations of the blood glucose concentrations of the diabetic animals as was suggested by the morning and evening blood glucose determinations (Table 1).

Blood and sciatic nerve *myo*-inositol specific activity. After the intraperitoneal injection of 2-^{3}H-*myo*-inositol, radioactivity was observed to rapidly appear in the blood of all groups of animals (Figure 1). Whereas the maximum mean blood *myo*-inositol specific activity was observed at 1 h in the untreated diabetic group and declined thereafter, it appeared to rise gradually throughout most of the study in the controls and the insulin-treated diabetics. However, within each group of animals, no statistically significant differences in the *myo*-inositol specific activities were observed at the different time periods. Thus, these data do not allow conclusions to be drawn concerning either the rates of absorption of 2-^{3}H-*myo*-inositol from the intraperitoneal space or its rate of peripheral disposal in the various groups of animals. It should be noted, however, that the mean blood *myo*-inositol specific activity of the diabetic animals (both treated and untreated) was higher than that of the control animals at all times. It is not clear whether this difference was due to more rapid absorption of 2-^{3}H-*myo*-inositol from the intraperitoneal space, to decreased gastrointestinal absorption of unlabeled *myo*-inositol, to decreased endogenous *myo*-inositol synthesis, to a contracted total exchangeable *myo*-inositol pool, or to a combination of these factors in the diabetic animals.

In a similar fashion, water-soluble radioactivity rapidly appeared in the sciatic nerve homogenates of all groups of animals after the intraperitoneal injection of 2-^{3}H-*myo*-inositol (Figure 1). The specific activity of the nerve *myo*-inositol was roughly an order of magnitude less than that of the whole blood, and (with the exception of the fourth hour) no differences in the nerve specific activity of the three groups was observed.

Sciatic nerve water-soluble radioactivity. The time course of recovery of water-soluble radioactivity from the sciatic nerve homogenates of the three groups of animals after the intraperitoneal injection of 2-^{3}H-*myo*-inositol is shown in Figure 2. In the control and the insulin-treated diabetic groups, the mean recovery increased for the first 2 h and remained relatively stable thereafter. In contrast, the maximal recovery of water-soluble radioactivity from the nerves of untreated diabetics was observed at 1 h, and it rapidly declined thereafter. The values observed in the untreated diabetics were statistically significantly lower than those of the insulin-treated diabetics at the third and fourth hours. We have no ready explanation for the temporal differences in the patterns of recovery of water-soluble radioactivity from the nerves of the three groups of animals. However, due to the experimental design, in none of the groups of animals were the sciatic nerves exposed to constant blood *myo*-inositol specific activities. As is evident in Figure 1, the blood *myo*-inositol specific activity tended to fall throughout the experiment in the untreated diabetics,

FIGURE 1. Mean blood and sciatic nerve water-soluble *myo*-inositol specific activities in the various groups of animals at intervals following the intraperitoneal injection of 2-^{3}H-*myo*-inositol. The controls are represented by the dot-dash lines, the untreated streptozotocin-diabetics by the dashed lines, and the insulin-treated diabetics by the solid lines.

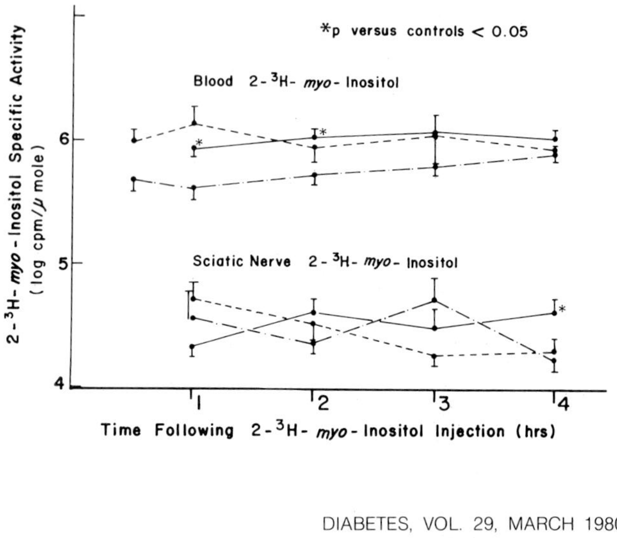

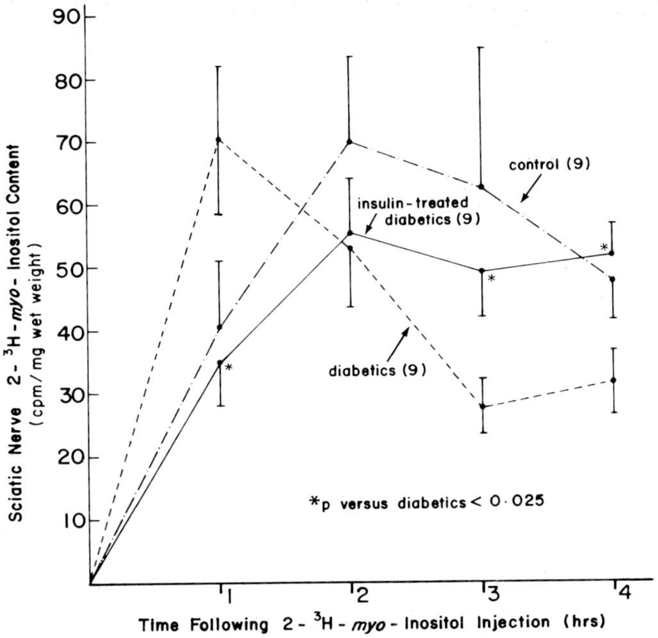

FIGURE 2. Recovery of water-soluble 2-^{3}H-*myo*-inositol from homogenates of sciatic nerves from control, diabetic, and insulin-treated diabetic rats at hourly intervals following the intraperitoneal injection of 2-^{3}H-*myo*-inositol. The number of animals in each group is given in the parentheses.

whereas it tended to rise in the other two groups of animals. That these differences may have influenced the patterns of the recoveries of water-soluble (as well as lipid-bound) radioactivity from the nerves is suggested by the trend observed to exist between the blood and nerve *myo*-inositol specific activities in both groups of diabetic animals ($r = 0.61$, $P < 0.1 > 0.05$).

If it is assumed that the epineurial and perineurial fluid space of the rat sciatic nerve constitutes approximately 20% of the wet weight of this tissue,[31] and if it is further assumed that the water-soluble 2-^{3}H-*myo*-inositol within this space is in equilibrium with that of the blood, the space of distribution of water-soluble *myo*-inositol within the nerve can be calculated from the data used to generate Figures 1 and 2. As shown in Table 3, within 1 h of the intraperitoneal injection of 2-^{3}H-*myo*-inositol, the calculated space of distribution of this material within the sciatic nerve exceeded both the rapidly equilibrating space as well as the total water space of the control nerve (assuming that the latter is approximately 64.6 ml/100 g wet wt[31]). Since the space of distribution of 2-^{3}H-*myo*-inositol within these nerves was approximately twice that of the water space of the tissue at the second and third hours of the experiment, this suggests a rapid accumulation of this material by the extravascular elements of the nerve. The present data do not, however, offer any information as to the cellular localization of this accumulation nor do they allow any conclusions to be drawn concerning the mechanisms responsible for this accumulation. In contrast, although the sciatic nerve 2-^{3}H-*myo*-inositol space rose to approximate the water space in the diabetic nerves, it did not exceed this space during the course of the experiment. This observation provides support for the recent suggestion that the transport of *myo*-inositol by the diabetic nerve may be impaired.[12] Furthermore, the slight but significant mean increase in the *myo*-inositol space in the sciatic nerves of the insulin-treated animals compared with that of the untreated diabetic animals may mean that insulin treatment slightly ameliorates this defect in neural *myo*-inositol accumulation.

TABLE 3
Sciatic nerve 2-^{3}H-*myo*-inositol space

	ml/100 g wet wt		
Time	Controls (9)	Diabetics (9)	Insulin-treated diabetics (9)
1 hour	96.5 ± 25.5	62.5 + 10.3	50.6 ± 9.8
2 hours	126.1 ± 24.2	72.2 ± 13.1	65.1 ± 10.1*
3 hours	131.5 ± 43.8	29.3 ± 4.7*	51.2 ± 7.5‡
4 hours	59.4 ± 7.6	45.4 ± 7.0	60.3 ± 5.9
Means	103.4 ± 4.8	52.4 ± 1.6†	56.8 ± 1.4†

* P versus controls < 0.05
† P versus controls < 0.001
‡ P versus untreated diabetics < 0.05

Sciatic nerve lipid-bound 2-^{3}H-*myo*-inositol. As shown in Figure 3, when expressed on the basis of nerve weight, the recovery of lipid-bound radioactivity was maximal 1 h after intraperitoneal 2-^{3}H-*myo*-inositol injection in the control animals and declined thereafter. Although the pattern of recovery of lipid-bound radioactivity from the sciatic nerves of the untreated diabetic animals was similar to that of the controls, the amount of radioactivity recovered from the nerve lipids was markedly decreased at all times. Initially, the recovery of lipid-bound radioactivity from the nerves of the insulin-treated diabetics was similar to that of the untreated diabetics, but it increased to approximate that of the controls during the third and fourth hours after injection. The explanation for the delayed appearance of radioactivity in the lipid fraction of the nerves of the insulin-treated diabetics is not apparent, but it may be related to the increased availa-

FIGURE 3. Recovery of lipid-bound radioactivity from homogenates of sciatic nerves of control, streptozotocin-diabetic, and insulin-treated diabetic rats at intervals following the intraperitoneal injection of 2-^{3}H-*myo*-inositol. The number of nerves studied is given between the parentheses.

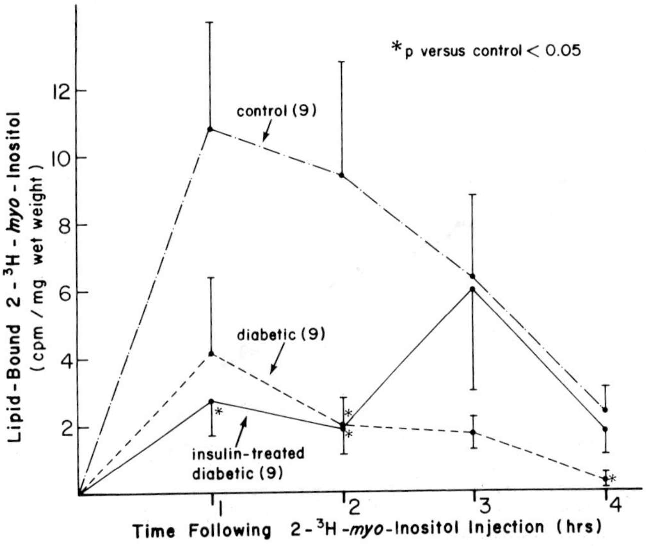

bility of water-soluble 2-^{3}H-*myo*-inositol substrate in the nerves of the insulin-treated animals during the second half of the experiment (see Figures 1 and 2).

Since it was possible that the decreased recovery of lipid-bound 2-^{3}H-*myo*-inositol from the nerves of the two groups of diabetic animals was a consequence of the decreased *myo*-inositol content of their nerves (Table 2) rather than a reflection of impaired phosphatidylinositol synthesis, the net incorporation of 2-^{3}H-*myo*-inositol into phospholipids was also calculated on the basis of the nerve *myo*-inositol specific activity. As shown in Figure 4, the net recovery of 2-^{3}H-*myo*-inositol from nerve lipids in the control animals increased during the first 2 h of the experiment and then declined. In both groups of diabetic animals, the net incorporation of radioactive *myo*-inositol into nerve lipids was markedly decreased during the first 2 h of the experiment. Thus, regardless of whether the recovery of lipid-bound radioactivity was expressed as a function of nerve weight or of the ambient 2-^{3}H-*myo*-inositol specific activity, a marked impairment in the incorporation of *myo*-inositol into the lipid fraction of the diabetic nerves was apparent.

Distribution of radioactivity among the phosphoinositides. In many of the nerve homogenates, the total amount of radioactivity recovered from the thin-layer plates was insufficient to determine the contribution of mono-, di-, and triphosphatidylinositol to the total lipid-bound radioactivity. Consequently, in only those samples in which the recovery of radioactivity from the thin-layer plates exceeded 10 cpm/mg wet wt of original homogenate was this distribution estimated. The in vivo data shown in Table 4 represent pooled results from the various time periods. As shown, phosphatidylinositol accounted for the majority of the lipid-bound radioactivity in both control and diabetic nerves, and the relative contribution of this entity was similar in the two groups. Whereas the contribution of diphosphatidylinositol to the total lipid-bound radioactivity was also similar in both groups, the recovery of triphosphatidylinositol-associated radioactivity was decreased in the nerves obtained from the diabetic animals. The information available concerning the distribution of radioactivity in these phospholipids is not adequate to draw any conclusions concerning the change of distribution of radioactivity with time. However, the decreased recovery of 2-^{3}H-*myo*-inositol in triphosphatidylinositol is consistent with the recently observed decrease in the activity of phosphatidylinositol 4-phosphate kinase (E.C. 2.7.1.68) in homogenates of nerves obtained from streptozotocin-diabetic rats.[13]

TABLE 4
Distribution of radioactivity among *myo*-inositol-containing phospholipids recovered from control and diabetic rat sciatic nerves in vivo and from nerve homogenates in vitro

Study group	Percent distribution of radioactivity		
	Phosphatidyl-inositol	Diphosphatidyl-inositol	Triphosphatidyl-inositol
In Vivo (1 to 4 h)			
Controls (N = 15)	73.6 ± 6.5	14.8 ± 4.3	12.5 ± 4.2
Diabetics (N = 5)	87.0 ± 7.7	11.1 ± 7.0	1.9 ± 1.9*
In Vitro (1 h)			
Controls (N = 10)	74.6 ± 0.9	10.8 ± 0.2	14.6 ± 0.9
Diabetics (N = 9)	85.9 ± 0.5†	10.8 ± 0.3	3.2 ± 0.4†

* P vs controls < 0.05
† P vs controls < 0.001

Sciatic nerve CDP-diglyceride:inositol transferase activity. Approximately 96% of the incorporation of 2-^{3}H-*myo*-inositol into lipid was found to depend on the presence of CDP-dipalmitate in both control and diabetic nerve homogenates, and this was presumed to represent CDP-diglyceride:inositol transferase activity. The incorporation of radioactivity into lipid in the presence of nerve homogenates was found to be linear with respect to time (for at least 120 min) and with respect to protein (below a concentration of 0.6 mg/ml in the assay system). Nonspecific exchange activity accounted for a minor fraction of the incorporation of *myo*-inositol into lipid and was similar in the nerve homogenates of both groups of animals. When considered as a function of nerve weight, CDP-diglyceride:inositol transferase activity was decreased by 44% in the nerves of the untreated diabetic animals (Table 5). Insulin treatment normalized the activity of this enzyme on both a weight and a protein basis (Table 5).

Although the rate of incorporation of 2-^{3}H-*myo*-inositol into phospholipids observed in the present study was higher than that observed by other workers,[13] this discrepancy can probably be explained by the differences in the assay conditions employed. Of more interest is the fact that the magnitude of the decrease in CDP-diglyceride:inositol transferase activity we observed 2 wk after the induction of severe diabetes (65 mg/kg body wt of SZ) was similar to that observed by Whiting et al. in nerves of rats after 12 wk of milder diabetes (35 mg/kg body wt of SZ).[13] It should be noted that our observations are not in agreement with those of Hothersall and McLean, who did not demonstrate any ef-

FIGURE 4. Incorporation of 2-^{3}H-*myo*-inositol into the phospholipids of nerves from control, streptozotocin-diabetic, and insulin-treated diabetic rats at timed intervals following the intraperitoneal injection of 2-^{3}H-*myo*-inositol. The calculation is based on the specific activity of the nerve's water-soluble *myo*-inositol at the time of study. The number of nerves obtained from each group of animals is given in parentheses.

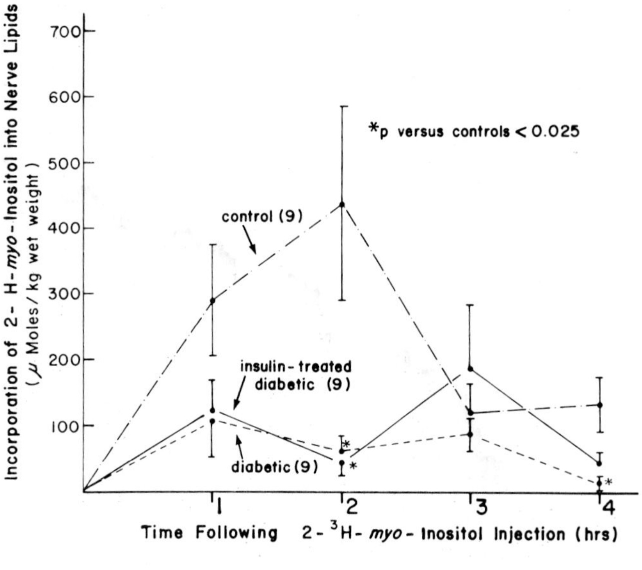

TABLE 5
CDP-diglyceride:inositol transferase activity in sciatic nerve homogenates from control, diabetic, and insulin-treated rats

Study group	Nerve protein content (μg/mg wet wt)	CDP-diglyceride:inositol transferase activity	
		nmol/h/mg wet wt	nmol/h/mg protein
Controls (N = 16)	89.8 ± 6.1	1.8 ± 0.2	20.0 ± 1.8
Diabetics (N = 8)	69.6 ± 6.9*	1.0 ± 0.1†	14.4 ± 0.9*
Insulin-treated diabetics (N = 7)	114.6 ± 10.0*‡	2.5 ± 0.2*‡	22.4 ± 1.9‡

* P versus controls < 0.05
† P versus controls < 0.01
‡ P versus diabetics < 0.01

fect of acute, short term diabetes on the CDP-diglyceride:inositol transferase activity of the particulate fraction of sciatic nerve homogenates.[12]

The pattern of incorporation of 2-^{3}H-*myo*-inositol into the phosphoinositides in the presence of nerve homogenates from control animals is shown in Table 4. In these experiments, the total recovery of 2-^{3}H-*myo*-inositol in the lipid fraction (on a protein basis) was reduced by 26% in the presence of diabetic nerve homogenates. The pattern of recovery of radioactivity in the individual phosphoinositides was remarkably similar to that observed in vivo. Thus, in the presence of the diabetic nerve homogenates, the proportion of lipid-bound radioactivity recovered as phosphatidylinositol was increased, whereas that recovered as triphosphatidylinositol was significantly decreased. These data suggest that the activities of both CDP-diglyceride:inositol transferase and phosphatidylinositol 4-phosphate kinase are decreased in nerve homogenates from diabetic animals (by 26% and 78%, respectively).

DISCUSSION

The experiments reported above have demonstrated that the induction of acute streptozotocin diabetes in the rat results in a number of abnormalities in the metabolism of *myo*-inositol and its phospholipid derivatives in the sciatic nerve. A 2-wk period of untreated diabetes was found to lower the nerve *myo*-inositol content, to decrease the space of distribution of 2-^{3}H-*myo*-inositol, to impair the incorporation of *myo*-inositol into nerve phospholipids, to decrease the total and specific activity of nerve CDP-diglyceride:inositol transferase, and to alter the pattern of incorporation of *myo*-inositol into the higher phosphoinositides. Obviation of hyperglycemia by twice daily injections of insulin was found to normalize the activity of sciatic nerve CDP-diglyceride:inositol transferase, to slightly increase the content and space of distribution of nerve water-soluble *myo*-inositol, but to have no effect on the incorporation of *myo*-inositol into nerve phospholipids.

The observation that acute streptozotocin diabetes resulted in a lowering of the sciatic nerve water-soluble *myo*-inositol content is in agreement with previous reports.[7–9,15,16] Since *myo*-inositol is actively accumulated by a number of mammalian tissues[32–35] and its uptake is competitively inhibited by elevated ambient glucose concentrations,[33–36] it seems reasonable to speculate that such a mechanism may have been responsible for the observed decrease in the free *myo*-inositol content of the diabetic nerves. Our observation that the 2-^{3}H-*myo*-inositol space of the normal rat nerve was larger than the entire wet weight of the tissue provides indirect evidence for the accumulation of *myo*-inositol by neural components that are beyond the space into which inulin can diffuse.[31] Thus, one could calculate that 2-^{3}H-*myo*-inositol accumulates within the aqueous portion of this space to a level 2.5 times that present within the vasculature within 2 h or 3 h of the intraperitoneal injection of this radioisotope. Furthermore, the loss of the capacity of the diabetic nerve to accumulate *myo*-inositol provides further evidence for a role of hyperglycemia in the production of this defect. However, the observation that careful insulin treatment only partially restored the nerve *myo*-inositol content and had a modest effect on the space of distribution of 2-^{3}H-*myo*-inositol renders this speculation dubious. It should be noted, however, that, despite our rigorous and often lethal attempts to maintain normoglycemia in the insulin-treated animals, their nerve glucose concentration at the time of sacrifice was nearly twice that of the controls. Therefore, it is possible that the nerves of the insulin-treated animals had been intermittently exposed to significant hyperglycemia throughout the course of treatment and that this exposure may have conditioned the defects in nerve uptake and content of *myo*-inositol in this experimental group. Alternatively, it is possible that the ambient glucose concentration has little direct effect on the uptake of *myo*-inositol by the peripheral nerve. Recent in vitro studies of the rat sciatic nerve have shown that, when normal whole cut nerves are incubated in the presence of high concentrations of glucose (30 mM) or galactose (20 mM), the incorporation of 2-^{3}H-*myo*-inositol into nerve phospholipids is not inhibited.[12] These data provide indirect evidence for the lack of a direct effect of hyperglycemia on nerve *myo*-inositol transport. Since the same workers demonstrated that exposure of the incubated nerve to insulin stimulated the incorporation of radioactive *myo*-inositol into phospholipid, they suggested that insulin may stimulate *myo*-inositol transport in this tissue.[12] This suggestion is open to question, since the transport of *myo*-inositol into this tissue was not directly measured and unphysiologic concentrations of insulin (250 mU/ml) were employed in these experiments.[12]

The possibility that the osmotic effect of the accumulation of polyhydric alcohols may be responsible (through an unknown mechanism) for the derangement in the regulation of nerve *myo*-inositol concentrations has been frequently considered.[7,12,15,16,22,36,37] The present studies do not provide support for this possibility, since a decreased nerve *myo*-inositol content and space of distribution was observed in the nerves of the insulin-treated animals, in which the sorbitol and fructose contents were within normal limits. Thus, the mechanisms responsible for the aforementioned abnormalities in the neural accumulation of free *myo*-inositol appear to be unrelated to either hyperglycemia or to the activity of the polyol pathway within this tissue. Although these defects appear to be directly related to the induction of experimental diabetes, both their localization within the various cellular components of the nerve as well as the mechanisms responsible for their development remain matters of speculation.

The observation that the activity of the enzyme responsible for phosphatidylinositol synthesis (CDP-diglyceride:inositol transferase) is profoundly reduced in the homogenates of diabetic rat nerves renders the impaired in vivo incorporation of radioactive *myo*-inositol into nerve phospholipids somewhat easier to explain. Thus, the 44% decrease in the activity of this enzyme (on a weight basis) could account, in large part, for the 69% decrease in recovery of lipid-bound 2-^{3}H-*myo*-inositol from diabetic nerves that was observed during the first 2 h after the injection of the tracer (Figure 3). One could further speculate that the somewhat greater decrease in recovery of lipid-bound radioactivity could have been due to the inability of the diabetic nerve to accumulate *myo*-inositol. However, this straightforward construct does not explain the abnormalities in phosphoinositide metabolism observed in the nerves of the insulin-treated diabetic animals. In this latter group, despite the fact that the activity of CDP-diglyceride:inositol transferase was normal, the in vivo recovery of lipid-bound radioactivity was reduced by 77% during the first 2 h of the experiment (Figure 3). Since the space of distribution of 2-^{3}H-*myo*-inositol was reduced to a similar degree in both groups of diabetic animals during this time, it is possible that the major factor responsible for impaired phosphoinositide synthesis in these animals was an inability to transport *myo*-inositol to the site of the enzyme rather than simply a deficiency in enzyme activity within the nerve. This speculation is supported by the in vitro observation that the incorporation of radioactive *myo*-inositol into nerve lipids in the whole nerve preparation is three orders of magnitude less than that observed in nerve homogenates.[12] Thus, although defective neural *myo*-inositol transport may be the predominant factor, the decreased activity of CDP-diglyceride:inositol transferase activity would also be expected to contribute to the decreased phosphatidylinositol synthesis within the nerve of the untreated diabetic animal.

The explanation for the decreased CDP-diglyceride:inositol transferase activity observed in the diabetic nerves is not apparent. Clearly, it is not due solely to the decreased protein content of the diabetic nerves, since the specific activity of the enzyme is also decreased. Furthermore, it is not the result of impaired antegrade axonal transport of this enzyme (Clements and Stockard, unpublished results). The most likely explanation is that the induction of streptozotocin diabetes may result in impaired synthesis of this enzyme within the nerve cell body. This possibility has not, as yet, been investigated.

Although we did not measure the activity of phosphatidylinositol 4-phosphate kinase in the various nerve homogenates, the pattern of incorporation of 2-^{3}H-*myo*-inositol into the phosphoinositides both in vivo and in vitro suggests that this enzyme is deficient in the diabetic nerve, a suggestion that is in agreement with the studies of Whiting et al.[13] The possibility that (as in the case of CDP-diglyceride:inositol transferase) insulin treatment might normalize the activity of phosphatidylinositol 4-phosphate kinase within the sciatic nerve of the diabetic rat has not been studied.

Finally, although numerous defects in the metabolism of *myo*-inositol and its phospholipid derivatives have been demonstrated in the nerve of the rat with acute experimental diabetes, the mechanisms by which insulin deficiency, hyperglycemia, or other factors give rise to these abnormalities have not been defined. However, the postulated relationship between phosphoinositide metabolism and nerve function[1–14] would suggest that these metabolic alterations may be responsible, in part, for the early changes in peripheral nerve function in human and experimental diabetes. The possibility that chronic alterations in phosphoinositide metabolism might underlie the eventual development of the structural and functional changes characteristic of diabetic polyneuropathy is, as yet, an untested question.

ACKNOWLEDGMENTS

This investigation was supported by the U.S. Public Health Service (RR-32 and AM-21065), the Medical Research Service of the Veterans' Administration, and the Diabetes Trust Fund. We appreciate the expert technical assistance of Barbara Poole, Nina Wampler, and Bradley Clements, as well as the excellent secretarial assistance of June Reid in the preparation of this manuscript.

REFERENCES

[1] Hawthorne, J. N., and Kai, M.: Metabolism of phosphoinositides in rat brain. *In* Handbook of Neurochemistry. Lajtha, A., Ed. New York, Plenum Press, 1970, pp. 491–508.

[2] Hendrickson, H. S., and Reinertsen, J. L.: Phosphoinositide interconversion: a model for control of Na^+ and K^+ permeability in the nerve axon membrane. Biochem. Biophys. Res. Commun. *44*:1258–64, 1971.

[3] Hawthorne, J. N.: Phospholipid metabolism and transport of materials across the cell membrane. *In* Form and Function of Phospholipids. Ansell, G. B., Hawthorne, J. N., and Dawson, R. M. C., Eds. Amsterdam, Elsevier Scientific Publishing Co., 1973, pp. 423–40.

[4] White, G. L., and Larabee, M. G.: Phosphoinositides and other phospholipids in sympathetic ganglia and nerve trunk of rats. Effects of neuronal activity and inositol analogs (β- and γ-hexachlorocyclohexane (lindane)) on (32P)-labelling, synaptic transmission and axonal conduction. J. Neurochem. *20*:783–98, 1973.

[5] White, G. L., Schellhase, H. U., and Hawthorne, J. N.: Phosphoinositide metabolism in rat superior cervical ganglion, vagus and phrenic nerve: effects of electrical stimulation and various blocking agents. J. Neurochem. *22*:149–58, 1974.

[6] Michell, R. H.: Inositol phospholipids and cell surface receptor function. Biochim. Biophys. Acta *415*:81–147, 1975.

[7] Greene, D. A., DeJesus, P. V., and Winegrad, A. I.: Effects of insulin and dietary myoinositol on impaired peripheral motor nerve conduction velocity in acute streptozotocin diabetes. J. Clin. Invest. *55*:1326–36, 1975.

[8] Winegrad, A. I., and Greene, D. A.: Diabetic polyneuropathy: the importance of insulin deficiency, hyperglycemia and alterations in myoinositol metabolism in its pathogenesis. N. Engl. J. Med. *295*:1416–21, 1977.

[9] Palmano, V. P., Whiting, P. H., and Hawthorne, J. N.: Free and lipid *myo*-inositol in tissues from rats with acute and less severe streptozotocin-induced diabetes. Biochem. J. *167*:229–35, 1977.

[10] Tret'jak, A. G., Limarenko, I. M., Kossova, G. V., Gulak, P. V., and Kozlov, Y. P.: Interrelation of phosphoinositide metabolism and ion transport in crab nerve fibres. J. Neurochem. *28*:199–205, 1977.

[11] Hawthorne, J. N., Pickard, M. R., and Griffin, H. D.: Phosphatidylinositol, triphosphoinositide and synaptic transmission. *In* Cyclitols and Polyphosphoinositides. Wells, W. W., and Eisenberg, F., Jr., Eds. New York, Academic Press, 1978, pp. 145–51.

[12] Hothersall, J. S., and McLean, P.: Effect of diabetes and insulin on phosphatidylinositol synthesis in rat sciatic nerve. Biochem. Biophys. Res. Commun. *88*:477–84, 1979.

[13] Whiting, P. H., Palmano, K. P., and Hawthorne, J. N.: Enzymes of *myo*-inositol metabolism and inositol lipid metabolism in rats with streptozotocin-induced diabetes. Biochem. J. *179*:549–53, 1979.

[14] Hawthorne, J. N., and Pickard, M. R.: Phospholipids in synaptic function. J. Neurochem. *32*:5–14, 1979.

[15] Ward, J. D., Baker, R. W. R., and Davis, B. H.: Effect of blood sugar control on the accumulation of sorbitol and fructose in nervous tissues. Diabetes *21*:1173–78, 1972.

[16] Ward, J. D.: The polyol pathway in the neuropathy of early diabetes. *In* Vascular and Neurological Changes in Early Diabetes. Camerini-Dávalos, R. A., and Cole, H. S., Eds. New York, Academic Press, 1973, pp. 425–32.

[17] Benjamins, J. A., and Agranoff, B. W.: Distribution and properties of CDP-diglyceride:inositol transferase from brain. J. Neurochem. *16*:513–27, 1969.

[18] Takenawa, T., and Egawa, K.: CDP-diglyceride:inositol transferase

from rat liver. J. Biol. Chem. *25*:5419–23, 1977.
[19] Gould, R. M., Lasek, R. J., and Spencer, P. S.: Phosphoinositide metabolism in peripheral axons. *In* Cyclitols and Polyphosphoinositides. Wells, W. W., and Eisenberg, F., Jr., Eds. New York, Academic Press, 1978, pp. 535–47.
[20] Gould, R. M.: Inositol lipid synthesis in axons unmyelinated fibers of peripheral nerve. Brain Res. *117*:169–74, 1976.
[21] Eliasson, S. G.: Nerve conduction changes in experimental diabetes. J. Clin. Invest. *43*:2353–58, 1964.
[22] Gabbay, K. H.: Role of sorbitol pathway in neuropathy. *In* Vascular and Neurologic Changes in Early Diabetes. Camerini-Dávalos, R. A., and Cole, H. S., Eds. New York, Academic Press, 1973, pp. 417–32.
[23] Jefferys, J. G. R., Palmano, K. P., Sharma, A. K., and Thomas, P. K.: Influence of dietary myoinositol on nerve conduction and inositol phospholipids in normal and diabetic rats. J. Neurol. Neurosurg. Psychiatry *41*:333–39, 1978.
[24] Brown, M. J., Iwamori, M., Kishimoto, Y., Rapoport, B., Moser, H. W., and Asbury, A. K.: Nerve lipid abnormalities in human diabetic neuropathy: a correlative study. Ann. Neurol. *5*:245–52, 1979.
[25] Slein, M. W.: D-glucose determination with hexokinase and glucose-6-phosphate dehydrogenase. *In* Methods of Enzymatic Analysis. Bergmeyer, H. U., Ed. New York, Academic Press, 1963, pp. 117–23.
[26] Clements, R. S., Jr., and Reynertson, R.: Myoinositol metabolism in diabetes mellitus: effect of insulin treatment. Diabetes *26*:215–21, 1977.
[27] Wells, W. W.: Gas-liquid chromatography of carbohydrates. *In* Clinical Biochemistry: Principles and Methods. Curtis, H. C., and Roth, M., Eds. Berlin, Walter de Gruyter, 1974.
[28] Clements, R. S., Jr., and Rhoten, W. B.: Phosphoinositide metabolism and insulin secretion from isolated rat pancreatic islets. J. Clin. Invest. *57*:684–91, 1976.
[29] Gonzalez-Sastre, F., and Folch-Pi, J.: Thin-layer chromatography of the phosphoinositides. J. Lipid Res. *9*:532–53, 1968.
[30] Lowry, O. H., Rosebrough, N. J., Farr, A. L., and Randall, R. J.: Protein measurement with the Folin phenol reagent. J. Biol. Chem. *193*:264–75, 1951.
[31] Bradbury, M. W. B., and Crowder, J.: Compartments and barriers in the sciatic nerve of the rabbit. Brain Res. *103*:515–26, 1976.
[32] Cotlier, E.: *Myo*-inositol: active transport by the crystalline lens. Invest. Ophthalmol. *9*:681–91, 1970.
[33] Varma, S. D., Chakraponi, B., and Reddy, V. N.: Intraocular transport of myoinositol. II. Accumulation in the rabbit lens in vitro. Invest. Ophthalmol. *9*:794–800, 1970.
[34] Hauser, G.: Energy and sodium-dependent uptake of inositol by kidney cortex slices. Biochem. Biophys. Res. Commun. *19*:696–701, 1965.
[35] Caspary, W. F., and Crane, R. K.: Active transport of *myo*-inositol and its relation to the sugar transport system in hamster small intestine. Biochim. Biophys. Acta *203*:308–16, 1970.
[36] Broekhuyse, R. M.: Changes in *myo*-inositol permeability in the lens due to cataractous condition. Biochim. Biophys. Acta *163*:269–72, 1968.
[36] Stewart, M. A., Sherman, W. R., Kurien, M. D., Moonsammy, G. I., and Wisgerhof, M.: Polyol accumulation in nervous tissue of rats with experimental diabetes and galactosemia. J. Neurochem. *14*:1057–66, 1967.
[37] Gabbay, K. H., and Snider, J. J.: Nerve conduction defect in galactose-fed rats. Diabetes *21*:295–300, 1972.

Effects of Exogenous Fatty Acid Concentration on Glucagon-induced Changes in Hepatic Fatty Acid Metabolism

J. DENIS McGARRY AND DANIEL W. FOSTER

SUMMARY

Studies were conducted to clarify the relationship between the external fatty acid concentration and glucagon in the regulation of hepatic fatty acid metabolism. Hepatocytes from fed rats were incubated with increasing concentrations of oleate (up to 1 mM) in the presence and absence of glucagon and the time sequence of changes in cellular malonyl-CoA levels, fatty acid synthesis, fatty acid oxidation, and ketogenesis were measured. At low concentrations of fatty acid the effect of glucagon was to abolish malonyl-CoA synthesis and lipogenesis and to produce a marked stimulation of fatty acid oxidation and ketogenesis. Similar effects were obtained with high concentrations of fatty acid in the absence of glucagon and, under these conditions, the additional presence of the hormone produced little further response. The results are consistent with the concept that the rate of fatty acid oxidation in liver is dictated largely by the relative concentrations of long-chain acyl-CoA (substrate for carnitine acyltransferase I) and malonyl-CoA (inhibitor of the transferase). They also indicate that the preemptive effect of fatty acids on glucagon-induced changes in fatty acid metabolism stems from their ability to reduce the tissue malonyl-CoA content, probably through long-chain acyl-CoA suppression of acetyl-CoA carboxylase. DIABETES 29:236–240, March 1980.

Evidence has been previously adduced that the ketogenic effect of glucagon on mammalian liver stems primarily from the ability of the hormone to switch the direction of fatty acid metabolism from synthesis to oxidation.[1–5] The key event in this metabolic transformation appears to be a cyclic AMP-mediated inactivation of key glycolytic enzymes (such as phosphofructokinase and pyruvate kinase) and acetyl-CoA carboxylase, which results in depletion of hepatic malonyl-CoA content and cessation of lipogenesis. Since malonyl-CoA is a potent inhibitor of carnitine acyltransferase I, the enzyme catalyzing the first step in fatty acid oxidation, a fall in its concentration serves to activate β-oxidation and thereby accelerate the production of acetoacetic and β-hydroxybutyric acids.

The above formulation was arrived at largely from studies in which the effects of glucagon on fatty acid metabolism were measured in hepatocytes from fed rats incubated with low concentrations of exogenous oleic acid (0.4 mM or less).[4,5] Under these conditions the hormone produced marked enhancement of fatty acid oxidation and ketogenesis. However, studies from other laboratories have demonstrated that the stimulatory effect of glucagon on fatty acid oxidation is much less pronounced when higher concentrations of fatty acid are employed.[6–8] Theoretically, this phenomenon might be explained as follows. Exposure of the liver to increasing concentrations of long-chain fatty acids produces concomitant elevation of intracellular levels of long-chain acyl-CoA.[9–11] The latter are potent inhibitors of acetyl-CoA carboxylase[12] and, as such, result in suppression of malonyl-CoA synthesis and lipogenesis.[6,11] Insofar as malonyl-CoA levels are reduced by this mechanism, the inhibitory effect of glucagon on fatty acid synthesis and its stimulatory effect on fatty acid oxidation should be preempted.

To test the validity of this thesis we felt it important to simultaneously examine rates of fatty acid synthesis, fatty acid oxidation, and ketogenesis together with changes in tissue malonyl-CoA levels in hepatocytes exposed to various concentrations of exogenous fatty acid, in the presence and absence of glucagon. The results obtained are entirely consistent with the predictions outlined above and emphasize the pivotal role of malonyl-CoA in regulating rates of hepatic fatty acid synthesis and oxidation.

From the Departments of Internal Medicine and Biochemistry, The University of Texas Health Science Center at Dallas, Dallas, Texas 75235
Address reprint requests to J. Denis McGarry, Department of Internal Medicine, University of Texas Health Science Center, 5323 Harry Hines Boulevard, Dallas, Texas 75235.
Received for publication 28 September 1979.

MATERIALS AND METHODS

Animals. Male Sprague-Dawley rats, weighing approximately 140 g at the time of experiments, were meal-fed a high sucrose, fat-free diet as previously described.[13] They were used for isolation of hepatocytes immediately after their last feeding.

Preparation of hepatocytes. Hepatocytes were prepared as described earlier[4] and were routinely adjusted to a cell density of 200 mg/ml in Krebs-Henseleit bicarbonate buffer (KHB).

Measurements of fatty acid oxidation, fatty acid synthesis, and cellular malonyl-CoA levels. Experiments were carried out at 37°C in 25-ml Erlenmeyer flasks. For studies of fatty acid oxidation the flasks initially contained 200 mg of hepatocytes in 2 ml of KHB with or without glucagon (10 μg).* After a preincubation period of 30 min, each flask received 0.5 ml of 14% defatted albumin in KHB containing sodium [1-^{14}C]-oleate (specific activity 0.4 μCi per μmol) in a concentration of 0, 1, 3, or 5 mM. This resulted in a final albumin concentration of 2.8% and final oleate concentrations of 0, 0.2, 0.6, or 1 mM in the incubation mixtures. The respective ν values (molarity fatty acid:molarity of albumin) were 0, 0.49, 1.48, and 2.46. When fatty acid synthesis and tissue malonyl-CoA levels were measured, radioactive oleate was replaced by nonradioactive fatty acid at the same concentrations. Fatty acid synthesis was assessed using ^3H_2O [4] and malonyl-CoA was assayed using a previously described radioisotopic method.[13] All other analytical procedures have been published.[4] In the text the term "fatty acid oxidation" will always refer to the conversion of labeled oleate into total acid-soluble products plus CO_2. The term "ketones" denotes the quantity of isotope from labeled oleate recovered in acetoacetate plus β-hydroxybutyrate.

Materials. The sources of all materials have been given previously.[3,4]

RESULTS

Figure 1 shows the effects of different oleate concentrations on the rate of fatty acid synthesis and the cellular malonyl-CoA content in hepatocytes from fed rats. As noted earlier,[4] in the absence of any additions the rate of fatty acid synthesis accelerated throughout the period of incubation (open circles, Figure 1A). This was accompanied by an initial rapid rise in the tissue malonyl-CoA level, which tended to plateau between the 30- and 60-min time points (Figure 1B). Both parameters were suppressed upon addition of oleate at 30 min, the degree of suppression increasing as the concentration of fatty acid was raised from 0.2 to 1 mM. Similarly, both began to revert toward control values as the added fatty acid was metabolized, though from the figure this is more obvious for malonyl-CoA concentrations than for the rate of fatty acid synthesis. In the presence of glucagon both the malonyl-CoA level and the rate of fatty acid synthesis were severely depressed during the initial 30 min of incubation. It is known that this action of the hormone results from inhibition of glycolysis and the acetyl-CoA carboxylase step, probably through cyclic AMP-mediated enzyme phosphorylation.[4,5,14] As expected on the basis of previous studies,[4] the effects of the hormone began to wane during the latter period of the experiment. In this case also, the effect of increasing the exogenous oleate concentration was to cause a proportional further suppression of malonyl-CoA synthesis and lipogenesis.

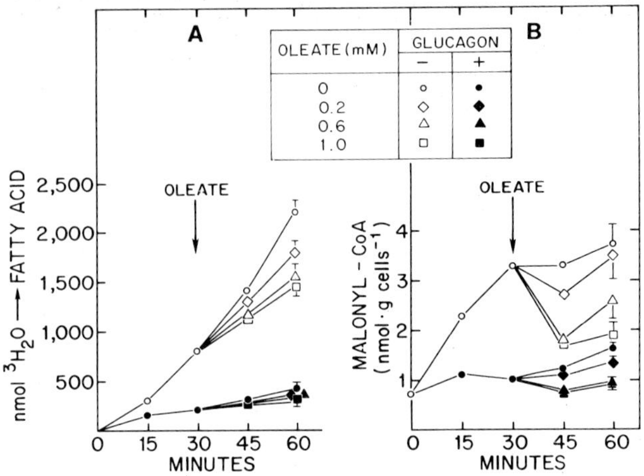

FIGURE 1. Effect of increasing concentrations of oleate on fatty acid synthesis and malonyl-CoA levels in hepatocytes from fed rats. Hepatocytes (200 mg) were initially incubated with 2 ml of Krebs-Henseleit bicarbonate buffer in the presence and absence of glucagon (10 μg) for the measurement of fatty acid synthesis (panel A) and cellular malonyl-CoA content (panel B), as described under MATERIALS AND METHODS. At 30 min 0.5 ml of 14% albumin in the same buffer, containing different concentrations of sodium oleate, was added to give the final concentrations of oleate indicated. Results are means ± SEM for 6–8 experiments.

Figure 2 shows the relationship between the average cellular content of malonyl-CoA between 45 and 60 min and the rate of fatty acid synthesis during this period. The expected linear plot was obtained. As routinely observed in this laboratory[4,5] such plots generally intersect the abscissa at a point equivalent to a tissue malonyl-CoA content between 0.5 and 0.7 nmol/g wet wt. We assume that this quantity of malonyl-CoA is bound to cellular macromolecules and is therefore unavailable for metabolic purposes.

Figure 3 shows the effects of glucagon on the rate of oxidation of [1-^{14}C]-oleate when the labeled fatty acid was added at the 30-min time point in the same concentrations as those employed in the experiments of Figure 1. From panel A it is evident that the degree of stimulation of overall fatty acid oxidation by glucagon decreased with increasing concentration of substrate. Qualitatively similar effects were seen as regards the rate of conversion of the labeled fatty acid into ketones (panel B). When the percent stimulation of oleate conversion into products over the 45–60-min interval was examined as a function of the concentration of fatty acid added at 30 min, the following relationships emerged. With 0.2, 0.6, and 1 mM oleate the stimulation of overall oxidation caused by glucagon was 167%, 93%, and 31%, respectively. Under the same conditions the hormone stimulated the conversion of oleate into ketones by 432%, 240%, and 115%, respectively. As pointed out earlier,[5] under these experimental conditions the stimulatory effect of glucagon on ketogenesis will always exceed the degree of enhancement of β-oxidation. The reason stems from the fact that by block-

* This pharmacologic concentration of glucagon was employed in order to obtain maximal effects of the hormone. As noted previously,[4] while much lower concentrations produce similar metabolic responses the effects are transient, probably as a result of hormone degradation by the hepatocytes.

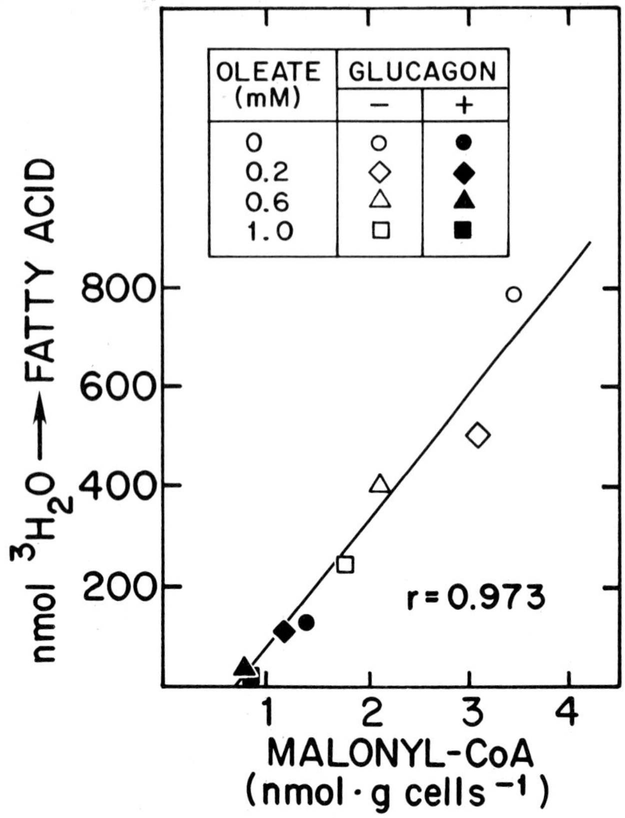

FIGURE 2. Relationship between the rate of fatty acid synthesis and cellular content of malonyl-CoA in hepatocytes from fed rats exposed to different concentrations of oleate. Taking the data from Figure 1, the rate of fatty acid synthesis has been plotted against the average tissue malonyl-CoA level between 45 and 60 min.

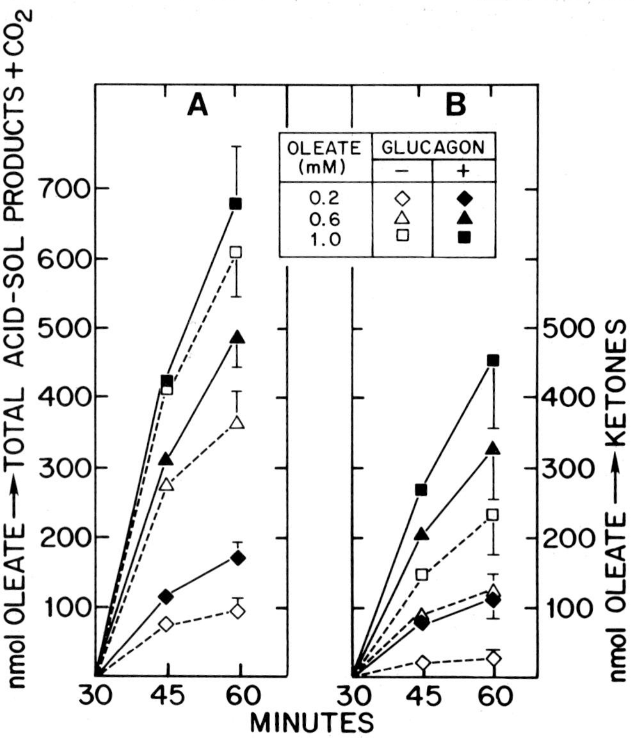

FIGURE 3. Effect of glucagon on the oxidation of different concentrations of oleate in hepatocytes from fed rats. Incubation conditions were identical with those described for Figure 1 except that radiolabeled oleate (1-^{14}C) was added at the 30-min time point. Oxidation products were measured as described under MATERIALS AND METHODS. Results are means ± SEM for four experiments.

ing endogenous pyruvate production, glucagon not only prevents the synthesis of malonyl-CoA but presumably also renders the cells deficient in oxaloacetate. As a result, in the presence of the hormone a much greater fraction of the acetyl-CoA generated through the β-oxidation process enters the ketogenic pathway rather than the tricarboxylic acid cycle.†

Figure 4 represents a combination of the data from Figure 1B and Figure 3 and shows the relationship between the ability of glucagon to lower the tissue malonyl-CoA level and the hormone's effect on fatty acid oxidation at the three concentrations of oleate used. Clearly, the higher the level of exogenous oleate, the less effective was the hormone in causing additional reduction of the malonyl-CoA concentration and further stimulation of the processes of β-oxidation and ketogenesis. Also evident from the figure is the extrapolation that had we used initial concentrations of oleate in excess of 1 mM, a point would presumably have been reached where glucagon would have produced no significant stimulation of fatty acid oxidation, while still causing a reduction in the tissue malonyl-CoA content of about 0.6–0.7 nmol/g. We assume that under such conditions the intracellular concentration of oleyl-CoA reaches a sufficiently high level to drive fatty acid oxidation maximally

† Carnitine was absent from all of the incubations reported here. However, had it been included together with glucagon, rates of fatty acid oxidation and ketogenesis would have reached values considerably higher than those seen with the hormone alone.[4,5]

FIGURE 4. Relationship between the stimulation of oleate oxidation and the fall in malonyl-CoA content caused by glucagon in hepatocytes from fed rats exposed to different concentrations of oleate. The data are taken from the 45–60-min intervals of Figures 1B and 3. Note that it is the fall in the average malonyl-CoA content that is plotted.

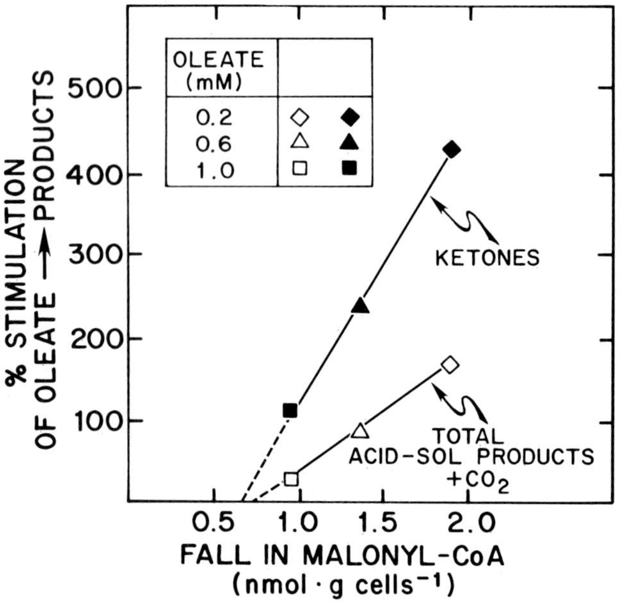

such that this additional small fall in malonyl-CoA concentration has no discernible effect.

DISCUSSION

The purpose of the present investigation was to clarify the biochemical basis underlying the observation that the stimulatory effect of glucagon on fatty acid oxidation in livers from fed animals diminishes with exposure of the tissue to increasing concentrations of long-chain fatty acids. As noted in the introduction, a plausible explanation for this phenomenon could be advanced on the basis of isolated reports, each of which dealt with different aspects of hepatic fatty acid metabolism. However, validation of the scheme proposed required that four key metabolic parameters, namely fatty acid oxidation, ketogenesis, fatty acid synthesis, and tissue malonyl-CoA levels, be measured simultaneously and shown to correlate in the predicted fashion in cells exposed to glucagon and various concentrations of fatty acids. This was accomplished in the current studies.

Of the many biochemical factors that could potentially influence the overall rate of fatty acid oxidation in liver, it seems reasonable to conclude that four will be of major importance. These are the extracellular concentration of fatty acid and the intracellular levels of long-chain acyl-CoA, carnitine, and malonyl-CoA. Considering first the situation in vivo, two extremes can be clearly distinguished. In the carbohydrate fed state (low [glucagon]:[insulin]) plasma free fatty levels are low,[15] as are the intrahepatic concentrations of long-chain acyl-CoA[9,10] and carnitine,[16] while the tissue content of malonyl-CoA is elevated.[10,13] Under these conditions fatty acid synthesis is brisk and the physiologic role of malonyl-CoA can be viewed as a mechanism to ensure unidirectional flow of carbon from glucose → fatty acids → triglycerides → very low density lipoproteins by inhibiting carnitine acyltransferase I, and thereby preventing the futile reoxidation of newly synthesized fatty acids. At the same time, the oxidation of exogenous fatty acids and the production of acetoacetic and β-hydroxybutyric acids is restricted. By contrast, in ketotic states (high [glucagon]:[insulin]) the liver carnitine concentration rises,[16,17] malonyl-CoA levels fall,[10,13] fatty acid synthesis is greatly depressed,[5,10] plasma free fatty acids are elevated,[15] intrahepatic concentrations of long-chain acyl-CoA rise,[9,10] and the processes of fatty acid oxidation and ketogenesis occur at high (uninhibited) rates.[4,5,15]

Studies in vitro, such as those presented here and by others,[6–8] allow one to examine situations that are analogous to or intermediate between the two extremes noted above. For example, incubation of hepatocytes from fed rats with low concentrations of oleate simulated the in vivo environment of the liver in fed animals. Although not measured directly, it is reasonable to assume that under these conditions the tissue level of long-chain acyl-CoA (substrate for carnitine acyltransferase I) was also low.‡ The prevailing high concentration of malonyl-CoA (inhibitor of the transferase) served to drive lipogenesis and to suppress fatty acid oxidation. The effect of glucagon was to abolish malonyl-CoA synthesis and lipogenesis and to cause a marked stimulation of fatty acid oxidation and ketogenesis.† The key event in this switch of hepatic fat metablism from synthesis to oxidation presumably was the glucagon-induced lowering of the malonyl-CoA level without significant change in the concentration of long-chain acyl-CoA (because fatty acid levels were held low experimentally). On the other hand, exposure of fed hepatocytes to high concentrations of oleate (which ordinarily would occur only after fasting or in uncontrolled diabetes) revealed an additional level of metabolic control. In keeping with reports from other groups[6–8] the stimulatory effect of glucagon on fatty acid oxidation and ketogenesis was now far less pronounced. In confirmation of the findings of Cook et al.[6] we observed a fall in the cellular content of malonyl-CoA as the concentration of oleate in the medium was raised. This was accompanied by a proportional fall in the rate of endogenous fatty acid synthesis. There can be little doubt that the operative mechanism was inhibition of acetyl-CoA carboxylase due to an increase in the intracellular concentration of long-chain acyl-CoA.[12,‡] The net effect was that the high extracellular concentration of fatty acid indirectly enhanced its own oxidation by feedback inhibition of malonyl-CoA synthesis and lipogenesis. Under these circumstances it might be expected that glucagon, which exerts its effects by blocking synthesis of malonyl-CoA, would have progressively less impact on rates of fatty acid synthesis and oxidation as the external concentration of fatty acid is raised. This is in fact what was observed. In the latter situation the driving force for fatty acid oxidation was presumably also an elevation of the [long-chain acyl-CoA]:[malonyl-CoA] ratio, induced not by glucagon but by a rise in fatty acyl-CoA levels as the initial event.

It is noteworthy that over the time period during which metabolic events were studied, the tissue malonyl-CoA level swung from about 0.7 to 3.5 nmol/g wet wt. with the various manipulations employed. This is a similar range to that observed in our earlier studies[4,5] and, taken together with the fact that the Ki for malonyl-CoA toward carnitine acyltransferase I is in the region of 1.5 μM,[2,3] is entirely compatible with the postulated regulatory role of this compound in hepatic fatty acid oxidation.

Finally, the question has been raised as to whether the glucagon-induced removal of the malonyl-CoA inhibition of hepatic fatty acid oxidation has any relevance for the enhancement of ketogenesis in ketotic states; the argument here was that the high plasma fatty acid level itself should be sufficient to suppress acetyl-CoA carboxylase activity and thus allow rapid rates of ketone body production.[6] While conceivable in principle, evidence from a number of in vivo studies is against such a possibility. For example, in both dogs and humans[18,19] suppression of insulin and glucagon secretion by somatostatin produced a marked curtailment in hepatic ketone production as compared with rates observed when the glucagon deficit was corrected by exogenous administration of the hormone. In both situations plasma free fatty acid levels remained elevated because of insulin deficiency. Along the same lines, we infused a triglyceride emulsion plus heparin into saline- and glucagon-treated fed rats and found that ketonemia developed far more rapidly in the latter group, despite the fact that equally high plasma free fatty acid concentrations were achieved in both.[20] Similar studies were carried out by Schade and Eaton[21] in diabetic humans receiving a saline or glucagon infusion. Again, the ketogenic response to acute elevation of circulat-

‡ Hepatic levels of long-chain acyl-CoA are known to fluctuate in parallel with the plasma fatty acid concentration.[9–11]

ing fatty acid levels was more pronounced in the individuals who were made hyperglucagonemic compared with the control group. Taken together, these observations suggest that in the intact animal the transformation of the liver from nonketogenic to ketogenic mode is initiated by elevation of the circulating [glucagon]:[insulin] ratio, independent of changes in the plasma free fatty acid concentration. As indicated by our studies with hepatocytes, the biochemical consequence of this hormonal perturbation at the level of the liver is glycogen depletion, reduction of the tissue malonyl-CoA content, and activation of the fatty acid oxidation machinery. High levels of plasma fatty acids, as would eventually be reached in prolonged fasting or uncontrolled diabetes, doubtlessly would contribute to the further suppression of lipogenesis and acceleration of the ketogenic process. However, we interpret this to be a secondary rather than the primary controlling mechanism.

ACKNOWLEDGMENTS

The expert technical assistance of Martha Bennett, Petra Contreras, and Murphy Daniels is gratefully acknowledged.

This work was supported by the United States Public Health Service Grant AM-18573. J. Denis McGarry was a recipient of Research Career Development Award 1-K04-AM0763.

REFERENCES

[1] McGarry, J. D., Mannaerts, G. P., and Foster, D. W.: A possible role for malonyl-CoA in the regulation of hepatic fatty acid oxidation and ketogenesis. J. Clin. Invest. *60*:265–70, 1977.

[2] McGarry, J. D., Mannaerts, G. P., and Foster, D. W.: Characteristics of fatty acid oxidation in rat liver homogenates and the inhibitory effect of malonyl-CoA. Biochim. Biophys. Acta *530*:305–13, 1978.

[3] McGarry, J. D., Leatherman, G. F., and Foster, D. W.: Carnitine palmitoyltransferase I—the site of inhibition of hepatic fatty acid oxidation by malonyl-CoA. J. Biol. Chem. *253*:4128–36, 1978.

[4] McGarry, J. D., Takabayashi, Y., and Foster, D. W.: The role of malonyl-CoA in the coordination of fatty acid synthesis and oxidation in isolated rat hepatocytes. J. Biol. Chem. *253*:8294–8300, 1978.

[5] McGarry, J. D., and Foster, D. W.: In support of the roles of malonyl-CoA and carnitine acyltransferase I in the regulation of hepatic fatty acid oxidation and ketogenesis. J. Biol. Chem. *254*:8163–68, 1979.

[6] Cook, G. A., King, M. T., and Veech, R. L.: Ketogenesis and malonyl coenzyme A content of isolated rat hepatocytes. J. Biol. Chem. *253*:2529–31, 1978.

[7] Heimberg, M., Weinstein, I., and Kohout, M.: The effects of glucagon, dibutyryl cyclic adenosine 3', 5'-monophosphate, and concentration of free fatty acid on hepatic lipid metabolism. J. Biol. Chem. *244*:5131–39, 1969.

[8] Christiansen, R. Z.: Regulation of palmitate metabolism by carnitine and glucagon in hepatocytes isolated from fasted and carbohydrate refed rats. Biochim. Biophys. Acta *488*:249–62, 1977.

[9] Bortz, W. M., and Lynen, F.: Elevation of long chain acyl-CoA derivatives in livers of fasted rats. Biochem. Z. *229*:77–82, 1963.

[10] Guynn, R. W., Veloso, D., and Veech, R. L.: The concentration of malonyl-CoA and the control of fatty acid synthesis in vivo. J. Biol. Chem. *247*:7325–31, 1972.

[11] Goodridge, A. G.: Regulation of fatty acid synthesis in isolated hepatocytes. J. Biol. Chem. *248*:4318–26, 1973.

[12] Bortz, W. M., and Lynen, F.: The inhibition of acetyl CoA carboxylase by long chain acyl CoA derivatives. Biochem. Z. *337*:505–9, 1963.

[13] McGarry, J. D., Stark, M. J., and Foster, D. W.: Hepatic malonyl-CoA levels of fed, fasted and diabetic rats as measured using a simple radioisotopic assay. J. Biol. Chem. *253*:8291–93, 1978.

[14] Beynen, A. C., Vaartjes, W. J., and Geelen, M. J. H.: Opposite effects of insulin and glucagon in acute hormonal control of hepatic lipogenesis. Diabetes *28*:828–35, 1979.

[15] McGarry, J. D., Meier, J. M., and Foster, D. W.: The effects of starvation and refeeding on carbohydrate and lipid metabolism in vivo and in the perfused rat liver. J. Biol. Chem. *248*:270–78, 1973.

[16] McGarry, J. D., Robles-Valdes, C., and Foster, D. W.: The role of carnitine in hepatic ketogenesis. Proc. Natl. Acad. Sci. USA *72*:4385–88, 1975.

[17] Parvin, R., and Pande, S. V.: Enhancement of mitochondrial carnitine and carnitine acylcarnitine translocase-mediated transport of fatty acids into liver mitochondria under ketogenic conditions. J. Biol. Chem. *254*:5423–29, 1979.

[18] Keller, U., Chiasson, J. L., Liljenquist, J. E., Cherrington, A. D., Jennings, A. S., and Crofford, O. B.: The roles of insulin, glucagon and free fatty acids in the regulation of ketogenesis in dogs. Diabetes *26*:1040–51, 1977.

[19] Gerich, J. E., Lorenzi, M., Bier, D. M., Schneider, V., Tsalikian, E., Karam, J. H., and Forsham, P. H.: Prevention of human diabetic ketoacidosis by somatostatin. N. Engl. J. Med. *292*:985–89, 1975.

[20] McGarry, J. D., Wright, P. H. and Foster, D. W.: Hormonal control of ketogenesis. Rapid activation of hepatic ketogenic capacity in fed rats by anti-insulin serum and glucagon. J. Clin. Invest. *55*:1202–9, 1975.

[21] Schade, D. S., and Eaton, R. P.: Glucagon regulation of plasma ketone body concentration in human diabetes. J. Clin. Invest. *56*:1340–44, 1975.

Rapid Publication

Nonaggregating Insulin Solutions for Long-Term Glucose Control in Experimental and Human Diabetes

A. MICHAEL ALBISSER, WILLIAM LOUGHEED, KUSIEL PERLMAN, AND ANDREJ BAHORIC

SUMMARY

A physiologic additive for dissolving insulin crystals for parenteral application has been found. Insulin crystals are relatively insoluble in simple aqueous solutions. They will dissolve, however, in highly acidic solutions, but these are not suitable for parenteral use. Both neutral and acid pH insulin solutions have a tendency for the dissolved hormone to reaggregate. Notwithstanding possible changes in biologic activity, such formed aggregates must be prevented because they interfere with the flow in portable insulin delivery devices and result in the loss of glycemic control. The addition of 1.5% autologous serum to the aqueous diluent for insulin has eliminated these difficulties and increased by 37% the apparent biologic activity of insulin solutions prepared in this way. With this additive, continuous uninterrupted intravenous insulin infusion has provided near ideal blood glucose control in four pancreatectomized dogs for 5 mo and four patients with juvenile-onset diabetes for 18–23 days. Serum apparently contains factor(s) that promote the dissolution of insulin and prevent the formation of peptide aggregates in dilute solutions. DIABETES 29:241–243, March 1980.

Subcutaneous insulin injections fail to normalize most of the metabolic derangements of diabetes mellitus. In contrast, insulin that is infused intravascularly by either closed-loop or open-loop insulin delivery mechanisms remarkably improves many of these abnormalities, even after short-term application of only 12–24 h.[1,2] Closed-loop systems[3,4] regulate insulin delivery on the basis of continuously measured blood glucose concentrations, while open-loop systems[5–8] regulate insulin delivery according to a carefully selected schedule usually involving a basal infusion rate, which is augmented at meal time. Almost complete metabolic and hormonal normalization can be achieved with preprogrammed intraportal insulin delivery in dogs.[9]

The development of an implantable artificial endocrine pancreas has been hampered not only by the lack of a suitable glucose sensor for the closed-loop system but also by the uniform and progressive propensity for insulin solutions to precipitate and/or gradually aggregate[10] in the reservoirs of the open-loop systems. Such aggregates interfere with the flow of insulin[11] and eventually result in clinically unacceptable blood glucose control, regardless of the pH of the infusate. These appear to be fundamental limitations to the realization of new methods of insulin delivery. All attempts to obtain physiologic diluents that prevent or slow this aggregation have been unsuccessful. However, it has been recognized that a physiologic solvent for insulin that also prevents its aggregation is urgently needed.

Curiously, natural crystals[12] dissolve rapidly in the blood after the secretion of insulin granules from the B-cell in the healthy pancreas. This apparent incongruity (zinc insulin crystals are usually only dissolved in acid media) led to a series of animal studies in which autologous serum was added to the insulin diluents. These experiments were designed to examine whether the addition of serum would prevent the formation of insulin aggregates, thereby facilitating long-term near ideal glycemic control in pancreatectomized dogs and adolescent patients with type I diabetes mellitus.

MATERIALS AND METHODS

Four pancreatectomized laboratory beagles were studied for 12–16 mo before and 5 mo after the addition of serum to their diluted insulin infusates. Each dog carried a portable insulin delivery system[13,14] weighing 630 g for the entire period. Initially, regular neutral porcine crystalline zinc insulin (Connaught Laboratories, Toronto, Canada) was dissolved to a final concentration of 1.24 U/ml in water for injection containing 1% benzyl alcohol as a bacteriostatic agent and adjusted to pH 7.4 using small amounts of ammonium hydroxide. This mixture was transferred aseptically through two cascaded 0.22-μm pore-size disposable bacte-

From the Hospital for Sick Children, Toronto, Canada.
Address reprint requests to Dr. A. M. Albisser, Biomedical Research, The Hospital for Sick Children, 555 University Avenue, Toronto M5G 1X8, Canada.
Received for publication 21 December 1979.

rial filters into an autoclaved plastic reservoir. The outlet of the reservoir entered a peristaltic pumping system, which, following flow rate calibration, was connected to an indwelling vascular catheter.[15]

Serum for the insulin diluent for each animal was prepared from fasting blood samples from that animal. For this purpose 8-ml blood samples were drawn without additives, transferred to centrifuge tubes, and refrigerated for 1–2 h to allow clotting. They were then rimmed, spun at 3500 rpm at 4°C for 12 min, the serum fraction was aspirated, and arbitrarily 3.0 ml added to 200 ml of the above bacteriostatic water with a resulting pH of 7.5. Insulin was added as before.

Fasting plasma glucose concentrations were measured daily and the basal rate of insulin delivery adjusted until normal values were obtained. Insulin waveforms and diet were as previously described.[8] After this initial adjustment, changes in the basal rates were not required. Pumps maintained their initial flow rate ± 1% and reservoirs were refilled through a combination of two bacterial filters every 3–5 days. Similar methods were used in four adolescent (14–17 yr) juvenile-onset diabetic patients who were infused for 18–23 days with similar insulin solutions but containing 3 U/ml.

RESULTS

It was remarkable to note an immediate and substantial reduction in the insulin requirements of the dogs infused with insulin solutions containing only 1.5% autologous serum, as shown in Figure 1. Mean ± SEM daily insulin requirements were 1.67 ± 0.11 U/kg/day without serum and 1.05 ± 0.10 U/kg/day with serum ($P < 0.006$). Mean ± SEM fasting plasma glucose levels were similar: 78 ± 2 mg/dl before and 77 ± 3 mg/dl after the addition of serum.

Equally impressive results were demonstrated by the four juvenile-onset diabetic volunteers studied using this improved method. Fasting glycemias of 75 ± 3 mg/dl (range 49–139) were obtained every morning for the duration of the study.

Some discoloration in the form of yellowing was noted and found to be lipid infiltration of the polyvinyl chloride plastic and silicone rubber materials used for the insulin reservoirs. Insulin aggregates were not seen in any of the studies. The flow of insulin was never interrupted, and the previous frequent loss of blood glucose control was not encountered.

FIGURE 1. Daily insulin requirements and mean fasting glycemias of four pancreatectomized dogs before and after the addition of autologous serum (1.5%) in bacteriostatic water containing 1.24 U/ml porcine crystalline zinc insulin.

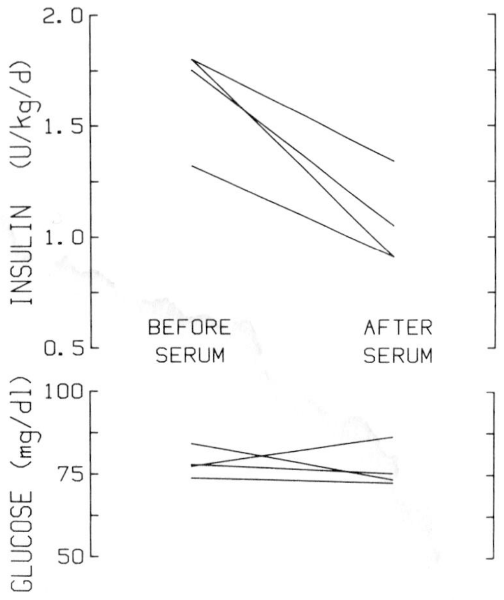

DISCUSSION

For 3 yr now, we have been using prototype, portable, open-loop insulin delivery devices on unrestrained pancreatectomized dogs[8,9] and volunteer insulin-requiring diabetics.[16] In spite of repeated efforts to incorporate suggested phosphate (pH 7.4), acetate (pH 3), and other physiologic buffers as diluents for crystalline zinc insulin, good blood glucose control was only achieved when the reservoirs and delivery components were replaced every 1–3 days. Otherwise, a tendency to unacceptable hyperglycemia prevailed. Insulin loss on surfaces was minimal (2–5%) due to the high concentrations of the hormone used (1000–3000 U/L). This was verified by immunoassay.[8]

Microscopic examination of the obstructions formed in the delivery system revealed amorphous and crystalline structures,[17] which subsequent assay indicated to be highly concentrated with immunoreactive insulin. Similar optical examination of the solutions, illuminated with polarized light, showed a suspension of crystalline and amorphous aggregates 1–100 μm in diameter. The size of these aggregates increased with time and eventually accumulated at and obstructed the entrances to the small (0.015 in. inside diameter) catheters used to convey the insulin from the pumps to the subjects. This rapidly resulted in hyperglycemia that could not be reversed by increasing the pumping rate because the flow path was obstructed by the accumulation of aggregates and there was the risk of hypoglycemia if the obstructions were dislodged by the increased pressure generated by the pump. Normoglycemia was always restored by disconnecting the pump, flushing the tubes, and/or replacing them. With the addition of serum no such aggregates were seen.

It appears as if serum contains a factor that promotes the dissolution of insulin or prevents the formation of aggregates in dilute solutions. Whether 1.5% serum is an optimal amount has not been established. To explore whether albumin was responsible for the effect, we conducted a clinical study with an insulin solution prepared as above, but containing 2% human serum albumin in place of the usual serum. In spite of the presence of albumin, glycemic control could not be maintained and insulin aggregates formed in the reservoirs within a short period of time. Although albumin is known to reduce insulin adsorption to glass and plastic containers, it does not appear to prevent the formation of aggregates in dilute solutions.

In the presence of small quantities of unfractionated serum the previously noted aggregates were not evident, and the biologic activity of the solution was significantly higher than similar solutions without serum. Whether this notable difference is a consequence of a more homogenous, monomeric solution is not known. In the dogs similar glycemic control was achieved but with 37% less insulin when serum was added. Fortunately, serum is readily available, easily isolated and processed, and can be returned to the same subject with minimal risk. Further work is indicated to isolate and characterize the factor(s) responsible for the prevention of aggregate formation in insulin solutions. In the mean time, experimental and clinical studies can now proceed unhampered by the uncertainties of variable insulin delivery. Early studies in adolescent diabetics indicate that it will be possible to explicitly define insulin requirements in the fasting and fed states and that open-loop insulin delivery devices for diabetes treatment may now be not only technologically but also biologically feasible.

ACKNOWLEDGMENTS

We acknowledge the help and advice given by Dr. E. Marliss, Dr. B. Zinman, Dr. R. E. Ehrlich, and Bill Wilson. This work was supported by contract no. NO1-AM-9-2201 from the National Institutes of Health.

REFERENCES

[1] Zinman, B., Stokes, E. F., Albisser, A. M., Hanna, A. K., Minuk, H. L., Stein, A. N., Leibel, B. S., and Marliss, E. B.: The metabolic response to glycemic control by the artificial pancreas in diabetic man. Metabolism *28*:511–18, 1979.

[2] Hanna, A. K., Marliss, E. B., Nakhooda, A. F., Minuk, H., Albisser, A. M., Leibel, B. S., and Zinman, B.: Insulin, glucagon and amino acid levels during glycemic control by the artificial pancreas in diabetic man. Metabolism, 1980. In press.

[3] Albisser, A. M., Leibel, B. S., Ewart, T. G., Davidovac, Z., Botz, C. K., and Zingg, W.: An artificial endocrine pancreas. Diabetes *23*:389–96, 1974.

[4] Albisser, A. M., Leibel, B. S., Ewart, T. G., Davidovac, Z., Botz, C. K., Zingg, W., Schipper, H., and Gander, R.: Clinical control of diabetes by the artificial pancreas. Diabetes *23*:397–404, 1974.

[5] Slama, G., Hautecouverture, M., Assan, M., and Tchobroutsky, G.: One to five days of continuous intravenous insulin infusion on seven diabetic patients. Diabetes *23*:732–38, 1974.

[6] Genuth, S., and Martin, P.: Control of hyperglycemia in adult diabetics by pulsed insulin delivery. Diabetes *26*:571–81, 1977.

[7] Service, F. J.: Normalization of plasma glucose of unstable diabetes: studies under ambulatory, fed conditions with pumped intravenous insulin. J. Lab. Clin. Med. *91*:480–89, 1978.

[8] Goriya, Y., Bahoric, A., Marliss, E. B., Zinman, B., and Albisser, A. M.: Glycemic regulation using a preprogrammed insulin delivery device. III. Long-term studies on diabetic dogs. Diabetes *28*:558–64, 1979.

[9] Albisser, A. M., Goriya, Y., Bahoric, A., Marliss, E. B., and Zinman, B.: Hormone and metabolite control in diabetic dogs with long term glucose normalization by portal open-loop insulin delivery. 10 IDF Satellite Symposium. Workshop on Artificial Beta Cell in Diabetes Research and Management. Advanced Postgraduate Course in Diabetes, Heviz, Hungary, September 1979. Acta Diabetol. Lat., 1980. In press.

[10] Poulsen J. E., and Deckert T.: Insulin preparations and the clinical use of insulin. *In* Insulin. Luft, R., Ed. Moindal. Sweden. A. Lindgren and Soner, AB, 1976.

[11] Irsigler, K., and Kritz, H.: Long-term continuous intravenous insulin therapy with a portable insulin dosage-regulating apparatus. Diabetes *28*:196–203, 1979.

[12] Arquilla, E. R., Packer, S., Tarmas, W., and Miyamoto, S.: The effect of zinc on insulin metabolism. Endocrinology *103*:1440–49, 1978.

[13] Jackson, W. S., Lougheed, W., Marliss, E. B., Zinman, B., and Albisser, A. M.: For insulin infusion: a miniature precision peristaltic pump and silicone rubber reservoir. Diabetes Care, 1980. In press.

[14] Ferguson, R. T., Zinman, B., Marliss, E. B., and Albisser, A. M.: An electronic flow rate controller for a portable insulin infusion pump. Submitted to Diabetes Care.

[15] Bahoric, A., Filler, R. M., Perlman, K., Jackman, W. S., and Albisser, A. M.: New devices and methods for long term vascular access for blood sampling and insulin infusion, Diabetes Care, 1980. In press.

[16] Hanna, A. K., Minuk, H., Albisser, A. M., Marliss, E. B., Ellman, J., Jackman, W., Leibel, B. S., and Zinman, B.: A portable system for continuous intravenous insulin delivery: characteristics and results in human diabetics. Diabetes Care *3*:01–08, 1980.

[17] Lougheed, W., and Albisser, A. M.: Insulin delivery and the artificial beta cell. Luminal obstructions in capillary conduits. Int. J. Artif. Organs, 1980. In press.

Organization Section

NEW BENEFITS FOR MEMBERS

Effective January 1, 1980, membership in the National Professional Section automatically confers membership in the member's appropriate Affiliate without payment of additional dues.

Members may choose between having their dues payment cover a calendar year (from January 1 through December 31) or having their membership extend forward for the twelve months following the effective date of their election. Members who choose the calendar year will be sent all back copies of publications for the calendar year in which they were elected; those choosing the flexible year will begin their subscriptions as of the effective date of their election, but they may purchase copies of any back issues that are still available.

Qualified professionals who have received their first professional degree, diploma, or certificate during the preceding five years are eligible for a special membership. Annual dues for these members will be one-half the regular amount for the balance of the five year period and, thereafter, the full amount.

NEW MEMBERS

The following were elected to the Professional Section as of January 1, 1980:

Ambjorn J.E. Agren, Uppsala, Sweden
Peter B. Arner, M.D., Huddinge, Sweden
Roberto T. Barcellos-Betti, M.D., Sorocaba, Brazil
Eugene J. Barrett, M.D., New Haven, CT
Michael M. Barsotti, M.D., Great Falls, MT
Nancy S. Bash, Templeton, CA
James C. Beard, M.D., Seattle, WA
C. Sabin Belknap, M.D., Portland, OR
Robert G. Biesbroeck, M.D., Seattle, WA
Izzi B. Blitz, M.D., Maracaibo, Venezuela
Geremia Bolli, M.D., Perugia, Italy
Michael A. Bolognese, M.D., Gaithersburg, MD
Frank W. Booth, Ph.D., Houston, TX
Rosemary Breedlove, R.N., Los Fresnos, TX
Marcello D. Bronstein, M.D., Sao Paulo, Brazil
Sergio D. Carvalho, M.D., Florianopolis, Brazil
Lawrence C.B. Chan, M.D., Houston, TX
Matthew Cohen, M.D., Melbourne, Australia
Larry Cousins, M.D., San Diego, CA
Richard W. Dame, M.D., Louisville, KY
Abram Drewiacki, M.D., Santos, Sao Paulo, Brazil
Frederick L. Dunn, M.D., Dallas, TX
Joseph C. Dvorak, M.D., Arlington, VA
Hussein E. El-Damasy, M.D., Cairo, Egypt
Mark B. Feigin, M.D., Ph.D., Chicago, IL
Sandra L. Fields, B.S.N., Sparks, NV
David Fitz-Patrick, M.D., Montreal, Canada
David L. Flores, B.S.N., Altus, OK
Robert O. Fuentes, M.D., Boston, MA
Elaine F. Galland, New York, NY
Morton H. Goldstein, M.D., Princeton, NJ
Martin M. Grajower, M.D., Bronx, NY
Raymond F. Gregory, M.D., Houston, TX
Rosalyn S. Gross, Northridge, CA
Rolf L. Gunnarsson, M.D., Huddinge, Sweden
Philippe A. Halban, Ph.D., Geneva, Switzerland
Beverly N. Halford, M.P.H., Hull, MA
Curtis E. Harris, M.D., Oklahoma City, OK
Maralee F. Harris, R.N., Oklahoma City, OK
Mildred Kaufman, Chapel Hill, NC
Avis M. Keslar, Cheyenne, WY
Gerald S. Kidd, II, M.D., Aurora, CO
Warren J. Kidson, M.D., Bellevue Hill, N.S.W., Australia
Johannes Kobberling, M.D., Goettingen, Germany
Alex Kutas, M.D., Long Beach, CA
Tai-Hee Lee, M.D., Kwangju, Chonnam, Korea
Sol Lopis, M.D., Johannesburg, South Africa
Robert T. Lyons, Ph.D., Rochester, NY
Stephen Marshall, Ph.D., Denver, Colorado
William F. Maurer, M.D., Park Ridge, IL
Soaira Mendoza, M.D., Los Andes Merida, Venezuela
Mary Jane Metzger, R.N., Scarsdale, NY
Ronald P. Mitchell, M.D., Newcastle, N.S.W., Australia
Alan C. Moses, M.D., Newton Lower Falls, MA
Barbara B. Nolen, B.S.N., Wichita, KS
Stephen P. Nozetz, M.D., Long Beach, CA
Madonna M. Pachota, B.S.N., Union Lake, MI
Sharon A. Penny-Hopkins, B.S.N., Roslyn Heights, NY
Julie M. Peterson, Houston, TX
Richard E. Quint, D.P.M., Tucson, AZ
Luis Antonio Raio-Granja, M.D., Sao Paulo, Brazil
Victor L. Roberts, M.D., Elmhurst, NY
Irwin Y. Rosenblum, Ph.D., Alamogordo, NM
Mindy F. Rosenblum, M.D., Philadelphia, PA
Peter S. Ross, M.D., Vienna, VA
Ewaldo M.K. Russo, M.D., Sao Paulo, Brazil
Arlene Samowich, Detroit, MI
Fausto Santeusanio, M.D., Perugia, Italy
John A. Scarlett, M.D., Philadelphia, PA
Robert F. Schatzle, Queens Village, NY
Joanne C. Scherr, M.D., Duarte, CA
Martha S. Sereday, M.D., Buenos Aires, Argentina
Ulf Smith, M.D., Gothenburg, Sweden
Cynthia F. Spence, R.N., Woodlawn, MD
Christine A. Stadell, Gainesville, FL
Bettie C.C. Stanislao, Ph.D., Fargo, ND
Alberta M. Stephens, M.S.N., Grinnell, KS
D. Parker Stokes, M.D., Florence, SC
Utoyo Sukaton, M.D., Jakarta, Indonesia
Frederick S. Sunderlin, Jr., M.D., Danville, PA
Stephen P. Swersie, M.D., Staten Island, NY
Robin Tefft, Copperas Cove, TX
Carol B. Teutsch, M.D., Tucker, GA
Edith Tucker, Brooklyn, NY
Anne L. Turner, M.S.N., Nashville, TN
Phillippe A. Vague, M.D., Marseille, France
Svetislav K. Vanov, M.D., Florham Park, NJ
E. Russell Weidman, M.D., Houston, TX
K. Charles Wright, M.D., Marquette, MI
Carlos A. Zapata, M.D., Birmingham, AL

TUMOR MATERIAL RESOURCES

In order to better utilize interesting and rare tumor material, a central clearing house is needed. The University of Chicago Diabetes Center offers to serve this role and will provide additional immunoassay data as well as coordinating materials for morphological and biochemical studies in other centers. Human islet or G.I. tract tumors producing any known hormone(s), but especially glucagon, somatostatin, VIP, or gastrin, as well as insulin, are of interest. Material (as much as possible) should be frozen immediately after excision and maintained at −70°C or below before and during shipment.

Please direct inquiries or notify either A. H. Rubenstein (312) 947-5536, D. F. Steiner (312) 753-3971, or H. S. Tager (312) 753-3974 concerning tumor material.

NEWS OF AFFILIATE ASSOCIATIONS

The North Dakota Affiliate, Inc. of the American Diabetes Association is hosting the fifth annual statewide symposium, "Diabetes Mellitus: The Problem Patient," on April 18–19, 1980 in Grand Forks, North Dakota, for physicians and health care professionals.

The symposium will feature guest speakers Barbara El-Beheri, R.D., Nutrition Program Coordinator for the American Diabetes Association in New York, Dr. Frederick Goetz, professor of medicine, Section of Endocrinology and Metabolism, University of Minnesota Medical School, and other distinguished speakers in the field.

The statewide symposium is sponsored by the North Dakota Affiliate, ADA; the University of North Dakota School of Medicine; and the Veterans Administration Center in Fargo, N.D. Continuing Education credits are available.

For further information or registration material, contact American Diabetes Association, North Dakota Affiliate, Inc., P.O. Box 234, Grand Forks, North Dakota 58201, phone (701) 746-4427.

HLA-DRw Antigens in Mexican-American and Black-American Diabetic Patients

ADINA ZEIDLER, JIMMY LOON, S. DOUGLAS FRASIER, DINESH KUMAR, ROBERT PENNY, AND PAUL TERASAKI

SUMMARY

HLA-A, -B, and -C antigens were studied in 67 Mexican-American and 38 black-American diabetic patients who had the onset of their disease before age 31 yr. Control populations consisted of 322 Mexican-American and 367 black-American subjects for HLA-A, -B, and -C antigens. In addition, HLA-DRw antigens were studied in 60 Mexican-American and 34 black-American diabetic patients. Control populations for HLA-DRw antigens consisted of 189 Mexican-American and 145 black-American subjects.

We found that juvenile-onset–diabetic patients of Mexican-American origin who had the onset of their disease before age 19 demonstrated a significant increase in HLA-DRw4. HLA-DRw4 was also significantly increased in black-American patients with juvenile-onset diabetes mellitus. HLA-DRw2 was not detected in any patient with juvenile-onset diabetes in either ethnic group. A significant association was found between HLA-B18 and HLA-DRw3 in Mexican-American juvenile-diabetic patients.

These findings, which are comparable to those in similar Caucasian patients, provide additional information to support the hypothesis that HLA-DRw antigens play a major role in determining the susceptibility to juvenile-onset diabetes mellitus. DIABETES 29:247–250, April 1980.

The genes that code for the histocompatibility complex of man occupy four separate loci on the short arm of chromosome 6.[1] Several alleles have been recognized for each locus. This human gene complex appears to be analogous to the H2 locus of the mouse, an area referred to as the immune region, which influences immunologic responses to a single synthetic antigen.[2] Additional evidence has accumulated to imply that the immune response and the susceptibility of laboratory animals to experimentally induced diseases such as autoimmune thyroiditis[3] and allergic encephalomyelitis[4] may be under the control of genes linked with the histocompatibility complex. These genes are thought to control the immune response and are termed Ir genes. Their products are referred to as immune region–associated, or Ia, antigens.[5]

The HLA-DRw locus is part of the human histocompatibility complex and is distinct from other HLA loci (A, B, C).[1] This locus has seven alleles, which are termed DRw1–DRw7.[6] The gene products of these alleles have been serologically detected on B lymphocytes, macrophages, sperm, and epithelial cells.[7–9] The HLA-A, -B, and -C loci code for glycoproteins, which are also serologically detectable by cytotoxicity assay methods.[10] The D locus has also been described, and the cell surface antigens coded at this locus have been detected by mixed lymphocyte culture (MLC) techniques.[11] There is controversy as to whether the DRw locus and D locus are the same or whether they represent separate genes coding for distinct cell surface antigens.[12]

Recent studies have clearly demonstrated an association between insulin-dependent diabetes mellitus and the HLA antigens B8, B15, B18, and Cw3 in Caucasians[13–18] and Bw54 in Japanese.[19] In Caucasian diabetic patients, a combination of B8 and B15 or B8 and B18 has been found to increase the susceptibility to the disease.[20] Juvenile-onset diabetes mellitus has also been found to be strongly associated with HLA-DRw3 and -DRw4.[12,21] In sharp contrast, the frequency of DRw2 is decreased or absent in Caucasian patients with juvenile-onset diabetes mellitus.[22]

Since HLA frequencies vary significantly with ethnic background, it was of interest to study the association of HLA-A, -B, -C, and -DRw antigens in diabetic patients of Mexican-American and black-American origins.

PATIENTS AND METHODS

Sixty-seven unrelated Mexican-American and thirty-eight unrelated black-American patients whose diabetes began

From the Departments of Medicine and Pediatrics, University of Southern California School of Medicine, Los Angeles County-USC Medical Center, and the Department of Surgery, University of California School of Medicine, Los Angeles, California.

Address reprint requests to Adina Zeidler, M.D., Raulston Research Laboratories 120, University of Southern California School of Medicine, 2025 Zonal Avenue, Los Angeles, CA 90033.

Received for publication 15 August and in revised form 30 October 1979.

before age 31 yr were studied for HLA-A, -B, and -C antigens. Sixty Mexican-Americans and thirty-four black-Americans were also studied for HLA-DRw antigens. The diabetic patients, all of whom received insulin, were divided into two groups. Group 1 consisted of juvenile-onset, insulin-dependent, ketosis-prone diabetic patients whose disease began before age 19; none were overweight. Group 2 consisted of insulin-treated patients whose diabetes began between ages 19 and 31; they were not prone to ketosis and they were more than 20% above their ideal weight. Control populations consisted of 332 Mexican-Americans for HLA-A, -B, and -C and 189 Mexican-Americans for HLA-DRw. Control populations consisted of 367 black-Americans for HLA-A, -B, and -C and 145 black-Americans for HLA-DRw.

HLA-A, -B, and -C antigens were determined on peripheral blood lymphocytes by the microdroplet lymphocyte cytotoxicity test.[23] The following HLA antigens were determined: HLA-A1, -A2, -A3, -A11, -A25 (10), -A26 (10), -A28, -A29, -Aw23 (9), -Aw24 (9), -Aw30, -Aw31, -Aw33, -Aw34, and -Aw36; HLA-B7, -B8, -B13, -B14, -B15, -B17, -B18, -B27, -B37, -B40, -Bw22, -Bw35, -Bw38, -Bw39 (16), -Bw44 (12), -Bw45 (12), -Bw49 (21), -Bw50 (21), -Bw51 (5), -Bw52 (5), -Bw53, and -Bw54 (22); and HLA-Cwl, -Cw2, -Cw3, and -Cw4.

The HLA-DRw antigen typing (DRw 1–5 and DRw7) was performed on B-cell–enriched lymphocyte populations by microtoxicity testing as previously described.[10]

Statistical analysis. Chi-square tests for significance and relative risk for the disease were calculated as described by Svejgaard et al.[24–25]

RESULTS

The frequencies of HLA-A, -B, and -C antigens among Mexican-American patients in groups 1 and 2 were compared with those found in a comparable control population. The frequencies of HLA-B and -C antigens in diabetic patients, which were found to deviate from those in control subjects, are shown in Table 1. Among the patients in group 1, the frequency of HLA-B18 was higher than it was in the control population but the difference was not statistically significant. Among patients in group 2, the frequency of HLA-B7 and -B8 was greater than it was in control subjects, but neither of these increases was statistically significant. Several HLA antigens were present in decreased frequency in diabetic patients. Among the diabetics in group 1, the frequencies of HLA-B14, -B40, and -Cw4 were decreased in comparison with control subjects. Among patients in group 2, the frequencies of HLA-B14, -Cw2, and -Cw4 were all decreased when compared with those of controls: None of these decreased frequencies in HLA antigens were statistically significant. There were no notable deviations in the frequency of any of the other HLA-A, -B, or -C antigens studied, when diabetic patients were compared to the control population.

TABLE 1
Frequency of HLA-B and -C antigens in Mexican-American control subjects and diabetic patients

	Controls N = 332	Group 1 N = 33			Group 2 N = 34		
Antigen	%	%	χ^2	P*	%	χ^2	P*
B7	8	8	0.02	NS	18	2.10	NS
B8	6	9	0.02	NS	18	4.25	NS
B14	11	6	0.43	NS	3	1.53	NS
B18	6	21	8.01	NS	6	0.10	NS
B40	21	9	1.91	NS	26	0.30	NS
CW2	8	12	0.15	NS	0	3.00	NS
CW4	31	15	2.80	NS	21	1.00	NS

* Corrected for number of antigens.

The frequency of HLA-DRw antigens in Mexican-American diabetic patients and the control population is shown in Table 2. The incidence of DRw4 was significantly increased among patients in group 1 as compared with normal control subjects (X^2 = 9.49; P = 0.016). A moderate increase in the frequency of DRw3 was also noted among patients in group 1; this difference was not statistically significant, however. No Mexican-American diabetic patient in group 1 demonstrated the presence of the HLA-DRw2 antigen. As shown in the table, the relative risk to develop diabetes in a Mexican-American who was positive for both DRw3 (RR = 2.013) and DRw4 (RR = 3.693) was increased, while the relative risk for diabetes was extremely small in Mexican-Americans positive for HLA-DRw2.

When the frequencies of HLA-A, -B, and -C antigens in black-American diabetic patients were compared to those in the appropriate control population, no notable differences were found. However, as shown in Table 3, there was a significant increase in HLA-DRw4 in group 1 black-American diabetic patients when they were compared with the suitable control population (X^2 = 30.6; P = 0.0001). There was also an increase in the frequency of DRw3 among patients in group 1, but this increase was not statistically significant. Again, HLA-DRw2 was not detected in any diabetic patient in group. 1. The relative risk of developing diabetes before age 19 was markedly increased in black-Americans positive for HLA-DRw4 (RR = 14.238) and extremely low for black-Americans positive for HLA-DRw2. In black-Americans there was also an increased risk of developing diabetes between the ages of 19 and 30 in individuals positive for HLA-DRw3 (RR = 3.560) or DRw4 (RR = 4.333).

Our data were analyzed for the presence of an association between all HLA-A, -B, -C and -DRw antigens studied. As shown in Table 4, there was an association between HLA-Bw35 and HLA-Cw4 in both Mexican-American and black-American diabetic subjects. However, this association is no different from that found in control populations of both ethnic groups. A significant association between HLA-B18 and HLA-DRw3 was also found in Mexican-American diabetic patients in group 1, which was notably different from any association between these antigens among either patients in group 2 or Mexican-American control subjects. Black-American patients in group 1 also showed an association between these two antigens, but the degree of association was not statistically significant. This association was not present in either black-American diabetic patients in group 2 or the appropriate control population. There was no association between HLA-B18 and HLA-DRw4 in either Mexican-American or black-American diabetic patients.

DISCUSSION

We have studied the frequencies of HLA-A, -B, -C, and -DRw antigens in Mexican-American and black-American diabetic patients and in control subjects of comparable ethnic background. We did not find an increased frequency of

TABLE 2
Frequency of HLA-DRw antigens in Mexican-American control subjects and diabetic patients

	Controls N = 189	Group 1 N = 30				Group 2 N = 30			
Antigen	%	%	χ^2	P*	RR†	%	χ^2	P*	RR†
DRw1	20	10	0.99	NS	0.518	7	2.10	NS	0.375
DRw2	15	0	3.88	NS	0.092	17	0.06	NS	1.209
DRw3	20	33	1.89	NS	2.013	23	0.03	NS	1.254
DRw4	38	70	9.49	0.016	3.693	33	0.08	NS	0.836
DRw5	15	3	2.08	NS	0.285	7	0.86	NS	0.492
DRw7	14	3	1.72	NS	0.312	13	0.00	NS	1.043

* Corrected for number of antigens.
† Relative risk.

HLA-B8, -B15, or -Cw3 in Mexican-American diabetics, as has been demonstrated in comparable Caucasian patients. This finding suggests the possibility that there is an ethnic difference in the HLA antigens associated with the development of insulin-dependent diabetes mellitus, particularly in patients who have the onset of their disease before age 19.

We were unable to demonstrate any differences in the frequency of HLA-A, -B, or -C antigens in black-American diabetic patients and in controls. This may also represent an ethnic difference in the HLA antigens associated with the development of diabetes mellitus or may be the result of the relatively small number of black-American patients studied. HLA typing is currently being carried out in larger groups of both black-American and Mexican-American diabetic patients.

The relative frequencies of HLA-DRw antigens in Mexican-American diabetic patients have not been reported previously, and only a preliminary report of the association between HLA-DRw antigens and diabetes in black-American patients has appeared.[26] Our data demonstrate a significant increase in the frequency of DRw4 in Mexican-American juvenile-onset–diabetic patients. The frequency of HLA-DRw3 was also increased in this group of patients, but the difference from control subjects was not statistically significant. HLA-DRw2 was completely absent in this group of young diabetics. These findings are in agreement with those reported for Caucasians with juvenile-onset diabetes mellitus by Farid et al.[12] and by Solow et al.[21] Black-American diabetics with an early onset of their disease also showed a significant increase of HLA-DRw4 and, again, DRw2 was not detected in any juvenile-onset black-American diabetic patient. We were unable to demonstrate a significant increase in the frequency of HLA-DRw3 in young black-American diabetics, probably because of the small number of patients studied. Our findings in black-Americans with diabetes mellitus are similar to those recently reported in preliminary form.[26]

Our results confirm the known association between HLA-Bw35 and HLA-Cw4 in both Mexican-American and black-American populations. This same association was detected in diabetic patients of both ethnic groups. An unexpected association between HLA-B18 and HLA-DRw3 was found in Mexican-American juvenile-onset–diabetic patients that was significantly different from the association of these antigens in older diabetics or in Mexican-American controls. A similar association, which did not reach the level of statistical significance, was found in young diabetics of black-American origin. We did not observe an association between HLA-B18 and HLA-DRw4, as has been noted in Caucasian diabetics.

Our findings add considerable support to the previously postulated importance of HLA-DRw antigens in relationship to the development of juvenile-onset diabetes mellitus. In Mexican-American and black-American populations, as well as in Caucasians, the presence of HLA-DRw4 and/or HLA-DRw3 may confer a susceptibility to the development of diabetes mellitus while the presence of HLA-DRw2 may in some way reduce the susceptibility. In all ethnic populations studied thus far, the presence of HLA-DRw4 and DRw3 and the absence of DRw2 appear to be important markers for the development of insulin-dependent diabetes mellitus.

Of particular importance in further elucidating these rela-

TABLE 3
Frequency of HLA-DRw antigens in black-American control subjects and diabetic patients

	Controls N = 145	Group 1 N = 21				Group 2 N = 13			
Antigen	%	%	χ^2	P*	RR†	%	χ^2	P*	RR†
DRw1	15	14	0.01	NS	1.047	8	0.10	NS	0.664
DRw2	36	0	9.26	0.016	0.042	8	3.02	NS	0.216
DRw3	30	38	0.24	NS	1.450	62	4.02	NS	3.560
DRw4	7	52	30.60	0.0001	14.238	23	2.30	NS	4.333
DRw5	24	5	2.95	NS	0.230	23	0.07	NS	1.047
DRw7	11	19	0.50	NS	2.034	23	0.01	NS	0.949

* Corrected for number of antigens.
† Relative risk.

TABLE 4
Association between HLA-B, -C, and HLA-DRw antigens in normal control subjects and diabetic patients of black-American and Mexican-American origin*

		Mexican			Black		
		Controls N = 142	Group 1 N = 30	Group 2 N = 30	Controls N = 178	Group 1 N = 22	Group 2 N = 13
HLA-BW35	HLA-CW4	0.85	0.64	0.60	0.73	0.89	0.54
HLA-B18	HLA-DRw3	0.15	0.71†	0.10	0.08	0.13	0.001
HLA-B18	HLA-DRw4	−0.03	−0.22	0.26	−0.05	−0.22	0.00

* The data are expressed as correlation coefficients.
† $P < 0.01$ when compared with control and with patients in group 1.

tionships are family studies of the distribution of HLA antigens in diabetic and nondiabetic family members. These studies are currently being pursued in both Mexican-American and black-American patients.

ADDENDUM

After our paper was submitted for publication, Rodey et al. reported data comparable to ours with regard to HLA-DRw antigens in black-American diabetic patients.[27]

ACKNOWLEDGMENT

Expert secretarial assistance was provided by Ms. Wilda Lyons. Mr. Joseph Draus provided technical assistance.

This work was supported by a grant from the National Institute of Arthritis, Metabolism, and Digestive Diseases (AM 2375).

REFERENCES

[1] Francke, U., and Pellegrino, M. A.: Assignment of the major histocompatibility complex to a region of the short arm of human chromosome 6. Proc. Natl. Acad. Sci. USA *74*:1147–51, 1977.

[2] Benacerraf, B., and McDevitt, H. O.: Histocompatibility-linked immune response genes. Science *175*:273–79, 1972.

[3] Vladutiu, A. O., and Rose, N. R.: Autoimmune murine thyroiditis: relation to histocompatibility (H-2) type. Science *174*:1137–39, 1971.

[4] Gasser, D. L., Newlin, C. M., Palm, J. et al.: Genetic control of susceptibility to experimental allergic encephalomyelitis in rats. Science *181*:872–73, 1973.

[5] Arbeit, R. D., Sachs, D. H., Amos, D. B., and Dickler, H. B.: Human lymphocyte alloantigen(s) similar to murine Ir region-associated (Ia) antigens. J. Immunol. *115*:1173–75, 1975.

[6] Bodmer, W. F.: Joint report of the seventh international histocompatibility workshop. *In* Histocompatibility Testing. Bodmer, W. F., Batchelor, J. R., Bodmer, J. G. et al., Eds. Copenhagen, Munksgaard, 1978, pp. 351–57.

[7] Winchester, R. J., Fu, S. M., Wernet, P. et al.: Recognition by pregnancy serums on non-HL-A alloantigens selectively expressed on B lymphocytes. J. Exp. Med. *141*:924–29, 1975.

[8] Rowden, G., Lewis, M. G., and Sullivan, A. K.: Ia antigen expression on human epidermal Langerhans cells. Nature *268*:247–48, 1977.

[9] Kamoun, M., Wiels, J., Lepage, V. et al.: Presence of Ia equivalent on human spermatozoa detected by specific reagents prepared by the absorption-elution technique on B cell lymphoid lines or PHA stimulated cells (abstract). Tissue Antigens *10*:245, 1977.

[10] Terasaki, P. I., Bernoco, D., Park, M. S., et al.: Microdroplet testing for HLA-A, -B, -C and -D antigens. Am. J. Clin. Pathol. *69*:103–20, 1978.

[11] Senzar, D. P. S., and Terasaki, P. I.: A semimicro mixed leukocyte culture test. Transplantation *11*:260–67, 1971.

[12] Farid, N. R., Sampson, L., Noel, P. et al.: HLA-D-related (DRw) antigens in juvenile diabetes mellitus. Diabetes *28*:552–57, 1979.

[13] Singal, D. P., and Blajchman, M. A.: Histocompatibility (HL-A) antigens, lymphocytotoxic antibodies and tissue antibodies in patients with diabetes mellitus. Diabetes *22*:429–32, 1973.

[14] Nerup, J., Platz, P., Andersen, O. O. et al.: HL-A antigens and diabetes mellitus. Lancet *2*:864–66, 1974.

[15] Thomsen, M., Platz, P., Andersen, O. O. et al.: MCL typing in juvenile diabetes mellitus and idiopathic Addison's disease. Transplant. Rev. *22*:125–47, 1975.

[16] Cudworth, A. G., and Woodrow, J. C.: HL-A system and diabetes mellitus. Diabetes *24*:345–49, 1975.

[17] Ludwig, H., Schernthaner, G., and Mayr, W. R.: Is HLA-B7 a marker associated with a protective gene in juvenile-onset diabetes mellitus? N. Engl. J. Med. *294*:1066, 1976.

[18] Solow, H., Hidalgo, R., Blajchman, M. et al.: HLA-A, B, C, and B-lymphocyte alloantigens in insulin-dependent diabetes. Transplant Proc. *9*:1859–61, 1977.

[19] Sasazuki, T., Kohno, Y., Iwamoto, I. et al.: HLA and Graves' disease or diabetes mellitus in Japan (letter). N. Engl. J. Med. *298*:630–31, 1978.

[20] Nerup, J., Cathelineau, Cr., Seignalet, J. et al.: HLA and endocrine diseases. *In* HLA and Disease. Dausset, J., and Svejgaard, A., Eds. Copenhagen, Munksgaard, 1977.

[21] Solow, H., Hidalgo, R., and Singal, D. P.: Juvenile-onset diabetes: HLA-A, -B, -C, and -DR alloantigens. Diabetes *28*:1–4, 1979.

[22] Ilonen, J., Herva, E., Tiilikainen, A. et al.: HLA-Dw2 as a marker of resistance against juvenile diabetes mellitus. Tissue Antigens *11*:144–46, 1978.

[23] Terasaki, P. I., McClelland, J., Park, M. S. et al.: Microdroplet lymphocyte cytotoxicity test. *In* Manual of Tissue Typing Techniques. Bethesda, NIH, 75-545, 1974, pp. 67–74.

[24] Svejgaard, A., and Ryder, L. P.: Associations between HLA and disease. Notes on methodology and a report from the HLA and disease registry. *In* HLA and Disease. Dausset, J., and Svejgaard, A., Eds. Copenhagen, Munksgaard, 1977, pp. 46–71.

[25] Svejgaard, A., Jersild, C., Nielson, L. S. et al.: HL-A antigens and disease. Statistical and genetical considerations. Tissue Antigens *4*:95–105, 1974.

[26] Rodey, G. E., White, N., Frazer, T. E. et al.: HLA association with juvenile onset diabetes (JOD) in American blacks. Evidence for the primary nature of D locus association with diabetes (abstract 204). Diabetes *28* (Suppl. 2):395, 1979.

[27] Rodey, G. E., White, N., Frazer, T. E. et al.: HLA-DR specificities among black Americans with juvenile-onset diabetes. N. Engl. J. Med. *301*:810–12, 1979.

Metabolic Activity of Diabetic Monocytes

MITSUO KITAHARA, HARMON J. EYRE, ROBERT E. LYNCH, MARVIN L. RALLISON, AND HARRY R. HILL

SUMMARY

There have been several reported abnormalities in the cellular components of the acute inflammatory response in diabetes mellitus. These studies have dealt primarily with polymorphonuclear leukocytes. In the present investigations, we have examined monocyte metabolic activity in diabetic patients and controls. Following particle ingestion, the microbicidal mechanisms of the monocyte are activated and excited molecular oxygen and carboxyl groups are generated. Upon decay to the ground state, these molecules emit photons, which can be measured as chemiluminescence. Chemiluminescence production was significantly increased in 27 patients with poorly controlled diabetes (blood glucose levels from 208 to 712 mg/dl). The mean peak in the diabetics was 31.3 $\pm$ 8.2 (SD) $\times$ 10^3 cpm versus 25.8 $\pm$ 3.8 $\times$ 10^3 cpm in controls. Hexose monophosphate shunt activity as determined by ^{14}C-I-glucose utilization was also increased (667 $\pm$ 284 percent increase in diabetics versus 425 $\pm$ 154 in controls). Superoxide dismutase-inhibitable superoxide production was also significantly augmented in diabetic monocytes (9.77 $\pm$ 3.06 nmol/10^6 monocytes/20 min versus 6.36 $\pm$ 1.10 nmol). Addition of glucose to whole blood from a normal individual, or to normal or diabetic monocyte suspensions, resulted in marked enhancement of chemiluminescence production. Increasing blood sugar levels appear, therefore, to be associated with monocyte metabolic activation in diabetic patients. Such activation could conceivably be detrimental to the diabetic host by contributing to cell damage through the release of toxic oxygen products. DIABETES *29*:251–256, April 1980.

From the Howard Hughes Medical Institute Laboratories, the Division of Clinical Immunology and Allergy, and the Division of Hematology and Oncology; Departments of Medicine, Pediatrics, and Pathology, University of Utah, Salt Lake City, Utah. Dr. Lynch is an Associate Investigator and Dr. Hill is an Investigator of the Institute.

Address reprint requests to Dr. Harry R. Hill, Division of Clinical Immunology and Allergy, Department of Pediatrics, University of Utah Medical Center, Salt Lake City, Utah 84132.

Received for publication 23 May 79 and in revised form 16 November 1979.

Although there is considerable controversy whether patients with diabetes mellitus have an increased frequency of infection, there is no question that infections are more severe and protracted in such individuals and certainly complicate control of blood sugar and ketosis.[1–4] Several investigators have reported abnormalities in the cellular components of the acute inflammatory response in diabetes. DaCosta[5] first reported defective phagocytic activity by normal leukocytes suspended in diabetic plasma. Bybee and Rogers,[6] using a visual assay of bacterial uptake by polymorphonuclear leukocytes (PMN), found a significant decrease in phagocytic activity for *Staphylococcus aureus* by the PMNs of diabetics with acidosis. Bagdade et al.,[7] observed a decrease in PMN phagocytic activity, which was correlated with fasting blood glucose levels. In contrast, Tan et al.[8] found no correlation between abnormal phagocytosis and blood glucose concentrations; however, their observations were done during the time of treatment. Mowat and Baum,[9] Hill and associates,[10] and Miller and Baker[11] have observed depressed in vitro chemotactic responses by neutrophils of both juvenile and adult diabetic patients. Diabetic PMN metabolism has also been investigated and reduced glycolysis has been detected in association with hypercholesterolemia.[12] Although a number of studies have reported data on insulin receptors in diabetic monocytes,[13,14] there have been no reports on monocyte functional or metabolic activity in diabetes mellitus. In the present investigations, we have studied diabetic monocyte metabolism in diabetics, employing chemiluminescence, superoxide generation, and hexose monophosphate shunt activity.

MATERIALS AND METHODS

Cell preparations. Heparinized (10 U/ml) whole blood was diluted with sterile phosphate-buffered saline (PBS: 4,500 ml distilled water, 5.2 g Na_2HPO_4, 0.9 g KCl, 0.9 g KH_2PO_4, and 36 g NaCl; pH 7.4), and mononuclear cells were separated by Ficoll-Paque[15] (Pharmacia Fine Chemicals, Piscataway, New Jersey). The mononuclear cell layer was removed and washed in PBS. The cells were then suspended in PBS with a monocyte concentration of 2.0×10^6 per milliliter for chemiluminescence (CL) and hexose monophosphate shunt activity determinations. The monocyte concentration was adjusted to 5×10^5 per milliliter in PBS for superoxide generation determinations.

Chemiluminescence assay. Zymosan particles (Schwartz-Mann, Orangeburg, New York) were washed once in PBS and 10 ml of normal serum was added to 100 mg of the zymosan pellet.[16] The mixture was vortexed well and rotated for 1 h at 37°C in a Rotorack (Fisher Scientific, Santa Clara, California). After centrifugation, the serum was removed and the particles were washed. The original volume was replaced with an equal volume of PBS.

Four-tenths milliliters of opsonized zymosan particles in PBS (10 mg/ml) were added to 0.5 ml of the monocyte suspension (2×10^6 per ml) and 2.6 ml of PBS (total volume = 3.5 ml). The mixture was made in Beckman (Fullerton, California) poly Q scintillation vials that had been wrapped in aluminum foil and stored in darkness for at least 18 h before use.[16,17] The vials were immediately capped, mixed, and placed in a Beckman LS-100c scintillation counter out of phase with one photomultiplier tube disconnected. Each reaction mixture was counted (starting at 0 min) at 5–10-min intervals for 60–90 min. Duplicate samples were performed for each variable and CL was expressed as mean counts per minute (cpm), unless otherwise indicated. Usually the CL peak value occurred between 15 and 25 min after addition of opsonized zymosan.

C-14-glucose utilization. Carbon-14 dioxide produced by oxidation of ^{14}C-labeled glucose was adsorbed on filter paper saturated with 20% sodium hydrooxide and suspended from the stopper in a flask containing 1×10^6 monocytes in the incubation mixture. The mixture also contained 1 μmol of glucose, 1 μCi of glucose-1-^{14}C (New England Nuclear, Boston, Massachusetts), 0.1 ml of preopsonized zymosan, and 0.5 ml of the 2×10^6/ml monocyte suspension.[18] After 20 min of incubation the stoppers were removed, and the filter paper was air dried. The filter paper was then placed in scintillation counting vials with 10 ml of scintillation counting fluid, Aquasol (New England Nuclear, Boston, Massachusetts). Since the lots of ^{14}C-glucose were different, the results were expressed as the percent increase above the baseline count.

Superoxide generation. Superoxide dismutase- (SOD) inhibitable reduction of ferricytochrome c by intact monocytes was employed as a measure of superoxide formation.[19] In this assay the standard reaction mixture contained 0.1 mM ferricytochrome c (Sigma Chemical Co., St. Louis, Missouri), 1 mg preopsonized zymosan, and 5×10^5 monocytes per ml in PBS. Paired reactions with and without added SOD (12 μg/ml, Sigma Chemical Co.) were employed. Zymosan was deleted for resting values. The reaction mixtures were incubated at 37°C in a water bath (oscillating at 80 times/min) for 20 min. The mixtures were then transferred to tubes from glass vials and the tubes were centrifuged at 4°C for 5 min at $1500 \times g$. Spectrophotometric measurements were made with a Cary M15 spectrophotometer (Varian Instrument Division, Cary Products, Palo Alto,

TABLE 1
Clinical and laboratory data on the 27 diabetic patients

Subject	Age	Blood glucose (mg/dl)	Cholesterol (mg/dl)	Treatment	Chemiluminescence (% of control)
1	43	250	ND*	Insulin	108
2	57	352	ND	"	141
3	26	312	ND	"	152
4	18	637	126	"	146
5	49	315	ND	"	130
6	62	236	196	"	115
7	57	340	224	"	136
8	72	712	193	"	188
9	73	208	192	"	137
10	54	230	268	Diet	112
11	58	215	ND	"	114
12	53	300	95	Insulin	155
13	64	276	285	"	136
14	46	375	ND	"	119
15	46	386	ND	"	109
16	63	482	ND	"	138
17	53	311	ND	"	111
18	42	215	376	"	123
19	52	293	220	"	100
20	57	270	100	"	109
21	51	270	160	"	89
22	42	215	140	"	99
23	74	226	ND	"	130
24	57	400	ND	Chlorpropamide	97
25	51	260	ND	Insulin	101
26	56	218	186	Chlorpropamide	107
27	51	229	229	Insulin	124

* Not determined.

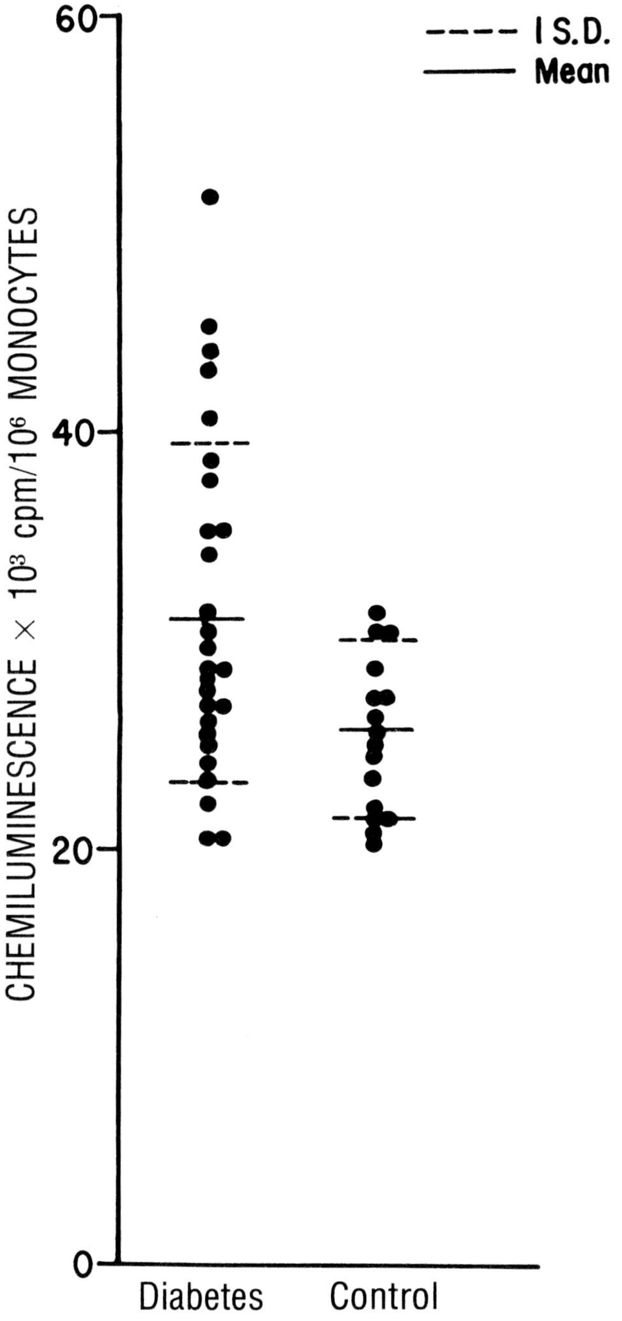

FIGURE 1. Chemiluminescence production by diabetic and control monocytes. P = 0.005 by the two-tailed, unpaired Student's *t* test.

California). Nanomoles of cytochrome c reduced were determined from the increase in the absorbance at 550 nm using E = 21.0 cm^{-1} mM^{-1}.[20] The results were expressed as nmole/10^6 monocytes/20 min.

Clinical material. Healthy nondiabetic controls consisted of male laboratory personnel, hospital workers, and medical students. All patients studied had uncomplicated diabetes mellitus (age range: 18–74 yr, mean 52.9 yr, Table 1). Twenty-three of the 27 patients were receiving insulin treatment at the time of leukocyte testing. Two patients (#16 and #17) were females; the rest were males. None were obese. The blood was drawn in the morning before insulin administration, while the patient was in the fasting state. At the time of blood collection these patients did not have evidence of acute infections or other inflammatory processes. The patients' glucose levels and chemical parameters are shown in Table 1. Blood glucose ranged from 208 to 712 mg/dl and cholesterol from 95 to 376 mg/dl; creatinine and BUN were in the normal range.

Statistical methods. The statistical methods employed were the two-tailed, paired and unpaired Student's *t* test as well as the Wilcoxon sign rank test. These are indicated in the text, tables, and figure legends.

RESULTS

The peak value of diabetic and control monocyte CL induced by opsonized zymosan is illustrated in Figure 1. A significant increase in monocyte CL production ($31.3 \pm 8.1 \times 10^3$ cpm) was observed in patients with diabetes mellitus when compared with the mean of the control value ($25.8 \pm 3.8 \times 10^3$ cpm, $P = 0.005$). While all of the controls were not age-matched, four were, including the one shown in Figure 2. Three of our patients were over 70 yr of age but all had CL peaks greater than the simultaneously tested controls (#8, #9, and #23). Unstimulated CL in controls and diabetics from 6000 to 8000 cpm did not differ between groups (background counts with a blank vial were 4000–5000 cpm). A number of patients with diabetes had markedly increased CL, and except for five instances, exceeded that of the simultaneously tested control (Table 1).

To determine if adequate control of the diabetic state affected monocyte CL production, we next examined a patient with significant hyperglycemia (BS 400 mg/dl) before and after insulin therapy. As shown in Figure 2, the patient's CL was significantly above that of the control (whose blood sugar was 90 mg/dl; $P < 0.02$). After insulin therapy, which corrected the blood sugar to 120 mg/dl, the patient's CL returned to normal levels.

Addition of insulin in a concentration of 100 μU/ml significantly lowered diabetic monocyte CL production ($P = 0.0002$) but had no effect on CL production of normal monocytes (Table 2).

Monocyte hexose monophosphate shunt activity as deter-

FIGURE 2. Monocyte chemiluminescence production by a poorly controlled diabetic with a fasting blood glucose of 400 mg/dl (△——△). Chemiluminescence after insulin treatment which resulted in a blood glucose of 120 mg/dl (▲——▲). Sex- and age-matched control chemiluminescence production (○——○) was identical at each study. Statistical analysis was by the paired, two-tailed Student's *t* test.

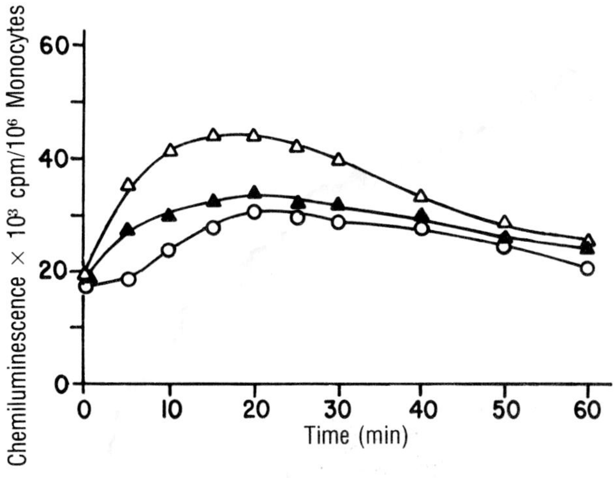

TABLE 2
Effect of insulin on diabetic and control monocyte chemiluminescence production

Peak CL production (cpm × 10³)					
Diabetics			Controls		
Subject	With insulin*	Without insulin*	Subject	With insulin†	Without insulin†
1	21.7	26.7	1	21.6	24.7
2	40.3	43.7	2	30.0	31.0
3	34.9	38.4	3	20.6	25.5
4	29.1	34.9	4	25.6	26.9
5	31.7	35.1	5	26.7	30.5
6	30.5	36.0	6	29.9	27.2

*P = 0.0002 by the two-tailed, paired Student's *t* test; † NSD.

mined by carbon-14 dioxide production from ^{14}C-1-glucose was also significantly increased when compared with controls (667 ± 284 percent increase in diabetics versus 425 ± 154; P = 0.018, Figure 3).

SOD-inhibitable superoxide production was also augmented in diabetic monocytes (9.77 ± 3.06 nmol/10^6 monocytes/20 min) when compared with controls (6.36 ± 1.10 nmol, P = 0.004, Figure 3). An association between diabetic monocyte CL production and blood glucose levels was observed (correlation coefficient r = 0.58, P < 0.01). There was no association between CL values and triglyceride, cholesterol, BUN, or creatinine levels.

FIGURE 3. $^{14}CO_2$ and superoxide generation by diabetic and control monocytes exposed to opsonized zymosan. P = 0.018 and 0.004, respectively, by the two-tailed, unpaired Student's *t* test.

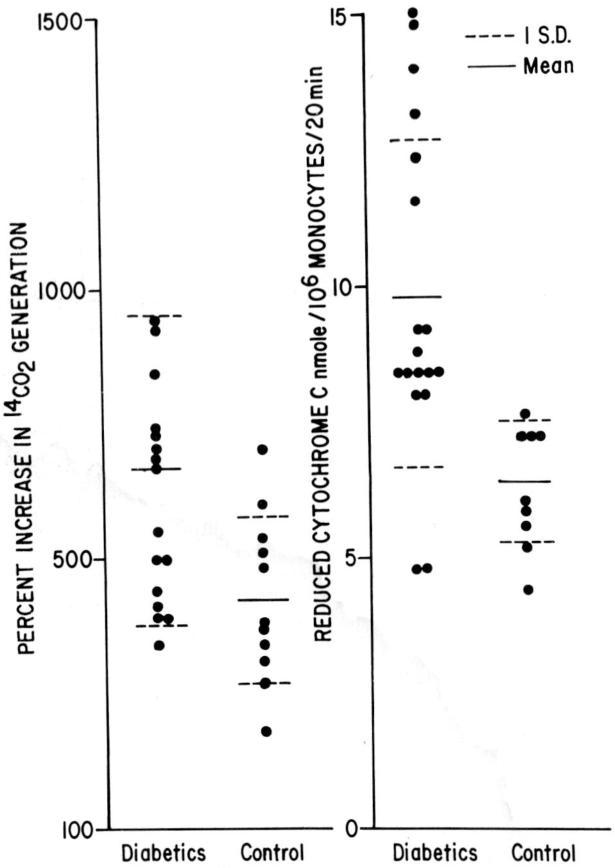

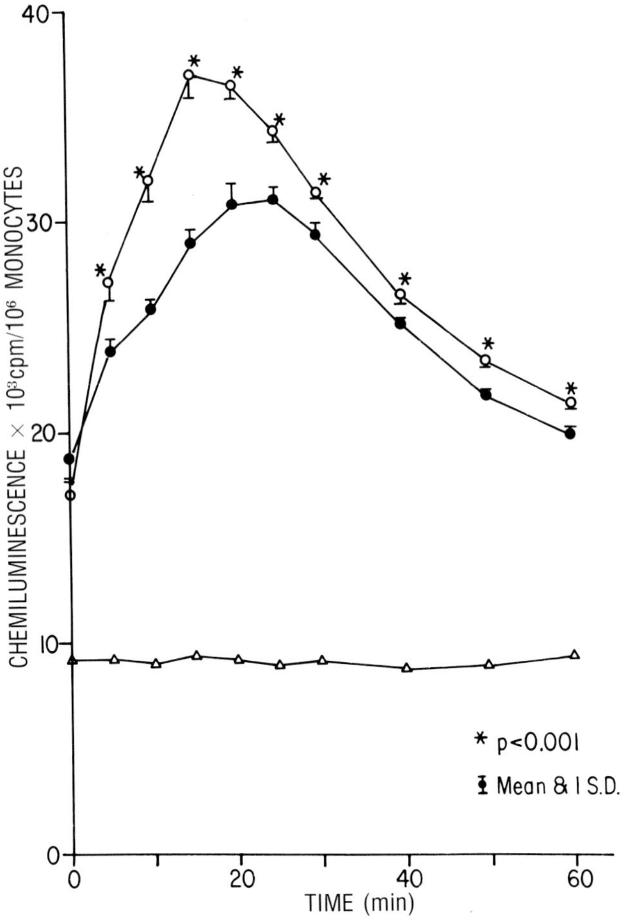

FIGURE 4. Effect of glucose addition to a whole blood sample from a nondiabetic individual on subsequent monocyte chemiluminescence production. The open circles represent chemiluminescence production of monocytes from whole blood samples incubated with added glucose (250 mg/dl) for 1 h. The solid dots are CL values produced by monocytes from whole blood samples without added glucose (140 mg/dl). The triangles represent unstimulated monocyte chemiluminescence. Chemiluminescence values are the mean of quadruplicate samples from a single individual.

Because increased monocyte CL production seemed to be associated with high blood glucose levels, we next sought to determine the effect of this carbohydrate on CL production in vitro. The effect of glucose on monocyte metabolic activity was investigated in two ways. (1) Whole blood from a nondiabetic individual was incubated with an appropriate concentration of glucose resulting in a final blood glucose level of 250 mg/dl, and (2) glucose was added directly to the phagocytic mixture before CL and superoxide generation determinations. Figure 4 shows normal monocyte CL with and without the addition of glucose (a final concentration of 250 mg/dl). At the time of this experiment the donor's 2-h postprandial blood glucose was 140 mg/dl. The monocytes incubated with added glucose showed significantly increased CL production when compared with the same cells to which no glucose had been added. The effect on CL of adding glucose (100 mg/dl) immediately before a study is illustrated in Figure 5. Again, CL production was markedly enhanced as well as superoxide generation (7.55 ± 1.12 nmol/10^6 monocytes/20 min versus 5.03 ± 1.30) (P < 0.05). This effect of glucose on CL was totally abolished by SOD (100 μg/ml). In contrast, glucose still exerted an enhancing effect on phagocytizing monocytes

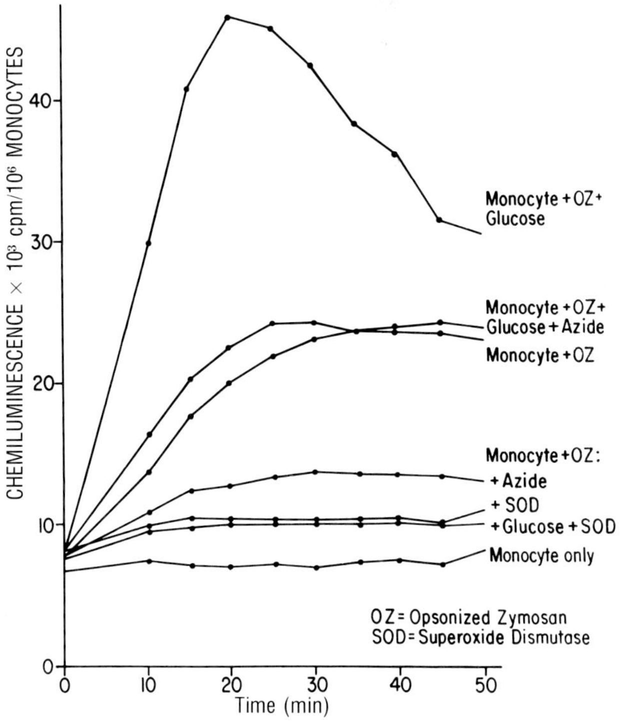

FIGURE 5. Effect of superoxide dismutase and azide on glucose-induced enhancement of monocyte chemiluminescence. Reported in a single experiment with duplicate samples for all variables.

in the presence of azide (1 mM), which is an inhibitor of myeloperoxidase[21] (Figure 5).

Glucose enhancement of zymosan induced monocyte CL production was observed in both normal and diabetic subjects (Table 3). As shown in Figure 6, the diabetic monocytes produced more CL than controls and responded to added glucose in concentrations ranging from 1 to 500 mg/dl. The normals also responded to these concentrations but did not reach equivalent peaks in CL production. Monocytes treated with 2-deoxyglucose (peak CL: 21×10^3 cpm) had approximately the same CL peak as that of untreated cells (peak CL: 20×10^3 cpm).

TABLE 3
Effect of glucose addition to the reaction mixture on monocyte chemiluminescence production

	Peak CL production (cpm × 10^3)		
Subject	Without glucose*	With glucose* (100 mg/dl)	Percent
Controls			
1	21.7	38.3	176
2	20.6	35.8	173
3	22.6	37.2	165
4	29.5	44.2	150
5	22.5	45.9	196
Diabetics			
1	23.3	37.9	163
2	26.9	46.4	172
3	21.3	32.6	153
4	20.8	31.9	153
Average	23.2	38.9	168

* Difference (Student's *t* test) between CL with and without added glucose. $P < 0.001$.

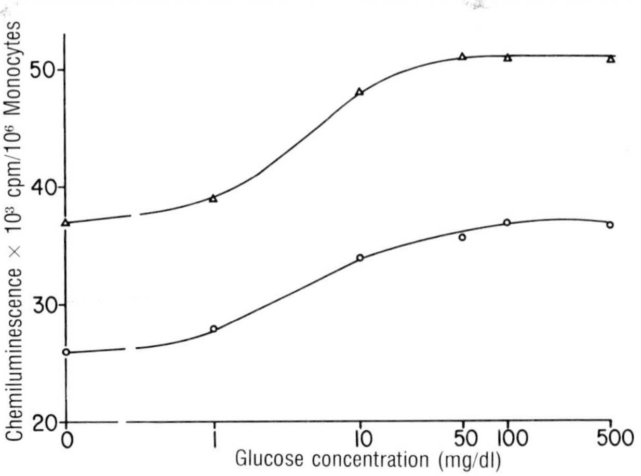

FIGURE 6. Dose-response effect of glucose on chemiluminescence production of normal (○——○) and diabetic (△——△) monocytes.

DISCUSSION

Metabolic disorders observed in diabetes mellitus have been felt to interfere with various defense mechanisms. PMN from diabetic patients exhibit diminished chemotactic activity, which is corrected by adding insulin.[9–11] Impaired bactericidal activity and fungicidal capacity in diabetes have also been demonstrated by several investigators.[5–7,22] In addition, Bagdade et al.[23] found defective granulocyte adherence, which seemed to be a reversible defect controlled by normalizing the blood glucose. Thus, functional defects in diabetic PMN seem to be well documented by several investigators.

The metabolic activity of diabetic PMN as measured by glucose utilization is more controversial, however. Martin et al.[24] and Munroe and Shipp[12] incubated PMN for 4 h and found reduced glucose utilization and glycolysis in moderately severe diabetics or in normoglycemic hypercholesterolemic diabetics. In contrast, Kalant and Schucher[25], using a 2-h incubation period, demonstrated a higher rate of glucose utilization and there was no difference between normals and diabetics under these circumstances. Smejkalova et al.[26] found depressed glucose utilization in diabetics. In the present studies, we have shown that monocyte metabolic activity as determined by hexose monophosphate shunt activity, superoxide generation, and CL production is significantly elevated compared with controls. Although controls were not always age-matched, none of the patients or controls were obese and only three of the patients were over 70 yr of age. Van Epps and co-workers[27] have found that CL does not vary with age except for being lower in neonates and patients greater than 70 yr of age. All three of our patients over 70 had CL peaks greater than simultaneously tested controls. The evidence of activated metabolism can perhaps be attributed to an intracellular metabolic disorder of the glycolytic pathway, resulting from a lack of insulin. Since diabetic monocytes have a relative deficiency of insulin, this may result in a diminution of energy production in the form of ATP.[28] The reduction of ATP as a source of energy could induce a compensatory increase in oxidative glycolysis through the hexose monophosphate shunt,[22] which would, therefore, generate more superoxide and similar excited molecular species. Treatment with insulin resulted in lower CL production by the monocytes of a patient who initially had a blood sugar level of 400 mg/dl. Similarly, insulin was found to depress monocyte CL production when added to diabetic cells in vitro. These results suggest that a relative deficiency of insulin may, in fact, contribute to the abnormality observed in diabetic monocytes.

What role might the enhanced production of toxic oxygen products by monocytes from diabetics have in the host defense abnormalities observed in this disease? At present, this is unknown but it is tempting to speculate. Baehner et al.[29] demonstrated that cellularly derived H_2O_2 could attenuate the phagocytic rate of PMNs. In addition, Bagdade et al.[30] observed that leukocyte phagocytic and microbicidal activity was impaired in diabetic subjects with hyperglycemia. These observations on granulocytes and ours on diabetic monocytes raise the possibility that oxidants produced through the hexose monophosphate shunt may be detrimental to the cell, causing phagocytic, chemotactic, and perhaps other defects. It is conceivable that antioxidants such as vitamin E may be capable of reversing such abnormalities, thus suggesting at least the possibility of pharmacologically modifying diabetic phagocyte function.

ACKNOWLEDGMENTS

This work was supported, in part, by U.S. Public Health Service grants AM21140 and AI13150 and a grant from the Thrasher Foundation.

REFERENCES

[1] Younger, D.: Infection and diabetes. Med. Clin. North Am. *49*:1005–13, 1965.

[2] Zaky, D. A., Bently, D. W., Lowy, K., Betts, R. F., and Douglas, R. G.: Malignant external otitis: a severe form of otitis in diabetic patients. Am. J. Med. *61*:298–302, 1976.

[3] Marble, A., White, H. J., and Fernald, A. T.: The nature of the lowered resistance of bacterial infection. J. Clin. Invest. *17*:423–30, 1938.

[4] Bauer, H., Flanagan, J. F., and Sheldon, W. H.: Experimental cerebral mucomycosis in rabbits with alloxan diabetes. Yale J. Biol. Med. *28*:29–36, 1955.

[5] DaCosta, J. C., and Beardsley, E. J. G.: The resistance of diabetics to bacterial infection. Am. J. Med. Sci. *136*:361–73, 1908.

[6] Bybee, J. D., and Rogers, D. E.: The phagocytic activity of polymorphonuclear leukocytes obtained from patients with diabetes mellitus. J. Lab. Clin. Med. *64*:1–13, 1964.

[7] Bagdade, J. D., Nielson, K. L., and Bulger, R. J.: Reversible abnormalities in phagocyte function in poorly controlled diabetic patients. Am. J. Med. Sci. *263*:452–56, 1972.

[8] Tan, J. S., Anderson, J. L., Watanakunakorn, C., and Phair, J. P.: Neutrophil dysfunction in diabetes mellitus. J. Lab. Clin. Med. *85*:26–33, 1975.

[9] Mowat, A. G., and Baum, J.: Chemotaxis of polymorphonuclear leukocytes from patients with diabetes mellitus. N. Engl. J. Med. *284*:621–27, 1971.

[10] Hill, H. R., Sauls, H. S., Dettloff, J. L., and Quie, P. G.: Impaired leukotactic responsiveness in patients with juvenile diabetes mellitus. Clin. Immunol. Immunopathol. *2*:395–403, 1974.

[11] Miller, M. E., and Baker, L.: Leukocyte function in juvenile diabetes mellitus: Hormonal and cellular aspects. J. Pediatr. *81*:979–82, 1972.

[12] Munroe, J. F., and Shipp, J. C.: Glucose metabolism in leukocytes from patients with diabetes mellitus with and without hypercholesterolemia. Diabetes *14*:584–90, 1965.

[13] Olefsky, J. M.: The insulin receptor: its role in insulin resistance of obesity and diabetes. Diabetes *25*:1154–62, 1976.

[14] Flier, J. S., Kahn, C. R., and Roth, J.: Receptors, antireceptor antibodies and mechanisms of insulin resistance. N. Engl. J. Med. *300*:413–19, 1979.

[15] Boyum, A.: Isolation of mononuclear cells and granulocytes from human blood. Isolation of mononuclear cells by one centrifugation and granulocytes by combining centrifugation and sedimentation at *lg*. Scand. J. Clin. Lab. Invest. *97* (Suppl):77–89, 1968.

[16] Hill, H. R., Hogan, N. A., Bale, J. F., and Hemming, V. G.: Evaluation of nonspecific (alternate pathway) opsonin activity by neutrophil chemiluminescence. Int. Arch. Allergy Appl. Immunol. *53*:490–97, 1977.

[17] Hemming, V. G., Hall, R. T., Rhodes, P. G., Shigeoka, A. O., and Hill, H. R.: Assessment of group B streptococcal opsonins in human and rabbit serum by neutrophil chemiluminescence. J. Clin. Invest. *58*:1379–87, 1976.

[18] Holmes, B., Page, A. R., and Good, R. A.: Studies of the metabolic activity of leukocytes from patients with a genetic abnormality of phagocytic function. J. Clin. Invest. *46*:1422–32, 1967.

[19] Rosen, H., and Klebanoff, S. J.: Chemiluminescence and superoxide production by myeloperoxidase-deficient leukocytes. J. Clin. Invest. *58*:50–60, 1976.

[20] Massey, V.: The microestimation of succinate and the extinction coefficient of cytochrome C. Biochem. Biophys. Acta *34*:255–56, 1969.

[21] Klebanoff, S. J., and Pincus, S. H.: Hydrogen peroxide utilization in myeloperoxidase deficient leukocytes: a possible microbicidal control mechanism. J. Clin. Invest. *50*:2226–29, 1971.

[22] Cech, P., Papathanapsion, A., Boreux, G., Roth, P., and Miescher, P. A.: Hereditary myeloperoxidase deficiency. Blood *53*:403–11, 1979.

[23] Bagdade, J. D., Stewart, M., and Walters, E.: Impaired granulocyte adherence. A reversible defect in host defense in patients with poorly controlled diabetes. Diabetes *27*:677–81, 1978.

[24] Martin, S. P., McKinney, G. R., Green, R., and Baker, C.: The influence of glucose, fructose and insulin on the metabolism of leukocytes of healthy and diabetic subjects. J. Clin. Invest. *32*:1171–74, 1953.

[25] Kalant, N., and Schucher, R.: Glucose utilization and insulin responsiveness of leukocytes in diabetes. Can. J. Biochem. Physiol. *40*:899–903, 1962.

[26] Smejkalova, E., Smejkal, V., and Skrha, F.: Comparative study of some metabolic deviations in diabetes mellitus and hyperthyroidism. Enzymologia *35*:289–97, 1968.

[27] Van Epps, D. E., Goodwin, J. S., and Murphy, S.: Age-dependent variations in polymorphonuclear leukocyte chemiluminescence. Infect. Immun. *22*:57–61, 1978.

[28] Weber, G., Stamm, N. B., and Fisher, E. A.: Insulin: inducer of pyruvate kinase. Science *149*:65–67, 1965.

[29] Baehner, R. L., Boxer, L. A., Allen, J. M., and Davis, J.: Autooxidation as a basis for altered function by polymorphonuclear leukocytes. Blood *50*:327–35, 1977.

[30] Bagdade, J. D., Root, R. K., and Bulger, R. J.: Impaired leukocyte function in patients with poorly controlled diabetes. Diabetes *23*:9–15, 1974.

Impaired Responses of Catecholamines, Growth Hormone, and Cortisol to Graded Exercise in Diabetic Autonomic Neuropathy

JANNIK HILSTED, HENRIK GALBO, AND NIELS JUEL CHRISTENSEN

SUMMARY

Six juvenile diabetics [age, 31 ± 2 yr ($\bar{x}$ and SEM); duration of diabetes, 15 ± 4 yr], who showed signs of autonomic neuropathy (decreased beat-to-beat variation in heart rate during deep breathing), and seven control patients of similar age (27 ± 1 yr) and duration of diabetes (14 ± 2 yr) performed graded exercise on an ergometer cycle 3 h after breakfast and subcutaneous administration of insulin.

Plasma epinephrine increased significantly in both patient groups and was not significantly different at exhaustion [0.43 ± 0.17 ng/ml (neuropathy) vs. 1.07 ± 0.28 ng/ml (controls), $P < 0.1$]. Plasma norepinephrine levels increased significantly in control patients but not in autonomic neuropathy, and they were significantly different at exhaustion [1.43 ± 0.34 ng/ml (neuropathy) vs. 2.51 ± 0.26 ng/ml (controls), $P < 0.05$]. The relationships between plasma norepinephrine and epinephrine levels, respectively, and relative work load (expressed as oxygen uptake—in per cent—of individual maximal oxygen uptake) were shifted to the right in patients with autonomic neuropathy, indicating impaired sympathetic activity.

A significant decrease in plasma glucagon levels was found at low work loads (50 W and 75 W) in control patients but not in patients with autonomic neuropathy. At exhaustion, plasma glucagon levels were similar to resting levels in both patient groups. At exhaustion, plasma growth hormone and cortisol levels were significantly above preexercise levels only in control patients (50.5 ± 7.9 mU/L and 23.5 ± 2.9 μg/100 ml, respectively), and they were higher in these patients, $P < 0.025$ and $P < 0.005$, respectively, than in patients with autonomic neuropathy (24.4 ± 8.4 and 12.8 ± 1.6, respectively). Metabolic responses were similar in the two patient groups, as judged from plasma concentrations of glucose, lactate, free fatty acids, glycerol, and beta-hydroxybutyric acid.

In conclusion, diabetics with decreased beat-to-beat variation in heart rate displayed impaired responses of catecholamines, indicating a defective sympathoadrenal outflow, and of other glucoregulatory hormones during graded exercise. DIABETES *29*:257–262, April 1980.

From the Institute of Medical Physiology B, University of Copenhagen; Hvidøre Hospital; and Medical Department F, Herlev Hospital, Denmark.
Address reprint requests to J. Hilsted, M.D., Institute of Medical Physiology B, Juliane Maries Vej 30, DK-2100 Copenhagen Ø, Denmark.
Received for publication 23 July and in revised form 19 November 1979.

We previously reported[1] that the capacity for graded exercise, expressed as both the maximally tolerable work load and the maximal oxygen uptake ($\dot{V}_{O_2}$ max), is reduced in insulin-dependent diabetics who show signs of autonomic neuropathy (decreased beat-to-beat variation in heart rate during hyperventilation,[2] which is considered to be caused by cardiac parasympathetic neuropathy). The findings of lower maximal heart rate and of deviation to the right of the relationships between heart rate and blood pressure, respectively, and relative work load, expressed as oxygen uptake—in per cent—of individual maximal oxygen uptake, indicated impaired activity in sympathetic nerves to the heart and to resistance vessels.

The aim of the present study was to determine whether sympathetic activity, as assessed by measurements of plasma concentrations of norepinephrine and epinephrine, in fact was lower in patients with autonomic neuropathy than in controls during these graded exercises.

The exercise-induced increase in plasma glucagon in rats can be blocked by adrenergic-blocking agents.[3,4] Accordingly, a possible sympathetic defect in patients with decreased beat-to-beat variation in heart rate might cause an altered glucagon-release pattern. Plasma levels of growth hormone and cortisol increase during graded exercise in man,[5–8] while glucagon levels initially decrease and subsequently return to preexercise levels.[9] As exercise-induced responses of individual hormones probably are closely interrelated,[10] we found it of interest to investigate whether the responses of glucagon, growth hormone, and cortisol are also altered during graded exercise in patients with diabetic autonomic neuropathy. Furthermore, by measuring plasma levels of glucose, lactate, free fatty acids (FFA), glycerol, and beta-hydroxybutyric acid (BOH), we estimated whether the metabolic exercise response, which is believed to be modulated by the hormonal response, is affected in diabetic autonomic neuropathy.

MATERIALS AND METHODS

Patients. Six juvenile diabetics [age, 31 ± 2 yr ($\bar{x}$ and SEM); duration of diabetes, 15 ± 4 yr], who showed signs of autonomic neuropathy (beat-to-beat variation 7 ± 1 min^{-1}) as well as of somatic neuropathy (sense of vibration, 33 ± 6 V[11]), and seven control patients of similar age (27 ± 1 yr) and duration of diabetes (14 ± 2 yr), who had no neuropathy according to these criteria (beat-to-beat variation, 31 ± 2 min^{-1}; sense of vibration, 11 ± 0.5 V), volunteered in the study (for details, see ref. 1). One patient with neuropathy had a slight orthostatic hypotension (140/90 lying, 120/90 standing), even after treatment with tablets of fludrocortisone (dose, 0.25 mg per day) and tablets of etilephrine (25 mg per day). No other clinical signs of neuropathy were found in the patients.

Mean daily dose of insulin was 41 ± 4 IU (neuropathy) and 40 ± 3 IU (controls). Apart from the patient with orthostatic hypotension, no patient received any medicine, except insulin. No patient had a history of angina pectoris, cardiac arrhythmias, or pulmonary disease. Auscultation of heart and lungs ECG in six precordial leads were normal in all patients. No patient had signs or symptoms of other endocrine disease. Hemoglobin was normal in both patient groups [9.2 ± 0.4 mmol/L (neuropathy) and 9.4 ± 0.2 (controls)]. Serum creatinine was normal in all patients [74 ± 3 μmol/L (neuropathy) and 87 ± 2 (controls)]. Two patients in each group had a slight proteinuria. Ophthalmoscopy, performed by an experienced ophthalmologist immediately before the exercise experiments, showed that no patient had proliferative retinopathy. Feet were intact in all patients, none of whom had ulcerations of feet or legs.

The patients were actively employed and did not participate in physical-training programs.

Methods. After a good night's sleep and at least 12 h of abstinence from tobacco and alcohol, the patients ate their usual breakfast and took their usual morning dose of insulin at 7 a.m. They arrived in the laboratory at 10 a.m. They were weighed and had a cannula inserted intravenously in the forearm, whereupon they rested supine on a couch for 30 min and in the sitting position for 15 min. Subsequently, the patients exercised on an ergometer cycle at increasing work loads until exhaustion, as previously described.[1] At rest and at the end of each work load, oxygen uptake was measured and blood samples were drawn for determination of concentrations of catecholamines, glucagon, growth hormone, cortisol, glucose, lactate, FFA, glycerol, and beta-hydroxybutyric acid and for determination of packed cell volume.

Due to subjective symptoms of hypoglycemia, two control patients and one patient with autonomic neuropathy were given 200 ml of apple juice in the rest period preceding their last exercise bout.

Blood samples were drawn without causing stasis; during the experiments, an average of 120 ml of blood was drawn. Blood glucose (mmol/L blood) was determined by the hexokinase method[12] and blood lactate (mmol/L blood) by means of the lactate-dehydrogenase method.[13] Free fatty acids (FFA) in serum (mEq/L serum) were determined spectrophotometrically as copper soaps.[14] Glycerol (mmol/L serum) was determined by an enzymatic spectrophotometric method[15] and beta-hydroxybutyric acid (mmol/L blood) by an enzymatic fluorometric method.[16] For catecholamine analysis, 18 ml blood was sampled in iced tubes, which contained 16 mg EDTA and 16 mg ascorbic acid. After centrifugation, the supernatant was deep-frozen (−20°C). Plasma norepinephrine and plasma epinephrine were determined by a double-isotope derivative assay[17] with certain modifications.[18] For glucagon determination, 6 ml blood was drawn. Glucagon was measured with radioimmunoassay after ethanol extraction of plasma.[19] The antiserum employed (AB 4305)[20] does not cross-react significantly with enteroglucagon and measures decreasing glucagon concentrations during the 100 g oral glucose tolerance tests. Detection limit is below 20 pg/ml, and within-assay coefficient of variation is about 5%. Measurements of glucagon concentration in plasma with added exogenous hormone

FIGURE 1. The relationships between plasma norepinephrine and epinephrine levels, respectively, and work load, given as oxygen uptake ($\dot{V}_{O_2}$) in per cent of $\dot{V}_{O_2}$ max. The points represent measurements of catecholamines at rest, at 50 W, 75 W, and 100 W, and at exhaustion in patients with neuropathy and at rest, at 50 W, 75 W, 100 W, and 125 W, and at exhaustion in control patients. One patient with neuropathy and two patients without neuropathy were able to work for more than 2 min at loads higher than that eliciting $\dot{V}_{O_2}$ max. Extrapolated $\dot{V}_{O_2}$ is used to describe these work loads. Asterisks (*) denote significant difference ($P < 0.05$) between the two patient groups; open circles (○) denote significant ($P < 0.05$) difference from resting levels.

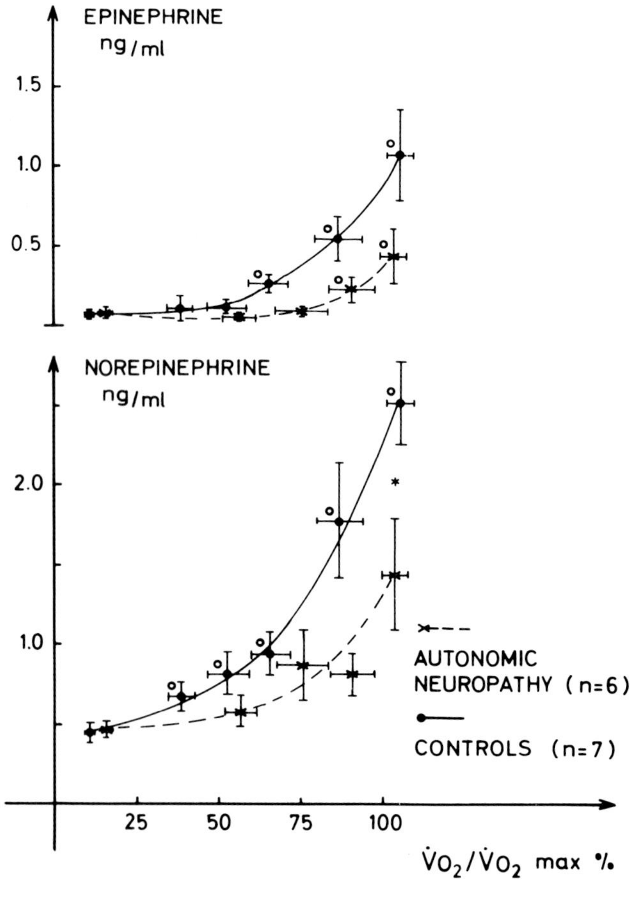

and in mixtures of plasma with different concentrations yielded results that deviated less than 10% from the expected values. Growth hormone (GH) and cortisol in serum were measured by commercially available solid phase radioimmunoassay kits (Phadebas and Byk-Mallinckrodt, respectively). One unit of GH equals 0.5 mg of the first international reference preparation of human GH (66/127) obtained from the National Institute for Biological Standards and Control, Holly Hill, London. The intra-assay coefficient of variation of the GH assay was 4% at 24 $\mu U \cdot ml^{-1}$, and the interassay coefficient of variation was 10%. The intra-assay coefficient of variation for the cortisol assay was 13% at 22 $\mu g \cdot 100\ ml^{-1}$, and the interassay coefficient of variation was 15%. Details concerning measurements of oxygen uptake and heart rate have been given elsewhere.[1] Packed cell volume was determined by the microhematocrit method.

Statistical evaluation was made by means of the Mann-Whitney U test for unpaired comparisons and by means of the Wilcoxon matched-pairs signed-ranks test for paired comparisons. Correlation analysis was made by means of the Spearman rank correlation coefficient test.[21] Differences were considered to be significant if P values less than 0.05 were obtained.

RESULTS

The relationships between relative work load, expressed as actual oxygen uptake in per cent of maximal oxygen uptake, and plasma norepinephrine and epinephrine levels, respectively, were shifted to the right in patients with autonomic neuropathy (Figure 1). A significant correlation was found between beat-to-beat variation and both plasma norepinephrine levels ($r_s = 0.66$, $P < 0.05$, $N = 13$) and plasma epinephrine levels ($r_s = 0.57$, $P < 0.05$, $N = 13$) at exhaustion. At exhaustion, plasma norepinephrine also correlated with threshold for sense of vibration ($r_s = -0.51$, $P < 0.05$, $N = 13$), and plasma epinephrine correlated with the blood glucose concentration ($r_s = -0.53$, $P < 0.05$, $N = 13$). An exponential relationship was found between heart rate and plasma norepinephrine as well as plasma epinephrine concentrations (Figure 2). During exercise the plasma concentrations of growth hormone and cortisol, but not of glucagon, increased significantly in control patients (Figure 3). No significant changes in these hormones were found in patients with autonomic neuropathy (Figure 3). At exhaustion, growth hormone levels correlated significantly with beat-to-beat variation ($r_s = 0.53$, $P < 0.05$, $N = 13$) as well as with threshold for sense of vibration ($r_s = -0.54$, $P < 0.05$, $N = 13$), and cortisol levels correlated significantly with the latter ($r_s = -0.61$, $P < 0.05$, $N = 12$). No significant differences in the concentrations of metabolites (Figures 4 and 5) were found between the two patient groups.*

The hematocrit rose significantly in both patient groups [from 46.3 ± 1.6% to 48.0 ± 1.5% (neuropathy) and from 49.7 ± 0.9% to 51.8 ± 1.1% (controls)]. The magnitude of plasma volume changes, as reflected by changes in hematocrit, was not sufficient to affect the interpretation of the results.

* In the three patients who were given apple juice, the responses of catecholamines, glucagon, growth hormone, cortisol, lactate, FFA, and glycerol were similar to those found in the other members of the respective group (controls or neuropathy). Blood glucose increased in the two control patients who were given apple juice (from 4.2 to 5.9 mmol/L and from 2.6 to 4.6 mmol/L, respectively) but not in the one patient with autonomic neuropathy. Beta-hydroxybutyric acid levels rose in all three patients after intake of apple juice but fell in the other patients throughout the experiments.

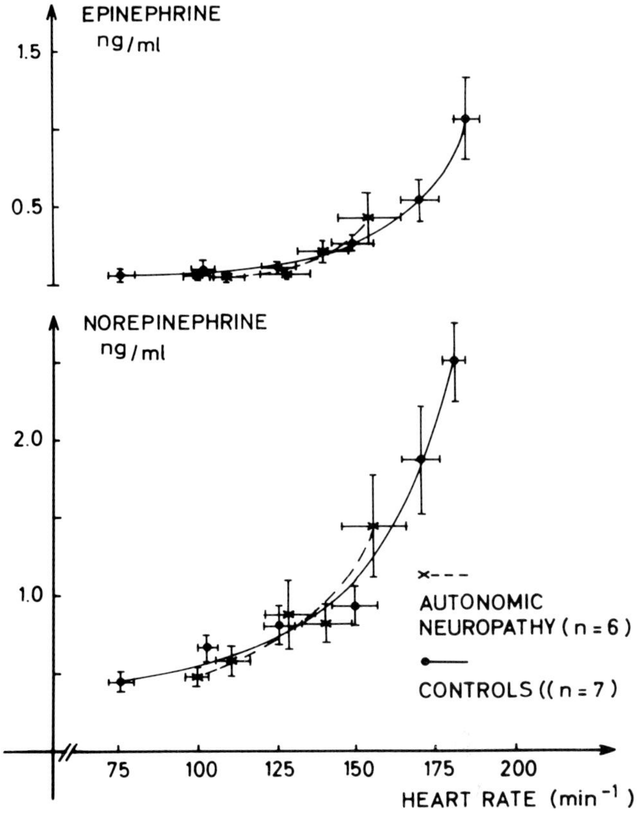

FIGURE 2. The relationship between heart rate and plasma catecholamine concentrations. For details, see legend to Figure 1.

DISCUSSION

In the present study, hormonal and metabolic responses to graded exercise were compared in diabetics with and without decreased beat-to-beat variation in heart rate during deep respiration. The main findings were diminished increments in plasma catecholamines and blunted responses of other glucoregulatory hormones in the patients with reduced beat-to-beat variation.

Mean plasma catecholamine levels tended to be higher in control patients than in patients with autonomic neuropathy at absolute work loads, but the differences were not significant. Nevertheless, evidence for impaired sympathetic function was found in patients with decreased beat-to-beat variation: For a given type of exercise in normals, the increased sympathetic outflow to the heart and to peripheral resistance vessels in the splanchnic area is more closely related to the oxygen uptake in per cent of the maximal oxygen uptake than to the actual load.[22,23] This is so, since the stress imposed by a certain work load depends on body size and degree of training. In diabetics with decreased beat-to-beat variation, the relationships between plasma norepinephrine and plasma epinephrine levels, respectively, and relative work load were shifted to the right compared with control patients (Figure 1). In other words, patients with decreased beat-to-beat variation had to be more

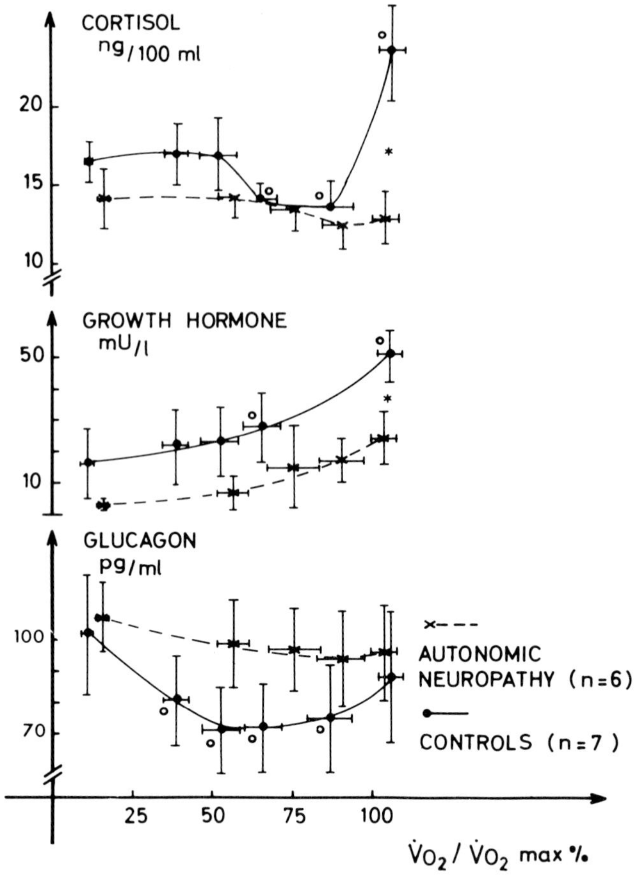

FIGURE 3. The relationship between glucagon, growth hormone, and cortisol levels in plasma, respectively, and work load, given as oxygen uptake ($\dot{V}_{O_2}$) in per cent of $\dot{V}_{O_2}$ max. For details, see legend to Figure 1.

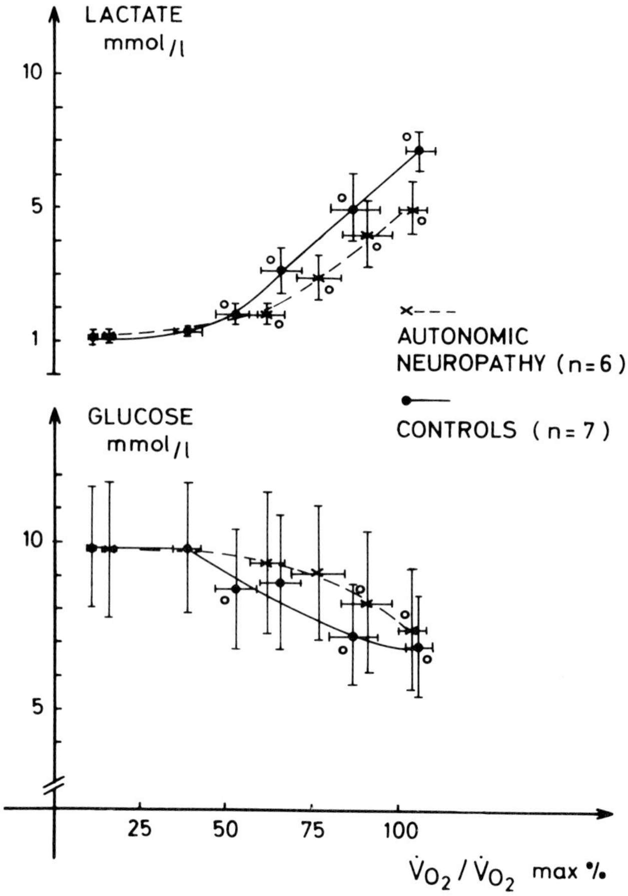

FIGURE 4. The relationship between blood glucose and lactate levels, respectively, and work load, given as oxygen uptake ($\dot{V}_{O_2}$) in per cent of $\dot{V}_{O_2}$ max. For details, see legend to Figure 1.

heavily stressed to reach a given plasma catecholamine level than did other patients.

The relationship between heart rate and plasma norepinephrine levels (Figure 2) in patients with autonomic neuropathy is not markedly different from the one found in control patients. This finding can be interpreted in three ways: (1) The patients with automatic neuropathy were not maximally loaded ($\dot{V}_{O_2}$ max was estimated too low); relative work load is, in that case, more correctly expressed by actual heart rate, (2) plasma norepinephrine (NE) is derived mainly from the heart; the shifts to the right of the relationships between NE concentrations (Figure 1) and heart rate (HR),[1] respectively, and relative work load then reflect the same phenomenon, namely, a decreased sympathetic outflow to the heart, (3) the sympathetic nerves to the heart and the sympathetic nerves from which plasma NE is derived (probably nerves to resistance vessels) are equally affected (if cardiac nerves were more affected, the NE/HR relationship would be shifted to the left; if, on the other hand, nerves producing circulating NE were more affected, the relationship would be shifted to the right in patients with autonomic neuropathy). Arguments for the assumption that a valid determination of maximal oxygen uptake was made have been given elsewhere.[1] Regarding the origin of circulating NE, it has been shown that the heart is not a major source of circulating NE.[24] The interpretation that sympathetic nerves to the heart and to resistance vessels are equally affected is supported by the previous finding of decreased tissue concentrations of catecholamines in heart as well as in arteries from deceased patients who had autonomic neuropathy.[25]

The relationship between plasma NE levels and relative work load (Figure 1) in control patients was similar to findings in normals, whereas the relationship between plasma epinephrine levels and relative work load was shifted to the left in control patients compared with normals (Galbo, H., and Christensen, N. J.; unpublished results). The increase in plasma epinephrine levels in control patients compared with normals is probably due to decreasing blood glucose levels in control patients (Figure 4) during the experiment, since decreasing blood glucose levels during exercise stimulate epinephrine secretion.[10] In normals, blood glucose levels remain constant or increase slightly during graded exercise.[7,9] The significant decrease in blood glucose levels in both patient groups is most likely explained by increased absorption of insulin from subcutaneous injection sites, as was previously reported in insulin-treated diabetics during exercise.[26]

A significant positive correlation was found between beat-to-beat variation (low values are considered a measure of cardiac vagal neuropathy[2]) and sympathetic activity, expressed as plasma NE and epinephrine concentrations at exhaustion, suggesting that dysfunction of the parasym-

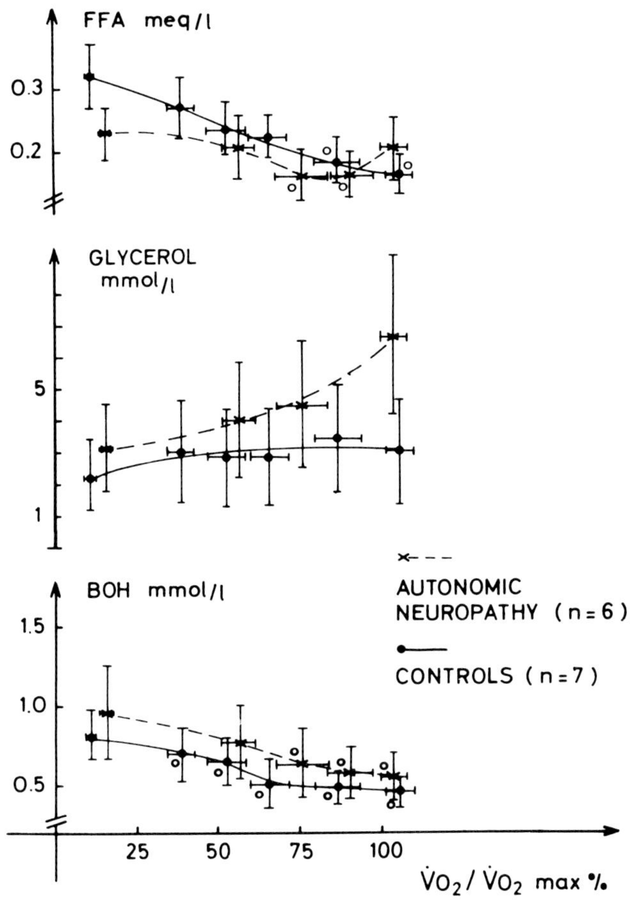

FIGURE 5. The relationship between FFA (serum), glycerol (serum), and blood beta-hydroxybutyric acid concentrations, respectively, and work load, given as oxygen uptake ($\dot{V}_{O_2}$) in per cent of $\dot{V}_{O_2}$ max. For details, see legend to Figure 1.

pathetic and the sympathetic nervous system in some respects may run parallel in patients with decreased beat-to-beat variation.

Also, the exercise responses of metabolites and of glucoregulatory hormones other than the catecholamines depend on body size and degree of training.[10,23] For this reason, responses of glucoregulatory hormones and metabolites are given as a function of relative work load (Figures 3–5). Plasma glucagon concentrations at exhaustion were not significantly different from resting levels in any of the two patient groups. This accords with previous findings[7,9] in normals during graded exercise. The observed differences in catecholamine responses found in this study, apparently, did not have any influence on glucagon responses to heavy exercise, a finding that is in accordance with the view that, in man, catecholamines have no major, enhancing effect on glucagon secretion during exercise.[27] In diabetics the growth hormone response to exercise can be suppressed by alpha-receptor blockade.[6] However, the lack of increase in growth hormone concentrations found in patients with decreased beat-to-beat variation in our study was not due to impaired peripheral sympathetic activity in these patients. This is so, since the alpha-adrenergic enhancement of growth hormone release is mediated by catecholamines released locally from neurons in the hypothalamus and not by peripherally secreted catecholamines.[28]

The increase in plasma cortisol levels found in this study in control patients is similar to that reported previously in normal man.[7,8] As previously stated,[1] the lower catecholamine levels in patients with autonomic neuropathy than in control patients may be due to lesions situated in central or peripheral neurons and in either afferent or efferent neurons. Growth hormone and cortisol responses to surgery have been shown to be mediated by impulses through afferent nerves.[29] Possibly, the impaired growth hormone and cortisol responses to exercise in patients with autonomic neuropathy are also due to neuronal damage. It has been suggested that glucoregulatory hormones may substitute for each other during exercise.[10] However, the reduced catecholamine levels found in the present study in patients with autonomic neuropathy were not accompanied by significant compensatory increments in growth hormone, glucagon, or cortisol.

Metabolic responses to graded exercise were similar in the two patient groups as judged from metabolite concentrations in plasma. This seems odd in the light of the differences in hormonal responses between the two groups. The dissociation between hormonal and metabolic responses may be interpreted as either a lack of essential influence of the measured hormones on the metabolic response to graded exercise or a change in sensitivity of adipose tissue and glycogen stores to the glucoregulatory hormones in patients with autonomic neuropathy.

ACKNOWLEDGMENTS

Glucagon antiserum was a gift from J. J. Holst, M.D., Institute of Medical Physiology C, University of Copenhagen.

Lisbeth Kall, Grethe Nielsen, Anne Boesen, and Else Stibolt Jensen gave skilled technical assistance.

Dr. Erik Lauritzen performed the ophthalmoscopic examinations.

The study was supported by grants from the Danish Medical Research Council and dr. med. Erik Garde and Elisabeth Gardes legat.

REFERENCES

[1] Hilsted, J., Galbo, H., and Christensen, N. J.: Impaired cardiovascular responses to graded exercise in diabetic autonomic neuropathy. Diabetes *28*:313–19, 1979.

[2] Hilsted, J., and Jensen, S. B.: A simple test for autonomic neuropathy in juvenile diabetics. Acta Med. Scand. *205*:385–87, 1979.

[3] Harvey, W. D., Faloona, G. R., Unger, R. H.: The effect of adrenergic blockade on exercise-induced hyperglucagonemia. Endocrinology *94*:1254–58, 1974.

[4] Luyckx, A. S., and Lefebvre, P. J.: Mechanisms involved in the exercise-induced increase in glucagon secretion in rats. Diabetes *23*:81–93, 1974.

[5] Hansen, Aa. P.: The effect of intravenous glucose infusion on the exercise-induced serum growth hormone rise in normals and juvenile diabetics. Scand. J. Clin. Lab. Invest. *28*:195–205, 1971.

[6] Hansen, Aa. P.: The effect of adrenergic receptor blockade on the exercise-induced serum growth hormone in normals and juvenile diabetics. J. Clin. Endocrinol. *33*:807–12, 1971.

[7] Bloom, S. R., Johnsen, R. H., Park, D. M., Rennie, M. J., and Sulaiman, W. R.: Differences in the metabolic and hormonal response to exercise between racing cyclists and untrained individuals. J. Physiol. (Lond.) *258*:1–18, 1976.

[8] Davies, C. T. M., and Few, J. D.: Effects of exercise on adrenocortical function. J. Appl. Physiol. *35*:887–91, 1973.

[9] Galbo, H., Holst, J. J., Christensen, N. J.: Glucagon and plasma catecholamine responses to graded and prolonged exercise in man. J. Appl. Physiol. *38*:70–76, 1975.

[10] Galbo, H., Richter, E. A., Hilsted, J., Holst, J. J., Christensen, N. J., and Henriksson, J.: Hormonal regulation during prolonged exercise. Ann. N.Y. Acad. Sci. *301*:72–90, 1977.

[11] Jerslid, M., and Lauritzen, E.: Sensibilité vibratoire chéz les diabetiques. Diabetes *6*:237–41, 1957.

[12] Schmidt, F. H.: Die enzymatische Bestimmung von Glucose und Fructose nebeneinander. Klin. Wochenschr. *39*:1244–47, 1961.

[13] Hohorst, H. J.: Methode der Enzymatische Analyse. Weinheim, Verlag Chemie, 1970, pp. 1425–29.

[14] Duncombe, W. G.: The colorimetric micro-determination of non-esterified fatty acids in plasma. Clin. Chim. Acta *9*:122–24, 1964.

[15] Eggstein, M., and Kreutz, F. H.: Eine neue Bestimmung der Neutralfette im Blutserum and Gewebe. Klin. Wochenschr. *44*:262–67, 1966.

[16] Olsen, C.: An enzymatic fluorimetric micromethod for the determination of acetoacetate, β-hydroxybutyrate, pyruvate and lactate. Clin. Chim. Acta *33*:293–300, 1971.

[17] Engelman, K., and Portnoy, B.: A sensitive double-isotope derivative assay for norepinephrine and epinephrine. Circ. Res. *26*:53–57, 1970.

[18] Christensen, N. J.: Plasma noradrenaline and adrenaline in patients with thyrotoxicosis and myxedema. Clin. Sci. *45*:163–71, 1973.

[19] Heding, L. G.: Radioimmunological determination of pancreatic and gut glucagon in plasma. Diabetologia *7*:10–19, 1971.

[20] Holst, J. J., and Aasted, B.: Production and evaluation of glucagon antibodies for radioimmunoassay. Acta Endocrinol. *77*:715–26, 1974.

[21] Siegel, S.: Non-parametric Statistics for the Behavioral Sciences. McGraw-Hill, Kogalenska, 1956.

[22] Clausen, J. P.: Effect of physical training on cardiovascular adjustments to exercise in man. Physiol. Rev. *57*:779–815, 1977.

[23] Horvath, S. M.: Review of energetics and blood flow in exercise. Diabetes *28*(Suppl. 1):33–38, 1979.

[24] Fisher Hansen, J., Christensen, N. J., and Hesse: B.: Determinants of coronary sinus noradrenaline in patients with ischaemic heart disease: coronary sinus catecholamine concentration in relation to arterial catecholamine concentration, pulmonary artery oxygen saturation and left ventricular end-diastolic pressure. Cardiovasc. Res. *12*:415–21, 1978.

[25] Neubauer, B., and Christensen, N. J.: Norepinephrine, epinephrine and dopamine contents of the cardiovascular system in long-term diabetics. Diabetes *25*:6–10, 1976.

[26] Berger, M., Halban, P. A., Assal, J. P., Offord, R. E., Vranic, M., and Renold, A. E.: Pharmacokinetics of subcutaneously injected tritiated insulin: effects of exercise. Diabetes *28*(Suppl. 1): 53–57, 1979.

[27] Galbo, H., Holst, J. J., Christensen, N. J., and Hilsted, J.: Glucagon and plasma catecholamines during beta-receptor blockade in exercising man. J. Appl. Physiol. *40*:855–63, 1976.

[28] Blackard, W. G., and Hubbell, G. J.: Stimulatory effect of exogenous catecholamines on plasma HGH concentrations in presence of beta adrenergic blockade. Metabolism *19*:547–52, 1970.

[29] Kehlet, H.: Influence of epidural analgesia on the endocrine-metabolic response to surgery. Acta Anaesthesiol. Scand. (Suppl. 70): 39–42, 1978.

Beta-Cell Electrical Activity in Response to High Glucose Concentration

PAUL M. BEIGELMAN AND BERNARD RIBALET

SUMMARY

Glucose-induced β-cell electrical activity, recorded with glass microelectrodes, is characterized by trains of fast action potentials ("spikes"). The membrane depolarizes before each train of spikes and then repolarizes. This pattern is termed a "burst." There is a characteristic biphasic response to a square wave of 11.1 mM glucose. Pulses at higher glucose concentrations (22.2 mM or more) evoke transient, constant spike activity. The duration of this activity is lengthened and the lag period shortened in proportion to the concentration and length of the glucose pulse. The lag period between removal of glucose and the cessation of spike activity is also proportional to the glucose concentration. DIABETES *29*:263–265, April 1980.

Mouse pancreatic β-cell electrical activity, recorded by using glass microelectrodes, is characterized by phasic response to glucose, which appears to be related to insulin secretion.[1-8]

In the present study, electrical responses to short pulses of glucose at varying concentrations are presented. It is shown that the duration of electrical activity is proportional to glucose concentration and duration of the glucose stimulus. As the glucose concentration was augmented, there was a decrease of the lag period between the beginning of the glucose pulse and the electrical response, as well as an increase of the persistence of "spike" activity after glucose removal.

A recent abstract by Atwater and Malaisse[9] reports the effects upon β-cell electrical activity of 56 mM glucose in 2–5-s pulses. A minimum pulse of 3 s was required to elicit an electrical response, which occurred 15 s after glucose perifusion. There was an increased duration of activity in response to higher glucose pulses or pulses of more prolonged duration and a shortened duration of the lag period, the decrease being proportional to glucose concentration and the duration of the pulse.

METHODS

The techniques used have been previously described in detail.[4-7] Partially dissected mouse pancreatic islets were perifused at 37°C with a Krebs-Ringer bicarbonate solution. The β-cells were impaled with glass microelectrodes. Addition of glucose was made without adjusting for changes in osmolarity so as to maintain constant sodium concentration. No effect upon electrical activity was noted due to an increased osmolarity of 100 mosmol using a nonpermeable carbohydrate, sucrose. Similar observations have been reported by Atwater and Malaisse.[9] The glucose concentrations varied from 11.1 to 111.2 mM. A 5–10-min control period without glucose always preceded glucose stimulation.

As previously reported, the β-cell electrical activity was identified in a solution containing 11.1 mM glucose.[1-6] The activity is described as a periodic, slow membrane depolarization (a), followed by a rapid depolarization (b), to a plateau where fast action potentials ("spikes") are elicited (c), and ending with membrane repolarization (d) (Figure 1). In this study, electrical activity has been designated as the first appearance of spikes > 5 mV.

Five seconds were required for a new solution to reach the chamber after change. Four seconds were required for a total exchange of solution in the chamber, the volume of the chamber being 0.6 ml and flow rate 5 ml/min. As an approximation of the appropriate correction factor, 5 s was subtracted from the observed lag time between change of solution and commencement of electrical activity (spikes) with elevated (22.2 mM or more) glucose, since the dilutional effect in such a small chamber would be negligible (less than 1 s). With 11.1 mM glucose, total exchange of solution within the chamber would be necessary to elicit spike activity, so 10 s was subtracted from the observed lag period.

From the Departments of Medicine and Pharmacology, University of Southern California School of Medicine, Los Angeles, California.
Address reprint requests to Paul M. Beigelman, M.D., Department of Medicine, University of Southern California School of Medicine, 2025 Zonal Avenue, Los Angeles, California 90033.
Received for publication 14 May and in revised form 23 October 1979.

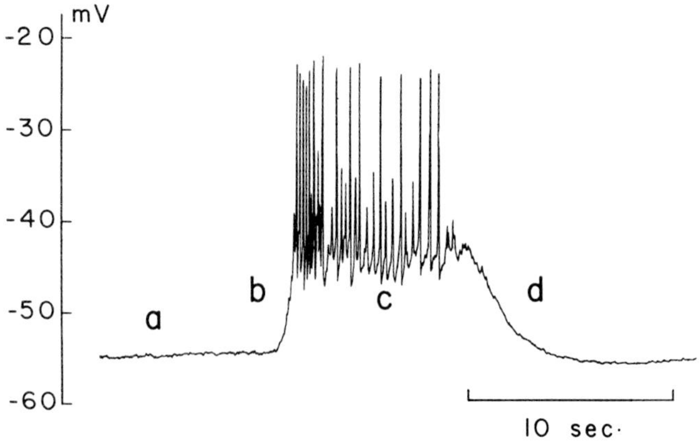

FIGURE 1. "Bursts" of "spikes" in a β-cell stimulated by 11.1 mM glucose. The burst begins with slow depolarization (a), followed by a rapid depolarization (b), to a plateau (c) with fast action potentials (spikes), and terminates with postburst silent hyperpolarization (d).

These corrections can be subjected to criticism since it is not possible to determine the precise concentration of glucose at the surface of the β-cell. Nevertheless, this variation should not exceed $^1/_{10}$ of the maximum time subtracted, about 1 s.

In each figure the arrows represent change of solution at the stopcock. The correction factors are used for the data given in the text.

RESULTS

The lag periods observed between the beginning of a glucose stimulus and the electrical responses of β-cells were compared at two glucose concentrations: 11.1 and 55.6 mM. In most experiments, the effects of 11.1 and 55.6 mM glucose were studied in the same cell, with alternating pulses at these two concentrations given in random succession. The experiments with 11.1 mM glucose were performed in 16 β-cells from 14 mice; 55.6 mM glucose was given in 10-s pulses in 12 cells and as a prolonged stimulus of 3–4 min in 4 cells. There was no significant difference between lag periods obtained with 55.6 mM glucose for a 10-s pulse compared with a square wave perifusion of 3–4 min. The mean lag periods were 105 ± 10 s for 11.1 mM glucose and 45 ± 5 s for 55.6 mM glucose ($P < 0.001$). Following a square wave of glucose, the continuation of spike activity after the removal of glucose was significantly greater at 55.6 mM glucose (175 ± 10 s) as compared with that at 11.1 mM glucose (25 ± 5 s) ($P < 0.001$). Shortening of the lag period and increased duration of spike activity proportionate to glucose concentration is indicated in Figure 2, which shows a cell stimulated with 20-s pulses of glucose. An 11.1-mM glucose pulse caused only slight depolarization, whereas 22.2 mM glucose evoked, following a 65-s lag period, 20 s of spike activity. A 33.3-mM glucose pulse caused shortening of the lag period to 40 s. Further decrease of the lag period to 30 s and increase of spike activity duration to 100 s was observed as the glucose was increased to 55.6 mM.

At 11.1 mM glucose, a minimum duration of 30 s for the pulse was required to elicit spike activity. However, pulses of shorter duration could evoke silent depolarization (Figure 3, upper panel). A 30-s pulse of 11.1 mM glucose elicited a 10-s response of small spikes and a few large spikes (Figure 3, upper panel). A 60-s pulse increased the duration of electrical response to 35 s, and 65 s of spike activity occurred after a 90-s pulse of 11.1 mM glucose (Figure 3, upper panel). The lag period between glucose stimulus and spike activity was 80–85 s. In the same cell, a 2-s pulse of 55.6 mM glucose was sufficient to evoke spike activity lasting 25 s; a lag period of 65 s was observed. A 4-s pulse of 55.6 mM glucose in this cell reduced the lag period to 55 s and increased the duration of spike activity to 80 s. A 6-s pulse further reduced the lag period to 50 s and increased spike activity to 105 s (Figure 2, lower panel).

Figure 4 shows the effects upon electrical activity of a square increase of glucose, at various concentrations, for longer periods of time. There was a normal biphasic response to 11.1 mM glucose, with a 70-s lag period until commencement of spike activity, and a 40-s period between removal of glucose and silent hyperpolarization. In the

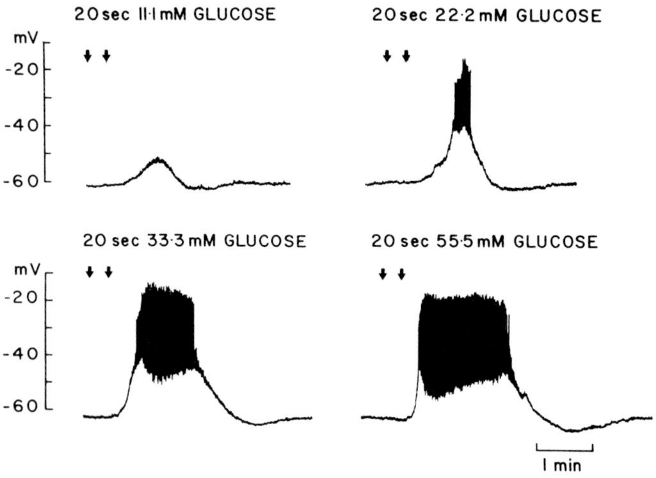

FIGURE 2. Effect upon electrical activity of a short pulse of glucose at varying concentrations. The double arrows enclose the 20-s pulse. All results were obtained in the same cell.

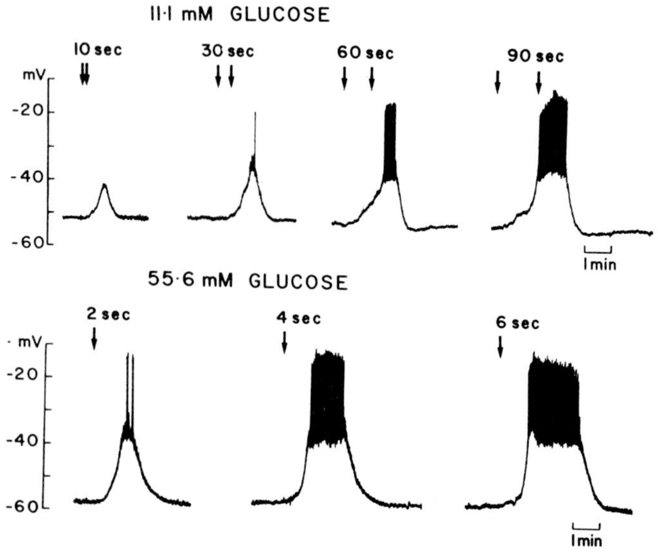

FIGURE 3. Effect of pulse duration upon electrical activity at 11.1 and 55.6 mM glucose. Upper panel represents pulses of 10-, 30-, 60-, and 90-s duration with 11.1 mM glucose. Lower panel depicts pulses of 2-, 4-, and 6-s duration with 55.6 mM glucose. All results were obtained in the same cell.

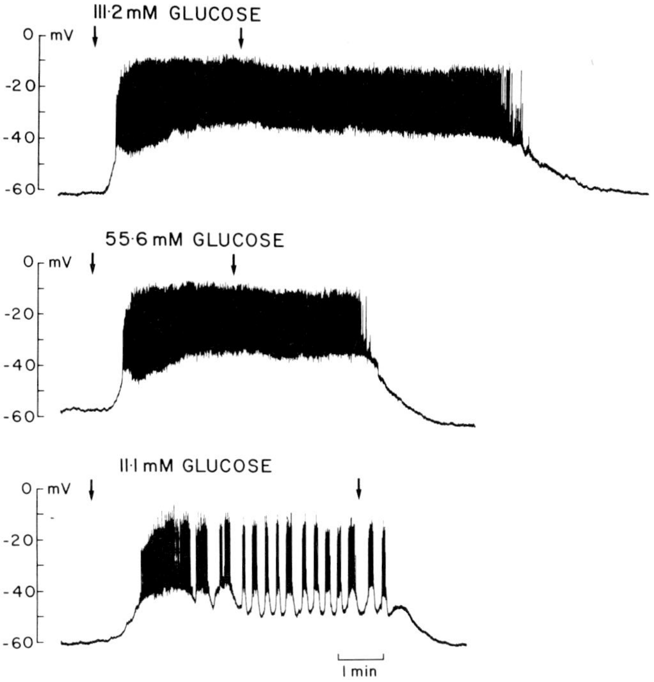

FIGURE 4. Effect of prolonged perifusion of varying glucose concentrations. Arrows indicate 4-min perifusion with 55.6 mM (middle panel) and 111.2 mM glucose (upper panel), and 10-min perifusion with 11.1 mM glucose (lower panel). All observations were made in the same cell.

same cell, a 55.6-mM square increase of glucose evoked electrical activity after a shortened lag period of 35 s. This activity persisted for 190 s after glucose removal. With 111.2 mM glucose, the lag period was further decreased to 25 s and constant spike activity continued for 380 s after removal of glucose.

DISCUSSION

Idahl[10] noted that an increase of intermediates of glucose metabolism, glucose-6-phosphate and fructose-1,6-diphosphate, significantly preceded insulin secretion in perifused mouse islets, with an increase to greater than one-half maximum of glucose-6-phosphate as early as 20 s after a square wave increase of peri-insular glucose concentration. The insulin release in response to 17 mM glucose was delayed not less than 80 s, which is comparable to our results with 11.1 mM glucose. As shown by Atwater et al.,[8] there is a definite time relationship between periodicity of spike activity and insulin secretion from an individual islet. Therefore, the shortened lag period and increased duration of activity noted at higher glucose concentrations may possibly indicate a contracted time span between application of glucose and increase of glucose metabolites, possibly related to the amount of metabolites. The increase of such metabolites, in turn, may decrease the time interval of insulin release.

There is a growing awareness of the physiologic importance of the lag period between application of a glucose stimulus and response of electrical activity and insulin release, particularly the shortening of the lag phase as prestimulus perifusion glucose concentration was elevated.[5,11,12] It has been proposed that a dual system may work in which there is (1) an effector of β-cell membrane surface receptor sites, with immediate response, and (2) substrate metabolism, causing a more delayed response.[12] This hypothesis is also consistent with our data and might indicate the reason for very high glucose having an almost immediate effect. The prolonged duration of electrical response to high glucose pulses suggests that very transient, even fleeting, elevations of serum glucose may profoundly affect the physiology of the normal β-cell.

ACKNOWLEDGMENTS

This work was suppored, in part, by grants from the American Diabetes Association and the Juvenile Diabetes Foundation.

REFERENCES

[1] Dean, P. M., and Matthews, E. K.: Glucose-induced electrical activity in pancreatic islet cell. J. Physiol. (Lond.) *210*:255–64, 1970.

[2] Meissner, H. P., and Schmelz, H.: Membrane potential of beta-cells in pancreatic islets. Pfluegers Arch. *351*:195–206, 1974.

[3] Meissner, H. P.: Electrical characteristics of the beta cells in pancreatic islets. J. Physiol. (Paris) *72*:757–67, 1976.

[4] Atwater, I., and Beigelman, P. M.: Dynamic characteristics of electrical activity in pancreatic β-cells: 1. Effects of calcium and magnesium removal. J. Physiol. (Paris) *72*:769–86, 1976.

[5] Beigelman, P. M., Ribalet, B., and Atwater, I.: Electrical activity of pancreatic beta cells: effects of glucose and arginine. J. Physiol. (Paris) *73*:201–17, 1977.

[6] Atwater, I., Ribalet, B., and Rojas, E.: Cyclic changes in potential and resistance of the β-cell membrane induced by glucose in islets of Langerhans from mouse. J. Physiol. (Lond.) *278*:117–39, 1978.

[7] Ribalet, B., and Beigelman, P. M.: Cyclic variation of K^+ conductance in pancreatic β-cells: Ca^{++} and voltage dependence. Am. J. Physiol. *237*:c137–46, 1979.

[8] Atwater, I., Rojas, E., and Scott, A.: Simultaneous measurements of insulin release and electrical activity in single microdissected islets of Langerhans. J. Physiol. (Lond.) *291*:57P, 1979.

[9] Atwater, I., and Malaisse, W.: Timing the stimulus-secretion coupling with glucose: glucoreceptor or metabolic by-product? Diabetologia *13*:379, 1977.

[10] Idahl, L. A.: Dynamics of pancreatic β-cell responses to glucose. Diabetologia *9*:403–12, 1973.

[11] Lenzen, S.: The immediate insulin-secretory response of the rat pancreas to glucose compared with tolbutamide and other secretagogues. Diabetes *27*:27–34, 1978.

[12] Vague, P., Ramahandridona, G., DiCampo, C., and Mahmoud, F.: Kinetics of early insulin response by the isolated and perifused rat pancreas. Suggestion for two different actions of glucose on the insulin releasing process. Horm. Metab. Res. *9*:453–56, 1977.

Effects of Acute Variation of Fetal Glycemia on Glycogen Storage and on Glycogen Synthase and Phosphorylase Activities in the Liver of the Rat Fetus

M. GILBERT AND J. BOURBON

SUMMARY

The effects of variations of glycemia from 1.7 to 35 mM on the activity of glycogen synthase and phosphorylase, on glycogen content, and on U-^{14}C-glucose incorporation into glycogen in the liver of the near-term rat fetus were investigated. Hypoglycemia did not affect the activities of phosphorylase and synthase; total glycogen content was not modified, but incorporation of labeled glucose was markedly decreased. This is consistent with a decreased glycogen synthesis. A slight hyperglycemia (about 5.5 mM) sharply decreased phosphorylase a (active) activity but increased slightly glycogen synthase a activity; liver glycogen content and labeled glucose incorporation were both enhanced. Higher levels of glycemia induced a decrease of phosphorylase a activity of the same order, but by contrast, glycogen synthase a activity increased progressively with increasing glycemia. Sequential study showed that hyperglycemia first induced the decrease of phosphorylase activity, then increased synthase activity. Marked hyperglycemia strongly enhanced liver glycogen content and labeled glucose incorporation. The fetal liver appears very responsive to acute variations of glycemia. The mechanisms seem to be oriented toward maximal glycogen accumulation. DIABETES 29:266–271, April 1980.

The fetal liver accumulates glycogen at the end of gestation. This accumulation is under hormonal control.[1] However, little is known about the influence of nutritional factors on glycogen accumulation. Severe starvation in the pregnant rat is associated both with decreased fetal glycemia and decreased fetal liver glycogen.[2–5] Glucose infusion to the pregnant starved rat increases fetal liver glycogen.[2]

From the Laboratoire de Physiologie du Développement du Collège de France, Paris.

Address reprint requests to M. Gilbert, Laboratoire de Physiologie du Développement, Collège de France, II, place Marcelin Berthelot, 75231 Paris Cédex 05, France.

Received for publication 13 September 1979 and in revised form 15 November 1979.

The present work is an attempt to determine to what extent variations of maternal glycemia affect glycogen accumulation in the fetal liver. We studied the effects of acute variations of plasma glucose (hypoglycemia, moderate hyperglycemia, and marked hyperglycemia) on glycogen storage and on synthase and phosphorylase activities in the liver of the fetuses of normal fed rats. These experimental conditions were obtained through maternal venous infusion of saline, insulin, or glucose solutions.

MATERIALS AND METHODS

The study was made on female rats of the Wistar strain weighing approximately 280–320 g and fed ad libitum. Gestation was verified 14 days after mating, by abdominal palpation, and the fetal age determined according to Jost and Picon.[1]

UDP-U-^{14}C-glucose (312 mCi/mmol) and D-U-^{14}C-glucose (3.05 mCi/mmol) came from the Radiochemical Centre (Amersham, Bucks, G.B.). UDP-glucose, glucose 6-phosphate, glucose 1-phosphate, and oyster glycogen were obtained from Calbiochem (San Diego, California). Amylo, α-1,4,α-1,6-glucosidase and glucose oxidase (Perid method) were provided by Boehringer (Mannheim, Germany). Other chemicals were obtained from Prolabo (Paris, France).

Pregnant rats were anesthetized with an intraperitoneal injection of sodium pentobarbital (30 mg/kg body wt). A primed steady state infusion technique was used. The rats were infused through the saphenous vein. For control fetuses, mothers were infused with saline solution (NaCl 0.9%); for hypoglycemic fetuses, infusion of insulin solution was used (5 iU/ml at a rate of 6 iU/h); and for hyperglycemic fetuses, infusion of glucose solution 30% w/v through the saphenous vein was given. A priming dose of 1 ml was rapidly infused (2 min), followed by a constant infusion. Fetal blood glucose levels in the range of from 5.5 to 32 mM were obtained by altering the infusion rate from 1.2 to 4.5 ml/h. In some experiments U-^{14}C-glucose was added in trace amount to the glucose, insulin, or saline infusions.

Fetal blood was collected from exteriorized fetuses, (whose placenta was left in situ) with a heparinized pipette at the level of the armpit vessels. The livers were immediately placed in liquid N_2 and stored at −20°C for enzymatic assays and glycogen determinations.

Glycogen synthase (EC 2.4.1.11) activity was measured by incorporation of U-^{14}C-glucose from UDP-U-^{14}C-glucose into glycogen. The incorporated radioactivity was measured after adsorption of an aliquot of incubation mixture on filter paper. Active synthase a (active) was measured by the method of De Wulf and Hers.[6] The liver was homogenized with 3 vol of ice-cold solution containing 150 mM sucrose and 100 mM glycylglycine buffer (pH 7.4); 0.02 ml of homogenate was incubated for 10 min at 20°C in a final volume of 0.2 ml containing 0.2 μmol of UDP-glucose + UDP-U-^{14}C-glucose (100 c.p.m./nmol), 1 mg of glycogen, 6 μmol of glycylglycine buffer (pH 7.4), 1 μmol of Na_2SO_4, and 0.5 μmol of EDTA. Then 0.1 ml of the mixture was placed on a piece (2 × 2 cm) of Whatman 31 ET chromatography paper (according to Thomas et al.[7]) and the reaction stopped by placing the paper in cold ethanol. The papers were washed three times (3 × 10 min) with 66% ethanol. Papers rinsed with acetone and dried were placed in vials containing 10 ml of scintillation liquid (P.C.S. Amersham, Searle). The radioactivity was measured in a Nuclear Chicago (Mark 1) liquid scintillation spectrometer. Activity was expressed in μmoles of glucose incorporated into glycogen per min/g wet liver (i.e., units/g wet liver). In a few cases, total (a + b) glycogen synthase activity was measured according to Devos and Hers.[8]

Phosphorylase (EC 2.4.1.1) was assayed by measuring Pi released during incorporation of glucose 1-phosphate into glycogen. Only the active form of phosphorylase a was determined according to Hue et al.[9] Pieces of liver were homogenized in 10 vol of ice-cold solution containing 100 mM NaF, 20 mM EDTA, 0.5% (w/v) glycogen, and 50 mM glycylglycine (pH 7.4). One-tenth milliliter of the homogenate was incubated for 30 min at 20°C, with an equal volume of a mixture containing 100 mM glucose 1-phosphate, 2% (w/v) glycogen, 0.3 mM NaF, and 1 mM caffeine (pH 6.1). The reaction was stopped by adding 0.5 ml of 10% (w/v) trichloroacetic acid. The mixture was centrifuged (16,000 × *g*, 2 min) and Pi assayed in the supernatant as described by Fiske and Subbarow.[10] The activity was expressed as μmoles Pi released/min/g wet liver (i.e., units/g wet liver).

The technique for glycogen determination in the fetal liver was that described by Roehrig and Allred.[11] When U-^{14}C-glucose was added to the 30% glucose or saline infusion, the glycogen content of the liver and radioactivity incorporated into glycogen were simultaneously determined according to the method of Chan and Exton.[12] Frozen liver was weighed and homogenized (2.5%) in twice distilled water with a glass teflon homogenizer. One-tenth milliliter of the homogenate was spotted on a piece (2 × 3 cm) of filter paper (Whatman 3 MM chromatography paper). The papers were dropped into a beaker containing 66% ethanol and washed three times (3 × 10 min). They were then briefly rinsed with acetone, dried, and placed in plastic tubes containing 0.4 ml acetate buffer (0.05 M, pH 4.5), 1.6 ml H_2O, and 0.02 ml of amylo,α-1,4,α-1,6-glucosidase (3 U). The tubes were placed at 55°C for 30 min to allow hydrolysis of glycogen. Glucose was determined in 0.1 ml of hydrolysate with the glucose oxidase method. Hydrolyzed oyster glycogen was used as the standard. One milliliter of the hydrolysate was placed in a vial containing 10 ml of scintillation liquid (P.C.S. Amersham, Searle, G.B.), and radioactivity was measured in the liquid scintillation spectrometer.

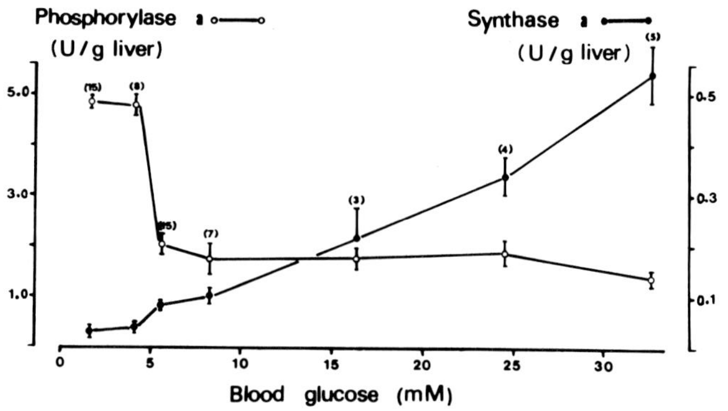

FIGURE 1. Effect of blood glucose concentration on glycogen synthase and phosphorylase activities in the fetal liver. On day 21.5 of pregnancy, maternal glucose or insulin infusion was sustained during 60 min. At the end of this time period the activity of phosphorylase (○——○) and synthase (●——●) was measured on the same liver. The activities have been measured at different fetal blood glucose concentrations (between 1.7 and 32 mM). Values are means ± SEM with the number of experiments in parentheses.

Means of the experimental series were compared by Student's *t* test.

RESULTS

Relation between fetal glycemia and enzyme activities. The activity of phosphorylase a and glycogen synthase a was measured at different blood glucose concentrations in 21.5-day-old fetuses. The maternal infusions of saline, insulin, or glucose were continued for 60 min in different experiments. Saline infusion did not modify fetal blood glucose level (Figure 3). Hypoglycemia between 3.5 and 1.7 mM did not affect the activity of phosphorylase and synthase. Hyperglycemia between 3.5 and 5.5 mM increased glycogen synthase and decreased phosphorylase activity. Higher levels of glycemia induced a decrease of the phosphorylase activity of the same order (Figure 1). By contrast, glycogen synthase activity increased progressively with increasing glycemia.

The activity of synthase was plotted versus the corresponding value of phosphorylase for each liver in Figure 2. There is an inverse correlation between the activities of these enzymes.

Sequential study of glycogen synthase and phosphorylase activities during glucose infusion (marked hyperglycemia). Glycogen synthase a and glycogen phosphorylase a activities were determined 15, 30, 60, and 150 min after the beginning of maternal infusion with 30% glucose solution (3 ml/h) on day 21.5 of gestation. Controls were obtained by saline infusion at the same rate. Saline infusion did not significantly modify fetal glycemia nor the enzymatic activities at any time.

Ten minutes after beginning glucose infusion, the fetal glycemia increased to 15 mM and afterward remained stable (Figure 3). Activity of glycogen synthase a was not modified for 15 min. A sharp increase occurred between 30 and 60 min, while between 60 and 150 min there was a decrease of enzymatic activity (Figure 3). A similar pattern was

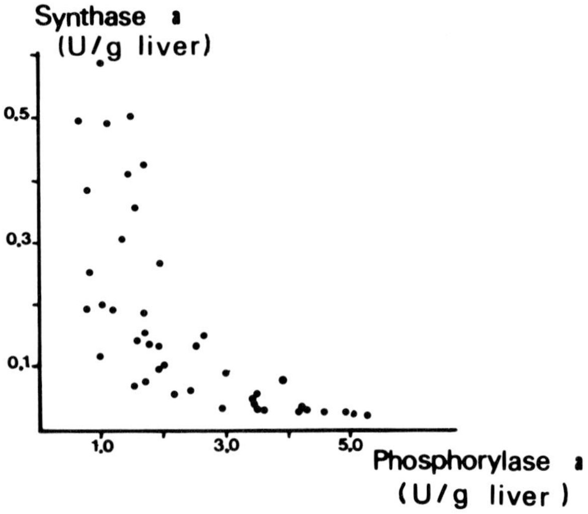

FIGURE 2. Correlation between the activity of synthase and phosphorylase in fetal liver. Values of glycogen synthase shown in Figure 1 have been plotted versus the corresponding values of glycogen phosphorylase.

observed in 18.5-, 19.5-, and 20.5-day-old fetuses (data not shown).

The increase of synthase a activity resulted from an activation of the enzyme, not from synthesis, since the total activity (a + b) was not enhanced (initial value = 1.18 ± 0.45 U/g liver; final value = 1.21 ± 0.40 U/g liver).

The activity of phosphorylase a decreased during the first 30 min and afterward remained practically unchanged (Figure 3). The same was observed on days 19.5 and 20.5. At 18.5 days, the decrease occurred only after 30 min and was transitory (data not shown).

Relation between fetal glycemia, liver glycogen content, and incorporation of labeled glucose into liver glycogen. On day 21.5 of gestation, maternal infusions of tracer amounts of U-^{14}C-glucose were made during 150 min under the following four experimental conditions: normoglycemia with saline infusion (2 μCi/ml, 2.2 ml/h); hypoglycemia with insulin infusion, 5 iU/ml (1.2 μCi/ml, 2.2 ml/h); moderate hyperglycemia with 30% glucose solution (3 μCi/ml, 1.2 ml/h); and marked hyperglycemia with 30% glucose solution (11 μCi/ml, 3 ml/h). Under these conditions specific radioactivities of blood glucose were approximately the same.

Fetal hypoglycemia did not modify the liver glycogen content compared with fetuses of normoglycemic mothers, but labeled glucose incorporation into glycogen was strongly decreased (Figure 4). Moderate hyperglycemia (about 5.5 mM) increased slightly but significantly the fetal liver glycogen content ($P < 0.01$) and glucose incorporation ($P < 0.001$) compared with fetuses of saline-infused mothers (Figure 4). Marked hyperglycemia (about 15 mM) strongly increased both fetal liver glycogen content and labeled glucose incorporation (Figure 4).

Effect of marked hyperglycemia on liver glycogen content as a function of fetal age. Fetal glycemia and liver glycogen were determined in 17.5–21.5-day-old fetuses under three experimental conditions: (1) immediately after anesthesia of the mother; (2) after a 150-min saline infusion to the mother; and (3) after a 150-min 30% glucose infusion to the mother. Fetal glycemia is reported in Table 1. After

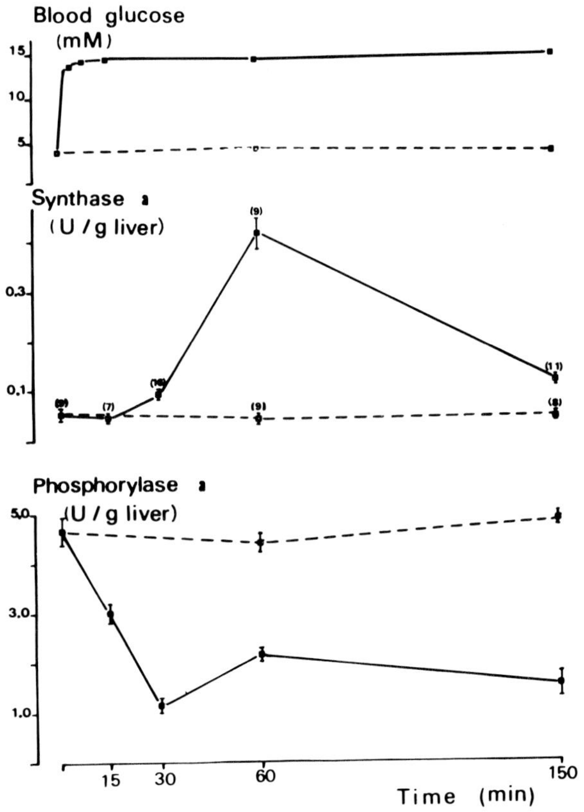

FIGURE 3. Sequential activation of glycogen synthase and inactivation of glycogen phosphorylase in the fetal liver on day 21.5 of gestation. The pregnant rat was infused with either saline (---) or glucose solution (——). At different time intervals after the beginning of maternal infusion, synthase and phosphorylase activities were measured in the same liver. Fetal hyperglycemia occurred only at 5, 15, 60, and 150 min. Values are means ± SEM of the number of determinations shown in parentheses.

glucose infusion, it was about 8–10 times higher than that of control fetuses (saline infusion) from day 17.5 to day 21.5. At all stages, there was no difference between the glycemia of fetuses taken at time zero and that of fetuses taken after saline infusion.

Liver glycogen is reported in Figure 5. Saline infusion did not affect glycogen content at any stage. In 17.5- or 18.5-day-old fetuses, liver glycogen concentration after glucose infusion was not modified compared with fetuses of saline-infused dams. In the liver of 19.5-, 20.5-, and 21.5-day-old fetuses, glycogen concentration was increased by about 30% after glucose infusion.

DISCUSSION

The results reported in Figure 1 indicate that a slight fetal hyperglycemia (5.5 mM) induced a decrease of glycogen phosphorylase activity as striking as that seen with very high glycemia (32 mM); the changes observed indicate that a slight increase of fetal blood glucose may be sufficient to control fetal liver glycogen metabolism.

By contrast, glycogen synthase activity progressively increased until glycemia reached 32 mM. Similar observations were obtained with glucose levels extending from 5 to 55 mM in the perfused adult rat liver,[13] in the isolated rat liver cells,[9] and in the liver of rats and mice in vivo.[14] The results plotted in Figure 2 indicates that the glycogen synthase activity is enhanced only in livers in which the level of

TABLE 1
Fetal glycemia (mM) immediately after anesthesia of the mother (controls) and after a 150-min maternal saline or glucose infusion at different stages of pregnancy

	Days of gestation				
	17.5	18.5	19.5	20.5	21.5
Controls		2.7 ± 0.3 (12)	2.4 ± 0.2 (25)	2.6 ± 0.2 (13)	3.6 ± 0.2 (32)
Saline infusion	1.1 ± 0.2 (14)	1.3 ± 0.1 (18)	1.8 ± 0.2 (12)	2.2 ± 0.3 (23)	3.3 ± 0.2 (18)
Glucose infusion	16.7 ± 0.2 (14)	14.3 ± 0.2 (20)	15.2 ± 0.1 (13)	13.1 ± 0.1 (22)	15.0 ± 0.1 (31)

Values are means ± SEM of the number of determinations shown in parentheses.

phosphorylase is lower than a value of 2 U. Since an increase of fetal blood glucose produced an inactivation of glycogen phosphorylase and an activation of glycogen synthase, this sequence of events might be the biochemical expression of the concept of hepatic threshold to glucose initially proposed by Soskin.[15]

Sustained fetal hyperglycemia (Figure 4) induced firstly an inactivation of the major part of the glycogen phosphorylase followed by an activation of the glycogen synthase. The same sequence has been observed in adult rats[14] and monkeys[16] as well as in the perfused liver[13,17] and in isolated hepatocytes.[9] The apparent existence of a threshold of phosphorylase activity for synthase activation suggests that the response of fetal liver to glucose obeys the pattern proposed by Hers and co-workers.[14] One can assume that, as shown in the adult rat liver, the primary effect of glucose is to bind to phosphorylase a[18] and to favor the conversion of this enzyme into phosphorylase b (inactive form) by phosphorylase phosphatase.[19] Since phosphorylase a is a strong inhibitor of glycogen synthase phosphatase,[20] its disappearance would be a prerequisite for the activation of glycogen synthase, which occurs in a second step. Thus, the difference in the response of the two enzymes may permit a better stimulation of glycogen synthesis when the degradation is diminished or stopped in the first step.

FIGURE 4. Relation between fetal glycemia, liver glycogen content, and incorporation of labeled glucose into liver glycogen. On day 21.5 of gestation, maternal infusions of U-^{14}C-glucose in trace amount were made during 150 min under four experimental conditions. For experimental details see text. Open bars, liver glycogen content; hatched bars, radioactivity in glycogen. *, significant statistical difference ($P < 0.01$); **, highly significant statistical difference ($P < 0.001$).

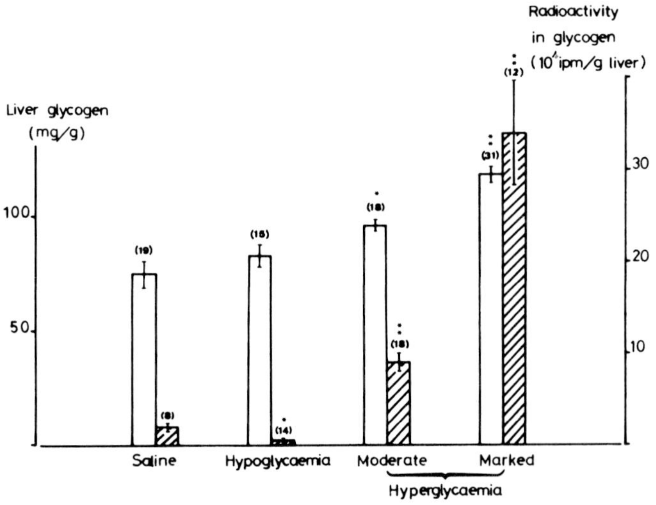

However, some findings which do not agree with this model have been reported in the adult rat. Nuttall et al.[21] in the rat liver in vivo and Gilboe and Nuttall[22] in acellular preparations of rat liver observed a significant glucose-induced synthase activation before a decrease of phosphorylase activity was detectable. In the fasted rat liver in vivo, glucose induced a striking activation of glycogen synthase without concomitant inactivation of phosphorylase, while phosphorylase inactivation occurred in the liver of the fed rat.[23] In a rat hepatocyte preparation, Ciudad et al.[24] reported a simultaneous increase of synthase and phosphorylase activity in the presence of fructose and postulated that inactivation of phosphorylase is not a prerequisite for synthase activation.

Roach and Larner[25] have proposed an alternative explanation for stimulation of glycogen synthesis: glycogen synthase activity depends on the phosphorylation state of the enzyme, and hormones modulate this phosphorylation state. However, metabolic activators such as glucose are able to induce an increase of activity at the same phosphorylation state without modifying it. In this model, inactivation of phosphorylase a, which inhibits synthase phosphatase, is not required, since activation can occur without dephosphorylation of synthase b by synthase phosphatase.

It is likely that in our fetal model (as in the adult rat liver) both mechanisms can occur: glucose might induce simultaneously a direct activation of synthase activity and an activation of synthase phosphatase through phosphorylase inactivation.

Recently Katz et al.[26] established the existence of two distinct systems of glycogen synthesis by isolated adult rat hepatocytes. In the first, glycogen is derived from gluconeogenic precursors, essentially lactate, pyruvate, and dihydroxyacetone;[27] glucose is produced concurrently with glycogen synthesis, and a high glucose concentration is not required to obtain glycogen accumulation. In the second system, synthesis of glycogen from glucose as sole substrate requires a high glucose concentration for a significant rate. In this second system only, glycogen accumulation is accompanied by a decrease of phosphorylase activity.

Since in the rat fetus the gluconeogenic pathway from lactate, pyruvate, and amino acids is not functional until birth,[28,29] one can assume that the first system cannot apply to our fetal model. Glucose of maternal origin is probably the main substrate for glycogen synthesis in the fetal rat liver. Consequently, glycogen synthesis in the liver of the rat fetus might be explained by Her's model. Any increase of maternal blood glucose would be of physiologic significance for glycogen storage in the fetal liver.

The possibility that the observed effect of glucose might

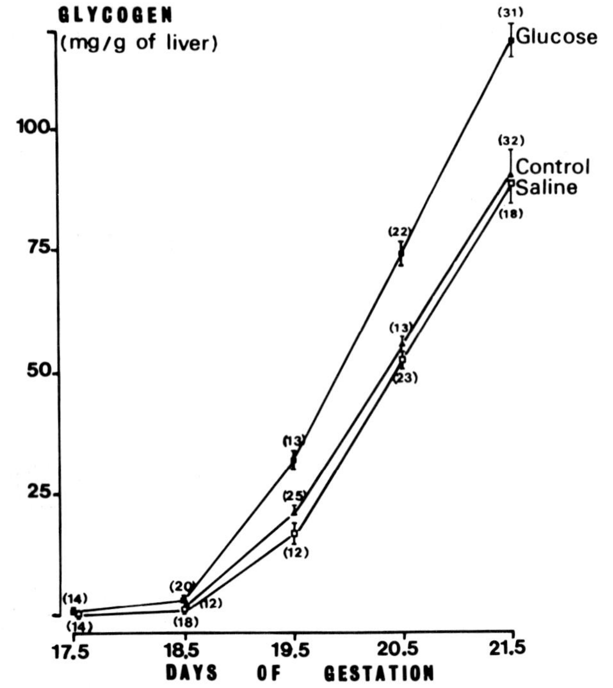

FIGURE 5. Effect of maternal glucose infusion on fetal liver glycogen concentration. Control fetuses (▲——▲) of nonperfused dams were studied immediately after maternal anesthesia. In fetuses of glucose-(■——■) and saline-perfused females (□——□), the liver glycogen was measured 150 min after the beginning of maternal infusion. Values are means ± SEM of the number of determinations shown in parentheses.

be mediated by insulin cannot be ruled out, since in the term rat fetus, an acute hyperglycemia stimulates insulin secretion.[30] However, in the perfused liver of the adult rat[13] and in isolated hepatocytes[9] as well as in adult rat liver in vivo,[14] the activation of glycogen synthase by high glucose concentrations does not depend on the presence of insulin. In preliminary experiments we injected insulin intravenously (40 mU) into the 21.5-day-old rat fetus. This rather high dose of insulin induced effects on glycogen synthesis qualitatively similar to those of glucose, but quantitatively lesser than those induced by a moderate increase of blood glucose from 3.8 to 5.5 mM. Therefore, it is unlikely that the glucose-induced increase of insulinemia is totally responsible for glycogen synthesis stimulation.

As expected from the effects on enzyme activities, fetal hyperglycemia increased glycogen content of the liver over a period of 150 min, i.e., it enhanced net glycogen synthesis. Since a moderate hyperglycemia (5.5 mM) was able to significantly enhance glycogen synthesis in the liver of the rat fetus, one can assume that physiologic increments of maternal glycemia as a result of nutritional state would affect fetal liver glycogen synthesis.

In contrast, acute fetal hypoglycemia was without effect on fetal liver glycogen content. No degradation of glycogen occurred, but, as shown by incorporation of labeled glucose, synthesis was markedly reduced. Girard et al.,[31] in similar experiments, observed reduced fetal insulinemia (half of the control value) after acute maternal hypoglycemia. In spite of the decrease, this level of fetal blood insulin might be high enough to protect glycogen against degradation.

Thus, the liver of the rat fetus seems to be able to resist an acute fall in maternal blood glucose, while it responds to slight maternal blood glucose increase by enhancement of glycogen synthesis. The mechanisms seem to be oriented toward maximal glycogen accumulation. Why this should be true is not known since, teleologically, glycogen breakdown would be expected during hypoglycemia.

As far as young gestational ages are concerned, the present study confirms previous results obtained in the rabbit fetus:[32] fetal hyperglycemia greatly enhances the rate of glucose incorporation into fetal liver glycogen only on and after a definite stage of gestation (19.5 days in the rat and 26 days in the rabbit). In the rat, the liver synthesizes glycogen from 18.5 days up to birth. Nevertheless, hyperglycemia is not sufficient to obtain an increase of glycogen storage before day 19.5. On days 17.5 and 18.5 other factors, such as hormone(s), are probably limiting for development of the physiologic maturation of hepatocytes necessary for glycogen accumulation.[1]

ACKNOWLEDGMENT

We thank Dr. F. Battaglia for helpful discussion and criticism.

Note added in proof. Hyperglycemic fetuses from 30% glucose-infused mothers were given an amount of anti-insulin serum from guinea pigs (through the vitellin vein) which was able to complex 2.5 mU of insulin; controls received normal guinea pig serum. This treatment did not affect either the increase of liver glycogen content or ^{14}C-glucose incorporation. Therefore, insulin suppression did not impair the increase of glycogen accumulation due to the rise of fetal blood glucose.

REFERENCES

1 Jost, A., and Picon, L.: Hormonal control of fetal development and metabolism. Adv. Metab. Disord. *4*:123–84, 1970.

2 Goodner, C. J., and Thompson, D. J.: Glucose metabolism in the fetus in utero. The effect of maternal fasting and glucose loading in the rat. Pediatr. Res. *1*:443–51, 1967.

3 Bossi, E., and Greenberg, R. E.: Sources of blood glucose in the rat fetus. Pediatr. Res. *6*:765–72, 1972.

4 Vinicor, F., Kohalmi, D., and Clark, C. M.: Characterization of carbohydrate metabolism in the isolated fetal rat heart. Effect of fasting and alloxan diabetes. Diabetes *23*:662–68, 1974.

5 Girard, J. R., Ferre, P., Gilbert, M., Kervran, A., Assan, R., and Marliss, E. B.: Fetal metabolic response to maternal fasting in the rat. Am. J. Physiol. *1*:E456–63, 1977.

6 De Wulf, H., and Hers, H. G.: The interconversion of liver glycogen synthetase a and b in vitro. Eur. J. Biochem. *6*:552–57, 1978.

7 Thomas, J. A., Schlender, K. K., and Larner, J.: A rapid filter paper assay for UDP glucose glycogen glucosyl transferase including an improved biosynthesis of UDP-^{14}C-glucose. Anal. Biochem. *25*:486–99, 1968.

8 Devos, P., and Hers, H. G.: Glycogen metabolism in the liver of the foetal rat. Biochem. J. *140*:331–40, 1974.

9 Hue, L., Bontemps, F., and Hers, H. G.: The effect of glucose and of potassium ions on the interconversion of the two forms of glycogen phosphorylase and of glycogen synthetase in isolated rat liver preparation. Biochem. J. *152*:105–14, 1975.

10 Fiske, C. H., and Subbarow, Y.: The colorimetric determination of phosphorus. J. Biol. Chem. *66*:375–80, 1925.

11 Roehrig, K. L., and Allred, J. B.: Direct enzymatic procedure for the determination of liver glycogen. Anal. Biochem. *58*:414–21, 1974.

12 Chan, T. M., and Exton, J. M.: A rapid method for the determination of glycogen content and radioactivity in small quantities of tissue or isolated hepatocytes. Anal. Biochem. *71*:96–105, 1976.

13 Glinsmann, W., Pauk, G., and Hern, E.: Control of rat liver glycogen synthetase and phosphorylase activities by glucose. Biochem. Biophys. Res. Commun. *39*:774–82, 1970.

14 Stalmans, W., De Wulf, H., Hue, L., and Hers, H. G.: The sequential inactivation of glycogen phosphorylase and activation of glycogen synthe-

tase in liver after the administration of glucose to mice and rats. The mechanism of the hepatic threshold to glucose. Eur. J. Biochem. *41*:127–34, 1974.

[15] Soskin, S.: The liver and carbohydrate metabolism. Endocrinology *26*:297–308, 1940.

[16] Curnow, R. T., Rayfield, E. J., George, D., Zenser, T. V., and De Rubertis, F.: Control of hepatic glycogen metabolism in the rhesus monkey: effect of glucose, insulin and glucagon administration. Am. J. Physiol. *228*:80–87, 1975.

[17] Buschiazzo, H., Exton, J. H., and Park, C. R.: Effects of glucose on glycogen synthetase phosphorylase and glycogen deposition in the perfused rat liver. Proc. Natl. Acad. Sci. USA *65*:383–87, 1970.

[18] Stalmans, W., Laloux, M., and Hers, H. G.: The interaction of liver phosphorylase a with glucose and AMP. Eur. J. Biochem. *49*:415–27, 1974.

[19] Stalmans, W., De Wulf, H., Lederer, B., and Hers, H. G.: The effect of glucose and of a treatment by glucocorticoids on the inactivation in vitro of liver glycogen phosphorylase. Eur. J. Biochem. *15*:9–12, 1970.

[20] Stalmans, W., De Wulf, H., and Hers, H. G.: The control of liver glycogen synthetase phosphatase by phosphorylase. Eur. J. Biochem. *18*:582–87, 1971.

[21] Nuttall, F. Q., Gannon, M. C., and Larner, J.: Oral glucose effect on glycogen synthetase and phosphorylase in heart, muscle and liver. Physiol. Chem. Phys. *4*:497–515, 1972.

[22] Gilboe, D. P., and Nuttall, F. Q.: The regulation of liver glycogen synthetase D phosphatase by ATP and glucose. Biochem. Biophys. Res. Communun. *53*:164–71, 1973.

[23] Goldstein, D. E., and Curnow, R. T.: Effect of starvation on hepatic glycogen metabolism and glucose homeostasis. Metabolism *27*:315–23, 1978.

[24] Ciudad, C. J., Massague, J., and Guinovart, J. J.: The inactivation of glycogen phosphorylase is not a prerequisite for the activation of liver glycogen synthase. FEBS Lett. *99*:321–24, 1979.

[25] Roach, P. J., and Larner, J.: Regulation of glycogen synthase: a relation of enzymic properties with biological function. T.I.B.S. *1*:110–12, 1976.

[26] Katz, J., Golden, S., and Wals, P. A.: Glycogen synthesis by rat hepatocytes. Biochem. J. *180*:389–402, 1979.

[27] Katz, J., Golden, S., and Wals, P. A.: Stimulation of hepatic glycogen synthesis by amino acids. Proc. Natl. Acad. Sci. USA *73*:3433–37, 1976.

[28] Yeung, D., and Oliver, I. T.: Gluconeogenesis from amino-acids in neonatal rat liver. Biochem. J. *103*:744–48, 1967.

[29] Yeung, D., and Oliver, I. T.: Development of gluconeogenesis in neonatal rat liver. Effect of premature delivery. Biochem. J. *105*:1229–33, 1967.

[30] Kervran, A., and Girard, J.: Glucose-induced increase of plasma insulin in the rat foetus in utero. J. Endocrinol. *62*:545–51, 1974.

[31] Girard, J. R., Kervran, A., Soufflet, E., and Assan, R.: Factors affecting the secretion of insulin and glucagon by the rat fetus. Diabetes *23*:310–16, 1974.

[32] Gilbert, M., and Jost, A.: Hyperglycemia and glycogen storage in the rabbit fetal liver. Role of age and hormonal status. Biol. Neonate *32*:125–31, 1977.

HbA$_1$ in Subjects with Abnormal Glucose Tolerance but Normal Fasting Plasma Glucose

GEREMIA BOLLI, PIETRO COMPAGNUCCI, MARIA G. CARTECHINI, FAUSTO SANTEUSANIO, CARLO CIROTTO, LUCIANO SCIONTI, AND PAOLO BRUNETTI

SUMMARY

HbA$_{1(a+b+c)}$(HbA$_1$) was determined chromatographically in 107 subjects with normal fasting plasma glucose (FPG) and 112 patients with overt diabetes. Subjects with normal FPG were divided into two groups based on their response to two oral glucose tolerance tests (OGTTs), at an interval of 2 mo. In 40 subjects with normal OGTT (group I), HbA$_1$ ranged from 5.2% to 7.2%, while in 67 subjects with abnormal OGTT (group II), it ranged from 6.3% to 9.6%. HbA$_1$ levels were significantly higher in group II than in group I (7.7 $\pm$ 0.09% versus 6.4 $\pm$ 0.08%, mean $\pm$ SEM, $P < 0.0005$), but 14 subjects of group II had HbA$_1$ levels less than 7.2%. No correlation was found between HbA$_1$ and FPG, OGTT peak, and curve area in either group. However, the correlation became significant in all 107 subjects with normal FPG (groups I + II). In patients with overt diabetes, HbA$_1$ ranged from 6.3% to 18% (11.9 $\pm$ 0.22%) and correlated with FPG ($r = 0.78$, $P < 0.0005$).

The traditional OGTT seems more sensitive than the HbA$_1$ measurement in detecting subjects with reduced carbohydrate tolerance. HbA$_1$ level, on the other hand, is known to be a more specific indicator of structural abnormalities following long-term hyperglycemia. Thus HbA$_1$ determination might be a helpful test along with OGTT to improve both selection and follow-up of subjects with true borderline diabetes. DIABETES 29:272–277, April 1980.

Many recent reports have thrown light on the structure[1–4] and characteristics of the human hemoglobin glycosylated A$_{1c}$ fraction. Glycosylated hemoglobin (HbA$_1$) is increased in diabetics[5] as a consequence of chronic hyperglycemia[6] and correlates closely with their blood level and urinary excretion of glucose.[7–9] Moreover, when glycemic control in diabetics is improved, the HbA$_1$ levels decrease in a few weeks.[10–13] Therefore, it is generally accepted that the determination of HbA$_1$ is useful in planning medical treatment and in carrying out follow-up studies of patients with clinically overt diabetes.[14]

At present, only a few results are available on HbA$_1$ levels in subjects with minor carbohydrate intolerance, as shown by an abnormal oral glucose tolerance test (OGTT) response.[15–18] However, it has not been established whether or not the HbA$_1$ measurement may be an indicator of preclinical diabetes. Moreover, because HbA$_1$ values obtained in subjects with normal fasting plasma glucose (FPG), who are not tested for carbohydrate tolerance, are usually considered as normal, the HbA$_1$ in patients with preclinical diabetes may have been also considered as normal.

To clarify whether slightly reduced carbohydrate tolerance influences the hemoglobin glycosylation rate, we determined the levels of HbA$_1$ in subjects with normal FPG and an abnormal response to two OGTTs at an interval of 2 mo. The values were compared with those obtained in subjects with a normal OGTT response as well as with insulin-dependent diabetics with different degrees of glycemic control.

PATIENTS AND METHODS

Two groups of subjects with FPG in the normal range (4.2–6.9 mmol/l) were studied. Group I consisted of 40 subjects with a normal plasma glucose OGTT response and group II of 67 subjects with an abnormal response. All subjects considered for the present study were healthy volunteers, except for four patients of group II (6%), whose reduced carbohydrate tolerance was associated with a particular clinical state—pheochromocytoma in one case (continual secretion of norepinephrine) and Cushing's syndrome in the other three. Plasma glucose OGTT response was considered abnormal if the 1- and 2-h values exceeded 10 and 7.8 mmol/l, respectively, in subjects under 50 yr.[19] These limits were each increased by 0.055 mmol/decade for subjects over 50 yr.[20] Subjects with only one of the two values above these normal limits were excluded from the present study.

From the Institutes of Medical Pathology, Clinical Medicine, and Histology and Embryology, University of Perugia, Italy.
Address reprint requests to Paolo Brunetti, Institute of Medical Pathology, University of Perugia, 06100 Perugia, Italy.
Received for publication 25 July 1979 and in revised form 17 October 1979.

TABLE 1
HbA_1 ($HbA_{1(a+b+c)}$) levels in subjects with normal fasting plasma glucose (FPG), divided according to their normal (group I) or abnormal (group II) response to two oral glucose tolerance tests (1 mmol/l = 18 mg/dl plasma glucose)

	Age (yr)	FPG (mmol/l)		Oral glucose tolerance test (OGTT) (plasma glucose) (mmol/1) 0	1 h	2 h	3 h	OGTT area (cm²)	HbA_1 (%)
Group I (N = 40)	41.5 ± 2.3* (15–70)†	4.6 ± 0.1 (3.3–6.1)	First‡	4.7 ± 0.2 (3.9–6.1)	6.7 ± 0.2 (4.4–9.3)	5.3 ± 0.2 (4.3–7.2)	4.6 ± 0.2 (3.1–6.4)	59.9 ± 1.5	6.4 ± 0.08 (5.2–7.2)
			Second‡	4.6 ± 0.9 (4.2–6.0)	6.9 ± 0.4 (5.8–8.6)	5.1 ± 0.3 (5.0–6.4)	4.9 ± 0.7 (4.4–5.8)	61.0 ± 2.2	6.3 ± 0.08 (5.3–7.1)
Group II (N = 67)	54.7 ± 1.6§ (21–85)	5.6 ± 0.1¶ (4.4–6.9)	First	5.5 ± 0.3¶ (4.3–6.1)	11.8 ± 0.3¶ (10.2–21.3)	10.1 ± 0.3¶ (7.8–20.3)	7.3 ± 0.3¶ (3.1–15.7)	102.0 ± 2.2¶	7.7 ± 0.09¶ (6.3–9.6)
			Second	5.6 ± 0.4¶ (4.6–6.0)	12.1 ± 0.3¶ (10.5–19.3)	10.9 ± 0.3¶ (8.0–21.2)	7.9 ± 0.4¶ (5.2–13.2)	100.0 ± 3.4¶	7.7 ± 0.09¶ (6.2–9.5)

* Mean ± SEM.
† Range.
‡ First and second OGTT.
§ $P < 0.01$ (χ^2 test) versus group I.
¶ $P < 0.001$ (χ^2 test) versus group I.

Each subject was instructed to eat a diet containing at least 300 g carbohydrate for 3 days before testing. Venous blood was drawn in the morning after an overnight fast and at the first, second, and third hour after 556 mmol glucose administration. The OGTT was repeated in each subject after 2 mo with the same protocol.

We determined HbA_1 also in 112 patients with clinically overt diabetes. These subjects all showed a good glycemic stability, resulting from four to six plasma glucose determinations (fasting and postlunch) and daily glycosuria during the 4 wk preceding HbA_1 measurement.

Heparinized venous blood for HbA_1 determination was drawn at the zero hour of each OGTT. $HbA_{1(a+b+c)}$ was measured chromatographically according to an improvement of the Kynoch and Lehmann method.[21] The red blood cells of each sample were washed with saline, hemolyzed with distilled water, and the ghosts centrifuged out at 40,000 *g* for 20 min at +4°C. The clear supernatant was immediately stored at +4°C for up to 4 days before chromatographic isolation in duplicate. Glass chromatographic columns (internal diameter 2 cm) were filled with Bio Rex 70 (Bio Rad, 200–400 mesh), 5 cm high, after careful equilibration in 41 mmol phosphate buffer, 10 mmol KCN, pH 6.75. Hemolysate (0.3–0.5 ml) was added to the top of the resin and eluted with the same buffer at 18–20°C. One hundred milliliters containing glycosylated fractions A_{1a}, A_{1b}, and A_{1c} was collected, while the A_0 fraction was eluted with 100 ml of phosphate buffer (0.15 mol, pH 6.40) and the absorbance determined at 410 nm. HbA_1 concentration was expressed as percent of total hemoglobin eluted. The interassay coefficient of variation of this method in our laboratory is 1.2% for the assay at high HbA_1 level (15%–16%) and 1.8% at low level (6%–7%), respectively.

Plasma glucose was measured by a Beckman glucose analyzer.

Statistical correlations were obtained by Pearson's r coefficient and the regression lines calculated by the least squares method. The comparison of the slopes of the regression lines was obtained by Student's *t* test for differences between regression slopes.[22]

RESULTS

Plasma glucose levels were highly reproducible in our subjects with normal FPG; no significant difference was observed between the first and second plasma glucose OGTT response at an interval of 2 mo (Table 1). The individual variation of glucose peak value and area under the OGTT curve was less than 15%. In group II, FPG was significantly higher than in group I ($\chi^2 = 43.08$, $P < 0.0005$), although all values of the two groups fell within the normal range. HbA_1 levels were 6.4 ± 0.08% (mean ± SEM) in group I (range 5.2%–7.2%). HbA_1 levels in group II (7.7 ± 0.09%, range 6.3%–9.6%) were significantly higher than in group I ($\chi^2 = 61.75$, $P < 0.0005$), as shown in Figure 1. HbA_1 was 7.9% in the patient with pheochromocytoma and 8.4%, 9.1%, and 8.4% in the patients affected by Cushing's syndrome. The significantly different distribution of HbA_1 values between subjects of groups I and II is shown in Figure 2. Fourteen subjects of group II (21%) had HbA_1 levels less than 7.2%, that is, they were in the normal range. Plasma glucose peak and OGTT area values of these 14 subjects did not differ significantly from those of the remaining 53 of group II, whose HbA_1 levels were more than 7.2%.

There was no significant correlation between the age of subjects and plasma glucose OGTT response in either groups I or II (Table 2). Similarly, there was no correlation between plasma glucose (FPG and OGTT plasma glucose response) and HbA_1. However, these correlations became significant when subjects were considered as a single group (groups I + II, N = 107), as shown in Figure 3. HbA_1 levels were less than 7.2% in subjects with FPG less than 4.4 mmol/l and more than 7.2% in subjects with FPG more than 6.1 mmol/l. Moreover, when FPG ranged between 4.4 and 6.1 mmol/l, HbA_1 levels were less than 7.2% in all subjects of group I and 14 subjects of group II, while in 39 subjects of group II they were more than 7.2%. The correlation

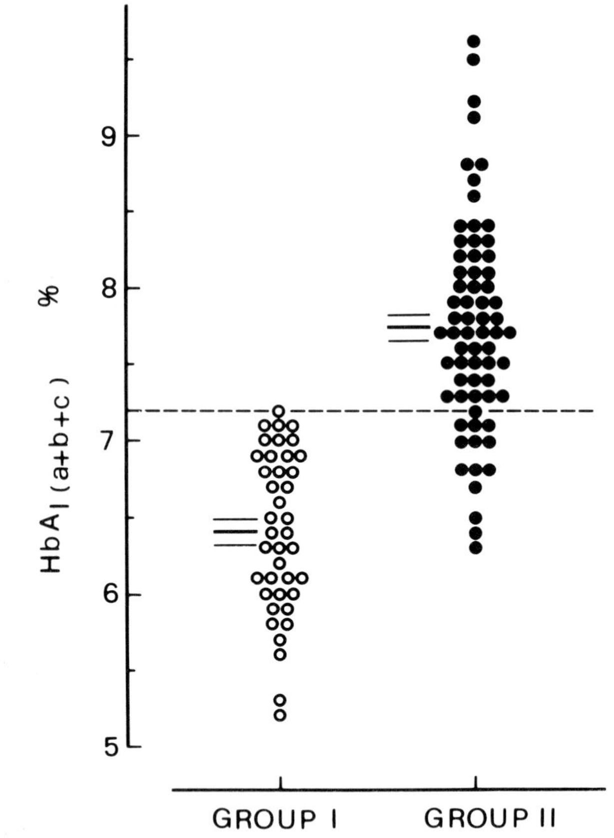

FIGURE 1. Glycosylated hemoglobin levels in subjects with normal fasting plasma glucose and normal (○, group I, N = 40) or abnormal (●, group II, N = 67) OGTT response.

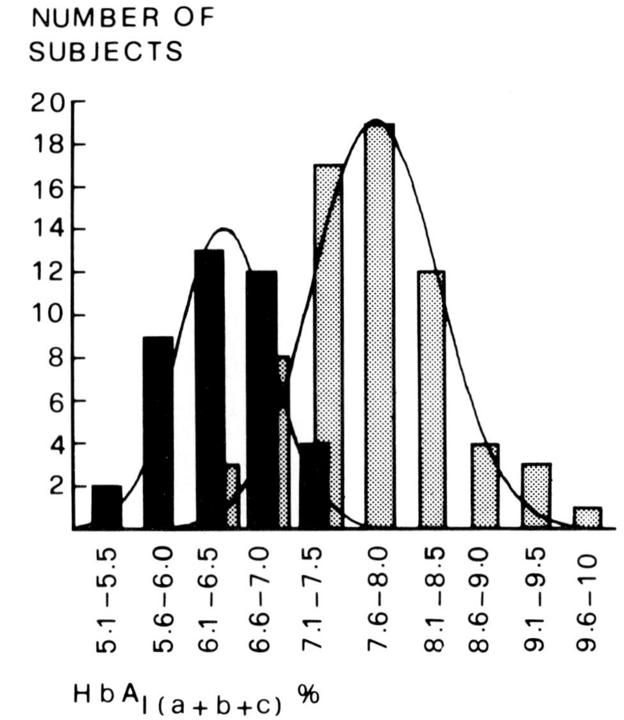

FIGURE 2. Distribution of glycosylated hemoglobin levels in subjects with normal fasting plasma glucose and normal (■) or abnormal (▨) OGTT response.

between HbA$_1$ and FPG showed a clear continuity of HbA$_1$ values between subjects with normal and abnormal OGTT responses. On the other hand, a distinction between HbA$_1$ values of the two groups was observed in the correlation of HbA$_1$ with plasma glucose peak levels and area under the OGTT curves. It is evident that, when plasma glucose peak was more than about 10 mmol/l and/or the OGTT area more than 78 cm^2, HbA$_1$ values suddenly rose over 7.2% in 54 subjects (79%) of group II. As the mean age of group II was significantly higher than that of group I ($\chi^2 = 19.8$, $P < 0.0005$), it might be suggested that the HbA$_1$ increase was age-related. However, no significant correlation between age and HbA$_1$ was found in groups I + II. Moreover, when subjects in the two groups were matched for each decade (21–70 yr; χ^2 test between groups = 8.9, P = NS), the HbA$_1$ levels remained significantly higher in group II than in group I ($\chi^2 = 52.2$, $P < 0.0005$).

In patients with clinically overt diabetes, HbA$_1$ values ranged from 6.3% to 18% (11.9 ± 0.22%) and a close correlation was found between HbA$_1$ (y, independent variable) and FPG (x, dependent variable) ($r = 0.78$, $P < 0.0005$). The slope of the regression line in diabetics was not significantly different from that of subjects with normal FPG (groups I + II) (Figure 4).

DISCUSSION

Our results confirm previous reports that the levels of glycosylated hemoglobin are higher in subjects with overt diabetes than in normals, the highest values (17%–18%) being observed in poorly controlled patients.[5,7,11,12,14] Because our diabetics with fairly good glycemic control showed low levels of HbA$_1$ (about 7%), the close correlation we found in 112 subjects with overt diabetes is highly significant throughout a wide range of glycosylated hemoglobin. This close relationship confirms that HbA$_1$ reflects blood glucose levels in diabetics and that it is a good indicator of glycemic control in patients with clinically overt diabetes.[10,14]

TABLE 2
Correlations in the subjects admitted to groups I and II

	(X) (Y)	Age FPG	Age OGTT peak	Age OGTT area	Age HbA$_1$	FPG HbA$_1$	OGTT peak HbA$_1$	OGTT area HbA$_1$
Group I (N = 40)		NS*	NS	NS	NS	NS	NS	NS
Group II (N = 67)		NS	NS	NS	NS	NS	NS	NS
Groups I + II (N = 107)		r = 0.20 (P < 0.05)	r = 0.35 (P < 0.001)	r = 0.36 (P < 0.001)	NS	r = 0.40 (P < 0.001)	r = 0.53 (P < 0.001)	r = 0.57 (P < 0.001)

* NS: not statistically significant.

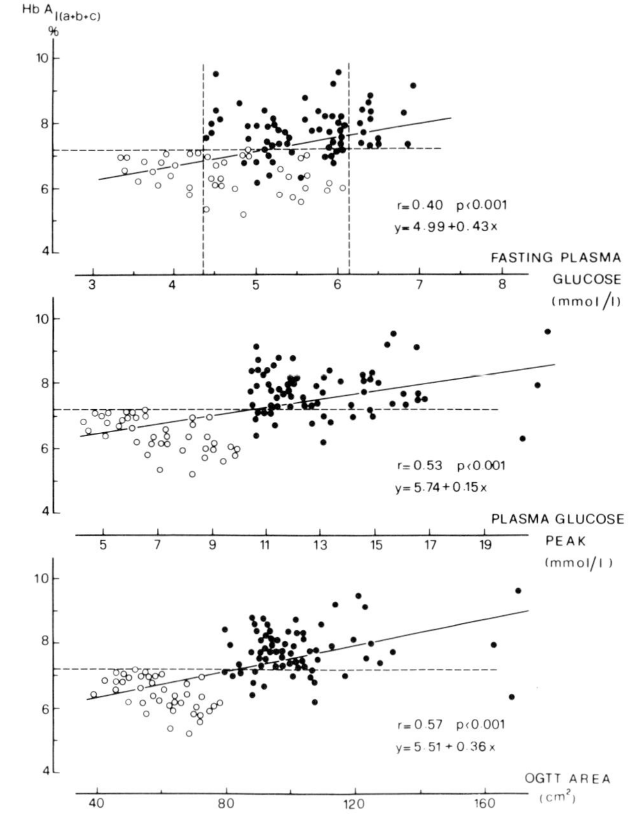

FIGURE 3. Correlations between glycosylated hemoglobin and plasma glucose (fasting, OGTT peak, and curve area) in 107 subjects with normal fasting plasma glucose and normal (○) or abnormal (●) OGTT response.

HbA_1 levels ranged from 5.2% to 7.2% in subjects tested twice for normal plasma glucose OGTT response. This range is narrower than previously reported by others in nondiabetic subjects[15,23,24] and subjects with normal OGTT response.[18] This could be due to the high specificity and reproducibility of our chromatographic method for determination of HbA_1 and to the careful selection of subjects with normal carbohydrate tolerance. On the other hand, the HbA_1 levels ranged from 5.2% to 9.6% in all subjects of groups I + II who showed normal FPG. It might be suggested, therefore, that HbA_1 values range more widely in subjects considered only for their normal FPG levels. Because normal FPG may be present in subjects with reduced carbohydrate tolerance, normal levels of HbA_1 should be obtained only in subjects carefully tested for "normal" carbohydrate tolerance. Our results suggest that HbA_1 concentrations in controls having normal carbohydrate tolerance include a narrower range than in individuals who are selected as controls because of a normal FPG concentration alone. Therefore, the absence of a significant correlation between HbA_1 and age, FPG, and plasma glucose OGTT response in our normal subjects may be mainly due to the narrow HbA_1 distribution range. Recently, Graf et al.[23] reported a significant correlation between HbA_1 and FPG in normals. Because these authors found the HbA_1 to range from about 5.8% to 11.5% in subjects with normal FPG who were not tested for glucose tolerance, the question arises as to whether they included subjects with carbohydrate tolerance in their group of normals. Our study, moreover, did not confirm the difference between the slopes of HbA_1 and FPG regression lines found by Graf et al. in diabetics and subjects with normal FPG, but this may well be due to differences in selecting normal subjects.

In our study HbA_1 levels were significantly higher in subjects with still normal FPG but abnormal OGTT than in normals. The HbA_1 increase might be due to the hyperglycemic peaks following carbohydrate consumption in subjects with reduced carbohydrate tolerance. Because these peaks may occur for only a few hours a day, the HbA_1 increase is slight but significant compared with normals. However, 14 subjects of group II (abnormal OGTT) had HbA_1 values in the normal range. The normal HbA_1 level of these 14 subjects cannot be explained by the different plasma glucose OGTT response compared with the other 53 subjects with elevated HbA_1 values. Because all subjects with FPG more than 6.1 mmol/l had HbA_1 levels of more than 7.2% and the 14 subjects with normal HbA_1 levels had FPG values less than 6.1 mmol/l, it might be suggested that FPG levels in the upper part of the normal range are associated with both reduced carbohydrate tolerance and elevated HbA_1 levels, while this does not necessarily occur when FPG is less than 6.1 mmol/l. Because plasma glucose OGTT response did not differ in subjects with FPG levels more or less than 6.1 mmol/l, high-ranging PFG, although still normal, might be important along with postlunch hyperglycemic peaks in determining increased HbA_1 levels in subjects with reduced carbohydrate tolerance.

In our study the traditional OGTT is more sensitive in detecting subjects with reduced carbohydrate tolerance than the HbA_1 determination. This result is quite in line with the recent report of Santiago et al.,[15] although HbA_1 levels were increased in 79% of subjects with abnormal OGTT response in our study and in 53% in Santiago's study.

While the OGTT seems more sensitive, the HbA_1 determination might be more specific in detecting subjects with reduced carbohydrate tolerance, since the HbA_1 levels can provide the proof of the "biological" abnormalities following long-term increase of blood glucose values.[14] At present, the nonphysiologic nature of the OGTT and its poor prognostic value are being emphasized.[25–27] Moreover, an abnormal OGTT response could reflect only a transient carbohydrate tolerance in subjects normoglycemic in their usual life.[18]

In conclusion, while increased HbA_1 levels are a consequence of long-term hyperglycemia, normal HbA_1 levels in subjects with an abnormal OGTT response might indicate only a more recent carbohydrate intolerance, although further investigation is needed. Thus, HbA_1 determination might be a helpful test along with OGTT to improve both selection and follow-up of subjects with true borderline diabetes.

Note added in proof. While this paper was submitted, Dunn et al.[28] reported the HbA_{1c} concentration in subjects tested for carbohydrate tolerance by an OGTT (USPHS criteria). Although the FPG levels in Dunn's patients appear higher than in ours, it should be stressed that the percentage of subjects showing both an impaired OGTT response and an increased glycosylated Hb level found by Dunn et al. is 63.5%, which is interestingly similar to that of our study (79%).

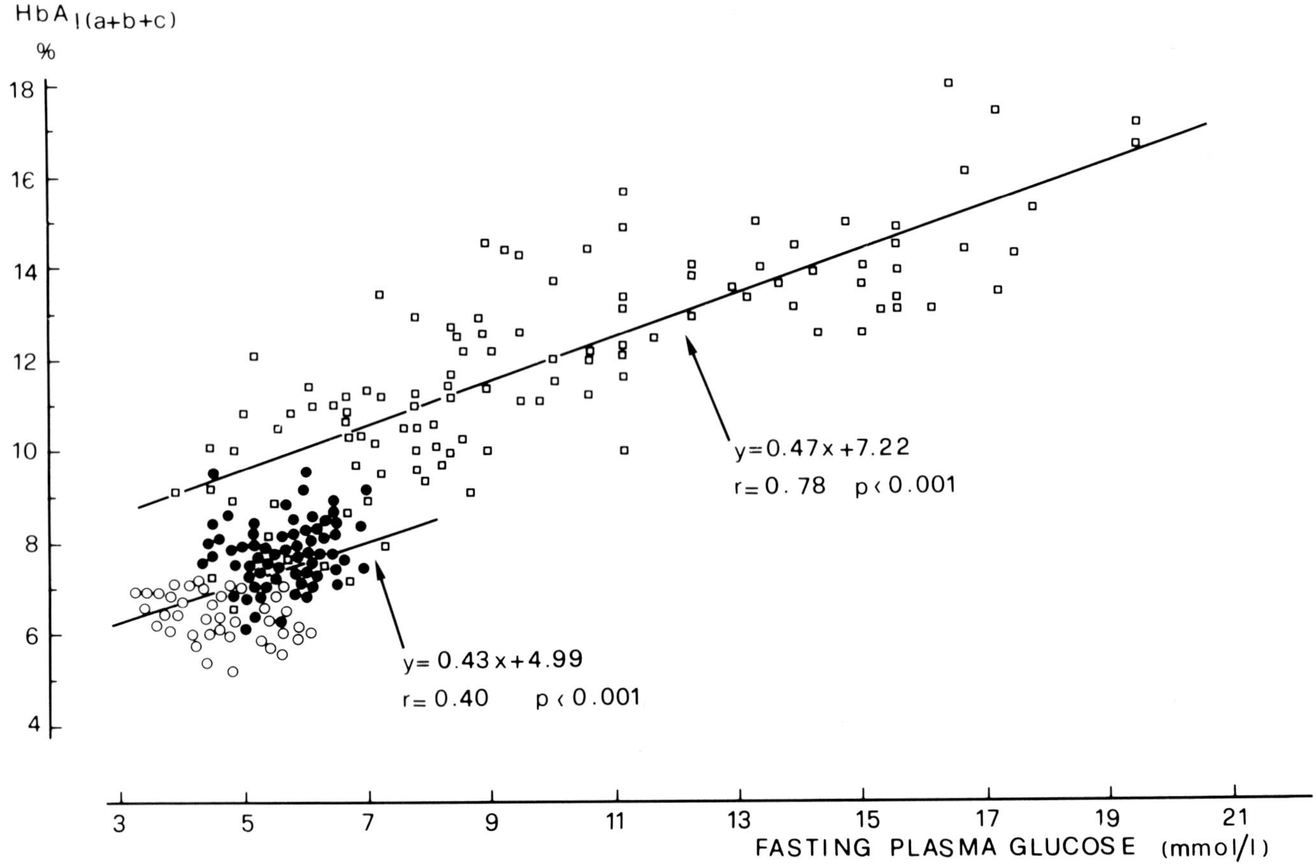

FIGURE 4. Correlations between glycosylated hemoglobin and fasting plasma glucose in 112 patients with overt diabetes (□) and 107 subjects with normal fasting plasma glucose and (○) normal or (●) abnormal OGTT response. There is no statistical difference between the slopes of the regression lines in diabetics and subjects with normal FPG (t = 0.0004).

ACKNOWLEDGMENTS

We wish to thank Dr. A. H. Rubenstein for reviewing the manuscript and for his valuable advice.

This work was supported by grant 78.02009.04 from the Italian National Research Council (C.N.R.).

REFERENCES

[1] Bunn, H. F., Haney, D. N., Gabbay, K. H., and Gallop, P. M.: Further identification of the nature and linkage of the carbohydrate in hemoglobin A_{1c}. Biochem. Biophys. Res. Commun. *67*:103–09, 1975.

[2] Bunn, H. F., Haney, D. N., Kamin, S., Gabbay, K. H., and Gallop, P. M.: The biosynthesis of human hemoglobin A_{1c} in vivo. J. Clin. Invest. *57*:1652–59, 1976.

[3] Haney, D. N., and Bunn, H. F.: Glycosylation of hemoglobin in vitro: affinity labeling of hemoglobin by glucose-6-phosphate. Proc. Natl. Acad. Sci. USA *73*:3534–38, 1976.

[4] Koenig, R. J., Blobstein, S. H., and Cerami, A.: Structure of carbohydrate of hemoglobin A_{1c}. J. Biol. Chem. *252*:2992–97, 1977.

[5] Trivelli, L. A., Ranney, H. M., and Lai, H.-T.: Hemoglobin components in patients with diabetes mellitus. N. Engl. J. Med. *284*:353–57, 1971.

[6] Fitzgibbons, J. F., Koler, R. D., and Jones, R. J.: Red cell age-related changes of hemoglobins A_{1a+b} and A_{1c} in normal and diabetic subjects. J. Clin. Invest. *58*:820–24, 1976.

[7] Koenig, R. J., Peterson, C. M., Kilo, C., Cerami, A., and Williamson, J. R.: Hemoglobin A_{1c} as an indicator of the degree of glucose intolerance in diabetes. Diabetes *25*:230–32, 1975.

[8] Gabbay, K. H., Hasty, K., Breslow, J. L., Ellison, R. C., Bunn, H. F., and Gallop, P. M.: Glycosylated hemoglobins and long-term blood glucose control in diabetes mellitus. J. Clin. Endocrinol. Metab. *44*:859–64, 1976.

[9] Gonen, B., Rubenstein, A. H., Rochman, H., Tanega, S. P., and Horwitz, D. L.: Haemoglobin A1: an indicator of the metabolic control of diabetic patients. Lancet *2*:734–37, 1977.

[10] Koenig, R. J., Peterson, C. M., Jones, R. L., Saudek, C., Lehrman, M., and Cerami, A.: Correlation of glucose regulation and hemoglobin A_{1c} in diabetes mellitus. N. Engl. J. Med. *295*:417–20, 1976.

[11] Ditzel, J., and Kjaergaard, J.-J.: Haemoglobin A_{1c} concentrations after initial insulin treatment for newly discovered diabetes. Br. Med. J. *1*: 741–42, 1978.

[12] Bolli, G., Cartechini, M. G., Compagnucci, P., Santeusanio, F., Massi-Benedetti, M., Calabrese, G., Puxeddu, A., and Brunetti, P.: Modification of glycosylated haemoglobin concentration during artificial endocrine pancreas treatment of diabetics: evidence for a short-term effect on HbA$_1$ levels. Diabetologia. In press, 1980.

[13] Fraser, D. M., Smith, A. F., Gray, R. S., Borsey, D. Q., Sinclair, M. E., Clarke, B. F., and Duncan, L. J. P.: Glycosylated haemoglobin concentrations in newly diagnosed diabetics before and during treatment. Br. Med. J. *1*: 979–81, 1979.

[14] Gonen, B., and Rubenstein, A. H.: Haemoglobin A1 and diabetes mellitus. Diabetologia *15*:1–8, 1978.

[15] Santiago, J. V., Davis, J. E., and Fisher, F.: Hemoglobin A_{1c} levels in a diabetes detection program. J. Clin. Endocrinol. Metab. *47*:578–80, 1978.

[16] Ditzel, J., Nielsen, N. V., and Berg, O.: Haemoglobin A_{1c} and fluorescein angiography in subjects with borderline diabetes. Diabetologia *14*:228, 1978. Abstract.

[17] Saibene, V., Brembilla, L., Bertoletti, A., and Pozza, G.: Combined OGTT and glycosylated haemoglobins detection for carbohydrate intolerance diagnosis. Diabetologia *14*:267, 1978. Abstract.

[18] Lev-Ran, A., and VanderLan, W. P.: Glycohemoglobins and glucose tolerance. JAMA *241*:912–14, 1979.

[19] Fajans, S. S., and Conn, J. W.: Early recognition of diabetes mellitus. Ann. N.Y. Acad. Sci. *82*:208–18, 1959.

[20] Whitehouse, F. W.: The diagnosis of diabetes—how to determine which patients to treat. Med. Clin. North Am. *62*:627–37, 1978.

[21] Kynoch, P. A. M., and Lehmann, H.: Rapid estimation (2½ hours) of glycosylated haemoglobin for routine purposes. Lancet *2*:16, 1977.

[22] Armitage, P.: Statistical Methods in Medical Research. Oxford, Blackwell Scientific Publications, 1971, pp. 131–34, 147–66, 279–88.

[23] Graf, R. J., Halter, J. B., and Porte, D., Jr.: Glycosylated hemoglobin in normal subjects and subjects with maturity-onset diabetes: evidence for a saturable system in man. Diabetes *27*:834–39, 1978.

[24] Davis, R. E., Nicol, D. J., McCann, V. J., and Calder, J. S.: Glycosylated haemoglobin levels in patients with diabetes mellitus. Med. J. Aust. *1*:530–32, 1978.

[25] Siperstein, M. D.: The glucose tolerance test: a pitfall in the diagnosis of diabetes mellitus. Adv. Intern. Med. *20*:297–323, 1975.

[26] O'Sullivan, J. B., and Mahan, C. M.: Prospective study of 352 young patients with chemical diabetes. N. Engl. J. Med. *278*:1038–41, 1968.

[27] Jarrett, R. J., Keen, H., Fuller, J. H., and McCartney, M.: Worsening to diabetes in men with impaired glucose tolerance ("borderline diabetes"). Diabetologia *16*:25–30, 1979.

[28] Dunn, P. J., Cole, R. A., Soeldner, J. S., and Gleason, R. E.: Reproducibility of hemoglobin A_{1c} and sensitivity to various degrees of glucose intolerance. Ann. Intern. Med. *91*:390–96, 1979.

Effect of Insulin, Glucose, and 2-Deoxy-glucose Infusion into the Third Cerebral Ventricle of Conscious Dogs on Plasma Insulin, Glucose, and Free Fatty Acids

G. J. TABORSKY, JR., AND R. N. BERGMAN

SUMMARY

Previous studies have demonstrated that exogenous insulin, injected into central cerebrospinal fluid cavities of dogs, stimulates the release of endogenous insulin from the pancreas. To determine whether this response was elicited by (1) insulin per se, (2) an effect of insulin on glucose transport, or (3) glucopenia in the cerebrospinal fluid, we measured plasma insulin, glucose, and free fatty acids during the infusion of insulin, glucose, and 2-deoxy-glucose (2DG), individually or in combination, into the third cerebral ventricle of conscious dogs. As expected, the third ventricular infusion of insulin alone elicited a small, but significant, rise of plasma insulin. Surprisingly, infusion of insulin with glucose produced a smaller increase of plasma insulin ($P < 0.05$) and the infusion of insulin with 2DG produced a much larger increase of plasma insulin ($P < 0.05$) than did the third ventricular infusion of insulin alone. The third ventricular infusion of either glucose alone or 2DG alone had no effect on the plasma levels of insulin. These data suggest that administration of insulin into the cerebral ventricles stimulates pancreatic insulin secretion but not by accelerating the transport of glucose into a chemosensitive area of the brain. **DIABETES 29:278–283, April 1980.**

The autonomic nervous system exerts a dual control over insulin secretion. The parasympathetic nervous system can augment insulin secretion: electrical stimulation of the vagus enhances glucose-induced insulin release.[1] The sympathetic nervous system can produce a net impairment of insulin release: electrical stimulation of the mixed pancreatic nerve during the infusion of atropine inhibits both basal[2] and glucose-induced insulin release.[2,3] The parasympathetic pathway may be under the central influence of the ventrolateral hypothalamus, since electrical stimulation in this area also augments insulin secretion.[4] The sympathetic pathway appears to be under the central influence of the ventromedial hypothalamus, since electrical stimulation of this area can inhibit insulin secretion.[5] The demonstration of chemoreceptors in these areas of the brain raises the possibility that the hypothalamus may do more than simply integrate signals from higher centers and peripheral afferents. For example, Oomura[6] has found hypothalamic neurons which alter their rate of firing in response to iontophoretic application of insulin, glucose, and 3-o-methylglucose. In addition, Havrankova et al.[7] have recently demonstrated the specific binding of insulin to hypothalamic as well as other brain tissue. These putative receptors appear to influence the neural input which the beta-cells receive, since Chen, Woods, and Porte[8,9] have shown that injection of insulin into the cerebrospinal fluid (CSF) of dogs stimulates the secretion of insulin from the pancreas. In these experiments, the injection of insulin decreased the glucose concentration of the CSF, leading Woods and Porte[9] to hypothesize that the secretion of insulin observed was stimulated by an increase of glucose uptake into some area of the brain. If this hypothesis were correct, the addition of glucose to the centrally administered insulin should augment the neural stimulation of insulin release. Conversely, the addition of 2-deoxy-glucose (2DG), a competitive inhibitor of glucose transport and phosphorylation,[10] to the centrally administered insulin should diminish the neural stimulation of insulin release. Therefore, we examined the effect of insulin, glucose, and 2-deoxy-glucose (2DG) infused individually or in combination into the third cerebral ventricle of conscious dogs on plasma insulin, glucose, and free fatty acids.

METHODS

Thirteen adult dogs of mixed German shepherd breed, weighing from 26 to 34 kg, were used in the 26 experiments performed. At least 3 days before the experiments, a blood-

Presented, in part, at the 36th Annual Meeting of the American Diabetes Association in San Francisco, California, June 20, 1976.
From the Department of Biomedical Engineering, University of Southern California, Los Angeles, California.
Address reprint requests to Gerald J. Taborsky, Jr., Ph.D., Division of Endocrinology and Metabolism (151), VA Medical Center, 4435 Beacon Avenue S., Seattle, Washington 98108.
Received for publication 6 September 1979.

sampling catheter was implanted in the right atrium of the heart, and an infusion catheter was implanted in the third ventricle of the brain. A 12-gauge polyvinyl chloride catheter was inserted into the right jugular vein and advanced to the right atrium of the heart. The catheter was tied into position, and the free end was passed beneath the skin of the back of the neck where it exited through a midline incision. The catheter was flushed with 20 ml of sterile saline, filled with 3 ml of saline containing 100 U/ml heparin, and capped. The third cerebral ventricle was catheterized by the technique of Maran and Yates, as described elsewhere.[11]

Before the experimental series was begun, the dogs were trained to lie quietly on a warm table for extended periods. Dogs were fasted for 18 h before the start of all experiments, which were performed with the dogs in a fully conscious, relaxed state. At the end of each experimental series, the dogs were killed and the placement of both catheters was verified as follows. One hundred microliters of fluorescein dye was infused into the brain via the cerebral catheter. The brain was removed, dissected along the midline, and examined under ultraviolet illumination. Ventricular catheterization was judged successful if the fluorescein dye stained both medial walls of the third ventricle. The catheterization was judged unsuccessful if the fluorescein dye was restricted to a "pocket" in brain tissue on either side of the third ventricle. With successful catheterization, the dye appeared to be most concentrated on the basal part of the third ventricular walls, directly adjacent to the ventromedial hypothalamus and progressively less concentrated downstream in the fourth ventricle (Figure 1). Dye was never observed upstream in the lateral ventricle. Thus, contact with high concentrations of infusate was presumably limited to medial brain areas at the level of the thalamus and below. After assessing the placement of the cerebral catheter, the chest was opened, the pericardium incised, and the right atrium palpated for the tip of the blood-sampling catheter.

Each experiment was divided into three periods—an adjustment period, a control period, and a test period. During the adjustment period (30 min), the dog was allowed to relax; no blood samples were drawn. During the control period (25 min), the dog received a third ventricular infusion of mock cerebrospinal fluid (MCSF) at a rate of 5 or 50 μl/min. MCSF has the following composition: NaCl, 125 mM; $NaHCO_3$, 25 mM; KCl, 3.5 mM; $CaCl_2$, 1.3 mM; $MgCl_2$, 1.14 mM; NaH_2PO_4, 0.51 mM; urea, 1.67 mM; and glucose, 3.38 mM.[12] During the test period (30–90 min), the dog received one of five cerebroventricular infusates, depending on the experiment: (1) insulin (200 mU/min); (2) insulin (200 mU/min) with glucose (0.225 mg/min); (3) insulin (200 mU/min) with 2DG (0.225 mg/min); (4) glucose (5.5 mg/min); or (5) 2DG (5.5 mg/min). Infusates 1, 2, and 3 were delivered at 5 μl/min; 4 and 5 were infused at 50 μl/min; all were dissolved in MCSF. Insulin (regular) was obtained from Eli Lilly (Indianapolis); glucose and 2DG were obtained from Sigma Chemicals (St. Louis).

FIGURE 1. Schematic illustration of the brain showing the position of the third ventricular catheter (needle) and the spread of infused dye (hatched area) observed after brain dissection.

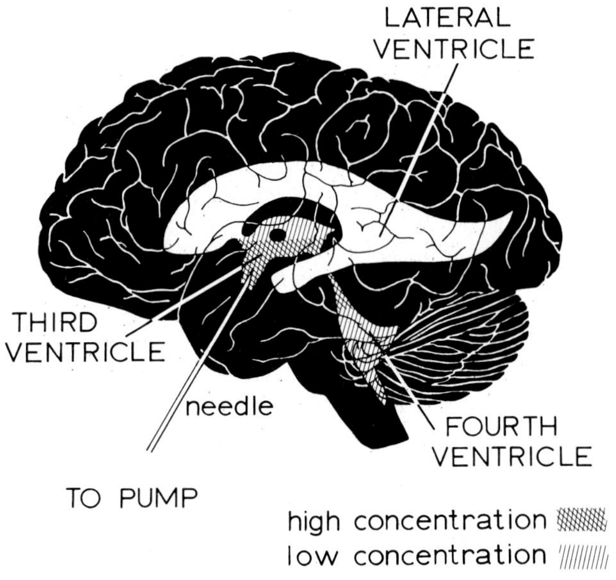

Blood samples of 2.5 ml were drawn at 5-min intervals during the control and test periods. Samples were placed in tubes containing heparin and NaF and then centrifuged; plasma was separated and frozen for later analysis. A maximum of 50 ml of blood (20 samples) was drawn during an experiment. No change of hematocrit was observed. Insulin was measured by radioimmunoassay using the dextran-charcoal separation method of Herbert et al.[13] Glucose was measured using a glucose analyzer (Beckman Instruments, Inc., Fullerton, California) by an automated modification of the glucose oxidase technique. Plasma free fatty acids (FFA) were measured by the colorimetric assay of Smith.[14] Mean values within a treatment group were compared using paired Student's *t* tests. Comparisons between treatment groups were performed using the two-sample Student's *t* test or the Welch *t* test[15] if the variances were significantly different.

RESULTS

During the infusion of MCSF into the third cerebral ventricle, plasma insulin averaged 32 ± 7 μU/ml ($\bar{x}$ ± SEM, N = 8, see Figure 2, Table 1). During the first half-hour of insulin infusion into the third ventricle (200 mU/min), the level of plasma insulin averaged 64 ± 9 μU/ml; during the second half-hour of insulin infusion into the third ventricle, plasma insulin averaged 51 ± 7 μU/ml. Both averages were significantly greater than those observed during the preceding intraventricular infusion of MCSF (both $P < 0.05$, see Figure 2, Table 1). Plasma glucose averaged 89 ± 3 mg/dl during the infusion of MCSF and did not change significantly during the intraventricular infusion of insulin (see Figure 2). Plasma FFA averaged 779 ± 74 μeq/l during the infusion of MCSF and decreased significantly ($P < 0.01$) to 641 ± 77 μeq/l during the second half-hour of the intraventricular insulin infusion (see Figure 2).

When glucose was infused into the third ventricle (0.225 mg/min) in combination with insulin (200 mU/min), a different pattern of plasma insulin concentration was observed: no significant change was noted during the first half-hour of infusion (see Table 1 and Figure 3). Neither plasma glucose nor plasma free fatty acids changed significantly during the third ventricular infusion of insulin plus glucose (see Figure 3). Infusions of glucose alone into the third cerebral ventricle at 5.5 mg/min, a rate over 20 times the previous one, had no effect on plasma insulin (see Tables 1 and 2). Likewise,

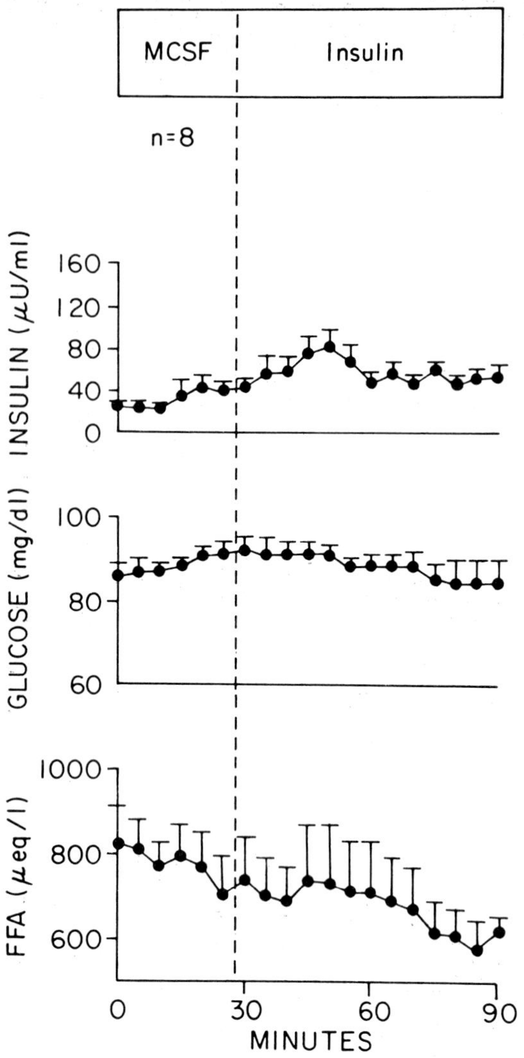

FIGURE 2. The effect of third ventricular infusions of mock cerebrospinal fluid (MCSF) (0–25 min) or insulin (200 mU/min, 30–90 min) on plasma insulin, glucose, and FFA ($\bar{x}$ ± SEM, N = 5).

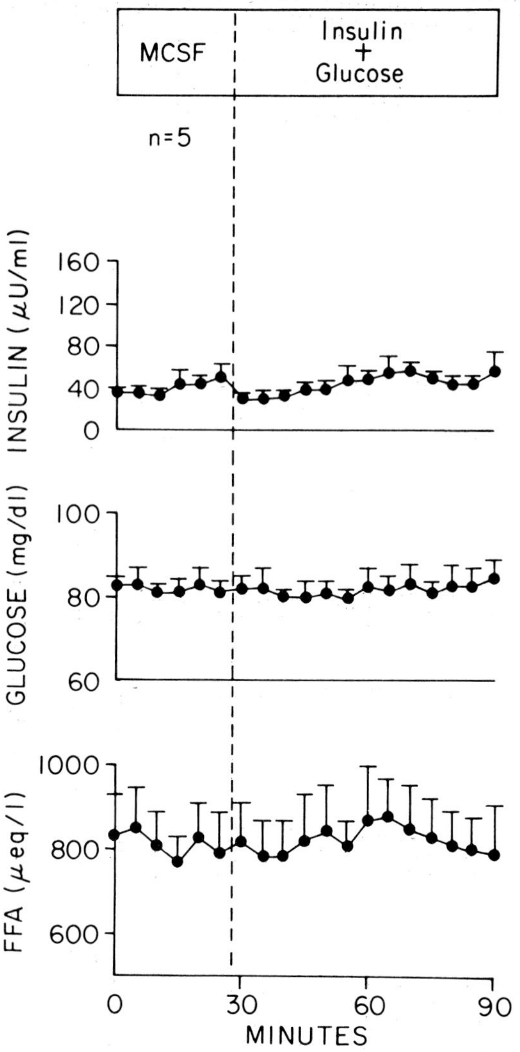

FIGURE 3. The effect of third ventricular infusions of MCSF (0–25 min) or insulin (200 mU/min) plus glucose (0.225 mg/min, 30–90 min) on plasma insulin, glucose, and FFA ($\bar{x}$ ± SEM, N = 5).

plasma glucose, which averaged 82 ± 2 mg/dl, and plasma FFA, which averaged 668 ± 38 μeq/L during the infusion of MCSF, did not change significantly during the hour-long third ventricular infusion of glucose alone (see Table 2).

TABLE 1
Average concentration of plasma insulin (μU/ml, mean ± SEM) during infusion of mock cerebrospinal fluid (MCSF) or combinations of insulin, glucose, and 2-deoxy-D-glucose (2DG) into the third cerebral ventricle of conscious dogs

	Treatment after MCSF				
	Insulin alone (N = 8)	Insulin + glucose (N = 5)	Insulin + 2DG (N = 5)	2 DG alone (N = 4)	Glucose alone (N = 4)
MCSF	32 ± 7	41 ± 5	34 ± 6	29 ± 6	28 ± 6
Treatment (1st ½ h)	64 ± 9	37 ± 6*	46 ± 6	28 ± 9*	28 ± 4*
Treatment (2nd ½ h)	51 ± 7	51 ± 10	150 ± 48*	26 ± 7*	27 ± 5*

* Significantly different from average value during treatment with insulin alone (0.01 < P < 0.05).

Third ventricular infusions of 2-deoxy-glucose (2DG) at 0.225 mg/min with insulin (200 mU/min) produced a large increase of plasma insulin during the second half-hour of infusion (see Figure 4), which was significantly greater than that produced by the infusion of insulin alone (P < 0.05, see Table 1). This rise of plasma insulin was accompanied by a progressive decrease of plasma glucose (P < 0.025) that averaged 18 ± 6 mg/dl below control during the second half-hour of infusion (see Figure 4). The apparent

TABLE 2
Average concentration ($\bar{x}$ ± SEM) of plasma insulin, glucose, and FFA during infusion of mock cerebrospinal fluid (MCSF) on glucose into the third cerebral ventricle of conscious dogs

	Plasma concentrations of:		
	Insulin (μU/ml)	Glucose (mg/dl)	FFA (μeq/L)
MCSF	28 ± 6	82 ± 2	668 ± 38
Glucose alone (1st ½ h)	28 ± 4	83 ± 2	667 ± 72
Glucose alone (2nd ½ h)	27 ± 5	85 ± 2	594 ± 87

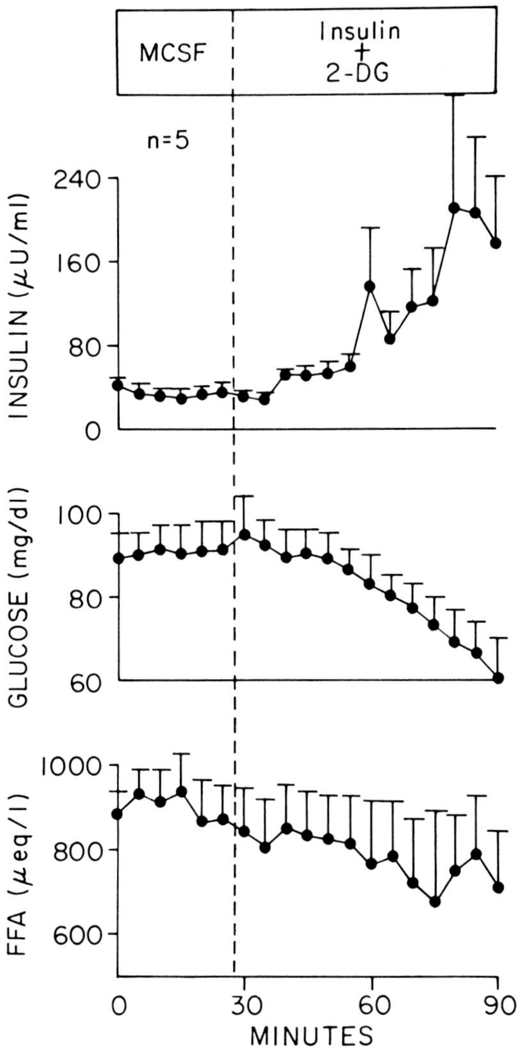

FIGURE 4. The effect of third ventricular infusions of MCSF (0–25 min) or insulin (200 mU/min) plus 2DG (0.225 mg/min, 30–90 min) on plasma insulin, glucose, and FFA ($\bar{x}$ ± SEM, N = 5).

decrease of plasma free fatty acids during the second half-hour of infusion did not reach statistical significance ($\Delta = -159 \pm 96$ μeq/L, P = 0.09). Infusions of 2DG alone into the third cerebral ventricle at 5.5 mg/min, over 20 times the previous dose, had no significant effect on plasma insulin (see Tables 1 and 3). Likewise, plasma glucose, which averaged 85 ± 2 mg/dl, and plasma FFA, which averaged

TABLE 3
Average concentration ($\bar{x}$ ± SEM) of plasma insulin, glucose, and FFA during infusion of mock cerebrospinal fluid (MCSF) or 2-deoxy-D-glucose (2DG) into the third cerebral ventricle of conscious dogs

	Plasma concentrations of:		
	Insulin (μU/ml)	Glucose (mg/dl)	FFA (μeq/L)
MCSF	29 ± 6	85 ± 2	813 ± 100
2DG alone (1st ½ h)	28 ± 9	85 ± 2	735 ± 97
2DG alone (2nd ½ h)	26 ± 7	85 ± 2	752 ± 128

813 ± 100 μeq/L during the infusion of MCSF, did not change significantly during the hour-long third ventricular infusion of 2DG alone (see Table 3).

DISCUSSION

These data on plasma insulin levels from conscious dogs are consistent with those from anesthetized dogs in which Chen, Woods, and Porte[8,9] showed that injection of insulin into the cerebrospinal fluid (CSF) stimulated the secretion of insulin via a vagal pathway. However, the present experiments were designed to test a separate hypothesis of Woods and Porte[9] that centrally administered insulin stimulates such a response by increasing the transport of glucose into a glucoregulatory area of the brain. If this latter hypothesis is correct, one might expect that the addition of glucose to an insulin infusate should increase glucose uptake further and, thus, produce a larger rise of plasma insulin than a third ventricular infusion of insulin alone. In contrast to expectations, the combination of insulin and glucose produced a significantly smaller increase in plasma insulin than did the third ventricular infusion of insulin alone. In accord with this paradoxic result, the combination of insulin and 2-deoxy-D-glucose, a competitive inhibitor of glucose transport and phosphorylation,[10] elicited a much larger rise of plasma insulin than did the third ventricular infusion of insulin alone. Thus, neither set of data supports the hypothesis that increased glucose uptake is the stimulus for neurally mediated insulin secretion. Rather, these data suggest that insulin has a direct effect on some population of central neurons and that glucose metabolism in these neurons can alter the effectiveness of insulin.

This effect of insulin may be on ionic flux. Insulin appears to increase potassium uptake[16] in various tissues, including skeletal muscle,[17] adipose tissue,[18] liver,[19] and perhaps brain.[20] Insulin also alters sodium flux in muscle[21] and phosphate flux in liver.[22] As might be expected from these observations, insulin is known to hyperpolarize the membrane potential of cells from both muscle[23] and adipose[24] tissues. In addition, either systemic[25] or local[6] administration of insulin alters the endogenous firing rate of certain hypothalamic neurons. Oomura has identified a group of hypothalamic neurons in which the insulin effect is accentuated by the simultaneous application of 2DG[6] and in which it is inhibited by the simultaneous application of glucose.[6] Thus, the known effect of insulin to alter the rate of ionic flux across the cell membranes of other tissue may also explain its ability to influence the central neurons that modulate insulin release. It should be pointed out, however, that alternative mechanisms, such as the acceleration of amino acid transport by insulin,[26] could mediate this central action.

Woods and Porte[9] reported that the intracisternal injection of insulin produced an acute hypoglycemia, which was presumably the result of the neurally mediated release of insulin. We observed a smaller increase of plasma insulin during the third ventricular infusion of insulin alone with no change of plasma glucose. Chen et al.,[8] in a companion study, also failed to observe acute hypoglycemia despite the substantial insulin release stimulated by the injection of insulin into the lateral ventricle. The reason for these discrepancies in glycemia is not clear. However, since Woods and Porte[9] have implicated the vagus in the neurogenic release of insulin, it is possible that a vagally mediated release of glucagon[27] also occurs. The ratio of insulin to glucagon secreted might determine the net effect on plasma glucose.

Recent work has convincingly demonstrated the presence of endogenous insulin in cerebrospinal fluid[28] as well as in brain tissue.[29] Others have recently reported the specific binding of insulin to various brain areas,[7,30] suggesting the presence of central receptors for insulin. Earlier, Oomura[6] had demonstrated a local effect of insulin by showing that iontophoretic application of minute amounts of insulin to the surface of certain hypothalamic neurons can change their rate of firing. Chen, Woods, and Porte[8,9] demonstrated that centrally administered insulin can influence the function of cells outside the brain by showing that insulin infused into the CSF activates a neural pathway, which in turn stimulates the release of insulin from the pancreas. Taken together, these studies outline a central system influencing insulin secretion. The data from the present study, however, would suggest that this system is activated more effectively by the combination of central insulin and glucopenia, which calls into question its potential physiologic significance. Thus, despite the presence of insulin and insulin-specific receptors in the brain, and despite the demonstration of both local and peripheral effects of centrally administered insulin, the physiologic role of central insulin in the regulation of the endocrine pancreas remains obscure.

The precise location of the central sites of insulin action has not been determined in the present studies. However, the results of our dye infusions would indicate that the infusate is restricted to the level of the third ventricle and below (see Figure 1). While penetration of hydrophilic protein molecules the size of insulin into brain tissue is thought to be minimal, the specific binding of insulin to circumventricular organs and the medial basal hypothalamus, which is adjacent to the third ventricle, has recently been demonstrated.[31] These areas represent possible sites for the central action of insulin.

In our experiments, glucose was infused into the third cerebral ventricle of conscious dogs and had no significant effect on the plasma level of glucose, confirming the findings of Sloviter et al.[32] and Coimbra et al.[33] In addition, this glucose infusion was without effect on the plasma level of insulin and FFA. Coimbra et al.[33] also reported no change of plasma insulin after the injection of glucose into the lateral cerebral ventricles of fasted rats; they did, however, observe a significant decrease of plasma FFA. Differences between their study and ours, either in the site of infusion (lateral ventricle versus third ventricle), the species of animal studied (rat versus dog), or the variability of FFA levels, may account for the differences in the observed effect of central glucose on plasma FFA.

In the present study, third ventricular infusion of 2DG alone had no significant effect on the plasma levels of insulin or FFA. Coimbra et al.[33] also reported no change of plasma insulin after the injection of 2DG into the lateral ventricle. They did, however, observe a significant increase of plasma FFA in fed rats. Difference in the observed effect of central 2DG on plasma FFA may be due to the experimental differences listed above as well as differences in the duration of fasting. Both Müller et al.[34] and Coimbra et al.[33] observed an increase of plasma glucose following the injection of 2DG into the lateral ventricle of rats. Frohman and Nagai[35] have observed a similar hyperglycemia following the infusion of 2DG into the lateral cerebral ventricle of conscious dogs. It is important to note, however, that the doses used in the present study are well below the minimum effective dose necessary to elicit this hyperglycemic response in the dog.[35] This comparison underscores the potency of these relatively small doses of 2DG and glucose to modulate the effects of intraventricular insulin on plasma insulin concentration.

In summary, infusions of insulin into the third cerebral ventricle of conscious dogs produce a small rise of plasma insulin, which is inhibited by the addition of glucose to the intraventricular infusate and enhanced by the addition of 2DG to the insulin infusate. These data suggest that glucopenia of certain brain cells potentiates the neurally mediated release of insulin after the administration of exogenous insulin to the CSF. It is suggested that central insulin may change the firing rate of those neurons that modulate insulin release by altering the flux of ions across their cell membranes, although other possible mediators, such as amino acids, cannot be excluded.

ACKNOWLEDGMENTS

The authors are grateful to Gary Ogawa for performing the assays; to Bobby Haller for demonstrating the ventricular catheterization technique; to Jeffrey Garfinkle, Bill Hagopian, and Peggy Taborsky for skilled technical assistance with the experiments; and to Joanne Ebert and Pat Jenkins for secretarial assistance.

This work was supported by NIH Grants AM-20443 and AM-18467. Dr. Taborsky was supported by a NIH Training Grant (GM-01724).

REFERENCES

[1] Bergman, R. N., and Miller, R. E.: Direct enhancement of insulin secretion by vagal stimulation of the isolated pancreas. Am. J. Physiol. *225*:481–86, 1973.

[2] Girardier, L., Seydoux, J., and Campfield, L. A.: Control of A and B cells in vivo by sympathetic nervous input and selective hyper- and hypoglycemia in dog pancreas. J. Physiol. (Paris) *72*:801–14, 1976.

[3] Porte, D., Jr., Girardier, L., Seydoux, J., Kanazawa, Y., and Posternak, J.: Neural regulation of insulin secretion in the dog. J. Clin. Invest. *52*:210–14, 1973.

[4] Steffens, A. B., Mogenson, G. J., and Stevenson, J. A. F.: Blood glucose, insulin and free fatty acids after stimulation and lesions of the hypothalamus. Am. J. Physiol. *222*:1446–52, 1972.

[5] Frohman, L. A., and Bernardis, L. L.: Effect of hypothalamic stimulation on plasma glucose, insulin, and glucagon levels. Am. J. Physiol. *221*:1596–1603, 1971.

[6] Oomura, Y.: Central mechanism of feeding. Adv. Biophys. *5*:65–142, 1973.

[7] Havrankova, J., and Roth, J.: Insulin receptors are widely distributed in the central nervous system of the rat. Nature *272*:827–29, 1978.

[8] Chen, M., Woods, S. C., and Porte, D., Jr.: The effect of cerebral intraventricular insulin upon pancreatic insulin secretion in the dog. Diabetes *24*:910–14, 1975.

[9] Woods, S. C., and Porte, D., Jr.: The effect of intracisternal insulin upon plasma glucose and insulin in the dog. Diabetes *24*:905–09, 1975.

[10] Cramer, F. B., and Woodward, G. E.: 2-deoxy-D-glucose as an antagonist of glucose in yeast fermentation. J. Franklin Inst. *253*:354–60, 1952.

[11] Maran, J. W., and Yates, F. E.: Cortisol secretion during intrapituitary infusion of angiotensin II in conscious dogs. Am. J. Physiol. *233*:E273–E285, 1977.

[12] Mitchell, R. A., Loeschcke, H. H., Massion, W. H., and Severinghaus, J. W.: Respiratory responses mediated through superficial chemosensitive areas on the medulla. J. Appl. Physiol. *18*:523–33, 1963.

[13] Herbert, V., Law, K. S., Gottlieb, C. W., and Bleicher, S. J.: Coated charcoal immunoassay of insulin. J. Clin. Endocrinol. *25*:1375–84, 1965.

[14] Smith, S. W.: A new salting-out technique for colorimetric-free fatty acid assays. Anal. Biochem. *67*:531–39, 1975.

[15] Afifi, A. A., and Azen, S. P.: Statistical Analysis: A Computer-oriented Approach. New York, Academic Press, 1972, pp. 65–66.
[16] Hiatt, N., Yamakawa, T., and Davidson, M. B.: Necessity for insulin in transfer of excess infused K to intracellular fluid. Metabolism *23*:43–49, 1974.
[17] Andres, R., Baltzan, M. A., Cader, G., and Zierler, K. L.: Effect of insulin on carbohydrate metabolism and on potassium in the forearm of man. J. Clin. Invest. *41*:108–15, 1962.
[18] Gourley, D. R. H., and Bethea, M. D.: Insulin effect on adipose tissue and potassium. Proc. Soc. Exp. Biol. Med. *115*:821–23, 1964.
[19] Burton, S. D., and Ishida, T.: Effect of insulin on potassium and glucose movement in perfused rat liver. Am. J. Physiol. *209*:1145–61, 1965.
[20] Ellison, R. J.: Changes in cerebral potassium during insulin hypoglycemia. Proc. Soc. Exp. Biol. Med. *98*:128–29, 1958.
[21] Creese, R., and Northover, J.: Maintenance of isolated diaphragm with normal sodium content. J. Physiol. (Lond.) *155*:343–57, 1961.
[22] Kastens, P. J., Haxhe, J. J., Lambotte, L., and Lambotte, C.: The effect of insulin on the uptake of potassium and phosphate by the isolate perfused canine liver. Metabolism *12*:941–50, 1963.
[23] Zierler, K. L.: Hyperpolarization of muscle by insulin in a glucose-free environment. Am. J. Physiol. *197*:524–26, 1959.
[24] Beigelman, P. M., and Hollander, P. B.: Effect of insulin upon resting electrical potential of adipose tissue. Proc. Soc. Exp. Biol. Med. *110*:590–95, 1962.
[25] Anand, B. K., Chhina, G. S., Sharma, K. N., Dua, S., and Singh, B.: Activity of single neurons in the hypothalamic feeding center: effect of glucose. Am. J. Physiol. *207*:1146–54, 1964.
[26] Kipnis, D. M., and Noall, M. W.: Stimulation of amino acid transport by insulin in the isolated rat diaphragm. Biochim. Biophys. Acta *28*:226–27, 1958.
[27] Kaneto, A., Miki, E., and Kosaka, K.: Effects of vagal stimulation on glucagon and insulin secretion. Endocrinology *95*:1005–10, 1974.
[28] Woods, S. C., and Porte, D., Jr.: Relationship between plasma and cerebrospinal fluid insulin levels of dogs. Am. J. Physiol. *233*:E331–E334, 1977.
[29] Havrankova, J., Schmechel, D., Roth, J., and Brownstein, M.: Identification of insulin in rat brain. Proc. Natl. Acad. Sci. USA *75*:5737–41, 1978.
[30] Posner, B. I., Kelly, P. A., Shiu, R. P. C., and Friesen, H. G.: Studies of insulin, growth hormone, and prolactin binding: tissue distribution, species variation, and characterization. Endocrinology *95*:521–31, 1974.
[31] VanHouten, M., Posner, B. I., Kopriwa, B. M., and Brawer, J. R.: Insulin-binding sites in rat brain: *In vivo* localization to the circumventricular organs by quantitative radioautography. Endocrinology *105*:666–73, 1979.
[32] Sloviter, H. A., and Sabata, K.: Inactivity of cerebrospinal fluid in the regulation of blood glucose concentration. Am. J. Physiol. *204*:153–56, 1963.
[33] Coimbra, C. C., Gross, J. L., and Migliorini, R. H.: Intraventricular 2-deoxy-glucose, glucose, insulin, and free fatty acid mobilization. Am. J. Physiol. *236*:E317–E327, 1979.
[34] Müller, E. E., Frohman, L. A., and Cocchi, D.: Drug control of hyperglycemia and inhibition of insulin secretion due to centrally administered 2-deoxy-D-glucose. Am. J. Physiol. *224*:1210–17, 1973.
[35] Frohman, L. A., and Nagai, K.: Central nervous system-mediated stimulation of glucagon secretion in the dog following 2-deoxy-D-glucose. Metabolism *25*:1449–52, 1976.

Altered Responsiveness to Cortisol, Epinephrine, and Glucagon in Insulin-infused Juvenile-onset Diabetics

A Mechanism for Diabetic Instability

HARRY SHAMOON, ROSA HENDLER, AND ROBERT S. SHERWIN

SUMMARY

To evaluate the mechanism of rebound and stress hyperglycemia in diabetes, cortisol, epinephrine, and glucagon were infused into normal and juvenile-onset diabetic subjects for 5–6 h in doses designed to simulate the increments observed in insulin hypoglycemia or severe stress. Plasma glucose and glucose kinetics were normalized in the diabetics before each experiment by infusion of insulin (0.25–1.0 U/h) for 4–6 h, which was then continued during anti-insulin hormone administration.

Infusion of cortisol and epinephrine produced comparable elevations in plasma cortisol (35–45 μg/dl) and plasma epinephrine (350–450 pg/ml) in normal and diabetic subjects. However, the increment in plasma glucose in diabetics after cortisol (86 ± 15 mg/dl) and epinephrine (129 ± 12 mg/dl) infusion was fivefold to sevenfold greater than it was in normals ($P < 0.001$), despite ongoing insulin infusion. Whereas cortisol failed to alter glucose production in normals, in diabetics there was a progressive 35% increase in glucose production ($P < 0.001$). Similarly, epinephrine produced only a transient (<90 min) 60% rise in glucose production in normal subjects, but caused a sustained 50%–90% rise in glucose production in diabetics throughout the entire 5-h study. In contrast, both cortisol and epinephrine infusion was accompanied by a 25%–40% ($P < 0.001$) decline in glucose clearance, no different than in normal and diabetic subjects. Glucagon infusion produced a transient 35%–40% rise in glucose production, which was of comparable magnitude and duration in normal controls and diabetics. However, the glucagon-induced rise in plasma glucose was threefold greater in the diabetics due to failure of endogenous insulin secretion and consequent lack of an increase in glucose clearance as observed in normal controls. When saline was administered to the insulin-infused diabetics, neither plasma glucose nor glucose production were altered from baseline values.

It is concluded that (1) the hyperglycemic effect of each of the anti-insulin hormones is increased in diabetics, in spite of prior normalization of plasma glucose concentration, by continuous insulin infusion and (2) hyperglycemia is particularly exaggerated by elevations of cortisol and epinephrine in diabetes as a consequence of an altered response of the liver to these hormones. DIABETES *29*:284–291, April 1980.

It is a long-standing clinical observation that stress induces a greater derangement in glucose regulation in diabetics than in normal humans with similar medical and surgical illnesses, despite usual insulin treatment.[1] Furthermore, in diabetes, paradoxic rebound hyperglycemia may result from hypoglycemia caused by excessive insulin treatment (Somogyi phenomenon).[2] While it has been suggested that anti-insulin hormone excess is involved in this brittleness,[2–4] it has not been previously determined whether insulin-treated diabetics actually exhibit excessive anti-insulin hormone secretion during stress or augmented sensitivity to normal increments in these hormones. The latter is, in fact, in keeping with the normal rise in plasma cortisol and epinephrine and the absent rise in plasma glucagon observed in nonketotic juvenile-onset diabetics during insulin-induced hypoglycemia.[5–7]

The importance of augmented sensitivity to anti-insulin hormones in the pathogenesis of diabetic instability remains to be established. While glucagon infusion[8] and chronic glucocorticoid administration[9] have been reported to cause an exaggerated rise in blood glucose in diabetics, an enhanced hyperglycemic response has not been noted in diabetics when either cortisol[9] or epinephrine[10,11] is given acutely (<90 min). Moreover, the former studies have generally involved insulin-withdrawn diabetics, and therefore insulin lack rather than altered tissue responsiveness to the

This study was presented in part at the 39th Annual Meeting of the American Diabetes Association, Los Angeles, June 10–12, 1979.
From the Department of Internal Medicine, Yale University School of Medicine, New Haven, Connecticut.
Address reprint requests to Robert S. Sherwin, M.D., Department of Internal Medicine, Yale University School of Medicine, 333 Cedar Street, New Haven, Connecticut 06510.
Received for publication 12 October 1979.

anti-insulin hormone may have contributed to these findings. This possibility is supported by data suggesting a normal hepatic response to glucagon infusion in insulin-withdrawn diabetics.[12,13] The influence of the diabetic state on the response of hepatic and peripheral tissues to cortisol and epinephrine has not been previously determined.

The present study was consequently undertaken to examine the effects of acute "stress-like" elevations of cortisol, epinephrine, and glucagon on plasma glucose and glucose kinetics in normal and diabetic humans. Plasma glucose and glucose turnover were normalized in the diabetics before each experiment with a continuous insulin infusion to minimize the effects of insulin deficiency per se. Our data indicate that diabetes increases the hyperglycemic actions of anti-insulin hormones, despite ongoing infusion of insulin in basal amounts. The exaggerated hyperglycemic effect of cortisol and epinephrine in diabetics is due to an augmented response of the liver, while the increased hyperglycemic effect of glucagon is due to a lack of a rise in peripheral glucose clearance, as observed in normal subjects.

METHODS

Subjects. Two groups of subjects were studied. The normal control group consisted of 22 healthy volunteers (13 males and 9 females) aged 19–32 yr. The diabetic group consisted of 16 ambulatory juvenile-onset diabetics (10 males and 6 females) who were receiving a total of 44 ± 4 U of insulin daily [in single (N = 6) or divided (N = 10) doses] for 12 ± 2 yr (mean ± SEM). They ranged in age from 18 to 34 yr. All subjects were within 15% of ideal body weight (based on 1959 Metropolitan Life Insurance Co. tables). They habitually consumed weight-maintaining diets containing at least 200 g of carbohydrate and were taking no drugs (other than insulin). None of the subjects had a history of liver or renal disease or evidence of an intercurrent medical illness at the time of study. The subjects were informed of the nature, purpose, and possible risks of the study before obtaining their written, voluntary consent to participate.

Procedures. All studies were performed in the morning (at 0730 h) after a 12–14-h overnight fast. A total of 52 experiments was performed (six controls and eight diabetics were studied on two to three occasions). The diabetic subjects received no intermediate-acting insulin for 24 h before the study. An indwelling catheter was inserted in an antecubital vein in each arm for blood sampling and for continuous infusion (Harvard Apparatus Co., Millis, Massachusetts) of glucoregulatory hormones and [3-^{3}H]-glucose.

In the normal control group, a 2-h equilibration period (t = −120 to 0 min) was employed, during which a primed continuous infusion of [3-^{3}H]-glucose (New England Nuclear, Boston, Massachusetts) was administered. The priming dose (35 μCi) was injected rapidly, followed by a constant infusion of 0.25 μCi/min, which was continued for the remainder of the study. In all subjects, the specific activity of [3-^{3}H]-glucose in plasma reached a stable plateau within 90 min.

In the diabetic group, the equilibration period was extended to reduce plasma glucose levels (128–263 mg/dl, preinfusion) to values comparable to those observed in normal controls. For this purpose, crystalline zinc insulin (Eli Lilly Co., Indianapolis, Indiana) was initially infused at a rate of 0.5–2.0 U/h until plasma glucose concentration approached normal values (< 135 mg/dl). The dose of insulin was then reduced to 0.25–1.0 U/h and a primed continuous infusion of [3-^{3}H]-glucose was begun and maintained throughout the entire experimental period. Three to four hours was allowed to elapse after the priming injection of the tracer to ensure that the specific activity of [3-^{3}H]-glucose had reached a plateau and that plasma glucose had stabilized within the normal range for at least 1 h before infusion of anti-insulin hormones or saline. The coefficient of variation of glucose specific activity and plasma glucose concentration in the diabetics before anti-insulin infusion (3.4 ± 0.5% and 2.7 ± 0.5%, respectively) was similar to that observed in normal controls (2.9 ± 0.4 and 1.3 ± 0.3, P = NS). The dose of insulin required to maintain normal plasma glucose levels in the diabetics during the stabilization period was no different in the various treatment groups (cortisol, 0.44 ± 0.10 U/h; epinephrine, 0.42 ± 0.09 U/h; glucagon, 0.37 ± 0.10 U/h; and saline, 0.39 ± 0.08 U/h). Thereafter, this insulin infusion dose was continued until the completion of the study. The duration of insulin infusion before counterregulatory hormone infusion was 4–6 h and did not differ between groups. None of the subjects exhibited hypoglycemia, i.e., plasma glucose < 60 mg/dl.

After the equilibration period, cortisol (11 controls and 6 diabetics), epinephrine (8 controls and 9 diabetics), glucagon (4 controls and 5 diabetics), or physiologic saline (5 controls and 4 diabetics) was infused for 5–6 h. Cortisol sodium succinate (Solucortef, The Upjohn Company, Kalamazoo, Michigan) was administered as a primed continuous infusion for 6 h. The priming dose was given over the initial 150-min period at twice the continuous infusion rate. The continuous infusion dose was 5 mg/m^2 body surface area per hour. Epinephrine (Adrenalin, Parke-Davis and Co., Detroit, Michigan) was infused at a rate of 1.2 μg/m^2 body surface area per minute for 5 h. Crystalline beef and pork glucagon (Eli Lilly and Co., Indianapolis, Indiana) was infused at a rate of 3 ng/kg body wt per minute for 5 h. The infusates were freshly prepared in sterile saline. Ascorbic acid (1 mg/ml) was added to the epinephrine solution to protect against oxidation. Human serum albumin (300 mg/dl) was added to the glucagon solution, and 2 ml of the subjects' whole blood was added to 50 ml of insulin infusate to prevent adherence to glassware and tubing.[14] Three blood samples were drawn at 15-min intervals before initiation of the cortisol, epinephrine, glucagon, or saline infusions and at 15–30-min intervals thereafter until the completion of the infusions at 5–6 h.

Analyses. Plasma glucose concentration was measured by the glucose oxidase method using a Beckman glucose analyzer (Beckman Instruments, Inc., Fullerton, California). The methods used for the determination of plasma immunoreactive insulin, plasma immunoreactive glucagon (using Unger antibody 30K), and glucose specific activity have been previously described.[5,15] Plasma epinephrine and norepinephrine were measured by an isotope derivative method[16] and plasma cortisol was determined fluorometrically.[17]

Calculations. Rates of endogenous glucose production and uptake were calculated in the steady state before hormone infusion by the isotope dilution equation and during nonsteady state conditions using Steele's equations in their derivative form.[18] Derivative functions were calculated using a polynomial-fitting procedure.[19] The value of 0.65 (pool fraction) was used to correct for noninstantaneous mixing within the entire glucose pool.[20] The measurement of glucose turnover rates, based on the primed continuous infusion of glucose tracer, the pool fraction technique, and polynomial equations, has been validated for both steady and nonsteady states.[21] Glucose clearance was calculated by dividing the rate of glucose uptake by the plasma glucose concentration.[22] Glucose clearance has been used as an index of the rate of glucose removal from plasma independent of the plasma glucose concentration.[23] All calculations were performed on an Olivetti P 6060 computer.

Statistical analyses were performed employing an analysis of variance with repeated measures design to compare the response of different treatment groups over time.[24] The unpaired Student's *t* test was used for comparison of specific time points, and the paired *t* test was used in comparing changes from baseline. Data in the text and figures are presented as the mean ± SEM.

RESULTS

Response to cortisol infusion in normal subjects. Figure 1 demonstrates the changes in plasma cortisol, plasma glucose, and glucose kinetics during infusion of cortisol in normal subjects. Plasma cortisol levels (13 ± 1 μg/dl, basal) increased rapidly, reaching a plateau 200%–250% above baseline values within 60 min. Plasma glucose (89 ± 2 mg/dl, basal) gradually increased by 10–15 mg/dl. At the completion of the study (6 h), plasma glucose levels were significantly higher in the cortisol-treated (102 ± 3 mg/dl) than in the saline-treated subjects (88 ± 2 mg/dl, $P < 0.001$). Glucose output (1.97 ± 0.11 mg/kg/min, basal) tended to decline during the cortisol infusion ($0.1 > P > 0.05$) but remained comparable to saline-treated subjects throughout the 6-h study period. On the other hand, glucose clearance decreased within 2 h after the onset of the cortisol infusion ($P < 0.05$), reaching values 25%–30% below baseline at 6 h ($P < 0.005$).

FIGURE 1. Effect of cortisol infusion on plasma cortisol concentration and glucose kinetics in normal subjects.

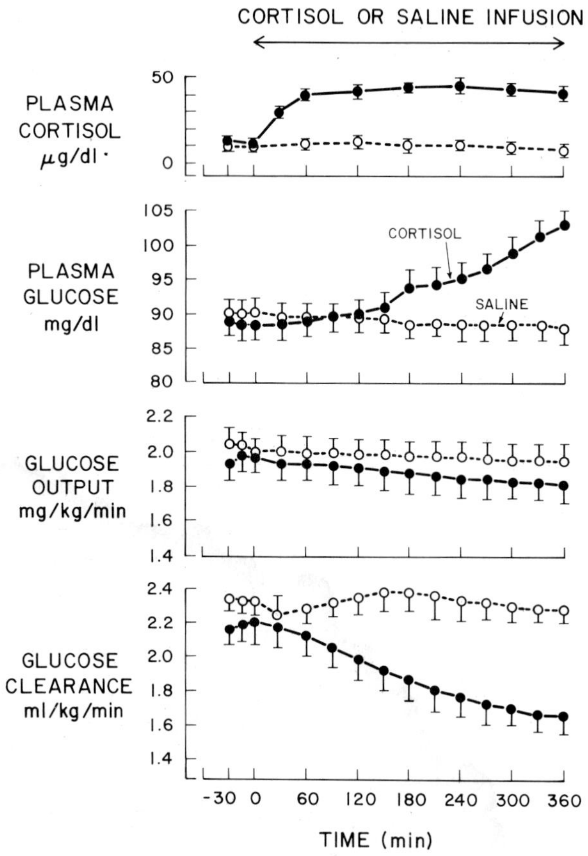

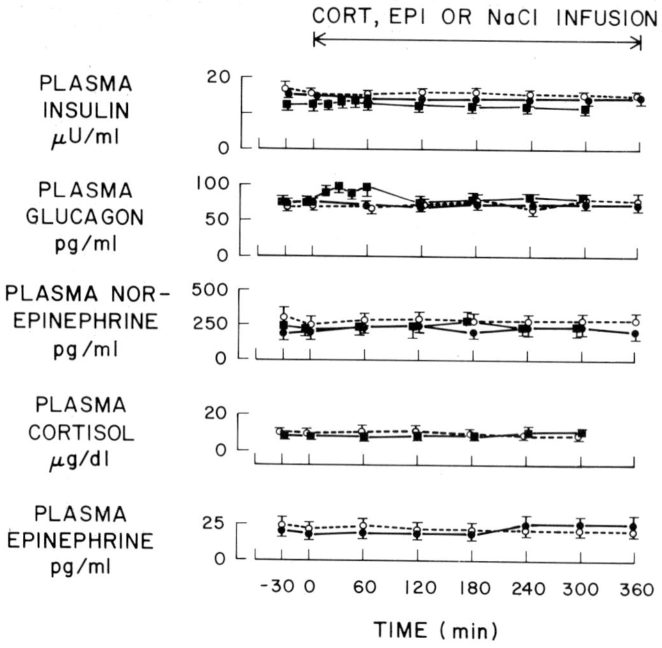

FIGURE 2. Effect of cortisol and epinephrine infusion on the plasma concentrations of other glucoregulatory hormones in normal subjects. ●, cortisol; ■, epinephrine; ○, saline.

As shown in Figure 2, the cortisol infusion had no effect on plasma insulin, plasma glucagon, plasma epinephrine, or plasma norepinephrine concentrations. Furthermore, the levels of these hormones were no different in cortisol- and saline-treated subjects (P = NS).

Influence of diabetes on the response to cortisol infusion. Figure 3 compares the metabolic response to cortisol administration in insulin-infused diabetics with that of normal controls and insulin-infused diabetics given saline. Plasma cortisol levels in the diabetics were comparable to those observed in normal subjects in the basal state (11 ± 1 μg/dl) and after (35–40 μg/dl) cortisol infusion (P = NS). Plasma cortisol concentration (10 ± 1 μg/dl, basal) remained constant in insulin-infused diabetics given saline. Before cortisol administration, plasma glucose levels in the insulin-infused diabetics (92 ± 1 mg/dl) were not significantly different from those observed in normal subjects. However, after cortisol infusion, the rise in plasma glucose was markedly exaggerated in the diabetic group, reaching values six- to sevenfold greater than in normal controls ($P < 0.001$). In contrast, plasma glucose levels decreased slightly (11 ± 5 mg/dl over 6 h), but not significantly, when saline was administered to insulin-infused diabetics.

The mechanism of the exaggerated hyperglycemic response to cortisol in diabetics becomes apparent when one examines glucose kinetics (Figure 3). Although endogenous glucose production was normalized in the diabetics

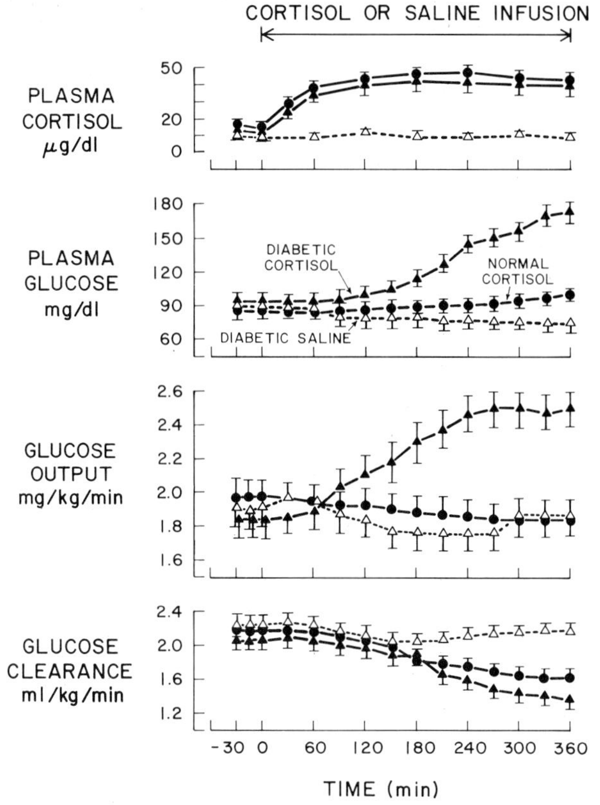

FIGURE 3. Influence of diabetes on the response of glucose kinetics to cortisol infusion. Plasma glucose, glucose production, and glucose clearance were normalized in the diabetics before cortisol administration by infusion of insulin, which was then continued for the remainder of the study. Changes in glucose kinetics in insulin-infused diabetics given cortisol (closed triangles) are compared with those observed in insulin-infused diabetics given saline (open triangles) and in normal subjects given cortisol (closed circles).

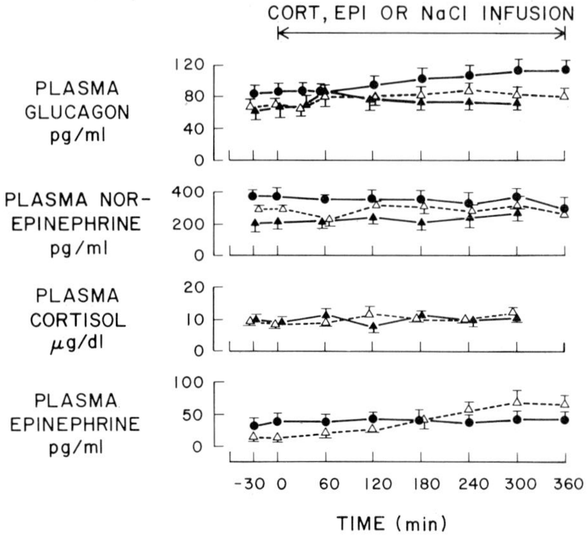

FIGURE 4. Effect of cortisol and epinephrine infusion on the plasma concentrations of other anti-insulin hormones in insulin-infused diabetic subjects. ●, cortisol; ▲, epinephrine; △, saline.

before cortisol administration (1.88 ± 0.13 versus 1.97 ± 0.11 mg/kg/min in controls, P = NS), hypercortisolemia produced a progressive and sustained rise in glucose production in the diabetic group. Glucose production rose by 35% (P < 0.001) within 270 min and then stabilized for the remainder of the study. In contrast, glucose output was not significantly altered in normals given cortisol or in insulin-infused diabetics given saline. Cortisol infusion also produced a progressive 30%–35% decline in glucose clearance (P < 0.001), which was no different from that observed in normal subjects.

The effect of the cortisol infusion on plasma glucagon, epinephrine, and norepinephrine concentrations in diabetic subjects is shown in Figure 4. Plasma glucagon concentration (84 ± 14 pg/ml, basal) increased slightly, reaching values significantly above baseline only in the final hour of study (35%–40%, P < 0.01). However, the plasma glucagon response to cortisol in the diabetics was not significantly different from that observed in saline-infused diabetic controls (P = NS). Plasma epinephrine levels were unchanged during the cortisol infusion but increased two- to threefold (P < 0.05) in the insulin-infused diabetics given saline. Plasma norepinephrine concentration remained constant in the cortisol-infused diabetics as well as in the various control groups.

Response to epinephrine infusion in normal subjects. Infusion of epinephrine in normal subjects produced a prompt increase in plasma epinephrine (24 ± 3 pg/ml, basal), which stabilized at levels of 375–425 pg/ml between 2 and 5 h (Figure 5). Plasma glucose (91 ± 2 mg/dl, basal) increased rapidly, reaching peak levels (125–130 mg/dl) between 45 and 150 min (Figure 5). Thereafter, plasma glucose gradually declined, but remained 24 ± 2 mg/dl above preinfusion values by 5 h. Glucose production rose by 60% (P < 0.001) within 15–30 min and then returned to baseline levels by 90 min. Glucose clearance progressively declined by 30% (P < 0.02).

The effect of the epinephrine infusion on the other glucoregulatory hormones is shown in Figure 2. Although epinephrine produced marked hyperglycemia, plasma insulin was not significantly altered. Plasma glucagon (95 ± 9 pg/ml, basal) tended to increase slightly (by 20%) at 30 min (0.1 > P > 0.05) but remained at basal levels thereafter. The epinephrine infusion had no effect on the plasma cortisol or norepinephrine concentrations.

Influence of diabetes on the response to epinephrine infusion. The effect of the epinephrine infusion on plasma epinephrine, plasma glucose, and glucose kinetics in insulin-infused diabetics is shown in Figure 6. In the diabetics, basal (27 ± 6 pg/ml) and postinfusion (300–450 pg/ml) epinephrine concentrations as well as basal glucose levels (88 ± 6 mg/dl) were comparable to those observed in normal subjects (P = NS). While plasma glucose initially rose at similar rates in diabetics and normals, beyond the first hour the rise in plasma glucose was markedly increased in the diabetics, reaching levels five- to sixfold greater than those observed in normal subjects (P < 0.001). In contrast saline infusion produced a slight decline in plasma glucose in insulin-treated diabetics (Figure 6).

Despite prior normalization of glucose output with insulin, the initial (0–60 min) rise in glucose production induced by epinephrine was 50%–100% greater in the diabetics than in the controls (P < 0.05). More important, epinephrine infusion produced a sustained rather than a transient rise in glucose production in the diabetics. Glucose production remained 50%–90% above preinfusion levels (P < 0.001),

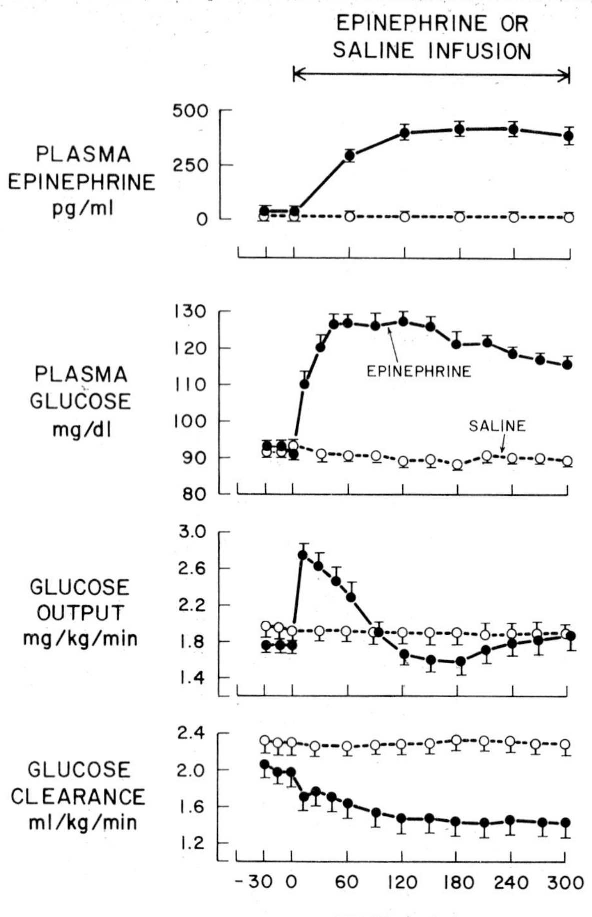

FIGURE 5. Effect of epinephrine infusion on plasma epinephrine concentration and glucose kinetics in normal subjects.

saline control levels (P < 0.001), or values observed in normal subjects (P < 0.002) between 1 and 5 h. Epinephrine infusion produced a comparable decline in glucose clearance in normal and diabetic subjects (P = NS). As shown in Figure 4, the infusion of epinephrine had no effect on plasma glucagon, norepinephrine, or cortisol concentrations in diabetic subjects.

Response to glucagon infusion in normal and diabetic subjects (Figure 7). Plasma glucagon concentrations in the basal state and after glucagon infusion were virtually identical in normal (96 ± 10 and 348 ± 39 pg/ml) and diabetic (91 ± 20 and 352 ± 42 pg/ml) subjects. Infusion of glucagon produced a threefold greater peak rise in plasma glucose concentration in the diabetic group (P < 0.01). Plasma glucose later declined in both groups but remained above baseline values only in the diabetics (P < 0.01) by 5 h. In marked contrast to cortisol and epinephrine, changes in glucose production during the glucagon infusion were of comparable magnitude and duration in normal and diabetic subjects. In both groups, glucose production (2.03 ± 0.04 in normals versus 2.14 ± 0.15 mg/kg/min in diabetics, P = NS) rose by 35%–40% (P < 0.001) within 15–30 min and then gradually returned to baseline levels by 2 h. Glucose clearance, on the other hand, increased by 15% (P < 0.05) in normal subjects but remained unchanged in the diabetics, thereby accounting for the increased hyper-

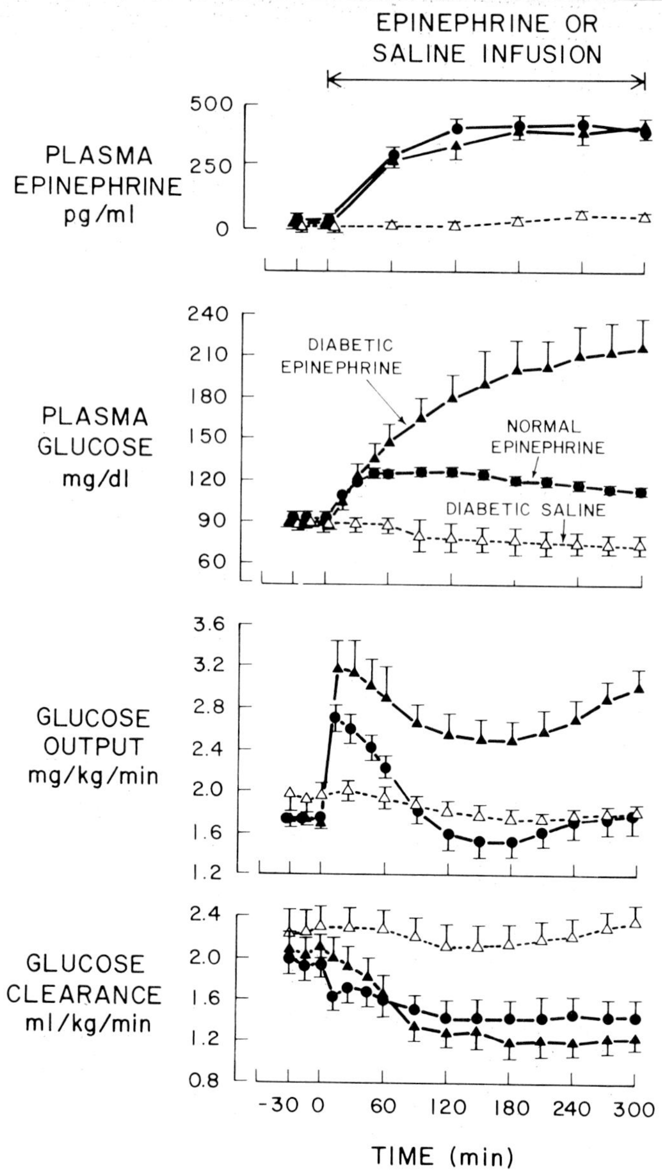

FIGURE 6. Influence of diabetes on the response of glucose kinetics to epinephrine infusion. Changes in glucose kinetics in insulin-infused diabetics given epinephrine (closed triangles) are compared with those observed in insulin-infused diabetics given saline (open triangles) and in normal subjects given epinephrine (closed circles).

glycemic response in diabetics. The rise in glucose clearance in normal subjects was accompanied by a 55%–90% elevation in plasma insulin concentration during the first hour of glucagon administration (11 ± 1 μU/ml in the basal state versus 17 ± 1, 20 ± 1, 19 ± 2, and 17 ± 2 μU/ml at 15, 30, 45, and 60 mins, respectively; P < 0.05 compared with preinfusion level). Plasma insulin levels subsequently returned to baseline values by 3 h (12 ± 3, 12 ± 3, and 11 ± 2 at 3, 4, and 5 h, respectively).

DISCUSSION

While it is well recognized that physiologic stress adversely affects blood glucose regulation to a much greater extent in juvenile-onset diabetics than in normal subjects, the mechanism underlying this phenomenon has not previously been determined. In the present study we demonstrate that each

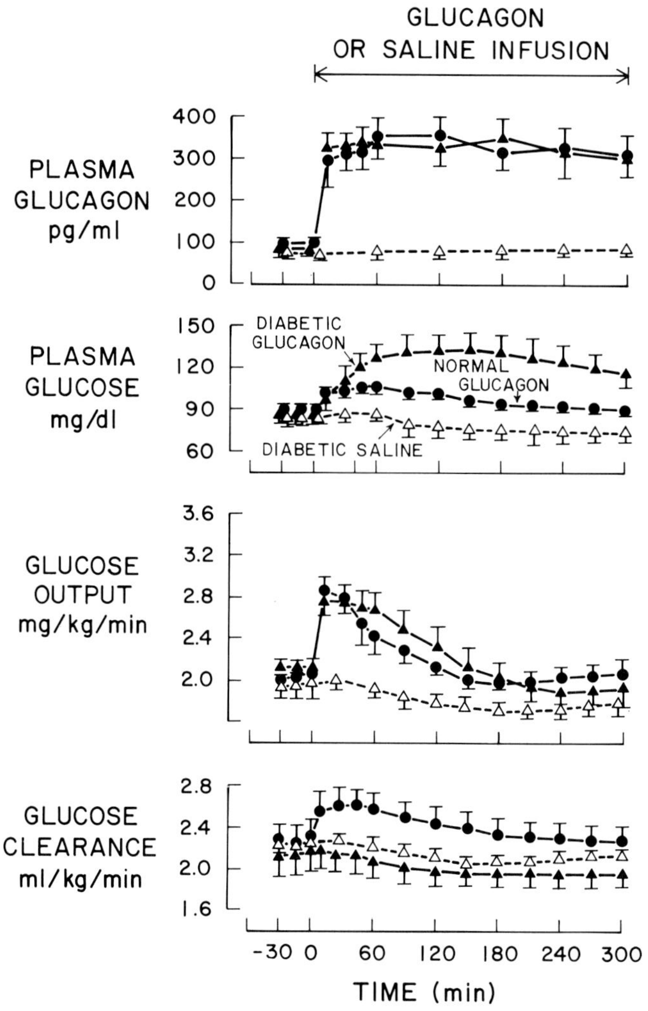

FIGURE 7. Changes in plasma glucagon concentration and glucose kinetics in response to the infusion of glucagon in normal (closed circles) and insulin-infused diabetic subjects (closed triangles).

of the "stress hormones," cortisol, epinephrine, and glucagon, causes an exaggerated rise in plasma glucose in juvenile-onset diabetics. This enhanced hyperglycemic action was most pronounced in response to cortisol and epinephrine and was demonstrable in the face of ongoing insulin infusion in doses that normalized plasma glucose concentration and glucose turnover before each experiment. Our data indicate that increased sensitivity to cortisol and epinephrine in diabetes is attributable to an alteration in the response of the liver to these hormones. Both cortisol and epinephrine reduced peripheral glucose clearance to a similar degree (25%–40%) in normal and diabetic subjects. The diabetic state, on the other hand, failed to alter the stimulatory action of glucagon on the liver. Enhanced hyperglycemia in this circumstance is due to a failure of endogenous insulin secretion and consequent lack of an increase in glucose clearance as observed in normal subjects.

The plasma concentrations of cortisol, epinephrine, and glucagon achieved in this study were comparable to or less than those reported during severe physiologic stress in humans. Three- to fourfold increases in plasma cortisol have been observed after insulin-induced hypoglycemia[25] and abdominal surgery[26] and are generally exceeded in diabetic ketoacidosis.[3,27] The levels of plasma epinephrine produced by infusion of epinephrine (350–450 pg/ml) were considerably lower than those reported during severe insulin hypoglycemia[25] and diabetic ketoacidosis[6] and similar to those observed during moderate hypoglycemia,[5] heavy exercise,[28] and in the perioperative period.[29] Finally, comparable increments in plasma glucagon have been reported in severe trauma,[30] cardiogenic shock,[31] and diabetic ketoacidosis.[3,32]

Previous studies concerning the acute effects of cortisol and epinephrine on blood glucose regulation in human diabetes have involved insulin-withdrawn rather than insulin-treated subjects. In those studies, neither hormone caused an exaggerated hyperglycemic response in diabetics.[9–11] The discrepancy between the current findings and those earlier reports may be more apparent than real when the duration of hormone treatment is considered. Our data demonstrate that the disparate responses of normal and diabetic subjects become evident only after 90–120 min of cortisol or epinephrine exposure, whereas blood glucose measurements were previously obtained over 60–90-min intervals.[9–11]

Our findings indicate that alterations in the hepatic response to cortisol and epinephrine can entirely account for the exaggerated hyperglycemic effect of these hormones in diabetes. While infusion of cortisol had no effect on hepatic glucose output in normals, identical elevations in plasma cortisol produced a progressive and sustained 35% increase in glucose production in the diabetics (Figure 3). Similarly, infusion of epinephrine produced only a transient (<90 min) rise in hepatic glucose output in normal subjects but caused a sustained 50%–90% increase in glucose production in diabetics (Figure 5). Inasmuch as glucose production remained at baseline levels in insulin-infused diabetics given saline, the enhanced response of the liver was due to the anti-insulin hormone rather than to an insufficient insulin infusion dose. Similar findings have not been previously reported in either diabetic animals or humans. In fact, a fall (rather than a rise) in hepatic glucose output has been observed in depancreatized dogs following glucocorticoid administration.[33]

With respect to the mechanism of the altered hepatic responsiveness in diabetics, this phenomenon cannot be accounted for by changes in endogenous glucagon secretion. Epinephrine had no effect on plasma glucagon levels, whereas cortisol produced only a small (30 pg/ml) delayed rise in glucagon concentration in diabetic subjects. The latter occurred 3 h after the onset of the rise in hepatic glucose output (Figure 4) and was similar to that observed in saline-infused diabetics (P = NS). In addition, the time course of the cortisol-induced change in hepatic glucose output is not in keeping with a glucagon-mediated effect. Cortisol induced a sustained elevation in glucose output, whereas greater increments in plasma glucagon had only a transient stimulatory effect on hepatic glucose output (Figure 7). While glucocorticoids[15] and epinephrine[34] have been previously reported to stimulate glucagon secretion in humans, in those studies adrenal steroids were given for more prolonged periods and the doses of epinephrine were threefold greater than in this report.

Although the insulin infusion doses employed were equivalent to normal basal systemic delivery rates[14,35] and to normalized plasma glucose concentration and glucose kinetics, a role for insulin deficiency in the altered hepatic response of diabetics cannot be excluded. Since insulin was infused peripherally, portal insulin deficiency may have occurred in spite of normal rates of hepatic glucose production. Reduced levels of insulin in the portal circulation may thus have rendered the liver more vulnerable to cortisol and epinephrine. It is also possible that the infusion of cortisol or epinephrine in normal subjects (but not diabetics) produced a rise in portal insulin concentration that was not detected by peripheral hormone measurements and thus diminished the hepatic response to these hormones in this group. However, this possibility is not supported by studies in normal humans employing somatostatin. When somatostatin and epinephrine are infused simultaneously, a transient rather than a sustained increase in glucose output occurs in spite of the fall in plasma insulin induced by somatostatin.[36] Alternatively, the relatively brief period (4–6 h) of insulin treatment may have been inadequate to normalize the responsiveness of the liver to these hormones. Regardless as to whether the magnitude or duration of insulinization in the diabetics was comparable to the normal state, the degree of insulinization is likely to be equal to or greater than that achieved in the clinical setting with conventional insulin treatment, where elevated glucose levels are usually present.

In contrast to the findings with cortisol and epinephrine, neither the time course nor the magnitude of the rise in hepatic glucose output induced by hyperglucagonemia was altered in the insulin-infused diabetics (Figure 7). These findings are in keeping with previous studies involving insulin-withdrawn diabetics[12,13] and suggest that the augmented hepatic response to cortisol and epinephrine is unlikely to be a nonspecific consequence of the diabetic state. It should be noted, however, that the glucagon-induced rise in plasma glucose concentration in diabetics was increased compared with normal controls. In normal subjects, glucagon infusion was accompanied by a rise in plasma insulin that enhanced peripheral glucose clearance and promoted the rapid disposal of glucose transiently released by the liver. In the diabetics, however, endogenous insulin deficiency precluded such an increase in glucose clearance, and thus the removal of glucose from the circulation was delayed. It should be noted that, in contrast to glucagon, infusion of cortisol and epinephrine to normal subjects had no significant effect on peripheral insulin concentration (Figure 2). The maintenance of basal insulin levels during epinephrine infusion can be attributed to the known suppressive effects of epinephrine on endogenous insulin secretion.[37] The failure of insulin to rise during cortisol administration may be related to the gradual nature of the plasma glucose increment or might alternatively be a consequence of a suppressive effect of acute hypercortisolemia on glucose-stimulated insulin release.[38]

The current observations have important clinical implications. The demonstration of enhanced responsiveness to physiologic elevations of anti-insulin hormones in insulin-infused diabetics provides a mechanism for the propensity of these patients to develop severe hyperglycemia during illness, despite usual insulin treatment. In addition, our findings may account for rebound hyperglycemia observed in diabetics (but not normal subjects) following insulin-induced hypoglycemia (the Somogyi phenomenon). The importance of altered hepatic sensitivity to cortisol and epinephrine in the latter circumstance is underscored by the fact that cortisol and epinephrine levels are similar in normal and diabetic subjects under conditions of insulin hypoglycemia,[5,6] whereas glucagon concentrations fail to increase in diabetics.[7] Finally, our data may have implications regarding the use of mechanical open-loop insulin delivery systems that administer insulin via the peripheral (rather that portal) route.[39–42] It is possible that these devices may not prevent marked hyperglycemia when cortisol or epinephrine secretion is increased. Whether more prolonged normalization of glucose homeostasis with peripheral infusion devices would normalize the response of the liver to cortisol and epinephrine remains to be determined.

ACKNOWLEDGMENTS

We thank Andrea Belous, Aida Groszman, Ralph Jacob, Hemma Mehta, and Annette Meyer for their expert technical help and Phyllis Strumpf and Barbara Hoxsie for their secretarial assistance. We are grateful to Mary Walesky, R.N., for her care of our patients and Dr. Philip Felig for his valued criticism.

This research was supported in part by grants AM 20495 and RR125 from the National Institutes of Health. Dr. Shamoon is the recipient of a Juvenile Diabetes Foundation Fellowship. Dr. Sherwin is the recipient of a Research Career Development Award (AM 00334) from the National Institutes of Health.

REFERENCES

1 Bondy, P. K., and Felig, P.: Disorders of carbohydrate metabolism. *In* Duncan's Diseases of Metabolism, 7th edit. Bondy, P. K., and Rosenberg, L. E., Eds. Philadelphia, W. B. Saunders Co., 1974, pp. 221–340.

2 Somogyi, M.: Exacerbation of diabetes by excess insulin action. Am. J. Med. *26*:169–91, 1959.

3 Schade, D., and Eaton, R. P.: The controversy concerning counterregulatory hormone secretion. A hypothesis for the prevention of diabetic ketoacidosis? Diabetes *26*:596–601, 1977.

4 Alberti, K. G. M. M., Christensen, N. J., Iverson, J., and Ørskov, H.: Role of glucagon and other hormones in development of diabetic ketoacidosis. Lancet *1*:1307–11, 1975.

5 Saccà, L., Sherwin, R., Hendler, R., and Felig, P.: Influence of continuous physiologic hyperinsulinemia on glucose kinetics and counterregulatory hormones in normal and diabetic humans. J. Clin. Invest. *63*:849–57, 1979.

6 Christensen, M. J.: Plasma norepinephrine and epinephrine in untreated diabetics during fasting and after insulin administration. Diabetes *23*:1–8, 1974.

7 Gerich, J. E., Langlois, M., Noacco, C., Karam, J. H., and Forsham, P. H.: Lack of glucagon response to hypoglycemia in diabetes: evidence for an intrinsic pancreatic alpha cell defect. Science *182*:171–73, 1973.

8 Sherwin, R. S., Fisher, M., Hendler, R., and Felig, P.: Hyperglucagonemia and blood glucose regulation in normal, obese and diabetic subjects. N. Engl. J. Med. *294*:455–61, 1976.

9 Schade, D., Eaton, R. P., and Standefer, J.: Glucocorticoid regulation of plasma ketone body concentration in insulin-deficient man. J. Clin. Endocrinol. Metab. *44*:1069–79, 1977.

10 Gerich, J. E., Lorenzi, M., Tsalikian, E., and Karam, J. H.: Studies on the mechanism of epinephrine-induced hyperglycemia in man. Evidence for participation of pancreatic glucagon secretion. Diabetes *25*:65–71, 1976.

11 Benson, J. W., Jr., Johnson, D. G., Palmer, J. P., Werner, P. L., and Ensinck, J. W.: Glucagon and catecholamine secretion during hypoglycemia in normal and diabetic man. J. Clin. Endocrinol. Metab. *44*:459–64, 1977.

12 Bomboy, J. D., Jr., Lewis, S. B., Lacy, W. W., Sinclair-Smith, B. C., and Liljenquist, J. E.: Transient stimulatory effect of sustained hyperglucagonemia on splanchnic glucose production in normal and diabetic man. Diabetes *26*:177–84, 1977.

13 Sherwin, R., Wahren, J., and Felig, P.: Evanescent effects of hypo- and hyperglucagonemia on blood glucose homeostasis. Metabolism *25*:1381–83, 1976.

[14] Sherwin, R. S., Kramer, K. J., Tobin, J. D., Insel, P. A., Liljenquist, J. E., Berman, M., and Andres, R.: A model of the kinetics of insulin in man. J. Clin. Invest. *53*:1481–92, 1974.

[15] Wise, J. K., Hendler, R., and Felig, P.: Influence of glucocorticoids on glucagon secretion and plasma amino acid concentrations in man. J. Clin. Invest. *52*:2774–82, 1973.

[16] Passon, P. G., and Peuler, J. D.: A simplified radiometric assay for plasma norepinephrine and epinephrine. Anal. Biochem. *51*:618–31, 1973.

[17] De Moor, P., Steeno, O., Rankin, M., and Hendrikx, A.: Fluorometric determination of free plasma 11-hydroxy corticosteroids in man. Acta Endocrinol. (Kbh) *33*:297–307, 1960.

[18] Steele, R.: Influences of glucose loading and of injected insulin on hepatic glucose output. Ann. N.Y. Acad. Sci. *82*:420–30, 1959.

[19] Eigler, N., Saccà, L., and Sherwin, R. S.: Synergistic interactions of physiologic increments of glucagon, epinephrine, and cortisol in the dog. A model for stress-induced hyperglycemia. J. Clin. Invest. *63*:114–23, 1979.

[20] Cowan, J. S., and Hetenyi, G., Jr.: Glucoregulatory responses in normal and diabetic dogs recorded by a new tracer method. Metabolism *20*:360–72, 1971.

[21] Radziuk, J., Norwich, K. H., and Vranic, M.: Experimental validation of measurements of glucose turnover in nonsteady state. Am. J. Physiol. *234*:E84–E93, 1978.

[22] Riggs, D. S.: The Mathematical Approach to Physiological Problems: A Critical Primer. Baltimore, Williams & Wilkins, 1963, pp. 196–98.

[23] Cherrington, A. D., Williams, P. E., and Harris, M. S.: Relationship between the plasma glucose level and glucose uptake in the conscious dog. Metabolism *27*:787–91, 1978.

[24] Winder, B. J.: Statistical Principles in Experimental Design, 2nd edit. New York, McGraw-Hill, 1979, pp. 21–26, 518–39.

[25] Garber, A. J., Cryer, P. E., Santiago, J. V., Haymond, M. W., Pagliara, A. S., and Kipnis, D. M.: The role of adrenergic mechanisms in the substrate and hormonal response to insulin-induced hypoglycemia in man. J. Clin. Invest. *58*:7–15, 1976.

[26] Plumpton, F. S., Besser, G. M., and Cole, P. V.: Corticosteroid treatment and surgery. An investigation of the indications for steroid cover. Anaesthesia *24*:3–11, 1969.

[27] Sperling, M. A., Bacon, G., Kenny, F. N., and Drash, A. L.: Cortisol secretion in acidotic and nonacidotic diabetes mellitus. Am. J. Dis. Child. *124*:690–92, 1972.

[28] Galbo, H., Holst, J. J., and Christensen, N. J.: Glucagon and plasma catecholamine response to graded and prolonged exercise in man. J. Appl. Physiol. *38*:70–76, 1975.

[29] Halter, J. B., Pflug, A. E., and Porte, D., Jr.: Mechanism of plasma catecholamine increases during surgical stress in man. J. Clin. Endocrinol. Metab. *45*:936–44, 1977.

[30] Lindsey, C. A., Santeusanio, F., Braaten, J., Faloona, G. R., and Unger, R. H.: Pancreatic alpha cell function in trauma. JAMA *227*:757–61, 1974.

[31] Willerson, J. T., Hutcheson, D., Leshin, S. J., Faloona, G. R., and Unger, R. H.: Serum glucagon and insulin levels and their relationships to blood glucose values in patients with acute myocardial infarction. Am. J. Med. *57*:747–53, 1974.

[32] Muller, W. A., Faloona, G. R., and Unger, R. H.: Hyperglucagonemia in diabetic ketoacidosis: its prevalence significance. Am. J. Med. *54*:52–57, 1973.

[33] Ninomiya, R., Forbath, N. F., and Hetenyi, G., Jr.: Effect of adrenal steroids on glucose kinetics in normal and diabetic dogs. Diabetes *14*:729–39, 1965.

[34] Gerich, J. E., Karam, J. H., and Forsham, P. H.: Stimulation of glucagon secretion by epinephrine in man. J. Clin. Endocrinol. Metab. *37*:479–81, 1973.

[35] Genuth, S. M.: Metabolic clearance of insulin in man. Diabetes *21*:1003–12, 1972.

[36] Rizza, R., Haymond, M., Cryer, P., and Gerich, J.: Transient hepatic but persistent peripheral effect on sustained hyperepinephrinemia on glucose homeostasis in man. Clin. Res. *26*:684A, 1978.

[37] Robertson, R. P., and Porte, D., Jr.: Adrenergic modulation of basal insulin secretion in man. Diabetes *22*:1–8, 1973.

[38] Kalhan, S. C., and Adam, P. A. J.: Inhibitory effect of prednisone on insulin secretion in man: model for duplication of blood glucose concentration. J. Clin. Endocrinol. Metab. *41*:600–10, 1975.

[39] Tamborlane, W. V., Sherwin, R. S., Genel, M., and Felig, P.: Reduction to normal of plasma glucose in juvenile diabetics by subcutaneous administration of insulin with a portable infusion pump. N. Engl. J. Med. *300*:573–78, 1979.

[40] Pickup, J. C., Keen, H., Parsons, J. A., and Alberti, K. G. M. M.: Continuous subcutaneous insulin infusion: an approach to achieving normoglycemia. Br. Med. J. *1*:204–07, 1978.

[41] Tamboriane, W. V., Sherwin, R. S., Genel, M., and Felig, P.: Restoration of normal lipid and aminoacid metabolism in diabetic patients treated with a portable insulin-infusion pump. Lancet *1*:1258–61, 1979.

[42] Santiago, J. V., Clemens, A. H., Clarke, W. L., and Kipnis, D. M.: Closed-loop and open-loop devices for blood glucose control in normal and diabetic subjects. Diabetes *28*:71–81, 1979.

Effects of Insulin and Pancreatic Polypeptide on Gastric Somatostatin Release

TSUTOMU CHIBA, TOMOHIKO TAMINATO, SEIZO KADOWAKI, HIROMI ABE, KAZUO CHIHARA, SHIGERU MATSUKURA, YASUO GOTO, YUTAKA SEINO, AND TAKUO FUJITA

SUMMARY

Effects of arginine and such pancreatic hormones as insulin and pancreatic polypeptide on gastric somatostatin release from the isolated perfused rat stomach were studied. The stomach was isolated from a fasted rat by a modification of the method of Lefébvre and was perfused with 4.6% dextran Krebs-Ringer bicarbonate buffer containing 5.5 mM glucose. Both insulin and pancreatic polypeptide (10^{-10}, 10^{-9}, and 10^{-8} M) caused a significant decrease in gastric somatostatin secretion. Insulin (10^{-10} M), furthermore, inhibited the glucagon (5×10^{-8} M)-induced somatostatin response. Arginine (10 and 19 mM) failed to elicit any significant change of somatostatin release.

These results suggest that gastric somatostatin release is affected by pancreatic hormones. DIABETES 29:292–295, April 1980.

Significant amounts of somatostatin have been found in the stomach by radioimmunoassay[1,2] as well as by immunocytochemical techniques.[3] The demonstration of gastric somatostatin secretion by the administration of various nutrients[4] suggests an important role of gastric somatostatin in carbohydrate metabolism as well as in nutrient homeostasis. In addition, increased gastric somatostatin content has been shown in hypoinsulinemic, streptozotocin-diabetic rats,[5,6] while spontaneously diabetic mice with hyperinsulinemia apparently have decreased gastric somatostatin content.[7]

These observations prompted us to investigate the direct effects of such pancreatic hormones as insulin and pancreatic polypeptide (PP) on gastric somatostatin secretion. Since arginine is known to stimulate pancreatic somatostatin release,[8–10] we also studied the effect of arginine on gastric somatostatin secretion using the isolated rat stomach.

From the Third Division, Department of Medicine, Kobe University School of Medicine, Kobe, the Department of Medicine, Shimane Medical College, Izumo, and the Second Division, Department of Medicine, Kyoto University School of Medicine, Kyoto, Japan.
Received for publication 5 September 1979.

METHODS

Male Wistar rats, weighing between 300 and 350 g, were maintained in a temperature-controlled and air-conditioned room under light-dark cycle, were fed Oriental laboratory chow (Oriental Yeast Co., Tokyo) and were given tap water ad libitum. The perfusion of rat stomach was performed with the method described by Lefébvre et al.[11] adapted to the rat.[12] Animals were anesthetized by intraperitoneal injection of 40 mg/kg of pentobarbital after an overnight fast. After a midline laparotomy, polyethylene cannulae were inserted into the left gastric artery and gastric vein. All other vessels and pancreas were carefully excluded by ligation. The cardia was ligated, and then a catheter was inserted into the stomach through the pyloric ring to drain gastric juice. All perfusions were accomplished with 4.6% dextran (mean mol wt = 70,000) Krebs-Ringer bicarbonate buffer containing 5.5 mM glucose (DKRBG). The perfusate was continuously gassed with 95% O_2 and 5% CO_2 and was maintained at pH 7.4 and Pa O_2 of 350 mm Hg. Both the perfusate and the stomach preparation were kept at 37°C throughout the experiment. The perfusate was infused into the left gastric artery by means of a peristaltic pump at a flow rate of 2 ml/min without recirculation, and the test materials were introduced via a side arm to give an appropriate final concentration.

In the first experiment, after the prestimulation period (20 min) of perfusion with DKRBG alone, rat insulin (10^{-10}, 10^{-9}, and 10^{-8} M) (Novo, Copenhagen), bovine PP (10^{-10}, 10^{-9}, and 10^{-8} M) (Lilly Laboratory, Indianapolis), and L-arginine (10 and 19 mM) (Nakarai Chemicals, Ltd., Kyoto) were infused for 30, 15, and 15 min, respectively. Rat insulin and bovine PP, L-arginine, and crystalline beef-pork glucagon were dissolved in 0.1 M acetic acid and then diluted with the perfusate immediately before use. The final pH of the perfusate of the test and control solutions were the same. In the control experiment, the stomach was perfused with solution free of test substances. In the second experiment, crystalline beef-pork glucagon (5×10^{-8} M) (Lilly Laboratory, Indianapolis) was infused for 15 min with or without 10^{-10} M rat insulin from the beginning of the preperfusion period.

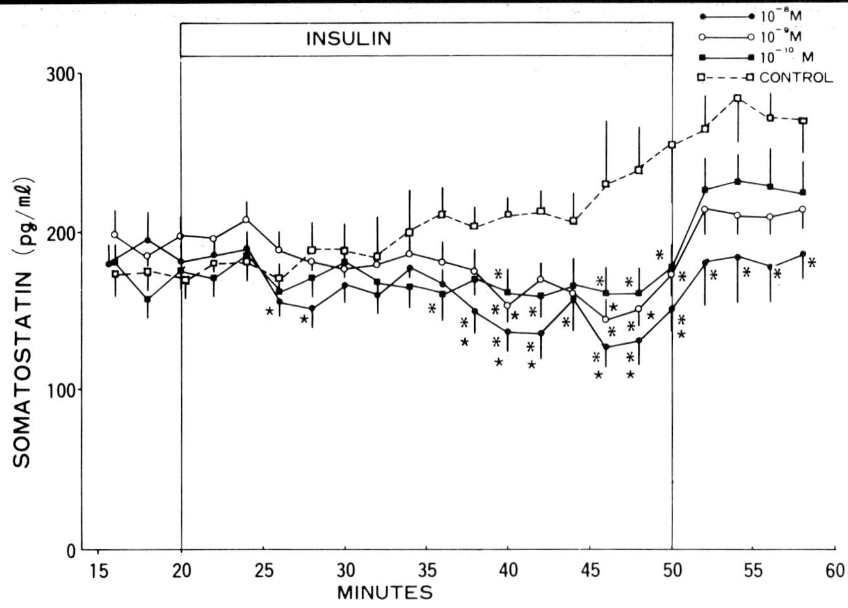

FIGURE 1. Effect of exogenous insulin on gastric somatostatin release. After equilibration for 20 min, insulin was infused for 30 min at the doses of 10^{-10}, 10^{-9}, and 10^{-8} M. All values are the x̄ ± SEM.
*** Significantly lower ($p < 0.05$) than control values.**
***Significantly lower ($p<0.05$) than baseline values.**

Only one perfusion was done in each stomach, and six perfusions were performed with each dose of each stimulus.

The venous effluents were collected every minute into chilled tubes containing a bacitracin (Sigma Chemical Co., St. Louis)–Trasylol (Bayer Leverkusen, Germany) mixture (2×10^{-5} M and 1000 KIU/ml, respectively), frozen immediately, and stored at −20°C until assayed.

Immunoreactive somatostatin (IRS) levels were measured by a specific radioimmunoassay utilizing antiserum RA-823, described previously.[12] Antiserum RA-823 was found not to cross-react with insulin, PP, glucagon, and arginine. The minimal detectable quantity of the assay was 10 pg/ml. Intra-assay and interassay variations were 5.4% and 8.5%, respectively. Immunoreactive insulin (IRI) was measured by polyethylene glycol radioimmunoassay[13] with rat insulin used as the standard. Immunoreactive glucagon (IRG) was determined by radioimmunoassay with the talcum-adsorption method[14] using antiserum 30K (purchased from University of Texas Southwestern Medical School, Dallas).

Statistical analysis was performed by unpaired Student's *t* test when two means were compared and by Duncan's new multiple range test when more than two means were compared.[15] For comparison within the group, the paired *t* test was used. Results are presented as the x̄ ± SEM.

RESULTS

In the first experiment, somatostatin release gradually increased with perfusion of control solution, as shown in Figure 1. The basal somatostatin level in the venous effluent at the end of the prestimulation period was 169 ± 12 pg/ml, and the final concentration of somatostatin at 60 min after the start of the preperfusion was 258 ± 11 pg/ml, a value significantly higher than the somatostatin concentration in the preperfusion period ($P < 0.02$).

The infusion of insulin caused a gradual but significant decrease of gastric somatostatin secretion (Figure 1). The nadirs obtained by the infusion of 10^{-10}, 10^{-9}, and 10^{-8} M insulin were 158 ± 14 pg/ml ($P < 0.05$ versus control), 146 ± 15 pg/ml ($P < 0.05$), and 127 ± 15 pg/ml ($P < 0.01$) at 22, 26, and 26 min after the beginning of insulin infusion, respectively. A rebound well above the baseline was observed immediately after cessation of insulin infusion ($P < 0.05$ versus baseline). IRG was not detected in any perfusate throughout the perfusion period. Bovine PP also elicited a prompt and significant decrease in gastric somatostatin secretion. The nadirs of 110 ± 28 pg/ml ($P < 0.05$), 86 ± 17 pg/ml ($P < 0.01$), and 75 ± 11 pg/ml ($P < 0.01$) were obtained by 10^{-10}, 10^{-9}, and 10^{-8} M of bovine PP at 2, 9, and 3 min after the start of infusion, respectively (Figure 2). No IRI or IRG was detectable in the perfusate. On the other hand, exogenous arginine (10 and 19 mM) exhibited no significant effects on gastric somatostatin release (Figure 3). IRI and IRG were not detected in any perfusate.

In the second experiment, 5×10^{-8} M glucagon elicited a

FIGURE 2. Effect of bovine PP on gastric somatostatin secretion. After preperfusion for 20 min, PP was infused for 15 min at the concentrations of 10^{-10}, 10^{-9}, and 10^{-8} M. All values represent the x̄ ± SEM.

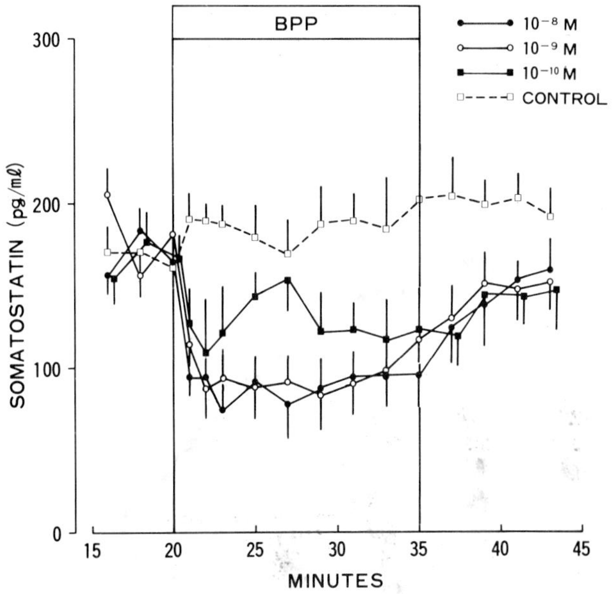

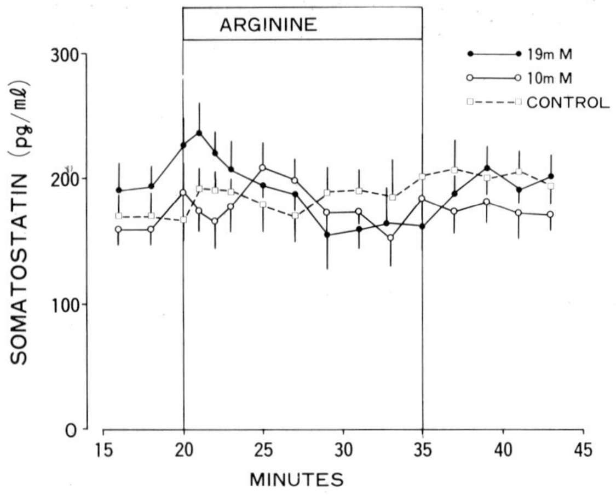

FIGURE 3. Effect of arginine on gastric somatostatin secretion. After preperfusion for 20 min, arginine was infused for 15 min at the doses of 10 and 19 mM. All values show the x̄ ± SEM.

TABLE 2
Total amounts of gastric somatostatin released during 15 min of infusion of 5×10^{-8} M glucagon, with and without 10^{-10} M insulin

Dose of insulin (M)	Somatostatin released* (pg/15 min)	Relative amounts of somatostatin released† (%)
0	19,970 ± 590	100.0
10^{-10}	14,350 ± 780 (a)	71.9

* Values represent the x̄ ± SEM (six animals).
† The relative amounts of somatostatin released (expressed as a percent of the amounts released without insulin).
(a) Significantly different from the amounts released without insulin ($P < 0.001$).

significant increase in gastric somatostatin secretion. This increase was significantly reduced, however, in the presence of 10^{-10} M insulin throughout the perfusion period (Figure 4).

The total amounts of somatostatin secreted during the stimulation periods in the first and the second experiments are shown in Tables 1 and 2, respectively.

DISCUSSION

The present study clearly shows that not only exogenous insulin but also PP suppresses gastric somatostatin secretion, and it further demonstrates that glucagon-induced gastric somatostatin release is reduced by exogenous insulin. In the present experiments, we also observed an abrupt rebound in somatostatin secretion immediately after the end of insulin infusion, suggesting an outpouring of previously blocked somatostatin secretory ability. These findings indicate the possible participation of these pancreatic hormones in the regulation of gastric somatostatin release.

Such inhibitory effect of insulin on gastric somatostatin release is quite different from that on pancreatic somatostatin secretion, which does not change significantly in response to insulin in vitro, as previously reported.[8,16] Two possibilities may be offered to explain such difference. Gastric somatostatin may be more readily inhibited by insulin than pancreatic somatostatin, since it has been reported already that secretion of gastric glucagon is suppressed by lower concentrations of insulin than of pancreatic glucagon.[17] Exogenous insulin, on the other hand, probably does not affect pancreatic somatostatin secretion, because pancreatic D cells are surrounded by a higher concentration of endogenous insulin than are gastric D cells. The fact that the acute insulin deficiency induced by the addition of anti-insulin antiserum promotes pancreatic somatostatin release[18] lends support to the second possibility. Furthermore, such suppression of gastric somatostatin release by insulin may be compatible with the previous observations in which hypoinsulinemic rats were found to have increased gastric soma-

TABLE 1
Total amounts of gastric somatostatin released during the infusion of various stimuli

	Dose of stimuli (M)	Gastric somatostatin released*	Relative amounts of somatostatin released† (%)
		pg/30 min	
Control	0	12,290 ± 920	100.0
Insulin	10^{-10}	10,250 ± 520 (a)	83.4
	10^{-9}	10,230 ± 690 (a)	85.0
	10^{-8}	9300 ± 260 (a,d)	75.7
		pg/15 min	
Control	0	5540 ± 230	100.0
PP	10^{-10}	3870 ± 290 (b)	69.9
	10^{-9}	2850 ± 260 (b,c)	51.4
	10^{-8}	2530 ± 310 (b,c)	45.7
Arginine	19×10^{-3}	5380 ± 160	97.1
	10×10^{-3}	5350 ± 180	96.6

* All values represent the x̄ ± SEM (six animals).
† The relative amounts of somatostatin released are expressed as a percent of the amounts released by the control.
(a) $P < 0.05$ as compared with the control.
(b) $P < 0.01$ as compared with the control.
(c) $P < 0.05$ as compared with 10^{-10} M of the same peptide.
(d) $P < 0.05$ as compared with 10^{-9} M of the same peptide.

FIGURE 4. Gastric somatostatin release in response to 5×10^{-8} M glucagon with (solid line) and without (dashed line) 10^{-10} M insulin throughout the perfusion period. Each value represents the x̄ ± SEM.

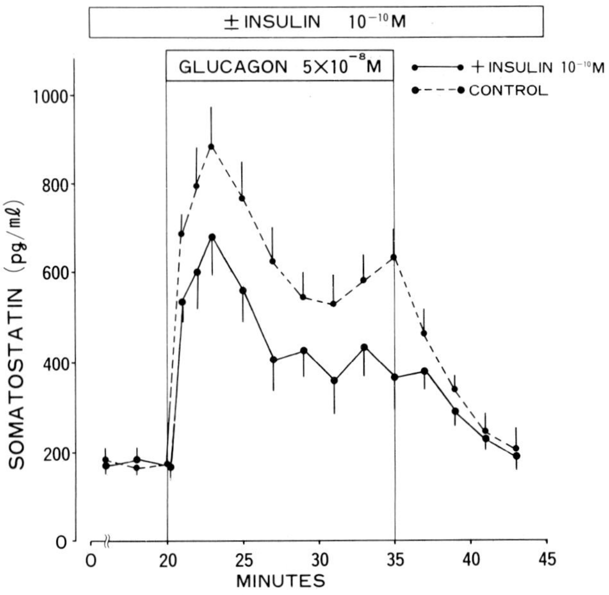

tostatin content,[5,6] while hyperinsulinemic mice were found to have decreased somatostatin content.[7]

The present study shows that PP clearly suppressed gastric somatostatin secretion. Although it has been suggested that PP has no acute effect on pancreatic D cells,[19] the infusion of a physiologic concentration of PP was shown to inhibit pancreatic secretion[20] and bile flow,[21] implying that PP may contribute primarily to the regulation of gastrointestinal function.

The failure to see the trophic effect of arginine on gastric somatostatin release contrasts with the previous studies, in which pancreatic somatostatin secretion was increased by arginine.[8-10] The reason for these conflicting results is not clear at present. Weir et al. suggested that arginine-stimulated pancreatic somatostatin release might be initiated by the paracrine secretion of glucagon.[8] Therefore, the unresponsiveness of gastric somatostatin secretion to arginine may possibly be explained by the fact that no glucagon was detected during the arginine infusion in the perfused rat stomach. Recently, Marre et al.[22] have reported that basal gastric glucagon is detectable and is enhanced by arginine stimulation using pancreatectomized rat in vivo. Differences in the results of their and our experiments might be caused by disparate experimental models.

The results suggest that the pancreatic responses of nutrient homeostasis may affect gastric somatostatin release rather than the converse.

ACKNOWLEDGMENTS

This work was supported, in part, by grants from the Ministry of Education, Science, and Culture and from the Ministry of Health and Welfare, Japan. We are grateful to Dr. R. E. Chance, Lilly Research Laboratories, for a generous gift of bovine pancreatic polypeptide. We wish to thank Miss A. Toyonaga for technical assistance and Miss S. Yanagihara for secretarial assistance.

REFERENCES

[1] Arimura, A., Sato, H., Dupont, A., Nishi, N., and Schally, A. V.: Somatostatin: abundance of immunoreactive hormone in rat stomach and pancreas. Science *189*:1007–09, 1975.

[2] Patel, Y. C., and Reichlin, S.: Somatostatin in hypothalamus, extrahypothalamic brain and peripheral tissues of the rat. Endocrinology *102*:523–30, 1978.

[3] Polak, J. M., Pearse, A. G. E., Grimelius, L., Bloom, S. R., and Arimura, A.: Growth-hormone release inhibiting hormone in gastrointestinal and pancreatic D cells. Lancet *1*:1220–22, 1975.

[4] Schusdziarra, V., Harris, V., Conlon, J. M., Arimura, A., and Unger, R. H.: Pancreatic and gastric somatostatin release in response to intragastric nutrients and HCl in the dog. J. Clin. Invest. *62*:509–18, 1978.

[5] Patel, Y. C., Cameron, D. P., Bankier, A., Malaisse-Lagae, F., Ravazzola, M., Studer, P., and Orci, L.: Changes in somatostatin concentration in pancreas and other tissues of streptozotocin diabetic rats. Endocrinology *103*:917–23, 1978.

[6] Berelowitz, M., Shapiro, B., Kronheim, S., and Pimstone, B. L.: Tissue somatostatin like immunoreactivity (SLI) in streptozotocin (SZ) diabetic rats—response to insulin replacement. Diabetes *27*(Suppl. 2):442, 1978.

[7] Patel, Y. C., Cameron, D. P., Stefan, Y., Malaisse-Lagae, F., and Orci, L.: Somatostatin: widespread abnormality in tissue of spontaneously diabetic mice. Science *198*:930–31, 1977.

[8] Weir, G. C., Samols, E., Loo, S., Patel, Y. C., and Gabbay, K. H.: Somatostatin and pancreatic polypeptide secretion: effects of glucagon, insulin, and arginine. Diabetes *28*:35–40, 1979.

[9] Patton, G. S., Ipp, E., Dobbs, R. E., Orci, L., Vale, W., and Unger, R. H.: Pancreatic somatostatin release. Proc. Natl. Acad. Sci. USA *74*:2140–43, 1977.

[10] Goto, Y., Seino, Y., Taminato, T., Kadowaki, S., Chiba, T., Note, S., and Imura, H.: Theophylline: potentiation of arginine-induced somatostatin release from the isolated rat pancreas. Diabetes *28*:457–59, 1979.

[11] Lefébvre, P. J., and Luyckx, A. S.: Factors controlling gastric-glucagon release. J. Clin. Invest. *59*:716–22, 1977.

[12] Chiba, T., Seino, Y., Goto, Y., Kadowaki, S., Taminato, T., Abe, H., Kato, Y., Matsukura, S., Nozawa, M., and Imura, H.: Somatostatin release from isolated perfused rat stomach. Biochem. Biophys. Res. Commun. *82*:731–37, 1978.

[13] Desbuquois, B., and Aurbach, G. D.: Use of polyethyleneglycol to separate free and antibody-bound peptide hormones in radioimmunoassays. J. Clin. Endocrinol. Metab. *33*:732–38, 1971.

[14] Sakurai, H., Kuzuya, H., Kurahachi, H., Fukase, M., and Imura, H.: A sensitive radioimmunoassay for glucagon using talc method. Jpn. J. Nucl. Med. *10*:135–36, 1973.

[15] Steel, R. D. G., and Torrie, J. H.: *In* Principles and Procedures of Statistics. New York, McGraw-Hill, 1966, p. 107.

[16] Kadowaki, S., Taminato, T., Chiba, T., Mori, K., Abe, H., Seino, Y., Matsukura, S., and Fujita, T.: Somatostatin release from isolated perfused rat pancreas: possible role of endogenous somatostatin on insulin release. Diabetes *28*:600–03, 1979.

[17] Lefébvre, P. J., and Luyckx, A. S.: Glucose and insulin in the regulation of glucagon release from the isolated perfused dog stomach. Endocrinology *103*:1579–82, 1978.

[18] Taminato, T., Seino, Y., Chiba, T., Abe, H., Kato, Y., Matsukura, S., and Imura, H.: Effects of endogenous and exogenous insulin on somatostatin release from the isolated pancreatic islets of rats. Diabetes *27*(Suppl. 2):507, 1978.

[19] Ipp, E., Dobbs, R. E., McCorkle, K., Harris, V., and Unger, R. H.: Further evidence for similar secretory responses of pancreatic somatostatin and insulin. Clin. Res. *26*:33A, 1978. (Abstract)

[20] Taylor, I. L., Solomon, T. E., Walsh, J. H., and Grossman, M. I.: Physiological blood levels of pancreatic polypeptide (PP) inhibit pancreatic secretion. Gastroenterology *74*:1102, 1978. (Abstract)

[21] Bloom, S. R., Greenberg, G. R., Adrian, T. E., Besterman, H. S., Mallinson, C. N., McCloy, R. F., Chadweck, V. S., and Baron, J. H.: Physiologic role of PP in man. Ir. J. Med. Sci. *146*(Suppl. 1):15, 1978.

[22] Marre, M., Bobbioni, E., Suarez, M., Reach, G., Dubois, M. P., and Assan, R.: Control of gastric glucagon secretion in the acutely pancreatectomized rat. Diabetes *28*:213–20, 1979.

Glycosylation of Plasma Protein and its Relation to Glycosylated Hemoglobin in Diabetes

D. K. YUE, K. MORRIS, S. McLENNAN, AND J. R. TURTLE

SUMMARY

Glycosylation of plasma proteins was studied in diabetic and normal subjects by an adaptation of a thiobarbituric acid method previously used for glycosylated hemoglobin. There was a highly significant correlation between the degree of glycosylation in vivo of plasma protein and hemoglobin. The process of glycosylation depended on time and temperature and was not mediated enzymatically. Plasma protein of all molecular sizes could be glycosylated. At 37°C, 4.6% of ^{14}C-glucose became attached to plasma protein after 24 h of incubation in vitro; no difference between normal and diabetic plasma protein could be demonstrated. After glycosylation, glucose dissociated from protein slowly; 72% remained attached after dialysis for 24 h. As an estimate of diabetic control, measurement of glycosylation of plasma protein is a suitable alternative to determination of glycosylated hemoglobin. Results of each method correlated equally well with the degree of diabetic control when this was assessed by calculation of the M-factor, mean plasma glucose concentrations, or variance of the plasma glucose determinations. In hemolytic anemia, hemoglobinopathy, and recent transfusion, measurement of glycosylation of plasma protein may be more accurate than that of glycosylated hemoglobin. It may also provide an estimate of diabetic control between that provided by short-term blood glucose determination and long-term glycosylated hemoglobin.
DIABETES *29*:296–300, April 1980.

The measurement of glycosylated hemoglobin (GHb) has improved significantly the objective assessment of diabetic control.[1] The glycosylation of hemoglobin depends on a nonenzymatic reaction occurring after the synthesis of hemoglobin. GHb is known to have an increased affinity for oxygen. The resultant tissue hypoxia has been incriminated as a cause of diabetic microangiopathy.[2] Glycosylation of rat and bovine lens crystallins has been reported and may be important in the genesis of cataracts in diabetes.[3] Glycosylation of serum albumin was also reported recently.[4] Glycosylation of other plasma proteins may likewise result in alterations of their functions. These may be important in producing the numerous metabolic and structural abnormalities known to occur in diabetes mellitus. This study was carried out to characterize further the process of glycosylation of plasma proteins.

From the Department of Medicine, University of Sydney, and the Department of Endocrinology, Royal Prince Alfred Hospital, Sydney, NSW, Australia.
Address reprint requests to Dr. D. K. Yue, Department of Medicine, University of Sydney, Sydney, N.S.W. 2006, Australia.
Received for publication 4 September 1979.

PATIENTS AND METHODS

Heparinized blood was obtained from 45 patients attending the Diabetic Clinic of the Royal Prince Alfred Hospital. Thirty-five patients were treated with insulin, seven patients by oral hypoglycemic agents, and three patients by dietary management. Routinely, plasma glucose levels were estimated at 10 a.m. and 2 p.m. during each clinic visit by the glucose-oxidase method. GHb was measured by cation-exchange chromatography using commercially available columns purchased from Isolab. The glycosylation of plasma protein was estimated by an adaptation of the thiobarbituric acid (TBA) method described by Flückiger et al.[5] for the measurement of GHb. The TBA reaction is specific for the detection of ketoamine-linked carbohydrate residues in proteins formed by the Amadori rearrangement[6] of protein-bound hexose. The 5-hydroxymethylfurfural (5-HMF) released by dehydration and hydrolysis of this linkage reacts with thiobarbituric acid to form a chromagen that has maximal absorbance at a wavelength of 443 nm. Plasma samples (2 ml) were separated from red cells immediately and free glucose was removed by dialysis for 12 h against 10 L of a buffer containing Na Hepes, 50 mmol/L, and NaCl, 0.15 mol/L, pH 7.4. Control experiments had shown that dialysis of this duration removed free glucose completely. To a 1-ml sample of dialyzed plasma was added 0.5 ml of oxalic acid (0.9 mol/L) and the mixture was boiled for 2 h in a water bath. After cooling to room temperature, 0.5 ml of 40% trichloroacetic acid (TCA) was added and immediately vortexed before centrifugation at 1000 *g* for 10 min. One milliliter of the supernatant was removed and incubated with 0.25 ml of thiobarbituric acid (0.05 mol/L) at 40°C for 40 min, and the absorbance was read at 443 nm. All estimations were performed in duplicate, and only unhemolyzed plasma samples were used. Results were correlated with GHb determined from samples obtained on the same day.

In 24 patients, there were eight or more plasma glucose determinations made during visits to the Diabetic Clinic in the preceding 2 yr (14 with 20 determinations, one with 18 determinations, two each with 12 and 10 determinations, and five with eight determinations). Using these blood glucose results, the degree of diabetic control in these 24 patients was estimated by the calculation of M-factor,[7] mean plasma glucose concentration, and variance of the plasma glucose concentrations. The M-factor was derived according to Schlichtkrull,[7] except that 8–20 blood glucose determinations formed the basis of the calculation. Each of these parameters of diabetic control was correlated individually with results of glycosylation of plasma protein and GHb.

In six diabetic plasma samples the glycosylation of protein was studied over a fourfold dilution of plasma. Results at each dilution were expressed as a percentage of the absorbance at 443 nm of the undiluted sample.

Glycosylation of plasma protein was studied in vitro by incubating 0.5 ml of plasma with 50 μl of 6-^{14}C-glucose (New England Nuclear) containing 20–40 nCi. The reaction was carried out in glass tubes (0.8 × 5.5 cm). The temperature of incubation was varied from 4°C to 45°C, time of incubation from 1 h to 48 h, and glucose concentration from 0.1 mmol/L to 278 mmol/L. After incubation, plasma proteins were precipitated by 0.5 ml of 20% TCA and then washed twice with 2 ml of 2.5% TCA. The precipitate was dissolved in 2 ml Instagel (Packard Instruments) and counted for 5 min in a Wallac-LKB beta liquid scintillation counter. Nonspecific binding of glucose was determined by adding labeled glucose of the same specific activity to plasma, incubated under identical conditions, immediately before precipitation of the protein by TCA, as described. Specific binding was calculated by subtracting the nonspecific binding from the counts precipitated after appropriate incubation and was expressed as a percentage of the total radioactivity present. Glycosylation of protein was compared in samples obtained from 10 diabetic patients and 10 normal individuals. The incubation was carried out routinely at 37°C for 24 h.

The glycosylated components of plasma were identified by the following experiments. Plasma (5 ml) was fractionated on a Sephacryl S-300 (Pharmacia) column of 60 × 2 cm. Elution was carried out with Na Hepes–NaCl buffer and fractions of 4 ml were collected. Another 5 ml aliquot of the same plasma was incubated at 37°C for 24 h with ^{14}C-glucose at a final concentration of 16 mmol/L and 7 μCi/ml. The incubated sample was applied on to the same Sephacryl S-300 column and was eluted under identical conditions. The protein content of the eluate was estimated by measurement of absorbance at 280 nm. The glycosylation of protein in each fraction was analyzed by the thiobarbituric acid method. The radioactivity of ^{14}C-glucose bound to protein was determined by counting a 0.5 ml aliquot of each fraction in 10 ml of Instagel for 5 min. The elution position of alpha-2 macroglobulin, haptoglobin, IgG, and IgM was determined by single immunodiffusion using Tripartigen plates obtained from Behringwerke. The elution position of albumin was monitored by double immunodiffusion using the Ouchterlony technique.

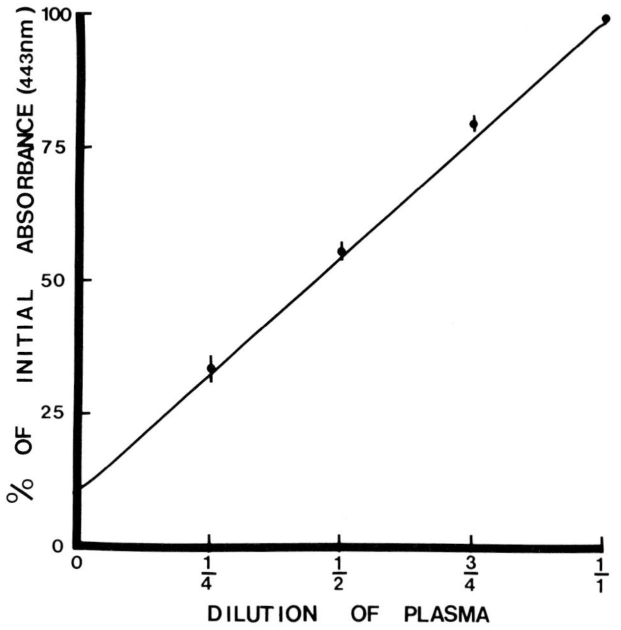

FIGURE 1. The relationship between measurement of glycosylation of plasma protein by the thiobarbituric acid method and dilution of plasma samples. The absorbance at 443 nm of each dilution is expressed as a percentage of the absorbance of the undiluted sample. Each point represents the $\bar{x} \pm$ SEM of six plasma samples; 100% corresponds to an absorbance of 0.41 ± 0.04.

In 30 of the plasma samples obtained from diabetic patients the fibrinogen concentrations were measured by an ammonium sulfate precipitation method[8] and alpha-2 macroglobulin and haptoglobin by single immunodiffusion. The galactose and mannose contents of plasma protein were analyzed by the anthrone reaction.[9] Results were correlated with glycosylated plasma protein and GHb.

All results were expressed as $\bar{x} \pm$ SEM. Linear correlations were calculated by the least squares' method.

RESULTS

The effect of serial dilution of plasma on measurement of glycosylation of plasma protein is shown in Figure 1. There is a linear relationship between absorbance at 443 nm and the amount of protein present over a fourfold dilution of the plasma samples. Eighty-five per cent (85%) of the specimens examined by the thiobarbituric acid method (38/45) had final optical density within this range. Serial dilution of a glucose solution (50 mmol/L) subjected to boiling in acid and analyzed by the thiobarbituric acid method also resulted in a proportional reduction in absorbance at 443 nm. The minimal glucose concentration tested that yielded a positive reading was 6.25 mmol/L, corresponding to an absorbance of 0.035 at 443 nm. The intra-assay coefficient of variation of the thiobarbituric acid method was 3.1%; the interassay coefficient of variation was 6.3%. The corresponding figures for the GHb measurements were 1.5% and 3.0%.

The highly significant correlation ($r = 0.74$, $p < 0.005$) between the degree of in vivo glycosylation of plasma protein and hemoglobin is shown in Figure 2. Each of these two

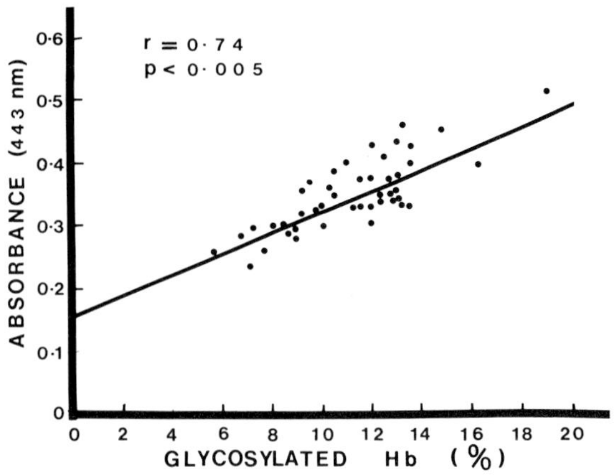

FIGURE 2. The correlation between glycosylation of plasma protein measured by the thiobarbituric acid method and glycosylated hemoglobin measured by cation-exchange chromatography.

parameters is correlated with three different estimates of diabetic control and the results are shown in Figure 3. There is a significant and similar correlation of each with M-factor, mean blood glucose levels, and variance of the blood glucose determinations. For each assay the correlations with M-factor and mean blood glucose concentrations are slightly better than that with the variance of blood glucose determinations.

The effects of temperature and duration of incubation on the in vitro glycosylation of protein is shown in Figure 4. The degree of glycosylation depends on time and temperature. At 37°C, glycosylation is detectable by 1 h, and it continues to rise slowly up to 48 h. After incubation with ^{14}C-glucose for 24 h at 37°C, the mean in vitro glycosylation in diabetic plasma was 4.6 ± 0.3% of the total radioactivity present, not significantly different from that in normal individuals of 4.5 ± 0.6%. There was no evidence of saturation of the glucose binding onto plasma protein, even at glucose concentrations of 278 mmol/L.

FIGURE 3. The correlation of glycosylation of plasma protein and glycosylated hemoglobin with M-factor, mean plasma glucose concentrations, and variance of the plasma glucose determinations in 24 diabetic subjects.

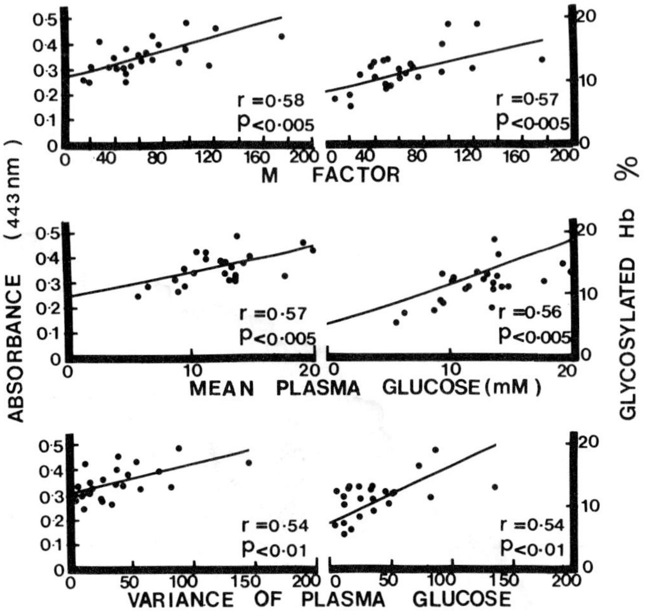

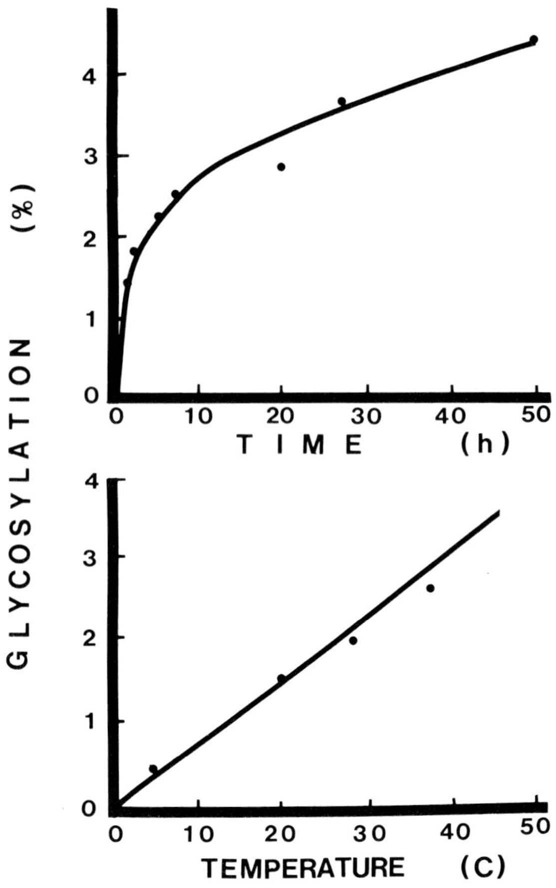

FIGURE 4. The in vitro glycosylation of plasma protein at different time and temperature of incubation. ^{14}C-glucose was present at a concentration of 0.1 mmol/L and 40–80 nCi/ml.

The elution pattern of plasma proteins on Sephacryl S-300 chromatography is shown in Figure 5. When plasma was incubated with glucose (16 mmol/L), increased glycosylation of proteins of all molecular sizes could be demonstrated by the thiobarbituric acid method. ^{14}C-labeled glucose was shown to bind to all protein components, but the major peak corresponded to the position of albumin. The radioactivity bound to protein was 2.2 ± 0.1% (mean of four experiments) of the total radioactivity present.

Fractions 25, 26, and 27 of the above experiment, containing the albumin peak, were pooled and dialyzed against Na Hepes–NaCl buffer at 4°C and 37°C. No difference in the rate of disappearance of 6-^{14}C-glucose from plasma proteins could be detected at these temperatures. In three experiments the mean radioactivity remaining attached to plasma protein after 6 h of dialysis was 87%; the corresponding figure of 24 h was 72%.

There was no significant correlation between the plasma concentration of haptoglobin, alpha-2 macroglobulin, and fibrinogen with glycosylation of plasma protein. The correlation coefficients were 0.10, 0.04, and 0.08, respectively. The total mannose and galactose concentrations of plasma protein also showed no correlation with glycosylation of plasma protein (r = 0.08). Similarly, no correlation between any of these measurements with GHb could be demonstrated. The

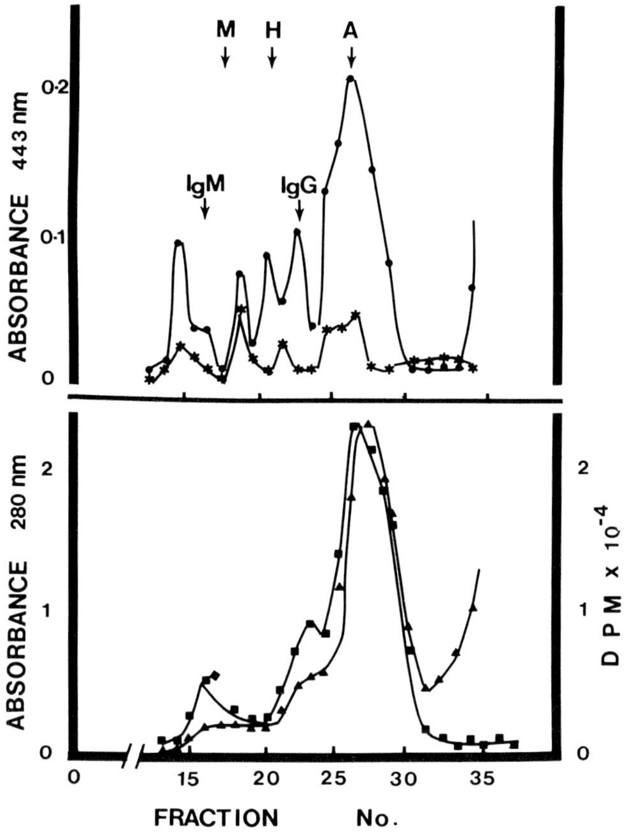

FIGURE 5. The elution profile of plasma protein on Sephacryl S-300 chromatography. The elution positions of IgM, IgG, alpha-2 macroglobulin (M), haptoglobin (H), and albumin (A) are indicated by arrows. Glycosylation of plasma protein with (●) and without (*) preincubation with glucose (16 mmol/L) is shown in the top panel. The radioactivity of ^{14}C-labeled glucose (▲) bound to plasma protein preincubated with radioactive glucose (7 μCi/ml) and the absorbance of eluate at 280 nm (■) are shown in the bottom panel.

corresponding correlation coefficients were 0.12, − 0.17, and 0.06, respectively.

DISCUSSION

The formation of GHb by a post-translational attachment of glucose to hemoglobin is now well established. Glycosylation of plasma proteins by similar mechanisms has been demonstrated in this study. The glycosylation process depends on temperature and time of incubation. Hyperglycemia, lasting for only a few hours at physiologic temperature, would result in readily detectable glycosylation. Similarly to the formation of GHb, glycosylation of protein appears not to be mediated by an enzymatic mechanism, as the process is relatively slow, nonsaturable even at high glucose concentrations, and is not reduced by incubation temperature higher than 37°C. The glycosylation of protein is only slowly reversible; 72% of glucose remained attached to protein after dialysis at physiologic temperature for 24 h. In vivo the net dissociation of glucose from protein could be expected to be even slower, as plasma always contains free glucose.

The GHb level is determined primarily by the mean blood glucose concentration in the preceding 2–3 mo.[1] The highly significant correlation between the in vivo glycosylation of plasma protein and hemoglobin observed in this study suggests that the mean glucose concentration is also the most important parameter in determining the extent of protein glycosylation. This is supported by the good correlation observed between glycosylation of plasma protein and mean blood glucose levels in diabetic patients. Plasma proteins of all molecular sizes can be glycosylated, but albumin was quantitatively the most important, presumably because of its high concentration in plasma. It is unlikely that the correlation between glycosylation of protein and hemoglobin can be explained by an increased de novo synthesis in glycoprotein in poorly controlled diabetes. When concentrations of such individual glycoproteins as fibrinogen, alpha-2 macroglobulin, and haptoglobin were analyzed, no correlation with glycosylation of plasma protein or GHb was observed. There is no evidence that plasma proteins from diabetic individuals are more likely to be glycosylated; we could not demonstrate any difference in the in vitro incorporation of ^{14}C-labeled glucose to plasma proteins from diabetic or normal subjects. Mannose and galactose are quantitatively the most important hexose constituents of plasma glycoprotein. As mannose and galactose can also be converted to 5-HMF and react with thiobarbituric acid, it is possible that the observed correlation between glycosylation of protein and hemoglobin is due to an increased mannose and galactose content of plasma glycoproteins. However, when the content of these two hexoses in plasma proteins was measured, no correlation with either glycosylation of plasma protein or GHb could be detected. Thus, the most likely explanation for the increased protein glycosylation in poorly controlled diabetes is a post-translational incorporation of glucose as a consequence of hyperglycemia. This would explain the detection of carbohydrate on albumin, which is known not to be a glycoprotein.[10,11] Many substances are transported while bound to albumin, and binding of certain drugs to alpha-1 acid glycoprotein has been reported.[12]

Our observation that albumin was quantitatively the most important glycosylated plasma component supports the finding of Day et al.[4] Our results also agreed well with a recent report by Kennedy et al.[13] that protein-bound hexose concentration was correlated with GHb level. In addition, we were able to demonstrate a correlation between the degree of protein glycosylation with M-factor, mean glucose levels, and variance of blood glucose concentrations, while they were unable to show such a relationship between protein-bound hexose with fasting glucose level, further evidence that a single glucose determination is not a good index of overall diabetic control. We were unable to show the correlation between haptoglobin concentration and the degree of glycosylation of either plasma protein or hemoglobin reported by Kennedy et al.[13]

The measurement of glycosylated plasma protein by the thiobarbituric acid method is reproducible, technically easy, and requires only readily obtainable chemicals. It can provide the same information as the measurement of GHb. The almost identical correlation of glycosylated protein and glycosylated hemoglobin with M-factor and with mean and variance of blood sugar levels indicate that these two methods are equally suitable as assessments of diabetic control. The better correlations of each with M-factor and mean blood glucose concentrations than with variance of blood glucose determinations suggest that they reflect more accurately persistent hyperglycemia rather than instability of diabetes. In such clinical conditions as hemolytic anemia, hemoglobinopathy, and recent transfusion the measurement of GHb is unreliable.[14] In these situations the assessment of diabetic control can be made by measuring the glycosylation of plasma protein. As the circulating half-lives of plasma proteins are only 2–3 days the monitoring of glycosylation of protein may represent a temporal assessment of diabetic control intermediate to that of blood sugar and GHb measurements.[10] It may provide an objective index of the efficacy of treatment in diabetes without waiting for the slow changes in GHb levels. It is possible that the binding and subsequent dissociation of glucose from plasma proteins may serve as a buffer against major fluctuations in blood sugar concentrations. However, in view of the slow nature of both the forward and reverse reactions, it seems unlikely that this will be of great physiologic significance in the minute to minute regulation of blood sugar concentration.

The affinity of GHb for oxygen is known to be greater than that of the native hemoglobin. This phenomenon is attributed to the steric hindrance of the additional glucose for the binding of 2,3-diphosphoglycerate onto the hemoglobin molecule. The glycosylation of plasma protein as a result of persistent hyperglycemia may similarly affect the functions of other plasma protein components. These possibilities remain to be explored. Glycosylation of tissue proteins may also account for such phenomena as basement membrane thickening, receptor dysfunction, and metabolic abnormalities, which are sequelae of long term diabetes mellitus.[15,16]

ACKNOWLEDGMENTS

This study was supported by the Coppleson Postgraduate Medical Institute of N.S.W., the John Claude Kellion Foundation, and the National Health and Medical Research Council of Australia.

REFERENCES

[1] Bunn, F. H., Gabbay, K. H., and Gallop, P. M.: The glycosylation of hemoglobin: relevance to diabetes mellitus. Science *200*:21–27, 1978.

[2] Ditzel, J.: Oxygen transport impairment in diabetes. Diabetes *25* (Suppl.2):832–38, 1976.

[3] Stevens, V. J., Rouzer, C-A., Monnier, V. M., and Cerami, A.: Diabetic cataract formation: potential role of glycosylation of lens crystallins. J. Biol. Chem. *75*:2918–22, 1978.

[4] Day, J. F., Thorpe, S. R., and Boynes, J. W.: Nonenzymatically glucosylated albumin. J. Biol. Chem. *254*:595–97, 1979.

[5] Flückiger, R., and Winterhalter, K. H.: In vitro synthesis of hemoglobin A1C. FEBS Lett. *71*:356–60, 1976.

[6] Gottschalk, Alfred: Glycoproteins. Their Composition, Structure and Function. Amsterdam, Elsevier, 1966, p. 96.

[7] Schlichtkrull, J., Munck, O., and Jersild, M.: The M-value, an index of blood-sugar control in diabetics. Acta Med. Scand. *177*:95–102, 1965.

[8] Fowell, A. A.: Turbidimetric method of fibrinogen assay. Am. J. Clin. Pathol. *25*:340–42, 1955.

[9] Graff, M. M., Greenspan, E. M., Lehman, I. R., and Holechek, J. J.: Estimation of nonglucosamine polysaccharides of the serum proteins with the anthrone reagent. J. Lab. Clin. Med. *37*:736–42, 1951.

[10] Jonsson, A., and Wales, J. K.: Blood glycoprotein levels in diabetes mellitus. Diabetologia *12*:245–50, 1976.

[11] Spiro, R. G.: Glycoproteins and diabetes. Diabetes *12*:223–30, 1963.

[12] Piafsky, K. M., Borga, O., Odar-Cederlof, I., Johansson, C., and Sjoqvist, F.: Increased plasma protein binding of propranolol and chlorpromazine mediated by disease induced elevation of plasma α_1 acid glycoprotein. N. Engl. J. Med. *299*:1435–39, 1978.

[13] Kennedy, A. L., Kandell, T. W., and Merimee, T. J.: Serum protein-bound hexose in diabetes: the effect of glycemic control. Diabetes *28*:1006–10, 1979.

[14] Bunn, H. F., Hamey, D. N., Kamin, S., Gabbay, K. H., and Gallop, P. M.: The biosynthesis of human hemoglobin A1C: slow glycosylation of hemoglobin in vivo. J. Clin. Invest. *57*:1652–59, 1976.

[15] Spiro, R. G.: Search for a biochemical basis of diabetic microangiopathy. Diabetologia *12*:1–14, 1976.

[16] Olefsky, J. M., and Reaven, G. M.: Decreased insulin binding to lymphocytes from diabetic subjects. J. Clin. Invest. *54*:1323–28, 1974.

Hagfish Insulin: The Discrepancy Between Binding Affinity and Biologic Activity

STEFAN O. EMDIN, OLE SONNE, AND JØRGEN GLIEMANN

SUMMARY

Hagfish insulin exhibits a binding affinity of about 25% of that of pig insulin in rat adipocytes and IM-9 lymphocytes, even though its relative biologic potency is only about 5% in adipocytes. The dissociation rate constant of hagfish insulin is about half that of pig insulin, and the association rate constant is about one eighth. A longer time is, therefore, required for hagfish insulin to reach a steady state of binding. Failure to reach steady state is the probable reason why some previous results suggested a relative binding affinity of hagfish insulin of the same magnitude as the relative biologic potency. DIABETES 29:301–303, April 1980.

In general, insulin analogues and insulins from different animal species exhibit parallel changes in binding affinity and biologic potency when compared with pig insulin.[1,2] Hagfish insulin was the first analogue to show a discrepancy; we found a relative biologic potency of 4.6% and a relative binding affinity of 23%.[3] However, Muggeo et al.[4] recently reported that the relative potency and binding affinity were both around 5%. The principal and potentially important question is whether or not an insulin analogue-receptor complex can convey a different (in casu less efficient) message to the effector system than standard pig insulin. In the attempt to resolve this question, we studied the kinetics of binding of ^{125}I-hagfish insulin.

MATERIAL AND METHODS

Hagfish insulin was prepared as described previously,[3] and its relative potency with respect to conversion of U-^{14}C-glucose to lipids in rat adipocytes was 5%. Hagfish insulin and pig insulin were iodinated in parallel to specific activities of about 70 μCi/μg.[3] Incubations with rat adipocytes (5% vol/vol) were carried out at 37°C, pH 7.4, in Krebs-Ringer Hepes buffer containing 5% (wt/vol) bovine serum albumin and 0.35 mM bacitracin. The incubation conditions and further manipulations with the cells have been described in detail elsewhere.[5] Incubations with IM-9 lymphocytes (1.5×10^6 cells/ml) were carried out under the same conditions as those used for adipocytes.

RESULTS AND DISCUSSION

We have previously established that the half-time for association and dissociation of tracer ^{125}I-pig insulin (i.e., total insulin concentration $\ll K_d$) is about 7 min and that a steady state can be maintained for several hours;[5] 45 min ($6-7 \times T_{1/2}$) is sufficient time, therefore, to obtain a steady state of binding of pig insulin. Under these conditions, $1.72 \pm 0.16\%$ (SD; $N = 6$) of 80 pM ^{125}I-pig insulin was specifically bound to adipocytes as compared with $0.44 \pm 0.03\%$ for 80 pM ^{125}I-hagfish insulin. In separate competition-inhibition experiments (not shown) it was found that the inhibition constant of pig insulin was the same (about 1.5 nM) when ^{125}I-pig insulin and ^{125}I-hagfish insulin were used as tracers. In other words, the two insulins were bound to the same receptors. Therefore, the fraction 0.44/1.72 (25.6%) is a direct measure of the affinity of hagfish insulin relative to pig insulin. This is in agreement with our previous results obtained from competition curves with unlabeled hagfish insulin,[3] but it is in contrast with the results obtained by Muggeo et al.[4]

In preliminary experiments (not shown) we found that tracer ^{125}I-pig insulin associated rapidly to IM-9 lymphocytes at 37°C; steady state is reached by about 4 min and can be maintained for hours. The concentration of pig insulin causing half-maximal displacement of ^{125}I-pig insulin was 2 nM. After 45 min of incubation the lymphocytes bound $1.90 \pm 0.10\%$ ^{125}I-pig insulin as compared with $0.56 \pm 0.09\%$ ^{125}I-hagfish insulin, i.e., the relative binding affinity of hagfish insulin in that system was 29%. Again, this is in contrast with the relative binding affinity of 5% reported by Muggeo et al.[4]

From the Department of Pathology, University of Umeå, S-901 87 Umeå, Sweden; the Institute of Medical Physiology C, University of Copenhagen, 3c Blegdamsvej, DK-2200 Copenhagen N, Denmark; and the Institute of Physiology, University of Århus, Universitetsparken, DK-8000 Århus C, Denmark.
Address reprint requests to S. O. Emdin, Department of Pathology, University of Umeå, S-901 87 Umeå, Sweden.
Received for publication 21 September 1979.

Experiments were designed in an attempt to explain the differences in results. It is well known that the steady state of binding of ^{125}I-pig insulin varies markedly with changes in pH. If the pH-dependence of binding of ^{125}I-hagfish insulin were different, one would anticipate different relative potencies in experiments carried out in buffers with just moderately different pH. However, we found the same relative potency for hagfish insulin in the pH range 7.0 to 7.9 (7.0, 30%; 7.3, 29%; 7.6, 28%; 7.9, 28%).

On the other hand, it turned out that the time course of association and dissociation was different for hagfish insulin and pig insulin. In spite of its lower affinity, bound hagfish insulin dissociated more slowly from the receptors than did bound pig insulin. Figure 1 (A and B) shows that the half-time of dissociation of 80 pM hagfish insulin is about 15 min as compared with 7 min for pig insulin. Likewise, as shown in Figure 1 (C and D), the half-time of association of 80 pM hagfish insulin is about 15 min. The fact that a longer time is needed to obtain steady state of binding of hagfish insulin is the most probable reason for the discrepancy between our results and those of Muggeo et al.[4] In the laboratory of the latter authors, binding of tracer ^{125}I-pig insulin to adipocytes at 37°C reaches a peak by 10 to 20 min.[6] The decline obtained at longer times is most probably due to extracellular degradation of the tracer.[5] In any case, it has now been established that a steady state of insulin binding to adipocytes can be maintained for several hours at 37°C.[5,7] Thus the ratio of binding of two different analogues with different time courses is only going to reflect the ratio of their affinities when steady state is obtained for both analogues. If binding is measured at peak value for the rapid analogue (pig insulin), the affinity of the slow analogue will be underestimated. The same mechanism may account for the apparent low affinity of hagfish insulin on IM-9 lymphocytes reported by Muggeo et al.[4] Their incubation time was 90 min at 15°C. This may hardly be sufficient time to obtain a steady state of binding of pig insulin, since 30% of the tracer still remains on the cells after dissociation for this time period in medium not containing insulin,[8] and it is almost certainly not sufficient time for hagfish insulin. In fact it has been observed that steady state for binding of ^{125}I-pig insulin at 15°C is obtained after 150–180 min, whereas binding of hagfish insulin is increasing almost linearly during this period (P. De Meyts, personal communication).

FIGURE 1. Time course of dissociation and association of ^{125}I-hagfish insulin to adipocytes. Panel A: Adipocytes (5% vol/vol) were incubated with 80 pM ^{125}I-hagfish insulin (○) or ^{125}I-pig insulin (●) for 45 min. Dissociation (time 0) was initiated by the addition of 3 μM unlabeled pig insulin. Panel B: The results are shown in a semilogarithmic plot (B_∞ = B/F 120 min) after the addition of unlabeled insulin. Panel C: The time course of association of 80 pM ^{125}I-hagfish insulin (○) or ^{125}I-pig insulin (●) to adipocytes (3.5% vol/vol). Panel D: The data are shown in a semilogarithmic plot (B_∞ = B/F at time 90 min).

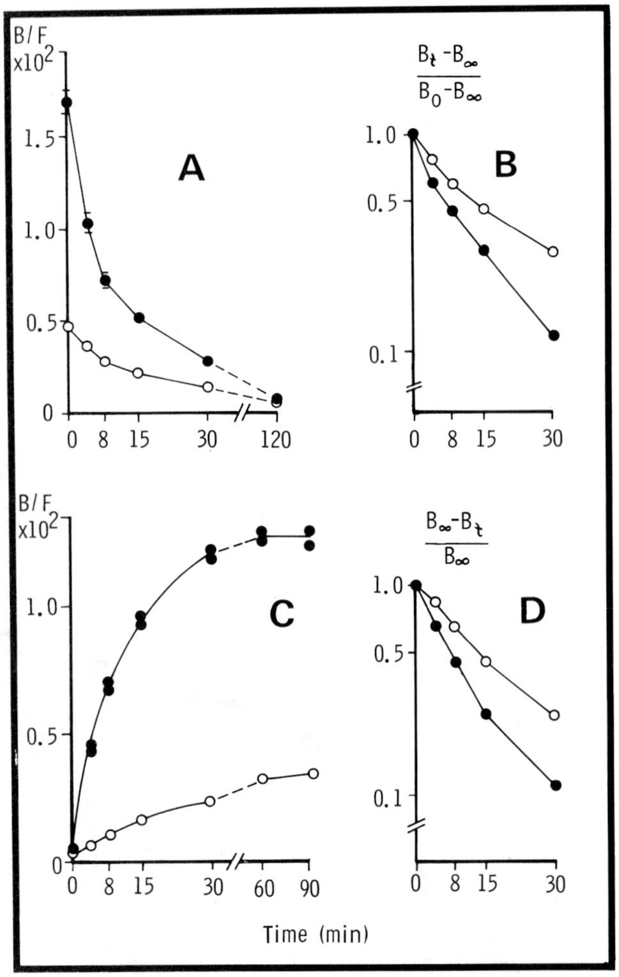

When ^{125}I-pig insulin is bound to adipocytes, radioactivity dissociates at 37°C as about 50% iodoinsulin and 50% iodotyrosine.[5] It seemed an attractive hypothesis, therefore, that the slower dissociation rate of hagfish insulin might be explained by a markedly reduced receptor-mediated degradation. In paired experiments we found that 38 ± 3% of bound ^{125}I-hagfish insulin was degraded to iodotyrosine as compared with 49 ± 2% (SD, N = 14) of bound pig insulin. Column chromatography showed that the degradation product of ^{125}I-hagfish insulin was iodotyrosine, as was shown before for pig insulin.[5] The difference in fractional degradation, although statistically significant, is of small magnitude and cannot explain the differences in total dissociation rates.

The present study confirms that the binding affinity of hagfish insulin is about 25% of that of pig insulin and shows that the relative affinity is of the same magnitude in IM-9 lymphocytes. Unexpectedly, the dissociation rate constant (k_{-1}) was about half that of pig insulin. If this was the only change, the affinity constant [K_a = (k + 1)/(k − 1)] would have doubled. Since K_a is actually decreased to about 25%, the association rate constant must be reduced to about 12% of that of pig insulin. As a general conclusion, it may be stated that the relative affinity of an analogue is not necessarily measured correctly under incubation conditions that are relevant for pig insulin. Longer times may be required to reach steady state of binding, even for analogues with reduced affinity.

It is generally agreed that the biologic potency of hagfish insulin is only 5% with respect to glucose transport in adipocytes, and the hagfish receptor complex must, therefore, be less efficient in conveying the message to the effector system. The present results do not provide an explanation for this phenomenon, but they do allow the exclusion of some possible mechanisms. Firstly, nearly the same fractions of receptor-bound hagfish and pig insulin were degraded. The attenuated efficiency of hagfish insulin seems, therefore, unrelated to receptor-mediated degradation. Secondly, previous studies on the time course of binding of pig insulin and activation of the biologic effect in adipocytes have shown that the activation brought about by submaximally stimulating concentrations is proportional to receptor occupancy.[9] This is incompatible with the hypothesis that the rate of association determines the biologic response. Therefore, the marked decrease in the association rate constant of hagfish insulin is probably not the reason for its disproportionally low potency. Thirdly, it seems at least theoretically possible that the state of activation at a given occupancy is proportional to the rate of dissociation from the receptor complexes. However, as shown by Simon et al.[10] in rat liver membranes and human lymphocytes, the dissociation rate constant of chicken insulin is also about half that of pig insulin, and, since the association rate constant is about the same, the affinity constant is increased.[10] We reproduced these findings in adipocytes, and we found a half-time of dissociation of chicken insulin of 15 min. In addition, the same fraction of bound pig insulin and chicken insulin was degraded (Sonne, O., Simon, J., and Gliemann, J., unpublished observations). Thus, the hormone receptor complex, once formed, is more stable for both chicken insulin and hagfish insulin than it is for pig insulin. The presence of a histidine in residue 8 of the A chain is the probable reason for the decreased dissociation rate constant of chicken insulin.[11] The mechanism may be similar in hagfish insulin, which also contains His_{A8}.[12] However, the decreased dissociation rate constant cannot be the reason for the disproportional decrease in the biologic potency of hagfish insulin, since the potency of chicken insulin is increased roughly in proportion to its increased affinity.[10,13] Since rate theories (association and dissociation) have to be dismissed, it must be concluded that hagfish insulin, while occupying the receptor, is less efficient in conveying a message to the glucose transport sites.

ACKNOWLEDGMENTS

This work was supported by grants from the Swedish Medical Research Council (project number 12X–718).

REFERENCES

1 Gliemann, J., and Gammeltoft, S.: The biological activity and binding affinity of modified insulins determined on isolated rat fat cells. Diabetologia *10*:105–14, 1974.

2 Gammeltoft, S., and Gliemann, J.: The binding of insulins from different animal species to rat fat cell receptors. Acta Physiol. Scand. *91*:7A–8A, 1974.

3 Emdin, S. O., Gammeltoft, S., and Gliemann, J.: Degradation, receptor binding affinity and potency of insulin from the Atlantic hagfish determined on isolated rat fat cells. J. Biol. Chem. *252*:602–08, 1977.

4 Muggeo, M., van Obberghen, E., Kahn, C. R., Roth, J., Ginsberg, B. H., De Meyts, P., Emdin, S. O., and Falkmer, S.: The insulin receptor of the Atlantic hagfish. Diabetes *28*:175–81, 1979.

5 Gliemann, J., and Sonne, O.: Binding and receptor-mediated degradation of insulin in adipocytes. J. Biol. Chem. *253*:7857–63, 1978.

6 Kahn, C. R., and Baird, K.: The fate of insulin bound to adipocytes. Evidence for compartmentalization and processing. J. Biol. Chem. *253*:4900–06, 1978.

7 Olefsky, J. M., Kobayashi, M., and Chang, H.: Interactions between insulin and its receptors after the initial binding event. Functional heterogeneity and relationships to insulin degradation. Diabetes *28*:460–71, 1979.

8 De Meyts, P., Bianco, A. R., and Roth, J.: Site-site interactions among insulin receptors: characterization of negative cooperativity. J. Biol. Chem. *251*:1877–88, 1976.

9 Gliemann, J., Gammeltoft, S., and Vinten, J.: Time course of insulin-receptor binding and insulin-induced lipogenesis in isolated rat fat cells. J. Biol. Chem. *250*:3368–74, 1975.

10 Simon, J., Freychet, P., Rosselin, G., and De Meyts, P.: Enhanced binding affinity of chicken insulin in rat liver membranes and human lymphocytes: relationship to the kinetic properties of the hormone-receptor interaction. Endocrinology *100*:115–21, 1977.

11 Märki, F., de Gasparo, M., Eisler, K., Kamber, B., Riniker, B., Rittel, W., and Sieber, P.: Synthesis and biological activity of seventeen analogues of human insulin. Hoppe-Seyler's Z. Physiol. Chem. *360*:1619–32, 1979.

12 Peterson, J. D., Steiner, D. F., Emdin, S. O., and Falkmer, S.: The amino acid sequence of the insulin from a primitive vertebrate, the Atlantic hagfish (Myxine glutinosa). J. Biol. Chem. *250*:5183–91, 1975.

13 Simon, J., Freychet, P., and Rosselin, G.: Chicken insulin: radioimmunological characterization and enhanced activity in rat fat cells and liver plasma membranes. Endocrinology *95*:1439–49, 1974.

Pancreatic Islets

A Tissue Rich in Serotonin

JANICE L. BIRD, EUGENE E. WRIGHT, AND JEROME M. FELDMAN

SUMMARY

Despite the fact that exogenous serotonin is an inhibitor of insulin secretion in a variety of species, many investigators doubt that endogenous serotonin plays a role in the regulation of insulin secretion. This is because, with the exception of the guinea pig, most animals do not demonstrate histochemical evidence of serotonin in their pancreatic islets. In this study, the serotonin content of collagenase-isolated golden hamster islets was compared with the serotonin content of other hamster tissues known to contain serotonin. In the serotonin assay, serotonin was converted to N-acetyl serotonin by N-acetyltransferase; the latter is converted to tritiated melatonin by hydroxyindole-o-methyltransferase and tritiated S-adenosylmethionine. In control hamsters, the mean ± SEM serotonin concentration in μmol/kg wet weight of islets (26.3 ± 9.00) was greater than that of pancreas (4.0 ± 0.84), anterior pituitary (6.3 ± 1.53), median eminence (2.5 ± 0.69), and cerebral cortex (1.9 ± 0.30). There was no significant increase in tissue serotonin after the administration of the monoamine oxidase inhibitor tranylcypromine. When the serotonin precursor 5-hydroxytryptophan alone was given to hamsters, there was a 22-, 31-, and fivefold increase in islet, pancreatic, and anterior pituitary serotonin, respectively. When 5-hydroxytryptophan was given to hamsters after tranylcypromine administration, there was a 58-, 73-, 14-, and 10-fold increase in islet, pancreatic, anterior pituitary, and median eminence serotonin, respectively. Tissue serotonin decreased after administration of reserpine but not after administration of p-chlorophenylalanine. Exposure to collagenase did not alter the serotonin concentration of pancreas or cerebral cortex in control or drug-treated hamsters. Hamsters receiving tranylcypromine plus 5-hydroxytryptophan had a higher plasma glucose concentration (266 ± 19 versus 116 ± 8 mg/dl), lower plasma insulin concentration (19 ± 3 versus 46 ± 8 μU/ml), and lower plasma insulin/glucose ratio (0.06 ± 0.01 versus 0.40 ± 0.06) than control hamsters. The present study demonstrates that animals whose islets do not have histochemical evidence of serotonin may have a high concentration of serotonin by chemical analysis and that large increases in islet serotonin concentration probably inhibit pancreatic insulin secretion. **DIABETES *29*:304–308, April 1980.**

From the Durham Veterans Administration Medical Center and Division of Endocrinology, Department of Medicine, Duke University Medical Center, Durham, North Carolina.

Address reprint requests to Jerome M. Feldman, M.D., Box 2963, Duke University Medical Center, Durham, North Carolina 27710.

Received for publication 17 May 1979 and in revised form 25 October 1979.

Monoamines were first identified by Falck and Hellmann in the pancreatic islet using a formaldehyde-induced histochemical fluorescence technique.[1] Further studies showed that, within the cells, monoamines were located in the insulin storage granules.[2] Consequently, the role of intracellular pancreatic islet monoamines in the regulation of insulin secretion has been the subject of many investigations. Pharmacologic manipulation of pancreatic islet serotonin and dopamine content in in vitro and in vivo systems has resulted in evidence for monoaminergic inhibition[3-9] and stimulation[10-12] of insulin secretion. These discrepancies may be the result of species variation in monoamine uptake and action or differences in experimental design.[5,13]

In the golden hamster in vitro pancreas system, it has been demonstrated that serotonin inhibits glucose-mediated insulin release.[3,4] Although the formaldehyde-induced histochemical fluorescence technique does not demonstrate the presence of serotonin in golden hamster islets,[14,15] there is some evidence that this technique may not accurately reflect the true tissue serotonin concentration.[16,17] Precise quantitation of pancreatic islet serotonin has been limited by the insensitivity of chemical analysis when applied to minute amounts of islet tissue. In the present study we have used a specific and sensitive radioenzymatic technique to compare the serotonin content of golden hamster pancreatic islets to that of other tissues known to contain serotonin. Drugs that alter monoamine synthesis and degradation were evaluated for their effect on tissue serotonin content.

MATERIALS AND METHODS

Materials. The following chemicals were purchased: 5-hydroxytryptamine creatinine sulfate complex (serotonin) (Calbiochem, San Diego, California); collagenase, class IV (Worthington Biochemical Co., Freehold, New Jersey); reserpine for injection, U.S.P. (Eli Lilly and Co., Indianapolis, Indiana); 5-hydroxy-L-tryptophan (5-HTP), N-acetyl-5-hydroxytryptamine (N-acetyl serotonin), DL-p-chlorophenylalanine (PCPA), L-norepinephrine bitartrate, L-epinephrine bitartrate, L-3,4-dihydroxyphenylethylamine HCl (dopamine), S-acetyl coenzyme A, N-acetyl-5-methoxytryptamine (melatonin) (Sigma Chemical, St. Louis, Missouri); S-adenosyl-L-methionine (methyl-^{3}H) (^{3}H-SAM) with specific activity of 7.5 Ci/mmol (New England Nuclear, Boston, Massachusetts); insulin radioimmunoassay kits (Amersham Corporation, Arlington Heights, Illinois); and male golden hamsters (100–125 g) (Engel Laboratory, Inc, Farmersburg, Indiana). The following chemicals were gifts: tranylcypromine sulfate (Tran) (Smith, Kline and French Laboratory, Philadelphia, Pennsylvania); N^1-(DL-seryl)-N^2-(2,3,4-trihydroxy benzyl), hydrazine (Ro-4-4602) (Hoffman-LaRoche Co., Nutley, New Jersey).

Preparation of hamster tissues. Hamsters were anesthetized with CO_2 and decapitated. Blood was collected in heparinized beakers and the plasma separated and frozen (−27°C). Anterior pituitary, median eminence, and samples of cerebral cortex and pancreas were immediately removed, weighed, and frozen (−27°C) until time of analysis. The islets (200–500/pancreas) were prepared by a modified collagenase digestion procedure[18] and frozen (−27°C) in 200 μl of 1:1 Hank's solution and 0.1 N HCl until time of analysis. The plasma glucose and insulin concentrations were determined on six hamsters in each experimental group.

The effect of collagenase on the measurement of serotonin in tissues was determined by dividing pancreas and cerebral cortex from individual animals into two aliquots. One aliquot was analyzed in the usual manner; the other was minced into small segments and incubated with collagenase solution in the same way that pancreas is incubated when islets are being isolated. The suspension of tissue was then poured into 25 ml of Hank's solution (5°C). The suspension was centrifuged at 2400 rpm and the supernatant was discarded. After being washed two additional times, the tissue was suspended in Hank's solution. Pancreas and cerebral cortex, prepared in the conventional manner and after collagenase exposure, were analyzed for serotonin. The protein content of the two types of tissue suspensions was determined by the Lowry method. The serotonin concentration of each collagenase-treated tissue was expressed as a percent of the serotonin concentration in its paired aliquot prepared without exposure to collagenase.

Some hamsters received medications by intraperitoneal injection. The dose and time of administration of drugs before the hamsters were killed were: reserpine 0.5 mg/kg at 72, 48, and 24 h; PCPA 100 mg/kg at 72, 48, and 24 h; Tran 25 mg/kg at 48 and 24 h; Ro-4-4602 500 mg/kg at 2 h; and 5-HTP 30 mg/kg at 1 h.

Analytical methods. The radioenzymatic assay for serotonin of Saavedra et al.[19] was used. Briefly, tissue homogenates were incubated with acetyl coenzyme A and N-acetyltransferase, which resulted in the acetylation of serotonin in the 5 position to form N-acetyl serotonin. Incubation was continued with the addition of ^{3}H-SAM and hydroxy-indole-o-methyltransferase (HIOMT). The ^{3}H-methyl group was transferred to the hydroxyl group of N-acetyl serotonin, which resulted in ^{3}H-melatonin. Melatonin was separated by differential solvent extraction and the radioactivity quantified in toluene counting solution.

The following specific modifications were made:

1. N-acetyltransferase was semipurified from hamster liver, dialyzed once, and frozen (−27°C) in 0.02 M sodium phosphate buffer, pH 7.2, for up to 2 wk.

2. Frozen tissues were homogenized in 0.1 N HCl. The assay was carried out on 25 μl of uncentrifuged tissue homogenate, with a final total volume of 110 μl.

3. Ro-4-4602 (0.1 mM) was included in the initial incubation.

4. Two milliliters of the organic phase containing ^{3}H-melatonin was evaporated in counting vials to dryness (10 min), resolubilized in toluene counting solution, and the radioactivity determined.

Each tissue was assayed with its own acetyl coenzyme A blank and internal standard of 100 pmol serotonin, because of the possible variability of tissue N-acetyl serotonin and nonradioactive SAM. The sensitivity of the assay, defined as 50% greater than blank, was 4–8 pmol serotonin/tube and linear up to 400 pmol serotonin/tube. The coefficients of variation for this assay were: intra-assay 13% and interassay 16%. The percent that various related compounds cross-reacted with serotonin in this assay were: 5-HTP less than 1% when Ro-4-4602 (0.1 mM) was included in the assay; dopamine and norepinephrine less than 1%; and epinephrine less than 7%. Lowry protein determinations[20] were made on each islet sample and ranged from 0.2 to 0.65 μg protein/islet because of variation in the size of islets obtained. The wet weight of the islets was estimated on the basis that their protein content represented 15% of their wet weight.[21] All values of tissue serotonin were expressed as μmol serotonin/kg wet weight.

Plasma glucose concentration was determined with a glucose oxidase method.[22] Plasma insulin concentration was determined with a double antibody radioimmunoassay method.[23] As pure hamster insulin was not available, beef insulin was used as the insulin standard. The ratio of plasma insulin to plasma glucose (I/G) was calculated by dividing the concentration of insulin in μU/ml by that of glucose in mg/dl. This ratio gives an estimate of the insulin responsiveness of the pancreatic islets to a glucose stimulus.[24]

Statistical methods. The basal serotonin concentration of the various tissues had a small variance; however, 5-HTP treatment resulted in a larger variance. Since the standard deviation in the original scale varied directly as the mean, the logarithmic transformation was used to stabilize the variance.[25] The logarithmically transformed data were tested for significance by analysis of variance and Scheffe's single-tailed multiple comparison test.[26] All data are expressed as the mean ± SEM, unless otherwise stated.

RESULTS

Serotonin levels. Tissue serotonin concentrations in μmol/kg wet weight are depicted in Figure 1 for cerebral cortex, anterior pituitary, and median eminence and in Figure 2 for pancreas and islets. In control hamsters, serotonin was present in measurable amounts in all tissues (cerebral cortex 1.94 ± 0.30, anterior pituitary 6.3 ± 1.53, median eminence 2.5 ± 0.69, pancreas 4.0 ± 0.84, and islets 26.3 ± 9.00). The highest concentration was found in the islets; this value was four times greater than that found in the anterior pituitary or pancreas.

The effect of pharmacologic manipulation on tissue serotonin content was evaluated. Monoamine oxidase (MAO), an enzyme in the major degradative pathway for serotonin, was blocked by the administration of Tran. The dose used had been shown to inhibit MAO activity 64%–88%.[27] As compared with the control group, in the anterior pituitary serotonin concentration decreased slightly; in all other tissues an insignificant increase was observed (cerebral cortex 2.6 ± 0.82, anterior pituitary 4.3 ± 0.86, median eminence 6.0 ± 0.83, pancreas 9.0 ± 2.46, and islets 40.0 ± 15.20).

The immediate precursor of serotonin, 5-HTP, was administered to normal hamsters to promote serotonin synthesis. There was a 22-, 31-, and fivefold increase in islet, pancreatic, and anterior pituitary serotonin, respectively. This was a significant increase over the serotonin concentration in tissues from control hamsters ($P < 0.01$).

When 5-HTP was administered to hamsters who had received Tran, there was a 58-, 73-, 14-, and 10-fold increase in islet, pancreatic, anterior pituitary, and median eminence serotonin, respectively. This was a significant increase over the serotonin concentration in tissues from control hamsters ($P < 0.01$). The serotonin content of cerebral cortex was not significantly increased by Tran plus 5-HTP administration. The islets of hamsters receiving Tran plus 5-HTP had a five times greater concentration of serotonin (1529 ± 287 μmol/kg wet wt) than the pancreas (293 ± 53 μmol/kg wet wt) and a 17 times greater concentration of serotonin than the anterior pituitary (88 ± 11 μmol/kg wet wt). Administration of the decarboxylase inhibitor, Ro-4-4602, to two hamsters treated with Tran plus 5-HTP inhibited the increase in serotonin concentration of the pancreas 52% and of the islets 85%.

To determine whether a decrease in the tissue serotonin concentration could be induced, reserpine, an inhibitor of serotonin re-uptake, was administered to two hamsters. All tissues, except the pancreas, demonstrated a decrease in serotonin concentration (cerebral cortex 32%, anterior pituitary 59%, median eminence 37%, pancreas 0%, islets 80%). PCPA, an inhibitor of serotonin synthesis, was also administered. Tissue serotonin concentration was not diminished in four hamsters.

The effect of collagenase on serotonin measurement in pancreas and cerebral cortex was determined on tissues from two control hamsters, two hamsters treated with 5-HTP, and two hamsters treated with Tran plus 5-HTP. The serotonin concentration of the collagenase-treated pancreas was 110 ± 13% of the serotonin concentration of the pancreas prepared for analysis in the conventional manner. The serotonin concentration of the collagenase-treated cerebral cortex was 112 ± 20% of the serotonin concentration of the cerebral cortex prepared for analysis in the conventional manner. Neither of these differences was statistically significant.

Plasma glucose and insulin. The plasma levels of glucose and insulin and the plasma insulin/glucose ratio in control hamsters and in hamsters receiving Tran, 5-HTP, or Tran plus 5-HTP are shown in Table 1. When given alone, neither Tran nor 5-HTP had any effect on the plasma glucose, plasma insulin, or plasma insulin/glucose ratio. When 5-HTP was administered to hamsters that were pretreated with

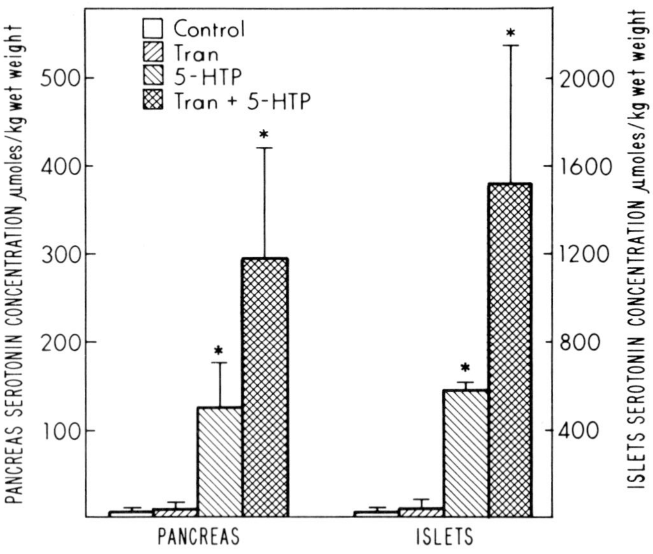

FIGURE 2. Serotonin concentration of pancreas and islets in control state and after the administration of pharmacologic agents. The concentration is expressed in μmol serotonin/kg wet weight. The bar represents the mean of five hamsters and the bracket represents the SEM. Scale for islets is four times greater than that for pancreas. The asterisk (*) groups are significantly different ($P < 0.01$) when compared with their respective control group.

FIGURE 1. Serotonin concentration of cerebral cortex, anterior pituitary, and median eminence in control state and after the administration of pharmacologic agents. The concentration is expressed in μmol serotonin/kg wet weight. The bar represents the mean of five hamsters and the bracket represents the SEM. The asterisk (*) groups are significantly different ($P < 0.01$) when compared with their respective control group.

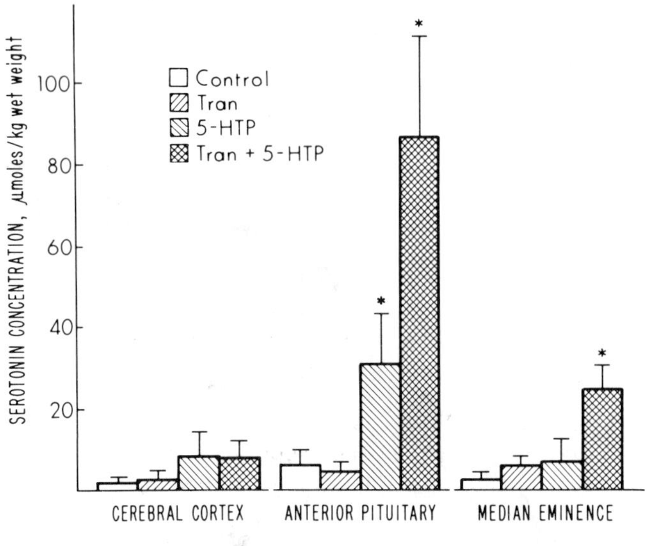

TABLE 1
Effect of administration of tranylcypromine (Tran) and 5-hydroxytryptophan (5-HTP) on plasma glucose, insulin, and insulin/glucose ratio of golden hamsters*

	Control	Tran	5-HTP	Tran + 5-HTP
Plasma glucose (mg/dl)	116 ± 8	111 ± 10	100 ± 6	266 ± 19‡
Plasma insulin (μU/ml)	46 ± 8	40 ± 6	46 ± 9	19 ± 3†
Plasma insulin/glucose ratio	0.40 ± 0.06	0.38 ± 0.05	0.48 ± 0.09	0.06 ± 0.01‡

* Each value is the mean ± SEM of six animals.
† $P < 0.05$ when compared with controls.
‡ $P < 0.01$ when compared with controls.

Tran, there was an increase in plasma glucose and a decrease in plasma insulin and the plasma insulin/glucose ratio.

DISCUSSION

In the present study we used a sensitive and specific radioenzymatic assay to demonstrate the presence of serotonin in the cerebral cortex, anterior pituitary, median eminence, pancreas, and pancreatic islets of the golden hamster. Under basal conditions, the islet serotonin concentration was at least four times greater than that of the other tissues measured. Pharmacologic manipulation resulted in the accumulation of serotonin in all tissues. 5-HTP was used to promote serotonin synthesis. As shown previously in the islet, the uptake of 5-HTP is three times greater than that of serotonin, and 5-HTP is readily converted to serotonin by the significant activity of islet aromatic amino acid decarboxylase.[28,29] Tran, a MAO inhibitor, was used to inactivate the major degradative pathway of islet serotonin.[30] Administration of Tran plus 5-HTP resulted in a significant increase in the serotonin concentration of all tissues, except the cerebral cortex. Islet serotonin concentration increased from 5 to 200 times greater than the other tissues. The high concentration of serotonin in islets was not due to exposure to collagenase, for collagenase exposure did not increase the serotonin concentration of pancreas or cerebral cortex.

The presence of significant amounts of other biogenic amines has also been demonstrated in the islets of the golden hamster. The norepinephrine concentration is 42.1 ± 8.07 μmol/kg wet wt, and the dopamine concentration is 7.5 ± 1.62 μmol/kg wet wt.[31] The specificity of the serotonin assay is derived from its less than 1% cross-reactivity with either norepinephrine or dopamine. To prevent cross-reactivity with 5-HTP, the decarboxylase inhibitor, Ro-4-4602, was employed to inactivate any decarboxylase present in enzyme or tissue preparations.

Histochemical fluorescence studies have demonstrated the presence of monoamines in the islets of several species, but have not identified serotonin in golden hamster islets.[14,15] Consequently, some investigators have questioned the physiological relevance of studies demonstrating inhibition of insulin secretion by serotonin in the in vitro golden hamster pancreas system.[32] Our present study demonstrates that serotonin is present in significant amounts in hamster islets. It has been previously noted that measurement of rat brain norepinephrine and dopamine by histochemical fluorescence did not always accurately reflect the content of these monoamines by quantitative chemical analysis.[16] The eye of the invertebrate *Aplysia* was recently demonstrated to have large amounts of serotonin measured by gas chromatography-mass spectrometry, which was not detected by histochemical fluorescence.[17] Therefore, although histochemical fluorescence data are valuable for assessing the role of monoamines, the results may be only semiquantitative in some tissues.

Studies using the in vitro hamster pancreas system demonstrated an inhibition of glucose-mediated insulin release in response to administration of serotonin.[8] In the present study, hamsters that received 5-HTP after pretreatment with Tran had significant hyperglycemia. This may, in part, be due to extrapancreatic effects, for serotonin stimulates hepatic glycogenolysis in rats and rabbits.[33] However, our hamsters had a decrease in plasma insulin concentration and the plasma insulin/glucose ratio, suggesting that there was an impairment of pancreatic insulin secretion in response to the hyperglycemia. This decrease in plasma insulin levels may be due to the increased serotonin concentration in the pancreatic islets. When electron microscopic autoradiography is used after the administration of tritium-labeled 5-HTP to the mouse, there is evidence of 5-HTP uptake in both the β-cells and the α-cells.[34] Neither the β- nor α-cells of the golden hamster contain serotonin when evaluated by histochemical techniques.[15] At this time no data are available on the uptake of tritium-labeled 5-HTP by specific cell types in the islets of the golden hamster. Thus, we cannot be certain that there is an increase in serotonin concentration specifically in the β-cells and that this increase is responsible for the hyperglycemia and impaired insulin secretion that we observed.

The present study demonstrates that, when a sensitive radioenzymatic technique is used, significant amounts of serotonin are measured in hamster islets, a tissue in which serotonin cannot be detected by histochemical fluorescence. The islet serotonin concentration is greater than other monoamine-containing tissues. Pharmacologic manipulation, which results in a significant increase in islet serotonin concentration, also induces hyperglycemia. These observations are consistent with an active role for serotonin in the regulation of islet insulin secretion.

ACKNOWLEDGMENTS

We sincerely appreciate the expert technical assistance of Charles Castleberry and the expert secretarial assistance of Cynthia Cox.

This study was supported by the Veterans Administration and NIH Chinese Hamster Program Project 08P1 AM 21933A01.

REFERENCES

[1] Falck, B., and Hellmann, B.: Evidence for the presence of biogenic amines in pancreatic islets. Experientia (Basel) *19*:139–40, 1963.

[2] Jaim-Etcheverry, G., and Zieher, L. M.: Electron microscopic cytochemistry of 5-hydroxytryptamine (5-HT) in the beta cells of guinea pig endocrine pancreas. Endocrinology *83*:917–23, 1968.

[3] Feldman, J. M., and Lebovitz, H. E.: Serotonin inhibition of in vitro insulin release from golden hamster pancreas. Endocrinology *86*:66–70, 1970.

[4] Feldman, J. M., and Lebovitz, H. E.: Specificity of serotonin inhibition of insulin release from golden hamster pancreas. Diabetes *19*:475–79, 1970.

[5] Quickel, K. E., Feldman, J. M., and Lebovitz, H. E.: Inhibition of insulin secretion by serotonin and dopamine: species variation. Endocrinology *89*:1295–1302, 1971.

[6] Lundquist, I., Ekholm, R., and Ericson, L. E.: Monoamines in the pancreatic islet of the mouse, 5-hydroxytryptamine as an intracellular modifier of insulin secretion, and the hypoglycemic action of monoamine oxidase inhibitors. Diabetologia *7*:414–22, 1971.

[7] Feldman, J. M., Boyd, A. E., III, and Lebovitz, H. E.: Structural determinants of catecholamine action on in vitro insulin release. J. Pharmacol. Exp. Ther. *176*:611–21, 1972.

[8] Feldman, J. M., Quickel, K. E., and Lebovitz, H. E.: Potentiation of insulin secretion in vitro by serotonin antagonists. Diabetes *21*:779–88, 1972.

[9] Feldman, J. M., and Lebovitz, H. E.: A serotonergic mechanism for the control of insulin secretion. Trans. Assoc. Am. Physicians *35*:279–94, 1972.

[10] Telib, M., Raptis, S., Schroder, K. E., and Pfeiffer, E. F.: Serotonin and insulin release in vitro. Diabetologia *4*:253–56, 1968.

[11] Lechin, F., Coll-Garcia, E., van der Dijs, B., Pena, F., Bentolila, A., and Rivas, C.: The effect of serotonin on insulin secretion. Acta Physiol. Lat. Am. *25*:339–46, 1975.

[12] Gagliardino, J. J., Zieher, L. M., Iturriza, F. C., Hernandez, R. E., and Rodriquez, R. R.: Insulin release and glucose changes induced by serotonin. Horm. Metab. Res. *3*:145–50, 1971.

[13] Feldman, J. M.: Species variation in the islets of Langerhans. Diabetologia *16*:1–4, 1979.

[14] Cegrell, L.: The occurrence of biogenic monoamines in the mammalian endocrine pancreas. Acta Physiol. Scand. Suppl. *314*:1–60, 1968.

[15] Cegrell, L.: Monoaminergic mechanisms in the pancreatic alpha cells. *In* The Structure and Metabolism of the Pancreatic Islets. Falkmer, S., Hellman, B., and Taljedal, I. B., Eds. Oxford, Pergamon Press, 1970, pp. 131–40.

[16] Kopin, I. J., Palkovitz, M., Kobayashi, R. M., and Jacobowitz, D. M.: Quantitative relationship of catecholamine content and histofluorescence in brain of rats. Brain Res. *80*:229–35, 1974.

[17] Corrent, G., McAdoo, D. J., and Eskin, A.: Serotonin shifts the phase of the circadian rhythm from the *Aplysia* eye. Science *202*:977–79, 1978.

[18] Feldman, J. M., and Chapman, B.: Preparation of islets of Langerhans from rabbits and hamsters by the collagenase digestion technique. Acta Diabetol. Lat. *12*:208–18, 1975.

[19] Saavedra, J. M., Brownstein, M., and Axelrod, J.: A specific and sensitive enzymatic-isotopic microassay for serotonin in tissues. J. Pharmacol. Exp. Ther. *186*:508–15, 1973.

[20] Lowry, O. H., Rosebrough, N. J., Farr, A. L., and Randall, R. J.: Protein measurement with Folin phenol reagent. J. Biol. Chem. *193*:265–75, 1951.

[21] Hellerstrom, C., and Brolin, S. E.: Biochemistry and biophysics of insulin secretion. *In* Handbook of Experimental Pharmacology, Vol. 34(2). Hasselbatt, A., and Bruchhausen, F. V., Eds. Berlin, Springer-Verlag, 1975, pp. 57–78.

[22] Saifer, A., and Gerstenfeld, B.: Photometric micro determination of blood glucose with glucose oxidase. J. Lab. Clin. Med. *5*:448–60, 1958.

[23] Hales, C. N., and Randle, P. J.: Immunoassay of insulin with insulin antibody precipitate. Biochem. J. *88*:137–46, 1963.

[24] Seltzer, H. S., Allen, E. W., Herron, A. L., and Brennan, M. T.: Insulin secretion in response to glycemic stimulus: relation of delayed initial release to carbohydrate intolerance in mild diabetes mellitus. J. Clin. Invest. *46*:323–35, 1967.

[25] Snedecor, G. W., and Cochran, W. G.: The logarithmic transformation. *In* Statistical Methods, 6th edit. Iowa, The Iowa State University Press, 1967, pp. 329–30.

[26] Zar, J. H.: Scheffe's multiple contrasts. *In* Biostatistical Analysis. Englewood Cliffs, N.J., Prentice-Hall, 1974, pp. 133–37, 159–61, 417.

[27] Feldman, J. M., Henderson, J. H., and Blalock, J. A.: Effect of pharmacological agents and fasting on pancreatic islet norepinephrine in the golden hamster. Diabetologia *17*:169–74, 1979.

[28] Mahony, C., and Feldman, J. M.: Species variation in pancreatic islet monoamine uptake and action. Diabetes *26*:257–61, 1977.

[29] Lebovitz, H. E., and Downs, R. W., Jr.: Catecholamine biosynthesis enzymes in pancreatic islet cells. *In* Frontiers in Catecholamine Research. Usdin, E., and Snyder, S. H., Eds. Great Britain, Pergamon Press, 1973, pp. 831–33.

[30] Bosin, T. R.: Metabolism of serotonin by monoamine oxidase. *In* Serotonin in Health and Disease, Vol. 1. Essman, W. B., Ed. New York, Spectrum Publications, 1978, pp. 198–223.

[31] Zern, R. T., Foster, L. B., Blalock, J. A., and Feldman, J. M.: Characteristics of the dopaminergic and noradrenergic systems of the pancreatic islets. Diabetes *28*:185–89, 1979.

[32] Lundquist, I., Sundler, F., Hakanson, R., Larsson, L.-I., and Heding, L. G.: Differential changes in the 5-hydroxytryptamine and insulin content of guinea pig B-cells. Endocrinology *97*:937–47, 1975.

[33] Erspamer, V.: Peripheral physiological and pharmacological actions of indolealkylamines. *In* 5-Hydroxytryptamine and Related Indolealkylamines. Erspamer, V., Ed. New York, Springer-Verlag, 1966, pp. 245–359.

[34] Ekholm, R., Ericson, L. E., and Lundquist, I.: Monoamines in the pancreatic islets of the mouse-subcellular localization of 5-hydroxytryptamine by electron microscopic autoradiography. Diabetologia *7*:339–48, 1971.

Impaired Granulocyte Adherence in Mildly Diabetic Patients

Effects of Tolazamide Treatment

J. D. BAGDADE AND E. WALTERS

SUMMARY

Granulocyte adherence in 10 of 15 untreated asymptomatic hyperglycemic diabetic outpatients (mean fasting glucose ± SEM, 289 ± 16 mg/100 ml) was 62 ± 7% of control values. After treatment (2–4 wk) with tolazamide (500 mg daily), adherence to the nylon fiber columns employed in this study returned to control levels in the seven patients whose fasting glucose levels fell, (mean, 192 ± 16 mg/100 ml) and deteriorated in the three in whom fasting hyperglycemia worsened. Results of this study indicate that, even in some mildly diabetic patients, a reduction in granulocyte adherence similar to that found in insulin-dependent diabetics may impair the inflammatory response. DIABETES *29*:309–311, April 1980.

Infection was a frequent cause of death in the diabetic before the availability of antimicrobial treatment and insulin. The fact that, even with these therapies, infection continues to occur frequently in diabetic patients has suggested that their susceptibility to infection is altered. There is little evidence that the capacity of the well controlled diabetic to resist infection is impaired. Recent studies, however, performed in poorly controlled diabetics before and after intensive management with insulin, have demonstrated abnormalities in the chemotaxis,[1–3] adherence,[4] phagocytosis,[5,6] and microbicidal function[7,8] of granulocytes, which could compromise their inflammatory response.

Most recent studies of host defense in diabetes have examined insulin-dependent patients with grossly disturbed glucose homeostasis. If the severity of these abnormalities, in fact, is related to the degree of insulin deficiency, as our previous studies have suggested,[4,5,8,9] then it is possible that granulocyte dysfunction also may be present in less severely diabetic patients. The following studies were undertaken to determine whether asymptomatic diabetic outpatients with fasting hyperglycemia have abnormalities in granulocyte adherence similar to those we found earlier in insulin-requiring patients,[4] and, if present, whether they are reversed by treatment with the oral sulfonylurea tolazamide.

From the Department of Medicine, University of Washington School of Medicine, and the Providence Medical Center.
Address reprint requests to J. D. Bagdade, M.D., Providence Medical Center, 500 17th Avenue, Seattle, Washington 98124.
Received for publication 30 April and in revised form 11 December 1979.

MATERIALS AND METHODS

Subjects studied. Heparinized blood samples were obtained from 15 patients at 8 a.m. on the days of study after an overnight fast during a period of poor control, and repeated after 2–4 weeks of diabetic treatment in the 10 patients who were found to have abnormal adherence when initially studied. Of the three patients whose treatment with tolazamide was a failure, two were studied a third time after insulin treatment. None had evidence of renal insufficiency, infection, or ketoacidosis or was taking medications known to alter leukocyte adherence.

On the days that diabetic patients were studied, blood samples were obtained under identical conditions from one or more healthy sex-matched controls. The same subjects served as controls for the same diabetic patients studied before and after treatment. Blood glucose was measured in all diabetic and control subjects at the time of each study.

The adherence assay system. Granulocyte adherence was studied according to the method of MacGregor et al. as recently described.[10] Briefly, 1 ml aliquots of each blood specimen were added to the tops of three Pasteur pipettes with uniform diameter and aperture to which preweighed nylon fiber had been packed with a column length of 15 mm. Each aliquot was allowed to filter through the columns at room temperature. The granulocytes were counted (Coulter counter) on each whole blood sample before addition to the columns (100 white cells are differentiated for each blood smear) and in the effluent blood. The granulocyte adherence was estimated by the following equation:

$$100\% - \frac{\text{PMN/ml in effluent}}{\text{PMN/ml in original sample}} \times 100 = \%\ \text{PMN adherence.}$$

The granulocyte adherence for a given specimen was defined as the mean value for three columns tested and was expressed as a percentage of control.

Since female subjects showed uniformly higher adherence to the fiber column, as previously shown,[4] columns containing less fiber (70 mg) were used for the females than males (80 mg). With their respective columns, 10 normal female subjects showed a granulocyte adherence of 58 ± 1%, mean ± SEM; 10 normal males demonstrated an average adherence of 67 ± 2% on the 80 mg fiber columns. The effects of incubation of whole blood for one hour from two control subjects with two concentrations of tolinase (10 and 50 mg/ml) were indistinguishable from those observed with saline alone.

RESULTS

Before treatment, granulocyte adherence was reduced in ten (groups II and III) and was comparable to control in five (group I) of the fifteen mildly diabetic patients studied (Table 1). After tolazamide treatment of the subnormal group, adherence increased in all seven patients in whom fasting glucose levels decreased; in all three tolazamide nonresponders whose glucose levels rose, adherence deteriorated ($P < 0.008$, Fisher's exact test). Two of these patients were treated for 2–3 wk with insulin after which fasting glucose concentrations fell slightly (in patient 1, from 380 to 366, and in patient 2, from 420 to 337 mg/100 ml) and adherence improved (in patient 1, from 32 to 48, and in patient 2, from 70 to 81% of control, group III, Table 1).

DISCUSSION

Resistance to infection may become impaired in some diabetic patients because of alterations in the normal mechanisms of host defense. In symptomatic diabetics, a number of disturbances in granulocyte function have been reported, which have been reversed when control was improved with insulin treatment.[4–6,8] The fact that their severity often has correlated with fasting glucose levels and that some infections occur frequently in mildly diabetic patients has suggested that host defenses also may be compromised when clinical manifestations of insulin deficiency are mild.

The nylon fiber column technique employed in this study is believed to be the best available experimental tool to estimate the adherence of granulocytes to vascular endothelium, the step in host defense that precedes diapedesis and exudate formation in extravascular tissues. Our results, showing that adherence measured by this technique may be impaired in some mildly diabetic patients, support the suggestion that the integrity of host defense mechanisms may be adversely affected even when insulin deficiency is not severe.

The metabolic basis for this abnormality is unclear. None of the patients studied were receiving alcohol or any anti-inflammatory agent which have been shown to inhibit adherence.[11] Granulocyte adherence and delivery have been shown by MacGregor and co-workers to be inhibited by cAMP[12] and epinephrine, a hormone that increases granulocyte cAMP levels. Since insulin can lower cAMP levels in a number of tissues, it is interesting to speculate that the improvement observed in our patients after tolinase treatment could reflect this insulin effect.

Similar to the improvement in adherence that we recently reported in more severely diabetic patients after treatment with insulin,[4] this disturbance also was reversed in these mildly insulinopenic subjects when improved control was achieved with sulfonylurea therapy. The reversibility of this defect in those patients in whom glucose homeostasis improved after treatment is consistent with the hypothesis that, when abnormalities in granulocyte function occur in diabetic patients, they may result from metabolic alterations related to insulin deficiency.[13]

It is also possible, however, that this functional defect may result from hyperglycemia itself. We have reported earlier[4] that, when whole blood from normal control subjects was incubated with glucose at concentrations encountered clinically, adherence was impaired. This in vitro effect, as well as the reduced performance we observed in granulocytes from diabetic patients, could result from the glycosylation of membrane and cellular proteins,[14] which might alter their capacity to adhere to the nylon fiber.

A number of points about the frequency of this abnormality in our patients are noteworthy. For one, adherence was not impaired in all subjects studied before treatment, including three patients who had fasting glucose levels exceeding 300 mg/100 ml. While the severity of granulocyte dysfunction we reported in previous studies in more severely diabetic patients has correlated closely with their fasting glucose levels,[8,9] in this adherence study we could not demonstrate this association.

This lack of a glucose adherence relationship may reflect the fact that basal glucose levels in adult-onset diabetics are a less precise estimate of insulin availability than they are in insulin-dependent patients. In this regard the measurement of the glycosylated hemoglobin A_{1c}, a more accurate index of long-term diabetic control than basal glucose,[14] might have provided a more useful basis for correlating with adherence. Unfortunately, however, this measurement was unavailable at the time this study was performed. Small sample size, their relatively mild diabetic

TABLE 1
Changes in granulocyte adherence and fasting glucose values in diabetic patients

	Glucose (mg/100 ml)	Adherence (% control)	Glucose (mg/100 ml)	Adherence (% control)
Group I: Untreated				
1	190	141		
2	280	127		
3	310	108		
4	340	162		
5	350	113		
Group II: Tolazamide Responders				
1	160	58	150	81
2	228	25	220	134
3	284	61	230	94
4	313	37	240	108
5	260	70	130	179
6	320	91	171	100
7	266	70	195	90
$\bar{x}$ ± SD	261.5 ± 54.8	58.9 ± 22.0	190.8 ± 42.0	112.3 ± 33.9
Group III: Tolazamide Nonresponders				
1	345	40	380	32
2	334	82	420	70
3	360	83	380	56
$\bar{x}$	346.3	68.3	393.3	52.7

state, and the presence of varying degrees of obesity-related insulin resistance, which would tend to raise glucose levels by retarding its assimilation by peripheral tissues, are other factors that might contribute to weakening this correlation in these patients.

Despite the high frequency of abnormal adherence found in the participants in this study, none had evidence of infection. This finding is consistent with clinical experience, which suggests that host defense mechanisms have considerable reserve and must be severely compromised before microbial invasion and dissemination can actually occur. If, however, because of metabolic dysfunction[13] related to insulin deficiency, there are associated abnormalities in granulocyte chemotaxis, phagocytosis, and intracellular killing, as have been described in poorly controlled diabetics, then a situation exists in which the development of infection is more likely. In light of the associations found between these disturbances in host defense and the availability of insulin, it would appear that good control of diabetic patients is the best means of minimizing the likelihood that they will acquire infection.

ACKNOWLEDGMENTS

This work was supported by grants R01 AM 17939 from the National Institute of Arthritis, Metabolism, and Digestive Diseases and from the Upjohn Company.

REFERENCES

[1] Mowat, A. G., and Baum, J.: Chemotaxis of polymorphonuclear leukocytes from patients with diabetes mellitus. N. Engl. J. Med. *284*:621–27, 1971.

[2] Hill, H. R., Sauls, H. S., Dettloff, J. L., and Quie, P. G.: Impaired leukocyte responsiveness in patients with juvenile diabetes mellitus. Clin. Immunol. Immunopathol. *2*:395–403, 1974.

[3] Miller, M. E., and Baker, L.: Leukocyte functions in juvenile diabetes mellitus: humoral and cellular aspects. J. Pediatr. *81*:979–82, 1972.

[4] Bagdade, J. D., Stewart, M., and Walters, E.: Impaired granulocyte adherence: a reversible defect in host defense in patients with poorly controlled diabetes. Diabetes *27*:677–81, 1978.

[5] Bagdade, J. D., Nielson, K. L., and Bulger, R.: Reversible abnormalities in phagocytic function in poorly controlled diabetic patients. Am. J. Med. Sci. *263*:451–56, 1972.

[6] Bagdade, J. D., Root, R. K., and Bulger, R. J.: Impaired leukocyte function in patients with poorly controlled diabetes. Diabetes *23*:9–15, 1974.

[7] Tan, J. S., Anderson, J. L., Watanakunakorn, C., and Phair, J. P.: Neutrophil dysfunction in diabetes mellitus. J. Lab. Clin. Med. *85*:26–33, 1975.

[8] Nolan, C. M., Beaty, H. N., and Bagdade, J. D.: Further characterization of impaired bactericidal function of granulocytes in patients with poorly controlled diabetes. Diabetes *27*:889–94, 1978.

[9] Bagdade, J. D.: Phagocytic and microbicidal function in diabetes mellitus. Acta Endocrinol. (Copenhagen) *83*(Suppl. 205):26–34, 1976.

[10] MacGregor, R. R., Spagnulo, P. J., and Lentnek, A. L.: Inhibition of granulocyte adherence by ethanol, prednisone, and aspirin, measured with an assay system. N. Engl. J. Med. *291*:642–46, 1974.

[11] MacGregor, R. R.: The effect of anti-inflammatory agents and inflammation on granulocyte adherence. Evidence of regulation by plasma factors. Am. J. Med. *61*:597–607, 1976.

[12] MacGregor, R. R., Macarac, E. J., and Kefalides, N. A.: Comparative adherence of granulocytes to endothelial monolayers and nylon fiber. J. Clin. Invest. *61*:697–702, 1978.

[13] Esmann, V.: The diabetic leukocyte. Enzyme *13*:32–55, 1972.

[14] Williamson, J. R., and Kilo, C.: Current status of capillary basement-membrane disease in diabetes mellitus. Diabetes *26*:65–73, 1977.

Glucose and Insulin Responses to Oral Glucose in Overt Non-insulin-dependent Diabetics With and Without the Islet Cell Antibody

R. S. GRAY, W. J. IRVINE, E. H. D. CAMERON, AND L. J. P. DUNCAN

SUMMARY

Plasma insulin, glucose, and insulin/glucose responses to a 50-g oral glucose tolerance test (OGTT) were compared in 14 islet cell antibody (ICAb) positive non-insulin-dependent diabetics (NIDDM), 14 matched ICAb negative NIDDM, and 14 ICAb negative nondiabetic controls. Both groups of NIDDM exhibited marked carbohydrate intolerance with insulinopenia. Despite having significantly higher plasma glucose concentrations during the study, the ICAb positive NIDDM had significantly lower insulin levels, and thus lower insulin/glucose ratios, than the ICAb negative NIDDM both in the fasting state and in response to the OGTT. Similarly, ICAb positive NIDDM had higher integrated glucose responses (ΔG), lower integrated insulin responses (ΔI), and lower $\Delta I/\Delta G$ values than ICAb negative NIDDM. Three ICAb negative and seven ICAb positive NIDDM subsequently required insulin treatment.

These findings show that ICAb positive NIDDM suffer from a greater disturbance of B-cell function than do matched ICAb negative NIDDM. **DIABETES 29: 312–316, April 1980.**

The presence of islet cell antibody (ICAb) in a non-insulin-dependent diabetic (NIDDM) implies a high risk of deteriorating carbohydrate tolerance, with the development of insulin dependency as evidence of relative or absolute insulin deficiency.[1,2] On the basis of this and other observations, ICAb positive NIDDM have been regarded as suffering from the same disease as insulin-dependent diabetics,[1,2] albeit in a less severe form. Under normal circumstances, the distinction between NIDDM and insulin-dependent diabetics (IDDM) is clinically derived and is based on the susceptibility of IDDM, but not NIDDM, to ketosis.[3]

Little attempt has yet been made to compare the metabolic disorder found in overt NIDDM with and without ICAb. Tiengo et al.[4] have shown that plasma glucagon and insulin responses to an intravenous arginine infusion are similar in overt diabetics with and without ICAb, but the diabetics were poorly matched in terms of treatment and duration of diabetes, the majority already insulin-dependent and therefore showing a very poor insulin response to this form of stimulus. The purpose of the present study was to determine the plasma glucose and insulin responses to an oral glucose tolerance test (OGTT) in ICAb positive and ICAb negative overt NIDDM, who were otherwise well matched in terms of weight, age, duration of diabetes, and treatment.

PATIENTS AND METHODS

Fourteen ICAb positive NIDDM were individually matched with 14 ICAb negative NIDDM (having been ICAb negative within 1 mo of diagnosis of diabetes) and 14 nondiabetic ICAb negative controls. The clinical and metabolic data of the ICAb positive and negative NIDDM are shown in Table 1. None had ever exhibited ketonuria. The median age of the controls (five males, nine females) was 51.5 yr (range, 30–70 yr) and their median percent ideal body weight was 96.5 (range, 91–103). There was no significant difference when comparing ICAb positive and negative NIDDM with respect to interval between diagnosis, symptomatic onset of diabetes and time of study, presenting plasma glucose, presenting percent ideal body weight, nor mean plasma glucose recorded at the time of six consecutive outpatient attendances before the study. ICAb positive and negative NIDDM were treated in a similar manner. ICAb negative NIDDM had a longer duration of diabetic symptoms before diagnosis than did ICAb positive NIDDM ($P < 0.05$). One ICAb positive NIDDM was known to suffer from pernicious anemia and another had previously been treated for thyrotoxicosis but was biochemically euthyroid at the time of study. Controls were normal laboratory or medical personnel. Informed consent was obtained from all subjects.

From the Diabetic Department, Endocrine Unit and Immunology Laboratories, Regional Hormone Assay Laboratory, and University Departments of Clinical Chemistry and of Medicine, Royal Infirmary, Edinburgh.
Address reprint requests to R. S. Gray, University of Colorado Health Sciences Center, 4200 East Ninth Avenue B151, Denver, Colorado 80262.
Received for publication 11 July 1979 and in revised form 10 December 1979.

TABLE 1
Clinical and metabolic characteristics of NIDDM studied

Subjects	Sex	Treatment*	Age (yr)	% Ideal body weight (at time of study)	Duration of symptoms (mo)	Interval between diagnosis and study (yr)	% Ideal body weight (at time of diagnosis)	Mean plasma glucose† (mmol/L)	Plasma glucose at diagnosis (mmol/L)	Follow-up‡ (yr)
ICAb positive NIDDM										
1	F	CP:Phen	63	61	2.0	15.0	62	10.5	15.4	1.8 (1.5)
2	F	CP:Met	67	94	4.0	0.6	90	15.3	17.1	2.2
3	F	Met	60	111	0.5	1.8	184	13.6	17.8	2.2 (1.1)
4	M	Glib:Met	49	112	12.0	8.3	109	10.9	17.5	2.2
5	M	CP	49	90	2.0	2.0	106	13.5	17.8	2.2 (0.4)
6	M	Glip	39	100	0.8	1.5	113	5.2	15.6	2.2 (0.3)
7	F	CP:Met	59	72	1.0	0.5	83	16.5	14.1	2.2 (0.3)
8	F	CP:Phen	60	105	1.8	1.1	99	9.7	22.8	1.8 (0.8)
9	F	CP	47	92	0.8	1.0	100	11.6	13.5	1.8
10	F	CP	76	81	3.0	0.5	88	9.5	18.0	1.7
11	M	—	21	113	0.0	1.3	126	11.7	7.5	1.0
12	F	CP	50	72	0.5	1.6	76	9.5	15.0	0.7 (0.1)
13	F	CP	59	101	3.0	0.6	93	13.8	9.8	0.7
14	M	CP	56	104	2.0	0.2	102	9.4	20.5	0.7
	Median and Range		57.5 (21–76)	97.0 (61–113)	1.9 (0–12)	1.2 (0.2–15.0)	99.5 (62–184)	11.2 (5.2–16.5)	16.4 (7.5–22.8)	2.0 (0.7–2.2)
ICAb negative NIDDM										
1	F	CP:Met	68	105	3.0	13.5	112	12.6	15.3	2.0
2	F	CP	70	103	6.0	0.8	100	12.9	18.6	2.2
3	F	CP	59	86	2.0	2.0	81	10.5	15.8	2.3 (0.8)
4	M	Glib:Met	50	85	12.0	8.2	96	9.8	20.8	2.2 (0.5)
5	M	CP:Met	45	94	0.0	2.5	96	10.6	18.3	2.2
6	M	CP:Phen	52	88	12.0	3.0	96	10.5	17.2	1.8 (1.0)
7	F	CP:Met	59	72	5.0	0.5	83	13.9	21.5	2.2
8	F	CP:Phen	60	105	4.0	0.5	99	9.7	17.0	2.2
9	F	CP:Met	57	118	10.0	1.5	117	13.1	22.0	1.8
10	F	Glip	77	100	9.0	0.5	100	11.4	13.3	1.5
11	M	—	38	120	1.3	1.8	126	5.9	14.8	0.7
12	F	CP	50	72	0.8	0.5	80	8.6	16.2	0.6
13	F	CP	59	100	2.5	0.6	103	9.2	26.0	0.7
14	M	CP	48	97	1.5	0.1	97	9.2	13.8	0.7
	Median and Range		58.0 (38–77)	98.5 (72–120)	3.5 (0–12)	1.2 (0.1–13.5)	98.5 (80–126)	10.5 (5.9–13.9)	17.1 (13.3–26.0)	1.9 (0.6–2.3)

* All NIDDM were taking a carbohydrate-restricted, weight-maintaining diet in addition.
† Mean plasma glucose of six consecutive outpatient attendances prior to study.
‡ Interval between time of study and subsequent requirement for insulin therapy in parentheses.
CP = chlorpropamide, Phen = phenformin, Met = metformin, Glib = glibenclamide, Glip = glipizide.

Each subject was studied after an overnight fast (12 h) having omitted taking all medications on the morning of the study. All subjects had been advised to take at least 200 g carbohydrate daily for the 3 days before the study. A basal venous blood sample was collected, after which each subject ingested 50 g glucose in 200 ml water over 2 min. Further blood samples were collected at 30, 60, 90, 120, and 150 min after glucose ingestion. Blood for glucose estimation was transferred immediately to fluoride oxalate-containing tubes and glucose was estimated by a standard glucose oxidase method.[5] Plasma for insulin assay was separated and stored at −20°C and insulin was measured by a specific radioimmunoassay with a double antibody separation step. ICAb was detected by indirect immunofluorescence as previously described.[6]

Statistical significance was assessed by means of the Wilcoxon test for paired differences, unless otherwise stated.

RESULTS

Table 2 shows that, by comparison with controls, both ICAb positive and negative NIDDM have marked carbohydrate intolerance, but ICAb positive NIDDM exhibit significantly higher plasma glucose levels than do ICAb negative NIDDM throughout the study. ICAb positive NIDDM have significantly lower insulin levels than do ICAb negative NIDDM at 0, 30, 60, 90, and 120 min and a lower insulinogenic index (insulin/glucose ratio) than do ICAb negative NIDDM throughout the study.

Table 3 shows ranked integrated insulin (ΔI), glucose (ΔG), and ΔI/ΔG responses of individual NIDDM in relation to ICAb status. The ICAb positive NIDDM have higher ΔG and lower ΔI/ΔG responses ($P < 0.05$, both cases) than do ICAb negative NIDDM when analyzed by the Wilcoxon rank sum test. Table 4 shows median and range ΔI, ΔG, and ΔI/ΔG responses of ICAb positive and negative NIDDM and controls. ICAb positive NIDDM had higher ΔG and lower ΔI and ΔI/ΔG responses ($P < 0.01$, < 0.05, and < 0.01, respectively) than did ICAb negative NIDDM.

Since the OGTTs were carried out, seven ICAb positive and three ICAb negative subjects have required insulin treatment because of weight loss, unacceptably high random plasma glucose levels, uncontrolled diabetic symptoms, and ±ketonuria. The decision to introduce insulin

TABLE 3
Ranked integrated 0–2 h insulin (ΔI), glucose (ΔG), and ΔI/ΔG responses to 50-g OGTT in NIDDM according to ICAb status

Rank	ΔI	ICAb	Rank	ΔG	ICAb	Rank	ΔI/ΔG	ICAb
1	488.0	−	1	259.3	+	1	5.18	−
2	419.8	−	2	207.6	+	2	4.64	−
3	369.6	+	3	198.5	+	3	4.25	−
4	295.0	−	4	190.0	−	4	3.86	−
5	272.5	−	5	184.5	+	5	3.69	−
6	241.6	−	6	179.5	+	6	3.32	+
7	156.6	+	7	176.0	+	7	1.64	+
8	139.8	−	8	168.9	−	8	1.01	−
9	131.9	+	9	168.8	+	9	0.92	−
10	121.0	−	10	167.8	−	10	0.91	−
11	115.7	−	11	164.5	+	11	0.89	+
12	77.8	+	12	153.2	−	12	0.57	+
13	56.2	+	13	151.4	+	13	0.56	−
14	55.8	−	14	137.2	+	14	0.37	+
15	55.7	+	15	131.9	−	15	0.36	+
16	55.2	−	16	128.8	−	16	0.33	−
17	46.2	+	17	126.4	−	17	0.31	+
18	45.4	−	18	125.7	+	18	0.27	−
19	44.9	+	19	122.2	−	19	0.25	+
20	42.5	+	20	114.6	−	20	0.24	−
21	41.4	+	21	111.2	+	21	0.22	+
22	36.9	−	22	108.6	+	22	0.22	−
23	35.0	−	23	98.8	−	23	0.22	−
24	33.9	+	24	81.0	−	24	0.19	+
25	27.2	+	25	80.6	+	25	0.16	+
26	26.7	−	26	69.5	−	26	0.14	+
27	16.0	+	27	65.5	−	27	0.13	+
28	13.8	+	28	58.7	−	28	0.10	+

TABLE 2
Plasma glucose, insulin, and insulin/glucose levels during 50-g OGTT in ICAb positive and negative NIDDM and in controls

		0′	30′	60′	90′	120′	150′
Glucose (mmol/L)	ICAb positive NIDDM	15.3 (5.0–24.0)	18.7 (9.2–29.0)	21.3 (11.7–34.0)	21.1 (11.9–36.4)	20.0 (10.0–36.5)	20.0 (7.5–35.0)
	ICAb negative NIDDM	9.7 (4.9–17.0)	14.2 (8.1–22.0)	17.7 (9.7–25.0)	17.0 (6.7–27.0)	16.0 (3.7–25.0)	15.5 (3.5–23.0)
	Controls	4.9 (3.1–5.6)	7.4 (4.7–11.2)	6.3 (2.8–7.2)	4.3 (2.8–5.3)	4.3 (2.3–6.4)	4.2 (3.5–5.3)
	P*	<0.02	<0.02	<0.05	<0.02	<0.01	<0.01
Insulin (mU/L)	ICAb positive NIDDM	4.6 (1.1–15.2)	5.7 (1.4–31.2)	6.5 (2.3–53.6)	6.5 (1.9–66.4)	6.4 (1.5–60.8)	6.6 (1.8–52.0)
	ICAb negative NIDDM	6.6 (2.7–14.4)	16.7 (3.2–73.6)	12.8 (3.5–59.2)	12.6 (3.5–96.0)	12.0 (3.6–60.8)	6.7 (3.5–25.6)
	Controls	4.2 (2.6–11.4)	34.0 (17.9–116.0)	32.0 (24.5–52.8)	14.5 (6.2–28.8)	7.2 (2.8–37.6)	4.5 (2.4–9.7)
	P*	<0.05	<0.02	<0.02	<0.01	<0.02	NS
Insulin/ glucose	ICAb positive NIDDM	0.29 (0.09–1.05)	0.28 (0.09–2.50)	0.30 (0.11–3.48)	0.26 (0.10–4.44)	0.28 (0.10–4.14)	0.31 (0.08–4.19)
	ICAb negative NIDDM	0.76 (0.27–2.69)	1.06 (0.17–5.18)	0.74 (0.19–5.76)	0.76 (0.19–8.60)	0.73 (0.22–6.67)	0.55 (0.16–4.0)
	Controls	0.83 (0.60–2.28)	4.73 (1.76–15.47)	5.31 (4.0–10.7)	3.11 (1.55–6.9)	1.68 (1.06–6.67)	1.08 (0.66–2.06)
	P*	<0.01	<0.02	<0.01	<0.01	<0.01	<0.01

* ICAb positive versus ICAb negative NIDDM. Results are expressed as median and range.

TABLE 4
Integrated 0–2-h insulin (ΔI), glucose (ΔG), and ΔI/ΔG responses to 50-g OGTT in ICAb positive and negative NIDDM and in controls

	ΔI	ΔG	ΔI/ΔG
ICAb positive NIDDM	45.6 (27.2–369.6)	170.3 (80.6–259.3)	0.275 (0.097–3.324)
P*	<0.01	<0.05	<0.01
ICAb negative NIDDM	118.4 (26.7–488.0)	124.3 (58.7–190.0)	0.915 (0.218–5.183)
Controls	201.8 (135.8–419.8)	44.9 (27.8–53.2)	4.32 (2.55–10.16)

* ICAb positive versus ICAb negative NIDDM. Results expressed as median and range.

treatment was made without prior knowledge of the patients' ICAb status.

DISCUSSION

The heterogeneity of insulin responses to an oral glucose load has been described in the context of potential abnormality of glucose tolerance[7] and impaired glucose tolerance.[8,9] Some workers claim that early chemical diabetes is accompanied by hyperinsulinemia and that subnormal insulin responses are found with increasing severity of diabetes.[8,10,11] High insulin responders rarely exhibit deteriorating carbohydrate tolerance[9,12] and the heterogeneity of the insulin response has been shown to correlate with variable peripheral insulin resistance.[13] In contrast, little is known about the insulin responses of subjects known to suffer from overt diabetes treated with oral hypoglycemic therapy.

Our findings illustrate that, in this last-mentioned group, there is also a marked heterogeneity of the insulin response to an oral glucose load. ICAb positive NIDDM have significantly lower insulin levels in response to the OGTT by comparison with ICAb negative NIDDM, and this is even more evident when the prevailing plasma glucose level is taken into account and the insulin response expressed as the insulinogenic index. Similarly, ICAb negative NIDDM have greater integrated insulin responses and greater ΔI/ΔG values than ICAb positive NIDDM. It is clear that insulinopenia, rather than peripheral insulin resistance, is responsible for the carbohydrate intolerance exhibited by ICAb positive NIDDM, and to this extent ICAb positive NIDDM and IDDM share a common underlying metabolic abnormality. Despite our attempts to match the two groups of NIDDM, the ICAb positive NIDDM clearly suffer from a greater degree of carbohydrate intolerance than do ICAb negative NIDDM. It is possible that high carbohydrate intake, for 3 days before the study, was responsible for the marked disparity in the degree of carbohydrate intolerance found in the two groups of NIDDM. This difference was not evident in terms of the random plasma glucose recorded at six outpatient attendances before this study, nor at the time of the patients' original presentation with diabetes. ICAb positive NIDDM thus suffer from severe carbohydrate intolerance as a consequence of profound insulin deficiency, which may result from autoimmune destruction of the pancreatic B-cell population.

Previous studies have failed to demonstrate a significant difference in the metabolic disorder found in ICAb positive and negative subjects, whether severely or mildly diabetic. Comparisons of ICAb positive and negative IDDM[4,15] and overt NIDDM[4] have shown similar glucagon responses to an intravenous infusion of arginine. The majority of IDDM, whether persistently ICAb positive (i.e., more than 4 yr from diagnosis of diabetes) or not, have no detectable C-peptide.[16–18] Interpretation of a comparison of insulin responses to an intravenous infusion of arginine in ICAb positive and negative overt NIDDM[4] is complicated by the small number of patients studied, the inadequate matching of the two groups of NIDDM, and the relatively weak stimulus of B-cell function employed. Tiengo et al. have also reported[4] that ICAb positive and negative subjects with impaired glucose tolerance do not differ in terms of plasma glucose and insulin response to a 100-g OGTT, but again only a small number of subjects was studied.

The earliest metabolic abnormality in the development of Type I diabetes has yet to be clearly defined. It remains to be seen whether it is also characterized by primary insulin deficiency, or whether peripheral insulin resistance initially leading to hyperinsulinemia and subsequent beta-cell exhaustion is found in this condition. In this context, the report of a flat glycemic response to an oral glucose load, accompanying a normal insulin response, in ICAb positive nondiabetics[4] would appear to imply a state of peripheral insulin sensitivity rather than resistance.

Our findings confirm the value of ICAb as a predictor of failure of oral hypoglycemic therapy as suggested by our previous studies.[1,2] The shorter duration of diabetic symptoms exhibited by ICAb positive NIDDM before diagnosis may also indicate a more rapid progression of the underlying disease process. Such evidence supports the view that ICAb positive NIDDM should be classified together with IDDM[1,2] and should be distinguished from the more common ICAb negative NIDDM in terms of prognosis and underlying metabolic disturbance.

The presence of ICAb in an NIDDM who is apparently satisfactorily controlled on the basis of random plasma glucose concentrations should alert the clinician to the considerable risk of subsequent deterioration of diabetic control. It could even be argued that ICAb positive overt diabetics should be treated with insulin from the outset, thereby avoiding the possible hazards of oral hypoglycemic therapy[19] and minimizing the risk of the development of ketoacidosis under stress. Insulin deficiency, of the degree shown by the ICAb positive NIDDM, may have other deleterious consequences including the development of microangiopathy[12] and increased lipolysis. Furthermore, the identification of an ICAb positive NIDDM may provide an opportunity for the treatment of the underlying disease process—rather than treating the metabolic consequences of that process—thereby possibly delaying or obviating the need for insulin therapy.[20]

ACKNOWLEDGMENT

The authors wish to acknowledge Dr. Robert Elton, Medical Statistics and Computing Department, University of Edinburgh, for his assistance with statistical analyses.

REFERENCES

1 Irvine, W. J., McCallum, C. J., Gray, R. S., and Duncan, L. J. P.: Clinical and pathogenic significance of pancreatic islet-cell antibodies in diabetics treated with oral hypoglycaemic agents. Lancet *1*:1025–27, 1977.

2 Irvine, W. J., Sawers, J. S. A., Feek, C. M., Prescott, R. J., and Duncan,

L. J. P.: The value of islet-cell antibody in predicting secondary failure of oral hypoglycaemic agent therapy in diabetes mellitus. J. Clin. Lab. Immunol. *2*:23–26, 1979.

[3] National Diabetes Data Group: Classification and diagnosis of diabetes mellitus and other categories of glucose intolerance. Diabetes *28*:1039–57, 1979.

[4] Tiengo, A., Del Prete, G. F., Nosadini, R., Betterle, C., Garotti, C., and Bersani, G.: Insulin and glucagon secretion in diabetic and non-diabetic patients with circulating islet-cell antibodies. Diabetologia *13*:451–58, 1977.

[5] Morley, G., Dawson, A., and Marks, J.: Manual and autoanalyser methods for measuring blood glucose using Guiacum and Glucose Oxidase. Proc. Assoc. Clin. Biochem. *5*:42–45, 1968.

[6] Irvine, W. J., McCallum, C. J., Gray, R. S., Campbell, C. J., Duncan, L. J. P., Farquhar, J. W., Vaughan, H., and Morris, P. J.: Pancreatic islet-cell antibodies in diabetes mellitus correlated with duration and type of diabetes, coexistent autoimmune disease, and HLA type. Diabetes *26*:138–47, 1977.

[7] Johansen, K., Soeldner, J. S., and Gleason, R. E.: Insulin, growth hormone, and glucagon in prediabetes mellitus: a review. Metabolism *23*:1185–99, 1974.

[8] Reaven, G., and Miller, R.: Study of the relationship between glucose and insulin responses to an oral glucose load in man. Diabetes *17*:560–69, 1968.

[9] Fajans, S. S., Floyd, J. C., Tattersall, R. B., Williamson, J. R., Pek, S., and Taylor, C. I.: The various faces of diabetes in the young. Arch. Intern. Med. *136*:194–202, 1976.

[10] Chiles, R., and Tzagournis, M.: Excessive serum insulin responses to oral glucose in obesity and mild diabetes. Diabetes *19*:458–64, 1970.

[11] Jackson, W. P. U., van Mieghem, W., and Keller, P.: Insulin excess as the initial lesion in diabetes. Lancet *1*:1040–44, 1972.

[12] Kosaka, K., Hagura, R., and Kuzuya, T.: Insulin responses in equivocal and definite diabetes, with special reference to subjects who had mild glucose intolerance but later developed definite diabetes. Diabetes *26*:944–52, 1977.

[13] Reaven, G. M., and Olefsky, J. M.: Relationship between heterogeneity of insulin responses and insulin resistance in normal subjects and patients with chemical diabetes. Diabetologia *13*:201–06, 1977.

[14] Clarke, B. F., and Campbell, I. W.: Long-term comparative trial of glibenclamide and chlorpropamide in diet-failed, maturity-onset diabetics. Lancet *1*:246–48, 1975.

[15] Gray, R. S., Irvine, W. J., Buchanan, K. D., and Duncan, L. J. P.: Glucagon response to arginine infusion in insulin dependent diabetics with and without the islet-cell antibody in the serum. J. Clin. Lab. Immunol. *1*:115–18, 1978.

[16] Theophanides, C. G., Pyke, D. A., and Watkins, P. J.: Islet function in diabetics with persistent islet-cell antibodies. Diabetes *27* (Suppl. 1):265–66, 1978.

[17] Irvine, W. J., Rubenstein, A. M., Toft, A. D., and Feek, C. M.: C-peptide secretion correlated with islet-cell antibody status in diabetes. J. Clin. Lab. Immunol. *2*:1979. In press.

[18] Hendriksen, C., Faber, O. K., Drejer, J., and Binder, C.: Prevalence of residual B-cell function in insulin-treated diabetics evaluated by the plasma C-peptide response to intravenous glucagon. Diabetologia *13*:615–19, 1977.

[19] University Group Diabetes Programme: A study of the effects of hypoglycemic agents on vascular complications in patients with adult-onset diabetes. Diabetes *19* (Suppl. 2):747–830, 1970.

[20] Irvine, W. J., Leslie, R. D. G., Jansen, F. K., Rossini, A., and Nerup, J.: The possibility of prevention of Type 1 diabetes. *In* The Immunology of Diabetes. Irvine, W. J., Ed. Edinburgh, Teviot Scientific Publications, 1979. In press.

Complement-mediated Cytotoxic Effects on Pancreatic Islets With Sera from Diabetic Patients

HARRY G. RITTENHOUSE, DALE L. OXENDER, SUMER PEK, AND DIANE AR

SUMMARY

Sera from 11/30 patients with juvenile-onset-type diabetes (JOD) had cytotoxic effects on isolated pancreatic islets from hamsters when guinea pig complement was present. The cytotoxic activity could be readily eliminated by heating the guinea pig complement at 56°C for 30 min, thus demonstrating a complement-dependent process. Complement-dependent cytotoxicity toward pancreatic islets was not observed with sera from 11 patients with maturity-onset-type diabetes, 4 nondiabetic hospital patient controls, and 28 healthy adult subjects. The presence of circulating complement-mediated cytotoxic factor(s) toward isolated islets indicates the potential importance of autoimmune pathogenic damage to pancreatic islets in some patients with diabetes. DIABETES *29*:317–322, April 1980.

The demonstration of autoantibodies specific for pancreatic islets in sera of diabetic patients has led to increased interest in possible autoimmune participation in diabetes mellitus. Immunofluorescence studies in several laboratories have provided evidence for the presence of specific islet cell autoantibodies (ICA) in the sera of more than 70% of newly diagnosed juvenile-onset-type diabetic (JOD) patients.[1–3] In contrast, fewer than 1% of normal subjects were found to have these circulating ICA.[4–6] The persistence of ICA is significantly greater in JOD patients with organ-specific polyendocrine autoimmune disease than in JOD patients with no other autoimmune abnormalities. Circulating ICA are uncommon in maturity-onset-type diabetes (MOD); when present, they may indicate future development of insulin-dependent diabetes.[5,7]

From the Mental Health Research Institute, Department of Biological Chemistry, and Department of Internal Medicine (Division of Endocrinology and Metabolism and the Metabolism Research Unit), University of Michigan, Ann Arbor, MI 48109.

Address reprint requests to Dale L. Oxender, 5319 Medical Science I, Ann Arbor, MI 48109.

Received for publication 16 July and in revised form 26 November 1979.

Using immunofluorescent techniques, ICA appear to be directed against cytoplasmic components of pancreatic islet cells from persons with blood type O, since a diffuse fluorescence throughout the islet cells is observed in histologic tissue sections. Circulating ICA, which are directed against surface components of islet cells, have also been detected by immunofluorescence using viable islet cells as substrate, including human insulinoma cells[8] and mouse or rat islet cell suspensions.[9] The latter study demonstrates that some JOD patients possess circulating cell-surface ICA that are not species-specific, which thus allows the convenient use of them as substrate of pancreatic islet preparations from animals.

The nature of the islet cell antigen(s) to which ICA are directed is not known at the present time, although the above studies suggest the presence of both cytoplasmic and cell-surface antigen(s).

The presence of organ-specific cell-surface autoantibodies in diabetic patients raises the question of what their role in immunopathogenic activity is toward pancreatic islets. In this report we summarize the results of our preliminary investigations on possible cross-species cytotoxic effects of sera from diabetic patients toward intact hamster islets.

MATERIALS AND METHODS

Pancreatic islets were prepared from male Syrian golden hamsters, aged 80 days to 120 days, by a modified method of Ballinger and Lacy.[10] Hamsters were killed by cervical dislocation. The pancreas was quickly excised, trimmed of fat, placed in 8 ml Hank's buffer (pH 7.4 at 4°C) in a small siliconized beaker, and thoroughly minced to 1–1.5 mm^3 with dissecting scissors. The minced tissue was transferred to a capped siliconized culture tube (16 × 125 mm) and was diluted with cold Hank's buffer. After one minute of sedimentation at gravity at 4°C, the supernatant portion was discarded, sedimentation was repeated, and collagenase [(Worthington type IV), 1000 U per pancreas, suspended in 1 ml] was added to the tube. The digestion mixture was shaken vigorously at 37°C for 7 to 9 min, then diluted with cold Hank's buffer to 10 ml, shaken vigorously, and centrifuged at 200 *g*, at 4°C, for one minute; the supernatant portion was discarded. The washing was repeated once. The tissue sediment was resuspended in 4 ml of 300 g per liter Ficoll 400 [(Sigma) dialyzed and lyophilized] in Hank's buffer to give a final concentration of 25% Ficoll. The suspension was transferred to a separate siliconized culture tube, and 2-ml portions of 23%, 20.5%, and 11% Ficoll were layered on top of it. The mixture was then centrifuged in a swinging bucket rotor at 250 *g*, at 4°C, for 12 min. Intact islets, essentially free of other tissue, were located at the 11% to 20.5% interface. The intact islets were removed with a siliconized capillary pipette and were washed twice with Hank's buffer at 4°C. Under a dissecting microscope, the islets were selected to be of uniform shape and size using a siliconized capillary pipette: approximately 200 usable islets per hamster were obtained.

Serum samples were taken from patients with juvenile-onset-type diabetes (JOD, insulin-dependent diabetes mellitus) and maturity-onset-type diabetes (MOD, not-insulin-dependent diabetes mellitus), ranging in age from 18 mo to 55 yr, with the duration of disease from one month to five years. Sera obtained from nondiabetic hospital patients and healthy adult subjects were used as controls. All sera were stored at −20°C until used.

The cytotoxicity assay was performed in duplicate for each serum sample. Each experiment included at least one known noncytotoxic human serum sample, as well as a serum sample obtained from a rabbit immunized against an homogenate of an hamster islet cell tumor. This rabbit antiserum directed against hamster islets had a complement-mediated cytotoxic effect on hamster islet cells, thus providing a positive control serum for these studies. Before use in the assay, serum samples were heat-inactivated at 56°C for 30 min and incubated with 4 μg of bovine insulin (Sigma) per 100 μl to saturate all binding sites on any endogenous insulin antibodies. Since the concentration of bound antibodies on the cell surface may be a critical variable in complement-mediated damage to cells,[11] a small number of islets per assay was employed routinely. Ten to twelve intact islets were suspended in 25 μl of Ham's medium containing 13% heat-inactivated fetal calf serum in 6-mm-diameter microtiter plates (Cook Engineering Co.) and incubated at 4°C for two days. Fetal calf serum was heat-inactivated, since, otherwise, islets incubated in the presence of untreated calf serum were occasionally damaged morphologically, and significant amounts of trypan blue entered the cells. The islets were incubated at 37°C in humidified 5% CO_2 in air for 2 h.

In a typical experiment, 50 μl of human serum was added to a well containing 10 to 12 pancreatic islets and the mixture was incubated at 37°C. After one hour, 20 μl of fresh guinea pig complement was added every hour to make a total of 100 μl by the end of 5 h. The mixture was then incubated for an additional 17 h at 37°C. One more aliquot of guinea pig complement was added and the mixture was incubated for two additional hours. When the incubation ended, the islet mixture was exposed to 0.4% trypan blue at 22°C for 4 min. The mixture was then placed as a wet mount on a microscope slide and was observed with a phase-contrast microscope within two minutes. The extent of damage to islets was evaluated both functionally, by assessing the cellular uptake of the vital dye trypan blue, and morphologically, by identifying the extent of disruption of the structure of the islets. Since each islet is composed of over 100 cells in a highly ordered structure, morphologic damage to the islets could be readily evaluated by phase-contrast microscopy. Photography was performed within five minutes from the time of addition of trypan blue.

Positive cytotoxicity in this assay was defined as the uptake of trypan blue by more than 90% of the outer cells of the islets (extending from the periphery of the islet to ⅓ the radius toward the center) plus morphologic damage to the normally compact, dense structure of the islet.

Serum samples included in the cytotoxicity assay were analyzed for cytoplasmic ICA using cryostat and/or fixed sections of fresh human O-type cadaveric pancreas. Serum-treated sections were stained indirectly with fluorescein isothiocyanate-conjugated goat anti-human immunoglobulin G, and immunofluorescence was determined by fluorescence microscopy.

RESULTS

Hamster islets, incubated in growth medium in the presence of guinea pig complement, remained morphologically identical to freshly prepared untreated islets (Figure 1A). Intact islets often appeared dark after photography because of their dense central core (Figure 1A-D). Nevertheless, cells that were stained with trypan blue could easily be distinguished from unstained cells using a phase-contrast miscrope. Figure 1B shows a photomicrograph of an islet incubated with a serum sample from a patient with maturity-onset-type diabetes. This serum caused no observable morphologic damage. The trypan blue–stained cells in this sample, as well as in other samples assessed as negative, were fewer than 5% of the total cell population. Also, control experiments, in which sera from two JOD patients were incubated in the absence of guinea pig complement, exhibited no cytotoxic or disruptive effects on islets (Figure 1C and D). In marked contrast, sera from the same two JOD patients dramatically affected the morphology of and trypan blue uptake by islet cells in the presence of guinea pig complement (Figure 1E and F). More than 90% of the cells of the islets were stained by trypan blue after treatment with these JOD serum samples. On the other hand, with normal human serum or with JOD serum in the absence of complement, fewer than 5% of cells were stained with trypan blue. The damage to islet morphology that occurred after incubation with JOD sera plus complement was dramatic: Many islets were severely fragmented, and some islets appeared to be undergoing dissolution. Control experiments revealed that islets always remained intact in the presence of guinea pig complement alone.

The cytotoxicity assay was applied to serum samples obtained from 30 patients with JOD, 11 patients with MOD, 4 nondiabetic control hospital patients, and 28 healthy adult subjects (Table 1). Complement-dependent cytotoxicity toward hamster islets was detected in 37% of samples from JOD patients. None of the serum samples from MOD patients induced cytolysis. One heat-inactivated serum sample from a JOD patient and one sample from a healthy subject were cytotoxic, regardless of whether fresh exogenous complement had been added or not. The nature of this complement-independent cytotoxic phenomenon is not apparent; the JOD patient has not been included among the 11 patients with complement-dependent cytotoxicity.

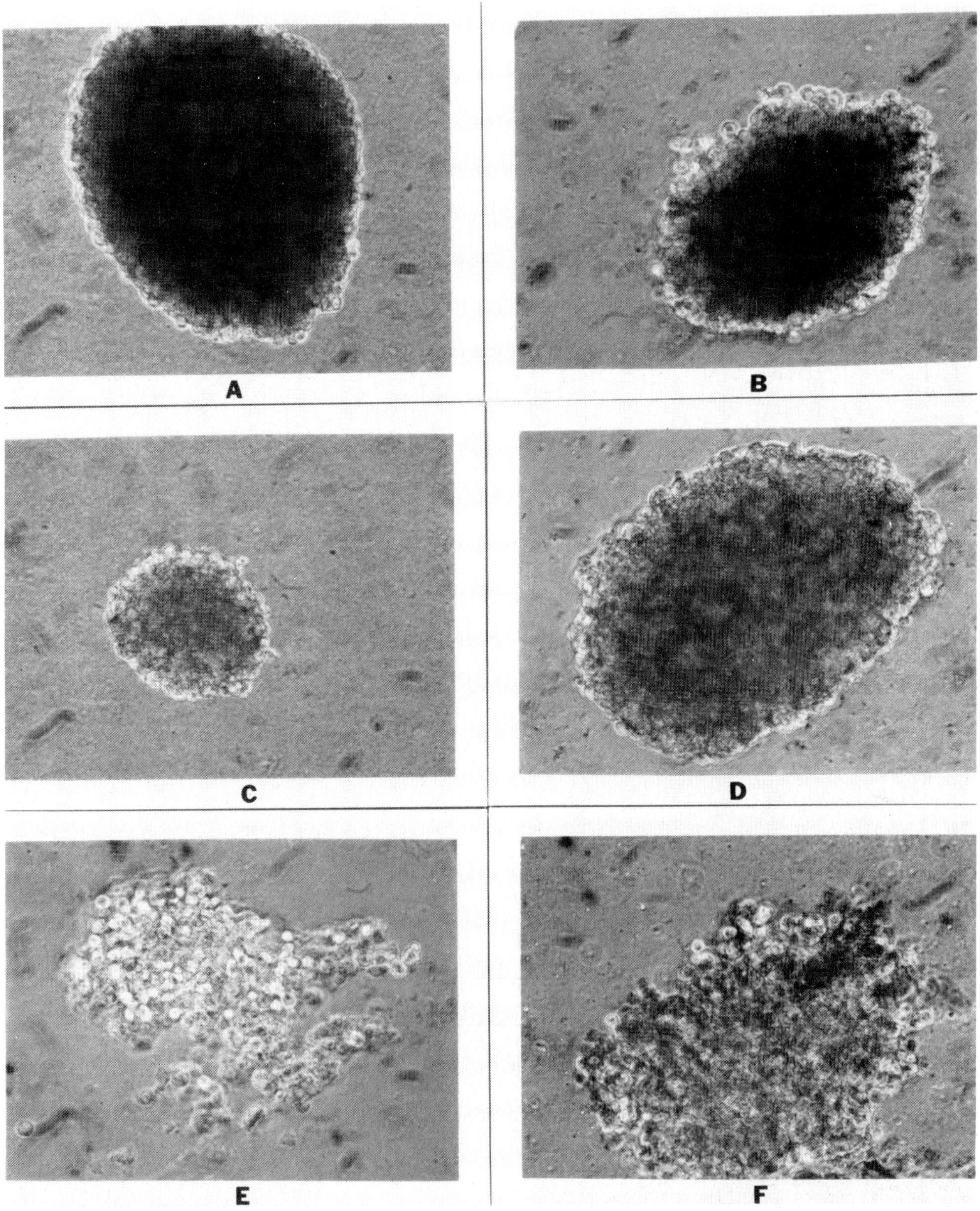

FIGURE 1. Cytotoxicity assay with hamster islets. A. culture medium and fresh guinea pig C′; B. culture medium, serum from a maturity-onset-type diabetic patient, and fresh guinea pig C′; C. culture medium, serum from a juvenile diabetic (RB), and heat-inactivated guinea pig C′; D. culture medium, serum from a juvenile-diabetic patient (RW), and heat-inactivated guinea pig C′; E. same as in C, except that fresh guinea pig C′ was added; F. same as in D, except that fresh guinea pig C′ was added.

TABLE 1
Results of complement-mediated cytolysis tests on isolated islets of hamster. All sera showing cytotoxicity represent a minimum of three separate experiments

Groups	Complement-dependent cytotoxicity	Complement-independent cytotoxicity
Juvenile-onset-type diabetes*	11/30	1/30
Maturity-onset-type diabetes	0/11	0/11
Nondiabetic Control Hospital Patients		
Juvenile short stature	0/2	0/2
Addison's disease	0/1	0/1
Crohn's disease	0/1	0/1
Healthy adult subjects	0/28	1/28

* Duration of disease, 1 mo to 20 yr.

Immunoglobulins from serum of a JOD patient (ND), previously shown to be positive in the cytotoxicity assay, were precipitated using 50% ammonium sulfate. The precipitate was dissolved in Hank's buffer to the original volume and was dialyzed against the same buffer at 4°C for 48 h; the buffer was changed several times. The gamma globulin fraction induced complement-dependent cytotoxicity to a degree similar to that seen with the unfractionated serum, while the supernatant fraction did not.

To assess whether the cytotoxic factor(s) was macromolecular, complement-mediated cytotoxic sera from three JOD patients (ND, SS, JG) were dialyzed against Hank's buffer. Dialysis did not eliminate the cytotoxic effect of these sera.

Twenty-three of the thirty JOD serum samples used in this study were evaluated for the presence of islet cell antibodies by the immunofluorescent technique (Table 2). Six of the seven serum samples from JOD patients that exhibited complement-dependent cytotoxicity were found to contain cytoplasmic islet cell antibodies. The noncytotoxic sample with positive immunofluorescence was from a patient with JOD and Addison's disease. The single JOD serum (CH) that exhibited a complement-independent cytotoxicity was also found to contain cytoplasmic ICA by immunofluorescent techniques. ICA was not detectable in any of the serum samples from 10 healthy adult subjects or 2 nondiabetic control patients.

Eleven of the thirty serum samples from JOD patients were screened for the presence of endogenous insulin antibodies. The samples were incubated for 3 days at 4°C in the presence of tracer amounts of radioiodinated insulin; the globulins were then precipitated with polyethylene glycol. Radioactivity in the precipitate, in amounts substantially greater than those seen in control sera, was detected in seven JOD samples, suggesting the presence of circulating

TABLE 2
Comparative evaluation of sera from diabetic patients and normal subjects using complement-dependent cytotoxicity of hamster pancreatic islets and immunofluorescence of thin sections of human type-O pancreas

	Patient code	Age (yr)	Sex	Time since diagnosis (yr)	Complement-dependent cytotoxicity	Complement-independent cytotoxicity	Immunofluorescence on thin sections
Juvenile-onset-type diabetes	NF	18	F	2	+	−	+
	RW	13	F	0.1	+	−	+
	RB	20	F	1.3	+	−	+
	BK	15	M	2	+	−	+
	RY	2.5	F	1	+	−	+
	SS	17	F	9	+	−	+
	JG	10	F	0.1	+	−	−
	PS	16	F	13	−	−	+
	CS	15	F	6	−	−	+
	VB	13	F	5.5	−	−	+
	DF	20	F	0.1	−	−	+
	EP	8	F	0.5	−	−	+
	KK	16	M	14	−	−	+
	DA	6	F	4	−	−	+
	VC	11	F		−	−	+
	ED	9	M	0.1	−	−	−
	AMM	12	M	0.1	−	−	−
	SD	10	M	0.1	−	−	−
	DC	13	F	9	−	−	−
	CH					+	+
Juvenile-onset-type diabetes with Addison's disease	LH	55	F	10	+	−	−
	LB	75	F	17	−	−	+
	DP	27	F	20	−	−	+
Addison's disease	MW				−	−	−
Crohn's disease	MT				−	−	−
Healthy adult subjects	DA				−	−	−
	PG				−	−	−
	AP				−	−	−
	BP				−	−	−
	CV				−	−	−
	FC				−	−	−
	JR				−	−	−
	JM					+	−

insulin antibodies. No correlation was found between the presence of insulin antibodies and the cytotoxic factor(s). Three of the four cytotoxic serum samples had insulin antibodies. On the other hand, insulin antibodies were also present in four of the seven samples without cytotoxicity.

DISCUSSION

The results of our study provide evidence that the serum from some juvenile-onset-type diabetic patients has a cytotoxic effect on isolated hamster pancreatic islets in vitro. The cytotoxic effect of the positive diabetic sera was evident by marked morphologic damage to the islets and by actual cytolysis of a majority of the cells located at the periphery of the islet. Although the biochemical nature of the cytotoxic factor has not yet been identified, it is apparently a complement-mediated process, since elimination of complement from the system prevents the cytotoxic effects.

The susceptibility of a high percentage of islet cells to cytolysis by diabetic serum, as observed with this assay and shown in Figure 1E and F, would indicate that multiple islet cell types are serving as targets for the cytotoxic factor. This would seem to argue against a similar pathogenic reaction occurring in vivo, since histologic studies of the pancreas in diabetic patients reveal that only the beta cells are extensively damaged.[12,13] An alternative explanation is that a cytotoxic factor, present in diabetic serum, selectively attacks beta cells and is followed by the release of intracellular components. Under the restricted confines of the microwell cytotoxicity assay used in this study, the liberated intracellular components from damaged beta cells may create a toxic environment for other islet cell types and result in further cytolysis.

Reproducible demonstration of complement-mediated cytotoxic effects of diabetic sera toward isolated hamster islets required careful observance of the assay conditions described above. In particular, the susceptibility of intact islets to the cytotoxic effects of JOD sera depended on the duration of incubation of the sera with islets and complement, the preincubation of islets in the growth medium, and on the proportion of the test serum to the number of islets in the assay mixture. For example, when experiments were performed with islets incubated in JOD serum for less than 3 h, if the islets were not incubated in growth medium before the assay or if more than 50 islets per 50 μl of test serum were used for the assay, complement-mediated cytotoxicity was only sporadically observed for any of the eleven JOD sera samples assessed as positive in this study. The need for prolonged incubation of diabetic serum with intact islets may be based on the highly organized and compact multicellular structure of islets delaying the penetration and action of the cytotoxic factor(s). The integrity of islet cell surface antigens may play a role in the full expression of the cytotoxic effect of the diabetic serum. Prior incubation of the islets in growth medium may have allowed the recovery of the antigen(s), which could have been damaged by collagenase during the preparation of islets.

An important consideration in the present study is the cross-species nature of our cytotoxicity assay. If the cytotoxic factor is an immunoglobulin, it would be expected that only human sera, which contain antibodies cross-reactive with hamster islets, would have the potential to exhibit cytotoxic effects. It is likely that not all the antigenic determinants of human islets exist on hamster islets. Thus, in our hamster islet system, the cytotoxic effect of human circulating ICA may be only partially evident. In our initial experiments, fresh human complement was used in place of guinea pig complement, without observable cytotoxic effects of diabetic serum toward pancreatic islets. This may have been due to the lability of human complement or the use of hamster islets as target tissue. Although islets from small animals have the obvious advantages of being both available and easy to isolate, the use of human islets as well as human complement may ultimately be necessary to define the prevalence and characteristics of the phenomenon of cytotoxicity and what implications it has in the diabetic disease process.

We are currently investigating whether the cytotoxic factor detected in this study is a circulating antibody. There is precedence for the presence of circulating antibodies which damage specific tissues by a complement-mediated mechanism in autoimmune-associated human diseases. The immunopathogenic effect of autoantibodies toward erythrocytes in patients with autoimmune hemolytic anemia demonstrates the in vivo importance of this type of mechanism.[14] Other in vitro and in vivo systems in which the binding of circulating antibodies to target tissue cells leads to tissue damage include Hashimoto's autoimmune thyroiditis,[15–17] multiple sclerosis,[18–20] and myasthenia gravis.[21] In general, the ability of these autoantibodies to damage their target cells in vivo has been difficult to establish. Recently, Lennon et al. provided evidence for the in vivo role of complement-mediated damage to the acetylcholine receptor in an experimental autoimmune myasthenia gravis system.[22]

In order to damage cell membranes, circulating autoantibodies and complement components must be accessible to the target tissue. Structured multicellular tissues may present physical barriers to potential cytotoxic antibodies. This may explain why passive transfer of sera from donors with experimental autoimmune thyroiditis to normal individuals in the same species is not easily achieved.[23,24]

At the present time, the potential role of circulating islet cell antibodies in the pathogenesis of insulin-dependent diabetes is conjectural. Antibodies directed toward cytoplasmic islet cell antigens are not likely to initiate immune damage in pancreatic islets; rather, they may serve to opsonize previously damaged tissue for removal by macrophages.[4] Islet cell surface antibodies, detected by immunofluorescence with viable islet cells,[9] are more likely candidates in immunopathogenic mechanisms.[25] Regardless of the origin of islet cell antibodies or their role in the etiology of diabetes, the presence of antibodies that are capable of damaging beta cells may have important harmful consequences in the survival of normal human pancreatic islets transplanted to diabetic patients.

In the present study, intact pancreatic islets, which have a highly organized multicellular structure, were found to be susceptible to a cytotoxic factor in diabetic sera. Apparently, the organized structure of the islets is not a sufficient barrier to prevent complement-mediated cell damage by diabetic serum. Future studies with perfused intact rat pancreas may allow for assessment of potential cytotoxic effects of diabetic serum at a higher level of tissue organization.

Independent immunofluorescent evaluation of the serum samples used in this study revealed a positive correlation of islet cell antibodies with the cytotoxic factor. If the complement-mediated cytotoxic factor present in diabetic patient sera is an immunoglobulin and possesses specificity toward pancreatic islets, evidence will be provided for the possible inclusion of autoimmune events in the immunopathogenesis of juvenile-onset-type diabetes in man.

ACKNOWLEDGMENT

We thank Dr. George E. Bacon of the Department of Pediatrics and Communicable Diseases for providing serum samples from juvenile diabetic patients, Dr. Michal Schwartz of the Mental Health Research Institute for helpful discussions, Dr. Dennis Martin and Ms. Barbara Torretti of the Biochemistry Core Facility of the Michigan Diabetes Research and Training Center (MDRTC) for immunofluorescence analysis of islet cell antibodies, and Ms. Sylvia Grauds of the Ligand Assay Core Facility of the MDRTC for the evaluation of insulin:anti-insulin complexes.

This study was supported, in part, by USPHS grant AM-20572 (MDRTC) from the National Institute of Arthritis, Metabolism, and Digestive Diseases as a pilot/feasibility study.

REFERENCES

[1] Lendrum, R., Walker, J. G., and Gamble, D. R.: Islet-cell antibodies in juvenile diabetes mellitus of recent onset. Lancet *I*:880–83, 1975.

[2] Bottazzo, G. F., Doniach, D., and Pouplard, A.: Humoral autoimmunity in diabetes mellitus. Acta Endocrinol. (Copenhagen) Suppl. *205*:55–62, 1976.

[3] Cudworth, A. G., Gamble, D. R., White, G. B. B., Lendrum, R., Woodrow, J. C., and Bloom, A.: Aetiology of juvenile-onset diabetes. Lancet *I*:385–88, 1977.

[4] Doniach, D., and Bottazzo, G. F.: Autoimmunity and the endocrine pancreas. Pathobiol. Annu. *7*:327–46, 1977.

[5] Irvine, W. J., McCallum, C. J., Gray, R. S., Campbell, C. J., Duncan, L. J. P., Farquhar, J. W., Vaughan, H., and Morris, J. P.: Pancreatic islet-cell antibodies in diabetes mellitus correlated with the duration and type of diabetes, coexistent autoimmune disease, and HLA type. Diabetes *26*:138–47, 1977.

[6] Lendrum, R., and Walker, G.: Serum antibodies in human pancreatic disease. Gut *16*:365–71, 1975.

[7] Irvine, W. J., McCallum, C. J., Gray, R. S., and Duncan, L. J.: Clinical and pathogenic significance of pancreatic islet-cell antibodies in diabetics treated with oral hypoglycaemic agents. Lancet *I*:1025–27, 1977.

[8] McLaren, N. K., Huang, Sh. W., and Fogh, J.: Antibody to cultured human insulinoma cells in insulin-dependent diabetes. Lancet *I*:997–99, 1975.

[9] Lernmark, A., Freedman, Z. R., Hofmann, C., Rubenstein, A. H., Steiner, D. F., Jackson, R. E., Winter, R. J., and Traisman, H. S.: Islet-cell surface antibodies in juvenile diabetes mellitus. N. Engl. J. Med. *299*:375–80, 1978.

[10] Ballinger, W. F., and Lacy, P. E.: Transplantation of intact pancreatic islets in rats. Surgery *73*:175–86, 1972.

[11] Jerne, N. K., and Nordin, A. A.: Plaque formation in agar by single antibody-producing cells. Science *140*:405, 1963.

[12] LeCompte, P. N.: Insulitis in early juvenile diabetes. Arch. Pathol. *66*:450–57, 1958.

[13] Orci, L., Baetens, D., Rufener, C., Amherdt, M., Ravazzola, M., Studer, P., Malaisse-Lagae, F., and Unger, R. H.: Hypertrophy and hyperplasia of somatostatin D-cells in diabetes. Proc. Natl. Acad. Sci. USA *73*:1338–42, 1976.

[14] Rubin, H.: Autoimmune hemolytic anemias; warm and cold antibody types. Am. J. Clin. Pathol. *68*(Suppl.5):638–42, 1977.

[15] Doniach, D., and Roitt, I. M.: Autoimmunity in Hashimoto's disease and its implications. J. Clin. Endocrinol. Metab. *17*:1293–1304, 1957.

[16] Doniach, D.: Humoral and genetic effects of thyroid autoimmunity. *In* Autoimmunity in Endocrine Disease. Irvine, W. J., Ed. Clin. Endocrinol. Metab. London, W. B. Saunders, 1957, pp. 267–85.

[17] Irvine, W. J.: Studies on the cytotoxic factor in thyroid disease. Br. Med. J. *1*:1444–49, 1962.

[18] Caspary, E. A.: Humoral factors involved in immune processes in multiple sclerosis and allergic encephalomyelitis. Br. Med. Bull. *33*:51–53, 1977.

[19] Abramsky, O., Lisak, R. P., Silberberg, D. H., and Pleasure, D.: Antibodies to oligodendroglia in patients with multiple sclerosis. N. Engl. J. Med. *297*:1207–11, 1977.

[20] Bornstein, M. B.: The immunopathogenesis of multiple sclerosis. Mt. Sinai J. Med. *41*:46–55, 1974.

[21] Toyka, K. V., Drachman, D. B., Griffin, D. E., Pestronk, A., Winkelstein, J. A., Fischbeck, K. H., Jr., and Kao, I.: Myasthenia gravis: study of humoral immune mechanisms by passive transfer to mice. N. Engl. J. Med. *296*:125–31, 1977.

[22] Lennon, V. A., Seybold, M. E., Lindstrom, J. M., Cochrane, C., and Ulevitch, R.: Role of complement in the pathogenesis of experimental autoimmune myasthenia gravis. J. Exp. Med. *147*:973–83, 1978.

[23] Vladntiu, A. O., and Rose, N. R.: Transfer of experimental autoimmune thyroiditis in mouse by serum. J. Immunol. *106*:1139–42, 1971.

[24] Rose, N. R.: Experimental autoimmune thyroiditis. *In* Textbook of Immunopathology. Miescher, P., and Muller-Eberhard, H. D., Eds. New York, Grune and Stratton, 1968, pp. 215–29.

[25] Kaldany, A.: Autoantibodies to islet cells in diabetes mellitus. Diabetes *28*:102–05, 1979.

Starvation-induced Changes of Somatostatin, Glucagon, and Insulin Secretion from the Isolated Perfused Rat Pancreas

SUSUMU SEINO, HIDEO SAKURAI, YUTAKA SEINO, KINSUKE TSUDA, KEIICHIRO TANIGAWA, HIDESHI KUZUYA, YASUO GOTO, AND HIROO IMURA

SUMMARY

The effect of 16- and 48-h fasting on pancreatic somatostatin, insulin, and glucagon secretion was studied, using the isolated perfused rat pancreas. In the presence of 4.4 mM glucose, basal somatostatin and insulin concentrations in the perfusate were significantly lower in 48-h fasted rats than in fed animals, whereas basal glucagon secretion was significantly elevated in fasted rats. The infusion of 19 mM arginine significantly augmented secretion of somatostatin and glucagon and attenuated insulin secretion in 48-h fasted rats. It is concluded that fasting causes a decrease in basal pancreatic somatostatin secretion in vitro, although the response to arginine is rather exaggerated. Insulin and glucagon secretion also changed during the fasting. These results suggest that not only insulin and glucagon, but also somatostatin contribute to nutrient homeostasis. DIABETES 29:323–325, April 1980.

Recent studies have demonstrated that pancreatic D-cells, secreting somatostatin, are located closely to the A-cells and B-cells within the pancreatic islet.[1,2] Orci and Unger[3] suggested the role of pancreatic somatostatin as a "paracrine" substance, acting locally on neighboring cells to regulate hormone secretion. On the other hand, several investigators have postulated that somatostatin plays an important role in the regulation of nutrient homeostasis,[3–7] by affecting gastrointestinal function and nutrient absorption. In this respect, somatostatin secretion under various nutritional conditions is of great interest. Starvation is known to cause changes in insulin and glucagon secretion.[8–12] The present study was designed to investigate the effect of fasting on somatostatin, glucagon, and insulin secretion from the isolated perfused rat pancreas.

From the Second Division, Department of Internal Medicine, Kyoto University School of Medicine, Radioisotope Research Center Kyoto University, and Shimane Medical School, Kyoto and Izumo, Japan.

Address reprint requests to Susumu Seino, M.D., Second Division of Internal Medicine, Kyoto University School of Medicine, Shogoin Kawahara-cho, Sakyo-ku, Kyoto 606, Japan.

Received for publication 30 July 1979 and in revised form 22 October 1979.

MATERIALS AND METHODS

Male Wistar rats weighing 250–300 g were housed for at least a week in a conditioned room and divided into three groups: fed ad libitum, and 16- and 48-h fasting before the experiment. Body weights in 16- and 48-h fasted rats were significantly lower than those of fed rats, with the mean loss of 5.9% and 12%, respectively. The pancreas was isolated and perfused by the procedure described by Grodsky et al.[13] with minor modifications;[14] the preparation includes the attached segment of duodenum and the splenic veins were ligated.

All perfusions were accomplished with 4.4 mM glucose with Krebs-Ringer bicarbonate buffer containing 0.25% bovine serum albumin and 4.6% dextran (mean mol. wt. 70,000). The medium was gassed with 95% O_2–5% CO_2 and maintained at pH 7.4 and 37°C.

The flow rate was kept constant at 1.9 ml/min. After an equilibration period of 20 min, L-arginine hydrochloride, to provide a final concentration of 19 mM, was introduced over 15 min through a side arm pump. Each 1-min effluent from the portal vein was collected in chilled tubes containing 1000 U of Trasylol, frozen immediately, and stored at −20°C until assayed.

Radioimmunoassays. Immunoreactive somatostatin was measured by a specific radioimmunoassay with a modification of the method described by Arimura et al.,[15] using antiserum T-316, which is specific for somatostatin. Antiserum T-316 was produced in a rabbit by repeated immunizations with synthetic cyclic somatostatin (Takeda Pharmaceutical Co., Osaka) coupled to crystallized bovine serum albumin. T-316 had no cross-reactivity with insulin, glucagon, gastrin, motilin, VIP, secretin, and substance-P. N-tyrosyl somatostatin was iodinated with ^{125}I-Na by the chloramine-T method[16] and subsequently purified on Sephadex G-25 (fine) column. The minimum detectable quantity of the assay was 10 pg/ml and serial dilutions of the perfusate gave a parallel curve to that of standard somatostatin. Immunoreactive insulin was measured by radioimmunoassay with the polyethylene glycol method.[17] Immunoreactive glucagon was determined by radioimmunoassay with a talcum absorption technique of Sakurai et al.,[18] using antiserum (Otsuka Assay Laboratory, Tokushima), which is specific for pancreatic glucagon.[19]

Statistical analysis was performed using Student's *t* test for unpaired groups.

RESULTS

Basal perfusate somatostatin concentrations in the presence of 4.4 mM glucose were significantly lower in 48-h fasted rats ($P < 0.005$) and tended to be lower, although not significantly, in 16-h fasted rats than in those of fed controls, as shown in Table 1. Basal perfusate insulin levels also decreased to the undetectable value in 48-h fasted rats compared with the mean value of 6 ± 1 μU/ml in fed animals. Conversely, basal perfusate glucagon concentrations were significantly higher in 48-h fasted rats ($P < 0.05$) and higher, although not significantly, in 16-h fasted rats than those in fed controls.

Arginine (19 mM) infusion in addition to 4.4 mM glucose promptly evoked somatostatin release in all three groups with the mean (± SEM) peak values of 55 ± 5 pg/ml, 55 ± 4 pg/ml, and 55 ± 4 pg/ml in fed, 16-h fasted, and 48-h fasted rats, respectively, which were not significantly different from each other (Figure 1).

However, when arginine-induced somatostatin response is expressed as the sum of increments above the basal level during the 15-min period (ΣΔIRS), somatostatin secretion in rats fasted for 48-h significantly increased, compared with that in the fed rats ($P < 0.05$), as shown in Figure 2. On the contrary, the integrated insulin secretion induced by arginine (ΣΔIRI) was reduced by starvation for 48 h compared with that in the fed group ($P < 0.005$), whereas glucagon secretion (ΣΔIRG) was markedly higher in the 48-h fasted than in the fed group ($P < 0.005$).

DISCUSSION

The present study demonstrates that 48-h fasting decreased basal somatostatin release from the isolated perfused rat pancreas, whereas arginine-induced somatostatin release was rather enhanced by starvation, considering the decrease in basal levels. The mechanism responsible for the decrease in basal somatostatin and the increase in stimulated somatostatin secretion by fasting, although not clear at present, deserves consideration.

TABLE 1
Basal somatostatin, insulin, and glucagon secretion in the presence of 4.4 mM glucose from the isolated perfused pancreas of fed, 16-h fasted, and 48-h fasted rats

		Body weight (g)	Somatostatin secretion (pg/ml)	Insulin secretion (μU/ml)	Glucagon secretion (pg/ml)
Fed	(6)	280 ± 16	33 ± 6	6 ± 1	56 ± 3
16-h fasted	(7)	261 ± 5	23 ± 6	8 ± 4	69 ± 4
48-h fasted	(5)	252 ± 9	15 ± 1*	< 3	81 ± 9†

Results are shown as mean ± SEM with numbers of rats in parenthesis.
* $P < 0.005$ versus fed group.
† $P < 0.05$ versus fed group.

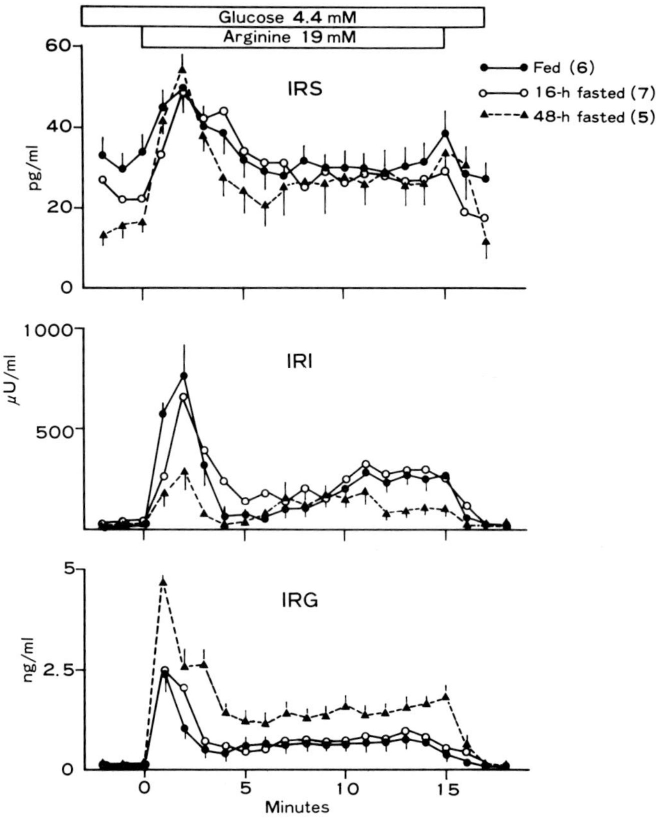

FIGURE 1. Somatostatin, insulin, and glucagon responses to 19 mM arginine in the presence of 4.4 mM glucose from the isolated perfused pancreas of fed, 16-h fasted, and 48-h fasted rats. Means ± SEM are shown in fed and 48-h fasted rats.

Recent studies have suggested that somatostatin may locally interact with regulation of insulin and glucagon secretion within the pancreatic islets as a "paracrine" mechanism.[1–3,20,21,23–26] Glucagon stimulates somatostatin release,[20,21] while there is evidence that insulin may inhibit somatostatin secretion.[24–26,29] Therefore, somatostatin secretion may be affected by the changes of endogenous glucagon or insulin secretion induced by fasting. However, as to the basal somatostatin levels, this seems unlikely because the present data showed that basal somatostatin levels were actually reduced despite the increased basal glucagon and the decreased basal insulin secretion by the starvation. On the contrary, the increase in arginine-stimulated somatostatin secretion by fasting may be due to endogenously enhanced glucagon or reduced insulin secretion, resulting from the interaction of somatostatin, glucagon, and insulin within the islets.

The present study confirms previous observations that arginine stimulates pancreatic somatostatin release[20–22] and further demonstrates that the 48-h fasting enhances arginine-induced somatostatin release, when decreased basal levels were taken into consideration. Recently, Shapiro et al.[28] reported that somatostatin-like immunoreactivity (SLI) in portal blood was decreased in 72-h fasted rats compared with that in the fed rats. Moreover, they also demonstrated that the decrease in basal SLI was associated with an increased tissue SLI, thus indicating the possibility of re-

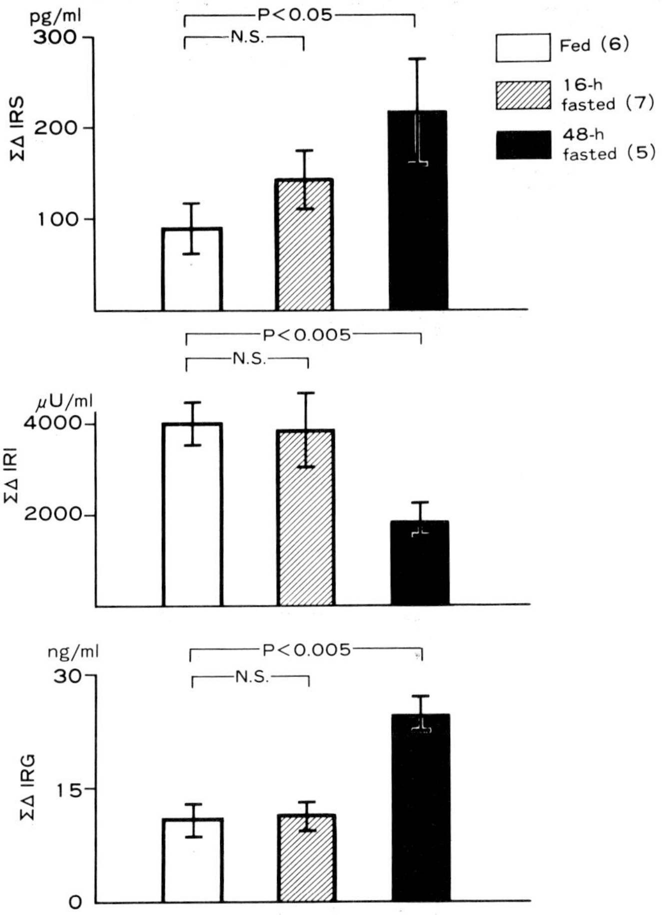

FIGURE 2. Somatostatin, insulin, and glucagon responses to 19 mM arginine in the presence of 4.4 mM glucose from isolated perfused pancreas, expressed as the sum of the increments above basal levels during arginine infusion. Abbreviations are shown as ΣΔIRS, ΣΔIRI, and ΣΔIRG.

duced secretion. On the other hand, Schauder et al.[29] observed an increase in stimulated somatostatin secretion from perifused isolated islets of 48-h fasted rats, although they used glucose as the stimulus. Our present data with low baseline and high stimulated somatostatin secretion seem to agree with the results of Shapiro et al. and Schauder et al., respectively. Further investigation should clarify the exact mechanism by which somatostatin secretion changes during fasting.

ACKNOWLEDGMENTS

The authors are grateful to Dr. Noboru Yanaihara, Shizuoka College of Pharmacy, for kindly giving the N-tyrosil somatostatin; to Dr. Tomoyoshi Nishino, Otsuka Assay Laboratory, for a generous gift of antiglucagon serum; and to Kyoko Masaki for her skillful technical assistance. Part of this study was conducted in the Radioisotope Research Center, Kyoto University.

REFERENCES

1 Luft, R., Efendic, S., Hofket, T., Tohansson, O., and Arimura, A.: Immunohistochemical evidence for the localization of somatostatin-like immunoreactivity in a cell population of the pancreatic islets. Med. Biol. (Helsinki) *52*:428–30, 1974.

2 Dubois, M. P.: Immunoreactive somatostatin is present in discrete cells of the endocrine pancreas. Proc. Natl. Acad. Sci. USA *72*:1340–43, 1975.

3 Orci, L., and Unger, R. H.: Functional subdivisions of islets of Langerhans and possible role of D-cells. Lancet *2*:1243–44, 1975.

4 Unger, R. H., Ipp, E., Schusdziarra, V., and Orci, L.: Hypothesis: physiologic role of pancreatic somatostatin and the contribution of D-cell disorders to diabetes mellitus. Life Sci. *20*:2081–86, 1977.

5 Schusdziarra, V., Harris, V., Conlon, J. M., and Arimura, A.: Pancreatic and gastric somatostatin response to intragastric and intraduodenal nutrients and HCl in the dog. J. Clin. Invest. *62*:509–18, 1978.

6 Schusdziarra, V., Rouiller, D., Harris, V., Conlon, J. M., and Unger, R. H.: The response of plasma somatostatin-like immunoreactivity to nutrients in normal and alloxan diabetic dogs. Endocrinology *103*:2264–73, 1978.

7 Schusdziarra, V., Harris, V., Arimura, A., and Unger, R. H.: Evidence for a role of splanchnic somatostatin in the homeostasis of ingested nutrients. Endocrinology *104*:1705–08, 1979.

8 Unger, R. H., Eisentraut, A. M., and Madison, L. L.: The effect of total starvation upon the levels of circulating glucagon and insulin in man. J. Clin. Invest. *42*:1031–39, 1963.

9 Malaisse, W. J., Malaisse-Lagae, F., and Wright, P. H.: Effect of fasting upon insulin secretions in the rat. Am. J. Physiol. *213*:843–48, 1967.

10 Buchanan, K. D., Vance, J. E., and Williams, R. H.: Effect of starvation on insulin and glucagon release from isolated islets of Langerhans of the rat. Metabolism *18*:155–62, 1969.

11 Grey, N. J., Goldring, S., and Kipnis, D. M.: The effect of fasting, diet, and actinomycin D on insulin secretion in the rat. J. Clin. Invest. *49*:881–89, 1970.

12 Bosboom, R. S., Zweens, J., and Bouman, P. R.: Effect of feeding and fasting on the insulin secretory response to glucose and sulfonylureas intact rats and isolated perfused rat pancreas. Diabetologia *9*:243–50, 1973.

13 Grodsky, G. M., Batts, A. A., Benett, L. L., Vcella, C., McWilliams, N. B., and Smith, D. F.: Effects of carbohydrates on secretion of insulin from isolated rat pancreas. Am. J. Physiol. *205*:638–44, 1963.

14 Goto, Y., Seino, Y., Taminato, T., et al.: Modulation by alloxan of glucagon and insulin secretion in the isolated perfused rat pancreas. Endocrinology *102*:1496–1500, 1978.

15 Arimura, A., Sato, H., Coy, D. H., and Schally, A. V.: Radioimmunoassay for GH-release inhibiting hormone. Proc. Soc. Exp. Biol. Med. *148*:784–89, 1975.

16 Hunter, W. M., and Greenwood, F. C.: Preparation of iodine-131 labelled human growth hormone of high specific activity. Nature *194*:495–96, 1962.

17 Desbuquois, B., and Aurbach, G. D.: Use of polyethylene glycol to separate free and antibody-bound hormones in radioimmunoassay. J. Clin. Endocrinol. Metab. *33*:732–38, 1971.

18 Sakurai, H., and Imura, H.: Radioimmunoassay of glucagon. Jap. J. Nucl. Med. *10*:135–36, 1976.

19 Imagawa, K., Nishino, T., Shin, S., Uehata, S., Hashimura, E., Yanaihara, C., and Yanaihara, N.: Production of anti-glucagon sera with a C-terminal fragment of pancreatic glucagon. Endocrinol. Jpn. *26*:123–31, 1979.

20 Patton, G. S., Ipp, E., Dobbs, R. E., Vale, W., Orci, L., and Unger, R. H.: Response of pancreatic immunoreactive somatostatin release to arginine. Life Sci. *19*:1957–60, 1976.

21 Weir, G. C., Samols, E., Loo, Y., Patel, C., and Gabbay, K. H.: Somatostatin and pancreatic polypeptide secretion: effects of glucagon, insulin, and arginine. Diabetes *28*:35–40, 1979.

22 Goto, Y., Seino, Y., Taminato, T., Kadowaki, S., Chiba, T., Note, S., and Imura, H.: Theophylline: potentiation of arginine-induced somatostatin release from the isolated rat pancreas. Diabetes *28*:457–59, 1979.

23 Kadowaki, S., Taminato, T., Chiba, T., Mori, K., Abe, H., Seino, Y., Matuskura, S., and Fujita, T.: Somatostatin release from isolated perfused rat pancreas: possible role of endogenous somatostatin on insulin release. Diabetes *28*:600–03, 1979.

24 Rothman, J., and Ignarro, L. J.: Effect of anti-insulin in pancreatic somatostatin release. Clin. Res. *26*:775A, 1978.

25 Rouiller, D., Schusdziarra, V., and Unger, R. H.: Effect of insulin upon pancreatic and gastric release of somatostatin-like immunoreactivity. Diabetes *28* (Suppl.):352, 1979.

26 Imura, H., Taminato, T., Kadowaki, S., Chiba, T., and Fujita, T.: Regulation of somatostatin secretion from endocrine pancreas and stomach in rat. Excerpta Medica. In press.

27 Patel, Y. C., Amherdt, M., and Orci, L.: Somatostatin secretion from monolayer cultures of neonatal rat pancreas. Endocrinology *104*:676–79, 1979.

28 Shapiro, B., Berelowitz, M., Pimstone, B. L., Kronheim, S., and Sheppard, M.: Tissue and serum somatostatin-like immunoreactivity in fed, 15-h fasted, and 72-h fasted rats. Diabetes *28*:182–84, 1979.

29 Schauder, P., McIntosh, C., Arends, J., and Frerichs, H.: Effect of fasting on the release of insulin and somatostatin from perifused islets of Langerhans. Diabetes *28*:204–07, 1979.

Rapid Publications

Diurnal Episodic Pattern of Insulin Secretion in the Dog

WALTER P. VANHELDER, ANNA SIREK, OTAKAR V. SIREK, KENNETH H. NORWICH, ZDENKA POLICOVA, AND TOMAS VANHELDER

SUMMARY

Sampling portal blood every 15 min by means of indwelling cannulae, we have found evidence that basal insulin secretion in nonanesthetized dogs takes place in six or seven major secretory episodes over a 24-h period. Reproducible patterns were obtained in four experiments conducted on three normal animals. When frequency of peaks was plotted against the log of insulin concentration, a normal distribution was obtained (lognormal distribution). The means and variances were nearly the same in the three animals. Low levels of insulin (10–25 μU/ml) alternated with peaks which were occasionally higher than 200 μU/ml. The average duration of a peak was 30 min and seemed to be independent of ambient glucose levels. It is suggested that these peaks are the result of surges in plasma growth hormone concentrations and/or spontaneous repetitive discharges along neuronal pathways functionally related to insulin secretion. DIABETES *29*:326–328, April 1980.

Pulsatile hormone secretion has been recognized as a characteristic secretory pattern for pituitary tropic hormones.[1–8] The release of these peptide hormones from the pituitary is governed by neural mechanisms that are responsible for the episodic secretion of specific hypothalamic releasing or inhibitory factors. In contrast to this, the secretion of insulin is thought to be regulated primarily by substrate availability and modulated by the autonomic nervous system and gastrointestinal hormones.

We should like to report now that basal insulin secretion measured "at source" in portal blood of conscious normal dogs shows a rhythmic pattern similar to that described for pituitary protein hormones.

From the Department of Physiology, Medical Sciences Building, University of Toronto, Toronto, Ontario M5S 1A8.
Address reprint requests to Dr. A. Sirek, Department of Physiology, Medical Sciences Building, University of Toronto, Toronto, Ontario M5S 1A8.
Received for publication 2 January 1980.

MATERIALS AND METHODS

Under general anesthesia (Nembutal, 35 mg/kg) and aseptic conditions, indwelling silastic catheters were placed into the portal vein through the cranial branch of the splenic vein in three young male dogs weighing 13–16 kg. The open end of each catheter was brought out through the skin of the back, out of reach of the dog. The catheters were filled and frequently flushed with heparinized saline (1:40). Two weeks after surgery, when the animals were fully recovered, the actual experiment was performed. Every 15 min over a 24-h period, 2-ml blood samples were withdrawn and immediately replaced by 2 ml of saline. Care was taken to maintain normal routine in that the animals were fed once a day and lights were turned off from 2100 to 800 h. Plasma glucose was determined in fresh samples by the Beckman Analyzer (true glucose) and insulin was determined in stored frozen plasma samples, after thawing, by the double antibody assay of Hales and Randle,[9] using the kit of Amersham Searle Corporation (Chicago, Illinois). Plasma samples giving values in excess of 100 μU/ml were suitably diluted and reassayed. Analyses of auto- and cross-correlations were carried out by standard procedures.[10] A probit analysis was carried out[11] using the natural logarithm of insulin concentration; the probit regression line was calculated in each case. Values obtained for the first 5 h after feeding were excluded from calculations so as to minimize the possibility of equalization by supplying the same type and amounts of nutrients.

RESULTS

The daily pattern of portal insulin and glucose concentrations of three dogs is shown in Figure 1. Dog N606 was studied under identical conditions on two separate occasions 1 wk apart. The cross-correlation analysis showed that insulin concentrations varied independently from glucose levels. With respect to insulin peaks, the analysis of auto-correlation gave no indication of regular cycling. The plot of probit against log concentrations gave an excellent straight line in every case, showing that the log of concentration was normally distributed. The results are comparable in all four experiments, and are shown in Figure 2.

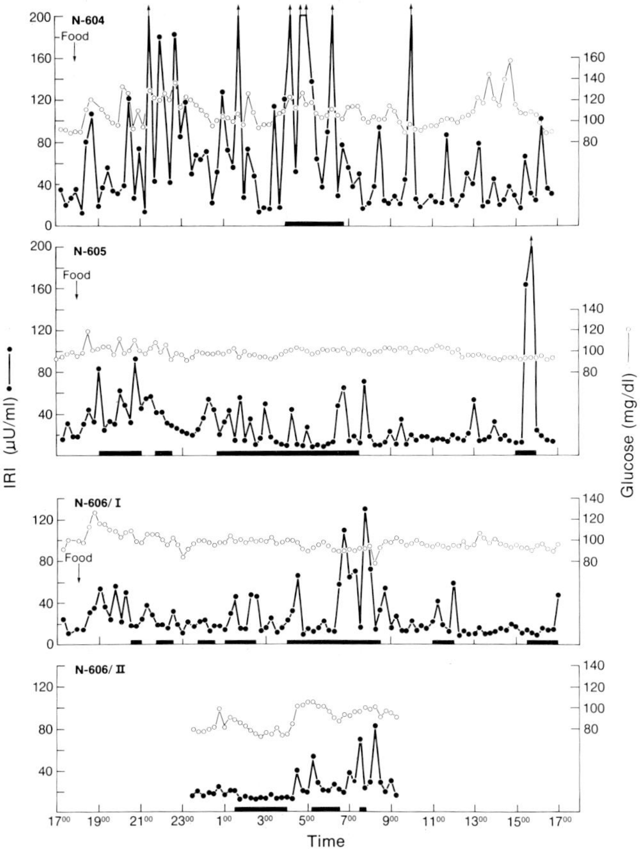

FIGURE 1. Twenty-four hour glucose and insulin profiles in portal blood of three normal dogs. N606 was studied again for 8 h one week later. Black lines along the abscissa indicate periods of sleep.

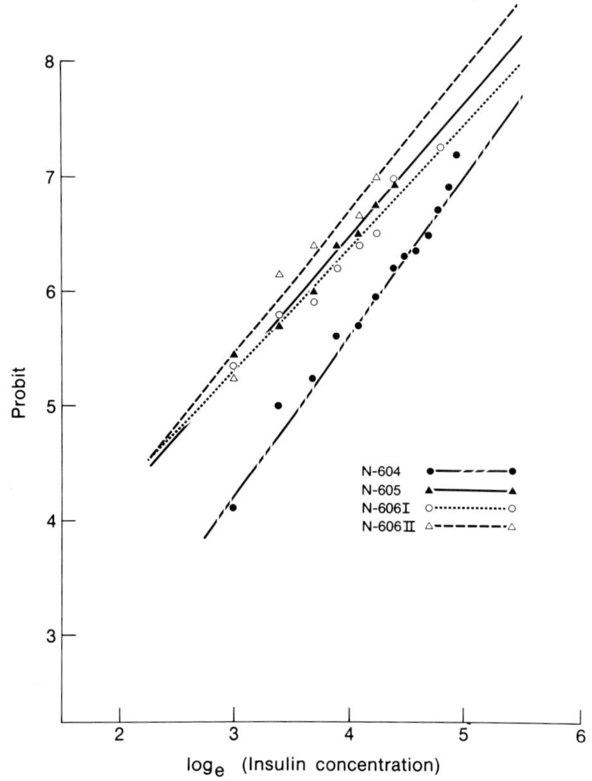

FIGURE 2. Frequency distribution of log$_e$ (insulin concentration). Designating a normal distribution with mean, x, and variance, s^2 by N ($\bar{x}$, s^2), we have, by probit analysis: dog N604, mongrel, N (3.55, 0.51); N605, beagle, N (2.69, 0.81); N606, beagle, I, N (2.72, 0.88); II, N (2.66, 0.64). Lines were fitted by least squares regression.

DISCUSSION

The results of our experiments provide, for the first time, evidence that insulin is secreted throughout the day and night in the form of intermittent bursts. The pronounced episodic secretion of insulin is reflected only in the portal vein. Except for a few hours after feeding, the peaks in insulin concentrations were not related to glucose levels. Also, spike concentrations were present during both periods of sleep and wakefulness.

It was reported that in arterial blood of conscious dogs, sampled every 0.1 to 2 min up to 10 h, insulin concentrations showed "no fluctuations or linear trends," unless the animals were infused with glucose.[12] However, in a subsequent communication from the same laboratory, it was concluded that "oscillations are part of the normal dynamics of the glucose/insulin system."[13] In fasting normal monkeys (but not in man) regular oscillations of insulin, glucagon, and glucose levels were observed in the vena cava.[14] Samples were taken at 2- or 5-min intervals for 30 min; the cycling period averaged 9 min and the secretion of insulin increased to 120% of the baseline values. Oscillations of glucose preceded those of insulin levels, suggesting a stimulus-secretory relationship.[14] Plasma C-peptide was found to cycle synchronously with insulin.[15] In humans, small oscillations in the plasma insulin concentration were found in peripheral venous blood when sampling was done every minute for 2 h. The length of a cycle was 11 to 15 min, the mean amplitude 1.4 μU/ml, and glucose cycled in advance of insulin.[16,17]

There are several basic differences between our study and the investigations from other laboratories. We are reporting on irregular episodic bursts of insulin secretion over a period of 24 h, and the surges that we saw are of a variable magnitude up to 20 times the baseline values. This is different from the results of short-term studies, showing oscillations with regular cycling and amplitudes seldom exceeding twice the baseline values. Furthermore, we were sampling "at source," in the portal vein, i.e., before passage through the liver, while in other studies sampling was done in the peripheral circulation where factors other than the rate of insulin secretion may have appreciably altered ambient hormone concentrations. Finally, the secretory bursts described by us were independent of plasma glucose concentrations, while the peripheral insulin oscillations described by others were related to preceding oscillations in plasma glucose concentrations. Thus, it is unlikely that regular peripheral insulin oscillations and irregular portal insulin surges would be governed by identical control mechanisms.

Since we have not concentrated on studying the relatively small oscillations in plasma insulin concentrations, we cannot exclude the possibility that we may have missed them on occasion by sampling every 15 min. However, it is highly unlikely that we missed a real burst in insulin secretion, because when sampling was done at 2-min intervals for 15-min periods at random, the results did not appreciably alter the pattern obtained by 15-min sampling. Thus the connecting of individual points by lines as done in Figure 1 appears to be justified. The rhythmicity of the pattern of secretion shows similarities in all three dogs. The nearly identical slopes of the probit lines (similar variances) are indicative of closely related patterns of basal insulin secretion.

Alterations in blood flow would be expected to produce fluctuations within the range that we have seen for plasma glucose levels, but it is difficult to visualize how blood flow could be responsible for a 20-fold increase in insulin concentration. Moreover, the similarity of insulin profiles, particularly in dog N606 in which almost identical patterns were seen on two separate occasions, argues against alterations in blood flow as a reasonable explanation.

Very high insulin concentrations were observed six to seven times over a 24-h period. The frequency of these peaks is similar to the frequency of surges in plasma growth hormone (GH) secretion observed in man[2,4] and in the rat.[18] We have shown earlier that a sudden increase of the plasma GH concentration in the dog results in an immediate release of insulin and glucagon from the pancreas.[19] Thus, it is attractive to speculate that the peaks in insulin are driven by preceeding surges in plasma GH. Since in the present series of experiments we have not determined GH levels, we can not make further comments at this time, nor exclude the possibility that the insulin surges are the result of a neural or neurohumoral stimulation originating from levels of the brain higher than the pituitary. Enhanced insulin release was observed after electrical stimulation of certain areas of the brain[20] and after injections of hypothalamic extracts.[21–23] Assuming that the control of basal insulin secretion is driven by such a central mechanism, the moving force would have to rest in the spontaneous firing of neuronal cells (i.e., in primary neural activation) and the neurohumor would reach the pancreatic beta cell either directly by release from local nerve endings, or indirectly through endocrine or paracrine communications. By considering the pancreatic beta cell as a neuroendocrine cell,[25] spontaneous activity becomes another possibility.[26] Further experiments are in progress to elucidate the mechanism underlying the pulsatile secretion of insulin.

ACKNOWLEDGMENTS

This study was supported by a grant from Denison Mines Limited of Toronto and by an operating grant from the Natural Sciences and Engineering Research Council of Canada. The expert secretarial assistance of S. Meredith is gratefully acknowledged.

REFERENCES

1 Hunter, W. M., and Rigal, W. M.: The diurnal pattern of plasma growth hormone concentration in children and adolescents. J. Endocrinol. *34*:147–53, 1966.

2 Quabbe, H. J., Schilling, E., and Helge, H.: Pattern of growth hormone secretion during a 24-hour fast in normal adults. J. Clin. Endocrinol. Metab. *26*:1173–77, 1966.

3 Spitz, I., Gonen, B., and Rabinowitz, D.: Growth hormone release in man revisited: spontaneous vs. stimulus-initiated tides. *In* Growth and Growth Hormone. Pecile, A., and Müller, E. E., Eds. Amsterdam, Excerpta Medica, 1972, pp. 371–81.

4 Finkelstein, J. W., Roffward, H. P., Boyar, R. M., Kream, J., and Hellman, L.: Age-related change in the twenty-four hour spontaneous secretion of growth hormone. J. Clin. Endocrinol. Metab. *35*:665–70, 1972.

5 Parker, D. C., and Rossman, L. G.: Sleep-wake cycle and human growth hormone, prolactin and luteinizing hormone. *In* Advances in Human Growth Hormone Research. Raiti, S., Ed. DHEW publication no. (NIH) 74-612, 1973, pp. 294–317.

6 Krieger, D. T., Allen, W., Rizzo, F., and Krieger, H. P.: Characterization of the normal temporal pattern of plasma corticosteroid levels. J. Clin. Endocrinol. Metab. *32*:266–84, 1971.

7 Van Haelst, L., Van Cauter, E., Degoute, J. P., and Golstein, J.: Circadian variations of serum thyrotropin levels in man. J. Clin. Endocrinol. Metab. *35*:479–82, 1972.

8 Boyar, R. L., Perlow, M., Hellman, L., Kapen, S., and Weitzman, E. D.: Twenty-four hour pattern of luteinizing hormone secretion in normal men with sleep stage recording. J. Clin. Endocrinol. Metab. *35*:73–81, 1972.

9 Hales, C. N., and Randle, P. J.: Immunoassay of insulin with insulin-antibody precipitate. Biochem. J. *88*:137–46, 1963.

10 Bloomfield, P.: Fourier Analysis of Time Series. New York, John Wiley and Sons, 1976.

11 Finney, D. J.: Probit Analysis. Cambridge University Press, 1971, 3rd ed.

12 Ookhtens, M., Marsh, D. J., Smith, S. W., Bergman, R. N., and Yates, F. E.: Fluctuations of plasma glucose and insulin in conscious dogs receiving glucose infusions. Amer. J. Physiol. *226*:910–19, 1974.

13 Yates, F. E., Gold, M. N., and Cohen, R. R.: Oscillations of plasma glucose: Dependence on periodicity of insulin secretion. Presented at the 61st Annual Meeting of the Endocrine Society, Anaheim, California, June 13–15, 1979.

14 Goodner, C. J., Walike, B. C., Koerker, D. J., Ensinck, J. W., Brown, A. C., Chideckel, E. W., Palmer, J., and Kalnasy, L.: Insulin, glucagon and glucose exhibit synchronous, sustained oscillations in fasting monkeys. Science *195*:177–79, 1977.

15 Koerker, D. J., Goodner, C. J., Hansen, B. W., Brown, A. C., and Rubenstein, A. H.: Synchronous, sustained oscillation of C-peptide and insulin in the plasma of fasting monkeys. Endocrinology *102*:1649–52, 1978.

16 Matthews, D. R., Lang, D. A., Peto, J., and Turner, R. C.: Cyclical variation ("hunting") of basal plasma glucose and insulin concentrations in normal and diabetic man. Diabetologia *15*:254, 1978.

17 Land, D. A., Matthews, D. R., Phil, D., Peto, J., and Turner, R. C.: Cyclic oscillations of basal plasma glucose and insulin concentrations in human beings. N. Engl. J. Med. *301*:1023–27, 1979.

18 Tannenbaum, G. S., and Martin, J. B.: Evidence for an endogenous ultradian rhythm governing growth hormone secretion in the rat. Endocrinology *98*:562–70, 1976.

19 Sirek, A., Vranic, M., Sirek, O. V., Vigas, M., and Policova, Z.: The effect of growth hormone on acute glucagon and insulin release. Am. J. Physiol. *6*:E107–E112, 1979.

20 Berthoud, H. R., Bereiter, D. A., and Jeanrenaud, B.: Role of the lateral hypothalamic area in insulin secretion and regulation of glycemia. Excerpta Medica No. 481, 10th Congress of The International Diabetes Federation, September 9–14, 1979.

21 Martin, J. M., Mok, C. C., Penfold, J., Howard, N. J., and Crowne, D.: Hypothalamic stimulation of insulin release. J. Endocrinol. *58*:681–82, 1973.

22 Lockhart-Ewart, R. B., Mok, C. C., and Martin, J. M.: Neuroendocrine control of insulin secretion. Diabetes *25*:96–100, 1976.

23 Hill, D. E., Mayes, S., DiBattista, D., Lockhart-Ewart, R., and Martin, J. M.: Hypothalamic regulation of insulin release in rhesus monkeys. Diabetes *26*:726–31, 1977.

24 Martin, J. M.: Neurohumoral regulation of insulin secretion and glucose utilization. *In* Obesity in Childhood. Cacciari, E., Laron, Z., and Raiti, S., Eds. Proc. Serono Symp. *17*:7–18, 1978.

25 Pearse, A. G. E., and Takor Takor, T.: Embryology of the diffuse neuroendocrine system and its relationship to the common peptides. Fed. Proc. *38*:2288–94, 1979.

26 Stagner, J., Samols, E., and Weir, G.: Detection of sustained insulin, somatostatin and glucagon oscillations in the isolated perfused canine pancreas. Presented at the 61st Annual Meeting of The Endocrine Society, Anaheim, California, June 13–15, 1979.

Phenformin Increases Insulin Binding to Human Cultured Breast Cancer Cells

D. COHEN, V. PEZZINO, R. VIGNERI, R. AVOLA, R. D'AGATA, AND P. POLOSA

SUMMARY

The effect of the hypoglycemic biguanide, phenformin, on the binding of insulin to MCF-7 cells, an in vitro line derived from a human breast cancer, has been investigated. Cells incubated for 24 h in the presence of 1.0 μg/ml of phenformin bound 62.2 $\pm$ 8.1% (mean $\pm$ SE) more ^{125}I-insulin than did controls. The phenformin effect was dose-dependent over the concentration range of 0.1 μg/ml to 10.0 μg/ml. The increased binding was due to an increase in receptor number without a change in binding affinity. This demonstration of increased receptor number in response to phenformin exposure provides support for the hypothesis that one action of phenformin is to enhance tissue sensitivity to insulin. DIABETES *29*:329–331, April 1980.

The mechanism underlying the hypoglycemic effect of biguanides, such as phenformin, that are still used in the treatment of non-insulin-dependent maturity-onset diabetes mellitus in various parts of the world, are incompletely understood.[1,2] There is evidence, however, that suggests that phenformin acts by increasing the physiologic responsiveness of human peripheral tissues to circulating insulin.[3–6] An effect of biguanides on the binding of insulin to the target cell, the initial step in insulin action,[7] was the possibility investigated in this study.

In order to exclude the possible interference of changing levels of circulating hormones and metabolites that could occur in in vivo studies, and to focus directly on the drug-target cell interaction, an in vitro model system was chosen. The MCF-7 cell line, derived from a human breast cancer, is suitable for studies of insulin action because it is responsive to physiologic concentrations of insulin, and because it has both well characterized, high affinity insulin receptors and an insulin degrading capacity.[8]

From the Istituto di Patologia Medica dell'Università di Catania, Ospedale Garibaldi, 95124-Catania, Italy and the Istituto di Chimica Biologica dell'Università di Catania, v. le A.Doria, Catania, Italy.
Address reprint requests to Riccardo Vigneri, Istituto di Endocrinologia, Via Ofelia 35, 95123-Catania, Italy.
Received for publication 7 February 1980.

METHODS AND MATERIALS

The MCF-7 cell line, derived from a human breast carcinoma and placed into tissue culture at the Michigan Cancer Foundation, was a gift from Dr. M. Lippman (NIH, Bethesda, Maryland). The cells were grown in continuous monolayer culture in Falcon tissue culture flasks using Eagle's Minimal Essential Medium (MEM) plus essential amino acids, penicillin, streptomycin, and 10% fetal calf serum (FCS). The insulin receptors, insulin degrading capacity, and insulin responsiveness (increased acetate, thymidine, and leucine incorporation in response to physiologic concentrations of insulin) have been previously characterized.[8]

Porcine insulin was purchased from Sigma (distributed by Mascia e Brunelli, Milan, Italy) and labeled with ^{125}I from the Amersham Radiochemical Center (Amersham, Great Britain) to a specific activity of 95–120 μCi/μg by the chloramine T method.[9] Phenformin (N-beta-phenetylbiguanide) was a gift from Boehringer Biochemia (Milan, Italy).

Binding studies were performed on cells 4 days after their implantation into tissue culture flasks, while they were in a state of semiconfluence (approximately 1.5 $\times$ 10^6 cells/flask). Twenty-four hours before the binding study, the medium in the flask was changed and phenformin was added.

To prepare cells for binding studies, the procedure of Osborne et al.[8] was followed. Briefly, the cells within the flasks were rinsed with Eagle's MEM (without FCS), rinsed again with a solution of 150 mM NaCl : 0.02% EDTA, and then harvested by a 5-min incubation in the same solution. The harvested cells were diluted with Eagle's MEM (without FCS), centrifuged at 250 $\times$ *g* for 3 min, resuspended in phosphate buffered (pH 7.6) physiologic saline, recentrifuged, and finally resuspended in the binding assay buffer (100 mM HEPES, 120 mM NaCl, 1.2 mM $MgSO_4$, 2.5 mM KCl, 15 mM $NaC_2H_3O_2$, 10 mM glucose, 1 mM EDTA, and 1% bovine serum albumin, pH 7.6) to a final concentration of 1 $\times$ 10^6 cells/ml.

Within an experiment, two to four flasks were pooled to obtain the cell suspension for each experimental group. All incubations were performed at 22°C. Cell viability, as determined by trypan blue exclusion, was typically greater than 90% at the termination of the incubation period. The concentration of ^{125}I-insulin was 0.4 ng/ml, and that of the unlabeled insulin was 100 μg/ml.

For the separation of bound and free hormone, triplicate 100-μl assay aliquots were layered over 200 μl of cold binding buffer in microfuge tubes, and centrifuged in a Beckman microfuge (Beckman Instruments, Palo Alto, California) for 2 min. The supernatants were collected for determination of insulin degradation by precipitation of intact hormone with 10% trichloroacetic acid. Cell pellets were then washed, the microfuge tips excised, and the radioactivity counted. Specific binding was calculated as the difference between the binding of the ^{125}I-insulin in the absence and presence of excess unlabeled insulin.

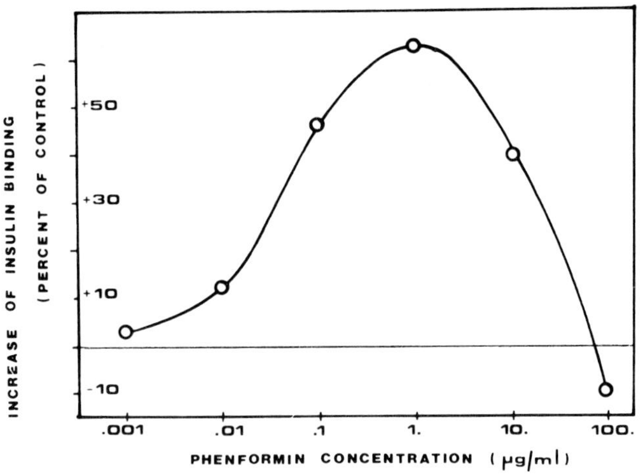

FIGURE 2. Effect of phenformin concentration on specific insulin binding to the MCF-7 cells. Cells were preincubated with phenformin for 24 h.

RESULTS

In a preliminary experiment, the binding of insulin was measured in cells that had been preincubated with 1.0 μg/ml of phenformin for 0, 3, 12, 24, and 48 h. An increase in insulin binding was detectable after 3 h of exposure to phenformin, and was maximal after 24 h (although there was no significant difference between the 12-, 24-, and 48-h time points). For convenience, 24 h was used as the standard period of preincubation with phenformin in the experiments that followed.

Cells incubated in the absence of phenformin specifically bound ^{125}I-insulin maximally between 4–6 h, and maintained a plateau until 8 h. Cells preincubated with 1 μg/ml of phenformin for 24 h produced a similarly shaped binding curve that demonstrated increased binding at all binding assay time points (Figure 1). In a series of seven separate experiments, preincubation of MCF-7 cells with 1 μg/ml of phenformin for 24 h produced an increase in insulin binding at a steady state of 62.2% ± 8.1 (mean ± SE, range of 35–96%) over the untreated cells. The degradation of ^{125}I-insulin was also slightly increased in cells preincubated with phenformin (22–30% of total in untreated cells; 25–36% of total in phenformin-treated cells).

At 24 h of preincubation, a small but reproducible effect of phenformin was detectable at 0.01 μg/ml, and a maximal effect was seen at 1.0 μg/ml. A concentration of 100 μg/ml proved to be cytotoxic, causing a lowering of the medium pH and a decrease in insulin binding (Figure 2).

A Scatchard analysis of the data (Figure 3) revealed that the phenformin-induced increase in insulin binding was due to an increase in the number of insulin binding sites without a significant change in binding site affinity.

DISCUSSION

These data demonstrate that preincubation of MCF-7 cells with phenformin significantly increases their ability to specifically bind insulin. The Scatchard analysis indicates that the enhanced insulin binding is primarily due to an increase in the number of insulin binding sites. This effect of phenformin is rapid (detectable after 3 h of drug exposure), and is dose-related over a concentration range (0.01–10 μg/ml) that includes the effective therapeutic concentration range in blood (0.05–0.1 μg/ml).[10]

Several mechanisms have been suggested to be responsible for the antihyperglycemic action of phenformin.

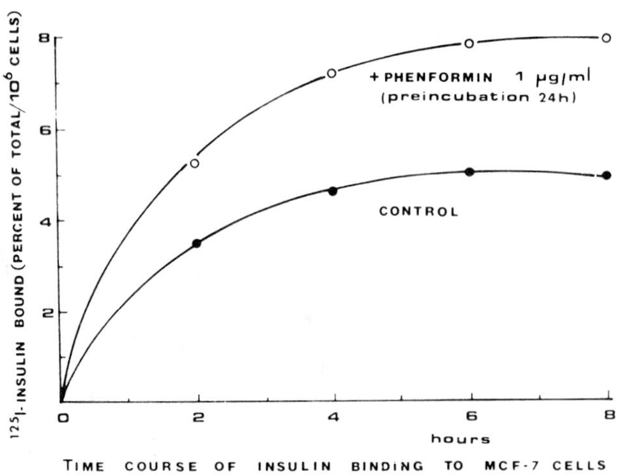

FIGURE 1. Insulin binding to the MCF-7 cells in the presence and absence of preincubation with phenformin.

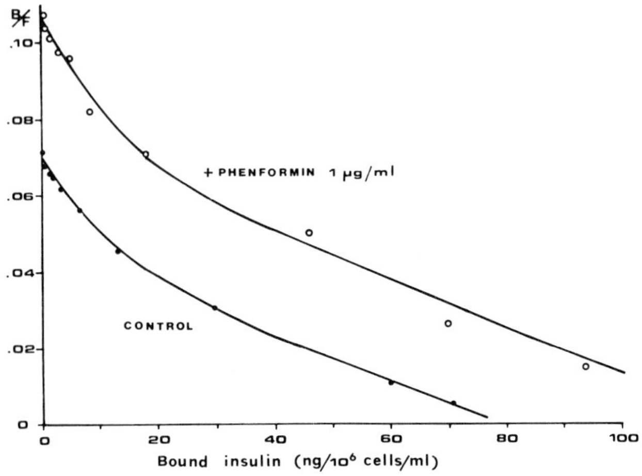

FIGURE 3. Scatchard plot of the binding data in MCF-7 cells with and without 24-h phenformin preincubation. Each point is the mean of three separate experiments.

Among these are decreased glucose absorption from the gut,[11] increased anaerobic glucose metabolism as a consequence of tissue hypoxia,[12] increased glucose metabolism as a consequence of decreased fatty acid oxidation,[13] and enhanced sensitivity of peripheral tissues to circulating insulin.[4–7] The observations reported here lend support to this last hypothesis.

If normal insulin target cells in vivo respond to phenformin by increasing their insulin binding capacity, as do these cells in vitro, then this effect may play a role in the therapeutic action of the drug. The consistency of this hypothesis will require the demonstration (currently under investigation) of an association between the increased insulin binding and the biologic response to insulin in these cells. In addition, the possibility that biguanides may well have multiple sites of action must be recognized.

Recently, the other major class of hypoglycemic agents, sulphonylureas, have been reported to increase the number of insulin receptors in mice[14] and humans.[15,16] These data were obtained in vivo, and thus the possibility that the changes were secondary to alterations in circulating insulin or metabolites cannot be excluded. The data reported here, in contrast, were obtained in vitro, and therefore suggest a direct effect of phenformin upon the target cell.

The process through which cells may increase their effective insulin receptor number in response to phenformin is unknown: structural modifications of the plasma membrane or changes in the insulin receptor turnover rate could conceivably be involved. It is of interest, in this regard, that preliminary experiments (unpublished) with the sulfonylurea glibenclamide (0.1 – 1.0 μg/ml) have also shown increased insulin binding to the MCF-7 cells, with increments ranging from 15–42% of controls.

ACKNOWLEDGMENTS

We thank Dr. I. D. Goldfine, of the University of San Francisco, California for helpful discussion. These studies were supported by grants from the CNR (National Council for Research, Italy, grant 79.01556.96) and from Boehringer Biochemia (Milano, Italy). Dr. D. Cohen was the recipient as a visiting scientist of CNR grant 206042/04/80317.

REFERENCES

[1] Shen, S. H., and Bressler, R.: Clinical pharmacology of oral antidiabetic agents. N. Engl. J. Med. *296*:493–97, 787–93, 1977.

[2] Cash, W. D.: Assessment of the metabolic effects of phenformin in relation to the problem of lactic acidosis. *In* Endocrinology and Metabolism Advisory Committee Meeting, October 12, 1976. Pharmaceutical Division, Ciba Geigy Corp., Summit, N.J., pp. 4–59.

[3] Butterfield, W. J. H., and Whichelow, M. J.: The hypoglycemic action of phenformin; effect of phenformin on glucose metabolism in peripheral tissues. Diabetes *2*:281–86, 1962.

[4] Whichelow, M. J., and Butterfield, W. J. H.: In vivo studies on the hypoglycemic action of phenformin. Postgrad. Med. J. (Suppl.)*45*:24–29, 1969.

[5] Stout, R. W., Brunzell, J. D., Bierman, E. L., and Porte, D.: Effect of phenformin on glucose-insulin interrelationships. Diabetes *23*:624–30, 1974.

[6] Halpern, A., Wajchenberg, B. L., and Fazia, A. I. M.: Mechanism of action of phenetylbiguanide (phenformin) in normal subjects. II. Intestinal absorbtion versus nonintestinal effects. Metabolism *23*:349–58, 1974.

[7] Vigneri, R., and Goldfine, I. D.: The mechanism of action of insulin. Min. Endocr. *2*:59–72, 1977.

[8] Osborne, C. K., Monaco, M. E., Lippman, M., and Kahn, C. R.: Correlation among insulin binding, degradation, and biological activity in human breast cancer cells in long-term tissue culture. Cancer Res. *38*:94–102, 1978.

[9] Goldfine, I. D., and Smith, G. J.: Binding of insulin to isolated nuclei. Proc. Natl. Acad. Sci. USA *73*:1427–31, 1976.

[10] Catellier, C., Fraser, E., Ayatte-Ferron, L., and Savoie, J. Y.: Blood levels of phenformin following a customary therapeutic dose. Union Med. Can. *106*:323–26, 1977.

[11] Hollobaugh, S. L., Rao, M. B., and Kruger, F. A.: Studies on the site of mechanism of action of phenformin. I. Evidence for significant "non-peripheral" effects of phenformin in glucose metabolism in normal subjects. Diabetes *19*:45–49, 1970.

[12] Muntoni, S.: Inhibition of fatty acid oxidation by biguanides: implications for metabolic physiopathology. Adv. Lipid Res. *12*:311–77, 1974.

[13] Corsini, G. H., Sirigu, F., Tagliamonte, P., and Muntoni, S.: Effects of biguanides on fatty acid and glucose oxidation in muscle. Pharmacol. Res. Commun. *6*:253–58, 1974.

[14] Feinglos, M. N., and Leibovitz, H. E.: Sulfonylureas increase the number of insulin receptors. Nature *276*:184–85, 1978.

[15] Olefsky, J. M., and Reaven, G. M.: Effects of sulfonylurea therapy on insulin binding to mononuclear leukocytes of diabetic patients. Am. J. Med. *60*:89–95, 1976.

[16] Beck-Nielsen, H., Pedersen, O., and Linskov, H. O.: Increased insulin sensitivity and cellular insulin binding in obese diabetics following treatment with glibenclamide. Acta Endocrinol. *90*:451–62, 1979.

Organization Section

NATIONAL DIABETES INFORMATION CLEARINGHOUSE

The National Diabetes Information Clearinghouse invites you to add your name to our mailing list for information about patient and professional education materials. You will receive annotated bibliographies on a variety of diabetes topics; our bi-monthly bulletin, *Diabetes Dateline;* and other timely information. If you would like to receive our materials, send your name and address (with zip code) to: The National Diabetes Information Clearinghouse, 805 15th St., N.W., Suite 500, Washington, DC 20005. This announcement is a service of the National Institute of Arthritis, Metabolism and Digestive Diseases of the National Institutes of Health.

WILDERNESS CHALLENGE—1980

"Wilderness Challenge—1980" provides unique camping experiences for young diabetics ages 16 through 18 years of age. Medically supervised programs have been developed to enhance the self-concept of young men and women with diabetes and promote outdoor skills, good fellowship and an appreciation for nature.

The programs include a wilderness canoeing experience in the Boundary Waters Canoe Area (BWCA) on the Minnesota-Canada border July 29–August 8; an ideal backpacking trip for beginning and intermediate campers in the Isle Royale National Park June 28–July 8; and an exciting challenge for the experienced backpacker in Wyoming's Big Horn Mountains July 17–27.

For further information, contact Donnell D. Etzwiler, M.D., Diabetes Education Center, 4959 Excelsior Boulevard, Minneapolis, Minnesota 55416 phone (612) 920-6742.

HORMONES AND CELL REGULATION

The Institut National des Sciences et de la Recherche Médicale and the Direction Générale à la Recherche Scientifique et Technique will sponsor its V Colloquium, "Hormones and Cell Regulation," on October 1–4, 1980.

For further information and registration materials, contact Professor B. Jeanrenaud, Laboratoire de Recherches Médicales, Université de Genève, Avenue de la Roseraie, 64, 1204 Geneve, Switzerland.

SYMPOSIUM ON INSULIN RECEPTORS

The 1st International Symposium on Insulin Receptors will be held in Rome on September 22–23, 1980. This symposium will be a satellite symposium of the EASD 1980 Congress of Athens.

For further information regarding the symposium and registration, contact D. Andreani, R. Lauro, or R. DePirro, II Clinica Medica, Policlinico Umberto 1°, 00100 Rome, Italy.

SYMPOSIUM ON ADVANCES IN PEDIATRIC RESEARCH

The Third International Symposium on Advances in Pediatric Research, "Current Views on the Etiology and Pathogenesis of Insulin-dependent Diabetes Mellitus," will be held at the Hospital for Sick Children in Ontario on October 20–23, 1980. Twenty-one invited speakers will discuss the morphologic, functional, and metabolic changes in insulin-dependent diabetes; autoimmunity; HLA system; virus and islet-cell antibodies in the etiology of the disease; insulin receptors and counterregulatory hormones; epidemiologic studies in various populations; and animal models of insulin-dependent diabetes.

Registration will be limited to 150 participants. For further information, contact Dr. Julio M. Martin, Research Institute, The Hospital for Sick Children, 555 University Avenue, Totonto, Ontario M5G 1X8, Canada.

COURSE IN TEAM MANAGEMENT OF DIABETES

The Diabetes Education Center (a component of the St. Louis Park Medical Center Research Foundation) will sponsor a comprehensive five-day program, "Clinical Experience in the Team Management of Diabetes Mellitus." The course is designed for health professionals, patients, and/or family members.

The dates of the classweeks for the second half of 1980 are as follows: July 7–11 (juvenile week), 14–18, July 28–August 1; August 18–22, 25–29; September 22–26 (adult week); October 13–17 (juvenile week), 27–31; November 10–14, 17–21; and December 1–5, 15–19.

Tuition is $250. The course is approved for 34 contact hours for physicians and nurses, and for 30 clock hours for dieticians, pharmacists, and others.

For further information, contact Carole Mensing, R.N., Health Professional Coordinator, Diabetes Education Center, 4959 Excelsior Boulevard, Minneapolis, Minnesota 55416, phone (612) 920-6742.

INTERNATIONAL SYMPOSIUM ON ISLET-PANCREAS-TRANSPLANTATION AND ARTIFICIAL PANCREAS

A satellite symposium to the 16th Annual Meeting of the European Association for the study of Diabetes (EASD) Congress will be organized on the subject of islet-pancreas-transplantation and artificial pancreas (dynamic insulin therapy systems: artificial beta cell, preprogrammed insulin infusions, pancreas- and islet cell-transplantation). This symposium is being organized by the Diabetes Center and the Artificial Pancreas Unit, Department of Clinical Therapeutics University of Athens, Greece; the center of Internal Medicine University of Ulm, Germany; and the center of Internal Medicine University of Giessen Germany, in collaboration with the Hellenic Society for Transplantation, and will take place from September 22–23, 1980 in Athens, Greece, immediately preceding the EASD Congress (September 24–27, 1980). This meeting will include invited lectures and a limited number of free communications. Deadline for receipt of abstracts (maximum 250 words) is May 15, 1980 (postmarked).

For further information, contact Professor S. Raptis M.D., P.O. Box 3127, Athens 606, Greece. Congress language is English. Abstracts should be sent to S.R., Athens, Greece.

CONFERENCE ON INSULINS AND GROWTH HORMONE

The Bureau of Drugs of the Food and Drug Administration will present a "State of the Art Conference on Insulins and Growth Hormone" on June 3–4, 1980 at the Masur Auditorium, Clinical Center, NIH, Bethesda, Maryland. Discussions will include current aspects of the use of purified insulins of animal origin as well as human insulin and growth hormone obtained through recombinant DNA technology. The program will consist of invited presentations on scientific and regulatory topics by leading investigators and officials from industry, academia, and government. The proceedings will be published.

For further information, contact John L. Gueriguian, M.D., Bureau of Drugs, Division of Metabolism and Endocrine Drug Products, FDA, 5600 Fishers Lane, Rockville, Maryland 20857.

NEW MEMBERS

The following were elected to the Professional Section as of February 1, 1980:

Yoshiharu Akazawa, M.D., Kyoto, Japan
Jerome E. Bodian, M.D., Englewood, NJ
Thomas A. Boyd, Ph.D., Hershey, PA
William H. Brooks, M.D., Kansas City, KS
Richard G. Daly, M.D., La Mesa, CA
Vincenzo Esposito, M.D., Napoli, Italy
Diane B. Friedman, M.D., Minneapolis, MN
Carol J. Gilmore, M.S., Los Angeles, CA
J. Ronald Graf, M.D., Tacoma, WA
Leslie A. Howard, R.D., Tulsa, OK
William C. Knowler, M.D., Phoenix, AZ
Kathleen L. Krauser, M.S.N., Indianapolis, IN
Dennis S. Krauss, M.D., Providence, RI
Michael N. Krupp, Ph.D., Baltimore, MD
Jane M. Lehan, B.S., Granada Hills, CA
William J. Levy, M.D., Cleveland, OH
Martin J. Luria, M.D., Long Branch, NJ
Karen McCarthy, B.S., Shelby, NC
Carey A. Mickel, M.D., Elberton, GA
George W. Moore, M.D., Keesler AFB, MS
Robert W. Murray, M.D., Milwaukee, WI
Jeffrey D. Neill, M.D., New Britain, CT
Maureen A. O'Connor, New Haven, CT
Pat Richardson, M.S.N., Decatur, GA
Debra S. Ruchin, R.D., West Hartford, CT
Cynthia W. Sanborn, M.S.N., Charlottesville, VA
Robert Schwartz, M.D., Providence, RI
Brahm Shapiro, M.C., Ch.B., Ann Arbor, MI
Jean J. Spence, R.D., Spartanburg, NC
Supartondo, M.D., Jakarta, Indonesia
John L. Swarner, M.D., Valparaiso, IN
Catherine D. Treadow, R.N., Manchester, CT
Robert W. Tuman, Ph.D., Chalfont, PA
M. Antonia Verso, M.D., Phoenix, AZ
Barbara H. Ward, M.A., Riverside, CT
Kathleen L. Wishner, M. D., Duarte, CA
Ina M. Young, Ph.D., London, England
Barbara L. Zinaman, B.S.N., Brookline, MA

Potentiation of Insulin Secretion to Nonglucose Stimuli in Normal Man by Tolbutamide

MICHAEL A. PFEIFER, JEFFREY B. HALTER, RON GRAF, AND DANIEL PORTE, JR.

SUMMARY

To determine how sulfonylureas affect beta cell function, insulin release in response to isoproterenol and arginine was assessed in 32 normal subjects before and during a tolbutamide infusion. When the plasma glucose was allowed to decrease during tolbutamide, the acute insulin response (AIR) to isoproterenol was not changed (ΔAIR = −4 ± 8 μU/ml, $\bar{x}$ ± SEM, n = 8, p = NS) and was enhanced slightly for arginine (ΔAIR = +61 ± 26 μU/ml, n = 6, $p < 0.05$). When plasma glucose levels were maintained by means of a concomitant variable glucose infusion during tolbutamide, the insulin responses to both isoproterenol and arginine were enhanced (isoproterenol: ΔAIR = +55 ± 15 μU/ml, n = 6, $p < 0.001$; arginine: ΔAIR = +137 ± 34 μU/ml, n = 8, $p < 0.001$). Regression analysis demonstrated a linear relationship between change in the prestimulus glucose level and the change in the AIR to isoproterenol during tolbutamide (r = 0.66, n = 14, $p < 0.02$). Since the slope of this relationship is not significantly different from a similar relationship in the absence of tolbutamide, the potentiating effect of tolbutamide is an amplification of an established physiologic relationship. We conclude that tolbutamide augments the insulin response to nonglucose stimuli. However, this potentiating effect of tolbutamide may be masked by a decrease in the prestimulus glucose level. DIABETES *29*:335–340, May 1980.

Sulfonylureas have been reported to have direct effects on pancreatic insulin secretion,[1] hepatic glucose output,[2] peripheral glucose utilization,[3] and insulin receptors.[4] Since basal insulin levels[5,6] and secretory responses to various stimuli appear to be unchanged[7–11] during chronic administration of sulfonylureas, the insulinotrophic effects have been considered to be transient. Thus, the decrease of fasting glucose levels during chronic sulfonylurea therapy has been ascribed to the nonpancreatic effects of the drug.

However, there is evidence in vivo in man and in studies in vitro that islet responses to such nonglucose stimuli as isoproterenol,[12] arginine,[13] GIP,[14] VIP,[15] and secretin[16] are modulated by the glucose level to which the islet is exposed. We have recently demonstrated that the insulin-secretory response to the beta adrenergic agonist, isoproterenol, is markedly potentiated in man by elevation of the circulating glucose level and is inhibited when the plasma glucose level is lowered.[12] Therefore, assessment of the action of sulfonylureas at the pancreatic level must consider the influence of any change in glucose levels induced by the drug. This study was designed to determine if sulfonylureas can enhance insulin secretion in response to nonglucose stimuli and to determine the relationship of these effects to prestimulus glucose level. Tolbutamide was chosen as the sulfonylurea agent because of its ready availability for intravenous use.

MATERIALS AND METHODS

Subjects. Thirty-two lean male volunteers (% IBW = 106 ± 2; $\bar{x}$ ± SEM) were studied: Average age was 34 yr, with a range of from 23 to 61. None of the subjects were using any medications at the time of the study, and none had a history of cardiovascular disease. All subjects has fasting plasma glucose levels of less than 105 mg/dl (95 ± 1) and had no family history of diabetes mellitus. All subjects were studied after an overnight fast. No cigarette smoking was allowed on the day of the study. Aspirin and aspirin-containing products were not allowed for a period of at least one week before the studies. All subjects were on an ad libitum diet before the study. Informed consent was obtained from all subjects.

Study protocol. All studies were performed on a metabolic ward. A 19-gauge butterfly needle was introduced into both

From the Department of Medicine, University of Washington School of Medicine, Division of Endocrinology and Metabolism, and the Geriatric Research, Education, and Clinical Center of the Veterans' Administration Medical Center, Seattle, Washington.
Address reprint requests to Michael A. Pfeifer, M.D., Medical Research Service (151), Bldg. 13, Rm. 113, VA Medical Center, 4435 Beacon Ave. S., Seattle, WA 98108.
Received for publication 27 August and in revised form 26 November 1979.

antecubital veins and each was kept patent by a slow infusion of 0.9% sodium chloride. Venous samples were obtained from one line for laboratory analyses after the line had been cleared of saline by withdrawing and discarding 1.5 ml of blood. The other intravenous line was used for administration of the drugs used during the study.

Two insulin secretagogues were used: the beta-adrenergic agonist, isoproterenol, and the amino acid, arginine. Isoproterenol was given rapidly (less than 3 s) at a dose (12 μg) determined to be a maximal stimulus for acute insulin release in man.[17] The acute insulin response to isoproterenol was calculated as the mean increase above prestimulus plasma insulin levels at 2, 3, and 4 min after the isoproterenol pulse. In other studies, 5 g of L-arginine monohydrochloride solution (10%) was given rapidly (less than 15 s) intravenously. This dose has also been determined to be a maximal stimulus for insulin secretion in man.[13] The acute insulin response to arginine was calculated as the mean increase above prestimulus plasma insulin levels at 2, 3, 4, and 5 min after the administration of the amino acid.

In all studies, a 45-min basal period was followed by a pulse of a secretagogue (isoproterenol or arginine). Venous samples were taken rapidly during the first 10 min after the pulse and then less frequently for an additional 20 min. Thirty minutes after the first secretagogue pulse, an infusion of tolbutamide was begun at a rate of 7.0 mg/m²/min. This dose was chosen because it caused a 20% fall of venous glucose levels over a one-hour period in preliminary studies without stimulating an increase of plasma catecholamine levels. After one hour of this infusion, a second pulse of the secretagogue was given.

In some studies, a variable glucose infusion was administered concomitantly during the tolbutamide infusion to prevent a change of plasma glucose level. The glucose infusion was begun at 100 or 200 mg/min ten minutes after the beginning of the tolbutamide infusion. The infusion rate was subsequently adjusted at five-minute intervals, depending on the results of bedside plasma glucose measurements, with a Beckman glucose analyzer. These results were available within two minutes of the time of blood sampling. An empirically derived formula based on preliminary studies[12] was used for calculating the glucose infusion rate. This variable glucose infusion was continued for the 50 min before the second secretagogue pulse and then maintained at the last rate before the pulse for the duration of the study.

The effect of sequential pulses of isoproterenol on insulin responses was determined by substituting a saline infusion for the tolbutamide infusion in four subjects. Sequential 5 g arginine pulses have been shown to have no effect on arginine-induced insulin secretion.[13]

Serum tolbutamide concentrations were determined one hour after the initiation of the tolbutamide infusion in all subjects. These measurements were performed by the Upjohn Company by use of a gas-liquid chromatographic method.[18]

Samples for measurement of plasma catecholamines were obtained five minutes before and immediately preceding all secretagogue pulses. The mean of these two measurements was used for data analysis. Five milliliter samples for measurement of plasma immunoreactive insulin (IRI) and glucose were anticoagulated by ethylenediaminetetraacetic acid (EDTA), kept on ice until the plasma was separated by centrifugation at 4°C, and subsequently frozen at −20°C for analysis at a later time. Two and one-half milliliter samples for measurement of plasma catecholamines (norepinephrine and epinephrine) were collected in chilled tubes containing ethyleneglycoltetraacetic acid (EGTA) for anticoagulation and glutathione to prevent oxidation, kept on ice until the plasma was separated by double centrifugation at 4°C (within 30 min), and subsequently frozen at −20°C for analysis at a later time.

Analytic methods. Plasma IRI levels were measured by a modification of the double antibody method of Morgan and Lazarow.[19] Plasma glucose was measured with the AutoAnalyzer ferricyanide method (Technicon Instruments). Bedside plasma glucose levels were determined by a glucose oxidase method (Beckman Instruments), but these measurements were not used for data analysis. Plasma norepinephrine and epinephrine levels were measured by the single isotope enzymatic assay of Peuler and Johnson.[20] Statistical analyses included paired Student's *t*-test, covariance of analysis with regression, and an F-test for parallelism.

RESULTS

Isoproterenol studies. Figure 1 depicts the acute insulin response to isoproterenol before and during an infusion of tolbutamide. Plasma glucose was allowed to decline during tolbutamide administration in the studies. The tolbutamide infusion caused both a gradual decrease in glucose (Δ glucose = −27 ± 1 mg/dl, n = 8, $p < 0.001$) and a rise in insulin (Δ insulin = +8 ± 2 μU/ml, n = 8, $p < 0.01$). The plasma insulin levels plateaued by 30 min and remained stable until the second pulse. The plasma glucose during tolbutamide was not associated with an increase of plasma norepinephrine or epinephrine (Table 1). The mean acute insulin response to isoproterenol during tolbutamide was not significantly different from the response to the first pulse (ΔAIR = −4 ± 8 μU/ml, n = 8, p = NS; see Table 1). Table 1 also

FIGURE 1. Insulin responses to two sequential 12 μg pulses of isoproterenol without and then during a 7 mg/m²/min tolbutamide infusion in eight normal subjects. There was no significant change in the acute insulin response.

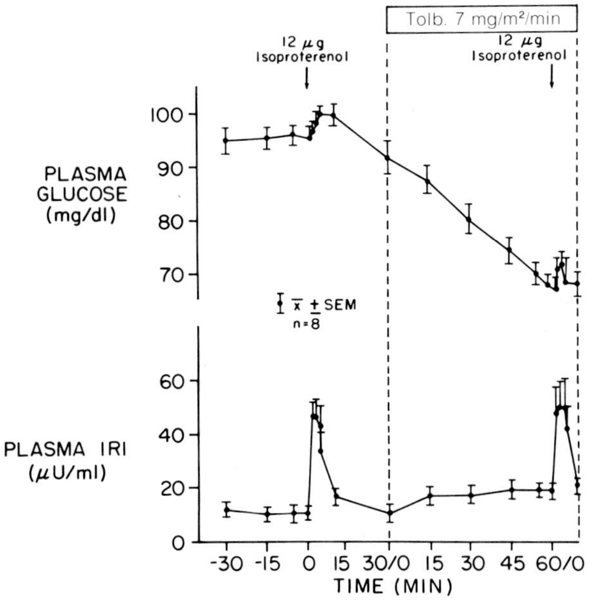

TABLE 1*
Glucose and insulin levels and responses to isoproterenol and arginine

	Prestimulus					Acute Insulin Response†
	Glucose (mg/dl)	IRI (μU/ml)	NE (pg/ml)	EPI (pg/ml)	TOLB (mg/dl)	(μU/ml)
Isoproterenol Studies						
Saline Protocol (n = 4)						
Baseline	98 ± 1	9 ± 2	231 ± 16	48 ± 9	—	39 ± 10
Saline	98 ± 2	9 ± 1	202 ± 24	40 ± 7	—	37 ± 9
p (saline vs. baseline)	NS	NS	NS	NS	—	NS
Tolbutamide Protocol (n = 8)						
Baseline	96 ± 1	11 ± 2	256 ± 38	77 ± 31	—	34 ± 6
Tolbutamide infusion	69 ± 2	19 ± 4	249 ± 28	54 ± 7	8.03 ± 0.96	30 ± 10
p (tolbutamide vs. baseline)	<0.001	<0.005	NS	NS	—	NS
Tolbutamide + Glucose Protocol (n = 6)						
Baseline	95 ± 1	10 ± 2	257 ± 43	41 ± 6	—	34 ± 6
Tolbutamide infusion + glucose	92 ± 5	36 ± 6	237 ± 32	38 ± 4	8.39 ± 1.06	89 ± 21
p (tolbutamide + glucose vs. baseline)	NS	<0.001	NS	NS	—	<0.001
p (tolbutamide + glucose vs. tolbutamide)	<0.005	<0.05	NS	NS	NS	<0.025
Arginine Studies						
Tolbutamide Protocol (n = 6)						
Baseline	96 ± 3	13 ± 2	343 ± 83	44 ± 15	—	47 ± 6
Tolbutamide infusion	74 ± 4	27 ± 3	391 ± 80	65 ± 26	8.05 ± 0.44	114 ± 20
p (tolbutamide vs. baseline)	<0.001	<0.001	NS	NS	—	<0.05
Tolbutamide + Glucose Protocol (n = 8)						
Baseline	93 ± 4	10 ± 3	285 ± 23	58 ± 7	—	44 ± 7
Tolbutamide infusion + glucose	95 ± 6	35 ± 8	334 ± 36	54 ± 9	7.59 ± 0.54	181 ± 20
p (tolbutamide + glucose vs. baseline)	NS	<0.001	NS	NS	—	<0.001
p (tolbutamide + glucose vs. tolbutamide)	<0.02	NS	NS	NS	NS	<0.05

* All values are $\bar{x}$ ± SEM
† $\bar{x}$ Δ 2-4′ IRI (isoproterenol studies)
$\bar{x}$ Δ 2-5′ IRI (arginine studies)

demonstrates that the insulin responses to sequential 12 μg isoproterenol pulses in the absence of tolbutamide are not significantly different (ΔAIR = −2 ± 3 μU/ml, n = 4, p = NS).

The effect of tolbutamide on isoproterenol-induced insulin secretion when the plasma glucose was maintained at basal levels by a variable glucose infusion (Δ glucose = −3 ± 5 mg/dl, n = 6, p = NS) is shown in Figure 2. There was an increase in insulin level during the combined infusion of tolbutamide and glucose, reaching a plateau by 30 min and remaining stable until the second pulse (Δ insulin = +25 ± 4 μU/ml, n = 6, p < 0.001). An increase of acute insulin response to isoproterenol (ΔAIR: +55 ± 15 μU/ml, n = 6, p < 0.001) occurred in all subjects during the tolbutamide infusion when compared with the baseline pulse (see Table 1).

There was no difference in the serum tolbutamide concentration during the tolbutamide alone infusion (8.03 ± 0.96 mg/dl, n = 8) and the combined infusion of tolbutamide and glucose (8.39 ± 1.06 mg/dl, n = 6, p = NS).

Regression analysis of the data from the studies with tolbutamide alone and tolbutamide plus variable glucose infusion demonstrates that a significant linear relationship exists between the change of glucose levels and the change of the acute insulin response to isoproterenol (r = 0.66, n = 14, p < 0.02, Figure 3). Therefore, the magnitude of the acute insulin response to isoproterenol during tolbutamide in normal subjects depends on the prestimulus level of glucose. In Figure 3, the regression line for the change in the acute insulin response to isoproterenol versus the change in the plasma glucose level for normal subjects in

FIGURE 2. Insulin responses to two sequential 12 μg pulses of isoproterenol without and, then, during a 7 mg/m²/min tolbutamide infusion in six normal subjects. Plasma glucose level during the tolbutamide infusion was maintained by a variable infusion of glucose and then continued at the last rate during the second pulse of isoproterenol. There was a significant increase in the AIR (p < 0.001).

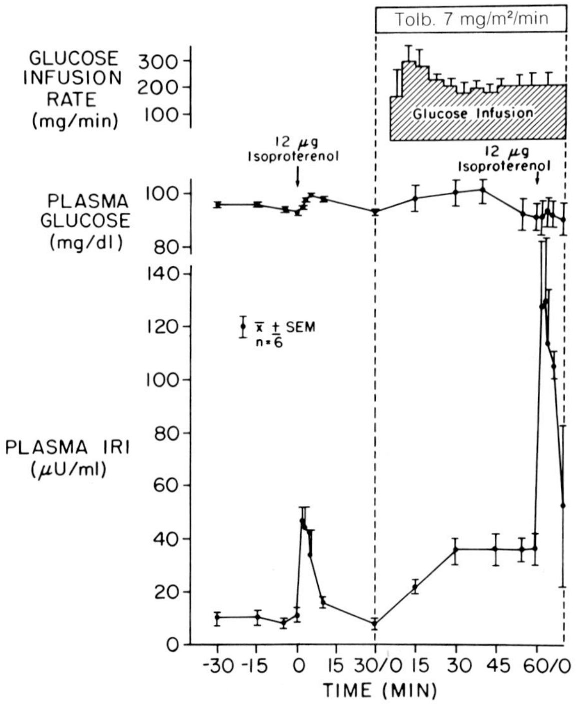

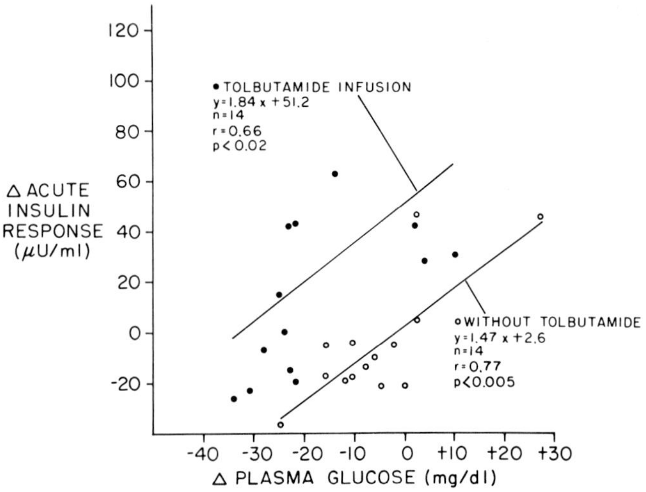

FIGURE 3. Regression lines for Δ plasma glucose (second pulse prestimulus level minus first pulse prestimulus level) vs. ΔAIR (second AIR − first AIR) with and without the presence of tolbutamide are compared.

the absence of tolbutamide, derived from our previous studies,[12] is compared with that obtained during the tolbutamide studies. The slopes of these regression lines are not significantly different (1.84 vs. 1.47, F = 0.24, p = NS), but the Y-axis intercepts are different (51.2 vs. 2.6, F = 18.44, $p < 0.01$).

Arginine studies. Similar studies were performed in 14 normal subjects using arginine as the secretagogue. The first pulse was once again followed by an infusion of tolbutamide (Figure 4) or tolbutamide plus glucose (Figure 5). The acute insulin response to arginine was enhanced by tolbutamide (ΔAIR = +61 ± 26 μU/ml, n = 6, p = 0.05) in spite of lower plasma glucose levels (Δ glucose = −22 ± 2 mg/dl, n = 6, $p < 0.001$). Further potentiation (ΔAIR = +137 ± 34 μU/ml, n = 8, p ± 0.001) was observed when plasma glucose levels were maintained at the basal level (Δ glucose = +2 ± 5 mg/dl, n = 8, p = NS). As shown in Table 1, no elevation of plasma catecholamines occurred during the arginine studies. The serum tolbutamide concentration was not significantly different in the two studies (tolbutamide = 8.04 ± 0.44 mg/dl, n = 6; tolbutamide and glucose = 7.59 ± 0.54 mg/dl, n = 8, p = NS).

FIGURE 4. Insulin responses to two sequential 5 g pulses of arginine are examined without and then during a 7 mg/m²/min infusion of tolbutamide in six normal subjects. An increase in the AIR was noted ($p < 0.05$).

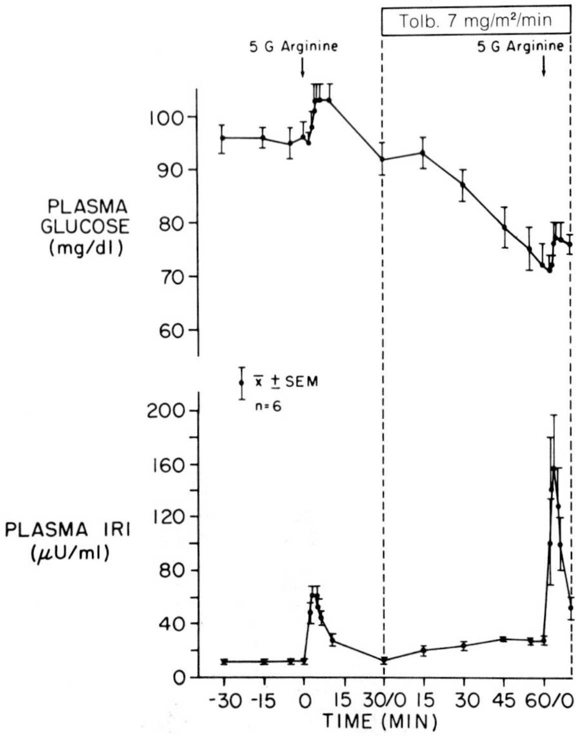

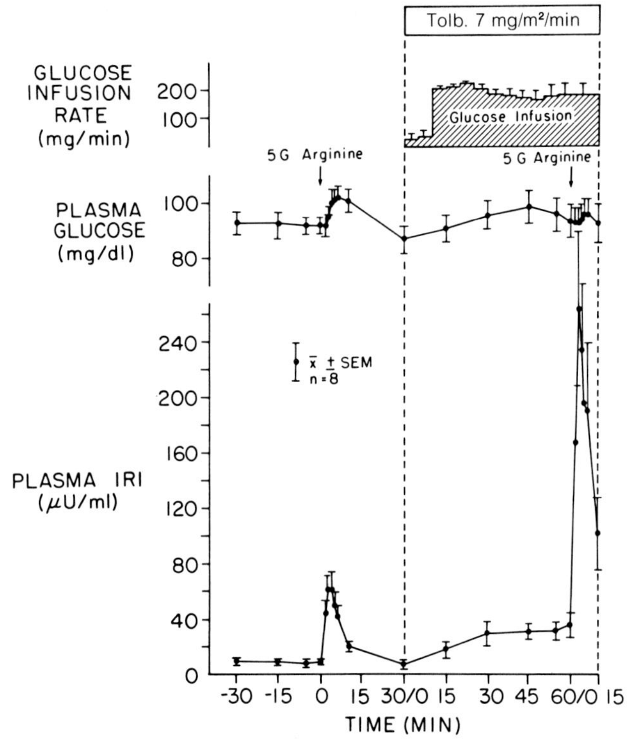

FIGURE 5. A similar protocol as in Figure 4 was performed. Plasma glucose level was maintained during the tolbutamide infusion by a concurrent variable glucose infusion and then continued at the last rate during the second pulse of arginine. A larger increase in the AIR was observed ($p < 0.05$) when compared with the protocol in Figure 4.

DISCUSSION

Studies in isolated perfused rat pancreas[21,22] and in vivo in normal man[23] have suggested that the effect of tolbutamide on insulin release depends on glucose. An examination of the insulin secretion data in Figure 1 appears to demonstrate that tolbutamide has no effect on isoproterenol-induced insulin secretion. However, the tolbutamide infusion also caused a decrease in prestimulus glucose levels. When glucose levels are maintained during the tolbutamide infusion (Figure 2), potentiation of the insulin responses occurs. The arginine studies add further validity to the concept that tolbutamide's effects on insulin release can be masked by accompanying falls of plasma glucose. Although there is a significant increase in AIR to arginine during the tolbutamide infusion (Figure 4), there was a greater increase in AIR when the glucose level was maintained

(Figure 5). Since the serum tolbutamide concentration and the plasma catecholamine levels are not significantly different, the augmentation is a result of the change in glucose level and not an alteration in adrenergic tone or an increase in tolbutamide level.

An alternative interpretation of these responses is that there is an increase of glucose uptake during the tolbutamide plus glucose study. This increase in intracellular glucose could be responsible for the increase in insulin secretion seen in these studies. However, in similar studies,[12] an infusion of insulin plus glucose showed no augmentation of the insulin response to isoproterenol. Thus, an increase in intracellular glucose is not responsible for the enhanced insulin responses observed when the plasma glucose is maintained.

Previous studies[12,13] have shown that insulin responses to isoproterenol and arginine depend on glucose in man. Figure 3 demonstrates that isoproterenol-induced insulin secretion is increased by tolbutamide at any level. Thus, even though there is no actual change in insulin secretion when tolbutamide is given alone, it is nonetheless greater than it would have been at the new lower glucose level; therefore, for that level of plasma glucose, there is a greater acute insulin response than would have occurred without tolbutamide being present.

It would appear that, like glucose, tolbutamide infusions can enhance nonglucose stimuli. The mechanism of this action is not known. Since the regression lines relating glucose level to the AIR to a nonglucose stimulus are parallel, it is possible that tolbutamide is simply amplifying the glucose potentiation signal. Alternatively, there is in vitro evidence that tolbutamide's effects are magnified at high glucose levels and are diminished at lower levels.[22] Such findings imply that the magnitude of the tolbutamide effect also depends on the level of glucose, suggesting a different mechanism of action for tolbutamide.

There has been much interest regarding the mechanism of the chronic effects of sulfonylurea therapy. Previous investigators have failed to find increases in basal insulin levels[5,6] or in insulin response to such secretagogues as standardized meals,[5,6,24] oral glucose,[7,8,25] intravenous tolbutamide,[11] or intravenous glucagon[11] during long-term treatment. Because of these findings, the direct effects of tolbutamide to alter hepatic glucose output,[2] peripheral glucose utilization,[3] insulin receptors,[4] and glucagon secretion[26,27] have been proposed to explain the lowered plasma glucose levels. However, the present studies suggest that important effects of sulfonylureas on islet function may have been overlooked when interpreting the insulin secretion studies. In diabetic as well as in normal subjects, insulin-secretory responses to a nonglucose stimulus depend on the circulating glucose level.[12] Thus, falls of plasma glucose accompanying chronic sulfonylurea therapy in diabetics could tend to mask insulin-secretory responses to nonglucose signals.

We hypothesize that long-term sulfonylurea use may continue to potentiate islet signals, thereby maintaining insulin responses, despite a fall in plasma glucose. Therefore, despite unchanged insulin levels, improved insulin-secretory ability may still contribute substantially to the sustained effectiveness of this drug in man. Studies of islet function during chronic sulfonylurea therapy will be required to further test this hypothesis.

ACKNOWLEDGMENTS

We wish to thank Mr. Howard Beiter, Ms. Barbara O'Neill, Ms. Karen Smith, and Ms. Connie Holmes for their technical assistance and Mrs. Pat Jenkins, Ms. Anne Bartlett, and Ms. Joanne Ebert for their secretarial assistance. We would also like to thank the Upjohn Company for measurement of the serum tolbutamide concentration and Mr. J. T. Keene and Mr. L. Helser of the Upjohn Company for their assistance.

This investigation was supported, in part, by a Public Health Service Special Emphasis Research Career Award (AM 00738-01) from the National Heart, Lung, and Blood Institute, by grants AM 12829, AM 20754, and AM 17047 from the National Institute of Arthritis, Metabolism, and Digestive Diseases, and by the Veterans' Administration.

REFERENCES

[1] Grodsky, G. M., Bennett, L. L., Smith, D., and Nemechek, K.: *In* Tolbutamide After Ten Years. New York, Excerpta Medica Foundation, 1967, p. 11.

[2] Tarding, F., and Schambaye, P.: The action of sulfonylureas and insulin on the glucose output from the liver of normal dogs. Endokrinologie *36*:223–28, 1958.

[3] Lebovitz, H. E., Feinglos, M. N., Bucholtz, H. K., and Lebovitz, F. L.: Potentiation of insulin action: a probable mechanism for the anti-diabetic action of sulfonylurea drugs. J. Clin. Endocrinol. Metab. *45*:601–04, 1977.

[4] Olefsky, J. M., and Reaven, G. M.: Effects of sulfonylurea therapy on insulin binding to mononuclear leukocytes of diabetic patients. Am. J. Med. *60*:89–95, 1976.

[5] Chu, P-C., Conway, M. J., Krouse, H. A., and Goodner, C. J.: The pattern of response of plasma insulin and glucose to meals and fasting during chlorpropamide therapy. Ann. Intern. Med. *68*:757–69, 1968.

[6] Shenfield, G. M., Logan, A., Shirling, D., and Baird, J.: Plasma insulin and glucose levels in maturity onset diabetics treated with chlorpropamide. Diabetologia *13*:367–71, 1977.

[7] Turtle, J. R.: Glucose and insulin secretory response patterns following diet and tolazamide therapy in diabetics. Br. Med. J. *3*:606–10, 1970.

[8] Reaven, G., and Dray, J.: Effect of chlorpropamide on serum glucose and immunoreactive insulin concentrations in patients with maturity-onset diabetes mellitus. Diabetes *16*:487–92, 1967.

[9] Sartor, G., Schersten, B., and Melander, A.: Effects of glipizide and food intake on the blood levels of glucose and insulin in diabetic patients. Acta Med. Scand. *203*:211–14, 1978.

[10] Seltzer, H. S., Allen, E. W., and Brennan, M. T.: Failure of prolonged sulfonylurea administration to enhance insulinogenic response to glycemic stimulus. Diabetes *14*:392–95, 1965.

[11] Barnes, A. J., Garbien, K. J. T., Crowley, M. F., and Bloom, A.: The effect of short and long term chlorpropamide treatment on insulin release and blood-glucose. Lancet *2*:69–72, 1974.

[12] Halter, J. B., Graf, R. J., and Porte, D., Jr.: Potentiation of insulin secretory responses by plasma glucose levels in man: evidence that hyperglycemia in diabetes compensates for impaired glucose potentiation. J. Clin. Endocrinol. Metab. *48*:946–54, 1979.

[13] Palmer, J. P., Walter, R. M., and Ensinck, J. W.: Arginine-stimulated acute phase of insulin and glucagon secretion. I. In normal man. Diabetes *24*:735–40, 1975.

[14] Dupre, J., Ross, S. A., Watson, D., and Brown, J. C.: Stimulation of insulin secretion by gastric inhibitory polypeptide in man. J. Clin. Endocrinol. Metab. *37*:826–28, 1973.

[15] Jensen, S. L., Fahrenkrug, J., Holst, J. J., Nielsen, O. V., and Schaffalitzky de Muckadell, O. B.: Secretory effects of VIP on isolated perfused porcine pancreas. Am. J. Physiol. *235*:E387–91, 1978.

[16] Lerner, R. L., and Porte, D., Jr.: Studies of secretin-stimulated insulin responses in man. J. Clin. Invest. *51*:2205–10, 1972.

[17] Halter, J. B., and Porte, D., Jr.: Mechanisms of impaired acute insulin release in adult onset diabetes: studies with isoproterenol and secretin. J. Clin. Endocrinol. Metab. *46*:952–60, 1978.

[18] Matin, S. B., and Rowland, M.: Determination of tolbutamide and chlorpropamide in biological fluids. J. Pharm. Pharmacol. *25*:186–88, 1973.

[19] Morgan, C. R., and Lazarow, A.: Immunoassay of insulin: two antibody system. Diabetes *12*:115–26, 1963.

[20] Peuler, J. D., and Johnson, G. A.: Simultaneous single isotope radioenzymatic assay of plasma norepinephrine, epinephrine and dopamine. Life Sci. *21*:625–36, 1977.

[21] Basabe, J. C., Lopez, N. L., Viktora, J. K., and Wolff, F. W.: Insulin secretion studied in the perfused rat pancreas. I. Effect of tolbutamide, leucine and arginine; their interaction with diazoxide, and relation to glucose. Diabetes *20*:449–56, 1971.

[22] Grodsky, G. M., Schmid, F. G., Manning, M., and Fanska, R.: Comparison of the independent and interrelated effects of glucose and sulfonylureas on insulin release in the perfused pancreas. *In* Pharmacology and the Future of Man. Proc. 5th Int. Congr. Pharmacol. *3*:230–38, 1972.

[23] Widström, A., and Cerasi, E.: On the action of tolbutamide in normal man. I. Role of adrenergic mechanisms in tolbutamide-induced insulin release during normoglycaemia and induced hypoglycaemia. Acta Endocrinol. (Copenhagen) *72*:506–18, 1973.

[24] Tsalikian, E., Dunphy, T. W., Bohannon, N. V., Lorenzi, M., Gerich, J. E., Forsham, P. H., Kane, J. P., and Karam, J. H.: The effect of chronic oral antidiabetic therapy on insulin and glucagon responses to a meal. Diabetes *26*:314–21, 1977.

[25] Sheldon, J., Taylor, K. W., and Anderson, J.: The effects of long-term acetohexamide treatment on pancreatic islet cell function in maturity-onset diabetes. Metabolism *15*:874–83, 1966.

[26] Samols, E., Tyler, J. M., and Mialhe, P.: Suppression of pancreatic glucagon release by the hypoglycaemic sulphonylureas. Lancet *1*:174–76, 1969.

[27] Grodsky, G. M., Epstein, G. H., Fanska, R., and Karam, J. H.: Pancreatic action of the sulfonylureas. Fed. Proc. *36*:2714–19, 1977.

Effects of Intraportal Islet Transplantation on the Transplanted Tissue and the Recipient Pancreas

I. Functional Studies

E. R. TRIMBLE, C. KARAKASH, F. MALAISSE-LAGAE, I. VASSUTINE, L. ORCI, AND A. E. RENOLD

SUMMARY

It is well known that, in diabetes, there is an abnormality of both pancreatic beta and alpha cell secretion. Since islet transplantation can markedly improve the diabetic state in streptozotocin-treated rats, we investigated the effects of intraportal transplantation on the beta and alpha cell secretion of the transplanted tissue. In addition we examined the effects of transplantation on the hormone content of both the transplanted tissue and the endogenous pancreas.

Animals were examined 6 and 20 wk after transplantation. Isolated perfusions of the islet-containing livers showed that both glucagon and insulin secretion could be promptly stimulated by arginine. The hormone content of the livers at death revealed that, while the insulin content of transplanted tissue was well maintained, there was a marked reduction in glucagon content. An increase in pancreatic glucagon content was found in rats with untreated diabetes of five months' duration; this was partially or fully prevented by islet transplantation. There was also a moderate increase in insulin content of the pancreases of animals that received islet transplants. DIABETES 29:341–347, May 1980.

In preliminary experiments carried out in this laboratory, it was noted that intraportally transplanted islets appeared to contain fewer glucagon-containing cells than islets within the normal pancreas. By contrast, increased glucagon content of pancreatic islets has been reported in streptozotocin diabetes.[1] Accordingly, we have undertaken a more detailed study of the changes occurring after transplantation in the glucagon and insulin content of both the transplanted islets and the pancreas of streptozotocin-diabetic rats. In addition, we used the isolated perfused liver system to make a direct assessment of the glucagon- and insulin-secretory capacity of the intraportally transplanted islets, since it is not clear how transplanted islets, which probably remain denervated,[2] should behave in an in vitro perfusion system. In vivo, selective denervation of the pancreas in otherwise intact dogs leads to reduced secretion of glucagon.[3] Furthermore, previous work suggested that insulin, but not glucagon, is secreted by intraportally transplanted rat islets,[4] even though measurable amounts of glucagon have been found in the venous outflow from allotransplanted pancreases of dogs in the early posttransplant period.[5,6]

MATERIALS AND METHODS

Animals. Inbred male Wistar-Lewis rats, obtained from the Charles River Breeding Laboratories, Wilmington, Mass., were used throughout. Animals, weighing 200–240 g, were made diabetic by the intravenous injection of streptozotocin (35–40 mg/kg) freshly dissolved in acidified saline (pH 4.5). Control animals received an intravenous injection of acidified saline. The injections were carried out under light ether anesthesia 12–16 h after food was withdrawn. The rats were kept singly in metabolic cages with free access to food and water. In general, there was at least a 3 wk period between streptozotocin injection and islet transplantation or sham operation.

Islets were isolated from donor rats, weighing 180–260 g, using a modification of the collagenase technique of Lacy and Kostianovsky.[7] After handpicking, the islets were suspended in modified Krebs-Ringer bicarbonate buffer. This buffer contained Na^+ 145.6, K^+ 6.0, Ca^{++} 2.0, Mg^{++} 2.4, Cl^- 127.8, PO_4^{--} 1.2, SO_4^{--} 2.4, HCO_3^- 24.6 meq per liter. To this was added glucose (5.5 mM) and bovine serum albumin (1%). An aliquot was taken from each batch of islets for measurement of the acid ethanol–extractable insulin and glucagon content (see below). After this, a known number of

Presented in part at the 28th Annual Meeting of the American Diabetes Association, June 1978, and published in abstract form in DIABETES *27* (Suppl. 2):440, 1978.
From the Institut de Biochimie Clinique, University of Geneva, Switzerland, the Laboratoires de Recherches Médicales, University of Geneva, Geneva, Switzerland, and the Institut d'Histologie et d'Embryologie, Medical School, University of Geneva, Switzerland.
Address reprint requests to E. R. Trimble, M.D., Institut de Biochimie Clinique, Sentier de la Roseraie, 1211 Geneva 4, Switzerland.
Received for publication 10 September and in revised form 14 December 1979.

islets (950–1200) was placed in a siliconized glass syringe with 0.2–0.3 ml modified Krebs-Ringer bicarbonate buffer. The syringe was then joined to a fine catheter, which terminated in a 23-F.G.* needle through which the islets were expelled into the portal vein. In some experiments, islets were directed to the right hepatic lobe by placing a clamp on the portal vein branches to the median, left, and caudate lobes immediately before discharging the islets. The concentration of islets in the right hepatic lobe in some experiments was carried out to facilitate subsequent morphometric immunocytochemical analysis of the transplanted tissue (to be reported elsewhere). After islet injection, the syringe, catheter, and needle were repeatedly flushed out with buffer. The islets that escaped injection, usually few in number, were counted so that the number of islets actually transplanted could be calculated. The time from killing the first donor until injection of islets was usually less than two hours.

For four of the transplantations to the right hepatic lobe, islets maintained for 46 h under tissue culture conditions were used instead of freshly isolated islets. The Eagle's minimal essential medium used for maintenance contained 10% heat-inactivated calf serum, 14 mM $NaHCO_3$, 8.3 mM glucose, 400 IU/ml sodium penicillin G, and 200 μg/ml streptomycin sulfate. The islets were placed in sterile plastic Petri dishes and kept at 37°C in an incubator gassed with an air-CO_2 mixture. The islets did not attach to the Petri dish and remained as individual islets throughout the 46-h maintenance period. At the end of this time the islets were washed with and suspended in Krebs-Ringer bicarbonate buffer and subsequently handled in the same way as islets transplanted immediately after collagenase isolation. Nondiabetic and diabetic control rats received an intraportal injection of Krebs buffer at sham operation.

After operation the urinary volume was measured daily for 7–14 days and at weekly intervals thereafter. Weight was measured at weekly intervals.

Intravenous glucose tolerance tests (i.v. GTT). The glucose dose was 0.5 g/kg. The tests were carried out on transplanted and nondiabetic control rats under sodium pentobarbital anesthesia, after 12–16 h of food withdrawal, during either the 6th or 20th week after operation. Blood samples obtained from the tail vein at 0, 5, 15, 30, and 45 min were used for measurement of plasma glucose and insulin concentrations.

Liver perfusions. Animals were anesthetized by intraperitoneal injection of pentobarbital and the liver was perfused in situ according to the method described by Assimacopoulos-Jeannet and colleagues.[8] The livers were perfused at a rate of 15 ml/min with Krebs-Ringer bicarbonate buffer, containing 3% dialyzed bovine serum albumin, 40% washed bovine erythrocytes, and Trasylol 250 KIU/ml, using the single flow-through technique. The basal buffer contained glucose 2.8 mM and was perfused during 30 min. Samples from the last 10 min of this period were taken for estimation of basal insulin and glucagon secretion rates. For the next 30 min arginine monohydrochloride 20 mM was added to the perfusate, following which the basal perfusate was reintroduced. Samples were immediately cooled to 4°C, centrifuged to remove the bovine erythrocytes, and stored at −20°C until the time of insulin and glucagon immunoassay.

Insulin and glucagon were measured at minute intervals during the basal period and the first 15 min of arginine stimulation; thereafter the measurements were made at five minute intervals.

Liver, pancreas, and islet extraction for the determination of insulin and glucagon content. Immediately after death the livers and pancreases were removed and insulin and glucagon were extracted by a modification of the Kenny technique.[9] The weighed tissues were placed in ice-cold acidified ethanol (0.7 M HCl/ethanol, 1:3 v/v) and homogenized. Twenty-four hours later the supernatant was decanted and tissue was resuspended in acidified ethanol for a similar time. The supernatants from each sample were pooled and kept at −20°C until hormonal measurements were performed, usually within 2–3 days of the time of extraction. Acidified ethanol was also used for the extraction of insulin and glucagon from the isolated islets.[10]

Assays. Plasma glucose concentrations were measured by the glucose oxidase method,[11] and insulin and glucagon by the method of Herbert et al.[12] Rat insulin standard and guinea-pig anti-pork insulin serum were used in the insulin assay. For the assay of glucagon, a pork glucagon standard and 30K antiserum were used. The minimum sensitivity of the insulin assay was 50 pg/ml and of the glucagon assay, 7 pg/ml.

Materials. Streptozotocin was a gift from Dr. W. J. Dulin, the Upjohn Company, Kalamazoo, Mich., and collagenase was obtained from Worthington Biochemical Corp., Freehold, N.J. Sodium penicillin G and streptomycin sulfate were bought from Chas. Pfizer and Co., N.Y., and Novo Industri A.S., Copenhagen, Denmark, respectively. Rat insulin was obtained from Dr. J. Schlichtkrull, Novo Research Institute, Bagsvaerd, Denmark, and guinea-pig anti-pork insulin serum was a gift from Dr. P. Wright, University of Indiana, Indianapolis. Pork glucagon standard was purchased from Novo Industri A.S., Copenhagen, Denmark, and 30K antiserum from Dr. Roger Unger, University of Texas Health Sciences Center, Dallas, Texas.

Statistics. Student's unpaired *t* test was used to evaluate differences between groups.

RESULTS

Urine volume. The diabetic rats used for transplantation or sham operation had preoperative urinary volumes of 110 ± 7 ml/24 h ($\bar{x}$ ± SEM) (range, 90–140 ml). In transplanted animals, this fell to 12 ± 2 ml two days after transplantation and to 6 ± 1 ml at two weeks. Thereafter the urinary volume remained stable until the time of killing at either 6 or 20 wk after transplantation. The urinary volume of nondiabetic rats was within the range 0.5 to 10 ml/24 h.

Weight gain (table 1). The net weight gain for the transplanted rats and the nondiabetic and diabetic control groups, from the time of transplantation or sham operation until death, is shown separately for those animals killed at 6 wk and those at 20 wk.

Random preoperative plasma glucose concentrations. Random nonfasting, midmorning plasma glucose concentration of the diabetic rats (before transplantation or sham operation) was 587 ± 20 mg/dl. The range for nondiabetic rats was 120–165 mg/dl (mean, 151 mg/dl).

* F.G. = French gauge.

TABLE 1
Net weight gain per rat between transplantation or sham operation and death (g, X̄ ± SEM). Parentheses indicate number of animals in each group.

	Transplanted animals	Nondiabetic controls	Diabetic controls
6 wk group	76 ± 3 (7)	78 ± 7 (7)	6 ± 4 (8)
20 wk group	175 ± 15 (8)	188 ± 16 (7)	17 ± 9 (5)

Intravenous glucose tolerance (table 2). Results are shown for 12 animals with islets transplanted to the right hepatic lobe, 3 animals with islets transplanted throughout the liver, and 12 nondiabetic controls. The test was carried out during the 6th postoperative week on five control rats and seven with islets transplanted to the right hepatic lobe; the remainder were tested during the 20th postoperative week. At no time during the i.v. G.T.T. did the plasma glucose values of the animals tested during the 6th week differ from those tested during the 20th week either in the control group or in the group with islets transplanted to the right hepatic lobe. In addition, the glucose tolerance of those animals that received islets maintained under tissue culture conditions before transplantation to the right hepatic lobe (n = 4, two tested at 6 and two tested at 20 wk) was similar to the glucose tolerance of those that received transplants of freshly isolated islets. On account of this the results for all rats receiving islets to the right hepatic lobe (n = 12) have been shown as one group. Fasting plasma glucose was normalized in animals with islets transplanted either to the right hepatic lobe or throughout the liver, although glucose tolerance was not fully normalized in either group. Fasting plasma insulin was normalized in rats with islets transplanted either to the right hepatic lobe or throughout the liver. However, the plasma insulin concentrations measured at 5 and 15 min were significantly higher in nondiabetic controls than in either of the transplanted groups; at 30 and 45 min there was no significant difference among the plasma insulin concentrations of the nondiabetic control and the two islet-transplanted groups.

Liver perfusions (figure 1). Perfusions were performed on seven rats with islets transplanted to the right hepatic lobe. Three perfusions were done during the 6th posttransplant week and four during the 20th week. No statistical difference was found between the secretion rates of either insulin or glucagon at these two postoperative times; hence the results have been pooled.

Arginine was used as the stimulus so that the stimulated output of both insulin and glucagon could be measured. Prompt stimulation of insulin secretion was obtained after exposure of the liver to perfusate containing arginine 20 mM. The insulin secretion rate in the first 10–15 min achieved a level approximately five times the basal rate. During 30 min of stimulation by arginine, approximately 2.4% of the total liver content of insulin was released. Prompt stimulation of glucagon secretion by arginine also occurred, with a clear falloff in secretion rate when arginine was withdrawn. The stimulated secretion rate was approximately twice that of the basal rate, and 1.5% of the total liver content of glucagon was secreted during the 30 min stimulation period. In control experiments, livers from nondiabetic control rats were perfused with glucagon, 250 pg/ml, in the presence of Trasylol, 250 KIU/ml. The recovery of glucagon in the perfusate after one passage through the liver was 104 ± 5% (n = 4). In the absence of Trasylol, glucagon recovery was only 83 ± 3% (n = 4). Trasylol did not prevent insulin degradation by the liver, which averaged 35% during a single transhepatic passage.

TABLE 2
Intravenous glucose tolerance tests (glucose 0.5 g/kg)

	Group	Time (minutes) 0′	5′	15′	30′	45′
Glucose (mg/dl, X̄ ± SEM)	Nondiabetic* (n = 12)	132 ± 3	382 ± 18	264 ± 13	177 ± 11	151 ± 7
	Transplant to*† right hepatic lobe (n = 12)	117 ± 6	361 ± 7	273 ± 8‡	240 ± 9∥	198 ± 13§
	Transplant throughout liver (n = 3)	122 ± 3	405 ± 26	321 ± 13∥	283 ± 2∥	248 ± 7∥
Insulin (ng/ml, X̄ ± SEM)	Nondiabetic (n = 12)	0.93 ± 0.14	4.83 ± 0.60	2.90 ± 0.42	1.87 ± 0.50	1.61 ± 0.25
	Transplant to right hepatic lobe (n = 12)	0.76 ± 0.09	1.56 ± 0.23∥	1.46 ± 0.18‡	1.43 ± 0.13	1.40 ± 0.15
	Transplant throughout liver (n = 3)	0.40 ± 0.10	0.90 ± 0.15§	0.82 ± 0.03‡	1.07 ± 0.12	1.03 ± 0.28

* Since the glucose tolerance of the animals tested 6 wk after sham operation or islet transplantation was similar to that of animals tested at 20 wk, the results for animals tested at 6 and 20 wk after operation have been pooled.
† This group includes animals receiving transplants of freshly isolated islets or islets maintained under tissue culture conditions before transplantation; the glucose tolerance of the two subgroups was similar and the results have, therefore, been pooled.
Comparison with nondiabetic controls: ‡ $p < 0.05$, § $p < 0.005$, and ∥ $p < 0.001$.

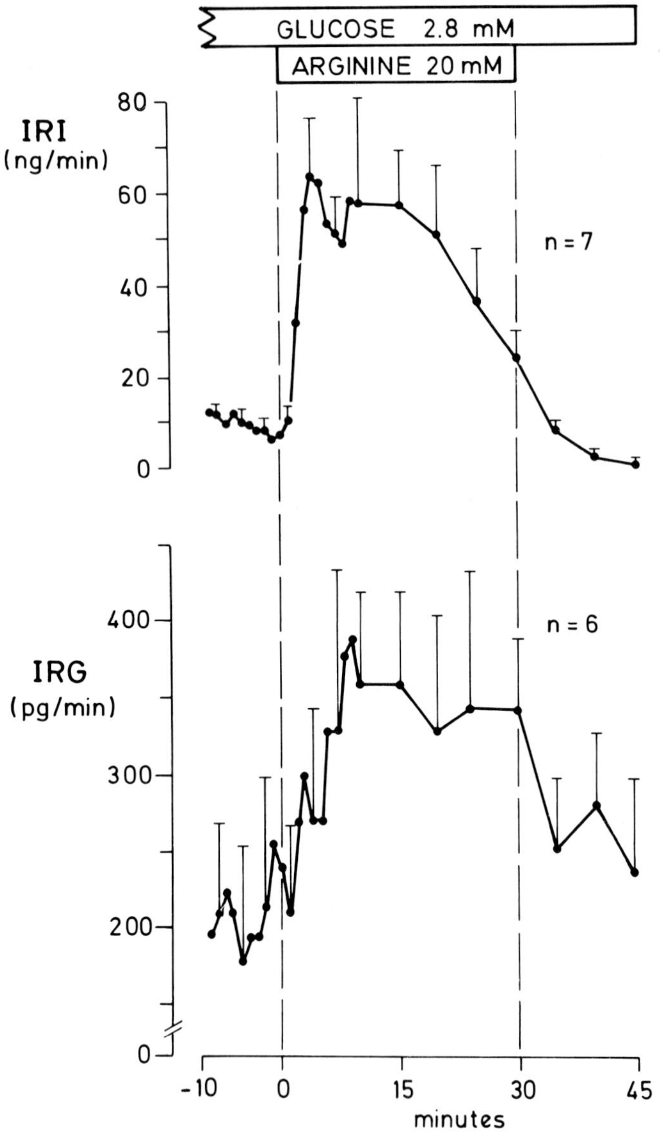

FIGURE 1. Insulin and glucagon secretion rates from perfused livers containing transplanted pancreatic islets (x̄ ± SEM). The livers were perfused for 30 min (−30–0 min) with basal perfusate containing glucose 2.8 mM. Basal samples were collected during the last 10 min of this period. Arginine monohydrochloride 20 mM was added to the perfusate for the nex 30 min (0–30 min). Following this the livers were again perfused with the basal perfusate for 15 min.

Insulin and glucagon content of isolated islets. The mean insulin and glucagon content of freshly isolated islets in this series was 63.6 ng and 5.1 ng, respectively, per islet. (For animals receiving islets throughout the liver, n = 3, the mean islet insulin content was 33.7 ng per islet, which was lower than the mean for the total group.) After 2 days' maintenance under tissue culture conditions the mean islet content was 12.4 ng and 1.4 ng for insulin and glucagon, respectively. However, it will be shown below that the hormone content of these two tissues became similar following transplantation.

Insulin and glucagon content of islets transplanted into the liver. Table 3 shows the hormone content of the liver at the time of death (a) in absolute terms and (b) as a percentage of the calculated total hormonal content of the number of islets transplanted per animal. For this calculation the mean insulin content of freshly isolated islets in this series was used. Thus it can be seen that the insulin contents of the livers at the time of killing were 70–90% of the content of the equivalent number of freshly isolated islets these animals received. Those animals that received islets after 2 days' maintenance under tissue culture conditions had hepatic insulin and glucagon contents in the same range as the animals that received freshly isolated islets. If the assumption is made that all islets which were transplanted survived until the animal was killed, the mean insulin content per transplanted islet fell from 63.6 ng to 46.1 ± 6.6 ng (n = 8) in animals receiving freshly isolated islets, and it rose from 12.4 ng to 56.4 ± 12.8 ng per islet (n = 4) in animals receiving tissue culture–maintained islets, respectively (the final content per islet equivalent was not statistically different between the two groups). This clearly indicates that the loss of insulin content which occurred during the tissue culture maintenance period (see previous section) was largely reversed after the islets were implanted in the liver.

TABLE 3
Insulin and glucagon content of the liver of transplanted rats at the time of killing (X̄ ± SEM).

Time of killing after transplantation	Group	No. of animals	Insulin (μg)*	Glucagon (μg)
6 wk	Transplant to right lobe liver	4	49.6 ± 9.6 (68%)†	0.8 ± 0.2 (12%)
20 wk	Transplant to right lobe liver	5	55.1 ± 10.2 (92%)	0.7 ± 0.1 (19%)
	Transplant throughout liver	3	29.7 ± 0.2 (86%)‡	

* Hormonal content in micrograms extracted from the whole liver.
† Parentheses denote the hormonal content of the liver compared with the content of the equivalent number of freshly isolated islets that the animals received.
‡ The mean insulin content of freshly isolated islets transplanted into this subgroup was less than that for the transplant series as a whole (the mean content was 33.7 ng per islet for this subgroup, whereas the mean content for the series as a whole was 63.6 ng per islet).

Calculations done from glucagon contents of transplanted livers showed that the content fell to 12–19% of the calculated initial value, using the content of freshly isolated islets to make the calculation. Thus, again assuming that all islets survived, the glucagon content per islet fell from 5.1 ng to 0.72 ± 0.12 ng (n = 8) in animals receiving freshly isolated islet transplants and from 1.4 ng to 0.72 ± 0.17 ng (n = 4) in animals receiving tissue culture–maintained islets.

PANCREATIC INSULIN AND GLUCAGON CONTENT

Insulin (Figure 2)

Nondiabetic control rats

The insulin content per pancreas was 125.5 ± 16.4 μg at 6 wk and 172.8 ± 15.6 μg 20 wk after sham operation.

Untreated diabetic control rats

The pancreases contained insulin 3.6 ± 0.8 μg at 6 wk and 2.8 ± 0.6 μg at 20 wk after sham operation (2.8% and 1.6%, respectively, of the nondiabetic control values for these time points).

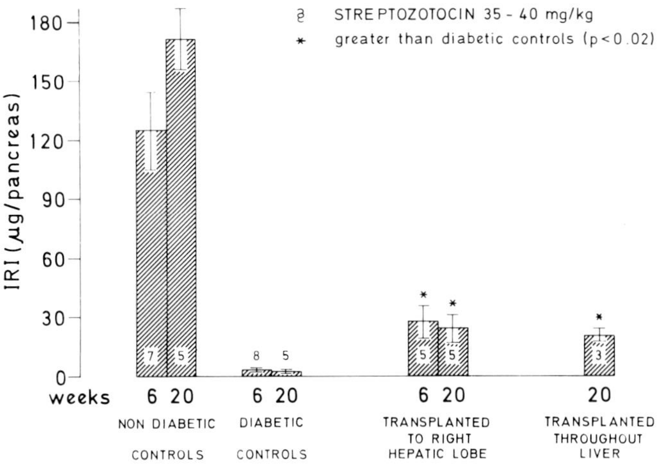

FIGURE 2. Pancreatic insulin content 6 or 20 wk after intraportal islet transplantation in streptozotocin-diabetic§ rats or after sham operation in nondiabetic and untreated diabetic controls ($\bar{x} \pm$ SEM).

Diabetic rats treated by islet transplantation

In all, 12 rats had islets transplanted to the right hepatic lobe. Four of seven killed at 6 wk and five of five killed at 20 wk had pancreatic hormonal extractions done. The insulin content at 6 wk was 27.7 ± 8.5 μg and, at 20 wk, it was 23.9 ± 6.9 μg per pancreas.

Three animals had islets transplanted throughout the liver. They were killed twenty weeks later, when the insulin content per pancreas was 20.2 ± 3.5 μg.

Glucagon (Figure 3)

Nondiabetic controls

Pancreatic glucagon content 6 wk after sham operation was similar to that at 20 wk (7.7 ± 1.1 μg and 7.6 ± 0.6 μg, respectively).

Untreated diabetic control rats

The pancreatic glucagon contents at 6 and 20 wk after sham operation were 8.7 ± 0.6 μg and 14.4 ± 3.1 μg, respectively, the latter result being significantly greater than that of the nondiabetic control animals of the same age.

Diabetic rats treated by islet transplantation

At the 6 wk time point the pancreases contained glucagon 2.4 ± 0.8 μg, which was significantly less than either age-matched nondiabetic or diabetic controls. At 20 wk the pancreases of rats with islets transplanted to the right hepatic lobe had a glucagon content of 6.7 ± 0.8 μg, which was significantly less than that of the diabetic controls and was similar to that of the nondiabetic controls. The three rats with islets transplanted throughout the liver had pancreatic glucagon contents which were midway between those of the nondiabetic and those of the diabetic controls.

FIGURE 3. Pancreatic glucagon content 6 or 20 wk after intraportal islet transplantation in streptozotocin-diabetic§ rats or after sham operation in nondiabetic and untreated diabetic controls ($\bar{x} \pm$ SEM).

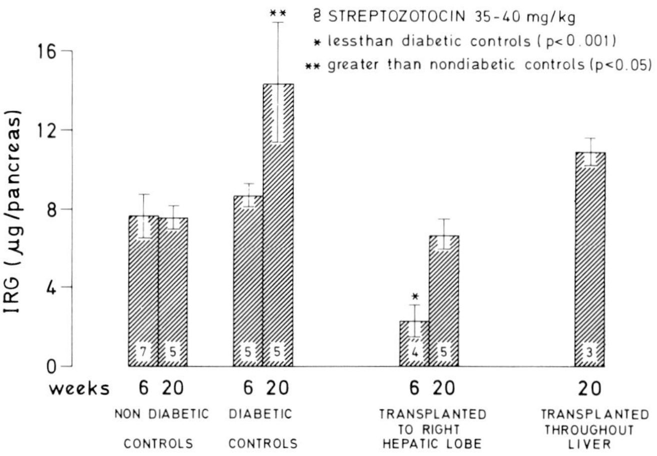

DISCUSSION

Transplantation of about 1000 islets resulted in normalization of body weight gain and of fasting plasma glucose and fasting plasma insulin concentrations. Intravenous glucose tolerance was not fully normalized, however, either in those rats with islets transplanted throughout the liver or in those with islets transplanted to the right hepatic lobe. In general terms, the effects of islet transplantation were similar whether the islets were concentrated in the right hepatic lobe or transplanted throughout the liver, except that the glucose tolerance of the former group was somewhat better than that of the latter. For those animals in which islets were transplanted throughout the liver, the mean insulin content of donor islets at the moment of transplantation was less than for those animals in which transplanted islets were concentrated in the right hepatic lobe. The amount of insulin, in absolute terms, extracted from the livers of this latter group was greater than that from the former group (see Table 3), which fact may at least partly explain the differences in glucose tolerance and glucose-induced insulin secretion found between the groups.

The insulin and glucagon content of islet tissue transplanted into the liver was similar, at the end of the experiment, in those rats that received freshly isolated islets and in those that received islets maintained under tissue culture conditions for 2 days before transplantation. The insulin and glucagon contents of islets maintained under tissue culture conditions were, at the time of transplantation, only 20–30% of those of freshly isolated islets. The reported changes in insulin content of islets maintained under tissue culture conditions have been variable.[13,14] In our laboratory, the insulin content, which is reduced after 2 days' maintenance, is partially or fully restored when the maintenance period is prolonged to 6 days.[10] This suggests that, under the conditions described, the initial loss of hormone content is caused by environmental factors and not by death of tissue. Moreover, the present results show restoration of insulin content to such tissue after transplantation. The peripherally located alpha cells of the islet are theoretically at greater risk from damage by collagenase digestion than are the more centrally located beta cells. It is not possible to be sure whether the fall in glucagon content during the maintenance period was caused by the culture conditions or was the result of damage by collagenase. The decrease by a further 50% in glucagon content of maintained islets after transplantation may be a result of such factors as even minimal damage by foreign-body–type fibrous reaction or to a feedback mechanism regulating total glucagon reserve.[15] The reported effects of implantation on tissue transplanted from adult animals have been variable,[15,16] with maintenance of or marked decrease in either insulin or glucagon contents being described.

Our liver perfusion results indicate that both the alpha

and beta cells of transplanted islets continue to secrete hormone and respond rapidly to arginine stimulation. These results differ from those of Charles et al.,[4] who, using a similar transplantation and perfusion system, found arginine to stimulate insulin but not glucagon secretion. These workers were also unable to detect basal glucagon secretion. However, like Charles et al., we have not demonstrated clear biphasicity of insulin and glucagon secretion from the transplanted tissue. Apart from those who have measured glucagon secretion in the venous outflow of pancreatic allotransplants in the early postoperative period,[5,6] there has been a report of glucagon secretion by the sheep pancreas autotransplanted to the neck.[17] In the latter report, glucagon secretion has been documented for periods of up to 4 yr after transplantation.

Since it has been reported that intraportally transplanted islets lodge mainly in the terminal radicles of the portal vein and are in close contact with hepatocytes,[18] it is probable that the insulin concentration measured in the hepatic effluent was somewhat less than the total amount secreted (since insulin is partially degraded by the liver), but that the glucagon measured represented the total amount released by the transplanted tissue. It is extremely difficult to decide the most appropriate comparison for secretion rates under these conditions. We have calculated that 2.4% and 1.5% of the total liver content of insulin and glucagon, respectively, were collected in the effluent during the 30 min stimulation with arginine. The amount of insulin and glucagon secreted by freshly isolated, perifused islets in the presence of the same glucose and arginine concentrations during 30 min was 1–3% of content (unpublished observations). The amount of insulin and glucagon secreted from the in vitro perfused transplanted islets would, therefore, appear to be similar to the secretion rates for freshly isolated islets under the conditions described here. However, since intraportally transplanted islets probably remain denervated[2] and selective denervation of the pancreas alone causes a marked reduction in plasma glucagon concentrations,[3] the amount of glucagon secreted from the islet-transplanted liver in vivo may be rather small. By contrast, selective denervation has much less effect on plasma insulin concentrations and, therefore, possibly less effect on in vivo insulin secretion from transplanted islets.

Streptozotocin-induced diabetes was associated with marked changes within the pancreas some of which were altered by intraportal islet transplantation. In streptozotocin diabetes, there is not only a reduction in the insulin content of the pancreatic islet, but also an increase of its glucagon content.[1] The total glucagon content of the pancreas in untreated diabetes has been reported to be normal,[15] increased,[16] or initially low with later restoration towards the normal.[19] When we measured the glucagon content of the whole pancreas, we found an increase in the total content in those animals with diabetes of five months' duration. This increase in total pancreatic glucagon content was either partially or fully prevented by intraportal islet transplantation. This would appear to be analogous to the reported effects of transplantation on plasma glucagon concentrations in diabetes, where normal levels were restored after transplantation,[4,15] except when the amount of tissue transplanted was much greater than the equivalent of an adult pancreas,[20] in which case both hyperinsulinemia and hyperglucagonemia were found after transplantation. Those animals killed 6 wk after transplantation had reduced pancreatic glucagon content compared with age-matched nondiabetic controls. A reduction in pancreatic glucagon content was seen 6 wk after the subcutaneous transplantation of duct-ligated pancreases into streptozotocin-diabetic mice[16] and also after intraportal transplantation of islets into streptozotocin-diabetic Lewis rats by Pipeleers-Marichal et al.[15] The latter group has already suggested the existence of a feedback mechanism regulating pancreatic glucagon content. If this is the case the effects in our series were seen most markedly in the pancreases of those animals killed 6 wk after transplantation. Reduction in glucagon content of transplanted tissue, however, could have arisen for any number of reasons, which have already been discussed above.

There were no spontaneous recoveries from diabetes in the diabetic control groups. At death 6 wk or 20 wk after sham operation, the pancreatic insulin content of untreated diabetic rats was 2% and 1% of age-matched nondiabetic controls, respectively. It is clear that the effect of the intravenous injection of streptozotocin (35–40 mg/kg) depends on many variables, one of which is probably the strain of rat. While this dose caused severe diabetes associated with weight loss in one strain,[21] the same dose in another strain caused a milder diabetes where weight gain was only reduced by 50%.[22] The effect of streptozotocin in the Wistar-Lewis strain was to give a moderately severe diabetes where the untreated diabetic rats were just able to maintain their body weight. However, *all* beta cells were not killed by the streptozotocin treatment, since some pancreatic insulin was measurable in untreated diabetic controls and the pancreatic insulin content increased after transplantation. Furthermore, the ability of streptozotocin to cause beta cell destruction is related to the dose.[22] Using a higher dose of streptozotocin (50 mg/kg) in the same strain of rat, we also found an increased pancreatic insulin content after successful islet transplantation but the phenomenon was less marked (mean pancreatic insulin content of untreated diabetic controls was 0.5 μg and that of transplanted rats, 2.5 μg, unpublished observations). The reported effect of successful pancreatic endocrine transplantation on the insulin content of the recipient pancreas has been to increase it[23] or to leave it unchanged.[15]

In conclusion, we have found that (1) both glucagon and insulin secretion could be stimulated from intraportally transplanted pancreatic islets, (2) after transplantation there was a reduction in the glucagon content of the transplanted tissue while the insulin content was better maintained, and (3) treatment by islet transplantation could partially or fully prevent the increase in pancreatic glucagon content associated with long-standing streptozotocin diabetes of moderate severity in the Wistar-Lewis strain of rat.

ACKNOWLEDGMENTS

We acknowledge with pleasure the expert technical assistance of Ms. L. Cavillier, T. Cuche, D. Duvillard, and H. Petersen. This work was supported by the Swiss National Science Foundation (grant no. 3.774. 0.76).

REFERENCES

[1] Patel, Y. C., and Weir, G. C.: Increased somatostatin content of islets from streptozotocin-diabetic rats. Clin. Endocrinol. 5:191–94, 1976.

[2] Pipeleers, D. G., Pipeleers-Marichal, M. A., Karl, I. E., and Kipnis, D. M.: Secretory capability of islets transplanted intraportally in the diabetic rat. Diabetes *27*:817–24, 1978.

[3] Girardier, L., Seydoux, J., Berger, M., and Veicsteinas, A.: Selective pancreatic nerve section. An investigation of neural control of glucagon release in the conscious unrestrained dog. J. Physiol. (Paris) *74*:731–35, 1979.

[4] Charles, M. A., Imagawa, W., Forsham, P. H., and Grodsky, G. M.: Islet transplantation into rat liver: in vitro secretion of insulin from the isolated perfused liver and in vivo glucagon suppression. Endocrinology *98*:738–42, 1976.

[5] Idezuki, Y., Maki, T., Kabaya, T., Kasahara, K., and Kajinuma, H.: Glucagon secretion of the pancreatic allograft in the dog. Surg. For. *23*:373–75, 1972.

[6] Brynger, H., Claes, G., and Lernmark, Å.: Glucagon and insulin release from the allografted canine pancreas. Eur. Surg. Res. *7*:170–80, 1975.

[7] Lacy, P. E., and Kostianovsky, M.: Method for the isolation of intact islets of Langerhans from the rat pancreas. Diabetes *16*:35–39, 1967.

[8] Assimacopoulos-Jeannet, F., Exton, J. H., and Jeanrenaud, B.: Control of gluconeogenesis and glycogenolysis in perfused livers of normal mice. Am. J. Physiol. *225*:25–32, 1973.

[9] Kenny, A. J.: Extractable glucagon of the human pancreas. J. Clin. Endocrinol. *15*:1089–1105, 1955.

[10] Halban, P. A., Wollheim, C. B., Blondel, B., Niesor, E., and Renold, A. E.: Perturbation of hormone storage and release induced by cyproheptadine in rat pancreatic islets in vitro. Endocrinology *104*:1096–1106, 1979.

[11] Bergmeyer, H. U., and Bernt, E.: *In* Methoden der enzymatischen Analyse. Weinheim/Bergstrasse, Verlag Chemie, 1970, p. 1172.

[12] Herbert, V., Lau, K.-S., Gottlieb, C. W., and Bleicher, S. J.: Coated charcoal immunoassay of insulin. J. Clin. Endocrinol. *25*:1375–84, 1965.

[13] Eff, C.: Insulin release, insulin content, and glucose utilization in isolated mouse islets maintained in tissue culture. Acta Endocrinol. *87*:535–42, 1978.

[14] Rabinovitch, A., Cuendet, G. S., Sharp, G. W. G., Renold, A. E., and Mintz, D. H.: Relation of insulin release to cyclic AMP content in rat pancreatic islets maintained in tissue culture. Diabetes *27*:766–73, 1978.

[15] Pipeleers-Marichal, M. A., Pipeleers, D. G., Cutler, J., Lacy, P. E., and Kipnis, D. M.: Metabolic and morphologic studies in intraportal islet-transplanted rats. Diabetes *25*:1041–51, 1976.

[16] Kramp, R. C., Cuche, R., Muller, W. A., and Renold, A. E.: Subcutaneous, isogeneic transplantation of duct-ligated pancreas in streptozotocin diabetic mice: relationships between recovery and hormone contents in transplants or host pancreas. Metabolism *25*:1007–16, 1976.

[17] Arcus, A. C., Beaven, D. W., Hart, D. S., and Holland, G. W.: Long-term hormonal secretion from the autotransplanted sheep pancreas. Diabetologia *16*:325–30, 1979.

[18] Griffith, R. C., Scharp, D. W., Hartman, B. K., Ballinger, W. F., and Lacy, P. E.: A morphologic study of intrahepatic portal-vein islet isografts. Diabetes *26*:201–14, 1977.

[19] McEvoy, R. C., and Hegre, O. D.: Morphometric quantitation of the pancreatic insulin-, glucagon-, and somatostatin-positive cell populations in normal and alloxan-diabetic rats. Diabetes *26*:1140–46, 1977.

[20] Weber, C. J., Hardy, M. A., Lerner, R. L., Felig, P., and Reemtsma, K.: Hyperinsulinemia and hyperglucagonemia following pancreatic islet transplantation in diabetic rats. Diabetes *25*:944–48, 1976.

[21] Henriksson, C., Bergmark, J., and Claes, G.: Metabolic response to isologous transplantation of small numbers of isolated islets of Langerhans in the rat. Eur. Surg. Res. *9*:411–18, 1977.

[22] Junod, A., Lambert, A. E., Stauffacher, W., and Renold, A. E.: Diabetogenic action of streptozotocin: relationship of dose to metabolic response. J. Clin. Invest. *48*:2129–39, 1969.

[23] Kramp, R. C., Cuche, R., and Renold, A. E., with the technical assistance of Gonet, J. C.: Subcutaneous, isogeneic transplantation of either duct-ligated pancreas or isolated islets in streptozotocin diabetic mice. Endocrinology *99*:1161–67, 1976.

Clearance Rates of Metabolizable and Nonmetabolizable Sugars in Insulin-infused Dogs and in Exercising Dogs

B. ISSEKUTZ, JR.

SUMMARY

Dogs with indwelling arterial and venous catheters were trained to run on a treadmill (slope, 15%; speed, 100 m/min). The clearance rates (CR) of ^{3}H-inulin, 3-^{3}H-glucose (G), ^{14}C-L-arabinose (L-A), ^{14}C-D-xylose (D-X), ^{14}C-3-methyl-O-glucose (3-m-G) and 2-deoxy-glucose (2-d-G) were measured using the primed constant infusion tracer technics. With the exception of glucose, all substances were excreted in the urine; therefore the CR is the sum of the urinary clearance rate (UCR) plus the tissue clearance rate (tCR). By measuring CR_{inulin} and the concentration of ^{3}H-inulin in the urine, the flow rate of urine and the UCR and tCR of the simultaneously infused ^{14}C-sugars were calculated. Infusion of insulin (1.5 mU/kg min) and glucose (6 mg/kg min) into the resting dog raised plasma insulin to 60–40μU/ml at normoglycemia. The tCR of all sugars was increased: G>2-d-G>3-m-G>D-X>L-A. There was a great discrepancy between the phosphorylable (G, 2-d-G) and the nonmetabolizable sugars (3-m-G, D-X, L-A). Insulin increased tCR of glucose almost threefold, and it was estimated that 27% of the increase could be ascribed to the unassisted direct effect of membrane-transport (3-m-G) and 55% if the glucose could be phosphorylated but not metabolized further (2-d-G). Exercise decreased plasma insulin by almost 50%, hepatic glucose production rose more than twofold, and the tCR-glucose more than 2½-fold. The tCR of L-A remained unchanged and that of the other sugar derivatives was increased by the run in the following order G>2-d-G>3-m-G>D-X. It was estimated that only 16% of the increase of tCR-glucose could be ascribed to the effect of exercise on the membrane-transport if it was not assisted by the hexokinase, and 53% with the help of the enzyme but without the accelerated glycolysis. It is concluded that, under physiologic conditions, a relatively small fraction (16–20%) of the two- to threefold increase of glucose utilization can be ascribed to a direct membrane effect if the activity of flux-generating steps towards either glycogen formation (insulin) or glycolysis (exercise) is accelerated.

DIABETES *29*:348–354, May 1980.

From the Department of Physiology and Biophysics, Dalhousie University, Halifax, Nova Scotia, Canada B3H 4H7.
Address reprint requests to B. Issekutz, Jr., Department of Physiology and Biophysics, Dalhousie University, Halifax, Nova Scotia, Canada B3H 4H7.
Received for publication 29 June and in revised form 12 December 1979.

It took almost three decades of research to clarify the rather complex nature of glucose utilization by the muscle, as well as the effects of insulin and contraction on the process. That includes the transport of glucose across the cell membrane and the concerted activities of at least two nonequilibrium enzymes—the hexokinase and the phosphofructokinase.[1] The classic work of Levine and his colleagues[2–4] demonstrated that, in eviscerated-nephrectomized dogs, both insulin[3] and the electrical stimulation of hind leg muscles[4] increased the volume of distribution of a number of nonmetabolizable sugars (galactose, D-xylose, L-arabinose). Since then, the attention was focused on the role of glucose transport in the metabolism of the working muscle. Subsequent investigations, using isolated muscle preparations[5] or the hind leg of rats or cats,[6–8] confirmed the original findings.

According to our present concept, the flux of glucose across the cell membrane is a "carrier-facilitated passive transport" which moves glucose along but not against a concentration gradient.[9] This concentration gradient is maintained by the low K_m hexokinases (K_m approximately 0.1 mM = 1.8 mg% glucose) present in the muscle.[10] The most important characteristic of these enzymes is that they are effectively inhibited by the product glucose-6-phosphate. The concentration of this latter in the working muscle depends on the relative activity of phosphorylase "a" (intramuscular glycogenolysis) and on that of phosphofructokinase (rate of glycolysis) as one of the most important flux-generating nonequilibrium glycolytic enzymes.[11]

In most of these studies, rather large doses of insulin (1–10 U/kg) and/or electrical stimulation were used and the experiments were carried out on eviscerated-nephrectomized animals, on perfused muscle groups, or on isolated muscles. While these studies provided basic information, they were not designed to clarify the relative importance of the various steps of glucose utilization under physiologic exercise conditions. During exercise, plasma insulin was shown to decrease[12–14] and plasma FFA to rise. Both changes appear to decrease[14] rather than to increase the glucose uptake of the muscle. It was felt that there was a need to investigate the role of (a) membrane transport, (b) phosphorylation, and (c) glycolysis in the elevated glucose utilization by the muscle exercising under the most physiologic condition in the running dog. The recent revival of exercise regimen in the management of diabetes mellitus (for literature, see reference 15) further underlined the importance of such studies.

Using the primed constant rate infusion tracer technics, the effect of insulin infusion and that of a two hour run was studied on the clearance rates (CR) of 3-^{3}H-glucose, two pentoses (^{14}C-L-arabinose and ^{14}C-D-xylose) and two glucose derivatives: ^{14}C-3-methyl-O-glucose (3-m-gl) and ^{14}C-2-deoxy-D-glucose (2-d-gl). The former is a nonmetabolizable sugar while the latter readily forms 2-deoxy-glucose-6-phosphate, but it cannot pass the phosphoglucose-isomerase[16] (in larger concentration, it actually inhibits the glucolysis at this step). All these sugars were extensively used to study the specificity and the binding characteristic of the membrane-carrier system in vitro and in perfusion experiments. D-glucose, 2-d-gl, and 3-m-gl were shown to have high affinity (low K_m) and similar transport kinetics; studies of competitive inhibition led to the conclusion that they shared the same transport system. The pentoses L-arabinose and D-xylose exhibited low affinity (high K_m) for the carrier; nevertheless they all responded to insulin and muscular activity (literature, see reference 9).

METHODS

Specially selected (good runners) adult male dogs (mongrels; body wt, 12–16 kg) were kept on a high protein and high CHO diet[17] and trained to run on 15% slope at a speed of 100 m/min for 3 h. Three or four days before the first experiment (in morphine-Pentothal anesthesia), indwelling Tygon catheters were placed into the left jugular vein and carotid artery.

Since all the ^{14}C-sugars tested were also excreted in the urine, to estimate the urinary clearance rates in most experiments, ^{3}H-inulin (specific activity, 100–500 mCi/g; New England Nuclear) was infused along with the carbon-labeled test substance. An exception was made only when 3-^{3}H-glucose (s.a.: 10–20 mCi/mmol; New England Nuclear) was used in combination with the ^{14}C-2-deoxy-glucose. The experiment started 18–20 h after the last feeding, and care was taken that the bladder should be empty. Then, at $t = 0$, a priming dose was given intravenously followed by the constant rate infusion. The priming dose consisted of a mixture of 2.5 μCi/kg of the tritiated compound (inulin or glucose) and 0.3 μCi/kg of the ^{14}C-substance.

The corresponding constant infusion rates were 30 and 4 nCi/kg min, respectively. The specific activities (s.a.) and the source of the ^{14}C-sugars were as follows: L-[1-^{14}C] arabinose, s.a. >45 mCi/mmol, Amersham; D-[U-^{14}C]xylose, s.a. >50 mCi/mmol, Amersham; 3-O-methyl-[^{14}C]-glucose, s.a. = 20–55 mCi/mmol, New England Nuclear; 2-deoxy-[U-^{14}C]-glucose, s.a. = 300 mCi/mmol, New England Nuclear.

In 11 experiments, arterial samples were taken at 5, 10, 15, 30, 45, and 60 min after the priming dose and then every 15 min until the end of the experiments. In 30 experiments, the sampling started at t_{60}. The former pattern served to estimate the volume of distribution of inulin (VD_{in}) and that of the test sugar (mainly 3-m-gl) (see CALCULATIONS).

Two types of experiments were conducted: Type A served to test the effect of a moderately elevated plasma insulin level under our experimental conditions. In this series (16 experiments), the baseline values were obtained between t_{60} and t_{105}. From t_{105} to t_{195}, a mixture of insulin (1.5 mU/kg min) and dextrose (6 mg/kg min) was infused, followed by a recovery period from t_{195} to t_{255}. At the end of the experiment, the bladder was catheterized and the urinary concentrations of ^{3}H-inulin and of ^{14}C-sugar were measured.

In type B series (25 experiments), the effect of exercise was studied on the CRs. After a 105 min resting period, urine was obtained by catheterization and the dog started to run on a slope of 15% at a speed of 100 m/min for 105 min; at the end of the exercise period, another urine sample was obtained. Sixteen dogs participated in both types of experiments.

Chemical analysis. The arterial blood samples were collected in chilled tubes using EDTA as anticoagulant. After the plasma was separated, deproteinized [$Ba(OH)_2$ and $ZnSO_4$], and centrifuged, 2-ml aliquots of the supernatant were evaporated to dryness in a vacuum oven at 70°C. The residue was redissolved in 1 ml water PCS solubilizer (Amersham) added and counted in a Packard liquidscintillation spectrometer using the double label–counting technics. The values were expressed in nanocuries per milliliter plasma. The urine was diluted to 1 : 100 and 1-ml aliquots were evaporated and processed as the supernatant. Plasma glucose was obtained with the glucose oxidase method, and the double antibody technics of Hales and Randle[18] served to measure the immunoreactive insulin level (IRI) in the plasma.

CALCULATIONS

In dynamic steady state, the infusion rate F (nCi/kg min) divided by the plasma concentration of the radioactive substance (r_p, nCi/ml) gives the clearance rate (CR, ml/kg min) of that substance, that is, the volume of plasma which can be cleared of the substance at a given concentration in a minute. Since all the ^{14}C-labeled sugars tested were also excreted in the urine, the total CR was the sum of the urinary clearance (UCR) plus tissue CR (tCR). To obtain the latter, one has to measure UCR, which requires the rate of urinary flow ($\dot{V}$, ml/kg min), because $UCR = (r_u \times \dot{V})/r_p$, where r_u is the concentration of the radioactive substance in the urine (nCi/ml). Since the complete collection of urine and the required rinsing of the bladder faced technical difficulties (especially in the running dog), ^{3}H-inulin was used to provide $\dot{V}$. Inulin remains extracellularly, and urinary excretion ($= r_{ui} \times \dot{V}$) is the only route of elimination. Therefore, $\dot{V} = (CR_i \times \bar{r}_{pi})/r_{ui}$, where CR_i is the steady state clearance rate of inulin, r_{ui} is the concentration of ^{3}H-inulin in the urine, and $\bar{r}_{pi}$ is the mean plasma concentration of inulin-radioactivity, $\bar{r}_{pi} = (\int_0^t r_{pi}dt)/t$, t being the time between the priming dose and urine collection. In three experiments, during the basal phase, $\dot{V}$ was measured directly with a close-to-complete urine collection (without rinsing) and was compared with that obtained by measuring CR_i. The former values proved to be about 10% lower than the indirect method.

Then the UCR of the ^{14}C-test sugar was calculated: $(r_{uc}\dot{V})/\bar{r}_{pc}$ and tCR = CR − UCR, where r_{uc} and r_{pc} are the concentrations of radiocarbon in the urine and in the plasma, respectively. In the case of ^3H-glucose, UCR is zero and tCR is generally called metabolic clearance rate (MCR).

In contrast with the nephrectomized dogs, this is an open system assumed to consist of two compartments: an extracellular (the volume of distribution of inulin) and an intracellular compartment.[19] The constant infusion into the plasma maintains a concentration gradient and, therefore, a flux of the substance. In other words, $F>(r_{uc} \times \dot{V})$. In 11 experiments, attempts were made to estimate the apparent size of the two compartments. This was done by calculating the difference between the amount of radioactivity which entered and left the system and dividing the difference by the average value of r_p (that is, r_{pi} or r_{pc}) during the baseline period (t = 105).

$$VD = \frac{Pr + tF - CR \int_0^t r_p\,dt}{\int_0^t r_p\,dt/t},$$

where Pr = priming dose; F = infusion rate; t = time (usually 105 min); CR = average clearance rate in steady state (usually, between t_{60} and t_{105}). The integral was obtained by first doing a least square fit of r_p to a single exponential function between t_5 and t_{60} (degree of freedom = 3) and to an interpolating polynomial for the period t_{60}–t_{105} (df = 1) and, then, integrating these curves. In case the four values obtained in the latter period did not deviate from the arithmetic mean by more than ±3%, then this mean was used (df = 3) instead of the polynomial. It is evident that a decrease of r_p indicates an increase of VD. Nevertheless, because of the dynamic nature of our model, changes of tCR were used to measure the effect of insulin and exercise. Finally, in steady state, the hepatic glucose production (mg/kg min) was calculated from the ratio F/SA, where SA is the specific activity of the 3-^3H-glucose in the plasma (nCi/mg). All statistical calculations were based on Fisher's *t* test,[20] with one exception. Because of the large individual differences in the response of urine flow to exercise, in addition to the *t* test, the nonparametric Wilcoxon test[21] was used (Table 3).

RESULTS

Type A experiments: effect of insulin. Figure 1 shows the effect of insulin + dextrose infusion on the average plasma levels of the various ^{14}C-sugars tested. Insulin level rose from 12 to 60 μU/ml, and then it leveled off at 40 μU/ml. The concomitant infusion of glucose kept plasma glucose around the 100 mg/dl mark, with a transient sharp decrease on cessation of the infusions. Insulin decreased the plasma concentration of the radioactive sugars to various degrees. L-arabinose proved to be the least responsive (−3%), while D-xylose and 3-methyl-glucose showed essentially the same degree of decrease, −16.7% and −15.7%, respectively. The two phosphorylable glucoses represented a different category, the partially metabolizable 2-deoxy-gl declined by 31% and the natural d-glucose by 50%.

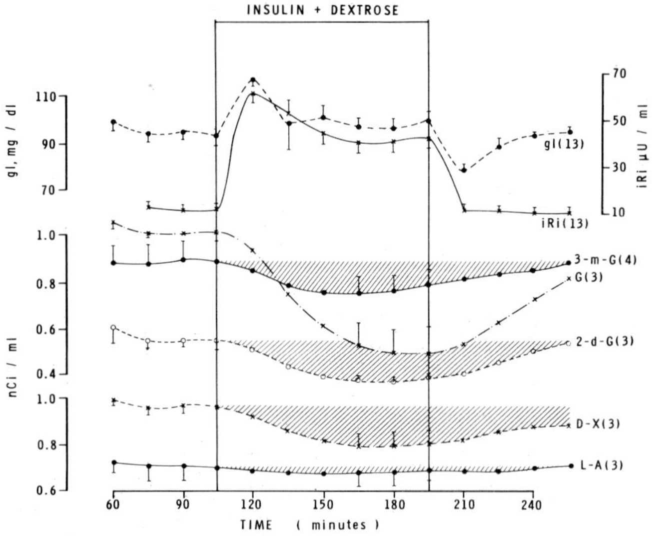

FIGURE 1. Effect of insulin (1.5 mU/kg min) plus dextrose (6 mg/kg min) infusions on plasma glucose levels (gl), on immunoreactive insulin (IRI) levels, and on the plasma concentration of radioactive sugar derivatives (nCi/ml). These latter values were corrected for the same infusion rate (4 nCi/kg min) of the radioactivity. Symbols: G, 3-^{3}H-glucose; 3-m-G, ^{14}C-3-methyl-O-glucose; 2-d-g, ^{14}C-2-deoxy-glucose; D-X, ^{14}C-D-xylose; and L-A, ^{14}C-L-arabinose. (n): number of experiments. Vertical lines: plus or minus SEM at points on which the values of Tables 1 and 2 are based.

Table 1 summarizes the baseline values. The average inulin space VD_{in} proved to be 18.5% of the body weight and 67.5% of the glucose space, as measured with the nonmetabolizable 3-m-glucose. This latter yielded a value of 27.4%, slightly higher than the 25% of body weight assumed by Radziuk et al.[22] in their recent study on glucose kinetics, and it was not significantly different from that found by Steele et al.[23] or that obtained in our laboratory using an entirely different approach (two tracer technics) to estimate the VD of glucose.[24] Perhaps it should be pointed out (although it may be just a coincidence) that the ratio VD_{in}/VD_{3-m-gl} = 0.675 is rather close to the so-called rapidly mixing pool fraction of glucose, 0.65, as suggested by Cowan and He-

TABLE 1
Baseline values

	VD		CR		UCR		tCR	
	$\bar{X}$	± SEM	$\bar{X}$	± SEM	$\bar{X}$	± SEM	$\bar{X}$	± SEM
Inulin	185	8.91	4.36	0.14	4.36	0.14	—	—
(n)		(10)		(30)		(30)		
L-arabinose			5.49	0.37	4.07	0.30	1.28	0.33
(n)				(7)		(6)		(6)
D-xylose			4.20	0.21	2.51	0.16	1.69	0.18
(n)				(7)		(7)		(7)
3-m-glucose	274	8.97	4.24	0.17	2.94	0.14	1.30	0.09
(n)		(9)		(12)		(10)		(10)
2-deoxy-gl	272	—	7.53	0.31	3.56	0.54	3.55	0.27
(n)	(2)			(13)		(7)		(7)
D-glucose	288		3.87	0.21	—	—	3.87	0.21
(n)	(1)			(11)				(11)

Urine flow $\dot{V}$ = 0.07 ± 0.01 ml/kg min; n = 30
VD: volume of distribution, ml/kg
CR, UCR, tCR: clearance rates, ml/kg min (total, urinary, and tissue)

TABLE 2
Effect of insulin (with dextrose) on tissue clearances (tCR). Deviations from baseline values.

	ΔtCR $\Delta\bar{X}$ ± SEM		% of glucose response	p <
L-arabinose (n)	0.29	0.07 (3)	4.3	0.05
D-xylose (n)	1.44	0.24 (3)	21.2	0.02
3-m-glucose (n)	1.81	0.28 (4)	26.7	0.01
2-deoxy-gl (n)	3.74	0.14 (3)	55.2	0.005
D-glucose (n)	6.78	1.20 (3)	100	0.005

tenyi.[25] In the present study, VD_{in} (= 185 ml/kg) was used to describe the course of the clearance rates in nonsteady state using a least square polynomial fit and the equation suggested by Steele et al.[23]

With the exception of 2-deoxy-gl, the CR of the tested sugars are in the relatively narrow range between 3.87 and 5.49 ml/kg min, rather close to the CR_{in} (4.36 = GFR). However, the calculations of tCR clearly separate two groups: the nonmetabolizable sugars have considerably lower tCR than those glucoses which can form gl-6-P. The 2-deoxy-gl has the highest CR, because its tCR is as high as that of D-glucose, and in addition it also has a UCR almost equal to that of inulin.

The effect of insulin is presented in Table 2. There was a statistically significant increase in the tCR of each sugar, although the effect on L-arabinose was almost negligible (22.6%). All other sugars which are known to respond to insulin in nephrectomized or perfused preparations[2–9] responded also in the intact dog, and, to the rather moderate rise of plasma insulin, tCR rose 90–180%. Nevertheless in terms of absolute increases of tCR, the two phosphorylable glucoses showed the biggest rise, and the flux of D-glucose rose considerably more than that of 2-deoxy-glucose. Based on ΔtCR of 3-m-glucose, 2-deoxy-glucose, and D-glucose, one may conclude that only about 27% of the insulin-induced rise of glucose uptake can be ascribed (at the measured levels of IRI) to the enhanced membrane transport per se, and this value is increased to 55% when the concentration gradient is maintained by phosphorylation. The rest of the increase is probably due to the well known stimulation of the glucosyltransferase system by insulin (for literature, see reference 1).

Type B experiments: effect of exercise. Figure 2 shows the average responses of plasma radioactivities (r_p, nCi/ml) to exercise. There was very little effect in experiments with L-arabinose and 3-m-glucose. D-xylose declined by about 15%, while 2-deoxy-glucose and D-glucose decreased by 33% and 58%, respectively. A somewhat different picture arose when the exercise-induced changes in urinary excretion or rather that of UCR were taken into account. Exercise always decreased the urine flow, $\dot{V}$. The decrease, however, was variable (see footnote in Table 3); therefore the *t* test showed a level of significance of $p < 0.05$, while according to the nonparametric Wilcoxon test, $p < 0.01$. Generally, the higher was the resting value of $\dot{V}$ the larger was the exercise-induced decrease.

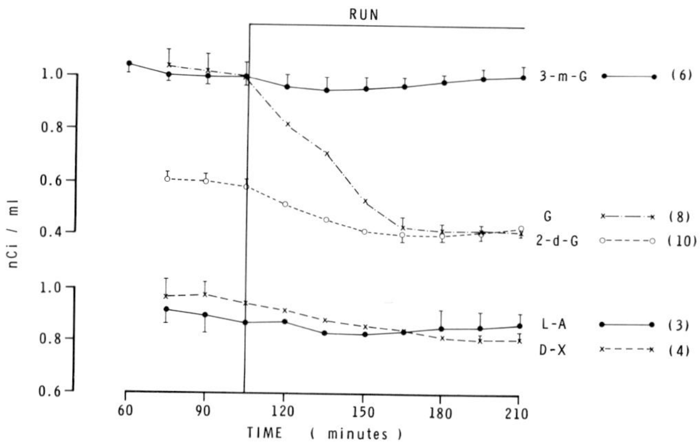

FIGURE 2. Effect of exercise (run, slope: 15%, speed: 100 m/min) on the plasma concentration of infused radioactive sugar derivatives (nCi/ml). For further information, see the legend of Figure 1.

Table 3 shows the effect of exercise on UCR and tCR of various sugars. The two pentoses responded but little to exercise. The CR-s of L-arabinose was not altered at all, and the rise of tCR of D-xylose, although statistically significant, proved to be less than 43%, about 0.7 ml/kg min. Surprisingly, the exercise hardly affected the total clearance rate of 3-m-gl. However, measurement of UCR and tCR revealed that the former was considerably decreased by the great reduction of $\dot{V}$ and that the latter was increased to the same extent during the run. On the other hand the tissue clearances of the two metabolizable glucoses rose considerably. Both 2-deoxy-glucose and D-glucose exceeded the exercise-induced rise of tCR of 3-m-G by factors of 3.5 and 6.5, respectively. In general, one may say that only about 16% of the exercise-induced rise of glucose uptake can be ascribed to the increased membrane transport per se, about 53% if the glucose phosphorylation maintains the concentration gradient, and the remaining 47% is probably a result of the greatly elevated glycolysis in the running dog.

Figure 3 shows the effect of a run on the course of the CR-s of glucose, 2-deoxy-gl, and 3-m-gl, as well as changes of plasma glucose and IRI levels. In experiments

TABLE 3
Effect of exercise on CR-s
Deviations from baseline (Δvalues)

	ΔUCR $\Delta\bar{X}$ ± SEM		ΔtCR $\Delta\bar{X}$ ± SEM		% of glucose response	*t* test p<
Inulin (n)	0.66	0.30 (17)	—	—		0.05
L-arabinose (n)	0.21	0.4	−0.38	0.24 (3)		NS
D-xylose (n)	0.50	0.35	0.72	0.16 (4)	10.6	0.02
3-m-glucose (n)	−1.02	0.30	1.07	0.46 (6)	15.8	0.05
2-deoxy-gl (n)	−0.34	0.21	3.58	0.52 (4)	52.8	0.001
D-glucose (n)	—	—	6.78	0.93 (8)	100	0.001

Change in urine flow (ΔV): −0.053 ± 0.021 ml/kg min, n = 17
$p < 0.05$ (*t* test); $p < 0.01$ (Wilcoxon test) (see CALCULATIONS)

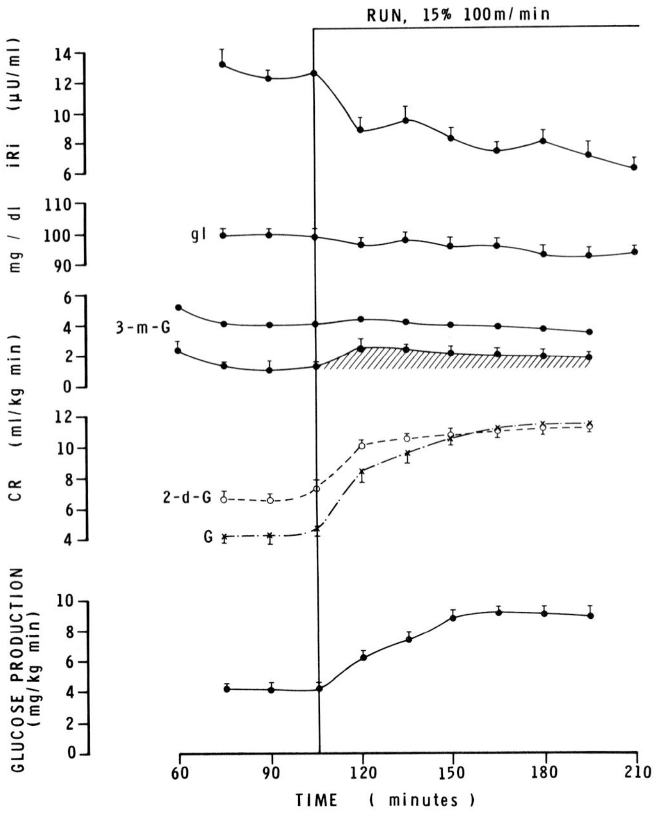

FIGURE 3. Effect of exercise on the average course of plasma insulin (IRI) and plasma glucose (gl) obtained in 18 experiments, the clearance rates of glucose (n = 8) and two glucose derivatives (3-m-G, n = 6; 2-d-G, n = 10), as well as on the rate of hepatic glucose production. The latter was obtained in experiments with 3-³H-glucose as tracer (n = 8).

with 3-³H-glucose as tracer, the rate of hepatic glucose output was also calculated. The more than twofold increase of glucose production and the even greater rise of the CR of glucose (the so-called metabolic clearance rate) was accompanied by a slight decline of plasma glucose (from 100 to 93 mg/dl) and by a considerable (some 50%) decrease of plasma insulin. During this time, the CR of 3-m-gl was not altered, but the tCR (shaded area) rose, although much less than that of the CR of 2-deoxy-glucose. At rest, the CR of 2-deoxy-glucose is always higher than that of D-glucose because of the urinary loss of the former. During exercise, however, they rise to about the same value.

Figure 4 shows the strict correlation between the CR-s of these two glucoses based on 80 samples obtained by simultaneous measurements in six experiments. For plotting purposes only, Figure 4 shows the means of ordered pairs. The regression coefficient 0.66 ± 0.05 is significant at the $p < 0.001$ level. The Y intercept, 3.92 ml/kg min, represents the UCR if tCR is zero, and it is not significantly different from the actually measured UCR, 3.56 ± 0.54, from experiments carried out with the combination of ³H-inulin and ¹⁴C-2-deoxy-glucose.

FIGURE 4. Correlation between the metabolic clearance rate (MCR) of glucose and the clearance rate (CR) of 2-deoxy-glucose. Each point represents the mean of eight values. Vertical and horizontal lines: plus or minus SEM of Y and X, respectively. UCR: measured urinary clearance rate of 2-d-glucose.

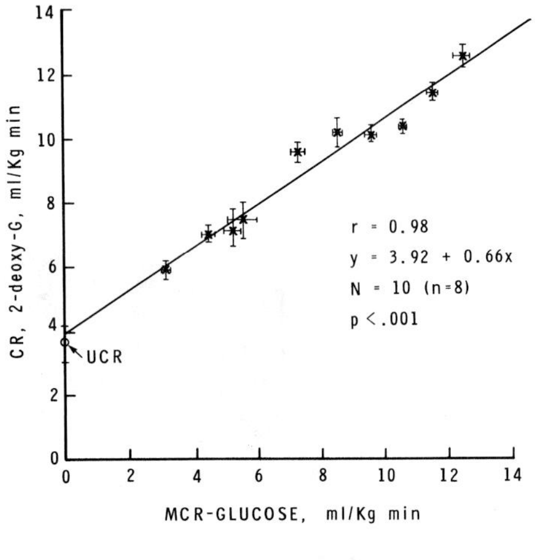

DISCUSSION

The presented results demonstrate that it is possible to study the transport of various sugars into the cells of the conscious dog under physiologic conditions, and that, by using radioactive sugars, one can do this without interfering with the normal flow of glucose utilization. It should be noted that, although the actual flux of the substance can be calculated (=CR × r_p), in this study the term clearance rate was preferred, because this is a measure of the ability of the kidneys (UCR) and extrarenal tissues (tCR) to remove the substance in question.[19] The effect of insulin infusion on the transport could clearly be demonstrated at plasma insulin levels (60–40 μU/ml) well within the physiologic range of the response to food intake. The order of responsivity of the various sugars generally agrees with the in vitro findings, that is, D-glucose>>D-xylose>L-arabinose.[9] However, the great difference between the 3-methyl-O-glucose (ΔtCR = 1.81 ml/kg min) and 2-deoxy-glucose (3.74 ml/kg min) was not expected. Only the latter can be phosphorylated and the more than twofold greater response seems to underline the importance of hexokinase activity in the overall effect of insulin. The observation that insulin increased the tCR (=MCR) of D-glucose even more than that of 2-deoxy-glucose may indicate that, in addition, other enzymes also participate in glucose uptake. One possible explanation is that a considerable part of the glucose is taken up by the liver, where the glucokinase phosphorylizes it to gl-6-P. The phosphorylation rate of 2-deoxy-glucose by glucokinase is less than 40% that of glucose.[26] In addition, when the administration of insulin is accompanied by infusion of glucose to prevent hypoglycemia, a large fraction of the utilized glucose enters the glycogenic pathways. However, the 2-deoxy-glucose is a poor substrate for that pathway. Nigam reported[27] that hepatoma cells incorporate 2-deoxy-glucose into glycogen at a rate only 3–5% that of glucose, while pigeon liver slices cannot form any glycogen from this substrate. Thus, the 2-deoxy-glucose-6-P, readily produced by the hexokinase, cannot be further metabolized, because both the glycolytic and the glycogenic pathways seem to be closed.

These findings and considerations led us to the conclusion that, under physiologic conditions, at plasma insulin and glucose levels within the normal range, the full effect of the hormone requires normal utilization of the glucose-6-P. In this respect, the stimulating effect of insulin on the enzyme UDPG-glucosyl transferase may play a crucial role (for literature, see page 191 in reference 1). Without this effect, the concentration of gl-6-P would rise with a concomitant inhibition of hexokinase, and the ΔtCR of glucose could be as low as that of 3-m-glucose. The membrane transport that is the carrier-assisted passive diffusion would slow down, because of the decrease of the extracellular versus intracellular concentration gradient. Considering that the K_m of hexokinase is less than 2% of the extracellular glucose concentration and that the enzyme may normally operate below its K_m value, it is understandable that the intracellular concentration of free glucose normally remains undetectable because of technical difficulties.

Experiments on exercising dogs yielded results somewhat similar to those obtained with insulin infusion. One should emphasize, however, two basic differences: (a) in type B series, plasma insulin level was only about 1/6th to 1/7th of that measured during insulin infusion; (b) during a run, both the activity of hexokinase and the rate of glycolysis are highly elevated (for flux-generating steps, see references 1 and 11).

Exercise increased the tCR-s of nonmetabolizable sugars much less than that of glucose and its phosphorylable derivative. L-arabinose did not respond at all, the tCR of D-xylose rose 43%, and that of 3-m-glucose, 82%. While these increases indicate that the rate of transport across the membrane can significantly rise even if it is not assisted by hexokinase activity, the actual increments of tCR (0.72 and 1.07 ml/kg min, respectively) are relatively small compared with those of D-glucose (6.8 ml/kg min) and 2-deoxyglucose (3.6 ml/kg min) (Table 3). The reason for the difference between these last two glucoses is not quite clear. Even though it is generally accepted that glucose, mannose, and 2-deoxyglucose are equally good substrates for hexokinases (with K_m values in the same order of magnitude), since these informations were obtained on brain, intestine, and kidney hexokinases (K_m = 0.027, 0.09, and 0.04 mM, respectively),[10,28,29] there is a distinct possibility that, in the skeletal muscle, 2-deoxy-glucose might have a lower affinity (higher K_m) to hexokinases than does D-glucose (unfortunately, there is no recent information concerning the K_m values of the various hexokinases in skeletal muscle for 2-d-glucose). On the other hand, it is also possible that the absence of both glycogenic and glycolytic pull in vivo slows down the phosphorylation of 2-deoxy-glucose. The strict correlation shown on Figure 4 could be explained by either mechanism or the combination of the two.

These observations seem to suggest that the exercise-induced two- to two-and-one-half-fold increase of glucose uptake requires a concerted control mechanism. In this mechanism, the increased membrane transport per se seems to play a minor role, yet it may stimulate the hexokinase activity provided the intracellular concentration of glucose-6-P does not rise, that is, the glycolytic pathway operates at a higher than normal rate. If the rate of formation of gl-6-P exceeds the rate of glycolysis, e.g. due to excessive glycogenolysis in the muscle, then gl-6-P accumulates, inhibiting the activity of hexokinase. Such an increase of glycogenolysis can be produced by epinephrine and the result is a rise of gl-6-P in the isolated muscle[30] and a decrease of the CR of glucose in the intact dog.[31,32] In electrically stimulated muscles, gl-6-P increases only with heavy exercise,[30,33] which greatly elevates lactate production. Under these circumstances, the intracellular concentration of free glucose becomes measurable,[32] indicating a discrepancy between the rate of membrane transport and of hexokinase activity. Whether such heavy exercise can be achieved in vivo is uncertain and certainly not for any length of time. Our well trained dogs ran at a highly elevated glucose turnover, but without increasing plasma lactate (Δlactate = 0.6 ± 1.1 mg/dl); therefore, the probability of an elevated gl-6-P is rather remote. Indeed, Towes et al.[33] showed that, during heavy exercise in man, there was no significant change in the concentration of glycolytic intermediates, including that of gl-6-P, even though the glycolytic flux increased 7- to 10-fold.

In conclusion, it seems to be possible to estimate the relative role of membrane transport of glucose, that of hexokinase, and the glycolytic flux during steady exercise by using 3-m-glucose, 2-deoxy-glucose, and 3-^{3}H-glucose. The elevated glucose utilization requires the acceleration of glycolysis below the level of the hexoseisomerase, possibly at the level of phosphofructokinase[11] or that of pyruvate dehydrogenase.[34] If this acceleration takes place, then the increase of the membrane transport contributes relatively little (about 16%) to the large (200–300%) rise of glucose utilization. The same seems to apply if plasma glucose is mainly used for glycogen synthesis, and this pathway is accelerated by insulin.

ACKNOWLEDGMENT

This study was supported by a grant from the Medical Research Council of Canada.

REFERENCES

1 Newsholme, E. A., and Start, C.: Regulation in Metabolism, chap. 3. London, John Wiley and Sons, 1973, pp. 88–132.

2 Levine, R., Goldstein, M. S., Huddleston, B., and Klein, S. P.: Action of insulin on the "permeability" of cells to free hexoses, as studied by its effect on the distribution of galactose. Am. J. Physiol. *163*:70–76, 1950.

3 Goldstein, M. S., Henry, W. L., Huddleston, B., and Levine, R.: Action of insulin on transfer of sugars across cell barriers: common chemical configuration of substances responsive to action of the hormone. Am. J. Physiol. *173*:207–11, 1953.

4 Goldstein, M. S., Mullick, V., Huddleston, B., and Levine, R.: Action of muscular work on transfer of sugars across cell barriers: comparison with action of insulin. Am. J. Physiol. *173*:212–16, 1953.

5 Nahara, H. T., and Özand, P.: Studies of tissue permeability. IX. The effect of insulin on the penetration of 3-methylglucose-H^3 in frog muscle. J. Biol. Chem. *238*:40–49, 1963.

6 Helmreich, E., and Cori, C. F.: Studies of tissue permeability. II. The distribution of pentoses between plasma and muscle. J. Biol. Chem. *224*:663–79, 1957.

7 Sacks, J., and Smith, J. F.: Effects of insulin and activity on pentose transport into muscle. Am. J. Physiol. *192*:287–89, 1958.

8 Morgan, H. E., Regen, D. M., and Park, C. R.: Identification of a mobile carrier-mediated sugar transport system in muscle. J. Biol. Chem. *239*:369–74, 1964.

9 Morgan, H. E., and Neely, J. R.: Insulin and membrane transport. *In* Handbook of Physiology, Section 7. Vol. 1, Endocrine Pancreas. Greep, R. O., and Astwood, E. B., Eds. Washington, D.C., Am. Physiol. Soc., 1972, pp. 323–31.

10 Colowick, S. P.: The hexokinases. *In* The Enzymes, vol. 9, third edit. Boyer, P. B., Ed. New York, Academic Press, 1973, pp. 1–48.

11 Newsholme, E. A.: The control of fuel utilization by muscle during exercise and starvation. Diabetes *28* (Suppl. 1):1–7, 1979.

12 Issekutz, B., Jr., Paul, P., and Miller, H. I.: Metabolism in normal and pancreatectomized dogs during steady state exercise. Am. J. Physiol. *213*:857–62, 1967.

13 Vranic, M., Kawamori, R., Pek, S., Kovacevic, N., and Wrenshall, G. A.: The essentiality of insulin and the role of glucagon in regulating glucose utilization and production during strenuous exercise in dogs. J. Clin. Invest. *57*:245–55, 1976.

14 Randle, P. J., Newsholme, E. A., and Garland, P. B.: Regulation of glucose uptake by muscle. 8. Effects of fatty acids, ketone bodies and pyruvate, and of alloxan diabetes and starvation, on the uptake and metabolic fate of glucose in rat heart and diaphragm muscles. Biochem. J. *93*:652–64, 1964.

15 Vranic, M., and Berger, M.: Exercise and diabetes mellitus. Diabetes *28*:147–63, 1979.

[16] Wick, A. N., Drury, D. R., Nakada, H. I., and Wolfe, J. B.: Localization of the primary metabolic block produced by 2-deoxyglucose. J. Biol. Chem. *224*:963–68, 1957.

[17] Issekutz, B., Jr.: Role of beta-adrenergic receptors in mobilization of energy sources in exercising dogs. J. Appl. Physiol.: Respirat. Environ. Exercise Physiol. *44*:869–76, 1978.

[18] Hales, C. N., and Randle, P. J.: Immunoassay of insulin with insulin antibody precipitate. Lancet *I*:200, 1963.

[19] Riggs, D. S.: The Mathematical Approach to Physiological Problems, chap. 8. Cambridge, Mass., MIT Press, 1970, pp. 193–200.

[20] Fisher, R. A.: Statistical Methods for Research Workers, 13th edit. New York, Hafner Publishing, 1963, pp. 129–42.

[21] Walphole, R.: Introduction to Statistics. New York, Macmillan, 1971, pp. 225–36.

[22] Radziuk, J., Norwick, K., and Vranic, M.: Experimental validation of measurements of glucose turnover in nonsteady state. Am. J. Physiol. *234*:E84–E93, 1978.

[23] Steele, R., Altszuler, N., Wall, J. S., Dunn, A., and DeBodo, R. C.: Influence of adrenalectomy on glucose turnover and conversion to CO_2: studies with C^{14} glucose in the dog. Am. J. Physiol. *196*:221–30, 1959.

[24] Issekutz, T. B., Issekutz, B., Jr., and Elahi, D.: Estimation of the hepatic glucose output in non-steady state. The simultaneous use of 2-^{3}H-glucose and ^{14}C-glucose in the dog. Can. J. Physiol. Pharmacol. *52*:215–24, 1974.

[25] Cowan, J. S., and Hetenyi, G., Jr.: Glucoregulatory responses in normal and diabetic dogs recorded by a new tracer method. Metabolism *20*:360–72, 1971.

[26] González, C., Ureta, T., Babul, J., Rabajille, E., and Niemeyer, H.: Characterization of isoenzymes of adenosine triphosphate: d-hexose 6-phosphotransferase from rat liver. Biochemistry *6*:460–68, 1967.

[27] Nigam, U. N.: Incorporation of 2-deoxyglucose into glycogen by intact Novikoff ascites-hepatoma. Arch. Biochem. Biophys. *120*:232–33, 1967.

[28] Sols, A., and Crane, R. K.: Substrate specificity of brain hexokinase. J. Biol. Chem. *210*:581–95, 1954.

[29] Lange, Ch. F., Jr., and Kohn, P.: Substrate specificity of hexokinases. J. Biol. Chem. *236*:1–5, 1961.

[30] Karpatkin, S., Helmreich, E., and Cori, C. F.: Regulation of glycolysis in muscle. II. Effect of stimulation and epinephrine in isolated frog sartorius muscle. J. Biol. Chem. *239*:3139–45, 1964.

[31] Issekutz, B., Jr., and Borkow, I.: Effect of catecholamines and dibutyryl-cyclic-AMP on glucose turnover, plasma free fatty acids, and insulin in dogs treated with methylprednisolone. Can. J. Physiol. Pharmacol. *50*:999–1006, 1972.

[32] Issekutz, B., Jr.: Energy mobilization in exercising dogs. Diabetes *28* (Suppl. 1):39–44, 1979.

[33] Berger, M., Haggs, S., and Ruderman, N. B.: Glucose metabolism in perfused skeletal muscle. Biochem. J. *146*:231–38, 1975.

[34] Towes, C. J., Ward, G. R., Leveille, R., Sutton, J. R., and Jones, N. L.: Regulation of glycogenolysis and pyruvate oxidation in human skeletal muscle in vivo. Diabetes *28* (Suppl. 1):100–02, 1979.

Effect of Adrenergic Agents on the Secretion of Gastrointestinal Immunoreactive Glucagon in Depancreatized Dogs

TOSHIHIDE YOSHIDA AND MOTOHARU KONDO

SUMMARY

To elucidate the mode of action of adrenergic agents on gastric A cells, the effects of infusion of adrenergic agonists and antagonists on the secretion of gastrointestinal immunoreactive glucagon (gastrointestinal IRG) from gastric A cells were investigated in 45 conscious, depancreatized dogs untreated with insulin.

Large amounts (0.6 μg/kg/min) of epinephrine, norepinephrine, and isoproterenol stimulated the release of gastrointestinal IRG, and catecholamine-induced gastrointestinal IRG release was completely abolished by simultaneous infusion of the specific beta receptor–blocking compound, propranolol, but not by alpha receptor blockade with phentolamine.

These findings suggest that, when adrenergic agonists are infused in large amounts, they may act through a beta receptor to increase the release of gastrointestinal IRG. DIABETES 29:355–360, May 1980.

Although high levels of circulating gastrointestinal immunoreactive glucagon (gastrointestinal IRG) have been demonstrated in totally depancreatized dogs untreated with insulin,[1–5] little is known about adrenergic regulation of the secretion of gastrointestinal IRG.

The present investigation was designed to examine the effect of exogenous alpha- and beta-adrenergic agonists and antagonists on the secretion of gastrointestinal IRG in conscious depancreatized dogs.

MATERIALS AND METHODS

Forty-five healthy mongrel dogs, weighing from 9.0 to 12.2 kg, were anesthetized with ketamine hydrochloride (Ketalar, Sankyo Co., Japan) and thiopental sodium (Ravonal, Tanabe Pharmaceutical Co., Japan). Total pancreatectomy was performed, and polyethylene catheters were inserted into the hilar region of the portal vein or into the femoral vein for blood sampling, and into the axillary vein for drug infusion. A C-type probe (5mmϕ*) (Narco Bio-Systems, Houston, Texas), used as the flow transducer, was fixed on the hilar region of the portal vein, and the dogs were maintained without insulin therapy for two or three days. All animals fasted for 24 h before the experiments. On the third or fourth day, ten conscious dogs were given infusions of epinephrine (Sankyo Co., Japan), norepinephrine (Sankyo Co., Japan), and isoproterenol (Protanol-L, Nikken Kagaku Co., Japan) for 30 min, respectively.

Figure 1 shows dose response curves of the secretion of gastrointestinal IRG induced by epinephrine, norepinephrine, or isoproterenol. Infusion of epinephrine or norepinephrine at a rate of 0.1 or 0.2 μg/kg/min had no effect on IRG levels, but infusion of 0.6 μg/kg/min showed a significant increase, which was further increased by the administration of 1.0 μg/kg/min. Infusion of isoproterenol, 0.2, 0.6, or 1.0 μg/kg/min, showed a significant increase of gastrointestinal IRG, but there was no increase at 0.1 μg/kg/min. To compare the relative intensity of effect, each drug was injected at a rate of 0.6 μg/kg/min.

Another ten dogs were given infusions of either phentolamine (Regitin, Ciba Pharmaceutical Co., Switzerland) at rates of 0.1, 0.2, and 0.4 μM/kg/min or propranolol (Inderal, ICI Ltd., England) at a rate of 0.1 μM/kg/min for 30 min, respectively.

The remaining 25 dogs were infused with adrenergic agonists plus antagonists at rates described above.

Urine, plasma glucose, and body weight were checked on the third or fourth day to assess the general condition of the animals. (Urolabstix-III, Ames Division of Miles-Sankyo Co. Ltd, Tokyo, Japan, was used for testing urine.) Urinary glucose was about 0.5% (++), urinary ketone bodies were (+), and urinary protein was about 30 mg/100ml (+). Plasma glucose levels were about 300 mg/dl and mean

* ϕ = diameter.

From the First Department of Internal Medicine, Kyoto Prefectural University of Medicine, Kamikyo-ku, Kyoto 602, Japan.
Address reprint requests to T. Yoshida M.D., First Department of Internal Medicine, Kyoto Prefectural University of Medicine, Kamikyo-ka, Kyoto 602, Japan.
Received for publication 16 July and in revised form 20 November 1979.

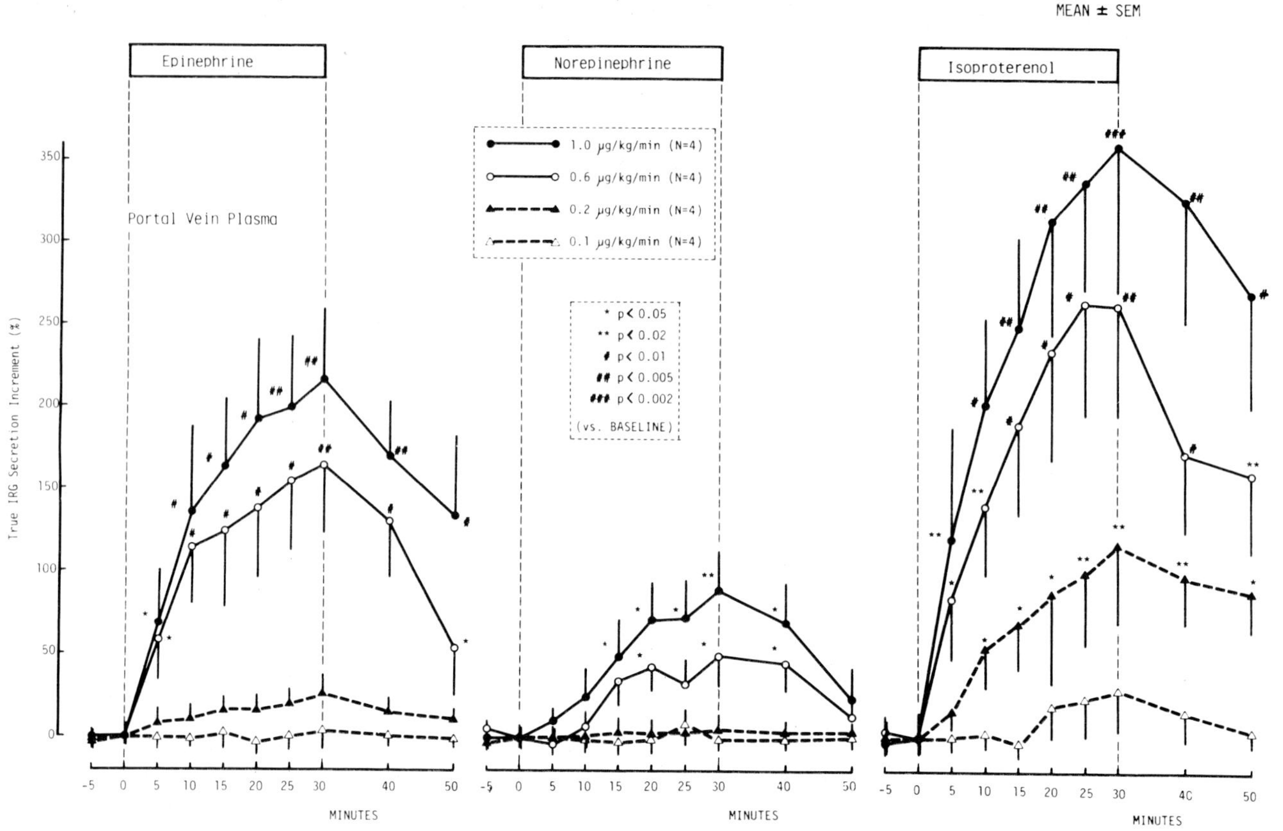

FIGURE 1. Dose response curves of the secretion of IRG induced by adrenergic agonists in depancreatized dogs.

body weight decreased by 15–20%, but consciousness was normal.

Blood was simultaneously withdrawn at appropriate intervals from the portal and femoral veins. Blood flow in the portal vein was measured by an electromagnetic flowmeter (Narcomatic-RT500, Narco Bio-Systems, Houston, Texas) with a C-type probe fixed on the portal vein. Blood flow increment was calculated as a percentage of the basal value. The blood sample was immediately transferred into a chilled tube containing 1.2 mg of ethylenediamine tetraacetate (Sigma Chemical Co., USA) and 1000 KIU of aprotinin (Trasylol, Bayer Co., Germany) per milliliter of blood. The sample was centrifuged immediately and the plasma was stored at −20°C until used. Glucagon (immunoreactive glucagon, IRG) was measured by radioimmunoassay using the C-terminal–specific glucagon antiserum, 30K (obtained from Dr. R. H. Unger, Dallas, Texas), by talc method to separate bound from free hormone.[6] The calculated plasma IRG value in the portal vein was corrected from the following formula:

$$\text{Calculated plasma IRG} = \text{plasma IRG concentration} \times \text{blood flow} \times \left(\frac{100 - \text{hematocrit}}{100}\right)$$

The value was further calculated and expressed as true IRG secretion increment in the percentage difference from the baseline value. Insulin (immunoreactive insulin, IRI) was measured by radioimmunoassay using the double-antibody method[7] and glucose was measured by the glucose-oxidase method.

All data are shown as mean ± SEM. Student's *t* test was used for statistical analysis and the measured values were compared with either basal levels or between the two groups.

RESULTS

EFFECT OF THE INFUSION OF EPINEPHRINE, NOREPINEPHRINE, OR ISOPROTERENOL ON THE SECRETION OF IRG, IRI, AND PLASMA GLUCOSE IN DEPANCREATIZED DOGS

Epinephrine. During infusion of epinephrine at a rate of 0.6 μg/kg/min for 30 min, the IRG level in femoral venous blood showed a significant increase from 255 ± 13 pg/ml to a peak of 373 ± 36 pg/ml at 30 min ($p < 0.02$). Plasma glucose levels increased from 330 ± 7 mg/dl to a maximum of 374 ± 16 mg/dl at 30 min ($p < 0.05$). No significant change was observed in IRI. In portal venous blood, the hematocrit showed no significant change, although the blood flow increment rose significantly to 35 ± 12% at 30 min ($p < 0.05$). The true IRG secretion increment showed a significant increase to a peak value of 164 ± 41% at 30 min ($p < 0.005$) (Figure 2).

Norepinephrine. During infusion of norepinephrine at a rate of 0.6 μg/kg/min for 30 min, a significant IRG response, similar to that elicited by the same rate of epinephrine, was observed either in femoral ($p < 0.02$) or in portal venous blood ($p < 0.05$). However, plasma glucose levels and IRI were unchanged (Figure 3).

Isoproterenol. During infusion of isoproterenol at a rate of 0.6 μg/kg/min for 30 min, a higher and significant IRG re-

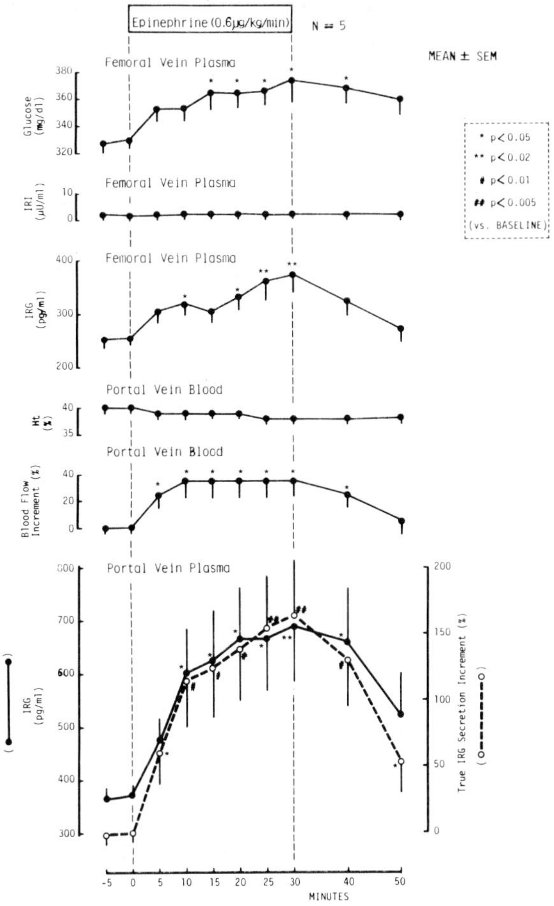

FIGURE 2. Effect of epinephrine on the secretion of IRG, IRI, and plasma glucose in depancreatized dogs.

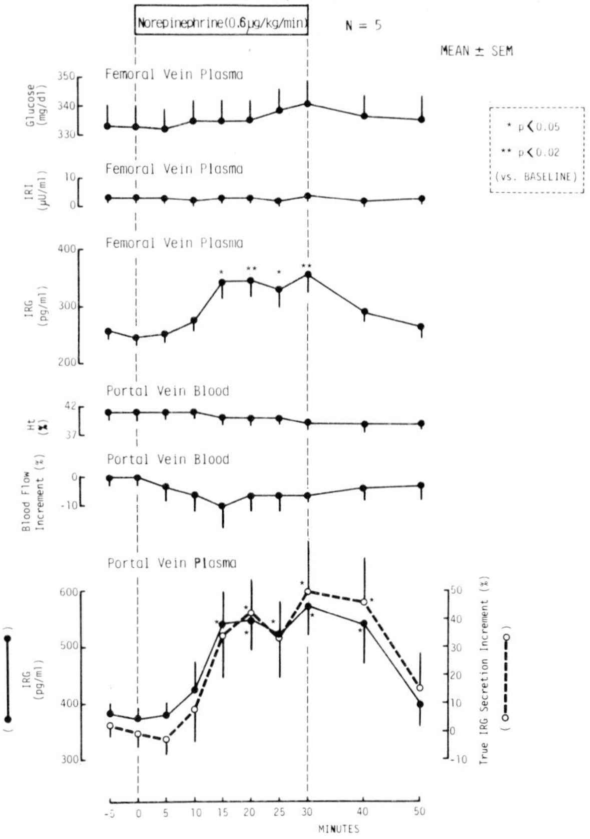

FIGURE 3. Effect of norepinephrine on the secretion of IRG, IRI, and plasma glucose in depancreatized dogs.

sponse, similar to that elicited by the same rate of epinephrine, was observed in both femoral ($p < 0.01$) and portal venous blood ($p < 0.005$). Plasma glucose levels also increased from the basal value of 317 ± 7 mg/dl to a peak of 380 ± 16 mg/dl at 30 min ($p < 0.01$), but IRI showed no change (Figure 4).

EFFECT OF THE INFUSION OF PHENTOLAMINE OR PROPRANOLOL ALONE ON THE SECRETION OF IRG, IRI, AND PLASMA GLUCOSE IN DEPANCREATIZED DOGS

When either phentolamine, at rates of 0.1, 0.2, and 0.4 μM/kg/min, or propranolol, at a rate of 0.1 μM/kg/min, was infused for 30 min, no significant changes were observed in IRG, IRI, and plasma glucose levels in femoral or in portal venous blood.

EFFECT OF PHENTOLAMINE OR PROPRANOLOL ON IRG RELEASE, AND PLASMA GLUCOSE RESPONSE INDUCED BY EPINEPHRINE, NOREPINEPHRINE, OR ISOPROTERENOL IN DEPANCREATIZED DOGS

Phentolamine. During the simultaneous infusion of phentolamine (0.1 μM/kg/min) and catecholamine (epinephrine norepinephrine, or isoproterenol at a rate of 0.6 μg/kg/min), no significant differences were found in responses of IRG and plasma glucose when compared with those obtained after catecholamine alone (Figure 5). The combined infusion of phentolamine at the increased rate (0.2 or 0.4 μM/kg/min) and catecholamine (epinephrine or norepinephrine, at a rate of 0.6 μg/kg/min, or isoproterenol, at a rate of 0.2 or 0.6 μg/kg/min) did not inhibit the release of IRG and plasma glucose when compared with the response induced by catecholamine alone.

Propranolol. Simultaneous infusion of propranolol (0.1 μM/kg/min) with epinephrine (0.6 μg/kg/min), norepinephrine (0.6 μg/kg/min), or isoproterenol (0.6 μg/kg/min) completely abolished catecholamine-induced IRG release and plasma glucose response ($p < 0.05$–0.005) (Figure 5).

DISCUSSION

IRG, originating mainly in the gastric fundus[8-10] and perhaps partly in the salivary gland,[11-13] has been reported to be the source of extrapancreatic glucagon, although glucagon has not been detected in the blood of eviscerated dogs.[14] Therefore, the main source of extrapancreatic glucagon in dogs was thought to be the gastric fundus.[9]

The regulation of gastrointestinal IRG has been reported previously. Gastrointestinal IRG secretion was inhibited in dogs by the infusion of insulin[1-3,15] and somatostatin.[16] It was stimulated by withdrawal of insulin therapy,[1,2] by the transplantation of the hypophysis in dogs,[4,5] by infusion of acetylcholine in dogs,[17] by vagal stimulation in rats[18] but not in dogs,[19] and by the administration of arginine in dogs[3,20,21] and rats.[18] When insulin deficiency was corrected in dogs, arginine infusion had no effect on gastrointestinal IRG secretion.[22]

In our study, we examined the effect of alpha- and beta-adrenergic substances on gastrointestinal IRG in conscious depancreatized dogs, which did not have severe ketoaci-

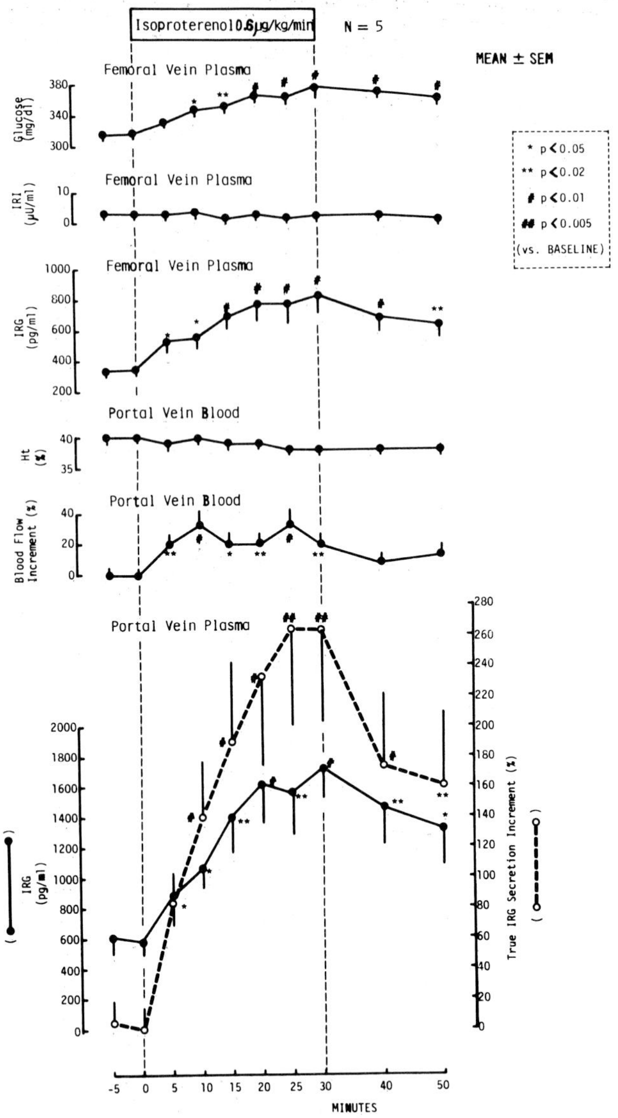

FIGURE 4. Effect of isoproterenol on the secretion of IRG, IRI, and plasma glucose in depancreatized dogs.

dosis or dehydration as measured by urinalysis and plasma glucose.

Epinephrine and isoproterenol, 0.05–0.2 µg/kg/min, are usually regarded as adequate infusions to induce alpha- and/or beta-agonism in metabolic studies.[23–25] However, we used 0.6 µg/kg/min of epinephrine, norepinephrine, and isoproterenol, which was calculated from dose response curves of gastrointestinal IRG shown in Figure 1.

Figures 2, 3, and 4 show that the secretion of gastrointestinal IRG was stimulated by the infusion of large amounts (0.6 µg/kg/min) of epinephrine, norepinephrine, or isoproterenol. The relative intensity of IRG secretion after catecholamine infusion was isoproterenol > epinephrine > norepinephrine. As shown in Figure 5, catecholamine-induced gastrointestinal IRG release was completely abolished by simultaneous infusion of the specific beta receptor–blocking compound, propranolol.

Alpha-adrenergic agonism of gastrointestinal IRG secretion was examined using combined infusions of catecholamine and alpha-blocking agents of varying concentrations. Combined infusion of the alpha-specific receptor–blocking compound, phentolamine, at rates of 0.1, 0.2, and 0.4 µM/kg/min, plus catecholamines (epinephrine at a rate of 0.6 µg/kg/min, norepinephrine at a rate of 0.6 µg/kg/min, or isoproterenol at a rate of 0.2 or 0.6 µg/kg/min) did not inhibit the release of gastrointestinal IRG that followed the infusion of catecholamine alone. However, the release of gastrointestinal IRG after norepinephrine infusion was inhibited completely when combined with beta-adrenergic receptor blockade. The high infusion rate of norepinephrine may have increased beta-agonism, which affected the release of gastrointestinal IRG. This needs further examination, because a direct alpha-adrenergic effect can not be excluded completely.

In this study, basal IRG before isoproterenol infusion in the portal vein was approximately 600 pg/ml (Figure 4), which was higher than in other experiments. (Figures 2 and 3). However, this may have been caused by the different testing days, because experiments with epinephrine and norepinephrine were done mainly on the third day after pancreatectomy, but studies with isoproterenol were carried out mainly on the fourth day. It has been shown that basal IRG increased daily after pancreatectomy in dogs without insulin therapy.[1–5]

There are conflicting reports about adrenergic effects on pancreatic A cells.[26,27] Iversen,[28] in 1973, found that pancreatic glucagon was stimulated by beta-adrenergic receptor agonists but was not influenced by alpha-adrenergic receptor agonists, while Samols and Weir,[29] in 1979, reported that there were alpha-adrenergic receptors on pancreatic A cells and that, in dogs, the secretion of glucagon was stimulated by either alpha- or beta-adrenergic receptor agonists. It has also been reported that the effect of alpha-adrenergic agonists on pancreatic A cell secretion was inhibitory in man[30] and dogs[31] and was stimulatory in man,[32] dogs,[29] ducks,[33] and rats.[34] Other experiments showed that beta-adrenergic agonists either inhibited glucagon secretion in man[32] and ducks[33] or stimulated glucagon in man,[30] dogs,[28,29] and rats.[35,36]

Botha et al.[37] examined the adrenergic effect on gastrointestinal IRG in a pancreatectomized patient and found that epinephrine caused a sharp fall in pancreatic glucagon-like immunoreactivity, which was overcome by either alpha or beta receptor blockade. It has been shown that gastrointestinal IRG increased daily in depancreatized dogs untreated with insulin,[1–5] but, in Botha's patient, insulin injection was only omitted for 24 h before examination, which may explain the difference in our results.

In this study, the infusion of epinephrine or norepinephrine at a rate of 0.1 or 0.2 µg/kg/min as shown in Figure 1 did not affect the secretion of gastrointestinal IRG. Possibly, gastric A cells were not influenced by the infusion of catecholamines in physiologic doses. These findings are consistent with the report of Vranic et al.[38] that in normal dogs plasma glucagon increased threefold during strenuous exercise, while in depancreatized dogs the concentration of plasma glucagon did not change during the same conditions. According to our knowledge, histologic examination of the sympathetic innervation of gastric A cells has not shown nerve terminals in close contact with gastric A cells.

Our study showed that large amounts (0.6 µg/kg/min) of

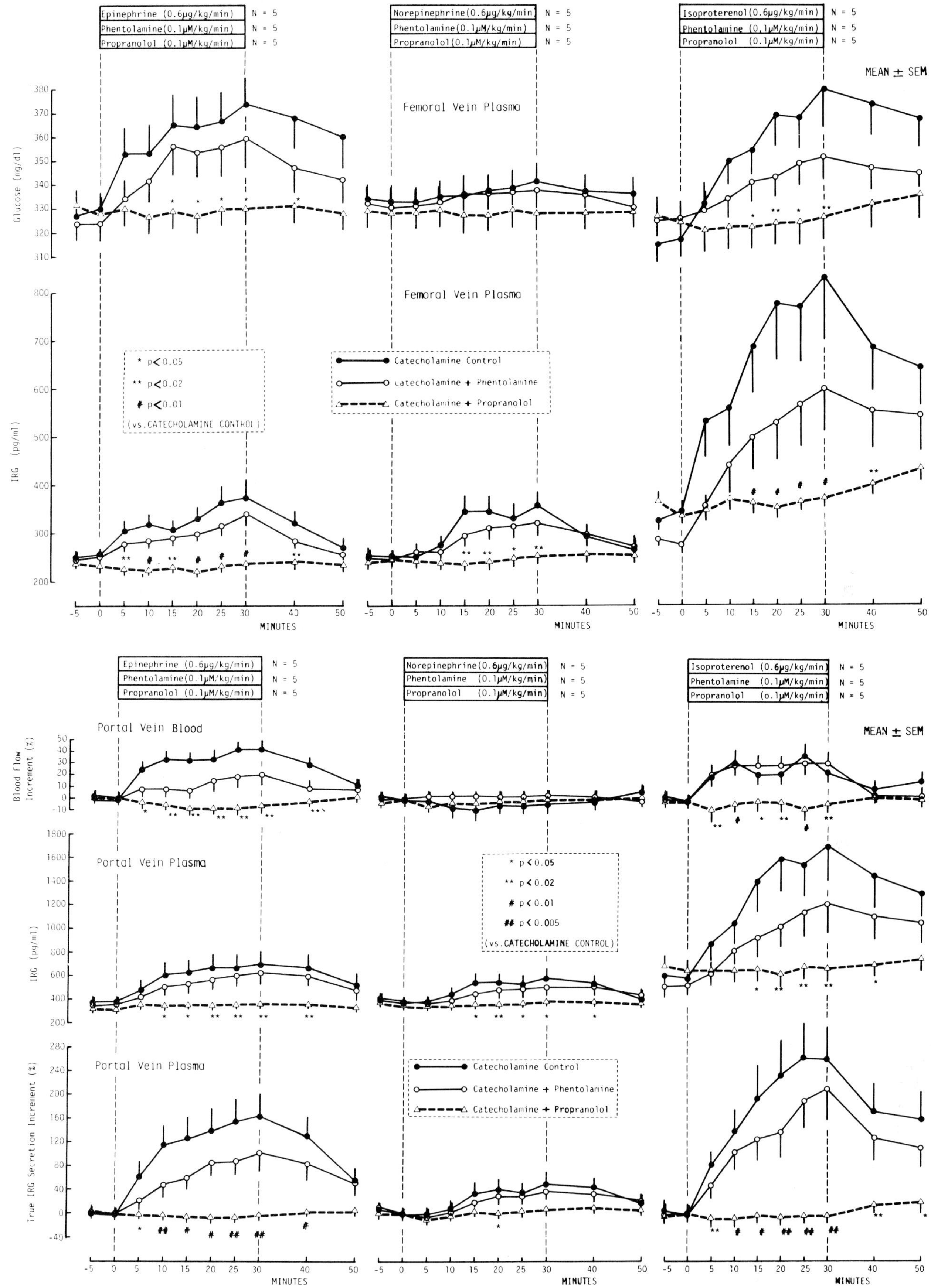

FIGURE 5. Effect of phentolamine or propranolol on IRG release, and plasma glucose response induced by epinephrine, norepinephrine, or isoproterenol in depancreatized dogs.

catecholamines increased the release of gastrointestinal IRG. It also suggested that they might act through a beta receptor, although a direct effect of alpha-adrenergic agonists on the release of gastrointestinal IRG could not be excluded.

ACKNOWLEDGMENTS

We thank A. Watanabe, M.D., for his excellent surgical assistance and Miss E. Okumura and Miss Y. Kuroi for their technical assistance.

This investigation was supported by grant 377270 from the Ministry of Education, Japan.

REFERENCES

[1] Matsuyama, T., and Foa, P. P.: Plasma glucose, insulin, pancreatic and enteroglucagon levels in normal and depancreatized dogs. Proc. Soc. Exp. Biol. Med. *147*:97–102, 1974.

[2] Vranic, M., Pek, S., and Kawamori, R.: Increased "glucagon immunoreactivity" in plasma of totally depancreatized dogs. Diabetes *23*:905–12, 1974.

[3] Mashiter, K., Harding, P. E., Chou, M., Mashiter, G. D., Stout, J., Diamond, D., and Field, J. B.: Persistent pancreatic glucagon but not insulin response to arginine in pancreatectomized dogs. Endocrinology *96*:678–93, 1975.

[4] Yoshida, T.: The effect of hypophysis upon gut glucagon. Folia Endocrinol. Jpn. *53*:1118–28, 1977.

[5] Yoshida, T., and Kondo, M.: The effect of hypophysectomy and hypophysis-transplantation on the secretion of gut glucagon immunoreactivity and gut glucagon-like immunoreactivity in depancreatized dogs. Endocrinol. Jpn. *27*(1): In press, 1980.

[6] Sakurai, H., Kuzuya, H., Kurahachi, H., Fukase, M., and Imura, H.: A sensitive radioimmunoassay for glucagon using talc method. Jpn. J. Nucl. Med. *10*: 135, 1973.

[7] Hales, C. N., and Randle, P. J.: Immunoassay of insulin with insulin antibody precipitate. Biochem. J. *88*:137–46, 1963.

[8] Sasaki, H., Rubalcava, B., Baetens, D., Blazquez, E., Srikant, C. B., Orci, L., and Unger, R. H.: Identification of glucagon in the gastrointestinal tract. J. Clin. Invest. *56*:135–45, 1975.

[9] Blazquez, E., Munoz-Barragan, L., Patton, G. S., Orci, L., Dobbs, R. E., and Unger, R. H.: Gastric A-cell function in insulin-deprived depancreatized dogs. Endocrinology *99*:1182–88, 1976.

[10] Larsson, L. I., Holst, J., Hakanson, R., and Sundler, F.: Distribution and properties of glucagon immunoreactivity in the digestive tract of various mammals: an immunohistochemical and immunochemical study. Histochemistry *44*:281–90, 1975.

[11] Silverman, H., and Dunbar, J. C.: The submaxillary gland as a possible source of glucagon. Bull. Sinai Hosp. Detroit *22*:192–93, 1974.

[12] Lawrence, A. M., Tan, S., Hojvat, S., and Kirsteins, L.: Salivary gland hyperglycemic factor: an extrapancreatic source of glucagon-like materials. Science *195*:70–72, 1977.

[13] Bathena, S. J., Smith, S. S., Voyles, N. R., Penhos, J. C., and Recant, L.: Studies on submaxillary gland immunoreactive glucagon. Biochem. Biophys. Res. Commun. *74*:1574–81, 1977.

[14] Lefebvre, P. J., and Luyckx, A. S.: Plasma glucagon after kidney exclusion: experiments in somatostatin-infused and in eviscerated dogs. Metabolism *25*:761–68, 1976.

[15] Lefebvre, P. J., and Luyckx, A. S.: Glucose and insulin in the regulation of glucagon release from the isolated perfused dog stomach. Endocrinology *103*:1579–82, 1978.

[16] Sakurai, H., Dobbs, R. E., and Unger, R. H.: The role of glucagon in the pathogenesis of the endogenous hyperglycemia of diabetes mellitus. Metabolism *24*:1287–97, 1975.

[17] Yoshida, T., and Kondo, M.: Effect of acetylcholine on the secretion of gut glucagon immunoreactivity and gut glucagon-like immunoreactivity in pancreatectomized dogs. Endocrinol. Jpn. *27*(1): In press, 1980.

[18] Marre, M., Bobbioni, E., Suarez, M., Reach, G., Dubois, M. P., and Assan, R.: Control of gastric glucagon secretion in acutely pancreatectomized rat. Diabetes *28*:213–20, 1979.

[19] Lefebvre, P. J., Luyckx, A. S., and Brassinne, A. H.: Vagal stimulation and its role in eliciting gastrin but not glucagon release from the isolated perfused dog stomach. Gut *19*:185–88, 1978.

[20] Matsuyama, T., Tanaka, R., Shima, K., Nonaka, K., and Tarui, S.: Lack of gastrointestinal glucagon response to hypoglycemia in depancreatized dogs. Diabetologia *15*:471–74, 1978.

[21] Muller, W. A., Girardier, L., Seydoux, J., Berger, M., Renold, A. E., and Vranic, M.: Extrapancreatic glucagon and glucagon like immunoreactivity in depancreatized dogs. A quantitative assessment of secretion rates and anatomical delineation of sources. J. Clin. Invest. *62*:124–32, 1978.

[22] Cherrington, A. D., Kawamori, R., Pek, S., and Vranic, M.: Arginine infusion in dogs. Model for the role of insulin and glucagon in regulating glucose turnover and free fatty acid levels. Diabetes *23*:805–15, 1974.

[23] Eigler, N., Sacca, L., and Sherwin, R. S.: Synergistic interactions of physiologic increments of glucagon, epinephrine and cortisol in the dog. J. Clin. Invest. *63*:114–23, 1979.

[24] Altszuler, N., Moraru, E., Gottlieb, B., and Hampshire, J.: Effect of isoproterenol on glucose turnover and insulin secretion in the normal dog. Biochem. Pharmacol. *27*:769–72, 1978.

[25] Winkler, B., Rathgeb, I., Bjerknes, C., Steele, R., and Altszuler, N.: Effect of norepinephrine on glycerol and glucose metabolism in the normal dog. Am. J. Physiol. *225*:81–84, 1973.

[26] Woods, S. C., and Porte, D., Jr.: Neural control of the endocrine pancreas. Physiol. Rev. *54*:596–619, 1974.

[27] Gerich, J. E., Charles, M. A., and Grodsky, G. M.: Regulation of pancreatic insulin and glucagon secretion. Annu. Rev. Physiol. *38*:353–88, 1976.

[28] Iversen, J.: Adrenergic receptors and the secretion of glucagon and insulin from the isolated, perfused canine pancreas. J. Clin. Invest. *52*:2102–16, 1973.

[29] Samols, E., and Weir, G.: Adrenergic modulation of pancreatic A, B, and D cells. J. Clin. Invest. *63*:230–38, 1979.

[30] Gerich, J. E., Langlois, M., Noacco, C., Schneider, V., and Forsham, P. H.: Adrenergic modulation of pancreatic glucagon secretion in man. J. Clin. Invest. *53*:1441–46, 1974.

[31] Miller, R. E., and Horton, E. S.: Neural release of glucagon is inhibited by hyperglycemia and enhanced by phentolamine. Diabetes *28*:762–68, 1979.

[32] Gerich, J. E., Karam, J. H., and Forsham, P. H.: Reciprocal adrenergic control of pancreatic alpha- and beta-cell function in man. Diabetes *21*(Suppl. 1):332–33, 1972. Abstract.

[33] Tyler, J. M., and Kajinuma, H.: Influence of beta adrenergic and cholinergic agents in vivo on pancreatic glucagon and insulin secretion. Diabetes *21*(Suppl. 1):332, 1972. Abstract.

[34] Harvey, W., Faloona, G., and Unger, R.: Effect of adrenergic blockade on exercise-induced hyperglucagonemia. Clin. Res. *20*:752A, 1972. Abstract.

[35] Luyckx, A. S., and Lefebvre, P. J.: Role of catecholamines in exercise-induced glucagon secretion in rats. Diabetes *21*(Suppl. 1):334, 1972. Abstract.

[36] Weir, G. C., Knowlton, S. D., and Martin, D. B.: Glucagon secretion from the perfused rat pancreas; studies with glucose and catecholamines. J. Clin. Invest. *54*:1403–12, 1974.

[37] Botha, J. L., Vinik, A. I., Child, P. T., Paul, M., and Jackson, W. P. U.: Pancreatic glucagon-like immunoreactivity in a pancreatectomized patient. Horm. Metab. Res. *9*:199–205, 1977.

[38] Vranic, M., Kawamori, R., Pek, S., Kovacevic, N., and Wrenshall, G. A.: The essentiality of insulin and the role of glucagon in regulating glucose utilization and production during strenuous exercise in dogs. J. Clin. Invest. *57*:245–55, 1976.

Duodenal Contribution to Pancreaticoduodenal Vein Islet Hormones During Stimulation of the Canine Pancreas with Calcium

K. HERMANSEN

SUMMARY

The possible influence of the duodenum on pancreatic hormones in the pancreaticoduodenal venous effluent of the canine pancreas was studied. The magnitude and dynamics of somatostatin, glucagon, and insulin responses during stimulation with 5 mM calcium were identical whether or not the duodenal remnant was excluded from the perfusion by clamping.

The results indicate that during perfusion with calcium the duodenal remnant is without any significant regulatory or contributory role on pancreatic hormone secretion from the isolated canine pancreas preparation. DIABETES *29*:361–364, May 1980.

The development of techniques for perfusing the pancreas initiated an era of increasing knowledge of the secretory mechanisms and dynamics of hormonal release. In most perfusion methods currently used, a portion of the duodenum remains attached.[1-3] The question has often been raised whether the endocrine cells of the duodenum might contribute to or modify the secretion of pancreatic somatostatin, glucagon, and insulin measured in the pancreatico-duodenal efflux.[4-7] This is obviously of considerable importance for the interpretation of many studies.

The present study was designed to determine if the duodenal remnant had any contributory significance for the hormone secretion from the isolated pancreaticoduodenal preparation. The responses of somatostatin, glucagon, and insulin during calcium stimulation were compared before and after exclusion from the perfusion of the duodenal remnant. Calcium was chosen as stimulus since it is a common key substance in the normal secretory process of the D,[3,8,9] A,[10-12] and B cells.[13,14]

From the Second University Clinic of Internal Medicine, Kommunehospitalet, DK-8000 Aarhus C, Denmark.

Address reprint requests to Dr. Hermansen.

Received for publication 28 September and in revised form 14 December 1979.

MATERIAL AND METHODS

Mongrel dogs, fasted overnight, weighing 18–25 kg, were used as pancreas donors. The techniques for isolation of the canine pancreas and the perfusion system have previously been described in detail.[1] In brief, the preparation consists of the pancreas and the proximal 10 cm of the attached duodenum. A non-recirculating medium of Krebs-Ringer bicarbonate buffer (pH 7.4) containing 40 g/L dextran (mol wt 75,000), 2 g/L bovine albumin, glutamate, fumarate, and pyruvate, each at a concentration of 5 mM, was pumped through the splenic and the celiac arteries, and the total portal effluent was collected every minute. Oxygenation of the Krebs-Ringer bicarbonate buffer was achieved by means of a rotating roller screen in an atmosphere of 94.4% O_2 and 5.6% CO_2.

Two types of experiments were performed—clamping and control experiments. During the entire perfusion in the control experiments and during the first half of the perfusion in the clamping experiments the duodenum was kept intact as previously described.[1] However, after the initial 40 min the duodenum was excluded from the perfusion circuit in the clamping experiments. To localize the outlet of the main pancreatic duct, the duodenum was cut through by a longitudinal incision on the side opposite the attachment of the pancreas. Two clamps were then applied close to each side of the main pancreatic duct, leaving the outlet patent and concomitantly excluding from the perfusion practically all the duodenum. At the end of each experiment, the preparation was perfused with methylene blue which colored the pancreas but not the duodenum. The perfusion flow was constant throughout the experiments (18–20 ml/min), except in two perfusion experiments where the flow rate decreased by about 5% after the exclusion of duodenum. The perfusion pressure (30–40 mm Hg) was kept constant throughout the experiments.

Somatostatin,[3,8] glucagon,[15] and insulin[15] were measured by specific radioimmunoassays, as described in detail previously. In the glucagon assay, an antibody was used which does not distinguish between glucagon-like immunoreactivity from the gut and pancreatic glucagon.

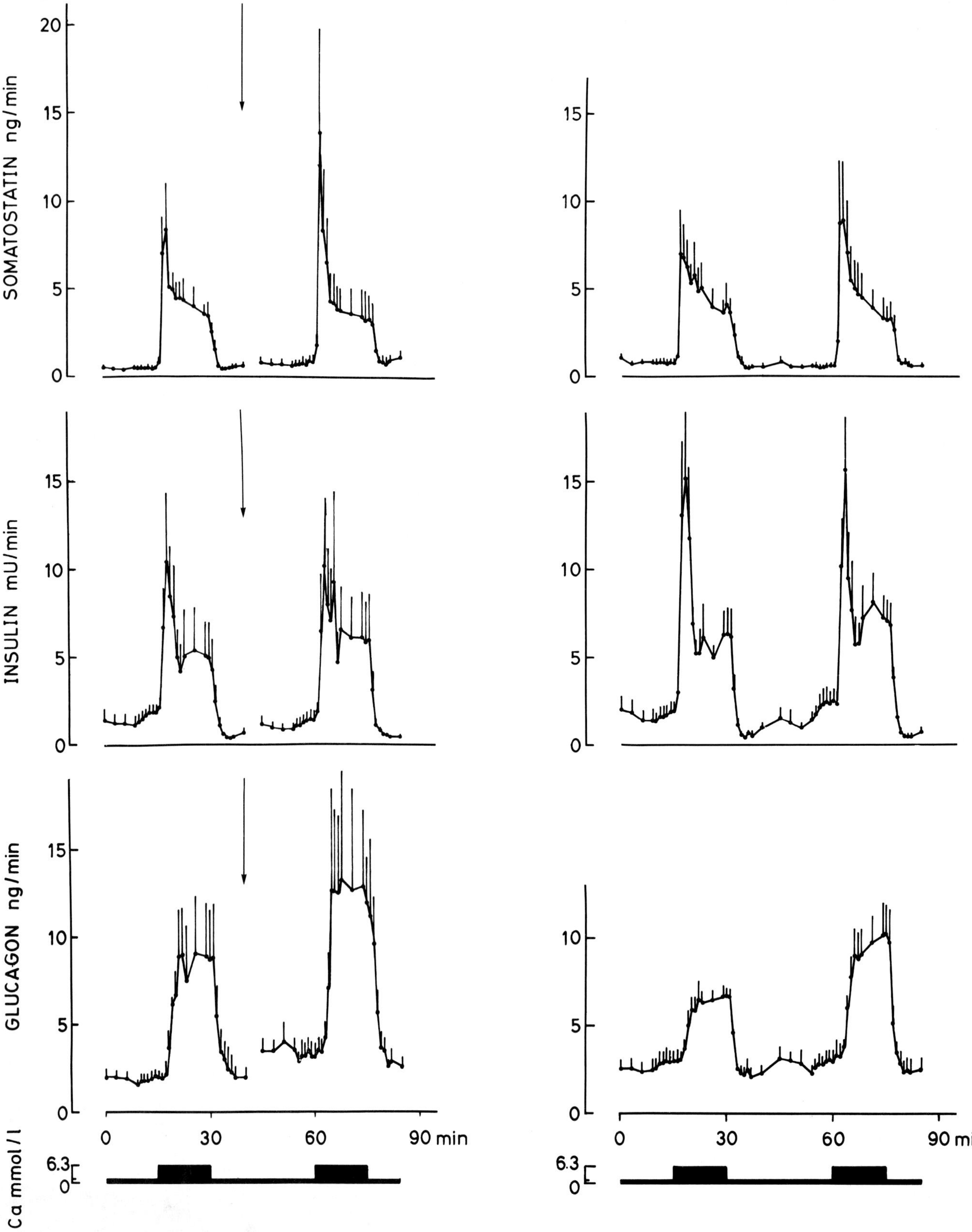

FIGURE 1. ***Left panel:*** **Lack of effect of duodenal exclusion on calcium (5 mmol/L)-stimulated somatostatin, glucagon, and insulin release from the isolated, perfused canine pancreas. The clamping off of the duodenum is indicated by arrows. Mean results ±SEM of four perfusion experiments.** ***Right panel:*** **Effect of 5 mmol/L calcium on somatostatin, glucagon, and insulin secretion in the control experiments with duodenum left intact. Mean results ±SEM of four perfusion experiments.**

Calculations. The incremental increase in hormone secretion in response to the second calcium stimulation was calculated as the average percentage increase above the basal level (±SEM). The basal hormone level was calculated as the mean of the last five one-minute values preceding the addition of high calcium. When comparing the two basal levels in each of the pancreas perfusions, the second of these was expressed in per cent of the first. Two-tailed Student's *t* tests were used for statistical evaluation of data employing a 5% limit of significance. Nonpaired tests were used for comparisons of results from control experiments with those from clamping experiments; otherwise, paired tests were used.

RESULTS

The effect of calcium on somatostatin, glucagon, and insulin release was tested before and after exclusion of the duodenum. During perfusion with a constant concentration of glucose (100 mg/100 ml perfusate), calcium was increased from 1.3 to 6.3 mM for 15 min. As illustrated in the left panel of Figure 1, this elicited an increase in the secretion of somatostatin, glucagon, and insulin whether or not the duodenum was included in the perfusion circuit. In both situations, somatostatin and insulin responses to an increase in calcium were immediate and biphasic, whereas glucagon responses were uniphasic.

After exclusion of the duodenal remnant, the total hormone output during the 15-min period with high calcium averaged (for somatostatin) 98 ± 25%, (for insulin) 107 ± 9%, and (for glucagon) 156 ± 11% of the total output obtained during the first calcium stimulation ($\bar{x}$ ± SEM, N = 4). For comparison, four control perfusions were performed in which no clamping was applied (Figure 1, right panel). As it can be seen, the patterns of response appeared similar to those obtained in the clamping experiments. Corresponding values in the controls were 98 ± 5% for somatostatin, 109 ± 5% for insulin, and 142 ± 18% for glucagon ($\bar{x}$ ± SEM, N = 4). There was no statistically significant difference between the two groups of experiments for any of the three hormones.

When the increments in hormone release were expressed as per cent above basal level ($\bar{x}$ ± SEM, N = 4), the somatostatin, insulin, and glucagon responses to high calcium following the clamping procedure were 709 ± 165%, 391 ± 103%, and 259 ± 92%, respectively. The analogous results in the control experiments were 886 ± 218% for somatostatin, 441 ± 103% for insulin, and 218 ± 18% for glucagon ($\bar{x}$ ± SEM, N = 4). The incremental increases in hormone output were not significantly different in the two types of experiments.

The basal levels for the three hormones did not change significantly during the perfusions (Figure 1). Glucagon levels tended to increase in both clamped and nonclamped experiments, but the change did not reach statistical significance.

DISCUSSION

Samols et al.[5,6] have repeatedly emphasized that it is important to use a duodenum-free preparation of pancreas in studying pancreatic hormone secretion since the duodenum contains somatostatin[16] and glucagon,[17] both of which, they thought, might contribute to changes in the hormone concentrations estimated in the pancreaticoduodenal efflux. They have accordingly termed their duodenum-free preparation 'the truly isolated pancreas preparation.' On the other hand, Unger et al.,[4] who employ an identical preparation to ours, have the opinion that the duodenal content of somatostatin and glucagon in the dog is so small as to be without significance for hormone release from the pancreaticoduodenal preparation. However, it has often proved fallacious to judge release activity from tissue content of hormones, since the latter reflects a balance between synthesis, storage, and release. We thought it of interest to try to settle the issue by excluding the duodenal remnant from the perfusion by clamping and to compare the magnitude and dynamics of the hormone release before and after exclusion. The results have been compared with those obtained in control experiments, where an exactly identical experimental protocol was followed, except that the clamping off of the duodenum was omitted. The present report shows that identical release patterns of hormones were obtained whether or not the duodenum was excluded both during basal conditions and during stimulation with calcium, which stimulates the A, B, and D cells of the pancreas. It therefore appears that the duodenal remnant does not contribute to or regulate hormone release in the perfused canine pancreas, at least under the circumstances examined in this study.

ACKNOWLEDGMENTS

Cyclic somatostatin for immunization and standards was kindly donated by Norman Grant, Wyeth Laboratories, Philadelphia, Pennsylvania; and Roger Guillemin, Salk Institute, La Jolla, California, generously gave us Tyr[11]-somatostatin for the iodination. Karen Just and Joan Hansen are thanked for expert technical assistance and Anette Larsen for typing the manuscript.

This work was supported by the Danish Medical Research Council, P. Carl Petersen Foundation, and a Novo research grant.

REFERENCES

1 Iversen, J., and Miles, D. W.: Evidence for a feedback inhibition of insulin on insulin secretion in the isolated perfused canine pancreas. Diabetes *20*:1–9, 1971.

2 Ipp, E., Dobbs, R. E., Arimura, A., Vale, W., Harris, V., and Unger, R. H.: Release of immunoreactive somatostatin from the pancreas in response to glucose, amino-acids, pancreozymin-cholecystokinin, and tolbutamide. J. Clin. Invest. *60*:760–65, 1977.

3 Hermansen, K., Christensen, S. E., and Ørskov, H.: Characterisation of somatostatin release from the pancreas. The role of calcium and acetylcholine. Diabetologia *16*:261–66, 1979.

4 Ipp, E., Dobbs, R. E., Arimura, A., Vale, W., and Unger, R. H.: The effects of gastrin, gastric inhibitory polypeptide, secretin and the octapeptide of cholecystokinin upon immunoreactive somatostatin release by the perfused canine pancreas. J. Clin. Invest. *60*:1216–19, 1977.

5 Samols, E., Weir, G. C., Ramseur, R., Day, J. A., and Patel, Y. C.: Modulation of pancreatic somatostatin by adrenergic and cholinergic agonism and by hyper- and hypoglycemic sulfonamides. Metabolism *27*(Suppl. 1):1219–21, 1978.

6 Samols, E., and Weir, G. C.: Adrenergic modulation of pancreatic A, B, and D cells. J. Clin. Invest. *63*:230–38, 1979.

7 Rehfeld, J. F.: Gastrointestinal hormones and somatostatin release. Gastroenterology *75*:540–41, 1978.

8 Hermansen, K., Christensen, S. W., and Ørskov, H.: Characterisation of somatostatin release from the pancreas: the role of potassium. Scand. J. Clin. Lab. Invest. *39*:717–22, 1979.

9 Hermansen, K., Christensen, S. E., and Ørskov, H.: The significance of the Na^+/K^+ pump for somatostatin release. Horm. Metab. Res. *12*:23–25, 1979.

[10] Iversen, J., and Hermansen, K.: Calcium, glucose, and glucagon release. Diabetologia *13*:297–303, 1977.

[11] Hermansen, K., and Iversen, J.: Effect of verapamil on pancreatic glucagon release from the isolated, perfused canine pancreas. Scand. J. Clin. Lab. Invest. *37*:139–42, 1977.

[12] Hermansen, K., and Iversen, J.: Dual action of Mn^{++} upon the secretion of insulin and glucagon from the isolated, perfused canine pancreas. Possible interactions with Ca^{++}. Diabetologia *15*:475–79, 1978.

[13] Grodsky, G. M., and Bennett, L. L.: Cation requirements for insulin secretion in the isolated, perfused pancreas. Diabetes *15*:910–13, 1966.

[14] Milner, R. D. G., and Hales, C. N.: The role of calcium and magnesium in insulin secretion from rabbit pancreas studies in vitro. Diabetologia *3*:47–49, 1967.

[15] Ørskov, H., Thomsen, H. G., and Yde, H.: Wick chromatography for rapid and reliable immunoassay of insulin, glucagon and growth hormone. Nature (Lond.) *219*:193–95, 1968.

[16] Polak, J. M., Pearse, A. G. E., Grimelius, L., Bloom, S. R., and Arimura, A.: Growth-hormone release-inhibiting hormone in gastrointestinal and pancreatic D cells. Lancet *I*:1220–22, 1975.

[17] Dobbs, R., Sakurai, H., Sasaki, G., Faloona, G., Valverde, I., Baetens, D., Orci, L., and Unger, R.: Glucagon: role in the hyperglycemia of diabetes mellitus. Science *187*:544–47, 1975.

Effects of Therapy on the Nature and Quantity of Fuels Oxidized During Diabetic Ketoacidosis

O. E. OWEN, V. E. TRAPP, G. A. REICHARD, JR., M. A. MOZZOLI, R. SMITH, AND G. BODEN

SUMMARY

We studied seven patients, in moderate to severe diabetic ketoacidosis (DKA), measuring respiratory exchanges of O_2, CO_2, and acetone and urinary excretion of nitrogen, ketone bodies, and glucose to calculate the respiratory quotient (RQ), nonprotein respiratory quotient (npRQ), metabolic requirements, and calories derived from fat, carbohydrate, and protein oxidation. Results from indirect calorimetry were related to circulating concentrations of glucose, free fatty acids, ketone bodies, and amino acids over a 14-h study consisting of a 2-h period I of rehydration with saline, a 4-h period II of rehydration and insulin therapy, and an 8-h period III of rehydration, insulin, and glucose administration.

During period I, of about 2 h of saline rehydration, the RQ (0.55–0.80) and npRQ (0.58–0.88) varied among the patients but in general was low. The caloric requirements were 1.24 kcal/min/1.73 m^2. Initially, fat contributed 78 ± 11%, glucose 17 ± 10%, and protein 5 ± 2% of the metabolic requirements. The circulating concentrations of fuels remained constant. During period II, after about 4 h of saline and insulin therapy, the RQ (0.62–0.88) and npRQ (0.55–0.91) remained rather stable, rising in only two of seven patients. Nevertheless, in all patients, saline and insulin therapy was associated with precipitous decreases in circulating concentrations of glucose, free fatty acids, acetoacetate, and beta-hydroxybutyrate and gradual decreases in plasma amino acids. During period III, after 8–12 h of insulin therapy, the RQ (0.68–0.92) and npRQ (0.48–1.01) increased, rising in five of six patients. Heightened RQ and npRQ values were observed only after plasma free fatty acid concentrations decreased to 0.44 ± 0.12 mM and plasma acetoacetate plus beta-hydroxybutyrate concentrations decreased to 5.27 ± 1.86 mM, while plasma glucose concentration remained elevated at 13.49 ± 3.67 mM because of intravenous glucose infusion.

Caloric requirements diminished progressively throughout the study, and after about 4 h of saline and insulin therapy a reciprocal relationship between the contributions of fat and glucose to metabolic requirements was evident. At the end of period III the caloric requirements were 0.77 kcal/min/1.73 m^2. Fat contributed 44 ± 16%, glucose 42 ± 22%, and protein 14 ± 8% of the metabolic requirements.

We have observed a dissociation between the decrease in plasma glucose, free fatty acids, ketone bodies, and amino acids and the nature of fuels oxidized. This suggests that, during the initial hours of therapy for DKA, the predominant effect of insulin is to promote fuel storage rather than to promote glucose and ketone body oxidation. It was 8–12 h in the course of therapy before the npRQ rose, reflecting heightened glucose oxidation and diminished fat oxidation. Metabolic requirements progressively decreased with therapy. DIABETES 29:365–372, May 1980.

From the Department of Medicine and General Clinical Research Center, Temple University Health Sciences Center, Philadelphia, and the Division of Research, Lankenau Hospital, Philadelphia, Pennsylvania.

Address reprint requests to Oliver E. Owen, M.D., Temple University Hospital, 3401 N. Broad Street, Philadelphia, Pennsylvania 19140.

Received for publication 15 October 1979.

Diabetic ketoacidosis (DKA) is characterized by the lack of reciprocity among the rates of hepatic glycogenolysis, gluconeogenesis, and ketogenesis, resulting in inappropriately elevated hepatic production rates of glucose and ketone bodies and subsequently hyperglycemia and hyperketonemia.[1] This, coupled with increased free fatty acid mobilization from adipose tissue and concurrent proteolysis, floods the bloodstream with an overabundance of fuels that compete as oxidative substrates for tissues.[1–3] Although these facts have been established, the exact nature and quantity of fuels consumed during DKA and the effects of therapy on this catabolic state are unknown.

The best method available for determining total body energy requirement and the nature of fuels oxidized is indirect calorimetry. Benedict and Joslin used these techniques to study diabetic patients during mild catabolic episodes and reported their results in 1912.[4] Their results were limited, and insulin therapy was not available. Recently, interest has

TABLE 1
Clinical characteristics of diabetic patients in ketoacidosis

Patient	Sex	Age (yr)	Height (cm)	Weight (kg)	Body surface area (m^2)	History of diabetes (yr)	Therapy prior to hospitalization (units of insulin)	Days without insulin	Concomitant disease
O.G.	M	23	170	71.5	1.82	7	NPH 40 + Reg 10	1	None apparent
W.B.	M	40	178	91.6	2.10	0	None		Obesity, hypertension
J.B1.	M	57	177	80.9	1.97	10	NPH 50 + Reg 25	6	Neuropathy
D.H.	F	18	155	43.5	1.38	17	Reg 40	3	None apparent
D.M.	F	31	155	48.0	1.48	1	NPH 16	4	Alcoholism
L.T.	F	49	150	39.0	1.27	10	NPH 22	5	Emaciation, pancreatic insufficiency
J.Ba.	F	69	145	52.0	1.42	36	NPH 40 + Reg 10	7	Organic heart disease
Mean (N = 7)		41	161	60.9	1.63	12			
±SEM		7	5	7.7	0.12	5			

focused on metabolic derangements during DKA and the responses of this disorder to corrective therapy.[5-9] Nevertheless, insight into the mechanisms responsible for the changes in concentrations of blood glucose, free fatty acids, and amino acids is restricted. Therefore, we studied seven patients who came to the hospital in DKA. We used the method of indirect calorimetry, coupled with techniques to measure blood substrate and hormone concentrations, to determine the nature and quantity of fuels oxidized during DKA and to define the effects of therapy on fuel metabolism during reversal of this catabolic state.

METHODS

Patients. Three male and four female adult patients in diabetic ketoacidosis were studied. Their clinical data are shown in Table 1. Although their average height, weight, and body surface area were normal, one male patient (W.B.) was obese and one female patient (L.T.) was emaciated. Table 2 shows their routine clinical laboratory data before therapy. Arterial pH, PCO_2, and HCO_3^- revealed that four patients (O.G., J.B1., D.H., and J.Ba.) were in severe and three patients (W.B., D.M., and L.T.) were in moderate states of acidosis. All patients were hyperglycemic and had positive plasma nitroprusside tests (Acetest or Ketostix, Ames Laboratories, Elkhart, Indiana). The patients were admitted to the General Clinical Research Center at Temple University Hospital after it was established that they were suffering from metabolic acidosis, hyperglycemia, and hyperketonemia and were clinically stable. Informed voluntary consent was obtained from all patients, and the protocol was approved by the Human Research Review Committee.

Experimental protocol. The patients were studied in the supine position in bed in a room equipped with an efficient ventilation system to maintain normal room air content. Intravenous catheters were placed in peripheral veins for collection of blood samples and for administration of water, electrolytes, insulin, and glucose. The study consisted of three parts: period I, rehydration with 0.45% or 9% saline; period II, rehydration and administration of insulin; period III, rehydration and administration of insulin and glucose. Appropriate supplementary electrolytes were administered.

The respiratory gaseous exchanges of O_2 and CO_2 and urinary excretion of nitrogen, glucose, and ketone bodies were periodically measured to calculate respiratory quotients (RQ), nonprotein respiratory quotients (npRQ), "corrected" nonprotein respiratory quotients ("corrected" npRQ), caloric requirements, and percentage of calories derived from protein, fat, and carbohydrate oxidation.

Blood was drawn to determine concentrations of plasma glucose, lactate, free fatty acids (FFA), glycerol, triglycerides, acetoacetate (AcAc), beta-hydroxybutyrate (β-OHB), acetone, alanine, glutamine, glutamate, urea nitrogen, glucagon, and serum insulin. The patients were all acutely ill, and the protocol was complex. Therefore, not all measurements could be done on each patient according to protocol. For instance, patient D.H. was too ill to obtain all the control specimens. She voided urine; respiratory gases and blood samples were obtained, and saline with insulin therapy was begun. Patient W.B. was investigated for only 4 h and patient O.G. for 8½ h after saline and insulin therapy was begun. The remaining four patients (J.B1., D.M., L. T., and J.Ba.) completed the study, which lasted approximately 14 h. Saline was infused intravenously at a rate of about 1 L/h during the initial several hours, insulin was infused intravenously at a minimal rate of 6 U/h, and glucose was infused intravenously at a minimal rate of about 15 g/h/70 kg

TABLE 2
Arterial blood pH, P_{CO_2}, and HCO_3^-, venous plasma glucose, and electrolytes

Patient	pH	P_{CO_2} (mmHg)	HCO_3^-(mM)	Glucose (mg/dl)	Na (meq/L)	K (meq/L)	Cl (meq/L)
O.G.	7.22	24	9.5	382	138	6.8	95
W.B.	7.32	21	10.5	476	129	2.8	92
J.B1.	7.19	10	3.6	484	129	3.8	83
D.H.	7.20	18	8.0	459	136	5.4	113
D.M.	7.29	20	8.7	480	133	3.3	84
L.T.	7.29	27	12.1	453	136	3.2	101
J.Ba.	7.09	25	7.3	966	145	3.0	109
Mean (N = 7)	7.23	21	8.5	528	135	4.0	97
±SEM	0.03	11	1.0	74	2	0.6	4

body wt during the final several hours. Respiratory gas and blood samples were collected nearly simultaneously, and urine collections were obtained approximately midway between collection of respiratory gas and blood samples. Collections were made at about hourly intervals between −2 h and +2 h and then at about 2-h intervals until about 12 h after initiating insulin therapy.

To determine respiratory exchanges of O_2 and CO_2, an open air-collecting system consisting of a plastic hood placed over the head of the patient was used. During each collection period, a constant, measured air flow of 35–55 L/min was maintained by a pump.[10] Samples of diluted expired air from the patient were collected in Douglas bags for subsequent analyses.

Calculations. The theory and equations for calculating RQ, npRQ, "corrected" npRQ, and nature and quantity of fuels oxidized are given in the Appendix.

Circulating substrate and hormone concentrations and urinary metabolites. The analytic methods and the precision for quantitating plasma, serum or urine AcAc, β-OHB, acetone, glucose, alanine, glutamine, glutamate, glycerol, triglycerides, FFA, glucagon, insulin, and nitrogen have been published.[11–13] The methods for measuring urine and breath acetone excretion have been published in detail.[13] Plasma and urine AcAc concentrations were measured immediately after the specimens were obtained to prevent loss from spontaneous decay. To prevent contamination from AcAc, β-OHB, and lactate, double-extracted plasma was used to determine FFA concentrations. All determinations were done in duplicate.

Respiratory O_2 and CO_2 analyses of the gaseous contents in the Douglas bags were performed using a calibrated Nyons diaferometer (Kipp at Zonen, Delft, Holland). This method has been shown to compare favorably with the micromethod of Scholander for gas analysis.[14] O_2 and CO_2 contents were corrected to STP, and O_2 consumption and CO_2 production were computed.

Data presentation and statistical analyses. The values are expressed as the mean ± SEM or as the mean and ranges. The ranges are used to depict the heterogeneity of the patient population. Individual patient data are presented to illustrate specific changes. Statistical differences among the periods were evaluated by using Student's t test for paired samples.[15]

RESULTS

Circulating substrate and hormone concentrations (Table 3). During period I (saline rehydration), blood was collected at −83 ± 12 and −10 ± 7 min before insulin therapy was begun. During this period the plasma concentra-

TABLE 3
Venous plasma and serum substrate and hormone concentrations during therapy for DKA

	Period I* Saline		Period II* Saline and insulin			Period III* Saline, insulin, and glucose			
	−83 12	−10 7	+68 3	+131 5	+246 4	+366 3	+480 4	+597 7	+728 4
Substrates									
AcAc (mM)	3.74	3.95	3.10	3.53	3.18	2.48†	1.82†	0.90†	0.66†
	0.79	0.40	0.58	0.56	0.59	0.78	0.55	0.38	0.27
β-OHB (mM)	12.07	12.54	9.44	8.64†	6.49†	4.52†	3.45†	1.69†	1.10†
	2.05	1.59	1.74	1.90	1.55	1.60	1.32	0.75	0.46
Acetone (mM)	5.02	5.38	3.55	4.89	5.31	4.51	3.89	2.58†	1.92
	1.55	0.78	0.75	0.99	1.00	1.04	1.28	0.96	1.20
FFA (mM)	1.74	1.88	0.97	0.72†	0.73†	0.45†	0.44†	0.63†	0.78†
	0.24	0.20	0.31	0.17	0.14	0.14	0.12	0.17	0.14
Glycerol (mM)	0.37	0.41	0.26†	0.23†	0.26	0.20†	0.20†	0.22†	0.27
	0.06	0.05	0.04	0.02	0.02	0.02	0.02	0.02	0.08
Triglycerides (mM)	2.35	3.13	2.64	2.51	2.22	1.65	1.65	1.53	1.27
	0.64	0.70	1.05	0.60	0.42	0.31	0.30	0.41	0.38
Glucose (mM)	25.08	25.32	14.60	14.06†	14.08†	15.58	13.49	11.82	9.95
	6.14	5.93	1.96	4.35	3.63	2.78	3.67	3.80	1.87
Lactate (mM)	2.42	2.43	2.02	2.20	1.95	1.93	1.70	1.53	1.60
	0.50	0.40	0.30	0.30	0.24	0.32	0.38	0.26	0.60
Alanine (μM)	477	506	489†	259†	326†	319†	320	376	239†
	91	76	87	68	60	80	97	134	52
Glutamine (μM)	499	483	469	419†	395	415	393†	330†	385†
	104	89	88	77	75	91	101	117	139
Glutamate (μM)	57	55	43	42†	40	33	30†	28†	21†
	9	10	16	8	11	8	6	10	8
Urea nitrogen (mg/dl)	31.7	33.3		27.9	24.5†	27.3	26.6		24.2†
	9.8	11.4		8.9	8.4	9.9	12.3		11.8
Hormones									
Glucagon (pg/ml)	393	435	284	270	289	198	160†		
	102	133	53	58	88	104	61		
Insulin (μU/ml)	42	29	563	449	376	630	223		
	16	10	288	217	246	223	22		

* Period times are given in minutes. Negative values indicate times before insulin therapy; positive values indicate times after insulin therapy. Values are means ± SEM.
† Significant difference from −10 ± 7 min time value during period I, $P < 0.05$.

tions of AcAc, β-OHB, acetone, FFA, glycerol, triglycerides, glucose, lactate, alanine, glutamine, and glutamate remained stable. All substrate concentrations, with the exceptions of glutamine and glutamate, were conspicuously elevated compared with normal values.[16] During period I, plasma glutamine concentrations were normal.[16] However, plasma glutamate concentrations were meaningfully depressed.[16] Previous work in patients with DKA has shown that rehydration decreases plasma glucose concentrations[5,17,18] while plasma ketone body concentrations remain constant.[18,19] The lack of a change in plasma glucose concentration in this study may have been due to the brevity of period I and the failure to achieve adequate rehydration or because only one blood sample was obtained from patient D.H. Plasma lactate concentrations ranged from 4.1 mM (J.Ba.) to 1.01 mM (L.T.). These values are comparable to those reported for patients in DKA[20] and are not responsible for the gross acidemia observed in these patients. Plasma alanine concentrations ranged from 902 μM (J.B1.) to 289 μM (W.B.). At the time patient J.B1. had the marked increase in plasma alanine, his plasma glucagon concentration was 468 pg/ml. Thus, lack of glucagon could not have been responsible for his high plasma alanine concentration. Plasma glucagon concentrations were elevated and agree with the data reported by others.[17,22] The serum insulin values shown for period I are probably spuriously elevated because of presumed insulin antibodies in the sera of patients previously treated with exogenous insulin. The serum IRI concentrations shown for periods I–III are displayed only to demonstrate relative differences in IRI concentrations before and after insulin therapy.

During period II (saline rehydration and insulin therapy) blood was withdrawn at 68 ± 3, 131 ± 5, and 246 ± 4 min. Plasma β-OHB, FFA, glycerol, glucose, alanine, glutamine, glutamate, and urea concentrations all decreased ($P < 0.05$) within this period. AcAc, acetone, triglycerides, lactate, and glucagon concentrations remained constant.

During period III (saline, insulin, and glucose therapy) blood was drawn at 366 ± 3, 480 ± 4, 597 ± 7, and 728 ± 4 min. Plasma concentrations of AcAc, β-OHB, acetone, FFA, glycerol, alanine, glutamine, and glutamate continued to decrease or decreased from the previous study periods. Plasma glucose concentration was maintained during period III between 15.58 and 9.95 mmol/L by continuous intravenous glucose administration. Plasma glucagon concentration progressively decreased throughout the study periods, becoming significantly ($P < 0.05$) reduced at 480 ± 4 min.

Renal excretion rates of nitrogen, glucose, and ketone bodies. During period I, urine was collected at −100 ± 8 and −30 ± 3 min before insulin therapy was begun. There were no differences in the excretion rates of the compounds measured. The average excretion rate of nitrogen was 10.6 ± 2.1 mg/min. Nitrogen excretion rate remained constant throughout the study. During control period I the average glucose excretion was 479 ± 90 μM/min. Glucose excretion fell to a minimal value of 171 ± 5 μM/min at 252 ± 10 min after saline and insulin therapy was started. Glucose excretion increased again to a value of 515 ± 203 μM/min at 447 ± 9 min during period III when glucose was infused intravenously together with saline, other electrolytes, and insulin. During period I the AcAc excretion rate was 51 ± 11 μM/min. There was a transient increase in urinary AcAc excretion at 30 ± 6 min to a maximal value of 64 ± 15 μM/min. However, this increase was not statistically significant. Thereafter renal excretion of AcAc declined. β-OHB excretion during period I was 277 ± 66 μM/min. There was a decrease in urinary β-OHB excretion between 138 ± 7 and 252 ± 10 min after insulin administration, but the change was not statistically significant. Acetone urinary excretion rate during the control period was 34 ± 7 μM/min and did not change significantly throughout the study. The lack of statistically significant changes in urinary ketone body excretion rates probably reflects the individual variations among the patients and the inability to obtain all the urine samples at every time period from all the patients and does not necessarily imply that the excretion rates of AcAc, β-OHB, and acetone did not decrease with time.

Respiratory gaseous exchanges and respiratory quotients (Table 4). To compare our results with different patient populations from the literature, the data in Table 4 were corrected to 1.73 m^2 body surface area. During period I, respiratory exchanges of CO_2, O_2, and acetone were measured at −124 ± 10 and −14 ± 6 min. The quantities of CO_2 and acetone expired and O_2 consumed were constant during this control period. The average rate of CO_2 expiration was 7.50 ± 0.40 mmol/min/1.73 m^2 and the average rate of O_2 inspiration was 11.00 ± 0.82 mmol/min/1.73 m^2. The average rate of acetone expiration was 150 ± 36 μmol/min/1.73 m^2. To simplify Table 3, only the mean ± SEM values for acetone are displayed. It should be reported, however, that there was a wide range of acetone excretion in the breath, varying from 37 μmol/min/1.73 m^2 (L.T.) to 364 μmol/min/1.73 m^2 (J.B1.). The acetone expiration rate depended primarily on the plasma concentration and the breath minute volume (data not shown). The average RQ and npRQ in period I were 0.70 ± 0.03 and 0.72 ± 0.03, respectively.* In all patients during period I the npRQ was corrected for urinary AcAc, β-OHB, and acetone excretion and breath acetone excretion. During period I the RQ was 0.70 or below in three patients (O.G., W.B., and D.H.). In these patients the npRQ was also corrected for glycosuria (see Appendix). There were no significant changes in the mean rates of exchanges of CO_2 and O_2 and in mean RQ values during periods II and III. Furthermore, since urinary nitrogen excretion remained approximately equal throughout the study (Table 4), the npRQ remained constant. Nevertheless, there were individual patients (O.G., D.H., and L.T.) who had higher RQ and npRQ values during the insulin therapy periods.

DISCUSSION

Respiratory quotients under any given circumstance are the result of numerous metabolic processes occurring simultaneously. Nevertheless, the RQ and the npRQ offer meaningful information on the composite nature and quantity of fuels oxidized and substrates stored. A wide range of RQ and npRQ has been reported.[23,24] During maximum lipogenesis

* It should be noted that the RQ and "corrected" npRQ are approximately equal during period I. This is due to several factors that cancel each other. If the RQ is below 0.79, which was the case in all patients except one (L.T.), the npRQ is less. Correcting the npRQ for acetone expiration increases the npRQ slightly. Furthermore, correcting the npRQ for ketonuria increases the npRQ more. If the RQ is greater than 0.79, which was the case in three patients (O.G., D.H., and L.T.) during periods II and III, the npRQ is higher.

TABLE 4
Respiratory gaseous exchanges and respiratory quotients during therapy for DKA

	Period I* Saline		Period II* Saline and insulin		Period III* Saline, insulin, and glucose		
	−124 10	−14 6	+86 9	+214 10	+475 8	+609 6	+728 5
CO_2 (mmol/min/1.73 m^2)							
O.G.	8.59	9.14	6.98	7.98	14.00	—	—
W.B.	7.55	7.33	6.09	6.67	—	—	—
J.B1.	6.91	7.02	5.50	5.71	5.77	5.49	5.60
D.H.	—	5.89	10.52	8.57	9.41	9.95	9.64
D.M.	9.68	8.95	8.93	5.22	6.48	6.83	6.60
L.T.	5.71	5.53	6.50	7.21	5.11	6.56	6.38
J.Ba.	—	7.66	7.94	7.77	6.03	—	—
Mean	7.69	7.36	7.49	7.02	7.80	7.21	7.06
±SEM	0.68	0.52	0.66	0.46	1.38	0.96	0.88
O_2 (mmol/min/1.73 m^2)							
O.G.	15.67	14.90	13.55	12.51	15.24	—	—
W.B.	12.30	11.69	10.77	10.80	—	—	—
J.B1.	9.85	9.51	7.70	7.88	8.40	7.64	7.41
D.H.	—	8.50	13.14	10.50	11.08	11.03	10.30
D.M.	12.88	12.65	11.41	7.01	8.18	8.93	8.68
L.T.	7.14	6.92	6.86	8.14	6.38	8.02	7.23
J.Ba.	—	9.84	10.88	11.10	7.72	—	—
Mean	11.57	10.57	10.62	9.70	9.50	8.90	8.40
±SEM	1.44	1.02	0.96	0.77	1.31	0.76	0.71
Acetone (μmol/min/1.73 m^2)							
Mean	159	144	119	120	105	51	66
±SEM	66	46	25	31	34	28	24
RQ							
O.G.	0.55	0.61	0.53	0.64	0.92	—	—
W.B.	0.61	0.63	0.57	0.62	—	—	—
J.B1.	0.70	0.74	0.72	0.73	0.68	0.72	0.76
D.H.	—	0.69	0.80	0.82	0.85	0.90	0.94
D.M.	0.75	0.71	0.78	0.74	0.79	0.76	0.76
L.T.	0.80	0.79	0.95	0.88	0.80	0.81	0.88
J.Ba.	—	0.78	0.73	0.70	0.78	—	—
Mean	0.68	0.71	0.72	0.73	0.80	0.80	0.84
±SEM	0.04	0.03	0.05	0.04	0.03	0.04	0.04
npRQ†							
Mean	0.70	0.73	0.71	0.72	0.79	0.80	0.82
±SEM	0.06	0.04	0.08	0.05	0.07	0.10	0.07

* Period times are given in min ± SEM. Negative values indicate times before initiating insulin therapy; positive values indicate times after initiating insulin therapy.
† See Appendix for calculations.

the RQ value occasionally exceeds 1.0,[25,26] and there are a few reports of patients during starvation[2,27] or in DKA[4,27] with RQ of less than 0.70.

In this study, throughout periods I, II, and III, the ranges of the RQ, npRQ, and "corrected" npRQ were wide, suggesting that heterogenous metabolic states existed in these patients (Table 4). Whereas the mixture of protein, fat, and glucose oxidized in these patients was diverse, their responses to insulin and glucose therapy were more uniform. During period II there were no increases in the RQ and npRQ in five patients (O.G., W.B., J.B1., D.M., and J.Ba.). Only two patients (D.H. and L.T.) increased their RQ and npRQ. This is remarkable because the circulating concentrations of β-OHB, FFA, glycerol, glucose, alanine, glutamine, and glutamate declined in all patients (Table 3). In contrast, during period III the RQ and npRQ increased in every patient (except for npRQ in J.B1.). The heightened RQ and npRQ values (Table 4) were observed late in the course of therapy when plasma FFA and ketone body concentrations had decreased, while plasma glucose concentration remained elevated (Table 3). Hyperglycemia persisted because of intravenous glucose infusion.

The relationships among the concentrations of circulating fuels and the "corrected" npRQ in one patient (O.G.) are illustrated in Figure 1. During the saline rehydration period, blood glucose, AcAc plus β-OHB, and plasma FFA concentrations remained reasonably constant. The addition of intravenous insulin therapy caused a sudden decrease in plasma glucose, AcAc, β-OHB, and FFA concentrations. Acetone concentration was little affected. Exogenous glucose was administered when the patient's plasma glucose decreased to 8.08 mmol/L (146 mg/dl). Thereafter the plasma glucose concentrations rose to a maximal value of 16.21 mmol/L (292 mg/dl), while plasma FFA and AcAc plus β-OHB concentrations continued to remain low or decreased. During the saline rehydration period, "corrected" npRQ (0.58–0.61) was also reasonably stable and suggested gluconeogenesis from fat.[23] The first clear-cut rise in npRQ occurred after 6 h of saline, insulin, and glucose therapy. From 1¼ to 8½ h, the npRQ increased from 0.42 to

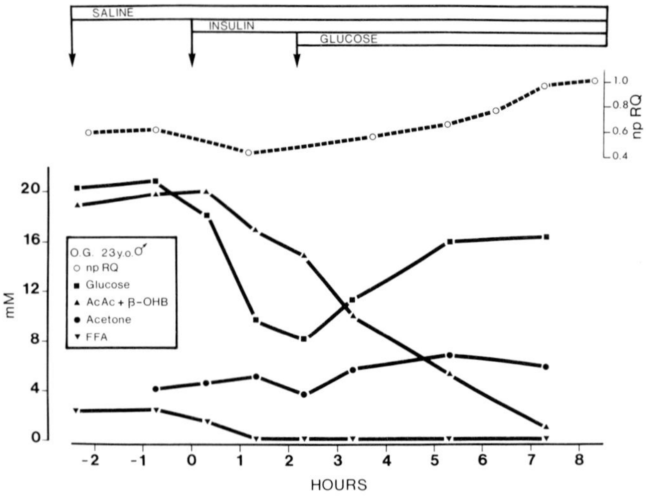

FIGURE 1. Relationships between the nonprotein RQ and plasma concentrations of glucose, acetoacetate (AcAc) plus beta-hydroxybutyrate (β-OHB), acetone, and free fatty acids (FFA) in one patient (O.G.) during the three periods of study. The bars at the top of the graph show when saline, insulin, and glucose were given.

1.01.* Oxidation of glucose, preformed AcAc, and β-OHB, and lipogenesis from glucose, AcAc, and β-OHB all increase the npRQ. Glucose oxidation was delayed and did not contribute to the early precipitous fall in plasma glucose. The results from this, and from the other patients, suggest that during the initial hours of fluid and insulin therapy for DKA the predominant effect of insulin is to promote fuel storage rather than glucose and ketone body oxidation.

The nature and quantity of fuels oxidized before and after insulin and glucose therapy are shown in Figure 2. At the beginning of period I the caloric requirements were 1.24 kcal/min/1.73 m^2. As the study progressed, there was a progressive decline in the metabolic requirements. After 12 h of therapy the caloric requirements had declined to 0.77 kcal/min/1.73 m^2. The initial high caloric expenditure was probably related to tachypnea, tachycardia, and other physical activities accompanying DKA. The depressed caloric expenditure observed at the end of the study was probably related to diminished circulating concentrations of thermogenic hormones in these catabolic diabetic[28] and emaciated patients.[29] Protein oxidation appeared to remain reasonably constant throughout the study. The apparent rise in protein contribution to the total metabolic requirements from 5 ± 2% to 14 ± 8% was partly due to the diminished total caloric requirements at the end of period III and to a "washout" of preformed nitrogenous waste products (see Table 3). Initially, fat contributed 78 ± 11% and glucose 17 ± 10% of the energy requirements. The relative contributions of the fuels to the diminishing caloric requirements did not change appreciably during the first 4 h of insulin therapy. Thereafter, a reciprocal change in the contributions of glucose and fat to metabolic requirements occurred. After 12 h of therapy, glucose contributed 42 ± 22% and fat 44 ± 16% of the total caloric requirements.

* The 1½-h npRQ could be spuriously low. Retained HCO_3^- in the patient's body HCO_3^- pool could cause a diminished respiratory excretion of CO_2. In the patient, however, the plasma total CO_2 concentration immediately before insulin therapy was 6.0 mM and after about 2 h of insulin therapy it was 7.0 mM. Therefore, apparent HCO_3^- retention did not significantly influence the 1½-h npRQ in this patient.

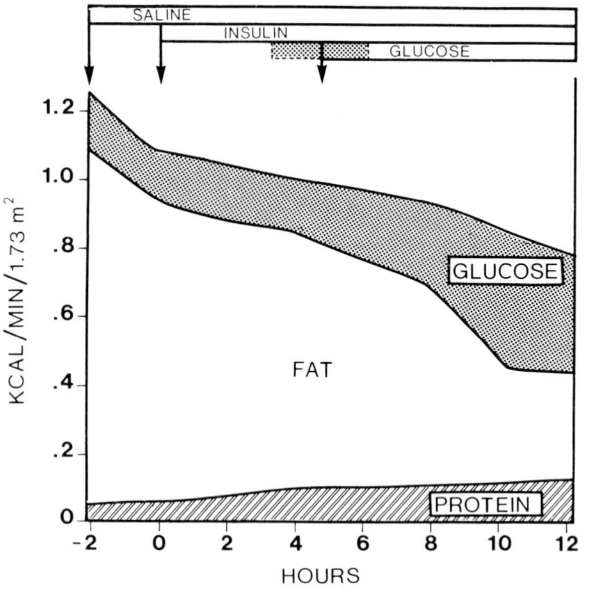

FIGURE 2. Nature and quantity of fuels during the three periods of therapy for DKA. The shaded area over the glucose bar reflects the SEM for giving intravenous glucose.

This study shows that, early in the therapy for DKA, insulin caused a precipitous decrease in plasma glucose, FFA, and ketone bodies without changing the nature of fuels oxidized. This suggests that one of the initial effects of insulin is to block hepatic glucose entry into the bloodstream and/or to promote glucose uptake and storage by tissues rather than to promote glucose oxidation. Another initial effect of insulin is to block the entry of FFA into the bloodstream. The removal of precursor FFA from plasma and changing the insulin-glucagon ratio diminish hepatic ketone body production.[30] The fall in plasma amino acid and urea concentrations during constant urinary nitrogen excretion suggests that more than one influence is operating simultaneously. While insulin is restraining proteolysis in peripheral tissues without completely shutting off the oxidation of amino acids, rehydration is permitting renal "washout" of preformed urea. Collectively, these processes of fuel storage or anabolism occur in the absence of heightened glucose oxidation, as indicated by unchanging npRQ. Late in the course of therapy the npRQ rose, reflecting heightened glucose oxidation and diminished fat oxidation.

The demonstration that glucose was translocated from the extracellular to the intracellular space but was not oxidized suggests that insulin may not affect glucose oxidation directly. With the information available from this study, it is reasonable to assume that insulin only influences the flux of fuels in and out of tissues and that cells of tissues have their own innate powers that determine the fate of available substrates. Once energy requirements are met, cells can store extra fuels and replete deficits. Increased glucose oxidation occurs when other preferred fuel competitors are removed while glucose and insulin remain available.

ACKNOWLEDGMENTS

This work was supported in part by U.S. Public Health Service grants AM25386, AM13527, and AM19397, and RR349, General Clinical Research Centers Branch, National Institutes of Health.

APPENDIX

In healthy humans the RQ and npRQ can be determined from measurements of the respiratory gaseous exchanges of O_2 and CO_2 and the urinary excretion of nitrogen. Under normal circumstances the quantity of protein undergoing catabolism to CO_2, water, and urea can be calculated from the amount of nitrogen excreted in the urine. According to Loewy's data, each gram of urinary N_2 represents the production of 4.75 L of CO_2 and the consumption of 6.02 L of O_2. Thus, the equations for calculations are:

$$RQ = \frac{CO_2 \text{ produced}}{O_2 \text{ consumed}} \quad (1)$$

$$npRQ = \frac{CO_2 \text{ produced} - (4.75 \times \text{g } N_2 \text{ excreted})}{O_2 \text{ consumed} - (6.02 \times \text{g } N_2 \text{ excreted})} \quad (2)$$

Special calculations apply when estimates for protein oxidation are derived from diabetic patients with glycosuria before insulin therapy is given. Amino acids mobilized from proteolysis can be oxidized in peripheral tissues or converted into glucose. In catabolic states, a reasonable estimate is that about 42% of the amino acid carbon skeletons mobilized from proteolysis can be oxidized directly, mainly in peripheral tissues, and the other 58% of the amino acid carbon skeletons can be converted to glucose before they are oxidized.[31] During severe diabetic ketoacidosis, very little or no glucose is oxidized to CO_2 and H_2O.[32–34] Once the renal threshold for glucose has been exceeded, glucose derived from amino acids can be excreted in the urine. Under such circumstances, none of the gluconeogenic amino acid carbon skeletons consume O_2 or produce CO_2. Therefore, Loewy's values for O_2 consumed and CO_2 produced based on urinary nitrogen excretion need to be corrected when glycosuria is present and the respiratory quotient is below 0.70, suggesting that no glucose is oxidized. If only 42% of the amino acid carbon skeletons, which are catabolized in muscle and other peripheral tissues, consume O_2 in the process of producing CO_2, then the equation for calculating the npRQ corrected for glycosuria is:

$$\text{corrected npRQ} = \frac{CO_2 \text{ produced} - (0.42)(4.75 \times \text{g } N_2 \text{ excreted})}{O_2 \text{ consumed} - (0.42)(6.02 \times \text{g } N_2 \text{ excreted})} \quad (3)$$

Other special considerations must be taken into account when estimates for fat oxidation are derived from diabetic patients with ketonuria and acetone expiration before insulin therapy is given. Oxygen is consumed for beta-oxidation of long-chain fatty acids in the liver when AcAc and β-OHB are produced. During diabetic ketoacidosis, large quantities of these ketone bodies are excreted in the urine. In addition, AcAc also undergoes spontaneous decarboxylation to acetone, which is excreted in urine and breath. For each mmole of AcAc, β-OHB, or acetone excreted in urine or breath, 1.5 mmole (33.6 ml) of O_2 is lost from the body. Furthermore, for each mmole of acetone formed, AcAc also produces 1 mmol (22.4 ml) of CO_2, which is expired during the tachypnea of diabetic ketoacidosis. Therefore, the quantities of oxygen lost during renal AcAc, β-OHB, and acetone excretion and the quantities of breath O_2 and CO_2 liberated from acetone formation must be taken into consideration when estimates for fat oxidation are calculated during diabetic ketoacidosis. The equation for the final "corrected" npRQ is:

$$\text{final "corrected" npRQ} = \frac{CO_2 \text{ produced} - [(0.42)(4.75 \times \text{g } N_2 \text{ excreted}) - CO_2 \text{ from AcAc decarboxylation})]}{O_2 \text{ consumed} - [(0.42)(4.75 \times \text{g } N_2 \text{ excreted}) - O_2 \text{ in urinary and breath ketone bodies})]} \quad (4)$$

This final "corrected" npRQ is referred to as the "corrected" npRQ in the text.

Insulin restrains hepatic glucose and ketone body production rates. The rapidity with which these processes occur during therapy for DKA is unknown. Furthermore, part of the ketone bodies lost from the body after insulin therapy is started are derived from preformed ketone bodies. Therefore, during periods II and III, we did not attempt to correct the npRQ for glucose or ketone body excretions.

After taking into account the quantities of O_2 consumed and CO_2 produced from protein catabolism, the caloric requirement of the patients during the three periods was estimated from the thermal equivalents of O_2 consumed and CO_2 produced across the respiratory system. The caloric values of a liter of oxygen at different npRQs as well as the percentages of fat and carbohydrate undergoing combustion were calculated from the different npRQ according to Cathcart and Cuthbertson.[24,34] Urinary nitrogen was equated to 26.4 cal × g N_2 excreted if the RQ was greater than 0.70 before insulin therapy. If the RQ was less than 0.70 before insulin administration, urinary nitrogen was equated to 26.4 cal × (0.42)(g N_2 excreted). After calculating the calories derived from protein oxidation, the nonprotein calories derived from fat and glucose oxidation were calculated from their relative percentages of the nonprotein calories.[24]

REFERENCES

1 Owen, O. E., Block, B. S. B., Patel, M., Boden, G., McDonough, M., Kreulen, T., Shuman, C. R., and Reichard, G. A., Jr.: Human splanchnic metabolism during diabetic ketoacidosis. Metabolism *26*:381–98, 1977.

2 Owen, O. E., Reichard, G. A., Jr., Boden, G., Patel, M. S., and Trapp, V. E.: Interrelationships among key tissues in the utilization of metabolic substrates. *In* Diabetes, Obesity and Vascular Disease. Metabolic and Molecular Interrelationships, Part 2. Katzen, H. M., and Mahler, R. J., Eds. New York, John Wiley & Sons, 1978, chap. 15.

3 Felig, P.: Amino acid metabolism in man. Annu. Rev. Biochem. *44*:933–55, 1975.

4 Benedict, F. G., and Joslin, E. P.: A study of metabolism in severe diabetes. Carnegie Institute of Washington, Publication No. 176, 1912.

5 Page, M., Alberti, K. G. M. M., Greenwood, R., Gumaa, K. A., Hockaday, T. D. R., Long, C., Nabarro, J. D. N., Pyke, D. A., Sonksen, P. H., Watkins, P. J., and West, T. E. T.: Treatment of diabetic coma in the continuous low dose infusion of insulin. Br. Med. J. *2*:687–90, 1974.

6 Felig, P.: Current concepts: diabetic ketoacidosis. N. Engl. J. Med. *290*:1360–63, 1974.

7 Kitabchi, A. E., Ayyagari, V., and Guerra, S. M. O.: The efficacy of low dose versus conventional therapy of insulin for treatment of diabetic ketoacidosis. Ann. Intern. Med. *84*:633–38, 1976.

8 Fisher, J. N., Shahshahnani, M. N., and Kitabchi, A. E.: Diabetic ketoacidosis: low dose therapy by various routes. N. Engl. J. Med. *297*:238–41, 1977.

9 Kreisberg, R. A.: Diabetic ketoacidosis: new concepts and trends in pathogenesis and treatment. Ann. Intern. Med. *88*:681–95, 1978.

10 Issekutz, B., Jr., Paul, P., Miller, H. I., and Bortz, W. M.: Oxidation of plasma FFA in lean and obese humans. Metabolism *17*:62–73, 1968.

11 Owen, O. E., and Reichard, G. A., Jr.: Human forearm metabolism during progressive starvation. J. Clin. Invest. *50*:1536–45, 1971.

12 Garber, A. J., Menzel, P. H., Boden, G., and Owen, O. E.: Hepatic ketogenesis and gluconeogenesis in humans. J. Clin. Invest. *54*:981–89, 1974.

13 Reichard, G. A., Jr., Haff, A. C., Skutches, C. L., Paul, P., Holroyde, C. P., and Owen, O. E.: Plasma acetone metabolism in the fasting human. J. Clin. Invest. *63*:619–26, 1979.

[14] Issekutz, B., Jr., and Rodahl, K.: Respiratory quotient during exercise. J. Appl. Physiol. *16*:606–10, 1961.

[15] Snedecor, G. W., and Cochren, W. G.: Statistical Methods, 6th edit. Ames, Iowa, Iowa State University Press, 1967.

[16] Owen, O. E., Mozzoli, M. A., Boden, G., Patel, M. S., Reichard, G. A., Jr., Trapp, V. E., Shuman, C. R., and Felig, P.: Substrate, hormone and temperature responses in males and females to a common breakfast. Metabolism. In press.

[17] Waldhausl, W., Kleinberger, G., Korn, A., Dudczak, R., Bratusch-Marrian, P., and Nowotny, P.: Severe hyperglycemia: effects of rehydration on endocrine derangements and blood glucose concentration. Diabetes *28*:577–84, 1979.

[18] Owen, O. E., Licht, J. H., and Sapir, D. G.: Renal function and effects of hydration during diabetic ketoacidosis. J. Clin. Invest. Submitted for publication.

[19] Sacks, H. S., Shahshahani, M. N., Kitabchi, A. E., and Gray, T. L.: Diabetic ketoacidosis: effects of intravenous fluid prior to insulin therapy. Clin. Res. *25*:624A, 1977.

[20] Watkins, P. J., Smith, J. S., Fitzgerald, M. G., and Malins, J. M.: Lactic acidosis in diabetes. Br. Med. J. *1*:744–47, 1969.

[21] Boden, G., Rezvani, I., Master, R. W., Trapp, V., Schwartz, M., and Owen, O. E.: Glucagon deficiency causes hyperaminoacidemia. Clin. Res. *27*:482A, 1979.

[22] Muller, W. H., Faloona, G. F., and Unger, R. H.: Hyperglucagonemia in diabetic ketoacidosis. Am. J. Med. *54*:52–57, 1973.

[23] Soskin, S., and Levine, R.: Carbohydrate Metabolism. Chicago, University of Chicago Press, 1952, pp. 138–43, 150–60.

[24] Best, C. H., and Taylor, N. B.: The Physiological Basis of Medical Practice. Baltimore, Williams & Wilkins Co., 1961, pp. 741–67.

[25] Passmore, R., and Swindells, Y. E.: Observations on the respiratory quotients and weight gain of man after eating large quantities of carbohydrate. Br. J. Nutr. *17*:331–39, 1963.

[26] Goldman, R. F., Haisman, M. F., Bynum, G., Horton, E. S., and Sims, E. A. H.: Experimental obesity in man: metabolic rate in relation to dietary intake. *In* Obesity in Perspective. Fogarty International Center Series and Preventative Medicine, Vol. 2, Part 2. Bray, G. A., Ed.

[27] Lusk, G.: The Elements of the Science of Nutrition. Philadelphia, W. B. Saunders Co., 1919.

[28] Pittman, C. S., Suda, A. K., Chambers, J. B., Jr., and Ray, G. Y.: Impaired 3,5,3′-triiodothyronine (T_3) production in diabetic patients. Metabolism *28*(4):333–38, 1979.

[29] Chopra, I. J., and Smith, S. R.: Circulating thyroid hormones and thyrotropin in adult patients with protein calorie malnutrition. J. Clin. Endocrinol. Metab. *40*:221–27, 1975.

[30] McGarry, J. D.: New perspectives in the regulation of ketogenesis. Diabetes *28*:517–23, 1979.

[31] Krebs, H. A.: The metabolic fate of amino acids. *In* Mammalian Protein Metabolism, Vol. 1. Munro, H. N., and Allison, J. B., Eds. New York, Academic Press, 1964, pp. 125–76.

[32] Shreeve, W. W., Baker, N., Miller, M., Shipley, R. A., Incefy, G. A., and Craig, J. W.: C^{14} studies in carbohydrate metabolism. II. The oxidation of glucose in diabetic human subjects. Metabolism *5*:22–33, 1956.

[33] Forbath, N., and Hetenyi, G., Jr.: Glucose dynamics in normal subjects and diabetic patients before and after a glucose load. Diabetes *15*:778–89, 1966.

[34] Cathcart, E. P., and Cuthbertson, D. P.: The composition and distribution of the fatty substances of the human subject. J. Physiol. *72*:349–60, 1931.

A Comparison of Basal and Insulin-stimulated Glucose Transport in Rat Adipocyte Plasma Membranes

CARL LUDVIGSEN AND LEONARD JARETT

SUMMARY

Specific D-glucose transport in plasma membranes prepared from control and insulin-treated rat adipocytes was measured using a recently developed dual isotope ([^{3}H]-D-glucose and [^{14}C]-L-glucose), rapid filtration assay which allowed measurements of initial rates at 1 s and 37°.[1] Plasma membranes from insulin-treated adipocytes showed an increase in glucose transport compared with control cells. Saturation kinetic data revealed that the plasma membranes from insulin-treated and control cells had the same K_m (26 mM) for glucose transport, whereas insulin treatment increased the V_{max} from 4433 pmol/mg protein/s to 9465 pmol/mg protein/s. Arrhenius plots showed no difference in the energy of activation between control and insulin-stimulated glucose transport states. The optimum pH of both control and insulin-stimulated glucose transport was 7.4. Lower or higher pHs progressively decreased both control and insulin-stimulated glucose transport proportionately. Calcium in the transport assay media did not affect basal or insulin-stimulated glucose transport. However, omission of calcium from the adipocyte incubation media significantly lowered the insulin stimulation by 24% while basal levels were not significantly affected. Insulin specifically bound to the plasma membrane was carried through the fractionation procedure, but removal of this insulin did not alter the stimulated glucose transport. Glucose transport by plasma membranes from control or insulin-treated adipocytes was equally (percentage) inhibited by N-ethylmaleimide, dithiothreitol, reduced glutathione, or cytochalasin B. No inhibition of control or insulin-stimulated transport was seen with cytochalasin D or oxidized glutathione. The data presented are consistent with insulin causing the formation of new transport sites similar to the existing basal sites. DIABETES *29:*373–378, May 1980.

This material was presented in part at the 29th Annual Meeting of the American Diabetes Association, 1979.
From the Division of Laboratory Medicine, Departments of Pathology and Medicine, Washington University School of Medicine and Barnes Hospital, St. Louis, Missouri 63110.
Address reprint requests to Dr. Jarett.
Received for publication 22 October 1979.

The ability of insulin to stimulate glucose transport is a well established phenomenon.[2–7] However, there is a controversy as to how insulin causes an increase in the facilitated diffusion of glucose. The answer to this question will reflect directly on insulin's mechanism of action. There appears to be at least three ways by which insulin could increase the transport of glucose. First, insulin may be increasing the number of glucose transport sites that are similar functionally to the existing basal glucose transport sites. Second, insulin could be increasing the number of glucose transport sites that are in some way different from the existing glucose transport sites. Third, insulin could be effecting a change in the existing glucose transport sites but not in number, which would favor a faster or more efficient flow of glucose.

Various studies support each hypothesis. The first hypothesis—insulin acting by increasing the number of glucose transport sites—is supported by the following studies. Olefsky[3] has shown insulin to increase the V_{max} but not the K_m of 2-deoxyglucose uptake in intact adipocytes. The parallel slopes of the Arrhenius analysis for both basal and insulin-stimulated glucose transport in those studies indicated that insulin had not changed the energy of activation for glucose transport. Olefsky deduced that insulin effects an increase in facilitated glucose transport by increasing the number of glucose transport sites which are identical to the existing basal glucose transport sites. This hypothesis is further supported by the study of Wardzala et al.[8] Their studies on the relationship of specific cytochalasin B binding and glucose transport activity, as modulated by insulin, indicate an increase in the number of cytochalasin B–bindable glucose transport sites with insulin treatment.

The second hypothesis (an increase in functionally different glucose transport sites) or third hypothesis (a change of characteristics of existing glucose transport sites) are supported by the studies of Whitesell and Gliemann,[4] Amatruda and Finch,[9] and Czech.[10] They have demonstrated, after insulin treatment, an increase in the V_{max} with no change in the K_m of glucose analogue transport, but with several other changes which distinguish basal from insulin-stimulated glucose transport. These include (1) a change in the temperature dependency of glucose transport with insulin treatment,[4,9,10] (2) a difference in the pH sensitivity of glucose transport with insulin treatment,[4] and (3) a difference in the degree of inhibition of basal or insulin-stimulated glucose transport by cytochalasin B after N-ethylmaleimide treatment.[10] These studies all point to a functional difference between basal and insulin-stimulated glucose transport systems. At present these investigators have not distinguished between the second hypothesis (the addition of functionally different sites) or the third hypothesis (a functional change in existing glucose transport sites).

In this study we compare glucose transport in plasma membranes prepared from control or insulin-stimulated adipocytes. A rapid glucose transport assay[1] which enables initial rates of specific D-glucose uptake to be measured was utilized. The kinetic parameters, temperature dependence, pH sensitivity, calcium requirement, as well as the effect of N-ethylmaleimide, dithiothreitol, cytochalasin B, cytochalasin D, and reduced and oxidized glutathione on both basal and insulin-stimulated glucose transport, were measured and compared. The data support the hypothesis that insulin effects an increase in glucose transport sites that are similar in nature to the existing basal glucose transport sites.

MATERIALS AND METHODS

Materials. Porcine insulin was a gift from Dr. R. Chance, Eli Lilly and Company, Indianapolis, IN. Radioactive isotopes, [^{3}H]-D-glucose (37 Ci/mmol) and [^{14}C]-L-glucose (54 mCi/mmol) were purchased from New England Nuclear, Boston, MA. Bovine serum albumin (fraction V) and collagenase were purchased from Sigma Chemical Co., St. Louis, MO. Sprague-Dawley rats (120–150 g) from Eldridge Laboratory Animals, Barnhart, MO, were used in all experiments. Millipore filters, type AAWP, 0.8 μm pore, were supplied by Millipore Corp., Bedford, MA. A metronome was purchased from the Franz Mfg. Co., New Haven, CT. ^{125}I-insulin (140 μCi/μg), prepared by a chloramine T method,[11] was a gift from Dr. G. T. Hammons, Laboratory Medicine, Washington University, St. Louis, MO.

Isolation of adipocytes and plasma membranes. Isolated adipocytes were prepared as recently described[1] by a collagenase digestion of epididymal fat pads from male Sprague-Dawley rats (120–150 g). The cells were washed twice with Krebs-Ringer phosphate buffer, pH 7.4, at 37° and were divided into two sets for a 15 min incubation at 37° under control and experimental conditions. Then the cells were washed twice at room temperature with 0.25 M sucrose, 10 mM Tris-HCl buffer (pH 7.4 at 4°) and fractionated in parallel as described by McDonald et al.[12] Protein content of plasma membrane preparations was determined by the method of Lowry et al.[13] using bovine serum albumin as a standard.

Glucose transport assays. The procedure for measuring glucose uptake into isolated plasma membrane vesicles has been described in detail.[1] Plasma membranes were resuspended in Krebs-Ringer phosphate to an approximate protein concentration of 1–1.5 mg/ml and sonicated in a Polar sonicator bath for 10 s. Plasma membranes (80 μl) were incubated with glucose solution (20 μl) of various concentrations for 20 min, at 37°C, to obtain glucose equilibrium. The assay was then begun by forcefully adding into the incubation 40 μl of a solution containing both [^{3}H] D-glucose (8 μCi) and [^{14}C] L-glucose (1.6 μCi) with one-fifth the D-glucose concentration, as was added to the plasma membranes for equilibration. The flux of tracer, under these equilibrium exchange conditions, was stopped by the addition of 2 ml of 2 mM $HgCl_2$ in KRP at 4° as previously described.[1] The "stopped" plasma membranes were then immediately decanted onto a 0.8 μm AAWP Millipore filter, held by a Gelman single port filtration apparatus, to which a Leeson vacuum pump was attached. The filters were then washed with 2 vol of 3 ml of the "stop" solution. The filters were placed in vials, dried, dissolved in 600 μl of ethylene glycol monomethyl ether, and counted after the addition of 10 ml of Aquasol II. The vials were counted with dual isotope settings and automatic quench correction. Filter retention of isotope was corrected for by subtracting counts determined by filtering the isotopic solution without tissue and washing the filter as usual. Nonspecific uptake was measured by L-glucose uptake, and data were corrected for this factor, unless indicated otherwise. The nonspecific uptake included diffusion, extracellular trapping, filter retention, and nonspecific absorption. This correction factor also would include any uptake into a subpopulation of unsealed vesicles. Thus the specific uptake of D-glucose by facilitated diffusion is represented by the D-L-glucose uptake values. The L-glucose value in these studies, as in the earlier study,[1] never exceeded half the total D-glucose value at the early time points used for measurement. L-glucose required at least 20 min to come to final equilibrium. The specific D-glucose value has been shown to reflect true facilitated diffusion, since it was totally inhibited by cytochalasin B,[1] which was confirmed in the present study (Table 1).

TABLE 1
Inhibition of glucose transport by sulfhydryl reagents

Plasma Membrane Treatment	Cell Treatment: Control (ratio of uptake)	Insulin
None	1	1
N-ethylmaleimide		
20 mM	0.24	0.22
10 mM	0.42	0.41
5 mM	0.55	0.61
1 mM	0.94	0.94
0.5 mM	0.94	0.98
Dithiothreitol		
15 mM	0.41	0.48
Glutathione (reduced)		
15 mM	0	0
5 mM	0.71	0.75
Glutathione (oxidized)		
5 mM	0.97	1.03
Cytochalasin B		
10^{-5} M	0.02	0.02
Cytochalasin D		
10^{-5} M	0.85	0.83

Plasma membranes were isolated from cells incubated 15 min at 37° with or without 100 μU insulin/ml. Isolated plasma membranes were then added to N-ethylmaleimide, dithiothreitol, glutathione (reduced or oxidized), cytochalasin B, and cytochalasin D (as indicated) for 15 min at 37°, and specific D-glucose uptake measured for 1 s. Uptake is expressed as the ratio of the uptake valve found with the test agent compared with the value without the agent. The data represent values from three experiments, with the SEM being less than 7% in all cases.

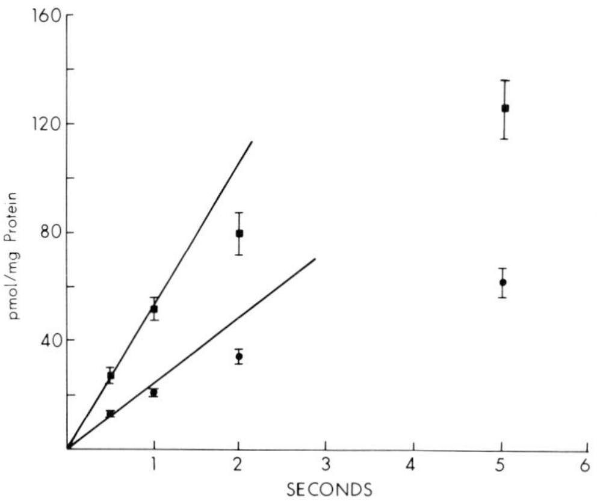

FIGURE 1. Early time course of specific D-glucose uptake. Plasma membrane vesicles isolated from control (●) or insulin (■)-treated (250 μU/ml) cells were assayed for glucose transport as described in MATERIALS AND METHODS. The data displayed represent the mean ± SE of three experiments, with each time point being performed in triplicate.

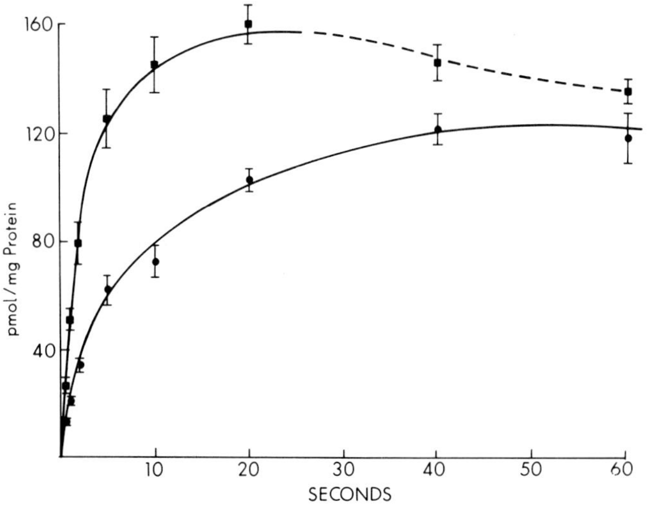

FIGURE 2. The time course of specific glucose (D-L) uptake of plasma membrane vesicles isolated from control (●) or insulin-treated (■) cells. Time courses of uptake were performed under equilibrium exchange conditions as described in MATERIALS AND METHODS. The data displayed represent the mean ± SE of three experiments, with each time point being performed in triplicate. The plateau of specific uptake for plasma membranes from insulin-treated cells is reached in 20 s. The dashed line represents a constant D-glucose value minus a steadily rising (with time) L-glucose value.

The timing of the 0.5, 1, 2, and 5 s periods of glucose uptake was accomplished by the use of a metronome. The anticipation of timing rather than the reaction to a clock or other signal provided a reproducible method, with standard errors of less than 5% in most cases with triplicate determinations.

Insulin-binding assay. Residual specific insulin binding to plasma membranes was measured by treating adipocytes with 10, 25, or 250 μU/ml ^{125}I-insulin for 15 min at 37°. Plasma membranes were isolated as usual and were resuspended in pH 6.0 or 7.4 KRP for 5 min at 24°. The membranes were centrifuged and resuspended in pH 7.4 KRP and an aliquot was taken for determination of residual radioactivity. Nonspecific binding of ^{125}I-insulin was determined by having 8 μM unlabeled insulin present during the 15 min, 37°, association period and by processing as above.

RESULTS

Kinetics of glucose transport. Glucose transport into plasma membranes isolated from control and insulin-treated cells was routinely assayed at 1 s. The 0.5, 1, 2, and 5 s points of specific glucose uptake (D-L-glucose) are displayed in Figure 1. Specific glucose uptake was defined as the difference between amounts of D- and L-glucose associated with the filtered membranes. In both basal and insulin-stimulated transports, the 1 s point of uptake was within 10% of a line through 0 and 0.5 s. The 2 s point deviated from that line by about 30% in both cases. The 1 s point was subsequently used as an estimate of initial rates. A complete time course of specific D-glucose uptake revealed that equilibrium was reached within 20 s in plasma membranes isolated from insulin-treated adipocytes and within 40 s in plasma membrane vesicles from control cells (Figure 2). The rapid equilibration of D-glucose in the plasma membranes from insulin-treated cells resulted in a drop in the specific glucose uptake curve between 20 and 60 s (Figure 2). This was caused by D-glucose rapidly reaching a constant equilibrium level while the L-glucose level continued to rise. The level of specific D-glucose uptake in both control and insulin-stimulated cases would eventually become zero, when the D-glucose and L-glucose spaces become equal. Insulin had no effect on L-glucose uptake values in any of these studies.

The variation in initial rates of uptake as a function of the concentration of glucose in the assay was used to determine kinetic parameters of glucose transport into plasma membranes from control and insulin-treated cells. Woolf-Hofstee analysis[14] of these data revealed a K_m of 26 mM for both basal and insulin-treated membranes, as determined from the slope of the line (Figure 3), while the V_{max} was increased from 4433 pmol/mg protein/s to 9466 pmol/mg protein/s after insulin treatment, as determined from the y-intercept. These data were derived from three complete saturation kinetic studies.

FIGURE 3. Woolf-Hofstee analysis of the saturation kinetics of specific D-glucose uptake. The relationship between initial rates (1 s uptake) of specific glucose (D-L) uptake and increasing glucose concentrations was studied in plasma membrane vesicles from control (●) and insulin-treated (■) cells. Initial rates of uptake of specific D-glucose uptake were measured as described in Figure 1. The data displayed represent the mean ± SE of three experiments, with each time point being performed in triplicate.

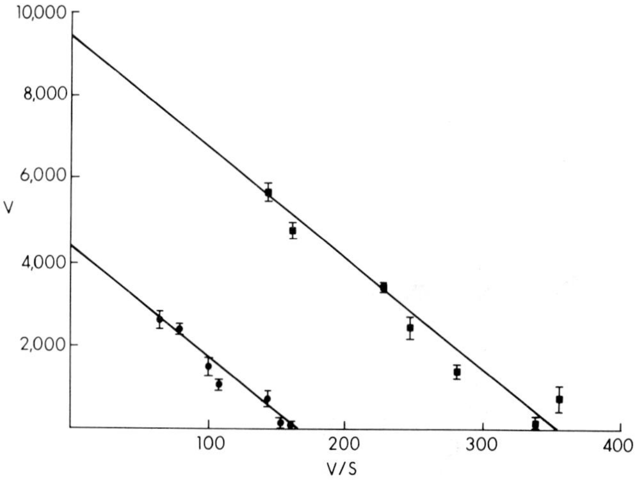

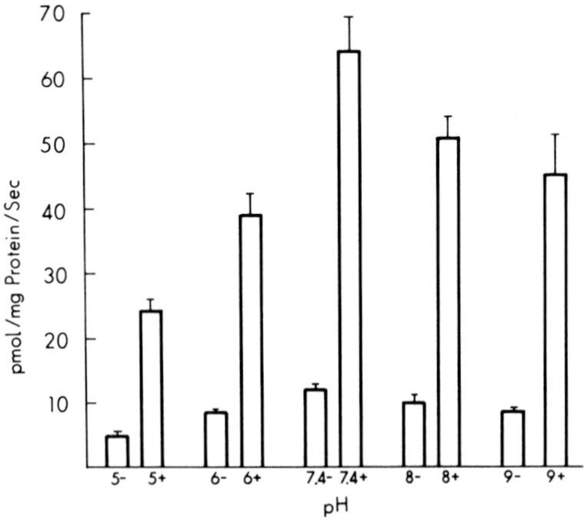

FIGURE 4. The effect of pH on basal (−) and insulin-stimulated (+) transport. Plasma membrane vesicles from control and insulin-stimulated cells were resuspended in KRP buffers of different pH. Initial rates of specific D-glucose uptake were measured as described in Figure 1. The data displayed represent the mean ±SE of three experiments, with each time point being performed in triplicate.

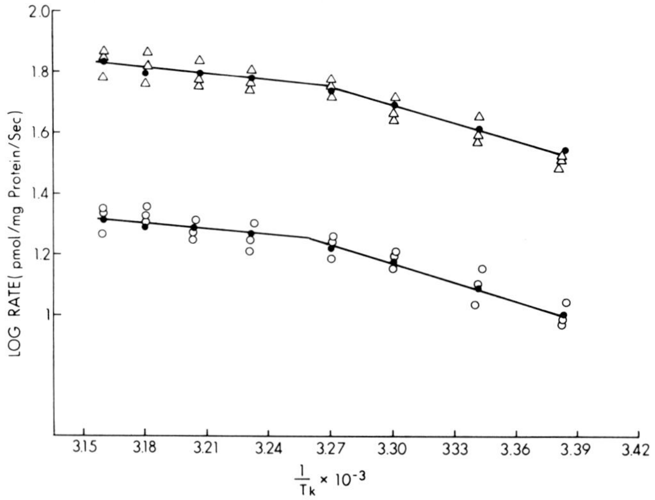

FIGURE 5. Arrhenius analysis of glucose transport by isolated plasma membrane vesicles from control (○) and insulin-stimulated (△) adipocytes. Initial rates of specific D-glucose uptake at various temperatures between 22° and 43° were measured as described in Figure 1. The solid points (●) represent a computer fit of a quadratic regression of the log rate of uptake as a function of temperature. The analysis indicated that the profiles for insulin-stimulated and control glucose transport were not significantly different. The statistical analysis performed does not rule out the postulate that the quadratic really is composed of an abrupt change between two linear portions. The lines drawn are by inspection to fit that postulate. The data displayed are representative of three similar experiments.

pH effects on glucose transport. The pH-sensitivity of glucose transport was determined by incubating five pairs of plasma membrane samples from control and insulin-treated cells in buffers of different pH and by determining initial glucose transport rates under these conditions (Figure 4). Glucose transport, in both the basal and insulin-stimulated state, exhibited an optimum pH of around 7.4. Glucose transport was inhibited to a greater extent at acidic than at alkaline pH. However, the ratio of insulin-stimulated to basal glucose transport remained approximately constant, regardless of pH. Changes in glucose transport due to pH reflected changes in specific D-glucose uptake since the uptake of L-glucose remained unchanged (data not shown).

Temperature effects on glucose transport. The effect of temperature on the initial rates of glucose transport was evaluated to help determine if the increase in glucose transport by insulin was due to (a) an increase in the efficiency of preexisting glucose transport sites or (b) an increase in the number of transport sites. An increase in the efficiency of transport would be indicated by a decrease in the energy of activation or slope of the Arrhenius plot from these data. However, basal and insulin-stimulated glucose transport showed parallel Arrhenius plots between 22° and 43°, with a change in slope occurring in both sets between 33° and 37° (Figure 5). The energy of activation was about 8 kcal/mol between 22° and 33° and about 4 kcal/mol at 37° to 43°. Therefore, the energy of activation for glucose transport was not decreased by insulin treatment.

Ca^{++} dependence of glucose transport. The effect of Ca^{++} concentration in the assay medium (on basal and insulin-stimulated glucose transport) was ascertained by resuspending four pairs of plasma membrane samples from control and insulin-treated cells at different Ca^{++} concentrations and by determining initial glucose transport rates. Assaying at 0, 0.01, 0.1, and 2.5 mM of added Ca^{++} in the medium had no significant effect on either basal or insulin-stimulated glucose transport (data not shown).

In contrast, the magnitude of the insulin stimulation of glucose transport by the isolated plasma membrane depended on the presence of Ca^{++} during incubation of the adipocytes with insulin. Initial rates of glucose transport were determined in plasma membranes from control and insulin-treated cells incubated with (1.4 mM) or without added Ca^{++}. There was a 24% decrease in the insulin stimulation of glucose transport in plasma membrane samples from cells incubated without added Ca^{++} compared with control samples (Figure 6): This effect was significant at the $P \leq 0.001$ level. Basal glucose transport was slightly decreased in samples not treated with Ca^{++} compared with control samples, but this difference was not significant.

FIGURE 6. The calcium dependence of the insulin stimulation of glucose transport. Intact adipocytes were resuspended in KRP with or without calcium (1.4 mM) and were treated with or without insulin (100 μU/ml). Plasma membrane vesicles were isolated from each set. Initial rates of specific D-glucose were isolated from each set. Initial rates of specific D-glucose uptake were measured as described in Figure 1. The data displayed represent the mean ±SE of three experiments, with each point being performed in triplicate.

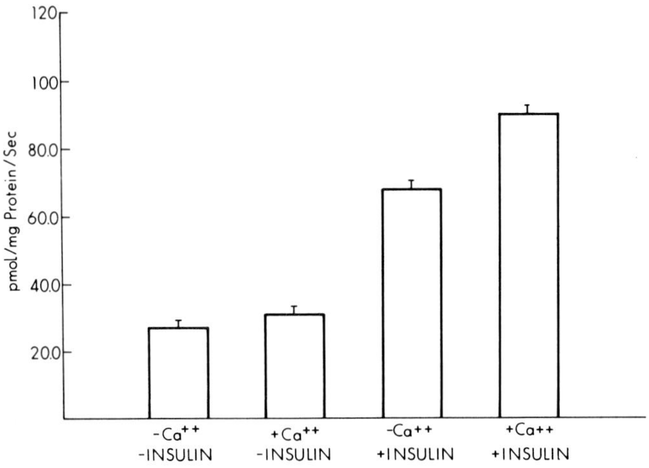

The effect of dissociating insulin from plasma membranes on glucose transport. The possibility was investigated that the stimulated glucose transport state in plasma membranes from insulin-treated cells was the result of residually bound insulin carried through the fractionation procedures. Despite extensive washing of the cells before fractionation and the multiple resuspensions and centrifugations needed in the membrane isolation procedure, a small (3.7 μU/mg protein) but significant amount of specifically bound ^{125}I-insulin was found associated with the isolated plasma membrane from cells treated with 250 μU ^{125}I-insulin/ml (40 μCi/μg). It was found that incubation of the plasma membranes at pH 6.0 for 5 min at 24° removed about two-thirds of the specifically bound insulin. Subsequent glucose uptake measurements at pH 7.4 were unaltered by this treatment. The plasma membranes from adipocytes treated with 10, 25, and 250 μU insulin/ml exhibited the same rates of uptake at pH 7.4 whether they had been pretreated at pH 6.0 or 7.4.

The effect of sulfhydryl and other agents on glucose transport. The work of Czech[10] and others[15,16] have indicated that disulfide bonds are important in the glucose transport system of adipocytes. Therefore, the effects of N-ethylmaleimide, dithiothreitol, reduced and oxidized glutathione, cytochalasin B, and cytochalasin D on basal and insulin-stimulated glucose transport by plasma membranes were measured. As shown in Table 1, these agents inhibited both basal and insulin-stimulated transport proportionately in every case; this effect depended on the concentration. Oxidized glutathione, which does not react with disulfide groups, had no effect. Cytochalasin B, a known inhibitor of glucose transport in the isolated plasma membrane system,[1,8,17] completely abolished both basal and insulin-stimulated glucose transport, while cytochalasin D had only a small effect at the same concentration.

DISCUSSION

In this study we compared glucose transport by plasma membranes from control and insulin-treated cells. There were several advantages over earlier studies using isolated plasma membranes[5,7,17] or the intact cell.[2–4,6,9,18] First, initial rates were determined for specific D-glucose transport by using a rapid assay technique,[1] developed for such measurements at physiologic temperatures. Thus, kinetic data could be derived. Second, temperature curves (Arrhenius plots), which depend on obtaining initial rates, were measured, with the time of incubation and length of insulin treatment being constant. Third, this approach used D-glucose and not a glucose analogue. Fourth, the plasma membranes used in this study were isolated without the use of EDTA, a metal chelator, which might cause structural and functional alteration of the membrane by the removal of Ca^{++} and Mg^{++}. Finally, the use of plasma membranes eliminated any metabolic effects that the intact cells may have on the measurements of glucose transport. This also allowed the effects of various agents to be studied directly on glucose transport and not on steps before or after the actual transport step.

Kinetic analysis revealed that the K_m for glucose transport by plasma membranes from insulin-treated cells was unchanged from the control. In contrast, the V_{max} of glucose transport by plasma membranes from insulin-treated adipocytes was double to triple that of membranes from control cells, on the average. The actual increase in the rate of glucose transport by membranes from insulin-treated cells compared with control ranged from a twofold to a sixfold increase, varying from experiment to experiment. Similar studies on 3-O-methylglucose transport by intact cells in this laboratory have revealed an average threefold to fourfold stimulation by glucose.[19] These findings are similar to the findings on intact adipocytes reported by others.[3,4,18] Other studies with isolated membranes[5–7] reveal an insulin stimulation of only the same magnitude as reported in the present study, all of which are less than those found with intact cell systems. It is probable that some of the insulin-generated transport sites are lost during fractionation. The value for the K_m of transport in this study, 26 mM, was higher than the value of 9 mM originally reported in studies using this rapid assay technique.[1] The only difference between the two studies was that in the present study there was a 15 min incubation of the cells before fractionation, whereas, in the previous studies, adipocytes were fractionated immediately after isolation. Repeating the immediate fractionation during the course of the present study still yielded the lower K_m value similar to that reported previously.[1] Thus, no ready explanation can be given for this difference in K_ms except for the effect of the incubation period. The data suggest that the facilitated transport system has lost some of its affinity for D-glucose. The K_m for D-glucose transport by the isolated plasma membrane can only be compared with whole cell studies, which used D-glucose, since other plasma membrane studies did not measure initial rates and therefore could not make kinetic analysis to provide a K_m. The whole cell studies by Whitesell and Gliemann[4] and Olefsky et al.[3] report the K_m to be 10 mM and 9 mM, respectively.

The increase in glucose transport induced by insulin could result from (1) the addition of new transport sites similar in nature to the existing basal glucose transport sites, (2) an addition of transport sites that are different from the existing basal glucose transport sites, or (3) an alteration in the existing transport sites, allowing more rapid transport to occur. The findings that the K_m of transport was unchanged while the V_{max} was increased by insulin were consistent with the first alternative. If alternatives 2 or 3 were correct, then it might be expected that the K_m would be lowered. Another approach at resolving this question was to look at the energy of activation of the transport process. Olefsky[8] found that insulin did not change the energy of activation of the glucose transport system in the intact cell. Vinten[18] found that the V_{max} of stimulated and nonstimulated 3-O-methylglucose transport showed the same temperature dependency between 18° and 37°. The present study confirms these findings with the isolated plasma membrane transport system. This further suggests that insulin causes an increase in the number of transport sites. This is supported by the recent finding of Wardzala et al.[8] that insulin treatment of adipocyte increases the binding of cytochalasin B to a specific site on the plasma membrane which they relate to the glucose transport system. They interpret this finding as indicative of insulin increasing the number of glucose transport sites. Thus, this body of evidence supports the concept that insulin causes formation of new transport sites.

The next major question to be addressed was whether the new transport sites generated by insulin are functionally similar to the transport sites in the control. All the major characteristics measured in this study would suggest that they are similar. Alteration of basal glucose transport caused by changes in pH of the assay media was proportionately similar to the changes in insulin-stimulated transport. Similarly, N-ethylmaleimide, dithiothreitol, cytochalasin B, cytochalasin D, and reduced and oxidized glutathione altered glucose transport in plasma membranes from control and insulin-treated cells identically. One apparent difference between the basal and insulin-stimulated transport is the partial dependency on extracellular Ca^{++} for obtaining maximal insulin stimulation. This partial dependency on calcium seems to be related to the mechanism by which insulin activates the glucose transport system, as this study shows no dependence of basal or insulin-stimulated glucose transport on the Ca^{++} concentration in the assay media. Bonne et al.[20] originally reported similar dependency on extracellular calcium for maximal insulin stimulation of glucose transport.

There are data from some intact cell studies[2,4,9] that do not agree with the present study or other intact cell studies[3,8] and would suggest that at least some of the insulin-stimulated transport sites are different from the basal sites. This idea is based primarily on observations that there is a greater temperature dependency (increased energy of activation) for insulin-stimulated 3-O-methyl or 2-deoxyglucose transport than for the control. This is opposite to what would be predicted from insulin facilitating glucose transport. The use of D-glucose instead of glucose analogues in the present study may explain the difference concerning temperature dependencies of transport in those whole cell studies. Also, making temperature changes with intact cells to derive Arrhenius plots may alter other metabolic processes, which could artifactually alter the resulting transport data. It is difficult to understand how accurate temperature curves can be obtained using whole cells to compare control and insulin-treated systems, since, to obtain insulin effects at low temperatures, excessively long incubations are required. These long incubations could cause alterations that would not be found in the shorter incubations used for the higher temperatures. The plasma membrane system avoids this problem, for the whole cells were incubated with insulin for 15 min and then isolated. Plasma membranes were incubated at different temperatures during glucose uptake studies but for equal lengths of time.

This study also demonstrated that specifically bound insulin was carried over with the isolated plasma membranes. Our data showed that removal of the residual specifically bound insulin did not alter the glucose-stimulated glucose transport by plasma membranes from insulin-treated cells. This would indicate that the alteration in glucose transport in the intact cell caused by insulin results in a stable alteration, which may include the formation of disulfide bonds, as suggested by Czech.[2,10] This suggestion has been further supported by the recent data from the laboratory of Lynn.[15,16] Consistent with this were the observations in the present study that sulfhydryl reagents, which reduce disulfide bonds or alkylate sulfhydryls, inhibited both basal and insulin-stimulated glucose transport to similar degrees. Further investigation into the nature of this permanently induced alteration may yield significant information about the mode of insulin action in stimulating glucose transport.

ACKNOWLEDGMENTS

We thank Mark Helfand for skillful technical assistance and Mrs. Dorothy DuBuque for preparation of the manuscript.

This work was supported by National Institutes of Health grants AM11892, AM20097, and GM07200.

REFERENCES

1 Ludvigsen, C., and Jarett, L.: A kinetic analysis of D-glucose transport by adipocyte plasma membranes. J. Biol. Chem. *254*:1444–46, 1979.

2 Czech, M.: Regulation of the D-glucose transport system in isolated fat cells. Mol. Cell. Biochem. *11*:51–63, 1976.

3 Olefsky, J. M.: Mechanism of the ability of insulin to activate the glucose-transport system in rat adipocytes. Biochem. J. *172*:137–45, 1978.

4 Whitesell, R. R., and Gliemann, J.: Kinetic parameters of transport of 3-O-methylglucose and glucose in adipocytes. J. Biol. Chem. *254*:5276–83, 1979.

5 Martin, D. B., and Carter, J. R.: Insulin stimulated glucose uptake by subcellular particles from adipose tissue cells. Science *167*:874–77, 1970.

6 Chandramoul, V., Milligan, M., and Carter, J. R.: Insulin stimulation of glucose transport in adipose cells, an energy-dependent process. Biochemistry *16*:1151–57, 1977.

7 Avruch, J., Carter, J. R., and Martin, D. B.: Insulin-stimulated plasma membranes from rat adipocytes: their physiological and physiochemical properties. Biochim. Biophys. Acta *288*:27–42, 1972.

8 Wardzala, L. J., Cushman, S. W., and Salans, L. B.: Mechanism of insulin action on glucose transport in the isolated rat adipose cell. J. Biol. Chem. *253*:8002–05, 1978.

9 Amatruda, J. M., and Finch, E. D.: Modulation of hexose uptake and insulin action by cell membrane fluidity. J. Biol. Chem. *254*:2619–25, 1979.

10 Czech, M. P.: Differential effects of sulfhydryl reagent on activation and deactivation of the fat cell hexose transport system. J. Biol. Chem. *251*:1164–70, 1976.

11 Hammons, G. T., and Jarett, L.: Characterization of lysosomal degradation of receptor bound ^{125}I-insulin by rat adipocytes and dissociation of lysosomal degradation of insulin from the short term biological effects of insulin. Diabetes (in press).

12 McDonald, J. M., Bruns, D. E., and Jarett, L.: Ability of insulin to increase calcium binding by adipocyte plasma membranes. Proc. Natl. Acad. Sci. USA *73*:1542–46, 1970.

13 Lowry, O. H., Rosebrough, N. J., Farr, A. L., and Randall, R. J.: Protein measurement with the folin phenol reagent. J. Biol. Chem. *193*:265–75, 1951.

14 Kotyk, A., and Janacek, K.: Cell Membrane Transport: Principles and Techniques. New York, Plenum Press, 1970, pp. 235–37.

15 Mukherjee, S. P., and Lynn, W. S.: Reduced nicotinamide adenine dinucleotide phosphate oxidase in adipocyte plasma membrane and its activation by insulin. Possible role in the hormone's effects on adenylate cyclase and the hexose monophosphate shunt. Arch. Biochem. Biophys. *184*:69–76, 1977.

16 Mukherjee, S. P., Lane, R. H., and Lynn, W. S.: Endogenous hydrogen peroxide and peroxidative metabolism in adipocytes in response to insulin and sulfhydryl reagents. Biochem. Pharmacol. *27*:2589–94, 1978.

17 Shanahan, M. F., and Czech, M. P.: Purification and reconstitution of the adipocyte plasma membrane D-glucose system. J. Biol. Chem. *252*:8341–43, 1977.

18 Vinten, J.: Cytochalasin B inhibition and temperature dependence of 3-O-methylglucose transport in fat cells. Biochim. Biophys. Acta *511*:259–73, 1978.

19 Ludvigsen, C., and Jarett, L.: The characterization of catecholamine stimulation of glucose transport by rat adipocytes and isolated plasma membranes. Endocrinology (In press).

20 Bonne, D., Belhadj, O., and Cohen, P.: Modulation by calcium of the insulin action and of the insulin-like effect of oxytocin on isolated rat lipocytes. Eur. J. Biochem. *75*:101–05, 1977.

Effects of Indomethacin on Acute Insulin Release in Man

ERIC TOPOL AND ROBERT G. BRODOWS

SUMMARY

Prostaglandin (PG) E_2 stimulates glucose-induced insulin release from isolated rat pancreatic islets but inhibits acute insulin release to intravenous (i.v.) glucose in man. Since PGs act as intracellular messengers, we have studied the effect of endogenous PG inhibition with indomethacin (a potent PG synthesis inhibitor) to clarify these differences. The acute insulin response (AIR) to 5 g and 20 g i.v. glucose, 5 g i.v. arginine, and 1 mg i.v. glucagon before and one hour after ingestion of 50 mg indomethacin (INDO) or placebo was studied in healthy lean subjects. INDO significantly lowered basal insulin levels (pre, 9.5 ± 1.6; post, 6.4 ± 1.8 μU/ml, $\bar{X}$ ± SE, $p < 0.02$, paired *t*-test) while placebo failed to alter basal insulin (pre, 8 ± 2.7; post, 6.9 ± 0.6 μU/ml). INDO substantially blunted the AIR to 5 g glucose (Δ3–5′ IRI pre, 20.3 ± 3; post, 8.4 ± 2.4 μU/ml, $p < 0.005$), 20 g glucose (Δ3–5′ IRI pre, 38.1 ± 9.7; post, 18.9 ± 8 μU/ml, $p < 0.005$), and 1 mg glucagon (0–10′ IRI area pre, 375 ± 73; post, 149 ± 30 μU · min/ml, $p < 0.05$), but it failed to influence arginine-stimulated AIR (0–10′ IRI area pre, 161 ± 34; post, 186 ± 31). Thus, PG inhibition with INDO lowers basal, glucose-, and glucagon-stimulated AIR, but it has no effect on arginine-stimulated AIR. Our data suggest that endogenous PGs enhance insulin secretion. DIABETES *29*:379–382, May 1980.

Prostaglandins (PG) are a ubiquitous group of cyclic fatty acids that may act as intracellular messengers or local hormones. Their presence in human pancreatic tissue has been documented by Karim,[1] and numerous in vitro and in vivo studies have attempted to elucidate the role of PGs in modulating insulin secretion. Some studies report PGs enhance insulin release in isolated rat islets and perfused rat pancreas,[2–4] while others find no effect on insulin secretion.[5,6] In vivo studies in various animal species have yielded equally discrepant data.[7,8] Recently, Robertson and Chen have reported that PGE_2 inhibits glucose-induced but not arginine-induced secretion in normal man.[9] Administration of drugs that inhibit endogenous prostaglandin synthesis has been observed to both augment and inhibit glucose-induced acute insulin response.[9,10] To clarify the role of PGs on beta cell physiology, in the present study we compared the effect of indomethacin, a potent PG synthetase inhibitor, on glucose-, glucagon-, and arginine-stimulated acute insulin release.

From the Endocrine-Metabolism Division, Genesee Hospital, and the Department of Medicine, University of Rochester School of Medicine and Dentistry, Rochester, New York 14607.
Address reprint requests to Robert G. Brodows, M.D., Department of Medicine, Genesee Hospital, 224 Alexander Street, Rochester, NY 14607.
Accepted for publication 27 December 1979.

METHODS

Study procedure. Normal volunteers with no personal or family history of diabetes mellitus were studied after a 12 h fast, between the hours of 8 a.m. and 12 noon. All subjects were within 10% of their ideal body weight (Metropolitan Life Insurance Tables). Written consent was obtained after a full explanation of the study. A scalp vein needle was placed in an antecubital vein and kept patent with 0.85% saline for blood sampling. Various insulin-stimulating substances were given in the antecubital vein of the contralateral arm. All studies were performed in a random order with an interval of at least three days between studies in each subject. On separate days, the acute insulin release to four stimuli was studied before and one hour after ingestion of 50 mg indomethacin or a placebo (blank hypodermic tablets, Lilly). Glucose stimulation was achieved by rapid intravenous (i.v.) boluses of 5 g (within 5 s) or 20 g (within 30 s) glucose with blood samples drawn before and 3, 5, 10, and 15 min after each pulsing. Arginine stimulation was provided by rapid (within 30 s) i.v. injection of 5 g of 10% arginine hydrochloride (Cutter), with samples being collected before and at 2, 4, 6, 10, and 15 min after each pulsing. Glucagon (Lilly) was injected at a dose of 1 mg, with blood being collected at 0, 2, 5, 10, 20, and 30 min.

Analytic methods. All blood was drawn into cold heparinized tubes, centrifuged immediately at 4°C, and plasma was separated and stored at −20°C for later glucose and insulin determinations. Glucose was determined by the AutoAnalyzer glucose oxidase method. Immunoreactive insulin (IRI) was determined in triplicate by a double antibody method (Amersham-Searle) specially modified to obtain accurate measurements of insulin below 10 μU/ml. Within assay and between assay variability were 6% and 10%, respectively. Indomethacin levels were kindly measured by Dr. Carl Stevenson, Merck Sharp and Dohme, in six subjects one hour after indomethacin ingestion.

Calculations. The acute insulin response to glucose was calculated as (1) the Δ3–5′ IRI: mean 3–5 min postglucose insulin values minus the insulin level immediately before the injection; (2) 0–10 min area: total incremental area above baseline (μU · min/ml) estimated by computing the sum of the partial areas under the response curve. Arginine- and glucagon-induced insulin responses were also calculated as total incremental area above preinjection insulin. All data are expressed as mean ± SE. Student's *t*-test and paired *t*-tests were used when applicable.

RESULTS

Effects of indomethacin on basal insulin and glucose levels. Indomethacin itself resulted in a small but significant decrease in IRI levels (preingestion, 9.5 ± 1.6; 60 min postingestion, 6.4 ± 1.8 μU/ml; n = 9, $p < 0.02$ by paired *t*-test) but there was no change in pre- and postbasal glucose levels (pre, 99 ± 2; post, 104 ± 4 mg/dl). Neither plasma insulin (8 ± 1.1 μU/ml vs 6.9 ± 0.6 μU/ml) nor plasma glucose (93 ± 4 mg/dl vs 97 ± 3 mg/dl) were significantly altered by placebo ingestion.

Effects of indomethacin on glucose-stimulated insulin release. The acute insulin response to a 5 g glucose pulse in nine subjects after indomethacin ingestion was markedly blunted (Figure 1) in the face of comparable glucose stimulation (Δ3–5′ glucose: pre, 32 ± 3.4; post, 31 ± 4 mg/dl). Significant inhibition of insulin release ($p < 0.005$) was evident from either Δ3–5′ IRI (20.3 ± 3 μU/ml vs 8.7 ± 2.3) or area (136 ± 24 μU · min/ml vs 65 ± 16) calculations. A similar inhibition of insulin release after indomethacin to the 20 g glucose injection is apparent in Figure 2; Δ3–5 min IRI fell from 38 ± 9.7 μU/ml to 18.9 ± 8 μU/ml ($p < 0.005$) and 0–10 min area from 235 ± 56 μU · min/ml to 117 ± 45 μU · min/ml ($p < 0.001$). Indomethacin levels one hour after drug ingestion of six subjects on the day of 5 g glucose pulse ranged from 1275 to 5900 ng/ml (3.6–17 μM).

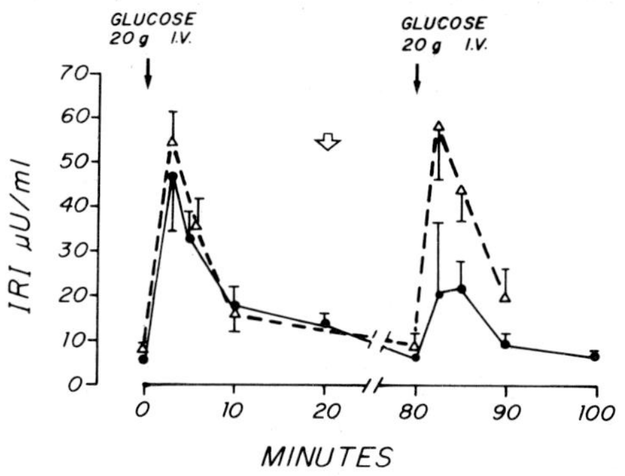

FIGURE 2. Plasma insulin response to 20 g glucose pulse, given before and after indomethacin (50 mg) (●), or placebo (△), given at 20 min (open arrow); x̄ ± SEM.

Placebo experiments failed to reveal significant alterations in the acute insulin response to either the 5 g (n = 9) or 20 g (n = 6) glucose pulse (Figures 1 and 2).

Effect of indomethacin on arginine- and glucagon-stimulated insulin release (Figures 3 and 4). During arginine pulsing, the peak insulin concentration (38.5 ± 6 vs 40.2 ± 6.7 μU/ml) and the incremental insulin area (161 ± 34 vs 186 ± 31 μU · min/ml) were similar before and after indomethacin (Figure 3). However, the acute insulin response to glucagon (Figure 4) was substantially decreased after indomethacin (0–10 min area: 375 ± 73 vs 149 ± 30 μU · min/ml, $p < 0.05$; peak: 55 ± 9 vs 25 ± 5 μU/ml, $p < 0.05$). The glucagon (n = 5) and arginine (n = 5) response was essentially unchanged after placebo administration.

DISCUSSION

The results of these studies clearly show that ingestion of indomethacin (50 mg) in normal subjects significantly decreases the acute phase of insulin release in response to either intravenous glucose or glucagon. Indomethacin itself also resulted in a small, but significant, fall in basal insulin levels. Of interest is the failure of a similar dose of indomethacin to alter insulin release in response to arginine. Indo-

FIGURE 1. Plasma insulin response to 5 g glucose pulse, given before and after indomethacin (50 mg) (●), or placebo (△), given at 20 min (open arrow); x̄ ± SEM.

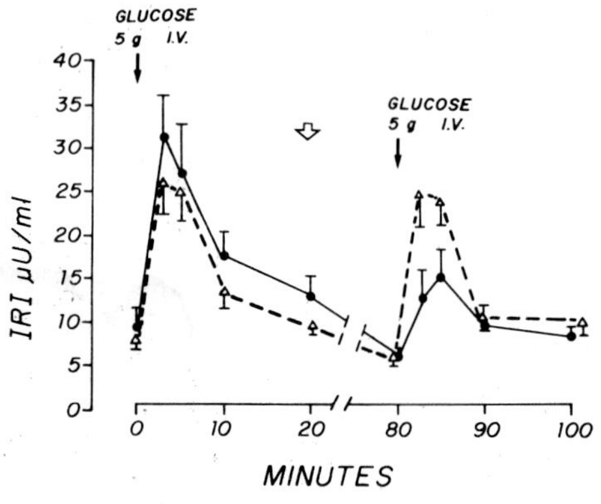

FIGURE 3. Plasma insulin response to 5 g arginine i.v., given before and after indomethacin (50 mg) (●), or placebo (△), given at 15 min (open arrow); x̄ ± SEM.

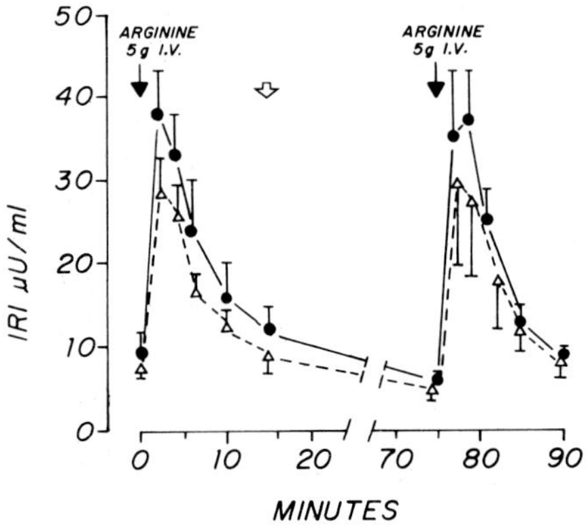

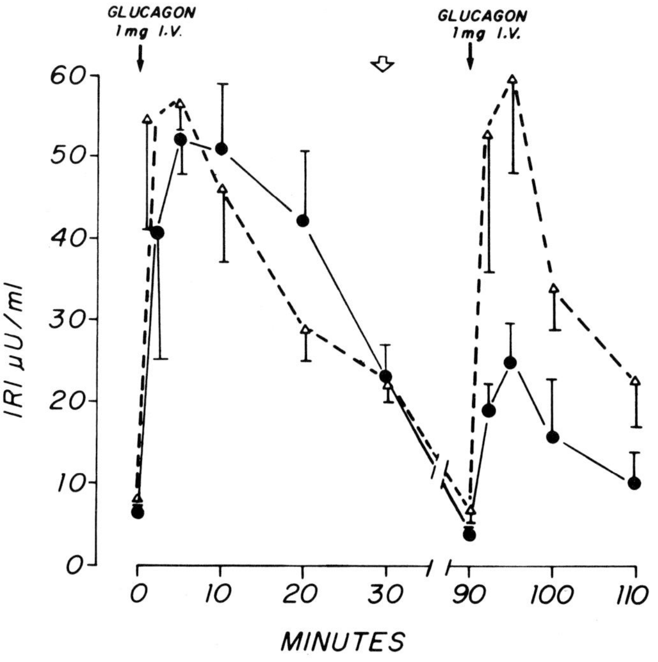

FIGURE 4. Plasma insulin response to 1 mg glucagon i.v., given before and after indomethacin (50 mg) (●), or placebo (△), given at 30 min (open arrow); x̄ ± SEM.

methacin inhibits PG synthesis by alterations in cycloöxygenase and phospholipase A_2 activity at concentrations similar to those achieved in our subjects.[11,12] In man, the action of similar agents may be demonstrated as rapidly as one hour after drug administration.[13] Indomethacin also inhibits phosphodiesterase and oxidative phosphorylation but at concentrations substantially higher than those achieved during our studies.[14,15] Thus, our results raise the possibility that endogenous PGs play a stimulatory role in insulin secretion. This is compatible with reports of PGs stimulating insulin release in both in vitro[2–4] and in vivo studies in which indomethacin (50 mg), given rectally and orally, inhibited acute phase insulin release.[10]

To further characterize the nature of the indomethacin-induced inhibition of insulin release, we studied the acute insulin response to glucagon and arginine after indomethacin ingestion. Since indomethacin did not inhibit insulin release to all stimuli, it is unlikely that indomethacin merely depleted the pool of insulin available for immediate release. The ability of indomethacin to inhibit glucagon-stimulated but not arginine-stimulated insulin release agrees with some, but not all, previous studies. In vitro, PGE_1 inhibits glucagon-evoked insulin release.[7] In man, Robertson and Chen failed to alter arginine-induced insulin release with PGE_2 infusion,[9] although augmented release may occur after acetylsalicylic acid ingestion.[16,17] It is known that glucagon releases insulin by adenylate cyclase activation,[18] while the insulinotropic action of arginine is probably related to potentiation of the glucose signal at a site between the glucose receptor and the cyclic AMP system.[19] Thus, in the present study, indomethacin inhibited insulin release only to secretagogues that induce insulin release via a rise in beta cell cyclic AMP. One could postulate that indomethacin, by inhibiting local islet cell PG concentrations, would lower cyclic AMP content and, thus, decrease the insulin response to glucose. This hypothesis is consistent with in vitro studies, in which prostaglandins increased islet cyclic AMP content,[20] and with current concepts, assigning a possible role to islet cyclic AMP generation in the process of glucose-induced insulin release.[21] Against such formulation is the recent finding that indomethacin may antagonize cyclic AMP directly, since it inhibits cyclic AMP–dependent protein kinase in ileal mucosal homogenates.[22] However, the exact effect of indomethacin in pancreatic tissue remains to be established.

Another possible explanation for the indomethacin-induced changes in insulin secretion might be that indomethacin altered either beta cell glucose receptors or receptor-linked glucose transport. In support of such a concept is a recent report by Olefsky that PGE_2 enhances insulin receptor–glucose transport interactions in isolated adipocytes.[23] It could be speculated that similar relationships exist between endogenous PGs and the glucose receptors in the beta cell.

Several studies in man, utilizing PG infusions,[9,24] salicylate infusions,[9,25] or aspirin ingestion,[16,17] suggest that PGs inhibit insulin release in man. The physiologic validity of i.v. PG administration may be questioned, since PGs act mainly as intracellular messengers, and various intermediary compounds and metabolites may be active in tissues. In addition, infusion of PGs may alter other metabolites and hormones known to influence insulin secretion.[24] The biologic actions of PGs often follow a bell-shaped dose-response curve;[26] thus, effects demonstrated at high concentrations may be absent or even reversed at low ones. Therefore, erroneous conclusions may be made if nonphysiologic PG levels are achieved. In most studies of the characteristics of drugs inhibiting PG biosynthesis, indomethacin is substantially more potent than aspirin or salicylate.[14,27] Since oral administration of PG inhibitors does not appear to suppress PG tissue levels in an organ-specific manner,[28] it is unlikely that differences between aspirin, salicylates, and indomethacin are related to selective pancreatic PG inhibition by any one of these drugs. It is possible that differences exist between these agents in regard to PG catabolism.[29] Finally, one cannot exclude that the pharmacologic effects of these drugs are unrelated to alterations in endogenous PG concentrations.[14] Although in no study has indomethacin been compared with aspirin in regards to insulin secretion, it is of note that aspirin and indomethacin have discrepant effects on growth hormone secretion.[30] Unfortunately, all current studies are hampered by the lack of an in vivo method of estimating the degree of intracellular PG synthesis inhibition achieved by the various aspirin-like drugs. It is obvious that further studies in man are necessary before a cohesive theory of PG-insulin relationships in health and disease can be proposed.

ACKNOWLEDGMENTS

The authors wish to thank Diane Nichols and Elaine Quincey for technical assistance and Elaine Rago for secretarial help.

This work is supported, in part, by grant AM21664 from the National Institutes of Health, the American Diabetes Association—Rochester Affiliate, and the Carroll C. Colgan Fund.

REFERENCES

[1] Karim, S. M., Sandler, M., and Williams, E. D.: Distribution of prostaglandins in human tissues. Br. J. Pharmacol. Chemother. *31*:340–44, 1967.

[2] Johnson, D. G., Fujimoto, W. Y., and Williams, R. H.: Enhanced release of insulin by prostaglandins in isolated pancreatic islets. Diabetes *22*:658–63, 1973.

[3] Pek, S., Tai, T. Y., Crowther, R., and Fajans, S. S.: Glucagon release precedes insulin release in response to common secretagogues. Diabetes *25*:764–70, 1976.

[4] Pek, S., Tai, T. Y., and Elster, A.: Stimulatory effects of prostaglandins E-1, E-2, and F2-alpha on glucagon and insulin release in vitro. Diabetes *27*:801–04, 1978.

[5] Saunders, R. M., and Moser, C. A.: Changes in vascular resistance induced by prostaglandins E2 and F2 in the isolated rat pancreas. Arch. Int. Pharmacodyn. Ther. *197*:86–92, 1972.

[6] Rossini, A. A., Lee, J. B., and Frawley, T. F.: An unpredictable lack of effect of prostaglandins on insulin release in isolated rat islets. Diabetes *20*(Suppl. 1):374, 1971.

[7] Sacca, L., Perez, G., Renzo, F., Pascuccui, I., and Conderelli, M.: Reduction of circulating insulin levels during the infusion of different prostaglandins in the rat. Acta Endocrinol. (Copenhagen) *79*:266–74, 1975.

[8] Hertelendy, F., Todd, H., Ehrhart, K., and Blute, R.: Studies on growth hormone secretion. IV. In vivo effects of prostaglandin E1. Prostaglandins *2*:79–91, 1972.

[9] Robertson, R. P., and Chen, M.: A role for prostaglandin E in defective insulin secretion and carbohydrate intolerance in diabetes mellitus. J. Clin. Invest. *60*:747–53, 1977.

[10] Widstrom, A.: Influence of indomethacin on glucose-induced insulin response in normal man—role of prostaglandins in the rapid insulin release? Horm. Metab. Res. *9*:172–75, 1977.

[11] Smith, W. L., and Lands, W. E. M.: Stimulation and blockade of prostaglandin biosynthesis. J. Biol. Chem. *246*:6700–02, 1971.

[12] Kaplan, L., Weiss, J., and Elsbach, P.: Low concentrations of indomethacin inhibit phospholipase A_2 of rabbit polymorphonuclear leukocytes. Proc. Natl. Acad. Sci. USA *75*:2955–58, 1978.

[13] Smith, J. B., and Willis, A. L.: Aspirin selectively inhibits prostaglandin production in human platelets. Nature, New Biol. *231*:235–37, 1971.

[14] Flowers, R. J.: Drugs which inhibit prostaglandin biosynthesis. Pharmacol. Rev. *26*:33–65, 1974.

[15] Flores, S., and Sharp, G.: Endogenous prostaglandins and osmotic water flow in the toad bladder. Am. J. Physiol. *223*:1392–97, 1972.

[16] Giugliano, D., Torella, R., Siniscalchi, N., Improta, L., and D'Onofrio, F.: The effect of acetylsalicylic acid on insulin response to glucose and arginine in normal man. Diabetologia *14*:359–63, 1978.

[17] Micossi, R., Pontiroli, A. E., Baron, S. H., Tamayo, R. C., Lengel, F., Bevilacqua, M., Raggi, U., Norbiato, G., and Foa, P. P.: Aspirin stimulates insulin and glucagon secretion and increases glucose tolerance in normal and diabetic subjects. Diabetes *27*:1196–1204, 1978.

[18] Turtle, J. R., and Kipnis, D. N.: An adrenergic receptor mechanism for the control of cyclic 3′5′ adenosine monophosphate synthesis in tissues. Biochem. Biophys. Res. Commun. *28*:797–802, 1967.

[19] Efendić, S., Cerasi, E., and Luft, R.: Arginine-induced insulin release in relation to the cyclic AMP system in man. J. Clin. Endocrinol. Metab. *34*:67–*72*; 1972.

[20] Kuo, W. N., Hodgkins, D. S., and Kuo, J. F.: Adenylate cyclase in islets of Langerhans. Isolation of islets and regulation of adenylate cyclase activity by various hormones and agents. J. Biol. Chem. *248*:2705–11, 1973.

[21] Rabinovitch, A., Grill, V., Renold, A. W., and Cerasi, E.: Insulin release and cyclic AMP in islets of fed and starved rats. J. Clin. Invest. *58*:1209–16, 1976.

[22] Kantor, H. S., and Hampton, M.: Indomethacin in submicromolar concentrations inhibits cyclic AMP-dependent protein kinase. Nature *276*:841–42, 1978.

[23] Olefsky, J. M.: Interaction between insulin receptors and glucose transport: effect of prostaglandin E_2. Biochem. Biophys. Res. Commun. *75*:271–76, 1977.

[24] Giugliano, D., Torella, R., Sgambato, S., and D'Onofrio, F.: Effect of α- and β-adrenergic inhibitions and somatostatin in plasma glucose, free fatty acids, insulin, glucagon, and growth hormone responses to prostaglandin E_1 in man. J. Clin. Endocrinol. Metab. *48*:302–08, 1979.

[25] Chen, M., and Robertson, R. P.: Restoration of the acute insulin response by sodium salicylate: a glucose dose-related phenomenon. Diabetes *27*:750–56, 1978.

[26] Horrobin, D. F.: Interaction between prostaglandins and calcium. The importance of bell-shaped dose-response curves. Prostaglandins *14*:667–77, 1977.

[27] Lands, W. E. M., and Rome, L. H.: Inhibition of prostaglandin biosynthesis. *In* Prostaglandins: Chemical and Biochemical Aspects. Karim, S. M. M., Ed. Baltimore, University Park Press, 1976, pp. 87–137.

[28] Fitzpatrick, F. A., and Synalda, M. A.: In vivo suppression of prostaglandin biosynthesis by non-steroidal anti-inflammatory agents. Prostaglandins *12*:1037–51, 1976.

[29] Pace-Asciak, C., and Cole, S.: Inhibitors of prostaglandin catabolism. I. Differential sensitivity of 9-PGDH, 13-PGR and 15-PGDH to low concentrations of indomethacin. Experientia *31*:143–45, 1975.

[30] Cavagnini, F., DiLandro, A., Invitti, C., Raggi, U., Alessandrini, P., Pinto, M., Girotti, G., and Vigo, P.: Effects of acetylsalicyclic acid and indomethacin on growth hormone secretion in man. Metabolism *26*:193–200, 1977.

Induction of Hyperglycemia with Insulin Antibodies to B-Chain Determinants

JOHN M. KELSO, IRENE Y. TAMAI, MICHAEL D. ROTH, IGNACIO VALDES, AND EDWARD R. ARQUILLA

SUMMARY

Insulin antibodies measured by a radioimmune method (AB_R) are significantly better inducers of hyperglycemia than are insulin antibodies measured by an immune hemolysis method (AB_H) when injected intraperitoneally into mice. The ability to induce hyperglycemia by an insulin antiserum can be predicted by the titer of AB_R measured. AB_R interact in vitro with determinants severely perturbed on nickel-insulin, partially perturbed on proinsulin and desasparagine-desalanine insulin, and unaffected on zinc-insulin or zinc-free monocomponent insulin. AB_H, on the other hand, interact in vitro with determinants severely perturbed on proinsulin and desasparagine-desalanine insulin but stabilized on nickel-insulin and zinc-insulin. Since the connecting peptide of proinsulin is probably in apposition to the A-chain residues on the solvent surface, the more effective reaction of proinsulin with AB_R than with AB_H is submitted as evidence that AB_R are directed toward residues on the B-chain surface of insulin. Because AB_R are more effective inducers of hyperglycemia than are AB_H, it is proposed that the degree of hyperglycemia induced by antibodies in vivo is a result of interactions with determinants on the B-chain surface of insulin. These results support the possibility that insulin in vivo is more accessible for interaction with antibodies directed to the B-chain of insulin. It is also possible that AB_R, which are directed to B-chain determinants, are of higher affinity than is the affinity between insulin and receptors or that the active site of insulin for maintaining euglycemia includes the B-chain surface residues. DIABETES *29*:383–390, May 1980.

Presented in abstract form at the annual meeting of the Federation of American Societies for Experimental Biology held at Dallas in April, 1979, and the Second International Insulin Symposium held at Aachen in September, 1979.
From the Department of Pathology, University of California—Irvine, California College of Medicine, Irvine, California.
Address reprint requests to Edward R. Arquilla, Department of Pathology, University of California Irvine Medical Center, 101 City Drive South, Orange, California 92668.
Received for publication 30 August 1979 and in revised form 9 January 1980.

Antisera used to measure insulin in immunoassay systems are composed of several populations of antibodies. Each population is in turn directed toward one of several determinants on the insulin molecule. Previous studies demonstrated that insulin derivatives with perturbed A-chain determinants exhibited higher relative immunologic activity in a radioimmune inhibition assay than in an immune hemolysis-inhibition assay.[1,2] From these results and the knowledge of the structure of insulin,[3] it was possible to propose that B-chain surface residues form determinants which interact with the antibodies operative in the radioimmune inhibition assay (AB_R).* In addition, it was possible to obtain evidence that the connecting peptide of proinsulin is in apposition to the surface residues of the A-chain of insulin and that antibodies operative in the immune hemolysis inhibition assay (AB_H) interact with determinants formed by A-chain surface residues.

The induction of hyperglycemia by guinea pig insulin antiserum injected into mice, rats, rabbits, cats, dogs, pigs, and sheep has been explained as being caused by the binding of the antibodies with endogenous insulin in the circulation.[4–6] The experiments presented in this report were designed to determine whether insulin in vivo—in circulation, on the cell membrane, or both—is oriented in a specific manner or is freely accessible to binding with all antibodies. Pools of insulin antisera were formed with antisera selected on the basis of the titer of AB_R or AB_H. By performing inhibition studies with five derivatives of insulin, additional evidence was obtained to further support the earlier studies[1,2] that AB_R are directed toward determinants formed by B-chain surface residues, whereas AB_H are directed toward determinants formed by A-chain surface residues.

When antisera were injected intraperitoneally into mice, a

* Abbreviations used in this paper are: AB_R, antibodies measured by the radioimmune system; AB_H, antibodies measured by the immune hemolysis system; AP, antiserum pool; Zn-insulin, zinc-insulin; MC-insulin, zinc-free monocomponent insulin; Ni-insulin, nickel insulin; DAA-insulin, desasparagine-desalanine insulin; RIIA, radioimmune inhibition assay; IHIA, immune hemolysis inhibition assay.

qualitatively superior ability to induce hyperglycemia by antisera with high titers of AB_R was observed as compared with the hyperglycemia induced by an antiserum pool with high titers of Ab_H. It is therefore possible to predict the ability of antisera to induce hyperglycemia by determining the level of AB_R present. It is proposed that the antibody binding to the B-chain determinants is of a higher affinity, is more readily accessible in vivo, or that the B-chain surface of insulin expresses its biologic activity.

MATERIALS AND METHODS

Preparation and characterization of insulin antiserum pools. Mongrel outbred guinea pigs were immunized with either monocomponent bovine insulin, fibrillar bovine insulin, or 10 times recrystallized Zn-bovine insulin (Novo Company) by a method previously described.[7] Each guinea pig received 0.125 mg of antigen in 0.20 ml of complete Freund's adjuvant in each paw pad. Fourteen days later, three equally spaced booster injections were given intradermally during a 7-day period. Each booster injection contained 0.1 mg of the antigen in 0.1 ml of buffered saline. Seven days later this procedure was repeated. Ten days after the booster injection, 1-ml blood samples were taken from the hind leg of each animal and titrated. When satisfactory antibody titers were obtained, the guinea pigs were exsanguinated immediately. Blood samples were allowed to clot at room temperature for 1 h and then overnight at 4°. The next day the serum was separated by centrifugation and stored at −80°.

The titer of AB_R and AB_H of the antiserum from each animal was measured by radioimmune titration and immune hemolysis titration,[2,8] respectively. The radioimmune titer is the dilution of antiserum of which 0.1 ml will bind 50% of 2×10^4 cpm of ^{125}I-monoiodoinsulin[9] (approximately 0.059 ng, sp act = 200 mci/mg) in a final volume of 0.3 ml. The immune hemolysis titer is the dilution of antiserum of which 0.1 ml will hemolyze 50% of 8.7×10^6 sheep red blood cells coated with Zn-insulin[10] in a final volume of 0.4 ml. In both titrations, antiserum and the insulin indicator were incubated for 1 h at 4°C. In the radioimmune titration, dextran-coated charcoal was added after the initial incubation to separate bound from free ^{125}I-monoiodoinsulin as previously described by Herbert.[11] In the immune hemolysis titration, excess complement was added after the initial incubation, the mixture was then incubated at 37° for 30 min, and the degree of specific immune hemolysis was determined as previously described.[7,10]

Three antiserum pools (AP) were prepared according to the radioimmune titers and immune hemolysis titers of the component insulin antisera. AP1 and AP2 were pools of antisera with high radioimmune titers and low immune hemolysis titers. AP3 was a pool containing antisera with low radioimmune titers and high immune hemolysis titers. AP1 and AP2 had high radioimmune titers and low immune hemolysis titers. AP3 had a low radioimmune titer and a high immune hemolysis titer (Table 1).

Insulin derivatives. MC-insulin was prepared from twice recrystallized bovine insulin (Elanco Co.) by chelation with EDTA and purification on a DEAE-Sephadex column equilibrated with 0.01M Tris, 0.01M glycine, 0.08M NaCl, and 7M urea buffer, pH 9.[9,12] The MC-insulin migrated as a single

TABLE 1
Radioimmune titer and immune hemolysis titer for each insulin antiserum pool (AP)

AP	Radioimmune titer*	Immune hemolysis titer†
AP 1	11,500	1,700
AP 2	9,000	405
AP 3	1,200	5,110

* Radioimmune titer is the antiserum dilution of which 0.1 ml will bind 50% of 2×10^4 cpm of ^{125}I-monoiodoinsulin (approximately 0.059 ng, sp act = 200 mCi/mg) in a final volume of 0.3 ml.
† Immune hemolysis titer is the insulin antiserum dilution of which 0.1 ml will hemolyze 50% of 8.7×10^6 sheep red blood cells coated with Zn-insulin aggregates in a final volume of 0.4 ml.

band in 15% acrylamide slab gel electrophoresis, indicating homogeneity and less than 2% contamination. The zinc content of the MC-insulin was analyzed by atomic absorption and was found to be less than one atom of zinc per 38 insulin molecules (UCIMC Laboratories, Orange, California). A single preparation of MC-insulin was used in the inhibition studies. In addition, this same preparation was used as the starter to prepare the Zn-insulin and Ni-insulin used in the inhibition studies.

Purified bovine proinsulin was a gift from Dr. Jorgen Schlichtkrull of the Novo Company, Dr. Ron Chance of the Eli Lilly Company, and Dr. Don Steiner, Dept. of Biochemistry, U. of Chicago. The three proinsulins were not significantly different from each other immunologically or by 15% acrylamide slab gel electrophoresis.

DAA-insulin was prepared by the exhaustive digestion of insulin with carboxypeptidase A[13] and was purified by column chromatography.[7]

MC-insulin, proinsulin, and DAA-insulin were all dissolved in 0.01N NaOH and were immediately diluted to approximately 1.74 μM in an equal volume of 0.22M phosphate buffer. The concentration was adjusted with sample buffer to exactly 1.74 μM spectrophotometrically (molar absorptivity at 276 nm = 5950).[2] All stock insulin solutions were stored at 4°C for no longer than 2 wk. The concentration was confirmed by molar absorptivity when used.

Zn-insulin and Ni-insulin were freshly prepared from MC-insulin stock. To 0.1 ml of 1 mg/ml (1.74 μM) MC-insulin stock, 0.02 ml of 0.523 mM $ZnSO_4$ or $Ni(NO_3)_2$ was added. The resulting 0.833 mg/ml (1.45 μM) Ni- and Zn-insulin solutions (approximately 0.6 atoms Zn or Ni per molecule of insulin) were then shaken at 175 rpm at 4°C for exactly 1 h. The Ni- and Zn-insulin solutions were used exactly 1 h after being diluted to the appropriate concentrations in either of the two immune inhibition assays.

Acrylamide slab gel electrophoresis. The acrylamide slab gel electrophoresis was a modification of the method of Laemmli.[14] An 11-cm-slab gel, containing 15% acrylamide and 0.4% N,N′-bis-methylene acrylamide, was used. Polymerizing agents employed were tetramethylethylenediamine and ammonium persulfate in a final concentration of 0.05%. Insulin (0.02 ml, 1.74 μM in 0.11M phosphate buffer, pH 7.4) and tracking dye (0.005 ml, 0.02% bromophenol blue and 50% glycerol) were run at 30 mA until tracking dye was 1 cm from the bottom of the gel. Staining and destaining were accomplished at 60°C. Staining solution was 0.1% coomassie blue (Sigma Co.), 7% acetic acid, and 10%

methanol. Destaining solution was 7% acetic acid and 10% methanol.

Immune inhibition assays. In the radioimmune inhibition assay (RIIA) and immune hemolysis inhibition assay (IHIA), a fixed dilution of insulin antiserum was reacted with a fixed concentration of the respective indicator insulin (^{125}I-monoiodoinsulin or Zn-insulin-coated sheep red blood cells) in the presence of varying concentrations of inhibitor.[2,8] The ability of a given insulin derivative to inhibit the binding of antibodies to indicator insulin in each assay system was measured.

For the RIIA and IHIA, each AP was diluted to its titer in the respective assay. For example, for AP1, the radioimmune titer was 11,500 and the immune hemolysis titer was 1,700. Therefore, in the RIIA, AP1 was diluted 1:11,500, while in the IHIA, AP1 was diluted 1:1,700. The amount of binding or lysis at these dilutions, when no inhibitor was added, was used as the maximum binding or lysis for the calculation of percent inhibition. The appropriately diluted antiserum (0.1 ml) was added to 0.1 ml of indicator insulin and 0.1 ml of the appropriate insulin derivative used as inhibitor. The assays were then run exactly as in the radioimmune or immune hemolysis titrations described above.

Measurement of diabetogenic activity. Male C57 B1/6 mice (Microbiological Associates), 8 to 12 wk of age, fed Purina mouse chow and water ad libitum, were injected intraperitoneally with one of the three antiserum pools (AP). Control groups received normal guinea pig serum. Groups of ten animals received one of four doses—0.05, 0.1, 0.2, or 0.4 ml of AP1, AP2, or AP3. Simultaneously, control groups of five or ten animals each received comparable doses of normal guinea pig serum.

Blood glucose was measured at 0, 15, 30, 45, 60, 90, 120, 180, and 240 min after injection. Blood samples (0.025 ml) were taken from the periorbital sinus, diluted 1:5 in distilled water, and glucose levels were determined by a glucose oxidase method with a glucose analyzer (YSI-model 23A). The diabetogenic activity was determined by calculating the difference between the area under the blood glucose vs. time curve for a given dose of a given AP and the area under the same curve for normal guinea pig serum and was expressed as mg glucose/dl × min during the four hours after injection.

The degree of correlation between diabetogenic activity and both radioimmune titer and immune hemolysis titer was calculated by the method of least squares for each of the antisera pools.

RESULTS

Binding characteristics of antibodies in the insulin antiserum pools. Inhibition studies in both immunoassay systems were performed with five insulin derivatives: MC-insulin, Zn-insulin, Ni-insulin, DAA-insulin, and proinsulin. Each antiserum pool was diluted to its respective titer for each immunoassay system. Therefore, the levels of antibodies in each AP equaled the amount of antibody that bound 50% of the ^{125}I-insulin in the radioimmune titration or that was capable of hemolyzing 50% of the Zn-insulin-coated red cells in the immune hemolysis titration. The amount of inhibitor (picomoles) required to inhibit 50% of the interaction between antibodies and the indicator (I^{125}-insulin or insulin-coated sheep red blood cells) in each of the respective assays was used to determine the relative degree of immunologic reactivity of each derivative.

The interaction of the five inhibitors with the insulin antibodies in each AP is presented in Figures 1 and 2 and Tables 2 and 3. Ni-insulin reacted poorest of the five derivatives with AB_R (Figure 1, Table 2). Approximately five times (20% cross reaction) as much Ni-insulin as MC-insulin was required to obtain 50% inhibition. Both DAA-insulin and proinsulin reacted about half as well as MC-insulin. Zn-insulin reacted as well as MC-insulin. It follows that the determinants on the insulin molecule that interact with AB_R are perturbed to the greatest degree on Ni-insulin, to a lesser degree on DAA-insulin and proinsulin, and not at all on Zn-insulin when compared with MC-insulin.

In contrast, Ni-insulin was the most reactive of the five inhibitors with AB_H (Figure 2, Table 3). An average of one fortieth as much Ni-insulin (40-fold greater reactivity) as MC-insulin was required for 50% inhibition. An enhanced reaction with Zn-insulin was also observed. Zn-insulin reacted approximately 10 times better than MC-insulin with AB_H. Proinsulin and DAA-insulin reacted poorest of the five inhibitors with AB_H, each reacting approximately one thirtieth as well as MC-insulin. The poor reactivity of proinsulin and DAA-insulin with AB_H suggests that the determinants with which they interact are perturbed to a greater degree on proinsulin and DAA-insulin than on the other three insulin derivatives tested.

The determinants on Ni-insulin with which the AB_R interact were found to be maximally perturbed. On the other hand, the determinants on Ni-insulin with which AB_H interact can best be described as more stable (most reactive) than these same determinants on any of the other derivatives tested. The determinants on Zn-insulin with which AB_R interact were not perturbed. The determinants on Zn-insulin with which AB_H interact were stabilized in a manner similar to Ni-insulin.

These observations are consistent with previous results.[2] The observations with Ni-insulin are new and are best explained as being caused by a marked perturbation of the B-chain surface determinants with which AB_R interact. Surprisingly and of interest was the augmented reactivity of Ni-insulin with AB_H, which is best explained by stabilization of the determinants on the A-chain surface (Figure 3).

The diabetogenic activity of insulin antiserum pools. The level and duration of the hyperglycemia induced was related to the radioimmune titer and the dose of AP injected. The plots of blood glucose vs. time for the 0.1-ml dose of each insulin antiserum pool are presented in Figure 4. The diabetogenic activity of the two insulin antiserum pools with high radioimmune but low immune hemolysis titers (AP1 and AP2) was qualitatively greater than that measured for the insulin antiserum pool with a low radioimmune titer and a high immune hemolysis titer (AP3). The calculated diabetogenic activities when 0.1 ml each of AP1 and AP2 were injected intraperitoneally were 36,713 and 30,433 (mg glucose/dl × min), respectively, compared with 6,721 when 0.1 ml of AP3 was injected. There was a slight difference in the hyperglycemia induced by AP1 and AP2. AP2 induced a steeper hyperglycemia, peaking at 60 min, with a quicker decline to normal levels, compared with AP1, where the

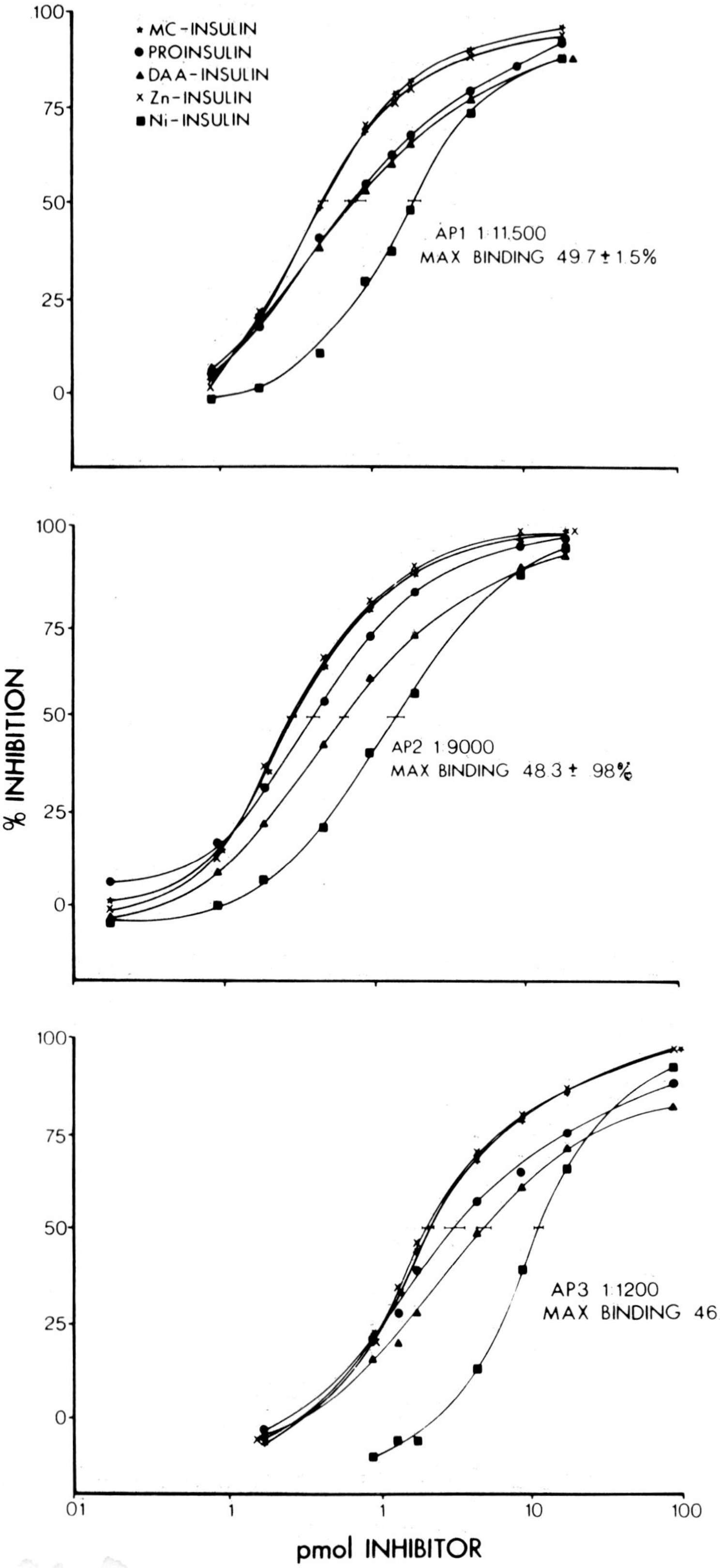

FIGURE 1. Radioimmune inhibition assay (RIIA). Percent inhibition vs. picomoles of inhibitor per tube for each insulin antiserum pool (AP). Each point represents a mean of at least three determinations. The $\bar{x} \pm$ SEM maximum binding obtained with the dilution of each AP in the absence of any inhibitor was determined from at least three experiments. The inhibitors were monocomponent insulin (MC-insulin), proinsulin, desalanine-desasparagine insulin (DAA-insulin), zinc-insulin (Zn-insulin), and nickel-insulin (Ni-insulin).

peak hyperglycemia was at 120 min followed by a more sustained hyperglycemia at 3 and 4 h. The antiserum pool with the low radioimmune titer (AP3) caused a hyperglycemia that peaked significantly lower at 60 min and was back to normal limits at 180 min, resulting in a qualitatively attenuated diabetogenic activity.

The diabetogenic activity was calculated from the differences in area between the respective hyperglycemia curves

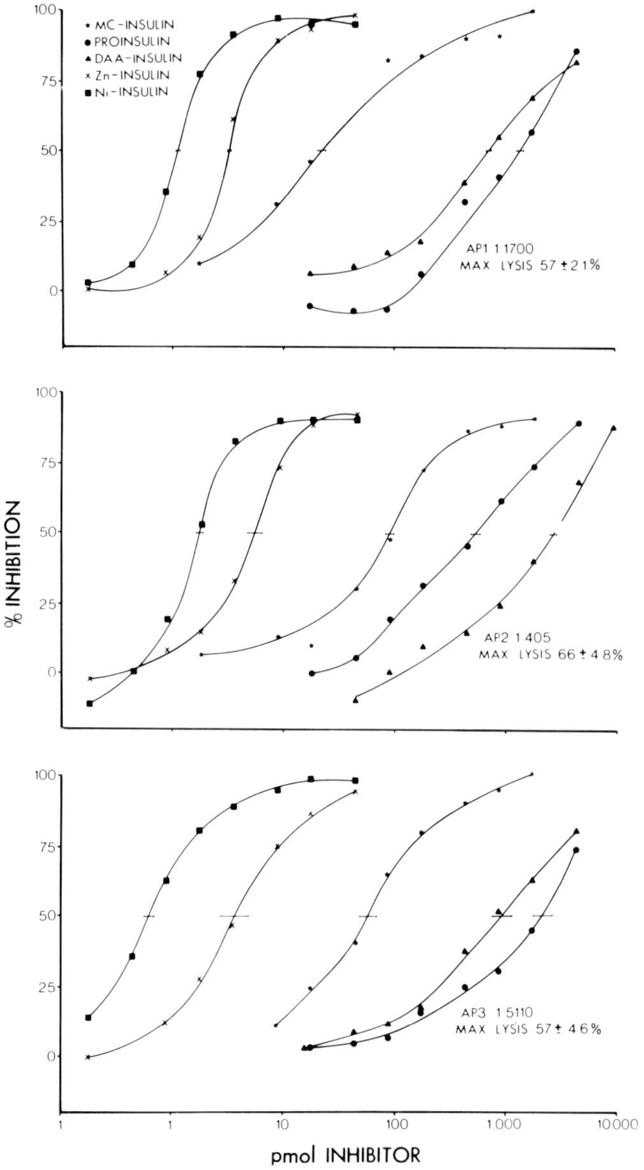

FIGURE 2. Immune hemolysis inhibition assay (IHIA). Percent inhibition vs. picomoles of inhibitor per tube for each insulin antiserum pool (AP). Each point represents at least three determinations. The $\bar{x}$ ± SEM maximum lysis obtained with the dilution of each AP in the absence of any inhibitor was determined from at least three experiments. The inhibitors were monocomponent insulin (MC-insulin), proinsulin, desalanine-desasparagine insulin (DAA-insulin), zinc-insulin (Zn-insulin), and nickel-insulin (Ni-insulin).

of each insulin antiserum pool for each of four doses and the curve obtained with normal guinea pig serum. The diabetogenic activity was linearly related to the 0.05- and 0.1-ml doses for all three pools of insulin antisera. A maximal diabetogenic activity was calculated at the 0.2-ml dose for AP1 and AP2, but it was linearly related to the 0.05-ml through 0.4-ml doses for AP3. The relative diabetogenic activity measured for each of the three antiserum pools (AP1 > AP2 > AP3) was maintained at each dose (Figure 5).

A maximum hyperglycemia (420 mg/dl) was obtained when 0.1 ml each of AP1 and AP2 were injected. The diabetogenic activity observed with higher doses (Figure 5) was caused by a sustained rather than an elevated hyperglycemia. The maximum hyperglycemia (380 mg/dl) induced with AP3 was observed only when 0.4 ml of antiserum was injected. Therefore, the increase of diabetogenic activity at higher doses for AP3 (Figure 5) reflected both an elevated and a sustained hyperglycemia.

A strong positive correlation ($r = 0.9868$, $P < 0.01$) between diabetogenic activity and radioimmune titer was observed (Figure 6). Figure 6 was generated from doses in the linear portion of the dose response curves for each AP (Figure 5; 0.05- and 0.1-ml doses). Although the correlation remained significant ($P < 0.01$) when higher doses were included in the calculation, both the slope and the correlation decreased (Table 4). This is best explained by the fact that, for high doses of AP1 and AP2 (0.2 and 0.4 ml), the blood glucose remained elevated at 4 h, when the experiment was terminated. Had the experiment been permitted to continue until glycemia returned to normal limits, it is likely that the diabetogenic activity vs. radioimmune titer plot would have had similar correlations and slopes when the higher doses were included in the calculations.

A negative correlation ($r = 0.8338$, $P < 0.01$) between diabetogenic activity and immune hemolysis was observed. This negative correlation was expected, since the antisera were selected to have inversely related radioimmune and immune hemolysis titers. In preliminary experiments, where the diabetogenic activity of insulin antisera was determined randomly, a positive correlation between diabetogenic activity and radioimmune titer and no correlation between diabetogenic activity and immune hemolysis titer were observed.

These observations are submitted as evidence that insulin in vivo—in the circulation, in the cell surface receptor, or

TABLE 2
Radioimmune inhibition assay (RIIA)
[picomoles of inhibitor required per tube for 50% inhibition of each antiserum pool (AP)]

Inhibitor	Antiserum Pool AP-1	AP-2	AP-3
MC-insulin	0.45 ± 0.02	0.28 ± 0.02	2.19 ± 0.10
Proinsulin	0.71 ± 0.04	0.37 ± 0.03	3.28 ± 0.52
DAA-insulin	0.77 ± 0.12	0.59 ± 0.03	4.82 ± 0.49
Zn-insulin	0.47 ± 0.04	0.28 ± 0.02	1.98 ± 0.04
Ni-insulin	1.88 ± 0.16	1.31 ± 0.16	11.60 ± 0.77

Results are presented as mean values ± SEM for at least three determinations.

TABLE 3
Immune hemolysis inhibition assay (IHIA)
[picomoles of inhibitor required per tube for 50% inhibition of each antiserum pool (AP)]

Inhibitor	Antiserum Pool AP-1	AP-2	AP-3
MC-insulin	22.10 ± 1.62	86.50 ± 9.22	56.20 ± 11.70
Proinsulin	1330.00 ± 76.70	528.00 ± 57.90	2150.00 ± 475.00
DAA-insulin	719.00 ± 47.50	2610.00 ± 174.00	916.00 ± 162.00
Zn-insulin	3.31 ± 0.10	5.22 ± 0.87	3.65 ± 1.04
Ni-insulin	1.17 ± 0.05	1.67 ± 0.12	0.64 ± 0.07

Results are presented as mean values ± SEM for at least three determinations.

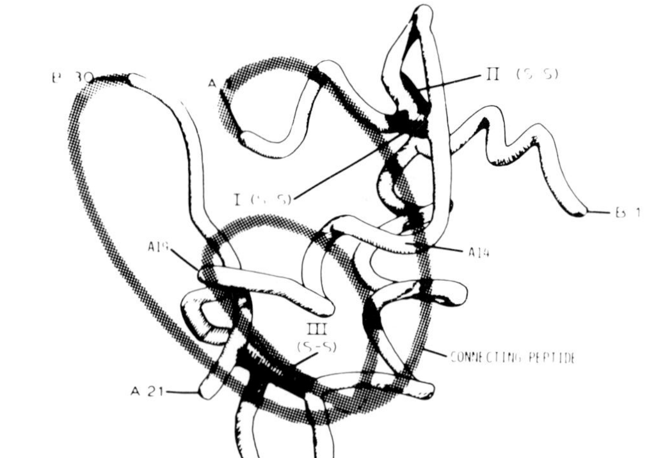

FIGURE 3. Views of the A- and B-chain surfaces of a worm model of insulin. The models were constructed from the alpha carbon coordinates (graciously supplied by Guy Dodson and Dorothy Hodgkin) of the 51 amino acid residues in insulin. The projection of the connecting peptide on the solvent surface is proposed from the data presented in the text. I (S-S) is the interchain disulfide bridge (A-6 to A-11). II (S-S) is the interchain disulfide bridge (A-7 to B-7). III (S-S) is the interchain disulfide bridge (A-20 to B-19). A-1 is the position of the alpha carbon of the N terminal Gly of the A-chain. B-1 is the position of the alpha carbon of the N terminal Phe of the B-chain. A-21 is the position of the alpha carbon of the C terminal Asp of the A-chain. A-14 and A-19 are the positions of the alpha carbons of the A-chain Tyr to which >90% of the iodine is substituted in the ^{125}I-monoiodotyrosylinsulin used in these experiments.

both—is accessible for interaction with insulin antibodies directed to determinants on the B-chain surface. These interactions may be of higher affinity or more accessible than

TABLE 4
Calculation of diabetogenic activity vs. radioimmune titer

Doses (ml) included	Correlation (R)	Significance (P)	Slope
0.05, 0.1	+0.9868	0.01	28
0.05, 0.1, 0.2	+0.9057	0.01	26
0.05, 0.1, 0.2, 0.4	+0.7480	0.001	21

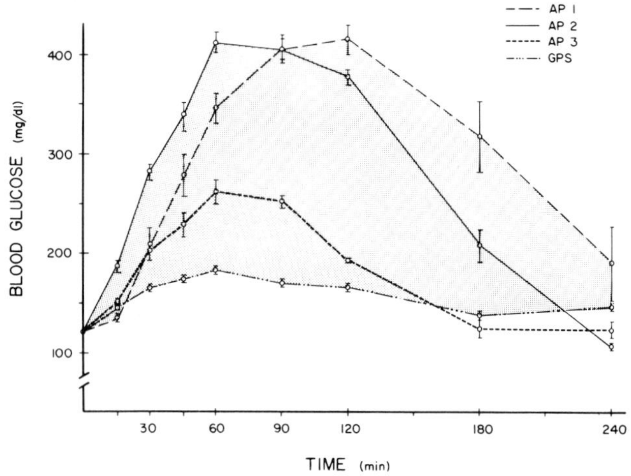

FIGURE 4. Blood glucose ($\bar{x} \pm$ SEM) vs. time after intraperitoneal injection of 0.1 ml of each insulin antiserum pool (AP) or normal guinea pig serum. N = 10 for each point on each AP curve through 120 min. N = 6 for the 180-min and 240-min points. The normal guinea pig serum curve is a composite of the four doses 0.05, 0.1, 0.2, and 0.4 (N = 20), since each dose elicited the same response. The area under this normal guinea pig serum curve was subtracted from the area under each AP curve for the determination of diabetogenic activity for each dose of each AP (Figure 5).

in vivo interactions with insulin antibodies directed to determinants on the A-chain surface.

DISCUSSION

In preliminary studies, a positive correlation between the level of AB_R in insulin antisera and the level of hyperglycemia induced was observed when the antisera were injected. In these same experiments, there was no correlation between the level of AB_H in the insulin antiserum and the level of hyperglycemia induced.

In the experiments described in this manuscript, we successfully predicted the hyperglycemia-inducing potency of three antiserum pools. We expected the two antiserum pools—AP1 and AP2—comprised of antisera with elevated levels of AB_R and low levels of AB_H to be significantly more potent inducers of hyperglycemia than the antiserum

FIGURE 5. Diabetogenic activity vs. dose for each insulin antiserum pool (AP). The diabetogenic activity (mg glucose/dl × min) was calculated from the difference in an area under the curve of hyperglycemia vs. time for each AP dose and the glycemia curve obtained with normal guinea pig serum (Figure 4).

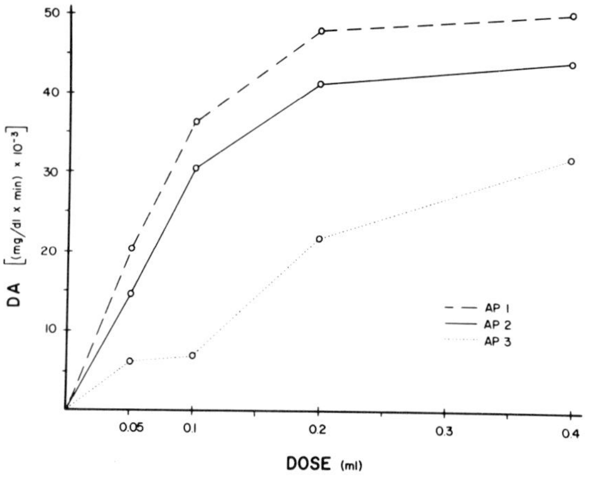

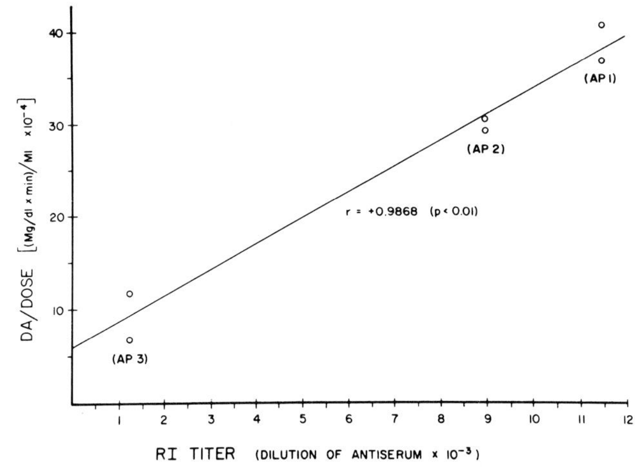

FIGURE 6. Diabetogenic activity (0.05- and 0.1-ml doses) vs. radioimmune titer for each antiserum pool (AP). The slope of this line of best fit is an estimate of the diabetogenic activity (see Figure 5) that can be expected when low doses ($<$0.1 ml) of insulin antiserum containing radioimmune antibody titers in the designated range are injected intraperitoneally into mice.

pool—AP3—comprised of antisera with low levels of AB_R and elevated levels of AB_H.

The positive correlation between radioimmune titer and diabetogenic activity in contrast with the lack of (or negative) correlation between immune hemolysis titer and diabetogenic activity is evidence that AB_R are more potent inducers of hyperglycemia than are AB_H. This supports the probability that insulin in vivo, either in circulation, on the cell surface, or both, is oriented to permit interaction with AB_R to a greater degree than is AB_H. There are at least three possible explanations for this phenomenon. First, AB_H may be of relatively low affinity compared with AB_R and, thus, less effective in causing hyperglycemia. Second, AB_H may be directed toward determinants on insulin, which are relatively less accessible in vivo than those to which AB_R are directed. Third, AB_H may be directed toward a site not essential for insulin's activity while AB_R may be directed toward an active site. None of these possibilities excludes the other nor do any of them separately or collectively negate the early interpretations[4–6] that the hyperglycemia induced by the injection of guinea pig insulin antibodies is a result of the interaction between antibodies and endogenous insulin in the circulation.

The difference in the two assays is best attributed to the reaction of antibody with the insulin indicator in each assay —^{125}I-monoiodoinsulin in the RIIA and sheep red blood cells coated with Zn-insulin aggregates in the IHIA. There are at least three differences in the indicator insulins. First, the insulin in the radioimmune system is soluble, while that in the immune hemolysis system is attached to an insoluble matrix. This may affect the affinity required for, and the kinetics of, the antibody-indicator interaction. Second, the Zn-insulin linked to red cells in the immune hemolysis system is at a concentration (1 mg/ml) that exists primarily in hexamers.[8] When these Zn-insulin hexamers are linked to red cells with bisdiazobenzadine, cross linking within the hexamer may occur, resulting in an indicator in which certain determinants are buried and unavailable for antibody binding.[2,8] Such determinants on the ^{125}I-monoiodoinsulin indicator in the radioimmune system would be accessible for antibody interaction. Third, the number of insulin molecules available for antibody interaction is four orders of magnitude greater in the immune hemolysis system than in the radioimmune system.

The immunologic reactivity of proinsulin with AB_R was 15-fold greater than that with AB_H (see Figures 1 and 2 and Tables 2 and 3). Therefore, AB_R are directed toward sites on the insulin molecule that are less perturbed on proinsulin than the sites to which AB_H are directed. Similar observations with other antisera have been previously reported.[2] It has been proposed[15,16] that the connecting peptide in proinsulin is in apposition to surface residues of the A-chain of the insulin molecule (Figure 3). It follows that, in proinsulin, the determinants least accessible for antibody interaction are on the A-chain surface. This logic supports the postulate that AB_H are directed toward A-chain surface determinants and AB_R are directed toward B-chain surface determinants (Figure 3).

Extending this logic, it is proposed that, on Ni-insulin, the poorest inhibitor of AB_R but the most effective inhibitor of AB_H, the B-chain determinants are severely perturbed. The A-chain determinants, on the other hand, are stabilized and immunologically more reactive than the other derivatives tested when each is compared with MC-insulin. The B-chain determinants on Zn-insulin are unperturbed and the A-chain determinants are markedly more stable than on MC-insulin. Both the B-chain and A-chain determinants are perturbed in DAA-insulin, although the A-chain determinants are more severely perturbed. These observations are submitted as additional evidence to the previous reports[2,4] that AB_R are directed to B-chain surface determinants and AB_H to A-chain surface determinants.

Since AB_R are more potent inducers of hyperglycemia than AB_H and because they are directed toward the B-chain determinants of insulin, it is proposed that antibody binding to the B-chain determinants of insulin is either of higher affinity, more readily accessible in vivo, or that this surface of insulin is needed to express its biologic activity. None of these possibilities excludes the other.

ACKNOWLEDGMENTS

This work was supported by grants from the United States Public Health Service (AM-13441-11) and from the Kroc Foundation.

REFERENCES

[1] Arquilla, E. R., Miles, P. V., and Morris, J. W. S.: Immunochemistry of insulin. *In* Handbook of Physiology, Section 7, Volume 1. Washington, D.C.; American Physiological Society, 1972, pp. 159–73.

[2] Arquilla, E. R., Dorio, R. J., and Brugman, T. M.: Structural studies of insulin and insulin derivatives using various immunologic indicators and antibody populations. Diabetes *25*:397–403, 1976.

[3] Blundell, T., Dodson, G., Hodgkin, D., and Mercola, D.: Insulin: the structure in the crystal and its reflections in chemistry and biology. Adv. Protein Chem. *26*:279–402, 1972.

[4] Moloney, P. J., and Coval, M.: Antigenicity of insulin: diabetes induced by specific antibodies. Biochem. J. *59*:179–85, 1955.

[5] Armin, J., Grant, R. J., and Wright, P. H.: Acute insulin deficiency provoked by single injections of anti-insulin serum. J. Physiol. *153*:131–45, 1960.

[6] Armin, J., Cunningham, N. F., Grant, R. T., Lloyd, M. K., and Wright, P. H.: Acute insulin deficiency provoked in the dog, pig and sheep by single injections of anti-insulin serum. J. Physiol. *157*:64–73, 1961.

[7] Brugman, T. M., and Arquilla, E. R.: Circular dichroic and immunologic studies of structure relationships of insulin and derivatives. Biochemistry *12*:727–32, 1973.

[8] Arquilla, E. R., Thiene, P., Brugman, T. M., Ruess, W., and Sugiyama,

R.: Effects of zinc ion on the conformation of antigenic determinants on insulin. Biochem. J. *175*:289–97, 1978.

[9] Sodoyez, J. C., Sodoyez-Goffaux, F., Goff, M. M., Zimmerman, A. E., and Arquilla, E. R.: (^{127}I) or carrier free (^{125}I) monoiodoinsulin. Preparation, physical, immunological, and biological properties and susceptibility to "insulinase" degradation. J. Biol. Chem. *250*:4268–77, 1975.

[10] Arquilla, E. R., and Finn, J.: Genetic control of combining sites of insulin antibodies produced by guinea pigs. J. Exp. Med. *122*:771–84, 1965.

[11] Herbert, V., Kam-Seng, L., Gottlieb, C. W., and Bleicher, S. J.: Charcoal immunoassay of insulin. J. Clin. Endocrinol. Metab. *25*:1374–84, 1965.

[12] Hamlin, J. L., and Arquilla, E. R.: Monoiodoinsulin. Preparation, purification, and characterization of a biologically active derivative substituted predominantly on tyrosine A14. J. Biol. Chem. *249*:21–32, 1974.

[13] Slobin, L., and Carpenter, F.: Action of carboxypeptidase A on bovine insulin: preparation of desalanine-desasparagine insulin. Biochemistry *2*:16–22, 1963.

[14] Laemmli, V. K.: Cleavage of structural proteins during the assembly of the head of bacteriophage T4. Nature *227*:680–85, 1970.

[15] Hodgkin, D. C.: The structure of insulin. Diabetes *21*:1131–50, 1972.

[16] Steiner, D., Wolfgang, K., Tager, H. S., and Peterson, J. D.: Proteolytic processing in the biosynthesis of insulin and other proteins. Fed. Proc. *33*:2105–15, 1974.

Integrated Concentration of Growth Hormone in Juvenile-onset Diabetes

JOHN T. HAYFORD, MARK M. DANNEY, JAMES A. HENDRIX, AND ROBERT G. THOMPSON

SUMMARY

Twenty-four-hour patterns of plasma growth hormone concentrations were evaluated during 50 studies of 42 subjects with juvenile-onset diabetes mellitus. Blood was sampled continuously over 24 h using a portable peristaltic pump under conditions in which subjects remained ambulatory and maintained their daily dietary and insulin regimens. All diabetics showed diurnal patterns characterized by frequent episodes of secretion of growth hormone. The mean 24-h concentration of growth hormone, designated the integrated concentration, was significantly higher among juvenile-onset diabetics ($P < 0.001$) than it was in age- and sex-matched nondiabetic populations. Juvenile-onset diabetics younger than 20 yr had significantly higher ($P < 0.005$) growth hormone integrated concentrations than did older juvenile-onset diabetics. There was no statistically significant correlation between the integrated concentrations of glucose and growth hormone; thus, the study failed to provide us with support for the hypothesis that elevated growth hormone concentrations in diabetics are a consequence of hyperglycemia. Variability of diurnal glucose concentrations was positively correlated ($P < 0.015$) with the growth hormone integrated concentration among juvenile-onset diabetics. Our observations indicate that rapid declines in plasma glucose concentration or episodes of absolute hypoglycemia were significant factors, contributing to both the elevated integrated concentration and the secretory spiking of growth hormone observed in the diabetic population. DIABETES 29:391–398, May 1980.

The role of growth hormone relative to the abnormal metabolism of diabetes is controversial, despite nearly 50 yr of investigation. As early as 1930, Houssay and Biasotti[1] reported that hypophysectomy ameliorated glucose intolerance in experimental diabetes, whereas reimplantation of the pars distalis reestablished abnormal glucose tolerance. Subsequent investigations have implicated growth hormone as a factor in the etiology of diabetes,[2,3] as a factor contributing to the abnormal glucose tolerance,[4] and as a factor in the pathogenesis of microvascular disease associated with diabetes.[3,5–8]

Many contradictions may be noted in the extensive literature relating growth hormone secretion to various aspects of the abnormal metabolism in diabetes and to the chronic complications of the disease. These contradictions are, in part, related to methods of assessment of growth hormone metabolism. In both normal and diabetic subjects, plasma growth hormone concentrations fluctuate markedly and unpredictably during 24 h. Measurement of plasma growth hormone concentrations in an unstimulated subject, even those measured in samples obtained under such standardized conditions as fasting, are highly variable among subjects and among samples from the same subject on different occasions. Although a variety of provocative tests, employing standardized stimuli (e.g., pharmacologic doses of secretagogues), has been used to evoke growth hormone secretion, all such tests disturb normal physiology. The relevance of such observations to an understanding of physiology in ambulatory, unstimulated subjects is unknown. These limitations have been circumvented, in part, by the intermittent sampling of blood over extended periods of time[9–13] without employment of pharmacologic stimuli.

The present report concerns observations of the 24-h patterns of plasma growth hormone concentration in ambulatory juvenile-onset diabetics. Blood samples were collected continuously in constant volume, timed aliquots over 24 h. Study conditions were designed to reflect, as closely as possible, the free living state: the patterns of food consumption, insulin therapy, and activity were set to mimic the subject's daily routines. The data reemphasize the abnormalities in growth hormone metabolism that occur in diabetes and indicate that the lability of blood glucose concentration is an important factor in inducing the elevation in growth

From the Department of Pediatrics, University of Iowa College of Medicine, Iowa City.
Address reprint requests to John T. Hayford, M.D., Department of Pediatrics, University of Iowa College of Medicine, Iowa City, Iowa 52242.
Received for publication 27 August and in revised form 20 December 1979.

hormone concentrations observed in this diabetic population.

MATERIALS AND METHODS

SUBJECTS

Diabetics. Forty-two subjects with newly diagnosed or previously diagnosed diabetes mellitus were enrolled for metabolic study using a continuous 24-h blood-sampling procedure. The study population was divided into two groups based on the previous therapy initiated for their glucose intolerance (Table 1):

1. Juvenile-onset diabetics with established treatment (JOD). The group consisted of 39 subjects (23 female, 16 male) with history of ketosis, with a requirement of exogenous insulin since diagnosis, and treatment for at least 2 mo. In 34 of the subjects, diagnosis was established before age 18 yr (mean age at diagnosis = 11.7 yr, SD = 5.5 yr). The JOD subjects were further divided for statistical analysis by sex and age at the time of study. None of the JOD group exceeded ideal weight for height by greater than 15%.[14] Insulin dose averaged 0.82 U/m²/day for the entire JOD group; however, the insulin dose for the younger JOD subjects (mean = 1.05, SD = 0.54 U/m²/day) was significantly greater ($P < 0.002$) than that for the older JOD subjects (mean = 0.57, SD = 0.15 U/m²/day).

2. Newly diagnosed juvenile-onset diabetics (NJOD). The group consisted of four subjects (three female, one male) diagnosed within 2 wk of study. All subjects had a previous history of ketosis, and one subject had been started on insulin therapy (subject 25b). Although all had significant hyperglycemia and intermittently showed ketonuria, neither ketonemia nor acidosis was present during the study period.

Subjects were enrolled from the pediatric and adult diabetes clinics or were referred from private physicians. Many subjects were experiencing difficulty in diabetic control, evaluation being prompted by excessive glycosuria or recurrent episodes of hypoglycemia. Although few of the study subjects could be classified as being under good diabetic control, all were active, functioning well within their social and employment environments, and are thus representative of an unselected diabetic population in our clinic population. Subjects 12 and 17 are exceptions, in that they were hospitalized for reeducation and regulation before admission to the study. Several subjects were studied on two or more occasions, criteria for restudy being based primarily on the subject's availability rather than prospectively established criteria.

PROTOCOL OF STUDY

Subjects were admitted to the Clinical Research Center on the day before study for a complete history and physical examination, explanation of the study protocol, and acclimatization to the clinic's facilities. The study protocol had been approved by the University of Iowa Committee on Human Investigation, and informed written consent was obtained from each subject and/or legal guardian. Subjects were maintained on their previous insulin or medicine regimens. Diet history was assessed by recall, and the dietary pattern while in hospital was designed to mimic home dietary patterns with respect to total caloric intake, to distribution of protein, fat, and carbohydrate calories, and to schedule of meal and snack consumption.

Between 0800 and 0900 h, after an overnight fast, the 24 h of continuous blood withdrawal was started using methods previously described.[15] An indwelling venous catheter, impregnated with an anticoagulant-binding resin, was placed in an antecubital vein under aseptic conditions and was connected to a constant speed, portable, continuous withdrawal pump (Cor-Med). Blood samples were collected in 30-min aliquots into iced 0.2 M EDTA-0.033 M benzamidine solutions (150 μl per milliliter blood). All samples were maintained at 4°C until centrifugation, and harvested plasma was frozen until assay. During the 24-h withdrawal period, subjects remained ambulatory within the Clinical Research Center.

ANALYTIC METHODS

Plasma glucose was determined with a semiautomated glucose oxidase system (Beckman glucose analyzer). Growth hormone was determined in triplicate by a double antibody radioimmunoassay.[16] Free and total insulin was assessed by radioimmunoassay using the extraction procedure of Gennaro and VanNorman.[17] Total insulin in subjects not treated with exogenous insulin was assessed by a double antibody radioimmunoassay[18] without prior extraction. The reported hormone and glucose concentrations were corrected for the 27% dilution resulting from collection in the anticoagulant-preservative solution.

ANALYSIS OF DATA

Glucose, insulin, growth hormone, and clinical demographic data were statistically analyzed using the SAS76[19] statistical package, available through the University's computing facilities. Each subject's hormone and glucose responses were characterized by several parameters: (1) Integrated concentration (IC)—the mean concentration of the 48 half-hourly plasma samples collected during the 24-h study. (2) Sequential variation (SV)—an expression of the lability of a hormone or substrate concentration, defined as the geometric mean change in concentration from the previous sample.[15] The lability of hormone or substrate concentration, due to either changes in amplitude or frequency, varies directly with sequential variation. Cumulative frequency distributions of the growth hormone concentration were calculated for each diabetic group, the concentration being coded in 1.25-ng/ml intervals.

Nondiabetic control population. Data for the growth hormone and glucose integrated concentrations in nondiabetic control populations, using an identical 24-h sampling procedure, were obtained from our previous publications[20–22] and unpublished data. The latter data base was obtained from a population of healthy adolescent and adult subjects receiving self-selected diets or formula diets prepared to reflect the calorie distributions observed in a free-living American population. Our data in nondiabetics were used for comparison statistics for the cumulative frequency distributions and sequential variation. Previous publications[20–22] have documented a significant influence of sex and age on the growth hormone integrated concentration; therefore, data from sex- and age-matched control populations were used for comparisons with the diabetic groups. In contrast, the glucose integrated concentration and the sequential variation in glucose concentration do not depend on age and sex; therefore, the results in diabetics were compared

TABLE 1
Demographic characteristics of study subjects, integrated concentrations of growth hormone (IC HGH) and glucose (ICG), and sequential variation of growth hormone (SV HGH) and glucose (SVG) observed during 24-h studies in the five subgroups of diabetics

	Subject number	Age (yr)	Duration (yr)	IC HGH (ng/ml)	ICG (mg/dl)	SV HGH (ng/ml)	SVG (mg/dl)
Juvenile-Onset Diabetics-Young Males (JOD-YM)							
	1	11.5	1.2	8.0	281	9.1	63.2
	2	13.2	4.2	8.5	255	9.7	50.9
	3	14.3	1.4	12.6	426	14.3	59.8
	4	15.0	0.3	20.3	268	21.3	37.2
	5A	15.0	4.0	5.7	276	5.2	31.3
	6	15.7	6.7	11.8	291	9.2	53.4
	7	16.0	12.0	13.7	278	6.8	60.8
	8	16.0	1.0	11.5	593	4.5	90.4
	9	16.0	6.0	8.0	407	5.4	51.5
	5B	16.9	5.9	8.6	347	7.8	60.2
Mean		14.9	4.3	10.9	342	9.3	55.9
SD		1.6	3.6	4.2	107	5.1	16.0
Juvenile-Onset Diabetics-Young Females (JOD-YF)							
	10A	12.3	5.3	9.8	354	11.4	45.9
	11	12.8	4.8	4.0	445	2.9	41.3
	10B	13.1	6.1	9.7	354	12.9	43.4
	12	14.7	0.2	9.5	320	10.3	69.4
	13	15.0	8.7	18.2	334	8.1	41.9
	14	15.8	7.0	16.9	176	13.6	34.5
	15	15.9	8.8	6.5	373	4.5	28.7
	16	15.9	8.9	12.7	256	10.3	34.9
	17	16.2	3.9	14.3	215	9.7	38.1
	18	16.7	2.2	13.3	447	10.3	57.8
	19	17.7	14.7	4.9	291	6.1	30.5
	20A	17.4	5.4	10.0	297	10.5	57.0
	20B	18.1	6.1	10.5	411	11.3	41.1
	21	18.7	7.7	5.3	408	3.3	40.7
Mean		15.5	6.4	10.4	334	8.9	43.2
SD		1.9	3.5	4.4	82	3.4	11.3
Juvenile-Onset Diabetics Younger than 20 yr (JOD-YM + JOD-YF)							
Mean		15.3	5.5	10.6	337	9.1	48.5
SD		1.8	3.6	4.2	91	4.1	14.6
N		24	24	24	24	24	24
Juvenile-Onset Diabetics-Adult Males (JOD-AM)							
	22	24.8	12.8	5.9	320	6.3	52.8
	23A	25.3	22.3	7.5	125	7.4	36.6
	23B	25.6	22.6	6.6	167	6.1	39.4
	24	26.0	7.5	7.5	182	3.1	31.4
	25A	26.6	0.3	2.7	205	2.1	34.9
	26	26.7	12.7	6.4	323	7.0	50.8
	27	26.7	4.7	2.7	137	2.9	27.7
	28A	40.8	19.8	7.1	111	9.4	30.4
	28B	40.9	19.9	2.2	147	2.3	27.7
Mean		29.3	13.6	5.3	191	5.2	36.9
SD		6.6	8.1	2.2	79	2.6	9.3
Juvenile-Onset Diabetics-Adult Females (JOD-AF)							
	29	21.0	2.0	7.9	281.6	8.2	32.1
	30	21.2	19.2	3.4	221.8	3.1	50.7
	31A	22.4	7.4	2.9	369.3	2.2	50.5
	32	23.0	10.0	3.7	254.0	4.0	34.0
	31B	23.1	8.1	4.7	294.4	5.9	51.0
	31C	23.8	8.8	3.1	259.0	3.3	90.1
	33	24.0	16.0	7.0	115.9	7.1	22.9
	34	26.0	18.0	20.2	138.3	22.4	50.7
	35	27.9	16.9	6.6	200.8	4.8	48.3
	36	28.2	18.2	6.2	291.4	6.8	34.7
	37	28.5	20.5	32.3	312.6	24.8	54.4
	38	31.0	17.0	5.0	178.9	4.5	23.5
	39	41.0	17.0	9.1	235.3	3.2	48.3
Mean		26.2	13.8	8.6	242.6	7.7	45.4
SD		5.4	5.8	8.4	71.4	7.3	17.3

TABLE 1 (Continued)

	Subject number	Age (yr)	Duration (yr)	IC HGH (ng/ml)	ICG (mg/dl)	SV HGH (ng/ml)	SVG (mg/dl)
Juvenile-Onset Diabetics Older than 20 yr (JOD-AM + JOD-AF)							
Mean		27.5	13.7	36.8	7.3	6.7	41.9
SD		6.0	6.7	9.4	6.7	5.9	14.9
N		22	22	22	22	22	22
Juvenile-Onset Diabetics (All Subjects)							
Mean		21	9.4	9.0	282	8.0	45.3
SD		7.5	6.7	5.7	102	5.7	15.0
N		46	46	46	46	46	46
Newly Diagnosed Juvenile-Onset Diabetics (NJOD)							
	40	8.3	0	1.9	301	2.1	51.0
	41	14.5	0	1.9	485	2.2	52.7
	42	22.5	0	6.8	230	6.2	24.0
	25B	26.0	0	3.0	270	3.4	37.7
Mean		17.8	0	3.4	322	3.5	41.4
SD		8.0		2.3	113	1.9	13.4

with population statistics obtained from the entire nondiabetic control group.

RESULTS

The mean glucose integrated concentration (IC) observed among the JOD groups (Table 1) was twofold to threefold higher than it was in the nondiabetic population (N = 124, mean glucose IC = 103, SEM = 0.84 mg/dl). In contrast with nondiabetic subjects, in whom age had no influence on glucose IC, young JOD subjects had significantly higher glucose IC ($P < 0.001$) than did the older JOD subjects.

In addition to the hyperglycemia, the glucose concentration from the sequential half-hourly samples fluctuated widely. The mean sequential variation (SV) of glucose among the diabetic groups encompassed the range from 36.8 to 55.9 mg/dl. The lability of glucose concentration among diabetics contrasts with the less fluctuating pattern of sequential glucose concentrations observed in the nondiabetic population (N = 72, glucose SV = 15, SEM = 0.34 mg/dl). Analogous to the results of glucose IC, there was significantly less fluctuation ($P < 0.05$) in the sequential glucose concentrations among the older JOD groups than in the younger JOD group. Sex of the subject, however, was not a significant factor on the glucose SV. The explanation for the lower glucose IC and the little variation of sequential glucose concentrations among older diabetic subjects cannot be resolved by our data, although exercise patterns, residual beta-cell activity, and dietary patterns may all contribute to these phenomena.

Growth hormone concentrations fluctuated widely between the half-hourly samples collected during the 24 h of study, showing multiple spikes in plasma concentration throughout the day and night. Diurnal patterns of growth hormone concentrations for individuals are not presented; however, they were qualitatively similar to patterns in diabetic subjects reported in previous publications.[9–12,23] A small percentage of growth hormone peaks occurred with coincident episodes of hypoglycemia (plasma glucose < 75 mg/dl); however, the majority were not correlated with obvious clinical events. Peaks in growth hormone concentration occurred during the initial 1 to 2 h of sleep in many diabetic subjects, but they were not as consistent an observation as in nondiabetics. Diurnal patterns of growth hormone concentrations in diabetic subjects differed from those observed in nondiabetic subjects by an increase in both the amplitude and the frequency of growth hormone peaks. None of the diabetic subjects had a 24-h pattern with persistently elevated, nonfluctuating concentrations of growth hormone. The sequential variation of growth hormone in JOD subjects (N = 46, growth hormone SV = 8.0, SEM = 0.8 ng/ml) was significantly higher ($P < 0.001$) than that in nondiabetic subjects (N = 85, growth hormone SV = 4.61, SEM = 0.27 ng/ml). There were no significant differences among JOD subjects when compared by sex or age.

The mean growth hormone integrated concentration for the four subgroups of JOD was significantly greater ($P < 0.001$) than that of the age-matched nondiabetic population (Figure 1). Two subjects in the JOD-AF had a growth hormone IC markedly elevated compared with other diabetics in this group. However, even if these two subjects are eliminated, the mean growth hormone IC for the JOD-AF group remains significantly higher ($P < 0.001$) than that of the age- and sex-matched nondiabetic population. Within each group there were several subjects with a growth hormone IC within the range for age- and sex-matched nondiabetic subjects; however, no clinical characteristics were noted that distinguished diabetic subjects with a normal growth hormone IC from the remainder of the diabetic subjects with growth hormone IC greater than that of a nondiabetic population. The juvenile diabetics younger than age 20 (JOD-YM and JOD-YF) had growth hormone IC significantly greater ($P < 0.005$) than the juvenile-onset diabetics older than age 20 (JOD-AM and JOD-AF). There was no significant difference between the growth hormone IC in males and females in each age category.

The diurnal patterns of growth hormone in newly diagnosed juvenile-onset diabetics (NJOD) contrast with the JOD subjects with established therapies. There was no sta-

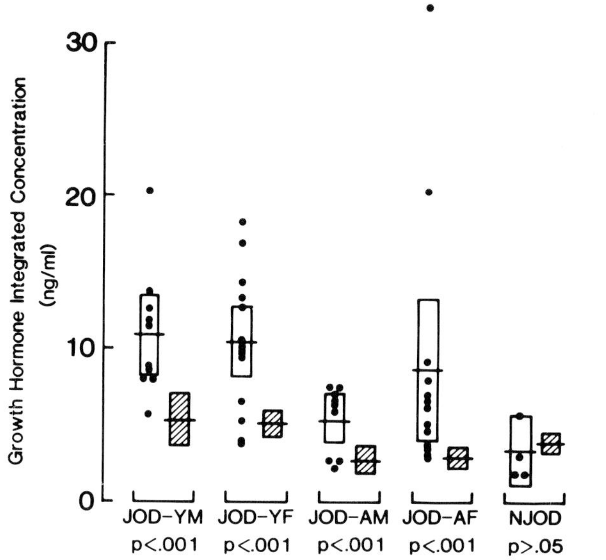

FIGURE 1. The individual and mean (±2 SEM) growth hormone integrated concentrations of the five groups of juvenile-onset diabetics are compared with the mean (±2 SEM) growth hormone integrated concentration for age- and sex-matched nondiabetic populations (shaded bars) abstracted from previous publications.[20-22] Subjects are grouped by age (less than 20 yr = JOD-Y, and over 20 yr = JOD-A) and sex (male = JOD-M, and female = JOD-F) or as newly diagnosed diabetics (NJOD).

tistically significant difference between the growth hormone IC of the NJOD subjects and the nondiabetic control population (Figure 1). Furthermore, although the degree of glucose intolerance as assessed by glucose IC and glucose SV was similar between the NJOD and JOD groups, the former group did not have an equivalent elevation in growth hormone IC.

Growth hormone concentrations greater than 5 ng/ml were observed in a greater percentage of half-hourly samples in the JOD group than in a nondiabetic population (Figure 2). Whereas growth hormone concentrations of more than 5 ng/ml occurred in only 28% of samples in a nondiabetic population, concentrations exceeding this limit were observed in 48% of the half-hourly samples in JOD subjects. In contrast, the cumulative frequency distributions of half-hourly growth hormone concentrations in NJOD more closely approximated the distribution in the nondiabetic population. It is of note that both groups of diabetics had a significant, although variable, percentage of samples with growth hormone concentration less than 2.5 ng/ml, indicating that growth hormone concentration in diabetics intermittently suppresses to the basal concentrations observed in nondiabetics.

Half-hourly samples in which growth hormone concentrations exceeded 5 ng/ml were observed twice as frequently in diabetics less than 20 yr of age as in the nondiabetic group (Figure 3). Among the two age subgroups of JOD, the cumulative frequency distributions of half-hourly growth hormone concentrations of the younger JOD showed the greatest discrepancy from that of the normal population. The cumulative frequency distribution of the adult female JOD group was skewed toward a greater frequency of growth hormone concentrations higher than 5 ng/ml compared with the adult male JOD group. In contrast, there was no significant difference in the cumulative frequency distributions between females and males in the younger JOD groups.

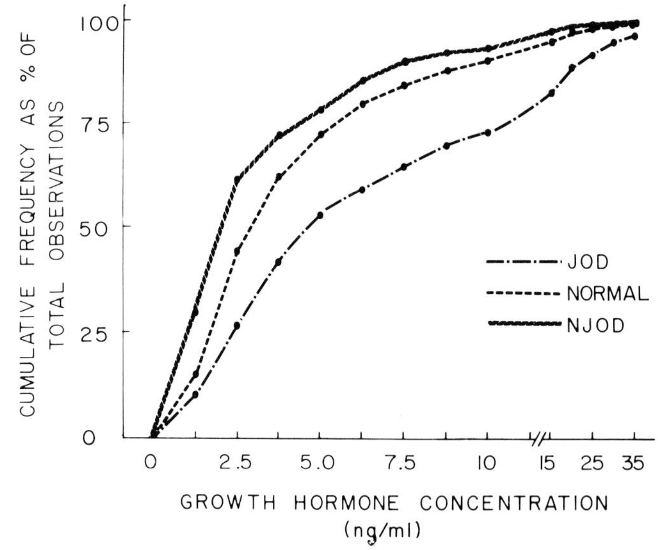

FIGURE 2. Cumulative frequency distributions of half-hour growth hormone concentrations for juvenile-onset diabetics with established therapy (JOD, N = 2025), newly diagnosed juvenile-onset diabetics (NJOD, N = 163), and a nondiabetic population (normal, N = 5094) (N represents the number of samples in each data group).

The integrated concentration of growth hormone was not significantly correlated with those of glucose, free insulin, or total insulin. However, there was a significant correlation ($P < 0.015$) between growth hormone IC and the lability of the diurnal glucose concentration, as expressed by glucose sequential variation.

This latter observation directed our analysis to evaluating whether the occurrence of a peak in growth hormone concentration was correlated with the glucose concentration either coincident with a peak or during the half hour preceding a peak in growth hormone concentration. Growth

FIGURE 3. Cumulative frequency distributions of half-hour growth hormone concentrations for age subgroups of juvenile-onset diabetics with established therapy. Juvenile-onset diabetics less than 20 yr old (JOD-Y, N = 1050) and those older than 20 years (JOD-A, N = 975) are contrasted with a nondiabetic population (normal, N = 5094) (N represents the number of samples in each group).

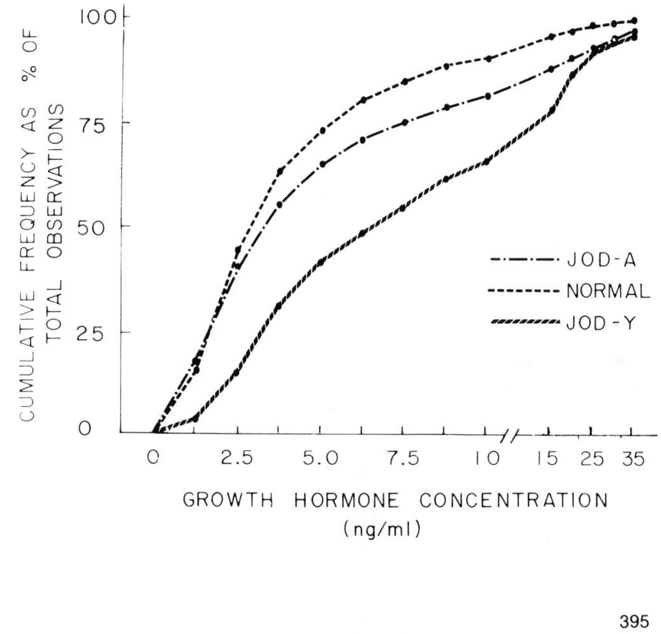

hormone peaks were identified within the entire set of data from the 46 JOD studies by an increase in growth hormone concentration greater than 2.5 ng/ml above the concentration of the sample obtained in the previous half hour and a concentration of more than 6 ng/ml. Restricting the analysis to this subset of samples associated with growth hormone peaks, no significant correlation was observed between the growth hormone concentration during a secretory peak and either the simultaneous glucose concentration, the glucose concentration from the preceding half-hourly sample, or the rate of change of glucose concentration.

The above analysis suggested no relationship between the magnitude of the growth hormone concentration and the magnitude of the glucose concentration or the rate of change in glucose concentration. However, parametric analysis is insensitive as a method to assess if a rise in growth hormone concentration of variable magnitude occurs when the glucose concentration reaches a critical threshold for stimulation of growth hormone secretion. To analyze this question, the growth hormone response at each half-hourly sample point for all JOD subjects was classified as either a secretory peak (growth hormone concentration greater than 6 ng/ml and rate of change from preceding sample greater than 2.5 ng/ml) or no secretory peak. The glucose response, either concentration or rate of change in concentration, for each sample was coded in 50-mg/dl intervals. The frequency of observed growth hormone peaks at each glucose interval was compared with the frequency of growth hormone peaks expected if such peaks were randomly distributed over the glucose concentration intervals, the ratio of the observed to expected occurrences being defined as the relative frequency of a peak growth hormone response. Random occurrence of growth hormone peaks, independent of the associated glucose concentration or rate of change of glucose concentration, would require that the relative frequency of a peak growth hormone response approximate unity.

Figure 4 shows that there is a progressive increase in the relative frequency of a peak growth hormone response as the rate of change in glucose concentration from the prior sample becomes more negative. This trend, of a growth hormone peak occurring in association with a falling glucose concentration, was statistically significant when analyzed within a contingency table ($x^2 = 46.35$, df = 7, $P < 0.005$). When the change in glucose concentration from the prior sample was positive, the relative frequency of a peak growth hormone response was less than 1.0 and was quite constant over the interval of a 0- to 150-mg/dl change. Nevertheless, the ratio did not approach zero, as would be expected in a nondiabetic population.

FIGURE 4. Relative frequency (observed/expected) of peaks in growth hormone (defined by an increase in growth hormone concentration greater than 2.5 ng/ml from the previous sample and a concentration greater than 6 ng/ml) correlated to the rate of change in glucose concentration. The interrupted line shows the frequency distribution of samples within each increment of glucose concentration change.

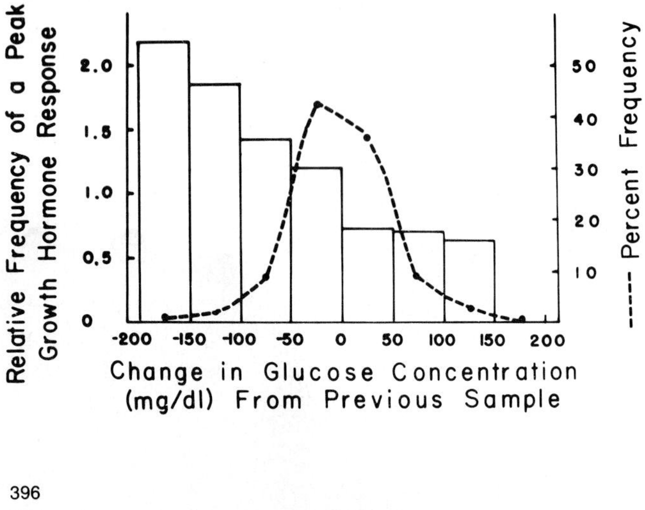

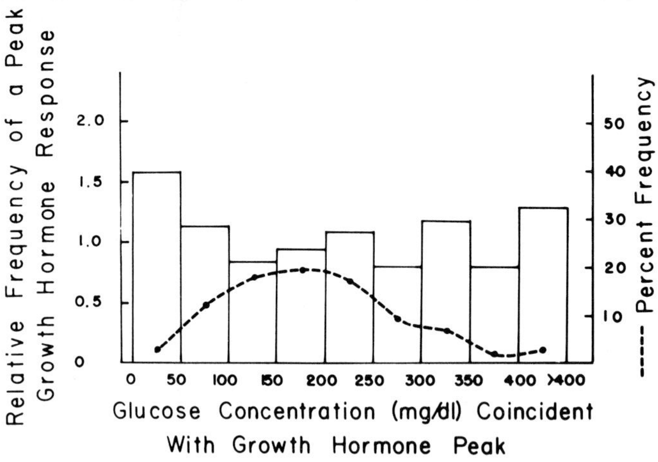

FIGURE 5. Relative frequency (observed/expected) of peaks in growth hormone (defined by an increase in growth hormone concentration greater than 2.5 ng/ml from the previous sample and a concentration greater than 6 ng/ml correlated to the glucose concentration coincident with the peak response. The interrupted line shows the frequency distribution of samples within each increment of glucose concentration.

A similar analysis, relating the relative frequency of a peak growth hormone response to the concurrent glucose concentration (Figure 5), shows a relatively uniform level over the range of glucose concentrations. Glucose concentrations less than 75 mg/dl were associated with a significant increase in the frequency of a simultaneous growth hormone peak when analyzed within a contingency table ($x^2 = 14.37$, df = 1, $P < 0.005$). No significant increase in the relative frequency of a peak growth hormone response was detected when the blood glucose concentration was analyzed during the half hour before the increase in growth hormone.

DISCUSSION

In this report, we extend and confirm data from previous reports[9–12,23–29] that plasma growth hormone concentrations are significantly higher in JOD subjects than in nondiabetic subjects. In addition, sequential growth hormone concentrations in JOD subjects observed over 24 h are more labile than those in nondiabetics. The elevated sequential variation of growth hormone concentration and the rightward shift in the cumulative frequency distributions indicate that JOD subjects have an increase in both the frequency of growth hormone peaks and the amplitude of growth hormone spikes compared with nondiabetic subjects.

Our observation of significantly elevated growth hormone IC among juvenile-onset diabetics compared with nondiabetics contrasts with the normal mean 24-h growth hormone concentration in diabetics reported by Merimee et al.[13] This discrepancy probably reflects differences in the composition of the two study populations, with respect to both age at the time of study and type of diabetes. Compared with the previous publication,[13] our group is significantly younger, 35 of the 39 JOD subjects being less than 30 yr old. In addition, all our subjects were ketosis-prone and insulin-dependent. Our observation that the growth hormone integrated concentration, in both nondiabetics[20-22] and diabetics, declines with age and the glucose lability is more pronounced among the younger diabetics provides a probable explanation of the differences between our data and that of Merimee et al.

The growth hormone IC in the newly diagnosed juvenile-onset diabetics is well within the normal limits for an age-matched nondiabetic population. Our observations in newly diagnosed diabetics are consistent with those of Winter et al.[23] who used an identical continuous blood-sampling technique. Whereas several investigators have reported that fasting,[3,25,26] exercise-stimulated,[26] and mean 24-h[30] growth hormone concentrations are significantly elevated in newly diagnosed diabetics compared with nondiabetics, this observation has not been universal.[23-31] The discrepancy between these previously published data and our observations reflects in large part methodologic differences in both the blood-sampling procedures and the metabolic status of the subjects during study. Although intermittent ketonuria was observed in several NJOD subjects, none had acetonemia or acidosis. These observations of normal growth hormone IC in our small population of newly diagnosed diabetics are not compatible with the hypothesis that disordered growth hormone secretion has a significant role in the etiology of juvenile-onset diabetes.

The elevation in growth hormone IC probably reflects an increase in growth hormone secretion rather than a change in growth hormone clearance rate or distribution space. Although data related to the distribution space are not available. Navalesi et al.[32] have previously reported no significant difference in the metabolic clearance rate of growth hormone in diabetics and in normals. In addition, the rate of growth hormone's decline in the sequential half-hourly samples among the diabetics was similar to our observations in our nondiabetic population.

The factors inducing the exaggerated and more frequent fluctuations of growth hormone concentrations observed in diabetics over 24 h or in response to provocative stimuli remain incompletely characterized. Both a primary disorder in hypothalamic-pituitary regulation of growth hormone and a secondary disorder in growth hormone metabolism associated with the abnormal carbohydrate metabolism of diabetes can be hypothesized in the pathogenesis. The former hypothesis is supported by the observations of exaggerated growth hormone secretion among diabetics to standardized provocative stimuli[3,25,26] and the lack of suppression of growth hormone concentrations despite the elevated glucose concentrations.[13] However, the suppression of growth hormone in diabetics by exogenous somatostatin[33,34] demonstrates that, at least to some suppressive stimuli, the hypothalamic-pituitary response is intact. In addition, our observations, and those of previous reports,[9-12] that growth hormone returns intermittently to basal concentrations (comparable to those in the normal) between peaks in the hormone's concentration, mitigate against the hypothesis that the diabetic has an abnormal hypothalamic-pituitary set point of growth hormone secretion.

The hypothesis that abnormalities in growth hormone metabolism among diabetics are a consequence of the abnormal carbohydrate metabolism has support from several lines of investigation. Carrall et al.,[30] Johansen et al.,[10] and Vigneri et al.[29] found that, among newly diagnosed diabetics, insulin regimens which lowered the mean glucose concentration toward or within the normal range improved the diurnal growth hormone concentration. In contrast, Hanssen et al.,[28] utilizing much more limited metabolic assessment, did not observe any significant correlation between mean blood glucose and mean growth hormone concentration in his study of 20 newly diagnosed diabetics before and after insulin replacement. Although the above reports suggest a link between elevated glucose concentrations and growth hormone concentrations, we found no statistically significant correlation between the degree of hyperglycemia (as expressed by the glucose integrated concentration) and the growth hormone integrated concentration. The independence of these variables was present in all the subgroups of subjects studied. Furthermore, among the subjects studied on multiple occasions, there is no observed correlation between glucose IC and growth hormone IC. The lack of correlation between the mean glucose and the mean growth hormone concentrations in previously treated diabetics has been alluded to previously,[28] although the data are based on a smaller study population.

In contrast with the lack of correlation between the integrated concentrations of glucose and growth hormone, there was a statistically significant ($P < 0.015$) correlation between variability in plasma glucose (as expressed by glucose SV) and growth hormone IC in the JOD group. The studies of diabetics by Molnar et al.,[12] using continuous blood glucose determinations and hourly growth hormone determinations, had suggested that lability of glucose might be a factor in etiology of the observed elevation of mean growth hormone concentration. These authors noted that diabetics with less glucose variability—defined by mean amplitude of glycemic excursions (MAGE)—had mean growth hormone concentrations not significantly different from those of controls.

The observation that variability of glucose is correlated with growth hormone IC complements our observation that a disproportionate number of peaks in growth hormone occurred in association with declining glucose concentrations (Figure 4). As the rate of fall of glucose concentration increased, there was a progressive increase in the relative frequency of a peak growth hormone response. Our observations that hypoglycemia (defined as plasma glucose less than 75 mg/dl) was associated with an increased occurrence of a peak in growth hormone concentration are consistent with those of Molnar et al.[35] They reported that hypoglycemia is a contributing factor, but not a sufficient explanation, for the observed elevation in growth hormone in diabetics. Our data suggest that rate of glucose decline is an equally important factor in the increased frequency and magnitude of growth hormone secretion among diabetics. The remaining factors, important to the augmented and fluctuating pattern in diabetics, are still uncharacterized.

The metabolic consequences of the elevated mean 24-h growth hormone concentration in diabetics compared with that observed in the nondiabetic population remain unknown. The recent report of Soman et al.,[36] demonstrating reduction in insulin binding to monocyte insulin receptors in response to growth hormone replacement in hypopituitary subjects, suggests that increased growth hormone concentration may induce relative insulin resistance by altering insulin receptor binding characteristics. Although monocyte binding was not assessed in our study population, there was a significant positive correlation between insulin dose (units per kilogram) and growth hormone IC ($r = 0.305$, $N = 46$, $P < 0.05$) among JOD subjects. The hypothesis that the elevated growth hormone concentration contributes to the microvascular disease of diabetes could not be evaluated from our data. However, the two diabetics (subjects 33 and 36) with significant retinopathy had growth hormone IC similar to other unaffected diabetic subjects without retinopathy on funduscopic exam. Obviously, the influence of chronicity of growth hormone evaluation and duration of diabetes cannot be assessed in our limited population with microvascular disease. Further research is needed to evaluate these questions as they relate the role of growth hormone to the sequelae of diabetes; however, these data suggest that the therapy designed to reduce the lability of glucose fluctuation and episodes of hypoglycemia in diabetes should also reduce the mean 24-h growth hormone concentration.

ACKNOWLEDGMENTS

We are indebted to Samuel J. Fomon, M.D., University of Iowa, for his review and comments, to Timothy Osweiler for his technical assistance, to Aline Autenrieth for her secretarial assistance, and to the cadre of nurses on the Clinical Research Center.

The work was supported in part by grants (AM-18439 and RR59) from the National Institutes of Health and a grant from the Iowa Affiliate, American Diabetes Association. Drs. Hayford and Hendrix were supported by National Research Service Award T32-AM07018.

REFERENCES

[1] Houssay, B. A., and Biosotti, A.: La diabetes pancreatica de los perros hipofisoprivos. Rev. Soc. Argent. Biol. *6*:251–96, 1930.

[2] Luft, R., and Cerasi, E.: Human growth hormone as a regulator of blood glucose concentration and as a diabetogenic substance. Diabetologia *4*:1–9, 1968.

[3] Baird, J. D., Hunter, W. M., and Smith, A. W. M.: The relationship between human growth hormone and the development of diabetes mellitus and its complications. Postgrad. Med. J. *49*:132–40, 1973.

[4] Ikkos, D., and Luft, R.: Aspects of the metabolic action of human growth hormone. *In* Human Pituitary Hormone. Ciba Foundation Colloquia on Endocrinology. Vol. 13. Wolstenholme, G. E. W., and O'Conner, C. M., Eds. London, 1960, pp. 106–34.

[5] Lundbaek, K., Jensen, V. A., Olsen, T. S. et al.: Diabetes, diabetic angiopathy, and growth hormone. Lancet *2*:131–33, 1970.

[6] Merimee, T. J.: A follow-up study of vascular disease in growth hormone deficient dwarfs with diabetes. N. Engl. J. Med. *298*:1217–22, 1978.

[7] Passa, P., Rousselie, F., Gauville, C. et al.: Retinopathy and plasma growth hormone levels in idiopathic hemochromatosis with diabetes. Diabetes *26*:113–20, 1977.

[8] Osterby, R., Seyer-Hansen, K., Gundersen, H. J. G. et al.: Growth hormone enhances basement membrane thickening in experimental diabetes. Diabetologia *15*:487–89, 1978.

[9] Hansen, A. P., and Johansen, K.: Diurnal patterns of blood glucose, serum free fatty acids, insulin, glucagon and growth hormone in normals and juvenile diabetics. Diabetologia *6*:27–33, 1970.

[10] Johansen, K., and Hansen, A. P.: Diurnal serum growth hormone levels in poorly and well controlled juvenile diabetics. Diabetes *20*:239–45, 1971.

[11] Hansen, A. P.: Serum growth hormone patterns in juvenile diabetes. Dan. Med. Bull. *19*:8–32, 1972.

[12] Molnar, G. D., Taylor, W. F., Langworthy, A. et al.: Diurnal growth hormone and glucose abnormalities in unstable diabetics: studies of ambulatory-fed subjects during continuous blood glucose analysis. J. Clin. Endocrinol. *34*:837–46, 1972.

[13] Merimee, T. J., Fitzgerald, C. R., Gold, L. A. et al.: Characteristics of growth hormone secretion in clinically stable diabetes. Diabetes *28*:308–12, 1979.

[14] Metropolitan Life Insurance Company, No. 380, L.W. (10-70), New York, 1969.

[15] Thompson, R. G., Hayford, J. T., and Danney, M. M.: Glucose and insulin responses to diet: effect of variations in source and amount of carbohydrate. Diabetes *27*:1020–26, 1978.

[16] Schalch, D. S., and Parker, M. C.: A sensitive double antibody immunoassay for human growth hormone in plasma. Nature (London) *203*: 1141–42, 1964.

[17] Gennaro, W. D., and VanNorman, J. D.: Quantification of free, total and antibody bound insulin in insulin-treated diabetics. Clin. Chem. *21*:873–79, 1975.

[18] Morgan, C. R., and Lazarow, A.: Immunoassay of insulin: two antibody system. Diabetes *12*:115–26, 1963.

[19] Barr, A. J., Goodnight, J. H., Sall, J. P. et al.: A User's Guide to SAS76. Raleigh, North Carolina, Sparks Press, 1976.

[20] Thompson, R. G., Rodriguez, A., Kowarski, A. et al.: Growth hormone: metabolic clearance rates, integrated concentrations and production rates in normal adults and the effect of prednisone. J. Clin. Invest. *51*:3193–99, 1972.

[21] Thompson, R. G., Rodriguez, A., Kowarski, A. et al.: Integrated concentrations of growth hormone correlated with plasma testosterone and bone age in preadolescent and adolescent males. J. Clin. Endocrinol. Metab. *35*:334–37, 1972.

[22] Plotnick, L. P., Thompson, R. G., Beitins, I. et al.: Integrated concentrations of growth hormone correlated with stage of puberty and estrogen levels in girls. J. Clin. Endocrinol. Metab. *38*:436–39, 1974.

[23] Winter, R. J., Plotnick, L. P., and Thompson, R. G.: Chemical diabetes in childhood. Integrated concentrations of glucose, insulin and growth hormone. Diabetes *27*:909–15, 1978.

[24] Drash, A., Field, J. B., Garces, L. Y. et al.: Endogenous insulin and growth hormone response in children with newly diagnosed diabetes mellitus. Pediatr. Res. *2*:94–102, 1968.

[25] Sabeh, G., Mendelsohn, L. V., Corredor, D. G. et al.: Growth hormone in insulin treated diabetes mellitus. Metabolism *18*:748–53, 1969.

[26] Hansen, A. P.: Abnormal serum growth hormone response to exercise in juvenile diabetics. J. Clin. Invest. *49*:1467–78, 1970.

[27] Sperling, M. A., Wollesen, F., and Delamater, P. V.: Daily production and metabolic clearance of growth hormone in juvenile diabetes mellitus. Diabetologia *9*:380–83, 1973.

[28] Hanssen, K. F.: Immunoreactive growth hormone in plasma and urine in juvenile diabetics before and during initial insulin treatment. Acta Endocrinol. (Copenhagen) *75*:50–63, 1974.

[29] Vigneri, R., Squatrito, S., Pezzino, V. et al.: Growth hormone levels in diabetes: correlation with clinical control of the disease. Diabetes *25*:167–72, 1976.

[30] Carrall, R. J., Hunter, W. M., Campbell, I. W. et al.: Reversal by insulin treatment of abnormal growth hormone patterns in newly diagnosed diabetes mellitus. Acta Endocrinol. (Copenhagen) *77*:115–21, 1974.

[31] Theodoridis, C. G., Chance, G. W., Brown, B. T. et al.: Growth hormone response to oral glucose load in untreated diabetic children. Arch. Dis. Child. *46*:117–19, 1971.

[32] Navalesi, R., Pilo, A., and Vigneri, R.: Growth hormone kinetics in diabetic patients. Diabetes *24*:317–27, 1975.

[33] Christensen, S. E., Hansen, A. P., Weeke, J., and Lundbaek, K.: 24-Hour studies of the effects of somatostatin on the levels of plasma growth hormone, glucagon, and glucose in normal subjects and juvenile diabetics. Diabetes *27*:300–06, 1978.

[34] Ward, F. R., Leblanc, H., and Yen, S. S. C.: The inhibitory effect of somatostatin on growth hormone, insulin and glucagon secretion in diabetes mellitus. J. Clin. Endocrinol. Metab. *41*:527–32, 1975.

[35] Molnar, G. D., Fatourechi, V., Ackerman, E. et al.: Growth hormone and glucose interrelationships in diabetes: studies of inadvertent hypoglycemic episodes during continuous blood glucose analysis. J. Clin. Endocrinol. *32*:426–37, 1971.

[36] Soman, V. J., Tamborlane, W., DeFronzo, R. et al.: Insulin binding and insulin sensitivity in isolated growth hormone deficiency. N. Engl. J. Med. *299*:1025–30, 1978.

Review

Insulin Action and the Regulation of Hexose Transport

MICHAEL P. CZECH

Current work in the area of insulin action relates directly to some of the most pressing unsolved questions in membrane biochemistry, including those related to receptor dynamics, transmembrane signaling, and the molecular mechanisms by which biologic transport systems operate. Thus, the well-recognized rapid action of insulin to modulate fluxes of both charged and neutral substances across cell surface membranes is of great interest. In the last few years experimental approaches have been developed which are now yielding structural information about cell surface membrane components involved in eliciting transport activation by insulin. These advances include affinity labeling of the insulin receptor[1-5] as well as solubilization and reconstitution of the hexose transport system from an insulin-sensitive cell type.[6,7] Of the known insulin-sensitive transport systems, which include transporters for cations[8-10] as well as amino acids[12,13] and anions,[11] the D-glucose transport systems have probably been the most actively studied. The classic target tissues in which hexose uptake is markedly enhanced by the hormone are muscle and fat (see ref. 14 for review). Hexose transport in these tissues is stereospecific and operates by facilitated diffusion such that the concentration gradient of D-glucose across the cell surface membrane provides the driving force for net influx. Thus, the insulin response in these systems may be viewed as a simple gating effect for an uncharged solute. This paper will focus attention on advances in our understanding of the molecular aspects of insulin action on hexose transport made over the past few years.

ASSAY METHODOLOGY FOR ADIPOCYTE HEXOSE TRANSPORT

An isolated cell type which is extraordinarily sensitive to insulin and has probably been most employed to study insulin action on D-glucose transport is the rat adipocyte. These cells are easily prepared from pieces of adipose tissue by digestion with a crude bacterial collagenase-protease mixture.[15] However, a persistent problem with this model system has been the difficulty in monitoring initial rates of D-glucose transport due to the small cytoplasmic volume relative to the cell surface area.[16] This morphologic attribute of the adipocyte usually leads to rapid equilibration of a nonmetabolizable analogue of glucose, requiring methods to analyze uptake in seconds. In spite of this, the early studies of Crofford et al.[17,18] indicated that hexose transport in adipose tissue occurred by facilitated diffusion and was activated by insulin. This conclusion agreed with the earlier work of Levine and his colleagues, which documented the effect of insulin on glucose utilization in intact animals to be related to activation of hexose transport rather than intracellular glucose metabolism.[19,20] However, until relatively recently, kinetic parameters of the D-glucose transport system of adipocytes have not been measured with confidence.

In order to circumvent the major problem impeding kinetic analysis of hexose transport in white fat cells, we initially employed brown fat cells which readily respond to insulin and have a large cytoplasmic space to total cellular volume ratio.[21] A rapid filtration method was devised to separate medium from cells.[22,23] These studies documented time-dependent, stereospecific uptake of 3-O-methylglucose by brown fat cells and a stimulatory effect of insulin which reflected enhancement of the apparent V_{max} with no detectable effect on apparent K_m.[22] More recently, this filtration method was utilized to monitor 3-O-methylglucose transport in white fat cells.[24] In these initial studies it was surprising that equilibration of the hexose across the adipocyte membrane in the presence of insulin occurred as late as 5 min or more.[24] Apparent linearity of uptake was observed through 30 s and initial rate measurements were monitored at various 3-O-methylglucose concentrations. The major conclusion from these kinetic measurements was that activation of adipocyte hexose transport by insulin represents an effect of the hormone on the V_{max} parameter rather than the K_m of transport.

An alternate method for the measurement of 3-O-methyl-

From the Section of Physiological Chemistry, Division of Biology and Medicine, Brown University, Providence, Rhode Island 02912.
Dr. Czech is the recipient of Career Development Award (AM-00249) from the United States Public Health Service.
Received for publication 26 December 1979.

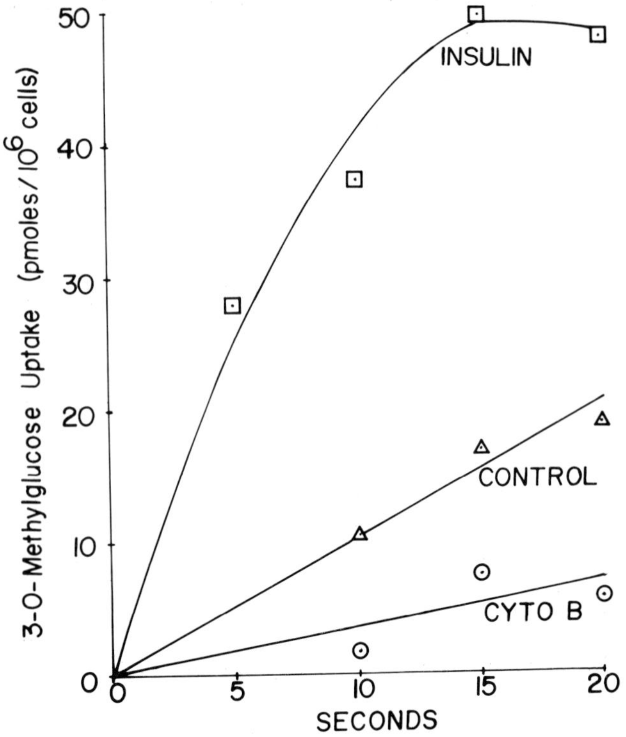

FIGURE 1. Time course of 3-O-(^{3}H)methylglucose uptake by intact adipocytes in the presence and absence of insulin or cytochalasin B. Fat cells (2×10^5 cells per tube) were incubated in 0.2 ml of Krebs-Ringer phosphate buffer for 15 min with 2.4 mU/ml insulin or 10 μM cytochalasin B or no addition before 0.05 mM 3-O-(^{3}H)methylglucose was added. Incubation was continued at room temperature and, at the times indicated, 3 ml of ice cold buffer was added to the cells. The reaction mixture was then rapidly decanted onto Whatman glass fiber filters under vacuum and washed with 9 ml ice cold buffer as previously described.[24] The filters were then dried and the radioactivity present determined by standard methods.[22]

glucose transport in adipocytes was developed by Vinten et al.[25] and involves modification of an oil flotation technique[26] for separation of fat cells from incubation medium. Data using this method[27,28] have indicated equilibration of 3-O-(^{3}H) methylglucose across the adipocyte plasma membrane by about 10 s under conditions where transport is activated by insulin. Thus, Vinten[27] and Whitesell and Gliemann[28] have claimed that the rapid filtration method of Czech underestimates the adipocyte 3-O-methylglucose transport rate by as much as 100-fold. In response to this discrepancy, we recently employed the filtration method exactly as it had been previously[24] to monitor the time course of 3-O-(^{3}H) methylglucose uptake in adipocytes prepared with collagenase lots currently obtained from Worthington. Figure 1 depicts typical experimental results with such cells, which indicate very rapid equilibration of the labeled hexose across the adipocyte membrane in the presence of insulin. These data do not differ greatly from those reported by Vinten et al.[25] and Whitesell and Gliemann,[28] indicating the filtration method itself provides reasonable estimates of hexose uptake. Therefore, the apparent discrepancy between the original data on initial rates of hexose uptake using the filtration technique[24] and data of others[26–28] and ours reported here (Figure 1), using the same filtration technique, does not reflect faulty methodology. Rather, the most probable explanation involves the variable collagenase preparations that were utilized. Indeed, the original report by Czech[24] on the D-glucose transport system activity of fat cells showed a five-fold difference in apparent V_{max} of transport between two representative experiments and emphasized this variability between cell preparations. Significant variability in absolute values of adipocyte glucose uptake and utilization among cell preparations is well known, although the apparent difference in hexose transport rates obtained originally by filtration[24] and now (Figure 1) is unusually large.

Probably the most compelling evidence that reasonable estimation of hexose transport rates can be obtained by both the rapid filtration method and the oil flotation technique is the similarity of conclusions reached by the different laboratories using these procedures. All three major conclusions in the original studies of Czech[24] using rapid filtration were subsequently confirmed by Vinten,[27] Vinten et al.,[25] and Whitesell and Gliemann.[28] These conclusions are (1) insulin increases V_{max} without markedly affecting K_m, (2) the K_m of adipocyte 3-O-methylglucose transport is in the low mM range (Czech[24] reported 1–3 mM while Whitesell and Gliemann[28] report 2.5–5 mM), and (3) adipocyte hexose transport is significantly more sensitive to temperature when activated by insulin than in the basal state. Conclusion (1) has also been confirmed in studies using arabinose as the glucose analog.[29] Recent advances in the oil flotation methodology[28] have allowed transport measurements to be made at earlier time points than have been attempted using rapid filtration and thus very precise estimations of transport kinetics have been obtained. However, it is important to recall that the fat cell preparation is an artifact of its own preparative procedure, which involves digestion of adipose tissue with a complex and variable mixture of degradative enzymes. Thus the absolute kinetic values obtained for its various functions are subject to variability and alterations relative to those which hold for native adipocytes in situ.

HEXOSE TRANSPORT REGULATION IN INTACT CELLS

Insulin action on hexose transport in both muscle and fat is rapid in onset and is readily observed in the presence of protein synthesis inhibitors such as cycloheximide. The rat adipocyte has been the most widely used model in studies designed to correlate the kinetics of binding of ^{125}I-insulin with initiation of biologic action on transport. It is well established that, at 37°C, within about 20–30 s after binding of ^{125}I-insulin to the number of adipocyte receptors required to elicit maximal activation of D-glucose transport, the transport activity is observed to be fully enhanced.[28,30] This lag period before maximal transport activation is achieved is temperature-dependent and increases to about 2 min at 22°C.[28] Deactivation of hexose transport activity following removal of insulin from adipocytes with or without the introduction of anti-insulin serum has been reported to be also very rapid at 37°C.[31,32] However, more recent data have suggested that deactivation is a much slower process than the activation mechanism and that the presence of glucose in the medium enhances the deactivation rate.[33] Further clarification of the kinetics of deactivation would be useful.

An intriguing feature of insulin-sensitive hexose transport systems is their responsiveness to a wide variety of membrane perturbations. Treatment of adipocytes with such diverse agents as oxidants,[22,34–39] polyamines,[40,41] hypertonicity,[42] sulfhydryl reagents,[43,44] lectins,[23,45–47] antireceptor antibodies,[48–54] anti-membrane antibodies,[55,56] proteases,[57] phospholipases,[58,59] and neuraminidase,[60,61] mimics the action of insulin to enhance D-glucose transport activity. The broad specificity that characterizes this group of reagents diminishes their usefulness in terms of providing insight into insulin action. The mechanisms involved in the actions of these various agents may or may not share common features with the mechanism of insulin action. A key point to be learned from the studies on the insulinomimetic agents cited above is their limited value as supportive evidence for specific hypotheses on insulin action. In spite of this problem, certain notable aspects of hexose transport activation and deactivation have emerged from studies of these agents.

One interesting class of agents used to mimic insulin action involve those that have multivalent binding sites for the adipocyte plasma membrane. These include such lectins as concanavalin A and wheat germ agglutinin, as well as antibodies against the insulin receptor or other membrane proteins. Czech and Lynn[23] first found that the lectins concanavalin A and lens culnarnaris agglutinin, which bind mannose-containing oligosaccharides, increase adipocyte glucose metabolism and demonstrated that this effect resulted from activation of D-glucose transport system activity using brown fat cells as a model system.[45] This stimulatory effect of concanavalin A on adipocyte glucose uptake was confirmed by Cuatrecasas and Tell[62] who also showed a similar effect of wheat germ agglutinin. Insulin action on fat cell lipolysis was also mimicked by the lectins. Other studies also indicated that the lectins bound cell surface insulin receptors, which suggested that their actions may be mediated via the insulin receptor.[46,63] However, Czech and Lynn[45] found that adipocytes subjected to trypsinization, to block insulin binding and action, remained almost fully responsive to concanavalin A and suggested that a nonreceptor mechanism mediates lectin action. The differential sensitivity to trypsin of adipocyte responsiveness to insulin versus lectins was also observed by Cuatrecasas.[46] Since concanavalin A was found to agglutinate adipocytes[45] and initiate patching of the lectin-bound sites on the surface membrane,[64] it seemed reasonable that such membrane perturbation might be involved in eliciting transport activation.

While the above proposal has not been tested directly, recent data on the actions of various antibodies on D-glucose transport and other cellular processes have provided useful insights into the mode of action of such divalent and multivalent agents. In a comprehensive series of studies performed by Kahn, Flier, and colleagues,[48–54] circulating antibodies in patients with a rare form of insulin resistance and acanthosis nigricans were shown to block ^{125}I-insulin binding to adipocytes and mimic insulin action. Antibodies raised in rabbits against purified insulin receptor were also found to activate hexose uptake in adipocytes.[65] Furthermore, antibodies raised in rabbits injected with adipocyte plasma membranes or intrinsic membrane proteins mimicked insulin action on hexose transport and lipolysis but did not block ^{125}I-insulin binding to adipocyte receptors.[55,56] At least for these antibodies, association with the insulin-binding site on the insulin receptor is not required for initiation of the biologic response.[55] The actions of these anti-membrane antibodies are similar to those of the lectins in that the antibodies readily activate transport in trypsinized cells, which exhibit little or no receptor binding to insulin itself.[56] The question of whether the anti-membrane antibodies bind to regions on the insulin receptor, which do not bind the hormone itself, has recently been addressed using antibody immobilized on Sepharose. When solubilized adipocyte membranes in sodium cholate were passed through columns of immobilized immunoglobulin from control or immunized rabbits, very little or no binding of insulin receptors to such columns was obtained (Pillion and Czech, unpublished data). These data demonstrate that membrane events elicited by multivalent agents, which bind to cell surface sites exclusive of insulin receptors, can result in transport activation.

An important issue associated with the above work relates to the possibility that lateral aggregation of membrane proteins caused by lectins or antibodies is an obligatory feature of their insulinomimetic action. Monovalent Fab fragments of either human anti-insulin receptor antibodies[54] or anti-membrane antibodies[56] were thus prepared and found to be devoid of biologic activity using isolated fat cells. Activation of transport activity could be achieved by monovalent anti-receptor[54] or anti-membrane[56] Fab fragments upon addition of anti-Fab antibody, which restores multivalency of the Fab fragments by cross-linking them. The interpretation of these studies is illustrated in Figure 2 which emphasizes the correlation between lateral membrane aggregation events and insulinomimetic action. In addition, Kahn et al.[66] have reported potentiation of the action of submaximal doses of insulin by addition of anti-insulin antibody, indicating aggregation of membrane receptors or other components may be involved in insulin action itself. However, it should be emphasized that although membrane cross-linking or aggregation phenomena appear to be involved in transport activation by antibody, even when the antigen is insulin bound to its receptor,[66] there is no direct evidence that such membrane events play a role in the action of insulin itself.

Another interesting series of experiments, conducted as a result of the observed insulin-like activity exhibited by oxi-

FIGURE 2. Requirement of multivalency for activation of hexose transport by anti-membrane protein antibodies in intact fat cells. This figure outlines results obtained with rabbit anti-intrinsic membrane protein Ig, monovalent Fab prepared from this Ig, or Fab plus anti-Fab on glucose utilization in adipocytes.[55,56] Provided above the schematized membrane are the incubation conditions employed and below are the respective biological responses on glucose uptake observed. The aggregation of intrinsic membrane proteins is expected to occur in response to intact antimembrane Ig or monovalent Fab plus divalent anti-FabIg, but not Fab fragments alone. The detailed mechanism whereby membrane aggregation events might trigger transport activation is unknown.

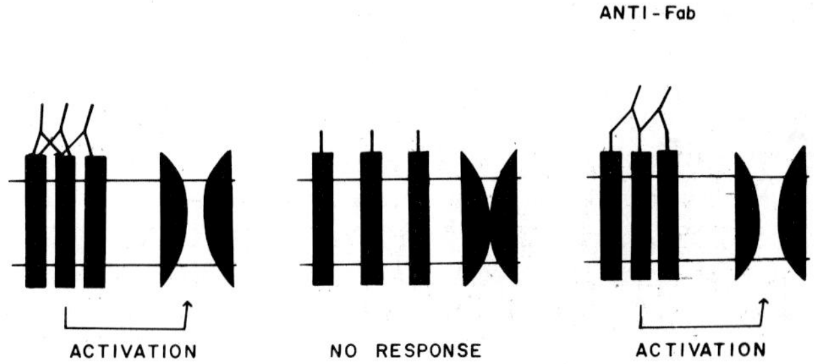

dants, have led to the hypothesis that membrane redox reactions may be involved in hexose transport activation by insulin.[34-39] The model proposed consisted of two basic features: (1) the chemical signal which triggers the activation of hexose transport system activity in response to insulin was proposed to be the oxidation of key membrane sulfhydryls to the disulfide form, and (2) fat cell transport activity under any condition was postulated to simply reflect the number of these key membrane proteins which are present in the activated, disulfide form. In other words, the hexose transport system, or a regulatory component thereof, was considered to exist in a reduced, inactive form or an oxidized, active state which could catalyze the facilitated diffusion of glucose across the cell surface membrane.

The data to support this hypothesis included the finding that oxidants such as H_2O_2 and diamide mimicked insulin action on hexose transport, and reductants inhibited transport activity.[35,67] Treatment of fat cells with N-ethylmaleimide was observed to inhibit insulin action while prior incubation of cells with the hormone completely protected transport activity from inhibition by the sulfhydryl reagent.[35,67] In addition, it was found that N-ethylmaleimide prevented the elevated transport activity of insulin-treated fat cells from returning to control levels upon trypsinization of cells, which destroys insulin receptors and normally terminates insulin action.[36] Thus, both activation and deactivation of the transport system were exquisitely sensitive to N-ethylmaleimide inhibition, while the transport system itself was completely resistant to the effects of the agent. This interaction between insulin and N-ethylmaleimide, presumably at the cell surface membrane, could be shown to reside at a site distinct from the insulin binding protein.[36] Indeed, in white fat cells N-ethylmaleimide has little effect on binding of insulin to specific cell surface receptors.[68] More recent studies have indicated that increased cellular H_2O_2 levels occur in response to insulin when glucose is present in the medium.[37-39] This thiol redox hypothesis has remained viable, yet no direct data have yet been obtained to prove the concept.

Another hypothesis which is currently under intense investigation involves the concept that cellular calcium flux may be involved in the action of insulin on hexose transport in both muscle and adipocytes. In this regard, it has been suggested that insulin action results in a rapid increase in intracellular free calcium pools.[69-75] Several groups have reported that the action of insulin on certain cellular responses, including hexose transport, requires the presence of calcium in the incubation medium.[69,76-81] The impact of these observations, however, is somewhat diminished by the incomplete inhibition of insulin action by the absence of calcium, and earlier studies,[82,83] which failed to observe inhibition of insulin action on glucose metabolism in the absence of this cation.

Recent reports have appeared indicating that insulin has dramatic effects on calcium flux in intact cell systems. Thus, increased $^{45}Ca^{2+}$ efflux was observed from adipose tissue[84] or isolated fat cells[85,86] which had been previously incubated with labeled calcium in the absence of insulin. Recent experiments by Clausen and co-workers have also indicated a significant increase in labeled calcium release from soleus muscles which had been preincubated in the presence of $^{45}Ca^{2+}$ before the addition of insulin.[87] In addition, Clausen[87] found that the calcium ionophore A23187 mimicked the activation of glucose uptake observed with insulin in soleus muscle by a mechanism requiring calcium in the medium. Similar actions of A23187 in myoblasts[88] and thymocytes[89] have also been observed. However, at least two groups have failed to observe insulinomimetic effects of the ionophore in fat cells and soleus muscle.[80,90] Verapamil and SKF525A, known inhibitors of calcium flux in adipocytes, have been reported to have no effect on glucose uptake.[80] The ionophore A23187 does indeed increase intracellular calcium levels in such experiments on fat cells, since Lawrence and Larner[91] reported clear effects of the ionophore on fat cell glycogen metabolism under similar conditions. However, in those experiments the ionophore acted to inhibit glycogen synthase rather than stimulate the enzyme as does insulin.

Other effects of insulin on calcium dynamics have been reported in fat cells. For example, McDonald et al.[92] observed an increase in the amount of $^{45}Ca^{2+}$ that plasma membranes prepared from insulin-treated adipocytes bound compared with controls. Markedly altered transport of Ca^{2+} in endoplasmic reticulum obtained from fat cells, which had been exposed to low levels of insulin, was also reported.[93,94] In addition, alterations in calcium content in various mitochondrial compartments were observed due to the action of insulin in intact cells.[95] The above studies indicating effects of insulin on calcium movements, under conditions which appear to be quite physiologic, clearly support a possible role of this cation in the regulation of hexose transport systems. However, it is still difficult to accommodate the somewhat confusing literature on calcium movements in response to insulin in a unified manner. Further data on this interesting hypothesis are required to clarify the potential role of calcium in insulin action.

There is also extensive but somewhat paradoxical data on the potential role of cellular ATP stores in muscle and fat cells in insulin action. This area has been recently reviewed by Gould[96] and will be only briefly outlined here. A large number of reports have indicated a coordinate inhibition of insulin action on hexose transport and depletion of intracellular ATP levels in both muscle and fat cells.[97-103] Exogenous ATP has been reported to initiate a return of insulin responsiveness to ATP-depleted muscles.[100] ^{125}I-insulin binding to muscle was reported to decrease in parallel with reduced cellular ATP stores,[101] but such effects of ATP depletion were not associated with decreased ^{125}I-insulin binding to fat cells.[102,103] The above studies have implicated a pathway involved in insulin action on hexose transport which may be energy-dependent and utilizes ATP.

On the other hand, several reports have indicated that exogenous ATP at quite low concentrations can inhibit the response of fat cell hexose transport to the hormone.[104,105] This inhibitory effect of ATP on insulin-activated hexose transport activity was found to parallel the labeling of two low molecular weight plasma membrane peptides when adipocytes were incubated with ^{32}P-ATP.[105] This labeling was substantially inhibited by the known glucose transport inhibitor phloretin. The above observations suggest that a phosphorylation step may be involved in the inhibition of insulin action on hexose transport. However, further work is needed to clarify the paradoxical results that endogenous ATP is required for insulin action, but exogenous ATP blocks activation of transport by the hormone.

HEXOSE TRANSPORT PROPERTIES IN PURIFIED ADIPOCYTE PLASMA MEMBRANES

With the advent of appropriate methodology to isolate the plasma membrane fraction of rat adipocytes,[107] several studies were performed on the capability of this vesicle preparation to transport D-glucose. Carter et al.[108] found that D-glucose transport into adipocyte plasma membranes was stereospecific and was inhibited by phloretin. The membrane vesicles equilibrated the labeled hexose rather rapidly, and true initial rates of uptake were not measured in these experiments. However, recent observations by Ludvigsen and Jarett[109] on D-glucose uptake by membranes at 0.5 and 1 s after addition of hexose indicated nearly linear uptake rates during this time. These studies allowed estimation of the K_m of transport to be 9.0 mM with a V_{max} of 3209 pmol/mg membrane protein/s. These data indicate that the D-glucose transport activity monitored in purified plasma membrane preparations exhibits all the characteristics expected of the native adipocyte hexose transporter.

One obstacle in studies on D-glucose transport regulation by insulin has been the general experience that insulin will not activate transport when added directly to purified plasma membrane preparations. However, Martin and Carter[110] made the important observation that membranes isolated from insulin-treated adipocytes exhibited greatly enhanced D-glucose transport activity compared with control membranes. Thus, when hexose transport is activated in intact adipocytes, cell disruption prevents deactivation of the system during membrane preparation. We refer to this phenomenon as the fossil effect, and it has sparked a search for other stable membrane alterations due to insulin which might relate to the activated transport system. To date, all physical properties measured in membranes derived from control versus insulin-treated adipocytes have not exhibited significant differences.[111] Treatment of fossilized membranes with anti-insulin serum did not lead to deactivation of transport activity,[111] indicating that insulin-receptor interaction need not persist in the membrane to retain activation of hexose transport activity. Furthermore, Pillion et al.[112] found that the increased hexose transport activity of membranes derived from cells incubated with insulin was also retained after elution of extrinsic membrane proteins off the membranes by dimethylmaleic anhydride extraction.

STRUCTURAL RELATIONSHIP BETWEEN THE HEXOSE TRANSPORTER AND INSULIN RECEPTOR

Recent studies by Jarett and colleagues[113–115] using preparations of ferritin-insulin have allowed visualization of insulin binding sites on adipocyte membranes using electron microscopy. The data presented indicated that insulin receptors exist on the cell surface in clusters or groups, which can be identified by their association with up to six or more monomeric ferritin-insulin complexes. These complexes do not appear to be aggregated in response to insulin binding and action since immobilization of the cell surface by cross-linking did not change the cluster disposition of ferritin-insulin on the membrane.[115] In an interesting series of experiments, cytochalasin B was shown to initiate the disaggregation of receptor clusters on adipocytes concomitant with its ability to block hexose transport activity.[116] Cytochalasin D, which does not block transport but does share the ability of cytochalasin B to alter general cell dynamics such as endocytosis, failed to modulate the disposition of ferritin-insulin on the fat cell surface. It was therefore proposed by these workers that insulin receptor complexes constituted hexose transporter pores in the surface membranes.[116] This hypothesis predicts that insulin binds directly to a complex containing the hexose transport system and that cytochalasin B blocks transport activity by dissociating this complex.

Another approach to the question of transporter structure and its relation to the insulin receptor involves attempts to isolate and purify these membrane components as a means of gaining insight into their chemical nature. In order to employ this approach, Shanahan and Czech developed methodology that allowed elution of extrinsic proteins from adipocyte membranes[117] and insertion of solubilized hexose transporter into artificial phospholipid vesicles, resulting in stereospecific D-glucose transport activity.[6] The method employed differed from that previously used for reconstituting the red cell hexose transporter[118] in that cholate was utilized instead of Triton X-100, and the formation of reconstituted membranes was accomplished on Sephadex G-50 columns. A freeze-thaw cycle and brief sonication step was employed in order to enlarge the volume of the reconstituted vesicles and facilitate assay of transport activity by rapid filtration.[117] The reconstitution procedure is outlined in Figure 3. D-(^{3}H)glucose transport into such reconstituted membranes was found to be inhibited by low concentrations of the known transport inhibitors phloretin and cytochalasin B and was greater than uptake of L-glucose. Vesicles reconstituted in the absence of adipocyte membrane protein did not exhibit these properties.

The development of this reliable reconstitution system has allowed chromatography of the cholate-solubilized adipocyte membrane proteins followed by assay of the fractions for transporting activity.[118] The data demonstrate that the adipocyte hexose transporter migrates with an apparent Stokes radius of 60–80 Å on Sepharose 6B, indicating it contains a region capable of spanning the plasma membrane. The transporter in cholate solution binds very tightly to DEAE or hydroxylapatite, and is not eluted from the former matrix using 1 M NaCl. Elution of a DEAE column with 4 M NaCl dissociates the transporter which can then be readily reconstituted into phospholipid vesicles.[119] Initial experiments indicated that a 94,000 mol wt glycoprotein fraction represented the major protein band present in cholate-solubilized intrinsic membrane proteins as visualized on dodecyl sulfate gels.[6] However, passage of this material through a column containing immobilized concanavalin A removed almost all the 94,000 and 78,000 mol wt glycoprotein fractions, while D-glucose transport activity eluted from the column.[118,119] Sequential use of immobilized lectin chromatography and gel filtration on Sepharose 6B yielded a fraction which appeared to be enriched by 25–50-fold in its ability to catalyze D-glucose uptake in reconstituted vesicles. These data indicate that none of the major membrane proteins of glycoproteins comprise the hexose transporter, but that it is present in the membrane in very small quanti-

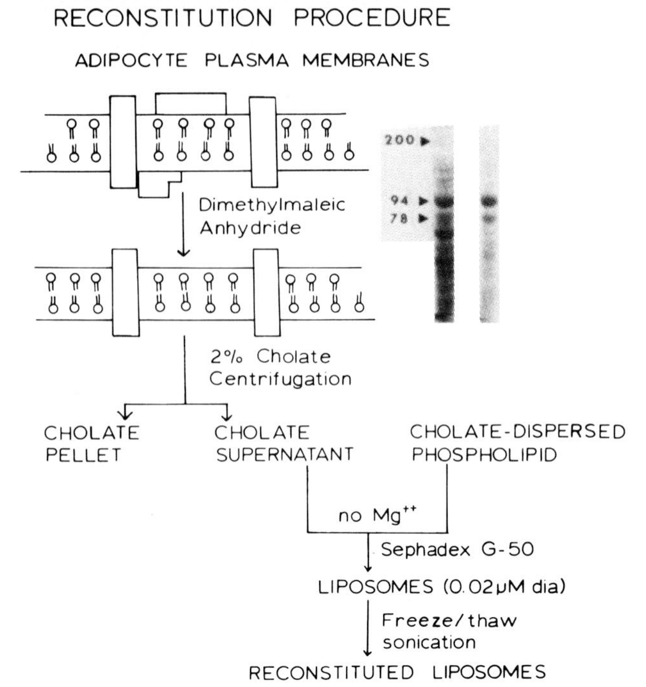

FIGURE 3. Procedure for reconstitution of the adipocyte D-glucose transport system into artificial phospholipid vesicles. The reconstitution method of Shanahan and Czech[6] is employed in concert with an extraction step[117] whereby adipocyte plasma membranes are incubated with dimethylmaleic anhydride to elute extrinsic membrane proteins from the membrane matrix. As can be visualized in the polyacrylamide gels shown, this extraction procedure simplifies the protein pattern of native membranes (left gel) to one where two glycoprotein fractions (94,000 and 78,000 mol wt) are the major residual components (right gel). The extracted membranes are then incubated in sodium cholate, centrifuged, and the soluble components combined in the absence of Mg^{2+} with cholate-dispersed phospholipids (usually phosphatidyl ethanolamine and phosphatidyl choline, 1:1) with[122] or without[6] cholesterol. Chromatography on Sephadex G-50 in the presence of Mg^{2+} results in reconstituted vesicle formation and the freeze-thaw cycle plus brief sonication enlarges the vesicles. The resultant vesicular preparation exhibits stereospecific hexose transport activity with all of the properties expected of the adipocyte transporter.

ties. It is interesting that the transport system does not bind to immobilized concanavalin A since this lectin markedly activates hexose transport in intact adipocytes.[45–47]

In another series of experiments, we have been able to develop an affinity-labeling technique to specifically insert a radioactive tag on high affinity insulin receptors. This methodology involves the cross-linking of ^{125}I-insulin to the hormone-binding subunit of the receptor using disuccinimidyl suberate which we synthesized.[2,3] This bifunctional reagent reacts rapidly with protein amino groups at physiological pH and thus can readily be used to covalently link ^{125}I-insulin to binding proteins in intact cells and isolated plasma membranes. Using this reagent, we[2,3] found that a membrane protein migrating at 125,000 apparent mol wt on reduced dodecyl sulfate polyacrylamide gels could be specifically labeled with ^{125}I-insulin. These data were in substantive agreement with results obtained using a photoaffinity analogue of insulin.[1,5] The extent of cross-linking of ^{125}I-insulin to this protein at various hormone concentrations paralleled the occupancy of the high affinity insulin receptor as determined by Scatchard analysis.[3] An important observation was that the labeled receptor migrated as an apparent 300,000 mol wt complex on nonreduced gels, indicating that the insulin receptor exists in the native adipocyte or liver membrane as a disulfide-linked complex containing at least one 125,000 mol wt insulin-binding monomer. A similar conclusion was recently reached by Jacobs and Cuatrecasas,[5] who reported a lower molecular weight protein also co-purified with the 125,000 receptor monomer.

The methodology that allows affinity-labeling insulin receptors and assay of D-glucose transport activity of solubilized proteins using the reconstitution method has enabled us to directly compare the chromatographic properties of these two membrane components. While both the labeled receptor and the hexose transporter migrate similarly on Sepharose 6B, marked differences were observed on these other chromatographic systems.[119,120] When ^{125}I-insulin was cross-linked to intact membranes before solubilization in sodium cholate, nearly all the labeled receptor eluted from hydroxylapatite with 0.1 M phosphate, while no transport activity was eluted at this phosphate concentration.[120] Elution of the hexose transporter with higher salt was accompanied by only small amounts of labeled receptor. Similar observations were made using DEAE chromatography. Furthermore, earlier observations indicated that the Triton X-100-solubilized insulin receptor binds tightly to immobilized lectins such as concanavalin A,[46,47] while hexose transport activity,

FIGURE 4. Current status of structural information on the high-affinity insulin receptor and the insulin-sensitive hexose transporter of adipocytes. While our knowledge of the protein chemistry of the adipocyte insulin receptor and D-glucose transport system is rudimentary at present, several important features of these components are now known. The receptor (left) resides in the native fat cell and liver-plasma membrane as a disulfide-linked complex containing at least one insulin-binding subunit with an apparent mol wt of about 125,000.[1–5] Experiments in which the labeled receptor was treated with low concentrations of reductant before electrophoresis in dodecyl sulfate revealed partially reduced receptor subunits of intermediate mol wt.[140,141] These data have been used to deduce a receptor structure proposed to contain four different disulfide-linked subunits,[140] based on a total mol wt in the 300,000 range. At least two kinds of subunits differing in mass compose the receptor—the 125,000 insulin-binding component and another smaller subunit.[140,141] Based on these recent observations, the simplest model is that shown here, which involves two 125,000 and two lower mol wt subunits of equal size. The insulin receptor appears to be a glycoprotein in that it binds to concanavalin A and wheat germ agglutinin[46,47] and exhibits changes in migration on gels following neuraminidase treatment.[141] The receptor has a region which, in Triton X-100, migrates on Sepharose 6B with an apparent Stokes radius of about 70 Å. The hexose transporter also contains a region of about this size when solubilized in sodium cholate,[118–120] but the subunit structure is presently completely unknown. The transporter appears devoid of mannose-like saccharides since it readily passes through immobilized concanavalin A.[118] The transport system is markedly sensitive to the membrane bilayer structure in which it resides.[122] The affinity-labeled insulin receptor displays chromatographic properties distinct from those characteristic of the hexose transporter in detergent solution as outlined in the text.[120] A transmembrane disposition of these components has not yet been proven.

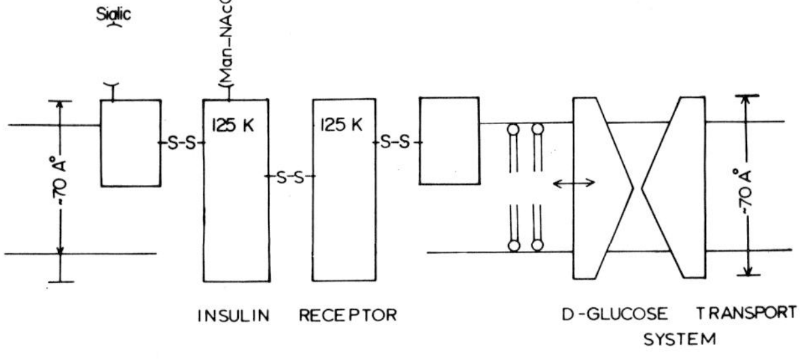

at least in sodium cholate, does not.[118] The impact of these data lead to the conclusion, summarized in Figure 4, that functional adipocyte hexose transporters in detergent solution exhibit chromatographic properties that are quite divergent from high affinity insulin receptors. Thus, these two activities are properties of two distinct polypeptide units, and hexose transport activation by the insulin-receptor complex must involve a membrane transduction mechanism. We have not ruled out the possibility that, in the native membrane, hexose transport protein(s) are associated with insulin receptor protein(s) by noncovalent means that are disrupted in mild detergents.

MEMBRANE MICROVISCOSITY AND INSULIN-SENSITIVE HEXOSE TRANSPORT ACTIVITY

The molecular mechanism or mechanisms involved in the transport of solutes across biologic membranes have not been elucidated in detail. Useful information about such transport mechanisms has been obtained from studies on the natural peptide ionophores. Two extreme models for solute transport are exemplified by the cage carrier and fixed channel concepts illustrated in Figure 5. The former type of transporter (e.g., valinomycin) binds to the solute to be transported (e.g., K^+) and diffuses within the membrane to effect transport in the direction of an electrochemical gradient. This mechanism is expected to be extremely sensitive to the viscosity or molecular motion of the membrane, and it has been demonstrated that transport catalyzed by such cage carriers is greatly inhibited upon converting a fluid phospholipid membrane to the ordered or "frozen" state by lowering temperature.[121] In contrast, fixed channel-type transporters such as gramacidin operate to transport cations (e.g., Na^+) as rigid pores. This mode of transport is, as expected, virtually unresponsive to the microviscosity of the membrane bilayer.[121] This relationship between the physical state of the membrane lipid bilayer and transport activity can thus provide some insight into the mechanism of membrane transporters.

FIGURE 5. Two different mechanisms by which ionophores operate to catalyze transfer of solutes across biological membranes. Cage-carrier ionophores such as valinomycin diffuse into and across a fluid membrane bilayer with bound ion and thereby facilitate the diffusion of water-soluble ions across the membrane (upper left). Activity of this transport mechanism is greatly decreased[121] when the membrane bilayer is ordered or "frozen" at low temperature (lower left). In contrast, the gramacidins exemplify a fixed channel mode of transport catalysis whereby specific ions diffuse through a rigid pore in the membrane formed by the ionophore (upper and lower right). Transport activity catalyzed by this mechanism is relatively insensitive to the microviscosity of the membrane bilayer in which it resides.[121]

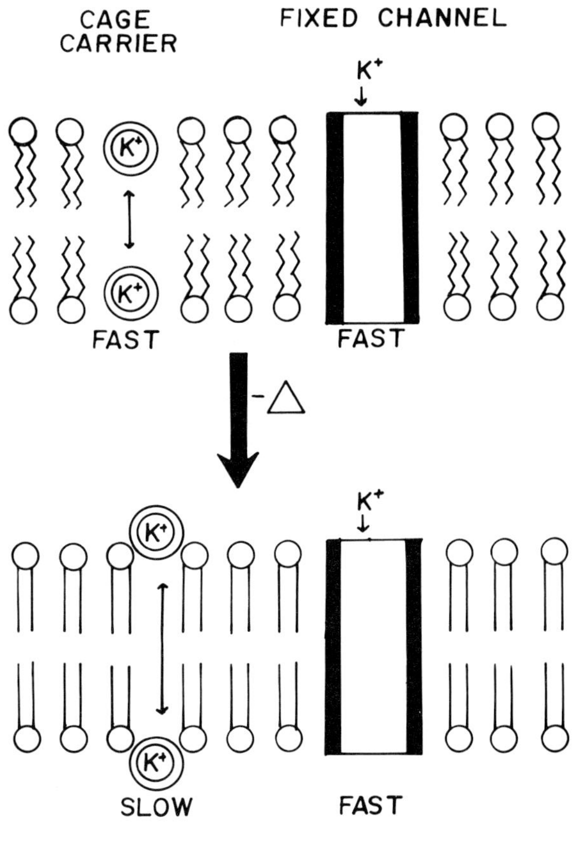

The availability of the reconstituted adipocyte hexose transport system has allowed investigation into its responsiveness to membrane structure, since pure phospholipids which undergo clear transitions from ordered to fluid states can be employed to prepare reconstituted vesicles. Melchior and Czech[122] observed virtually total inhibition of hexose transport activity at 0°C in such vesicles prepared from membrane protein and egg phosphatidylethanol and 1-stereayl-2-oleoyl phosphatidylcholine when the membrane was in the ordered or crystalline state. Increasing temperature enhanced hexose transport activity concomitant with bilayer melting until at about 30°C melting was complete and transport activity increased less markedly. That this coordinate pattern of membrane fluidizing and transport activation was causally related was suggested by experiments showing the transport temperature sensitivity could be shifted according to the melting properties of the resident phospholipid in the vesicle bilayer. Furthermore, the correlation of transport activity and membrane microviscosity also held when reconstituted membranes were prepared with cholesterol, which abolished the endothermic transitions of the membrane phospholipid.[122] At 0°C, where vesicles without cholesterol would be mostly in the ordered state, hexose transport was enhanced when cholesterol was present in the membranes. At 23°C, the presence of cholesterol decreased the activity of the transporter, concomitant with an expected increase in microviscosity. Taken together, these studies demonstrate that the adipocyte hexose transport system is quite responsive to the physical state of its bilayer environment. Furthermore, molecular motion in the membrane seems required for the expression of hexose transport activity, and it is concluded that the transporter does not operate as a rigid, fixed channel.

The experiments cited above were recently extended to the native adipocyte plasma membrane. Previous studies have shown that incubation of mammalian plasma membranes with such unsaturated fatty acids as cis-vaccenic or oleic acids leads to partitioning of these agents into the membrane with a concomitant decrease in microviscosity as evidenced by the fluorescence polarization of diphenylhexatriene[124] or immunofluorescence labeling.[125] When this procedure was performed with purified plasma membranes from adipocytes, a dramatic activation of hexose transport activity was observed in response to the incorporation of cis-vaccenic or oleic acids.[123] These studies represent the only reported instance in which hexose transport activity in the isolated, native fat cell membrane has been activated by direct addition of an agent. The data suggest that the adipocyte transporter is not fully active in the native membrane, and that its restraint can be released upon provision of a more fluid bilayer environment.

The possibility that regulation of adipocyte hexose transport activity might involve the participation of membrane microviscosity in some manner has recently been addressed. The hypothesis that hexose transport activation by insulin or other agents might reflect increased fluidity in the microenvironments of the transporter predicts that membrane fluidizers such as cis-vaccenate would not further activate transport in membranes derived from insulin-treated cells. On the other hand, this insulin-activated transport activity might be expected to respond to decreased motion in the membrane caused by incubation with saturated fatty acids. However, the basal transport system in control membranes, residing in immobilized regions, might not be sensitive to further increases in microviscosity. All of these predictions have been experimentally sustained.[123] Incubation of cis-vaccenic acid with membranes derived from insulin-treated cells resulted in no further increase in hexose transport activity. In contrast, incorporation of stearate into the membrane decreased the insulin-activated transport rate to control levels, but was ineffective in altering the hexose transporter in control membranes. The data suggest that basal hexose transport is unaffected by increased microviscosity. Insulin-activated transport is unaffected by decreased microviscosity but inhibited by increased microviscosity.

While these data represent only indirect evidence, they are consistent with two possible mechanisms for the action of insulin: (1) insulin increases bilayer fluidity in localized membrane regions in which the transporter resides, or (2) insulin increases the partition coefficient of the hexose transporter for more fluid regions of the adipocyte membrane. Consistent with the second of these working hypotheses, studies in the reconstituted system indicated that the basal glucose transporter partitioned more favorably into the ordered regions of phospholipid bilayers.[122] Thus, in vesicles containing egg phosphatidylcholine and egg phosphatidylethanolamine, D-glucose transport was fully inactivated when only 50% of the bilayer was in the ordered or crystalline state.[122] The temperature-sensitivity of the insulin-activated system following reconstitution is currently being investigated. It is interesting to note that experiments in other systems have demonstrated rapid effects of agents such as α-agonists[126] and lectins[127] on the methylation of phosphatidylethanolamine to phosphatidylcholine in target cells, an effect which might increase membrane fluidity. Also, insulin has been reported to increase desaturase activity,[128] increase phospholipase activity,[129] and increase the levels of unsaturated fatty acids in adipocyte membrane phospholipids.[130] However, the data cited above must be considered indirect with respect to the two hypotheses presented, and further studies are needed in this area.

TRANSPORT SYSTEM ACTIVATION VERSUS UNMASKING IN RESPONSE TO INSULIN

A central problem in the area of transport regulation by insulin is whether the actual number of transporter complexes in the membrane changes during activation. Two general models of increased hexose transport activity are consistent with the observed enhancement of V_{max} with no change in K_m. Insulin action could increase the number of operational hexose transporters such that transport activity under conditions of zero, suboptimal, or maximal doses of insulin would simply reflect the number of transporters converted from the precursor or inactive to the active state. Recruitment of transporters from other cellular compartments into the plasma membrane would also increase the number of transporters. The characteristics of the transport activity observed (temperature dependence, response to protein reagents, etc.) should be identical in basal or insulin-activated cells according to this model. Alternatively, if V_{max} changes in individual membrane transporter proteins occur in response to insulin, the V_{max} of transport observed under any condition should reflect the average V_{max} of all the V_{max} values exhibited by the transporters present in the membrane. This hypothesis predicts that the structure of the transporters or their membrane microenvironments are altered by insulin, and that basal transport activity may therefore exhibit different properties compared with insulin-stimulated hexose transport activity.

Early results on Na^+-K^+ ATPase stimulation due to insulin appeared to indicate that increased numbers of transport sites were elicited by the hormone, since insulin enhanced labeled ouabain binding to intact skeletal muscle.[131,132] Unmasking of latent Na^+ pumps by the hormone was proposed to explain these results. However, data have more recently emerged demonstrating an enhanced rate of (^{3}H)ouabain binding to soleus muscle and fat cells due to insulin, but no change was observed in the total number of ouabain binding sites.[133] It appears that the earlier studies were not performed after binding equilibrium had been achieved. These results therefore suggest that increased K^+ uptake in response to insulin reflects the activation of a given number of Na^+-K^+ ATPase enzyme complexes present in the membrane, rather than an unmasking effect.

Recently, a similar approach has been employed to address this question with respect to hexose transport in adipocyte membranes, but the conclusion differed from that on the Na^+-K^+ ATPase. In these studies,[134] (^{3}H)cytochalasin B binding was used as previously described in the human red cell[135] to assess D-glucose transporters. A very small but significant fraction of the total (^{3}H)cytochalasin B binding to adipocyte membranes was inhibited by 500 mM D-glucose plus 500 mM L-glucose compared with 500 mM L-glucose alone.[134] These studies were carried out in the presence of 2 μM cytochalasin E, which does not block hexose transport but inhibits nonspecific (^{3}H)cytochalasin B binding. Earlier studies performed in the absence of this cytochalasin analog failed to detect significantly decreased (^{3}H)cytochalasin B binding to fat cell plasma membrane due to 100 mM D-glucose.[136] Wardzala et al.[134] reported an increase in the D-glucose-sensitive fraction of (^{3}H)cytochalasin B binding sites in plasma membranes prepared from insulin-treated adipocytes compared with controls. These workers concluded that insulin acts to increase hexose transport activity by enhancing the number of functional transporters in the membrane. However, at least two instances of divergent properties of control versus insulin-stimulated hexose transport have been reported. Several groups have found a much greater temperature sensitivity of insulin-activated 3-O-methylglucose transport activity compared with control transport rates in intact cells,[24,136–138] although others have failed to make this observation.[27,139] In addition, the differential sensitivity of hexose transport activity in membranes from control versus insulin-treated adipocytes to both unsaturated and saturated fatty acids described in the previous section indicates very different properties of these systems.

These latter observations and the data on the Na^+-K^+ ATPase oppose the concept that the simple unmasking or recruitment of latent transporters identical to those which catalyze basal transport activity characterizes insulin action. It is possible that ion transport is regulated very differently from hexose transport. A stable change in the hexose transporter itself or in its membrane microenvironment due to insulin action seems more consistent with the data available, however. This alternative seems difficult to reconcile with the observed enhancement in the (^{3}H)cytochalasin B binding due to insulin.[134] However, it has not yet been directly demonstrated that the D-glucose-sensitive cytochalasin B binding sites actually relate to the number of hexose transporters which operate in the cell surface membrane. It is also possible that insulin action employs a more complex mechanism, which involves expression of new hexose transporters differing in certain properties from the basal transporters or which exists in different regions of the plasma membrane system. Unfortunately, we still do not have a direct answer to whether any of the mechanisms discussed above are actually employed in transport activation by insulin. It is encouraging that the methodologies currently available to approach this problem, especially functional reconstitution of the solubilized transporter, should prove quite powerful in future studies.

REFERENCES

1 Yip, C. C., Yeung, C. W. T., and Moule, M. L.: Photoaffinity labeling of insulin receptor of rat adipocyte plasma membrane. J. Biol. Chem. *253*:1743–45, 1978.

2 Pilch, P. F., and Czech, M. P.: Interaction of cross-linking agents with the insulin effector system of isolated fat cells. J. Biol. Chem. *254*:3375–81, 1979.

3 Pilch, P. F., and Czech, M. P.: The subunit structure of the high-affinity insulin receptor. Evidence for a disulfide-linked receptor complex in fat cell and liver plasma membranes. J. Biol. Chem. In press.

4 Sahyoun, N., Hock, R. A., and Hollenberg, M. D.: Insulin and epidermal growth factor-urogastrone: affinity crosslinking to specific binding sites in rat liver membranes. Proc. Natl. Acad. Sci. USA *75*:1675–79, 1978.

5 Jacobs, S., Hazum, E., Schechter, Y., and Cuatrecasas, P.: Insulin receptor: covalent labeling and identification of subunits. Proc. Natl. Acad. Sci. USA *76*:4918–21, 1979.

6 Shanahan, M. F., and Czech, M. P.: Purification and reconstitution of the adipocyte plasma membrane D-glucose transport system. J. Biol. Chem. *252*:8341–43, 1977.

7 Czech, M. P., Pillion, D. J., and Shanahan, M. F.: Resistance of the intact and reconstituted adipocyte hexose transport system to irreversible inhibition by sulfhydryl and amino reagents. J. Supramol. Struct. *9*:363–71, 1978.

8 Gavryck, W. A., Moore, R. D., and Thompson, R. C.: Effect of insulin upon membrane bound Na^+-K^+ ATPase extracted from frog skeletal muscle. J. Physiol. *252*:43–58, 1975.

9 Clausen, T., and Hansen, O.: Active Na^+-K^+ transport and the rate of ouabain binding, the effect of insulin and other stimuli on skeletal muscle and adipocytes. J. Physiol. *270*:415–30, 1977.

10 Clausen, T., and Kohn, P. G.: The effect of insulin on the transport of sodium and potassium in rat soleus muscle. J. Physiol. *265*:19–42, 1977.

11 Hepp, D., Challoner, D. R., and Williams, R. H.: Studies on the action of insulin in isolated adipose tissue cells. I. Stimulation of incorporation of ^{32}P-labelled inorganic phosphate into mononucleotides in the absence of glucose. J. Biol. Chem. *243*:4020–26, 1968.

12 Manchester, K. L.: The control by insulin of amino acid accumulation in muscle. Biochem. J.*117*:457–65, 1970.

13 Fehlman, M., Le Cam, A., and Freychet, P.: Insulin and glucagon stimulation of amino acid transport in isolated rat hepatocytes. Synthesis of a high affinity component of transport. J. Biol. Chem. *254*:10431–437, 1979.

14 Morgan, H. E., and Whitfield, C. F.: Regulation of sugar transport in eucaryotic cells. Curr. Top. Membr. Transp. *4*:255–303, 1973.

15 Rodbell, M.: Metabolism of isolated fat cells. I. Effects of hormones on glucose metabolism and lipolysis. J. Biol. Chem. *239*:375–80, 1964.

16 Angel, A., and Farkas, J.: Structural and chemical compartments in adipose cells. *In* Hormone and Metabolic Research, Supplement 2. Adipose Tissue, Regulation and Metabolic Functions. Jeanrenaud, B., and Hepp, D., Eds. New York, Academic Press, 1970, pp. 152–61.

17 Crofford, O. B., and Renold, A. E.: Glucose uptake by incubated rat epididymal adipose tissue. Rate-limiting steps and site of insulin action. J. Biol. Chem. *240*:14–21, 1965.

18 Crofford, O. B., and Renold, A. E.: Glucose uptake by incubated rat epididymal adipose tissue. Characteristics of the glucose transport system and action on insulin. J. Biol. Chem. *240*:3237–44, 1965.

19 Levine, R., Goldstein, M., Klein, S., and Huddlestun, B.: The action of insulin on the distribution of galactose in eviscerated nephrectomized dogs. J. Biol. Chem. *179*:985, 1949.

20 Levine, R., Goldstein, M. S., Huddlestun, B., and Klein, S. P.: Action of insulin on the 'permeability' of cells to free hexoses, as studied by its effect on the distribution of galactose. Am. J. Physiol. *163*:70–76, 1950.

21 Fain, J. N., Reed, N., and Saperstein, R.: The isolation and metabolism of brown fat cells. J. Biol. Chem. *242*:1887–94, 1967.

22 Czech, M. P., Lawrence, J. C., Jr., and Lynn, W. S.: Hexose transport in isolated brown fat cells. A model system for investigating insulin action on membrane transport. J. Biol. Chem. *249*:5421–27, 1974.

23 Czech, M. P., Lawrence, J. C., and Lynn, W. S.: Activation of hexose transport by concanavalin A in isolated brown fat cells. Effects of cell surface modification with neuraminidase and trypsin on lectin and insulin action. J. Biol. Chem. *249*:7499–505, 1974.

24 Czech, M. P.: Regulation of the D-glucose transport system in isolated fat cells. Mol. Cel. Biochem. *11*:51–63, 1976.

25 Vinten, J., Gliemann, J., and Østerlind, K.: Exchange of 3-O-methylglucose in isolated fat cells. J. Biol. Chem. *254*:794–800, 1976.

26 Gliemann, J., Østerlind, K., Vinten, J., and Gammeltoft, S.: A procedure for measurement of distribution spaces in isolated fat cells. Biochim. Biophys. Acta *286*:1–9, 1972.

27 Vinten, J.: Cytochalasin B inhibition and temperature dependence of 3-O-methylglucose transport in fat cells. Biochim. Biophys. Acta *511*:259–73, 1978.

28 Whitesell, R. R., and Gliemann, J.: Kinetic parameters of transport of 3-O-methylglucose and glucose in adipocytes. J. Biol. Chem. *254*:5276–83, 1979.

29 Foley, J. E., Cushman, S. W., and Salans, L. B.: Glucose transport in isolated rat adipocytes with measurements of L-arabinose uptake. Am. J. Physiol. *3*:E112–E119, 1978.

30 Häring, H. U., Kemmler, W., Renner, R., and Hepp, H. D.: Initial lag-phase in the action of insulin on glucose transport and cAMP levels in fat cells. FEBS Lett. *95*:177–80, 1978.

31 Gliemann, J., Gammeltoft, S., and Vinten, J.: Time course of insulin-receptor binding and insulin-induced lipogenesis in isolated rat fat cells. J. Biol. Chem. *250*:3368–74, 1975.

32 Crofford, O. B.: Time course termination of the glucose transport action of insulin in adipocytes. J. Biol. Chem. *250*:7089–92, 1975.

33 Ciaraldi, T. P., and Olefsky, J. M.: Relationship between deactivation of insulin-stimulated glucose transport and insulin dissociation in isolated rat adipocytes. J. Biol. Chem. *255*:327–30, 1980.

34 Czech, M. P., Lawrence, J. C., and Lynn, W. S.: Evidence for an electron transfer reaction involved in the Cu^{++}-dependent thiol activation of fat cell glucose utilization. J. Biol. Chem. *249*:1001–06, 1974.

35 Czech, M. P., Lawrence, J. C., and Lynn, W. S.: Evidence for the involvement of sulfhydryl oxidation in the regulation of fat cell hexose transport by insulin. Proc. Natl. Acad. Sci. USA *71*:4173–77, 1974.

36 Czech, M. P.: Differential effects of sulfhydryl reagents on activation and deactivation of the fat cell hexose transport system. J. Biol. Chem. *251*:1164–70, 1976.

37 Mukherjee, S. P., and Lynn, W. S.: Reduced nicotinamide adenine dinucleotide phosphate oxidase in adipocyte plasma membrane and its activation by insulin. Possible role in the hormone's effects on adenylate cyclase and the hexose monophosphate shunt. Arch. Biochem. Biophys. *184*:69–76, 1977.

38 May, J. M., and de Haen, C.: Insulin-stimulated intracellular hydrogen peroxide production in rat epididymal fat cells. J. Biol. Chem. *254*:2214–20, 1979.

39 May, J. M., and de Haen, C.: The insulin-like effect of hydrogen peroxide on pathways of lipid synthesis in rat adipocytes. J. Biol. Chem. *254*:9017–21, 1979.

40 Lockwood, D. H., Lipsky, J. J., Meronk, F., Jr., and East, L. E.: Actions of polyamines on lipid and glucose metabolism of fat cells. Biochem. Biophys. Res. Commun. *44*:600–17, 1971.

41 Lockwood, D. H., and East, L. E.: Studies of the insulin-like actions of polyamines on lipid and glucose metabolism in adipose tissue cells. J. Biol. Chem. *249*:7717–22, 1974.

42 Clausen, T., Elbrink, J., and Martin, B. R.: Insulin controlling calcium distribution in muscle and fat cells. Acta Endocrinol. *191*(Suppl.):137–43, 1974.

[43] Carter, J. R., and Martin, D. B.: The effect of sulfhydryl blockade on insulin action and glucose transport in isolated adipose tissue cells. Biochim. Biophys. Acta *177*:521–26, 1969.
[44] Minemura, T., and Crofford, O. B.: Insulin-receptor interaction in isolated fat cells. I. The insulin-like properties of *p*-chloromercuribenzene sulfonic acid. J. Biol. Chem. *244*:5181–88, 1969.
[45] Czech, M. P., and Lynn, W. S.: Stimulation of glucose metabolism by lectins in isolated white fat cells. Biochim. Biophys. Acta *297*:386–77, 1973.
[46] Cuatrecasas, P.: Interaction of concanavalin A and wheat germ agglutinin with the insulin receptor of fat cells and liver. J. Biol. Chem. *248*:3528–34, 1973.
[47] Katzen, H. M., and Soderman, D. D.: Interaction of carbohydrate binding sites on concanavalin A-agarose with receptors on adipocytes studied by buoyant density method. Biochemistry *14*:2293–98, 1975.
[48] Jarrett, D. B., Roth, J., Kahn, C. R., and Flier, J. S.: Direct method for detection and characterization of cell surface receptors for insulin by means of ^{125}I-labeled autoantibodies against the insulin receptor. Proc. Natl. Acad. Sci. USA *73*:4115–19, 1976.
[49] Kahn, C. R., Flier, J. S., Bar, R. S., Archer, J. A., Gorden, P., Martin, M. M., and Roth, J.: The syndromes of insulin resistance and acanthosis nigricans. Insulin-receptor disorders in man. N. Engl. J. Med. *294*:739–45, 1976.
[50] Flier, J. S., Kahn, C. R., Roth, J., and Bar, R. S.: Antibodies that impair insulin receptor binding in an unusual diabetic syndrome with severe insulin resistance. Science *190*:63–65, 1975.
[51] Flier, J. S., Kahn, C. R., Jarrett, D. B., and Roth, J.: Characterization of antibodies to the insulin receptor: a cause of insulin-resistant diabetes in man. J. Clin. Invest. *58*:1442–49, 1976.
[52] Flier, J. S., Kahn, C. R., Jarrett, D. B., and Roth, J.: The immunology of the insulin receptor. Immunol. Comm. *5*:361–73, 1976.
[53] Kahn, C. R., Baird, K., Flier, J. S., and Jarrett, D. B.: Effects of autoantibodies to the insulin receptor on isolated adipocytes. Studies of insulin binding and insulin action. J. Clin. Invest. *60*:1094–106, 1977.
[54] Kahn, C. R., Baird, K. L., Jarrett, D. B., and Flier, J. S.: Monovalent anti-receptor antibodies regain insulinomimetic actions when crosslinked by a second antibody. Diabetes *27*(Suppl. 2):449, 1978.
[55] Pillion, D. J., and Czech, M. P.: Antibodies against intrinsic adipocyte plasma membrane proteins activate D-glucose transport independent of interaction with insulin binding sites. J. Biol. Chem. *253*:3761–64, 1978.
[56] Pillion, D. J., Grantham, J. R., and Czech, M. P.: Biological properties of antibodies against rat adipocyte intrinsic membrane proteins. Dependence on multivalency for insulin-like activity. J. Biol. Chem. *254*:3211–20, 1979.
[57] Kono, T., and Barham, F. W.: Insulin-like effects of trypsin on fat cells. Localization of the metabolic steps and the cellular site affected by the enzymes. J. Biol. Chem. *246*:6204–09, 1971.
[58] Rodbell, M.: Metabolism of isolated fat cells. II. The similar effects of phospholipase C and of insulin on glucose and amino acid metabolism. J. Biol. Chem. *241*:130–39, 1966.
[59] Blecher, M.: Action of insulin on a glucose transport mechanism in the plasma membrane of the isolated adipose cell. Participation of membrane phospholipids and cyclic adenosine monophosphate in the transport processes. Gumma Symposia on Endocrinology *5*:145–61, 1968.
[60] Rosenthal, J. W., and Fain, J. N.: Insulin-like effect of clostridial phospholipase C. neuraminidase, and other bacterial factors on brown fat cells. J. Biol. Chem. *246*:5888–95, 1971.
[61] Cuatrecasas, P., and Illiano, G.: Membrane sialic acid and the mechanism of insulin action in adipose tissue cells. Effect of digestion with neuraminidase. J. Biol. Chem. *246*:4938–46, 1971.
[62] Cuatrecasas, P., and Tell, G. P. E.: Insulin-like activity of concanavalin A and wheat germ agglutinin—direct interactions with insulin receptors. Proc. Natl. Acad. Sci. USA *70*:485, 1973.
[63] Cuatrecasas, P.: Interaction of wheat germ agglutinin and concanvalin A with isolated fat cells. Biochemistry *12*:1312–23, 1973.
[64] Solomon, S. S., King, L. E., and Hashimoto, K.: Studies of the biological activity of insulin, cyclic nucleotides and concanavalin A in the isolated fat cell. Horm. Metab. Res. *7*:297–304, 1975.
[65] Jacobs, S., Chang, K., and Cuatrecasas, P.: Antibodies to purified insulin receptors have insulin-like activity. Science *200*:1283–85, 1978.
[66] Kahn, C., Baird, K., Baird, R., Jarrett, D. B., and Flier, J. S.: Direct demonstration that receptor cross-linking or aggregation is important in insulin action. Proc. Natl. Acad. Sci. USA *75*:4209–13, 1978.
[67] Czech, M. P.: Current status of the thiol redox model for the regulation of hexose transport by insulin. J. Cell. Physiol. *89*:661–68, 1976.
[68] Cuatrecasas, P.: Properties of the insulin receptor of isolated fat cell membranes. J. Biol. Chem. *246*:7265–74, 1971.
[69] Bihler, I.: Ionic effects in the regulation of sugar transport in muscle. *In* The Role of Membranes in Metabolic Regulation. Mehlman, M. A., and Hanson, R. W., Eds. New York, Academic Press, 1972, pp. 411–22.
[70] Bihler, I.: Mechanisms regulating the membrane transport of sugars in the myocardium. *In* Recent Advances in Studies on Cardiac Structure and Metabolism. Dhalla, N. S., Ed. Baltimore, University Park Press, 1974, pp. 209–216.
[71] Clausen, T., Elbrink, J., and Martin, B. R.: Insulin controlling calcium distribution in muscle and fat cells. Acta Endocrinol. 77(Suppl. 191):137–43, 1974.
[72] Clausen, T.: The role of calcium in the action of insulin, FEBS 11th Meeting Copenhagen 1977, Vol. 45, Symposium A4. Membrane Proteins, 1977.
[73] Clausen, T.: Calcium, glucose transport and insulin action. Biochemistry of Membrane Transport, FEBS Symposium No. 42. Semenza, G., and Carafoli, E., Eds. New York, Springer-Verlag, 1977.
[74] Kissebah, A. H., Hope-Gill, H., Vydelingum, N., Tulloch, B., Clarke, P., and Fraser, T. R.: Mode of insulin action. Lancet *1*:144–47, 1975.
[75] Fraser, T., and Russell, M. D.: Is insulin's second messenger calcium? Proc. Roy. Soc. Med. *68*:785–91, 1975.
[76] Holloszy, J. O., and Narahara, H. H.: Enhanced permeability to sugar associated with muscle contraction. J. Gen. Physiol. *50*:551–62, 1966.
[77] Holloszy, J. O., and Narahara, H. H.: Studies in tissue permeability: X. Changes in permeability to 3-O-methylglucose associated with contraction of isolated frog muscle. J. Biol. Chem. *240*:3493–3500, 1967.
[78] Gould, M. K., and Chaudry, I. H.: The action of insulin on glucose uptake by isolated rat soleus muscle. I. Effects of cations. Biochim. Biophys. Acta *215*:247–49, 1970.
[79] Jacobs, B. O., and Krahl, M. E.: The effects of divalent cations and insulin on protein synthesis in adipose cells. Biochim. Biophys. Acta *319*:410–15, 1973.
[80] Bonne, D., Belhadj, O., and Cohen, P.: Modulation by calcium of the insulin action and of the insulin-like effect of ocytocin on isolated rat adipocytes. Eur. J. Biochem. *75*:101–05, 1977.
[81] Bonne, D., Belhadj, O., and Cohen, P.: Calcium as modulator of the hormonal-receptors-biological-response coupling system. Eur. J. Biochem. *86*:261–66, 1978.
[82] Letarte, J., and Renold, A. E.: Ionic effects on glucose transport and metabolism by isolated mouse fat cells incubated with or without insulin. I. Lack of effect of medium Ca^{2+}, Mg^{2+} or PO_4^{3-}. Biochim. Biophys. Acta *183*:350–56, 1969.
[83] Rihan, Z., Jarett, R. J., and Keen, H.: EDTA and insulin: a study of the effect of salts of EDTA upon insulin action in vivo and in vitro. Diabetologia *3*:449–52, 1967.
[84] Clausen, T.: Role of insulin in ion transport in muscle and adipose tissue. Yugoslaw. Physiol. Pharmacol. Acta *5*:363–68, 1969.
[85] Hope-Gill, H., Kissebah, A., Tulloch, B., Clarke, P., Vydelingum, N., and Fraser, T. R.: The effects of insulin on adipocyte calcium flux and the interaction with the effects of dibutyryl cyclic AMP and adrenaline. Horm. Metab. Res. *7*:195–96, 1975.
[86] Hope-Gill, H. F., Kissebah, A. H., Clarke, P., Vydelingum, N., Tulloch, B., and Fraser, T. R.: Effects of insulin and procaine hydrochloride on glycogen synthetase activation and adipocyte calcium flux. Evidence for a role of calcium in insulin activation of glycogen synthetase. Horm. Metab. Res. *8*:184–90, 1976.
[87] Clausen, T., and Martin, B. R.: The effect of insulin on the washout of (^{45}Ca) calcium from adipocytes and soleus muscle of the rat. Biochem. J. *164*:251–55, 1977.
[88] Schudt, C., Gaertner, U., and Pette, D.: Insulin action on glucose transport and calcium fluxes in developing muscle cells in vitro. Eur. J. Biochem. *68*:103–11, 1976.
[89] Reeves, J. P.: Calcium-dependent stimulation of 3-O-methylglucose uptake in rat thymocytes by the divalent cation ionophore A 23187. J. Biol. Chem. *250*:9428–30, 1975.
[90] Grinstein, S., and Erlij, D.: Action of insulin and cell calcium: effect of ionophore A-23187. J. Membr. Biol. *29*:313–28, 1976.
[91] Lawrence, J. C., Jr., and Larner, J.: Effects of insulin, methoxamine, and calcium and glycogen synthase in rat adipocytes. Molec. Pharmacol. *14*:1079–91, 1978.
[92] McDonald, J. M., Bruns, D. E., and Jarett, L.: Ability of insulin to increase calcium binding by adipocyte plasma membranes. Proc. Natl. Acad. Sci. USA *73*:1542–46, 1976.
[93] Bruns, D. E., McDonald, J. M., and Jarett, L.: Properties of passive binding of calcium to endoplasmic reticulum from adipocytes. J. Biol. Chem. *252*:927–32, 1976.
[94] McDonald, J. M., Bruns, D. E., and Jarett, L.: Ability of insulin to increase calcium uptake by adipocyte endoplasmic reticulum. J. Biol. Chem. *253*:3504–08, 1977.
[95] McDonald, J. M., Bruns, D. E., and Jarett, L.: The ability of insulin to alter the stable calcium pools of isolated adipocyte subcellular fractions. Biochem. Biophys. Res. Comm. *71*:114–21, 1976.
[96] Gould, M. K.: Multiple roles of ATP in the regulation of muscle sugar transport. *In* TIBS, January 1979. New York, Elsevier-North Holland Biomedical Press, 1979, pp. 10–13.
[97] Walaas, E., and Walaas, O.: Effect of insulin on rat diaphragm under anaerobic conditions. J. Biol. Chem. *195*:367–73, 1952.
[98] Kono, T., Tetsuro, S., and Colowick, S. P.: Stereospecific sugar transport caused by uncouplers and SH-inhibitors in rat diaphragm. Arch. Biochem. Biophys. *93*:514–19, 1961.
[99] Korbl, G. P., Sloan, I. G., and Gould, M. K.: Effect of anoxia, 2,4-dinitrophenol and salicyclate on xylose transport by isolated rat soleus muscle. Biochim. Biophys. Acta *465*:93–109, 1977.
[100] Yu, K. T., and Gould, J. K.: Permissive effect of ATP on insulin-stimulated sugar transport by rat soleus muscle. Am. J. Physiol. *234*(4):E407–16, 1978.

[101] Yu, K. T., and Gould, M. K.: Insulin-stimulated sugar transport and ^{125}I-insulin binding by rat soleus muscle: permissive effect of ATP. Biochem. Biophys. Res. Commun. *77*:203–10, 1977.

[102] Chandramouli, V., Milligan, M., and Carter, R. J.: Insulin stimulation of glucose transport in adipose cells. Biochemistry *16*:1151–58.

[103] Kono, T., Robindon, F. W., Sarver, J. A., Vega, F. V., and Pointer, R. H.: Actions of insulin in fat cells. J. Biol. Chem. *252*:2226–33, 1977.

[104] Chang, K.-J., and Cuatrecasas, P.: Adenosine triphosphate-dependent inhibition of insulin-stimulated glucose transport in fat cells. Possible role of membrane phosphorylation. J. Biol. Chem. *249*:3170–80, 1974.

[105] Chang, K.-J., Marcus, N., and Cuatrecasas, P.: Cyclic adenosine monophosphate-dependent phosphorylation of specific fat cell membrane proteins by an endogenous membrane-bound protein kinase. J. Biol. Chem. *249*:6854–64, 1974.

[106] Loten, E. G., Regen, D. M., and Park, C. R.: Transport of D-allose by isolated fat cells. J. Cell. Physiol. *89*:651–60, 1976.

[107] McKeel, D. W., and Jarett, L.: Preparation and characterization of a plasma membrane fraction from isolated fat cells. J. Cell. Biol. *44*:417–32, 1970.

[108] Carter, J. R., Avruch, J., and Martin, D. B.: Glucose transport in plasma membrane vesicles from rat adipose tissue. J. Biol. Chem. *247*:2682–88, 1972.

[109] Ludvigsen, C., and Jarett, L.: A kinetic analysis of D-glucose transport by adipocyte plasma membranes. J. Biol. Chem. *254*:1444–46, 1979.

[110] Martin, D. B., and Carter, J. R.: Insulin-stimulated glucose uptake by subcellular particles from adipose tissue cells. Science *167*:873–74, 1970.

[111] Avruch, J., Carter, J. R., and Martin, D. B.: The effect of insulin on the metabolism of adipose tissue. *In* Handbook of Physiology, Section 7, Volume I. Greep, R. O., and Astwood, E. B., Eds. Washington, D.C., American Physiological Society, 1972, pp. 545–62.

[112] Pillion, D. J., Shanahan, M. F., and Czech, M. P.: Retention of insulin-stimulated D-glucose transport activity by adipocyte plasma membranes following extraction of extrinsic proteins. J. Supramol. Struct. *8*:269–77, 1978.

[113] Jarett, L., and Smith, R. M.: Ultrastructural localization of insulin receptors on adipocytes. Proc. Natl. Acad. Sci. USA *72*:3526–30, 1975.

[114] Jarett, L., and Smith, R. M.: Electron microscopic demonstration of insulin receptors on adipocyte plasma membranes utilizing a ferritin-insulin conjugate. J. Biol. Chem. *249*:7024–31, 1974.

[115] Jarett, L., and Smith, R. M.: The natural occurrence of insulin receptors in groups on adipocyte plasma membranes as demonstrated with monomeric ferritin-insulin. J. Supramol. Struct. *6*:45–59, 1977.

[116] Jarett, L., and Smith, R. M.: Effect of cytochalasin B and D on groups of insulin receptors and on insulin action in rat adipocytes. Clin. Invest. *6*:571–79, 1979.

[117] Shanahan, M. F., and Czech, M. P.: Partial purification of the D-glucose transport system in rat adipocyte plasma membranes. J. Biol. Chem. *252*:6554–61, 1977.

[118] Carter-Su, C., Pillion, D. J., and Czech, M. P.: Reconstituted D-glucose transport from the adipocyte plasma membrane. Chromatographic resolution of transport activity from membrane glycoproteins using immobilized concanavalin A. Biochemistry. In press.

[119] Czech, M. P., Carter-Su, C., and Pilch, P. F.: Chromatographic properties of the adipocyte hexose transport system in detergent solution and its resolution from the insulin receptor. *In* Proceedings of the Second International Insulin Symposium. In press.

[120] Carter-Su, C., Pilch, P. F., and Czech, M. P.: Chromatographic resolution of the adipocyte insulin-sensitive D-glucose transporter from the high-affinity insulin receptor. Submitted for publication.

[121] Krasne, S., Eisenman, G., and Szabo, G.: Freezing and melting of lipid bilayers and the mode of action of nonactin, valinomycin and gramicidin. Science *174*:412–15, 1971.

[122] Melchior, D. L., and Czech, M. P.: Sensitivity of the adipocyte D-glucose transport system to membrane fluidity in reconstituted vesicles. J. Biol. Chem. *254*:8744–47, 1979.

[123] Pilch, P. F., Thompson, P. A., and Czech, M. P.: Coordinate modulation of D-glucose transport activity and bilayer fluidity in plasma membranes derived from control and insulin-treated adipocytes. Proc. Natl. Acad. Sci. USA. *77*:915–18, 1980.

[124] Hanski, E., Rimon, G., and Levitzki, A.: Adenylate cyclase activation by the β-adrenergic receptors as a diffusion-controlled process. Biochemistry *18*:846–53, 1979.

[125] Schaeffer, B. E., and Zadunaisky, J. A.: Stimulation of cloride transport by fatty acids in corneal epithelium and relation to changes in membrane fluidity. Biochim. Biophys. Acta *556*:131–43, 1979.

[126] Hirata, F., Strittmatter, W. J., and Axelrod, J.: β-adrenergic receptor agonists increase phospholipid methylation, membrane fluidity, and β-adrenergic receptor-adenylate cyclase coupling. Proc. Natl. Acad. Sci. USA *76*:368–72, 1979.

[127] Hirata, F., Axelrod, J., and Crews, F. T.: Concanavalin A stimulates phospholipid methylation and phosphatidylserine decarboxylation in rat mast cells. Proc. Natl. Acad. Sci. USA *76*:4813–16, 1979.

[128] Prasad, M. R., and Joshi, V. C.: Regulation of rat hepatic stearoyl conenzyme A desaturase. J. Biol. Chem. *254*:997–99, 1979.

[129] Bereziat, G., Wolf, C., Colard, O., and Polonovski, J.: Phospholipases of plasmic membranes of adipose tissue. Possible intermediates of insulin action. Adv. Exptl. Biol. Med. *101*:191–99, 1978.

[130] Murray, D. K., and Nelson, D. H.: Insulin action on the fatty acid composition of phospholipids of isolated fat cell ghosts. 61st Annual Meeting of the Endocrine Society, Abstract 6, 1979, p. 74.

[131] Erlij, D., and Grinstein, S.: The number of sodium ion pumping sites in skeletal muscle and its modification by insulin. J. Physiol. *259*:13–31, 1976.

[132] Manery, J. F., Dryden, E. E., Still, J. S., and Madapallimattam, G.: Enhancement (*by ATP, insulin, and lack of divalent cations) of ouabain inhibition of cation transport and ouabain binding in frog skeletal muscle; effect of insulin and ouabain on sarcolemmal (Na + K) Mg-ATPase. Can. J. Physiol. *55*:21–33, 1977.

[133] Clausen, T., and Hansen, O.: Active Na^+-K^+ transport and the rate of ouabain binding; the effect of insulin and other stimuli on skeletal muscle and adipocytes. J. Physiol. *270*:415–30, 1977.

[134] Wardzala, L. J., Cushman, S. W., and Salans, L. B.: Mechanism of insulin action on glucose transport in the isolated rat adipose cell. J. Biol. Chem. *253*:8002–05, 1978.

[135] Lin, S., and Spudich, J. A.: Biochemical studies on the mode of action of cytochalasin B. Cytochalasin B binding to red cell membrane in relation to glucose transport. J. Biol. Chem. *249*:5778–83, 1974.

[136] Amatruda, J. M., and Finch, E. D.: Modulation of hexose uptake and insulin action by cell membrane fluidity. J. Biol. Chem. *254*:2619–25, 1979.

[137] Kono, T., Robinson, F. W., Sarver, J. A., Vega, F. V., and Pointer, R. H.: Action of insulin in fat cells. Effects of low temperature, uncouplers of oxidative phosphorylation, and respiratory inhibitors. J. Biol. Chem. *252*:2226–33, 1977.

[138] Whitesell, R. R., and Gliemann, J.: Kinetic parameters of transport of 3-O-methylglucose and glucose in adipocytes. J. Biol. Chem. *254*:5276–83, 1979.

[139] Olefsky, J. M.: Mechanisms of the ability of insulin to activate the glucose-transport system in rat adipocytes. Biochem. J. *172*:137–45, 1978.

[140] Czech, M. P., Massague, J., Pilch, P. F., and Carter-Su, C.: Structural aspects of the insulin effector system. N.Y. Acad. Sci. In press.

[141] Jacobs, S., Hazum, E., and Cuatrecasas, P.: The subunit structure of rat liver insulin receptor: antibodies directed against the insulin binding subunit. Submitted for publication.

Rapid Publications

Pirogliride: An Oral Hypoglycemic Drug Which Accelerates Glucose Usage and Insulin Secretion by Islets of Langerhans

WALTER S. ZAWALICH, VICTORIA A. WEILL, AND FRANZ M. MATSCHINSKY

SUMMARY

Pirogliride potentiates glucose-induced insulin secretion from isolated islets. This effect is accompanied by a facilitated glucose metabolism. Pirogliride partially prevents the known inhibitory effects of mannoheptulose on glucose-induced secretion and utilization. Pirogliride might be useful not only to probe the underlying mechanism of stimulated insulin secretion but also in the therapy of those diabetics who have an impaired β-cell responsiveness to glucose. DIABETES *29*:410–412, May 1980.

Impaired secretion of insulin in response to glucose appears to be a major defect in diabetes.[1–4] It is, therefore, a reasonable goal to develop therapeutic agents that stimulate insulin secretion by themselves or normalize the β-cells' response to glucose and possibly other physiologic stimuli as well. Orally effective sulfonylurea derivatives, which elevate serum insulin levels, have been used extensively to treat diabetics, but their safety and long-term efficacy has been questioned.[5] Recently, pirogliride [N-(1-methyl-2-pyrrolidinylidene)-N′-phenyl-1-pyrrolidinecarboximidamide] has been shown to be orally effective in producing hypoglycemia in experimental animals.[6,7] Pharmacologic studies with this drug suggested an involvement of the pancreatic β-cells, since the hypoglycemic effect was abolished in totally pancreatectomized dogs. We therefore decided to investigate whether pirogliride directly stimulates the secretion of insulin from islet tissue in vitro. The possible effect of pirogliride on glucose usage by isolated islets was also determined since the rate of glucose utilization by the tissue appears to control the rate of insulin secretion.[8–13] The results demonstrate that pirogliride (1) potentiates glucose-induced insulin secretion from isolated rat islets; (2) facilitates glucose metabolism by this tissue; and (3) partly overrides the effects of mannoheptulose, a seven-carbon sugar which in islets blocks glucose phosphorylation, glucose utilization, and glucose-induced insulin secretion.[14–17]

From the Departments of Physiology/G4, Biochemistry and Biophysics, and the Diabetes Research Center, University of Pennsylvania School of Medicine, Philadelphia, Pennsylvania.

Address reprint requests to Walter S. Zawalich, Department of Physiology/G4, University of Pennsylvania School of Medicine, Philadelphia, Pennsylvania 19104.

Received for publication 19 February 1980.

MATERIALS AND METHODS

Islets of Langerhans isolated from the pancreases of male rats fed ad lib were used. The methodology for the islet isolation with collagenase, perifusion, and metabolic studies has been previously published.[10] Briefly, groups of 50 islets were usually perifused for 30 min with 2.75 mM glucose to establish basal secretory rates and then stimulated with 5.5 mM glucose in the presence or absence of various concentrations of pirogliride, mannoheptulose, tolbutamide, or combinations of these compounds. In one group of experiments, the inslets were first perifused for 30 min without added substrate and then for an additional 30 min with 10 mM fructose, with or without pirogliride. Insulin secretion was measured by radioimmunoassay using rat insulin as standard. After the perifusion, the metabolic capacity of these islets was determined by measuring the rate of ^3H_2O formation from [5-^{3}H] glucose or [5-^{3}H] fructose (purchased from New England Nuclear, Boston, Massachusetts). The composition of the medium used for studying insulin secretion in the perifusion system, and for measuring hexose metabolism in the subsequent incubations, was the same except that the radioactive tracer was included during the incubation. While this type of sequential analysis has its shortcomings,[19] this methodology has yielded useful information on the capacity of islets to utilize various substrates and how this relates to insulin release. Most importantly, the physiologic integrity of the islets can be established (by determining the islets' secretory response) before subjecting them to the metabolic analysis.

RESULTS

When the glucose concentration in the perifusion medium was raised from 2.75 to 5.5 mM, the secretion of insulin was increased two- to fourfold (Figure 1A). The addition of 100 μM pirogliride together with 5.5 mM glucose greatly en-

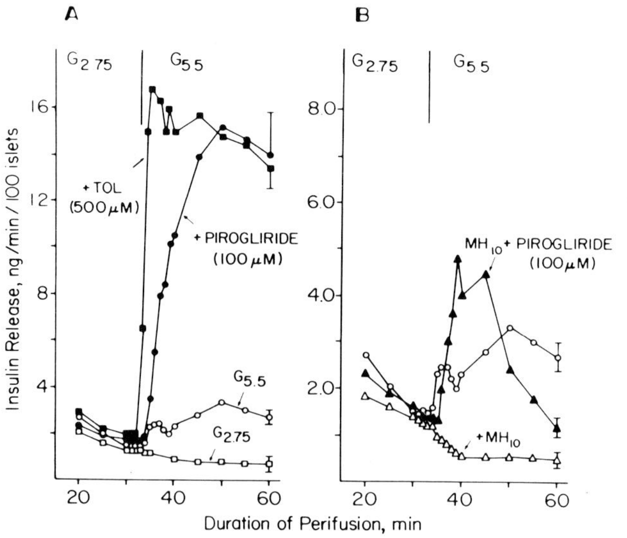

FIGURE 1. Effects of pirogliride, tolbutamide (TOL), and mannoheptulose (MH) on glucose-induced insulin release from isolated islets. (A) Groups of 50 islets were perifused for 30 min with 2.75 mM glucose. Islets were then exposed to 5.5 mM glucose alone (N = 8) or in combination with TOL (N = 3) or pirogliride (N = 7). (B) The islets were exposed to 10 mM MH with (N = 6) or without (N = 5) 100 μM pirogliride. The control response to 5.5 mM glucose is also shown for comparison. Note change in scale from (A) to (B).

hanced the secretion of insulin from islet tissue. Insulin secreted into the perifusion medium was significantly greater ($P < 0.05$, Student's *t* test) at all time points, except for the first minute of the response. With the drug present, insulin secretion was approximately fivefold greater than that observed with 5.5 mM glucose alone. In the absence of any added glucose, pirogliride at 50 or 100 μM failed to stimulate the secretion of insulin from islet tissue (N = 4 for each concentration, results not shown).

Experiments were conducted to compare pirogliride and the sulfonylurea tolbutamide. Although comprehensive dose-response studies were not performed, it was found that the insulin response to 5.5 mM glucose plus 500 μM tolbutamide resulted in a more pronounced first phase of insulin release when compared to that observed with 100 μM pirogliride (Figure 1A). The second phase release was similar with both drugs at the dosages used.

Mannoheptulose (MH) is a potent inhibitor of glucose-induced insulin secretion.[14–17] At 10 mM, MH completely blocked the insulin response to 5.5 mM glucose (Figure 1B). When 100 μM pirogliride was added together with MH, the β-cell response to glucose was partly preserved. Although insulin secretion diminished as the perifusion progressed, the total integrated insulin response to 5.5 mM glucose in the presence of 10 mM MH and 100 μM pirogliride (75 ± 10 ng/26 min/100 islets, N = 6) was comparable to that observed with 5.5 mM glucose alone (73 ± 12 ng/26 min/100 islets, N = 8).

Comparable experiments were performed with tolbutamide, glucose, and mannoheptulose. In the absence of any added glucose, 500 μM tolbutamide evoked a transient phase of insulin release (results not shown). The peak response occurred 3 min after stimulation and averaged 3.2 ± 0.3 ng/min/100 islets (N = 4) at this time point. Release quickly subsided to prestimulatory control values. In the presence of 5.5 mM glucose and 500 μM of the sulfonylurea, insulin release was greatly enhanced (see Figure 1A). The further addition of 10 mM MH to 5.5 mM glucose and 500 μM tolbutamide eliminated the potentiating effect of glucose and release was comparable to that obtained with tolbutamide alone. Peak release with this combination occurred 3 min after stimulation and averaged 3.0 ± 0.4 ng/min/100 islets (N = 4) at this time point.

Metabolic studies subsequently performed demonstrated that glucose utilization by islet tissue increased when the glucose concentration was elevated from 2.75 to 5.5 mM and that pirogliride significantly ($P < 0.05$) potentiated glucose usage at the latter concentration (Table 1, lines 3 and 4). No such acceleration of glucose metabolism was observed with 500 μM tolbutamide (Table 1, lines 5 and 6), although the insulin secretory response was comparable to that evoked by pirogliride. In addition to stimulating insulin secretion from mannoheptulose-blocked islets, pirogliride also significantly blunted the inhibitory effects of MH on glucose metabolism (Table 1, lines 7 and 8). In this group of experiments, the rates of glucose metabolism were measured in islets which were perifused with 2.75 mM glucose for 30 min and then removed for the metabolic analysis with the indicated additions. This was done because the insulin release due to this combination displayed kinetic characteristics that differed from those typical for glucose or glucose plus pirogliride. The insulin responses shown in Figure 1B were obtained in parallel experiments. In contrast to pirog-

TABLE 1
Effects of pirogliride, tolbutamide, and mannoheptulose (MH) on islet cell hexose metabolism

Substrate	N	Additions	Substrate usage, (pmol/islet) × h (mean ± SEM)
1. Glucose, 2.75 mM	8	—	32.0 ± 2.0
2. Glucose, 5.5 mM	8	—	52.2 ± 0.8
3. Glucose, 5.5 mM	3	Pirogliride, 50 μM	61.2 ± 0.9
4. Glucose, 5.5 mM	7	Pirogliride, 100 μM	66.6 ± 1.0
5. Glucose, 5.5 mM	3	Tolbutamide, 100 μM	50.3 ± 1.6
6. Glucose, 5.5 mM	3	Tolbutamide, 500 μM	50.0 ± 2.3
7. Glucose, 5.5 mM	5	MH, 10 mM	33.0 ± 2.0*
8. Glucose, 5.5 mM	6	MH, 10 mM + pirogliride, 100 μM	53.3 ± 2.0*
9. Glucose, 5.5 mM	4	MH, 10 mM + tolbutamide, 500 μM	31.5 ± 2.6*
10. Fructose, 10 mM	5	—	10.8 ± 0.3
11. Fructose, 10 mM	4	Pirogliride, 100 μM	10.4 ± 0.3

Batches of 50 islets were perifused for 30 min with 2.75 mM glucose and, in most cases, for an additional 30 min with the indicated substrate and additions (see Figure 1). In the fructose experiments, sugar was omitted from the initial 30 min period. After the perifusion, substrate usage was determined during an hour incubation with the stated additions.

* These groups of islets were perifused for 30 min with 2.75 mM glucose and then incubated with the stated additions to determine substrate usage.

liride, tolbutamide has no effect on the rate of glucose usage by mannoheptulose-treated islets (lines 7 and 9). Pirogliride did not alter the usage of 10 mM fructose by islet tissue (lines 10 and 11).

DISCUSSION

The data demonstrate that pirogliride is a potent potentiator of glucose-induced insulin secretion. Pirogliride is capable of attenuating mannoheptulose inhibition of glucose-induced insulin secretion. When compared with tolbutamide, a widely used hypoglycemic compound which is capable of weakly stimulating secretion in the absence of glucose,[20] pirogliride is effective only if glucose is present.

Perhaps the most intriguing aspect of the present report is the observation that pirogliride facilitated the utilization of glucose by islet tissue. While it might be argued that this facilitated metabolism results secondarily from an increased energy demand due to stimulated secretion, the results with tolbutamide hardly support this contention. In the presence of 5.5 mM glucose, insulin release was substantial with either 100 μM pirogliride or 500 μM tolbutamide. Only in the pirogliride-treated islets, however, is glucose usage increased. This, and the fact that pirogliride did not increase the usage of 10 mM fructose by islet tissue suggest, perhaps, that pirogliride is a specific accelerator of glucose metabolism.

While a considerable body of evidence has accumulated which supports the theory that glucose-induced insulin secretion is the result of glucose catabolism by the β-cell,[8–13] the precise nature of the intracellular trigger has, however, not been defined. The present report might be construed as evidence to support this theory. By accelerating the metabolism of glucose, pirogliride might amplify the metabolic signal normally produced by the hexose. There is evidence that pirogliride stimulates glucose oxidation of isolated muscle tissue in vitro.[21] The biochemical basis for this effect on glucose metabolism in both islet cells and peripheral tissue has yet to be elucidated.

Three pharmacologic actions of the drug fulfill the requirements of an ideal hypoglycemic agent: (1) effectiveness when administered orally, (2) potentiation of glucose-induced insulin release, and (3) direct activation of glucose metabolism. Future studies will have to be concerned with the biochemical mechanism of drug action, long-term efficacy, and with therapeutic safety.

ACKNOWLEDGMENTS

This work was supported by USPHS grants P-30 AM 19525-02S1-08 (funded through the Diabetes Research Center), ROI-AM 22122 S1, and the American Diabetes Association. Dr. Zawalich is the recipient of the 1978–1979 Elliott P. Joslin Award from the American Diabetes Association. Dr. Matschinsky is an Established Investigator of the American Diabetes Association.

Pirogliride was kindly donated by Dr. Gene Tutwiler, McNeil Laboratories, Fort Washington, Pennsylvania.

REFERENCES

[1] Brunzell, J. D., Robertson, R. P., Lerner, R. L., Hazzard, W. R., Ensinck, J. W., Bierman, E. L., and Porte, D., Jr.: Relationships between fasting plasma glucose levels and insulin secretion during intravenous glucose tolerance tests. J. Clin. Endocrinol. Metab. *42*:222–29, 1976.

[2] Cerasi, E., Luft, R., and Effendic, S.: Decreased sensitivity of the pancreatic beta cell to glucose in prediabetic and diabetic subjects. A glucose dose-response study. Diabetes *21*:224–34, 1972.

[3] Robertson, R. P., and Porte, D.: The glucose receptor. A defective mechanism in diabetes mellitus distinct from the beta adrenergic receptor. J. Clin. Invest. *52*:870–76, 1973.

[4] Palmer, J. P., Benson, J. W., Walter, R. M., and Ensinck, J. W.: Arginine-stimulated acute phase of insulin and glucagon secretion in diabetic subjects. J. Clin. Invest. *58*:565–70, 1976.

[5] The University Group Diabetes Program: A study of the effects of hypoglycemic agents on vascular complications in patients with adult-onset diabetes. Diabetes *19* (Suppl. 2):787–830, 1970.

[6] Tutwiler, G. F., Kirsch, T., and Bridi, G.: A pharmacologic profile of McN-3495 [N-(1-methyl-2-pyrrolidinylidene)-N′-phenyl-1-pyrrolidinecarboximidamide], a new orally effective hypoglycemic agent. Diabetes *27*:856–67, 1978.

[7] Tutwiler, G. F., and Birdi, G.: Comparison of McN-3495[N-(1-methyl-2-pyrrolidinylidene)-N′-phenyl-1-pyrrolidinecarboximidamide], a new orally effective hypoglycemic agent with biguanides. Diabetes *27*:868–76, 1978.

[8] Matschinsky, F. M., and Ellerman, J. E.: Metabolism of glucose in the islets of Langerhans. J. Biol. Chem. *243*:2730–36, 1968.

[9] Ashcroft, S. J. H., Bassett, J. M., and Randle, P. J.: Insulin secretion mechanisms and glucose metabolism in isolated islets. Diabetes *21* (suppl. 2):538–45, 1972.

[10] Hellman, B., Sehlin, J., and Täljedal, I.-B.: Effects of glucose and other modifiers of insulin release on oxidative metabolism of amino acids in micro-dissected pancreatic islets. Biochem. J. *123*:513–21, 1971.

[11] Hedeskov, C. J., and Capito, K.: The effect of starvation on insulin secretion and glucose metabolism in mouse pancreatic islets. Biochem. J. *140*:423–33, 1974.

[12] Malaisse, W. S., Sener, A., Koser, M., and Herchuelz, A.: Stimulus-secretion coupling of glucose-induced insulin release. Metabolism of α and B-D-glucose in isolated islets. J. Biol. Chem. *251*:5936–43, 1976.

[13] Zawalich, W. S., Rognstad, R., Pagliara, A. S., and Matschinsky, F.: A comparison of the utilization rates and hormone-releasing actions of glucose, mannose, and fructose in isolated pancreatic islets. J. Biol. Chem. *252*:8519–23, 1977.

[14] Coore, H. G., and Randle, P. J.: Regulation of insulin secretion studied with pieces of rabbit pancreas incubated in vitro. Biochem. J. *93*:66–78, 1964.

[15] Malaisse, W. S., Lea, M. A., and Malaisse-Lagae, F.: The effect of mannoheptulose on the phosphorylation of glucose and the secretion of insulin by islets of Langerhans. Metabolism *17*:126–32, 1968.

[16] Ashcroft, S. J. H., Hedeskov, C. J., and Randle, P. J.: Glucose metabolism in mouse pancreatic islets. Biochem. J. *118*:143–54, 1970.

[17] Zawalich, W. S., Pagliara, A. S., and Matschinsky, F. M.: Effects of iodoacetate, mannoheptulose, and 3-0-methylglucose on the secretory function and metabolism of isolated pancreatic islets. Endocrinology *100*:1276–83, 1977.

[18] Zawalich, W. S., and Matschinsky, F. M.: Sequential analysis of the releasing and fuel function of glucose in isolated pancreatic islets. Endocrinology *100*:1–8, 1977.

[19] Zawalich, W. S.: Intermediary metabolism and insulin secretion from isolated rat islets of Langerhans. Diabetes *28*:252–62, 1979.

[20] Grodsky, G. M., Bennet, L. L., Smith, D. F., and Nemechek, K: The effect of tolbutamide and glucose on the timed release of insulin from the isolated perifused pancreas. *In* Tolbutamide—After 10 Years. Butterfield, W. J. H., and Westering, V., Eds. Amsterdam, Excerpta Medica, International Congress Series no. 149, 1967, pp. 11–20.

[21] Tutwiler, G. F.: The hypoglycemic agent McN-3495[N-(1-methyl-2-pyrrolidinylidene)-N′-phenyl-1-pyrrolidinecarboximidamide]: Effect on glucose and fat metabolism in normal and diabetic tissue. Fed. Proc. *37*:745, 1978.

Nonenzymatically Glycosylated Serum Protein: Spurious Elevation Due to Free Glucose in Serum

ALLAN LAURENCE KENNEDY, THOMAS D. MEHL, AND THOMAS J. MERIMEE

SUMMARY

The presence of free glucose in serum was found to interfere with accurate measurement, by a colorimetric method, of nonenzymatically glycosylated serum proteins. A mean elevation to 241% of basal levels was observed in the serum of 11 nondiabetic subjects to which glucose, in a concentration of 300 mg/dl, had been added immediately before assay. After dialysis of serum samples to remove glucose, levels of nonenzymatically glycosylated serum proteins were 0.27 ± 0.11 and 0.79 ± 0.24 nmol 5-hydroxymethylfurfural/mg protein (mean ± SD), respectively, in 57 nondiabetic and 62 type I diabetic subjects. Levels observed before dialysis of serum were approximately two to three times higher. These studies indicate that removal of free sugar from serum is necessary for accurate measurement of glycosylated protein by the colorimetric method, and this can be achieved by overnight dialysis of serum against normal saline.

DIABETES 29:413–415, May 1980.

The recognition that hemoglobin undergoes postsynthetic, nonenzymatic glycosylation in vivo led to speculation that other proteins may be similarly affected.[1] Subsequently, glycosylation of lens crystallins,[2] collagen,[3] erythrocyte membrane proteins,[4] albumin, and other serum proteins [5,6] has been shown to occur in vivo.

It is known that glycosylated hemoglobin reflects the degree of glycemia in the preceding weeks to months, since erythrocytes have a half-life of approximately 60 days.[1] It has been postulated that nonenzymatic glycosylated serum protein (N.G.S.P.) levels may indicate the status of glycemia during the 1–2-wk period before measurement because serum proteins have a much shorter half-life than erythrocytes.[5] If measurement of N.G.S.P. is to be useful clinically, it is obviously important that the prevailing level of serum glucose should not interfere with its accurate measurement.

We have investigated the effect of artificially elevating the serum glucose level, just before assay, on the measurement of N.G.S.P. by a recently described method.[5] We have also investigated the effect on the measurement, in diabetic and control subjects, of removing glucose from serum by dialysis before assay. Our results show that free glucose in serum leads to spurious elevation of N.G.S.P. and that previously reported levels in diabetic and control subjects are falsely high.

METHODS

Serum was separated from venous blood samples obtained from 62 ambulatory, active, type I (juvenile-onset) diabetic and 57 normal control subjects after an overnight fast. N.G.S.P. was measured in each serum sample before and after dialysis against normal saline (18 h, serum/saline ratio of 1/350). Serum protein, both before and after dialysis, was measured by the Biuret method. Glucose was measured by a standard glucose oxidase method. Glucose was added, in increments of up to 300 mg/dl, to 11 control sera just before assay to determine whether the presence of free glucose would influence the measurement of N.G.S.P.

The method used for determinating N.G.S.P. was the one recently described by McFarland et al.[5] Glucose bound nonenzymatically to serum protein is released, by hydrolysis with 1 M oxalic acid at 100°C for 5 h, as 5-hydroxymethylfurfural (HMF), which is quantified colorimetrically by measuring the absorbance at 443 nm after reaction with thiobarbituric acid. Every sample was run in duplicate and assayed against its own blank in which the ketoamine protein derivative was reduced to a nonreactive form by $NaBH_4$.[7] The N.G.S.P. was calculated as nmol HMF/mg protein using pure 5-hydroxymethylfurfuraldehyde (Sigma Chemical Company) as standard, whereas McFarland et al. used glycosylated human albumin as standard.

From the Department of Medicine, Endocrinology Division, University of Florida, Gainesville, Florida.
Address reprint requests to T. J. Merimee, Department of Medicine, Division of Endocrinology and Metabolism, University of Florida, Box J-226, JHM Health Center, Gainesville, Florida 32610.
Received for publication 10 March 1980.

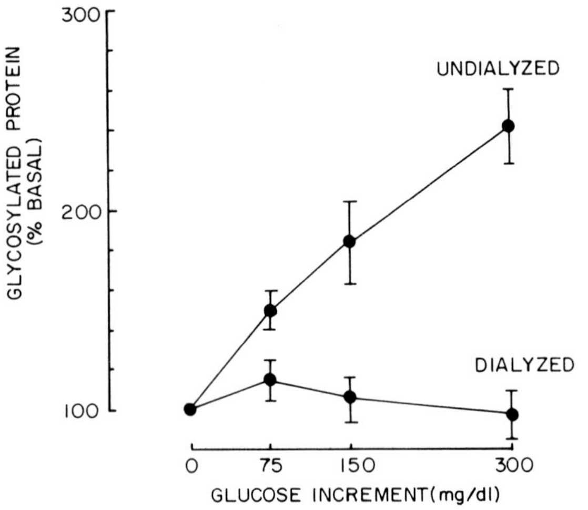

FIGURE 1. Effect on measurement of N.G.S.P. of adding glucose, in increasing concentration immediately before assay, to serum from nondiabetic control subjects. The points represent the mean values, as percent basal (no added glucose), in 11 subjects. The bars represent SEM. The lower line shows the effect of dialyzing the serum against normal saline to remove the added glucose before assay.

RESULTS

The effect of acutely increasing the glucose concentration on the measurement of N.G.S.P. in control serum is illustrated in Figure 1. There was a clear increase with increasing glucose concentration, so that in the presence of an added 300 mg/dl of glucose, artifactual elevations of 200–300% were observed. After dialysis to remove the added glucose no such increase was observed.

Serum glucose levels in the controls ranged from 51 to 108 mg/dl and in the diabetics from 27 to 538 mg/dl with a median value of 180 mg/dl. After overnight dialysis against normal saline, all serum glucose values were less than 12 mg/dl, and there was no significant difference between the levels in controls and diabetics. Mean serum protein levels before and after dialysis did not differ significantly. Figure 2 shows the levels of N.G.S.P. measured in the serum of control and diabetic subjects before and after dialysis against normal saline. Before dialysis, the mean ± SD N.G.S.P. was 0.93 ± 0.26 nmol HMF/mg protein in controls and 1.80 ± 0.63 nmol HMF/mg protein in diabetic subjects. After dialysis of serum, these values were 0.27 ± 0.11 and 0.79 ± 0.24 nmol HMF/mg protein, respectively, in control and diabetic subjects.

The intra-assay coefficient of variation for the complete N.G.S.P. assay procedure, including dialysis of serum, was 11%. The interassay coefficient of variation was 13%.

DISCUSSION

We have demonstrated that free glucose in the serum at the time of assay will cause spurious elevation of the level of N.G.S.P. as measured by the current method. It has been shown that nonenzymatic glycosylation of protein in vitro is dependent on the glucose concentration to which the protein is exposed, the length of time of exposure, and the temperature of incubation.[8] During the assay for N.G.S.P., serum and oxalic acid are incubated together for 5 h at 100°C in order to release the nonenzymatically bound glucose as 5-HMF. We would postulate that at this temperature

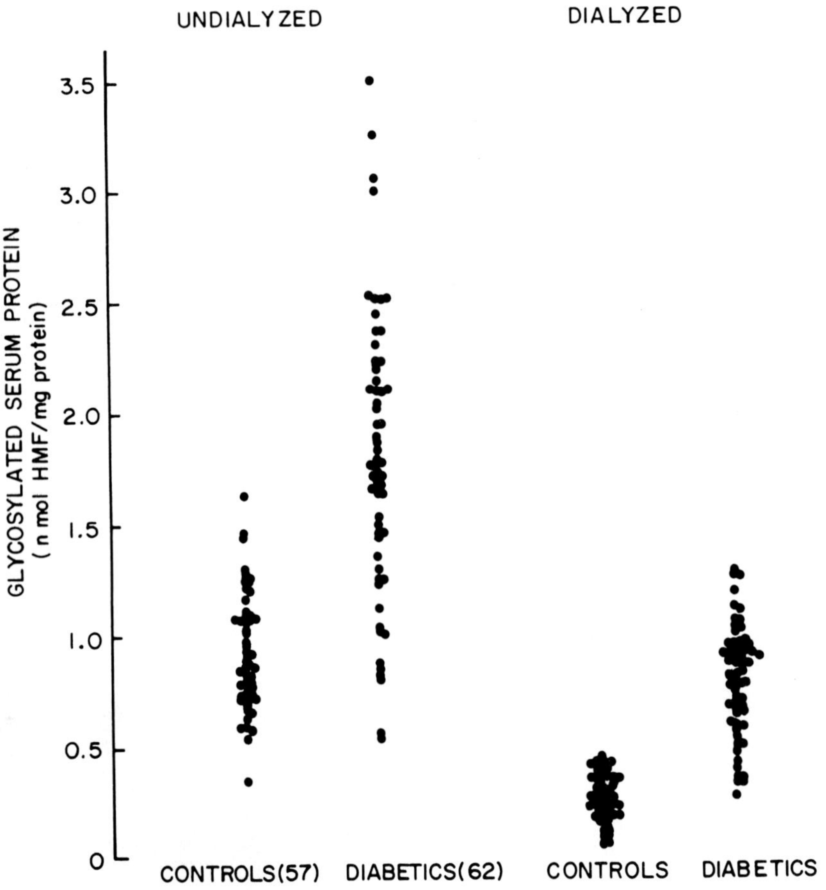

FIGURE 2. N.G.S.P. levels in 62 type I diabetic subjects and 57 age-matched controls. Sera were assayed before (left) and after (right) dialysis against normal saline.

further rapid glycosylation of protein by free sugar in the serum is enhanced, with subsequent hydrolysis and release of 5-HMF. This error can be circumvented by first dialyzing the serum to remove free glucose (Figure 1).

The ranges of values for N.G.S.P. we observed in the undialyzed serum of control and diabetic subjects were remarkably similar to those found by McFarland et al., despite the use of a different standard. However, whereas they found no overlap between diabetic and control values, 20 (32%) of our diabetics had N.G.S.P. values for undialyzed serum that were less than the highest value seen in controls. The explanation for this difference probably lies in the fact that only 3 (10%) of the South Carolina group's diabetic patients had serum glucose values of <100 mg/dl compared with 17 (27%) of ours. Therefore, there was probably less artifactual elevation of N.G.S.P. levels in those diabetic patients with low blood sugar levels. It is interesting that after dialysis of the serum to remove glucose, we found much less overlap between our control and diabetic subjects, with only 7 diabetics (11%) having values lower than the highest value in controls.

We do not dispute the conclusions of McFarland et al. that N.G.S.P. levels probably reflect the level of glycemia in the preceding 1–2 wk, as we have found a good correlation between dialyzed N.G.S.P. levels and glycosylated hemoglobin and fasting serum glucose (unpublished data). However, we believe that the actual ranges of values that we have observed in dialyzed serum are more correct. In support of this claim are the findings of Pecoraro et al.,[9] using a similar colorimetric method and 5-HMF as standard, that glycosylated hemoglobin levels range from approximately 1.3 to 5.5 nmol HMF/mg Hb in diabetic subjects. That is approximately a fourfold increase in the range that we found for glycosylated serum protein in diabetics, which would be expected since the half-life (and hence exposure to glucose) of hemoglobin is approximately four times that of serum proteins.

The main significance of our findings relates to the potential use of N.G.S.P. measurements as another index of glycemia, analogous to glycosylated hemoglobin, but reflecting glycemia over a shorter time. If the measurement is subject to error due to the prevailing level of glucose at the time the sample is drawn, then it would be of no value in many diabetic patients, particularly those with type I diabetes, where considerable perturbations of serum glucose levels may occur in minutes to hours and where successive fasting glucose levels may vary considerably without necessarily any real difference in the overall glycemia of the preceding 24 h. This problem can be overcome by dialyzing the serum before assay, a step that unfortunately, but unavoidably, lengthens the complete assay procedure. On the other hand, since many samples can be processed in one assay, measurement of N.G.S.P. has definite clinical and research potentials.

ACKNOWLEDGMENTS

We wish to thank Betty Russell for her skilled technical assistance and Dorothy Hellman for typing the manuscript.

This work was supported, in part, by grants from the National Institutes for Health, Division of Arthritis, Metabolism, and Digestive Diseases (AM-18130) and grants from the Florida Citrus Commission and the General Clinical Research Centers Program of the Division of Research Resources, National Institutes of Health (RR-00082).

REFERENCES

[1] Peterson, C. M., and Jones, R. L.: Minor hemoglobins, diabetic "control" and diseases of postsynthetic protein modification. Ann. Intern. Med. *87*:489–91, 1977.

[2] Stevens, V. J., Rouzer, C. A., Monnier, V. M., and Cerami, A.: Diabetic cataract formation: potential role of glycosylation of lens crystallins. Proc. Natl. Acad. Sci. USA *75*:2918–22, 1978.

[3] Robins, S. P., and Bailey, A. J.: Age related changes in collagen: the identification of reducible lysine-carbohydrate condensation products. Biochem. Biophys. Res. Commun. *48*:76–84, 1972.

[4] Bailey, A. J., Robins, S. P., and Tanner, M. J. A.: Reducible components in the proteins of human erythrocyte membrane. Biochem. Biophys. Acta *434*:51–57, 1976.

[5] McFarland, K. F., Catalano, E. W., Day, J. F., Thorpe, S. R., and Baynes, J. W.: Nonenzymatic glucosylation of serum proteins in diabetes mellitus. Diabetes *28*:1011–14, 1979.

[6] Dolhofer, R., and Wieland, O. H.: Glycosylation of serum albumin: elevated glycosyl-albumin in diabetic patients. FEBS Lett. *103*:282–86, 1979.

[7] Holmquist, W. R., and Schroeder, W. A.: A new terminal blocking group involving a Schiff base in hemoglobin A_{1c}. Biochemistry 5:2489–2503, 1966.

[8] Day, J. F., Thornburg, R. W., Thorpe, S. R., and Baynes, J. W.: Nonenzymatic glucosylation of rat albumin. J. Biol. Chem. *254*:9394–9400, 1979.

[9] Pecoraro, R. E., Graf, R. J., Halter, J. B., Beiter, H., and Porte, D., Jr.: Comparison of a colorimetric assay for glycosylated hemoglobin with ion-exchange chromatography. Diabetes *28*:1120–25, 1979.

Organization Section

NEW MEMBERS

The following were elected to the Professional Section on March 1, 1980:

Genrose J. Alfano, M.A., Freeport, NY
Denis G. Baskin, Ph.D., Redmond, WA
Helen C. Beaty, M.Ed., Harker Heights, TX
Otto Bellmann, M.D., Bonn, Germany
Robert S. Boltax, M.D., Derby, CT
Charles R. Bowden, Ph.D., Ft. Washington, PA
Sylvia J. Brown, B.S., Somerville, MA
Jane L. Bryant, B.S., Lexington, KY
Gery J. Cardamone, B.S., Fort Lauderdale, FL
Jose F. Caro, M.D., Rochester, NY
Margaret W. Catlin, B.S.N., Tucson, AZ
Timothy M. Chan, Ph.D., Nashville, TN
Wendy Citrin, M.S.W., Miami, FL
George E. Dailey, III, M.D., La Jolla, CA
Denis Daneman, M.B., B.Ch., Pittsburgh, PA
Brenda E. Davis, B.S.N., Macon, GA
Betty J. Diegel, B.S., Hillsdale, MI
Mary F. Donner, R.N., R.D., Santa Barbara, CA
June A. Downs, L.P.N., Brooklyn, CT
John A. Edwards, M.D., Anniston, AL
Amy D. Eliezer, M.S., Briarcliff Manor, NY
Lora N. Fairley, B.S., McAllen, TX
Barbara A. Felton, M.S., Lexington, KY
Merton C. Flom, Ph.D., Oakland, CA
Geraldine L. Francis, B.S., San Antonio, TX
Victor P. Frattali, Ph.D., Bethesda, MD
Jo Ann Greenwald, B.S.N., Hamden, CT
Neil I. Kaminsky, M.D., Albuquerque, NM
Richard C. Karl, M.D., Chicago, IL
Alan G. Kenien, M.D., Fargo, ND
James J. Lahey, M.B.A., Miami, FL
Jamie S. Lawson, Kansas City, KS
Wijdan Ali Luqman, M.B., Ch.B., Tacoma, WA
Carolé Mensing, R.N., Minneapolis, MN
Nadine E. Miller, B.S., Hollywood, FL
Gayle L. Myers, B.S.N., West Covina, CA
Takahide Nomura, M.D., Indianapolis, IN
Josephine O'Doherty, Ph.D., Greenfield, IN
Ronald P. Painton, M.D., Oklahoma City, OK
Thomas L. Paquette, Ph.D., Seattle, WA
Theodore S. Roosevelt, M.D., Glendora, CA
Frank J. Scarpa, M.D., Derby, CT
Deborah Siegler, B.H.S., Miami, FL
Linda M. Siminerio, R.N., Pittsburgh, PA
Rebecca M. Smith, B.S., North Little Rock, AR
Jan M. Smulovitz, M.D., Eugene, OR
Victor J. Stevens, Ph.D., New York, NY
Patrick A. Sullivan, M.B., B.Ch., Los Angeles, CA
Eva Tsalikian, M.D., Pittsburgh, PA
George H. West, M.D., Mason City, IA
Betty J. Whatley, M.S., Georgetown, KY
Charles A. Winterling, M.D., Concord, NH
Leonard A. Wisneski, M.D., Bethesda, MD
William F. Woodside, Ph.D., Albuquerque, NM
Marjorie A. Zigo, M.S., N. Miami, FL

TUMOR MATERIAL RESOURCES

In order to better utilize interesting and rare tumor material, a central clearing house is needed. The University of Chicago Diabetes Center offers to serve this role and will provide additional immunoassay data as well as coordinating materials for morphological and biochemical studies in other centers. Human islet or G.I. tract tumors producing any known hormone(s), but especially glucagon, somatostatin, VIP, or gastrin, as well as insulin, are of interest. Material (as much as possible) should be frozen immediately after excision and maintained at −70°C or below before and during shipment.

Please direct inquiries or notify either A. H. Rubenstein (312) 947-5536, D. F. Steiner (312) 753-3971, or H. S. Tager (312) 753-3974 concerning tumor material.

COURSE IN TEAM MANAGEMENT OF DIABETES

The Diabetes Education Center (a component of the St. Louis Park Medical Center Research Foundation) will sponsor a comprehensive five-day program, "Clinical Experience in the Team Management of Diabetes Mellitus." The course is designed for health professionals, patients, and/or family members.

The dates of the classweeks for the second half of 1980 are as follows: July 7–11 (juvenile week), 14–18, July 28–August 1; August 18–22, 25–29; September 22–26 (adult week); October 13–17 (juvenile week), 27–31; November 10–14, 17–21; and December 1-5, 15–19.

Tuition is $250. The course is approved for 34 contact hours for physicians and nurses, and for 30 clock hours for dieticians, pharmacists, and others.

For further information, contact Carole Mensing, R.N., Health Professional Coordinator, Diabetes Education Center, 4959 Excelsior Boulevard, Minneapolis, Minnesota 55416, phone (612) 920-6742.

CONFERENCE ON INSULINS AND GROWTH HORMONE

The Bureau of Drugs of the Food and Drug Administration will present a "State of the Art Conference on Insulins and Growth Hormone" on June 3–4, 1980 at the Masur Auditorium, Clinical Center, NIH, Bethesda, Maryland. Discussions will include current aspects of the use of purified insulins of animal origin as well as human insulin and growth hormone obtained through recombinant DNA technology. The program will consist of invited presentations on scientific and regulatory topics by leading investigators and officials from industry, academia, and government. The proceedings will be published.

For further information, contact John L. Gueriguian, M.D., Bureau of Drugs, Division of Metabolism and Endocrine Drug Products, FDA, 5600 Fishers Lane, Rockville, Maryland 20857.

POSTGRADUATE COURSE IN DIABETES MANAGEMENT

The Society for Continuing Medical Education in association with the American Diabetes Association will present a postgraduate course on the physiologic basis for the practical management of problems in diabetic patients. This course will be held on July 13–20, 1980 in Brussels, Belgium. Free communication is also welcome.

For further information, contact Erwin Witkin, M.D., Society for Continuing Medical Education, Suite 208, Baltimore, Maryland 21215, phone (301) 358-1541.

DIABETES AND OBESITY: CHANGING LIFESTYLES

The Professional Health Workers' Section of the Canadian Diabetic Association and the Division of Continuing Education in the Health Sciences of the University of British Columbia will present an Interprofessional Continuing Education Program entitled "Diabetes and Obesity: Changing Lifestyles" on June 9–11, 1980 at the Holiday Inn, 1133 West Hastings Street, Vancouver, British Columbia. The program is intended for all health care professionals concerned with the care of diabetic or obese patients.

For further information regarding fees and registration, contact Diabetes and Obesity: Changing Lifestyles, Room 105, I.R.C. Building, 2194 Health Sciences Mall, University of British Columbia, Vancouver, B.C., Canada V6T 1W5, phone (604) 228-2626.

BRANCHED CHAIN AMINO AND KETOACIDS

An international symposium on "Branched Chain Amino and Ketoacids: Metabolism and Clinical Implications" will be held at Kiawah Island, Charleston, South Carolina on November 15–16, 1980. The symposium's organizers are Dr. M. Walser and Dr. J. R. Williamson.

For further information, contact Beth McNamara, Department of Pharmacology, Johns Hopkins University School of Medicine, Baltimore, Maryland 21205 or Gayle Viale, Department of Biochemistry/Biophysics, University of Pennsylvania School of Medicine, Philadelphia, Pennsylvania 19104.

NEWS OF AFFILIATE ASSOCIATIONS DIABETES UPDATE 1980

The American Diabetes Association, Inc., Iowa Affiliate and Des Moines Area Community College will cosponsor "Diabetes Update 1980," a two-day educational symposium, on May 14–15, 1980, at Des Moines Area Community College, Ankeny, Iowa. Education of the diabetic and his/her family will be stressed during this symposium, which has been approved for 1.0 continuing education credits by the Iowa Nurses Association and for 10 Category 1 credit hours of the Physician's Recognition Award of the AMA.

For further information on registration, contact Alan Evan-Schwartz, American Diabetes Association, Iowa Affiliate, Professional Plaza, 5270 North Park Place NE, Cedar Rapids, Iowa 52402, phone (319) 377-4615.

Increased Glycosylation of Serum Albumin in Diabetes Mellitus

R. DOLHOFER AND O. H. WIELAND

SUMMARY

The level of glycosylated albumin has been determined in the serum of normal and diabetic subjects after purification of the albumin to apparent homogeneity. The sugar was released from the albumin preparations as 5-hydroxymethylfurfural (HMF) after 24 h of hydrolysis in 2 N acetic acid at 92°C, and it was assayed by the thiobarbituric acid reaction. The mean value for glycosylated albumin, expressed as picomoles of HMF per nanomole of albumin, obtained from 10 normal control and 65 diabetic subjects, was 64 and 124, respectively. The level of glycosylated albumin correlates with the mean blood glucose concentration ($n = 55$, $r = 0.715$), but not with the fasting blood sugar concentrations. Moreover, a linear relationship was observed between the amounts of glycosylated hemoglobin (HbA_{Ia-c}) and glycosyl-albumin ($n = 74$, $r = 0.88$). In an insulin-treated diabetic patient, there was a different temporal relationship between blood glucose concentrations and glycosylated hemoglobin and albumin levels. While HbA_{Ia-c} was lowered by only 15% after 20 days, glycosylated albumin had dropped by more than 50% during the same time. Our results indicate that glycosylated albumin might provide a valuable tool to assess the average blood sugar levels between shorter intervals, since the turnover of serum albumin is considerably faster than that of HbA_{Ia-c}, DIABETES 29:417–422, June 1980.

The development of the late complications of diabetes is widely thought to depend on careful metabolic control. Therefore, methods that are not subject to rapid fluctuations of the blood glucose level, but rather reflect the mean blood glucose level prevailing over a longer period of time, are of clinical significance. The glycosylated hemoglobins (HbA_{Ia-c}) have now become a widely used tool for assessing the long-term control of glycemia in diabetic patients.[1] However, because of the long survival time of hemoglobin, corresponding to the life span of the erythrocyte, HbA_{Ia-c} levels may remain elevated for many weeks after successful therapeutic control of blood sugar has been achieved. Searching for another more flexible parameter which might permit an evaluation of the degree of blood sugar control within shorter periods of time, we have found, in agreement with another report,[2] that, analogous to hemoglobin, serum albumin is also glycosylated nonenzymatically.[3]

These and other studies from this laboratory[4] also provided first evidence that the amount of glycosyl-albumin is increased in diabetic patients. It was the aim of the present work to substantiate our earlier finding and to establish if glycosyl-albumin levels are a function of blood glucose concentration. Such a relationship would suggest the possibility of using glycosyl-albumin as a tool for the semi–long-term control of diabetes, since the half-life of human serum albumin is much shorter (about 20 days[5]) than that of HbA_{Ia-c}.

MATERIALS

Human serum albumin, polyspecific and monospecific antisera, and M-Partigen immunoplates were from Behringwerke, Marburg. Affi-Gel Blue was from Bio-Rad, Munich. Whatman DE 52 cellulose was obtained from Hormuth & Vetter, Wiesloch. 2-Thiobarbituric acid, 5-hydroxymethyl-2-furancarboxaldehyde, D(+) glucose, and all other chemicals were from Merck, Darmstadt.

METHODS

Serum or plasma was obtained from 65 diabetic patients (ranging between 13 and 90 yr of age) and from 10 normal healthy persons (21–48 yr old).

Albumin was purified by DEAE-cellulose and Affi-Gel Blue chromatography as described,[3] except that the DEAE-cellulose was washed with 0.045 M K^+-phosphate buffer, pH 8.0, until A_{280} was near zero before the albumin was

From the Klinisch-chemisches Institut and Forschergruppe Diabetes, Städtisches Krankenhaus München-Schwabing, Kölner Platz 1, D-8000 München 40, FRG.
Address reprint requests to Prof. O. H. Wieland.
Received for publication 15 October 1979.

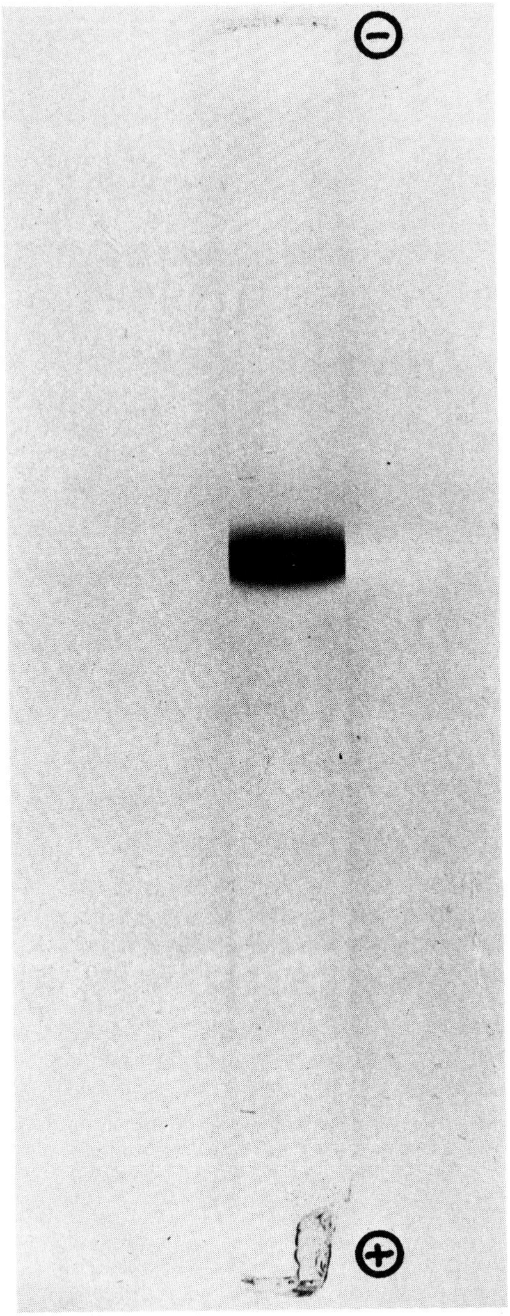

FIGURE 1. Polyacrylamide gel electrophoresis of human albumin. Albumin from a diabetic's serum was purified as described in the MATERIALS AND METHODS section, before 30 μg of protein in 0.01 ml 0.9% NaCl was applied on the gel. Electrophoresis according to the system 6 was performed as described by Maurer.[18] The gel was stained with amido black 10 B.

eluted with 0.1 M K^+-phosphate buffer, pH 8.0. For the assay of glycosyl-albumin, 0.4 ml of albumin solution (corresponding to 4 mg protein) was mixed with 0.06 ml glacial acetic acid[6] and was incubated for 24 h at a constant temperature of 92°C on an Eppendorf heating block (thermostat model 3401). Earlier studies had shown that the recovery of HMF is greatly increased at longer times of hydrolysis.[4] After cooling for about 5 min in an icebath, 0.1 ml of 3 M trichloroacetic acid (TCA) was added, and the sample was centrifuged for 5 min (Eppendorf model 5412). To 0.4 ml of the supernatant, 0.2 ml of 0.05 M thiobarbituric acid (TBA) was added, the mixture was incubated for 30 min at 40°C, and the extinction at 443 nm was measured. The concentration of 5-hydroxymethylfurfural (HMF) was calculated using a molar extinction coefficient of 4×10^4, as given by Keeney and Bassette[7] and confirmed in our laboratory. Immunoelectrophoresis was carried out according to Grabar and Wil-

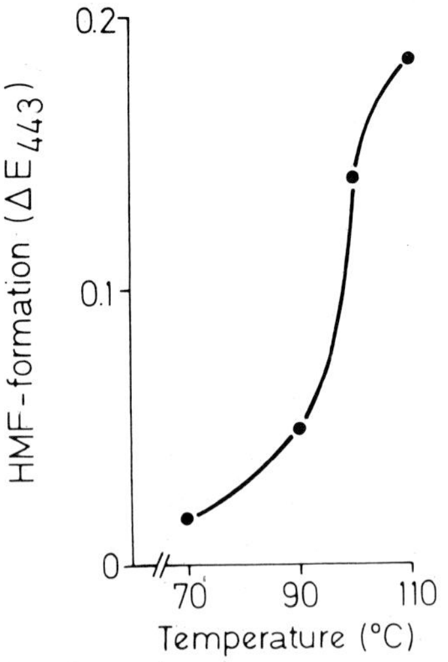

FIGURE 2. Formation of 5-hydroxymethylfurfural (HMF) as a function of temperature during hydrolysis. Commercial human albumin (10 mg/ml) was hydrolyzed in 2 N acetic acid for 24 h at the temperatures indicated before the thiobarbituric acid assay for HMF was performed as described in the MATERIALS AND METHODS section.

FIGURE 3. Formation of 5-hydroxymethylfurfural (HMF) as a function of protein concentration. Purified albumin from diabetic's serum was hydrolyzed at the protein concentrations indicated and analyzed for HMF-formation as described in the MATERIALS AND METHODS section.

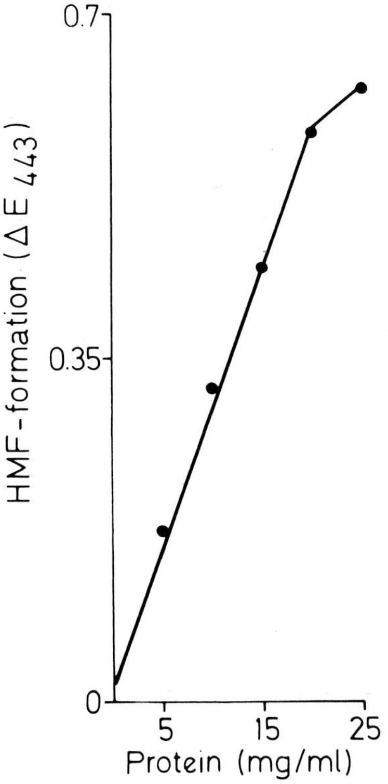

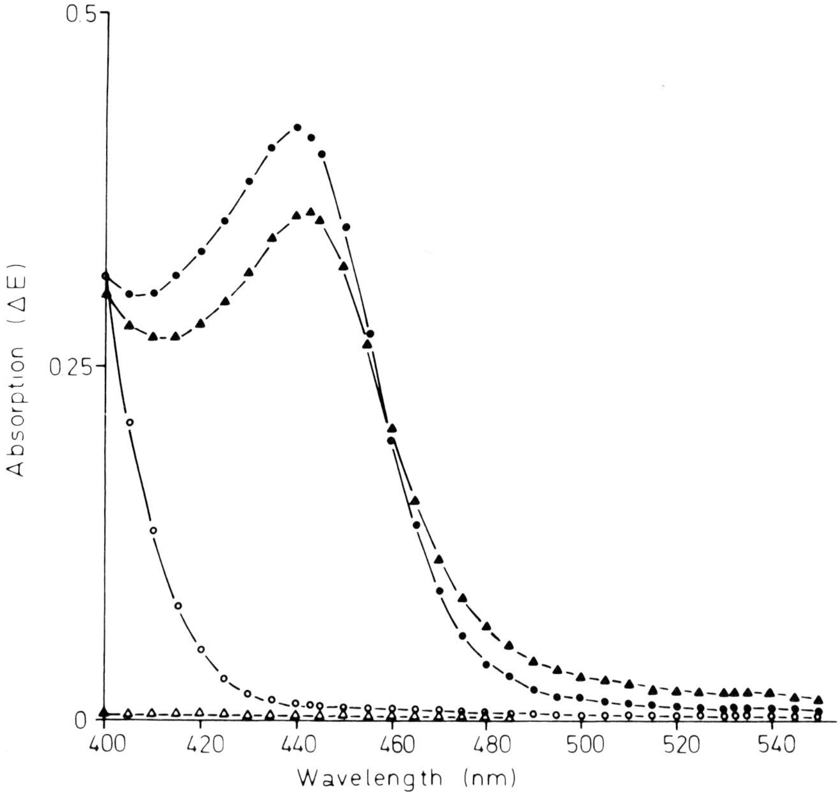

FIGURE 4. Absorption spectrum of (▲) 5-hydroxymethylfurfural(HMF)-thiobarbituric acid (TBA) adduct, prepared as described in the MATERIALS AND METHODS section, after hydrolysis of purified human albumin for 24 h in 2 N acetic acid; (●) reaction product of an HMF standard with TBA; (○) TBA, 50 mM; and (△) HMF standard, 25 μM.

liams.[8] Quantification of albumin and α_1-antichymotrypsin in purified albumin preparations was performed with M-Partigen plates according to the supplier's instruction.

Blood sugar was determined by the glucose-dehydrogenase UV method[9] (Merck, Darmstadt) and cholesterol and triglycerides enzymatically with test kits from Calbiochem (Lahn)[10] and Boehringer (Mannheim),[11] respectively. Hemoglobins A_{Ia-c} (HbA_{Ia-c}) were measured by the microcolumn method (Quick Sep, Panchem, Kleinwallstadt) according to the supplier's instruction. Protein was determined by the biuret method.[12] Serum albumin concentration was calculated from the total protein content of serum and the percentage of albumin obtained after electrophoresis of the serum on cellulose acetate. Statistical evaluation was performed according to the instructions in reference 13.

RESULTS

The determination of glycosyl-albumin in normal and diabetic sera depends on the fact that glycosyl-albumin does not behave differently from albumin during the purification procedures employed. Our studies with commercial human albumin showed that glycosylation in vitro with [^{14}C]-glucose affected neither the precipitation by $(NH_4)_2SO_4$ nor the elution patterns from DEAE-cellulose or Affi-Gel Blue, respectively (results not shown).

The purification procedure from both normal and diabetic sera yielded highly purified albumin preparations. Electrophoresis on polyacrylamide gels showed a single protein band (Figure 1). Analysis by immunoelectrophoresis displayed only trace amounts of contaminating protein. Using monospecific antisera, this was identified and quantified to be α_1-antichymotrypsin, amounting to 0.68 ± 0.07% ($\bar{x}$ ± SEM, n = 73). Previous work has shown that glucose is incorporated in vitro nonenzymatically into albumin in a form that yields HMF after acid hydrolysis.[3] The conditions of the formation of this TBA-reactive material have been studied now in more detail. The HMF-formation during 24 h proved to be extremely dependent on the incubation temperature, as shown on Figure 2. We have chosen a temperature of 92°C (precision < 0.5°C, provided by our Eppendorf equipment), because, under these conditions, all albumin samples—irrespective of the degree of glycosylation—could be assayed at the same protein concentrations, the absorption of the TBA reaction product remaining within the linear range of the standard curve. It should be noted in this context that the formation of HMF depends also on the duration of hydrolysis[4] and on the nature of the acid used.[6] Thus the HMF determined by the TBA assay represents a relative rather than an absolute value of protein glycosylation, depending on the experimental conditions.

As illustrated in Figure 3 the amount of HMF was a function of the albumin concentration employed, being linear up to 20 mg/ml. Thus, our routine assays at 10 mg/ml protein were well within the linear range. Figure 4 illustrates that the absorption spectrum of the TBA-reactive material released

TABLE 1
Levels of glycosyl-albumin (expressed as picomoles of HMF per nanomole of albumin) in normal and diabetic subjects

	n	pmol HMF / nmol Alb. ($\bar{x}$ ± S.D.)	Range
Normal controls	10	64 ± 4.6	56–72
Diabetic subjects	65	124 ± 37	61–255

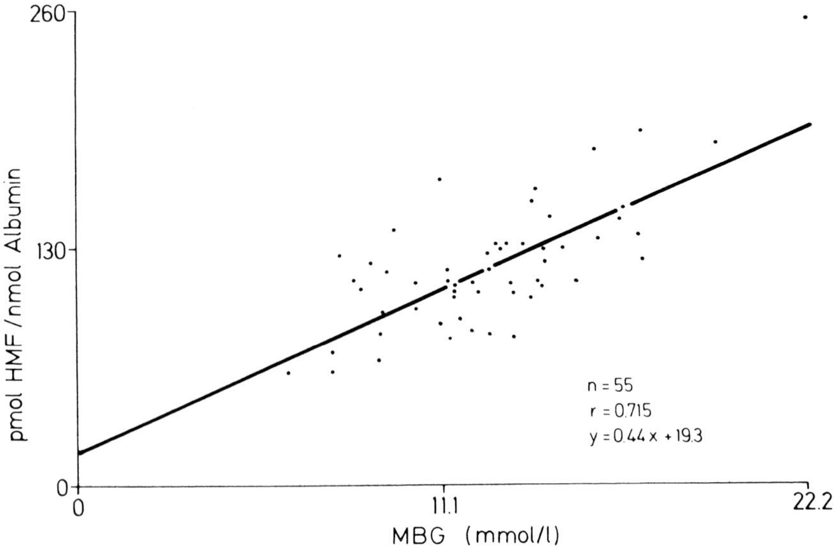

FIGURE 5. Glycosyl-albumin levels in diabetic subjects. MGB is the mean blood glucose level of the preceding 4 or 5 days. For further details, see text.

from albumin was nearly identical to that obtained from an HMF standard.

Our previous finding,[3,4] that the level of glycosyl-albumin is increased in the serum from diabetics, is substantiated by the data recorded in table 1. The amount of glycosyl-albumin, expressed as picomoles of HMF per nanomole of albumin, ranged from 56–71 and 61–255 in normal and diabetic sera, respectively. The highest degree of albumin glycosylation was displayed by the patients suffering from diabetic coma ($\bar{x} \pm SD = 187 \pm 8$ pmol HMF per nanomole of albumin, $n = 5$). The relationship between glycosyl-albumin and blood glucose within the diabetic group is illustrated in Figure 5. The mean blood glucose (MBG) level, shown on the abscissa, was calculated from all blood sugar determinations (usually taken at 0530 h, 0900 h, 1300 h, 1600 h, and 2300 h) within 4 or 5 days before blood was withdrawn for albumin analysis. Statistical analysis of the data from our diabetic patients (excluding those suffering from diabetic coma) revealed a clear correlation ($r = 0.715$, $n = 55$) between the mean blood glucose level and albumin glycosylation. This finding is comparable to a similar interrelationship already demonstrated between the degree of glycemia and the level of HbA_{Ia-c}.[14,15] It was therefore of interest to investigate whether increased albumin glycosylation is associated with elevated levels of HbA_{Ia-c}. The analysis of blood from 74 subjects, with respect to both parameters, established the regression line ($r = 0.88$) in Figure 6. In contrast with our results on the basis of MBG, no such correlation was demonstrable between glycosyl-albumin and the fasting blood sugar ($r = 0.3$, $n = 28$). However, nearly the same result as with MBG was obtained when the amount of glycosyl-albumin was correlated ($r = 0.733$, $n = 57$) with the highest single value of blood glucose found in the preceding interval of 4 or 5 days. The level of glycosyl-albumin was apparently independent of the age and body weight of the patients, the duration and therapy of their diabetes, and the blood levels of cholesterol and triglycerides. Moreover, glycosyl-albumin and total serum albumin contents were not interrelated.

Because of the relatively short half-life of serum albumin, the determination of glycosyl-albumin could be expected to provide a more flexible means of diabetes control than could HbA_{Ia-c}. This view is supported by the data summarized in Figure 7, obtained from a patient whose HbA_{Ia-c} and glycosyl-albumin levels were followed in parallel during insulin therapy for the indicated period of time. While HbA_{Ia-c} was decreased only slightly (from 20.7 to 17.5%) within 20 days of therapy, a marked lowering of glycosyl-albumin (from 208 to 91 pmol HMF per nanomole of albumin) occurred within the same time period.

DISCUSSION

The measurement of glycosyl-albumin as a tool to assess the semi-long-term control of diabetes appears reasonable, since albumin can be purified relatively easily from

FIGURE 6. Correlation between the levels of HbA_{Ia-c} and glycosyl-albumin in 10 normal and 64 diabetic subjects. The purification of albumin and the measurement of HbA_{Ia-c} were performed as described in the MATERIALS AND METHODS section.

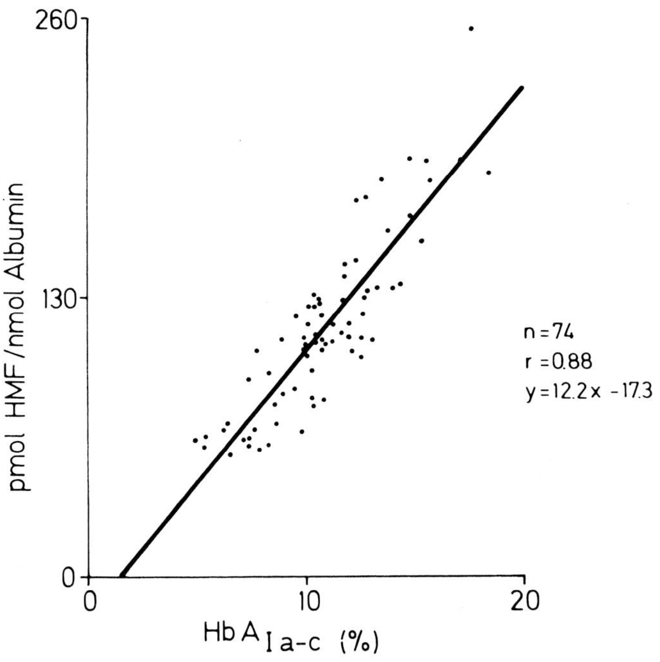

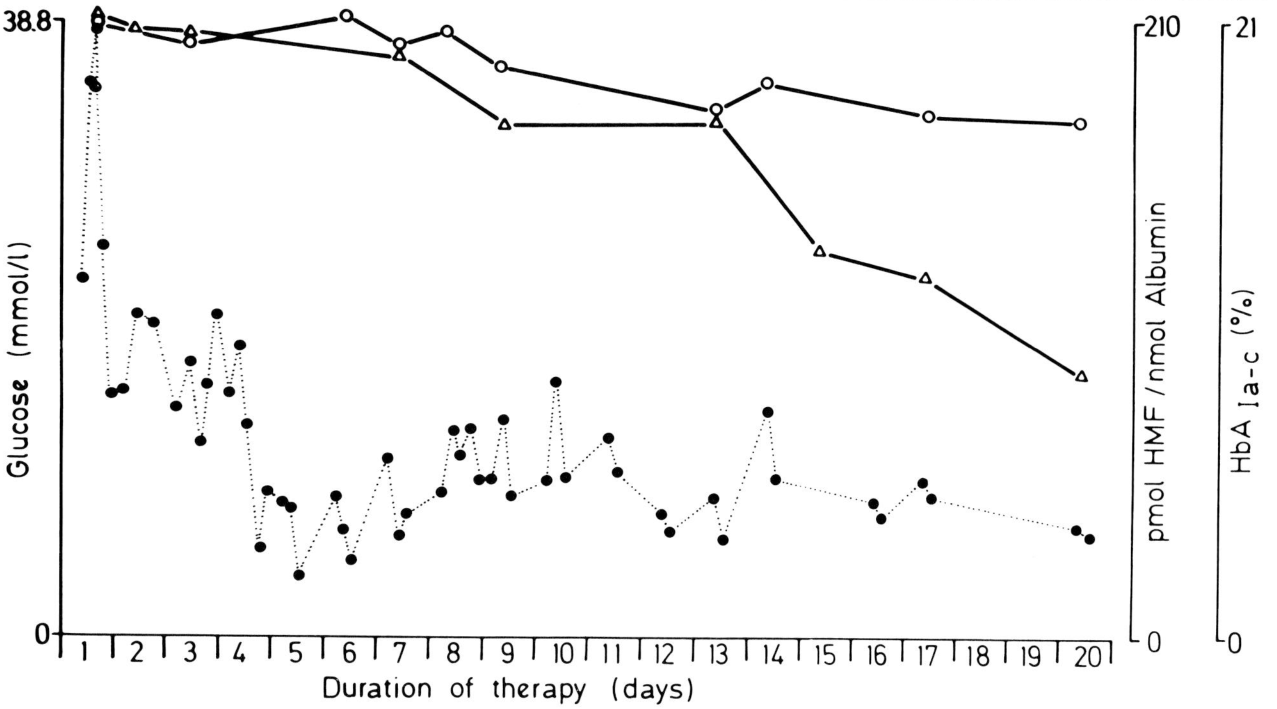

FIGURE 7. Temporal relationship between the levels of blood glucose (●), HbA_{Ia-c} (○), and glycosyl-albumin (△) in a diabetic patient during insulin therapy. For experimental details, see the MATERIALS AND METHODS section.

serum, and the TBA-reaction provides a simple and rapid means for the determination of HMF derived from glycosyl-albumin. As we have reported elsewhere, HMF can also be determined by high performance liquid chromatography using electrophoretically purified albumin samples from 100 μl serum or less.[4] Perhaps most important in this connection, however, is the fact that the circulating half-life of human serum albumin is about 20 days.[5] Although it has not been specified so far whether this rate of turnover is characteristic for both the glycosylated and the nonglycosylated forms of human albumin, it is worthwhile to note that, in any case, it is much faster than that of HbA_{Ia-c}. (For rat serum albumin, which has a half-life of 2 days, no difference in turnover was found between glycosylated and nonglycosylated forms.[16])

As to the sensitivity of albumin to monitor an increase in blood sugar, Figure 5 clearly shows that the level of glycosyl-albumin is already significantly increased at blood sugar concentrations of 8.3–11.1 mmol/l. Moreover, it is noteworthy that the level of glycosyl-albumin is a linear function of the mean blood glucose, at least up to 16.6 mmol/l. From this fact, and the data shown in Figure 7, it appears that the measurement of glycosyl-albumin may become a useful diagnostic tool capable of monitoring the state of glycemia during shorter yet still long enough periods of therapy. After submission of this paper, we became aware of the most recent results by McFarland et al.[17] on glucosylation of total serum protein. Apart from the fact that, in agreement with our earlier findings,[3] albumin was reported to represent the most abundant but not the only glycosylated serum constituent, these authors found that the degree of serum protein glycosylation is significantly correlated to the level of HbA_{Ia-c} and also to the fasting blood sugar concentration. While our results agree with respect to the correlation with HbA_{Ia-c}, we could not demonstrate a significant correlation between glycosyl-albumin and fasting blood glucose levels. The reason for this discrepancy is not known.

ACKNOWLEDGMENTS

This work was supported by the Deutsche Forschungsgemeinschaft, Bad Godesberg. The skillful technical assistance of Miss M. Schotsch and A. Militz is gratefully acknowledged. We also thank Professor H. Mehnert and his staff of the Third Medical Department of the Schwabing City Hospital for their cooperation in the studies of diabetic patients.

REFERENCES

1 Bunn, H. F., Gabbay, K. H., and Gallop, P. M.: The glycosylation of hemoglobin: relevance to diabetes mellitus. Science *200*:21–27, 1978.

2 Day, J. F., Thorpe, S. R., and Baynes, J. W.: Non-enzymatically glucosylated albumin. J. Biol. Chem. *254*:595–97, 1979.

3 Dolhofer, R., and Wieland, O. H.: Glycosylation of serum albumin: elevated glycosyl-albumin in diabetic patients. FEBS Lett. *103*:282–86, 1979.

4 Wieland, O. H., Dolhofer, R., and Schleicher, E.: Glycosylation of hemoglobin and of serum albumin in diabetes. 10th Congr. Int. Diabetes Fed. Vienna 1979, in press.

5 Schultze, H. E., and Heremans, J. F.: Molecular Biology of Human Proteins, Vol. 1. Amsterdam, New York; Elsevier/North-Holland, 1966, p. 475.

6 Gottschalk, A.: Some biochemically relevant properties of N-substituted fructosamines derived from amino-acids and N-arylglucosylamines. Biochem. Z. *42*:455–60, 1952.

7 Keeney, M., and Bassette, R.: Detection of intermediate compounds in the early stages of browning reaction in milk products. J. Dairy Sci. *42*: 945–60, 1959.

8 Grabar, P., and Williams, C. A.: Méthod permettant l'étude conjugée des propriétés électrophorétiques et immunochimiques d'un mélange de proteines Application du sérum sanguin. Biochim. Biophys. Acta *10*:193–94, 1953.

9 Dolhofer, R., Weiss, L., and Wieland, O. H.: Erfahrungen mit der Glucose-Dehydrogenase-UV-Methode zur Bestimmung der Blutglucose. J. Clin. Chem. Clin. Biochem. *14*:415–17, 1976.

[10] Allain, C. C., Poon, L., Chan, S. G., Richmond, W., and Fu, P.: Enzymatic determination of total cholesterol. Clin. Chem. *20*:470–75, 1974.

[11] Bucolo, G., and David, H.: Quantitative determination of serum triglycerides by the use of enzymes. Clin. Chem. *19*:476–82, 1973.

[12] Beisenherz, G., Boltze, H. J., Bücher, T., Czok, R., Garbade, K. H., Meyer-Arendt, E., and Pfleiderer, G.: Diphosphofructose-Aldolase, Phosphoglyceraldehyd-Dehydrogenase, Milchsäure-Dehydrogenase und Pyruvat-Kinase aus Kaninchenmuskulatur in einem Arbeitsgang. Z. Naturforsch. *8b*:555–77, 1953.

[13] Sachs, L.: Angewandte Statistik. Berlin, Heidelberg, New York; Springer-Verlag, 1974, pp. 298–344.

[14] Koenig, R. J., Peterson, C. M., Jones, R. L., Saudeck, C., Lehrman, M., and Cerami, A.: Correlation of glucose regulation and hemoglobin A_{Ic} in diabetes mellitus. N. Engl. J. Med. *295*:417–20, 1976.

[15] Dolhofer, R., Städele, A., and Wieland, O. H.: Clinical and biochemical studies on the significance and formation of hemoglobins A_{Ic} and A_{Ia+b} in diabetes mellitus. Klin. Wochenschr. *55*:945–54, 1977.

[16] Day, J. F., Thornburg, R. W., Thorpe, S. R., and Baynes, J. W.: Nonenzymatic glucosylation of rat albumin. J. Biol. Chem. *254*:9394–9400, 1979.

[17] McFarland, K. F., Catalano, E. W., Day, J. F., Thorpe, S. R., and Baynes, J. W.: Nonenzymatic glucosylation of serum proteins in diabetes mellitus. Diabetes *28*:1011–14, 1979.

[18] Maurer, H. R.: Disk-Elektrophorese. Berlin, Walter de Gruyter & Co., 1968, pp. 42–43.

Properdin Factor B(Bf) Allele Bf^{F_1} Specifies an HLA-B18 Diabetogenic Haplotype

JOHN DORNAN, PATRICIA ALLAN, ELKE P. NOEL, BODIL LARSEN, AND NADIR R. FARID

SUMMARY

We found the rare properdin factor B(Bf) variant F_1 to be present in 11% of 72 patients suffering from insulin-dependent diabetes (IDDM) compared with 2% among 150 normal controls. Bf^{F_1} thus confers a relative risk for IDDM of 5.55. All eight patients and three controls who were Bf^{F_1} positive were also HLA-B18 positive, reflecting the strong linkage disequilibrium between these two factors. We suggest that Bf^{F_1} marks a 'diabetogenic' B18-bearing HLA haplotype. Studies of unselected families with one or more affected members suggest that the B18, Bf^{F_1} does not necessarily segregate with IDDM phenotype. This study provides further evidence for the genetic heterogeneity of IDDM. DIABETES 29:423–427, June 1980.

The description of associations of HLA antigens[1,2] with insulin-dependent diabetes mellitus (IDDM) has reawakened a great interest in the genetics of this variety of the diabetes syndrome. These association studies have uncovered the heterogeneity of the disorder;[3,4] this heterogeneity becomes even more remarkable when differences in season of onset,[2-4] presence or absence of anti-islet cell antibodies[5] or of antibodies against therapeutic insulin,[6] and the progression of late complications are considered.[7] Two modes of inheritance have been forwarded by different workers: recessive[8,9] and 'overdominant';[2,10] however, polygenic inheritance cannot be excluded.[11] Attempts at linkage of a putative diabetogenic gene in the HLA region are fraught with problems—mainly of the necessary selection of multiplex families for such studies and the apparently high rate of nonpenetrance.[8,9] The relatively low expressivity probably reflects the fact that several genes as well as environmental factors are at play.[11]

From the Thyroid Research and Immunology Laboratories, Health Sciences Center, Memorial University of Newfoundland, St. John's, Newfoundland.
Reprint requests should be addressed to Dr. N. R. Farid, Thyroid Research Laboratory, 300 Prince Phillip Drive, St. John's, Newfoundland, Canada A1B 3V6.
Received for publication 9 October 1979.

In most Caucasian populations studied, an increased incidence of HLA-B8, -B15, -B18, -D(R)w3, and -D(R)w4 was found whereas -B7 and -D(R)w2 appeared to be protective against IDDM.[2,4,10,12] The D(DR) locus antigens show stronger association with IDDM than the B antigens with which they are in linkage disequilibrium i.e. DRw3 versus B8.[2,4,10] In contrast with the many studies of the HLA antigens per se, limited investigations of the association of gene products of loci that map within the major human histocompatibility complex (MHC), e.g. properdin factor B(Bf),[13,14] second and fourth complement (C_2 and C_4) components[15] with IDDM were performed. In this report we investigate the genetic polymorphism of Bf in a group of patients with IDDM and relate it to their HLA phenotypes in an attempt to confirm whether this is indeed a useful genetic marker for the disease,[16-18] quite independent from HLA.

MATERIALS AND METHODS

Seventy-two patients suffering from IDDM and 150 controls were studied for HLA antigens and Bf allotypes. We also studied 16 consecutive families in which one or more members had IDDM; in two of these families, the Bf^{F_1} allele was identified.

HLA antigens were determined by microcytotoxicity methods,[19,20] whereas Bf alleles were identified by high voltage gel electrophoresis followed by immunofixation.[21] The polymorphisms of C_2 and glyoxalase I (GLO) were determined by previously described methods.[22,23]

Relative risk and estimates of mean risk based on pooled data were calculated as described by Svejgaard et al.[24,25]

RESULTS

Eight patients with IDDM (11.1%) were found to be Bf^{F_1} positive compared with 2% of controls. Seven of these eight patients were phenotypically F_1S whereas one was F_1S_1; two of three controls were F_1S and the third, F_1S_1. The Bf gene frequencies for the IDDM group and the control group are shown in Table 1. The χ_2^2, comparing gene frequencies of these two populations, was highly significant (12.968, $P<0.001$). In view of the small numbers in the expected Bf^{F_1}

TABLE 1
Bf phenotypes and gene frequencies in controls and IDDM groups

	No. tested	Bf Phenotypes							Gene Frequencies			
		SS	FS	FF	SS_1	FS_1	F_1S	F_1S_1	Bf^S	Bf^F	Bf^{F_1}	Bf^{S_1}
Controls	150	102	38	3	2	2	2	1	0.82	0.153	0.01	0.0167
IDDM	72	49	14	—	1	—	7	1	0.833	0.0972	0.056	0.0139

The expected frequency of the Bf alleles was calculated from these gene frequencies in controls as they apply to the number of patients studied, 72. Because the expected numbers in the S_1 and F_1 cells were small, $\chi_2{}^2$ for the combinations of S_1 and F_1 was performed. This results in a $\chi_2{}^2$ of 10.01 ($P < 0.005$), with F_1 making the major contribution to this difference.

and Bf^{S_1} categories, these were combined. The difference in Bf^{F_1} and Bf^{S_1} made the major contribution to that χ^2 value (10.01). In both the controls and patients, Bf phenotypes conformed to that expected for Hardy-Weinberg equilibrium ($P > 0.2$ and $P > 0.3$, respectively).

The relative risk calculated for Bf^{F_1} amounted to 5.553 ($\chi^2 = 6.1136$, $P < 0.01$). Table 2 shows similar calculations made for the results of Raum et al.,[16] Bertram et al.,[17] and Kirk and his co-workers.[18] The estimated mean relative risk for the pooled data is 5.233 (95% confidence limits = 3.33 to 8.20), with no apparent significant heterogeneity between four sources of data.

We then examined the HLA antigens with which Bf^{F_1} was

TABLE 2
Combined estimate of the relative risk (x) of IDDM in Bf^{F_1}-positive versus Bf^{F_1}-negative individuals

	x	y	w	wy	wy^2
Present study (n = 72)	5.553	1.7144	2.08005	3.5660	6.1136
Raum et al.[16] (n = 106)	15.043	2.1711	3.8797	8.4232	18.2877
Bertram et al.[17] (n = 448)	3.373*	1.216	7.0771	8.60573	10.4648
Kirk et al.[18] (n = 239)	6.171	1.820	5.948	10.823	19.694
			18.985	31.418	54.560

If a = number of patients positive for Bf^{F_1} when b = number negative and c = number of controls positive for Bf^{F_1} when d = number negative, then relative risk (x) $= \frac{(2a + 1)(2d + 1)}{(2b + 1)(2b + 1)}$ (Haldane's modification), $\log_e$ of x = y, and variance of y is $\frac{a + b}{a \times b} + \frac{c + d}{c \times d}$; 1/variance of y = w.

The significance of y for individual studies is defined by calculating χ^2 for each study (= wy^2) with one degree of freedom. χ^2 values (or wy^2) for individual studies are summed to give total χ^2 (= Σwy^2), with degrees of freedom equaling the number of studies combined. The pooled χ^2 tests the significance of the deviation of the mean value of x from unity, = $(\Sigma wy)^2/\Sigma w$, and has one degree of freedom.

Heterogeneity of χ^2 tests consists of departure of individual values of x from the overall mean and $= \Sigma wy^2 - \frac{(\Sigma wy)^2}{\Sigma w}$, with degrees of freedom one less than the number of studies being combined.

The weighted estimated mean value of x = nat antilog $\Sigma wy/\Sigma w$ and its SE = nat antilog of $\sqrt{1/\Sigma w}$. 95% confidence limits of x = nat antilog $\Sigma wy/\Sigma w \pm (1.96 \times \sqrt{1/\Sigma w})$. *In this table,* combined mean estimate of x = 5.233, with pooled $\chi_3{}^2 = 51.99$ ($P < 0.0005$), 95% confidence limits of x = 3.33 − 8.20 and $\chi_2{}^2$ heterogeneity = 2.567, $P > 0.30$.

* Because they reported only gene frequencies, this estimate was made with the assumption that all Bf^{F_1}-positive patients and controls were heterozygous.

associated. Eleven diabetics were B18 positive; of these, eight were Bf^{F_1} positive. By comparison, 14 controls were B18 positive, only three of whom were also positive for Bf^{F_1}. We encountered no patients or controls in whom Bf^{F_1} was associated with a B antigen other than B18. Table 3 details the HLA phenotypes of the Bf^{F_1} positive patients. In only two of the eight patients was family data available for us to be certain that Bf^{F_1} B18 segregated on the same haplotype.

We previously found that HLA B18 confers[4] a moderate relative risk (2.7) for the susceptibility to IDDM, which contrasts with a value of 5.55 for Bf^{F_1}. To establish statistical comparisons between risks contributed by each factor, we tested the presence and the absence of one of the two factors (B18 and Bf^{F_1}) in patients and controls with and without the other antigen.[24] It is quite clear that (Table 4), when the influence of Bf^{F_1} was neutralized, B18 had little effect on the susceptibility to the disease. In contrast, when the influence of B18 was neutralized, it was clear that the effect of Bf^{F_1} on the susceptibility was completely restricted to B18 + ve individuals. The fact that no patients or controls were B18 − ve Bf^{F_1} + ve attests to the strong linkage disequilibrium between these two alleles.

Figure 1 shows two families studied in whom a family member was found to be positive for Bf^{F_1}. The diabetic offspring in the first family was not included in the series of 72 patients in view of the difference in the ascertainment methods. Apart from positivity for B18 and Bf^{F_1}, the components of the haplotypes in the two families were quite distinct. In one family, the diabetic child inherited the B18, Bf^{F_1} and DRw3 haplotype; in the second family, the B18 Bf^{F_1} was not transmitted to the diabetic child.

DISCUSSION

Until recently, only passing mentions were made to Bf alleles in IDDM or else MHC data of families with the disorder

TABLE 3
Phenotypes of the eight B18 Bf^{F_1}-positive patients

HLA −	A	B	C	DRw	Bf
# 1	2,_	17, 18, w4, 6	_,_	3,7	F_1S
# 2	2, 11	18, w21	ND	3,7	F_1S_1
# 3	2, w30	15, 18 w6	3,_	4,5	F_1S
# 4	2, w26	18, 40 w6	3,_	4,_	F_1S
# 5	11, 28	13, 18 w4, 6	2,5	5,7	F_1S
# 6	2, w32	18, 40	ND	ND	F_1S
# 7	1, w30	8, 18	ND	ND	F_1S
# 8	1, 9	8, 18	ND	ND	F_1S

ND = Not done.
Haplotypes associated with B18/Bf^{F_1} in controls were A28, B18; Aw30, B18; and Aw30, B18.

TABLE 4
Association of Bf^{F_1} and HLA B18 with insulin-dependent diabetes mellitus

		IDDM	Controls	χ^2	χ_2^2 sig.	χ_2^2 hetero
Bf^{F_1} +ve	B18 +	8	3*	0.00		
	B18 −	0	0			
Bf^{F_1} −ve	B18 +	3	11	0.2009		
	B18 −	61	136			
Totals				0.2009	0.7647 (P > 0.60)	0.6025 (P > 0.70)
B18 +	Bf^{F_1} +	8	3	4.6616		
	Bf^{F_1} −	3	11			
B18 −	Bf^{F_1} +	0	0	0		
	Bf^{F_1} −	61	136			
Totals				4.6616	6.4674 (P < 0.025)	0.6778 (P > 0.60)

To determine primacy of association, we examined the relation of Bf^{F_1} with IDDM after dividing the patients and controls into B18+ and B18− subgroups (upper panel) and that of HLA B18 with IDDM after dividing the patients and controls into Bf^{F_1} + and Bf^{F_1} − subgroups (lower panel).

* Haldane's modification for small numbers and reference 24 were used to calculate relative risk (x).

were detailed without comment.[26–28] Thus, Cudworth[26] noted that Bf^S is increased in IDDM, whereas a perusal of Rubenstein's[27,28] data indicates an increased incidence of the rare allele Bf^{F_1} in IDDM families. More recently, Raum et al.[16] reported that Bf^{F_1} was found in 22.6% of patients with IDDM compared with 1.9% of controls. On the basis of these findings as well as family data, they postulated a diabetogenic gene linked to Bf and in strong linkage disequilibrium with Bf^{F_1}. Unfortunately, these authors have not detailed their HLA data; this would have been of particular interest, as their high Bf^{F_1} gene frequency is probably explicable by the high proportion of Bostonians of Mediterranean extraction and, therefore, with high HLA B18 frequency. Independently, Bertrams et al.[17] reported a significant increase in the gene frequency of Bf^{F_1} in IDDM patients compared with controls; moreover, this difference became much more marked when the incidence of the haplotype B18, Bf^{F_1} was compared. Although Kirk et al.[18] typed their patients for HLA, they only reported a negative association between Bf^{F_1}, Bf^{S_1}, and BF^F with HLA B8; they did comment on the association of the former allele with B18.

The present study concurs with the previous reports,[16–18] in showing that Bf^{F_1} is increased in IDDM. We found 11% of these patients to be positive for Bf^{F_1} compared with a figure of 22.6% in Boston, 11.7% in Melbourne, and 6.0% in the German study (control frequency of Bf^{F_1} was about 1.9% in all four studies). No significant heterogeneity was found between these three sets of data. Our findings agree with those of Bertrams et al.[17] in that a greater increase of B18 Bf^{F_1} haplotype was observed—in fact, all eight Bf^{F_1}-positive individuals were positive for B18. The greater degree of haplotypic association observed by these authors probably reflects the increase in B18 and Bf^{F_1} in the IDDM group compared with controls. In two of four of these studies,[17,*] no significant increase in Bf^{S_1} was observed in patients suffering from IDDM, whereas Kirk et al.[18] commented on such an increase. Bf^{S_1} is in linkage disequilibrium with HLA B12 and B21.[21] Altogether, these findings from populations with different ethnic backgrounds suggest that the increase in the gene frequency of Bf alleles among patients suffering from IDDM reflects the MHC haplotypes in linkage disequilibrium. In this study, six of the eight patients who were positive for B18 Bf^{F_1} were of English or Irish origin and two were of French background.

* The data reported here.

The nature of the association of Bf^{F_1} with IDDM then becomes a matter for interpretation: is this Bf allele primarily associated with IDDM or is it secondary to the increase of B18 in IDDM? The statistical treatment of the data (Table 4) shows that Bf^{F_1} was more strongly associated with IDDM than was B18, the apparent association of the latter antigen being due to its strong linkage disequilibrium with Bf^{F_1}. Bf^{F_1} has been described to maintain strong linkage disequilibrium with B18 in several populations.[21,29–32] The question then becomes: is there a diabetogenic gene close to the Bf locus, which appears to be very close indeed to the HLA-B locus,[14,15] or does Bf^{F_1} mark specific B18-bearing haplotypes that are particularly diabetogenic? The statistical demonstration of the apparent primacy of Bf^{F_1} does not answer this question. However, the fact that Bf^{F_1} rarely occurs in B18-negative haplotypes supports our contention that B18 Bf^{F_1} haplotype is specifically diabetogenic, as has been shown for B8, DRw3 and B15, DRw4 haplotypes.[4] This would not be surprising, in view of preliminary evidence from this laboratory, suggesting that unusual HLA haplotypic arrangements are encountered in autoimmune endocrine diseases.[33,34] This includes distortion of C_2 alleles/HLA-B association in Graves' disease[33] and the concurrence of B8 with Bf^F in polyglandular autoimmune syndromes comprising Graves' disease.[34]

This finding of an association of Bf^{F_1} with IDDM raises an issue as to the mechanism of its action. Bf is crucial to the activation of the alternate complement pathway.[13–15,34] To our knowledge, there has been no indication that specific Bf allelic gene products are biologically more effective than

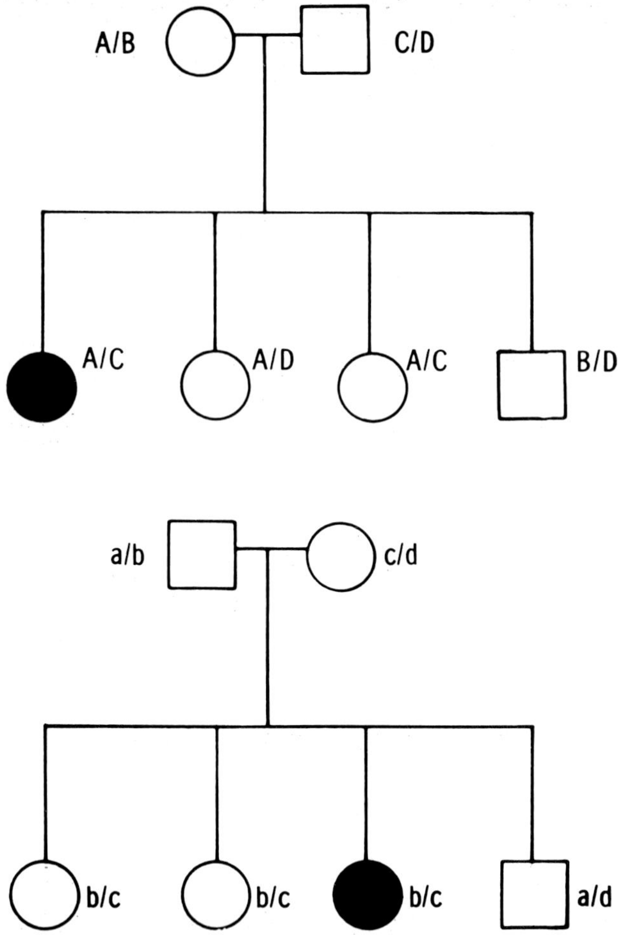

FIG. 1. The families with Bf^{F_1} identified: ○ female, □ male, and ● IDDM.

Haplotypes are as follows:
A = A30, B18, Cw-, DRw3, Bf^{F_1}, C_2^1, GLO^1
B = A2, Bw38, Cw-, DRw7, Bf^S, C_2^1, GLO^1
C = A24, B35, Cw4, DRw5, Bf^S, C_2^1, GLO^2
D = A3, B7, Cw-, DRw2, Bf^S, C_2^1, GLO^1

a = A2, B18, Cw-, DRw_, Bf^{F_1}, GLO^2
b = A3, B7, Cw-, DRw4, Bf^S, GLO^2
c = A2, B40, Cw2, DRw3, Bf^S, GLO^2
d = A2, B40, Cw3, DRw4, Bf^S, GLO^2

others nor that certain HLA antigens affect the level of Bf biologic activity.

HLA-B18 is the antigen most frequently associated with C_2 deficiency;[36] however, the haplotype active in that disorder comprises D(R)w2, an antigen rarely encountered in IDDM.[4,10,12] Indeed, its presence in the genotype appears to protect against IDDM.[4,10] In this study we did not find any DRw2-positive individuals among the B18 Bf^{F_1} patients. Therefore, if B18 is required to determine serum Bf level, a haplotypic arrangement other than B18/DRw2 may be necessary.

Our results in the two families in which one parent was positive for B18 Bf^{F_1} serve to remind us that this haplotype is not a necessary accompaniment to the IDDM phenotype in such families; in only one of the two families did Bf^{F_1} B18 pass on to an affected family member. Thus, one such family was encountered among 16 consecutive simplex or multiplex families studied, which compares well with an incidence of Bf^{F_1} positivity of 11% among the population of juvenile diabetics studied. It may be speculated that the dissociation between B18 Bf^{F_1} and IDDM in the second family was likely related to the fact that haplotypes b/c (Figure 1) ensured an HLA phenotype (DRw3/DRw4 heterozygote) associated with an enhanced susceptibility to IDDM.[4]

Our findings that, in family 1, the diabetic child was B18 and Bf^{F_1} as well as DRw3 positive led us to examine HLA DRw phenotypes of the B18 Bf^{F_1} patients to see whether this diabetogenic haplotype may be further specified by the associated DRw allele. Our data are limited in that respect; however, it would be important to examine the haplotypic arrangement of B18, Bf^{F_1}, DRw alleles in data from larger series of patients to answer this question. In a preliminary report by Deschamp et al.,[37] the finding that the Bf^{F_1} is a component of the haplotype Aw30, Cw5, B18, Bf^{F_1}, DRw3 observed in significantly higher frequency and linkage disequilibrium, at least in French IDDM patients, is informative in this context. Our results in this and previous studies[4] do not conflict with the proposals by Raum et al.[16] for a recessive or dominant diabetogenic gene linked to Bf^{F_1} and which is incompletely penetrant. Sibpair studies, which show that some two-thirds of such pairs are HLA identical as well as the increased risk attached to DRw3/DRw4 heterozygosity, suggest that, for the susceptibility to IDDM to be expressed, both parental haplotypes may be necessary,[2–4,10,26] only one of which will be B18, Bf^{F_1} (in view of the rarity of this allele), and that in only 11% of patients. It is apparent that the possible HLA phenotypes of diabetic patients are numerous indeed. Taken with the additive influence of certain HLA alleles on disease susceptibility, the difference in seasonal variation, presence and persistence of anti–B cell antibodies, and reported association with retinopathy[2–4] further underscores the heterogeneity of the genetic basis of IDDM.

ACKNOWLEDGMENTS

We wish to thank Dr. William H. Marshall and Ruth Grandy for carrying out C_2 allotyping, Dr. Ronald Payne for Glo typing, and Roxanne Butler for secretarial assistance. John Dornan and Patricia Allan were supported by Faculty of Medicine Summer Studentships.

This work was supported by a grant from the National Foundation–March of Dimes (7-127).

REFERENCES

[1] Nerup, J., Platz, P., Ortved Anderson, O., Christy, M., Lyngsøe, J., Poulsen, J. E., Ryder, L. P., Staub Nielsen, L., Thomsen, M., and Svejgaard, A.: HLA antigens and diabetes mellitus. Lancet *2*:864–66, 1974.

[2] Nerup, J., Cathelineau, C. R., Seignalet, J., and Thomsen, N.: HLA and endocrine diseases. *In* HLA and Disease. Dausset, J., and Svejgaard, A., Eds. Copenhagen, Munksgaard, 1977, pp. 46–71.

[3] Rotter, J. I., and Rimoin, D. L.: Heterogeneity in diabetes mellitus—update 1978. Evidence for further genetic heterogeneity within juvenile-onset insulin-dependent diabetes mellitus. Diabetes *27*:599–608, 1978.

[4] Farid, N. R., Sampson, L., Noel, P., Barnard, J. M., Davis, A. J., and Hillman, D. A.: HLA-D–related (DRw) antigens in juvenile diabetes mellitus. Diabetes *28*:552–57, 1979.

[5] Irvine, W. J., McCallum, C. J., Gray, R. S., Campbell, C. J., Duncan, L. J. P., Farquhar, J. W., Vaughan, H., and Morris, P. J.: Pancreatic islet-cell antibodies in diabetes mellitus correlated with the duration and type of diabetes, coexistent autoimmune disease, and HLA type. Diabetes *26*:138–47, 1977.

[6] Bertrams, J., Janse, F. K., Gruneklee, D., Reis, H. E., Drost, H., Gries,

F. A., and Kuwert, E.: HLA antigens and immunoresponsiveness to insulin in insulin-dependent diabetes mellitus. Tissue Antigens *8*:13–19, 1976.

[7] Barbosa, J., Noreen, H., Emme, L., Goetz, F., Simmons, R., de Leiva, A., Najarian, J., and Yunis, E. J.: Histocompatibility (HLA) antigens in diabetic microangiopathy. Tissue Antigens *7*:233–37, 1976.

[8] Rubinstein, P., Suciu-Foca, N., and Nicholson, J. F.: Genetics of juvenile diabetes mellitus. A recessive gene closely linked to HLA D and with 50 percent penetrance. N. Engl. J. Med. *297*:1036–40, 1977.

[9] Barbosa, J., King, R., Noreen, H., and Yunis, E. J.: The histocompatibility (HLA) system in juvenile insulin dependent diabetic multiplex kindreds. J. Clin. Invest. *60*:989–98, 1977.

[10] Thomson, M., Platz, P., Christy, M., Nerup, J., Ryder, L. P., and Svejgaard, A.: HLA-D-associated resistance and susceptibility to insulin-dependent diabetes mellitus. Transplant. Proc. *11*:1307–08, 1979.

[11] Neel, J. V.: The genetics of juvenile-onset-type diabetes mellitus (Editorial). N. Engl. J. Med. *297*:1062–63, 1977.

[12] Ilonen, J., Herva, E., Tillikainen, A., Åkerbolm, H. K., Loivukangas, T., and Kouvalainen, K.: HLA Dw2 as a marker of resistance against juvenile diabetes mellitus. Tissue Antigens *11*:144–46, 1978.

[13] Alper, C. A., Boenisch, T., and Watson, L.: Genetic polymorphism in human glycine-rich beta-glycoprotein. J. Exp. Med. *135*:68–80, 1972.

[14] Allen, F. H., Jr.: Linkage of HL-A and GBG. Vox Sang. *27*:382–84, 1974.

[15] Lachman, P. J., and Hobart, M. J.: Complement genetics in relation to HLA. Br. Med. Bull. *34*:247–52, 1978.

[16] Raum, D., Alper, A. C., Stein, R., and Gabbay, K. H.: Genetic marker for insulin dependent diabetes mellitus. Lancet *1*:1208–10, 1979.

[17] Bertrams, J., Baur, M. P., Grüneklee, D., and Gries, F. A.: Association of Bf^{F}1, HLA-B18 and insulin-dependent diabetes mellitus. Lancet *2*:98, 1979.

[18] Kirk, R. L., Theophilus, J., Whitehouse, S., Court, J., and Zimmet, P.: Genetic susceptibility to diabetes mellitus: the distribution of properdin factor B(Bf) and glyoxalase (GLO) phenotypes. Diabetes *28*:949–51, 1979.

[19] Mittal, K. K., Mickey, M. R., Singal, D. P., and Terasaki, P. I.: Serotyping for homotransplantation. XVIII. Refinement of microdroplet lymphocyte cytotoxicity test. Transplantation *6*:913–27, 1968.

[20] Farid, N. R., Sampson, L., Noel, E. P., Barnard, J. M., Mandeville, R., Larsen, B., Marshall, W. H., and Carter, N. D.: A study of human leukocytes D locus related antigens in Graves' disease. J. Clin. Invest. *63*:108–13, 1979.

[21] Larsen, B., Arnason, A., Barnard, J. M., Buehler, S. K., Edwards, J. H., and Marshall, W. H.: Bf types of HLA haplotyped individuals in an isolated Newfoundland population. Tissue Antigens *10*:403–09, 1977.

[22] Meo, T., Atkinson, J., Bernoco, M., Bernoco, D., and Cepellini, R.: Mapping of HLA locus controlling C2 structural variants and linkage disequilibrium between C_2^2 and Bw15. Eur. J. Immunol. *6*:916–19, 1976.

[23] Parr, W., Bagster, I., and Welch, S. G.: Human red cell glyoxalase I polymorphism. Biochem. Genet. *15*:109–33, 1977.

[24] Svejgaard, A., Jersild, C., Staub-Nielsen, L., and Bodmer, W. F.: HLA antigens and disease. Statistical and genetical considerations. Tissue Antigens *4*:95–105, 1974.

[25] Svejgaard, A., and Ryder, L. P.: Associations between HLA and disease. Notes on methodology and a report from the HLA and disease registry. *In* HLA and Disease. Dausset, J., and Svejgaard, A., Eds. Copenhagen, Munksgaard, 1977, pp. 46–71.

[26] Cudworth, A. G.: Type I diabetes mellitus. Diabetologia *14*:281–91, 1978.

[27] Rubinstein, P., Suciu-Foca, N., Nicholson, J. F., Fotino, M., Molinaro, A., Harisiadis, L., Hardy, M. A., Reemstma, K., and Allen, F. H., Jr.: The HLA system in the families of patients with juvenile diabetes mellitus. J. Exp. Med. *143*:1277–82, 1976.

[28] Suciu-Foca, N., and Rubinstein, P.: Complete HLA and Bf typing in families: II Bf and the structure of the HLA region. Transplant. Proc. *9* (Suppl. 1):83–86, 1977.

[29] Rittner, C., Grosse-Wilde, H., Rittner, B., Metzel, B., Scholz, S., Lorenz, H., and Albert, E. D.: Linkage group HL-A-MLC-Bf (properdin factor B). Humangenetik *27*:173–83, 1975.

[30] Bijnen, B. B., Schreuder, I., Khan, P. M., Allen, F. H., Giles, C. M., Lost, W. R. T., Volkers, W. S., and van Rood, J. J.: Linkage relationship of the loci of the major histocompatibility complex in families with a recombination in the HLA region. J. Immunogenet. *3*:171–83, 1976.

[31] Marcelli-Barge, A., Benjam, A., Poirier, J. C., Nunez-Roldan, A., and Dausset, J.: Observation of an HLA-Cw5, B18, Bf^{F}1 linkage disequilibrium in women. Tissue Antigens *10*:228, 1977.

[32] Arnason, A.: Personal communication, 1977.

[33] Noel, E. P., Sampson, L., Pepper, B. M., and Farid, N. R.: Polymorphism of the second component of complement (C2) in Graves' disease. Hum. Hered. (in press) 1980.

[34] Farid, N. R., Larsen, B., Payne, R., Noel, E. P., and Sampson, L.: Polyglandular autoimmune disease and HLA. Tissue Antigens (in press) 1980.

[35] Fearon, D. T., Austen, K. F., and Ruddy, S.: Properdin factor D: characteristics of its active site and isolation of the precursor form. J. Exp. Med. *139*:355–66, 1974.

[36] Day, N. K., L'Esperance, P., Good, R. A., Michael, A. F., Hansen, J. A., Dupont, B., and Jersild, C.: Hereditary C2 deficiency: genetic studies and association with the HL-A system. J. Exp. Med. *141*:1464–69, 1975.

[37] Deschamps, L., Lestradet, H., Marcelli-Barge, A., Benajam, A., Busson, M., Hors, J., and Dausset, J.: Properdin factor B alleles as markers for insulin-dependent diabetes. Lancet *2*:793, 1979.

Low Plasma Levels of Pancreatic Polypeptide in Obesity

VÉRONIQUE LASSMANN, PHILIPPE VAGUE, BERNARD VIALETTES, AND MARIE-CHRISTINE SIMON

SUMMARY

Plasma levels of pancreatic polypeptide (PP) were studied in a group of 22 normal and 22 obese subjects after an overnight fast. In a second group of 10 normal and 13 obese adults, PP secretion was stimulated by a protein-rich meal. The results indicate lower fasting PP values in the obese subjects and a decreased response during the second phase of the meal-induced secretion. This could suggest a possible role of PP in obesity. DIABETES *29*:428–430, June 1980.

Pancreatic polypeptide (PP) was identified during purification of insulin in the chicken[1] and in mammalians.[2] Although the structure of PP and the factors leading to its secretion are fairly well known at present, its role in physiologic and pathologic conditions is still unclear. PP may contribute to the regulation of satiety: in ob-ob mice it has been shown that injection of bovine PP results in reduction of both food intake and weight gain.[3] Similarly, complete regression of the obesity-hyperglycemia-hyperinsulinism syndrome has been observed in NZO mice after intraperitoneal injection of PP.[4]

Based on these experimental data in animals, the aim of this study was to see whether plasma levels of PP are modified in human obesity. For this purpose, plasma levels of PP in the fasting state and after stimulation by a protein-rich meal were compared in obese and normal adults.

METHODS

Subjects and test procedures. After an overnight fast, plasma PP levels were measured at 0800 h in 22 normal volunteers (6 males and 16 females) and in 22 obese adults (5 men and 17 women) (mean weight excess, 65%), with normal glucose tolerance, aged 20 to 40 yr.

In another series of 10 normal healthy (five men and five women) and 13 obese adults (2 men and 11 women), (mean weight excess, 73%) with normal glucose tolerance, of mean age 30.1 and 28.8 yr, respectively (no significant age difference), provocative testing was performed.

In the two series, all subjects were on the same standard hospital diet (9.2 kJ, 300 g carbohydrate) before testing. A protein-rich breakfast (2.5 kJ, 80 g protein) consisting of cheese (100 g), ham (50 g), powdered milk (40 g), bread (30 g), tea, and sugar (10 g) was rapidly ingested. Plasma PP, insulin, glucagon, glucose, and free fatty acid (FFA) levels were determined 15 min before, at the onset, and 5, 10, 20, 30, 60, 120, 180, and 240 min after ingestion.

Assays. Plasma PP was determined by radioimmunoassay using human PP as a standard and bovine PP as a tracer after labeling by I^{125} with chloramine-T followed by purification on Biogel P2 and P10 columns. Binding was achieved using rabbit anti-hPP serum (lot 615-1054 B-248-19). These products were the generous gift of Dr. R. Chance. Bound and free fractions were separated by precipitation with anti-rabbit serum.

Plasma glucose was determined using an AutoAnalyzer, FFA according to Dole's method, and plasma insulin and glucagon were measured with commercial radioimmunoassay kits (kits from Sorin and Hypolab).

Statistical analysis. Differences in plasma values between obese and control subjects were analyzed using the Student's *t* test.

RESULTS

Fasting plasma PP levels were significantly lower ($P < 0.001$) in the obese subjects (14.49 ± 2.75 pmol/L) compared with controls (27.1 ± 2.6 pmol/L).

Figure 1 shows the results obtained after ingestion of the protein-rich breakfast:

–Control subjects displayed a biphasic response with an initial rise in plasma PP reaching 118.5 ± 16.1 pmol/L after 5 min, followed by a decrease to 88.5 ± 19.0 pmol/L at 30 min. A second prolonged rise in plasma PP was then observed, extending to 240 min, with a maximum of 144.7 ± 17.3 pmol/L at 180 min.

From the Internal Medicine Unit, University Hospital Michel Lévy, Marseille, France.
Address reprint requests to V. Lassmann.
Received for publication 14 November 1979.

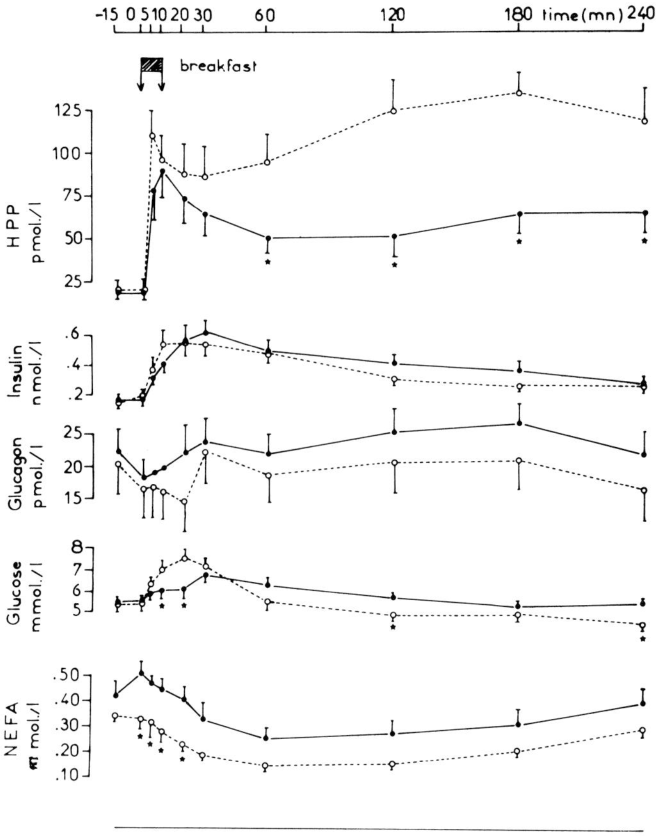

FIGURE 1. Hormonal and metabolic responses to protein-rich meal in 10 normal weight (○---○) and 13 obese (●—●) subjects; asterisks denote statistically significant differences ($P < 0.05$).

Males had slightly higher basal PP levels than females, but over the entire test, they displayed a lower rise in plasma PP levels. So, we considered males and females as a whole for the control group.

–A similar PP secretion pattern was found in the obese group. Nevertheless, although the first plasma peak was not significantly different from that in the controls (spike at 10 min; mean value, 96.6 ± 16.6 pmol/L), plasma PP values throughout the second rise were significantly lower (P between 0.02 and 0.002) in the obese subjects.

–Regarding the other measured plasma components, insulin and glucagon levels were not significantly different between obese and control subjects, whereas glucose levels in the obese group were slightly lower ($P < 0.05$ at 10 and $P < 0.01$ at 20 min) during the first 60 min after ingestion and slightly higher ($P < 0.01$ at 120 and 240 min) thereafter.

Plasma FFA levels were higher in the obese subjects than in the controls [significant difference ($P < 0.02$) at 0, 5, 10, and 20 min after ingestion], but both groups displayed parallel patterns during the test.

DISCUSSION

Results of this study show that plasma PP levels in obese individuals after an overnight fast and during the second phase of secretory response to a protein-rich meal are lower than in nonobese healthy adults.

Plasma PP levels increase with age,[5] but in our series obese and normal weight subjects had the same age range and mean. Lower PP levels in females than in males have been reported.[6] An excess of female representation in the obese group cannot explain the results observed in our study. Indeed, the sex ratio was the same among the control (6 M, 16 F) and obese subjects (5 M, 17 F) in whom basal PP levels were compared.

In the provocative test study, the control group comprised a lower proportion of females (5/10) than did the obese group (11/13). Normal females had, in fact, slightly lower basal PP levels than did normal males. But these levels increased more than those of males after stimulation at all times of sampling (statistical analysis was not performed because of the small number of subjects of the two sexes). Therefore, the larger number of females in the obese group cannot be responsible for the decreased poststimulative PP levels observed.

Decreased PP levels found in the obese could be the result of increased metabolic clearance. However, PP is not metabolized but is eliminated in its active form by the kidney.[7] Even though glomerular flow is slightly increased in the obese, this phenomenon does not suffice to account for these lower PP levels.

Accordingly, we are led to suggest the presence of decreased secretion of PP in the obese. As previously described by Fajans,[8] Adrian,[9] and Schwarz,[10] a biphasic PP secretory response is observed. The first phase seems to be mainly under vagal control.[11] Conversely, the second secretory phase would depend not only on vagal control but also on poorly recognized metabolic or hormonal factors.[9,11] It is interesting to note that the difference we observed between control and obese subjects was found during this second secretory phase.

This difference in plasma PP levels does not seem to be related to any of the other hormonal parameters studied, since the latter did not differ between the two groups.

Hypoglycemia stimulates and hyperglycemia suppresses PP secretion.[12] The slightly higher plasma glucose levels in the obese group during the second secretory phase might account for suppressed PP secretion in these cases. However, the slight difference in plasma glucose levels between obese and control subjects (5.78 ± 0.16 versus 4.99 ± 0.28 mmol/L at 120 min and 5.56 ± 0.11 versus 4.64 ± 0.23 mmol/L at 240 min) is not sufficient to explain the significant differences found in PP levels. Accordingly, the decreased PP response in the obese does not seem to be secondary to hyperglycemia.

Conversely, a possible influence of FFA levels cannot be excluded.

In obese animals, it is difficult to confirm the presence of an increased or decreased number of PP-secreting cells. A decreased number of pancreatic PP cells has been reported in the Zucker rat, which is genetically obese.[13] Malaisse-Lagae reported[3] a relatively decreased number of PP cells among the increased total cell population of the islets of the ob-ob mice. However, Gingerich[14] found that the PP content of the pancreas in ob-ob mice was greater than that in control mice. Likewise, the number of PP cells per islet was increased in the ob-ob mice. Nevertheless, it should be noted that these mice present islet hyperplasia and that the relative volume of the PP cells within the islets is less than normal.

Studies of plasma PP levels have been rarely reported in animal experiments, undoubtedly because of the difficulties in measuring plasma PP values in rodents. Nevertheless, Gates[4] reported that plasma PP is decreased in the NZO mouse.

The hypothesis, suggesting the existence of a circulating satiety factor, was advanced after the parabiosis experiments of Coleman in ob-ob mice.[15,16] These animals seem to possess a functioning satiety center, which remains sensitive to the satiety factor produced by lean mice.

Finally studies, showing that injections of PP induce weight reduction and decrease appetite in the ob-ob mouse[3] and reduce hyperglycemia, hyperinsulinism, and weight gain in the NZO mouse,[4] seem to indicate that PP may be needed in the regulation of food intake in certain types of genetic obesity in animals.

Our results, showing decreased PP levels after fasting and during the late postprandial phase in obese adults, are compatible with the suggestion that PP may somehow be active in satiety and may be reduced to a variable degree in certain types of human obesity. However, it should be kept in mind that factors other than PP may be different in obese subjects and the differences observed in normal and obese individuals may not necessarily play a causative role in the pathogenesis of the obesity.

REFERENCES

[1] Kimmel, J. R., Pollock, H. J., and Hazelwood, R. L.: A new pancreatic polypeptide hormone. Fed. Proc. *30*:1318, 1971. (Abstr.)

[2] Chance, R. E., and Jones, W. E.: Polypeptides from bovine, ovine, human and porcine pancreas. US Patent Office Pat. 3,842,063: 1974.

[3] Malaisse-Lagae, F., Carpentier, J. L., Patel, Y. C., Malaisse, W. J., and Orci, L.: Pancreatic polypeptide: a possible role in the regulation of food intake in the mouse. Hypothesis. Experientia *33*:915–16, 1977.

[4] Gates, R. J., and Lazarus, N. R.: The ability of pancreatic polypeptide (APP and BPP) to return to normal the hyperglycemia, hyperinsulinemia and weight gain of New Zealand obese mice. Horm. Res. *8*:189–202, 1977.

[5] Floyd, J. C., Jr., Fajans, S. S., Pek, S., and Chance, R. E.: A newly recognized pancreatic polypeptide: plasma levels in health and disease. Recent Prog. Horm. Res. *33*:519–70, 1977.

[6] Bakir, S. M., Gates, R. J., and Lazarus, N. R.: Low levels of pancreatic polypeptide in non-diabetic obese women. 10th IDF Congr., Vienna 1979. Amsterdam/New York, Excerpta Medica Publ., ICS 481, Abstract 34.

[7] Boden, G., Master, R. W. P., and Owen, O. E.: Hepatic and renal extraction of endogenous human pancreatic polypeptide (HPP). Scand. J. Gastroenterol. *13* (Suppl. 49):28, 1978. (Abstr.)

[8] Floyd, J. C., Jr., and Fajans, S. S.: A newly recognized human pancreatic islet polypeptide: concentrations in healthy subjects and in patients with diabetes mellitus. Diabetes *25* (Suppl. 1):330, 1976. (Abstr.)

[9] Adrian, T. E., Bloom, S. R., Besterman, H. S., Barnes, A. J., Cooke, T. J., Russel, R. C., and Faber, R. G.: Mechanism of pancreatic polypeptide release in man. Lancet *1*:161–63, 1977.

[10] Schwartz, T. W., and Rehfeld, J. J.: Mechanism of pancreatic polypeptide release. Lancet *1*:697–98, 1977.

[11] Schwartz, T. W., Stadil, F., Chance, R. E., Rehfeld, J. E., Larson, L. I., and Moon, N.: Pancreatic polypeptide response to food in duodenal ulcer patients before and after vagotomy. Lancet *1*:1102–05, 1976.

[12] Marco, J., Hedo, J. A., and Villanueva, M. L.: Relationship between plasma glucose and human pancreatic polypeptide (HPP) concentrations in normal subjects. Diabetologia *13*:216, 1977. (Abstr.)

[13] Larsson, L. I., Boder, G. B., and Shaw, W. N.: Changes in the islets of Langerhans in the obese Zucker rat. Lab. Invest. *36*:593–98, 1977.

[14] Gingerich, R. L., Gersell, D. J., Greider, M. H., Finke, E. H., and Lacy, P. E.: Elevated levels of pancreatic polypeptide in obese-hyperglycemic mice. Metabolism *27*:1526–31, 1978.

[15] Coleman, D. L.: Effects of parabiosis of obese with diabetes and normal mice. Diabetologia *9*:294–98, 1973.

[16] Coleman, D. L.: Obese and diabetes: two mutant genes causing diabetes-obesity syndromes in mice. Diabetologia *14*:141–48, 1978.

The Stimulus-secretion Coupling of Amino Acid-induced Insulin Release

Metabolism and Cationic Effects of Leucine

WILLY J. MALAISSE, JOHN C. HUTTON, ANGELO R. CARPINELLI, ANDRÉ HERCHUELZ, AND ABDULLAH SENER

SUMMARY

When isolated rat pancreatic islets are exposed to L-leucine (20 mM), the rate of NH_4 production is close to the summed rates of L-[1-^{14}C] leucine decarboxylation and α-ketoisocaproate production, whereas the rates of acetoacetate production and L-[U-^{14}C]-leucine oxidation are compatible with the conversion of each mole of the amino acid to one mole of acetoacetate and three moles of CO_2. ATP content, ATP/ADP ratio, and adenylate charge are maintained at normal values by L-leucine, whereas the NADH/NAD$^+$ ratio (but not the NADPH/NADP$^+$ ratio) is significantly increased. The release of insulin evoked by L-leucine is potentiated by 2-ketoisovalerate, unaffected by L-valine, and inhibited by menadione. L-leucine mimicks the effect of D-glucose on $^{86}Rb^+$ and $^{45}Ca^{2+}$ handling by the islets. However, relative to its rate of oxidation, the insulinotropic effect of L-leucine is less marked than that of D-glucose. This may be due, in part at least, to a decrease in the oxidation of endogenous nutrients. It is concluded that the metabolic, cationic, and secretory effects of L-leucine in isolated islets are not incompatible with the fuel hypothesis for insulin release. DIABETES *29*:431–437, June 1980.

L-leucine stimulates insulin release in vivo[1,2] and in vitro.[3-11] Although this amino acid is transported[12-14] and metabolized[15-17] in islet cells and although it affects the consumption of O_2[18] and the islet content of adenine[16] and pyridine nucleotides,[17,19,20] the relevance of its metabolism (see Figure 7) to its insulinotropic action was questioned by several authors.[21-24] The aim of the present series of studies is to further investigate the possible coupling between the metabolic, cationic, and secretory effects of L-leucine in isolated rat pancreatic islets.

From the Université Libre de Bruxelles, Laboratoire de Médecine Expérimentale, Boulevard de Waterloo, 115; 1000 Bruxelles, Belgium.
Address reprint requests to Dr. W. J. Malaisse.
Received for publication 13 August and in revised form 29 November 1979.

MATERIAL AND METHODS

All experiments were performed with isolated islets removed from fed female albino rats.[25] The methods used to measure the release of insulin,[26] the oxidation of exogenous nutrients,[27] the production of $^{14}CO_2$ from islets prelabeled with [U-^{14}C]palmitate,[28,29] the production of acetoacetate[30] and α-ketoisocaproic acid,[31] the incorporation of ^{14}C-nutrient in islet lipids and protein,[30] the content of free ^{14}C-labeled amino and α-keto acids,[30,31] the content of adenine and pyridine nucleotides,[32] the net uptake of ^{45}Ca[33] and ^{86}Rb[34] in incubated islets, the efflux of ^{45}Ca[35] and ^{86}Rb,[36] and the release of insulin[37] from perifused islets were all described in detail in prior publications.

For the measurement of NH_4^+ production, groups of 50 islets each were incubated for 120 min in 60 μl of the usual bicarbonate-buffered incubation medium, except for the absence of albumin. The NH_4^+ content of the incubation medium was then measured according to the method of Chaykin.[38]

All results are expressed at the mean (±SEM) together with the number of individual determinations (n), comparison of control and experimental values being restricted to data collected within the same experiment(s).

RESULTS

Metabolic variables. L-leucine accumulated in the islet cells. After 30 min of incubation in the presence of L-[1-^{14}C]leucine (20 mM), the intracellular pool of free ^{14}C-amino acids averaged 148 ± 27 pmol per islet (Table 1). Taking into account the intracellular H_2O space (approximately 3 nl per islet; see ref. 34), the content of ^{14}C-amino acids corresponded to an intracellular/extracellular concentration ratio close to 2.5.

Exposure of the islets to L-leucine caused an increased production of NH_4^+ (Figure 1). In the presence of 20 mM L-leucine and within the same series of experiments, the output of NH_4^+ exceeded the rate of L-[1-^{14}C]leucine decarboxylation by 30.2 ± 6.0 pmol/120 min per islet (degree of free-

TABLE 1
Effect of 2-ketoisovalerate on insulin release and islet content of intracellular ^{14}C-amino acid (pmol/islet) and ^{14}C-keto acid (pmol/islet) in islets incubated in the presence of L-leucine (20 mM). Insulin release was measured over 90 min of incubation. The intracellular content of radioactively labeled amino and keto acids was determined after 30 min of exposure to L-[1-^{14}C]leucine (20 mM) and is expressed as picomoles of leucine residue per islet.

2-ketoisovalerate (mM)	—	10
Insulin release (μU/90 min per islet)	72.0 ± 5.4 (31)	98.6 ± 5.5 (34)
Intracellular ^{14}C-amino acid	148.1 ± 27.2 (8)	132.6 ± 21.2 (9)
Intracellular ^{14}C-keto acid	5.6 ± 0.7 (8)	19.4 ± 2.4 (9)

dom = 24; $P < 0.001$).* This finding is consistent with the accumulation of 2-ketoisocaproic acid both within the islet cells (Table 1) and in the incubation medium. At the same concentration of L-leucine, 20 mM, the total production of 2-ketoisocaproic acid (islets + incubation medium) averaged 35.8 ± 5.0 pmol/120 min per islet (n = 16).

The islets contain a branched chain amino acid aminotransferase enzyme, which is a site of interaction between branched chain amino acids and corresponding keto acids.[30,31] The participation of such an enzyme in the metabolism of L-leucine is supported by the finding that 2-ketoisovalerate (10 mM) increased both the intracellular content of ^{14}C-keto acids in islets exposed to L-[1-^{14}C]leucine (20 mM) and the secretory response to the amino acid (Table 1). By contrast, L-valine (10 mM) failed to significantly enhance L-leucine–induced insulin release, the increment in secretion rate attributable to L-valine averaging no more than 21.0 ± 12.2% (degree of freedom = 47) of the control's output caused by L-leucine (20 mM) alone.

As expected from the pathway of 2-ketoisocaproate metabolism in the islets,[30] the rate of L-[1-^{14}C]leucine decarboxylation exceeded the rate of L-[U-^{14}C]leucine oxidation, when expressed as leucine residues. In the presence of L-leucine (20 mM), the rate of [U-^{14}C]leucine oxidation represented 49.1 ± 2.4% (n = 11) of the mean rate of [1-^{14}C]leucine decarboxylation, both measurements being performed within the same experiment(s). The output of acetoacetic acid was increased by L-leucine (20 mM) from a basal value

* The production of $^{14}CO_2$ from L-[1-^{14}C]leucine is taken to indicate decarboxylation; the production of $^{14}CO_2$ from L-[U-^{14}C]leucine is interpreted as oxidation (see Figure 7).

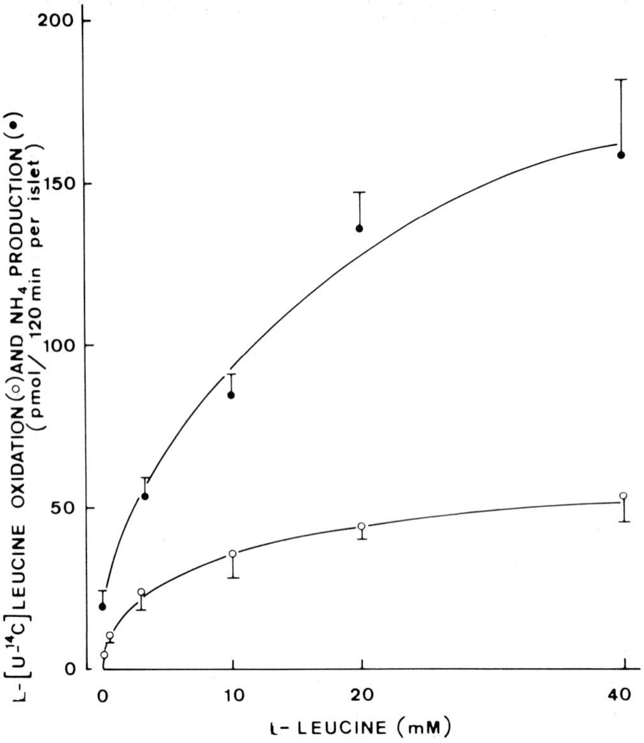

FIGURE 1. Dose-action relationship for L-[U-^{14}C]leucine oxidation (n = 24 ± 8) and NH_4^+ production (n = 9 ± 1) by islets exposed to increasing concentrations of the amino acid.

of 8.4 ± 2.0 (n = 7) to 88.9 ± 5.5 (n = 16) pmol/120 min per islet. The leucine-induced increment in acetoacetate production (80.5 ± 8.6 pmol/120 min per islet) represented close to twice the rate of L-[U-^{14}C]leucine oxidation (43.9 ± 3.8 pmol/120 min per islet; n = 61).

The rate of both L-[U-^{14}C]leucine oxidation and NH_4 production increased in a hyperbolic manner at increasing concentrations of the amino acid (Figure 1).

The rates of L-[U-^{14}C]leucine incorporation into islet lipids (7.1 ± 3.7 pmol/120 min per islet; n = 8) and protein (2.0 ± 0.7 pmol/120 min per islet; n = 8) were low relative to the rate of oxidation of the amino acid.

L-leucine (20 mM) caused a marked reduction in $^{14}CO_2$ output from islets prelabeled with [U-^{14}C]palmitate (Table 2), suggesting that the amino acid may interfere with the utilization of endogenous nutrients.

When islets are incubated in the absence of exogenous nutrient, their ATP content, ATP/ADP ratio, and adenylate charge are decreased.[16,39] L-leucine (20 mM) prevented

TABLE 2
Effect of L-leucine and antimycin A on $^{14}CO_2$ output from islets prelabeled with [U-^{14}C]palmitate. The incorporation of [U-^{14}C]palmitate (0.27 mM) into the islets during preincubation averaged 2.76 ± 0.22 pmol/islet per 120 min (n = 28). The output of $^{14}CO_2$ is expressed at cpm/120 min per islet (line 1) or in percent of the final radioactive content of the islet (line 3); in line 4, the latter values are normalized relative to the control data found in the absence of any agent. The $^{14}CO_2$ output in the presence of antimycin A represents mostly the labeled bicarbonate present in the islets at the onset of the final incubation.[29]

L-Leucine (mM)	—	20.0	—
Antimycin A (mM)	—	—	0.01
$^{14}CO_2$ output (cpm/120 min per islet)	138 ± 18 (10)	97 ± 8 (12)	36 ± 3 (6)
^{14}C content (cpm/islet)	3742 ± 722 (10)	3426 ± 190 (12)	2972 ± 333 (6)
$^{14}CO_2$ output/^{14}C content (percent)	4.10 ± 0.39 (10)	2.87 ± 0.17 (12)	1.24 ± 0.10 (6)
$^{14}CO_2$ output/^{14}C content (normalized)	100.0 ± 9.5 (10)	70.0 ± 4.1 (12)	30.2 ± 2.4 (6)

TABLE 3
Effect of L-leucine on the adenine and pyridine nucleotide content of pancreatic islets incubated for 30 min in the absence or presence of the amino acid

Leucine (mM)	—	20	P
ATP + ADP + AMP (pmol/islet)	10.7 ± 1.0 (8)	13.4 ± 1.5 (8)	NS
ATP (%)	54.4 ± 1.6 (8)	63.6 ± 3.5 (8)	<0.05
ADP (%)	30.6 ± 1.7 (8)	23.0 ± 1.0 (8)	<0.005
AMP (%)	15.0 ± 1.8 (8)	13.4 ± 3.4 (8)	NS
ATP/ADP (ratio)	1.84 ± 0.16 (8)	2.81 ± 0.23 (8)	<0.005
Adenylate charge (ratio)	0.696 ± 0.014 (8)	0.766 ± 0.024 (8)	<0.05
NAD⁺ (fmol/islet)	854 ± 78 (7)	814 ± 55 (7)	NS
NADH (fmol/islet)	52 ± 7 (7)	101 ± 8 (7)	<0.001
NADH/NAD⁺ (ratio)	0.060 ± 0.004 (7)	0.128 ± 0.014 (7)	<0.001
NADP⁺ (fmol/islet)	123 ± 9 (7)	101 ± 7 (7)	NS
NADPH (fmol/islet)	136 ± 19 (7)	136 ± 7 (7)	NS
NADPH/NADP⁺ (ratio)	1.140 ± 0.115 (7)	1.380 ± 0.129 (7)	NS
NADH + NADPH (fmol/islet)	188 ± 26 (7)	237 ± 12 (7)	NS

such a phenomenon, the ATP content, the ATP/ADP ratio, and the adenylate charge being significantly higher in islets exposed for 30 min to L-leucine than in the islets incubated in the absence of exogenous nutrient (Table 3). L-leucine augmented the NADH content and NADH/NAD⁺ ratio in the islets, but failed to increase significantly the NADPH/NADP⁺ ratio (Table 3).

Cationic variables. L-leucine caused a time- and dose-related stimulation of ^{45}Ca net uptake by the islets (Figure 2). L-leucine mimicked the effect of glucose to decrease ^{45}Ca fractional outflow rate from prelabeled islets perifused in the absence of extracellular Ca^{2+} (Figure 3, upper panel). In the presence of extracellular Ca^{2+}, the initial fall in ^{45}Ca efflux was soon masked by a secondary increase in ^{45}Ca efflux (Figure 3, middle panel). L-leucine, like D-glucose, caused a dramatic decrease in the fractional outflow rate of ^{86}Rb (Figure 4) and stimulated ($P < 0.001$) $^{86}Rb^+$ net uptake. Thus, the net uptake of ^{86}Rb, when expressed as picomoles of K^+ (using the same $^{86}Rb/^{39}K$ ratio as in the incubation medium), averaged 332 ± 17 (n = 30) and 407 ± 11 (n = 45) pmol/90 min per islet in the absence and presence of L-leucine, respectively.

FIGURE 2. Time-course and dose-action relationship for the effect of L-leucine on ^{45}Ca net uptake. The concentration of L-leucine used in the time-course study amounted to 20 mM (n = 14 in each case). The length of incubation used in the dose-action study amounted to 90 min (n = 26 ± 5).

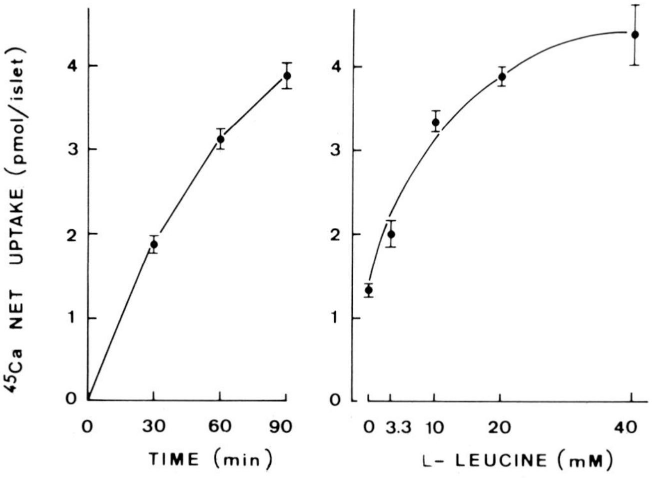

Secretory variables. In static experiments, L-leucine, in concentrations exceeding 3 mM, caused a dose-related increase in insulin release (Figure 5, left panel). The relation-

FIGURE 3. Effect of L-leucine (20 mM), administered during the period in-between the vertical dotted lines, on ^{45}Ca fractional outflow rate (F.O.R.) and release of insulin from islets prelabeled with ^{45}Ca (n = 5). The experiments were performed in the absence of extracellular Ca^{2+} and presence of EGTA (0.5 mM; upper panel) or at normal extracellular Ca^{2+} concentration (1.0 mM; middle and lower panels).

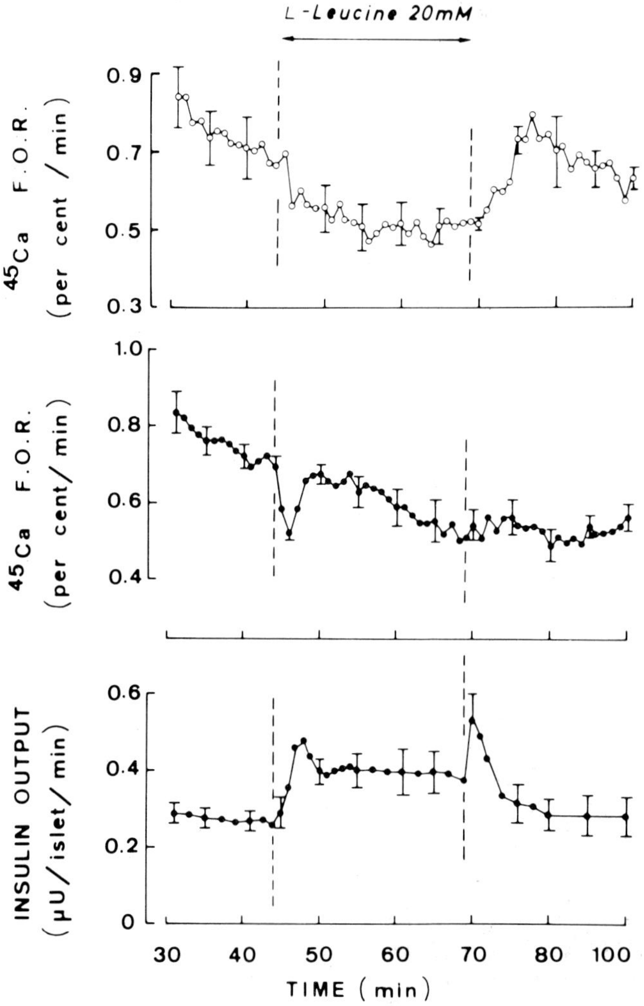

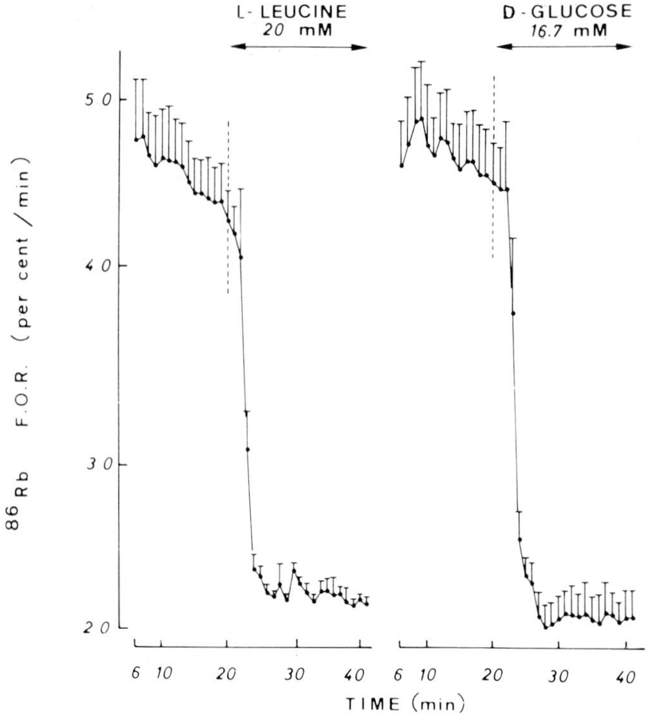

FIGURE 4. Effect of L-leucine (20 mM) or D-glucose (16.7 mM) on ^{86}Rb fractional outflow rate (F.O.R.) from islets prelabeled with ^{86}Rb (n = 4 in each case). The vertical dotted lines correspond to the time at which the nutrient was added to the perifusion medium.

ship between insulin output and net uptake of ^{45}Ca was characterized by the existence of a threshold value for the stimulant action of calcium on insulin release (Figure 5, right panel). In a dynamic system, the secretory response to L-leucine (20 mM) was characterized by an early peak followed by a period of steady-state stimulation (Figure 3, lower panel). A transient "off-response" was noted upon removal of L-leucine from the perifusate.

Comparison between L-leucine and D-glucose. L-leucine (20 mM) significantly augmented insulin release at all glucose concentrations in the range between zero and 16.7 mM. At high glucose concentrations, the effect of L-leucine

FIGURE 5. Dose-action relationship for the effect of L-leucine on insulin release (left panel; n = 22–40). Relationship between insulin release and ^{45}Ca net uptake at increasing concentrations of the amino acid (right panel).

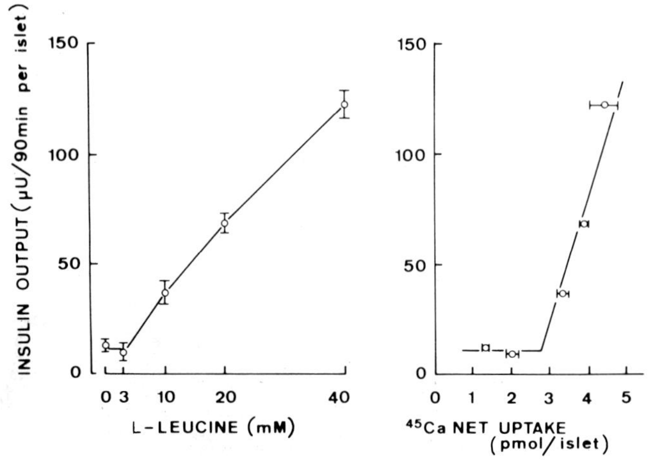

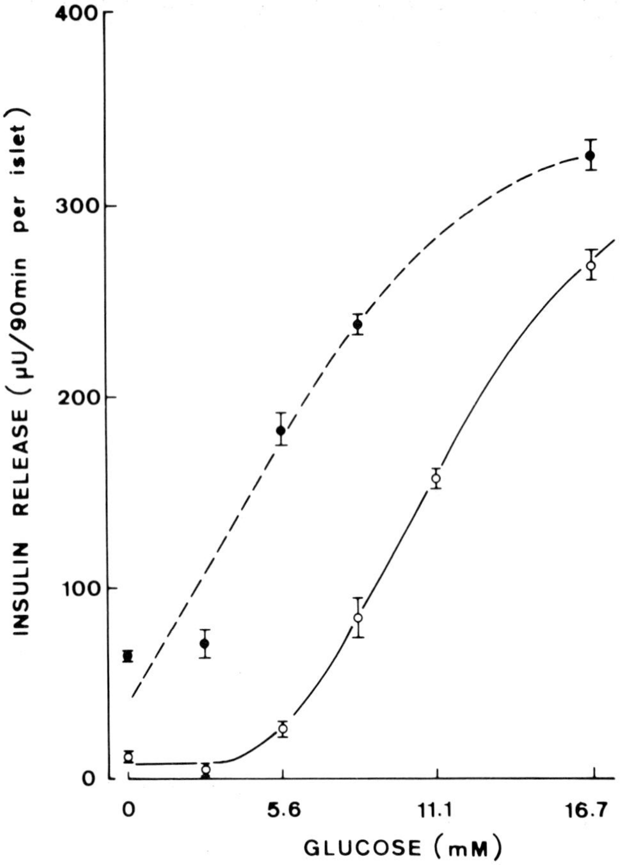

FIGURE 6. Insulin release evoked by increasing concentrations of D-glucose in the absence (open circles) and presence (closed circles) of L-leucine 20 mM (n = 19–29). The dotted line illustrates a shift of the sigmoidal curve (solid line) to the left, corresponding to the effect of an increase in D-glucose concentration of 6.4 mM.

was compatible with a shift to the left of the sigmoidal curve relating insulin output to glucose concentration (Figure 6). By reference to the abscissa of Figure 6, the magnitude of such a shift suggested that the insulinotropic effect of 20 mM L-leucine was comparable to that of 6.4 mM glucose. However, 20 mM L-[U-^{14}C]leucine was oxidized at the same rate as 11.1 mM D-[U-^{14}C]glucose (Table 4). These comparisons indicate that, relative to the oxidation rate, the insulinotropic potency of L-leucine was significantly lower than that of D-glucose. This is confirmed by the observation that, when tested within the same experiment, the release of insulin evoked by 20.0 mM L-leucine in the presence of 5.6 mM glucose (157.6 ± 3.5 μU/90 min per islet) was identical to

TABLE 4
Reciprocal effects of L-leucine and D-glucose on their oxidation rate (picomoles of substrate oxidized/120 min per islet). These data were used to calculate total oxidation of exogenous nutrients in the presence of both D-glucose and L-leucine.

L-[U-^{14}C]leucine (20.0 mM)	34.9 ± 4.7 (8)
L-[U-^{14}C]leucine (20.0 mM) + D-[U^{12}C]glucose (5.6 mM)	33.9 ± 3.4 (16)
D-[U-^{14}C]glucose (5.6 mM) + L-[U-^{12}C]leucine (20.0 mM)	17.5 ± 1.9 (6)
D-[U-^{14}C]glucose (11.1 mM)	33.8 ± 2.4 (15)
D-[U-^{14}C]glucose (11.1 mM) + L-[U-^{12}C]leucine (20.0 mM)	34.4 ± 4.2 (8)

that evoked by 11.1 mM D-glucose alone (156.9 ± 5.0 μU/90 min per islet), despite the fact that the total oxidation rate was significantly higher ($P < 0.02$) in the former (308 ± 35 pmol of $^{14}CO_2$/120 min per islet) than in the latter experimental condition (203 ± 14 pmol of $^{14}CO_2$/120 min per islet). The release of insulin evoked by L-leucine (20 mM), like that evoked by glucose (11.1 mM),[40] was inhibited by menadione (10 μM) from a control value of 43.7 ± 9.5 to 20.8 ± 4.6 μU/90 min per islet (n = 10 in each case; $P < 0.05$).

DISCUSSION

The aim of the present study was to investigate to what extent the process of L-leucine–induced insulin release could be ascribed to a sequence of metabolic and cationic events analogous to that thought to mediate the process of glucose-induced insulin secretion.[41]

The present data are compatible with the view that L-leucine is actively metabolized in the islet cells along a pathway which includes (1) the desamination of L-leucine by a branched chain amino acid aminotransferase, a process coupled with the conversion of a suitable 2-keto acid to the corresponding amino acid (e.g. the conversion of 2-ketoisovalerate to valine or that of α-ketoglutarate to L-glutamate); (2) the production of NH_4^+; (3) the generation of 2-ketoisocaproate, which, in part, accumulates in the islet cells and is liberated in the extracellular milieu; (4) the decarboxylation of 2-ketoisocaproate to form isovaleryl coenzyme A; and (5) the production of acetoacetate and acetyl coenzyme A, the latter being then oxidized to generate 2 mol of CO_2 per mole of L-leucine (Figure 7). The lower segment of this metabolic pathway in the islet cells, from 2-ketoisocaproate to acetoacetate and CO_2, was recently characterized in full detail.[30]

The metabolism of L-leucine was associated with the maintenance of a normal ATP/ADP ratio and adenylate charge in the islets, despite an apparent reduction in the utilization of endogenous nutrients, as judged by the output of $^{14}CO_2$ from islets prelabeled with [U-^{14}C]palmitate. Exposure of the islets to L-leucine resulted in a more reduced state of the NADH/$NADP^+$ system, whereas the NADPH/$NADP^+$ ratio was not significantly increased.

Since in the pathway of leucine metabolism in the islets CO_2 is incorporated into 3-methylcrotonyl coenzyme A, it could be argued that the leucine-induced reduction in $^{14}CO_2$ output from islets prelabeled with [U-^{14}C]palmitate does not correspond to a true decrease in oxidation of endogenous nutrients. This hypothesis is unlikely, however, since α-ketoisocaproate does not exert any obvious effect on $^{14}CO_2$ output from the prelabeled islets.[30] Moreover, in pancreatic islets removed from ob-ob mice,[18] the increase in O_2 consumption evoked by 10 mM L-leucine (+25.6% above basal value) is similar to that evoked by 5.6 mM D-glucose (+25.3% above basal value), whereas the present data indicate that the output of $^{14}CO_2$ is at least twice as high in the presence of 10 mM L-[U-^{14}C]leucine than of 5.6 mM D-[U-^{14}C]glucose. At the latter low glucose concentration, glucose does not affect $^{14}CO_2$ output from the islets prelabeled with [U-^{14}C]palmitate,[42] and the increment in O_2 consumption evoked by glucose 5.6 mM in the present system (0.89 pmol of O_2/min per islet; see ref. 43) is close to the rate of conversion of [U-^{14}C]glucose (5.6 mM) to $^{4}CO_2$ (0.88 pmol of CO_2/min per islet). Therefore, the contrasting situations

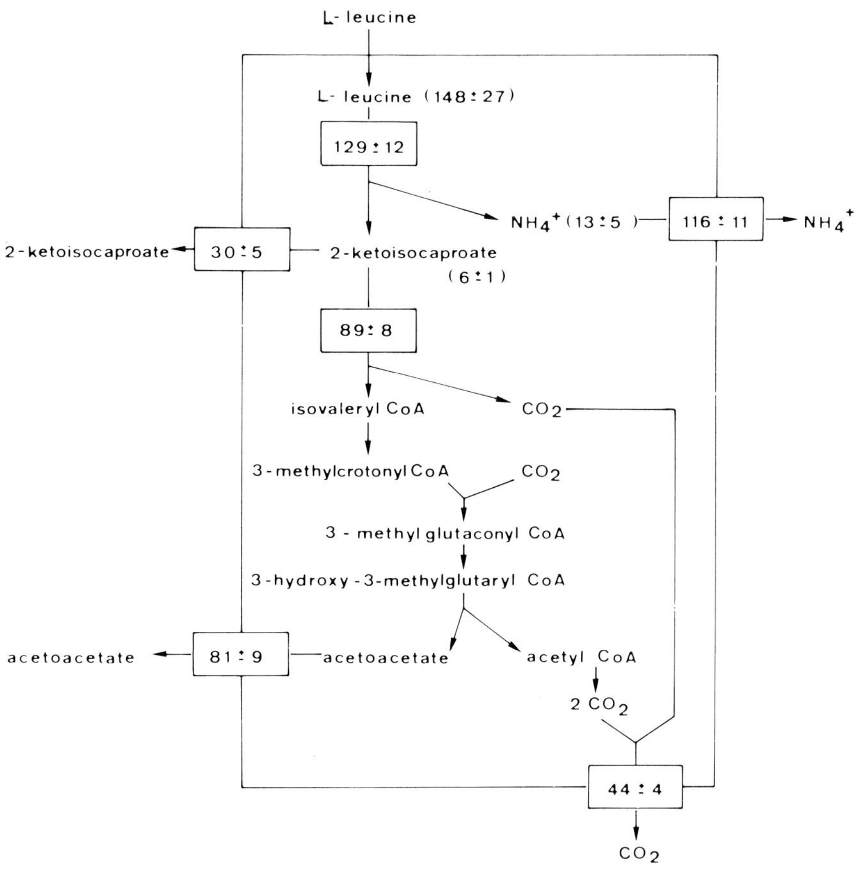

FIGURE 7. Quantification of L-leucine metabolism in isolated islets exposed to the amino acid at a 20 mM extracellular concentration. Intracellular contents are shown in parentheses and are expressed as picomoles per islet. Flow rates are shown in rectangles and are expressed as picomoles per 120 min per islet. The values for NH_4 content and production and acetoacetate production are corrected for basal values. The rate of L-leucine deamination is taken as the sum of the NH_4 content and the rate of NH_4 production. The rate of 2-ketoisocaproate output is taken as the difference between the total production of 2-ketoisocaproate (islets + incubation medium) and the amount of 2-keto acid recovered in the islets. The rate of 2-ketoisocaproate oxidative decarboxylation is judged from the rate of $^{14}CO_2$ output in islets exposed to L-[1-^{14}C]leucine. The rate of radioactive CO_2 output from islets exposed to L-[U-^{14}C]leucine is expressed as picomoles of L-leucine residues. It was previously shown that the C atom in the carboxyl group of acetoacetate is not derived from the α-ketoisocaproate carbon skeleton.

found in the presence of glucose 5.6 mM and L-leucine 10 mM strongly suggest that the amino acid indeed decreases the utilization of endogenous nutrients. Incidentally, this is the opposite situation of that found with the leucine analog 2-aminonorbornane-2-carboxylic acid, which, although probably not metabolized, increases glucose oxidation[44] and O_2 consumption[45] in the islets.

In several respects, L-leucine mimicked the effect of D-glucose on islet function. First, and as already reported,[3] L-leucine shifted to the left the sigmoidal curve relating insulin release to the ambient glucose concentration. The magnitude of such a shift suggested that the effect of 20 mM leucine was comparable to that of glucose at a concentration of approximately 6.4 mM. Second, L-leucine, like D-glucose, caused an initial fall and a secondary rise in ^{45}Ca efflux from prelabeled islets and stimulated the net uptake of ^{45}Ca by the islets. By comparison with data reported elsewhere,[46] the magnitude of the changes in ^{45}Ca efflux induced by L-leucine 20 mM was again similar to that seen at a glucose concentration between 5.6 and 8.3 mM. Last, L-leucine decreased $^{86}Rb^+$ fractional outflow rate, as already reported elsewhere,[47] and stimulated $^{86}Rb^+$ net uptake. In this respect, 20 mM L-leucine was as potent as 16.7 mM glucose; this is not surprising, since the effect of glucose itself to reduce K^+ conductance reaches a close to maximal magnitude at concentrations far below those required to cause a maximal-secretory response.[48]

These similarities suggest that the remodeling of cationic fluxes, evoked by either D-glucose or L-leucine, might be caused by common coupling factors generated by the metabolism of these nutrients. For instance, the possible participation of a change in redox potential in the process of leucine-induced insulin release is supported by the inhibitory effect of menadione on such a process. It was previously shown that leucine-induced insulin release is inhibited by iodoacetate (a likely inhibitor of α-ketoisocaproate dehydrogenase) and the absence of extracellular calcium,[49,50] whereas it is enhanced by theophylline and cytochalasin B.[3,51,52]

Taken as a whole, these findings suggest that the metabolic, cationic, motile, and secretory effects of L-leucine in isolated islets are compatible with the fuel hypothesis for insulin release, as defined elsewhere.[41] However, it should be emphasized that, in some respects, the situation found with L-leucine differed from that encountered in islets exposed to D-glucose. First, L-leucine affected the output of $^{14}CO_2$ from islets prelabeled with [U-^{14}C]palmitate much more severely than did D-glucose. Second, and possibly due to the just-mentioned phenomenon, the rate of insulin release relative to the rate of oxidation of the nutrient was significantly lower with L-leucine than with D-glucose. Third, in contrast to D-glucose[42] or 2-ketoisocaproate,[53] L-leucine failed to significantly increase the $NADPH/NADP^+$ ratio. And last, the metabolism of L-leucine in islet cells was associated with an increased production of NH_4^+. Since exogenous NH_4^+ is a potent inhibitor of insulin release,[54] the question may be raised whether the generation of endogenous NH_4^+ may not have altered the magnitude of the secretory response to L-leucine relative to the rate of oxidation of the amino acid. Such a possibility is scrutinized in greater detail in the next report in this series.[55]

ACKNOWLEDGMENTS

This work was supported in part by grants from the Belgian Foundation for Scientific Medical Research. We wish to thank J. Schoonheydt, A. Tinant, and M. Urbain for technical assistance and C. Demesmaeker for secretarial help.

REFERENCES

[1] Floyd, J. C., Fajans, S. S., Conn, J. W., Knopf, R. F., and Rull, J.: Stimulation of insulin secretion by amino acids. J. Clin. Invest. *45*:1487–1502, 1966.

[2] Floyd, J. C., Fajans, S. S., Knopf, R. F., and Conn, J. W.: Evidence that insulin release is the mechanism for experimentally-induced leucine hypoglycemia in man. J. Clin. Invest. *42*:1714–19, 1963.

[3] Malaisse, W. J., and Malaisse-Lagae, F.: Stimulation of insulin secretion by noncarbohydrate metabolites. J. Lab. Clin. Med. *72*:438–48, 1968.

[4] Milner, R. D. G.: The mechanism by which leucine and arginine stimulate insulin release in vitro. Biochim. Biophys. Acta *192*:154–56, 1969.

[5] Lambert, A. E., Jeanrenaud, B., Junod, A., and Renold, A. E.: Organ culture of fetal rat pancreas. II. Insulin release induced by amino acid and organic acids, by hormonal peptides, by cationic alterations of the medium and by other agents. Biochim. Biophys. Acta *174*:540–53, 1969.

[6] Edgar, P., Rabinowitz, D., and Merimee, T. J.: Effects of amino acids on insulin release from excised rabbit pancreas. Endocrinology *84*:835–43, 1969.

[7] Lernmark, A.: Specificity of leucine stimulation of insulin release. Hormones *3*:14–21, 1972.

[8] Schönborn, J., Westphal, P., and Panten, U.: Insulin release from the isolated perfused rat pancreas induced by L-leucine, 2-aminonorbornane-2-carboxylic acid and α-ketoisocaproic acid. Horm. Metab. Res. *7*:127–31, 1975.

[9] Landgraf, R., Landgraf-Leurs, M. M. C., and Hörl, R.: L-leucine and L-phenylalanine induced insulin release and the influence of D-glucose. Diabetologia *10*:415–20, 1974.

[10] Pek, S., Santiago, J. C., and Tai, T.-Y.: L-leucine-induced secretion of glucagon and insulin, and the "off-response" to L-leucine in vitro. I. Characterization of the dynamics of secretion. Endocrinology *103*:1208–18, 1978.

[11] Tai, T.-Y., Pek, S., and Santiago, J. C.: L-leucine-induced secretion of glucagon and insulin, and the "off-response" to L-leucine in vitro. II. The role of D-glucose. Endocrinology *103*:1219–26, 1978.

[12] Hellman, B., Sehlin, J., and Täljedal, I.-B.: Uptake of alanine, arginine and leucine by mammalian pancreatic β-cells. Endocrinology *89*:1432–39, 1971.

[13] Hellman, B., Sehlin, J., and Täljedal, I.-B.: Transport of L-leucine and D-leucine into pancreatic β-cells with reference to the mechanisms of amino acid-induced insulin release. Biochim. Biophys. Acta *266*:436–43, 1972.

[14] Cooperstein, S. J., and Lazarow, A.: Uptake of amino acids by islets of Langerhans and other tissues of the toadfish. Am. J. Physiol. *233*:E19–27, 1977.

[15] Hellman, B., Sehlin, J., and Täljedal, I.-B.: Effects of glucose and other modifiers of insulin release on the oxidative metabolism of amino acids in micro-dissected pancreatic islets. Biochem. J. *123*:513–21, 1971.

[16] Ashcroft, S. J. H., Weerasinghe, L. C. C., and Randle, P. J.: Interrelationships of islet metabolism, adenosine triphosphate content and insulin release. Biochem. J. *132*:223–31, 1973.

[17] Panten, U., Kriegstein, E. V., Poser, W., Schönborn, J., and Hasselblatt, A.: Effects of L-leucine and α-ketoisocaproate acid upon insulin secretion and metabolism of isolated pancreatic islets. FEBS Lett. *20*:225–28, 1972.

[18] Hellerström, C., Westman, S., Marsden, N., and Turner, D.: Oxygen consumption of the β-cells in relation to insulin release. *In* The Structure and Metabolism of the Pancreatic Islets. Falkmer, S., Hellman, B., and Täljedal, I.-B., Eds. Oxford, Pergamon Press, 1970, pp. 315–28.

[19] Panten, U., Christians, J., Kriegstein, E. V., Poser, W., and Hasselblatt, A.: Studies on the mechanisms of l-leucine and α-ketoisocaproic acid-induced insulin release from perifused isolated pancreatic islets. Diabetologia *10*:149–54, 1974.

[20] Ammon, H. P. T., Hoppe, E., Akhtar, M. S., and Niklas, H.: Effect of leucine on the pyridine nucleotide contents of islets and on the insulin released. Interactions in vitro with methylene blue, thiol oxidants, and p-chloromercuribenzoate. Diabetes *28*:593–99, 1979.

[21] Knopf, R., Fajans, S. S., Floyd, J. C., and Conn, J. W.: Comparison of experimentally induced and naturally occurring sensitivity to leucine hypoglycemia. J. Clin. Endocrinol. *23*:579–87, 1963.

[22] Christensen, H. N., Hellman, B., Lernmark, A., Sehlin, J., Tager, H. S., and Täljedal, I.-B.: In vitro stimulation of insulin release by non-metabolizable transport-specific amino acids. Biochim. Biophys. Acta *241*:341–48, 1971.

[23] Matschinsky, F. M., Ellerman, J., Stillings, S., Raybaud, F., Pace, C., and Zawalich, W.: Hexoses and insulin secretion. *In* Insulin (part 2). Hasselblatt, A., and Bruchhausen, F. V., Eds. Berlin, Springer-Verlag, 1975, pp. 79–114.

[24] Panten, U., Holze, S., and Lenzen, S.: Changes of function and metabolism of the pancreatic B-cell caused by amino acids and related compound. Horm. Metab. Res. in press, 1980.

[25] Lacy, P. E., and Kostianovsky, M.: Method for isolation of intact islets of Langerhans from the rat pancreas. Diabetes *16*:35–39, 1967.

[26] Malaisse, W. J., Brisson, G. R., and Malaisse-Lagae, F.: The stimulus-secretion coupling of glucose-induced insulin release. Interaction of epinephrine and alkaline earth cations. J. Lab. Clin. Med. *76*:895–902, 1970.

[27] Malaisse, W. J., Sener, A., and Mahy, M.: The stimulus-secretion coupling of glucose-induced insulin release. XVIII. Sorbitol metabolism in isolated islets. Eur. J. Biochem. *47*:365–70, 1974.

[28] Sener, A., Kawazu, S., Hutton, J. C., Boschero, A. C., Devis, G., Somers, G., Herchuelz, A., and Malaisse, W. J.: The stimulus-secretion coupling of glucose-induced insulin release. XXXIII. Effect of exogenous pyruvate on islet function. Biochem. J. *176*:217–32, 1978.

[29] Malaisse, W. J., Kawazu, S., Herchuelz, A., Hutton, J. C., Somers, G., Devis, G., and Sener, A.: The stimulus-secretion coupling of glucose-induced insulin release. XXXIV. Effect of lactate upon islet function. Arch. Biochem. Biophys. *194*:49–62, 1979.

[30] Hutton, J. C., Sener, A., and Malaisse, W. J.: The metabolism of 4-methyl-2-oxopentanoate in rat pancreatic islets. Biochem. J. *184*:291–301, 1979.

[31] Hutton, J. C., Sener, A., and Malaisse, W. J.: Interaction of branched chain amino acids and keto acids upon pancreatic islet metabolism and insulin secretion. J. Biol. Chem. in press, 1980.

[32] Malaisse, W. J., Hutton, J. C., Kawazu, S., and Sener, A.: The stimulus-secretion coupling of glucose-induced insulin release. XXXI. Metabolic effects of menadione in isolated islets. Eur. J. Biochem. *87*:121–30, 1978.

[33] Malaisse-Lagae, F., and Malaisse, W. J.: The stimulus-secretion coupling of glucose-induced insulin release. III. Uptake of ^{45}calcium by isolated islets of Langerhans. Endocrinology *88*:72–80, 1971.

[34] Malaisse, W. J., Boschero, A. C., Kawazu, S., and Hutton, J. C.: The stimulus-secretion coupling of glucose-induced insulin release. XXVII. Effect of glucose on K^+ fluxes in isolated islets. Pflügers Arch. *373*:237–42, 1978.

[35] Herchuelz, A., and Malaisse, W. J.: The dual regulation of calcium efflux from pancreatic islets. Horm. Metab. Res. in press, 1980.

[36] Boschero, A. C., and Malaisse, W. J.: The stimulus-secretion coupling of glucose-induced insulin release. XXIX. Regulation of $^{86}Rb^+$ efflux from perifused islets. Am. J. Physiol. *236*:E139–46, 1979.

[37] Herchuelz, A., and Malaisse, W. J.: Regulation of calcium fluxes in pancreatic islets: dissociation between calcium and insulin release. J. Physiol. (London) *283*:409–24, 1978.

[38] Chaykin, S.: Assay of nicotinamide deamidase. Determination of ammonia by the indophenol reaction. Anal. Biochem. *31*:375–82, 1969.

[39] Malaisse, W. J., Sener, A., Levy, J., and Herchuelz, A.: The stimulus-secretion coupling of glucose-induced insulin release. XXII. Qualitative and quantitative aspects of glycolysis in isolated islets. Acta Diabetol. Lat. *13*:202–15, 1976.

[40] Malaisse, W. J., Sener, A., Boschero, A. C., Kawazu, S., Devis, G., and Somers, G.: The stimulus-secretion coupling of glucose-induced insulin release. XXX. Cationic and secretory effects of menadione in the endocrine pancreas. Eur. J. Biochem. *87*:111–20, 1978.

[41] Malaisse, W. J., Sener, A., Herchuelz, A., and Hutton, J. C.: Insulin release: the fuel hypothesis. Metabolism *27*:373–86, 1979.

[42] Malaisse, W. J., Hutton, J. C., Kawazu, S., Herchuelz, A., Valverde, I., and Sener, A.: The stimulus-secretion coupling of glucose-induced insulin release. XXXV. The links between metabolic and cationic events. Diabetologia *16*:331–41, 1979.

[43] Hutton, J. C., and Malaisse, W. J.: Dynamic of O_2 consumption in rat pancreatic islets. Diabetologia in press, 1980.

[44] Gylfe, E.: Glucose oxidation and contents of free acids in pancreatic β-cells stimulated by a non-metabolizable leucine analogue. Biochim. Biophys. Acta *343*:584–89, 1974.

[45] Hellerström, C., Andersson, A., and Welsh, M.: Respiration of the pancreatic B-cell: effects of glucose and 2-aminonorbornane-2-carboxylic acid. Horm. Metab. Res. in press, 1980.

[46] Herchuelz, A., and Malaisse, W. J.: Regulation of calcium fluxes in pancreatic islets. Dissociated responsiveness to glucose of two distinct calcium movements. Am. J. Physiol. *238*:E87–95, 1980.

[47] Henquin, J. C.: The potassium permeability of pancreatic islet cells: mechanisms of control and influence on insulin release. Horm. Metab. Res. in press, 1980.

[48] Henquin, J. C.: D-glucose inhibits potassium efflux from pancreatic islet cells. Nature *271*:271–73, 1978.

[49] Sener, A., Pipeleers, D. G., Levy, J., and Malaisse, W. J.: The stimulus-secretion coupling of glucose-induced insulin release. XXVI. Are the secretory and fuel functions of glucose dissociable by iodoacetate? Metabolism *27*:1505–17, 1978.

[50] Malaisse-Lagae, F., Brisson, G. R., and Malaisse, W. J.: The stimulus-secretion coupling of glucose-induced insulin release. VI. Analogy between the insulinotropic mechanisms of sugar and amino acids. Horm. Metab. Res. *3*:374–78, 1971.

[51] Landgraf-Leurs, M. M. C., Landgraf, R., Daffner, R., and Hörl, R.: The stimulatory and inhibitory function of theophylline on amino acid-induced insulin release: studies with the perfused rat pancreas. Endocrinology *97*:1416–23, 1975.

[52] Levy, J., Herchuelz, A., Sener, A., Malaisse-Lagae, F., and Malaisse, W. J.: Cytochalasin B-induced impairment of glucose metabolism in islets of Langerhans. Endocrinology *98*:429–37, 1976.

[53] Hutton, J. C., Sener, A., Herchuelz, A., Atwater, I., Kawazu, S., Boschero, A. C., Somers, G., Devis, G., and Malaisse, W. J.: Similarities in the stimulus-secretion coupling mechanisms of glucose- and 2-keto acid-induced insulin release. Endocrinology *106*:203–19, 1980.

[54] Sener, A., Hutton, J. C., Kawazu, S., Boschero, A. C., Somers, G., Devis, G., Herchuelz, A., and Malaisse, W. J.: The stimulus-secretion coupling of glucose-induced insulin release. XXXII. Metabolic and functional effects of NH_4^+ in rat islets. J. Clin. Invest. *62*:868–78, 1978.

[55] Sener, A., and Malaisse, W. J.: The stimulus-secretion coupling of amino-acid induced insulin release. II. Sensitivity to K^+, NH_4^+ and H^+ of leucine-stimulated islets. Diabete Metab. in press, 1980.

Immunohistochemical Localization of Aldose Reductase

I. Enzyme Purification and Antibody Preparation—Localization in Peripheral Nerve, Artery, and Testis

MARK A. LUDVIGSON AND ROBERT L. SORENSON

SUMMARY
Aldose reductase (AR) was purified from rat and bovine seminal vesicles using DEAE-cellulose, hydroxylapatite, and Sephadex-gel column chromatography. The purification resulted in the obtention of an AR pool and a contaminating pool. Antibodies were raised in rabbits against both enzymes by subcutaneous injection of the AR pool. The antisera was judged to be specific for AR by immunoprecipitation of AR activity and by Ouchterlony double immunodiffusion and immunoelectrophoretic methods. Antibodies against rat AR were used in the unlabeled antibody-enzyme (PAP) technique to demonstrate the cellular location of the enzyme in a number of tissues known to be sites of diabetic lesions. Antibodies against bovine AR were not cross reactive with the rat enzyme, as determined by Ouchterlony and competitive protein-binding studies. AR was localized in rat tissues to the Schwann cell sheath of peripheral nerve, arterial endothelium, and the sustentacular (Sertoli) cells and mature spermatids of the testis. DIABETES 29:438–449, June 1980.

Aldose reductase (alditol: NADP oxidoreductase, EC 1.1.1.21) is one of two enzymes, the other being sorbitol dehydrogenase (L-iditol: NAD oxidoreductase, EC 1.1.1.14), which together constitute the polyol (sorbitol) pathway. Polyol pathway activity results in the conversion of a number of aldose sugars to the corresponding ketose sugars through a polyol intermediate and has a net production of NADP and NADH. Such hyperglycemic conditions as those encountered in diabetes and galactosemia result in enhanced pathway activity and subsequent accumulation of pathway substrates in a number of tissues.[1–4] The intracellular accumulation of polyols and cofactors under these conditions has implicated the polyol pathway in the etiology of diabetic complications.

van Heyningen[5,6] first postulated the association between intralenticular polyol accumulation and formation of sugar cataracts in diabetic and galactosemic rats. Kinoshita and others[7,8] have, in turn, shown that increased polyol activity results in the formation of sugar cataracts. This theory has been extended to other sites of diabetic complications.[1–4]

Previous attempts to localize the polyol pathway were restricted to the use of biochemical and histochemical techniques. Of particular interest, polyol pathway activity was demonstrated in lens,[5,6,9,10] peripheral nerve,[11–13] aorta,[14–16] kidney,[14,17,18] retina,[18–20] the male reproductive tract,[21–26] and islets of Langerhans.[18,27,28]

Our purpose in this study was to demonstrate the specific cellular location of AR in tissues known to be sites of diabetic lesions to provide a morphologic basis for the interpretation of the vast biochemical data which exists regarding polyol pathway activity and its possible role in the pathogenesis of diabetic complications. We report here the development of an immunohistochemical technique for the cellular localization of AR and the application of this technique to selective rat tissues. Portions of this work were reported previously.[29,30]

MATERIALS AND METHODS

Aldose reductase isolation. A modified version of the purification procedure reported by Gabbay and Cathcart[18] was used in the purification of seminal vesicle AR in this investigation. All purification steps, from tissue homogenization to the final enzyme preparation, were done at 4°C in the presence of 5mM mercaptoethanol and 0.02% chlorobutanol. Approximately 200-g quantities (130-145 sets of rat seminal vesicles) of fresh frozen seminal vesicles were trimmed of excess fat and fascia, cubed into small (2- or 3-cm square) pieces, and homogenized in a Waring commercial blender (high speed, 3 or 4 min) with a volume of tris phosphate buffer (pH 7.4) sufficient to produce a 2:1

This work was presented in part at the 38th Annual Meeting of the American Diabetes Association held at Boston, Massachusetts, on 13 June 1978.
From the Department of Anatomy, University of Minnesota School of Medicine, Minneapolis.
Address reprint requests to Mark A. Ludvigson, Ph.D., Department of Anatomy, 4-135 Jackson Hall, 321 Church Street S.E., Minneapolis, MN 55455.
Received for publication 29 October 1979.

(vol:wt) ratio. The tissue slurry was centrifuged (20 min at 46,000 *g*), the pellets were discarded, and solid ammonium sulfate was added to the supernatant to produce a 40%-saturated solution. The solution was magnetically stirred for 30 min, centrifuged (30 min at 15,000 *g*), and the pellet was discarded. The supernatant was then made 75% saturated by the addition of solid ammonium sulfate. The pellets thus obtained were dissolved in small (5–15 ml) amounts of tris phosphate buffer, pooled, and dialyzed (Spectropore #2, 45 mm in diameter, 12,000–14,000 mol wt cutoff) against four changes of a volume of buffer 20 times the dialysate volume. The dialysate (340 ml) was applied to a DEAE-cellulose column (2.6 × 45 cm) equilibrated in tris phosphate buffer. The column was washed with 500 ml of tris phosphate buffer and then eluted with 1200 ml of a 0 to 250 mM linear NaCl gradient; 15-ml fractions were collected.

The pooled and dialyzed fractions (200 ml) were loaded on the hydroxylapatite column (1.5 × 30 cm), which was subsequently washed with 200 ml of 5mM phosphate buffer (pH 6.8); 10-ml fractions were collected. The column was eluted with 800 ml of a 5- to 400-mM phosphate buffer gradient (pH 6.7). Fractions containing AR activity were pooled and applied to a Sephadex G-100 column (2.6 × 100 cm). The sample was eluted with tris phosphate buffer; 10-ml fractions were collected. Fractions containing AR activity were pooled, concentrated by pressure dialysis, and rechromatographed on Sephadex G-100. The pooled AR fractions from the second column run constituted the final, purified form of the enzyme. The enzyme serving as antigen was injected as the concentrated pool from the second Sephadex G-100 run; the enzyme being stored for future use as an immunohistochemical control was first dialyzed against tris phosphate buffer to remove the mercaptoethanol and preservative and was then stored frozen (−20°C).

Enzyme activity analysis. Aldose reductase activity was determined according to the method of Gabbay and O'Sullivan.[12] To properly identify AR and to distinguish it from hexonate dehydrogenase, glyceraldehyde and glucuronate were routinely utilized as substrates. The final concentrations of the constituents in the assay were 1mM glyceraldehyde or 10mM glucuronate, 70mM NADPH, and 5mM mercaptoethanol in phoshate buffer (67mM, pH 6.2).

Isolated enzyme was characterized by electrophoresis in 7.5% polyacrylamide gels (PAGE) using coomassie blue for protein stain. Protein bands containing AR activity were determined as such by end-point activity analysis of fractionated, eluted gel columns. Gels for enzyme determination were fractionated with a Gilson fractionator and were eluted in the enzyme activity media. Samples were incubated overnight at 4°C before being read at 340nm in a Beckman model 25 spectrophotometer. Fractions containing AR activity were indicated by a loss of NADPH absorbency at 340 nm.

Antibody preparation and characterization. Antibodies were raised against AR isolated from both bovine and rat seminal vesicles. The enzyme was injected into Dutch Pelt rabbits using Freund's complete adjuvant (1:1 vol/vol) for the initial inoculation (0.5 mg AR/animal). In subsequent injections, Freund's incomplete adjuvant was used (1:1 vol/vol, 0.25 mg/animal). The rabbits were bled 10 days after the fourth injection. Ouchterlony double immunodiffusion (pattern C plates, Hyland, Costa Mesa) and immunoelectrophoresis (Hyland) were used to characterize the antibody.

A competitive protein-binding system was developed to further determine the binding characteristics of the antibody. Bovine AR was labeled with I-125 using a modification of the lactoperoxidase method.[31] Labeled AR (10,000 cpm/0.5 ml) was used in competition for binding with various antisera against unlabeled bovine or rat AR. Antisera was diluted 1:100 in 1% BSA-borate buffer, pH 8.3. All samples were tested in triplicate. Complexes of antibody-bound enzyme were precipitated by the addition of 1 vol of polyethylene oxide (PEO, 25 g/75 ml H_2O). 100μl horse serum (50%) was added to each tube as carrier.

The ability of the various antisera to immunoprecipitate enzymatic activity was tested under enzyme activity assay conditions to further characterize the antisera. Aliquots of either bovine (0.004 ΔOD/min-25 μg protein) or rat (0.009 ΔOD/min-10 μg protein) enzyme were incubated overnight at 4°C with 100 μl of undiluted anti-bovine or anti-rat AR sera in a final volume of 200 μl. Some samples developed a notable flocculent precipitate. All reaction tubes were centrifuged at 10,000 *g* for 30 min. Enzyme activity was determined for both the supernates and pellets of tubes containing immunoprecipitates and for the incubate solutions of tubes where no precipitate was formed.

Procedures for immunohistochemical staining. Tissues were fixed in Bouin's fixative by immersion or by vascular perfusion with either picric acid formalin or with 4% paraformaldehyde (with or without 0.1% glutaraldehyde) in Sorenson's (0.2M) or cacodylate (0.2M) buffers, pH 7.2. Tissues were routinely dehydrated in a graded series of alcohols, embedded in paraffin, and sectioned at a thickness of 5 μm. The working dilution of the AR antisera was determined empirically on tissue sections. A 1:2000 dilution of antiserum in borate-buffered saline containing 10% normal sheep serum was found to give optimal immunohistochemical staining. The antiserum was employed in the unlabeled antibody-enzyme (PAP) technique[32] used throughout the study. Controls routinely consisted of omission of the primary antisera and preincubation of the primary working antisera with equal amounts (50 μg protein/ml) of either AR or the contaminating pool B. Localization of AR was considered positive only for those sites where immunostaining was abolished by preincubation of the antisera with AR but not by preincubation with the contaminating pool.

RESULTS

Purification and characterization of rat AR. Numerous purification trials for both bovine and rat AR were necessary to obtain sufficient amounts of enzyme to meet the immunization injection schedule and to serve as antigen in the subsequent immunohistochemical controls. Since the ultimate goal of this study was the immunohistochemical localization of AR in rat tissues, the purification of AR from rat seminal vesicle and the characterization of the anti-rat AR sera are reported here.

DEAE-cellulose column chromatography of the dialyzed 40–75% pellet obtained by ammonium sulfate fractionation of the crude extract of rat seminal vesicle resulted in both the removal of a large amount of unwanted protein in the column wash and the resolution of two aldose-reducing activities (Figure 1, upper). The first enzyme peak eluted essentially in the column wash (NaCl concentrations of 5mM). The ratio of glyceraldehyde/glucuronate-reducing activity was 1:3.4. The elution pattern and substrate specificities of this peak indicated it to be hexonate dehydrogenase.[33,34] The second enzyme peak eluted in the ionic gradient at 60 mM NaCl and exhibited a trailing shoulder with glyceraldehyde as substrate. The ratio of glyceraldehyde/glucuronate-reducing activity (5:1), and its elution in the ionic gradient, identified this peak as AR. It represented 13% of the total protein in the DEAE-column sample.

DEAE-cellulose column fractions containing AR activity were pooled and dialyzed and subjected to further column chromatographic separation on hydroxylapatite (Figure 1, middle). This column isolated a sharp protein peak containing AR activity, which eluted early in the ionic gradient and represented 9% of the total protein in the hydroxylapatite column sample. No protein was removed in the column wash. The ratio of glyceraldehyde/glucuronate-reducing activity in the AR peak was 2.5:1. There was no evidence of AR isozyme separation by hydroxylapatite, as was reported by Gabbay and Cathcart[18] for bovine kidney AR.

Repeated gel filtration chromatography of the pooled and concentrated hydroxylapatite fractions containing AR activity resulted in the final purified AR pool subsequently used as the antigen for antibody production and in the immunohistochemical absorption controls (Figures 1 lower, and 2). The second gel chromatographic run (Figure 2) resulted in the isolation of AR activity to a sharply defined protein peak (A) with a more slowly eluting, contaminating shoulder (B) not possessing AR activity. Because of concern for enzyme yield and stability, no further passages were made through Sephadex G-100 in an attempt to resolve the contaminating shoulder as a definitive protein peak. Fractions containing AR activity (peak A) were serially pooled, with the exception of those fractions constituting part of the contaminating shoulder (which represented only 6% of the total AR activity). Pool A was concentrated by ultrafiltration to 6.3 mg protein/10 ml tris phosphate buffer and thus served as the purified AR preparation used for antibody production and in immunohistochemical absorption controls. Pool A represented 26% of the total protein in the first Sephadex G-100 sample.

Fractions constituting the contaminating shoulder (including those fractions containing minor AR activity as described above) were also pooled and concentrated (to 3.4 mg protein/10 ml tris phosphate buffer) and were later used in additional immunohistochemical absorption controls to ensure positive AR localization. Pool B represented 14% of the total protein in the first Sephadex G-100 sample.

Molecular weight estimates for AR were determined by comparison of Sephadex G-100 chromatography profiles of standard molecular weight markers with the elution profile of AR activity. Rat seminal vesicle AR has a molecular weight of 36,500 ± 2000, as was determined by this method in the presence of 5mM mercaptoethanol. A representative summary of the purification procedure for AR is given in the purification table (1).

The purified AR pool contained five bands by PAGE (Figure 2) in the presence of 5mM mercaptoethanol. Three of these bands (with R_f values of 0.36, 0.40, and 0.43) comigrated as a slowly electrophoresing triplet cluster and were

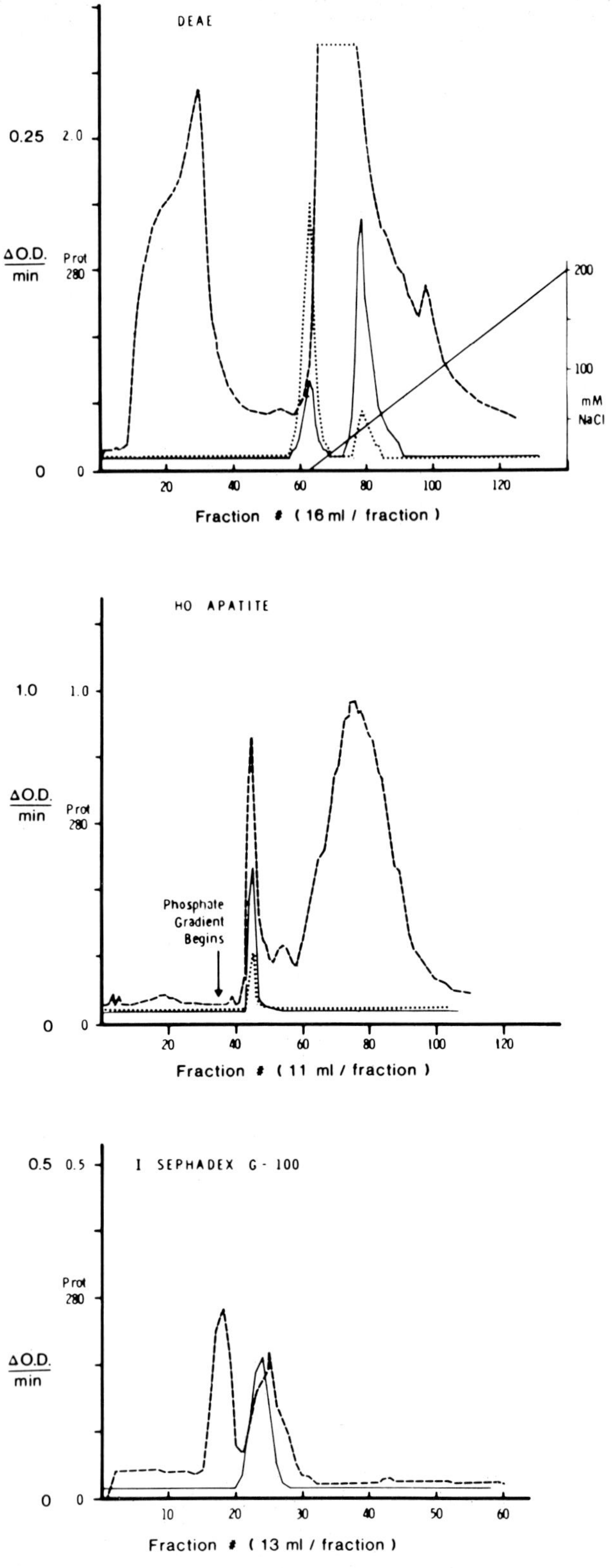

FIGURE 1. Chromatographic purification of AR by three successive columns—DEAE-cellulose (upper), hydroxylapatite (middle), and Sephadex G-100 (lower). DEAE-cellulose column chromatography resulted in the separation of hexonate dehydrogenase (in the column wash) and AR (60mM NaCl) activities. Sephadex G-100 column fractions containing AR activity were pooled and rechromatographed, as shown in figure 2. (- - -) Protein profile as determined spectrophotometrically at 280 nm; (····) enzymatic activity with glucuronate as substrate; (——) enzymatic activity with glyceraldehyde as substrate.

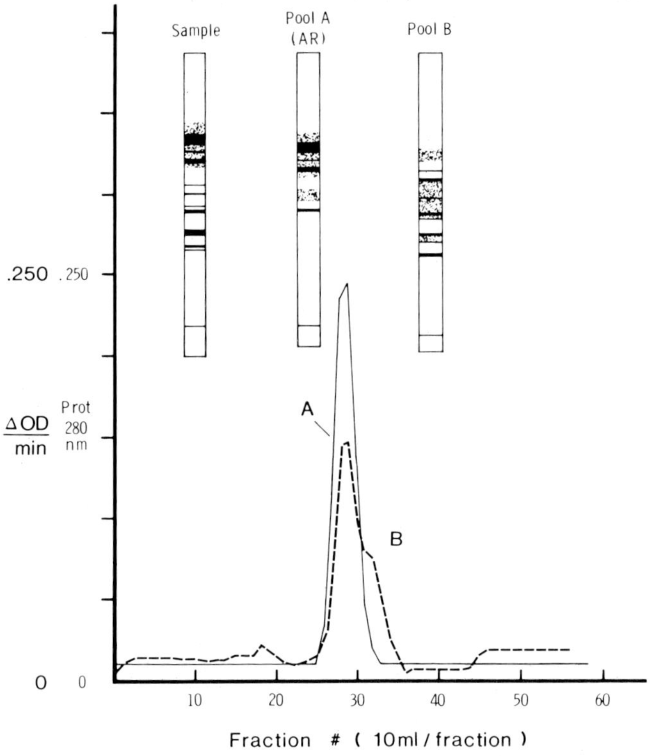

FIGURE 2. Repeated Sephadex G-100 column chromatography of AR. The rechromatographed AR pool from the first Sephadex column run (figure 1) produced the AR pool (A) and contaminating pool (B) subsequently used as antigen for the immunohistochemical localization of AR in rat tissues. Schematic representations of the gel electrophoretograms for the column sample, AR pool, and contaminating pool are included. (----) Protein profile as determined spectrophotometrically at 280 nm; (——) enzymatic activity with glyceraldehyde as substrate.

also present as a cluster in the column sample electrophoretogram, but not in the contaminating pool electrophoretogram. Since AR activity was measurable in both the column sample and AR pool, but not in the contaminating pool, one or more of the bands in this triplet was suspected to represent AR. Jedziniak and Kinoshita[35] report that bovine lens AR exists as three bands by PAGE in the presence of mercaptoethanol, with activity present only in the slowest migrating band. They report that the omission of mercaptoethanol or inclusion of AR inhibitors (TMG, $NADP^+$) in the samples for PAGE results in the shift of the active band to the inactive bands. Attwood and Doughty[36] report similar findings for bovine liver AR, where the enzyme is shown by PAGE to be present as two bands which are antigenically similar, but only one of which possesses activity.

To determine which band(s) represented AR activity in this present study, an end-point activity analysis (Figure 3) was done on duplicate gel columns of identical length. It was found that both the Sephadex column sample and the AR pool contain NADPH-oxidizing activity (taken to be AR activity), which possesses a peak migration factor (R_f) of 0.36, corresponding with the R_f value for the slowest migrating band of the triplet. In both the Sephadex column sample and AR pool, six gel fractions contained NADPH-oxidizing activity (1.2 cm of gel), and they accounted for the entire cluster of three bands. A slight NADPH-oxidizing activity, with an R_f = 0.36, was also present in the contaminating pool (B) and was interpreted to be the fraction of AR activity included in the contaminating shoulder pool (B). The evidence from this study suggests that rat seminal vesicle AR exists as three bands by PAGE in the presence of mercaptoethanol, one of which contains enzymatic activity with a migration factor of 0.36 in 7.5% gels. Sheaff and Doughty[10] show a similar R_f for bovine lens AR, although their findings indicate that the enzyme exists monomerically as a single band by PAGE and SDS-PAGE.

The AR pool, purified to the extent shown in Figure 2, served as the antigen for antibody formation and, along with the contaminating pool, was also employed as antigen for the preabsorption controls used in the immunohistochemistry. In the latter case, each pool was first dialyzed against 5 mM tris phosphate buffer, pH 7.4, to remove preservative and mercaptoethanol before they were frozen and stored at −20°C.

Characterization of AR antisera. Both the AR pool and the contaminating pool were used in double immunodiffusion and immunoelectrophoresis studies of anti-rat AR sera (Figure 4). Both pools were dialyzed to remove mercaptoethanol and concentrated to 1mg/ml for storage, after they were purified, and were used, as such, in these studies.

In the double immunodiffusion study, two components present in both the AR pool and the contaminating pool formed immunoprecipitin bands with the anti-rat AR serum (#4919) eventually used for immunohistochemistry (Figure 4A). In either case, one band predominated as a major component. The precipitin band patterns obtained with these

TABLE 1
Purification of rat seminal vesicle aldose reductase

	Total activity*	Total protein†	Specific activity‡	Yield (%)	Purification (-fold)
Crude extract	10.23	3031	0.0033	100	1
40% Ammonium sulfate supernatant	15.19	2826	0.0053	148	1.6
Sample for DEAE	—	—	—	—	—
Sample for HO-apatite	8.49	266	0.031	83	9.4
Sample for 1st G100	3.7	24	0.154	36	46.6
Sample for 2nd G100	3.6	13	0.276	35	83.6
Pool A (AR)	—	6.3	—	—	—
Pool B	—	3.4	—	—	—

* Micromoles NADPH oxidized per minute.
† Expressed as milligrams.
‡ Micromoles NADPH oxidized/mg protein-min.

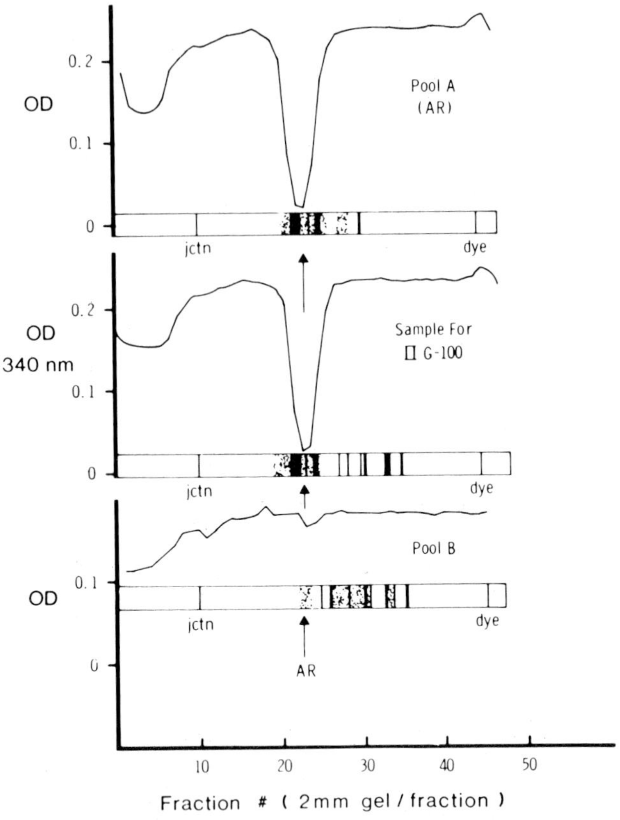

FIGURE 3. PAGE analysis of AR purification. The second (II) G-100 column sample and the resulting purified AR pool (pool A) and contaminating shoulder (pool B) were electrophoresed in duplicate. In each case, one gel was stained by coomassie blue for protein determination and the other gel was fractionated and analyzed for AR activity. The NADPH-oxidizing activity for each gel column is plotted above the corresponding PAGE electrophoretogram. Dye migration (bromophenol blue) was toward the anode.

two pools seem to be simply reversed in intensity, since they both appear at the same distance between the serum and antigen wells and have the same relative (straight and curved) shapes. Antisera from the other rabbits gave similar results for both pools, as is indicated by the lines of identity for the contaminating pool (Figure 4A).

Immunoelectrophoresis was used in an attempt to elucidate the nature of these two precipitin bands. Both pools were electrophoresed and allowed to diffuse against anti-rat AR serum (#4919). The AR pool produced one crisp immunoprecipitin band; two bands were produced by the contaminating pool, the major band comigrating with—and appearing similar in shape to—the AR band (Figure 4B).

As seen in table 2, anti-rat serum immunoprecipitated essentially all AR enzymatic activity when incubated overnight with the rat enzyme solution (0.009 ΔOD/min-10 μg protein). Furthermore, the loss of activity from the supernatant was accounted for in the pellet. The control serum (from a rabbit injected with tris-phosphate and adjuvant) did not produce a precipitate and AR activity was still measurable in the incubate. Nonspecific decay of NADPH in the assay system was determined to be 0.0016 ΔOD/min.

Antisera against bovine AR from two different rabbits were also characterized using bovine AR. These antisera both produced single immunoprecipitin bands when diffused against bovine AR in double immunodiffusion plates and both were capable of immunoprecipitating bovine AR activity. A preliminary antibody-binding study utilizing labeled bovine AR showed that both antisera were also capable of precipitating the labeled enzyme. The results of the competitive-binding study, in which the labeled bovine AR was displaced by the unlabeled bovine or rat enzyme, are shown in Figure 5. Labeled bovine enzyme was effectively displaced from either anti-bovine AR serum by 1.5-15 μg of unlabeled bovine AR (Figure 5A), whereas equal amounts of unlabeled rat enzyme were incapable of displacing radioactivity from the system (Figure 5B). The conclusion that AR from bovine and rat seminal vesicles are not cross immunoreactive is supported by the findings that no immunoprecipitin bands were formed in double immunodiffusion studies using undiluted anti-bovine AR and rat AR at concentrations of 60 μg/ml or 630 μg/ml.

IMMUNOHISTOCHEMICAL LOCALIZATION OF AR

Seminal vesicle. AR was localized exclusively to the epithelial lining of the seminal vesicle, (Figure 6), as may be expected for the demonstration of a glandular enzyme involved in the synthesis of the secretory products of that gland. The cellular staining pattern indicated that AR is distributed in the cytoplasmic compartment of the cell. In cells cut in their longitudinal extent through the nucleus, the staining pattern was seen to extend homogeneously throughout the cell, except for the areas of the nucleus and the apical accumulation of secretory vesicles, which appeared as negative images. No stromal elements of the seminal vesicle stained for AR.

Peripheral nerve. AR immunoreactivity was localized exclusively to the Schwann cell cytoplasm in peripheral nerve. Axons were devoid of immunoreactivity. In tissue sections where the knife plane passed through the nuclear area of a Schwann cell (Figure 7A), the staining image appeared as a "signet ring", with dense staining surrounding the negative image of the nucleus and tapering off on either side as a diminished ring circling the perimeter of the transected nerve fiber. Punctated, or delicately ringed, immunoreactivity was also present, encircling the negative image of the axon cylinder in numerous nerve fiber cross sections.

In longitudinal nerve sections (Figure 7B), the outer cuff of Schwann cell cytoplasm could be seen as densely stained, parallel bands delimiting the boundaries of the nerve fiber. Occasional spikes of immunoreactivity were seen to pass from the cytoplasmic cuff for varying distances into the area of the (extracted) myelin sheath and were interrupted to be Schmidt-Lanterman clefts containing cytoplasm contiguous with the outer cytoplasmic sleeve. The densely staining outer cytoplasmic sleeve curved inward at paranodal regions of the nerve fiber, participating in the formation of nodes of Ranvier. These same images were seen in sections of trigeminal nerve, indicating that AR is localized exclusively to the Schwann cell cytoplasm in cranial nerves as well.

Blood vessels. AR was shown to be present in the endothelial lining of the aorta (Figure 8A) and muscular arteries (Figure 8B). In some instances, the tunica media also showed faint immunoreactive staining, which was abolished by preincubation of the antiserum with AR, but it occurred inconstantly and was always extremely faint compared with the intensity of the endothelial staining. Furthermore, the AR

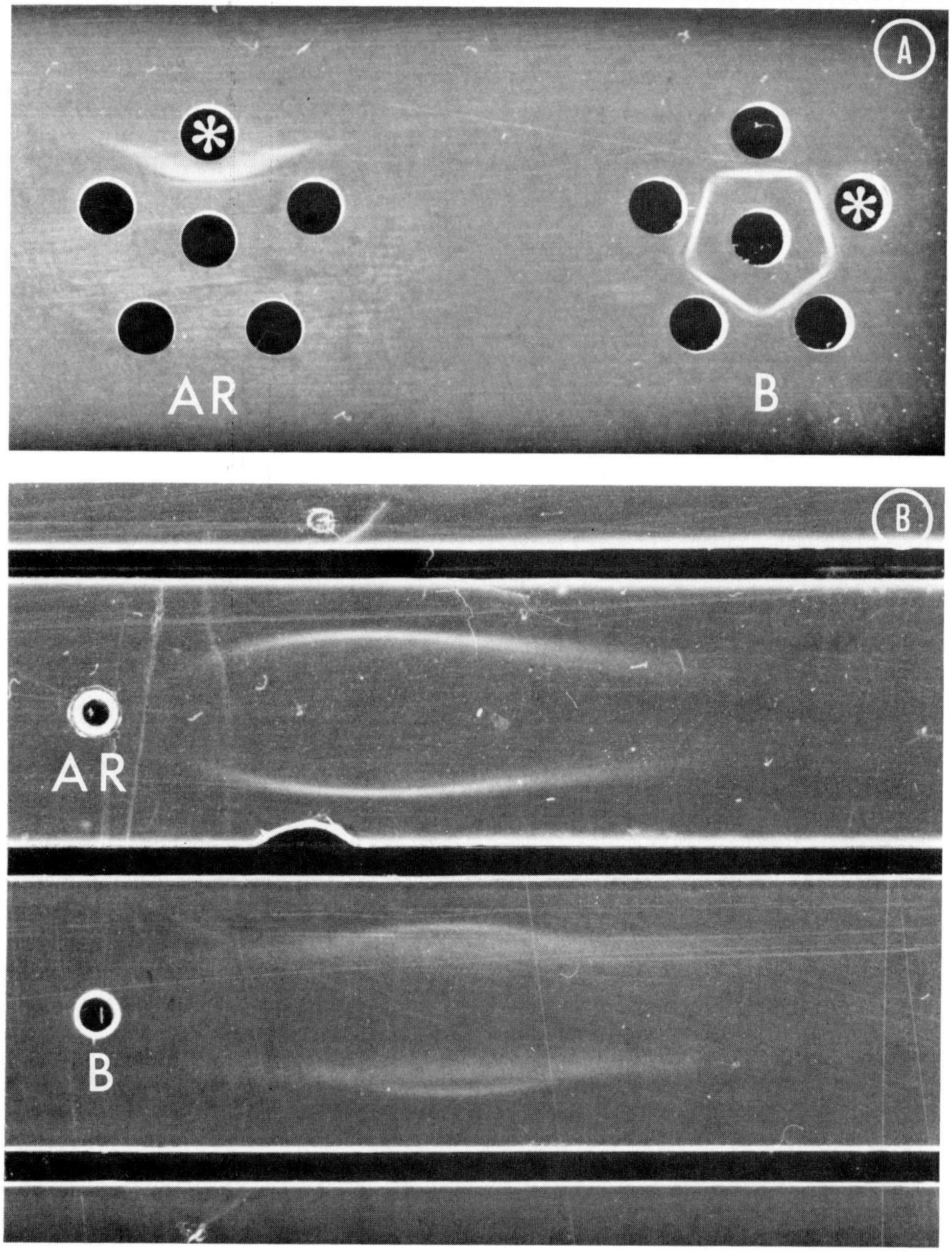

FIGURE 4. Double immunodiffusion and immunoelectrophoretic studies of anti-rat AR serum. (Upper panel, A) Two immunoprecipitin bands were formed by both the AR pool (AR) and the contaminating pool (B) with antiserum used for immunohistochemistry (#4919, serum well is designated by the asterisk). (Lower panel, B) One immunoprecipitin band was formed with the AR pool and two with the contaminating pool when incubated with antiserum in the immunoelectrophoretic study.

positivity of the endothelium was a constant feature of the vessel wall irrespective of the fixation method or vessel type (i.e., muscular or elastic), whereas the stainability of the tunica media followed no apparent pattern with respect to vessel type or fixation method. AR positivity was also demonstrated in the paranuclear cytoplasm of adipocytes found in the adnexa bordering the aorta (Figure 8B).

TABLE 2
Precipitation of rat AR activity by anti-rat AR serum

Serum	Precipitate	AR (△OD/min)	
		Supernatant	Precipitate
Control	none	0.004	----
Anti-rat AR	light flocculent suspension	0.0016	0.009

Testis. In this tissue, Sertoli cells contained AR. Longitudinal and cross sections through the wall of the seminiferous tubule (Figure 9A) showed dense basal staining of Sertoli cell cytoplasm which branched repeatedly and became more diffuse toward the luminal surface. Tangential sections through the abluminal aspect of a seminiferous tubule wall (Figure 9) demonstrated the mosaic staining pattern of numerous prominent Sertoli cell bases and the profiles of sheetlike cytoplasmic basal extensions. Participation of adjacent Sertoli cells in the formation of the blood-testis barrier, which separates basal and abluminal compartments of the tubule wall, was evident in numerous sections (Figure 9 A,C,E), where delicate immunoreactive cytoplasmic extensions of adjacent Sertoli cells were seen to bridge the negative images of the germ cell epithelium (spermatogonia).

Careful study of the staining patterns seen for various

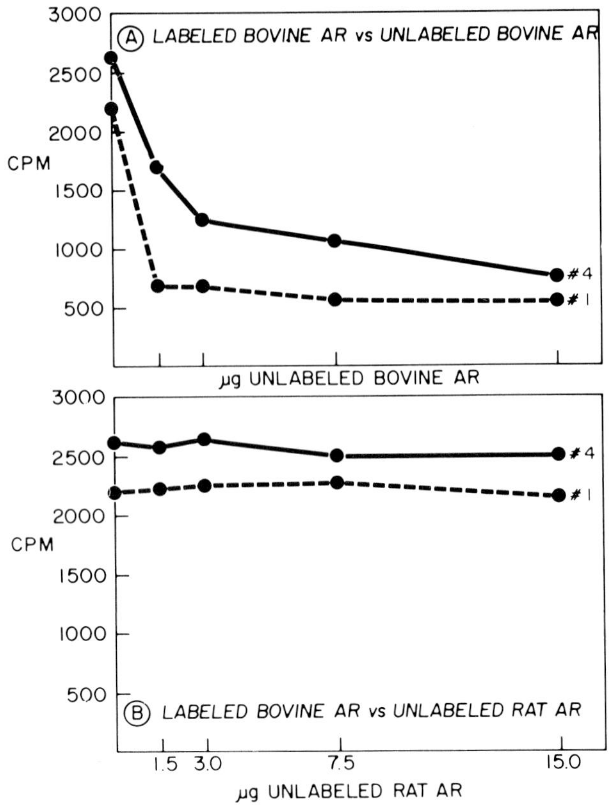

FIGURE 5. Anti-bovine AR competitive-binding study. Unlabeled bovine AR (1.5 to 15.0 µg) displaced labeled bovine enzyme bound by two different anti-bovine AR sera (A), whereas equal amounts of unlabeled rat enzyme did not (B).

seminiferous tubular profiles suggests that late stage, mature spermatids or residual body cytoplasm also contain immunoreactive AR. This conclusion was based on the observation (Figure 9 C,D) of a dense luminal ring of immunostaining present only in tubular profiles of late stage spermatogenesis, where adjacent serial sections, stained for morphology, showed numerous mature spermatids superficially embedded in the apical Sertoli cell cytoplasm. The staining pattern seen for tubular profiles of early stage spermatogenesis consistently lacked the luminal ring of immunoreactivity, and delicate, diffuse branches of AR-positive Sertoli cell cytoplasm reached the luminal surface (Figure 9 E,F). These relationships were consistently observed for all tubular profiles.

These data suggest that AR appears late in the developing germ cells. No immunoreactivity was demonstrated in spermatogonia, spermatocytes, or in early spermatid cell types. In addition, AR was not found in any interstitial cellular elements. We conclude that AR is localized exclusively in Sertoli cells and in mature spermatids or residual bodies.

DISCUSSION

The purification procedure resulted in the obtention of purified rat seminal vesicle AR, which was thought to exist as a cluster of triplet bands on PAGE. This conclusion was based on the fact that the presence of the triplet cluster, in both the column sample and AR pool, but not in the contaminating pool, coincided with assayable enzyme activity in those two pools. This conclusion is supported by the reported presence of three bands by PAGE for bovine lens AR.[35] In both instances, the slowest migrating band in the triplet contained AR activity. Other investigators have also shown AR from a number of tissues to exist as antigenically similar multiple bands, only one of which contained AR activity.[18,26,37]

The estimated molecular weight for rat seminal vesicle AR of 36,500 is in actual (or close) agreement with the molecular weight reported by Clements et al.[38] for human placental AR (36,500), by Gabbay[19] for bovine retinal AR

FIGURE 6. Immunoperoxidase photomicrographs of rat seminal vesicle. Tissue sections were incubated with anti-rat AR serum (#4919) at 1:1000 dilution (A) and, with the same dilution, were preabsorbed with 25 µg protein/ml of AR (B). Only the epithelial lining stained for AR. All subsequent immunohistochemistry was done with 1:2000-dilution antiserum and, with the same dilution, was preabsorbed with 50 µg protein/ml of AR. 222×.

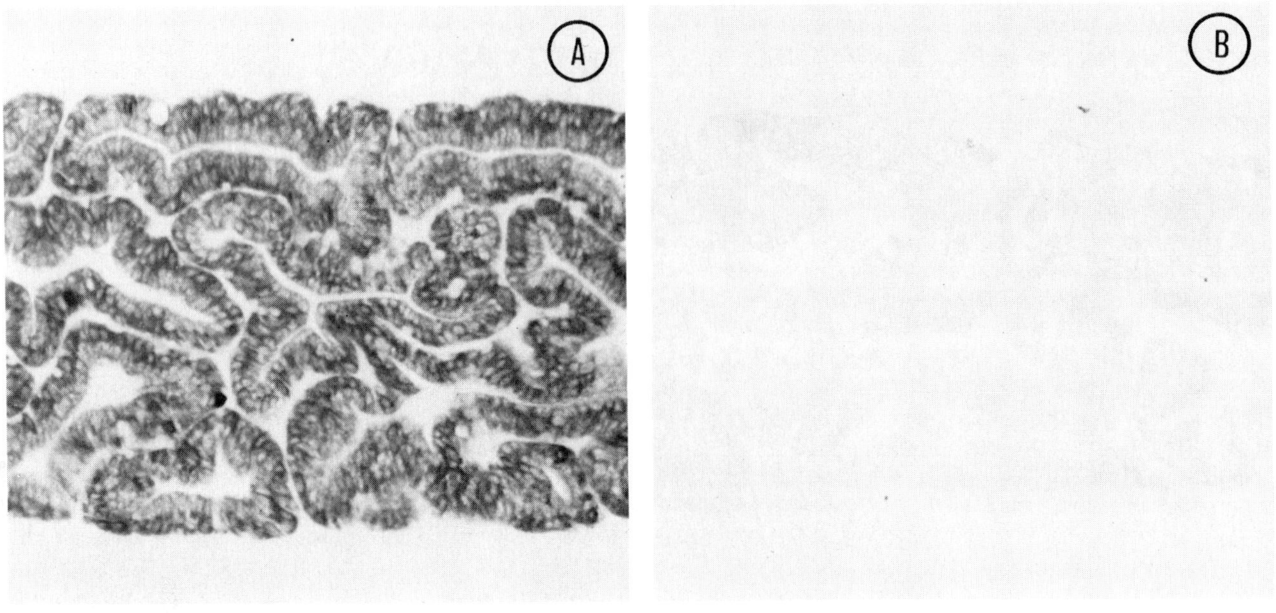

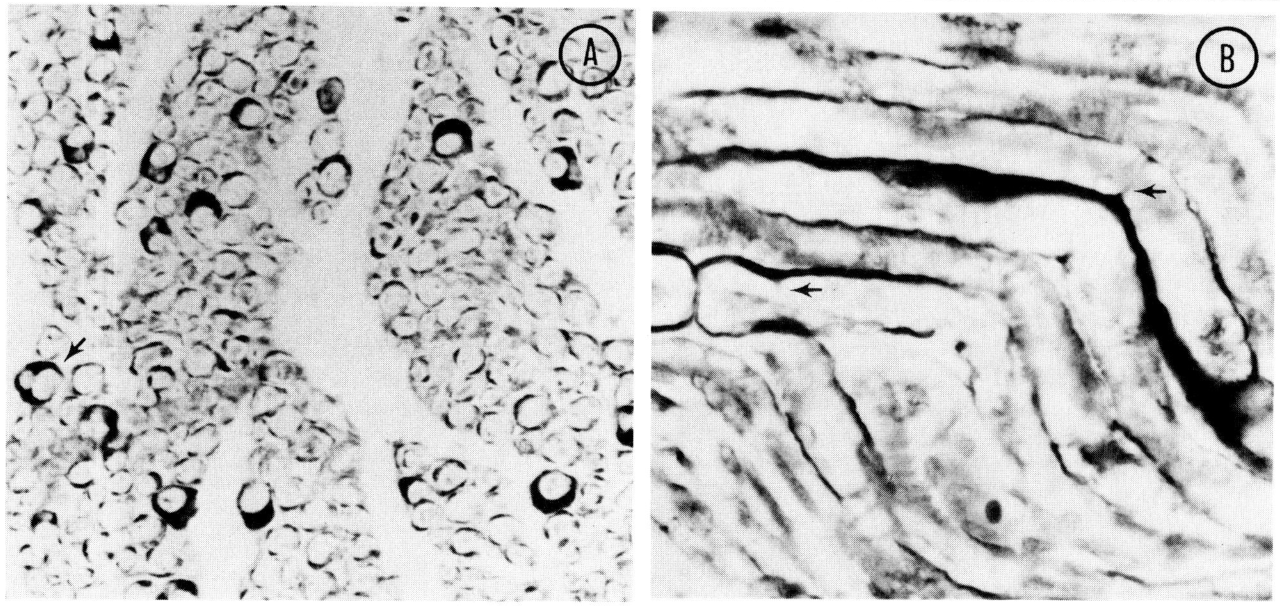

FIGURE 7. Immunoperoxidase photomicrographs of transverse (A) and longitudinal (B) sections of rat sciatic nerve. The characteristic "signet ring"–staining image is seen for Schwann cell cytoplasm in transverse sections through the nucleus (arrow, A, 496 ×). Occasional spikes of immunopositive cytoplasm, representing Schmidt-Lanterman clefts, are seen in B (arrows, 840 ×). (C) Preabsorption control for B, 840 ×.

(32,000), by Gabbay and Cathcart[18] for bovine kidney AR (32,000), and by Sheaff and Doughty[10] for bovine lens AR (37,000). The presence of multiple AR activity peaks on hydroxylapatite column chromatography, reported as isozymes by Gabbay and Cathcart,[18] was not demonstrated for seminal vesicle AR in this study.

The presence of two immunoprecipitin bands, formed by both the AR pool and the contaminating pool in the double immunodiffusion study, suggests that two antigens may be present in each pool in reciprocal concentrations, that is, each pool slightly contaminates the other.

This observation is corroborated by the results of the PAGE end-point activity analysis, where some activity is present in the contaminating pool. The generation of a single immunoprecipitin band, obtained with the AR pool in the immunoelectrophoretic study, was unexpected, given the outcome of the double immunodiffusion studies. A possible explanation for this apparent discrepancy may be that AR exists in equilibrium as a loosely associated monomer/dimer and that antibodies were raised against different determinants of both forms. In an electrophoretic field, the equilibrium may be such that only the monomer is present, thus accounting for one immunoprecipitin band, whereas in the passive immunodiffusion system, both monomer and dimer are present, thus precipitating two bands.

Although cross immunoreactivity for AR from different tissues in the rat was evident in the immunohistochemical demonstration of the enzyme, AR from rat and bovine seminal vesicles do not cross immunoreact, as demonstrated by double immunodiffusion and competitive protein-binding studies. Although the absence of immunoprecipitin bands in the double immunodiffusion studies utilizing anti-bovine AR and rat AR may be explained by an inability of the antigen-antibody ratios to reach an equilibrium point at the concentrations used, the same negative results were obtained with rat AR at two concentrations an order of magnitude apart. Furthermore, the results of the competitive-binding study corroborate this conclusion, where the precipitation of

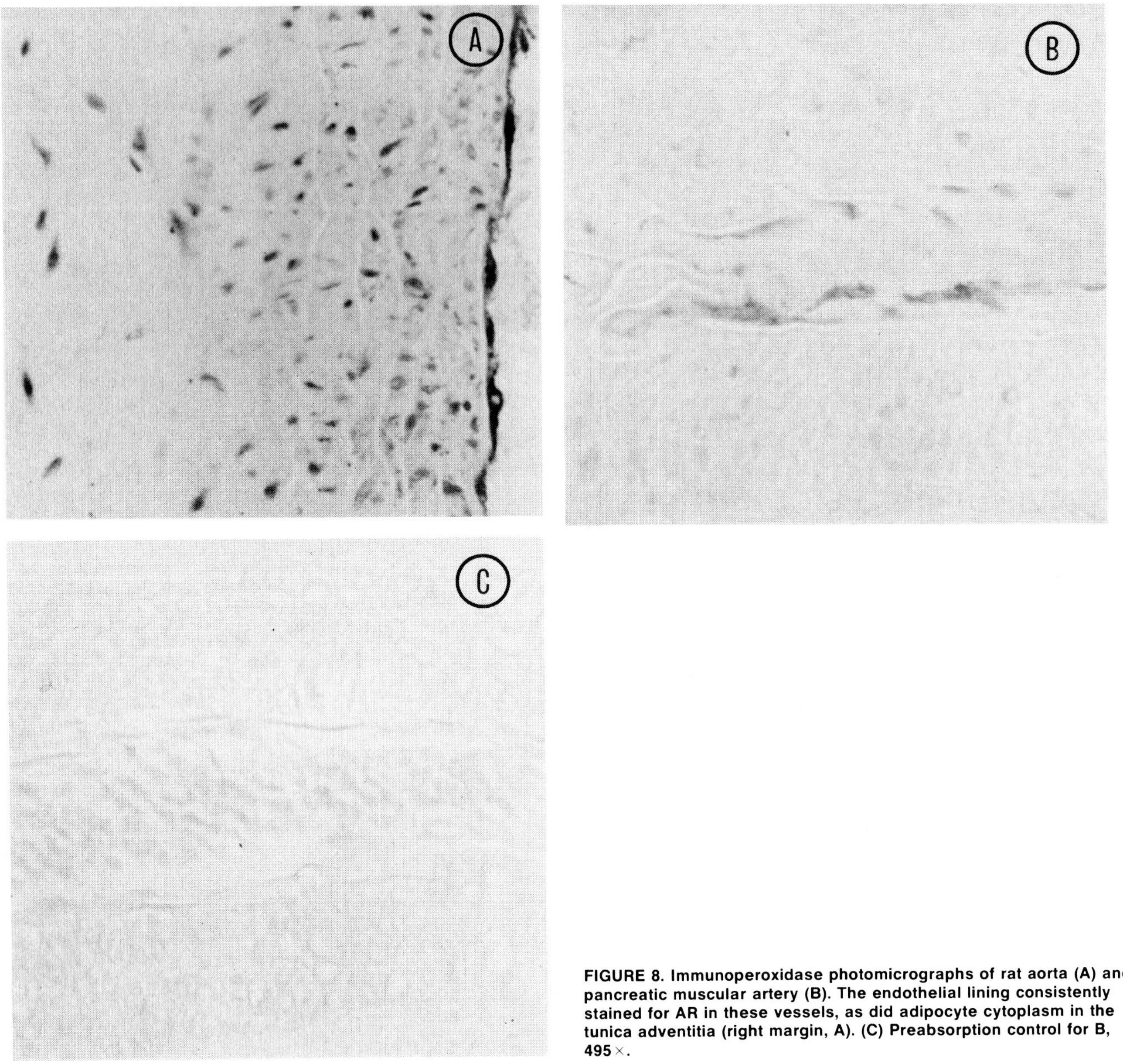

FIGURE 8. Immunoperoxidase photomicrographs of rat aorta (A) and pancreatic muscular artery (B). The endothelial lining consistently stained for AR in these vessels, as did adipocyte cytoplasm in the tunica adventitia (right margin, A). (C) Preabsorption control for B, 495×.

antigen-antibody complexes relies on polyethylene oxide and not on the presence of a precipitating antibody.

The specific nature of the AR-staining patterns obtained in this study for various tissues are in close correlation with the results obtained from biochemical and histochemical studies. Although some discrepancy exists concerning the number of immunoprecipitin bands obtained using this antiserum in Ouchterlony double immunodiffusion and immunoelectrophoretic systems, it remains clear that (1) antibodies were obtained specific to AR (enzymatic activity), (2) AR blocks the staining reaction, and (3) the contaminating pool does not. The compartmentalization of AR immunoreactivity to Schwann cell cytoplasm is in good agreement with the conclusion reached by Gabbay and O'Sullivan[12] and Gabbay[2] from their studies of pathway enzyme activity changes produced by wallerian degeneration. In addition, studies of impaired motor nerve conduction, brought about by enhanced polyol pathway activity in hyperglycemic states, also suggest Schwann cell involvement.[2,4,41–43]

The conclusion that mature spermatids (or residual body cytoplasm) contain AR in addition to the Sertoli cell is supported by reports of the histochemical demonstration of that

FIGURE 9. Immunoperoxidase photomicrographs of the seminiferous tubules of rat testis. (A) Immunopositive Sertoli cells are seen cut both in longitudinal extent and transversely through their bases as the tubule leaves the plane of section. (B) Preabsorption control for A, 185×. (C and D) Serial sections of late stage spermatogenesis tubules stained for AR (C) and for morphology (D), demonstrating the presence of a punctated, spiked luminal ring of immunostain, consistently noted in tubular profiles containing superficially embedded mature spermatids. Delicate spikes of immunoreactivity extend into the lumen in register with spermatid tail pieces (arrows), 472×. (E and F) Serial sections of early stage spermatogenesis tubules stained for AR (E) and for morphology (F). The absence of a luminal ring of immunostain was consistently noted in tubular profiles where immature spermatids are embedded deep in the Sertoli cell. Numerous immunopositive Sertoli cells are extending throughout the wall of the tubule, 472×.

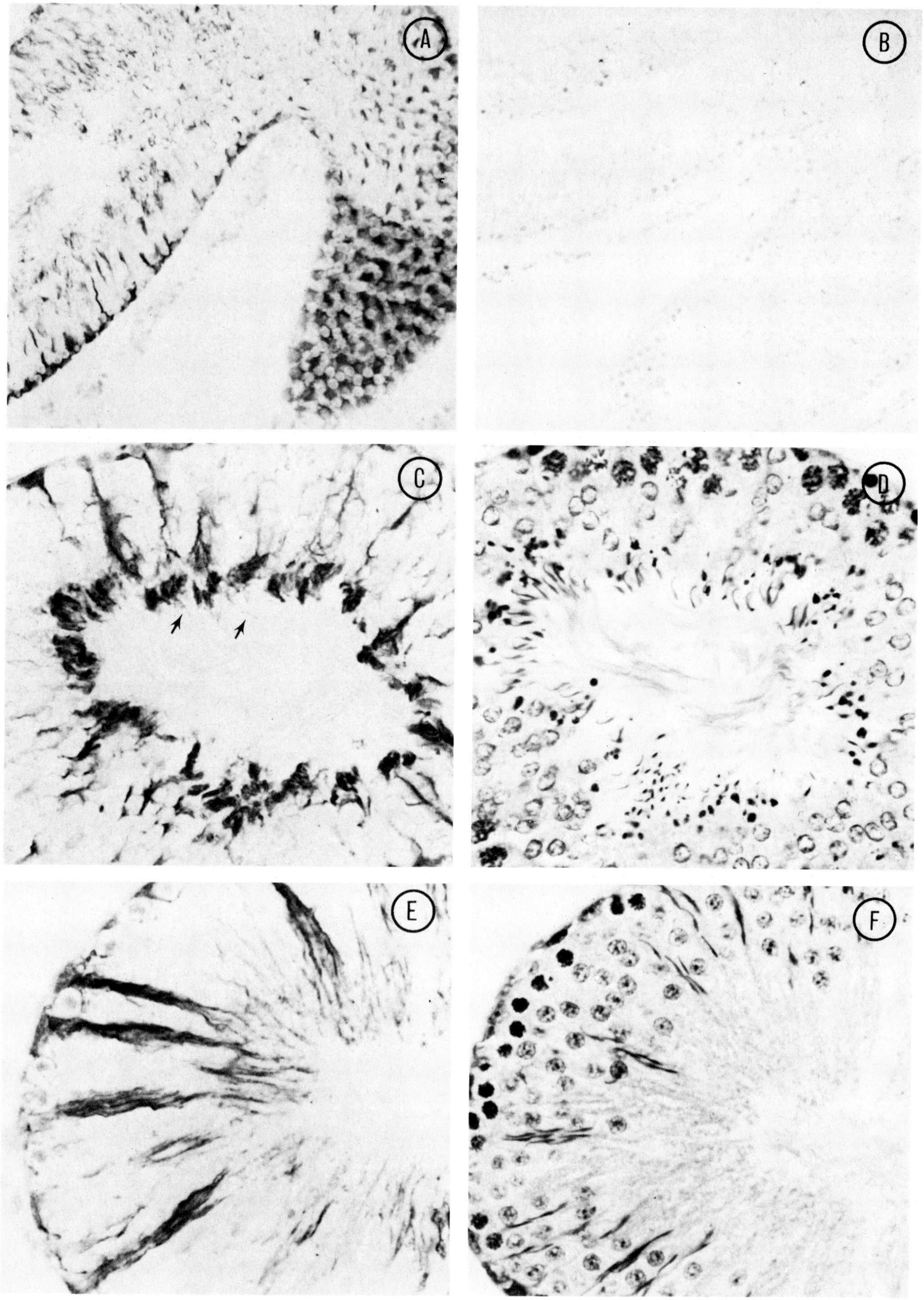
A
B
C
D
E
F

enzyme in mature spermatids.[26] Data suggesting the presence of sorbitol dehydrogenase in late stages of germinal epithelial cell differentiation[23,24] are also circumstantial evidence for the presence of the polyol pathway and, hence, AR. The claim for AR's presence in mature spermatids is based on the consistent demonstration of a luminal ring of stain only in those seminiferous tubules exhibiting late stage spermatogenesis, in which spermatids are superficially embedded in Sertoli cells. The possibility that this staining pattern may represent a maximal stainability of apical Sertoli cell cytoplasm, reflecting perhaps the trophic role this cell plays in response to spermatids in late stages of spermatogenesis (Y. Clermont, personal communication), cannot be ruled out at present, although this possibility seems unlikely from a morphologic point of view.

Rat pancreas was also investigated in this study. Immunoreactive AR was absent from all cellular elements except arterial endothelium. AR has been partially purified from rat pancreas and is immunologically identical to rat kidney medullar AR.[18] Accumulation of polyol pathway substrates occurs in isolated rat islets incubated in high glucose medium,[27,28] and Gabbay[2] demonstrated the presence of AR by the Ouchterlony technique in a human insulinoma using a monospecific antibody to human placental AR. Repeated attempts to immunostain rat pancreas, islets, or beta cell adenomata (courtesy of Dr. P. K. Dixit) for AR were unsuccessful in the present study. Although these results suggest that AR is not present in the pancreas, the literature is overwhelmingly at odds with this conclusion, and we must assume that the antiserum used in this study does not recognize immunologic determinants for pancreatic AR. There are reports that AR from sheep seminal vesicle and placenta do not cross react with antibodies directed against the other enzyme,[39,40] and it is possible that AR from rat seminal vesicle and pancreas do not share immunologic determinants, as well. Calculations based on the purification data suggest that the anti-rat AR serum, used at a dilution of 1:2000 in the unlabeled antibody-enzyme PAP technique, is capable of demonstrating the presence of picogram amounts of AR per cell, an antigen concentration approximately 1000 times less than that of such a typically stored hormone as insulin.[48]

The most direct consequence of this study is that the accurate knowledge of the cellular distribution of AR calls for a reassessment of the potentially pathogenic osmotic force generated by a given amount of polyol accumulation within a tissue. Only three tissues—lens, peripheral nerve, and kidney papilla—have, thus far, been shown to contain sufficiently high concentrations of polyols (10–80 μmol/g tissue) to be of possible osmotic importance in diabetes and galactosemia.[1,2] Ward[13] estimated that the osmotic pressure generated by increased pathway activity in the nerves of early diabetics will not exceed 5% if the pathway substrates are evenly distributed throughout the water compartment of the nerve. However, this is now known not to be the case, since AR is sequestered in Schwann cell cytoplasm, which represents only a fraction of the total nerve water compartment. Similarly, the accumulation of sorbitol in aortic wall incubated in 20mM and 50mM glucose medium, as reported by Morrison et al.[16] and Winegrad et al.,[46] is considered to be grossly insufficient to account for the swelling observed in terms of an osmotic mechanism.[2,47] However, if the accumulated sorbitol content (up to 50 nmol/g tissue) is limited to the endothelial lining, the osmotic force generated in this reduced volume may be sufficient to alter the permeability of the endothelium for diffusion of oxygen and nutrients to the interior of the vessel wall.

In conclusion, knowledge of the cellular distribution of AR in tissues known to be sites of diabetic complications allows for a reassessment of the large body of information at hand concerning the polyol pathway and the consequences of increased pathway activity in hyperglycemic states. However, these newly attained morphologic data must themselves be assessed in light of the available biochemical data, because the immunohistochemical demonstration of AR does not necessarily demonstrate enzymatically active AR. The morphologic and biochemical data must be interpreted simultaneously to obtain a proper appreciation of the microscopic extent of the arena in which the polyol pathway exerts a pathogenic influence.

ACKNOWLEDGMENTS

The scientific advice of Dr. Robert P. Elde and Dr. James B. Howard is gratefully acknowledged.

This investigation was supported by USPHS diabetes training grant AM07196.

REFERENCES

1 Gabbay, K. H.: The sorbitol pathway and the complications of diabetes. N. Engl. J. Med. *288*:831–36, 1973.

2 Gabbay, K. H.: Hyperglycemia, polyol metabolism, and complications of diabetes mellitus. Annu. Rev. Med. *26*:521–36, 1975.

3 Winegrad, A. I., Clements, R. S., and Morrison, A. D.: Insulin-dependent pathways of carbohydrate metabolism. *In* Handbook of Physiology; Endocrinology, Vol. 1, Steiner, D. F., and Freinkel, N., Eds. Washington, D.C., Am. Physiol. Soc., 1972, pp. 457–71.

4 Winegrad, A. I., Morrison, A. D., and Clements, R. S.: The polyol pathway: a model for biochemical mechanisms by which hyperglycemia may contribute to the pathogenesis of the complications of diabetes mellitus. *In* Diabetes. Proc. 8th Congr. IDF. Malaisse, W. J., and Pirart, J., Eds. Amsterdam and New York, Excerpta Medica/American Elsevier, 1974, pp. 387–95.

5 van Heyningen, R.: Formation of polyols by the lens of the rat with 'sugar' cataract. Nature (London) *184*:194–95, 1959.

6 van Heyningen, R.: The sorbitol pathway in the lens. Exp. Eye Res. *1*:396–404, 1962.

7 Kinoshita, J. H.: Cataracts in galactosemia. The Jonas S. Friedenwald memorial lecture. Invest. Ophthalmol. *4*:786–99, 1965.

8 Chylack, L. T., and Kinoshita, J. H.: A biochemical evaluation of a cataract induced in a high-glucose medium. Invest. Ophthalmol. *8*:401–12, 1969.

9 Kinoshita, J. H., Futterman, S., Satoh, K., and Merola, L. O.: Factors affecting the formation of sugar alcohols in ocular lens. Biochim. Biophys. Acta *74*:340–50, 1963.

10 Sheaff, C. M., and Doughty, C. C.: Physical and kinetic properties of homogeneous bovine lens aldose reductase. J. Biol. Chem. *251*:2696–2702, 1976.

11 Gabbay, K. H., Merola, L. O., and Field, R. A.: Sorbitol pathway: presence in nerve and cord with substrate accumulation in diabetes. Science *151*:209–10, 1966.

12 Gabbay, K. H., and O'Sullivan, J. B.: The sorbitol pathway: enzyme localization and content in normal and diabetic nerve and cord. Diabetes *17*:239–43, 1968.

13 Ward, J. D.: The polyol pathway in the neuropathy of early diabetes. Adv. Metab. Disord. *2*(Suppl. 2):425–532, 1973.

14 Clements, R. S., Weaver, J. P., and Winegrad, A. I.: The distribution of polyol:NADP oxidoreductase in mammalian tissues. Biochem. Biophys. Res. Commun. *37*:347–53. 1969.

15 Clements, R. S., Morrison, A. D., and Winegrad, A. I.: Polyol pathway in aorta: regulation by hormones. Science *166*:1007–08, 1969.

16 Morrison, A. D., Clements, R. S., and Winegrad, A. I.: Effects of elevated glucose concentrations on the metabolism of the aortic wall. J. Clin. Invest. *51*:3114–23, 1972.

17 Gabbay, K. H., and O'Sullivan, J. B.: The sorbitol pathway in diabetes and galactosemia: enzyme and substrate localization and changes in kidney. Diabetes *17*:300, 1968. (Abstr.)

18 Gabbay, K. H., and Cathcart, E. S.: Purification and immunologic identification of aldose reductases. Diabetes *23*:460–68, 1974.

[19] Gabbay, K. H.: Purification and immunological identification of bovine retinal aldose reductase. Isr. J. Med. Sci. *8*:1626–29, 1972.

[20] Buzney, S. M., Frank, R. N., Varma, S. D., Tanishima, T., and Gabbay, K. H.: Aldose reductase in retinal mural cells. Invest. Ophthalmol. *16*:392–96, 1977.

[21] Hers, H. G.: L'aldose-reductase. Biochim. Biophys. Acta *37*:120–26, 1960.

[22] Williams-Ashman, H. G., and Banks, J.: The ketose reductase of rat liver and accessory sexual organs. Arch. Biochm. Biophys. *50*:513–15, 1954.

[23] Bishop, D. W., Schrank, W. W., Musselman, A. D., and Muecke, E. C.: Testis sorbitol dehydrogenase and activity changes during induced aspermatogenesis and cryptorchidism. Fed. Proc. *26*:646, 1967. (Abstr.)

[24] Bishop, D. W., Tang, F. Y., Walker, P. S., and Ketner, G.: Sorbitol dehydrogenase and its substrates in mammalian testes. Fed. Proc. *29*:248, 1970. (Abstr.)

[25] Germino, N. I., Micucci, M., Grau, V., Rama, F., and Castellano, M. A.: Location of iditol:NAD oxidoreductase (sorbitol tetrazolium reductase or ketose-reductase) in the genital tract of the bull. J. Endocrinol. *47*:111–15, 1970.

[26] Micucci, M., Rama, F., Castellano, M. A., and Germino, N. I.: The histochemical distribution of fructose metabolism enzymes in bovine spermatogenesis. J. Anat. *109*:209–14, 1971.

[27] Morrison, A. D., Winegrad, A. I., Fink, C. J., and Lacy, P. E.: Sorbitol synthesis in isolated rat pancreatic islets. Biochem. Biophys. Res. Commun. *38*:491–95, 1970.

[28] Gabbay, K. H., and Tze, Wah Jun: Inhibition of glucose-induced release of insulin by aldose reductase inhibitors. Proc. Natl. Acad. Sci. USA *69*:1435–39, 1972.

[29] Ludvigson, M. A.: Immunohistochemical localization of aldose reductase in the rat. Anat. Rec. *190*:465–66, 1978. (Abstr.)

[30] Ludvigson, M. A., and Sorenson, R. L.: Immunohistochemical localization of aldose reductase in the rat. Diabetes *27*(Suppl. 2): 463, 1978. (Abstr.)

[31] Thorell, J. I., and Johansson, B. G.: Enzymatic iodination of polypeptides with ^{125}I to high specific activity. Biochim. Biophys. Acta *251*:363–69, 1971.

[32] Sternberger, L. A., Hardy, P. H., Cuculis, J. J., and Meyer, H. G.: The unlabeled antibody enzyme method of immunohistochemistry. Preparation and properties of soluble antigen-antibody complex (horseradish peroxidase-antihorseradish peroxidase) and its use in identification of spirochetes. J. Histochem. Cytochem. *18*:315–33, 1970.

[33] Moonsammy, G. I., and Stewart, M. A.: Purification and properties of brain aldose reductase and L-hexonate dehyrogenase. J. Neurochem. *14*:1187–93, 1967.

[34] Hayman, S., Lou, M. F., Merola, L. O., and Kinoshita, J. H.: Aldose reductase activity in the lens and other tissues. Biochim. Biophys. Acta *128*:474–82, 1966.

[35] Jedziniak, J. A., and Kinoshita, J. H.: Activators and inhibitors of lens aldose reductase. Invest. Ophthalmol. *10*:357–66, 1971.

[36] Attwood, M. A., and Doughty, C. C.: Purification and properties of calf liver aldose reductase. Biochim. Biophys. Acta *370*:358–68, 1974.

[37] Dons, R. F., and Winegrad, A. I.: Isolation and characterization of aldose reductase from calf brain. Biochim. Biophys. Acta *452*:1–12, 1976.

[38] Clements, R. S., and Winegrad, A. I.: Purification of alditol:NADP oxidoreductase from human placenta. Biochem. Biophys. Res. Commun. *47*:1473–79, 1972.

[39] Hastein, T., and Velle, W.: Purification and properties of aldose reductases from the placenta and the seminal vesicle of the sheep. Biochim. Biophys. Acta *178*:1–10, 1969.

[40] Velle, W.: Aldose reductase from seminal vesicle and placenta of ruminants. Methods Enzymol. *41*:165–70, 1975.

[41] Gabbay, J. H., and Snider, J. J.: Nerve conduction defect in galactose-fed rats. Diabetes *21*:295–300, 1972.

[42] Ward, J. D., Baker, R. W. R., and Davis, B. H.: Effect of blood sugar control on the accumulation of sorbitol and fructose in nervous tissues. Diabetes *21*:1173–78, 1972.

[43] Stewart, M. A., Sherman, W. R., Kurien, M. M., Moonsammy, G. I., and Wisgerhof, M.: Polyol accumulations in nervous tissue of rats with experimental diabetes and galactosemia. J. Neurochem. *14*:1057–66, 1967.

[44] Whereat, A. F.: Recent advances in experimental and molecular pathology. Atherosclerosis and metabolic disorder in the arterial wall. Exp. Mol. Pathol. *7*:233–47, 1967.

[45] Haust, M. D.: Injury and repair in the pathogenesis of atherosclerotic lesions. *In* Atherosclerosis. Proc. Second Int. Symp. Jones, R. J., Ed. Berlin, Springer, 1970, p. 12.

[46] Winegrad, A. I., Morrison, A. D., and Clements, R. S.: Alterations in the composition and metabolism of the inner aortic wall associated with increased polyol pathway activity. Horm. Metab. Res. (Suppl. 4):169–71, 1974.

[47] Rasio, E. A., and Morrison, A. D.: Glucose-induced alterations of the metabolism of an isolated capillary preparation. Diabetes *27*:108–13, 1978.

[48] Ludvigson, M. A.: Immunohistochemical localization of aldose reductase in the rat. Ph.D. Thesis. University of Minnesota at Minneapolis, 1979.

Immunohistochemical Localization of Aldose Reductase

II. Rat Eye and Kidney

MARK A. LUDVIGSON AND ROBERT L. SORENSON

SUMMARY

Aldose reductase (AR) was purified from rat seminal vesicles. Specific antibodies to this enzyme were prepared in rabbits and were used in the unlabeled antibody-enzyme (PAP) technique to localize AR in a number of tissues known to be sites of diabetic lesions. AR was localized in the following structures in the eye: lens epithelial lining and cortical lenticular fibers; corneal endothelium; the inner, nonpigmented layer of ciliary body epithelium and its extension as the posterior surface of the iris; and neuroglial (Müller) cells in the retina. Retinal capillary endothelium did not contain immunoreactive AR.

In the kidney, staining was intense in the inner medulla. Specific structures included thin limbs of the loop of Henle, collecting tubules deep in the inner medulla, and transitional epithelial cells lining the pelvic space: structures in the cortex included glomerular podocytes and distal convoluted tubules. Collecting tubules in the outer medulla and cortex, as well as proximal convoluted tubules and glomerular capillary endothelium did not contain immunoreactive AR.

DIABETES 29:450–459, June 1980.

The polyol or sorbitol pathway consists of two enzymatic reactions which together convert a number of aldose sugars to their corresponding ketose sugars through a polyol intermediate and yield a net production of NADP and NADH. Aldose reductase (alditol:NADP oxidoreductase, EC 1.1.1.21, or AR) is responsible for the production of the polyol intermediate; thus, in mammalian metabolism, the principle aldose sugar, glucose, is converted to sorbitol. Enhanced pathway activity occurs in such hyperglycemic conditions as diabetes and galactosemia, and the subsequent intracellular accumulation of polyols and cofactors under these conditions has implicated the polyol pathway in the etiology of diabetic complications.[1–4]

An understanding of the cellular distribution of AR in tissues known to be sites of diabetic complications would aid in the assessment of the polyol pathway's role in the etiology of these complications. Toward that end, antibodies generated against rat seminal vesicle AR[22] were used in the unlabeled antibody-enzyme (PAP) technique to determine the cellular location of the enzyme in rat eye and kidney. The development of the immunohistochemical technique as well as the cellular distribution of AR in the arterial wall, peripheral nerve, and testis have been reported.[22]

MATERIALS AND METHODS

The purification of rat seminal vesicle AR and the obtention and characterization of the antiserum was described previously.[22] The antiserum was determined to be specific for AR by immunoprecipitation of the enzyme (with AR activity recoverable in the precipitate) and by Ouchterlony double immunodiffusion and immunoelectrophoretic methods.

The tissues were fixed either in Bouin's fixative by immersion, or by vascular perfusion with either picric acid formalin or 4% paraformaldehyde (with or without 0.1% glutaraldehyde) in Sorenson's (0.2M) or cacodylate (0.2M) buffers, pH 7.2. Tissues were processed for paraffin embedment and were sectioned at 5μm. The working dilution of the AR antiserum was determined empirically on tissue sections. A 1:2000 dilution in borate-buffered saline containing 10% normal sheep serum was found to be optimal. The unlabeled antibody-enzyme (PAP) technique was used throughout the study.[25] Thus, tissue sections were consecutively incubated with anti-rat AR serum (overnight at 4°C), sheep anti-rabbit immunoglobulin (1:200, one hour, 22°C), and rabbit peroxidase-antiperoxidase (1:500, one hour, 22°C). Each incubation was followed with a wash in borate-buffered saline to remove the unreacted agents. The presence of AR was indicated by the precipitation of diaminobenzidine. Controls

This work was presented in part at the 38th Annual Meeting of the American Diabetes Association held at Boston, Massachusetts, on 13 June 1978.
From the Department of Anatomy, University of Minnesota School of Medicine, Minneapolis.
Address reprint requests to Mark A. Ludvigson, Ph.D., Department of Anatomy, 4-135 Jackson Hall, 321 Church Street S.E., Minneapolis, MN 55455.
Received for publication 29 October 1979.

routinely consisted of omission of the primary antiserum and preincubation of the primary working antiserum with 50 μg antigen protein/ml.

RESULTS

In general, the simplest fixation procedure gave the best immunohistochemical results; immersion in Bouin's fixative produced excellent AR localization. Other procedures, such as vascular perfusion with picric acid formalin or with paraformaldehyde, also gave acceptable localization results, although staining intensity was usually reduced. Picric acid formalin and 4% paraformaldehyde in phosphate buffer both tended to vacuolate and shrink the tissue. However, 4% paraformaldehyde with 0.1% glutaraldehyde in cacodylate buffer fixed kidney tissue most suitably for the delicate localization of AR immunoreactivity in cortical structures. None of the procedures successfully prepared lens nucleus.

The eye. The presence of AR was demonstrated in numerous cell types in the lens, cornea, iris, ciliary body, and retina. The lens epithelial lining stained heavily for AR (Figure 1A). Cortical lenticular fibers also contained AR, but the staining intensity was markedly reduced when compared with the lens epithelium. In the bow region of the lens, where the epithelial cells become greatly elongated to form lens fibers, the staining intensity was intermediate and blended with the extremes in intensity seen with the lens epithelium and cortical lens fibers. Although immunohistochemical quantitative estimates of antigen concentration are, at best, subjective values, these results suggest that the lenticular cellular content of AR may remain relatively constant, with the enzyme concentration inversely proportionate to cell volume.

AR is localized exclusively in the endothelial lining of the cornea. No immunoreactivity was demonstrated in either the stroma or epithelium (Figure 1C,D).

The inner, nonpigmented layer of the ciliary body epithelium and its extension as the posterior surface of the iris stained heavily for AR (Figures 1C and 2A). The outer epithelial layer of the ciliary body, as well as the vascular linings of small vessels contained in the ciliary body, did not stain for the enzyme (Figure 2A).

The immunostaining pattern for AR included elements in three layers of the retina; namely, the nerve fiber and ganglion cell layer, the inner plexiform layer, and the inner nuclear layer (Figure 3A–C). Toward the anterior margins of the retina, in the region of the ora serrata (Figure 3A), the inner nuclear layer was seen to contain densely stained, AR-positive cell bodies which extended fine immunopositive processes across the inner plexiform layer to end in the ganglion cell layer. A dense network of immunoreactive fibrous elements was a consistent finding in the ganglion cell layer. The position of the cell bodies and orientation of their processes indicated these cells to be neuroglial supporting cells (of Müller). The immunostaining pattern seen for these cells is identical to that seen in the histochemical demonstrations of Müller cells by dehydrogenase histochemistry (T. Kuwabara, personal communication). In the regions of the retina close to the optic papilla (Figure 3C), the immunostaining pattern was not as striking, and the fine cellular processes traversing the inner plexiform layer could not be demonstrated. Immunostaining of Müller cell paranuclear cytoplasm and basal arborizations (resting on the inner limiting membrane) were consistently noted throughout the extent of the retina from the optic papilla to the ora serrata.

The specific localization of AR to elements in the nerve fiber and ganglion cell layers is somewhat hampered by the dense immunoreactive-staining pattern produced by the complex neuroglial network of Müller cell processes. Careful study, however, leads to the conclusion that endothelial cells lining the central artery and constituting retinal capillaries do not contain immunoreactive AR. In Figure 3C, we demonstrate this to be the case for central artery endothelium. The endothelium of a large capillary in Figure 3B is clearly devoid of immunopositive staining, while the basal arborizations of Müller cells surrounding it contain immunoreactive AR. Also shown in Figure 3B is a small capillary whose endothelium stands out in negative image against the immunopositivity of the Müller cell cytoplasm.

Immunoreactive AR was also demonstrated in the optic nerve as it leaves the retina and passes through the posterior pole of the eye (Figure 3C). The staining pattern in the nerve tended to be diffuse and not well defined to specific cellular elements, but was abolished by preincubation of the antiserum with AR.

In conclusion, AR was demonstrated in the following structures in the eye: lens epithelium and cortical fibers, corneal endothelium, inner layer of the ciliary body epithelium, retinal Müller cells, and optic nerve. No vascular endothelial cells contained AR.

The kidney. The immunoreactive AR staining pattern seen for portions of the kidney was extremely difficult to interpret, largely because of the complex morphology of this organ, but also because the immunohistochemical demonstration of AR in kidney areas other than the inner medulla appeared to depend on the fixation method used. The order of staining intensity of reactive elements in various kidney zones consistently followed the decreasing progression: inner medulla > inner stripe of the outer medulla > outer stripe of the outer medulla and cortex. Although inner medullary elements stained convincingly for AR regardless of the fixation method employed, cortical and outer medullary structures were demonstrated only in kidney fixed by vascular perfusion of 4% paraformaldehyde–0.1% glutaraldehyde in cacodylate buffer. Under optimal fixation and staining conditions, most of the difficulty in staining interpretation centered around the sites of AR localization in the inner stripe of the outer medulla.

In the kidney cortex, AR was localized to convoluted portions of the distal tubule (Figure 4 A,B) and to the visceral layer (podocytes) of Bowman's capsule in the glomerulus (Figure 4B). Glomerular capillary endothelium did not stain for AR, nor did the parietal layer of Bowman's capsule. Podocytes generally stained best at the periphery of the glomerulus and no glomerular profile seemed to show a full complement of podocyte cytoplasm staining for the enzyme. In addition, the enzyme appeared to be present in the straight portions of the distal tubule in the cortex, although the possible identity of these occasional immunopositive tubular profiles as cortical collecting ducts could not be ruled out.

In the inner stripe of the outer medulla, immunopositive staining was noted in a limited number of tubular profiles within medullary rays which resembled thick and thin seg-

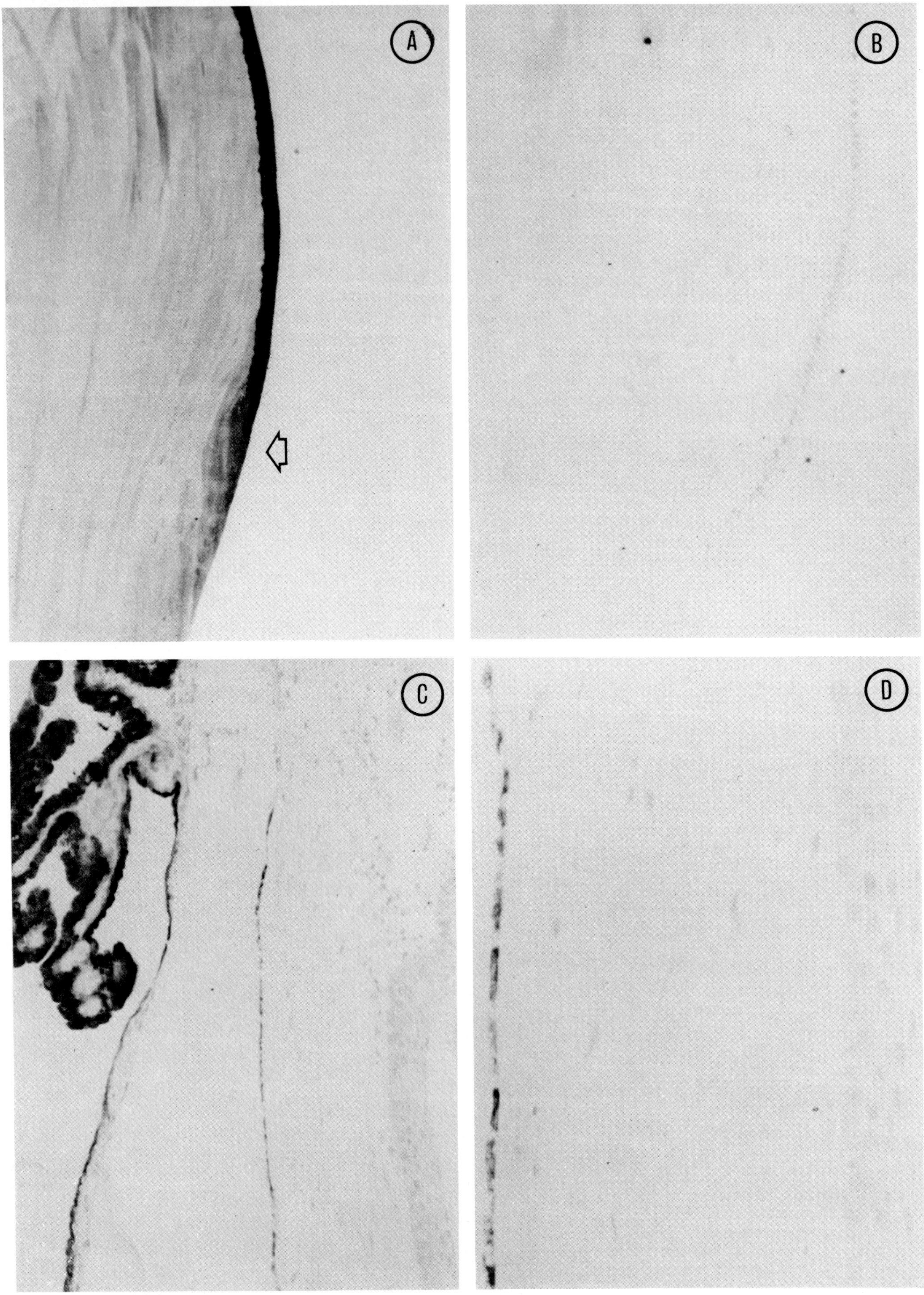
A
B
C
D

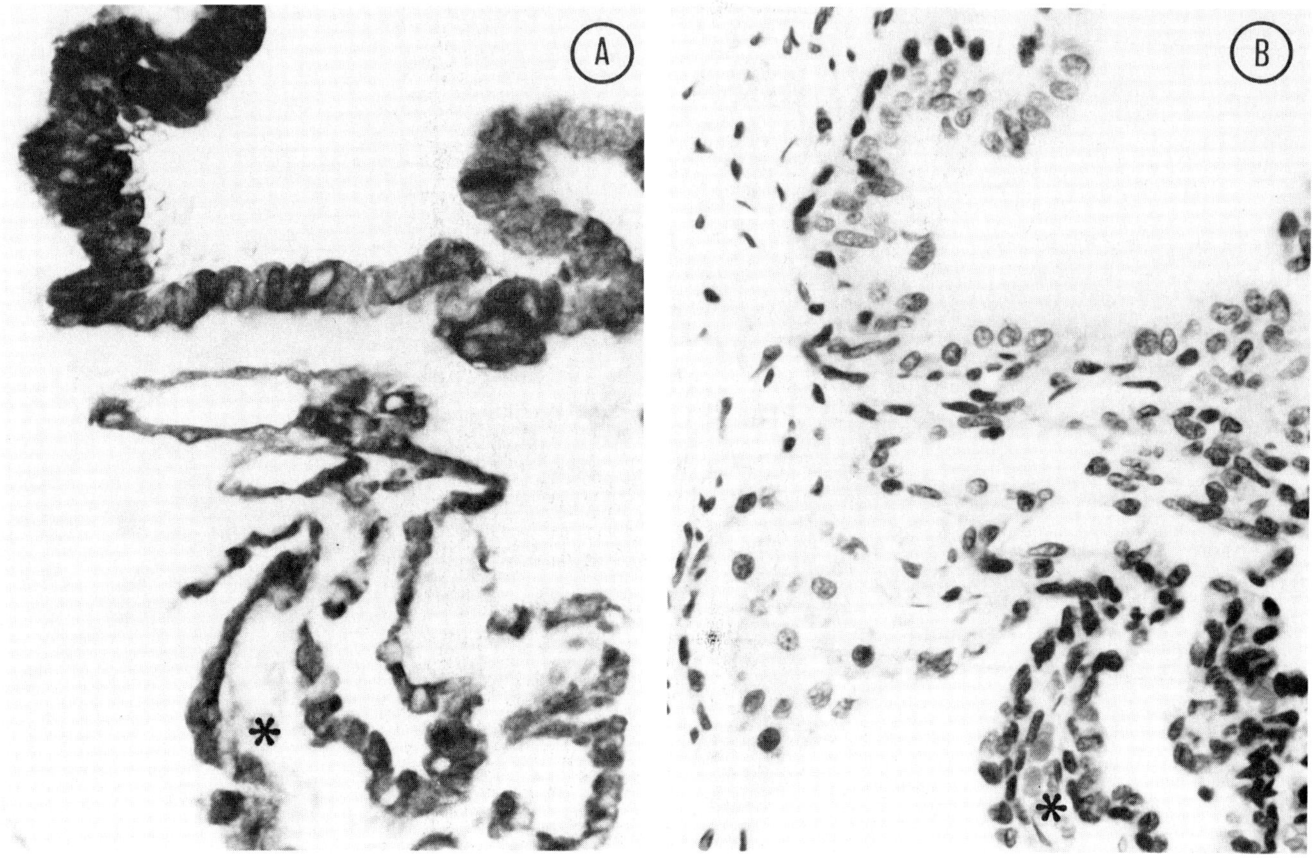

FIGURE 2. Photomicrographs of rat ciliary body cut in serial section and stained for AR (A) and for morphology (B). Immunoreactive AR is present in ciliary epithelium only in the inner layer of (columnar) cells; the outer layer is devoid of stain. Note also the absence of immunostain in the endothelial lining of blood vessels within the ciliary body (asterisk). 488 ×.

ments of the loop of Henle (Figure 4C,D). The identity of the profiles as thin segments, and not as vascular elements, is supported by their caliber, by the small size of their epithelial cells (as indicated by the relatively large number of nuclei seen per tubular profile), and by their position outside the vasa recta bundles (4C,D). It is rare that positive thin segments in the outer medulla can be traced to the inner medulla, where numerous thin segment profiles contain AR.

The staining pattern consistently observed at the junction of the inner and outer medulla was the abrupt immunopositive staining of thin segments in the inner medulla at precisely the junction line, while thin segments situated just opposite the junction, in the outer medulla, did not stain (Figure 5 A,D). In rare instances, immunoreactive thin segments from the outer medulla trailed into the inner medulla. This staining pattern demonstrates the junction of thin segments and ascending thick segments of the loop of Henle at the interface of the outer and inner medulla and suggests that only ascending thin limbs contain AR. However, this is contradicted by the demonstration of some immunoreactive thin segments in the outer medulla, which, by virtue of their location, must be descending thin limbs.

Interpretation of the staining pattern for AR in the inner medulla is less difficult. In the outer third of the inner medulla (Figure 5A–D), AR was present in thin limbs of the loop of Henle. Collecting tubules were clearly devoid of immunoreactive AR in this region. Figure 5D is also a demonstration of the absence of AR in endothelial cells of the inner medulla. The same staining pattern was seen in the middle third of the inner medulla (Figure 5E): thin segments stained heavily for AR. In addition, however, collecting tubules stained for the enzyme in this region, at first in isolated cells and then in small cell clusters and, finally, in the inner third of the inner medulla, the papillary ducts stained intensely for the enzyme (Figure 5F). In this region, as elsewhere in the inner medulla, thin segments stained for AR and can be seen to curve occasionally as the tips of the loops of Henle. In addition, some AR immunoreactivity is seen in the interstitial cells deep in the inner medulla; also, the transitional epithelium lining the papillary tip demonstrated immunoppositive staining.

In conclusion, AR was shown to be present with certainty in the following nephron structures: podocytes, distal convoluted tubules, thin segments of the loop of Henle, collecting tubules and papillary ducts in the inner medulla, and transitional epithelium in the pelvic space. No immunoreac-

FIGURE 1. Immunoperoxidase photomicrographs of structures in the rat eye. (A) Anterior cortical and bow regions of the rat lens. Note the dense staining of the lens epithelium, which blends in the bow region (arrow) with the less intense staining of the cortical fibers. 203 ×. (B) Preabsorption control for A. (C) Corneoscleral junction, showing immunoreactivity in the inner layer of the ciliary body epithelium and its extension as the posterior surface of the iris, and the endothelial lining of the cornea. 195 ×. (D) Higher magnification view of cornea in C. 488 ×.

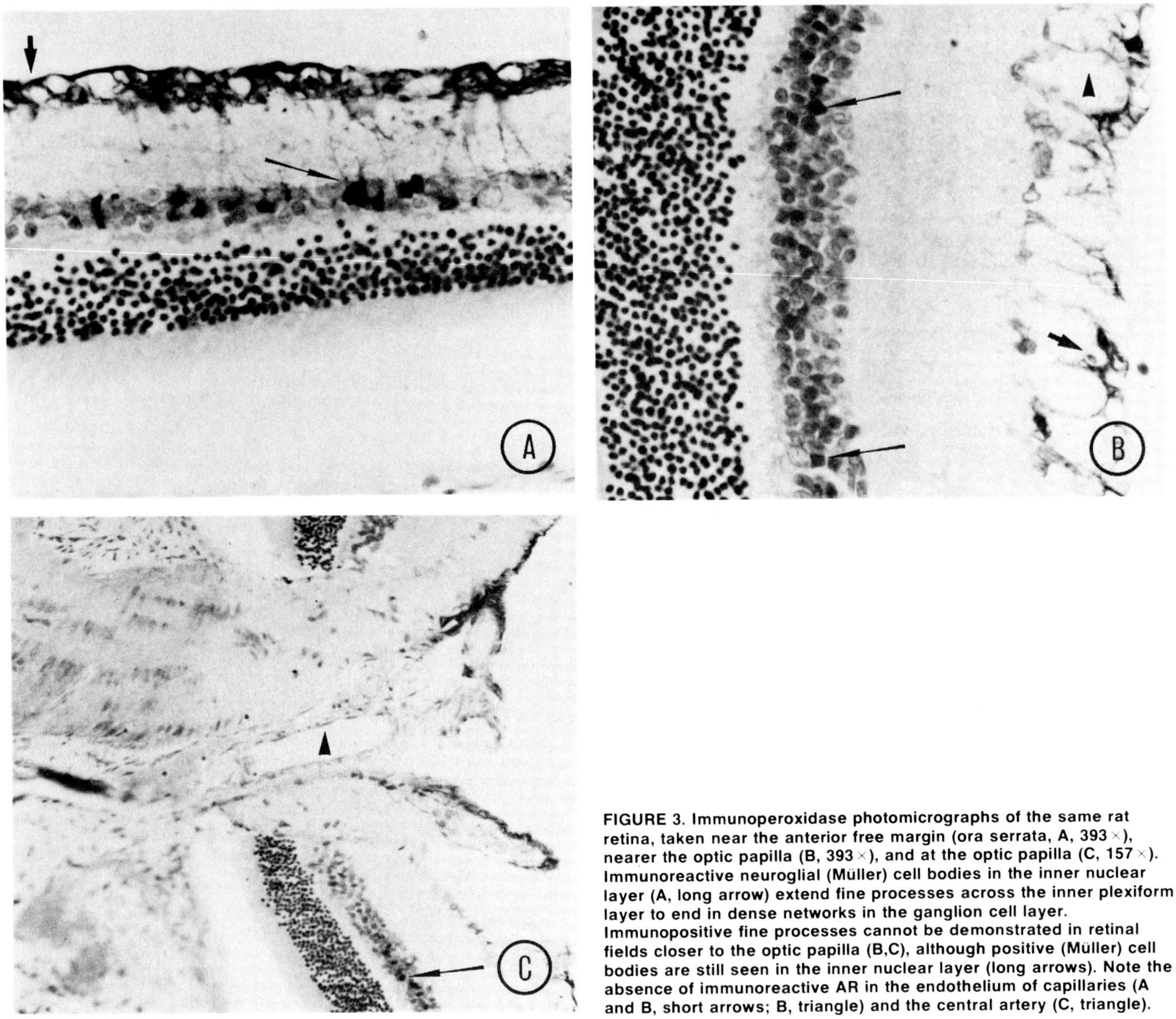

FIGURE 3. Immunoperoxidase photomicrographs of the same rat retina, taken near the anterior free margin (ora serrata, A, 393 ×), nearer the optic papilla (B, 393 ×), and at the optic papilla (C, 157 ×). Immunoreactive neuroglial (Müller) cell bodies in the inner nuclear layer (A, long arrow) extend fine processes across the inner plexiform layer to end in dense networks in the ganglion cell layer. Immunopositive fine processes cannot be demonstrated in retinal fields closer to the optic papilla (B,C), although positive (Müller) cell bodies are still seen in the inner nuclear layer (long arrows). Note the absence of immunoreactive AR in the endothelium of capillaries (A and B, short arrows; B, triangle) and the central artery (C, triangle).

tive AR was detected in glomerular capillary endothelium or vascular endothelium in the medulla.

DISCUSSION

The immunohistochemical localization of AR to specific cell types in the kidney and eye offers a new perspective for assessing the consequences of polyol pathway activity in these tissues under experimental and disease conditions. The cellular distribution of AR shown in this study largely agrees with observations of numerous other investigators who studied polyol pathway activity in eye and kidney.

The staining patterns seen for the lens indicate compartmentalization of AR activity primarily in the lens epithelium, as was suggested by biochemical[18,21,26] and histochemical[27] studies.

The loss of demonstrable immunopositive Müller cell processes, spanning the inner plexiform layer in regions of the retina close to the optic papilla, may be explained as a "dilution" phenomenon; although the Müller cells are present throughout the extent of the retina, their relative density, and hence immunoreactive stainability, is diminished in retinal fields farther removed from the ora serrata by the accumulation of greater numbers of nervous elements destined for the optic papilla.

There is evidence to support the conclusion of this study that immunoreactive AR is not present in rat retinal capillary endothelial cells. Buzney et al.[20] have shown that radioimmunoassayable AR is present in whole retina and in cultured pericytes (mural cells) from rhesus monkey retinal capillaries, but it is essentially undetectable in freshly iso-

FIGURE 4. Immunoperoxidase photomicrographs of rat kidney. In the cortex (A and B), immunoreactive AR is present in distal convoluted tubules and podocytes, but is absent in proximal convoluted tubules (indicated by triangles). A, 205 ×; B, 514 ×. Occasional immunopositive tubular profiles were seen in the inner stripe of the outer medulla (C and D) and were thought to represent thick (long arrows) and thin (short arrows) segments of the loop of Henle. No immunoreactivity was noted in vascular elements in the vasa recta (position denoted by asterisks). C and D, 218 ×.

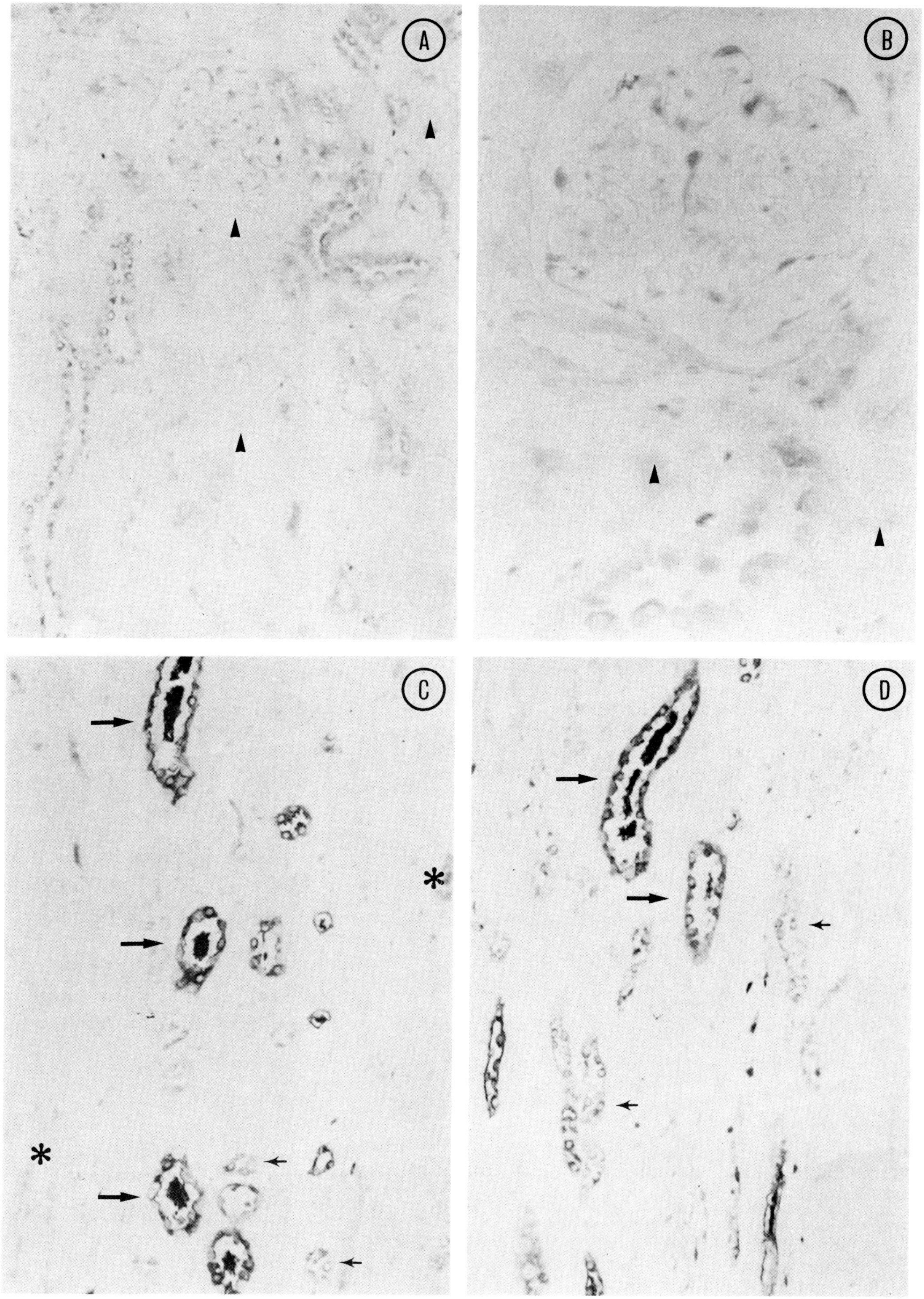

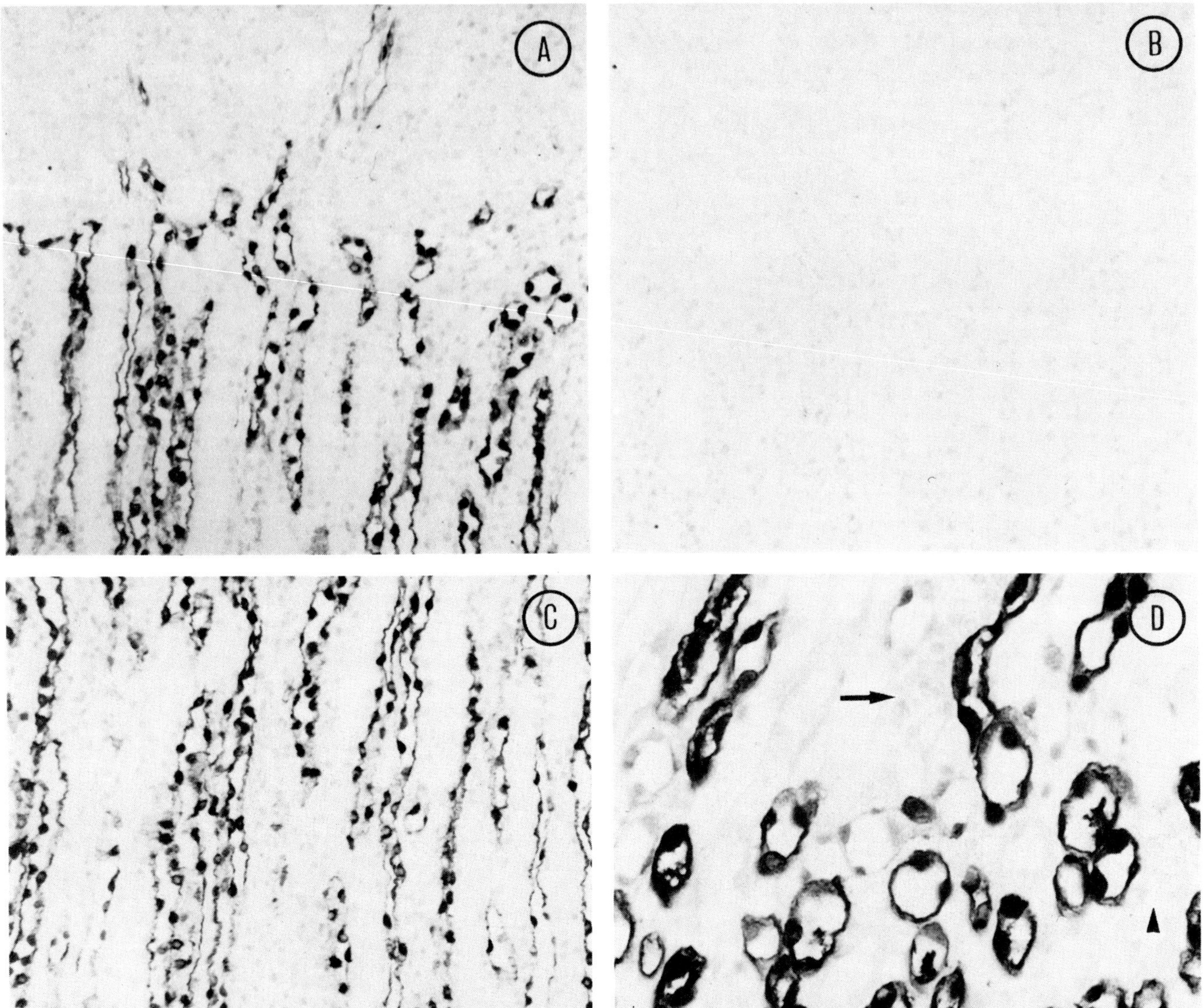
A
B
C
D
E
F

lated retinal capillaries, presumably because of the small number of pericytes compared with the total capillary tissue present. Furthermore, they support this claim by noting that pericytes remain viable when cultured in low glucose medium but not in high glucose medium. In addition, they note that pericytes are lost from diabetic retinal capillaries, while the endothelial cells survive and often proliferate. Whether capillary pericytes stain for AR cannot be determined with certainty from the data obtained in the present study, although there is some indication that they do in Figure 3A,B, where occasional focused or punctate immunostain deposits may be seen close to capillary lumina. The conclusion that AR is absent from rat retinal capillary endothelium is interesting in light of the fact that the laboratory rodent represents a poor animal model for the experimental pathogenesis of retinopathy (J. H. Kinoshita, private communication).

Knowledge of the cellular distribution of AR in the retina calls for a reassessment of the potentially pathogenic osmotic force generated by a given amount of polyol accumulation in this tissue. Hutton et al.[29] report that the sorbitol accumulation (1.5 μmol/g protein) observed in chemically diabetic rat retinas is osmotically insignificant if evenly distributed throughout the retina. However, the results of this study indicate that AR is sequestered in specific cellular locations, and evaluations of the osmotic force generated by the accumulated retinal sorbitol must be recalculated using a cell volume appropriate for the Müller cell population of the retina.

The general staining pattern seen in the kidney—with the greatest intensity found in the inner medulla and papillary tip—is similar to the work of other investigators. In the only known immunohistochemical study of AR done before this study, Gabbay and Cathcart[30] report heavy immunofluorescence in the papillary tip. Various biochemical studies also indicate that the highest AR activity and pathway substrate accumulations in the kidney are found in the papilla.[2,15,31]

The localization of AR to some specific nephronic segments is difficult to elucidate. Advantage was taken of the fact that, in the unilobar kidney of the rat, different segments of one nephron are in register with corresponding segments of neighboring nephrons. Thus, the structural feature which separates the outer medulla into outer and inner stripes is the abrupt change of the descending straight portion of the proximal tubule to the descending thin segment of the loop of Henle. By this rationale, it follows that kidney fields containing both thick and thin segment profiles of the loop of Henle are found only in the inner stripe of the outer medulla, and that the thick segment profiles in this area must therefore be those of the ascending straight portions of the distal tubule. In addition, the border between inner and outer medulla is formed by the abrupt junction of ascending thin segments of the loop of Henle with ascending straight portions of the distal tubule. Therefore, the inner medulla of the rat kidney contains only profiles of thin segments of the loop of Henle, collecting ducts, and blood vessels. These facts must be kept in mind while attempting to identify AR-positive nephronic segments.

Thick segments identified in the outer medulla were differentiated from collecting tubules on the basis of tubule caliber, lumen diameter, and the low cuboidal morphology of the cells constituting the tubule wall. However, the noted absence of AR in collecting tubule profiles within the first third of the inner medulla supports the conclusion that these profiles in the inner stripe of the outer medulla are not collecting tubules. Nevertheless, the identities of these tubules were difficult to determine. None of the tubular profiles exhibited continuity with positive profiles in the cortex and only rarely were they continuous with thin segments in the inner medulla. Only a small percentage of the total number of tubular profiles seen in the inner stripe of the outer medulla stained positively for AR. Therefore, regardless of the identity of the tubular profiles containing AR in the inner stripe, they account for only a small percentage of the total number of nephrons in the kidney. It is possible that the tubular profiles present in the inner stripe represent segments of the juxtamedullary nephrons, which account for only a small proportion of the total nephrons, and to which belong the thick and thin segments of the loop of Henle found deep in the inner stripe of the outer medulla and in the inner medulla. However, while there may be sufficient numbers of thin segment profiles to account for the juxtamedullary nephrons, there are clearly not enough thick segment profiles to support this contention.

There is little helpful information in the literature to aid in the interpretation problems encountered in the outer medulla. Hutton and colleagues[31] investigated the presence of polyol pathway intermediates in various kidney zones and report that measurable levels of sorbitol are formed in cortical and especially in medullary tubules in chemically diabetic rats. They reported no measurable sorbitol or fructose in glomeruli from diabetic rats or from normal rats whose glomeruli were incubated in high glucose medium. They have also shown the accumulation of polyol pathway substrates in monolayer cell cultures of monkey kidney epithelial cells derived from the cortex, but the specific origin of the cells is not known.[32] The findings of Corder et al.[33] for AR and sorbitol dehydrogenase distribution in the rat kidney disagree with all other investigations, including the present report, and are not readily interpretable.

The data taken as a whole suggest a peculiar enzyme distribution in the nephron, as shown in Figure 6. Farber and colleagues[34–36] demonstrated a similarly discontinuous but repetitive distribution of three oxidative enzymes in the kidney nephron by dehydrogenase histochemistry. Their data indicate that the nephronic distribution of succinate dehydrogenase and DPN diaphorase is influenced by kidney zone (e.g., junction of outer and inner medulla) as well as by nephronic substructure (e.g., thick versus thin segments of the loop of Henle).

FIGURE 5. Immunoperoxidase photomicrographs of rat kidney inner medulla. (A) Junction of outer (upper third of photograph) and inner medulla, illustrating the abrupt commencement of immunopositive thin segments in the inner medulla. 174×. (B) Preabsorption control for A. 174×. (C) Only thin segments of the loop of Henle stain for AR in regions of the inner medulla near the junction with outer medulla. 186×. (D) Tissue section of the junction between outer (upper third of photograph) and inner medulla, oriented at right angles to the view in A, illustrating the absence of immunoreactive AR in blood vasculature (arrow) and collecting tubules at this level (triangles). 462×. (E and F) In regions approaching the papillary tip, collecting tubules stain for AR, at first in isolated cell clusters and then intensely as papillary ducts. Immunopositive thin segments are seen throughout the field, many curving out of the plane of section (F) as the tip of the loop of Henle. 186×.

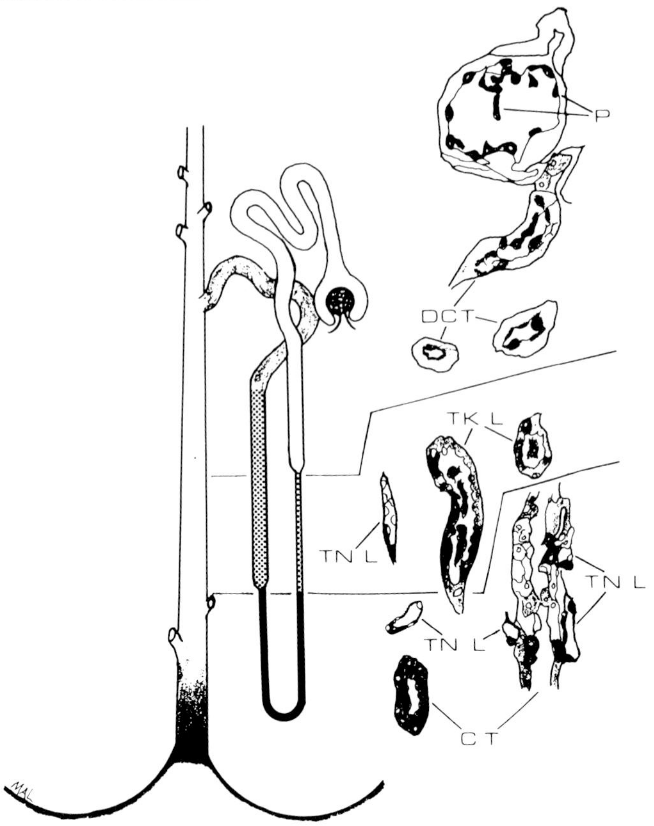

FIGURE 6. Schematic representation of AR distribution in the rat nephron. Camera lucida drawings of kidney structures containing AR are shown on the right. The presence of AR in the nephron is indicated by shaded areas; the stippling represents the uncertainty encountered in the outer medulla, as described in the text. P, podocytes; DCT, distal convoluted tubule; TK L, thick limb of the loop of Henle; TN L, thin limb of the loop of Henle; CT, collecting tubule.

Immunohistochemical localizations for AR were performed using tissues obtained from both normal and diabetic rats. No differences were seen in the staining patterns of normal and diabetic tissues fixed in similar fashion. This observation is not surprising if one considers that the pathway is known to exist normally in a wide variety of mammals and must be present before the hyperglycemic events to produce a pathogenic effect. What cannot be determined from the immunohistochemical results is the nature of the enzymatic activity of the localized AR. The immunostain deposits seen in tissue sections cannot ensure the presence of active AR or of AR localization in privileged sites containing metabolizable sugar. Possible differences in enzymatic activity brought about by the diabetic condition are likewise not differentiated by this localization method unless the differences include conformational or allosteric alterations, which change the antigenicity of the enzyme molecule.

An observation which has become evident from the results of the immunohistochemical localization studies reported here and earlier[22] is that AR appears to be associated in part with cells which provide a supportive or trophic role. Examples of this observation include the Schwann cell in peripheral nerve,[22] the glial cells (of Müller) in the retina, the Sertoli cells in the testis,[22] and also, possibly, the pericytes in capillaries. Investigations are under way to determine whether oligodendroglia in the central nervous system also contain AR. It is uncertain what ramifications this localization may have in diabetes beyond the obvious fact that these cells are essential for the well-being and proper functioning of the tissues with which they are associated. Perhaps more attention should be given to these "passive" supportive cells in research designed to determine the etiology of diabetic complications.

ACKNOWLEDGMENTS

The scientific advice of Dr. Robert P. Elde and Dr. J. B. Longley is gratefully acknowledged.

This investigation was supported by USPHS diabetes training grant AM07196.

REFERENCES

[1] Gabbay, K. H.: The sorbitol pathway and the complications of diabetes. N. Engl. J. Med. *288*:831–36, 1973.

[2] Gabbay, K. H.: Hyperglycemia, polyol metabolism, and complications of diabetes mellitus. Annu. Rev. Med. *26*:521–36, 1975.

[3] Winegrad, A. I., Clements, R. S., and Morrison, A. D.: Insulin-dependent pathways of carbohydrate metabolism. *In* Handbook of Physiology, Endocrinology, Vol. 1. Steiner, D. F., and Freinkel, N., Eds. Washington, D.C., Am. Physiol. Soc., 1972, pp. 457–71.

[4] Winegrad, A. I., Morrison, A. D., and Clements, R. S.: The polyol pathway: a model for biochemical mechanisms by which hyperglycemia may contribute to the pathogenesis of the complications of diabetes mellitus. *In* Diabetes. Proc. Eighth Congr. IDF. Malaisse, W. J., and Pirart, J., Eds. Amsterdam and New York, Excerpta Medica/American Elsevier, 1974, pp. 387–95.

[5] van Heyningen, R.: Formation of polyols by the lens of the rat with 'sugar' cataract. Nature (London) *184*:194–95, 1959.

[6] van Heyningen, R.: The sorbitol pathway in the lens. Exp. Eye Res. *1*:396–404, 1962.

[7] Kinoshita, J. H.: Cataracts in galactosemia. The Jonas S. Friedenwald memorial lecture. Invest. Ophthalmol. *4*:786–99, 1965.

[8] Chylack, L. T., and Kinoshita, J. H.: A biochemical evaluation of a cataract induced in a high-glucose medium. Invest. Ophthalmol. *8*:401–12, 1969.

[9] Gabbay, K. H.: Role of sorbitol pathway in neuropathy. Adv. Metab. Disord. *2* (Suppl. 2):417–24, 1973.

[10] Stewart, M. A., Sherman, W. R., Kurien, M. M., Moonsammy, G. I., and Wisgerhof, M.: Polyol accumulations in nervous tissue of rats with experimental diabetes and galactosemia. J. Neurochem. *14*:1057–66, 1967.

[11] Ward, J. D., Baker, R. W. R., and Davis, B. H.: Effect on blood sugar control of the accumulation of sorbitol and fructose in nervous tissues. Diabetes *21*:1173–78, 1972.

[12] Clements, R. S., Morrison, A. D., and Winegrad, A. I.: Polyol pathway in aorta: regulation by hormones. Science *166*:1007–08, 1969.

[13] Morrison, A. D., Clements, R. S., and Winegrad, A. I.: Effects of elevated glucose concentrations on the metabolism of the aortic wall. J. Clin. Invest. *51*:3114–23, 1972.

[14] Winegrad, A. I., Morrison, A. D., and Clements, R. S.: Polyol pathway activity in aorta. Adv. Metab. Disord. *2* (Suppl. 2):117–27, 1973.

[15] Gabbay, K. H., and O'Sullivan, J. B.: The sorbitol pathway in diabetes and galactosemia: enzyme and substrate localization and changes in kidney. Diabetes *17*:300, 1968. (Abstr.)

[16] Kinoshita, J. H., Futterman, S., Satoh, K., and Merola, L. O.: Factors affecting the formation of sugar alcohols in ocular lens. Biochim. Biophys. Acta *74*:340–50, 1963.

[17] Sheaff, C. M., and Doughty, C. C.: Physical and kinetic properties of homogeneous bovine lens aldose reductase. J. Biol. Chem. *251*:2696–2702, 1976.

[18] Gabbay, K. H. and Cathcart, E. S.: Purification and immunologic identification of aldose reductase. Diabetes *23*:460–68, 1974.

[19] Gabbay, K. H.: Purification and immunological identification of bovine retinal aldose reductase. Isr. J. Med. Sci. *8*:1626–29, 1972.

[20] Buzney, S. M., Frank, R. N., Varma, S. D., Tanishima, T., and Gabbay, K. H.: Aldose reductase in retinal mural cells. Invest. Ophthalmol. *16*:392–96, 1977.

[21] Clements, R. S., Weaver, J. P., and Winegrad, A. I.: The distribution of polyol: NADP oxidoreductase in mammalian tissues. Biochem. Biophys. Res. Commun. *37*:347–53, 1969.

[22] Ludvigson, M. A., and Sorenson, R. L.: Immunohistochemical localization of aldose reductase. I. Enzyme purification and antibody preparation—localization in peripheral nerve, artery, and testis. Diabetes *29*:xxx–xxx, 1980.

[23] Ludvigson, M. A.: Immunohistochemical localization of aldose reductase in the rat. Anat. Rec. *190*:465–66, 1978. (Abstr.)

[24] Ludvigson, M. A., and Sorenson, R. L.: Immunohistochemical localization of aldose reductase in the rat. Diabetes *27* (Suppl. 2):463, 1978. (Abstr.)

[25] Sternberger, L. A., Hardy, P. H., Cuculis, J. J., and Meyer, H. G.: The unlabeled antibody enzyme method of immunohistochemistry. Preparation and properties of soluble antigen-antibody complex (horseradish peroxidase –antihorseradish peroxidase) and its use in identification of spirochetes. J. Histochem. Cytochem. *18*:315–33, 1970.

[26] Hayman, S., Lou, M. F., Merola, L. O., and Kinoshita, J. H.: Aldose reductase activity in the lens and other tissues. Biochim. Biophys. Acta *128*:474–82, 1966.

[27] Collins, J. G., and Corder, C. N.: Aldose reductase and sorbitol dehydrogenase distribution in substructures of normal and diabetic rat lens. Invest. Ophthalmol. *16*:242–43, 1977.

[28] Corkey, R. F., Corkey, B. E., and Gimbrone, M. A., Jr.: Hexose transport and sorbitol accumulation in cultured human endothelial cells. Diabetes *27* (Suppl. 2):446, 1978. (Abstr.)

[29] Hutton, J. C., Schofield, P. J., Williams, J. F., and Hollows, F. C.: Sorbitol metabolism in the retina: accumulation of pathway intermediates in streptozotocin induced diabetes in the rat. Aust. J. Exp. Biol. Med. Sci. *52*:361–73, 1974.

[30] Gabbay, K. H., and Cathcart, E. S.: Immunochemical localization of aldose reductase. J. Clin. Invest. *49*:31a–32a, 1970. (Abstr.)

[31] Hutton, J. C., Schofield, P. J., Williams, J. F., and Hollows, F. C.: The localization of sorbitol pathway activity in the rat renal cortex and its relationship to the pathogenesis of the renal complications of diabetes mellitus. Aust. J. Exp. Biol. Med. Sci. *53*:49–57, 1975.

[32] Hutton, J. C., Williams, J. F., Schofield, P. J., and Hollows, F. C.: Polyol metabolism in monkey kidney epithelial cell cultures. Sorbitol synthesis. Eur. J. Biochem. *49*:347–53, 1974.

[33] Corder, C. N., Collins, J. G., Brannan, T. S., and Sharma, J.: Aldose reductase and sorbitol dehydrogenase distribution in the rat kidney. J. Histochem. Cytochem. *25*:1–8, 1977.

[34] Farber, E., Sternberg, W. H., and Dunlap, C. E.: Histochemical localization of specific oxidative enzymes. I. J. Histochem. *4*:254–65, 1956.

[35] Sternberg, W. H., Farber, E., and Dunlap, C. E.: Histochemical localization of specific oxidative enzymes. II. J. Histochem. *4*:266–83, 1956.

[36] Farber, E., Sternberg, W. H., and Dunlap, C. E.: Histochemical localization of specific oxidative enzymes. III. J. Histochem. *4*:284–94, 1956.

Acute Changes in Brain Tryptophan and Serotonin After Carbohydrate or Protein Ingestion by Diabetic Rats

ELIZABETH A. CRANDALL AND JOHN D. FERNSTROM

SUMMARY

In normal, fasting rats, intubation with glucose did not alter serum tryptophan, but it did reduce serum concentrations of the large neutral amino acids, tryptophan's competitors for brain uptake. The serum ratio of tryptophan to the sum of these competitors, which predicts brain tryptophan uptake, was thus increased. Brain tryptophan, serotonin (which is synthesized from tryptophan), and 5-hydroxyindoleacetic acid levels also increased. Such increases in brain serotonin are potentially important, since serotonin is a neurotransmitter. Changes in its level may indicate altered release by neurons and, thus, modified brain function. In contrast, glucose intubation of fasting streptozotocin-diabetic rats elicited only a small increase in the serum tryptophan ratio. Brain tryptophan increased slightly; no changes occurred in brain serotonin or in 5-hydroxyindoleacetic acid. Similar effects were noted when fasting diabetic rats consumed a single, carbohydrate meal. However, brain indoles *did* increase after carbohydrate ingestion in diabetic rats that received an insulin injection at the time food was presented.

Effects of ingesting a protein-containing meal were also studied. In normal rats, consumption of this meal increased the serum tryptophan ratio slightly. Brain tryptophan and serotonin levels were unchanged. In diabetic rats, ingestion of the protein-containing meal often lowered the serum tryptophan ratio. Brain tryptophan also fell in diabetic rats when the serum tryptophan ratio was reduced, but brain 5-hydroxyindoles did not fall.

The data demonstrate that the absence of a carbohydrate-induced increment in brain indole levels follows indirectly from the absence of the insulin-induced rise in the serum tryptophan ratio. The diabetic rat's inability to experience normal carbohydrate-induced increments in brain serotonin suggests that brain functions, normally dependent on such neurochemical signals, may be abnormal. DIABETES 29: 460–466, June 1980.

From the Laboratory of Brain and Metabolism, Department of Nutrition and Food Science, Massachusetts Institute of Technology, Cambridge, Massachusetts 02139.

Address reprint requests to Dr. John D. Fernstrom, M.I.T., Room 56-137, Cambridge, Massachusetts 02139.

Received for publication 22 October 1979.

Brain uptake of the large neutral amino acids tryptophan (Trp), tyrosine (Tyr), phenylalanine (Phe), leucine (Leu), isoleucine (Ile), and valine (Val) occurs via a single, saturable transport system at the blood-brain barrier. Transport kinetics follow the rules of competitive inhibition.[1,2] Thus, the rate of transport of any one neutral amino acid, such as tryptophan, depends not only on its own level in blood, but also on the blood concentrations of its competitors for brain uptake (i.e., Tyr, Phe, Leu, Ile, and Val). In rats consuming single meals, hour-to-hour changes in brain tryptophan concentrations usually do not correlate with alterations in serum tryptophan levels alone; instead, they *do* correlate with the changes in serum ratio of tryptophan to the sum of the other large neutral amino acids (Trp/Tyr + Phe + Leu + Ile + Val).[3,4] This serum tryptophan ratio expresses the competition between tryptophan and the other large neutral amino acids for brain uptake.[4]

The serum tryptophan ratio, brain tryptophan level, and brain serotonin concentration (and synthesis) are all increased soon after normal animals begin to consume carbohydrates.[5,6] The rise in brain indoles depends on the increase in the serum tryptophan ratio,[7] which is a consequence of insulin secretion (insulin lowers blood concentrations of the aromatic and branched-chain amino acids and increases or does not alter blood tryptophan levels[3,8]).

Because diabetic rats cannot secrete insulin, carbohydrate ingestion should not alter significantly the serum pattern of the large neutral amino acids, i.e., the serum tryptophan ratio should not increase. Therefore, brain tryptophan and 5-hydroxyindoles should not change either. The present experiments tested this hypothesis. Data were also obtained on the effect of ingesting a protein-containing meal on the serum tryptophan ratio and on brain indoles.

MATERIALS AND METHODS

Animals. Male Sprague-Dawley rats (125 g; Charles River Laboratories, Wilmington, MA) were housed 6–10 in a cage and were acclimated to our animal quarters for 3–7 days before diabetes was induced. Food and water were provided ad libitum (Charles River rat, mouse, and hamster maintenance formula), and lights were on from 8 a.m. to 8 p.m. daily. Diabetes was induced by a single, intracardiac injection (65 mg/kg) of streptozotocin (Sigma Chemical Co., St. Louis, MO) in a 2% solution of cold, 0.1 M citrate buffer (pH 4.5). Onset of diabetes occurred rapidly and was identified by polydipsia, polyuria, and urine glucose concentrations greater than 2% (2 g/100 ml). Fasting serum glucose levels in diabetic rats ranged from normal (110 mg/100 ml) to as high as 575 mg/100 ml; Table 5 gives post-sugar blood glucose values (~900 mg/100 ml). Serum insulin levels were also measured, to confirm the absence of insulin secretion. Ketone bodies were not detectable in fresh urine samples from normal or streptozotocin-treated rats, as determined using Ketostix reagent strips (Ames Co., Miles Laboratories, Elkhart, IN). The absence of significant amounts of ketone bodies in the urines of streptozotocin-diabetic rats is a typical finding when a dose of 65 mg/kg is used, as it was in the present studies.[9] During the period between streptozotocin injection and experimentation (5–10 days), diabetic rats gained about 1.6 g body weight/day, while normal rats (controls) gained about 5 g/day. At least 5 days elapsed between appearance of diabetic symptoms and experimentation.

Groups of six normal and diabeic rats were deprived of food, but not water, at 5 p.m. the night before an experiment; experiments were begun at 10 a.m. the next morning. In the first study, groups of normal and diabetic rats received a 2 M solution of glucose (1 ml/100 g body weight) by stomach tube and were killed 30, 60, or 120 min later. In the diet experiments, groups of six animals were housed two to a cage, fasted overnight, and the next morning were presented with either a 0% or an 18% casein diet. The rats were allowed to eat freely for 2 h and then were killed. During this 2-h period, normal rats each consumed 8–10 g food and diabetic rats 13–16 g; control groups of normal and diabetic rats continued to fast. When insulin (Iletin, U-40; Eli Lilly and Co., Indianapolis, IN; 4 IU/kg, diluted in saline 1:10) was administered to diabetic rats, it was injected intraperitoneally (i.p.) at the time food was presented; control rats received saline alone. Saline-treated rats each ate 9–12 g food and insulin-treated rats 13–15 g. All animals were killed 2 h later.

Animals were killed by decapitation. Brains were quickly removed, the cerebella separated from the remaining brain tissue, and both parts were frozen on dry ice. Blood was collected from the cervical wound and allowed to clot at 4°C. Brain tissue was stored at −70°C and sera at −20°C until assayed.

Experimental diets. The 18% casein diet contained 180 g casein, 226 g dextrin, 226 g dextrose, 183 g sucrose, 150 g Mazola oil, 35 g agar, and 1000 g water. The 0% protein diet contained 289 g dextrose, 289 g dextrin, 237 g sucrose, 150 g Mazola oil, 35 g agar, and 1000 g water.

Assay methods. Urine glucose was estimated visually using glucose enzymatic test paper (Tes-Tape; Eli Lilly and Co., Indianapolis, IN). Serum total tryptophan levels were measured by the method of Denckla and Dewey,[10] as modified by Bloxam and Warren.[11] Tryptophan concentrations in the cerebella were determined by the same technique, as modified by Lehman.[12] Cerebellar tryptophan levels have been shown to mirror accurately whole brain tryptophan concentrations in such diet studies.[6] Serum insulin levels were measured by radioimmunoassay,[13] using purified rat insulin as the reference preparation (kindly provided by Dr. R. Chance, Lilly Research Laboratories, Eli Lilly and Co., Indianapolis, IN). Brain serotonin and 5-hydroxyindoleacetic acid (5-HIAA) levels were measured by the method of Curzon and Green.[14] The serum levels of amino acids other than tryptophan were measured with a Beckman model 119C amino acid analyzer. Serum samples were prepared by adding 50 mg 5-sulfosalicylic acid to 1 ml serum and centrifuging at 3000 rpm for 30 min. The clear supernatants were stored at −20°C. Before being applied to the analyzer, the thawed supernatants were respun at 3000 rpm for 15 min and filtered (HAWP 01300; Millipore Corp., Bedford, MA).

Statistics. Data were analyzed by two-way analysis of variance, in which some combination of two of the following factors was used, depending on the experiment: normal vs. diabetic, time, and treatment.[15] When variances were significantly heterogeneous (F_{max} test),[16] log transformation of the data was performed before analysis. Differences between individual animal (normal vs. diabetic), time, or treatment (e.g., glucose, diet, or insulin) groups were then tested by one-way analysis of variance and the Neuman-Keuls test or by *t* test.[17]

RESULTS

In fasting diabetic rats, serum concentrations of branched-chain amino acids were consistently above normal (Tables 1 and 3), while those of other large neutral amino acids were usually unchanged. Fasting serum insulin levels were normal. The fasting serum tryptophan ratio was reduced (Tables 1 and 3), as was brain tryptophan (Tables 2 and 4). Fasting brain 5-HIAA (but not 5-HT) levels were reduced somewhat in diabetic rats (Tables 2 and 4). These changes are consistent with those reported by others for diabetic rats.[18–21]

When *normal* fasting rats were intubated with glucose, serum insulin levels increased substantially (Table 1). Serum concentrations of the aromatic amino acids—and particularly the branched-chain amino acids—fell significantly during the 120-min test period. Serum tryptophan levels were not significantly affected; thus, the serum tryptophan ratio increased considerably (Table 1). Brain tryptophan levels increased significantly at 60 and 120 min, and brain 5-HT and 5-HIAA levels were significantly elevated at 120 min (Table 2). When fasting *diabetic* rats were intubated with glucose, serum insulin levels did not increase significantly. Reductions in serum concentrations of branched-chain and aromatic amino acids were small (Table 1). No significant change in serum tryptophan was noted. Consequently, the serum tryptophan ratio increased only slightly. The brain levels of tryptophan, 5-HT, and 5-HIAA did not change significantly during the 120 min after glucose was intubated (Table 2).

Using the brain tryptophan, serum tryptophan, and serum tryptophan ratio values from each animal, plots of brain tryptophan vs. the serum ratio or serum tryptophan alone were

TABLE 1
Effects of glucose intubation of fasting normal or diabetic rats on serum neutral amino acid levels*

	Minutes after glucose intubation			
Amino acid	0	30	60	120
		(nmol/ml serum)		
Tryptophan†				
Normal rats	102 ± 4	90 ± 4	96 ± 4	98 ± 3
Diabetic rats	86 ± 5§	74 ± 8	88 ± 7	95 ± 8
Tyrosine‡				
Normal rats	86 ± 3	67 ± 5‖	58 ± 4‖	56 ± 2‖
Diabetic rats	69 ± 5§	51 ± 5§	63 ± 4	64 ± 6
Phenylalanine†‡				
Normal rats	68 ± 3	51 ± 1‖	49 ± 2‖	61 ± 2
Diabetic rats	78 ± 5	69 ± 4§	68 ± 7§	75 ± 6§
Leucine†‡				
Normal rats	167 ± 8	72 ± 5‖	57 ± 3‖	67 ± 5‖
Diabetic rats	273 ± 23§	240 ± 40§	167 ± 15§	245 ± 8§
Isoleucine†‡				
Normal rats	106 ± 6	49 ± 3‖	37 ± 2‖	43 ± 3‖
Diabetic rats	164 ± 15§	135 ± 18§	104 ± 10§	178 ± 56§
Valine†				
Normal rats	200 ± 11	108 ± 7‖	90 ± 5‖	85 ± 8‖
Diabetic rats	357 ± 29§	363 ± 66§	248 ± 25§	315 ± 11§
Tryptophan ratio†‡¶				
Normal rats	0.16 ± 0.01	0.26 ± 0.01‖	0.34 ± 0.03‖	0.30 ± 0.02‖
Diabetic rats	0.09 ± 0.01§	0.10 ± 0.02§	0.14 ± 0.01§	0.13 ± 0.04§
Insulin (μU/ml)†‡				
Normal rats	11 ± 2	78 ± 9‖	55 ± 5‖	24 ± 4‖
Diabetic rats	9 ± 2	7 ± 2§	13 ± 2§	9 ± 3§

* Groups of five male normal or diabetic rats were fasted overnight and then intubated with a 2 M glucose solution (1 ml/100 g). Diabetic rats had been treated with streptozotocin several days earlier. Animals were killed at the times indicated. Data are expressed as means ± standard errors. Data were analyzed by two-way analysis of variance.
† These values were significantly affected by diabetes ($P < 0.05$). Log transforms of all branched-chain amino acid values were performed before the two-way analysis of variance.
‡ These values were significantly affected by time ($P < 0.05$).
§ These values differed significantly ($P < 0.05$) from the corresponding normal values using Student's *t* test.
‖ These values differed significantly ($P < 0.05$) from time 0 using the Neuman-Keuls test.
¶ The serum tryptophan ratio was calculated using the serum concentrations of the amino acids named: Trp/Tyr + Phe + Leu + Ile + Val.

made (Figure 1). As previously reported,[4] higher serum ratios usually correlated with elevated brain tryptophan levels in normal animals. The same relationship was seen for diabetic animals, but both the serum ratio and the brain tryptophan values were substantially below normal. The points for both groups approximated a single line. In contrast, no clear correlation emerged when brain tryptophan was plotted against serum tryptophan alone (Figure 1).

Similar results were obtained when fasting rats were allowed to consume the 0% protein diet for 2 h (Tables 3 and 4). Insulin secretion by normal rats was associated with reductions in serum levels of all neutral amino acids except

TABLE 2
Effects of glucose intubation of fasting rats on brain tryptophan and 5-hydroxyindole levels in normal and diabetic rats*

	Minutes after glucose intubation			
Indole	0	30	60	120
		(nmol/g)		
Brain tryptophan†‡				
Normal rats	26.50 ± 2.00	30.90 ± 2.00	31.90 ± 0.50§	36.30 ± 0.50§
Diabetic rats	13.70 ± 1.50‖	11.30 ± 1.50‖	18.10 ± 1.00‖	15.70 ± 2.00‖
Brain serotonin				
Normal rats	4.11 ± 0.07	4.14 ± 0.13	4.10 ± 0.13	4.48 ± 0.05§
Diabetic rats	4.16 ± 0.18	4.13 ± 0.18	4.05 ± 0.14	4.30 ± 0.07
Brain 5-HIAA†‡				
Normal rats	3.47 ± 0.14	3.84 ± 0.04	3.86 ± 0.11	4.38 ± 0.18§
Diabetic rats	2.95 ± 0.13‖	2.95 ± 0.13‖	2.82 ± 0.10‖	3.25 ± 0.15‖

* Data are from the same experiment as in Table 1 and are expressed as means ± standard errors. Data were analyzed by two-way analysis of variance.
† These values were significantly affected by time ($P < 0.05$).
‡ These values were significantly affected by diabetes ($P < 0.05$).
§ These values differed significantly ($P < 0.05$) from time 0 using the Neuman-Keuls test.
‖ These values differed significantly ($P < 0.05$) from the corresponding normal values using the Student's *t* test.

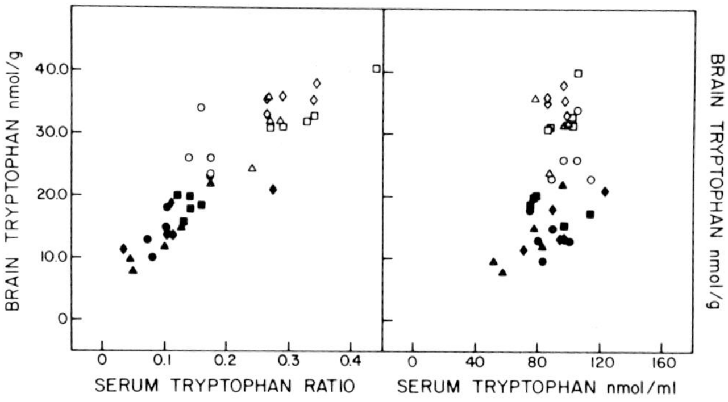

FIGURE 1. Data are from the same experiment shown in Tables 1 and 2. Points depicted are from individual rats. Symbols for normal rats are: 0 min (○), 30 min (△), 60 min (□), and 120 min (◇). Symbols for diabetic rats are: 0 min (●), 30 min (▲), 60 min (■), and 120 min (◆). A significant correlation was found between brain tryptophan concentration and the serum tryptophan ratio (r = 0.90); there was no significant correlation between brain tryptophan and serum tryptophan concentrations (r = 0.39).

tryptophan. Also, the serum tryptophan ratio and the brain concentrations of tryptophan and 5-HT increased significantly (brain 5-HIAA did not increase). In diabetic animals, insulin secretion in response to carbohydrate ingestion was greatly suppressed and often absent (Tables 3 and 4); therefore, serum neutral amino acid levels were seldom reduced, and only a small increase occurred in the serum tryptophan ratio (Table 3). Brain tryptophan and 5-HT levels were not significantly elevated (Tables 3 and 4); in this particular study, brain 5-HIAA rose significantly (Table 4), although it did not do so in other studies (Tables 2 and 5).

In other, similar experiments, fasting diabetic rats received a single injection of insulin (4 IU/kg, i.p.) or saline at the same time they were given free access to a carbohydrate meal (Table 5). This insulin dose did not cause hypoglycemia. When killed 2 h later, diabetic animals that had received insulin showed significant increments in the serum tryptophan ratio and in brain tryptophan and 5-HIAA (Table 5). In contrast, diabetic rats injected with saline showed no increments in the ratio, brain tryptophan, 5-HT, or 5-HIAA, as we anticipated (Table 5).

When normal rats consumed the protein-containing diet, no remarkable change occurred in the serum level of any large neutral amino acid (Table 3). Thus, the serum tryptophan ratio was not significantly changed, nor were brain tryptophan or 5-HT levels (Table 4); a significant reduction was noted in brain 5-HIAA levels.

When diabetic animals consumed the protein-containing meal, serum levels of the *aromatic* amino acids increased slightly; serum tryptophan increased twofold (Table 3). Serum concentrations of the *branched-chain* amino acids increased about threefold. Thus, the overall effect was to re-

TABLE 3
Effects of food ingestion by fasting normal or diabetic rats on serum neutral amino acid levels and on brain tryptophan concentrations*

Serum amino acid	Fasting	Carbohydrate	18% Casein
		(nmol/ml)	
Tryptophan†‡			
Normal rats	117 ± 7	105 ± 10	136 ± 8
Diabetic rats	43 ± 5	66 ± 6§‖	84 ± 7§‖
Tyrosine†			
Normal rats	91 ± 8	61 ± 6§	113 ± 5§
Diabetic rats	83 ± 11	55 ± 8	100 ± 12
Phenylalanine†‡			
Normal rats	79 ± 7	59 ± 3§	80 ± 3
Diabetic rats	92 ± 11	86 ± 6‖	102 ± 4‖
Leucine†‡			
Normal rats	204 ± 15	89 ± 5§	168 ± 4§
Diabetic rats	389 ± 59‖	347 ± 30‖	1253 ± 186§‖
Isoleucine†‡			
Normal rats	136 ± 17	55 ± 3§	98 ± 2§
Diabetic rats	237 ± 29‖	190 ± 12‖	701 ± 106§‖
Valine†‡			
Normal rats	267 ± 21	123 ± 7§	236 ± 4
Diabetic rats	569 ± 80‖	518 ± 45‖	1821 ± 215§‖
Tryptophan ratio†‡¶			
Normal rats	0.16 ± 0.01	0.27 ± 0.02§	0.20 ± 0.01
Diabetic rats	0.04 ± 0.01‖	0.06 ± 0.01§‖	0.03 ± 0.01‖
Insulin (μU/ml)†‡			
Normal rats	16 ± 3	45 ± 6§	67 ± 8§
Diabetic rats	1 ± 1‖	2 ± 1‖	5 ± 3‖
Brain tryptophan (nmol/g)†‡			
Normal rats	23.5 ± 1.2	33.0 ± 2.2§	22.1 ± 0.7
Diabetic rats	16.4 ± 1.6‖	14.6 ± 1.3‖	10.6 ± 0.8§‖

* Groups of six male normal or diabetic rats were fasted overnight, were presented with one of the experimental diets, and were killed 2 h later. Data were analyzed by two-way analysis of variance.
† These values were significantly affected by the diet ingested ($P < 0.05$).
‡ These values were significantly affected by diabetes ($P < 0.05$).
§ These values differ significantly ($P < 0.05$) from those in fasted controls using the Neuman-Keuls test.
‖ These values differ significantly ($P < 0.05$) from the corresponding normal values using the Student's *t* test.
¶ The serum tryptophan ratio is calculated using the serum concentrations of the amino acids named: Trp/Tyr + Phe + Leu + Ile + Val.

TABLE 4
Brain tryptophan and 5-hydroxyindole levels in normal and diabetic rats after food consumption*

Indole	Fasted	0% Protein	18% Protein
		(nmol/g)	
Brain tryptophan†‡			
Normal rats	18.1 ± 0.8	27.8 ± 0.7§	19.3 ± 0.6
Diabetic rats	13.4 ± 0.7‖	15.6 ± 0.9‖	11.4 ± 0.6‖
Brain serotonin‡			
Normal rats	3.03 ± 0.24	3.78 ± 0.15§	3.04 ± 0.06
Diabetic rats	2.96 ± 0.13	2.90 ± 0.24‖	2.94 ± 0.11
Brain 5-HIAA†‡			
Normal rats	3.02 ± 0.03	3.20 ± 0.14	2.29 ± 0.09§
Diabetic rats	1.83 ± 0.15‖	2.51 ± 0.11‖§	2.08 ± 0.10
Serum insulin (μU/ml)†‡			
Normal rats	9.8 ± 1.6	48.6 ± 6.3§	50.7 ± 9.7§
Diabetic rats	8.4 ± 1.1	10.6 ± 2.3‖	± 0.7‖

* Data are from a different experiment than that described in Table 3, but the protocols of the two experiments were the same (i.e., rats were killed 2 h after food was presented; n = 8). Data are expressed as means ± standard errors. Data were analyzed by two-way analysis of variance.
† These values were significantly affected by diet ($P < 0.05$).
‡ These values were significantly affected by diabetes ($P < 0.05$).
§ These values differed significantly from those in fasted controls ($P < 0.05$) using the Neuman-Keuls test.
‖ These values differed significantly from the corresponding normal values ($P < 0.05$) using Student's *t* test.

duce slightly the serum tryptophan ratio (Table 3). In this experiment (Table 3), brain tryptophan levels went significantly below fasting values; in another study, however, they fell only slightly (Table 4). Brain 5-HT and 5-HIAA levels in this latter experiment did not change significantly (Table 4).

The data from these diet studies were used to plot the individual values for brain tryptophan, the serum tryptophan ratio, and serum tryptophan alone (Figure 2). All values, from both diabetic and normal animals, approximated a single line when brain tryptophan was plotted with the serum ratio. When a similar plot of brain vs. serum tryptophan was constructed, the correlation was less impressive (Figure 2).

DISCUSSION

These data demonstrate that brain tryptophan and 5-hydroxyindole levels do not increase in diabetic rats soon after ingestion of glucose or a carbohydrate meal. These effects seem to be related to the lack of insulin secretion rather than to some other effect of streptozotocin-induced diabetes, since insulin administration to diabetic rats consuming carbohydrates significantly increased brain indoles (Table 5). The insulin dose used was somewhat higher than that used previously (i.e., 2 IU/kg[5,8]). This amount was selected because the fasting blood levels of branched-chain amino acids in diabetic animals were well above those in normal animals; a larger dose was considered necessary to reduce blood competitor levels sufficiently to favor brain tryptophan uptake. This insulin dose did not cause hypoglycemia (Table 5).

Insulin secretion (or injection) in normal animals elevates brain tryptophan (and 5-hydroxyindole) levels by stimulating tryptophan uptake. Insulin accomplishes this indirectly, by lowering serum levels of the amino acids that compete with tryptophan for brain uptake[3,22] while not reducing (and often increasing) serum tryptophan.[8] Consequently, tryptophan attains a competitive advantage over the other large neutral amino acids (i.e., the serum tryptophan ratio is elevated), leading to increased brain tryptophan transport.[3,4] If these notions are correct, then it should be possible to show that, in diabetic rats, glucose or carbohydrate ingestion does not increase the serum tryptophan ratio, brain tryptophan, or brain 5-hydroxyindoles. Such was indeed the case (Tables 1–5); moreover, it was also possible to reverse this refractoriness to carbohydrate ingestion by injecting insulin (Table 5). (Glucose intubation actually did increase the tryptophan ratio in diabetic rats at 60 min [Table 1]; however, this increase was quite small compared with that in normal rats and was associated with only an insignificant rise in brain tryptophan. The ratio's increase was the result of a modest, but significant, decline in blood levels of branched-chain amino acids at 60 min. We presently lack a clear explanation for this effect, although it might conceivably result from secretion of residual amounts of insulin and/or glucagon.)

Figures 1 and 2 show that changes in the serum tryptophan ratio (i.e., competitive uptake), not serum tryptophan levels alone, most reliably predict alterations in brain tryptophan (and 5-hydroxyindole) levels. In each study, the serum tryptophan ratio, not serum tryptophan alone, correlated best with brain tryptophan levels. While thus confirming the importance of competitive uptake for transport of tryptophan into brain, this result does not imply that, under some conditions (e.g., L-tryptophan injection), changes in serum trypto-

TABLE 5
Effect of insulin injection on brain indoles, blood glucose and insulin, and the serum tryptophan ratio in diabetic rats consuming a carbohydrate meal*

	Fasting	Saline	Insulin
Brain indoles (nmol/g)			
Tryptophan	14.1 ± 0.6	17.1 ± 0.6	27.3 ± 1.3†
5-HT	3.16 ± 0.15	3.15 ± 0.06	3.27 ± 0.10
5-HIAA	1.96 ± 0.07	2.04 ± 0.05	2.83 ± 0.12†
Serum tryptophan ratio	0.181 ± 0.013	0.194 ± 0.023	0.464 ± 0.042†
Serum glucose (mg/100 ml)	102.0 ± 9.0	966.0 ± 28.0	832.0 ± 50.0†
Serum insulin (μU/ml)	12.6 ± 1.7	7.2 ± 1.6	276.4 ± 83.5

* Groups of seven diabetic rats, fasted overnight, in the morning were either given free access to the carbohydrate meal or continued on their fast. Just after food was presented, two groups received injections of saline or insulin (4 IU/kg, i.p.). All animals were killed 2 h after food was given. Data are presented as means ± standard errors.
† $P < 0.01$ compared with saline or fasted group.

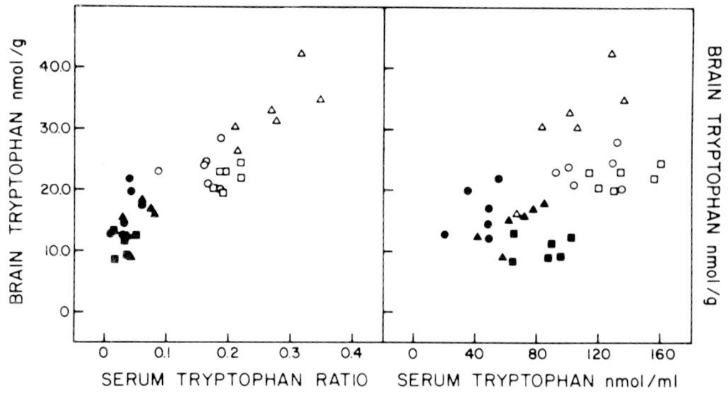

FIGURE 2. Data are from the experiment shown in Table 3. Points depicted are from individual rats. Symbols for normal rats are: fasting (○), 0% protein (△), and 18% protein (□). Symbols for diabetic rats are: fasting (●), 0% protein (▲), and 18% protein (■). A significant correlation was found between brain tryptophan concentration and the serum tryptophan ratio (r = 0.85); there was no significant correlation between brain tryptophan and serum tryptophan concentrations (r = 0.52).

phan alone cannot predict alterations in brain tryptophan—they can. Rather, our data support the notion that serum tryptophan is not the *only* determinant of brain tryptophan uptake. Consistent with this notion regarding diabetic rats are the recent findings of MacKenzie and Trulson,[23] who noted that such animals require larger doses of L-tryptophan to induce the same change in brain tryptophan produced by a smaller dose in normal rats. The most likely cause of this diminished responsiveness of brain tryptophan is increased blood levels of branched-chain amino acids in diabetes,[21,24,25] which enhance competition with tryptophan for brain uptake. Hence, in diabetic rats, higher tryptophan doses are required to overcome this increased competition, a possibility suggested by the investigators.[23] A similar effect may also hold for other amino acids that gain access to the brain via the large neutral amino acid carrier. In diabetics, higher doses of the neutral amino acid α-methyldopa (Aldomet; a centrally acting, antihypertensive agent), for example, may be necessary to elicit the same reduction in blood pressure obtained with smaller doses in nondiabetic hypertensive patients. Increased doses of L-dopa may also be required to treat diabetic subjects with Parkinson's disease. Both Aldomet and dopa have already been shown to be less efficacious in nondiabetics when consumed with high-protein meals (which elevate serum levels of the natural large neutral amino acids).[26-29]

Threefold increases were noted in serum branched-chain amino acid levels when diabetic rats ingested the 18% protein diet. Compared with the values in normal rats ingesting this diet, the difference was sevenfold to ninefold (Table 3). A similar effect of protein ingestion has been noted in human diabetics,[26] although the magnitude of increase was somewhat smaller than it was in rats. As a consequence, the serum ratio of each branched-chain amino acid probably also is abnormally high. Since the brain level of each large neutral amino acid correlates with its respective blood competitor ratio in normal rats after food ingestion,[4] the brain level of each branched-chain amino acid increases above normal in diabetic rats consuming protein meals. The functional significance to the brain of high branched-chain amino acid levels is unknown, but the brain does contain significant amounts of branched-chain amino acid transaminase activity,[30,31] and transamination appears somewhat precursor-dependent.[32] Hence, it seems possible that, if the brain levels of these amino acids increase soon after protein ingestion in the diabetic rat, their transamination rates may also increase.

Brain levels of serotonin and/or 5-HIAA invariably increase in normal rats soon after tryptophan injection or ingestion of sugars.[3,5,7,33] Both treatments rapidly raise brain tryptophan levels. In each case, it has been possible to demonstrate that the actual in vivo rate of tryptophan hydroxylation (an index of 5-HT synthesis[34]) is increased.[6] In the present studies, glucose intubation and carbohydrate ingestion each raised brain tryptophan and serotonin levels in normal rats (glucose administration also raised brain 5-HIAA), thus confirming earlier findings.[5,6] New support for these notions comes from the observation that, in diabetic rats, glucose or carbohydrate ingestion, which failed to raise brain tryptophan, also did not increase brain 5-HT or 5-HIAA (Tables 2–5). And, insulin administration to diabetic rats, at the time they began to consume carbohydrates, restored the normal rise in brain tryptophan and also increased brain 5-HIAA levels (suggesting that total flux through the pathway was increased, since 5-HT levels did not fall). These data are all consistent with the notion that 5-HT formation in brain depends on the brain tryptophan concentration.

Whether or not these increments in brain 5-hydroxyindoles ultimately enhance 5-HT release from nerve terminals is a topic of current investigation. Tryptophan-induced increments in brain 5-HT synthesis have been associated with increased growth hormone release,[35] improved sleep,[36] and analgesia.[37] In addition, drugs that enhance transmission across serotonin synapses in brain, as well as producing many of the same effects as tryptophan,[35,38,39] also influence appetite (for example, Wurtman and Wurtman[40] found that serotonin agonists and reuptake blockers selectively increase the rat's appetite for carbohydrates). If diet-induced (or insulin-induced) increases in brain tryptophan levels and serotonin synthesis can ultimately be shown to affect these brain functions in a similar manner, then ingestion of foods (especially carbohydrates) will constitute an important, *normal* modulator of brain chemistry and function. If such a relationship can be established, the *absence* of food-induced changes in brain 5-HT formation in diabetics may then be construed as an important *abnormality* of brain metabolism. Many studies are necessary before any conclusions can be drawn regarding the functional importance of the present findings in diabetics. However, the chemical effects presented here highlight a new, potentially important difference between the normal and diabetic brain.

ACKNOWLEDGMENTS

These studies were supported in part by grants from the American Diabetes Association, the Sugar Association, the National Institute of Mental Health, and the National Aeronautics and Space Administration. Dr. Fernstrom is the recipient of an NIMH Research Scientist Development Award. Ms. Crandall is supported by a training grant from the NIMH.

REFERENCES

1 Blasberg, R., and Lajtha, A.: Substrate specificity of steady-state amino acid transport in mouse brain slices. Arch. Biochem. Biophys. *112*: 361–77, 1965.

[2] Pardridge, W. M.: Kinetics of competitive inhibition of neutral amino acid transport across the blood brain barrier. J. Neurochem. 28:103–08, 1977.

[3] Fernstrom, J. D., and Wurtman, R. J.: Brain serotonin content: physiological regulation by plasma neutral amino acids. Science 178:414–16, 1972.

[4] Fernstrom, J. D., and Faller, D. V.: Neutral amino acids in the brain: changes in response to food injestion. J. Neurochem. 30:1531–38, 1978.

[5] Fernstrom, J. D., and Wurtman, R. J.: Brain serotonin content: increase following ingestion of carbohydrate diet. Science 174:1023–25, 1971.

[6] Colmenares, J. L., Wurtman, R. J., and Fernstrom, J. D.: Effect of ingesting a carbohydrate-fat meal on the levels and synthesis of 5-hydroxyindoles in various regions of the rat central nervous system. J. Neurochem. 25:825–29, 1975.

[7] Fernstrom, J. D., Faller, D. V., and Shabshelowitz, H.: Acute reduction of brain serotonin and 5-HIAA following food consumption: correlation with the ratio of serum tryptophan to the sum of competing neutral amino acids. J. Neural Transm. 36:113–21, 1975.

[8] Fernstrom, J. D., and Wurtman, R. J.: Elevation of plasma tryptophan by insulin in the rat. Metabolism 21:337–42, 1972.

[9] Rerup, C. C.: Drugs producing diabetes through damage of the insulin secreting cells. Pharmacol. Rev. 22:485–518, 1970.

[10] Denckla, W. D., and Dewey, H. R.: The determination of tryptophan in plasma, liver, and urine. J. Lab. Clin. Med. 69:160–69, 1967.

[11] Bloxam, D. L., and Warren, W. H.: Error in the determination of tryptophan by the method of Denckla and Dewey, a revised procedure. Anal. Biochem. 60:621–25, 1974.

[12] Lehman, J.: Light—a source of error in the fluorometric determination of tryptophan. J. Lab. Clin. Invest. 28:49–55, 1971.

[13] Arnold, M. A., and Fernstrom, J. D.: Salicylate reduces serum insulin concentrations in the rat. Life Sci. 19:813–17, 1976.

[14] Curzon, G., and Green, A. R.: Rapid method for the determination of 5-hydroxytryptamine and 5-hydroxyindoleacetic acid in small regions of rat brain. Br. J. Pharmacol. 39:653–55, 1970.

[15] Snedecor, G. W., and Cochran, W. G.: Statistical Methods. Ames, Iowa State University Press, 1967.

[16] Sokal, R. R., and Rohlf, F. J.: Biometry. San Francisco, W. H. Freeman & Co., 1969.

[17] Zivin, J. A., and Bartko, J. J.: Statistics for disinterested scientists. Life Sci. 18:15–26, 1976.

[18] Frayser, R., and Buse, M. G.: Branched chain amino acid metabolism in the retina of diabetic rats. Diabetologia 14:171–76, 1978.

[19] MacKenzie, R. G., and Trulson, M. E.: Does insulin act directly on the brain to increase tryptophan levels? J. Neurochem. 30:1205–08, 1978.

[20] MacKenzie, R. G., and Trulson, M. E.: Effects of insulin and streptozotocin-induced diabetes on brain tryptophan and 5-HT metabolism in rats. J. Neurochem. 30:205–11, 1978.

[21] Curzon, G., and Fernando, J. C. R.: Drugs altering insulin secretion: effects on plasma and brain concentrations of aromatic amino acids and on brain 5-hydroxytryptamine turnover. Br. J. Pharmacol. 60:401–08, 1977.

[22] Crofford, O. B., Felts, P. W., and Lacy, W. W.: Effect of glucose infusion on the individual plasma free amino acids in man. Proc. Soc. Exp. Biol. Med. 117:11–14, 1964.

[23] MacKenzie, R. G., and Trulson, M. E.: Regional accumulation of tryptophan and serotonin metabolism following tryptophan loading in diabetic rats. J. Neurochem. 31:157–60, 1978.

[24] Berger, M., Zimmerman-Telschow, H., Berchtold, P., Drost, H., Müller, W. A., Gries, F. A., and Zimmerman, H.: Blood amino acid levels in patients with insulin excess (functioning insulinoma) and insulin deficiency (diabetic ketosis). Metabolism 27:793–99, 1978.

[25] Carlsten, A., Hallgren, B., Jagenburg, R., Svanborg, A., and Werko, L.: Amino acids and free fatty acids in plasma in diabetes. I. The effect of insulin on the arterial levels. Acta Med. Scand. 179:361–70, 1966.

[26] Wahren, J., Felig, P., and Hagenfeldt, L.: Effect of protein ingestion on splanchnic and leg metabolism in normal man and in patients with diabetes mellitus. J. Clin. Invest. 57:987–99, 1976.

[27] Markovitz, D., and Fernstrom, J. D.: Diet and uptake of aldomet by the brain: competition with natural large neutral amino acids. Science 197:1014–15, 1977.

[28] Sved, A. F., and Fernstrom, J. D.: Diet alters the antihypertensive potency of methyldopa. Pharmacologist 20:189, 1978.

[29] Mena, I., and Cotzias, G. C.: Protein intake and the treatment of Parkinson's disease with levodopa. N. Engl. J. Med. 292:181–84, 1975.

[30] Benuck, M., Stern, F., and Lajtha, A.: Transamination of amino acids in homogenates of rat brain. J. Neurochem. 18:1555–67, 1971.

[31] Swaiman, K. F., and Milstein, J. M.: Oxidation of leucine, isoleucine, and related ketoacids in developing rabbit brain. J. Neurochem. 12:981–86, 1965.

[32] Chaplin, E. R., Goldberg, A. L., and Diamond, I: Leucine oxidation in brain slices and nerve endings. J. Neurochem. 26:701–07, 1976.

[33] Moir, A. T. B., and Eccleston, D.: The effects of precursor loading on the cerebral metabolism of 5-hydroxyindoles. J. Neurochem. 15:1093–1108, 1968.

[34] Carlsson, A., Kehr, W., Lindqvist, M., Magnussen, T., and Atack, C. V.: Regulation of monoamine metabolism in the central nervous system. Pharmacol. Rev. 24:371–84, 1972.

[35] Arnold, M. A., and Fernstrom, J. D.: Tryptophan injection stimulates growth hormone (GH) release in rats. Proc. 61st Meeting Endocr. Soc., Anaheim, Ca, 1979, p. 223.

[36] Hartmann, E.: L-tryptophan: a rational hypnotic with clinical potential. Am. J. Psychiatry 134:366–70, 1977.

[37] Fernstrom, J. D., and Lytle, L. D.: Corn malnutrition, brain serotonin, and behavior. Nutr. Rev. 34:257–62, 1976.

[38] Messing, R. B., Phebus, L., Fisher, L., and Lytle, L. D.: Analgesic effect of fluoxetine HCl (Lilly 110140), a specific uptake inhibitor for serotoninergic neurons. Psychopharmacol. Commun. 1:511–21, 1975.

[39] Samanin, R., Bernasconi, S., and Quattrone, A.: Antinociceptive action of quipazine: relation to central serotoninergic receptor stimulation. Psychopharmacologia (Berlin) 46:219–22, 1976.

[40] Wurtman, J. J., and Wurtman, R. J.: Drugs that enhance central serotoninergic transmission diminish elective carbohydrate consumption by rats. Life Sci. 24:895–904, 1979.

Critical Factors in the Chromatographic Measurement of Glycohemoglobin (HbA_1)

M. SIMON AND J. EISSLER

SUMMARY

Measurement of glycohemoglobin has been proposed as a criterion for the management of diabetes mellitus. We evaluated various conditions critical to the accuracy and precision of the cation-exchange method.

Tolerance limits for each variable were defined as follows: phosphate-eluding buffer (0.06 ± 0.005 mol/L ph 6.70–6.72), column temperature (19–21°C), and resin equilibration (to phosphate buffer, 0.07 mol/L, pH 6.70 ± 0.01). Hemoglobin absorbance measured in the Sorét region (approximately 416 nm) of the first chromatographic fraction divided by that of the total hemolysate provided the most accurate and precise result. Overall between-run precision expressed as coefficient of variation (CV, in percent) of normal and diabetic pools was 4.8% and 5.1%, respectively. When purified HbA_{1c} was added to hemolysates, recovery was 90–95%. Results were linear to at least 18% glycohemoglobin. Hemoglobin F (HbF) interfered with the method, whereas HbC and HbS did not. Red cells could be stored frozen for at least 6 days, thus easing transport of outpatient samples. A reference range of 6.0–8.8% glycohemoglobin was established from 85 nondiabetic adults (ages 23–65 yr). In a clinical study, only 4 of 13 treated diabetic patients believed to be in good control showed glycohemoglobin results within the normal range. All of the 19 treated diabetics in fair or poor control showed glycohemoglobin results greater than 10% of total Hb, ie., well above the normal range. DIABETES 29:467–474, June 1980.

It has been shown recently that the hyperglycemia of diabetes mellitus may be reflected in the formation of glycohemoglobin (glycosylated or fast hemoglobin, HbA_1). Glycosylation of hemoglobin (Hb) appears to occur concurrently with glycosylation of other proteins, and these changes may be responsible for nephropathy, retinopathy, and other complications.[1] Thus, measurement of glycohemoglobin may prove an important criterion for the clinical management of diabetic patients.[2] Several methods have been proposed for measurement of glycohemoglobin and most of these are based on cation-exchange separation of hemoglobin fractions.[3–5] Published descriptions have not included standards or procedures for preparing quality control pools. Lacking those conventional mechanisms for controlling accuracy and precision, the likelihood of long-term drift in the assay results is high.[6] Such assay drift would preclude long-term studies of the relationship of glycohemoglobin to the onset and progression of chronic complications.

HbA_{1c} was purified in the present study and was used with stabilized quality control pools to determine the critical conditions in a cation-exchange method for measurement of glycohemoglobin. While "glycohemoglobin" may be used to indicate *all* carbohydrate-containing hemoglobins,[10,11] glycohemoglobin here refers to the fast eluting chromatographic fraction (HbA_1), including HbA_{1a+b+c} and HbF (if present). Other chromatographic fractions comprised HbA_0 (the major adult hemoglobin $\alpha_2\beta_2$) and HbA_2 ($\alpha_2\delta_2$).

MATERIALS AND METHODS*

Purification of standard. HbA_{1c} was purified from the red cells of a diabetic donor using preparative methods;[12] about 67% of the original HbA_{1c} was recovered. The homogeneity of this preparation was examined using an isoelectric-focusing technique designed to separate the HbA_1 components.[13] Focusing yielded a single band of HbA_{1c}.

Equilibration of resin. The cation-exchange resin employed in this study was obtained in several lots from Bio-Rad Laboratories (Richmond, California) as Bio-Rex-70, 200–400 mesh. It was washed once with distilled water by

From the Research Department, Bio-Science Laboratories, Van Nuys, California.
Address reprint requests to M. Simon, Ph.D., Research Department, Bio-Science Laboratories, 7600 Tyrone Avenue, Van Nuys, California 91405.
Received for publication 5 September and in revised form 19 November 1979.

* Accurate preparation of the buffers and adequate chromatographic performance require ambient temperatures of 19–21°C. This temperature is maintained by placing the columns in an LKB Combi-Cold, or equivalent, cabinet.

stirring the resin using a glass rod with 2 vol of water. After allowing 15 min for settling, the fines were removed by pouring off the supernatant. The resin was converted from the sodium form by adding glacial phosphoric acid to a 1:3 (vol/vol) aqueous slurry of the resin until the pH reached 6.7. The resin was then washed twice with 2 vol of 0.5M buffer, pH 6.70 ± 0.02. The resistance of this buffer was found to be 30–35 Ω using a conductivity bridge (Yellow Springs Instrument, cell constant = 1.0). The resin was equilibrated against each batch with 0.05M sodium phosphate in 0.01M KCN (pH 6.70–6.72, resistance 220–240 Ω) until the pH of the supernatant matched that of the buffer. The resin was then equilibrated with 4-vol batches of 0.07M sodium phosphate in 0.01M KCN (pH 6.70–6.72, resistance 172–182 Ω) until the resistance and the pH of the supernatant exactly matched the buffer.

Routine method. One milliliter of red cells [separated from heparin or ethylenediaminetetraacetate (EDTA) plasma by centrifugation] was lysed by shaking with 2 ml of distilled water and 3 ml of carbon tetrachloride. After centrifuging 15 min at 1000 *g*, the upper phase (hemolysate) was removed fo use.

Disposable polyethylene transfer pipets (Scientific Products no. 5214-10, 6-in. size) were converted into columns by cutting off the top of the pipet bulbs to form reservoirs and tamping small cotton plugs into the tips.

Resin, batch-equilibrated with the cyanide-containing phosphate buffers just described, was slurry packed into disposable polyethylene transfer pipets to a bed height of 3 in.

Hemolysate (20 μl) was applied to the surface of the resin bed, and 200 μl eluting buffer (0.06M sodium phosphate containing 0.01M KCN, pH 6.70–6.72, resistance = 230–210 Ω) was used to rinse the sample into the bed. Eluting buffer (5 ml) was added to the reservoir and the entire eluate was collected (fast fraction). The flow rate was roughly 0.05 ml/min. We calculated the percent fast hemoglobin by dividing the absorbance of the fast fraction at 416 nm by that of 1:2000 aqueous dilution of the hemolysate. The performance of the method was monitored by including the purified A_{1c} standard as well as the nondiabetic and diabetic hemolysates (stored at −70°C and used as quality control pools) in each batch of samples.

Clinical range studies. Heparin, EDTA, or oxalated whole blood was obtained from 85 consenting adults (ages 23–65 yr) presenting no history of hyperglycemia. Thirty-four diabetics (ages 26–33 yr) attending an outpatient clinic were evaluated to be in good, fair, or poor control according to criteria used by Tze.[14]

RESULTS

Optimization of assay variables. The effects of chromatographic conditions on the separation of glycohemoglobin from HbA_0 were examined by comparing purified A_{1c} recovery and pool results when each parameter was varied independently. Under conditions where there was little resolution of the individual A_1 hemoglobins, separate bands could not be seen as the column was eluting and the main A_0 hemoglobin band merged with the fast eluting hemoglobins: this observation is termed A_0 breakthrough in this report. In the first experiment, shown in Figure 1, the resin was equilibrated to pH 6.72 with phosphate buffer (0.05M containing 0.01M potassium cyanide) and eluting buffers of pH 6.2 to pH 8.5 were examined using a nondiabetic hemolysate pool. In accord with other reports,[3] pH 6.72 buffer provided good recovery of HbA_{1c} with little HbA_0 contamination. The elution depended highly on pH, and the pH tolerance of the buffer was less than 0.05 pH units.

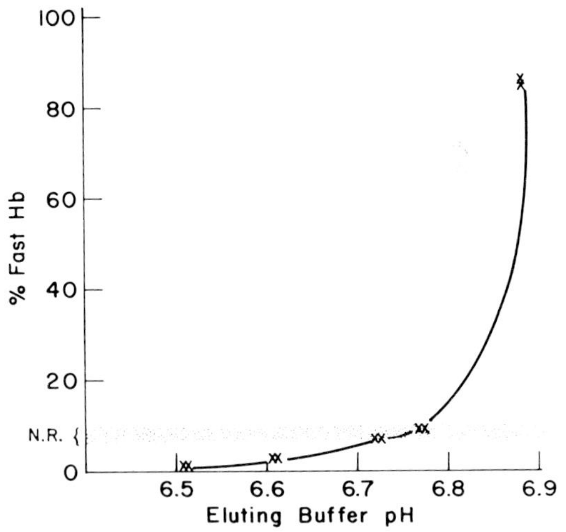

FIGURE 1. Effect of elution buffer pH on the percent hemoglobin recovered in the glycohemoglobin fraction using 20 μl of a nondiabetic hemolysate. All buffers were 0.05M sodium phosphate with 0.01M KCN. The resin was equilibrated to the same phosphate buffer (pH 6.70 ± 0.02). The normal range is indicated by the shaded area (N.R.).

In Figure 2 are the results of a nondiabetic hemolysate chromatographed at several different eluting buffer ionic strengths with a constant pH of 6.70 and 0.01M KCN. The elution of hemoglobin in the first 5 ml depended highly on the molarity of the phosphate buffer used. At 0.025M, little hemoglobin eluted, while at 0.1–0.15M almost *all* hemoglobin fractions eluted in the first 5 ml of buffer.

The results of experiments using purified HbA_{1c} and a nondiabetic hemolysate in which the ionic strength was varied

FIGURE 2. Effect of elution buffer ionic strength on the percent hemoglobin recovered in the glycohemoglobin fraction using 20 μl of a nondiabetic hemolysate. All buffers were sodium phosphate, pH 6.70–6.72, with KCN. The resin was equilibrated to 0.05M sodium phosphate containing 0.01M KCN, pH 6.70–6.72. The normal range is indicated by the shaded area (N.R.).

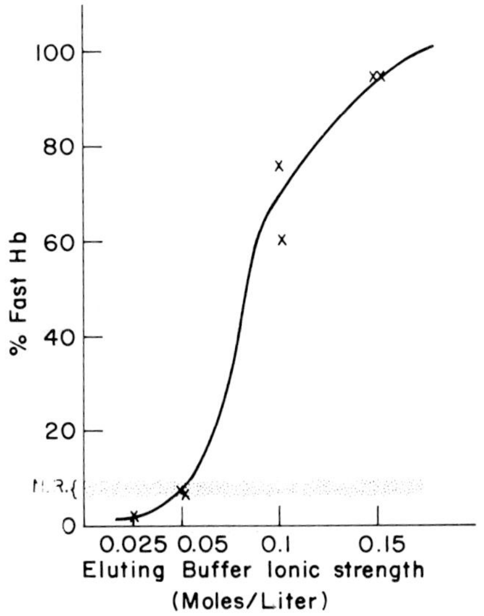

TABLE 1
Effect of molarity of phosphate buffers (pH 6.70) on elution of the glycohemoglobin fraction and purified HbA_{1c}

Molarity	Elution	0.05	0.05	0.06	0.065	0.05	0.06	0.07	0.083
	Resin	0.05	0.06	0.06	0.065	0.07	0.07	0.07	0.083
Resistance (Ω)	Elution	225	230	205	187	230	205	175	155
	Resin	235	205	205	187	175	175	175	155
Recovery A_{1c} (%)		6	<5	82	82	87	92	>100	>100
Pool Fast Hb (%)		2.4	<5	5.3	5.3	7.1	7.7	>15	>15
Observations		A_{1c} not eluted in 5 ml				visible bands		merged bands A_0 breakthrough	

Resin was initially equilibrated to 0.05M buffer.

within the narrow range of 0.05M to 0.08M are shown in Table 1. Also in these experiments, we varied the ionic strength used to equilibrate the resin from 0.05M to 0.07M. The resistance of each buffer (at 19–21°C, see below) was recorded to provide an indication of ionic strength independent of weighing errors in the buffer preparation. The results shown in Table 1 indicate that a combination of equilibration and elution buffer molarities was found that would provide full recovery of the A_{1c} peak with separate bands of A_{1a+b}, A_{1c}, A_0, and A_2 visually apparent during elution and no contamination of the fast fraction with A_0. The elution profile using these optimal conditions is shown in Figure 3. This system, composed of resin equilibrated to 0.07M buffer and to 0.06M elution buffer (both pH 6.70–6.72 containing 0.01M KCN), was used for all subsequent studies.

Figure 4 shows the effect of increasing the elution volume on the percent recovery of purified A_{1c} and on the hemoglobin appearing in the glycohemoglobin fraction from the normal pool. In the system described above, HbA_{1a} began to elute after approximately 1.5 to 2.1 ml, followed by A_{1b}. The figure shows that, by 4 ml, recovery of A_{1c} was virtually complete.

FIGURE 3. Elution pattern of 416-nm absorbance as a function of elution volume using a nondiabetic hemolysate. The first peak was HbA_{1a+b}; the second peak was HbA_{1c}.

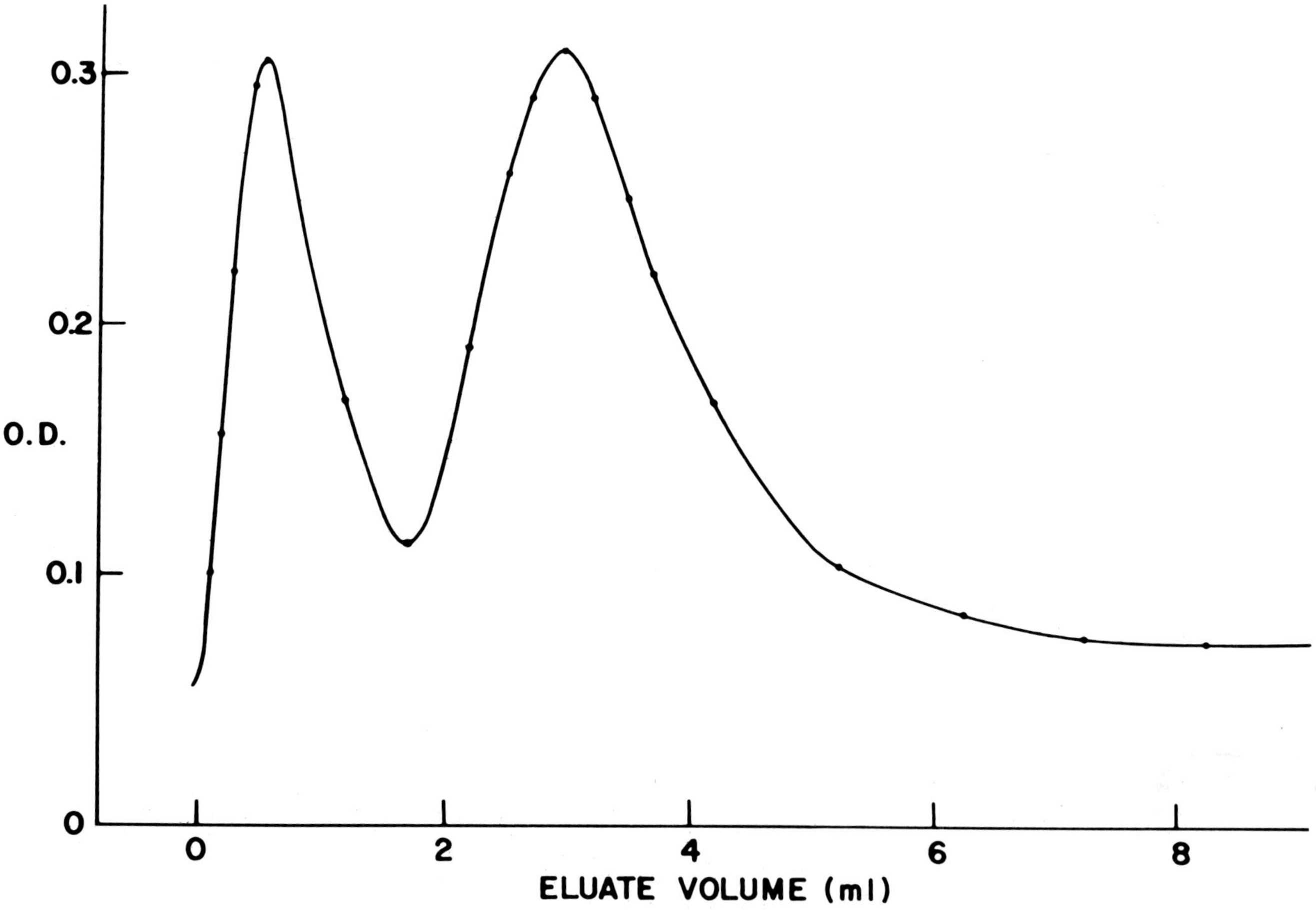

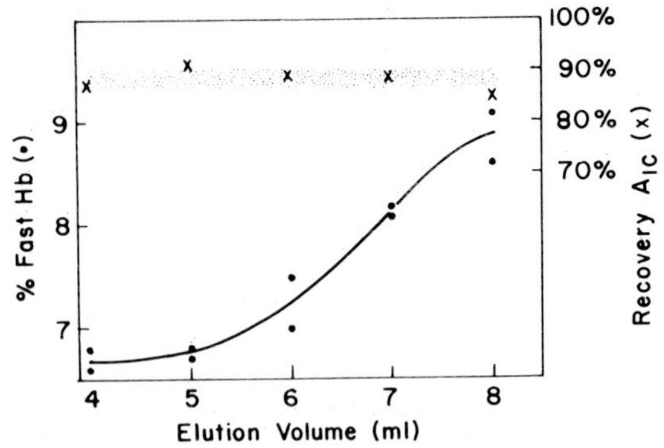

FIGURE 4. Effect of increasing elution volumes on the percent hemoglobin recovered in the glycohemoglobin fraction using 20 μl of a nondiabetic hemolysate (different patient than the one used in Figures 1 and 2) and on the recovery of purified A_{1c}. Other details are are described in the text.

A highly critical factor in the behavior of the small columns was temperature, as shown in Figure 5. At 7°C, purified A_{1c} remained at the top of the column and was not recovered at all in the fast fraction (5 ml). Conversely, at temperatures above 25°, substantial A-breakthrough was observed. Maximum recovery of A_{1c} without A_0 contamination required temperatures be kept between 19° and 21°C.

Several versions of quantitating percent glycohemoglobin after chromatography have been described.[3] In some methods, a second fraction (containing A_0 and possibly A_2) is eluted by a high phosphate, low pH buffer (0.25M, pH 6.4). Results can be calculated using the absorbances at 416 or 540 nm (see below) of the first and second fractions or of the first fraction and the total hemolysate (without chromatography): the glycohemoglobin absorbance is divided

FIGURE 5. Effect of temperature on the elution of hemoglobin into the glycohemoglobin fraction from a diabetic sample and on the recovery of purified A_{1c}. Other method parameters are described in the text.

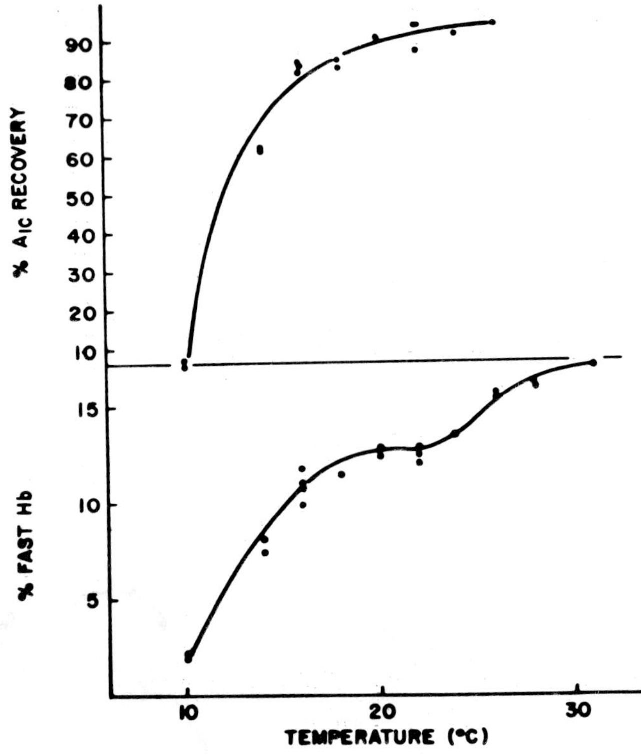

TABLE 2
Relative precision of absorbance measurements and calculations of percent glycohemoglobin (N = 5)

Wavelength (nm)	Calculation	Mean result (%)	Preliminary CV (%) (inter-run)
416	F/A	8.1	8.1
	F/T	7.2	10.2
540	F/A	7.4	18.9
	F/T	6.6	17.2

either by the sum of the absorbances of the first and second fractions (F/A) or by the absorbance of the total hemolysate (F/T). Table 2 is a list of the mean pool values and the precision using these calculations, the absorbances being determined on a Beckman 25 spectrophotometer. Precision of the 416-nm measurements was greater than that of the 540-nm measurements on the same sample. The F/T was less than the F/A ratio, because the total hemolysate included the A_2 fraction, which may not elute fully in the second fraction. These precision estimates differ from the final method precision described below, because the elution temperature was not controlled in this experiment; the data in Table 2 should be considered a comparative study. We found that the absorbance of the diluted hemolysate should be determined within one hour, because a rapid loss of absorbance occurs at high dilution.

The linearity of the method was determined by adding increasing amounts of purified A_{1c} to a normal hemolysate. Figure 6 demonstrates that linearity in precent glycohemoglobin extends from 7.6% to at least 18.2%. Recovery of the A_{1c} spiked to pools was about 90–95%.

The precision of the method was evaluated using prepared hemolysates stored at −70°C for up to 90 days. In independent runs over 10 days, the within-run coefficient of variation (C.V.) was 2.2% and the between-run C.V. was 4.8% using a nondiabetic adult pool (mean = 7.5% glycohemoglobin). Similarly, in a diabetic hemolysate (mean = 12.3% glycohemoglobin), within-run C.V. was 3.4% and the between-run C.V. was 5.1%.

Interference studies. Red cells from heparinized cord blood (containing high HbF) were centrifuged, washed three times with saline, and lysed by adding 1 vol of water and 2 vol of carbon tetrachloride; 20 μl of this hemolysate was added to the columns and eluted as described in ROUTINE METHOD. Almost *all* cord blood hemoglobin appeared in the glycohemoglobin fraction (80–94%). A normal pool containing 8% glycohemoglobin was diluted 1 + 1 with the cord blood hemolysate. Elution of the spiked pool showed one abnormal band eluting before HbA_{1a} and HbA_{1b} and another before HbA_{1c}; the glycohemoglobin fraction contained 30% of the total hemoglobin. Therefore, HbF appeared to be measured with the glycohemoglobin fraction, resulting in an elevation in the calculated percentage of HbA_1.

A human hemolysate containing HbC and HbS was prepared as described in METHODS, and 3.3% of the hemoglobin eluted in the fast fraction. This hemolysate was mixed (1 + 1) with a normal pool (7.9% glycohemoglobin). The fast fraction contained 6% of the hemoglobin in the mixture. This compared well with a theoretic yield of 5.6% in the gly-

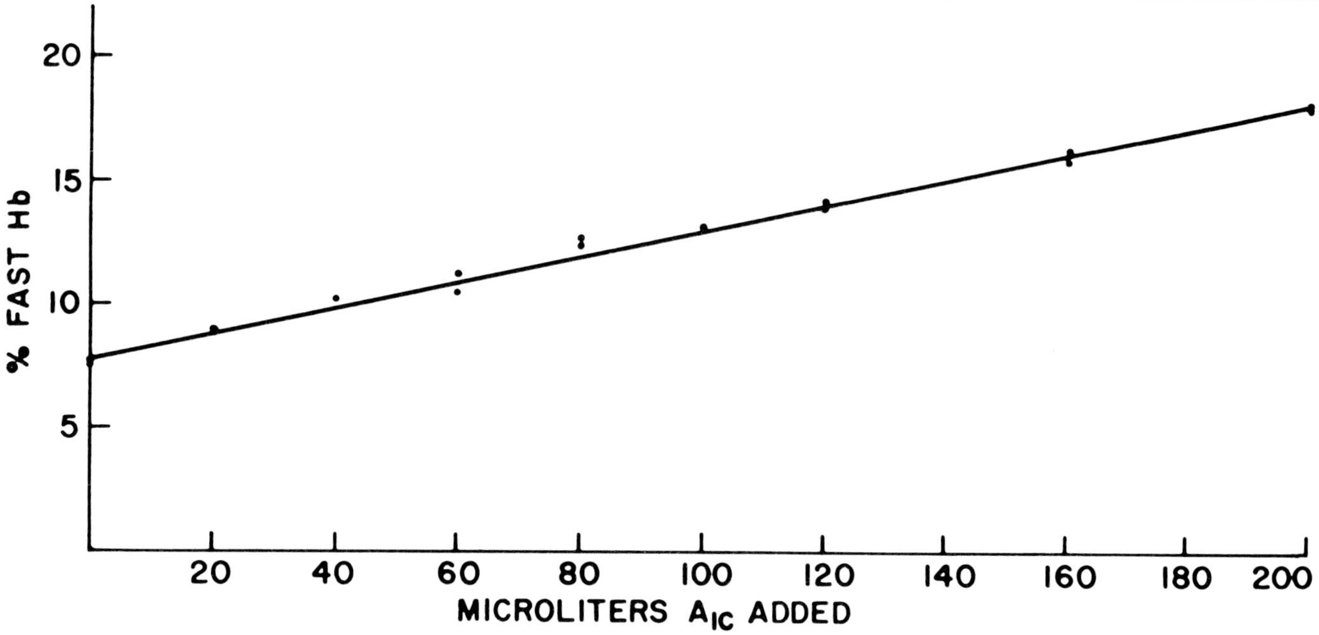

FIGURE 6. Linearity in percent glycohemoglobin with increasing amounts of purified A_{1c} added to a nondiabetic hemolysate. Elution conditions are described in the text.

cohemoglobin fraction, consistent with no interference. The abnormal hemoglobins remained at the top of the column with the A_0 and did not interfere in the fast fraction. Because the method did not depend on complete elution of a second fraction from the column, as required in other procedures,[3] no methodologic interference was observed by HbC and HbS.

The effect of high bilirubin in blood on glycohemoglobin was tested by adding 3.4 μg of bilirubin from a blood sample containing high bilirubin to the column; it eluted entirely in the glycohemoglobin fraction. The glycohemoglobin result increased from 9.5% to 10.8% in the normal pool when 20 μl of a high bilirubin serum was added to the hemolysate.

FIGURE 7. Distribution of the glycohemoglobin results in nondiabetic adults: 95% confidence limits indicate a range of 6.08–8.8% (mean, 7.2%) glycohemoglobin.

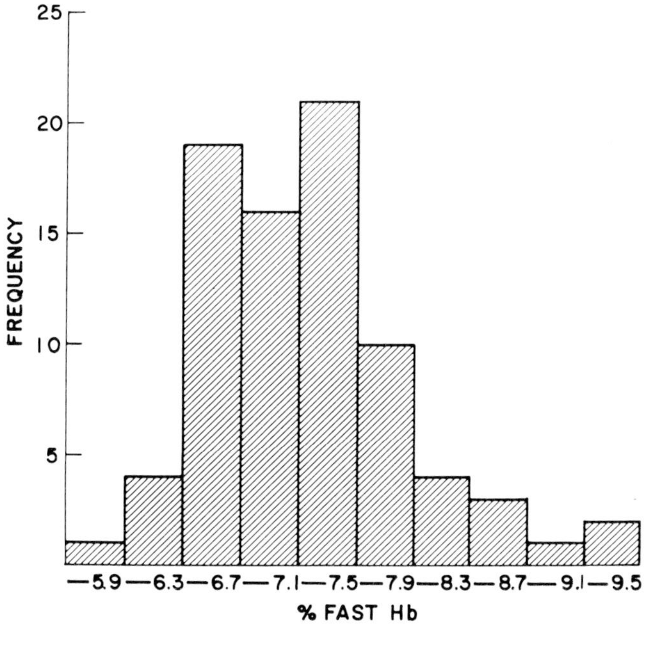

Reference range. The distribution of the glycohemoglobin results from 85 nondiabetic adults is shown in Figure 7. The data fit an arc sinh distribution with a non-Gaussian reference range estimate[15] of 6.0–8.8%. A trend toward increasing glycohemoglobin with increasing age is shown in Figure 8.

Clinical study. The results of a small study of treated diabetics attending an outpatient diabetes clinic are shown in Figure 9. A few patients in the group, rated as well controlled, exhibited glycohemoglobin results within the normal range. No overlap to the normal range was found in the less well-controlled groups of patients.

Sample stability. Other glycohemoglobin methods reported to date require fresh specimens or refrigerated storage (4°C). Since this storage condition is not convenient

FIGURE 8. Percent glycohemoglobin as a function of age in nondiabetic subjects. Correlation coefficient = 0.46.

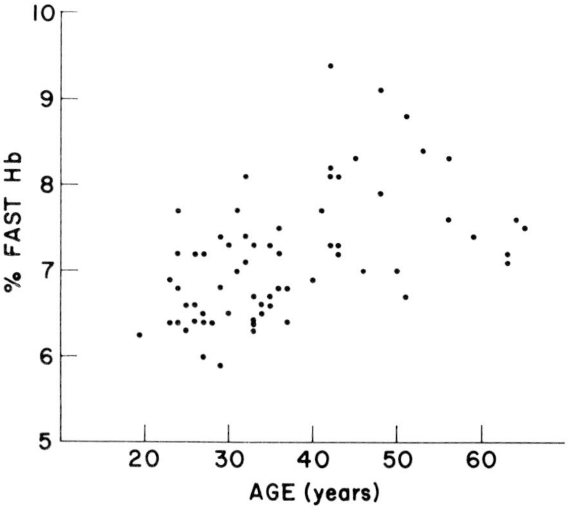

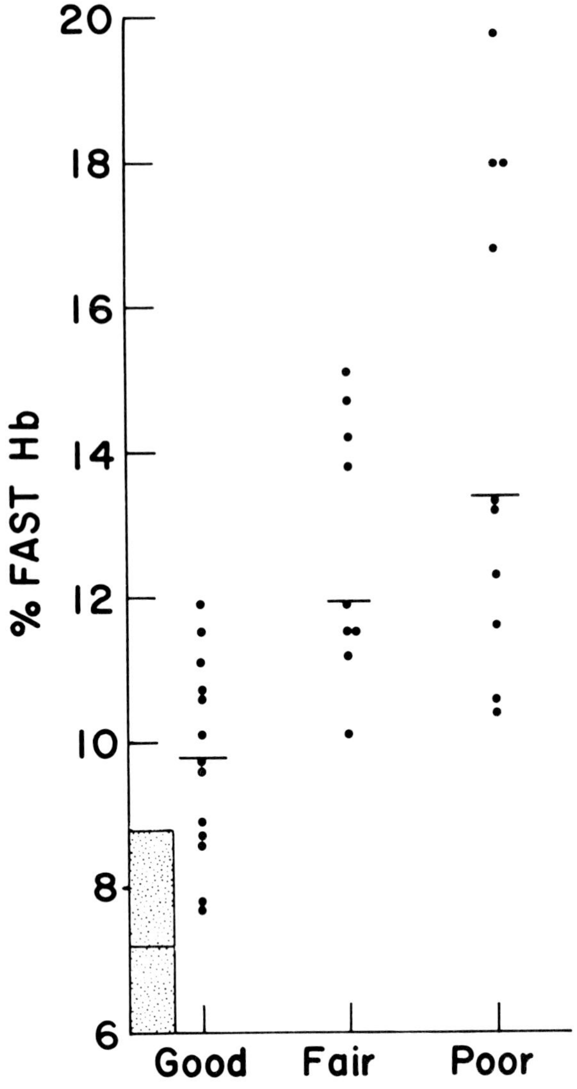

FIGURE 9. Distribution of glycohemoglobin results from 32 diabetics rated to be in good, fair, and poor control compared with the nondiabetic range. Group medians are indicated by the horizontal lines.

TABLE 3
Storage effects on glycohemoglobin in a single sample and recovery of purified HbA_{1c}

		% Glycohemoglobin				
			After storage* at			
Anti-coagulant	Sample	Day 0	30°C	4°C	−20°C	−70°C
Heparin	Whole blood	6.8	13.5	8.5	11.0	8.9
	Hemolysate		16.5	7.7	11.6	7.2
EDTA	Whole blood	7.0	18.5	8.0	10.6	9.0
	Hemolysate		29.3	7.5	11.9	7.4
Oxalate	Whole blood	7.5	11.8	7.8	10.5	8.7
	Hemolysate		16.5	7.6	13.3	7.8
		Percent recovery				
	Purified A_{1c}	94	67	93	95	94

* A_{1c} for 5 days, whole blood for 7 days, hemolysate for 10 days.

for monitoring diabetic outpatients, other stable conditions were sought (Table 3). These preliminary results suggested that whole blood samples stored at 30°C, −20°C, or −70°C would show elevated results. The red cell hemolysates shown in Table 3 appeared to be stable for at least 10 days stored at 4° or −70°C. Subsequently hemolysate pools stored at −70°C were used to monitor the precision of the assay (see above) and did not show any signs of deterioration for at least 3 mo.

In contrast with results from stored whole blood, storing the separated *red cells* frozen at −20°C (Figure 10) for 6 days did not affect glycohemoglobin results in samples drawn from normal and diabetic adults (N = 31). None of the results of the 31 samples tested was significantly affected by frozen storage of the red cells before hemolysate preparation.

DISCUSSION

The chromatographic separation of the glycohemoglobin fraction (A_{1a}, A_{1b}, and A_{1c}) from the main hemoglobin peak (A_0) was exquisitely sensitive to several variables: pH, ionic strength, temperature, and elution volume, as suggested by recent communications.[16] These variables must be rigorously and consistently controlled, i.e., the pH to ±0.02 units, and an operating temperature range of 19–21°C must be maintained. It is recommended that the resistance of all buffers (at controlled temperatures) be used to monitor and adjust ionic strength within the limits defined in METHODS. Even within the tolerances defined, the effects of these variables are observed as trends in the daily quality control pool results. Workers who have not controlled these variables report difficulties in achieving reproducible results.[6,16,17]

The good separation of A_{1a+b} from A_{1c} shown in Figure 3 represents a significant improvement over the single merged A_1 peak previously thought to be characteristic of small column methods.[16] The separation characteristics of the columns can be observed visually during elution and are fundamental to the accuracy and precision of glycohemoglobin determinations because the potential interference by HbA_0 is not apparent in the absorbance characteristics of the fractions.

During development of the method, we discovered that intact cells elute in the fast fraction and the resulting turbidity caused the percentage of glycohemoglobin to be biased high by as much as twofold. The effect of this turbidity on the absorbance could be removed by centrifugation of the eluates or by the more complete hemolysis obtained in the present procedure.

HbF was nearly completely recovered in the fast fraction. Glycohemoglobin determinations, therefore, may not be useful in monitoring pregnant patients, since HbF may be produced in varying amounts throughout pregnancy. This finding has also been reported in other chromatographic methods in which correction for HbF was applied.[8] This procedure is hampered by the poor precision of HbF measurements.[20] While no methodologic interference was apparent in the hemolysate containing HbC and HbS, the glycohemoglobin was low (well below the normal range); this may mean that HbS and/or HbC were not glycosylated at the same rate as A_0, or that the glycosylated S or C did not elute in the glycohemoglobin fraction, or that red cell survival was reduced in the patient.[18] Therefore, there may be a physio-

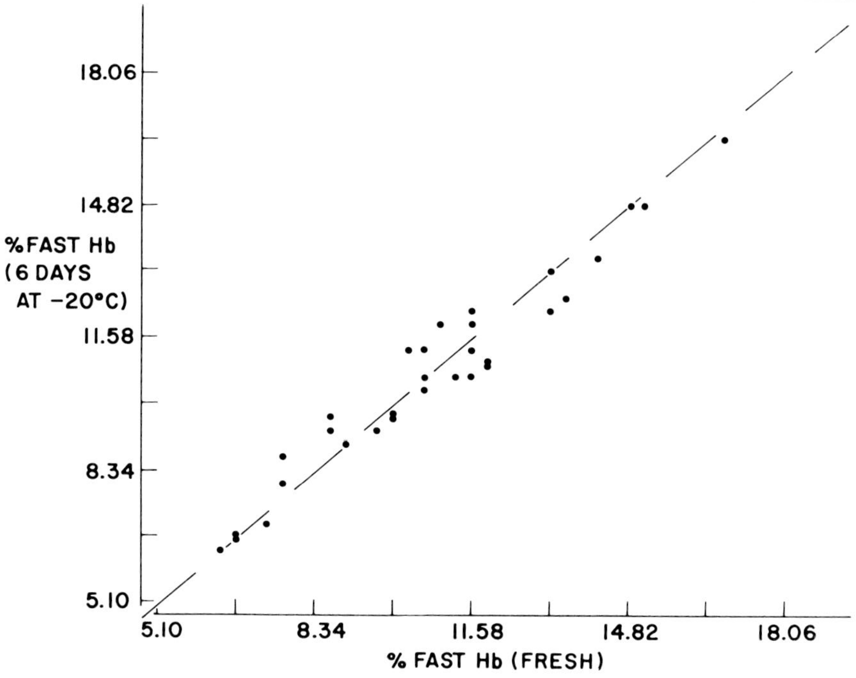

FIGURE 10. A comparison of glycohemoglobin results obtained from hemolysates of fresh red cells and of red cells frozen for 6 days at −20°C using diabetic and normal samples. A slope of 1.0 is shown by the dashed line.

logic (in vivo) interference from HbC and HbS, leading to difficulties in interpreting such results. However, results from such patients could be compared with previous determinations for long term clinical monitoring.

In accord with other reports,[19] a trend was found in which glycohemoglobin increased with age in nondiabetics. This factor may partly explain the differences in the normal ranges reported and in the degree of overlap of diabetic and nondiabetic results[15,19] (and see below).

The glycohemoglobin found in 34 treated diabetic patients grouped according to hyperglycemic control shows that values from only four patients believed to be in good control fell within the nondiabetic range. None of the patients rated fair or poor overlapped the reference range, and group medians reflected control ratings. The discrimination among groups was somewhat better than in the previous reports[15,19] and may be a result of our control of methodologic variables. Substantial overlap occurred among the diabetic groups and probably reflected the acknowledged difficulty in accurately assessing the status of many diabetics on the basis of clinical judgment and conventional laboratory testing.[2]

Sample stability is a potentially serious problem in routine patient monitoring that has received little attention in other reports. The statistical significance of published results has not been presented, even for the most commonly suggested storage condition of whole blood at 4°C. Based on the preliminary studies described, storage of whole blood for seven days did not appear promising at any temperature, with the possible exception of 4°C. The elevation in the glycohemoglobin fraction observed after storage of whole blood or hemolysates at 30°C could be attributed to hemoglobin breakdown products that co-elute with A_{1a+b}. These contaminants may begin to appear after as early as a few hours at room temperature.[7] This artifactual elevation in glycohemoglobin would interfere with the interpretation of samples from outpatients or other patients not in close proximity to the laboratory, because there is no way a priori to distinguish between a real elevation in the fast fraction and an artifactual elevation secondary to improper sample storage.

The demonstration that red cells could be stored at −20°C for at least six days before analysis (Figure 10) allowed convenient storage, especially for samples likely to encounter some delay in reaching the laboratory. As shown in Table 3, the stability of frozen whole blood was highly questionable and was not pursued. We have observed that hemolysates may be stored at −70°C for several months without apparent deterioration and are useful as quality control pools. The prepared A_{1c} standard was dialyzed against the cyanide-containing eluting buffer after chromatographic purification, and it was relatively stable in this form, except at 30°C.

In summary, the variables affecting the accuracy and precision of the chromatography and the quantitation of glycohemoglobin were examined in an effort to avoid methodologic artifacts so that the proper role of this laboratory test in the management of diabetic patients could be evaluated. The method described has been optimized with respect to those variables and has been fully characterized by linearity, recovey, precision, and interference studies. Particular attention has been directed toward stability questions, and the method was successfully applied to a small group of diabetic patients.

ACKNOWLEDGMENT

We thank Dr. Mayer Davidson for his evaluation of the diabetic patients tested.

REFERENCES

1 Peterson, C. M., and Jones, R. L.: Minor hemoglobins, diabetic "control," and diseases of postsynthetic protein modification. Ann. Intern. Med 87:489–91, 1977.

2 Cerami, A., Koenig, R. J., Peterson, C. M., and Stevens, V. J.: Forma-

tion of HbA_{1c} as a biochemical model for sequelae of diabetes. *In* Progress in Clinical and Biological Research, Vol. 21, 4th International Conference on Red Cell Metabolism and Function. Brewer, G. J., Ed. New York, Alan R. Liss Inc., 1978, pp. 33–45.

[3] Trivelli, L. A., Ranney, H. M., and Lai, H. T.: Hemoglobin components in patients with diabetes mellitus. N. Engl. J. Med. *284*:353–57, 1971.

[4] Allen, D. W., Schroeder, W. A., and Balog, J.: Observations on the chromatographic heterogeneity of normal adult and fetal human hemoglobin: a study of the effects of crystallization and chromatography on the heterogeneity and isoleucine content. J. Am. Chem. Soc. *80*:1628–34, 1958.

[5] Huisman, T. H. J., and Meyering, C. A.: Studies on the heterogeneity of hemoglobin. I. The heterogeneity of different human hemoglobin types in carboxy methycellulose and in Amberlite IRC-50 chromatography: qualitative aspects. Clin. Chim. Acta *5*:103–23, 1960.

[6] Wajcman, H., Dastugue, B., and Labie, D.: Quantitations of hemoglobin A_{1c}: a rapid, automated precision-chromatography technique. Clin. Chim. Acta *93*:33–39, 1979.

[7] Huisman, T. H. J., and Horton, B. F.: Studies on the heterogeneity of hemoglobin. VIII. Chromatographic and electrophoretic investigations of various minor hemoglobin fractions present in normal and in vitro modified red blood cell hemolysates. J. Chromatogr. *18*:116–25, 1965.

[8] Schwartz, H. C., King, K. C., Schwartz, A. L., Edmunds, D., and Schwartz, R.: Effects of pregnancy on hemoglobin A_{1c} in normal, gestational diabetic, and diabetic women. Diabetes *25*:1118–22, 1976.

[9] Bunn, H. F., Gabbay, K. H., and Gallop, P. M.: The glycosylation of hemoglobin: relevance to diabetes mellitus. Science *200*:21–27, 1978.

[10] McDonald, M. J., Shapiro, R., Bleichman, M., Solway, J., and Bunn, H. F.: Glycosylated minor components of human adult hemoglobin. J. Biol. Chem. *253*:2327–32, 1978.

[11] Bunn, H. F., Shapiro, R., Garrick, L. M., McDonald, M. J., Gabbay, K. H., and Gallop, P. M.: Heterogeneity of human hemoglobin A_0 due to non-enzymatic glycosylation. Fed. Proc. *37*:1390, 1978.

[12] Koenig, R. J., Blobstein, S. H., and Cerami, A.: Structure of carbohydrate of hemoglobin A_{1c}. J. Biol. Chem. *252*:2992–97, 1977.

[13] Spicer, K. M., Allen, R. C., and Buse, M. G.: A simplified assay of hemoglobin A_{1c} in diabetic patients by use of isoelectric focusing and quantitative microdensitometry. Diabetes *27*:384–88, 1978.

[14] Tze, W. J., Thompson, K. H., and Leichter, J.: HbA_{1c}—an indicator of diabetic control. J. Pediatr. *93*:13–16, 1978.

[15] Harris, E. K., and De Mets, D. L.: Estimations of normal ranges and cumulative proportions by transforming observed distributions to gaussian form. Clin. Chem. *18*:605–12, 1972.

[16] Welch, S. G., and Boucher, B. J.: A rapid micro-scale method for the measurement of hemoglobin $A_{1(a+b+c)}$. Diabetologia *14*:209–11, 1978.

[17] Ryall, R. G., and Graham, J. J.: Routine measurement of glycosylated hemoglobin. Lancet *1*:739, 1978.

[18] Makarem, A.: Hemoglobins, hemoglobin derivatives and hemoglobin binding proteins. *In* Clinical Chemistry. Principles and Technics, 2nd edit. Henry, R. J., Cannon, D. C., and Winkelman, J. W., Eds. New York, Harper and Row, 1974, pp. 1162–80.

[19] Dunn, P. J., Soeldner, J. S., and Wacks, M.: Measurement of glycosylated hemoglobins. Lancet *1*:838, 1978.

[20] Brosious, E. M., and Schmidt, R. E.: Quantitation of hemoglobin F. An interlaboratory study. Am. J. Clin. Pathol. *72*:421, 1979.

Lysosomal Degradation of Receptor-bound ^{125}I-labeled Insulin by Rat Adipocytes

Its Characterization and Dissociation from the Short-term Biologic Effects of Insulin

GLENN T. HAMMONS AND LEONARD JARETT

SUMMARY

In this study we used chloroquine to characterize the internalization and lysosomal degradation of receptor-bound ^{125}I-insulin by rat adipocytes and to determine the role of lysosomal processing of insulin in the short-term biologic effects of the hormone. Chloroquine inhibited the degradation of ^{125}I-insulin bound to adipocytes by both association and dissociation experiments. In the former experiments, chloroquine caused a time- and concentration-dependent increase in specifically bound insulin owing to an increase in intact insulin and a decrease in degradation products, as determined by trichloroacetic acid precipitability and gel chromatographic analysis of material extracted from the cells. In the dissociation experiments, 50 μM chloroquine decreased the rate of degradation by two thirds, as reflected in the release of degradation products from the cells. Chloroquine had no effect on the amount of ^{125}I-insulin specifically bound to or degraded by isolated plasma membranes, on the degradation of ^{125}I-insulin by proteases in the incubation medium, or on the endocytotic uptake of receptor-bound insulin. Quantitative electron microscopy, using monomeric ferritin-insulin, showed 50 μM chloroquine doubled the number of lysosomal structures containing ferritin. These findings are consistent with an inhibition by chloroquine of lysosomal degradation of internalized receptor-bound insulin. Chloroquine, at these same concentrations, had no effect on the ability of insulin to stimulate glucose transport and oxidation or to inhibit epinephrine-stimulated lipolysis. In these studies, we show that lysosomal degradation of internalized receptor-bound insulin is not necessary for insulin to cause short-term biologic effects in the adipocyte. DIABETES 29:475–486, June 1980.

Extensive investigation has established that the biologic responses to insulin are initiated by the binding of the hormone to receptors on the plasma membrane of target cells.[1] Terris and Steiner[2,3] first showed that a portion of receptor-bound insulin was degraded by hepatocytes and suggested that degradation followed internalization and localization to lysosomes. It is now accepted that a portion of bound insulin is internalized by hepatocytes and fibroblasts through receptor-mediated endocytosis.[4–9] Internalized insulin preferentially localizes to lysosomes in the hepatocyte.[10–12] Several investigators have shown that bound insulin is degraded by the adipocyte[13–16] and in several studies have demonstrated compartmentalization and, thus, possible internalization of bound insulin by the cell.[14,16–18] The plasma membranes of both hepatocytes[19,20] and adipocytes[15] contain insulin-degradative activity, and Dial et al.[20] have shown bound insulin to be an efficient substrate for degradation by mouse liver membranes. This membrane degradation must account for some of the degradation of bound insulin by intact cells. The destination and fate of insulin internalized by the adipocyte has not been established nor has the function of internalization been determined. It has been suggested that internalization of bound insulin and possibly its degradation at the plasma membrane or within the cell may be important in the mechanism by which insulin elicits its characteristic biologic effects in its target cells,[2,3,10,13,18,21] or, the mechanism by which downregulation of the insulin receptor occurs.[10,22] In this work we employed both biochemical and morphologic techniques using chloroquine, an inhibitor of lysosomal degradation of macromolecules[23–25] that include low-density lipoprotein[26] and epidermal growth factor,[27] to study the internalization and lysosomal degradation of receptor-bound ^{125}I-insulin by isolated adipocytes and to determine if lysosomal degradation of insulin participates in the short-term biologic effects of the hormone.

This study was presented, in part, at the Annual Meeting of the Federation of American Societies for Experimental Biology held in Dallas, Texas, in April, 1979, and at the 39th Annual Meeting of the American Diabetes Association, Inc., held in Los Angeles, California, in June, 1979.

From the Division of Laboratory Medicine, Departments of Pathology and Medicine, Washington University School of Medicine and Barnes Hospital, St. Louis, Missouri 63110.

Address reprint requests to Dr. Leonard Jarett, Division of Laboratory Medicine, Washington University School of Medicine, St. Louis, Missouri 63110.

Received for publication 19 November 1979.

MATERIALS

Porcine insulin (lot 615-1082B-108-I) was a gift from Dr. Ronald Chance of Eli Lilly; male Sprague-Dawley rats, weighing 120–180 g, were purchased from Eldridge Laboratory Animals, Barnhart, MO; collagenase, bovine serum albumin (fraction V), 3-O-methylglucose, and chloroquine diphosphate from Sigma Chemical Co., St. Louis, MO; silicone fluid (catalog no. 6428-R15) from Arthur H. Thomas Co., Philadelphia, PA; ammonium chloride from Mallinckrodt Chemical Works, St. Louis, MO; dinonyl phthalate and potassium azide from Eastman Kodak Co., Rochester, NY; potassium cyanide from Fisher Scientific Co., Fairlawn, NJ; [^{14}C]sucrose, 3-O-[methyl-^{3}H]glucose, D-[1-^{14}C]glucose, and L-[l-^{14}C]glucose from New England Nuclear, Boston, MA; carrier-free ^{125}I from New England Nuclear and Amersham, Arlington Heights, IL; glass fiber GF/C filters from Whatman, Ltd., England; epinephrine HCl from Parke-Davis, Detroit, MI; Enzymobead Radioiodination Kit (catalog no. 170-6002) from Bio-Rad Laboratories, Richmond, CA. Other reagents and chemicals were from standard sources.

METHODS

Preparation of ^{125}I-insulin. Iodination of insulin was carried out by either a chloramine-T[28] or a lactoperoxidase method[29] using the Enzymobead Radioiodination Kit[30] to a specific activity of 120–180 μCi/μg and was purified over a Sephadex G-50 column. The resulting ^{125}I-insulin contained an average of less than 0.5 atoms of ^{125}I per insulin molecule. Such preparations have been demonstrated to be predominantly monoiodinated and to retain full biologic activity.[28,31] Specific activity of the ^{125}I-insulin was 1200–1600 cpm/fmol.

Preparation of ^{125}I-BSA. Iodination of BSA* was carried out by the same chloramine-T method used for iodination of insulin, except BSA was substituted for insulin on a molar basis. The iodinated material eluting just after the void volume of a G-50 Sephadex column was taken to be ^{125}I-BSA.

Preparation of isolated adipocytes. Adipocytes were isolated from epididymal fat pads of male Sprague-Dawley rats, weighing 120–180 g, by a modification[32] of the method of Rodbell[33] using 0.5 mg/ml collagenase in KRP-AG or KRH-AG buffer. KRH buffer contained 125 mM NaCl, 5.9 mM KCl, 2.5 mM $CaCl_2$, 1.25 mM $MgSO_4$, 2.5 mM NaH_2PO_4, and 20 mM Hepes. KRP buffer contained 128 mM NaCl, 5.1 mM KCl, 1.4 mM $CaCl_2$, 1.4 mM $MgSO_4$, and 10 mM NaH_2PO_4. The pH of each buffer was adjusted to 7.4 with NaOH.

Preparation of adipocyte plasma membranes. Isolated plasma membranes were prepared by the method of Jarett[34] with minor modifications.[35] The membranes were resuspended in KRP buffer and the protein content was determined by the method of Lowry.[36]

Determination of cell-associated label. Recent evidence has shown that bound ^{125}I-insulin in adipocytes consists not only of intact insulin but also of higher and lower molecular weight compounds.[6,10,13,14,16] Thus, the term cell-associated label more aptly describes this spectrum of labeled compounds and will be used occasionally in this report. Use of the term bound insulin will also connote cell-associated label and will not imply that the radioactivity measured represents only intact insulin. Cell-associated label or ^{125}I-insulin binding was measured by the microfuge separation method of Gammeltoft and Gliemann,[37] substituting silicone oil for dinonyl phthalate or diluting with cold buffer and centrifuging through silicone oil, as described by Gliemann and Sonne.[13]

^{125}I-labeled insulin binding and degradation. All binding studies with cells were performed at 37°, except as noted in KRH-AG buffer at pH 7.4. The final concentration of cells was 10^5–10^6/ml. Cells were preincubated for 10 min with or without chloroquine or ammonium chloride, and ^{125}I-insulin was then added to a final concentration of 330 pM. Cell-associated label was determined at prescribed intervals. Nonspecific binding was the amount of ^{125}I-insulin bound in parallel incubations, to which unlabeled insulin, at a final concentration of 8.0 μM, was added simultaneously with the ^{125}I-insulin. The degradation of insulin was followed by measuring the TC precipitability of the label in the incubation medium. This technique with adipocytes parallels two more sensitive measures of insulin degradation—immunoprecipitability and rebinding to membranes.[15] A 50-μl aliquot was taken from the infranatant of each microfuge tube used to measure cell-associated ^{125}I-insulin, and precipitability of the aliquot with 10% TC was determined. When the effects of potassium azide or potassium cyanide on ^{125}I-insulin binding and degradation were being measured, these agents were added at the beginning of the preincubation.

^{125}I-insulin binding to adipocyte plasma membranes. Suspensions of plasma membranes, at a final concentration of 600–900 μg protein/ml, were incubated at 37° in KRP with 1% BSA, pH 7.4, in the presence or absence of chloroquine. After 30 min, ^{125}I-insulin was added for a final concentration of 330 pM and the incubation was continued for 40 min. Each incubation was terminated by layering 100 μl of the incubation suspension over 250 μl of ice cold 0.25 M sucrose in KRP in a 400-μl microfuge tube and centrifuging 1 min at 10,000 *g*. The tips of the microfuge tubes containing the membrane pellets were cut off and counted to determine membrane-associated radioactivity. Specific binding of ^{125}I-insulin to plasma membranes was determined by subtracting from total binding the amount of nonspecifically bound label in parallel triplicate incubations to which 8.0 μM unlabeled insulin was added simultaneously with the ^{125}I-insulin. As with cells, degradation of ^{125}I-insulin was followed by measuring TC precipitability of a 50-μl aliquot of supernatant.

Extraction and analysis of cell-bound ^{125}I-insulin. Adipocytes were incubated with labeled insulin and chloroquine and were separated from incubation medium by centrifugation through silicone oil, as described for binding studies. The cells were then immediately extracted with 4M urea, 1M acetic acid, and 0.1% Triton X-100, and the recovery of cell-associated counts was more than 90%. Aliquots of the extracts were analyzed by precipitation in 10% TC or gel chromatography using Sephadex G-50. The column (0.9 × 55 cm) was equilibrated and eluted at room temperature with 1M acetic acid containing 0.9% NaCl.

Dissociation of bound ^{125}I-insulin and analysis of bound and released labeled material. Adipocytes were incubated at 37° for 10 min in the presence or absence of chloro-

* The abbreviations used are TC, trichloroacetic acid; BSA, bovine serum albumin (fraction V); Hepes, 4-(2-hydroxyethyl)-1-piperazine ethane sulfonic acid; KRH, Krebs Ringer Hepes buffer; KRH-AG, Krebs Ringer Hepes buffer with 3% BSA and 11 mM glucose, pH 7.4; KRP, Krebs Ringer phosphate buffer; KRP-AG, KRP with 3% BSA and 11 mM glucose; 3-O-MG, 3-O-methylglucose; 3-O-[^{3}H]MG, 3-O-[methyl-^{3}H]glucose; EGF, epidermal growth factor.

quine; 670 pM ^{125}I-insulin was added and the incubation was continued for 45 min. Cells were centrifuged and the infranatant was aspirated. The cells were then washed twice in incubation buffer and resuspended in fresh incubation buffer at 37° containing 8.0 μM unlabeled insulin. Each set of cells was washed and resuspended in buffer that contained the same concentration of chloroquine as was in the initial incubation. At intervals during dissociation, aliquots of the incubation were analyzed by microfuge separation through silicone oil. The cell layer above the oil was immediately extracted with urea, acetic acid, and Triton X-100, was counted, and aliquots were analyzed by TC precipitation and gel column chromatography, as described above, to determine the amount and nature of labeled material remaining with the cells at each time point. A 50-μl aliquot of the infranatant from each microfuge tube was quickly added to 200 μl of the extraction mixture and was subsequently analyzed by TC precipitation to determine the nature of labeled material released from the cells during dissociation.

Determination of ^{125}I-BSA and [^{14}C]sucrose bound to and taken up by adipocytes. Incubation of ^{125}I-BSA with cells in the presence or absence of chloroquine and the determination of cell-associated label were carried out exactly as described above for ^{125}I-insulin by use of microfuge centrifugation through oil to separate cells from incubation medium. Incubation of [^{14}C]sucrose with cells was carried out in the same manner, except that the amount of trapped labeled sucrose was also measured. Cells were incubated at 37° with or without chloroquine for 10 min, labeled sucrose was then added to the incubations, and cell-associated labeled sucrose was determined at selected times during the incubation. Cell-associated [^{14}C]sucrose measured immediately after addition of the labeled sugar was taken to represent label trapped in extracellular water. This value for the trapped labeled sucrose was subtracted from cell-associated label at each later time point to determine the amount of label accumulated by cells during the incubation.

Morphologic studies on adipocytes using ferritin-insulin. Isolated adipocytes were incubated with monomeric ferritin-insulin at 37° for 45 min in the presence and absence of 50 μM chloroquine. The monomeric ferritin-insulin was the same preparation used in previous studies.[38] After incubation the cells were washed and processed for electron microscopy, as previously described.[39] This experiment was repeated twice, and electron mcrographs of more than 100 lysosomal structures in randomly selected cells were obtained for each experimental condition. The micrographs were analyzed for the presence of ferritin in each lysosomal structure without knowledge of the experimental conditions. Lysosomal structures included multivesicular bodies as well as dense bodies, as defined by others.[10]

Assays of glucose oxidation, 3-O-methylglucose transport, and epinephrine-stimulated lipolysis in adipocytes. The effect of chloroquine on basal and insulin-stimulated glucose oxidation was determined by adding 5×10^4 cells to vials that contained various concentrations of chloroquine (from 0 to 100 μM) in a final volume of 2 ml. After 15 min at 37°, 130 or 330 pM insulin was added to appropriate vials; the incubation was continued for 15 min, when D-[1-^{14}C]glucose (5.0 μM) was added to all vials, which were immediately capped. After incubation for another 60 min at 37°, the $^{14}CO_2$ released was determined as described by Gliemann.[40]

The effect of chloroquine on basal and insulin-stimulated transport of 3-O-MG into adipocytes was measured using a rapid filtration assay described previously,[41] substituting KRH buffer for KRP and KRB. Cells were preincubated for 10 min at 37° in plastic tubes in the presence of chloroquine at concentrations of 0–100 μM; then insulin (at 1.7 nM) was added to appropriate tubes and the incubation was continued for 40 min: 3-O-[methyl-^{3}H]glucose (0.5 mM) was then added for a 15-s incubation, which was terminated by the addition of ice-cold 2 mM $HgCl_2$. The cells were immediately collected by filtration, and the 3-O-[^{3}H]MG taken up by cells was determined as described.[41] The uptake of L-[1-^{14}C]glucose was simultaneously determined in each tube, and this value was used to correct for the nonspecific uptake of 3-O-[^{3}H]MG and for labeled sugar trapped in extracellular water.

The ability of insulin to inhibit epinephrine-stimulated lipolysis was measured in the presence and absence of chloroquine by a modification of a previously published procedure.[42] Adipocytes were incubated with chloroquine, at 0–100 μM, for 10 min at 37° with or without 0.7 μM epinephrine. Insulin, at 670 pM, was then added to appropriate tubes and the incubation was continued for 45 min. The reactions were terminated by the addition of 3M $HClO_4$ and the mixture was centrifuged. Aliquots of each infranatant were neutralized with $KHCO_3$ and glycerol was determined on each aliquot by the method of Lowry et al.[43]

RESULTS

Effect of chloroquine and NH_4Cl on ^{125}I-insulin binding to adipocytes and adipocyte-isolated membranes. Figure 1 is a demonstration of the effect of chloroquine on specific binding of ^{125}I-insulin by adipocytes. In the control preparations, specific binding reached a steady state level by 20 min of incubation, which was maintained for at least 2 h. Chloroquine caused a concentration-related increase in specifically bound insulin. In the presence of 5 μM chloro-

FIGURE 1. The effect of chloroquine on specific binding of ^{125}I-insulin to adipocytes. Adipocytes were incubated at 37° with 330 pM ^{125}I-insulin in the absence (●) or presence of 5 μM (▲), 20 μM (○), or 100 μM (△) chloroquine, and specific binding was determined at the indicated time points as described in METHODS. This was a representative experiment from a set of four. Each point represents the mean of four samples, with each SEM less than 7% of the corresponding mean.

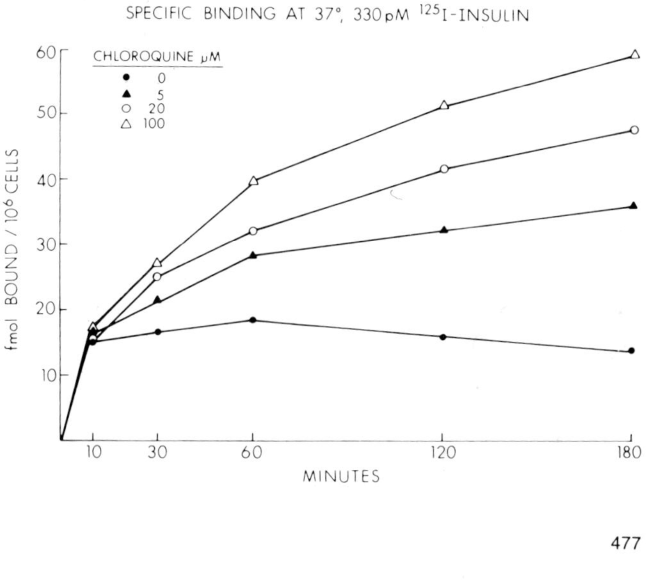

quine, the lowest concentration tested, specific binding was 130% of control at 30 min of incubation and was twice the control's by 120 min. Increasing the concentration of chloroquine to 100 μM increased specific binding of insulin to 164% of control at 30 min of incubation and to more than triple the control value at 120 min. Chloroquine, at 20 μM, caused intermediate effects. For each chloroquine concentration tested, the amount of specifically bound ^{125}I-insulin increased steadily with time of incubation and did not reach a plateau or steady state level, suggesting that chloroquine caused a time-dependent process of accumulation of specifically bound insulin in the adipocyte. Nonspecific binding of ^{125}I-insulin was constant from 10 through 180 min of incubation and was not affected by chloroquine (data not shown).

NH_4Cl, like chloroquine, inhibits lysosomal degradation of macromolecules, including EGF in fibroblasts[27] and human chorionic gonadotropin in Leydig cells.[44,45] Specific binding of 330 pM ^{125}I-insulin to adipocytes incubated for 45 min at 37° was increased to 123% and 131% of control in the presence of NH_4Cl at 20 and 50 mM, respectively. Nonspecific binding was not affected.

Chloroquine had no effect on degradative activity released into the incubation medium. Cells were incubated for 2 h in KRH-AG buffer at 37° in the absence of both chloroquine and insulin. The cells were then removed by centrifugation, leaving buffer containing degradative activity released from the cells. Aliquots of this buffer, containing released degradative activity, were incubated with various concentrations of chloroquine up to 2500 μM and 170–330 pM ^{125}I-insulin, and degradation of ^{125}I-insulin was followed by TC precipitability over 3 h. The amount of ^{125}I-insulin degraded to TC-soluble labeled material did not differ from control for any concentration of chloroquine tested at any time (data not shown).

The effect of chloroquine on plasma membrane binding and degradation of insulin was tested. Specific binding of ^{125}I-insulin to plasma membranes was determined after up to 40 min of incubation in the presence of chloroquine at concentrations of 0–250 μM. In each experiment, chloroquine caused small increases or decreases in specific binding relative to control, and the total pattern over four experiments was that chloroquine had no effect on specific binding of ^{125}I-insulin to plasma membranes. Chloroquine also did not affect either nonspecific binding or degradation of ^{125}I-insulin by adipocyte plasma membranes (data not shown).

Degradation of ^{125}I-insulin by suspensions of adipocytes can occur in the incubation medium, at the plasma membrane, or within the cell after internalization. The combined effects of these degradative processes were determined by measuring the amount of TC-soluble labeled material in the incubation medium in the experiments shown in Figure 1. A progressive decrease in the TC-soluble material was found in the incubation medium from cells treated with increasing concentrations of chloroquine (Table 1). The decrease was significantly different statistically from control in the 20 μM and 100 μM chloroquine conditions. Similar small, but statistically significant, decreases in the amount of TC-soluble labeled material present in the incubation medium after incubations of several hours were seen in other similar experiments. Since chloroquine did not alter the degradative activity present in the medium or the degradation by plasma membranes, the decrease in degradation products in the medium must reflect a decrease in the amount of ^{125}I-insulin degraded through chloroquine-sensitive intracellular mechanisms. The amount of the decrease suggests that the chloroquine-insensitive degradative pathways accounted for the majority of the degradation in these incubations.

TABLE 1
The effect of chloroquine on degradation of ^{125}I-insulin by adipocytes after 180 min of incubation at 37°

Chloroquine (μM)	TC soluble (%)	Significance (P)
0	21.1 ± 0.3	—
5	20.1 ± 0.3	<0.1
20	18.8 ± 0.3	<0.005
100	18.5 ± 0.1	<0.001

Data are from the same experiment shown in Figure 1. After 180 min of incubation, cells were removed as described in METHODS. Aliquots of incubation medium were precipitated with 10% TC, and the soluble counts in the supernatant were quantitated and expressed as the percent of total counts present at the start of the incubation to derive a measure of ^{125}I-insulin degraded during the 3-h period. Statistical significance relative to control was determined by the unpaired *t* test. Results are shown as $\bar{x}$ ± SEM of quadruplicate samples. These results are representative of three such experiments.

Effect of chloroquine on nonspecific uptake of [^{14}C]sucrose, ^{125}I-BSA, and ^{125}I-insulin. The influence of chloroquine on nonspecific endocytosis, including fluid phase endocytosis, was investigated by measuring the uptake of [^{14}C]sucrose and ^{125}I-albumin by adipocytes and by determining nonspecific binding of ^{125}I-insulin. Sucrose is taken into cells from the extracellular medium by nonspecific fluid phase endocytosis, enters the lysosome, and accumulates there without being degraded until residual lysosomal contents are expelled from the cell.[46] In Table 2, we show that the amount of [^{14}C]sucrose accumulated by chloroquine-treated cells was not significantly different statistically from controls at any concentration tested, but the data suggest there is a small concentration-dependent stimulation by chloroquine. The magnitude of this increase was small com-

TABLE 2
Effect of chloroquine on accumulation of [^{14}C] sucrose for 60 min by adipocytes at 37°

Chloroquine (μM)	[^{14}C] sucrose accumulated (% of mean control value)
0	100 ± 9 (12)
20	104 ± 9 (14)
50	116 ± 11 (9)
100	129 ± 11 (14)

Adipocytes were incubated at 37° with [^{14}C] sucrose in the presence of the indicated concentrations of chloroquine, and the amount of [^{14}C] sucrose accumulated over 60 min was determined as described in METHODS. The experiment was performed three times. Within each experiment, each experimental value was expressed as the percent of the mean of control values for that experiment, allowing data from all three experiments to be compared statistically. The values in this table represent the mean and SEM for each set of data, with the number of observations in parentheses. None of the experimental values was statistically significant compared with control (P > 0.05) by the unpaired *t* test.

pared with the increase in specific binding of ^{125}I-insulin at 60 min in the presence of these concentrations of chloroquine (Figure 1), and it cannot explain the effect of chloroquine on specific binding of ^{125}I-insulin to adipocytes. Similar experiments showed that concentrations of chloroquine of up to 1000 μM had no significant effect on the amount of ^{125}I-albumin associated with the cells at incubations of up to 120 min (data not shown). The lack of any effect of chloroquine on nonspecific binding of ^{125}I-insulin in repeated experiments was the most direct evidence against the stimulation of nonspecific uptake of insulin by chloroquine.

Effect of lowered temperature and inhibitors of energy generation on the action of chloroquine. If chloroquine inhibits processing of internalized ^{125}I-insulin at the level of the lysosome, then preventing the internalization of ^{125}I-insulin should prevent the accumulation of cell-bound ^{125}I-insulin seen in the presence of chloroquine. This was tested through two approaches, designed to block internalization by inhibiting energy-requiring endocytosis of receptor-bound ^{125}I-insulin. The effect of lowering the incubation temperature is shown in Table 3. At 37°, 20 μM chloroquine caused a 242% increase in specific binding at 180 min of incubation. At 24°, this same chloroquine concentration stimulated specific binding by only 53% at 210 min, and it had no effect at 14°. It should be noted that specific binding to control cells increased as the temperature decreased. The requirement of an energy-dependent uptake system for internalization of specifically bound ^{125}I-insulin before the site of the chloroquine effect was further tested by the use of potassium cyanide and sodium azide, metabolic inhibitors that deplete adenosine triphosphate (ATP) in the adipocyte.[17,47] Neither of these agents had a significant effect on specific or nonspecific insulin binding in the absence of chloroquine (data not shown). However, both agents caused a concentration-related inhibition of the increase in specific binding of labeled insulin caused by 50 μM chloroquine. In the absence of inhibitors, 50 μM chloroquine caused a 107% increase over control in specific binding of 330 pM ^{125}I-insulin after 45 min of incubation. In the presence of 5 mM potassium azide or 5 mM potassium cyanide, 50 μM chloroquine stimulated specific binding by only 23% and

TABLE 3
Effect of 20 μM chloroquine on specific binding of ^{125}I-insulin to adipocytes at 37°, 24°, and 14°

Temperature	Specific Binding: Control (fmol bound/10^6 cells)	Specific Binding: 20 μM chloroquine (fmol bound/10^6 cells)	Increase with chloroquine (%)
14°	34.6 ± 1.7	33.5 ± 2.5	0
24°	24.7 ± 1.8	37.7 ± 0.7	53
37°	14.0 ± 0.5	48.0 ± 2.0	242

Cells were incubated with or without 20 μM chloroquine for 10 min at 37°, then quickly cooled to final incubation temperature. ^{125}I-insulin, at 330 pM, was added and the incubation was continued for 180 min (14° and 37°) or 210 min (24°); specific binding was determined as in METHODS. Nonspecific binding was not affected by chloroquine at any temperature and did not vary significantly with temperature. These data are representative of two or more experiments at each temperature. Each value represents x̄ ± SEM of quadruplicate samples.

TABLE 4
Effect of chloroquine on TC precipitability of bound label extracted from adipocytes incubated with ^{125}I-insulin for 45 min at 37°

Chloroquine (μM)	Total bound (cpm/100 μl extract)	TC precipitable (%) (cpm/100 μl extract)	TC soluble (%) (cpm/100 μl extract)
0	295	236 ± 4 (80)	59 ± 3 (20)
5	356	299 ± 5 (84)	57 ± 2 (16)
20	417	366 ± 19 (88)	51 ± 1 (12)
100	528	483 ± 10 (91)	45 ± 2 (9)

Adipocytes were incubated with 330 pM ^{125}I-insulin for 45 min at 37°C in the absence or presence of chloroquine. Cells were separated from incubation medium, extracted, and analyzed as described in METHODS. This is a representative experiment from a set of three. Each value of TC-precipitable and TC-soluble counts is represented as x̄ ± SEM of quadruplicate samples and as percent of total bound at that chloroquine concentration.

40%, respectively. These results are consistent with a site of chloroquine action distal to an energy-requiring internalization step, such as receptor-mediated endocytosis.

Nature of cell-associated insulin. The effect of chloroquine on the nature of cell-associated ^{125}I-insulin was determined by TC precipitation and by gel chromatography of extracted cell-bound label. In Table 4, we demonstrate the effect of chloroquine, at 20–100 μM, on the TC precipitability of labeled material extracted from cells incubated for 45 min with 330 pM ^{125}I-insulin. As seen previously (Figure 1), increasing chloroquine concentrations caused a progressive increase in total cell-bound iodinated insulin. The TC-precipitable material accounted for this increase in total binding, so that at the highest chloroquine concentrations the TC-precipitable label was a greater percent of the total bound, suggesting a build-up of intact insulin and an inhibition of degradation. Degraded ^{125}I-insulin is rapidly expelled from the cell,[2,10,13,14,16] so that, even in the absence of chloroquine, only a minor component of cell-bound counts represents degraded material. Nevertheless, chloroquine caused a significant decrease in TC-soluble counts extracted from the cells.

The effect of chloroquine on cell-associated insulin was examined further by gel filtration analysis of the cell-extracted material. Figures 2A, B, and C illustrate the effect of 20, 50, and 100 μM chloroquine, respectively, on the composition of bound labeled material at 45 min of incubation. Consistent with the changes seen in TC precipitability of bound labeled material, increasing chloroquine concentrations caused a progressive increase in extracted material eluting with intact insulin and a corresponding decrease in low molecular weight degradation products. The number of counts eluting in the ^{125}I-insulin peak was 163%, 179%, and 184% of control for cells incubated with 20, 50, and 100 μM chloroquine, respectively. The sum of counts eluting in the peaks succeeding the ^{125}I-insulin peak, which represent degradation products, fell to 77%, 77%, and 57% of control as chloroquine was increased to 20, 50, and 100 μM, respectively. The number of counts eluting before the insulin peak did not show consistent changes with chloroquine.

Morphologic studies on the effects of chloroquine on the lysosomal content of ferritin-insulin. In recent elec-

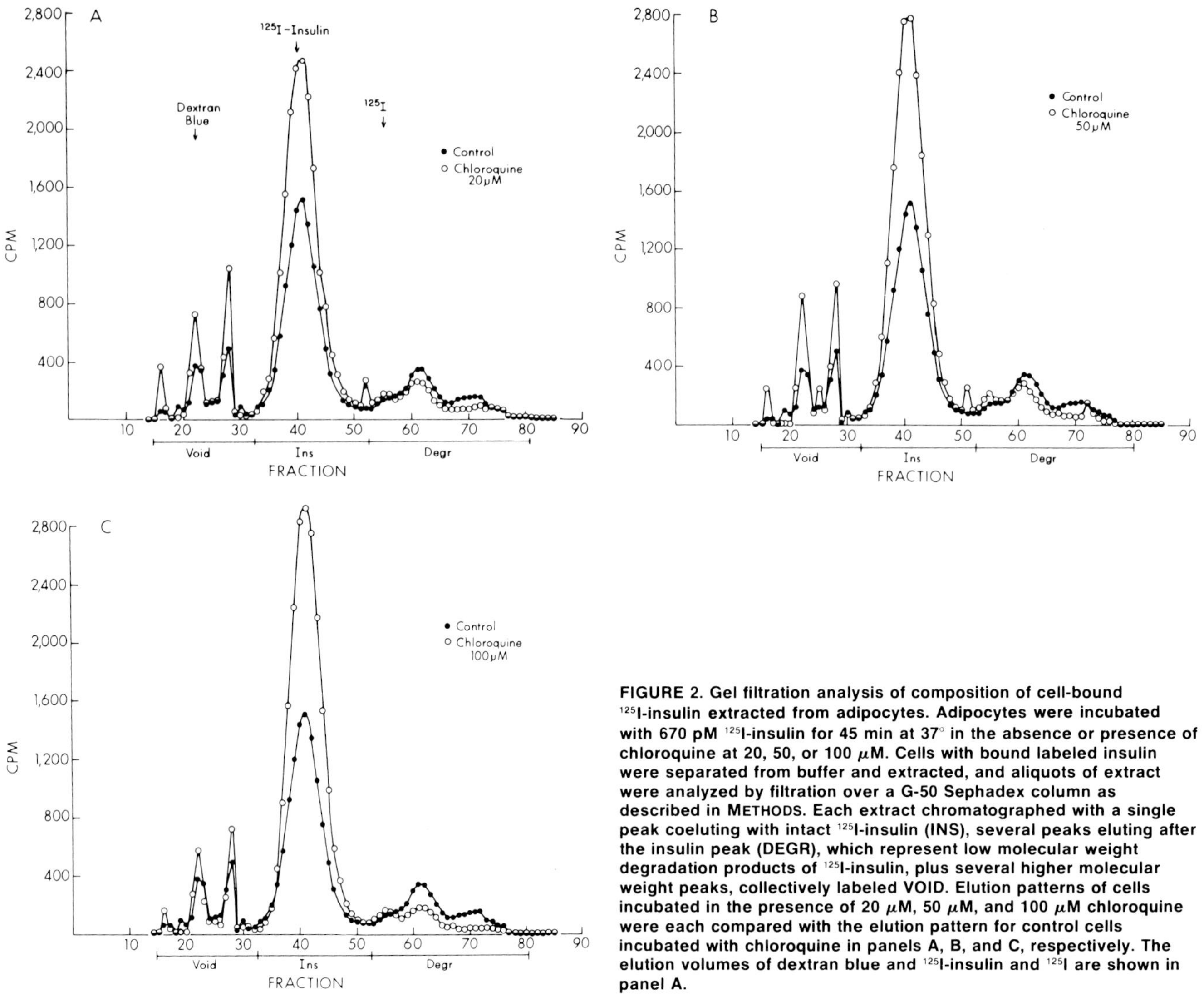

FIGURE 2. Gel filtration analysis of composition of cell-bound ^{125}I-insulin extracted from adipocytes. Adipocytes were incubated with 670 pM ^{125}I-insulin for 45 min at 37° in the absence or presence of chloroquine at 20, 50, or 100 μM. Cells with bound labeled insulin were separated from buffer and extracted, and aliquots of extract were analyzed by filtration over a G-50 Sephadex column as described in METHODS. Each extract chromatographed with a single peak coeluting with intact ^{125}I-insulin (INS), several peaks eluting after the insulin peak (DEGR), which represent low molecular weight degradation products of ^{125}I-insulin, plus several higher molecular weight peaks, collectively labeled VOID. Elution patterns of cells incubated in the presence of 20 μM, 50 μM, and 100 μM chloroquine were each compared with the elution pattern for control cells incubated with chloroquine in panels A, B, and C, respectively. The elution volumes of dextran blue and ^{125}I-insulin and ^{125}I are shown in panel A.

tron-autoradiographic studies using ^{125}I-insulin, internalized insulin associated specifically with the lysosome of the hepatocyte.[10] In morphologic studies of the adipocyte using ferritin-insulin, the hormone specifically localized to the glycocalyx coating of the plasma membrane and in the numerous surface invaginations and related microvesicles.[39] Lysosomal structures were rarely seen nor were looked for in those studies. In our experiments here, we photographed lysosomes in adipocytes incubated with monomeric ferritin-insulin in the presence or absence of 50 μM chloroquine for 45 min. Figure 3 is an electron micrograph of a chloroquine-treated cell showing a lysosomal structure (heterophagosome or multivesicular body). Structures resembling endocytotic vesicles are seen inside this organelle as well as numerous ferritin-insulin particles associated with the vesicles or with glycocalyx-like amorphous material. By quantitative analysis, we showed that, while only 35% of the lysosomal structures from control cells contained ferritin, 68% of them from chloroquine-treated cells contained the particles ($P < 0.01$ by *t* test). Other electron micrographs showed microvesicles containing ferritin-insulin fusing with the lysosomal structures, indicating the route of entry of ferritin-insulin into the cell. These microvesicles were not coated nor were the invaginations that gave origin to the vesicles. This morphologic study supports the biochemical data, suggesting that chloroquine inhibits the degradation by lysosomes of internalized insulin and the hormone accumulates in the organelle.

Effect of chloroquine on dissociation of bound ^{125}I-insulin from adipocytes. Dissociation experiments were performed to further characterize the effect of chloroquine on the degradation of internalized ^{125}I-insulin. These experiments allowed us to determine the rate of degradation of cell-bound ^{125}I-insulin when extracellular degradation was absent and to analyze the nature of the labeled material both released from the cell and remaining with the cell during dissociation. Figure 4A shows the amount and the TC precipitability of the ^{125}I-insulin remaining in the cells during the course of dissociaton, after an original 45-min incubation in the presence and absence of 50 μM chloroquine. The time required for dissociation of half the labeled insulin bound at the beginning of dissociation was definitely increased by chloroquine (8 min vs. 28 min). The dissociation was virtually complete for control cells by 120 min, and less than 10% remained with the cells at 60 min. In contrast, 37% and 26% of initial counts remained bound to chloroquine-

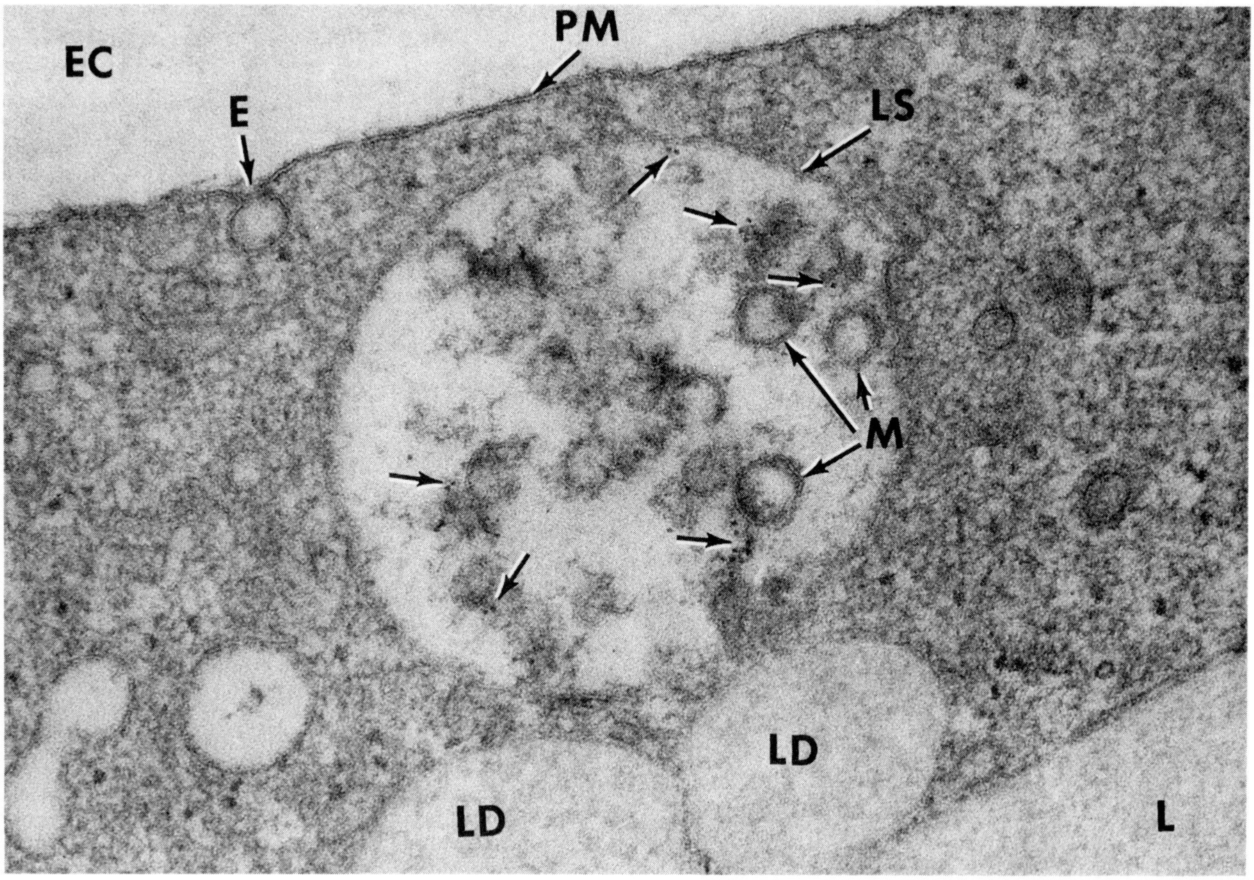

FIGURE 3. Electron micrograph demonstrating ferritin in an adipocyte lysosomal structure. Adipocytes were incubated for 45 min at 37° with 500 μU/ml monomeric ferritin-insulin in the presence of 50 μM chloroquine. In this micrograph, we demonstrate a lysosomal structure (LS)—a multivesicular body or heterophagosome—in an adipocyte. Electron-dense ferritin particles (unlabeled arrows) are present within the lysosomal structure, which also contains several microvesicles (M) and amorphous material resembling glycocalyx. An endocytotic invagination (E) is seen at the plasma membrane (PM) surface. Also labeled are the lipid depot (L) of the adipocyte with several cytoplasmic lipid droplets (LD) and the extracellular space (EC).

treated cells at 60 and 120 min, respectively. Even at 180 min, 21% of initial counts remained bound to the chloroquine-treated cells.

Other workers showed[2,10,13,14] that both intact and degraded labeled material dissociated from or was released by cells that had been allowed to bind ^{125}I-insulin, were washed and resuspended in fresh medium. We performed such experiments in the presence and absence of chloroquine. In Figures 4B and C, we illustrate the amounts of TC-precipitable and TC-soluble labeled material released into the dissociation medium by control (B) and chloroquine-treated cells (C). Since degradation products do not accumulate in cells[2,10,13,14,16] (Table 4 and Figure 4A), the rate of release of degradation products from cells into the medium during dissociation should reflect the rate of degradation of ^{125}I-insulin by the cells. The release of degraded material by control (B) and chloroquine-treated (C) adipocytes is also shown in Figure 4. The most striking effect of chloroquine was the distinct reduction in the amount of TC-soluble material released by chloroquine-treated cells compared with that by control at the early time points. The amount of TC-soluble material dissociating from the chloroquine-treated cells was less than half that of the control at 30 s or 10 min. The rate of appearance of TC-soluble material over the first 10 min can be taken as an estimate of the initial rate of total cellular degradation of ^{125}I-insulin by the cell. Using this assumption, the rate of degradation in control cells was 0.28 fmol/min/10^6 cells compared with 0.10 fmol/min/10^6 cells in chloroquine-treated cells. By this kinetic analysis, the rate of degradation in chloroquine-treated cells was only 36% of that in control cells. The amount of ^{125}I-insulin specifically bound to chloroquine-treated cells at the beginning of the dissociation was approximately twice as much as the amount bound initially to control cells. If specifically bound insulin is the substrate for uptake and degradation, then the rate of degradation should be corrected for differences in initial binding by normalizing all data (using the initial counts bound as 100%) for each set of cells. Using this corrected or normalized data, the rate of degradation for chloroquine-treated cells over the first 10 min was only 20% of control.

The number of TC-precipitable counts which dissociated from chloroquine-treated cells and controls was roughly equal at early time points. However, the release of TC-precipitable labeled material from control cells was almost completed at 10 min, while TC-precipitable material continued to dissociate from chloroquine-treated cells until at least 60 min. The amount of TC-precipitable labeled material which dissociated from chloroquine-treated and control cells was compared using normalized data, in which the number of initial counts bound was set at 100% for each set of cells. This showed that 49% of counts initially bound to

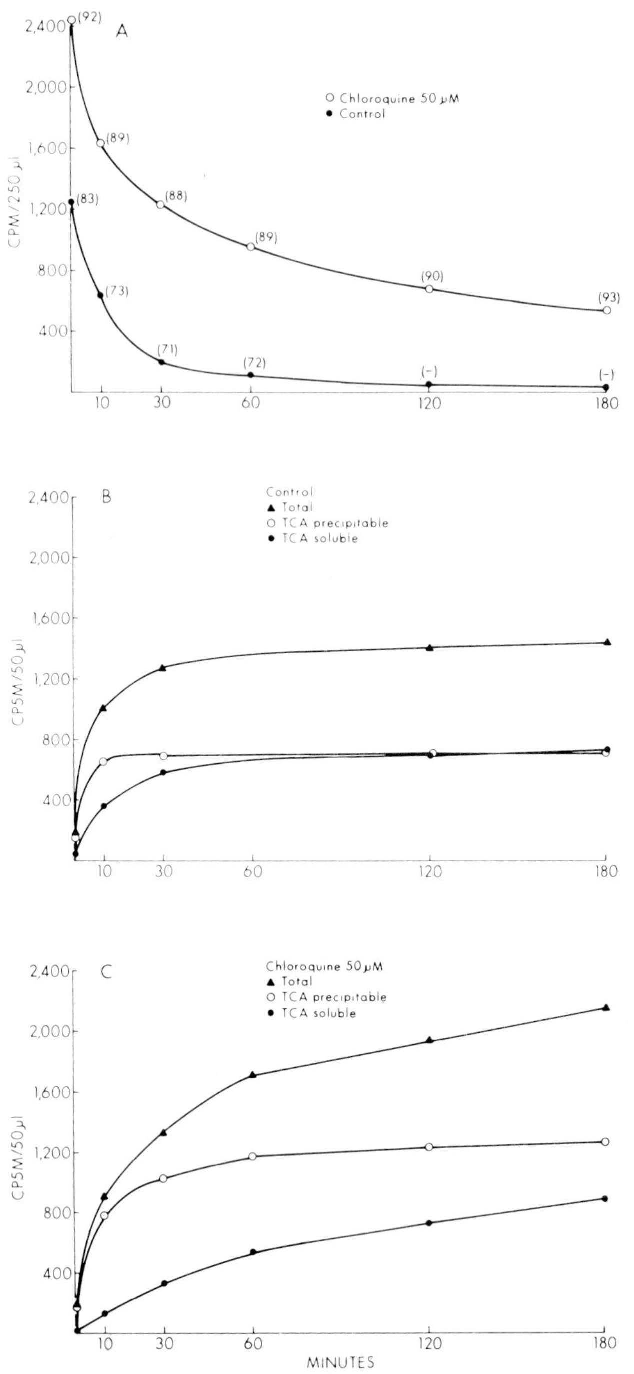

FIGURE 4. Effect of chloroquine on dissociation of ^{125}I-insulin bound to adipocytes. Adipocytes were incubated with 670 pM ^{125}I-insulin for 45 min at 37° with or without 50 μM chloroquine, separated from incubation buffer, washed twice, and resuspended in fresh buffer. The amount and TC precipitability of labeled material remaining with the cells and released or dissociated into the medium were assessed during dissociation, as described in METHODS. In A, we show the amount of label remaining with both chloroquine-treated (●) and control cells (○) during dissociation. The TC precipitability (%) of counts extracted from the cells is shown above each point, except the 120-min and 180-min points for control cells, in which there were too few counts to accurately determine TC precipitability. The amount and composition of labeled material released into the incubation medium during dissociation is shown for control cells (in B) and chloroquine-treated cells (in C). The amount of dissociated label precipitable (○) and soluble (●) and the total amount dissociated (▲) are plotted. Points represent the mean of at least three determinations.

control cells had dissociated as TC-precipitable material through 180 min. Illustrating the fact that dissociation of TC-precipitable material from control cells was nearly completed by 10 min, 44% and 47% of initial counts had dissociated as TC-precipitable material at 10 and 30 min, respectively. The dissociation of TC-precipitable counts from chloroquine-treated cells was essentially complete at 60 min, with 45% and 48% of initial counts being released at 60 and 180 min. The release of TC-precipitable counts was somewhat slowed by 50 μM chloroquine, with 30% and 39% of initial counts being dissociated at 10 and 30 min. The reduction in the rate of release of bound ^{125}I-insulin on TC-precipitable material was much smaller than the striking reduction in the rate of release of degraded ^{125}I-labeled material from chloroquine-treated cells.

The labeled material remaining with the cells during the dissociation process was predominantly TC precipitable for both chloroquine-treated and control cells (Figure 4). These cell extracts were further analyzed by gel filtration (data not shown). The amount of material eluting after the insulin peak, thus representing degraded material, was only a small portion of the total cell-associated counts at all times, confirming that degraded material exits rapidly from the cell. The size of the ^{125}I-insulin peak was much larger for chloroquine-treated cells than for control at the time dissociation began. The extremely small amount of material in the degradation product region for the chloroquine-treated cells explains why about 90% of the total cell-associated material during dissociation was TC precipitable. The amount of material in the degradation region for the control was equal to that for the chloroquine-treated cells, but the lower amount of intact insulin in control cells correlates with the lower TC precipitability of the total material extracted from control cells compared with chloroquine-treated cells. The rapid dissociation of bound ^{125}I-insulin from control cells was also analyzed by gel chromatography. At 30 min of dissociation, only a small amount of label remained with the cells, and this was accounted for almost entirely by counts eluting in the higher molecular weight peaks, suggesting the processing of ^{125}I-insulin to high molecular weight species as well as to low molecular weight degradation products. Essentially no counts remained with control cells after 60 (or 120) min of dissociation.

As expected, dissociation was much less rapid from chloroquine-treated cells, with a substantial amount of counts remaining in each set of peaks at 30 min. The number of counts in the insulin peak decreased to 41% of the initial amount, but the amount of high molecular weight material did not change. Even after 180 min of dissociation, a fourth of the counts initially bound remained with chloroquine-treated cells. Labeled material eluting before the ^{125}I-insulin peak accounted for 58% of the total compared with 21% at 0 min. Counts eluting in the ^{125}I-insulin peak accounted for only 21% of the total at 180 min compared with 67% at 0 min, reflecting the relatively rapid rate of dissociation of intact ^{125}I-insulin. In other experiments, in which dissociation was carried beyond 3 h, residual bound counts were entirely accounted for by peaks preceding the insulin peak. For both chloroquine-treated and control cells, the last labeled material to dissociate was the high molecular weight species eluting before intact insulin.

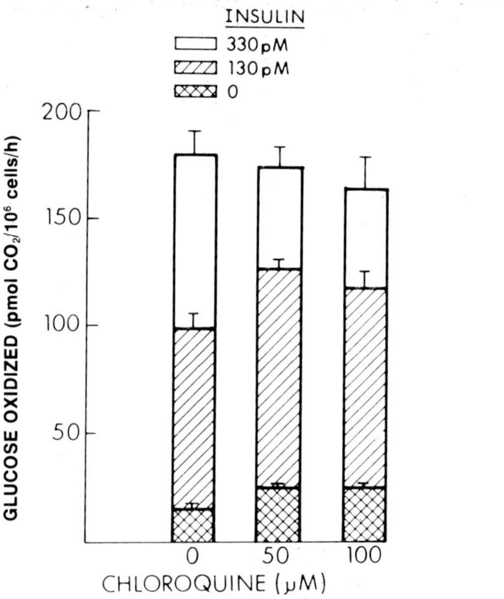

FIGURE 5. The effect of chloroquine on the insulin stimulation of glucose oxidation by adipocytes. The amount of $^{14}CO_2$ released over the 60 min of incubation was determined as described in METHODS. Each value represents the mean of quadruplicates, with vertical bars representing the SEM. These results are representative of three such experiments.

Effects of chloroquine on the stimulation of glucose oxidation by insulin. Insulin stimulates the oxidation of glucose to CO_2 by adipocytes by both increasing the transport of glucose into the cell and altering the activities of rate-limiting enzymes within the cell.[48] The effect of chloroquine on the stimulation of glucose oxidation by insulin was tested at two insulin concentrations, one a concentration causing maximal or near maximal stimulation of glucose oxidation (330 pM) and a submaximal concentration (130 pM). In Figure 5, we demonstrate that chloroquine, at either 50 or 100 μM, had no significant effect on insulin-stimulated glucose oxidation at either insulin concentration.

Effect of chloroquine on the stimulation of 3-O-MG transport by insulin. The effect of chloroquine on the ability of insulin to directly stimulate glucose transport, a membrane response, was more directly tested through the use of 3-O-MG, a nonmetabolizable glucose analogue that utilizes the same transport system as glucose.[49] In Figure 6, we demonstrate the effect of chloroquine, at 0–100 μM, on 3-O-[^{3}H]MG transport by adipocytes in the presence of 1.7 nM insulin. At the concentrations tested, chloroquine did not inhibit insulin-stimulated 3-O-MG transport. In addition, chloroquine did not effect the uptake of L-[1-^{14}C]glucose in these experiments, a fact which provides evidence that chloroquine did not cause an increase in simple diffusion.

Effect of chloroquine on the ability of insulin to inhibit epinephrine-stimulated lipolysis. In the experiments concerning glucose oxidation and 3-O-MG transport, we examined the effect of chloroquine primarily on an insulin-sensitive membrane response. The ability of insulin to block epinephrine-stimulated lipolysis was chosen as a way in which we could determine whether chloroquine had any effects on insulin-sensitive intracellular metabolic processes. Epinephrine stimulates lipolysis of stored triglyceride in the rat adipocyte through stimulation of the activity of hormone-sensitive lipase,[50] and insulin inhibits this lipolytic effect of epinephrine.[51] In Figure 7, we illustrate the effect of chloroquine on these processes. The stimulation of lipolysis by 0.7 μM epinephrine was not affected by chloroquine. Insulin, at 660 pM, reduced the rate of epinephrine-stimulated lipolysis by about 50%. Insulin's inhibition of the epinephrine effect was not influenced by chloroquine at any concentration tested.

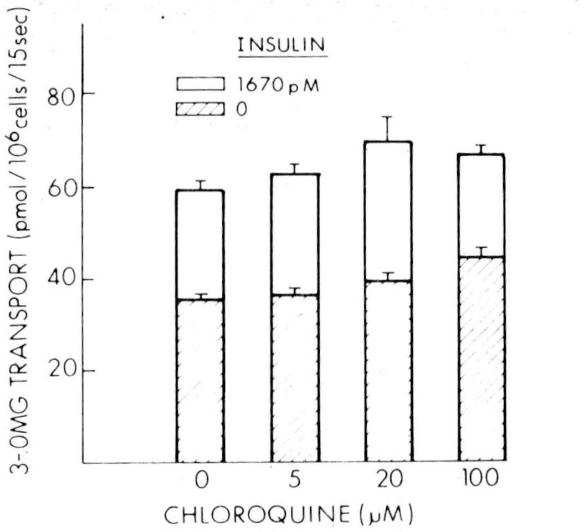

FIGURE 6. The effect of chloroquine on the insulin stimulation of 3-O-methylglucose transport in adipocytes at 37°. The uptake of 3-O-[methyl-^{3}H]glucose during a 15-s interval was determined as described in METHODS. Each value represents the mean of quadruplicates, with vertical bars indicating the SEM. These results are representative of three such experiments.

DISCUSSION

In the present report, we employed both biochemical and morphologic techniques to investigate the process of uptake, degradation, and release of receptor-bound insulin by adipocytes, and, through the use of chloroquine, we established the role of the lysosome in the degradation of internalized insulin. The data reported are consistent with the following model. A portion of ^{125}I-insulin specifically bound

FIGURE 7. The effect of chloroquine on the inhibition of epinephrine-stimulated lipolysis by insulin. The amount of glycerol released in each tube was determined as described in METHODS. Each result is the mean of quadruplicate determinations, with vertical bars representing the SEM.

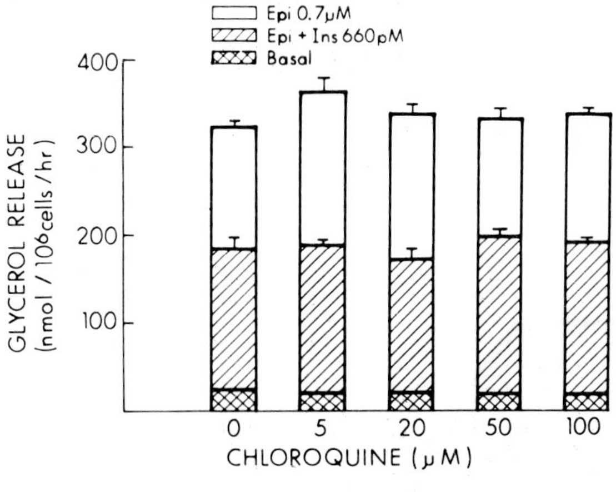

to its surface receptor was internalized by the cell through an energy-dependent process involving noncoated invaginations and endocytotic microvesicles, i.e., receptor-mediated endocytosis.[8,10] Some or all of this internalized insulin became localized to lysosomal structures through fusion of the endocytotic microvesicles with the lysosomes. Degradation then occurred in the lysosome with rapid expulsion of the small molecular weight degradative products from the cell. These studies further showed that lysosomal degradation of internalized receptor-bound insulin was not necessary for insulin to cause its short-term biologic effects.

Chloroquine, an agent known to accumulate in lysosomes of fibroblasts and to inhibit degradation of macromolecules by the lysosome, caused an inhibition of degradation of specifically bound insulin by adipocytes and a resultant increase in specifically bound, labeled material, shown to be primarily intact insulin. The inhibition of insulin degradation was demonstrated directly and most convincingly by the dissociation studies. The decreased initial rate of appearance of TC-soluble degradation products in the incubation media of chloroquine-treated cells showed that chloroquine greatly decreased the rate of degradation of insulin by the adipocyte. The analysis of the ^{125}I-labeled material extracted from cells during the association phase provided additional evidence of decreased degradation. Analysis by both TC precipitation and gel filtration chromatography demonstrated that, in the presence of chloroquine, the increase in cell-associated insulin was accounted for by a large increase in the amount of intact insulin and the amount of degradation products present in the cell was less than that in controls. The small amounts of degradative products found in both control and chloroquine-treated cells reflected the rapid explusion of these low molecular weight products from the cell. The large increase in intact insulin found in chloroquine-treated cells is consistent with the concept that a rapid turnover of internalized material occurred in control cells, so that the inhibition of degradation by chloroquine caused intact insulin to build up in the cell. Finally, the finding that chloroquine resulted in a significantly lower amount of TC-soluble material in the incubation medium of chloroquine-treated cells compared with that in controls at the end of a 3-h incubation of adipocytes with labeled insulin provided further support for the conclusion that chloroquine inhibited insulin degradation. These experiments support the conclusion that the inhibition of degradation of specifically bound insulin by chloroquine was due to an inhibition of lysosomal processing of internalized insulin.

If chloroquine interfered with some step in the uptake of insulin by the adipocyte before degradation by the lysosome, then results similar to those reported here might be found. Experiments were performed to rule out this possibility. First, chloroquine did not alter the degradation of insulin by proteolytic activity present in the incubation medium. Second, stimulation of nonspecific endocytosis by chloroquine, if it occurs, did not explain the effect of chloroquine on specific binding of ^{125}I-insulin to cells. Third, experiments showed that inhibitors of generation of intracellular energy, which reduce the rate of receptor-mediated endocytosis, caused a decreased accumulation of specifically bound ^{125}I-insulin in the presence of chloroquine. This supports the hypothesis that the effect of chloroquine on processing of intracellular insulin occurred at a point distal to the endocytotic step, at the level of the lysosome. Fourth, chloroquine did not affect specific binding of ^{125}I-insulin to or degradation by plasma membranes. Finally, electron microscope studies showed that chloroquine did not interfere with the fusion of endocytotic microvesicles and lysosomes, since twice the number of lysosomes contained ferritin-insulin in the presence of chloroquine than in its absence. A second agent reported to inhibit lysosomal degradation in several cell types—NH_4Cl—also caused a concentration-dependent increase in specific binding of ^{125}I-insulin to adipocytes.

The electron microscope studies provided morphologic evidence concerning the route of uptake into the cell of specifically bound insulin and its localization to the lysosome. Ferritin-insulin was associated with the glycocalyx coating on the cell surface in noncoated surface invaginations and with microvesicles in the cytoplasmic matrix and in lysosomal structures. In addition, microvesicles containing ferritin-insulin were observed fusing with lysosomal structures, suggesting that insulin is internalized by the adipocyte through a system of noncoated endocytotic microvesicles with subsequent localization to the lysosomes. These observations demonstrate morphologically the receptor-mediated endocytotic process suggested by the biochemical data. These morphologic observations are similar to those reported for EGF uptake by human carcinoma cells A-431.[52] Despite intensive searching for coated pits on the adipocyte surface, they were rarely found and showed no preferential localization of ferritin-insulin. The lack of participation of coated pits and coated vesicles in the uptake of ferritin-insulin into the adipocyte is consistent with recent observations by Carpentier et al.,[10] who were unable to demonstrate any association of bound ^{125}I-insulin with coated pits of hepatocytes. Haigler et al.[52] found EGF was taken up by invaginations and microvesicles that were predominantly not coated, as well. Finally, the finding that chloroquine doubled the fraction of lysosomes containing ferritin-insulin was consistent with the biochemical data, suggesting that chloroquine's main site of action was at the lysosomal level. These morphologic data would support the theory that the intact insulin was accumulating in the lysosome in the presence of chloroquine.

The ability of chloroquine to increase the specific binding of ^{125}I-insulin at reduced incubation temperatures was investigated to demonstrate that lowered temperature would reduce the rate of endocytosis and, thus, prevent the chloroquine effect. The difference in bound ^{125}I-insulin between chloroquine-treated and control cells was reduced or eliminated at lower temperatures, but not in the same manner as by inhibitors of intracellular energy generation. These inhibitors did not affect the amount of binding to control cells but did reduce the binding to chloroquine-treated cells, whereas lowering the temperature increased the level of cell-associated label in control cells to that seen in chloroquine-treated cells. This suggests that, at lowered temperature, control cells may function like chloroquine-treated cells. Thus, lowered incubation temperature may have inhibited lysosomal degradation to a greater extent than it inhibited receptor-mediated endocytosis with a resulting increase in cell-associated ^{125}I-insulin. Preliminary morphologic experiments showed that more lysosomal structures contained ferritin-insulin at 15° than at 37° (L. Jarett and R. M. Smith, unpublished observations), consistent with this interpretation.

Gel chromatography of labeled material extracted from cells under all conditions tested revealed the presence of large molecular weight material eluting with or just after the void volume. The amount or composition of high molecular weight material extracted from cells incubated with ^{125}I-insulin did not vary in a consistent way with increasing concentrations of chloroquine (Figure 2). Chromatographic analysis of labeled material remaining with cells during the dissociation experiments showed that the void volume material dissociated more slowly from the cell than did either intact ^{125}I-insulin or degradation products, in both the presence and absence of chloroquine. Labeled material retained by chloroquine-treated cells after 4 h of dissociation was accounted for entirely by counts eluting before the ^{125}I-insulin peak. Other investigators[10,13,14,16] have noted high molecular weight material in extracts of cells incubated with ^{125}I-insulin, and Hammond and Jarett[15] found such material after incubating ^{125}I-insulin with a cytosolic fraction from rat adipocytes. The nature and function, if any, of this high molecular weight material is not known.

The work reported here, coupled with previous work by several investigators,[2,3,10,12–18,53] strongly supports the conclusion that, in two important target cells for insulin—hepatocytes and adipocytes—a portion of receptor-bound insulin enters the cell by receptor-mediated endocytosis through noncoated surface invaginations and vesicles, localizes to lysosomes, and is degraded and released from the cell. Internalization and lysosomal processing of bound insulin could serve one or more general physiologic functions.[6,8] Internalization and lysosomal processing could (1) enable the hormone or a piece of it to elicit a biologic response and, thereby, function, at least in part, as its own second messenger, (2) allow degradation of insulin and, thereby, possibly control the immediate duration of response to the ligand, or (3) control the number of receptors for the hormone, so as to maintain a homeostatic balance under chronic or large changes in circulating levels of the hormone.

Data from this study demonstrated that internalization and lysosomal processing of receptor-bound insulin is not a necessary step in the mechanism by which insulin elicits several short term biologic responses. Under conditions in which chloroquine progressively inhibited insulin degradation by the lysosome, the agent had no effect on insulin's alteration of glucose transport, glucose oxidation, or epinephrine-stimulated lipolysis. Other studies support this conclusion. Insulin, concanavalin A, and antireceptor antibody, added directly to a plasma membrane–mitochondria mixture, were reported to cause a specific plasma membrane–mediated stimulation of pyruvate dehydrogenase activity of isolated mitochondria, suggesting the generation of insulin's second messenger by this subcellular system without the need for internalization and lysosomal processing.[54–56] LeCam et al.[57] report that internalization of bound insulin by hepatocytes is not necessary for insulin to stimulate transport of α-amino isobutyric acid. Kono et al.[18] recently reported that insulin's stimulation of glucose transport in adipocytes is not blocked by chloroquine. Ascoli and Puett[44,45] studied the effect of several lysosomotropic agents on the stimulation of steroidogenesis in Leydig cells by human chorionic gonadotropin. They found that chloroquine did not prevent stimulation by the hormone. The possible importance of internalization and lysosomal degradation of bound insulin for longer term responses by the cell, such as increased DNA synthesis, remains unknown. Gliemann[13] suggested that degradation at the membrane of receptor-bound insulin may be a fundamental step in the mechanism of insulin's action in the cell. The role of plasma membrane degradation has not been extensively investigated. However, with the development of an adipocyte plasma membrane preparation which demonstrates a biologic response to the direct addition of insulin,[54–56] the role of degradation at the plasma membrane in the mechanism of action of insulin can be investigated.

ACKNOWLEDGMENTS

This study was supported in part by U. S. Public Health Service grants AM 11892 and AM 20097.

G. T. Hammons received partial support by a postdoctoral fellowship from the Juvenile Diabetes Foundation.

The authors are indebted to Mr. Robert M. Smith for the electron micrographs and to Mrs. Dorothy DuBuque for preparation of the manuscript.

REFERENCES

[1] Kahn, C. R.: Membrane receptors for hormones and neurotransmitters. J. Cell Biol. *70*:261–86, 1976.

[2] Terris, S., and Steiner, D. F.: Binding and degradation of ^{125}I-insulin by rat hepatocytes. J. Biol. Chem. *250*:8389–98, 1975.

[3] Terris, S., and Steiner, D. F.: Retention and degradation of ^{125}I-insulin by perfused livers from diabetic rats. J. Clin. Invest. *57*:885–96, 1976.

[4] Gorden, P., Carpentier, J.-L., Freychet, P., LeCam, A., and Orci, L.: Intracellular translocation of ^{125}I-labeled insulin: direct demonstration in isolated hepatocytes. Science *200*:782–85, 1978.

[5] Bergeron, J. J. M., Sikstrom, R., Hand, A. R., and Posner, B. I.: Binding and uptake of ^{125}I-insulin into rat liver hepatocytes and endothelium. J. Cell Biol. *80*:427–43, 1979.

[6] Jarett, L., and Smith, R. M.: Binding and uptake of protein hormones into cells. The mechanism of the uptake process and its role in hormone action. *In* Transport of Macromolecules in Cellular Systems. Silverstein, S. C., Ed. Berlin, Dahlem Konferenzen, 1978, pp. 117–32.

[7] Schlessinger, J., Schechter, Y., Willingham, M. C., and Pastan, I.: Direct visualization of binding, aggregation, and internalization of insulin and epidermal growth factor on living fibroblastic cells. Proc. Natl. Acad. Sci. USA *75*:2659–63, 1978.

[8] Goldstein, J. L., Anderson, R. G. W., and Brown, M. S.: Coated pits, coated vesicles and receptor-mediated endocytosis. Nature (London) *279*:679–85, 1979.

[9] Maxfield, F. R., Schlessinger, J., Schechter, Y., Pastan, I., and Willingham, M. C.: Colllection of insulin, EGF, and α-macroglobulin in the same patches on the surface of cultured fibroblasts and common internalization. Cell *14*:805–10, 1978.

[10] Carpentier, J.-L., Gorden, P., Freychet, P., LeCam, A., and Orci, L.: Lysosomal association of internalized ^{125}I-insulin in isolated rat hepatocytes. J. Clin. Invest. *63*:1249–61, 1979.

[11] Ward, W. F., and Mortimore, G. E.: Evidence for a role of lysosomes in insulin degradation in liver. Diabetes *27* (Suppl. 2): 450, 1978. (Abstr.)

[12] Terris, S., Hoffman, C., and Steiner, D. F.: Mode of uptake and degradation of ^{125}I-labeled insulin by isolated hepatocytes and H4 hepatoma cells. Can. J. Biochem. *57*:459–48, 1979.

[13] Gliemann, J., and Sonne, O.: Binding and receptor-mediated degradation of insulin in adipocytes. J. Biol. Chem. *253*:7857–63, 1978.

[14] Olefsky, J. M., Kobayashi, M., and Chang, H.: Interactions between insulin and its receptors after the initial binding event. Diabetes *28*:460–71, 1979.

[15] Hammond, J. M., and Jarett, L.: Insulin degradation by isolated fat cells and their subcellular fractions. Diabetes *24*:1011–19, 1975.

[16] Kahn, C. R., and Baird, K.: The fate of insulin bound to adipocytes: evidence for compartmentalization and processing. J. Biol. Chem. *253*:4900–06, 1978.

[17] Kono, T., Robinson, F. W., Sarver, J. A., Vega, F. U., and Pointer, R. H.: Actions of insulin in fat cells: effects of low temperature, uncouplers of oxidative phosphorylation, and respiratory inhibitors. J. Biol. Chem. *252*:2226–33, 1977.

[18] Suzuki, K., and Kono, T.: Internalization and degradation of fat cell-bound insulin. J. Biol. Chem. *254*:9786–94, 1979.

[19] Freychet, P., Kahn, R., Roth, J., and Neville, D. M., Jr.: Insulin interactions with liver plasma membranes: independence of binding of the hormone and its degradation. J. Biol. Chem. *247*:3953–61, 1971.

[20] Dial, L. K., Miyamoto, S., and Arquilla, E. R.: Modulation of ^{125}I-insulin degradation by receptors in liver plasma membranes. Biochem. Biophys. Res. Commun. *74*:545–52, 1977.

[21] Steiner, D. F.: Insulin today (Banting Memorial Lecture 1976). Diabetes *26*:322–40, 1977.

[22] Catt, K. J., Harwood, J. P., Aguilera, G., and Dufau, M. L.: Hormonal regulation of peptide receptors and target cell responses. Nature (London) *280*:109–16, 1979.

[23] Lie, S. O., and Schofield, B.: Inactivation of lysosomal function in normal cultured human fibroblasts by chloroquine. Biochem. Pharmacol. *22*:3109–14, 1973.

[24] DeDuve, C., DeBarsy, T., Poole, B., Trouet, A., Tulkens, P., and Van Hoof, F.: Lysosomotropic agents. Biochem. Pharmacol. *23*:2495–2531, 1974.

[25] Wibo, M., and Poole, B.: Protein degradation in cultured cells. II. The uptake of chloroquine by rat fibroblasts and the inhibition of cellular protein degradation and cathepsin B_1. J. Cell Biol. *63*:430–40, 1974.

[26] Goldstein, J. L., Burnschede, G. Y., and Brown, M. S.: Inhibition of the proteolytic degradation of low density lipoprotein in human fibroblasts by chloroquine, concanavalin A, and Triton WR 1339. J. Biol. Chem. *250*:7854–62, 1975.

[27] Carpenter, G., and Cohen, S.: ^{125}I-labeled human epidermal growth factor: binding, internalization, and degradation in human fibroblasts. J. Cell Biol. *71*:159–71, 1976.

[28] Freychet, P., Roth, J., and Neville, D. M., Jr.: Mono-iodoinsulin: demonstration of its biological activity and binding to fat cells and liver membranes. Biochem. Biophys. Res. Commun. *43*:400–08, 1971.

[29] Hamlin, J. L., and Arquilla, E. R.: Monoiodoinsulin. J. Biol. Chem. *249*:21–32, 1974.

[30] Product Information #1060. Radioiodination of proteins with enzymobeads. Richmond, CA, Bio-Rad Laboratories, 1978.

[31] Schneider, B., Straus, E., and Yalow, R. S.: Some considerations in the preparation of radioiodoinsulin for radioimmunoassay and receptor assay. Diabetes *25*:260–67, 1976.

[32] Ludvigsen, C., and Jarett, L.: A kinetic analysis of D-glucose transport by adipocyte plasma membranes. J. Biol. Chem. *254*:1444–46, 1979.

[33] Rodbell, M.: Metabolism of isolated fat cells. I. Effects of hormones on glucose metabolism and lipolysis. J. Biol. Chem. *239*:375–80, 1964.

[34] Jarett, L.: Subcellular fractionation of adipocytes. Methods Enzymol. *31*:60–71, 1974.

[35] McDonald, J. M., Bruns, D. E., and Jarett, L.: Ability of insulin to increase calcium binding by adipocyte plasma membranes. Proc. Natl. Acad. Sci. USA *73*:1542–46, 1976.

[36] Lowry, O. H., Rosebrough, N. J., Farr, A. L., and Randall, R. J.: Protein measurement with the Folin phenol reagent. J. Biol. Chem. *193*:265–75, 1951.

[37] Gammeltoft, S., and Gliemann, J.: Binding and degradation of ^{125}I-labelod insulin by isolated rat fat cells. Biochim. Biophys. Acta *320*:16–32, 1973.

[38] Jarett, L., and Smith, R. M.: The natural occurrence of insulin receptors in groups on adipocyte plasma membranes as demonstrated with monomeric ferritin-insulin. J. Supramol. Struct. *6*:45–59, 1977.

[39] Jarett, L, and Smith, R. M.: Ultrastructural localization of insulin receptors on adipocytes. Proc. Natl. Acad. Sci. USA *72*:3526–30, 1975.

[40] Gliemann, J.: Assay of insulin-like activity by the isolated fat cell method. I. Factors influencing the response to crystalline insulin. Diabetologia *3*:382–88, 1967.

[41] Ludvigsen, C., Jarett, L., and McDonald, J.: The characterization of catecholamine stimulation of glucose transport by rat adipocytes and isolated plasma membranes. Endocrinology (in press).

[42] Jarett, L., and Smith, R. M.: Effect of cytochalasin B and D on groups of insulin receptors and on insulin action in rat adipocytes. J. Clin. Invest. *63*:571–79, 1979.

[43] Lowry, O. H., Passonneau, J. V., Hasselberger, F. X., and Schulte, D. W.: Effect of ischemia on known substrates and cofactors of the glycolytic pathway in brain. J. Biol. Chem. *239*:18–30, 1964.

[44] Ascoli, M., and Puett, D.: Degradation of receptor-bound human choriogonadotropin by murine Leydig tumor cells. J. Biol. Chem. *253*:4892–99, 1978.

[45] Ascoli, M., and Puett, D.: Inhibition of the degradation of receptor-bound human choriogonadotropin by lysosomotropic agents, protease inhibitors, and metabolic inhibitors. J. Biol. Chem. *253*:7832–38, 1978.

[46] Pittman, R. C., and Steinberg, D.: A new approach for assessing cumulative lysosomal degradation of proteins or other macromolecules. Biochem. Biophys. Res. Commun. *81*:1254–59, 1978.

[47] Silverstein, S. C., Steinman, R. M., and Cohn, Z. A.: Endocytosis. Annu. Rev. Biochem. *46*:669–722, 1977.

[48] Olefsky, J. M.: Effect of insulin on glucose oxidation independent of glucose transport. Biochem. Biophys. Res. Commun. *71*:106–13, 1976.

[49] Vinten, J., Gliemann, J., and Osterlind, K.: Exchange of 3-O-methyl glucose in isolated fat cells. Concentration dependence and effect of insulin. J. Biol. Chem. *251*:794–800, 1976.

[50] Steinberg, D., and Khoo, J. C.: Hormone sensitive lipase of adipose tissue. Fed. Proc. *36*:1986–90, 1977.

[51] Steinberg, D., Mayer, S. E., Khoo, J. C., Miller, E. A., Miller, R. E., Fredholm, B., and Eichner, R. E.: Hormone regulation of lipase, phosphorylase and glycogen synthase in adipose tissue. *In* Advances in Cyclic Nucleotide Research, Vol. 5 Drummond, G. I., Greengard, P., and Robison, G. A., Eds. New York, Raven, 1975, p. 549.

[52] Haigler, H. T., McKanna, J. A., and Cohen, S.: Direct visualization of the binding and internalization of a ferritin conjugate of epidermal growth factor in human carcinoma cells A-431. J. Cell Biol. *81*:382–95, 1979.

[53] Gammeltoft, S., Kristensen, L. O., and Sestoft, L.: Insulin receptors in isolated rat hepatocytes. J. Biol. Chem. *253*:8406–13, 1978.

[54] Seals, J. R., McDonald, J. M., and Jarett, L.: Insulin effect on protein phosphorylation of plasma membranes and mitochondria in a subcellular system from rat adiopocytes. I. Identification of insulin-sensitive phosphoproteins. J. Biol. Chem. *254*:6991–96, 1979.

[55] Seals, J. R., McDonald, J. M., and Jarett, L.: Insulin effect on protein phosphorylation of plasma membranes and mitochondria in a subcellular system from rat adipocytes. II. Characterization of insulin-sensitive phosphoproteins and conditions for observation of the insulin effect. J. Biol. Chem. *254*:6997–7001, 1979.

[56] Seals, J. R., and Jarett, L.: Activation of pyruvate dehydrogenase by direct addition of insulin to an isolated plasma membrane-mitochondria mixture: evidence for generation of insulin's second messenger in a subcellular system. Proc. Natl. Acad. Sci. USA (in press).

[57] LeCam, A., Maxfield, F., Willingham, M., and Pastan, I.: Insulin stimulation of amino acid transport in isolated rat depatocytes is independent of hormone internalization. Biochem. Biophys. Res. Commun. *88*:873–82, 1979.

Lilly Lecture 1979
Role of Insulin in the Regulation of Protein Synthesis

LEONARD S. JEFFERSON

Nitrogen imbalance was one of the earliest recognized metabolic disturbances associated with diabetes mellitus. This imbalance was first observed as tissue wasting and then as increased nitrogen excretion and increased concentrations of blood amino acids. All these changes are the ultimate result of an imbalance in protein turnover, with the rate of protein degradation exceeding the rate of synthesis. Soon after its discovery in the early 1920s, insulin was shown to correct the nitrogen imbalance in diabetics. Although there was early speculation that this action of insulin was due to effects on protein synthesis and/or protein degradation, a definitive demonstration of an effect of insulin on these pathways is only a recent occurrence and the biochemical mechanism(s) involved is still not understood.

We have investigated the action of insulin on protein turnover in heart, skeletal muscle, and liver. Protein turnover in heart is obviously important for the survival of the organism. Protein turnover in skeletal muscle is important because this tissue comprises approximately 45% of the body weight and provides the bulk of amino acids which become substrates for gluconeogenesis and, in diabetes, contribute to the hyperglycemic condition. Protein turnover in liver is important because this tissue also contributes amino acids for gluconeogenesis. In addition, most of the plasma proteins are synthesized in liver. To investigate protein turnover in these tissues, we have employed isolated perfused preparations of rat heart,[1] skeletal muscle,[2,3] and liver,[4] as well as isolated liver cells.[4] We have established the conditions and methodology for determining accurate rates of protein synthesis and degradation, and we have developed approaches for identifying the biochemical steps involved in the control of these pathways.[5,6] The purpose of this lecture is to review our recent studies on the role of insulin in the control of protein synthesis. A discussion of the role of insulin in the control of protein degradation is beyond the scope of this lecture and will not be presented.

From the Department of Physiology, College of Medicine, The Pennsylvania State University, Hershey, Pennsylvania.
Address reprint requests to Leonard S. Jefferson, Department of Physiology, College of Medicine, The Pennsylvania State University, Hershey, Pennsylvania 17033.

POSSIBLE SITES OF INSULIN ACTION ON PROTEIN SYNTHESIS

A schematic presentation of the pathway of protein synthesis is shown in Figure 1. A detailed presentation of each biochemical step involved in this pathway is not possible since not all the reactions have been identified and characterized. The pathway involves the transport of amino acids into the cell, the activation of intracellular amino acids to form aminoacyl-tRNA derivatives, and the polymerization of activated amino acids into protein. The latter process involves a series of ribosome-catalyzed reactions and results in the translation of the genetic code contained in specific messenger RNA's. The translation process is conveniently considered as peptide-chain initiation, elongation, and termination, each of which is a complex sequence of reactions involving a variety of enzymes and protein factors as well as GTP and ATP. The partial reactions of peptide-chain initiation in eukaryotic cells are best characterized in the cell-free system derived from rabbit reticulocytes. Seven or eight initiation factors (eIF's) have been purified from reticulocyte lysates and are partially characterized.[7-9] The first step in initiation is the formation of a ternary complex consisting of methionyl-$tRNA_f^{Met}$ (met-$tRNA_f^{Met}$), GTP, and the initiation factor designated eIF-2. Ternary complex formation is essential for the binding of met-$tRNA_f^{Met}$ to the 40S ribosomal subunit. Subsequent partial reactions permit the association of the met-$tRNA_f^{Met}$ complex with messenger RNA (mRNA) to form a 40S initiation complex followed by the addition of the 60S ribosomal subunit to form an 80S initiation complex. The elongation and termination processes require elongation factors (EF's) and releasing factors (RF's), respectively, and result in the synthesis and release of the completed protein.[10] After the termination step, the 40S and 60S ribosomal subunits and mRNA are available to recycle in the ribosome-catalyzed reactions.

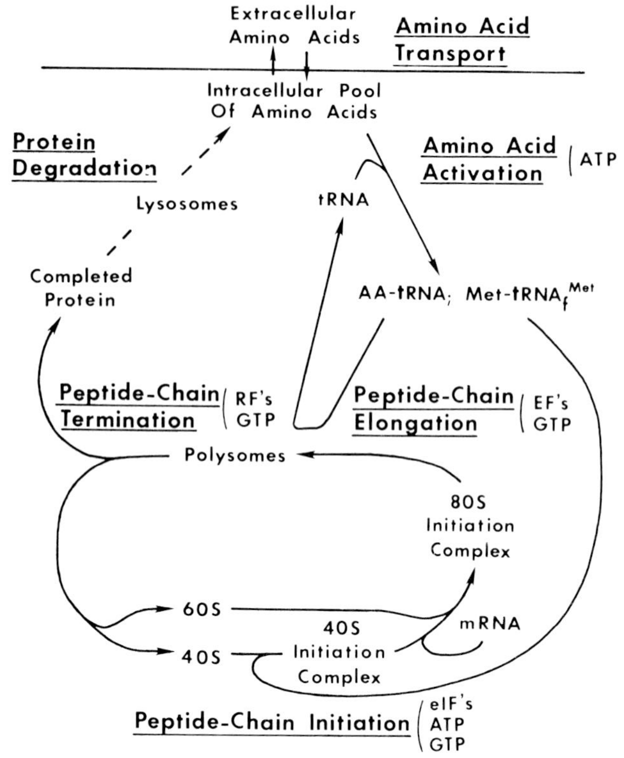

FIGURE 1. Pathway of protein turnover. The figure schematically depicts the major steps involved in protein synthesis and suggests that lysosomes may be involved in protein degradation. Abbreviations used are as follows: ATP, adenosine triphosphate; GTP, guanosine triphosphate; tRNA, transfer RNA; AA-tRNA, aminoacyl-transfer RNA; Met-tRNA$_f^{Met}$, the initiator methionyltransfer RNA; eIF's, eukaryotic initiation factors; mRNA, messenger RNA; EF's, elongation factors; RF's, releasing factors; 40S and 60S, the small and large ribosomal subunits, respectively.

While regulation at the level of translation would seem to be the most effective means of controlling overall rates of protein synthesis, the synthesis of specific proteins is probably modulated by the availability of the mRNA for the particular protein in question. The amount of translatable mRNA in the cytoplasm of a cell is the end result of a number of processes occurring in the nucleus and the cytoplasm.[11] After nuclear transcription, the pre-mRNA is processed to become translatable mRNA by steps involving addition of protein, splicing and cleavage of heterogeneous nuclear RNA transcripts, formation of 5′-terminal cap structures, internal methylation, and addition of poly (A) to the 3′ end. In addition, degradation of the mRNA could conceivably occur at any step after transcription. Thus, there are a number of sites at which the level of a specific translatable mRNA could be regulated. In addition to determining the amount of mRNA transcribed, the nuclear process of transcription is also responsible for the formation of ribosomal RNA and transfer RNA (tRNA), two essential components of the cell's protein synthesis machinery. The amount of synthesis and degradation of ribosomal RNA and tRNA can also be regulated, thus influencing the cell's overall capacity to carry out protein synthesis.

Insulin could regulate protein synthesis by modulating (1) the availability of amino acids, ATP, and GTP as substrates; (2) the availability of ribosomes, tRNA, mRNA, and enzymes that catalyze peptide-bond formation; and (3) the activity of

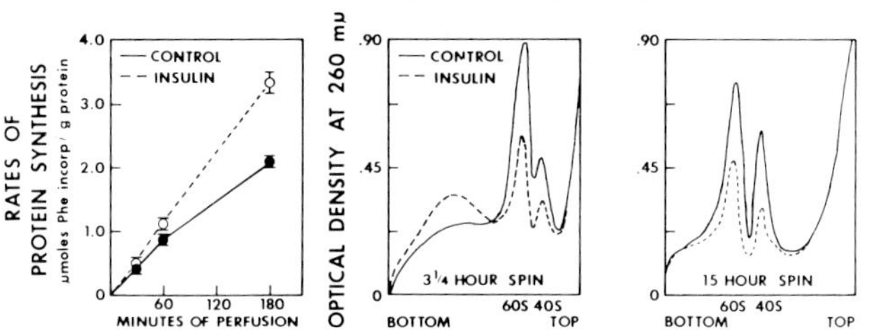

FIGURE 2. Effects of perfusion and insulin on protein synthesis and ribosomal aggregation in perfused rat heart. Hearts were perfused for 30–180 min with buffer containing 0.4 mM phenylalanine and normal plasma levels of the other amino acids, 15 mM glucose, 3% bovine serum albumin (Fraction V) and, where indicated, 1 μg/ml insulin. Estimates of protein synthesis (left panel), as μmol of phenylalanine incorporated per g protein, were calculated by dividing the dpm incorporated per g muscle by the specific activity of the intracellular phenylalanine precursor pool. Sucrose gradient analysis of polysomes and ribosomal subunits (center and right panels) was performed using unperfused hearts from fed rats and hearts perfused for 180 min. Muscles were homogenized in 3 volumes of 10 mM Tris-HCl buffer, pH 7.4, containing 250 mM KCl and 2 mM $MgCl_2$. The postmitochondrial supernatants were layered onto sucrose gradients (0.4–2.0 M) and the gradients were centrifuged at 200,000 × *g*. Centrifugation was continued 3.25 or 15 h to better resolve polysomes or ribosomal subunits, respectively. Polysome and subunit profiles in sucrose gradients were resolved by monitoring the UV absorbance at 260 mμm. Positions of the 60S and 40S ribosomal subunits are indicated. Polysome and subunit profiles from unperfused hearts are not shown, but were identical to those seen in hearts perfused for 180 min in the presence of insulin. The data are adapted from Jefferson et al.[12]

factors affecting rates of peptide-chain initiation, elongation, and termination. The physiologic significance of an effect of insulin on any of these parameters is dependent on the role of that particular parameter in restricting the rate of protein synthesis.

IDENTIFICATION OF THE SITE OF INSULIN ACTION ON PROTEIN SYNTHESIS IN HEART AND SKELETAL MUSCLE

When the isolated rat heart was perfused in vitro with buffer containing normal plasma levels of amino acids and glucose, the rate of protein synthesis was linear during the first hour, but then declined sharply during the second and third hours (Figure 2, left panel). Addition of insulin to the perfusate had little, if any, effect during the first hour, but maintained the initial rate of protein synthesis during the last 2 h of perfusion. Early studies attributed the effects of insulin on protein synthesis to an accelerated rate of amino acid transport[13,14] and increased formation of aminoacyl-tRNA.[15,16] Further investigation indicated that the hormone response illustrated in Figure 2 was not due to an increased intracellular supply of amino acids.[17] In rat hearts perfused for 3 h with buffer containing normal plasma levels of amino acids and 15 mM glucose, insulin reduced the intracellular levels of nine amino acids even though protein synthesis was accelerated.

Insulin could have accelerated protein synthesis by maintaining higher levels of high-energy phosphates. However, in both the presence and absence of the hormone, heart rate and ventricular pressure development were stable for 3 h of perfusion.[18] Furthermore, ATP levels did not decline significantly from unperfused tissue levels during 4.5 h of perfusion.[17] In hearts perfused for 1.5–3 h, creatine phosphate was elevated in the presence of insulin compared with control tissue. The significance of this observation with respect to the effect of the hormone on protein synthesis is not presently understood.

The alterations in the rate of protein synthesis produced by perfusion for time periods greater than 1 h and by insulin were accompanied by changes in the levels of polysomes and ribosomal subunits (Figure 2, center and right panels). An accumulation of ribosomal subunits and a fall in polysomes in association with the decline in the rate of protein synthesis indicated that a restraint on peptide-chain initiation had developed during perfusion and that this step had become rate-limiting for protein synthesis. Addition of insulin prevented this inhibition as evidenced by maintenance of the initial rate of protein synthesis and in vivo levels of polysomes and ribosomal subunits.

Virtually identical results were obtained in skeletal muscle perfused in the hemicorpus preparation. In skeletal muscle perfused for up to 1 h (Figure 3, panels A and D), ribosomal subunit levels were maintained at the low levels of the unperfused condition. Polysomes were also maintained at the preperfusion level.[19] For perfusions within this time period, the presence of insulin in the medium was not effective in increasing the rate of protein synthesis or in altering levels of ribosomal subunits or polysomes. With extension of perfusion time to 2 (panels B and E) or 3 h (panels C and F), the rate of protein synthesis declined from the rate that was measured during the first hour of perfusion, and levels of ribosomal subunits were markedly elevated from the unperfused level (polysomes decreased from the preperfusion level). The decline in the rate of protein synthesis, therefore, resulted from a restraint on peptide-chain initiation which developed after 1 h of perfusion. The presence of insulin in the initial buffer or addition of insulin after 2 h of perfusion (panels C and F) effectively stimulated protein synthesis within 1 h. This stimulation was brought about by the complete reversal of the restraint of peptide-chain initiation as evidenced by the return of ribosomal subunit and polysome levels to those observed in the unperfused condition. The ability of insulin to prevent or reverse the development of a restraint on peptide-chain initiation was not blocked by actinomycin D (unpublished data), suggesting that RNA synthesis is not essential for the hormone effect on initiation.

From these studies, it is evident that protein synthesis in heart and skeletal muscle is limited in perfusion-induced insulin deficiency at the level of peptide-chain initiation. It would be expected, therefore, that the reactions of peptide-chain initiation would also be limiting in muscle taken from diabetic animals. To test this possibility, the rates of protein synthesis in different muscles from diabetic rats were measured during the first hour of perfusion before the onset of perfusion-induced insulin deficiency. The results of synthesis measurements in the heart and in two skeletal muscles, the gastrocnemius and soleus, are shown in Figure 4. In the gastrocnemius, an example of muscle with mixed red and white fiber distributions, diabetes of 2 days' duration resulted in the anticipated reduction in the rate of protein synthesis. This decrease was due to both loss of tissue RNA and reduced translational efficiency, i.e., synthesis per unit

FIGURE 3. Rates of protein synthesis and levels of ribosomal subunits in perfused skeletal muscle of the rat. Rates of protein synthesis during the indicated time intervals were determined in the gastrocnemius muscle of the perfused hemicorpus as described in Figure 2. Levels of 60S and 40S ribosomal subunits were determined on samples of postmitochondrial supernatant from homogenized psoas muscle taken at the indicated times of perfusion as described in Figure 2. Preparations were perfused with Krebs-Henseleit bicarbonate buffer containing 3.0% bovine serum albumin (Fraction V), 15 mM glucose, 5× normal plasma levels of phenylalanine (0.4 mM), 1× normal plasma levels of other amino acids, and 30% washed bovine erythrocytes (control) or with the above medium containing 1 μg/ml insulin (insulin, shaded bars) added at the start of perfusion (0′) or after 120 min of perfusion (120′). Protein synthesis rates are expressed as nmol of phenylalanine incorporated per h per g muscle. Values are means ± SEM. The levels of ribosomal subunits seen in Panel D are equal to the levels found in unperfused muscle. The data are adapted from Jefferson et al.[19]

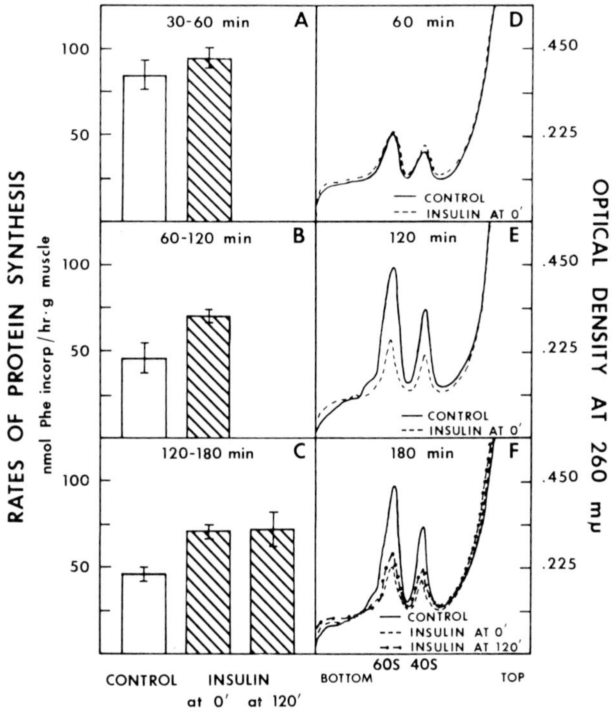

FIGURE 4. Effects of diabetes and insulin on rates of protein synthesis in perfused muscles of the rat. Rates of protein synthesis were determined by measuring the incorporation of ^{14}C-phenylalanine into muscles perfused for 60 min as described in Figure 2. Gastrocnemius and soleus muscles were perfused in the isolated hemicorpus preparation[3] with a Krebs-Henseleit bicarbonate buffer containing 4.5% bovine serum albumin (Fraction V), 15 mM glucose, 0.8 mM phenylalanine and the normal plasma levels of other amino acids. Hearts were perfused in a modified Langendorff preparation[1] with the buffer described above with the exception that 3.0% bovine serum albumin (Fraction V) was used. Two days before the experiment rats (200–300 g) were injected intravenously with 0.9% NaCl (control) or made diabetic by the injection of alloxan monohydrate (60 mg/kg, i.v.) after an overnight fast (diabetic). The effect of insulin in vitro was tested by the inclusion of insulin in the initial perfusion medium at a concentration of 1 μg/ml (shaded bars). The data for skeletal muscle are adapted from Flaim et al.[20]

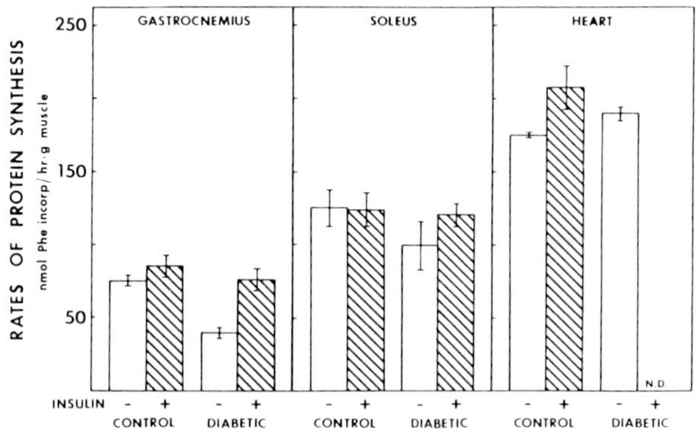

RNA. In contrast, in the soleus, a muscle with primarily red fibers, protein synthesis was much less affected by diabetes. The reduction in protein synthesis in this muscle was due entirely to reduced concentrations of RNA, as no decrease in translational efficiency was detected. Similarly, the rate of protein synthesis in the heart was not altered in animals with diabetes of 2 days' duration. In the gastrocnemius, addition of insulin to the perfusion medium restored protein synthetic efficiency to the same level as that observed in muscle of normal animals. The tissue RNA concentration was not changed by the presence of insulin in the medium. Therefore, only the gastrocnemius could acutely respond to insulin, since this was the only muscle of the three in which translational efficiency was impaired in diabetes.

To gain a better understanding of the differential responses of these muscles to diabetes, the in vivo levels of ribosomal subunits were determined. The results of these studies are shown in Figure 5. In the gastrocnemius and psoas, muscles with a mixed fiber distribution, ribosomal subunit levels indicated that polysomal disaggregation occurred in the diabetic state. Inhibition of peptide-chain initiation, then, was the cause of the reduced translational efficiency determined in vitro (Figure 4) and in vivo.[21] However, the subunit levels in heart muscle from diabetic rats were not elevated and, therefore, did not indicate an impaired peptide-chain initiation process. Subunit levels in soleus muscle were indicative of only a small degree of polysomal disaggregation. Therefore, the in vitro data indicating no block in translational efficiency in the heart and soleus of 2-day diabetic rats were accurately reflected in the state of polysomal aggregation in these muscles. It appears that muscles with more oxidative fibers are less susceptible to a block in peptide-chain initiation caused by the insulin deficiency of diabetes. Insulin deficiency of longer duration, however, does eventually lead to an impaired translational efficiency in these muscles which is not attributable to a block in initiation.[20]

These studies indicate that there is some process or factor that protects oxidative muscle in short-term diabetes from the inhibition of protein synthesis caused by insulin deficiency. It has been proposed that the high levels of circulating fatty acids seen in diabetics are responsible for maintaining the translational efficiency in heart muscle of rats with diabetes of 2 days' duration.[12] Indeed, in heart muscle perfused for 3 h, the presence of a fatty acid (e.g., palmitate) in the perfusate was as effective as insulin in maintaining the rates of protein synthesis (Figure 6, panel A). Other studies showed that in addition to palmitate, provision of lactate, pyruvate, acetoacetate, β-hydroxybutyrate, or oleate was also effective in maintaining protein synthesis.[22]

As was the case with insulin, addition of palmitate to the perfusate not only maintained the initial rate of protein synthesis, but also maintained polysomes and ribosomal subunits at levels found in vivo during 3 h of perfusion (Figure 6, panels B and C). In other experiments, the fatty acid was shown to reverse the perfusion-induced impairment in initiation. Provision of physiologic levels of oleate, lactate, pyruvate, acetoacetate, β-hydroxybutyrate, or acetate had a sim-

FIGURE 5. Effect of diabetes on the in vivo levels of ribosomal subunits in muscles of the rat. 60S and 40S ribosomal subunits were isolated by sucrose density gradient centrifugation as described in Figure 2. Control and diabetic rats were prepared as described in Figure 4. Tissue RNA concentrations (mg RNA per g muscle) in control rats were approximately 1.4 in psoas and gastrocnemius and 1.7 in soleus and heart. RNA concentrations in diabetic rats were approximately 1.1 in psoas and gastrocnemius and 1.5 in soleus and heart.

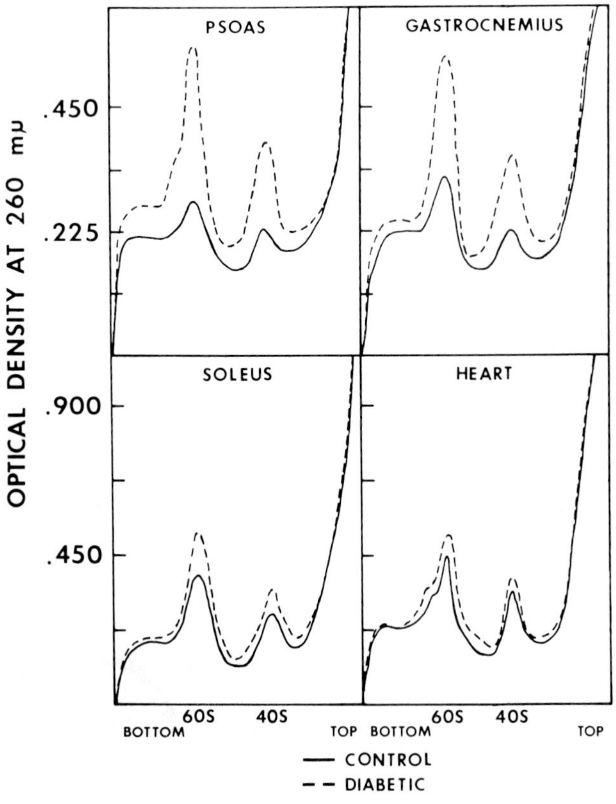

FIGURE 6. Effects of palmitate on protein synthesis and ribosomal aggregation in perfused rat heart and skeletal muscle. Hearts were perfused for 30–180 min with buffer described in Figure 4 and, where indicated, 1.5 mM palmitate bound to albumin. Skeletal muscle was perfused in the rat hemicorpus for 90 min with the same buffer containing 30% washed bovine erythrocytes. Protein synthesis was estimated by measuring phenylalanine incorporation (panel A and D) as described in Figure 2. Sucrose gradient analysis of polysomes and ribosomal subunits was conducted as described in Figure 2 using hearts that had been perfused for 180 min (panels B and C) and skeletal muscle perfused for 90 min (panels E and F). The data are adapted from Jefferson et al.[12]

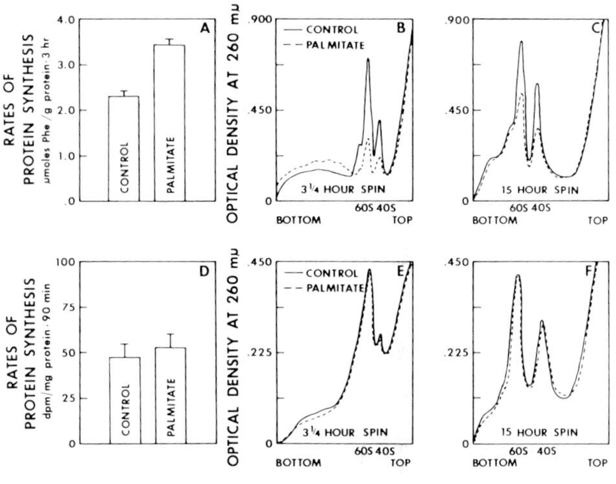

ilar effect in preventing the development of a restraint on peptide-chain initiation in hearts supplied with glucose alone.[22] These findings suggest that a metabolic product common to all of these substrates may be responsible for the stimulation of the synthetic pathway. Maintenance of peptide-chain initiation in heart muscle of diabetic animals, therefore, may be due to a protective effect of fatty acids.

In contrast to the situation in heart muscle, palmitate had no effect on protein synthesis (Figure 6, panel D) or ribosomal aggregation (Figure 6, panels E and F) in perfused skeletal muscle of mixed fiber distribution. Absence of an effect of fatty acids in mixed skeletal muscle allowed a reduction in the rate of protein synthesis in insulin deficient states (e.g., diabetes and starvation) and contributed to a net loss of protein from these tissues. Since fatty acids are effective in protecting the heart from the development of an impairment in peptide-chain initiation during insulin deficient states, they may also exert this effect in oxidative skeletal muscle. However, the effects of fatty acids on the rate of protein synthesis and the levels of ribosomal subunits in slow-twitch red skeletal muscle, e.g., the soleus, remain to be determined. In diabetes of longer duration, the fat stores of the animal would be depleted and peptide-chain initiation in heart may not be maintained.

Estimates of the rates of protein synthesis and levels of polysomes and ribosomal subunits supply information that localize the effects of hormones and other factors to groups of reactions within the ribosome cycle; however, they provide no indication of the mechanism of these effects. Both initiation and elongation, as defined in these studies, combine many steps that require specific protein factors, tRNA, ribosomes, mRNA, and the binding and hydrolysis of GTP.

The partial reactions of peptide-chain initiation have been investigated in only a preliminary way in heart and skeletal muscle. Since the formation of a ternary complex of met-$tRNA_f^{Met}$, GTP, and the initiation factor eIF-2 is an early step in the pathway,[7-9] possible alterations at this step were first studied. The properties of the eIF-2 factor from heart and skeletal muscle are similar to those of the factor that has been implicated in the physiologic control of initiation in cell-free systems derived from rabbit reticulocytes. Formation of the ternary complex requires GTP, is inhibited by GDP, Mg^{2+}, spermine, spermidine, and aurintricarboxylic acid, and is specific for initiator tRNA.[23] The ability of postribosomal supernatants from both the psoas and heart to form this ternary complex was reduced in muscles removed from 48-h fasted rats.[23] The fasted condition represents an insulin deficient state, and levels of ribosomal subunits isolated from the psoas are indicative of an impairment in peptide-chain initiation. In contrast, initiation in heart is not affected under these conditions and, therefore, the observed alterations in the amount of complex formed did not parallel changes in initiation. Furthermore, the formation of ternary complex by postribosomal supernatants taken from perfused muscles was not increased by the presence of insulin in the perfusion medium even though peptide-chain initiation was stimulated under the same conditions.[23] These experiments do not support the concept that the effect of insulin on initiation involved an alteration in ternary complex formation. However, an effect of insulin on this reaction cannot be ruled out, since the binding assay used to determine activity measured total eIF-2 and may not distinguish between in vivo active and inactive forms of the factor. Furthermore, interconversion of active and inactive forms during tissue preparation and assay may occur. It is interesting to note that eIF-2 is subject to phosphorylation and dephosphorylation.[24-26] While opinions are divided as to the physiologic significance of this covalent modification,[27-33] it may represent a means by which the activity of the factor could be regulated by insulin and other agents.

The partial reactions of peptide-chain initiation have been studied most extensively in cell-free systems derived from reticulocyte lysates. In the lysate systems, the initiation step was identified as the rate-limiting step in protein synthesis under a number of conditions including the following: (1) in the absence of added hemin,[34-36] (2) in the presence of oxidized glutathione[37,38] or low levels of double-stranded RNA,[39] (3) in lysates depleted of low molecular weight components by gel filtration,[40] and (4) in the presence of inhibitors of oxidative phosphorylation.[41-43] In contrast, a variety of phosphorylated sugars plus $NADP^+$ stimulated initiation in lysates prepared from glucose-starved or ATP-depleted cells,[42,43] while a similar stimulatory effect was observed with glucose, citrate, and fructose-1,6-diphosphate in lysates depleted of low molecular weight components by gel filtration.[40] These observations implicated a role for phosphorylated sugars, and possibly NADPH production, in the maintenance of the initiation step in reticulocyte lysates. A recent study demonstrated a direct role for glucose-6-phosphate in the regulation of peptide-chain initiation in reticulocyte lysates.[44] This report presented evidence that the effect of glucose-6-phosphate was unrelated to its ability to generate NADPH or to its metabolism in glycolysis or the pentose phosphate pathway, suggesting that the compound may act as an allosteric regulator of some step in the initiation process.

A similar role for glucose-6-phosphate in the regulation of peptide-chain initiation may exist in heart and skeletal muscle. While this proposal is only speculative at this time, it should be noted that the levels of this intermediate in muscle are known to change in a manner consistent with such a role. For example, the maintenance of initiation in hearts of diabetic rats was associated with elevated levels of glucose-6-phosphate (Figure 7). In contrast, the impairment in initiation that developed in skeletal muscle of diabetic rats was associated with no increase in levels of glucose-6-phosphate (Figure 7). Hearts perfused in the presence of glucose and palmitate contained higher glucose-6-phosphate levels than those perfused in the presence of glucose alone,[46] suggesting that the effect of fatty acids on protein synthesis may be related to their ability to cause an elevation in the concentration of this metabolic intermediate. Fatty acids were identified as the major oxidative substrates of heart muscle,[47] accounting for 75–90% of cardiac oxygen consumption. Provision of fatty acids decreased glucose utilization in the heart by inhibiting phosphofructokinase,[48] leading to an accumulation of glucose-6-phosphate which, in turn, inhibited hexokinase[49] and membrane transport of glucose.[50] Attempts to demonstrate a similar relationship between fatty acid utilization and glucose metabolism in mixed skeletal muscle were unsuccessful,[2,51] although findings in slow-twitch red skeletal muscle[52] suggested that

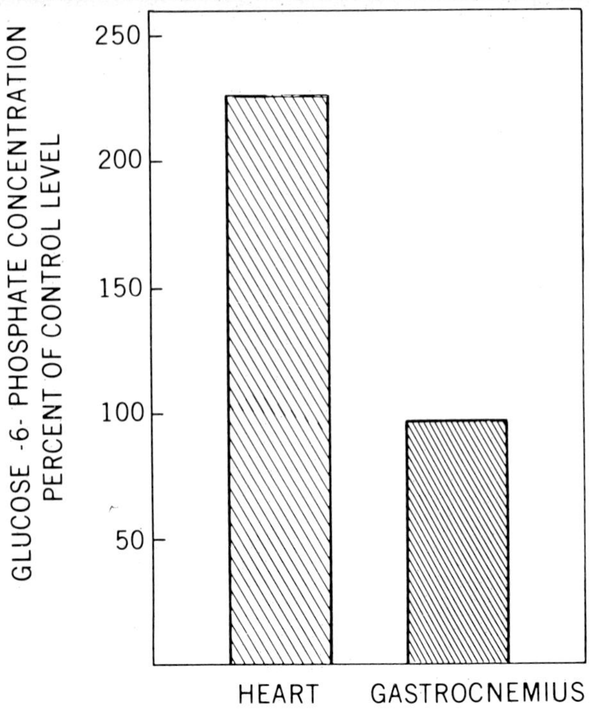

FIGURE 7. Effect of diabetes on the concentrations of glucose-6-phosphate in heart and skeletal muscle. Determinations of glucose-6-phosphate concentrations in heart and gastrocnemius muscle were made 2 days after induction of diabetes with alloxan (60 mg/kg, i.v.). Following induction of anesthesia (Nembutal, 50 mg/kg) muscles were quick-frozen and pulverized at the temperature of liquid nitrogen. Glucose-6-phosphate concentrations in acid-soluble extracts were determined as previously described[45] and are expressed as a percentage of the levels found in control tissues.

it may be more like heart muscle in this respect. Thus, the abilities of various muscles to utilize fatty acids and elevate glucose-6-phosphate levels may determine the extent to which an impairment in peptide-chain initiation develops in diabetes and starvation.

Glucose-6-phosphate levels were also elevated in heart and skeletal muscle perfused with glucose plus insulin compared with muscles perfused with glucose alone,[53] raising the possibility that glucose-6-phosphate may mediate the effects of insulin on protein synthesis. However, insulin stimulated peptide-chain initiation in skeletal muscle perfused in the absence of substrate.[19] Insulin was also effective at stimulating initiation but did not elevate glucose-6-phosphate levels in hearts perfused with pyruvate as substrate (unpublished data). Therefore, insulin appears capable of regulating initiation by a mechanism independent of glucose-6-phosphate levels.

On the basis of these findings, regulation of peptide-chain initiation appears to be similar to the model proposed for the control of glycogen synthase.[54] In this model, glycogen synthase is activated by glucose-6-phosphate via a mechanism involving the activation of a phosphoprotein phosphatase. Insulin is proposed to act independently of glucose-6-phosphate, by a mechanism involving an inhibition of a protein kinase. Whether glucose-6-phosphate and insulin act to control the state of phosphorylation of a component of the peptide-chain initiation process is yet to be established.

IDENTIFICATION OF THE SITE OF INSULIN ACTION ON PROTEIN SYNTHESIS IN LIVER

Early reports indicated that diabetes resulted in reduced rates of protein synthesis in perfused livers of diabetic rats[55,56] and that addition of insulin to the perfusion medium stimulated protein synthesis in livers from mildly diabetic animals.[56] However, in these studies, the specific activity of amino acid precursor pools was not monitored and thus reliable measurements of protein synthesis could not be obtained. The results of these studies were later questioned when it was demonstrated that insulin has a marked inhibitory effect on protein degradation in the perfused liver.[57] This inhibition would reduce the dilution of labeled amino acids within the liver by unlabeled amino acids derived from protein degradation and could lead to erroneous conclusions as to the effect of diabetes or insulin in the liver perfusion system. Indeed, when dilution of the specific activity of the labeled amino acid precursor was taken into account, it was not possible to demonstrate an effect of insulin on protein synthesis in perfused normal liver.[57]

Recently, we examined the effect of diabetes on hepatic protein synthesis in the perfused liver using conditions that minimized changes in precursor pool specific activity.[6] The results of these experiments are summarized in Figure 8. Hepatic protein synthesis was only slightly reduced 2 days

FIGURE 8. Effects of diabetes and insulin treatment on the synthesis of retained (intracellular) proteins by the perfused liver of the rat. Rates of protein synthesis were determined by measuring the incorporation of ^{3}H-leucine into total liver protein in 90-min perfusions. To obtain the amount of leucine incorporated per unit time, the dpm incorporated into liver protein per h per g body weight was divided by the specific activity of leucine in the perfusate. Based on an average leucine content in total hepatic protein of 9% (g/g) the rate of protein synthesis in mg was then calculated. No correction has been made for the small contribution made by labeled secretory proteins within the liver at the time the liver sample was taken. Livers were perfused in situ with a recirculating Krebs-Henseleit bicarbonate buffer containing 3.0% bovine serum albumin (Fraction V), 10 mM glucose, 5 mM leucine, 7.5 times normal plasma levels of other amino acids, and 30% washed bovine erythrocytes. Two or three days before the experiment, rats (100–120 g) were injected intravenously with 0.9% NaCl (control) or made diabetic as described in Figure 4 (diabetic). Insulin treatment (shaded bars) consisted of a single subcutaneous injection of 3 U of Lente insulin 24 h before perfusion. Values are means ± SEM. The data are adapted from Peavy et al.[6]

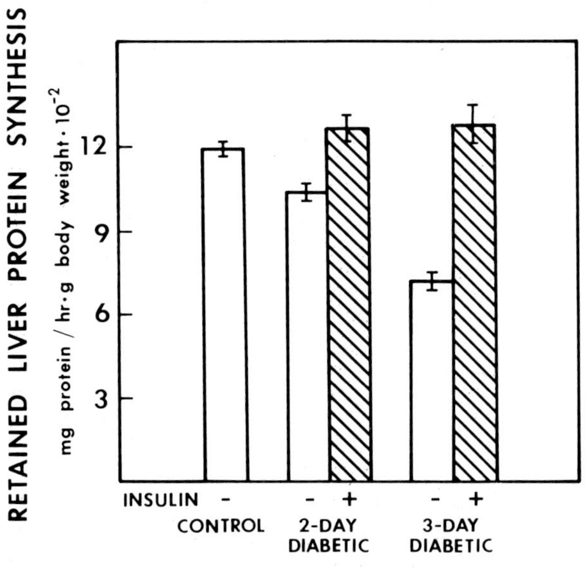

after the induction of diabetes, a result which is consistent with in vivo determinations using a constant infusion method.[21] In contrast, protein synthesis was significantly reduced in livers of 3-day (Figure 8) and 7-day (data not shown) diabetic rats. Thus, an impairment in synthesis of hepatic intracellular proteins was manifested in perfused liver after a longer period of diabetes. This difference may manifest itself only under in vitro conditions or it may be related to more prolonged and/or more severe diabetes. These experiments demonstrate that the defect was related to insulin deficiency, since treatment of diabetic animals with insulin restored the level of protein synthesis to that observed in livers of normal animals.

The results in Figure 8 are primarily indicative of the synthesis of intracellular liver proteins. Earlier indications that diabetes and insulin may influence the synthesis of hepatic secretory proteins came from studies in which it was shown that albumin secretion was reduced in perfused livers of alloxan-diabetic rats,[58] and from studies in which changes in cellular ultrastructure were apparent in livers of alloxan- or streptozotocin-diabetic rats.[59–62] In electron micrographs, the rough endoplasmic reticulum normally appeared as orderly rows of membrane-bound polyribosome structures, but in livers of diabetic animals, this ordered structure was severely disrupted.[59–62] Because secretory proteins are primarily synthesized by ribosomes on the rough endoplasmic reticulum, a disruption of this structure in livers of diabetic animals might be indicative of an impairment in the synthesis and secretion of secretory proteins. Our recent studies have shown that this is the case.[6] In these studies, livers of normal, diabetic, and insulin-treated diabetic animals were perfused and the absolute rates of albumin and total protein secretion were determined. As shown in Figure 9, albumin secretion was markedly reduced in livers of diabetic rats. Two days after the induction of diabetes, albumin secretion was reduced to about one half of the rate observed in livers from control rats, and by 3 days, the secretion rate was reduced further to about 10% of the control level. If the effect of diabetes on albumin secretion is compared to its effect on secretory protein production as a whole, it is evident that the effect of diabetes is relatively specific to albumin. The production of total secretory protein was impaired to a lesser extent than was the secretion of albumin, as illustrated by expressing albumin secretion as a percentage of total protein secretion. In normal animals, albumin accounted for approximately 40% of the protein secreted by the liver (calculated from Figure 9). The selective impairment of albumin secretion reduced this value to 13% in livers of 3-day diabetic rats. Thus, in perfused livers of diabetic animals, secretory protein synthesis is reduced to a much greater extent than is the synthesis of intracellular proteins (compare Figures 8 and 9) and impairment of albumin synthesis accounts for most of the effect on secretory protein synthesis.

Insulin treatment of diabetic rats increased both albumin and total protein secretion from perfused livers (Figure 9). The ability of insulin treatment to restore protein secretion rates to normal or near-normal levels lends support to the argument that the observed effect of diabetes is due to the insulin-deficient state of the animals, rather than to a direct cytotoxic effect of alloxan on the liver.

In contrast to skeletal muscle, peptide-chain initiation in liver is not altered as a result of diabetes. Total unfractionated polysomes isolated from diabetic rats were the same size as those isolated from normal rats.[63] Albumin-synthesizing polysomes, as determined by the binding of ^{125}I-antialbumin antibody to total polysomes, were also the same size in both diabetic and normal rats. These data suggested that diabetes did not selectively affect the rate of peptide-chain initiation or elongation. Only a coordinate and identical rate change in both translational processes could account for these findings. Such a possibility was eliminated by an independent measurement of elongation rates which revealed no alteration resulting from diabetes (unpublished data). Quantitation of the relative number of albumin-synthesizing polysomes demonstrated a reduction of the same magnitude as the relative decrease in albumin synthesis rates. A reduction in the number of albumin-synthesizing polysomes suggested a loss in the amount of active albumin mRNA. This possibility was investigated directly by examining albumin mRNA levels in livers of normal, diabetic, and insulin-treated diabetic rats. The results of these determinations, in which albumin mRNA was quantitated by translation and hybridization assays, are summarized in Figure 10. Albumin mRNA content was reduced in diabetic rats in a manner parallel to the changes observed in albumin synthesis in vivo and in perfused livers. The relatively good agreement between the translation and hybridization assays indicated that there was an actual re-

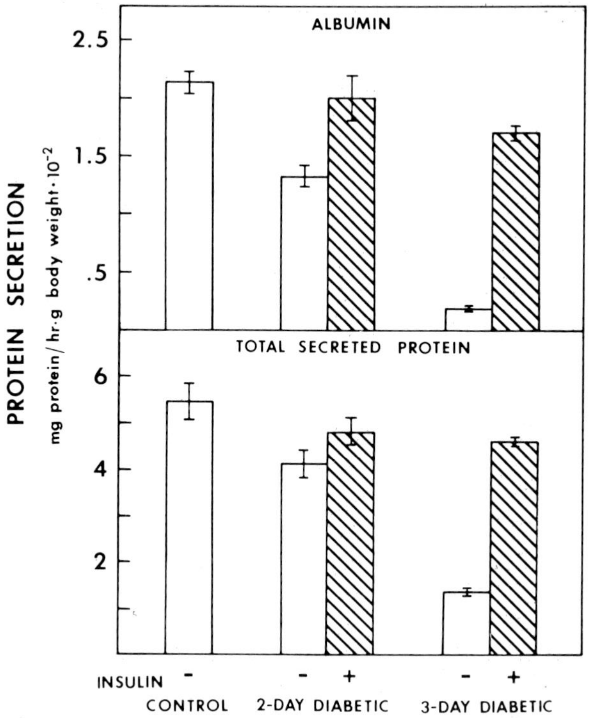

FIGURE 9. Effects of diabetes and insulin treatment on albumin and total protein secretion by the perfused liver of the rat. Livers were perfused as described in Figure 8. Samples of the perfusion medium were taken at intervals during the 90-min perfusion and the radioactivity in albumin was determined with a specific antibody and total secreted protein was determined by trichloroacetic acid precipitation. Rates of protein secretion were calculated in a manner analogous to that described for liver tissue proteins as presented in Figure 8. Alloxan and insulin treatments were as in Figures 4 and 8. Values are means ± SEM. The data are adapted from Peavy et al.[6]

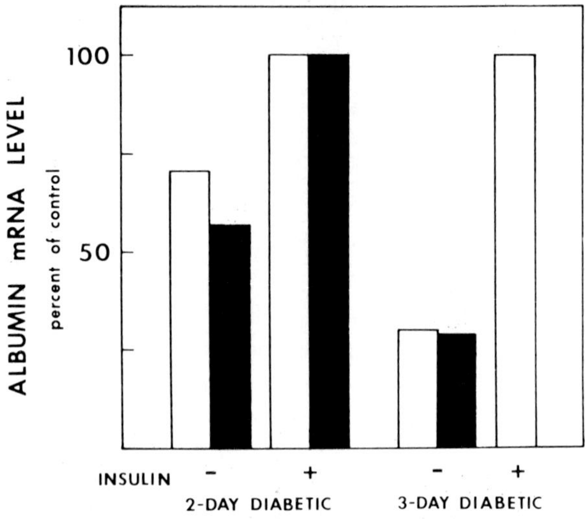

FIGURE 10. Effects of diabetes and insulin on albumin mRNA levels in the liver of the rat. Total poly(A)-containing RNA was isolated from unfractionated liver homogenates by phenol/chloroform extraction and affinity chromatography on poly(U)-Sepharose. The albumin mRNA content of the samples was determined by hybridization analysis utilizing a specific ^{3}H-labeled complementary DNA (cDNA) to rat albumin mRNA (open bars). Albumin mRNA activity of the poly(A)-containing samples was determined in a cell-free protein synthesizing system utilizing mRNA-dependent rabbit reticulocyte lysates (solid bars). The results of the assays are expressed relative to the results obtained with samples from livers of control (normal) animals. Rats were made diabetic as described in Figure 4. Insulin treatment was of two types. (1) Two-day diabetic animals were injected with 3 U of Lente insulin followed 24 h later by removal of the liver and extraction of poly(A)-containing RNA. (2) Three-day diabetic rats were injected daily with 1.6 U protamine-zinc insulin for 3 days before extraction of poly(A)-containing RNA. The data are adapted from Peavy et al.[6]

duction in albumin mRNA content in livers of diabetic rats, rather than conversion of active mRNA to a nonfunctional form. Treatment of diabetic rats with insulin, as shown in Figure 10, restored albumin mRNA to control levels. The correlation between albumin mRNA levels and the relative albumin production rates observed in normal, diabetic, and insulin-treated diabetic rats (Figures 9 and 10) suggests that the decrease in hepatic albumin production in diabetes is the result of decreased albumin mRNA levels, although a direct cause and effect relationship has not been firmly established at this time.

As indicated earlier, there are a number of possible sites at which the amount of translatable albumin mRNA could be regulated, such as transcription, processing or turnover of mRNA. The half-life of albumin mRNA was similar in livers of normal and diabetic rats,[63] suggesting that the major defect in diabetes with regard to albumin production lies in transcription of the albumin gene or in processing of albumin mRNA precursors. The mechanism by which diabetes and insulin affects the synthesis of other hepatic proteins, either secretory or intracellular proteins, may also involve changes in the levels of specific mRNA's or may be a more generalized effect involving some step in translation, although as discussed above, current information tends not to support this latter possibility.

CONCLUSION

During the past few years, a number of developments have contributed to an advance in our understanding of the role of insulin in the control of protein synthesis. These include (1) a vast improvement in the knowledge of the chemical reactions in the pathway of protein synthesis; (2) development of methods for obtaining accurate measurements of synthetic rates; (3) development and modification of procedures for in vitro perfusion of liver, heart, and skeletal muscle; (4) development of methods for measurement of intermediates in the synthetic pathway; (5) development of methods for quantitating the synthesis of individual proteins; and (6) development of techniques for measuring mRNA levels for specific proteins. These developments have led to the establishment of an anabolic role for insulin in the regulation of protein turnover and have permitted, in some instances, the identification of specific reactions or groups of reactions as the site of action of the hormone.

Specifically, two major control mechanisms have been implicated in the anabolic effect of insulin. One mechanism has been demonstrated in muscle tissue and one in liver. In skeletal muscle of mixed fiber types, diabetes results in a marked reduction in the synthesis of total protein, which is due to a decrease in both the number of ribosomes as well as their translational efficiency. The latter decrease, which is rapidly corrected by insulin, corresponds with changes in rates of peptide-chain initiation. In soleus, a skeletal muscle of slow-twitch red fiber type, and in the heart, an impairment in initiation does not develop in diabetes. However, perfused heart does develop an impairment, which can be rapidly reversed by insulin, fatty acids, or noncarbohydrate substrates. While insulin can act independently, the noncarbohydrate substrate effect, which may be mediated through glucose-6-phosphate, is probably responsible for the maintenance of normal rates of initiation in the hearts of diabetic animals. In the liver, diabetes results in a marked reduction in the synthesis of specific secretory proteins, especially albumin, while synthesis of intracellular protein is affected to a lesser extent. Synthesis of albumin and total hepatic protein is restored to normal levels by insulin. At a molecular level these alterations in albumin synthesis correspond with changes in albumin mRNA levels.

Future work on the role of insulin in the regulation of protein synthesis is dependent upon further definition and characterization of the individual components involved in the synthetic pathway. The individual enzymes catalyzing reactions in the synthetic pathway must be identified and characterized so that regulation can be understood at the molecular level. Although our knowledge of the sequence of reactions and factors involved in protein synthesis has progressed rapidly in recent years as a result of extensive studies in prokaryotes and reticulocytes, extrapolation of this information to tissues such as muscle and liver must be done with caution. Many more control mechanisms are likely to be operative in muscle and liver, resulting in a more complex situation than that which exists in the systems studied thus far. It is also clear that peptide hormones such as insulin can regulate protein synthesis by modifying gene expression. This opens up an area of study to which can be applied many of the existing techniques and approaches currently available to the molecular biologist. Thus, the stage is set for rapid advances in our understanding of the mechanism(s) of insulin action in the control of protein synthesis.

ACKNOWLEDGMENTS

The studies reported here were supported in part by grants AM15658 and AM13499 from the National Institute of Arthritis, Metabolism and Digestive Diseases. The collaborative support of Drs. Howard E. Morgan, John M. Taylor, Daniel E. Peavy, and Kathryn E. Flaim is also gratefully acknowledged.

L. S. Jefferson is an Established Investigator of the American Diabetes Association.

REFERENCES

[1] Morgan, H. E., Earl, D. C. N., Broadus, A., Wolpert, E. B., Giger, K. E., and Jefferson, L. S.: Regulation of protein synthesis in heart muscle. I. Effect of amino acid levels on protein synthesis. J. Biol. Chem. *246*:2152–62, 1971.

[2] Jefferson, L. S., Koehler, J. O., and Morgan, H. E.: Effect of insulin on protein synthesis in skeletal muscle of an isolated perfused preparation of rat hemicorpus. Proc. Natl. Acad. Sci. USA *69*:816–20, 1972.

[3] Jefferson, L. S.: A technique for perfusion of an isolated preparation of rat hemicorpus. Meth. Enzymol. *39*:73–82, 1975.

[4] Feldhoff, R. C., Taylor, J. M., and Jefferson, L. S.: Synthesis and secretion of rat albumin *in vivo*, in perfused liver, and in isolated hepatocytes: Effects of hypophysectomy and growth hormone treatment. J. Biol. Chem. *252*:3611–16, 1977.

[5] Rannels, D. E., Li, J. B., Morgan, H. E., and Jefferson, L. S.: Evaluation of hormone effects on protein turnover in isolated perfused organs. Meth. Enzymol. *37*:238–50, 1975.

[6] Peavy, D. E., Taylor, J. M., and Jefferson, L. S.: Correlation of albumin production rates and albumin mRNA levels in livers of normal, diabetic and insulin-treated diabetic rats. Proc. Natl. Acad. Sci. USA *75*:5879–83, 1978.

[7] Benne, R., and Hershey, J. W. B.: The mechanism of action of protein synthesis initiation factors from rabbit reticulocytes. J. Biol. Chem. *253*:3078–87, 1978.

[8] Schreier, M. H., Erni, B., and Staehelin, T.: Initiation of mammalian protein synthesis. I. Purification and characterization of seven initiation factors. J. Mol. Biol. *116*:727–53, 1977.

[9] Trachsel, H., Erni, B., Schreier, M. H., and Staehelin, T.: Initiation of mammalian protein synthesis. II. The assembly of the initiation complex with purified initiation factors. J. Mol. Biol. *116*:755–67, 1977.

[10] Weissbach, H., and Ochoa, S.: Soluble factors required for eukaryotic protein synthesis. Ann. Rev. Biochem. *45*:191–216, 1976.

[11] Revel, M., and Groner, Y.: Post-transcriptional and translational controls of gene expression in eukaryotes. Ann. Rev. Biochem. *47*:1079–126, 1978.

[12] Jefferson, L. S., Rannels, D. E., Munger, B. L., and Morgan, H. E.: Insulin in the regulation of protein turnover in heart and skeletal muscle. Fed. Proc. *33*:1098–104, 1974.

[13] Kipnis, D. M., and Noall, M. W.: Stimulation of amino acid transport by insulin in the isolated rat diaphragm. Biochim. Biophys. Acta *28*:226–27, 1958.

[14] Wool, I. G., and Krahl, M. E.: Incorporation of C^{14}-amino acids into protein of isolated diaphragms: An effect of insulin independent of glucose entry. Am. J. Physiol. *196*:961–64, 1959.

[15] Davey, P. J., and Manchester, K. L.: Isolation of labeled aminoacyl transfer RNA from muscle studies of the entry of labeled amino acids into acyl transfer RNA linkage *in situ* and its control by insulin. Biochim. Biophys. Acta *182*:85–97, 1969.

[16] Manchester, K. L.: The control by insulin of amino acid accumulation in muscle. Biochem. J. *117*:457–65, 1970.

[17] Rannels, D. E., Kao, R., and Morgan, H. E.: Effect of insulin on protein turnover in heart muscle. J. Biol. Chem. *250*:1694–701, 1975.

[18] Neely, J. R., Liebermeister, H., Battersby, E. J., and Morgan, H. E.: Effect of pressure development on oxygen consumption by isolated rat heart. Am. J. Physiol. *212*:804–14, 1967.

[19] Jefferson, L. S., Li, J. B., and Rannels, S. R.: Regulation by insulin of amino acid release and protein turnover in the perfused rat hemicorpus. J. Biol. Chem. *252*:1476–83, 1977.

[20] Flaim, K. E., Copenhaver, M. E., and Jefferson, L. S.: Effects of diabetes on protein synthesis in fast- and slow-twitch rat skeletal muscle. Am. J. Physiol. In press.

[21] Pain, V. M., and Garlick, P. J.: Effect of streptozotocin diabetes and insulin treatment on the rate of protein synthesis in tissues of the rat *in vivo*. J. Biol. Chem. *249*:4510–14, 1974.

[22] Rannels, D. E., Hjalmarson, A. C., and Morgan, H. E.: Effects of noncarbohydrate substrates on protein synthesis in muscle. Am. J. Physiol. *226*:528–39, 1974.

[23] Rannels, D. E., Pegg, A. E., Rannels, S. R., and Jefferson, L. S.: Effect of starvation on the initiation of protein synthesis in skeletal muscle and heart. Am. J. Physiol. *235*:E126–E133, 1978.

[24] Farrell, P. J., Balkow, K., Hunt, T., Jackson, R. J., and Trachsel, H.: Phosphorylation of initiation factor eIF-2 and the control of reticulocyte protein synthesis. Cell *11*:187–200, 1977.

[25] Kramer, G., Cimadevilla, J. M., and Hardesty, B.: Specificity of the protein kinase activity associated with hemin-controlled repressor of rabbit reticulocyte. Proc. Natl. Acad. Sci. USA *73*:3078–82, 1976.

[26] Levin, D. H., Ranu, R. S., Ernst, V., and London, I. M.: Regulation of protein synthesis in reticulocyte lysates: Phosphorylation of methionyl-$tRNA_f$ binding factor by protein kinase activity of translational inhibitor isolated from heme-deficient lysates. Proc. Natl. Acad. Sci. USA *73*:3112–16, 1976.

[27] Clemens, M. J., Henshaw, E. C., Rahamimoff, H., and London, I. M.: Met-$tRNA_f^{Met}$ binding to 40S ribosomal subunits: A site for the regulation of initiation of protein synthesis by hemin. Proc. Natl. Acad. Sci. USA *71*:2946–50, 1974.

[28] Datta, A., deHaro, C., Sierra, J. M., and Ochoa, S.: Role of 3':5'-cyclic-AMP-dependent protein kinase in regulation of protein synthesis in reticulocyte lysates. Proc. Natl. Acad. Sci. USA *74*:1463–67, 1977.

[29] deHaro, C., Datta, A., and Ochoa, S.: Mode of action of the hemin-controlled inhibitor of protein synthesis. Proc. Natl. Acad. Sci. USA *75*:243–47, 1978.

[30] deHaro, C., and Ochoa, S.: Mode of action of the hemin-controlled inhibitor of protein synthesis: Studies with factors from rabbit reticulocytes. Proc. Natl. Acad. Sci. USA *75*:2713–16, 1978.

[31] Lenz, J. R., and Baglioni, C.: Inhibition of protein synthesis by double-stranded RNA and phosphorylation of initiation factor, eIF-2. J. Biol. Chem. *253*:4219–23, 1978.

[32] Pinphanichakarn, P., Kramer, G., and Hardesty, B.: Partial reaction of peptide initiation inhibited by the reticulocyte hemin-controlled repressor. Biochem. Biophys. Res. Commun. *73*:625–31, 1976.

[33] Ranu, R. S., London, I. M., Das, A., Dasgupta, A., Majumdar, A., Ralston, R., Roy, R., and Gupta, N. K.: Regulation of protein synthesis in rabbit reticulocyte lysates by the heme-regulated protein kinase: Inhibition of interaction of Met-$tRNA_f^{Met}$ binding factor with another initiation factor in formation of Met-$tRNA_f^{Met}$ 40S ribosomal subunit complexes. Proc. Natl. Acad. Sci. USA *75*:745–49, 1978.

[34] Adamson, S. D., Herbert, E., and Godchaux, W., III: Factors affecting the rate of protein synthesis in lysate systems from reticulocytes. Arch. Biochem. Biophys. *125*:671–83, 1968.

[35] Rabinovitz, M., Freedman, M. L., Fisher, J. M., and Maxwell, C. R.: Translational control in hemoglobin synthesis. Cold Spring Harbor Symp. Quant. Biol. *34*:567–78, 1969.

[36] Zucker, W. V., and Schulman, H. M.: Stimulation of globin-chain initiation by hemin in the reticulocyte cell-free system. Proc. Natl. Acad. Sci. USA 59:582–89, 1968.

[37] Kosower, N. S., Vanderhoff, G. A., Benerofe, B., Hunt, T., and Kosower, E. M.: Inhibition of protein synthesis by glutathione disulfide in the presence of glutathione. Biochem. Biophys. Res. Commun. *45*:816–21, 1971.

[38] Kosower, N. S., Vanderhoff, G. A., and Kosower, E. M.: Glutathione. VIII. The effects of glutathione disulfide on initiation of protein synthesis. Biochim. Biophys. Acta *272*:623–37, 1972.

[39] Ehrenfeld, E., and Hunt, T.: Double-stranded poliovirus RNA inhibits initiation of protein synthesis by reticulocyte lysates. Proc. Natl. Acad. Sci. USA *68*:1075–78, 1971.

[40] Hunt, T.: Control of globin synthesis. Br. Med. Bull. *32*:257–61, 1976.

[41] Freudenberg, H., and Mager, J.: Studies on the mechanism of the inhibition of protein synthesis induced by intracellular ATP depletion. Biochim. Biophys. Acta *232*:537–55, 1971.

[42] Giloh (Freudenberg), H., and Mager, J.: Inhibition of peptide-chain initiation in lysates from ATP-depleted cells. I. Stages in the evolution of the lesion and its reversal by thiol compounds, cyclic AMP or purine derivatives and phosphorylated sugars. Biochim. Biophys. Acta *414*:293–308, 1975.

[43] Giloh (Freudenberg), H., Schochot, L., and Mager, J.: Inhibition of peptide chain initiation in lysates from ATP-depleted cells. II. Studies on the mechanism of the lesion and its relation to similar alterations caused by oxidized glutathione and hemin deprivation. Biochim. Biophys. Acta *414*:309–20, 1975.

[44] Ernst, V., Levin, D. H., and London, I. M.: Evidence that glucose-6-phosphate regulates protein synthesis initiation in reticulocyte lysates. J. Biol. Chem. *253*:7163–72, 1978.

[45] Lang, G., and Michal, G.: D-glucose-6-phosphate and D-fructose-6-phosphate. *In* Methods of Enzymatic Analysis, Vol. 3, Bergmeyer, H. U., Ed., New York, Academic Press, 1974, pp. 1238–42.

[46] Neely, J. R., Whitfield, C. F., and Morgan, H. E.: Regulation of glycogenolysis in hearts: Effects of pressure development, glucose and FFA. J. Physiol. *219*:1083–88, 1970.

[47] Bing, R. J., Siegal, A., Ungar, I., and Gilbert, M.: Metabolism of the human heart. II. Studies on fat, ketone and amino acid metabolism. Am. J. Med. *16*:504–15, 1954.

[48] Newsholme, E. A., Randle, P. J., and Manchester, K. L.: Inhibition of the phosphofructokinase reaction in perfused rat heart by respiration of ketone bodies, fatty acids and pyruvate. Nature *193*:270–71, 1962.

[49] England, P. J., and Randle, P. J.: Effectors of rat-heart hexokinase and the control of rates of glucose phosphorylation in the perfused rat heart. Biochem. J. *105*:907–20, 1967.

[50] Neely, J. R., Bowman, R. H., and Morgan, H. E.: Effect of ventricular pressure development and palmitate on glucose transport. Am. J. Physiol. *216*:804–11, 1969.

[51] Goodman, M. N., Berger, M., and Ruderman, N. B.: Glucose metabolism in rat skeletal muscle at rest. Effect of starvation, diabetes, ketone bodies and free fatty acids. Diabetes *23*:881–88, 1974.

[52] Rennie, M. J., and Holloszy, J. O.: Inhibition of glucose uptake and glycogenolysis by availability of oleate in well-oxygenated perfused skeletal muscle. Biochem. J. *168*:161–70, 1977.

[53] Regen, D. M., Davis, W. W., Morgan, H. E., and Park, C. R.: The regulation of hexokinase and phosphofructokinase activity in heart muscle. J. Biol. Chem. *239*:43–49, 1964.

[54] Lawrence, J. C., Jr., and Larner, J.: Activation of glycogen synthase in rat adipocytes by insulin and glucose involves increased glucose transport and phosphorylation. J. Biol. Chem. *253*:2104–13, 1978.

[55] Green, M., and Miller, L. L.: Protein catabolism and protein synthesis in perfused livers of normal and alloxan diabetic rats. J. Biol. Chem. *235*:3202–08, 1960.

[56] Penhos, J. C., and Krahl, M. E.: Stimulus of leucine incorporation into perfused liver protein by insulin. Am. J. Physiol. *204*:140–42, 1963.

[57] Mortimore, G. E., and Mondon, C. E.: Inhibition by insulin of valine turnover in liver. J. Biol. Chem. *245*:2375–83, 1970.

[58] Marsh, J. B.: The effects of fasting and alloxan diabetes on albumin synthesis by perfused rat liver. Am. J. Physiol. *201*:55–57, 1961.

[59] Morgan, C. R., and Jersild, R. A., Jr.: Alterations in the morphology of rat liver cells influenced by insulin. *Anat. Rec.* *166*:575–86, 1969.

[60] Pain, V. M., Lanoix, J., Bergeron, J. J. M., and Clemens, M. J.: Effect of diabetes on the ultrastructure of the hepatocyte and on the distribution and activity of ribosomes in the free and membrane-bound populations. Biochim. Biophys. Acta *353*:487–98, 1974.

[61] Peterson, D. T., Alford, F. P., Reaven, E. P., Ueyama, I., and Reaven, G. M.: Characteristics of membrane-bound and free hepatic ribosomes from insulin-treated rats. I. Acute experimental diabetes mellitus. J. Clin. Invest. *52*:3201–11, 1973.

[62] Reaven, E. P., Peterson, D. T., and Reaven, G. M.: The effect of experimental diabetes mellitus and insulin replacement on hepatic ultrastructure and protein synthesis. J. Clin. Invest. *52*:248–62, 1973.

[63] Peavy, D. E., Taylor, J. M., and Jefferson, L. S.: Regulation of hepatic albumin and total protein synthesis in normal and diabetic rats. Diabetes *28*:390, 1979.

Rapid Publication

Monolayer Cultures of Adult Pancreatic Islet Cells on Osmotically Disrupted Fibroblasts

P. MEDA, E. L. HOOGHE-PETERS, AND L. ORCI

SUMMARY

A simple method that permits the attachment of fully dissociated adult pancreatic islet cells to culture dishes, using osmotically disrupted fibroblasts, is described. Using this system, monolayer cultures consisting of either isolated or clustered adult endocrine islet cells can be readily established in standard culture media. DIABETES *29*:497–500, June 1980.

Several methods have been devised to establish monolayer cultures of endocrine islet cells from fetal and newborn pancreas.[4,7] The development of similar cultures using either whole or partially disrupted adult islets[1,5] has been complicated by the fact that only restricted regions of true monolayer form and, often, these are rapidly overgrown by fibroblasts. These limitations can be partially overcome by culturing whole, isolated islets in the presence of the phosphodiesterase inhibitor IBMX.[12] However, up to now, no method has been available for the preparation of monolayer cultures of adult islet cells without this drug and/or starting from a suspension of single islet cells. Dissociated islet cells have been consistently reported to adhere poorly to a variety of culture supports and to reaggregate, rapidly and spontaneously, into free-floating clumps.[5,13]

We describe here a simple method to promote the attachment of dissociated endocrine cells from islets of adult rats. According to the cell density selected at the time of plating, this system can be used to prepare monolayers in which the attached islet cells are either cultured isolated from each other or in which they have reaggregated to form large clusters.

From the Institute of Histology and Embryology, University of Geneva Medical School, 1211 Geneva 4, Switzerland.
Address reprint requests to P. Meda, M.D., Institute of Histology and Embryology, University of Geneva Medical School, CH-1211 Geneva 4, Switzerland.
Received for publication 18 March 1980.

MATERIALS AND METHODS

Isolation of islet cells. Islets of Langerhans were isolated by collagenase digestion[6] from the pancreas of male Wistar rats weighing 250–350 g. The isolated islets were first incubated for 60 min at 37°C in a Krebs-Ringer-bicarbonate (KRB) Ca^{2+}-free medium containing 16.7 mM glucose, 0.5% BSA, and 3 mM EGTA (Fluka AG, Buchs, Switzerland). At the end of the incubation, the islets were transferred into a KRB Ca^{2+}-free medium without EGTA but containing 16.7 mM glucose, 0.1% BSA, and 0.1% trypsin (Difco, 1:250) and disrupted at room temperature by 10 aspirations through three pipettes of decreasing tip diameter. The islet cell suspension (consisting of, at that stage, single cells and cell clumps) was then suspended in 10 ml of the trypsin-containing medium and incubated at 37°C in a spinner flask. Samples of this preparation were taken every 2 min and examined under a phase contrast microscope to check for the complete dissociation of islet cells. The incubation was stopped after 6–7 min by adding to the cell suspension a large volume of cold (4°C) sterile tissue culture medium 199 (Grand Island Biol. Co., Grand Island, New York) containing 16.7 mM glucose, 10% heat-inactivated fetal calf serum, 400 U/ml penicillin, and 200 μg/ml streptomycin (standard culture medium). The single cell suspension was then centrifuged at 700 *g* at room temperature for 8 min and the cell pellet resuspended in 10 ml of standard culture medium. The latter procedure was repeated twice more before plating the cells.

Preparation of fibroblasts. Fibroblasts were obtained from the first decantation of the enzymatically disrupted newborn rat pancreas used to prepare islet cell monolayer cultures according to Lambert et al.[7] Fibroblasts were grown to confluence in standard culture medium and then detached from the Petri dishes by a 3-min incubation at 37°C in Ca^{2+}- and Mg^{2+}-free PBS, followed by a 3–5-min incubation in the same PBS containing 5 mg/ml of trypsin (Difco, 1:250). The cells were then centrifuged at 1600 *g* for 10 min, resuspended in standard medium, and grown to confluence in 35-mm Petri dishes (Falcon Plastics, Oxnard, California). This procedure was repeated at least twice to eliminate the rare nonfibroblastoid cells present before the fibroblasts were used for the islet cell cultures.

Preparation of Petri dishes. Confluent fibroblasts at a passage number of 3–9 were used as substratum for islet cell culture. The culture medium was aspirated and the cells exposed for 3 min at room temperature to distilled, sterile water. The water was then removed and the dishes, still covered with the sheet of osmotically disrupted cells, were stored at 4°C for up to 1 mo.

Preparation of fibroblast-conditioned medium. Confluent pancreatic fibroblasts were washed with standard medium and subsequently cultured in the same medium for 3 days. The medium was aspirated, filtered through a 0.22-μm millipore filter (Millipore Corp., Bedford, Massachusetts), and stored at 4°C for up to 1 wk.

Culture of islet cells. The single cell suspension was plated either in standard culture medium on fibroblast-coated dishes or in fibroblast-conditioned medium on uncoated dishes. Under both conditions, 6×10^4 cells (i.e., the equivalent of about 20 islets) or 5×10^5 cells (i.e., the equivalent of about 150 islets) in 2 ml of medium, were cultured in each 35-mm Petri dish to produce low and high density cultures, respectively. The cells were cultured at 37°C in a humidified incubator gassed with air and CO_2, the CO_2 content being automatically regulated to maintain medium pH at 7.4. The medium was changed twice per week.

Immunofluorescence staining. Seven-day-old cultures were fixed overnight in Zamboni's fluid and subsequently stained by the indirect immunofluorescence technique[2] using a monospecific guinea pig anti-insulin serum (a gift from Dr. P. H. Wright) at a dilution of 1:50. After incubation with the antiserum, the cultures were washed in PBS, exposed to fluorescein-labeled sheep anti-guinea pig Ig (Pasteur Institute, Paris, France), counterstained with 0.01% Evans blue, and examined in a Zeiss ICM 405 inverted microscope equipped with an incident light excitation device (2 FL).

RESULTS

At the time of plating, the islet cell suspensions used in these experiments consisted almost exclusively of fully dissociated, single cells (Figure 1). After culture for up to 1 wk, these cells failed to attach to standard, uncoated plastic Petri dishes. Some of the unattached cells remained isolated and displayed degenerative changes. The others spontaneously reaggregated, first forming linear aggregates and then clumps. Similar results were obtained by seeding the single-cell preparation on collagen-coated dishes prepared as described in ref. 3.

FIGURE 1. Dark-field photograph of the dissociated islet cells at the time of plating. Note that a large proportion of the cells are present as single cells. (×50)

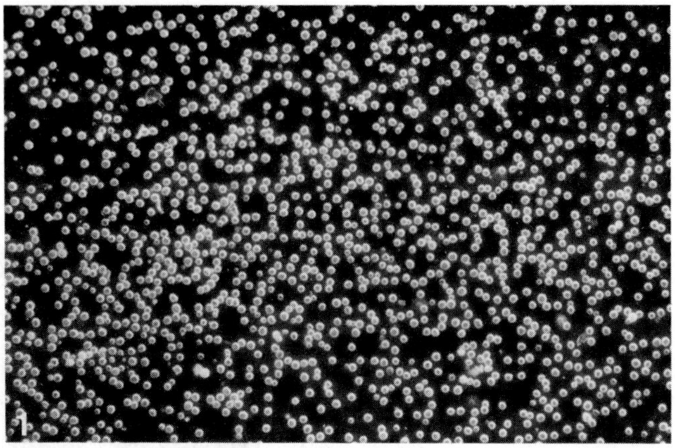

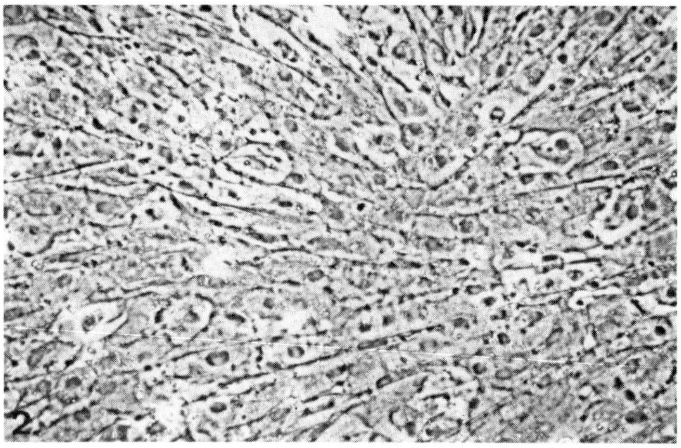

FIGURE 2. Appearance of the fibroblast monolayer after exposure to distilled water and storage at 4°C. (×130)

In contrast, when cultures were established on monolayers of osmotically disrupted fibroblasts (Figure 2), a large proportion of the seeded single islet cells firmly attached to the dish within 3 days of culture (first change of the medium), irrespective of the cell density plated. At that time, the cultures established by seeding a high density of single cells consisted mainly of attached islet cells, which had formed large clusters, while the cultures prepared by plating a low density of cells consisted mostly of attached but isolated cells. After 7 days, the clustered endocrine cells observed in high density cultures (Figure 3) were more flattened than after 3 days, while most of the isolated islet cells found in low density cultures still had a spherical shape (Figure 5). At that stage, the dead fibroblasts of the substratum had partially lifted off the culture dishes.

Most of the endocrine cells were clearly stained with the immunofluorescence technique using a specific anti-insulin serum in both high (Figure 4) and low density (Figure 6) cultures. Electron microscopy confirmed that these cells were fully differentiated B-cells containing a variable, but usually high number of typical secretory granules. Ultrastructurally, these cells appeared well preserved throughout the culture irrespective of whether they were isolated from each other or had formed clusters. In the latter case, numerous intercellular junctions were observed between adjacent cells (not shown). Immunofluorescence with monospecific antisera and electron microscopy demonstrated that fully differentiated, well-granulated glucagon-, somatostatin-, and pancreatic polypeptide-containing cells were also present in high and low density cultures (not shown).

To determine whether the presence of killed fibroblasts was necessary for the cell attachment observed, single-cell suspensions from adult islets were plated in a fibroblast-conditioned medium on uncoated Petri dishes. Although the fibroblast-conditioned medium slightly enhanced the attachment of adult islet cells, as compared with standard culture medium, it was markedly less effective than a sheet of dead fibroblasts in promoting such an effect.

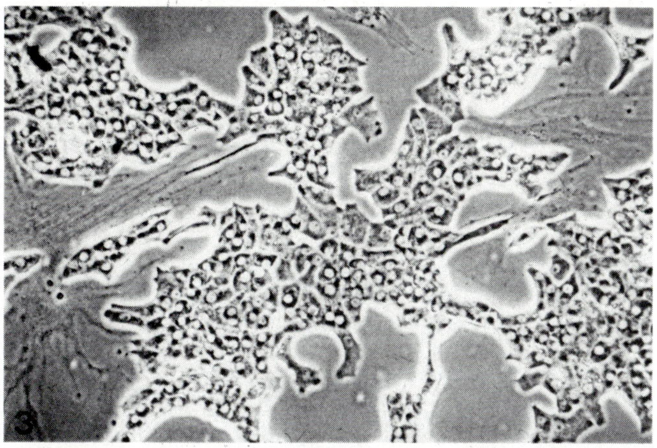

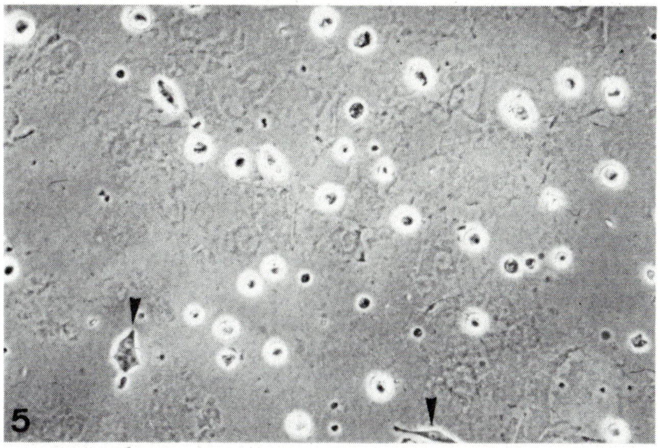

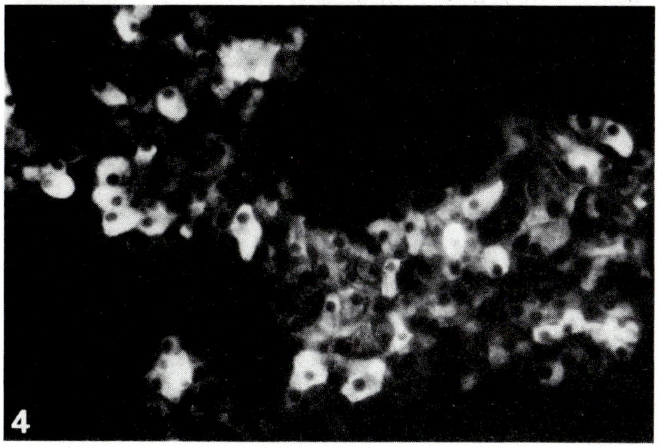

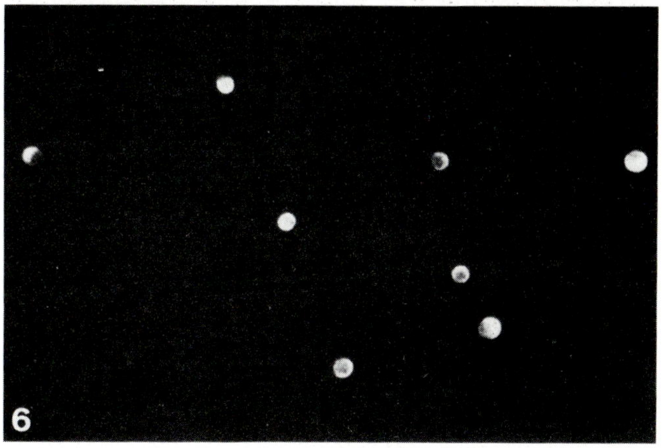

FIGURES 3 and 4. Adult islet cells cultured for 7 days on osmotically disrupted fibroblasts (high density culture). Figure 3: Large cluster of islet cells. Note that the osmotically disrupted fibroblasts have partially lifted off the dish surface and that living fibroblasts are rare. (×130) Figure 4: A cluster of endocrine islet cells has been stained by the indirect immunofluorescence technique for insulin. The intensity of the stain varies from cell to cell, probably reflecting their different content in secretory granules. (×170)

FIGURES 5 and 6. Adult islet cells cultured for 7 days on osmotically disrupted fibroblasts (low density culture). Figure 5: The islet cells attached to the Petri dish are separated from each other. Most of them maintain a spherical shape while others (arrowheads) are flattened. (×130) Figure 6: Isolated islet cells are clearly stained with the indirect immunofluorescence technique for insulin. (×215)

DISCUSSION

The cells of adult islets of Langerhans, like other adult differentiated cells, adhere poorly to a variety of culture supports when fully dissociated and, usually, rapidly reaggregate into free-floating clumps.[5,13] This behavior has prevented the culture of adult islet cells as single cells and may be responsible for the progressive dedifferentiation observed with time in free-floating islet cell cultures.[13] Living or killed fibroblasts have been reported to enhance the attachment and survival of specialized cells in primary cultures and to partially preserve their differentiation.[3,9,15] The results reported here show that the attachment of fully dissociated adult islet cells is markedly promoted on a sheet of osmotically disrupted fibroblasts.

Using this substratum, monolayer cultures of adult islet cells were readily established in a standard culture medium whatever the density of isolated cells plated. At a high density, the dissociated islet cells reaggregated to form monolayer clusters which, in our hands, were usually larger than the clusters obtained, from a similar amount of islet tissue, with previously described culture methods.[5,12] In contrast, at a low density, the dissociated islet cells attached to the disrupted fibroblasts without reaggregation and remained well separated from each other throughout the culture period. This type of culture provides, for the first time, a system to study single islet cells under well-defined conditions, since the cells can recover from the isolation procedure and be subsequently studied for several days on a support that prevents their reaggregation.

Morphologic characterization showed that both high and low density cultures included the four main types of endocrine cells that are found in whole rat islets.[8] At all times studied, the cells appeared well preserved and virtually identical to the corresponding cells observed in the islets. In particular, both isolated and clustered cultured islet cells stored their characteristic hormone and contained typical secretory granules.

It is uncertain why the sheet of disrupted fibroblasts improved the attachment of adult single islet cells more efficiently than the fibroblast-conditioned medium which, in other systems, markedly promoted cell attachment.[10,11] Work is now in progress to determine whether the factor(s) required for islet cell attachment is(are) soluble and whether, therefore, a conditioned medium prepared under particular conditions may totally replace the cell-derived substratum. In this context, it is nevertheless worth mentioning that fibroblast-conditioned medium has been reported to enhance the survival of B-cells in whole adult rat islets without promoting the adhesion of such islets to the culture dishes throughout 4 wk of culture.[14]

In summary, we have shown that the attachment of adult dissociated islet cells is markedly promoted using a substratum of osmotically disrupted fibroblasts. This system greatly facilitates the establishment of monolayers of clustered islet cells and allows the preparation of cultures in which islet cells are maintained isolated from each other for several days.

ACKNOWLEDGMENTS

It is a pleasure to thank Dr. M. Amherdt for providing the pancreatic fibroblasts and C. Curut, H. Geser, M. Sidler-Ansermet, and N. Maalaoui for technical assistance. This work was supported by the Swiss National Science Foundation, grant 3.120.77, and by a grant-in-aid from Hoechst AG, Frankfurt, West Germany.

REFERENCES

[1] Andersson, A., Hellerström, C., and Petersson, B.: Phase-contrast microscopy of fresh and cultured pancreatic islet cells of guinea-pigs. Z. Zellforsch. *82*:110–17, 1967.

[2] Coons, A. H., Leduc, E. H., and Connolly, J. M.: Studies on antibody production. I. A method for the histochemical demonstration of specific antibody and its application to a study of hyperimmune rabbit. J. Exp. Med. *102*:49–60, 1955.

[3] Hawrot, E.: Cultured sympathetic neurons: Effects of cell-derived and synthetic substrata on survival and development. Dev. Biol. *74*:136–51, 1980.

[4] Hilwig, I., Schuster, S., Heptner, W., and Wasielewski, E. V.: Über das wachstum der Pankreaszellen von Säugetieren als monolayer cultures. I. Züchtungsmethode, Morphologie und Insulingehalt. Z. Zellforsch. *90*:333–46, 1968.

[5] Kostianovsky, M., McDaniel, M. L., Still, M. F., Codilla, R. C., and Lacy, P. E.: Monolayer cell culture of adult rat islets of Langerhans. Diabetologia *10*:337–44, 1974.

[6] Lacy, P. E., and Kostianovsky, M.: Method for the isolation of intact islets of Langerhans from the rat pancreas. Diabetes *16*:35–39, 1967.

[7] Lambert, A. E., Blondel, B., Kanazawa, Y., Orci, L., and Renold, A. E.: Monolayer cell culture of neonatal rat pancreas: light microscopy and evidence for immunoreactive insulin synthesis and release. Endocrinology *90*:239–48, 1972.

[8] Larsson, L.-I., Sundler, F., and Håkanson, R.: Pancreatic polypeptide —a postulated new hormone: identification of its cellular storage site by light and electron microscopic immunocytochemistry. Diabetologia *12*:211–26, 1976.

[9] Michalopoulos, G., Russell, F., and Biles, C.: Primary cultures of hepatocytes on human fibroblasts. In Vitro *15*:796–806, 1979.

[10] Millis, A. J. T., Hoyle, M., and Field, B.: Human fibroblast conditioned media contains growth-promoting activities for low density cells. J. Cell Physiol. *93*:17–24, 1977.

[11] Moore, E. G.: Cell to substratum adhesion-promoting activity released by normal and virus-transformed cells in culture. J. Cell Biol. *70*:634–47, 1976.

[12] Ohgawara, H., Carroll, R., Hofmann, C., Takahashi, C., Kikuchi, M., Labrecque, A., Hirata, Y., and Steiner, D. F.: Promotion of monolayer formation in cultured whole pancreatic islets by 3-isobutyl-1-methylxanthine. Proc. Natl. Acad. Sci. USA *75*:1897–1900, 1978.

[13] Ono, J., Takaki, R., Okano, H., and Fukuma, M.: Long-term culture of pancreatic islet cells with special reference to the β-cell function. In Vitro *15*:95–102, 1979.

[14] Rabinovitch, A., Russell, T., and Mintz, D. H.: Factors from fibroblasts promote pancreatic islet B cell survival in tissue culture. Diabetes *28*:1108–13, 1979.

[15] Stoker, M., O'Neill, C., Berryman, S., and Waxman, V.: Anchorage and growth regulation in normal and virus-transformed cells. Int. J. Cancer *3*:683–93, 1968.

MAY 1980 VOLUME 29 SUPPLEMENT 2

diabetes

PROGRAM

40th Annual Meeting

SCIENTIFIC PROGRAMS

Sunday, June 15

Monday, June 16

Tuesday, June 17

1980

SHERATON WASHINGTON HOTEL
Washington, D.C.

DIAEAZ 29 (Supplement 2)
1A-143A (1980)

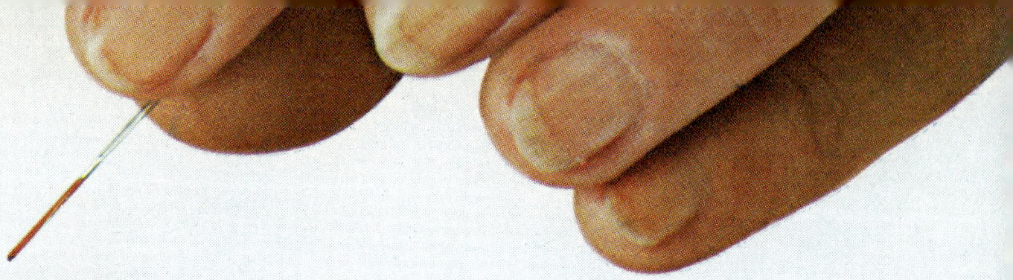

Upjohn

ON THE FRONTIERS OF DIABETIC RESEARCH...

What is Diabetes?

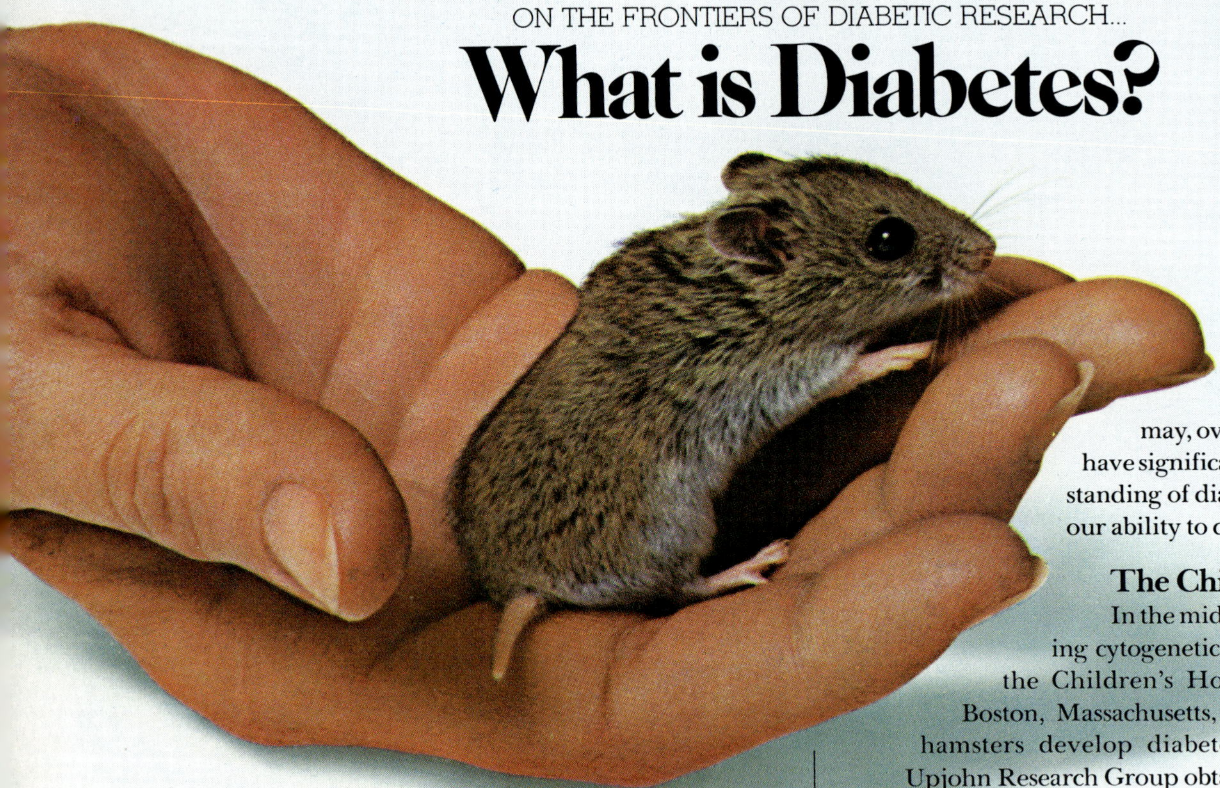

Although a medical scribe of ancient Egypt first made reference to diabetes mellitus in man, today, nearly 4000 years later, only meager specific knowledge exists as to the basic cause of the disease. Without such knowledge it has been possible to provide for limited control only *after* diabetes manifests itself in the form of elevated blood glucose. The possibility of prevention or even cure of diabetes, however, must depend on a full understanding of the genetic defect and/or defects underlying the disease. Our current understanding of diabetes may be compared to our former understanding of another disease of metabolic abnormality, phenylketonuria; only when the genetic lesion of that disease was discovered did it become possible to institute current programs of treatment.

Basic Diabetes Research at Upjohn

For more than fifteen years the Diabetes and Atherosclerosis Research Group at The Upjohn Company (W. E. Dulin, Manager; G. C. Gerritsen; A. Y. Chang) has addressed itself, in a series of unique experiments, to the very basic question: What is diabetes? As with all such fundamental research, practical results are slow in coming and the work of the Group has at times raised more questions than it has been able to answer. It appears now, however, that the research is moving toward important conclusions which may, over the next several years, have significant bearing on our understanding of diabetes and, hopefully, on our ability to control it.

The Chinese Hamsters

In the middle fifties, a group studying cytogenetics in Chinese hamsters at the Children's Hospital Medical Center, Boston, Massachusetts, discovered that certain hamsters develop diabetes spontaneously. The Upjohn Research Group obtained some of these hamsters in 1962, and by controlled inbreeding, succeeded over the years in producing large numbers of diabetic animals for study. To assure continuity of the research in the event of a catastrophe, duplicate breeding stock of all the inbred families are maintained at another site. These are the only such colonies in the United States today. In the course of the research, Upjohn has cooperated with scientists in academic

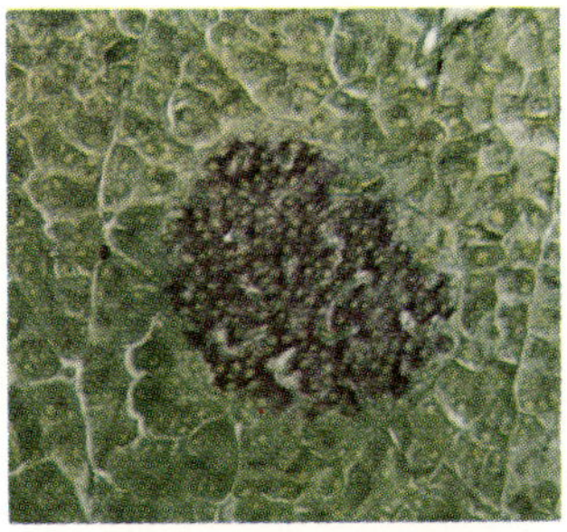

Normal Chinese hamster, pancreatic tissue. Note blue-stained insulin granules which appear within the beta cells of the islet of Langerhans.

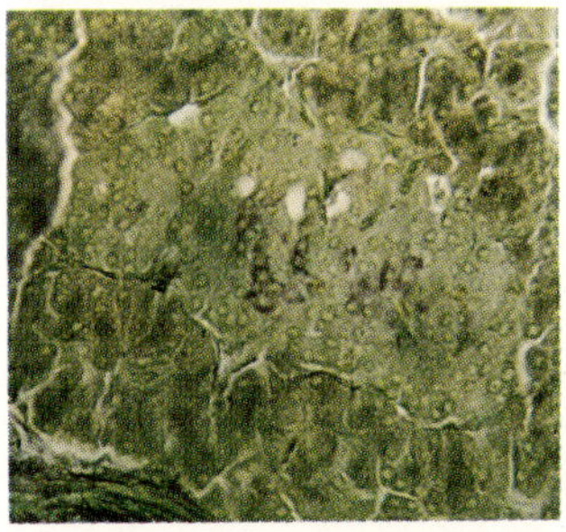

Diabetic Chinese hamster, pancreatic tissue. Insulin granules are almost totally absent. Though beta cells are present, there is some degranulization and vacuolization. The diabetic process is similar to that observed in human pancreatic tissue.

PROCEEDINGS OF A CONFERENCE ON PANCREAS TRANSPLANTATION
JUNE 8 AND 9, 1979, LOS ANGELES, CALIFORNIA

INTRODUCTION v

Adult Whole Pancreas or Segment

Early Experiments in Human Pancreas Transplantation FREDERICK C. GOETZ 1

Segmental Pancreatic Transplantation with Duct Ligation or Drainage to a Jejunal Roux-en-Y Loop in Nonuremic Diabetic Patients C. G. GROTH, G. LUNDGREN, R. GUNNARSSON, P. ARNER, B. BERG, AND J. ÖSTMAN 3

Clinical Segmental Pancreas Transplantation without Duct Anastomosis in Diabetic Renal Allograft Recipients DAVID E. R. SUTHERLAND, FREDERICK C. GOETZ, AND JOHN S. NAJARIAN 10

Adult Islets

Isolating the Elusive Islet DAVID W. SCHARP, RICHARD DOWNING, RONALD C. MERRELL, AND MARIE GREIDER 19

Transplantation of Dispersed Pancreatic Islet Tissue in Humans: Autografts and Allografts DAVID E. R. SUTHERLAND, ARTHUR J. MATAS, FREDERICK C. GOETZ, AND JOHN S. NAJARIAN 31

Alternatives in Pancreatic Islet Transplantation: Tissue Culture Studies KEITH REEMTSMA, COLLIN J. WEBER, F. XAVIER PI-SUNYER, ROGER L. LERNER, AND MARK A. HARDY 45

Evaluating the Benefits of Human Islet Transplantation FREDERICK C. GOETZ

DISCUSSION: SECTIONS ON WHOLE-ORGAN AND ISLET TRANSPLANTATION 56

Human Fetal Pancreas

Perifusion and Culture of Human Fetal Pancreas JANICE E. MAITLAND, DAVID G. PARRY, AND JOHN R. TURTLE 57

Human Fetal Pancreas: Culture and Function in Vitro A. ÅGREN, A. ANDERSSON, C. BJÖRKÉN, C. G. GROTH, R. GUNNARSSON, C. HELLERSTRÖM, G. LINDMARK, G. LUNDQVIST, B. PETERSSON, AND I. SWENNE 64

Cryopreservation of Human Fetal Pancreas JOSIAH BROWN, JOHN A. KEMP, SUSAN HURT, AND WILLIAM R. CLARK 70

Transplantation of Human Fetal Pancreas: Experience in Thymusaplastic Mice and Rats and in a Diabetic Patient K. H. USADEL, U. SCHWEDES, G. BASTERT, U. STEINAU, I. KLEMPA, W. FASSBINDER, AND K. SCHÖFFLING 74

Transplantation of Fetal Pancreatic Microfragments via the Portal Vein to a Diabetic Patient C. G. GROTH, A. ANDERSSON, C. BJÖRKÉN, R. GUNNARSSON, C. HELLERSTRÖM, G. LUNDGREN, B. PETERSSON, I. SWENNE, AND J. ÖSTMAN 80

DISCUSSION: SECTIONS ON HUMAN FETAL PANCREAS 84

Rejection and Donor Treatment

Immunologic Problems in Islet Transplantation CLYDE F. BARKER, ALI NAJI, AND WILLYS K. SILVERS 86

Effect of Culture on Islet Rejection PAUL E. LACY, JOSEPH M. DAVIE, AND EDWARD H. FINKE 93

Successful Allotransplantation of Mouse Pancreatic Islets to Nonimmunosuppressed Recipients KERRY M. BOWEN, LINDA ANDRUS, AND KEVIN J. LAFFERTY 98

The Effects of Oxygen, Temperature, and Time of Culture on the Survival of Mouse Thyroid and Pancreas Allografts DAVID W. TALMAGE	**105**
Suppression of Rejection of Allogeneic Islet Tissue in the Rat P. J. MORRIS, D. R. FINCH, J. F. GARVEY, M. D. POOLE, AND P. R. MILLARD	**107**
Specific Immunosuppression for Fetal Pancreas Allografts in Rats YOKO MULLEN	**113**
Immunosuppression and Organ Transplantation Tolerance Using Total Lymphoid Irradiation SHIMON SLAVIN, SAMUEL STROBER, ZVI FUKS, AND HENRY S. KAPLAN	**121**
DISCUSSION: SECTIONS ON REJECTION AND DONOR TREATMENT	**125**
INDEX	**126**

Early Experiments in Human Pancreas Transplantation

FREDERICK C. GOETZ

The first systematic trials of human pancreas transplantation began in late December 1966, although there had been occasional attempts to implant islet tissue before this in the form of benign insulin-secreting tumors. This report will briefly summarize the first phase of human pancreas transplantation, in which part or all of the gland was transplanted with direct vascular connections in the recipient.

The first such transplant was carried out by Kelly, Lillehei, and associates in late 1966.[1] The general anatomy of the transplant is shown in Figure 1. The body and tail of the pancreas (and also a kidney) from a patient who died during heart surgery were transplanted into a 20-yr-old woman who had had diabetes for 19 yr. An attempt to solve the problem of the digestive secretion was made by ligating the pancreatic duct and oversewing the cut end of the pancreas. Irradiation with cobalt 60 was given to the region of the graft.

This patient tolerated withdrawal of insulin for about 6 days before rising blood sugars necessitated resumption of insulin injections. Pancreas and kidney grafts remained in place for about 2 mo and then were removed. The patient died soon thereafter of venous complications, which were probably related to the grafting procedure.

Although the method of handling the digestive secretion was modified immediately by Lillehei,[2] Gliedman,[3] and others, the total of 49 pancreas grafts reported through 1975[4] usually followed the same general approach as described here. The principal modification introduced by Lillehei was the inclusion of at least a small portion of the donor duodenum to provide a conduit for the digestive juice either to the abdominal wall or to the small intestine.

A brief summary of the major points learned from whole-organ pancreas transplantation may be useful as an introduction to this symposium. The summary is based especially on the experience of Kelly and Lillehei or of Lillehei alone in 14 transplant cases at the University of Minnesota.

1. Hormonal effectiveness in some cases is striking. More than one-half of the Minnesota patients were able to maintain near-normal fasting and postmeal glucose values and essentially normal glucose tolerance test results (Figure 2) without insulin injections for periods from 1 to 11 mo.

2. Mortality and morbidity, by contrast, have been very high. The longest survival time for patients in the Minnesota experience was 11 mo and in the world experience a little over 4 yr.[5] Complications and causes of death varied but, in general, included sepsis, failure of the simultaneous kidney graft, and in some cases necrosis of the duodenal portion of the graft.

3. Uremia may be a necessary prerequisite for prolonged acceptance of a pancreas graft. The grafts of three Minnesota patients with moderately advanced kidney disease showed initially a highly favorable course, followed by abrupt failure at 1–12 wk, possibly through immune rejection. The patients survived the removal of the graft. Nonuremic patients can accept a pancreas graft but may reject it more readily at an early stage (3 mo or less).

Thus, it was clear by 1974 that highly effective endocrine function from transplantation of the pancreas was possible and that direct vascular anastomosis of a single pancreas was probably adequate to reverse the obvious metabolic features of diabetes. The risk of the procedure remained high. As transplantation of a kidney as a separate treatment for diabetic nephropathy gained ground, justification for the more experimental, simultaneous pancreas and kidney transplantation was difficult to maintain. It must be emphasized that transplantation of the endocrine pancreas at best is not a life-saving procedure but serves the purpose only of ameliorating the diabetic state. The challenge is to provide something clearly better than conventional insulin treatment.*

From the Section of Endocrinology and Metabolism, Department of Medicine, University of Minnesota Hospitals and Medical School, Minneapolis, Minnesota 55455.
Address reprint requests to F. C. Goetz, M.D., Box 93, University Hospitals, Minneapolis, Minnesota 55455.

*Detailed summaries of work up to 1974 will be found in references 6 and 7.

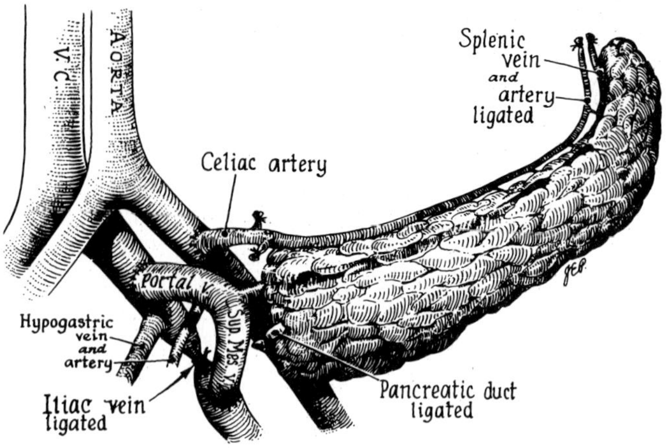

FIGURE 1. General surgical anatomy of the first human transplantation of the pancreas. Effluent blood from the duct-ligated pancreas segment flows into the iliac vein of the recipient. (Reproduced with permission of author and publisher, from Kelly et al., Surgery *61*:827–37, 1967.)[1]

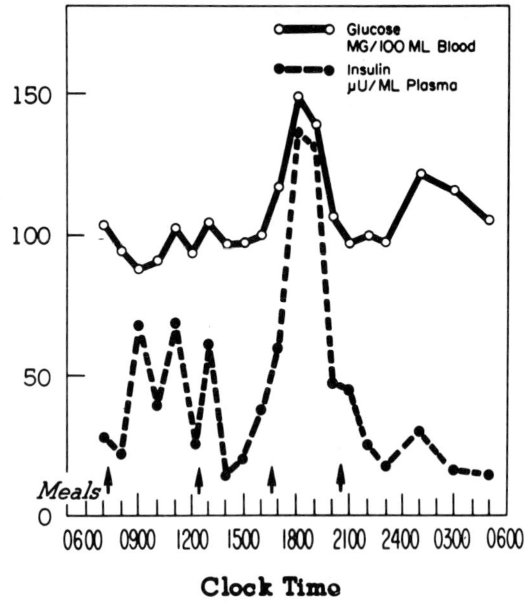

FIGURE 2. Plasma glucose and insulin levels before and after meals in a juvenile diabetic patient with a functioning whole-pancreas graft. (From the case records of R. C. Lillehei and F. C. Goetz.)

REFERENCES

[1] Kelly, W. D., Lillehei, R. C., Merkel, F. K., Idezuki, Y., and Goetz, F. C.: Allotransplantation of the pancreas and duodenum along with the kidney in diabetic nephropathy. Surgery *61*: 827–37, 1967.

[2] Lillehei, R. C., Idezuki, Y., Kelly, W. D., Najarian, J. S., Merkel, F. K., and Goetz, F. C.: Transplantation of the intestine and pancreas. Transplant. Proc. *1*:230–38, 1969.

[3] Gliedman, M. L., Gold, M., Whittaker, J., Rifkin, H., Soberman, R., Freed, S. Z., and Tellis, V. A.: Clinical segmental pancreatic transplantation with ureter-pancreatic duct anastomosis for exocrine drainage. Surgery *74*:171–80, 1973.

[4] Bergan, J. J.: American College of Surgeons/National Institutes of Health Organ Transplant Registry. Newsletter No. 16, April 1976.

[5] Gliedman, M. L., Tellis, V. A., Soberman, R., Rifkin, H., and Veith, F. J.: Long-term effects of pancreatic transplant function in patients with advanced juvenile-onset diabetes. Diabetes Care *1*:1–9, 1978.

[6] Goetz, F. C.: Conference on beta cell function, transplantation, and implantable glucose sensors: a summary. Metabolism *23*:875–84, 1974.

[7] Barker, C. F.: Transplantation of the islets of Langerhans and the histocompatibility of endocrine tissue. Report of a conference. Diabetes *24*:766–75, 1975.

Segmental Pancreatic Transplantation with Duct Ligation or Drainage to a Jejunal Roux-en-Y Loop in Nonuremic Diabetic Patients

C. G. GROTH, G. LUNDGREN, R. GUNNARSSON, P. ARNER, B. BERG, AND J. ÖSTMAN

SUMMARY

The results of seven segmental pancreas transplantations in diabetic patients, using a jejunal Roux-en-Y loop for drainage of digestive enzymes, are presented. An initial case with pancreatic duct ligation is also included. The patients ranged in age from 30 to 45 yr, with duration of diabetes from 8 to 24 yr, and were incapacitated but not uremic. Immunosuppression was attempted with azathioprine, prednisone, and antilymphocyte globulin, and, in one patient, thoracic duct drainage was added. The pancreas tolerated at least 16 min of warm ischemia and at least 4 h of cold storage; flushing with a balanced electrolyte solution was optimal. Six of the grafts provided control of blood glucose for 7–51 days, and, in one patient, an intravenous glucose tolerance test was normal at 7 and 21 days. Five of the grafts failed due to rejection 7–51 days after transplantation, and one was removed at 14 days, while still functioning, due to bleeding. In one case, early detection of rejection by a rise in postprandial blood glucose was treated and reversed by corticosteroid administration. Two failed in the immediate postoperative period from vascular thrombosis. Drainage of pancreatic secretions from a fistula was a common problem. DIABETES *29* (Suppl. 1):3–9, 1980.

Pancreas transplantation as a means of providing the diabetic patient with normally functioning B cells now has a 13-yr history.[1] Whereas the early workers used a pancreaticoduodenal transplant,[1–3] most investigators today favor a segmental, body and tail, pancreatic graft. This segment contains enough islets to correct diabetes and has its own blood supply from the splenic vessels. The chief advantages of this approach are (1) easy harvesting of the graft, (2) simple two-vessel revascularization, and (3) dispensation with the need to transplant bowel as well as the glandular tissue. This technique was pioneered by Gliedman and co-workers,[4] who performed transplantation in uremic diabetics and provided for exocrine drainage by pancreatic duct-to-ureter anastomosis. In two recipients, graft function exceeded 1 yr. An additional case in which the ureter was used as a conduit has been reported by Merkel and co-workers.[5]

The use of an intestinal Roux-en-Y loop for exocrine drainage from a segmental pancreatic graft was first reported by Groth and associates.[6] Experience with this technique has since been reported by Largiadér[7] and Gliedman[8] and their collaborators.

The purpose of this communication is to report the experience we have gained from seven segmental pancreatic transplantations using a jejunal Roux-en-Y loop for drainage. Reference will also be made to an initial transplantation where no provision was made for exocrine drainage but where the pancreatic duct was ligated. Emphasis is placed on aspects of organ preservation, surgical technique, and graft rejection. Findings concerning islet autoantibodies and insulin antibodies will also be reported.

PATIENTS AND METHODS

The patients. Our series consists of eight attempts at segmental pancreatic transplantation in six nonuremic diabetic patients; there were thus two second attempts. The patients ranged in age from 30 to 45 yr. They had had diabetes for between 8 and 24 yr. The indications for transplantation differed (Table 1). All patients were severely incapacitated by the disease, but none of them was uremic.

Graft function and patient survival. Within the first two postoperative days, one first-time graft developed venous thrombosis and one second-time graft developed arterial thrombosis. Six of the grafts provided control of blood glucose for 7–51 days (Table 1). While the grafts were functioning, an intravenous glucose tolerance test (25 g) was carried out in two patients; in one it was normal (Figure 1), while in the other it was abnormal with a prolonged period of hyperglycemia. Five of the grafts failed owing to rejection

From the Departments of Surgery and Medicine, Karolinska Institute, Huddinge Hospital, Stockholm, Sweden.
Address reprint requests to Dr. C. G. Groth, Department of Surgery, Huddinge Hospital, S-141 86 Huddinge, Sweden.

TABLE 1
Segmental pancreas transplantations at Huddinge Hospital, Stockholm

Transplant no.	Pt.	Sex	Age (yr)	Date of transplant	Indication for transplant	Duration of graft function (days) Cause of failure
Duct ligation						
1	H.T.	M	31	5/4/74	Hyperlabile diabetes	41 Graft rejection
Pancreaticojejunostomy						
2	H.E.	M	43	24/9/74	Labile diabetes and progressive angiopathy	1 Venous thrombosis
3	H.N.	M	39	23/1/75	Loss of vision due to optic nerve atrophy	35 Graft rejection
4	M.S.	F	35	4/11/75	Labile diabetes and sensory neuropathy	7 Graft rejection and wound abscess
5	H.N. (2nd)	M	40	13/3/76		0 Arterial thrombosis
6	H.E. (2nd)	M	45	19/11/76		14 Arterial bleeding*
Ductojejunostomy						
7	T.J.	M	32	5/4/78	Progressive angiopathy	51 Graft rejection
8	C.G.	F	30	27/10/78	Progressive angiopathy and sensory neuropathy	43 Graft rejection†,*

* Patient died.
† After withdrawal of immunosuppression.

(Figure 2, top) and one had to be removed while still functioning (Figure 2, bottom) because of potentially fatal arterial bleeding. Four of the six patients are still living after removal of the nonfunctioning graft. The patient with severe bleeding (H. E., second transplant) had a stormy course with pneumonia, septicemia, and gastrointestinal hemorrhage and eventually died. Patient C. G. suffered anoxic brain damage from continuous epileptic seizures 4 wk after transplantation and died in a coma a few weeks later. In the meantime, the immunosuppressive drugs were withdrawn and the graft was subsequently rejected.

FIGURE 1. Intravenous glucose tolerance test (25 g) before and 7 and 21 days after segmental pancreas transplantation. In the two last tests, the *k* value is normal (>1.1). Normal fasting blood glucose is 3.1–5.6 mmol/l.

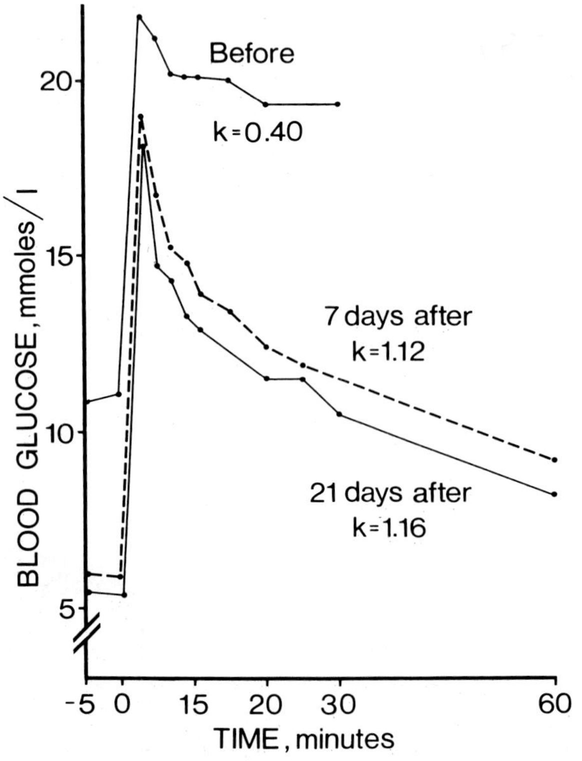

Graft procurement and preservation. The body and tail of the pancreas were removed from cadaver donors after circulation had stopped. A technique for rapid harvesting of the pancreatic segment under such conditions has been described earlier.[9] Cold perfusion was introduced through the celiac axis.

In the first six instances, a balanced electrolyte solution containing dextran 40 was used; on the last two occasions, a hyperosmolar intracellular type of electrolyte solution, as described by Sacks,[10] was used. The normothermic ischemia time before cooling could be started, the time of cold storage, and the time required for revascularization are presented in Table 2.

The four grafts cooled with the balanced electrolyte solution and not developing early thrombosis showed excellent immediate graft function, with control of blood glucose and only a minimal increase in serum amylase (Figure 3). In contrast, the two patients who had received grafts perfused with the intracellular type of electrolyte solution both showed a delay in the control of blood glucose and a marked elevation of serum amylase during the first postoperative days (Figure 4). These changes were especially marked in the last patient, where the graft had been stored cold for over 8 h; here, an insulin injection was required on the day after transplantation in order to control the blood glucose. Nonetheless, in these patients the fasting blood glucose levels returned to normal or nearly normal after 5 and 10 days, respectively. Another indication of the delayed onset of graft function in the last case was the presence of a low C-peptide[11] level immediately after transplantation. The level gradually increased during the next 3 wk (Figure 5).

The surgical technique. The splenic artery of the branch-ligated celiac axis of the graft was anastomosed end-to-end to the internal iliac artery of the recipient. In the first transplantations, the splenic vein of the graft was sutured end-to-side to the left external iliac vein; in the subsequent six operations, a segment of the portal vein of the graft was used for the anastomosis. The graft was placed extraperitoneally

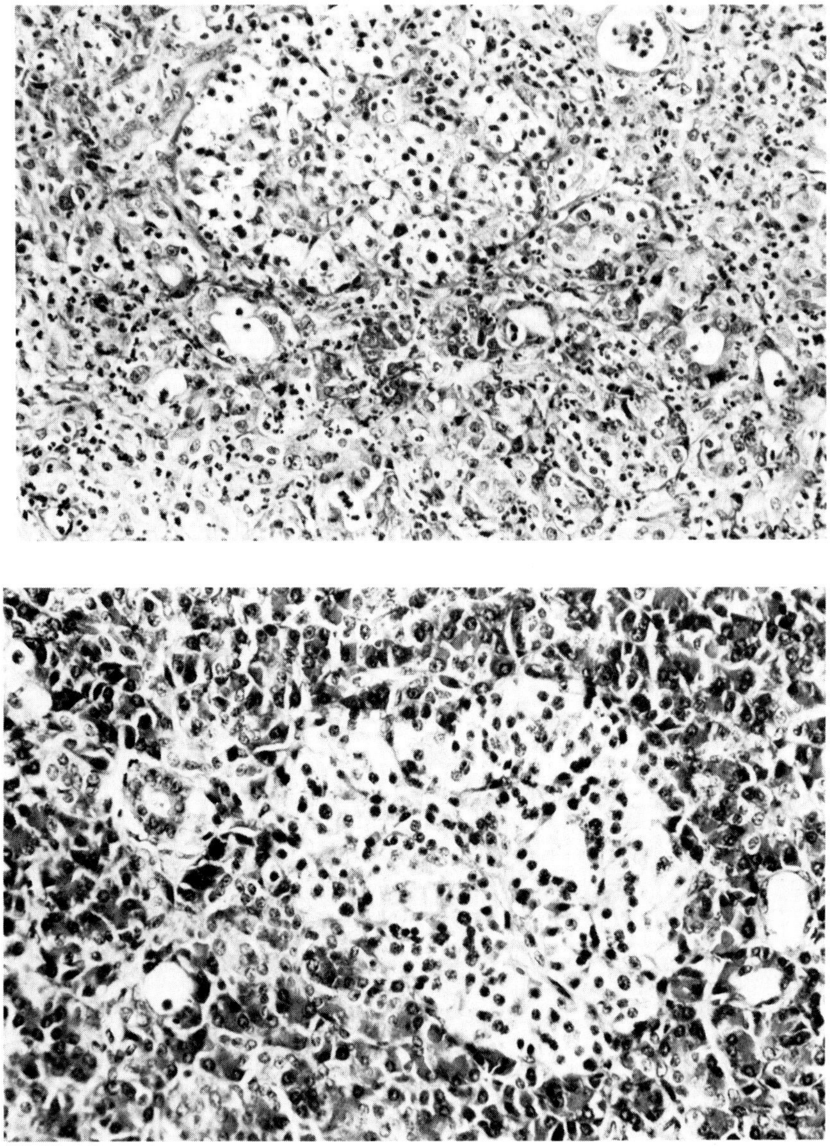

FIGURE 2. (Top) Allograft removed after irreversible rejection and destruction of the graft in 7 days. Note dense infiltration in the exocrine portion of gland by lymphocytes and granulocytes. The islet shows only unspecific degeneration. (hematoxylin and eosin.) (Bottom) Pancreas allograft removed 14 days after transplantation while still functioning; removal was necessitated by profuse bleeding from the artery. The histologic picture is essentially normal.

in the pelvis. In the first patient, no provision was made for exocrine drainage; instead, the pancreatic duct was ligated and a large ligature was placed around the graft at its transected end. In the subsequent five transplantations, exocrine drainage was provided by double-layer suturing of the transected end of the graft to the end of a jejunal Roux-en-Y loop brought 5 cm or so outside the peritoneum (Figure 6). In the last two operations, the distal end of the jejunal Y-loop was closed, and an end-to-side ductojejunostomy was created (Figure 7).

RESULTS

Pancreatic fistula. A few days after the transplantation, the patient receiving a graft with duct ligation developed a pancreatic fistula, which persisted until the graft was destroyed by rejection.

In the three recipients of grafts with a pancreaticojejunostomy that functioned for more than 1 wk, there was leakage of amylase-rich fluid from the wound. At reoperation, the fistula was located at the suture line in two cases and around a tube jejunostomy in one. In one of the former cases a

TABLE 2
Pancreas graft preservation, type of perfusate, and ischemia times

Transplant no.	Perfusate for cooling	Normothermic ischemia	Cold storage (5°C)	Time required for revascularization
1–6	Balanced electrolyte solution, with Dextran 40	4–16 min	3 h 25 min to 4 h 33 min	26–34 min
7 and 8	Hyperosmolar intracellular type of solution (Sacks)	7 and 10 min	3 h 31 min and 7 h 22 min	22 and 23 min

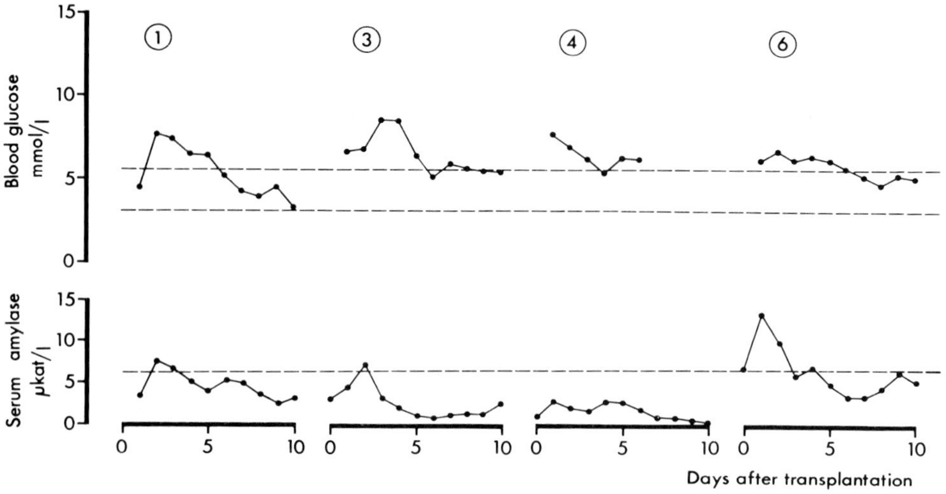

FIGURE 3. Blood glucose and serum amylase levels in four recipients of pancreas grafts perfused with balanced electrolyte solution. There was immediate control of the blood glucose concentration. Horizontal lines denote normal range.

successful repair was made. The first recipient of a graft with a ductojejunostomy also developed a pancreatic fistula after high-dose steroid therapy for a rejection episode. The leak was located at the suture line attaching the bowel to the graft capsule. In the second patient with a ductojejunostomy, no pancreatic fistula developed. Some 10 days after transplantation there was, however, a discharge of amylase-poor but bacteria-contaminated fluid from the wound.

Histocompatibility. In the case of the first six pancreatic transplantations, no attention was paid to histocompatibility matching, but in the two most recently treated patients it was decided to accept only grafts with one compatible HLA-DR antigen. The number of HLA-A and -B donor-recipient incompatibilities was one in one instance, two in two instances, three in three instances, and four in two instances. The last two recipients had one HLA-DR antigen in common with their donors, but in neither of them was the relative response in mixed lymphocyte cultures low (Table 3).

Immunosuppression. The drugs used for postoperative immunosuppression were azathioprine, prednisone, and antilymphocyte globulin (Behring). In one of the patients (no. 8) thoracic duct drainage was provided as an adjunct.[12] The

FIGURE 4. Blood glucose and serum amylase levels in two recipients of pancreas grafts perfused with hyperosmolar intracellular-type solution. Note hyperamylasemia and delayed control of the blood glucose. Horizontal lines denote normal range.

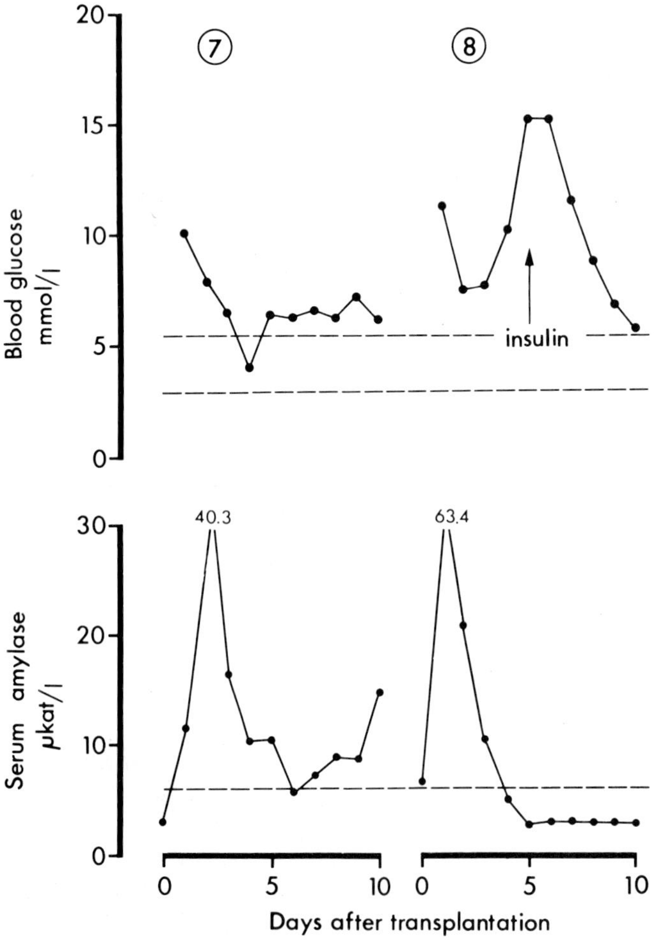

FIGURE 5. C-peptide index as a measure of graft function in one of the recipients of a graft perfused with the hyperosmolar intracellular type of electrolyte solution (transplant no. 8). The index increased gradually during the first 3 wk.

$$\text{C-peptide index} = \frac{\text{C-Peptide (nmol/L)}}{\text{Blood glucose (mmol/L)} - 2.5}$$

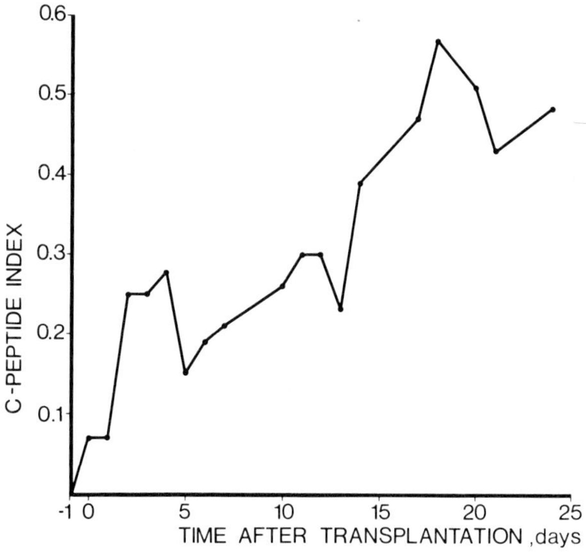

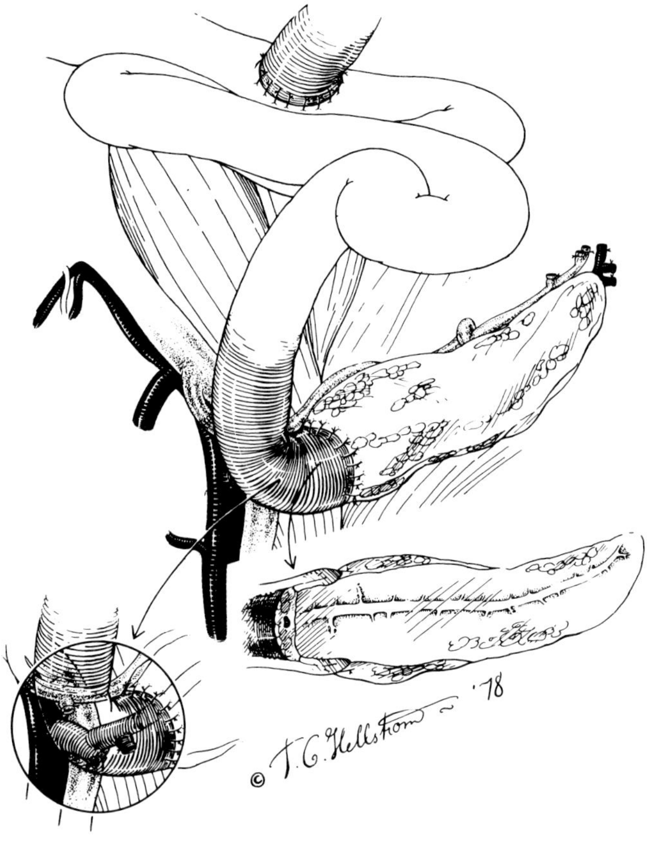

FIGURE 6. Segmental pancreas transplantation with vascular anastomoses to the left iliac vessel, and exocrine drainage provided for by end-to-end pancreaticojejunostomy to a Roux-en-Y loop.

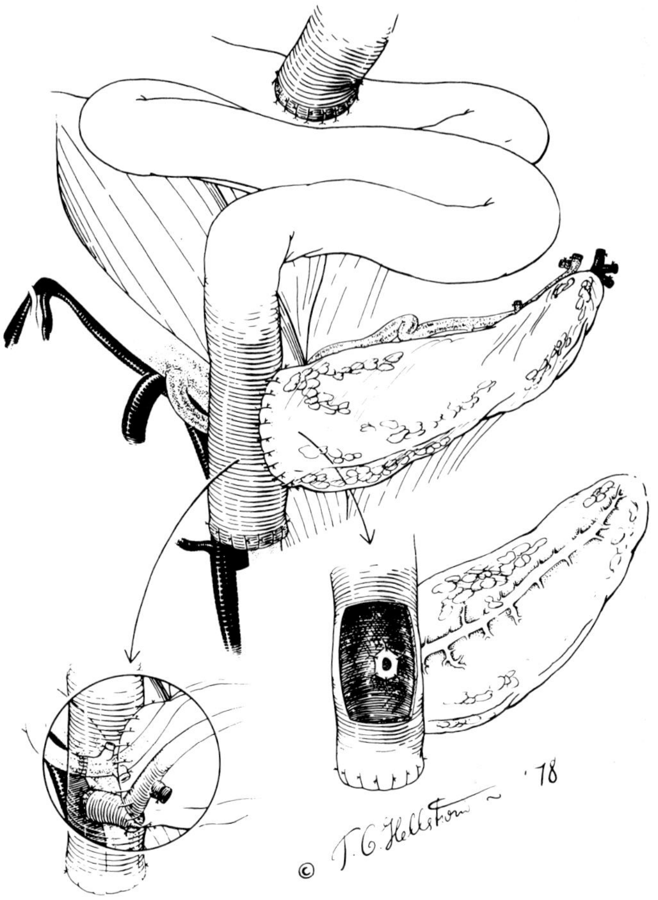

FIGURE 7. Segmental pancreas transplantation with vascular anastomoses to the left iliac vessel, and exocrine drainage provided for by end-to-side ductojejunostomy to a Roux-en-Y loop.

fistula was started on day 5 and left open for 30 days, during which time 44 L of lymph drained. At the end of this period, the reactivity of the peripheral blood lymphocytes in mixed lymphocyte culture was greatly depressed towards donor cells and third-party cells.[13] During the thoracic duct drainage, a rejection episode was successfully reversed with 6.5 g of methylprednisolone given intravenously.

Graft rejection. Five grafts failed due to rejection. In one patient there was a violent rejection episode 7 days after transplantation. In another, irreversible rejection with graft thrombosis developed after withdrawing the immunosuppressive treatment. In three recipients the rejection occurred while the patient was on maintenance immunosuppression, 3–6 wk after transplantation. In two of these patients (transplantations no. 1 and 7), the diagnosis of rejection was based on a sudden rise in the fasting blood glucose level (Figure 8). In one of the two, no attempt was made to treat the rejection because of a persistent pancreatic fistula. In the other there was no contraindication, and high-dose steroid therapy was given, but this resulted in only a temporary improvement in the blood glucose level (Figure 8). On retrospective analysis it was found that, in both these patients, the postprandial blood glucose level was elevated for about 1 wk before the rise in the fasting blood glucose concentration, indicating earlier evidence of a deterioration of graft function. In the last patient (no. 7) of this trio, an increase in the postprandial glucose level was taken as an early sign of rejection, and high-dose steroid therapy was instituted. There was no rise in the fasting blood glucose level and the postprandial value returned to normal after about 1 wk (Figure 8). In this patient, a decline in B cell function during rejection was disclosed by a fall in plasma C-peptide. A plot of C-peptide against blood glucose concentration showed an essentially normal C-peptide response before and after rejection, but practically no response during the actual episode (Figure 9).

Graft rejection was accompanied by only minor elevations in the serum amylase (Figure 8).

Histologic examination of the five grafts that had undergone rejection disclosed extensive necroses in two instances. In two grafts there were marked, and in one mild, histologic changes in the exocrine tissue typical of allogeneic rejection, with dense infiltration of inflammatory cells.

TABLE 3
HLA-DR antigen match and stimulation in mixed lymphocyte culture (MLC) in two pancreas transplantations

Transplant no.	HLA-DR antigens		Relative response in MLC (%)
	Recipient	Donor	
7	W3, W7?	W3, W4	104
8	W4, x	W4, x	76

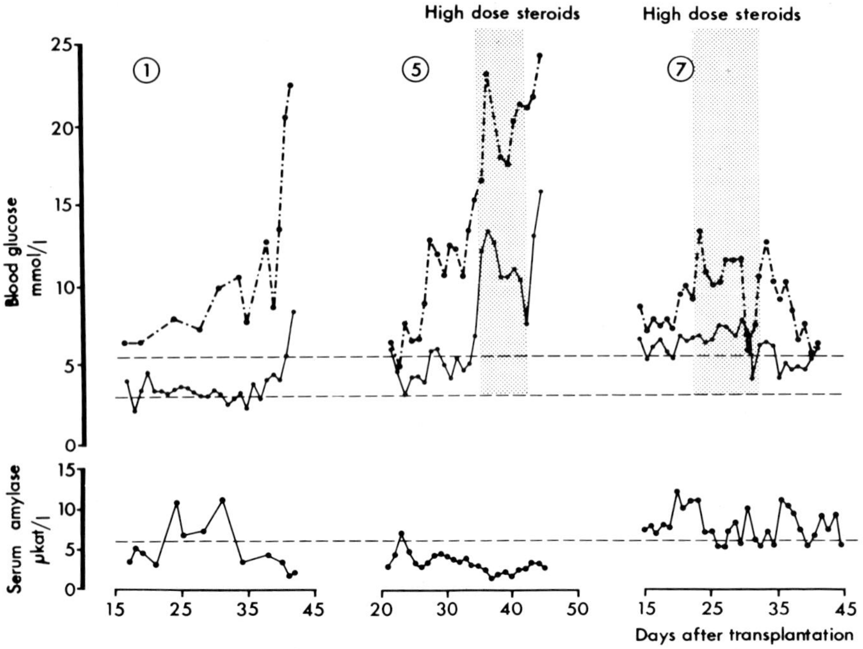

FIGURE 8. Changes in the fasting (——) and postprandial (---) blood glucose levels occurring during rejection of the pancreas graft in three recipients (transplantations no. 1, 5, and 7). Horizontal lines denote normal range. Note the increase in the postprandial level that preceded the increase in the fasting level in the recipients of transplants no. 1 and 5. In the latter, high-dose steroid therapy (*shaded area*) was instituted when the fasting blood glucose level was elevated but the rejection could not be reversed. In the recipient of transplant no. 7, such treatment was given from the time when an increase in the postprandial blood glucose occurred and rejection was reversed.

The cells of the islets of Langerhans showed evidence of mild degeneration but no cellular infiltration (Figure 2).

Islet autoantibodies. In the last two patients of our series, islet cell[14] and islet cell surface[15] antibodies were searched for by the immunofluorescence technique. Islet cell antibodies were not detected either at transplantation or postoperatively, including during rejection. There were no morphologic signs of insulitis. In the patient where islet cell surface antibodies were looked for, a clearly positive reaction was observed some hours after transplantation; it was still weakly positive 5 days later, becoming negative after 2 wk and remaining so.

Insulin antibodies. In all the recipients, the titers of insulin antibodies were repeatedly measured.[16] After exogenous insulin had been discontinued, a rapid fall in the titers, independently of the concentrations of total IgG, was observed in all the patients (Figure 10). The rate of disappearance of the insulin antibodies was about the same as for human IgG; this suggests that the formation of insulin antibodies ceased completely at transplantation when administration of porcine insulin was discontinued.

FIGURE 9. The correlation between plasma C-peptide and blood glucose level before, during, and after rejection (transplant no. 7). Before and after rejection the C-peptide response was excellent, indicating good B cell function; during rejection there was almost no response.

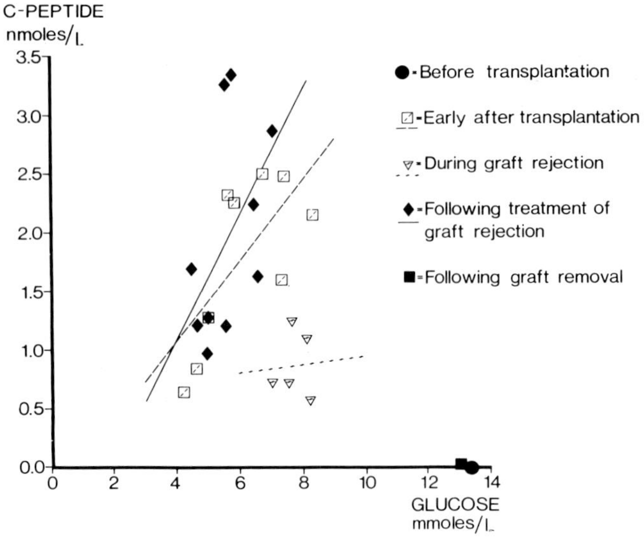

FIGURE 10. Insulin antibodies (insulin binding to IgG) and total IgG in plasma before and several times after pancreas transplantation and also after graft removel (transplant no. 7). The insulin antibodies decreased exponentially after transplantation, independently of the concentrations of total IgG. Four months after graft removal and reintroduction of insulin therapy, both insulin antibodies and total IgG had returned to original levels.

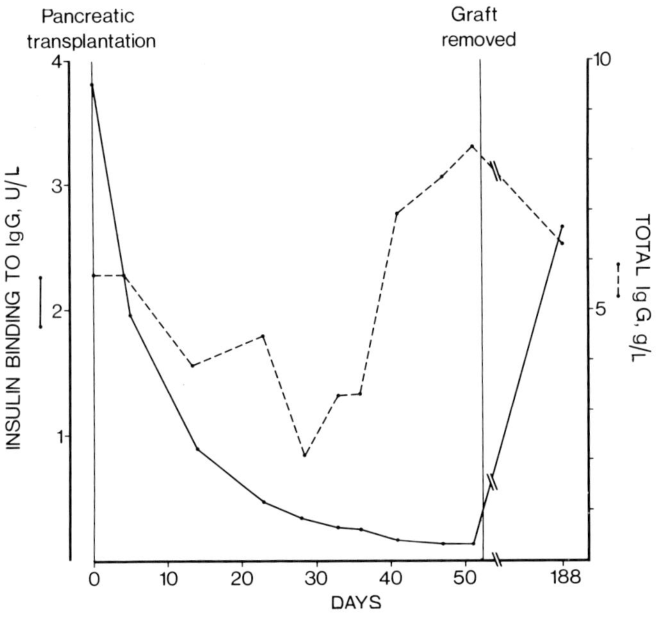

COMMENTS

While these results of segmental pancreatic transplantation might seem discouraging, several important lessons have been learned—lessons that should improve the prospects of long-term success in future patients.

It is evident that the pancreas tolerates at least 16 min of warm ischemia and at least 4 h of cold storage. For flushing, a balanced electrolyte solution seems preferable to a hyperosmolar solution with an intracellular electrolyte composition. When ischemic injury occurred, it was manifested as pronounced hyperamylasemia and delayed control of the blood glucose concentration.

The handling of the pancreatic juice has presented a major problem in this series of patients. Because of disappointing results obtained with end-to-end pancreaticojejunostomy, we now use ductojejunostomy, an approach that seems to offer valuable technical advantages.[17]

Our experience strongly underlines the fact that the pancreatic allograft is a target of rejection. The incidence and time of occurrence are not unlike those for cadaveric renal grafts. While it is disappointing that rejection was not avoided by using an HLA-DR, one-antigen–matched graft and thoracic duct drainage, it is encouraging to find that pancreatic graft rejection could be reversed by conventional steroid medication. One consistent early sign of pancreatic graft rejection was an elevated postprandial level of blood glucose; the fasting value rose only when the graft was badly damaged. The plasma C-peptide provided a direct measure of islet-cell function and might well serve as a useful guide in detecting rejection and also aid in differentiating between rejection and hyperglycemia resulting from high-dose steroid therapy.

It is reassuring that no islet cell antibodies appeared; otherwise, pancreatic transplantation in diabetic patients might be futile, since the graft would suffer the same fate as the autologous B cells.

Insulin-treated diabetics almost invariably develop antibodies against insulin. Had the insulin antibodies remained after transplantation, they would have inactivated released hormone, which would have increased the load on the transplanted islet cell tissue. The observed rapid disappearance of insulin antibodies was, therefore, encouraging.

If pancreatic transplantation is to become clinically worthwhile, it must be undertaken before the multiple organ damage has occurred; this was the reason for selecting nonuremic patients for our trials. We consider that the results to date justify further attempts along the present lines in carefully selected patients, for there would seem to be no fundamental reason why the chance of success should be smaller for pancreas than for kidney transplantation.

ACKNOWLEDGMENTS

This research was supported by the Swedish Medical Research Council, the Swedish Diabetes Association, the Edla Johansson Foundation, and Nordisk Insulinfond.

REFERENCES

[1] Lillehei, R. C., Simmons, R. L., Najarian, J. S., Weil, R., Uchida, H., Ruiz, J. O., Kjellstrand, C. M., and Goetz, F. C.: Pancreatico-duodenal allotransplantation: experimental and clinical experience. Ann. Surg. *172*:405–36, 1970.

[2] Connolly, J. E., Martin, D. C., Steinberg, T., Gwinup, G., Gazzaniga, A. B., and Barlett, R. H.: Clinical experience with pancreatiocoduodenal transplantation. Arch. Surg. *106*:489–94, 1973.

[3] Largiadèr, F., Uhlschmid, G., Binswanger, U., and Zaruba, K.: Pancreas rejection in combined pancreaticoduodenal and renal allotransplantation in man. Transplantation *19*(2):185–87, 1975.

[4] Gliedman, M. L., Gold, M., Whittaker, J., Rifkin, H., Soberman, R., Freed, S., Tellis, V., and Veith, F. J.: Clinical segmental pancreatic transplantation with ureter-pancreatic duct anastomosis for exocrine drainage. Surgery *74*:171–80, 1973.

[5] Merkel, F. K., Ryan, W. G., Armbruster, K., Seim, S., and Ing, T. S.: Pancreatic transplantation for diabetes mellitus. Illinois Med. J. *144*:477–79, 1973.

[6] Groth, C. G., Lundgren, G., Arner, P., Collste, H., Hårdstedt, Ch., Lewander, R., and Östman, J.: Rejection of isolated pancreatic allografts in patients with diabetes. Surg. Gynecol. Obstet. *143*(6): 933–40, 1976.

[7] Largiadèr, F.: Farewell to pancreatic organ transplantation? Eur. Surg. Res. *9*(6): 399–402, 1977.

[8] Gliedman, M. L., Tellis, V. A., Soberman, R., Rifkin, H., and Veith, F. J.: Long-term effects of pancreatic transplant function in patients with advanced juvenile-onset diabetes. Diabetes Care *1*:1–9, 1978.

[9] Björkén, C., Lundgren, G., Ringdén, O., and Groth, C. G.: A technique for rapid harvesting of cadaveric renal and pancreatic grafts after circulatory arrest. Br. J. Surg. *63*(7): 517–19, 1976.

[10] Sacks, S. A., Petritsch, P. H., and Kaufman, J. J.: Canine kidney preservation using a new perfusate. Lancet *1*:1024–28, 1973.

[11] Heding, L. G.: Radioimmunological determination of human C-peptide in serum. Diabetologia *11*:541–48, 1973.

[12] Groth, C. G., Lundgren, G., Gunnarsson, R., Arner, P., Berg, B., and Östman, J.: Segmental pancreatic transplantation in nonuremic diabetic patients. *In* Transplantation and Clinical Immunology X. Excerpta Medica, Amsterdam, 1979, pp. 196–201.

[13] Lundgren, G., Berg, B., Bieberfeldt, P., Konori, T., Ringdén, O., and Groth, C. G.: Analysis of the immunological effect of lymph drainage in organ transplant recipients. Scand. J. Urol. Nephrol. In press, 1979.

[14] Bottazzo, G. F., Florin-Christensen, A., and Doniach, D.: Islet-cell antibodies in diabetes mellitus with autoimmune polyendocrine deficiencies. Lancet *2*:1270–83, 1974.

[15] Lernmark, Å., Freedman, Z. R., Hofmann, C., Rubenstein, A. H., Steiner, D. F., Jackson, R. L., Winter, R. J., and Traisman, H. S.: Islet-cell-surface antibodies in juvenile diabetes mellitus. N. Engl. J. Med. *299*(8):375–80, 1978.

[16] Christiansen, A. H.: Radioimmunoelectrophoresis in the determination of insulin binding to IgG. Horm. Metab. Res. 5: 147–54, 1973.

[17] Dickerman, R. M., Twiest, M. W., Crudup, J. W., and Turcotte, J. G.: Transplantation of the pancreas into a retroperitoneal jejunal loop. Am. J. Surg. *129*(1):48–54, 1975.

Clinical Segmental Pancreas Transplantation Without Duct Anastomosis in Diabetic Renal Allograft Recipients

DAVID E. R. SUTHERLAND, FREDERICK C. GOETZ, AND JOHN S. NAJARIAN

SUMMARY

Segmental pancreatic allografts with unligated ducts were transplanted intraperitoneally to five diabetic patients who had received renal allografts more than 2 yr earlier. One patient is alive with a functioning graft 10.5 mo later. Two patients rejected their grafts at approximately 2 and 3 mo but are alive 8–9 mo later after resumption of exogenous insulin therapy. In both patients, carbohydrate metabolism was nearly normal during the period of graft function. Two patients died of infectious complications between 1 and 2 mo after transplantation. The main hazard of pancreas transplantation relates to the immunosuppression necessary to prevent rejection, setting the stage for infectious complications. Technically, pancreas transplantation is a feasible and efficient procedure, and, if better methods are developed for preventing rejection, it should be applicable to patients prone to develop secondary complications of diabetes. DIABETES 29 (Suppl. 1):10–18, 1980.

Clinical application of pancreas transplantation has been difficult. The details of 50 pancreas transplants in 47 diabetic patients have been published.[1–10] An additional 14 cases, the details of which have not been published, have been reported to the American College of Surgeons/National Institutes of Health Organ Transplant Registry.[11] In most instances the grafts were rejected or failed for technical reasons within a few weeks or months of transplantation.

Four patients had pancreas grafts that functioned for 1–4 yr until they died of complications unrelated to the pancreas transplant.[2,4,10] Although the transplants were done in an attempt to influence the progression of diabetic microangiopathy, in most patients the secondary complications of diabetes were far advanced at the time of transplantation. These cases showed that pancreatic grafts could restore carbohydrate metabolism to nearly normal without the need for exogenous insulin, but the high failure rate and morbidity from technical complications has inhibited widespread application.

Islet transplantation is an alternative to pancreas transplantation.[12] However, free grafts of islets are highly susceptible to rejection,[13] and it is much more difficult to prepare islets from human than from animal pancreases.[14] For these reasons, pancreas transplantation may still be a more efficient approach for total endocrine replacement therapy in human diabetes mellitus.

The major technical problem with transplantation of immediately vascularized pancreatic grafts is related to handling of the pancreatic duct and its secretions. Anastomoses of the duct are prone to leak, and exposure to enterokinase activates the pancreatic enzymes. Duct-ligated grafts have been successfully transplanted in animals,[15] and this approach has been taken in a few human cases of pancreas transplantation to retroperitoneal space of the iliac fossa.[1,8,9,16] However, pancreatitis, retroperitoneal fluid accumulation, fistula formation, and secondary infections have uniformily occurred. Dubernard et al.[17] were able to avoid establishing duct drainage by a technique designed to selectively suppress exocrine function. They obliterated the entire duct system by injection of Neoprene, a synthetic polymer that hardens after injection. They have reported the outcome of transplantation in eight patients.[10] Although complications were few and minor, most grafts ceased to function within a few months, either from rejection or from sclerosis induced by the Neoprene.

The various maneuvers designed to avoid duct drainage may not be necessary. Kyriakides et al.[18] transplanted segmental pancreatic grafts with unligated ducts intraperitoneally in pigs. They showed that free drainage of pancreatic secretions into the peritoneal cavity did not lead to complications. In the absence of enterokinase, the pancreatic enzymes were not activated, and the peritoneal cavity reabsorbed the pancreatic juice. We confirmed these results in

From the Departments of Surgery and Medicine, University of Minnesota Health Sciences Center, Minneapolis, Minnesota 55455.
Address reprint requests to Dr. D. E. R. Sutherland, Box 253 Mayo Memorial Building, University of Minnesota, 420 Delaware Street, S. E., Minneapolis, Minnesota 55455.

dogs and found that pancreatic grafts with unligated, nonanastomosed ducts maintained good endocrine function over several months of observation.[19] On the basis of this experience, we have placed cadaveric segmental pancreatic allografts with unligated ducts into the peritoneal cavity of five diabetic patients. All five patients have previously received renal allografts for treatment of end-stage diabetic nephropathy. The indications for pancreas transplantation were poor control of diabetes and a demonstrated propensity for developing the secondary complications of diabetes.

PATIENT POPULATION AND METHODS

Biographical information on the five patients is given in Table 1. They were dependent on exogenous insulin injections for 20 or more years, and each had received a renal allograft more than 2 yr before pancreas transplantation. All of the patients had diabetic retinopathy, but useful vision was present in at least one eye at the time of pancreas transplantation. Each patient had various other complications of diabetes (see case histories). All patients were taking prednisone and either azathioprine or cyclophosphamide to prevent rejection of their renal allografts.

After pancreas transplantation, each patient received horse antilymphoblast globulin intravenously (30 mg/kg/day) for a total of 14 doses. The dose of prednisone was increased to 2 mg/kg/day and then tapered to a maintenance dose over the next several weeks or months.

The pancreases were obtained from brain-dead cadaver donors that shared two or more HLA antigens of the A and B loci with the recipients. The technique of removing the body and tail of the pancreas from the donor was similar to that described by Gliedman et al.[16] The splenic artery and vein of the donor pancreas were anastomosed to the left iliac vessels of the recipient through a midline laparotomy incision, and the pancreatic duct was left open so that the pancreatic secretions drained freely into the peritoneal cavity.

In four cases the pancreases were transplanted immediately after removal from the donor, while in one instance (no. 4) the graft was stored for 6 h in Cold Electrolyte Solution for Preservation (Travenol Laboratories, Deerfield, Illinois) before transplantation. This graft was the only one that functioned poorly immediately after transplantation. In one case (no. 5) the pancreas graft was obtained from a donor with a gastrostomy. A Gram stain of the gastrostomy was negative. However, an infection with microorganisms cultured from the donor gastrostomy at the time of pancreatectomy was subsequently responsible for the death of the recipient.

Metabolic studies in varying detail were performed on all patients before and after transplantation. Blood glucose, amylase, and lipase concentrations were determined in our or other hospital laboratories by their routine methods. Before 1 November 1978, serum amylase levels in our hospital were determined by a method that expressed results as Somogyi units (SU) per deciliter. After 1 November 1979, a different method was used, so that serum amylase results were given in international units (IU) per liter. The first three patients had their transplants performed before 1 November 1978. The results of serum amylase determinations done after this date in these patients have been converted to SU per deciliter by multiplying the value in IU per liter by a factor of 2. Serum amylase levels obtained at other hospitals (after the patients had returned home) were also converted to SU per deciliter if different methods were used. The last two patients received pancreatic grafts after 1 November 1978, and serum amylase levels in these patients are given in IU per liter.

Insulin antibody, insulin, C-peptide, and glucagon concentrations in serum or plasma were measured in our Clinical Research Center Laboratory using standard immunoassay techniques.[20–23] Serum insulin was measured only if the patient's serum bound <3% of labeled insulin. The antibody used for serum C-peptide determination was obtained from Calbiochem-Behring Corporation, La Jolla, California (Antibody II, lot no. 86A099). Unger's "30K" rabbit antibody was used for the glucagon assay.

RESULTS

Three of the five patients are alive and well 8½–10½ mo after pancreas transplantation (Table 1). Two patients died of infectious complications, one at 7 wk (patient no. 4) and one at 1 mo (patient no. 5) after transplantation. In four of the five patients the need for exogenous insulin was completely obviated immediately after transplantation. One of the four (patient no. 1) has maintained good graft function for more than 10 mo. Two patients (no. 2 and no. 3) rejected their grafts approximately 2 and 3 mo after transplantation and have resumed exogenous insulin therapy. One patient (no. 5) had a functioning graft removed at 3 wk because of peritonitis caused by microorganisms cultured from the donor. The other patient (no. 4) had poor graft function (presumably

TABLE 1
Summary of pancreas transplant experience in five diabetic recipients of renal allografts

Case	Sex	Age (yr)	Duration of diabetes (yr)	Date of kidney transplant	Date of pancreas transplant	Outcome as of 8 June 1979
1	F	31	23	11/20/72	7/25/78	Normoglycemic with functioning graft at 10.5 mo.
2	F	35	26	8/23/73	8/12/78	Normoglycemic until rejection at 100 days. Alive after resumption of exogenous insulin therapy.
3	M	32	20	5/3/76	9/25/78	Normoglycemic until rejection at 7 wk. Alive after resumption of exogenous insulin therapy.
4	M	28	24	3/6/75	11/8/78	Poor function of graft. Developed cytomegalovirus and *Staphylococcus aureus* sepsis and died at 7 wk.
5	F	35	31	3/3/76	12/6/78	Normoglycemic until functioning graft removed at 3 wk because of peritonitis secondary to bacterial contamination from donor at time of transplant. Died at 1 mo.

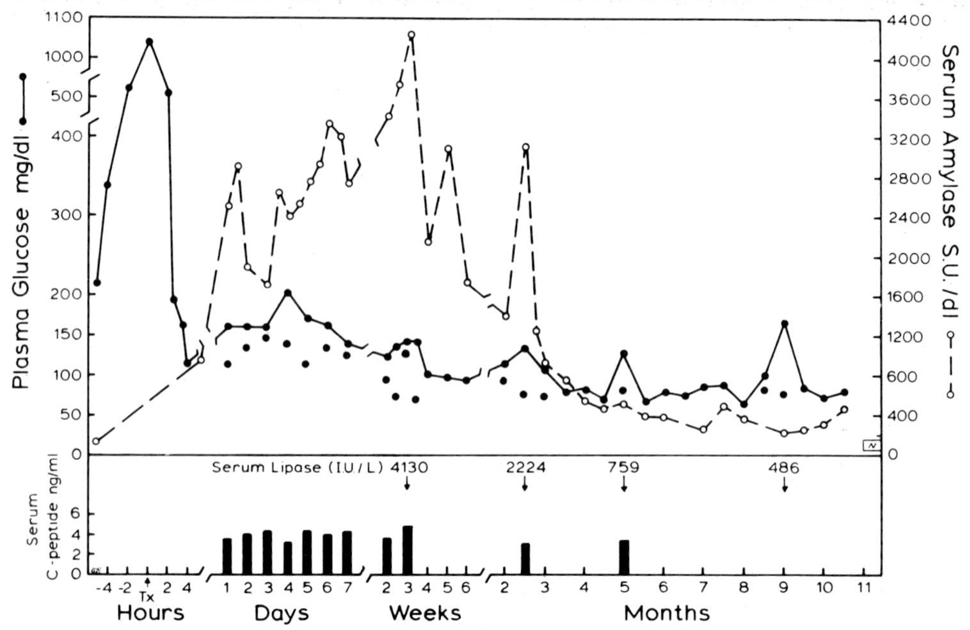

FIGURE 1. Blood glucose, C-peptide, amylase, and lipase levels after pancreas transplantation in patient no. 1. Line (•——•) connects highest glucose values, and unconnected dots represent low values recorded on the same day. The patient received a constant intravenous infusion of glucose solution during the first week.

because of ischemic damage during the period of preservation) and continued to need insulin after transplantation, although serum C-peptide concentration was increased.

The transplants were performed without technical complications in the first three patients. They had mild or no abdominal pain for 2 wk. Ascites was absent or minimal and fistulas or peritonitis did not occur. Pancreatic enzyme activity in the blood was elevated, reflecting the absorption of pancreatic juice from the peritoneal cavity.

Metabolic studies showed good pancreatic graft function in all but one patient, but minor abnormalities of carbohydrate metabolism were present. The results of the metabolic studies are given with the individual case histories.

Patient no. 1. This patient received a pancreas transplant 5.7 yr after a kidney transplant from her mother. She took 10–30 U of insulin per day and had extremely labile blood sugar concentrations. She was blind in the right eye and had involutional retinopathy on the left, but corrected visual acuity was 20/30. A biopsy of the grafted kidney had been done 4 yr after renal transplantation and showed early diabetic nephropathy: mild hyalinosis of afferent and efferent arterioles and linear staining for albumin on tubular basement membrane, lesions that were not present in the kidney at the time of transplantation. The patient had never been treated for rejection, and serum creatinine at the time of pancreas transplantation was 0.9 mg/dl.

The patient has needed no exogenous insulin since pancreas transplantation. Blood glucose, C-peptide, amylase, and lipase concentrations over this period are summarized in Figure 1. Serum amylase and lipase levels have gradu-

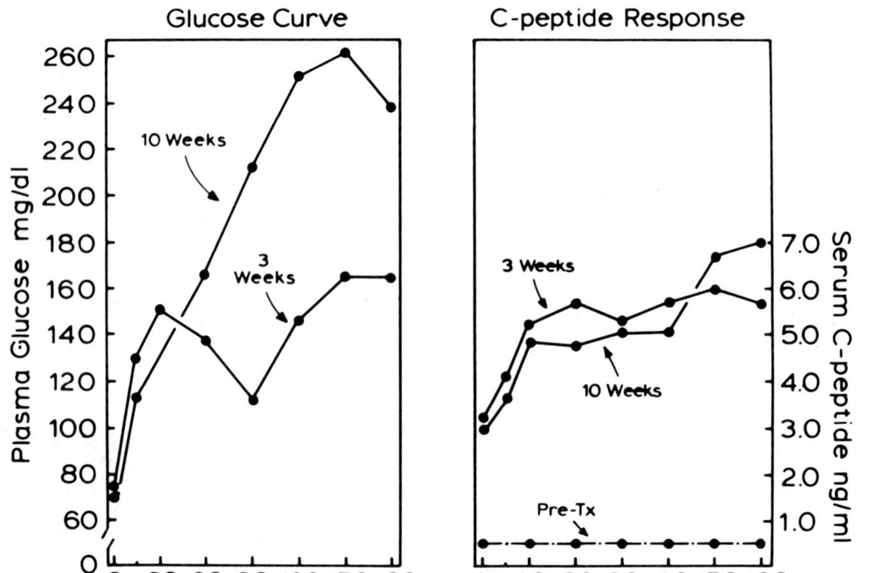

FIGURE 2. Results of oral glucose tolerance tests 3 and 10 wk after pancreas transplantation in patient no. 1.

ally declined, but the concentrations are still above normal. Plasma glucose levels have been normal or near normal since the first month after transplantation.

Plasma glucose concentrations did not return to baseline during the 3 h of sampling during oral glucose tolerance tests performed at 3 and 10 wk (Figure 2); however, C-peptide concentrations increased progressively over the periods of testing (Figure 2). In addition, plasma glucagon fell from 152 pg/ml before to 96 pg/ml by 3 h after glucose injection during the test at 10 wk. Serum insulin was not measured, because it was assumed that insulin antibodies were present. However, subsequent testing showed binding of insulin by the patient's serum to be <3%, and a glucose tolerance test at 5 mo included measurement of serum insulin (Table 2). This was carried out for 5 h. There was a delayed return of plasma glucose to baseline, but by 5 h the patient was hypoglycemic. Serum insulin concentration remained elevated for at least 3 h. Plasma glucagon declined appropriately during the glucose tolerance test.

Although the results of the oral gucose tolerance test at 5 mo were not completely normal, the metabolic profile over a day of normal meals and activity at this time (Figure 3) was not much different from that reported for normal individuals.[24] A metabolic profile at 9 mo was similar (Table 3). C-peptide concentrations during the 24-h profile at 5 mo ranged from 2.2 to 3.5 ng/ml and showed the same fluctuations in relation to meals as did the insulin levels, although the magnitude of the changes was less.

Since pancreas transplantation, the patient has returned to work as a social worker. Examination of the good left eye at 9 mo showed no changes in visual acuity and no progression of retinopathy. Menses, which had been absent for 4 yr, resumed 6 mo after pancreas transplantation. The patient reported subjective improvement in sensory preception in her feet. A biopsy of the transplanted kidney at 9 mo after pancreas transplantation did not show any changes from the biopsy taken 2 yr before. At this point it is too early to assess the influence of pancreas transplantation on the secondary complications of diabetes in this patient.

Patient no. 2. This patient received a pancreas transplant 5 yr after a kidney transplant from her mother. She had never been treated for rejection, and serum creatinine at the time of pancreas transplantation was 1.6 mg/dl. She took 50 U of insulin per day. She had had several major complications of her eyes, including proliferative diabetic retinopathy, vitreous hemorrhage, and cataract formation. Phacovitrectomies had been performed between 2 and 3 yr previously, and, at the time of pancreas transplantation, she had corrected visual acuity of 20/60 in both eyes.

After pancreas transplantation, the patient received no exogenous insulin until rejection occurred at 100 days (Figure 4). Plasma glucose levels were moderately elevated for the first few weeks but, by 1 mo, were normal. Serum amy-

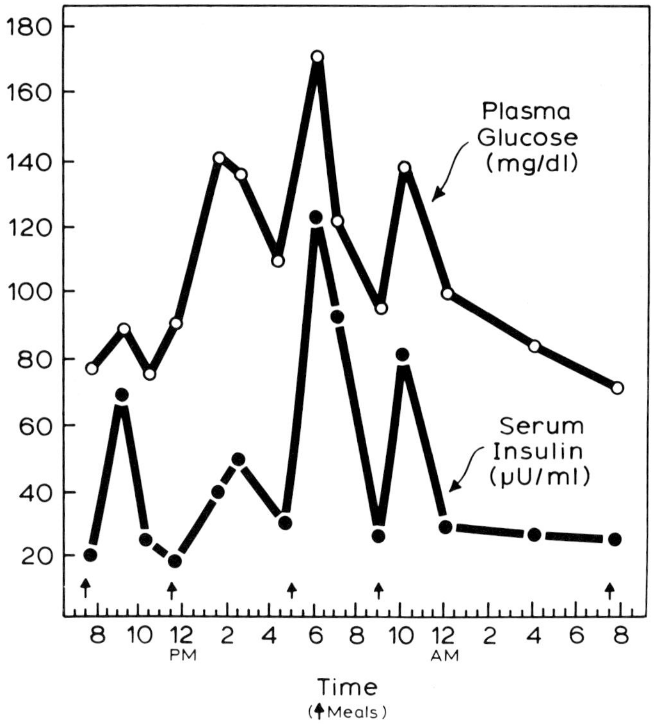

FIGURE 3. Metabolic profile during a 24-h period of normal meals and activity 5 mo after pancreas transplantation in patient no. 1.

TABLE 2
Oral glucose tolerance test* 5 mo after pancreas transplantation in patient no. 1

Minutes	Plasma glucose (mg/dl)	Serum insulin (μU/ml)	Serum† C-peptide (ng/ml)	Serum glucagon (pg/ml)
−10	83	19	2.8	186
−5	79	21	2.6	166
+15	116	82	3.2	
+30	143	97	3.4	117
+60	165	138	4.0	100
+90	180	194	4.7	
+120	202	214	4.5	91
+150	176	215	5.3	
+180	179	200	5.4	73
+240	121			
+300	48			

* Glucose 1.75 mg/kg ideal body weight. Total dose of glucose at 0 min: 85.6 g.

† Pretransplant C-peptide was <0.5 ng/ml.

TABLE 3
24-Hour metabolic profile 9 mo after pancreas transplantation in patient no. 1

Time		Plasma glucose (mg/dl)	Serum insulin (μU/ml)
0745	15 min before breakfast	76	9
0900	1 h after breakfast	157	70
1010	2 h after breakfast	132	58
1200	15 min before lunch	82	14
1300	1 h after lunch	123	28
1400	2 h after lunch	131	24
1645	15 min before supper	110	17
1800	1 h after supper	131	37
1900	2 h after supper	105	34
2051	15 min before h.s. snack	98	21
2233	1 h after h.s. snack	169	61
0002		119	41
0400		85	18
0745	15 min before breakfast	81	18

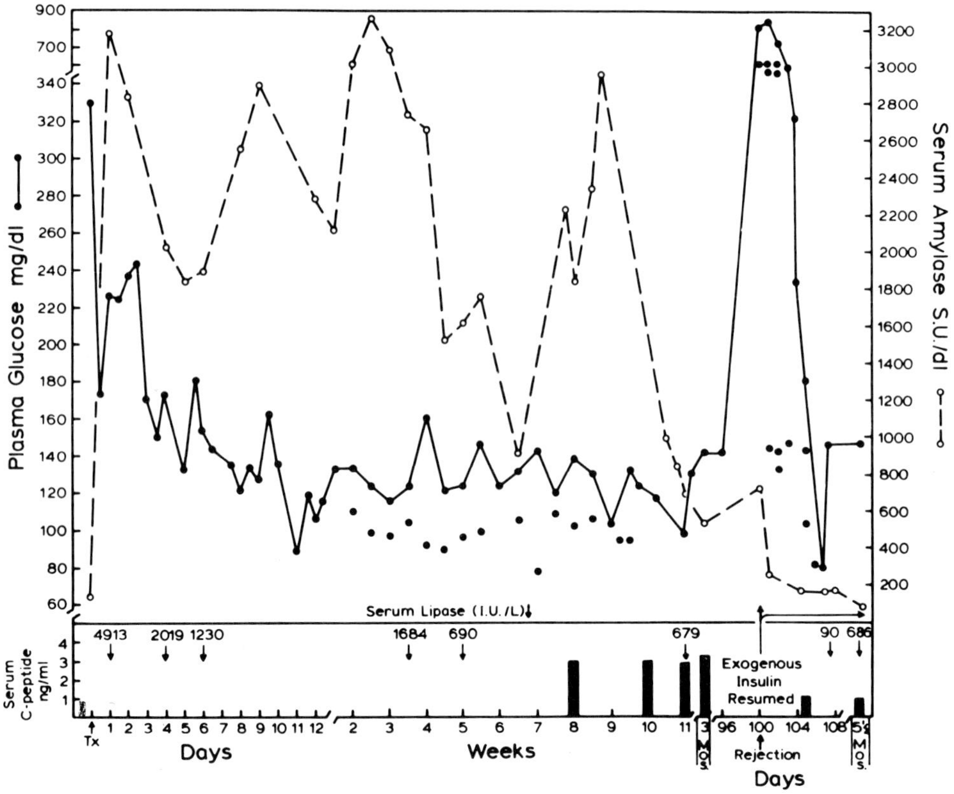

FIGURE 4. Blood glucose, C-peptide, amylase, and lipase levels after pancreas transplantation in patient no. 2. Dots are low glucose values recorded on same days as highest values connected by the solid line. The patient received intravenous glucose solutions for the first 10 days.

lase and lipase levels were elevated until rejection occurred.

During the second month after transplantation, the patient had intermittent fever, and urine cultures were positive for cytomegalovirus. Prednisone dose was reduced because of the cytomegalovirus infection and the patient improved. In addition, the patient developed erythematous nodular lesions of the legs and buttocks. A biopsy of one of the lesions on the buttocks showed subcutaneous fat necrosis. The elevation of serum lipase was probably responsible for the fat necrosis.

The patient was admitted to our Clinical Research Center (CRC) for metabolic studies approximately 3 mo after transplantation. Fasting plasma glucose concentrations were increased over the values obtained during the previous 2 mo, but postprandial plasma glucose levels during a day of normal meals and activity were not abnormal (Table 4). Serum C-peptide concentrations did not increase significantly after eating.

An oral glucose tolerance test was also performed at 3 mo. There was only a modest increase in plasma glucose concentration during the test, but levels had not returned to baseline by 5 h. Serum C-peptide levels were stable during the test (Table 5).

The minor abnormalities in carbohydrate metabolism detected at 3 mo may have been secondary to an ongoing rejection process, because 9 days after the patient was discharged from the CRC her plasma glucose rose to 805 mg/dl. Serum amylase and lipase levels fell to normal, concomitant with occurrence of hyperglycemia (Figure 4). The patient had no local or systemic symptoms associated with loss of pancreatic allograft function. She was given exogenous insulin to lower plasma glucose, and antirejection

TABLE 4
Metabolic profile during 2 days of normal meals and activity 3 mo after pancreas transplantation in patient no. 2

Time		Plasma glucose (mg/dl)	Serum C-peptide (ng/ml)	Plasma glucagon (pg/ml)
0845	before breakfast	122	2.8	282
1030	½ h after breakfast	120	3.0	
1130	½ h before lunch	135	2.9	
1350	1 h after lunch	123	2.8	
1630	½ h before supper	133	3.2	
1820	1 h after supper	123	2.8	
2200		120	2.8	
0730	before breakfast	109	2.6	231

TABLE 5
Oral glucose tolerance test* 3 mo after pancreas transplantation in patient no. 2

Minutes	Plasma glucose (mg/dl)	C-peptide (ng/ml)†
−10	117	2.9
+15	113	2.9
+60	120	3.0
+120	133	3.3
+180	131	3.2
+240	141	—
+300	134	—

* Glucose 1.75 g/kg of ideal body weight. Total dose of glucose at 0 min: 98.4 g.

† Pretransplant C-peptide was 0.9 ng/ml.

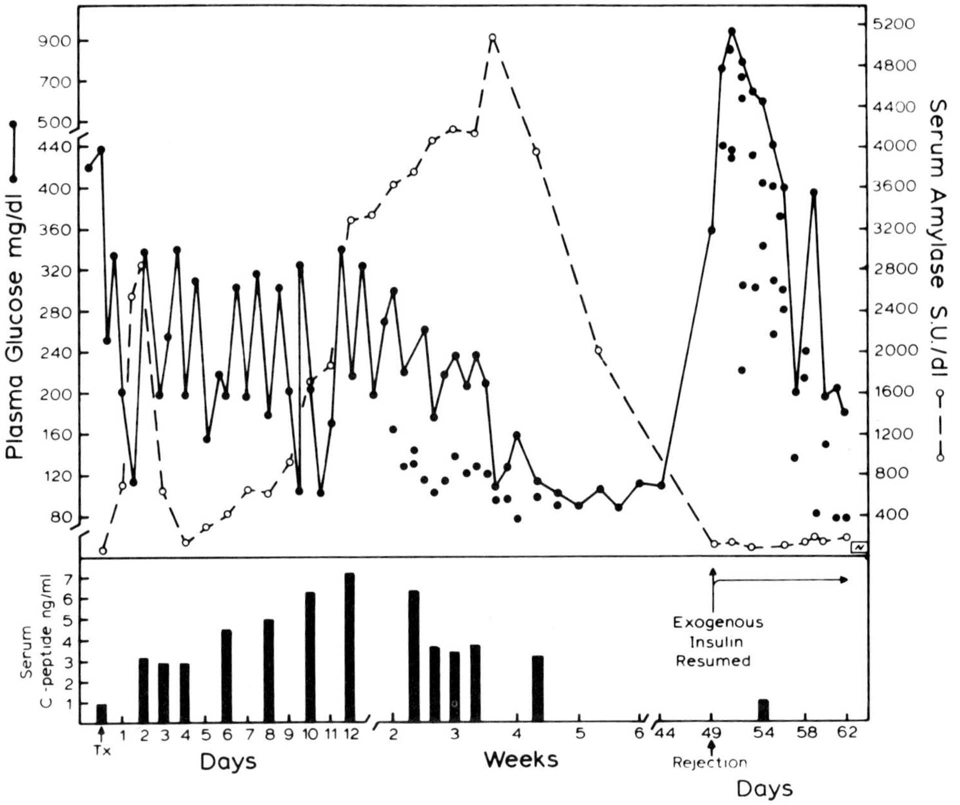

FIGURE 5. Blood glucose, C-peptide, and amylase levels after pancreas transplantation in patient no. 1. Unconnected dots represent low glucose values recorded on the same day as highest values connected by the solid line. The patient received intravenous glucose solution for the first 8 days.

treatment with oral prednisone was initiated. Antirejection treatment was not successful in restoring endocrine function of the grafted pancreas.

It was anticipated that the nodular lesions on the legs would improve after rejection; however, they have persisted. Serum lipase levels, although normal 8 days after rejection, were again elevated when measured 2 mo later (Figure 4). It is possible that the pancreatic allograft, which was not removed, has retained some exocrine function, although serum amylase levels have remained normal.

Since rejection of the pancreatic graft, the patient has developed deterioration of vision in the right eye, probably the result of cytomegalovirus retinitis. Renal allograft function has not changed. The patient currently takes 35 U of insulin per day, slightly less than before pancreas transplantation.

Patient no. 3. This patient received a pancreas transplant 2.3 yr after a kidney transplant from a cadaver. He had had no rejection episodes of the kidney, and his serum creatinine concentration at the time of pancreas transplantation was 1.1 mg/dl. He took 65 U of insulin per day but was persistently hyperglycemic on this dose. He had involutional retinopathy and corrected visual acuity of 20/25 in both eyes at the time of transplantation. After pancreas transplantation, the patient needed no exogenous insulin until rejection occurred at 7 wk (Figure 5). However, plasma glucose levels, particularly postprandial, were elevated above normal for the first 3 wk after transplantation. Serum amylase levels were only moderately elevated for the first 2 wk, but thereafter they were very high until rejection occurred (Figure 5). Serum C-peptide also increased after the first week and remained within the normal range until rejection occurred.

Oral glucose tolerance test at 1 mo showed a late rise in plasma glucose concentration, a small, but progressive increase in serum C-peptide concentration, and a small decrease in plasma glucagon concentration (Table 6). Plasma glucose concentration returned to baseline by 5 h.

The patient had no complications after transplantation, except for the development of oral thrush. Because of this problem, prednisone was rapidly reduced to maintenance levels. The patient returned to work after discharge from the hospital. Forty-four days after pancreas transplantation, fasting plasma glucose concentration was 111 mg/dl and 5 days later it was 359 mg/dl. Serum amylase declined to nor-

TABLE 6
Oral glucose tolerance test* 1 mo after pancreas transplantation in patient no. 3

Minutes	Plasma glucose (mg/dl)	Serum C-peptide (ng/ml)†	Plasma glucagon (pg/ml)
−10	90	3.1	115
−5	87	3.3	162
+5	92	3.2	—
+15	112	3.2	—
+30	141	3.3	153
+60	131	3.3	156
+120	125	3.6	127
+180	161	3.8	133
+240	203	—	—
+300	105	—	—

* Glucose 1.75 g/kg of ideal body weight. Total dose of glucose at 0 min: 133.2 g.

† Pretransplant C-peptide was 1.0 ng/ml.

mal concomitantly with occurrence of hyperglycemia, and serum C-peptide returned to pretransplant levels (Figure 5). Antirejection treatment with oral prednisone was unsuccessful in restoring pancreatic allograft function. There were no local or systemic symptoms associated with rejection, and the graft was not removed. The patient resumed exogenous insulin therapy and currently takes 44 U/day. Renal allograft function has remained normal.

Patient no. 4. This patient received a pancreas transplant 3.7 yr after a kidney transplant from his sister. Serum creatinine at the time of pancreas transplantation was 1.0 mg/dl. He took 26 U of insulin per day. Complications of diabetes included vascular disease and retinopathy. He had undergone photocoagulation treatments and a pituitary ablation 8 yr previously. At the time of pancreas transplantation he was blind in the right eye and visual acuity was 20/300 in the left eye. His right leg had been amputated after the kidney transplantation because of arterial occlusive disease. In addition, he had multiple scattered, nonhealing, superficial cutaneous ulcers. The patient received a pancreas graft that had been stored in the cold for 6 h, and the graft never functioned satisfactorily. Serum amylase activity increased from 50 IU/L before transplantation to 265 IU/L 1 day after transplantation, but thereafter it returned to normal (<88 IU/L). Some graft function was present. Serum C-peptide concentration at 1 mo was 2.3 ng/ml, compared with 1.2 ng/ml before transplantation; however, during this period, between 4 and 24 U of insulin was administered daily to prevent hyperglycemia.

Culture of the patient's urine at the time of transplant grew cytomegalovirus (CMV). At 2 wk after transplantation, blood cultures were positive for both CMV and *Staphylococcus aureus*. A central venous catheter was removed and found to be infected with *S. aureus*. Azathioprine administration was stopped and prednisone was tapered to maintenance levels, but the patient continued to run a septic course; a pulmonary embolus occurred, and the patient died 7 wk after transplantation. Autopsy was limited to examination of the grafted pancreas and kidney. Both organs had scattered local abscesses, consistent with hematogenous bacterial dissemination. Although the vascular anastomoses were patent, the splenic artery and vein within the substance of the grafted pancreas were thrombosed, and there were large areas of lobular necrosis throughout the pancreatic parenchyma.

Patient no. 5. This patient received a kidney transplant 2.8 yr ago from her brother. She was never treated for rejection, but during the 6 mo before pancreas transplantation her serum creatinine increased from 1.3 to 2.1 mg/dl. She had diabetic retinopathy and a previous vitreous hemorrhage in the left eye. At the time of pancreas transplantation visual acuity was 20/400 in the left and 20/40 in the right eye. She took 36–40 U of insulin daily.

After pancreas transplantation, the patient received no exogenous insulin until the graft was removed 17 days later. Representative blood glucose, amylase, and C-peptide levels during this period are summarized in Table 7. This patient received the graft from the donor with a gastrostomy. She had no fever or abdominal pain, but at 2 wk she developed ascites. Gram staining of the peritoneal fluid revealed no organisms, but *Enterobacter cloacae* and *Candida albicans* grew on culture—the same organims present in the donor gastrostomy. The pancreas graft was removed; immunosuppression was stopped, and peritonitis and acute renal failure were treated by peritoneal dialysis with antibiotics added to the dialysis fluid. After pancreatectomy the patient required more than 100 U of insulin daily to control hyperglycemia. Over the next week, peritoneal lavage fluid cultures became sterile, but the patient developed severe respiratory failure and died 1 mo after pancreas transplantation.

TABLE 7
Plasma glucose and serum amylase levels after pancreas transplantation in patient no. 5*

Days posttransplant	Plasma glucose (mg/dl) a.m./p.m.	Serum amylase† (IU/L)
1	128/142	1340
2	175/159	1136
3	169/146	1625
4	157/	1823
5	123/144	1711
6	/158	
7	113/127	906
8	248/159	780
9	/152	794
10	126/148	662
11	118/167	797
12	120/147	877
13	148/154	849
14	91/106	634
15	79/64	362
16	150/159	422
17	108/pancreatectomy	378
18	918/578 on insulin	116
19	219/237 on insulin	131

* Serum C-peptide 0.9 ng/ml pretransplant, and 4.6–5.6 ng/ml posttransplant while graft was in place.
† Normal 18–88 IU/L.

The connective tissue and fat on the surface of the excised pancreatic allograft was inflamed, but there was no cellular infiltrate within the pancreatic parenchyma. On microscopic examination, the epithelium of some ducts was flattened, but both acinar tissue and islets appeared normal (Figure 6).

DISCUSSION

The unknown nature of the outcome and the risks associated with pancreas transplantation have influenced the selection of patients for this procedure. Ideally, the pancreas transplant should be done before the secondary complications of diabetes appear. However, not all patients with diabetes mellitus develop secondary complications, and clinicians are reluctant to subject a patient, who might otherwise do well without transplantation, to the hazards of transplantation.

For that reason, we believe pancreas transplantation is mainly applicable at this time to diabetic patients who are clearly prone to develop morbid and life-threatening secondary complications and who already require immunosuppressive therapy. Diabetic patients who have previously received renal allografts fit these criteria. If more specific immunosuppressive therapy is developed in the future, the indications for transplantation can be broadened.

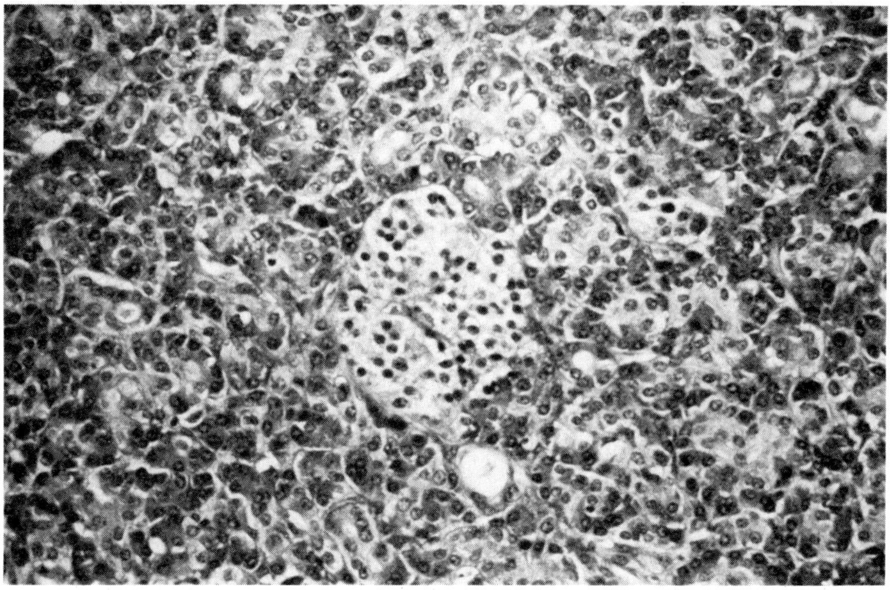

FIGURE 6. Microscopic section of pancreatic allograft removed from patient no. 5 at 17 days after transplantation. (Hematoxylin and eosin, ×250.)

Technically, pancreas transplantation by the open duct method is not difficult. Only vascular anastomoses are required, and the procedure is safe if infectious complications can be avoided. Both of our patients who died did so of infections. In each case the outcome could have been prevented. Patient no. 4 had cytomegalovirus in the urine and cutaneous ulcers that were probably the source of the *Staphylococcus aureus* sepsis that developed after transplantation. A patient with these problems should not be a candidate for transplantation because the increase in immunosuppression necessary to prevent rejection will exacerbate the infectious process. The other patient (no. 5) who developed a lethal infection did so because microorganisms were transferred from a donor gastrostomy at the time of transplantation. This complication could have been avoided by better donor selection and points out the hazard of enteric contamination at the time of pancreas transplantation.

In the first three cases, the pancreas transplants were performed without technical mishaps. Two patients rejected the grafts. In both of these cases their immunosuppression had been tapered faster than usual to reduce the risks of exacerbating mild infections that appeared after transplantation. In the one patient (no. 1) who received a normal course of immunosuppression, rejection has not occurred.

The results of metabolic studies in these patients have not been entirely normal. In two patients, the studies were carried out shortly before the grafts were totally rejected, and the rejection process may have been underway much earlier than recognized. It is interesting that, in patient no. 2, fasting plasma glucose levels were elevated, while postprandial levels were normal during the period before rejection became obvious. This observation is just the opposite of that made by Groth et al.[9]

In the patient who has not rejected the graft, the results of oral glucose tolerance tests show a prolonged elevation of plasma glucose concentration followed by a tendency to develop hypoglycemia. The venous effluent of the pancreas graft drains into the systemic circulation, bypassing the liver, and this arrangement is a possible explanation. However, experiments with pancreatic autotransplantation in dogs by Collins et al.[25] have not shown a metabolic disadvantage if secreted insulin initially bypasses the portal circulation. Alternatively, the abnormalities may be due to the administration of prednisone. Whether these abnormalities are important or not in relationship to the ultimate objective for pancreas transplantation—to prevent the occurrence of progression of secondary complications—is a question that cannot be answered at this time.

In summary, pancreas transplantation is a procedure that restores carbohydrate metabolism to nearly normal in selected diabetic patients. At this time, the procedure is more efficient than islet transplantation.[12] The main risk of pancreas transplantation is related to the immunosuppressive therapy necessary to prevent rejection, a problem that certainly is not any less for islet transplantation. If safer and more effective immunosuppressive therapy is developed, it should be possible to broaden the application of pancreas transplantation to patients who have not yet developed advanced complications of diabetes.

ADDENDUM

Note added in proof. Patient no. 1 has now been followed for 16 mo, and she remains normoglycemic without need for exogenous insulin. Five additional patients have received segmental pancreas transplants since submission of the manuscript, and all are alive and well. Three of the five patients no longer require exogenous insulin. Venous thrombosis developed in one graft, and it was removed. One graft was removed because the patient developed progressive ascites. The other three grafts are functioning at 1, 4, and 5 mo after transplantation.

ACKNOWLEDGMENTS

The authors acknowledge Beryl Greenberg for performing the insulin, C-peptide, and glucagon assays. Jerry Vincent prepared the illustrations, and Janet Sanders the manuscript.

This work was supported by USPHS grant AM19269, by a grant from the American Diabetes Association, Minnesota Chapter, and by NIH Grant RR-400 from the General Clinical Research Center Branch. Dr. Sutherland is the recipient of USPHS Research Career Development Award K04AM00161.

REFERENCES

[1] Kelly, W. D., Lillehei, R. C., Merkel, F. K., Idezuki, Y., and Goetz, F. C.: Allotransplantation of the pancreas and duodenum along with the kidney in diabetic nephropathy. Surgery *61*:827–37, 1967.

[2] Lillehei, R. C., Ruiz, J. O., Acquino, C., and Goetz, F. C.: Transplantation of the pancreas. Acta Endocrinol. *83* (Suppl. 205):303–20, 1976.

[3] Merkel, F. K., Poticha, S. M., Nudelman, E. J., Colwell, J. A., and Bergan, J. J.: Pancreas transplantation in man. I. The donor and recipient operation. Arch. Surg. *103*:205–10, 1971.

[4] Gliedman, M. L., Tellis, V. A., Soberman, R., Rifkin, H., and Veith, F. J.: Long-term effects of pancreatic transplant function in patients with advanced juvenile-onset diabetes mellitus. Diabetes Care *1*:1–9, 1978.

[5] Connolly, J. E., Martin, D. C., Steinberg, T., Gwinup, G., Gazzaniga, A. B., and Bartlett R. H.: Clinical experience with pancreaticoduodenal transplantation. Arch. Surg. *106*:489–94, 1973.

[6] Merkel, F. K., Ryan, W. G., Armbruster, K., Seim, S., and Ing, T. S.: Pancreatic transplantation for diabetes mellitus. Ill. Med. J. *144*:477–79, 1973.

[7] Largiader, F., and Kolb, E.: Rejection of pancreatic allografts: experimental and clinical results. *In* Transplantation and Clinical Immunology. X. Amsterdam, Excerpta Medica, 1979, pp. 240–44.

[8] Brynger, J., Blohme, G., Claes, G., Gustafsson, A., and Gelin, L. E.: Transplantation of a duct-ligated pancreatic allograft to a diabetic patient. Scand. J. Urol. Nephrol. *24* (Suppl.):59–62, 1975.

[9] Groth, C. G., Lundgren, G., Gunnarsson, R., Arner, P., Berg, B., and Östman, J.: Segmental pancreatic transplantation in nonuremic diabetic patients. *In* Transplantation and Clinical Immunology. X. Amsterdam, Excerpta Medica, 1979, pp. 196–201.

[10] Traeger, J., Dubernard, J. M., Touraine, J. L., Neyra, P., Malik, M. C., Pelissard, C., and Ruitton, A.: Pancreatic transplantation in man: a new method of pancreas preparation and results on diabetes correction. Transplant Proc. *11*:331–35, 1979.

[11] Gerrish, E. W.: Final newsletter, American College of Surgeons/National Institutes of Health Organ Transplant Registry, Chicago. June 30, 1977.

[12] Sutherland, D. E. R., Matas, A. J., and Najarian, J. S.: Pancreatic islet cell transplantation. Surg. Clin. North Am. *58*:365–82, 1978.

[13] Naji, A., Reckard, C. R., Ziegler, M. M., and Barker, C. F.: Vulnerability of pancreatic islets to immune cells and serum. Surg. Forum *26*:459–61, 1975.

[14] Najarian, J. S., Sutherland, D. E. R., and Steffes, M. W.: Isolation of human islets of Langerhans for transplantation. Transplant. Proc. *7*:611–13, 1975.

[15] Verschoor, L., Hulsmans, H. A. M., de Gruyl, J., Westbroek, D. L., and MacDicken, I.: Endocrine function of the canine pancreas: the effect of duct ligation and transplantation of the total duct ligated pancreas. Acta Endocrinol. *80*:302–18, 1975.

[16] Gliedman, M. L., Gold, M., Whittaker, J., Rifkin, H., Soberman, R., Freed, S., Tellis, V., and Veith, F. J.: Pancreatic duct to ureter anastomosis in pancreatic transplantation. Am. J. Surg. *125*:245–52, 1973.

[17] Dubernard, J. M., Traeger, J., Neyra, P., Touraine, J. L., Traudiant, D., and Blanc-Brunat, N.: A new method of preparation of segmental pancreatic grafts for transplantation: trials in dogs and in man. Surgery *84*:633–39, 1978.

[18] Kyriadides, G. K., Nuttall, F. Q., and Miller, J.: Segmental pancreatic transplantation in pigs. Surgery *85*:154–58, 1979.

[19] Kyriakides, G. K., Sutherland, D. E. R., Olson, L., Miller, J., and Najarian, J. S.: Segmental pancreatic transplantation in dogs. Transplant. Proc. *11*:530–32, 1979.

[20] Skom, J. H., and Talmage, D. W.: Nonprecipitating insulin antibodies. J. Clin. Invest. *37*:783–36, 1958.

[21] Goetz, F. C., Greenberg, B. Z., Ells, J., et al.: A simple immunoassay for insulin: application to human and dog plasma. J. Clin. Endocrinol. Metab. *23*:1237–46, 1963.

[22] Melani, F., Rubenstein, A. H., Oyer, P. E., and Steiner, D. F.: Identification of proinsulin and C-peptide in human serum by a specific immunoassay. Proc. Natl. Acad. Sci. U.S.A. *67* (1):148–55, 1970.

[23] Herbert, V., Lav, K. S., Gottlieb, C. W., et al.: Coated charcoal immunoassay of insulin. J. Clin. Endocrinol. *25*:1375–84, 1965.

[24] Molnar, G. D., Taylor, W. F., and Ho, M. M.: Day to day variation of continuously monitored glycaemia: a further measure of diabetes instability. Diabetologia *8*:342–48, 1972.

[25] Collins, J., Taylor, R. M. R., and Johnston, I.: Portal or systemic venous drainage for pancreatic transplantation: a physiological study. Ann. R. Coll. Surg. Engl. *58*:236, 1976.

Isolating the Elusive Islet

DAVID W. SCHARP, RICHARD DOWNING, RONALD C. MERRELL, AND MARIE GREIDER

SUMMARY

The lack of a technique that allows mass isolation of intact, viable human islets is part of the reason that islet transplantation has not become available to the human diabetic. This report outlines the history of islet isolation and presents two new technical modifications that have been developed in the dog. Many of the current problems in islet isolation are presented, including the difficulty in obtaining enough human pancreatic tissue with minimal warm-ischemia time; inadequate distention of the pancreas to provide sufficient disruption for maximal enzymatic reaction to release intact islets; inefficient chopping methods; the use of collagenase of variable composition; different digestion methods for obtaining isolated islets; and inefficient methods for separating and purifying the islets from the ductal, acinar, and fibrous components. The first new modification involves distention of the dog pancreas through the venous system of the gland rather than the ductal system. This results in improved intralobular disruption, which improved the yield of isolated dog islets by permitting more efficient collagenase digestion. The second new modification eliminates the concept of isolating intact islets: the dog pancreas is digested by trypsin to a single-cell preparation that is partially purified by Ficoll gradients; further purification of the endocrine cells results from selective aggregation using rotational culture. This process produces pseudoislets that contain all the islet cell types and can be kept in culture for up to 4 wk, releasing their hormones in response to appropriate stimuli. These modifications may assist in the struggle to isolate the elusive human islet for safe and effective islet transplantation in the diabetic patient. DIABETES *29* (Suppl. 1):19–30, 1980.

Isolation of viable islet cells from the pancreas of animals has provided information on the physiology of hormone release and material for recombinant DNA investigation and has allowed feasibility studies on the potential for islet transplantation for the treatment of diabetes. The majority of islet tissues for these studies and others has come from the rodent, since Moskalewski[1] first reported his technique for islet isolation in the guinea pig. A veritable explosion of studies has followed, and the majority of our experimental knowledge of islet cell function has been based on rodent tissue. While it is likely that the results are valid when using data on rodents to answer similar questions in man, certain anatomic and physiologic differences between rodent and human islets may invalidate these assumptions. In the area of islet transplantation especially, it would seem that one must have a human source of islets if one is going to be able to apply the successful results observed in rodents to human diabetics, but, to date, mass isolation of intact, viable human islets has not become a reality. The isolation techniques that work so well in the rodent are not effective in isolating large numbers of human islets. This report outlines the history of islet isolation from adult animal sources and presents two new modifications that we have recently been examining in an attempt to improve the yields of viable islet tissue from the larger mammalian pancreas.[2,3]

In 1911, Bensely[4] demonstrated that intravascular injection of a variety of dyes in the guinea pig would selectively stain pancreatic islets, thus identifying them so that they could be picked out by hand for study. This technique resulted in very small yields of islets in spite of some later modifications but, nevertheless, was an important beginning. Hellerstrom[5] in 1964 developed a freehand microdissection technique, which he applied in the obese hyperglycemic mouse. While this technique increased the yield of islets, its practical application was limited to this strain of mouse due to its uniquely large islets. Taking the lead from Banting and Best,[6] Kean[7] ligated the pancreatic duct in the rat before attempting islet isolation, reducing the amount of exocrine tissue by the progressive fibrosis of the

From the Departments of Surgery and Pathology, Washington University School of Medicine, St. Louis, Missouri 63110.

R. Downing's present address is Department of Surgery, Queen Elizabeth Hospital, Edgebaston, Birmingham, B15-2TH, England.

Dr. Merrell's present address is Department of Surgery, Stanford Medical Center, Boswell Building, Room A220, Stanford University, Stanford, California 94305.

gland. More recently, Payne et al.[8] have fibrosed the nonendocrine portion of the gland by feeding rats D-L-ethionine for several weeks before islet isolation; but questions have been raised by several investigators[9–11] as to whether the fibrosis which seems to make the isolation easier may also be affecting the islets by causing metabolic abnormalities in islet cell function as well.

The major breakthrough for islet isolation began, as mentioned, in 1965 when Moskalewski utilized an enzymatic technique to separate intact islets from the chopped guinea pig pancreas. He used the enzymatic complex called collagenase, incubated chopped pancreatic pieces at 37°C, and separated the released islets by sedimentation. All currently used modifications are based on this initial method. Lacy and Kostianovsky[12] in 1967 determined that mechanical disruption of the pancreas by ductal injection of a salt solution permitted increased enzymatic contact and improved the yield of isolated islets. Malaisse et al.[13] further reduced the digestion time by increasing the degree of agitation during the digestion process.

Handpicking the islets from the digestate was the only way at that time to recover the islets from the acinar debris. While this was tedious, it permitted the multitude of functional, anatomic, and other types of studies that have been conducted on the rodent islets. It was not, however, an attractive approach for the large-scale purification of isolated islets for transplantation studies since it required a lengthy time ex vivo to pick enough islets for transplantation. Lacy[12] successfully used a sucrose gradient to separate the islets from the digestate but found no insulin release in response to a glucose challenge in vitro. Jonsson[14] had suggested that sucrose damaged isolated rat peritoneal mast cells after examining the use of centrifugation gradients of sucrose, albumin, and Ficoll, a high-molecular-weight polymer of sucrose. Lindall et al.[15] demonstrated that Ficoll could be used to successfully isolate islets but did not study their ability to release insulin. Wallach and Kamat[16] in 1964 had reported that Ficoll contained varying amounts of sodium chloride, potassium, and low-molecular-weight polymers of sucrose that damage cell membranes. Jarett,[17] also working with cell membranes, dialyzed the Ficoll for his studies and obtained improved preparations. When our laboratory examined the ability of islets to release insulin after Ficoll isolation, we found that many lots from the supplier damaged the islets; but we reported in 1973 that insulin release was normal if the Ficoll was dialyzed before its use.[18] Collagenase digestion and Ficoll purification became the standard islet isolation technique for several years, especially for transplantation studies in rats.

With the feasibility of islet transplantation demonstrated by the rat portal vein model,[19–25] attention obviously turned to application of this technique to man. It soon became clear that the fairly standardized rat isolation techniques would not work in the more compact mammalian pancreases, including the human pancreas. Several investigators have reported isolating small numbers of islets using these techniques and have done limited studies on them. For example, Espinosa et al.[26] in 1971 reported studying human fetal islets, while Ashcroft et al.,[27] Ballinger and Lacy,[28] and Sutherland et al.[29] reported insulin response to a glucose challenge in isolated adult human islets. But mass isolation of purified, viable human islets has not as yet been reported.

With the recognition of this impasse to human islet isolation, we began to investigate the collagenase technique to determine if it could be improved. The primary problem with collagenase is the fact that it is an enzyme complex produced by bacteria. To date, there is no apparent control over the production of different component enzyme concentrations in each batch. The only practical method for determining an efficient batch seems to be by trial and error. Thus, with the standardized rat isolation technique, one would determine the optimal single digestion time which would give the maximal number of isolated islets with each new batch and pick one that gave the highest yield. But this is theoretically an inefficient method for isolating islets in man.

By looking for a single digestion end-point that releases the maximum number of islets, one loses islets that are released early in the digestion and kept in the enzyme mixture due to their breakdown by collagenase. One also loses islets that are still contained within the chopped pieces when the reaction is stopped at the end-point, which can be confirmed by examining histologically the remaining chopped pieces. In addition, the single end-point is determined by the appearance of the preparation—a skill that must be developed from experience—which varies between batches of collagenase and between strains, species, and ages of donors. Theoretically, if one could remove the islets from the digestate once they were liberated, one could protect them from breakdown, digest the entire gland to completion, and, thus, increase the yield of islets. Our laboratory developed a device that begins to accomplish this by incorporating a stainless steel filter of 260-μm pore size that permits passage of the liberated islets from the digestate. By doing repeated 1-min digestions, we were able to increase the yield of islets in the rat and eliminate the need to try to learn what an end-point should look like.[30,31] All of our transplantation studies since then have used this digestion-filtration device, and other investigators have confirmed its usefulness.[32,33] We then began examining the pancreas of other higher mammals, including the human pancreas. For the first time we began seeing isolated monkey and human islets in some numbers but, unfortunately, not in great enough numbers to produce effective islet transplantation. An advantage of the digestion-filtration method is that one need not try to determine a single end-point. This would be especially difficult in the human pancreas, since it is nearly impossible to gain enough experience with the digestion appearance to determine a digestion end-point at which the maximum number of islets are released. Unfortunately, different batches of collagenase continue to yield different results and must be tried for their effectiveness in isolating islets.

With this difficulty remaining in isolating human islets, many investigators have turned to another approach, which Mirkovitch[34] first reported. This method does not release isolated islets; instead, one chops the distended pancreas, incubates it with collagenase for 20 min, and then transplants these softened, chopped pieces containing islets into animals. While the initial work in dogs was troublesome, with a high degree of portal vein obstruction, human transplantation is continuing with no apparent difficulty.[35–37] This method and its results are summarized by David Sutherland in this supplement. We do not have enough data at present to compare the results using chopped pancreatic pieces with those of the isolated islets transplanted in the portal vein in our laboratory.

We have now returned to examining the islet isolation problem in the larger mammal by taking two new approaches. In the first, we have examined a new method of distending the pancreas which seems to give an improved intralobular disruption of the pancreas, resulting in increased numbers of isolated, intact islets being released by the collagenase.[2,38,39] The second method eliminated the concept of isolating intact islets. It consists of digesting the chopped, distended pancreas completely to a single cell suspension, concentrating the endocrine cells by Ficoll gradients, and forming pseudoislets by selective aggregation using a rotational culture technique.[3] Presentation of these two methods and some preliminary results will complete this report.

The basis of the first method of improving the distention of the gland came from the observation that ductal distention of the more organized and compact mammalian pancreas of the dog, cow, pig, monkey, or human did not give the same result as did ductal distention of the rat pancreas. The result after ductal distention of the left lobe of the dog pancreas is shown in Figure 1. While the distention initially may look excellent, one can observe that the predominant disruption of the pancreas is really interlobular and not the intralobular disruption that one needs to permit the islets to be released by collagenase. The rat pancreas, on the other hand, develops excellent interlobular and intralobular disruption by ductal distention. Since Lacy[12] had shown that mechanical disruption by ductal distention in the rat had improved the yield of islets, it seemed logical that this lack of effective disruption by ductal injection could be part of the reason for such a poor yield of islets from the higher mammalian pancreas.

There appears to be only four ways that one can distend a pancreas: (1) by direct injection of solution via a needle into the substance of the gland, (2) by ductal distention, (3) by injection of distention fluid through the arterial supply of the gland, and (4) by injection of fluid through the venous supply. While direct injection worked well for mouse islet isolation,[40] it had not been effective in our previous attempts in the dog, human, or monkey pancreas and was not further evaluated. Ductal injection had the problems previously described plus the obvious drawback of low islet yields. The next possible method examined was the injection of the arterial supply. Arterial injection of the pancreas via the splenic artery results in an excellent disruption of the gland with marked intralobular distention as compared with ductal distention, but, histologically, the islets are nearly completely destroyed by the pressure of the injection.

We next injected the venous supply of the pancreas via the splenic vein, which also gave an excellent intralobular disruption but did not seem to damage the islets. The mechanical separation around the islets achieved by venous disruption and the lack of this spacing achieved by ductal disruption are shown in Figure 2. Further evidence of this effect is found in more definitive reports of this technique in different animals.[38,41,42] The anatomic explanation of this species difference may be that the higher mammalian pancreatic duct simply cannot withstand the pressure generated by the rapid distention of solutions against the firm resistance of the stronger and more fibrous lobules of this type of pancreas. Thus, the duct may give way before the lobule can be adequately expanded, resulting in predominant interlobular disruption and not the needed intralobular disruption. In the rat, there is little fibrous resistance in the lobules, and, thus, the ducts seem to hold the pressure, resulting in excellent intralobular disruption.

The difference between the effects on the islets after arterial and venous distention is not surprising, but it is interesting in the light of an islet-to-acinar vascular portal circulation first described by Wharton in 1932 and confirmed by others to be present in many species, including man.[43–46] The islets receive afferent arterioles and have multiple efferent arterioles that go to the exocrine capillary system before joining into the portal circulation. This suggests an islet cell hormone function for the exocrine pancreas, which other investigators are beginning to examine. It has been reported that the efferent arterioles possess sphincters. When one injects solution through the arterial supply, one mechanically

FIGURE 1. Distal left lobe of the canine pancreas after ductal distention of Hank's balanced salt solution demonstrating the predominately interlobular disruption achieved.

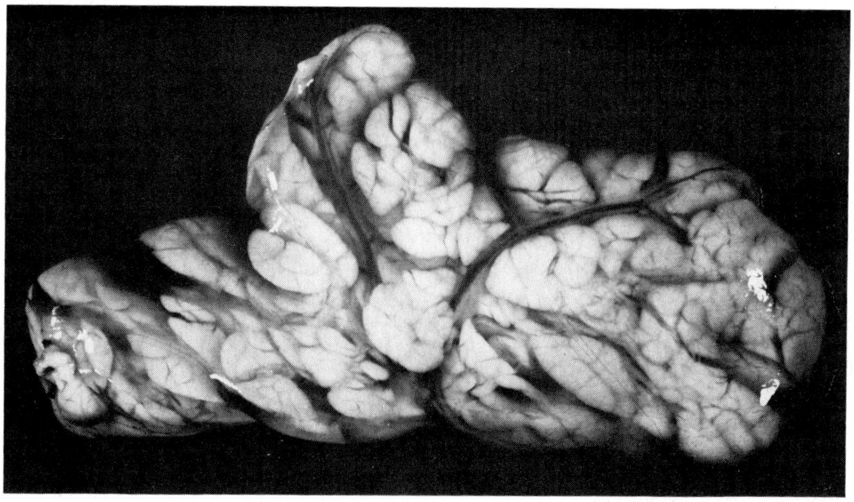

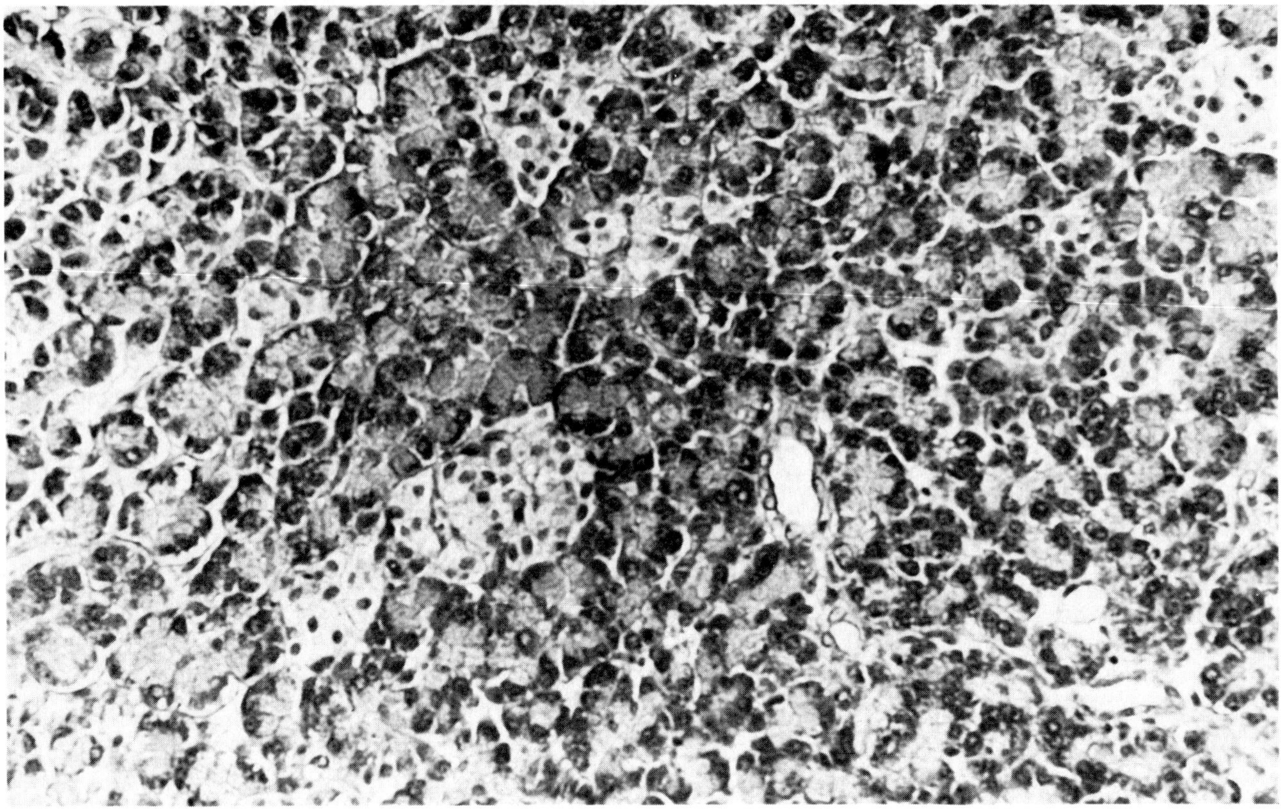

A

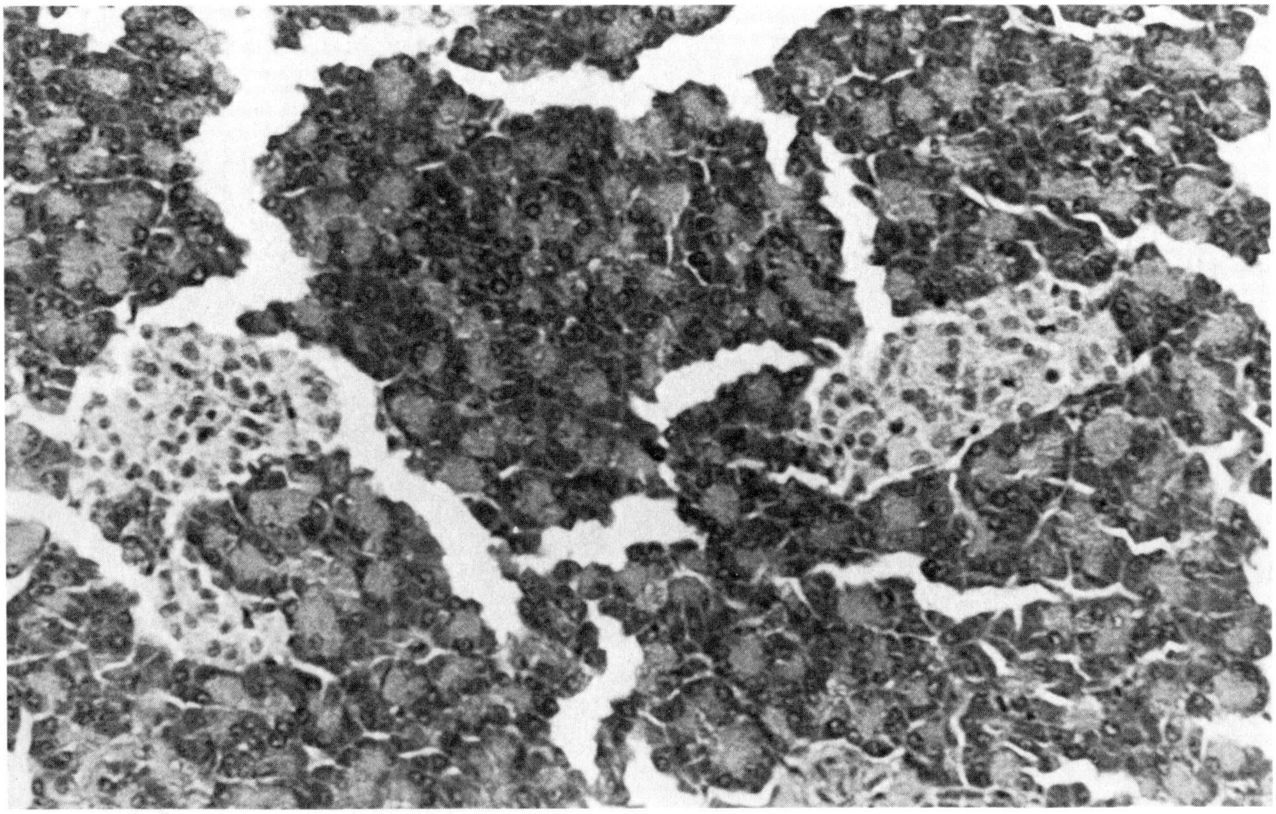

B

FIGURE 2. (A) Ductal distention. Microscopic appearance of the canine pancreas after ductal distention showing the lack of intralobular disruption. (Hematoxylin-eosin ×500.) (B) Venous distention. Demonstration of improved intralobular disruption causing mechanical spacing between the islets and the acinar tissue. (Hematoxylin-eosin ×500.)

destroys the islets, which would happen especially if the efferent sphincter system provides resistance to the injection. When one injects through the venous system, the islets are not destroyed. Perhaps the efferent sphincters are protecting the islets from this back-pressure, or perhaps the pressure generated is simply dispersed throughout the exocrine capillary system.

Another problem was encountered in attempting to isolate dog islets. Identification of rat islets in the final preparation by using dissecting microscopes is fairly easy, but we were unable to reliably identify dog islets without the assistance of neutral red to selectively stain the islets. While Bensley[4] had described the use of this dye, Lacy[12] and our laboratory[30] previously had placed neutral red in the distention fluid, giving excellent staining. This method was not successful in the dog, so an arterial perfusion system was developed which gave excellent selective staining of the islets.[38,42] We were thus able to quantitate more reliably the yield of islets after the two methods of distention.

The method used for the isolation of dog islets consisted of surgically preparing the dog's pancreas by isolating the arterial and venous supplies to the pancreas. Then neutral red (6 mg/dl) was mixed with blood cannulated from the femoral artery and returned to the splenic artery for a 20-min perfusion by a double-pump system with the celiac artery clamped. This gave selective staining to the islets while it prevented significant pancreatic edema. With the arterial supply still clamped, the portal vein, inferior and superior mesenteric veins, and left gastric veins were clamped and Hank's salt solution was rapidly and forcibly injected into the splenic vein, which effectively distended the pancreas. The gland was removed and finely chopped with scissors. Then 6 ml of the chopped pieces were loaded into each stainless steel basket (260-μm pore size) that had been prepared to fit into a 50-ml syringe barrel. A stopper was positioned over the open end and the tubing connected. Collagenase (Sigma Chemical Co.) was placed in the chamber with an initial concentration of 1000 U/ml of chopped pancreas. A series of digestions was done at 37°C in a shaker water bath, flushing the chamber between digestions to remove the liberated islets, which were collected, rinsed, and held on ice. There were two 2-min digestions using 1000 U of collagenase per milliliter of chopped pancreas. Then four 1-min digestions were done, reducing the collagenase concentration by half each time. The final islet preparation was loaded onto Ficoll discontinuous gradients (11, 20, 23, and 25%) and spun at 800 $\times$ g for 15 min. The islets were collected from the 11–20% layer and examined under the dissecting microscope where they could be identified by their staining produced by the neutral red. Histologic confirmation demonstrated that the red-stained structures were islets and, thus, they could be counted. These isolated islets from the distal left lobe of the pancreas under various staining techniques are shown in Figure 3.

While detailed data on the yields of islets, hormone extractions, and hormone release are presented in the referenced publications, the yields of isolated canine islets expressed as the number per milliliter of chopped pancreas and demonstrating a two- to threefold increase in the total yields after venous distention are shown in Figure 4. Part A illustrates the numbers of isolated islets at each digestion time and confirms the concept that the digestion-filtration technique is able to release islets throughout the digestion period, regardless of the type of canine pancreas distention. The increased numbers of isolated islets released at each digestion time after venous distention suggest that the improved intralobular disruption by venous distention is simply exposing more islets for collagenase release. Part B illustrates the accumulated number of islets released during the digestion procedure and also demonstrates the total increase in isolated islets achieved after venous distention. This type of data also demonstrates that there is a digestion time that gives a maximal number of isolated islets, but, if one had stopped the digestion at 5 min, for example, as one would with a single digestion end-point technique, an additional 150 islets per milliliter that were still trapped in the chopped pieces would have been lost. If one had stopped at 7 min, for example, many of the islets released at 2 and 4 min would have been lost due to the collagenase digestion of the isolated islets. Thus, the combination of venous distention with digestion-filtration gives us the maximal amount of isolated and purified islets for study. While this technique seems a promising improvement in the dog, other species, including man, are being investigated to determine if the same increase in islet yield can be achieved.

Even with this kind of increase, there are many significant problems remaining in the isolation of intact, viable islets as listed in Table 1. Human donor pancreas is rather limited due to the apparent requirement of a brief, warm ischemia time to keep autolysis at a minimum before attempting to isolate islets. At least, unpublished data in our laboratory suggest that the ability to isolate islets in animals is greatly reduced within minutes of the death of the donating animal. This area has not been thoroughly investigated, however. Perhaps techniques such as rapid cold perfusion, anti-trypsin inhibitor perfusion, or early degranulation of the exocrine pancreas by pilocarpine soon after death may provide additional valuable time in stabilizing the pancreas before isolation techniques. This report has presented a new method of pancreas distention in the dog that seems to be an improvement. Whether this method will work in human isolation is not yet known. Effective chopping of the entire pancreas by hand is difficult and inefficient. Several prototypes of automatic choppers, which are modifications of a

TABLE 1
Problems isolating intact islets

1. Donor tissue
   - A. Limited human source
   - B. Short warm ischemia time
2. Pancreas distention
   - A. Ductal vs. venous
3. Pancreas chopping
   - A. Hand vs. automatic
4. Digestion conditions
   - A. Collagenase
   - B. Single end point
   - C. Digestion-filtration
   - D. Continuous method
5. Purification
   - A. Sedimentation
   - B. Hand-picking
   - C. Ficoll gradients
   - D. Percoll gradients
   - E. Other gradients

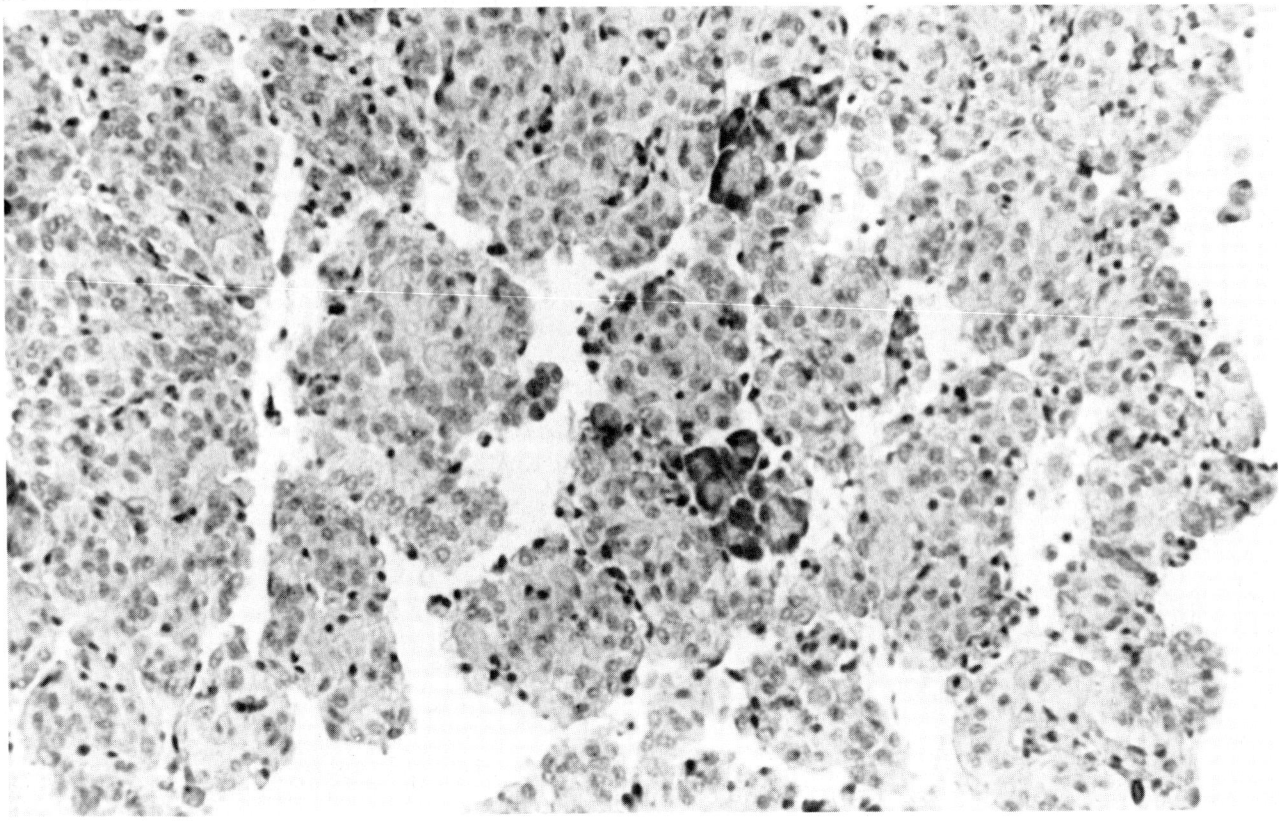

A

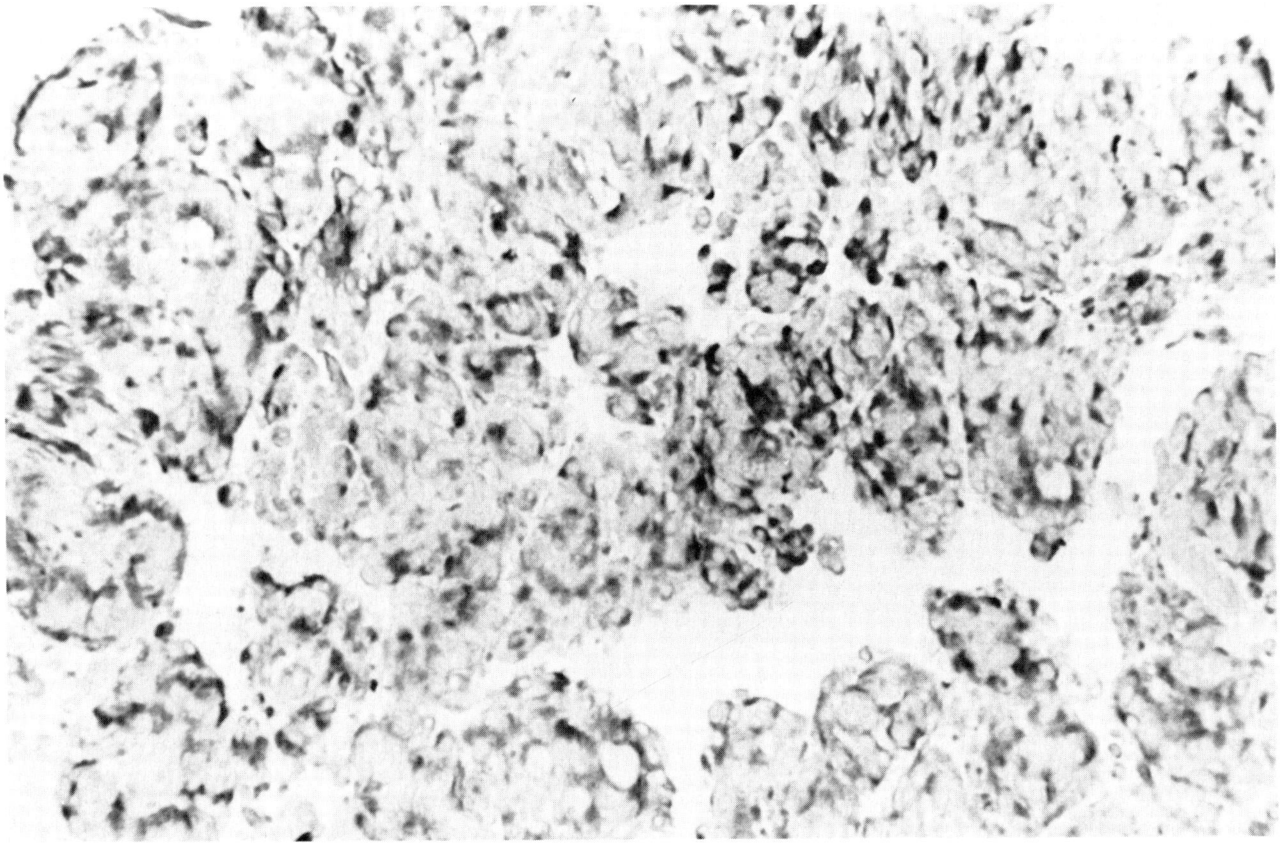

B

FIGURE 3. Isolated canine islets after venous distention, collagenase digestion-filtration, and Ficoll purification. These islets were handpicked off the Ficoll layers using the neutral red staining to distinguish them from the acinar debris which also comes up to the 11–20% layer. The arrows point to small aggregates of exocrine tissue included with the islets. (×500.) (A) Hematoxylin-eosin staining; (B) aldehyde fuchsin; (C) insulin antibody; (D) glucagon antibody.

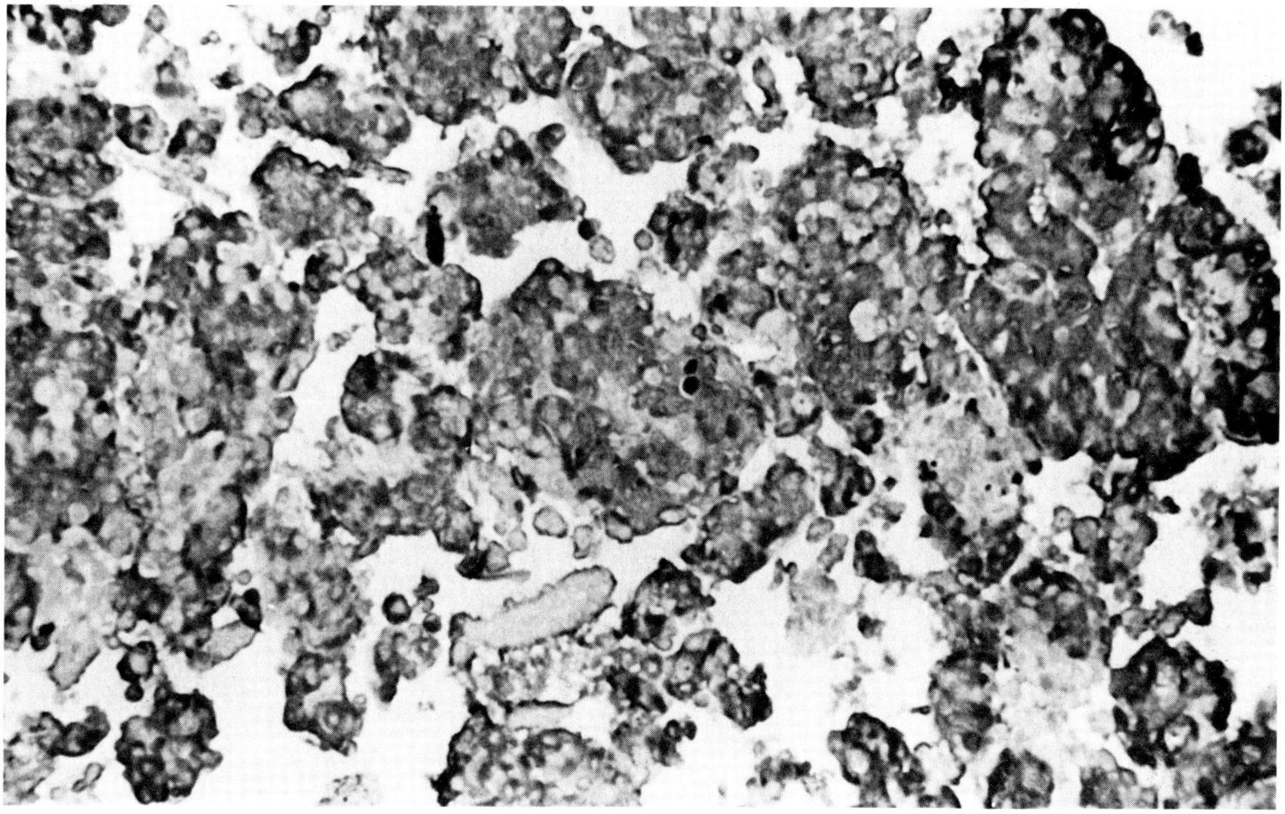

C

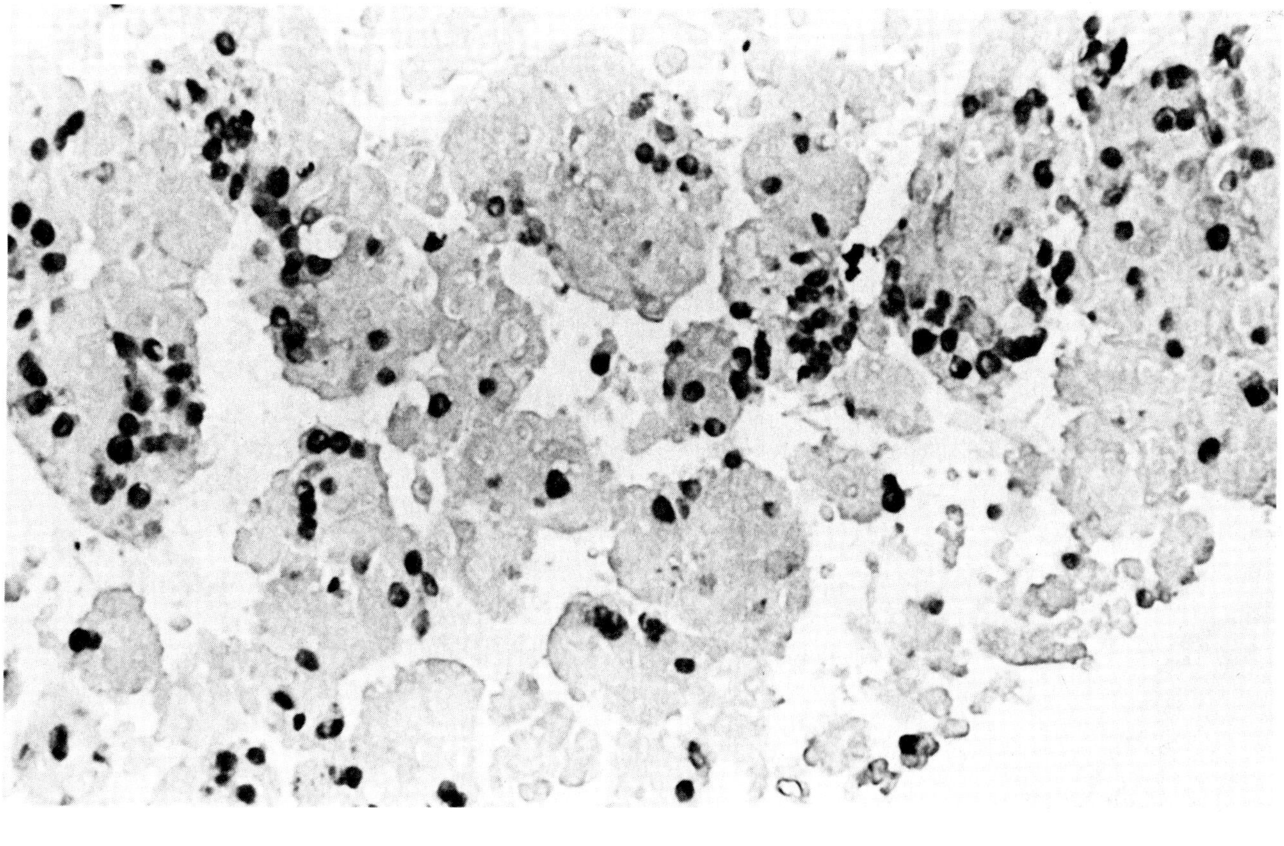

D

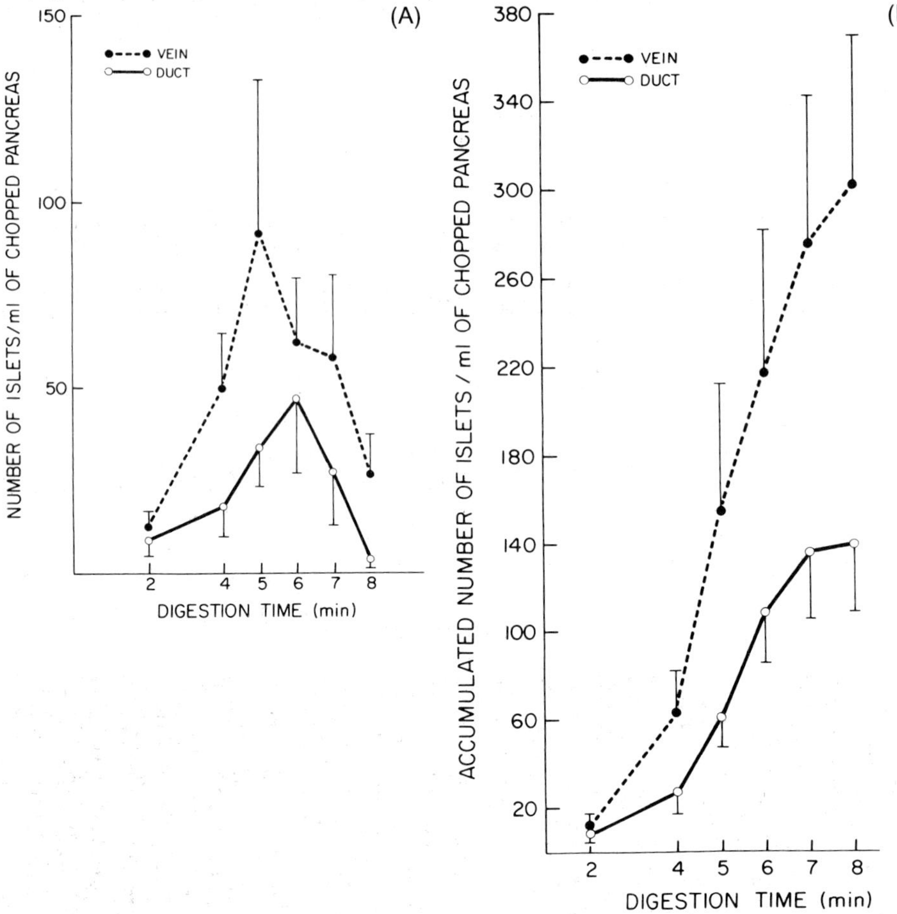

FIGURE 4. (A) The number of isolated canine islets per milliliter of chopped pancreas that were released at each digestion time by the digestion-filtration technique after either venous distention (●) or ductal distention (○) of the pancreas. x ± SEM; N = 5. (B) The accumulated total number of islets released during the digestion process after either venous distention (●) or ductal distention (○) of the pancreas. x ± SEM; N = 5.

design by Bruce Gray, are being used in various laboratories.[47,48] While their design seems to be good, further investigation is needed. A primary problem remains in the method of collagenase digestion. Even with digestion-filtration, different batches of collagenase can give completely different results, as can different concentrations of the enzymes. This makes studies on isolation methodology even more difficult. Perhaps continuous, automatic methods will have to be developed before standardization can be achieved. If companies such as Worthington or Sigma could supply a standard concentration of enzyme constituents, perhaps more uniform results would be realized. While Ficoll gradients result in fairly purified rat preparations, they give contaminated preparations of dog, monkey, and human islets. Even though the islets can be concentrated by using this gradient, the amount of acinar debris that stays with them is prohibitive. With the findings of Lacy et al.,[49,50] using immunoalteration techniques in tissue culture requiring totally pure islets, handpicking now may be required. New approaches such as handpicking as described by Finke et al.[51] may be needed in order to accomplish purification of the type required to alter the tissue before transplantation, but modifications of available centrifugation gradients may also result in such purification. Thus, with all these problems in isolating purified islets, it is understandable that many investigators have looked for other methods for obtaining islets for transplantation in man. Answers to these difficulties in islet isolation seem to be technical, however, and methodologic studies are definitely worthy of continued investigation.

While these studies on pancreatic distention were in progress for intact islet isolation, we were also examining another totally different method of islet cell isolation and purification in the dog. Since there has been so much difficulty isolating intact islets from the larger mammalian pancreas, we wondered if one could completely digest the gland to a single-cell preparation, find some way to purify the islet cells, and then form new islets again. The component techniques of such an approach are already available. Single-cell preparation from the pancreas has been a technique used for many years by several investigators for preparing tissue culture monolayers.[52,53] Moscona[54] has extensively studied selective aggregation using rotational culture techniques to examine different types of single-cell preparations under these culture conditions. We had already tried his rotational culture technique on isolated islets with interesting preliminary results.[55] Thus, we began the following study to determine if we could combine these two methods and form new islets from single-cell preparations of the intact pancreas.

We initially distended the dog pancreas by several methods; the type of distention used does not result in much difference in the final preparation. We have, therefore, used ductal distention for the studies that follow. The gland is finely chopped and 5 ml is placed in each 50-ml Erlenmeyer flask containing 15 ml of a 100–150 mg/dl trypsin solution

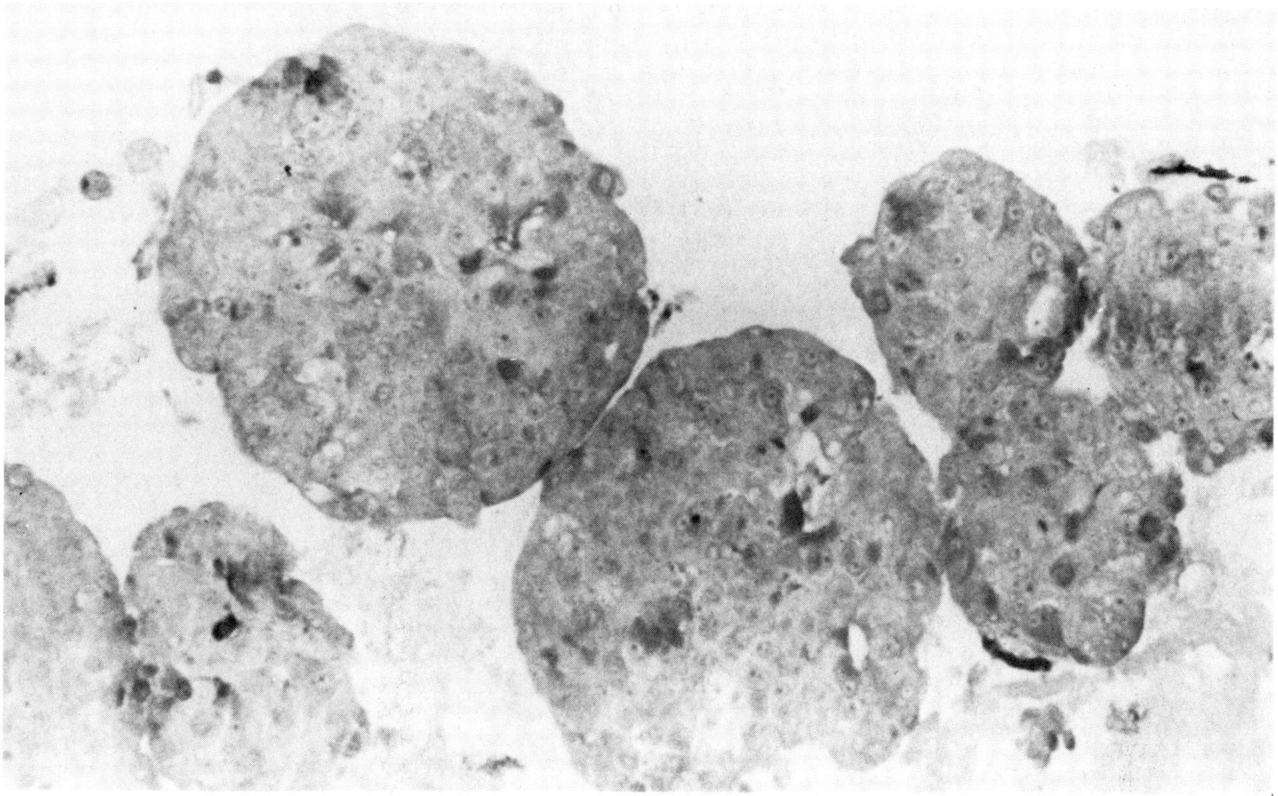

A

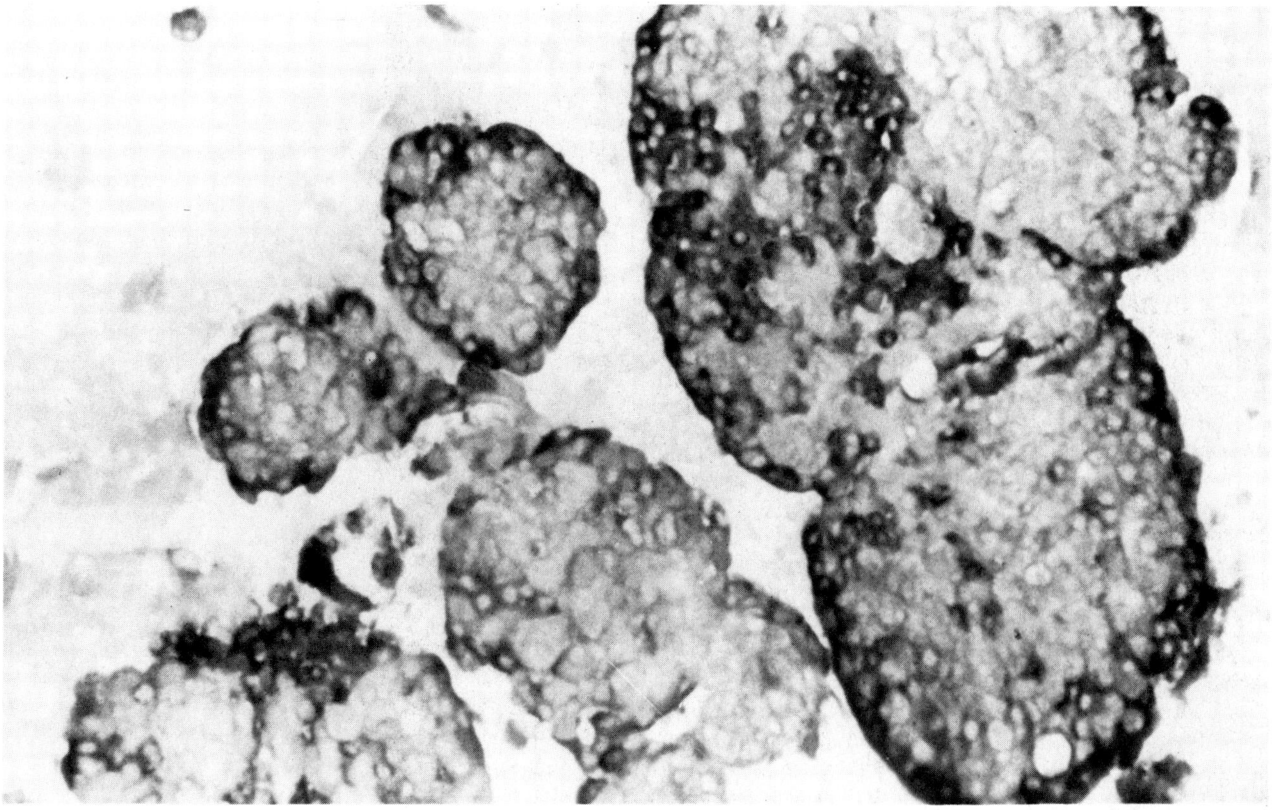

B

FIGURE 5. Pseudoislets after 8 days of tissue culture. These were formed by trypsin digestion of the canine pancreas to a single-cell preparation, Ficoll purification, and selective aggregation by rotational culture. (×500.) (A) Aldehyde fuchsin; (B) insulin antibody stain; (C) glucagon antibody stain.

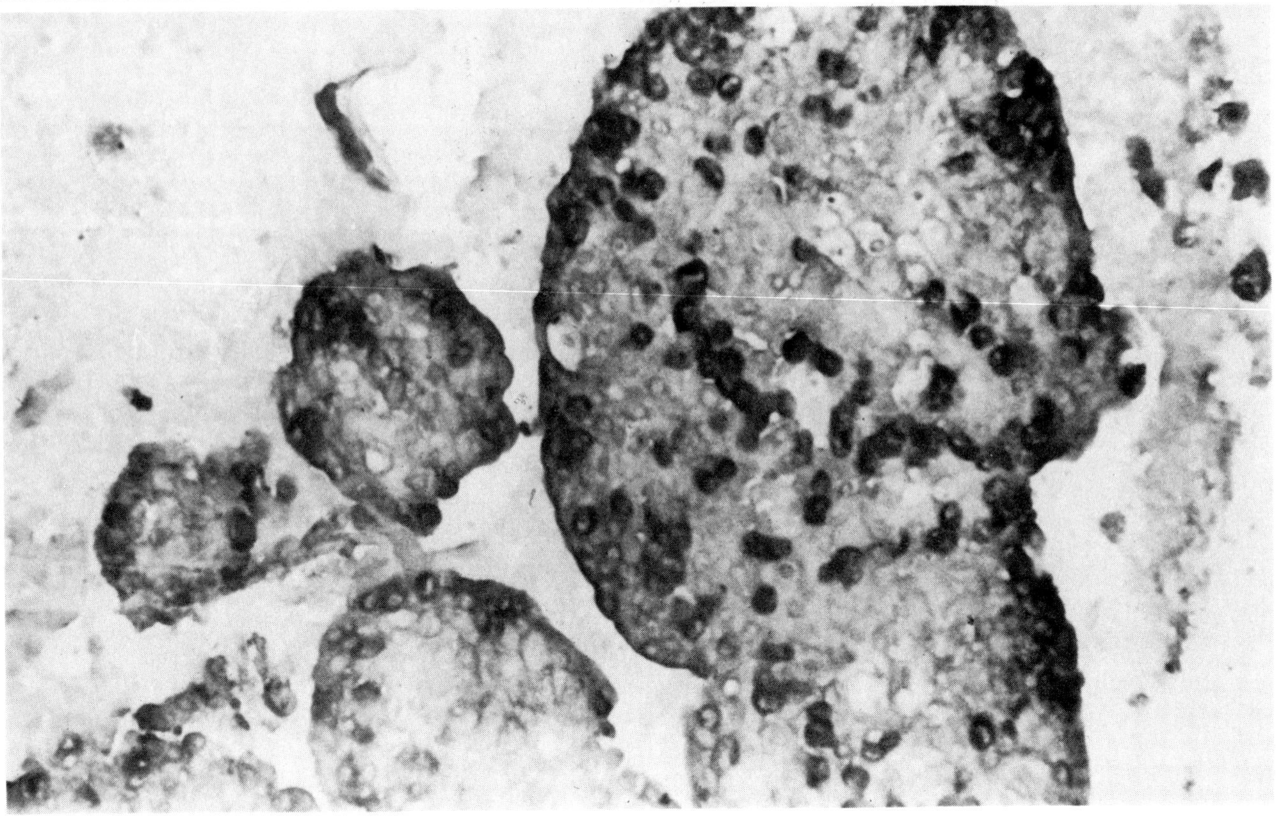

C

FIGURE 5. (continued)

in a Ca^{2+}-, Mg^{2+}-free, NaCl (8.0 g/L), KCl (0.2 g/L) salt solution with glucose (1 g/L), 25 mM Hepes, 0.02% EDTA, 100 U of penicillin per milliter, 100 μg of streptomycin per milliliter, and 5% calf serum. An initial 5-min digestion at 37°C is done in a Dubenoff shaker water bath at a slow speed, followed by several 1-min digestions. Between each digestion period, the flask is removed from the water bath, and the tissue is forced through a long, 14-gauge needle on a syringe to break up the tissue. The suspension is then removed and placed in an enzyme stop solution containing 10% calf serum at 4°C. This single-cell preparation is lightly centrifuged, filtered to remove larger pieces, and held at 4°C in the enzyme stop solution until completion of the digestion procedure. A total cell count is then taken with trypan blue exclusion performed for viability. The yield of cells at this point is variable but is in the range of 10^6–10^7 single cells per milliliter of chopped pancreas with a cell viability of over 90%. The cells are then placed on Ficoll discontinuous gradients and spun at 800 × *g* for 15 min. Each layer is removed and a cell count obtained, and the islets are washed in media. Then 1 × 10^6 cells are placed in 10-ml micro-Fernbach flasks containing 4 ml of Media 199 supplemented with Earle's salts, 150 mg/dl glucose, 2 mM glutamine, 100 U of penicillin per milliliter, 100 μg of streptomycin per milliliter, 10% fetal calf serum, and 25 mM Hepes. These flasks are placed in a rotational culture bath (New Brunswick, G76) at 110 rpm and 37°C. Media changes are performed every 2 or 3 days and in vitro glucose challenges done weekly. Initial aggregation takes place in several hours, but a firm, solid aggregate is not complete until about 4 days. The aggregates have been kept on culture for 4 wk with functional insulin output demonstrated during this period.[3]

The histologic appearance of these aggregates after 8 days of culture is shown in Figure 5. We have found aldehyde fuchsin staining to be unreliable, since it seems to stain acinar cells more readily than beta cells in this preparation. We therefore have used hormone antibody staining methods[56] to confirm the presence of the different islet cell types in the aggregates. As seen in the figure, one sees the stained beta cells and alpha cells in a more peripheral location within each aggregate. Immunostaining for pancreatic polypeptide cells demonstrates that these are found more centrally. Immunostaining for somatostatin has been inconsistent because of antibody difficulties, but preliminary results suggest the presence of these cells in a more central location as well. Contamination of these aggregates by acinar or duct cells in more recent experiments is reduced to the 10–30% level, as suggested by Figure 5A. With demonstration of the major islet cell types in this preparation, we have decided to call these aggregates pseudoislets. An example of their insulin production during the 4-wk culture period is shown in Figure 6.

This new method of pseudoislet formation offers several interesting possibilities for their use. One may be able to affect the percentage composition of the islet cell types by varying the isolation and culture conditions. For example, the Ficoll gradients appear to have little effect on beta cell purification from the single cell preparation but appear to be concentrating alpha cells on the lower levels.[57] Perhaps

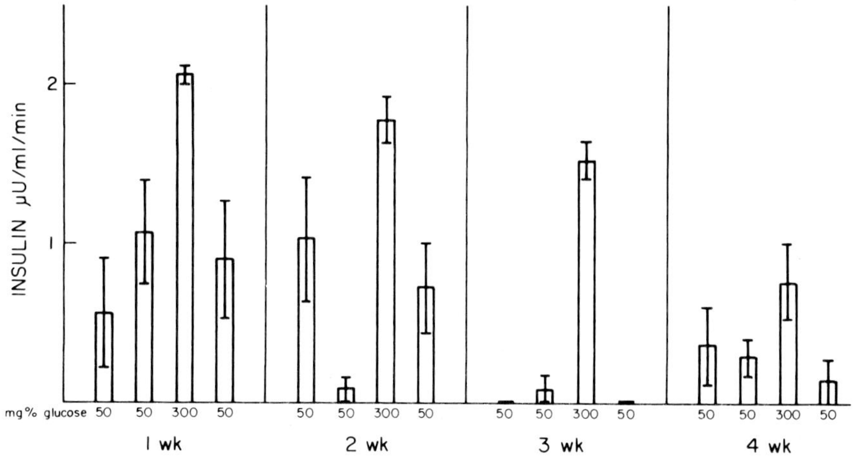

FIGURE 6. Pseudoislet insulin responsiveness after in vitro glucose stimulation during 4 wk of tissue culture. These aggregates were collected from the 11–15% Ficoll layer, cultured in Medium 199 with 159 mg/dl glucose rotational culture. Overnight media were removed from the flasks. The pseudoislets were washed, and fresh media containing either 50 mg/dl glucose or 300 mg/dl glucose were replaced with samples of insulin collected at the end of each challenge period. x̄ ± SEM.

by selective trypsinization of these pseudoislets, one may be able to obtain pure preparations of each of the different cell types. Such preparations as well as recombinations of the different cell types may provide interesting studies on the islet-to-islet cell interactions on islet cell hormone release. The use of pseudoislets as a source for transplantation tissue is also being considered. Our preliminary experience with this preparation so far suggests that the yields of islet tissue may be too small to consider single-donor transplantation, but the quantitation of the amount of islet tissue formed into pseudoislets per adult pancreas is currently being determined. We also do not have any information as yet as to whether pseudoislets will survive after transplantation. While their size can be varied by the culture conditions, they do not contain any capillaries, which transplanted intact isolated islets possess. Whether this will affect their survival after transplantation remains to be determined.

In conclusion, this report has attempted to summarize progress to date in the isolation of islet tissue from the adult pancreas. We have also presented two new methods that may increase our yield of viable islet tissue for transplantation. The studies by Lacy, Lafferty, and Talmadge that are included in this symposium suggest that immunoalteration of islet tissue may provide islet transplantation for diabetics without immunosuppression. With this possibility a step closer, we need to be able to develop rapid, efficient methods of obtaining islet tissue for transplantation from the human pancreas or perhaps even from nonhuman donors. The two new approaches presented here may lead to such an effective method and help capture the elusive islet for successful transplantation in the diabetic patient.

ACKNOWLEDGMENTS

We appreciate the technical assistance of L. Drummer, M. Feldmeier, L. Gardner, D. Kiske, B. Olack, R. Ross, and C. Scharp in these studies and the clerical skills of J. Metz in the preparation of the manuscript.

D. Scharp is the recipient of the NIH Research Career Development Award AM 00318. Other funding came from The Kroc Foundation and NIH grants AM 21966, AM 25585, and AM 18235.

REFERENCES

[1] Moskalewski, S.: Isolation and culture of the islets of Langerhans of the guinea pig. Gen. Comp. Endocrinol. *5*:324–53, 1965.

[2] Downing, R., Scharp, D. W., Greider, M., and Ballinger, W. F.: Mass isolation of islets of Langerhans from the dog pancreas. Diabetes *28*:426, 1979.

[3] Scharp, D. W., Merrell, R. C., Feldmeier, M. M., Downing, R., and Ballinger, W. F.: Pseudo-islet formation and culture from canine isolated pancreatic cells. In Vitro *15*:216, 1979.

[4] Bensley, R. R.: Studies on the pancreas of the guinea pig. Am. J. Anat. *12*:297–388, 1911

[5] Hellerström, C.: A method for the microdissection of intact pancreatic islets of mammals. Acta. Endocrinol. *45*:122–322, 1964.

[6] Banting, F. G., and Best, C. H.: The effect of pancreatic extract (insulin) on normal rabbits. Am. J. Physiol. *62*:162–176, 1922.

[7] Kean, H., Sells, R., and Jarrett, R. J.: A method for the study of the metabolism of isolated mammalian islets of Langerhans and some preliminary results. Diabetologia *1*:28–32, 1965.

[8] Payne, W. D., Sutherland, D. E. R., Matas, A. J., and Najarian, J. S.: Amelioration of diabetes in rats by transplantation of islet tissue from a single donor to multiple recipients. Surg. Forum *28*:301–04, 1977.

[9] Bergan, J. J., Hoehn, J. G., Porter, N., and Dry, L.: Total pancreatic allografts in pancreatectomized dogs. Arch. Surg. *90*:521–26, 1977.

[10] Chaya, E., Appert, H. E., and Howard, J. M.: Canine allografts of (homografts) of islet cell tissue. Arch. Surg. *93*:598–605, 1966.

[11] Seddon, J. A., and Howard, J. M.: The endocrine function of the homotransplanted pancreas. Surgery *59*:235–42, 1966.

[12] Lacy, P. E., and Kostianovsky, M.: Method for the isolation of intact islets of Langerhans from the rat pancreas. Diabetes *16*:35–39, 1967.

[13] Malaisse, W. J., Malaisse-Lagae, F., Walker, M. O., and Lacy, P. E.: The stimulus-secretion coupling of glucose-induced insulin release. V. The participation of a microtubular-microfilamentous system. Diabetes *20*:257–65, 1971.

[14] Jonsson, A. R., and Moran, N. C.: Comparison of several methods for isolation of rat peritoneal mast cells. Proc. Soc. Exp. Biol. Med. *123*:886–89, 1966.

[15] Lindall, A., Steffes, N., and Sorenson, R.: Immunoassayable insulin content of subcellular fraction of rat islets. Endocrinology *85*:218–23, 1969.

[16] Wallach, D. F. H., and Kamat, V. B.: Plasma and cytoplasmatic membrane fragments from Ehrlich ascites carcinoma. Proc. Natl. Acad. Sci. USA *52*:721–28, 1964.

[17] Jarrett, L. B.: Personal communication. Department of Pathology, Washington University School of Medicine, St. Louis, Missouri, 1972.

[18] Scharp, D. W., Kemp, C. B., Knight, M. J., Ballinger, W. F., and Lacy, P. E.: The use of ficoll in the preparation of viable islets of Langerhans from the rat pancreas. Transplantation *16*:686–89, 1973.

[19] Kemp, C. B., Knight, M. J., Scharp, D. W., Ballinger, W. F., and Lacy, P. E.: Effects of transplantation site on the results of pancreatic islet isografts in diabetic rats. Diabetologia *9*:486–91, 1973.

[20] Amamoo, D. G., Woods, J. E., and Donovan, J. L.: Preliminary experience with pancreatic islet-cell implantation. Mayo Clin. Proc. *49*:289–92, 1974.

[21] Naji, A., Reckard, C. R., Ziegler, M. M., and Barker, F. C.: Vunerability of pancreatic islets to immune cells and serum. Surg. Forum *26*:459–61, 1975.

[22] Mauer, S. M., Steffes, M. W., Sutherland, D. E. R., Najarian, J., Michael, A., and Brown, D.: Studies on the rate of regression of the glomerular

lesions in diabetic rats treated with pancreatic islet transplantation. Diabetes 24(3):280–85, 1975.

[23] Weber, C., Zatriqi, A., Weil, R., McIntosh, R., Hardy, M., and Reemtsma, K.: Pancreatic islet isografts, allografts and xenografts: comparison of morphology and function. Surgery 79:144–51, 1976.

[24] Griffith, R. C., Scharp, D. W., Hartman, B. K., Ballinger, W. F., and Lacy, P. E.: A morphologic study of intrahepatic portal-vein islet isografts. Diabetes 26:201–14, 1977.

[25] Pipeleers-Marichal, M., Pipeleers, D. G., Cutler, J., Lacy, P., and Kipnis, D.: Metabolic and morphologic studies in intraportal-islet-transplanted rats. Diabetes 25:1041–51, 1976.

[26] Espinosa, M. M. A., Driscoll, S. G., and Steinhe, J.: Insulin release from isolated human fetal pancreatic islets. Science 168:1111–12, 1970.

[27] Ashcroft, S. J. H., Randle, P. J., and Basset, J. T.: Isolation of human pancreatic islets capable of releasing insulin metabolizing glucose in vitro. Lancet 1:888, 1971.

[28] Ballinger, W. F., and Lacy, P. E.: Transplantation of intact pancreatic islets in rats. Surgery 72:175–86, 1972.

[29] Sutherland, D. E. R., Steffes, M. W., Bauer, G. E., McManus, D., Noe, B. D., and Najarian, J. S.: Isolation of human and porcine islets of Langerhans and islet transplantation in pigs. J. Surg. Res. 16:102–11, 1974.

[30] Scharp, D. W., Murphy, J. J., Newton, W. T., Ballinger, W. F., and Lacy, P. E.: Transplantation of islets of Langerhans in diabetic rhesus monkeys. Surgery 77:100–105, 1975.

[31] Scharp, D. W., Murphy, J. J., Newton, W. T., Ballinger, W. F., and Lacy, P. E.: Application of an improved technique for islet transplantation in primates and rats. Transplant. Proc. 7:739–41, 1975.

[32] Shibata, A., Ludvigsen, C. W., Jr., Naber, S. P., McDaniel, M. L., and Lacy, P. E.: Standardization of a digestion-filtration method for isolation of pancreatic islets. Diabetes 25:667–721, 1976.

[33] Orsetti, A., Puech, A. M., Zouari, N., Guy, Ch., and Passebois, F.: Isolement d'ilots de langerhans intacts au moyen de chambres de digestion filtration. J. Annu. Diabetol. Hotel Dieu, Paris, pp. 66–75, 1977.

[34] Mirkovitch, V., and Campiche, M.: Successful intrasplenic autotransplantation of pancreatic tissue in totally pancreatectomized dogs. Transplantation 21:265–66, 1976.

[35] Najarian, J. S., Sutherland, D. E. R., and Steffes, M. W.: Isolation of human islets of Langerhans for transplantation. Transpl. Proc 7:611–13, 1975.

[36] Matas, A. J., Sutherland, D. E. F., Steffes, M. W., and Najarian, J. S.: Short-term culture of adult pancreatic fragments for purification and transplantation of islets of Langerhans. Surgery 80:183–91, 1976.

[37] Najarian, J. S., Sutherland, D. E. R., Matas, A. J., Steffes, M. W., Simmons, R. L., and Goetz, F. C.: Human islet transplantation: a preliminary report. Transpl. Proc. 9:233–36, 1977.

[38] Downing, R., Scharp, D. W., and Ballinger, W. F.: An improved technique for the isolation and identification of mammalian islets of Langerhans. Transplantation. In press, 1980.

[39] Downing, R., Scharp, D. W., Merrell, R. C., Greider, M., and Ballinger, W. F.: Venous versus ductal distention of the dog pancreas for isolation of islets. Surg Forum 30:422–24, 1979.

[40] Eff, C.: Insulin release, insulin content and glucose utilization in isolated mouse islets maintained in culture. Acta Endocrinol. 87:535–42, 1978.

[41] Downing, R., Scharp, D. W., Merrell, R. C., and Nunnelley, S.: An improved method for the isolation of mammalian islets of Langerhans. I. The rat pancreas. Submitted for publication, 1979.

[42] Downing, R., Scharp, D. W., Merrell, R. C., Nunnelley, S., and Greider, M.: An improved method for the isolation of mammalian islets of Langerhans. II. The dog pancreas. Submitted for publication, 1979.

[43] Wharton, G. K.: The blood supply of the pancreas with special reference to that of the islands of Langerhans. Anat. Rec. 53:55–82, 1932.

[44] Andreassi, V. G.: Die blutversorgung der Langerhansschen Inseln der menschlichen Bauchspeicheldruse. Anat. Anz. 119:421–26, 1966.

[45] Fujita, T.: Insulo-acinar portal system in the horse pancreas. Arch. Histol. Jpn. 35:161–71, 1973.

[46] Fujita, T., and Murakami, T.: Microcirculation of monkey pancreas with special reference to the insulo-acinar portal system. A scanning electron microscope study. Arch. Histol. Jpn. 35:225–63, 1973.

[47] Matas, A. J., Sutherland, D. E. R., Steffes, M. W., and Najarian, J. S.: Short-term culture of adult pancreatic fragments for purification and transplantation of islets of Langerhans. Surgery 180:183–91, 1976.

[48] Gray, B. N., Carusco, G., Alford, F., and Chisholm, D.: Insulin and glucagon response of transplanted intrasplenic islets. Arch. Surg. 114:96–99, 1977.

[49] Lacy, P. E., Davie, J. M., Finke, E., and Scharp, D. W.: Prolongation of islet allograft survival. Transplantation 27:171–175, 1979.

[50] Lacy, P. E., Davie, J. M., and Finke, E. H.: Prolongation of islet allograft survival following in vitro culture (24°C) and a single injection of ALS. Science 204:312–13, 1979.

[51] Finke, E. H., Lacy, P. E., and Ono, J.: Use of reflected green light for specific identification of islets in vitro after collagenase isolation Diabetes 28:613, 1979.

[52] Lambert, A. E., Blondel, B., Kanazawa, Y., Orci, L., and Renold, A.: Monolayer cell culture of neonatal rat pancreas; light microscopy and evidence for immunoreactive insulin synthesis and release. Endocrinology 90:239–48, 1972.

[53] Chick, W.: Beta cell replication in rat pancreatic monolayer cultures. Effects of glucose, tolbutamide, glucocorticoid, growth hormone, and glucagon. Diabetes 22:687–93, 1973.

[54] Moscona, A. A.: Recombination of disassociated cells and the development of cell aggregates. In Cells and Tissues in Culture. E. N. Willner, ed. New York, Academic Press, 1965, p. 489.

[55] Scharp, D., Merrell, R. C., Feldman, S. D., Ruwe, E. A., Feldmeier, M. M., Ballinger, F. W., and Lacy, P. E.: Long term culture of islets of Langerhans utilizing a rotational culture method. In Vitro 13:174, 1977.

[56] Steinberger, L. A.: The unlabelled antibody enzyme method. *In* Immunocytochemistry. Englewood Cliffs, New Jersey, Prentice-Hall, 1977, p. 1974.

[57] Merrell, R., Scharp, D. W., Gingerich, R., Feldmeier, M., Greider, M., and Downing, R.: New approaches to the separation of islet cells. Surg. Forum 30:303–05, 1979.

Transplantation of Dispersed Pancreatic Islet Tissue in Humans
Autografts and Allografts

DAVID E. R. SUTHERLAND, ARTHUR J. MATAS, FREDERICK C. GOETZ, AND JOHN S. NAJARIAN

SUMMARY

Islet transplantation is successful in animals and holds considerable promise as endocrine replacement therapy for patients with diabetes mellitus, but clinical application to diabetic patients has been difficult. We have shown the technical feasibility of human islet transplantation by autotransplantation of dispersed pancreatic islet tissue into the portal vein in three patients with chronic pancreatitis and incapacitating, intractable pain who underwent near-total (>97%) pancreatectomy. In all three patients, the excised pancreas was dispersed by collagenase digestion, but no effort was made to purify the islets. Islet yield, as judged by tissue insulin content, ranged from 24 to 55%. The first patient, who never received insulin after the pancreatectomy and islet autotransplantation, had a normal oral glucose tolerance test by 3 wk and has remained normoglycemic for over 2 yr. In the second patient, viable islets were histologically identified in the liver parenchyma. The third patient was treated with hyperalimentation for 3 wk after the pancreatectomy and islet autotransplantation and, during this period, required insulin. After cessation of hyperalimentation and initiation of oral feedings, the patient was withdrawn from insulin. Although abnormalities of carbohydrate metabolism were present, the patient did not require insulin for more than 1 yr.

Seven diabetic renal allograft recipients have received allografts of dispersed pancreatic islet tissue prepared in the same way. No patients were cured of diabetes, although transient evidence of islet function —increase in serum or urinary C-peptide levels or decrease in exogenous insulin requirements— occurred in some. Although rejection was probably responsible for most of the failures, transplantation of allogeneic human islet tissue as a free graft is metabolically inefficient. With the current state of immunosuppressive therapy, the primary role of islet transplantation may be in a situation where rejection cannot occur: as an autograft to obviate the occurrence of diabetes after extensive pancreatectomy for benign disease. **DIABETES *29* (Suppl. 1):31–44, 1980.**

From the Departments of Surgery and Medicine, University of Minnesota Health Sciences Center, Minneapolis, Minnesota 55455.

Address reprint requests to Dr. Sutherland, Box 253 Mayo Memorial Building, University of Minnesota, 420 Delaware Street, SE, Minneapolis, Minnesota 55455.

Islet transplantation was originally conceived as an alternative to pancreas transplantation because of the difficulty of the latter procedure. Some of the problems with pancreas transplantation may be solved, but islet transplantation is still an attractive alternative.

In the earliest attempts to transplant free grafts of allogeneic islets to diabetic patients, the islet tissue was derived from fetal or stillborn infant pancreases or islet adenomatous tissue obtained at operation.[1] Transplantation was into intramuscular or subcutaneous sites; no patients were relieved of diabetes, and evidence of even transient function was unconvincing. Hegre and Lazarow[2] have summarized the historical aspects of islet transplantation.

The modern era of islet transplantation began in the early 1970s with several reports of successful transplantation in animals, with islet tissue prepared in a variety of ways from adult, neonatal, or fetal sources.[3–9] Attempts to adapt these new techniques for islet allotransplantation in diabetic humans have not been very successful.[10–13] There are a number of reasons why the attempts failed to cure diabetes: (1) transplantation of too few viable islets, (2) increased susceptibility to rejection, (3) an unfavorable environment created by administration of corticosteroids to prevent rejection, or (4) transplantation to inappropriate sites.

We have previously reported on the results of the 10 islet transplant procedures in seven diabetic patients who had received renal allografts several months or years before for treatment of diabetic nephropathy.[10,11] In our first series, a small number of purified adult islets derived from a single donor or dispersed pancreatic tissue derived from a single infant donor were transplanted to intraperitoneal, intramuscular, or portal vein sites. The adult islets were obtained by collagenase digestion and Ficoll-gradient separation. The infant islets were obtained by collagenase digestion alone of the exocrine-poor neonatal pancreas. No patients were cured of diabetes, although in some instances the amount of exogenous insulin that was administered could be reduced. On the other hand, no patients were harmed by the procedure. Peritonitis did not occur after intraperitoneal transplantation, and portal vein pressure and the results of liver function tests were stable after intraportal transplantation. In addition, rejection episodes were not induced in the previously transplanted kidneys.

Although rejection may have occurred, most or all of the grafts probably failed to cure diabetes for technical reasons. These results are not surprising. In order to ameliorate diabetes in animals with purified adult islets, multiple donors are required because the yield from one pancreas is low.[5] Multiple donors are also required for efficient transplantation of dispersed neonatal pancreatic islet tissue.[9] Our average yield of islets from adult human pancreases was less than 5%.[14] Similarly, the quantitiy of islet tissue that remained after collagenase digestion of the infant human pancreases averaged less than 7% of the normal adult islet mass.[15]

Subsequent to our initial attempt at clinical islet transplantation, it was shown in dogs that dispersed pancreatic islet tissue could be transplanted as free grafts to the spleen or portal vein without islet purification and that contaminating exocrine enzymes did not exert a deleterious effect.[16–20] Collagenase digestion alone was sufficient to prepare canine pancreatic islet tissue for transplantation. By eliminating the purification process, a larger quantity of islet tissue was available for transplantation, and islets derived from one donor pancreas could ameliorate diabetes.

In a second series of eight islet transplants in seven diabetic patients, we used this new approach and transplanted unpurified dispersed pancreatic islet tissue. Again, no patients were cured of diabetes, but, in two instances, exogenous insulin administration could be stopped for a few days and some evidence of islet function was obtained in a few of the other patients. Rejection was thought to be the ultimate cause of failure in these patients.

The failure to ameliorate diabetes in the diabetic islet allograft recipients was not entirely technical because we have been able to obviate the occurrence of diabetes in two patients by autotransplantation of islets derived from the resected pancreas after near-total pancreatectomy for treatment of chronic pancreatitis. In the cases of pancreatic islet autotransplantation, the outcome could not be influenced by the possibility of rejection. Our experience with islet autotransplantation after near-total pancreatectomy for chronic pancreatitis in three patients is detailed in this paper, and the outcome of transplantation of dispersed pancreatic islet tissue in our second series of allografts is summarized.

Metabolic studies were carried out in our Clinical Research Center. Insulin, C-peptide, and glucagon assays were done using standard immunoassay techniques.[21–24] C-peptide was not measured in urine samples collected before September 1977. C-peptide measurements on serum or plasma samples were evaluated for only some patients through 1977 and for all patients since 1978. The antibody used for urinary C-peptide and some serum C-peptide determinations (Antibody "C" from Calbiochem-Behring Corporation, La Jolla, California) was exhausted in May 1978, and subsequent serum C-peptide assays were performed using Antibody II (lot no. 86A049 also supplied by Calbiochem). Because we were unable until recently to perform satisfactory urinary C-peptide assays using Antibody II, no C-peptide data are given on urine samples collected after May 1978.

ISLET AUTOTRANSPLANTATION AFTER NEAR-TOTAL PANCREATECTOMY FOR CHRONIC PANCREATITIS

Total or near-total pancreatectomy is the surest way to relieve the pain of chronic pancreatitis,[26] but it is rarely applied because the metabolic consequences are so severe. More than 80% of patients with chronic pancreatitis who require operative treatment do not have diabetes at that time.[27] A variety of surgical procedures can be tried that will preserve pancreatic tissue, but pancreatectomy may be the only alternative for small-duct disease or where procedures to improve duct drainage have failed. Diabetes is a predictable event after major pancreatic resection,[25] and, when more than 95% of the gland is removed, all patients become insulin dependent.[28]

In an effort to obviate the need for exogenous insulin, we performed intraportal islet autotransplantation in three patients after near-total pancreatectomy for chronic pancreatitis. The patients were not diabetic before surgery, although one patient (no. 3) had minor abnormalities of carbohydrate metabolism. All three patients had been hospitalized repeatedly for abdominal pain from pancreatitis, and all required narcotics. Either previous procedures to relieve pain and correct anatomic abnormalities had failed, or, the patients had small pancreatic ducts and pancreatic resection was the only treatment possible.

We performed a near-total pancreatectomy with preservation of the duodenum[28] in all three patients. All pancreatic tissue was resected, except for a nubbin at the junction of the common duct and duodenum. In each case, the pancreatic remnant was less than 1.5 cm^3 by direct measurement. According to the weight of the excised pancreas, this remnant represented less than 4% of the total pancreatic mass before operation.

Dispersed pancreatic islet tissue was prepared for transplantation immediately after excision of the pancreas. The technique of tissue preparation was similar to that used in our experiments in dogs.[20] The arterial supply to the pancreas was flushed with cold Ringer's lactate solution. The pancreatic duct was injected under pressure with cold Medium 199. The pancreas was minced in a mechanical tissue chopper[29] until the fragments would pass through a 15-gauge needle. The pancreases were fibrotic but were not calcified, and the mincing procedure was not difficult. After mincing, the tissue was digested in Hank's solution with 1440–2176 U of collagenase (Worthington, 60 U/mg) per gram of tissue in a volume 2.5–5.0 times the weight of the pancreas (final collagenase concentration, 0.28–0.26%). Digestion took place in a shaking water bath at 37°C for 20 mins, the best digestion time according to our experiments in dogs.[18] After digestion, the tissue was washed four times at 4°C and suspended in 300 ml of cold Medium 199 for transplantation.

The islet mass of the transplanted tissue was estimated by measuring the insulin content of an aliquot of the tissue. The yield of islets from the pancreas was estimated by calculating the total insulin content of the pancreatic tissue before and after processing. Insulin content was measured in aliquots of the pancreatic tissue after mincing and in the washes collected after chopping and after collagenase digestion. The total pancreatic insulin content before processing was calculated by adding the "post-chop" tissue-insulin and "post-chop" wash-insulin contents or by adding the "post-chop" and "post-digestion" washes and "post-digestion" tissue-insulin contents. Islet yield was expressed as a percentage by dividing the "post-digestion" tissue-insulin content by the total pancreatic insulin content before processing. This method of estimating islet yield was based on previous work by Leonard et al.,[30] showing that tissue-insulin content is proportional to islet mass. The degree of contamination with exocrine enzymes of the transplanted tissue was similarly estimated by measuring amylase content in the pancreatic tissue and in the washes before, during, and after processing. Tissue amylase content also has been shown to parallel the content of other exocrine enzymes.[30] A colorimetric technique was used for amylase determination.[31] We have previously published the details of our application of these techniques for estimation of the relative proportion of islet and exocrine tissue in human pancreases before and after processing.[15]

The results of the measurement of pancreatic tissue insulin and amylase content in our three cases of autotransplantation after pancreatectomy are summarized in Table 1. Less insulin than amylase was lost during the processing of the tissue for transplantation, and the estimated final yield of islets in the transplanted tissue ranged from 24 to 55%. The proportion of islets that were viable was not determined, and the number of islets that was actually engrafted was almost certainly less than the number transplanted. Our experiments in dogs had shown that, for transplantation to be effective, there must be an optimal balance between the degree of tissue dispersal obtained by collagenase digestion and the quantity of islet tissue remaining after dispersion.[32] A collagenase digestion protocol associated with a high yield may not result in an effective transplant because the tissue may not be dispersed adequately for engraftment. We do not know if we used the optimal digestion protocol for dispersion of the human pancreases.

In each case the dispersed pancreatic islet tissue was returned to the operating room within 2.5 h after pancreatectomy. It was slowly infused into the portal vein of the pancreatectomized patients. Portal pressure was measured during infusion and never rose more than 14 cm of water above baseline.

The outcome was different for each patient. The first patient was mildly hyperglycemic immediately after pancreatectomy and autotransplantation but never required insulin. She was normoglycemic by 3 wk and has remained normoglycemic during nearly 2.5 yr of follow-up. The second patient died of a perforated intestinal ulcer 10 days after pancreactomy and islet autotransplantation; histologic examination showed numerous islets in the liver. The third patient was hyperglycemic while receiving intravenous infusion and required exogenous insulin during the first 3 wk after islet transplantation, but then became normoglycemic and did not need exogenous insulin for more than 1 yr. The details of metabolic studies in these patients are given with their individual case histories.

Patient no. 1. This 39-yr-old female patient had a 20-yr history of abdominal pain. She had undergone multiple abdominal operations and had repeated episodes of hyperamylasemia and hyperamylasuria. She did not drink alcohol and had no biliary tract disease; two uncles had pancreatitis. During the year before pancreatectomy, the pain increased in severity. Serum amylase levels were not elevated, but the patient had pancreatic exocrine deficiency, and her fecal fat content was 22%. However, pancreatic endocrine function was excellent. Fasting plasma glucose levels ranged from 70 to 79 mg/dl and postprandial levels up to 149 mg/dl before pancreatectomy. The results of two oral glucose tolerance tests before pancreatectomy were within normal limits (Figure 1). Plasma insulin levels increased to high levels during a glucose tolerance test 1 wk before operation (Table 2).

On 14 February 1977, the patient underwent a near-total pancreatectomy. Most of the excised pancreas was processed for islet autotransplantation, using 1440 U of collagenase per gram of tissue for dispersal (collagenase concentration, 0.3%). A small portion of the pancreas was examined histologically and showed chronic pancreatitis. Acinar tissue was replaced with broad bands of fibrous tissue containing dilated ducts, but there was a large number of islets present.

One and one-half hours after pancreatectomy the dispersed pancreatic islet tissue was infused into a mesenteric vein. Portal pressure rose from 10 to 14 cm of water. A blood sample drawn immediately before pancreatectomy showed a plasma glucose concentration of 195 mg/dl and a plasma insulin level of 8 μU/ml. During the interval between pancreatectomy and islet autotransplantation, plasma insulin declined to less than 4 μU/ml, and plasma glucose rose to 287 mg/dl. Plasma insulin concentration immediately after islet transplantation was 14 μU/ml, and values at 20, 60, and 135 min were 166, 34, and 126 μU/ml, respectively. Plasma

TABLE 1
Islet recovery and exocrine enzyme contamination in dispersed pancreatic tissue autotransplanted to pancreatectomized recipients

Patient	Weight of pancreas (g)	Total tissue insulin content (μg)	Total tissue amylase content (mg)	Insulin content of transplanted tissue (μg)	Amylase content of transplanted tissue (mg)	Islet* yield (%)	Amylase† retention (%)
1	42	17,860	77	9877	20	55	26
2	60	13,895	29	3326	4	24	13
3	82	13,118	561	7247	281	55	50

* Insulin content of transplanted tissue/total tissue insulin content of pancreas.
† Amylase content of transplanted tissue/total tissue amylase content of pancreas.

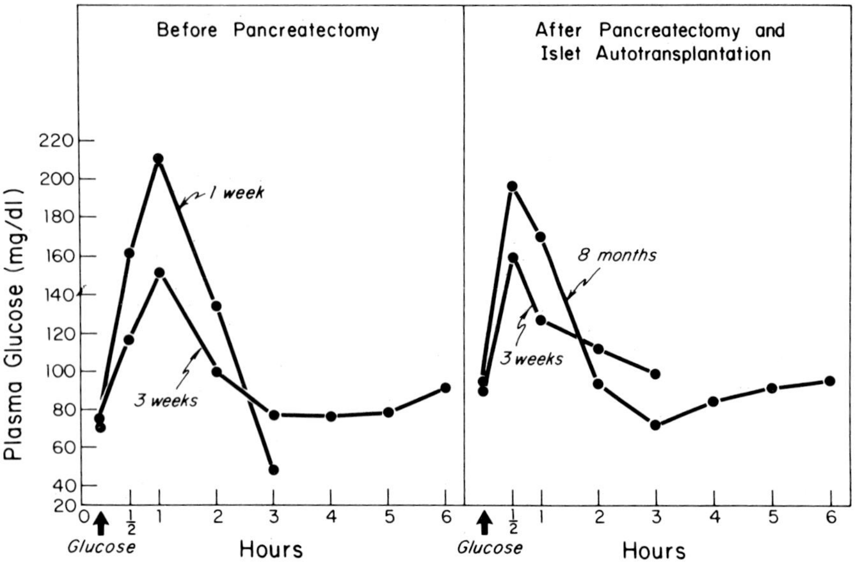

FIGURE 1. Results of oral glucose tolerance tests before and after pancreatectomy and islet autotransplantation in patient no. 1 with chronic pancreatitis.

insulin levels over the next 12 h ranged between 12 and 16 μU/ml, and twice daily measurements over the next 3 wk showed values that ranged from 4 μU/ml when fasting to 20 μU/ml postprandial.

An intravenous bolus of a 20% glucose solution was given at the time of islet transplantation, and the highest plasma glucose level recorded after islet autotransplantation was 352 mg/dl at ½ h. For the first 4 days after islet transplantation, plasma glucose levels ranged between 144 and 284 mg/dl. Levels then declined to between 100 and 195 mg/dl for the next 2 wk. Between 3 and 4 wk after transplantation, fasting plasma glucose levels ranged from 77 to 104 mg/dl and postprandial levels from 110 to 146 mg/dl. At 3 wk, glucose tolerance test results were within normal limits (Figure 1), although the magnitude of the insulin response was less after pancreatectomy and islet autotransplantation than before the operation (Table 2).

Liver function tests were minimally altered after the islet autotransplant procedure. Before the operation, serum bilirubin was 0.2 mg/dl, glutamic oxaloacetic transaminase (SGOT) 10 IU/L, and alkaline phosphatase 101 IU/L. The highest values during the first 3 wk after operation were 0.6 mg/dl for bilirubin, 49 IU/L for SGOT, and 314 IU/L for alkaline phosphatase. At 4 wk the respective values were 0.5 mg/dl, 18 IU/L, and 256 IU/L, all within normal limits except for a slight elevation of alkaline phosphatase.

The patient's pain was relieved by the operation, but she continued to take narcotics because of an addiction. She also took pancreatic extract (pancreatin) for treatment of pancreatic exocrine deficiency. Without the extract, the patient's fecal fat content was 26%, but, with pancreatin, her fecal fat content ranged from 4 to 7%.

She was discharged from the hospital 4 wk after operation and has since been cared for by her family physician. Six months after operation she had been successfully withdrawn from narcotics. At 9 mo, the results of an oral glucose tolerance test were normal and nearly identical to the one performed just before operation (Figure 1). Two years after pancreatectomy her physician reported that she weighed 133 lb, a gain of 36 lb since pancreatectomy. Blood sugar levels ranged from 85 to 97 mg/dl, and she required no exogenous insulin.

TABLE 2
Plasma insulin concentration during oral glucose tolerance tests before and after pancreatectomy and islet autotransplantation in patient no. 1

Time after glucose ingestion	Insulin concentration (μU/ml)	
	1 wk before	3 wk after
Pre	4	4
½ h	168	98
1 h	206	68
2 h	224	12
3 h	16	6

Patient no. 2. This 35-yr-old male patient, a bartender, had acute, relapsing pancreatitis. Hyperamylasemia and hyperamylasuria and abdominal pain persisted even during prolonged hospitalization and abstinence from alcohol. Retrograde pancreatic ductogram showed a normal duct of Wirschung and a mild dilation of the duct of Santorini. Sphincteroplasty of both ducts was performed on 13 July 1977. The pancreas was edematous and inflamed at that time. The operation was unsuccessful. The patient continued to require hospital care. Echograms and computerized radiotomograms showed a persistently enlarged, edematous pancreas. It was apparent that the only possible treatment to relieve pain would be pancreatectomy.

The patient was not diabetic. Plasma glucose levels during the year preceding pancreatectomy ranged from 75 to 179 mg/dl (mean ± SD, 102 ± 22 mg/dl, 26 determinations). Oral glucose tolerance tests were performed in September and November 1977; fasting plasma glucoses were 86 and 91 mg/dl, and values at 30 min and at 1, 2, and 3 h after glucose ingestion were 132, 135, 152, and 112 mg/dl during the first test and 113, 136, 122, and 127 during the second test. The results of the tests are moderately abnormal, but the patient was not able to eat a high-carbohydrate diet before the tests because oral feedings of any kind exacerbated his abdominal pain. The results of an intravenous glucose tolerance test 1 day before pancreatectomy were within normal limits. Preinjection plasma glucose levels were 89 and 88 mg/dl; values at 5, 10, 15, 20, 30, 40, and 50 min after glucose injection were 468, 396, 351, 300, 230, 203, and 179 mg/dl, respectively (T ½ = 32 min; K = −2.17% per minute). Corresponding plasma insulin values were 2 μU/ml before glucose injection, and 88, 97, 101, 87, 77, 99, and 88 μU/ml postinjection.

On 22 November 1977, a near-total pancreatectomy was performed. The pancreas was even more edematous and inflamed than at the first operation. A small portion was examined histologically and showed septal fibrosis, lobular disarray, chronic inflammation, and scattered areas of fat necrosis. Islets appeared to be normal, although in one section they were markedly enlarged.

The excised pancreas was digested with 2176 U of collagenase per gram of tissue (collagenase concentration, 0.28%). The dispersed pancreatic islet tissue was infused into the portal vein without a rise in portal pressure. In the immediate posttransplant period, plasma glucose was >400 mg/dl, and the patient received 22 U of insulin over 24 h. Plasma glucose levels then stabilized at <200 mg/dl, and the patient received no insulin for the next 24 h while on a constant intravenous infusion of 10% dextrose. Over the next 7 days, the infusion of 10% dextrose was continued, and 0–2 U of insulin was administered every 1–4 h to maintain plasma glucose levels between 150 and 250 mg/dl.

Seven days after operation, the patient suddenly developed abdominal pain. Exploratory laparotomy showed an acute perforation of an ulcer in the transverse colon. The transverse colon was resected, but the patient developed severe peritonitis and died 3 days later. This complication did not appear to be related to the islet transplant. The sudden death 10 days after pancreatectomy prevented us from performing metabolic studies to investigate the function of the transplanted islets, but an autopsy was performed. Histologic examination of the liver showed numerous islets in the deep parenchyma of both the right and left lobes (Figure 2). The islets were located within portal venule vascular space and within portal triades of the liver. Although some islets were surrounded by thrombi, the islets appeared viable. Masson-trichrome stain showed granulated endocrine cells. Granulation tissue around the islets contained viable red blood cells, showing that neovascularization had already occurred. Using a specific antisera for each hormone, an immunoperoxidase staining technique[33] identified insulin-containing beta cells (Figure 2C) and glucagon-containing alpha cells (Figure 2D) within the liver. The histologic findings showed that free grafts of human islet tissue will survive after intraportal transplantation to the liver.

Patient no. 3. This 57-yr-old, nonalcoholic female patient had a 4-yr history of chronic abdominal pain and intermittent hyperamylasemia and hyperamylasuria. A cholecystec-

FIGURE 2. Pancreatic islet tissue in liver after pancreatectomy and islet autotransplantation in patient no. 2 with chronic pancreatitis. (A) Hematoxylin-eosin stain, showing intact islet, ×40. (B) Masson-trichrome stain shows alpha cells with orange granules and degranulated bluish beta cells; red blood cells are interspersed in capillaries, showing that neovascularization has occurred, ×390. (C) Immunoperoxidase stain with anti-insulin antibody; insulin within beta cells is stained brown, ×415. (D) Immunoperoxidase stain with antiglucagon antibody; glucagon with alpha cells is stained brown, ×415. Magnifications shown are original magnifications.

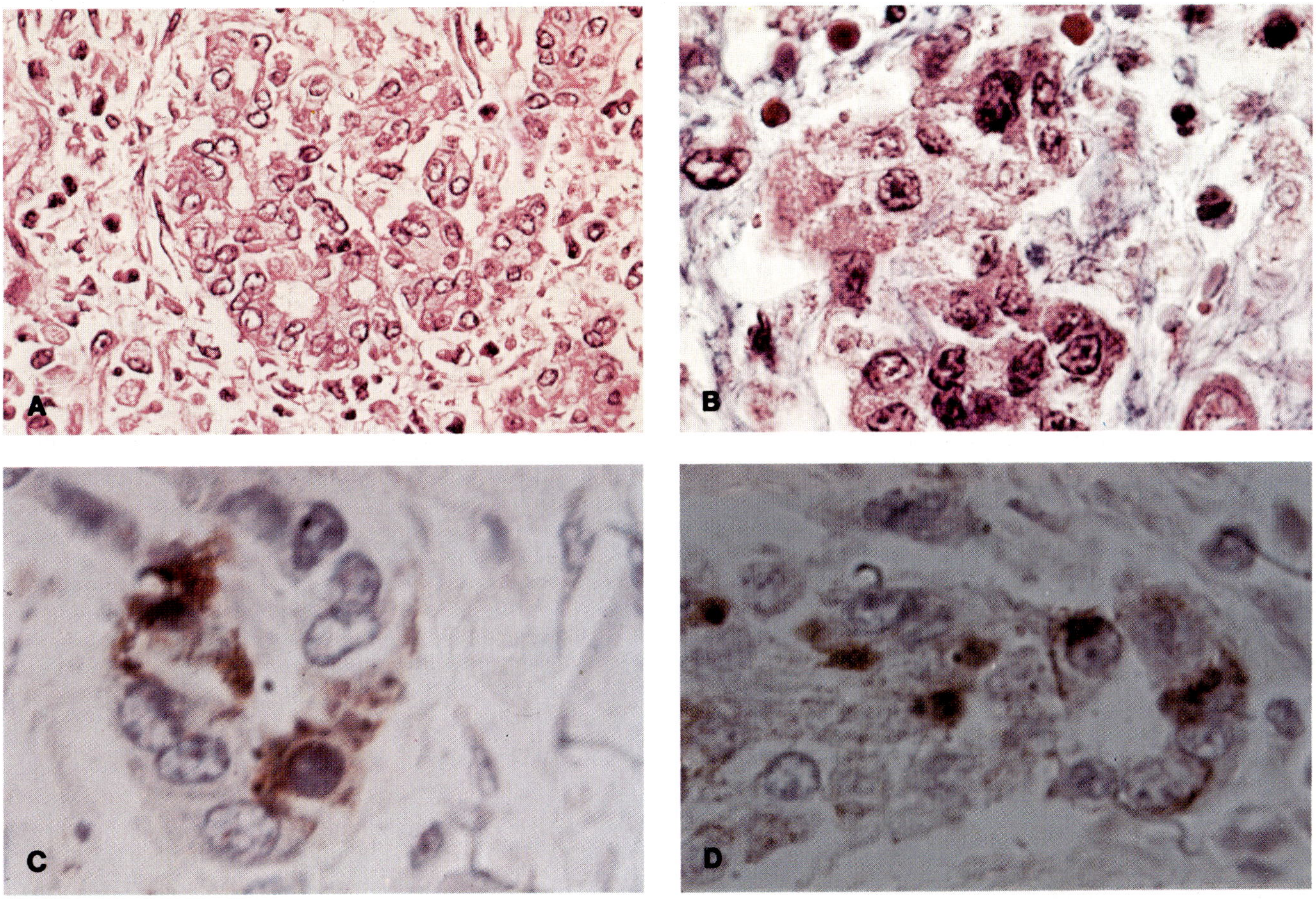

tomy did not relieve her symptoms or her hyperamylasemia. A dilated pancreatic duct could not be demonstrated on retrograde ductography. She ate very little because eating exacerbated her pain. During the year preceding pancreatectomy she had lost 10 lb.

She was not diabetic before pancreatectomy (fasting plasma glucose levels ranged from 91 to 115 mg/dl), but she did have some glucose intolerance. During an oral glucose tolerance test 18 mo before pancreatectomy, fasting plasma glucose concentration was 115 mg/dl, and values at ½, 1, 2, and 3 h after glucose ingestion were 119, 278, 233, and 114 mg/dl. Oral glucose tolerance test results at 1 and 2 wk before pancreatectomy showed an increase in plasma glucose concentration from 108 and 104 mg/dl before glucose ingestion to peak values of 283 mg/dl at 60 min in the first test and 285 mg/dl at 30 min in the second test. The peak glucose concentrations during the tests were abnormally high, but the patient was unable to eat a high-carbohydrate diet before the tests, and values at 2 h after glucose ingestion were 130 mg/dl in the first and 102 mg/dl in the second test. During the last glucose tolerance test before pancreatectomy, serum insulin levels increased from 2 μU before to 132, 126, 10, and 4 μU/ml at 30, 60, 120, and 180 min after glucose ingestion, respectively. Serum C-peptide concentration increased from 1.8 before to a peak of 4.2 ng/ml at 2 h after glucose ingestion. Urinary C-peptide excretion levels were normal before pancreatectomy (50–105 μg/24 h). Plasma glucagon levels before pancreatectomy ranged from 56 to 139 pg/ml, but the highest values, paradoxically, occurred during the first hour after ingestion of glucose during oral glucose tolerance testing. Of the three islet autograft recipients, this patient was studied in the greatest detail before and after pancreatectomy.

On 23 February 1978, a near-total pancreatectomy was performed. Histologic examination of a small portion of the excised pancreas revealed chronic inflammation, although there was little loss of acinar tissue. Only a few islets were seen, but they appeared normal. The rest of the pancreas was digested with 2000 U of collagenase per gram of tissue (collagenase concentration, 0.46%). The dispersed pancreatic tissue was infused into the portal vein 2 h and 20 min after pancreatectomy. Portal vein pressure rose from 8 to 22 cm of water.

The results of plasma insulin measurements taken immediately before pancreatectomy, between pancreatectomy and islet autotransplantation, and after islet autotransplantation are shown in Figure 3. Plasma insulin concentrations ranged from 8 to 15 μg/ml before pancreatectomy. Fifteen minutes after pancreatectomy, plasma insulin was less than 2 μU/ml, and no insulin could be detected in eight consecutive samples drawn every 15 min until the islets were infused, 140 min after pancreatectomy. These results confirmed the completeness of pancreatectomy. Ten minutes after infusion of the islet tissue, plasma insulin concentration was 153 μU/ml, and 35 min after infusion it was 310 μU/ml. Whether these high concentrations represented a physiologic release of insulin from the transplanted islets in response to the hyperglycemic state or were a consequence of free insulin escaping from damaged islets could not be determined, but plasma insulin rapidly declined to a stable level. Fifty to 160 min after islet transplantation, insulin concentrations ranged from 7 to 13 μU/ml, essentially the same intraoperative values as before pancreatectomy and a definite contrast to the results of measurements on the samples taken between pancreatectomy and transplantation.

Plasma glucose concentration rose from 231 to 585 mg/dl during the apancreatic period, but, by 3 h after islet transplantation, it had declined to 285 mg/dl. At this point, the patient was started on a constant intravenous infusion of insulin. This treatment was based on observations in rats by Brown et al.[34] that the results of islet transplantation were improved when the recipients were temporarily treated with exogenous insulin.

The first 80 days of this patient's course after pancreatectomy and islet autotransplantation are depicted in Figure 4. For the first 25 days she received intravenous dextrose and hyperalimentation solutions. During this interval, exogenous insulin doses were continuously adjusted in an attempt to

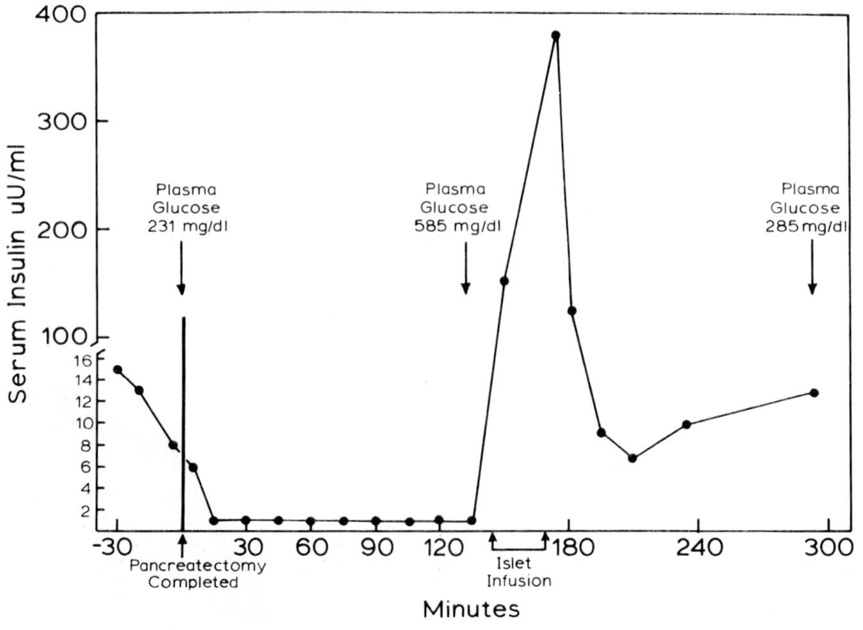

FIGURE 3. Plasma insulin concentrations immediately before pancreatectomy, between pancreatectomy and islet autotransplantation, and after islet autotransplantation in patient no. 3 with chronic pancreatitis.

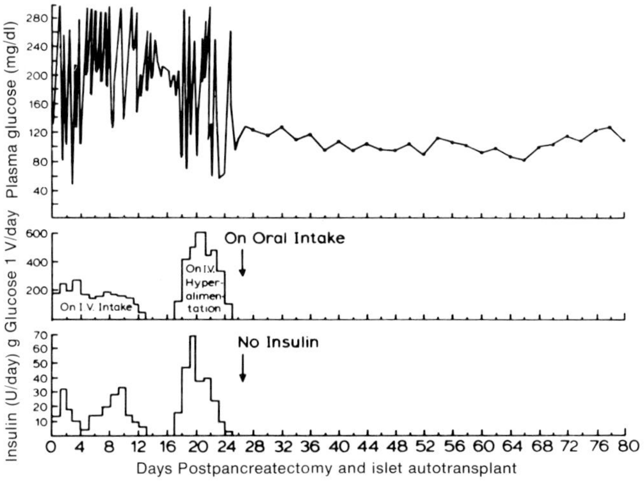

FIGURE 4. Postoperative treatment and plasma glucose levels during first 80 days after pancreatectomy and islet autotransplantation in patient no. 3 with chronic pancreatitis.

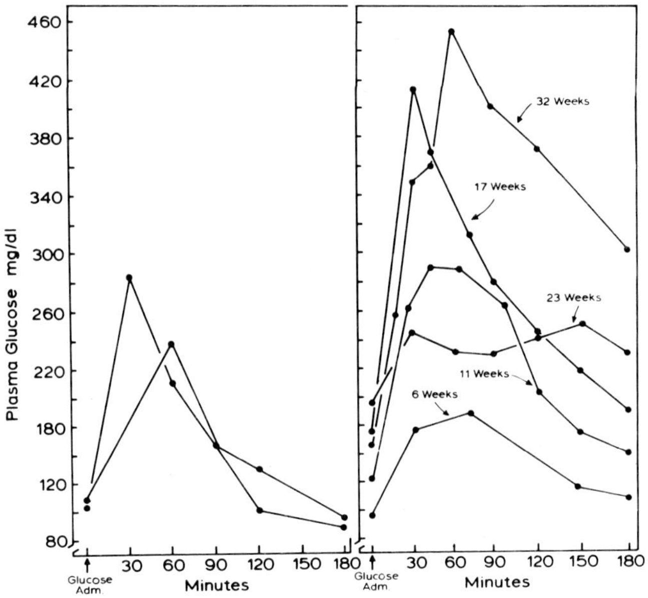

FIGURE 5. Results of oral glucose tolerance tests before (left) and during first 32 wk after (right) pancreatectomy and islet autotransplantation in patient no. 3 with chronic pancreatitis.

keep her plasma glucose concentration around 200 mg/dl. Her plasma glucose levels were extremely variable, however, until the intravenous fluids were stopped and oral feedings were begun. After that change, the patient required no insulin injections. Plasma glucose levels from the beginning of the second through the fourth month after pancreatectomy and islet transplantation ranged from 92 to 169 mg/dl (mean ± SD, 113 ± 21 mg/dl, 31 determinations). After 4 mo her plasma glucose levels increased. Between five and 14 mo after pancreatectomy and islet autotransplantation, plasma glucose levels ranged from 120 to 274 mg/dl (mean ± SD, 184 ± 33 mg/dl, 53 determinations), indicating that some deterioration in carbohydrate metabolism had occurred.

Plasma glucagon levels during the first 4 mo after pancreatectomy and islet autotransplantation ranged from 223 to 675 pg/ml, much higher than before operation. At 8 mo, plasma glucagon levels increased from 142 to 301 pg/ml during glucose tolerance testing. We do not know why glucagon levels were increased or the contribution of this increase to the abnormalities of carbohydrate metabolism observed after pancreatic islet autotransplantation. Glucagon levels at 1 yr ranged from 70 to 97 pg/ml.

Numerous oral glucose tolerance tests have been performed in this patient. In Figure 5, the results of glucose tolerance tests before pancreatectomy are compared with five tests done between 6 and 32 wk after pancreatectomy and islet autotransplantation. Beginning at 17 wk, peak glucose values were generally higher and there was a delayed return to baseline. In spite of these abnormalities, there was no need for exogenous insulin administration.

Plasma insulin concentrations could not be measured, because the patient had developed antibodies to insulin during the first month after islet autotransplantation, a time when the patient did receive exogenous insulin. However, plasma C-peptide levels were measured during the glucose tolerance tests. C-peptide levels were not as high as before pancreatectomy, but fasting plasma C-peptide levels of 1.3 and 1.8 ng/ml and peak values of 2.7 and 2.9 ng/ml occurred during oral glucose tolerance tests performed 11 and 17 wk after islet autotransplantation (Figure 6). C-peptide response during glucose tolerance tests at 23 and 32

FIGURE 6. Serum C-peptide concentrations during oral glucose tolerance tests before (left) and after (right) pancreatectomy and islet autotransplantation in patient no. 3 with chronic pancreatitis.

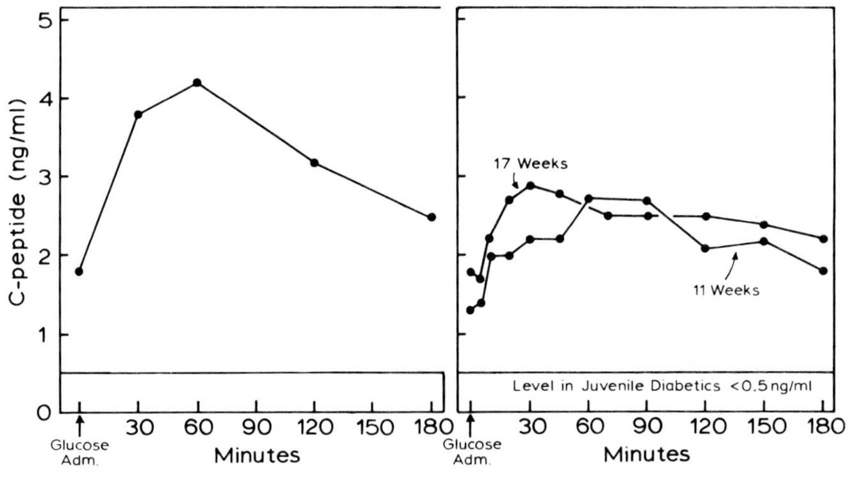

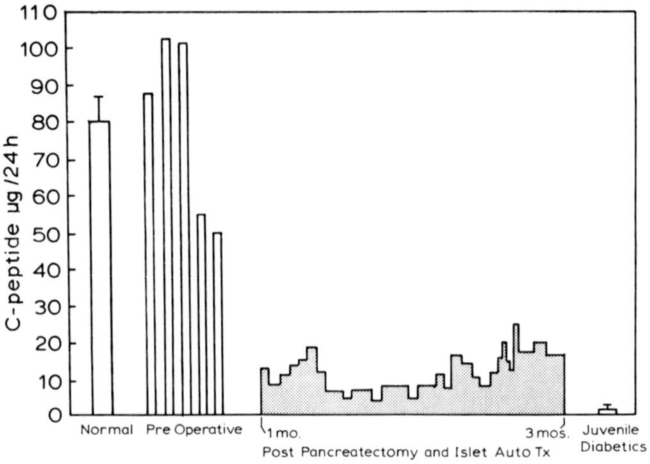

FIGURE 7. Urinary C-peptide excretion (24-h) before and after pancreatectomy and islet autotransplantation in patient no. 3 with chronic pancreatitis. Comparison is made with mean values from studies in normal and diabetic individuals.

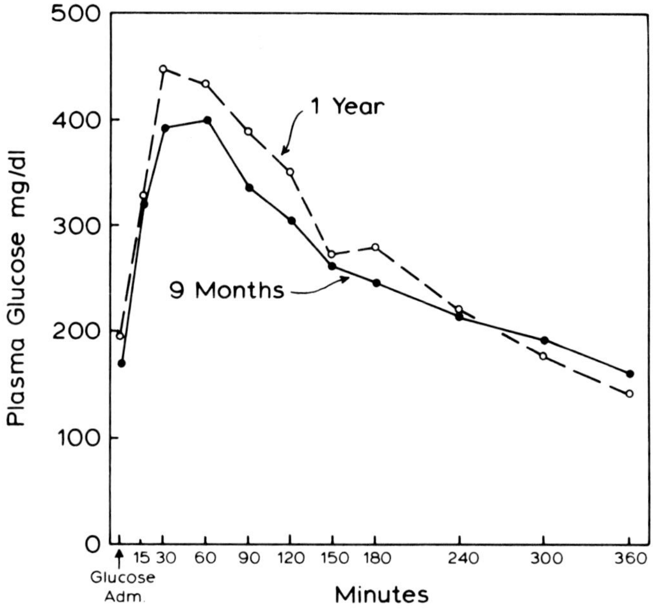

FIGURE 8. Results of oral glucose tolerance tests at 9 mo and at 1 yr after pancreatectomy and islet autotransplantation in patient no. 3 with chronic pancreatitis.

wk and at 1 yr were similar, with basal plasma levels ranging from 1.3 to 1.9 and peak levels from 2.0 to 2.5 ng/ml.

Urinary C-peptide excretion levels before and for the first 3 mo after pancreatectomy and islet autotransplantation were also measured (Figure 7). Twenty-four-hour values after operation averaged around 20% of her preoperative values. The results of urinary C-peptide determinations after May 1978 (between 4 and 16 mo after islet autotransplantation) are not yet available because of technical problems with our urinary C-peptide assay.

The patient's course after pancreatectomy and islet autotransplantation has been satisfactory. Again, intraportal embolization of autologous unpurified pancreatic islet tissue did not result in any serious impairment of liver function. Serum bilirubin, SGOT, and alkaline phosphatase values before operation were 0.3 mg/dl, 10 IU/L, and 135 IU/L, respectively. The values were 0.6 mg/dl, 54 IU/L, and 143 IU/L 1 day postoperative. Except for alkaline phosphatase, these were the highest values after the islet transplant. Three weeks after operation, bilirubin was 0.3 mg/dl, SGOT 8 IU/L, and alkaline phosphatase 221 IU/L. By 4 wk, alkaline phosphatase was 154 IU/L, and all values have remained within the normal range during 16 mo of follow-up.

The mild glucose intolerance that occurred at 4 mo after pancreatectomy and islet autotransplantation has remained stable. Figure 8 shows the results of oral glucose tolerance tests at 9 mo and at 1 yr. Peak plasma glucose levels were high, but plasma glucose levels returned to baseline by 5 or 6 h. However, because plasma glucose concentrations, particularly postprandial, persistently were in the range of 200 mg/dl, at 15 mo the patient was begun on 10 U of Lente insulin per day. With this treatment, she has had no glycosuria, and postprandial plasma glucose levels have ranged from 137 to 173 mg/dl.

The patient has been rehabilitated since pancreatectomy. Her abdominal pain has relented, and she has been withdrawn from narcotic medications. She takes pancreatic extract (Viokase) for exocrine deficiency. She is now able to eat, and her weight has increased by 8 lb.

Comments. These cases show that endocrine function can be preserved by islet autotransplantation to the portal vein after near-total pancreatectomy. The availability of such a technique provides greater versatility in the choice of therapy for chronic pancreatitis. Islet transplantation is not the only alternative; Hogle and Reemtsma[35] have successfully autotransplanted an excised pancreatic segment, with vascular anastomosis to the femoral vessels, of a patient with chronic pancreatitis.

The most significant aspect of the islet autograft experience, however, is the demonstration that islet transplantation is technically feasible in humans. We now know what could be achieved in diabetic patients after allotransplantation of unpurified islets derived from a single donor pancreas, providing the immunologic problems can be solved.

The best result was obtained in our first patient. The transplanted islets have obviated the need for exogenous insulin for nearly 2½ yr, and a glucose tolerance test at 9 mo showed that there had been no deterioration of islet function.

The second patient, unfortunately, died too soon after pancreatectomy and islet autotransplantation for the functional status of the transplanted islets to be adequately studied. However, the autopsy findings confirm that human islets can survive and become neovascularized within the liver.

The third patient was studied in the greatest detail. In her case, plasma insulin was undetectable immediately after pancreatectomy, in spite of elevated plasma glucose levels, attesting to the completeness of pancreatectomy.[21] Circulating insulin reappeared after islet autotransplantation. It is almost certain that pancreatic endocrine function after operation was derived from the transplanted islets. Carbohydrate metabolism for the first 4 mo was satisfactory, although it was not as good as that achieved by transplantation of immediately vascularized segmental pancreatic allografts in diabetic patients.[36] Thus, islet transplant from a single donor may not be as efficient as pancreas transplantation for treatment of diabetes, even if the immunologic problems are solved. Furthermore, after 4 mo this patient's carbohydrate metabolism deteriorated. Although she could survive without exogenous insulin, small doses were begun 15 mo after operation. There are several possible explanations for the deterioration of islet function. Unpurified islets derived from a pancreas with chronic inflammation may be damaged because of their continued association with exocrine pancreatic fragments. On the other hand, the quantity of islets that actually engrafted may have been marginal in this patient, and the deterioration could reflect an inadequate islet mass.

Cameron et al.[37] have performed intraportal islet autotransplants after near-total pancreatectomy in at least three patients with chronic pancreatitis. The outcome in one of their patients was described in detail. The need for exogenous insulin was completely obviated, and the results of glucose tolerance tests were nearly normal and identical to those obtained before pancreatectomy and islet autotransplantation. In addition, an intravenous glucose tolerance test performed with blood samples drawn simultaneously from hepatic and portal veins conclusively demonstrated secretion of insulin from the liver. There was sudden loss of islet function at 6 mo, however, and the patient required exogenous insulin. In our third case, deterioration of islet function was much less dramatic and of less magnitude, and the need for exogenous insulin was not mandatory. How often islet function will deteriorate after islet transplantation cannot be predicted until more experience is gained. Cameron et al.[37] have two other patients in whom islet autotransplants have been functioning for more than 6 mo with no evidence of deterioration, and the outcome in our first case was similar.

In summary, the results after autotransplantation of human islets are variable, just as they are in dogs.[20] Transplantation of unpurified dispersed pancreatic islet autografts can obviate the need for insulin in totally pancreatectomized dogs, but glucose tolerance test results are not completely normal.[16,18] Nevertheless, even this degree of islet function is a vast improvement over that in ketoacidosis-prone diabetics. Attempts to adapt this technique of transplantation of unpurified dispersed pancreatic islet tissue derived from single normal allogeneic donors to selected diabetic patients are justified if the risks can be minimized.

ALLOTRANSPLANTATION OF DISPERSED PANCREATIC ISLET TISSUE TO DIABETIC RENAL ALLOGRAFT RECIPIENTS

Seven diabetic patients have received intraportal allografts of unpurified dispersed pancreatic islet tissue derived from single donors. One patient received allografts of unpurified islets on two separate occasions. Another patient had previously received a transplant of purified islets in our first series of 10 transplants in seven patients.[14,15] Thus, to date, we have done 18 islet transplant procedures in 13 patients.

In our second series of eight transplants in seven patients, all but one of the transplants were performed several months or years after successful renal allotransplantation. One patient received an islet transplant simultaneously with a kidney transplant from the same cadaver donor.

The age of the donors ranged from 6 to 45 yr. All of the donors shared at least two HLA antigens of the A and B loci with the recipients. In five instances, the donor was tissue typed and the recipient was selected and prepared for islet transplantation before donor pancreatectomy. In three instances, the donor pancreatectomy was done before or concomitant with tissue typing, and the dispersed pancreatic islet tissue was stored at 4°C in Medium 199 from 4 to 18 h before transplantation. The dispersed pancreatic islet tissue for allotransplantation was prepared by collagenase digestion according to the same technique described for the islet autotransplant recipients. Tissue insulin amylase contents before, during, and after dispersion were also calculated as described previously. The results of these analyses are summarized in Table 3. Islet yield after pancreatic dispersal ranged from 20 to 60%. The percent yield did not necessarily reflect the amount of islet tissue transplanted, because some pancreases were smaller than others and had less pancreatic tissue insulin content. Again, the yield does not tell the adequacy of the preparation, since the degree of tissue dispersal is also important.[32]

All patients received horse antihuman lymphoblast globulin (10–30 mg/kg/day) for 10–14 days after islet transplantation. The six patients with previous renal allografts were taking maintenance doses of azathioprine (2–2.5 mg/kg/day) and prednisone (0.2–0.3 mg/kg/day). After islet transplantation, azathioprine was continued in the same dose. Four patients had their prednisone dose increased to

TABLE 3
Islet recovery and exocrine enzyme contamination in dispersed pancreatic tissue transplanted to diabetic allograft recipients

Patient	Weight of pancreas (g)	Total tissue insulin content (μg)	Total tissue amylase content (mg)	Insulin content of transplanted tissue (μg)	Amylase content of transplanted tissue (mg)	Islet* yield (%)	Amylase† retention (%)
1	37	9320	261	3230	29	35	11
2A	41	4821	225	1533	18	32	8
B	42	7474	65	3860	32	52	49
3	29	24,050	149	14,578	55	60	37
4	49	9062	228	2369	36	42	16
5	51	14,608	389	2490	64	20	16
6‡	25	7329	108	1529	22	21	20
7	33	4215	42	2135	17	51	40

* Insulin content of transplanted tissue/total tissue insulin content of pancreas.
† Amylase content of transplanted tissue/total tissue amylase content of pancreas.
‡ For patients 6 and 7, pancreas was dispersed using 4800 U collagenase per gram tissue. In all other cases, 1440–1660 U/g tissue was used.

2 mg/kg/day for 3 days and then gradually tapered to maintenance levels. Two other patients had their prednisone dose increased to 1 mg/kg/day and then rapidly tapered to pretransplant levels. The recipient with the simultaneous islet and kidney transplant received azathioprine 5 mg/kg/day and prednisone 2 mg/kg/day, and the dosages were tapered to maintenance levels according to our usual schedule after cadaveric renal allotransplantation.[38]

No patients were permanently ameliorated of diabetes after islet transplantation. Two recipients were withdrawn from exogenous insulin therapy for a short time, one (no. 2) between the second and fourth day and one (no. 6) between the 13th and 17th day after transplantation. During these intervals, plasma glucose levels were nearly normal, but hyperglycemia then recurred and exogenous insulin was resumed.

The outcome after the other six islet transplant procedures was variable. Two patients were able to reduce the dose of exogenous insulin; urinary C-peptide secretion was measured in one of these, and it was temporarily increased. In the other patients, there were minimal or no discernable effects of the islet transplantation on their diabetic condition.

There were no serious complications from intraportal transplantation of unpurified allogeneic pancreatic islet tissue. In one instance (the second transplant for patient no. 2), a significant elevation of portal pressure occurred during the infusion of the pancreatic islet tissue. This patient (no. 2) is the one that received unpurified allogeneic islets on two separate occasions. The portal pressure rose from 7 cm of water before infusion to 60 cm water at the end of infusion, but there were no sequelae from this elevation. During the other seven islet transplant procedures, mean (± SD) portal pressure before infusion was 7 ± 5 cm of water, and mean (± SD) portal pressure after infusion was 16 ± 5 cm water. The mean increase in portal pressure from the preinfusion value to the last measurement after islet infusion was 10 ± 6 cm of water.

Liver function tests were not significantly altered by intraportal islet transplantation (Table 4). Slight elevation of serum bilirubin, SGOT, and alkaline phosphatase occurred in some patients within the first few days after islet transplantation, but the values generally were within the normal range and they returned to baseline by the time of discharge from the hospital. The course of each patient is summarized in individual case histories.

Patient no. 1. This 22-yr-old male patient had been diabetic for 18 yr. One and one-half years before, he had received a cadaver renal allograft for treatment of end-stage diabetic nephropathy. His serum creatinine levels have been normal (0.7–1.4 mg/dl) since kidney transplantation, and he has had no rejection episodes. At the time of islet transplantation, he took 98 U of insulin daily for control of diabetes. Islet transplantation was performed on 27 February 1977. After collagenase digestion, the dispersed pancreatic islet tissue was stored in Medium 199 for 18 h at 4°C before transplantation. Portal pressure was increased by 5 cm of water after infusion of the pancreatic islet tissue. The patient continued to require exogenous insulin for control of plasma glucose levels. Two weeks after transplantation, the total insulin dose was reduced to 86 U, and there has been no change over the 26 mo since transplantation. No measurements of C-peptide were done in this patient. Mean (± SD) plasma glucose level during the 18 mo before transplantation was 287 ± 147 mg/dl (156 determinations); since transplantation, mean plasma glucose levels have been 258 ± 112 mg/dl (70 determinations). The patient performed qualitative tests for urine glucose four times daily before and after islet transplantation and states that glycosuria is less severe and less frequent than before transplantation. We have not documented this subjective assessment by quantitative urinary glucose measurements.

TABLE 4
Results of liver function tests (mean ± SD) before and after eight cases of intraportal allotransplantation of dispersed pancreatic islet tissue

Test serum	Pretransplant	Highest value after transplant*	Value at discharge†
Bilirubin (mg/dl)	0.4 ± 0.3	0.6 ± 0.4	0.3 ± 0.2
SGOT (IU/L)	12 ± 3	25 ± 12	14 ± 3
Alkaline phosphatase (IU/L)	184 ± 134	232 ± 108	182 ± 80

* Usually first or second day posttransplant.
† Approximately 2 wk posttransplant.

Patient no. 2. This 30-yr-old female patient had been diabetic for 22 yr. Four and one-half years before her first islet transplant, she had received a kidney transplant from her mother. Serum creatinine at the time of the first islet transplant was 0.9 mg/dl, and she had never been treated for rejection. For the 3 yr before islet transplantation, she took 32 U of insulin daily. Mean (± SD) plasma glucose during the 3 yr before islet transplantation was 238 ± 126 mg/dl (71 determinations). She received an islet transplant on 21 March 1977. The dispersed pancreatic tissue was stored at 4°C for 18 h before transplantation. Portal pressure rose from 2 cm of water before to 7 cm of water after islet infusion. Exogenous insulin could not be discontinued after islet transplantation, but plasma glucose concentrations and insulin requirements became exceedingly labile. Between 1 and 3 mo after islet transplantation, plasma glucose concentrations ranged from 40 to 435 mg/dl, and she took 4–20 U of insulin per day. The patient adjusted her own insulin dosage according to plasma glucose levels. She would take small doses of insulin for several days with good control of plasma glucose. Hyperglycemia would then occur, and she would increase the insulin dosage. Plasma glucose levels would stabilize for a few days, but then hypoglycemia would recur and the patient would decrease her insulin dose. This pattern would then repeat itself.

On 8 July 1977, the patient received a second islet transplant. In this instance, the pancreatic islet tissue was transplanted immediately after collagenase digestion. This is the only case where portal pressure rose significantly, by 53 cm of water. From the second through the fourth days after islet transplantation, plasma glucose levels ranged from 72 to 242 mg/dl (mean 168 ± 53 mg/dl, 17 determinations). Plasma glucose then abruptly rose to 358 mg/dl, and exogenous insulin was resumed. The patient then resumed the pattern seen before the second transplant of labile plasma glucose levels and a variation of insulin dose between 4 and 20 U/day.

Over the next year, her mean (±SD) plasma glucose level was 264 + 134 mg/dl (132 determinations). On 25 July 1978, the patient received an intact segmental pancreatic graft with vascular anastomoses. The graft functioned well and the patient was completely withdrawn from insulin and has maintained normal plasma glucose levels for more than 10 mo.[36] The pancreas graft was placed intraperitoneally; at the time of laparotomy, there were no findings to suggest that the portal hypertension after islet transplantation had persisted, although portal pressure was not measured at this time.

Patient no. 3. This 36-yr-old male patient had been diabetic for 20 yr. Three and one-half years before islet transplantation, he received a renal allograft from his brother. He had no rejection episodes of the kidney, and at the time of islet transplantation his serum creatinine was 1.3 mg/dl. He took between 55 and 65 U of insulin per day. During the 10 mo before islet transplantation, mean (±SD) plasma glucose level was 239 ± 109 mg/dl (67 determinations). On 27 September 1977, the patient received an intraportal transplant of dispersed pancreatic islet tissue. There were technical difficulties with the tissue preparation. The motor of our mechanical chopper[29] malfunctioned, and we had to mince most of the tissue by hand, which added an hour to the procedure; the interval between donor pancreatectomy and islet infusion was 3½ h. There were no other technical difficulties of the transplant procedure. Portal pressure rose 8.5 cm of water after islet tissue infusion.

Although there was evidence of temporary function of the transplanted tissue, it was inadequate to ameliorate the diabetic state. Before islet transplantation, urinary C-peptide excretion ranged from 1.2 to 3.3 μg for 24 h. From the second through the fourth weeks after islet transplantation, urinary C-peptide excretion ranged from 4.5 to 11.0 μg/24 h (mean ±SD of 6.9 ± 22 μg for 24 h).

During the fourth week after islet transplantation, the patient received 34 U of insulin per day. On this regimen, mean (±SD) plasma glucose level was 175 ± 58 mg/dl. The patient then developed a fever and symptoms characteristic of cytomegalovirus (CMV) infection. He ultimately sero-converted to CMV. Simultaneous with development of the fever, plasma glucose levels increased. The patient returned to his previous dose of 55–65 U of insulin per day, and urinary C-peptide levels fell to the range of 1.5–3.5 μg/24 h by 2 mo after transplantation.

For the first month after transplantation, the islets seemed to function but not sufficiently to ameliorate diabetes. A combination of an inadequate beta cell mass, the diabetogeneic action of the prednisone, and the occurrence of CMV infection may have contributed to the inability of the transplanted islets to obviate the need for exogenous insulin. Rejection may ultimately have occurred.

Patient no. 4. This 26-yr-old female patient had been diabetic for 12 yr. She had received a kidney transplant from her brother 5 yr before and had no rejection episodes. Serum creatinine levels ranged from 0.5 to 1.0 mg/dl. Two and one-half years before transplantation of unpurified dispersed pancreatic islet tissue, she had received an intraportal transplant of purified islets.[11] Before the first islet transplant, she took 72 U of insulin per day; by 2 mo after the first islet transplant, her insulin dose had been reduced to 36 U, and at 18 mo she took 32 U per day. This is the only patient in the first series in which a sustained reduction in insulin dose was possible. At 2 yr, her insulin dose was increased, and, at the time of the transplant of unpurified islet tissue on 4 October 1978, she took 50 U of insulin per day. During the 6 mo before transplantation, her mean (±SD) plasma glucose level was 212 ± 116 mg/dl (70 determinations). After preparation, the dispersed pancreatic islet tissue was stored at 4°C for 4 h before intraportal transplantation. During infusion of the islet tissue, portal pressure rose from 10 to 20 cm of water. At 2 wk after islet transplantation the patient was receiving 20 U of insulin per day. Plasma glucose level during the second and third weeks after islet transplantation was 222 ± 124 mg/dl (40 determinations). Urinary C-peptide excretion was 1.5 to 2.8 μg/24 h. The patient then had a series of complications. First, she fell and broke her hip. In addition she developed a fever, and blood cultures of her blood grew CMV. Immunosuppressive drug doses were immediately tapered to maintenance levels. By 4 wk after transplantation, she required her pretransplant dose of insulin to control hyperglycemia, and there was no evidence that the transplanted islets were functioning.

Patient no. 5. This 31-yr-old male patient had been diabetic for 23 yr. Three years before, he had received a renal allograft from his sister. He had no rejection episodes and at the time of islet transplantation his serum creatinine was 1.4 mg/dl. He took 56 U of insulin per day. During the 3 yr before islet transplantation, his mean (±SD) plasma glucose level was 267 ± 167 mg/dl (135 determinations). On 30 April 1978, the patient received an islet transplant. During the first 6 mo he took the same dose of insulin as before islet transplantation. Mean plasma glucose levels during this interval were 194 ± 113 mg/dl (418 determinations). At 6 mo there was a sudden decrease in insulin requirements, and over the past 7 mo he has taken 37 U of insulin per day. During that interval, mean plasma glucose levels have been 152 ± 81 mg/dl (31 determinations). The change at 6 mo coincided with the reduction of his prednisone dose to maintenance levels. Urine collections for C-peptide before islet transplantation had not been done over a 24-h period, but C-peptide excretion during a short-term collection was 1.42 μg/g of creatinine. Twenty-four hours after islet transplantation, urinary C-peptide excretion was 12 μg/g of creatinine and 18 μg/24 h. During the first 3 mo after islet transplantation, mean (±SD) urinary C-peptide excretion was 5 ± 2 μg/g creatinine and 8 ± 4 μg/24 h (28 determinations). On days when urinary glucose excretion (measured only on 15 of the collections) was <1 g for 24 h, urinary C-peptide ranged from 1.8 to 4.6 μg/24 h, mean (±SD) 5 ± 2 μg (10 determinations). On days when urinary glucose excretion was >1 g/24 h, urinary C-peptide excretion ranged from 4.4 to 16.4 μg for 24 h (mean 12 ± 5 μg, five determinations). These determinations were made during the early posttransplant period, when high doses of prednisone were used. C-peptide urinalyses subsequent to this time have not been completed. Serum C-peptide levels before transplantation were less than 0.5 ng/ml. Multiple serum C-peptide determinations since transplantation have all been in the range of 1.1–1.2 ng/ml, well below the normal range. There is minimal evidence of function of the transplanted islets in this patient.

Patient no. 6. This 42-yr-old female patient had been diabetic for 25 yr. Three years before, she had received a kidney transplant from her sister. She had one severe rejection episode 10 mo posttransplant. Treatment with high doses of corticosteroids reversed the rejection episode, and her serum creatinine stabilized between 2 and 3 mg/dl. Mean (±SD) plasma glucose level for the year preceding islet transplantation was 328 ± 180 mg/dl (52 determinations). She took 40–50 U of insulin daily. Serum C-peptide concentrations before transplantation ranged from 0.8 to 1.0 mg/ml. On 12 July 1978, she received an islet transplant. At 13 days after transplantation she was withdrawn from insulin. Mean plasma glucose for the next 5 days was 148 ± 60 mg/dl. Serum C-peptide was 2.9 ng/ml. On the 18th day after transplantation, she had an abrupt elevation of plasma glucose to >400 mg/dl. Exogenous insulin therapy was resumed, and, since that time, she has continued to take insulin at the same dose as before transplantation. Serum C-peptide levels after this time were less than 1.1 ng/ml. Mean (±SD) plasma glucose level for the next 11 mo was 179 ± 90 mg/dl (131 determinations). Although there was some evidence that the transplanted islets functioned for a few days within the first 2½ wk after transplantation, the effect was not sustained, and rejection probably occurred.

Patient no. 7. This 37-yr-old man received a kidney and islet transplant simultaneously from the same cadaver donor. He had been diabetic for 30 yr before transplantation and took 42 U of insulin daily. Mean (±SD) plasma glucose levels during the 5 mo before islet transplantation were 334 ± 168 mg/dl. A serum C-peptide level before transplantation was 0.9 ng/ml. The transplant was performed on 6 October 1978. There was no change in the insulin dose during the first month after transplantation. Mean (±SD) plasma glucose level during this interval was 280 ± 136 mg/dl. Serum C-peptide levels ranged from 1.0 to 1.5 ng/ml. At 1 mo he had an elevation of his serum creatinine. A kidney biopsy showed acute rejection. Antirejection treatment with prednisone was followed by a return of serum creatinine to normal. During the course of antirejection treatment, his insulin dose was increased to 68 U/day. Serum C-peptide concentration after completion of antirejection treatment was 0.5 ng/ml. Mean (±SD) plasma glucose concentration during the 7 mo since completion of antirejection treatment has been 210 ± 103 mg/dl (52 determinations). This patient had only minimal evidence of islet function after transplantation; no increase in exogenous insulin dose was necessary in spite of the high dose of steroids. After rejection, his insulin requirements increased, the usual situation after kidney transplantation and treatment with prednisone.

Comments. The results of our experience with allotransplantation of unpurified dispersed pancreatic islet tissue are disappointing, especially in view of the relative success achieved with islet autotransplantation after pancreatectomy. The difficulty with application of islet allotransplantation in humans is similar to that experienced with islet transplantation in animals: success in the isogeneic situation is easy to achieve, while allografts are often rejected before function can even be established.[6,11]

Two other groups of investigators have described their attempts at intraportal islet allotransplantation in humans. Largiader and Kolb[12] simultaneously transplanted a kidney and unpurified dispersed pancreatic islet tissue from single cadaver donors to the portal vein of four uremic diabetic patients. Their method of tissue preparation—collagenase digestion—was similar to ours and was one they had found suitable for islet autotransplantation in dogs.[19] The procedure was well tolerated, but they could detect no benefit to the diabetic condition, and the patients continued to need exogenous insulin. One patient rejected the kidney transplant and returned to dialysis; the renal allograft functioned in two patients for at least a few months, although it was not reported whether rejection episodes occurred. In four unpublished cases by Largiader et al. (personal communication, June 1979), dispersed pancreatic islet tissue from cadaver donors was implanted in the spleen simultaneously with a kidney transplant. In three patients the need for exogenous insulin was not obviated, although one patient had a decrease in insulin requirements at 6 mo. One patient was gradually withdrawn from insulin between 7 and 8 mo; exogenous insulin administration was stopped 9 mo after intrasplenic islet allotransplantation, and the patient has received no insulin for at least 2 mo. This case represents the best result of a human islet allotransplant procedure to date.

Groth et al.[13] transplanted fetal pancreatic microfragments to the portal vein of a diabetic patient. The microfragments were obtained from several fetuses and preserved in tissue culture for a few hours to several days before transplantation. This patient has had an increase in serum and urinary C-peptide levels, but has continued to require exogenous insulin during 2 mo of follow-up.

Our cases show that islet allotransplantation is a safe but metabolically inefficient procedure. The failure to successfully ameliorate diabetes for more than a brief period raises the question of technical problems versus rejection. The high doses of steroids given to the patients may also produce a diabetogeneic effect sufficient to mask any graft function that may have occurred before rejection. Our results with transplantation of unpurified dispersed pancreatic islet tissue in totally pancreatectomized dogs were similar.[39,40] Autotransplantation alone of pancreatic tissue digested for 20 min uniformly ameliorated diabetes. Treatment of the autotransplant recipients with steroids had a deleterious effect on the results. Islet allotransplantation to pancreatectomized dogs that were immunosuppressed with corticosteroids and azathioprine ameliorated diabetes in only 8 of 24 dogs. Thus, even in a good experimental model, the results of islet autotransplantation could not be duplicated by allotransplantation.

Technical problems, such as prolonged cold or warm ischemia, occurred in some of our eight cases. In our experiments in dogs, autotransplantation of dispersed pancreatic islet tissue, preserved in the cold, ameliorated diabetes only half the time.[39] At this point, preservation in the cold is unreliable. Another technical problem may have been inadequate dispersal of the pancreatic tissue. The tissue insulin contents after collagenase digestion of the human pancreases were generally higher than measured insulin contents after the optimal period of collagenase digestion in our experiments in dogs.[32] While this collagenase digestion protocol was sufficient to achieve a satisfactory effect in our cases of islet autotransplantation, in the autotransplant situation, the transplanted islets did not have to overcome the diabetogeneic effect of steroids, and there was no possibility of rejection before the grafts became established.

SUMMARY AND CONCLUSIONS

Isolation of purified islets from human pancreas is difficult.[14] Unpurified dispersed pancreatic islet tissue prepared by collagenase digestion alone can successfully ameliorate diabetes after intrasplenic or intraportal transplantation in totally pancreatectomized dogs.[16-20] We adapted this technique for intraportal islet autotransplantation and allotransplantation in humans.

In three patients who underwent near-total pancreatectomy for treatment of chronic pancreatitis, pancreatic endocrine function was preserved by islet autotransplantation. In one patient the carbohydrate metabolism has been normal for nearly 2.5 yr. One patient died 10 days after the operation, but islets were found in the liver. In the other patient, carbohydrate metabolism was impaired, but sufficient islet function was present to obviate the need for exogenous insulin for over 1 yr.

Application of this technique for allotransplantation to diabetic renal allograft recipients has not been successful. Logistic and technical problems, the diabetogeneic action of steroids, and susceptibility to rejection probably all contributed to failure.

The efficiency of preparation for transplantation of tissue from a single pancreas needs to be improved, but the relative success of human islet autotransplantation in a situation where rejection cannot occur emphasizes the need for efforts to focus on the immunologic aspects of clinical islet allotransplantation. At this point, the primary application of human islet transplantation is as an autograft to preserve endocrine function after total or near-total pancreatectomy for benign disease. However, if the rejection problem can be solved, islet transplantation is a potentially safe and effective treatment for patients with diabetes mellitus.

ADDENDUM

Note added in proof. Since submission of the manuscript, five additional patients with chronic pancreatitis have undergone total or near total pancreatectomy and islet autotransplantation. One patient does not require exogenous insulin, two are receiving 6–8 U/day, and two require >20 U/day.

ACKNOWLEDGMENTS

This work was supported by USPHS grant AM19269, by a grant from the American Diabetes Association, Minnesota Chapter, and by NIH grant RR-400 from the General Clinical Research Center Branch. Dr. Sutherland is a recipient of USPHS Research Career Development Award KO4 AM 00161. Darlene McManus, Elizabeth Frenzel, Phyllis Gorecki, June Eckhardt, and Marie Wiklund helped with the preparation of human islet tissue and performed the analyses of tissue insulin and amylase contents. Beryl Greenberg performed the insulin, C-peptide, and glucose assays on blood and urine samples from the islet transplant recipients. Jerry Vincent prepared the illustrations and Janet Sanders the manuscript. The authors express their appreciation to Dr. Arthur C. Rubenstein, University of Chicago, for his advice and help in the performance and interpretation of the C-peptide assays.

REFERENCES

1 Brooks, J. R.: Endocrine Tissue Transplantation. Springfield, Illinois, Charles C Thomas, 1962, pp. 3–103.

2 Hegre, O. D., and Lazarow, A.: Islet cell transplantation. *In* The Diabetic Pancreas. New York, Plenum Press, 1977, pp. 517–50.

3 Ballinger, W. F., and Lacy, P. E.: Transplantation of intact pancreatic islets in rats. *Surgery 72*:175–86, 1972.

4 Leonard, R. J., Lazarow, A., and Hegre, O. D.: Pancreatic islet transplantation in the rat. Diabetes *22*:413–28, 1973.

5 Kemp, C. B., Knight, M. J., Scharp, D. W., Ballinger, W. F., and Lacy, P. E.: Effect of transplantation site on the results of pancreatic islet isografts in diabetic rats. Diabetologia *9*:486–91, 1973.

6 Reckard, C. R., Ziegler, M. M., and Barker, C. F.: Physiological and immunological consequences of transplanting isolated pancreatic islets. Surgery *74*:91–99, 1973.

7 Brown, J., Molnar, I. G., Clark, W., and Mullen, Y.: Control of experimental diabetes mellitus in rats by transplantation of fetal pancreas. Science *184*:1377–79, 1974.

8 Mauer, S. M., Sutherland, D. E. R., Steffes, M. W., Leonard, A. J., Najarian, J. S., Michael, A. F., and Brown, D. M.: Pancreatic transplantation: effects on the glomerular lesions of experimental diabetes in the rat. Diabetes *23*:748–53, 1974.

9 Matas, A. J., Sutherland, D. E. R., Steffes, M. W., and Najarian, J. S.: Islet transplantation using neonatal rat pancreata: quantitative studies. J. Surg. Res. *20*:143–47, 1976.

10 Najarian, J. S., Sutherland, D. E. R., Matas, A. J., Steffes, M. W., Simmons, R. L., and Goetz, F. C.: Human islet transplantation: a preliminary report. Transplant. Proc. *9*:233–36, 1977.

11 Sutherland, D. E. R., Matas, A. J., and Najarian, J. S.: Pancreatic islet cell transplantation. Surg. Clin. North Am. *58*:365–382, 1978.

12 Largiader, F., and Kolb, E.: Rejection of pancreatic allografts. Experimental and clinical results. *In* Transplantation and Clinical Immunology X, Amsterdam, Excerpta Medica, 1979, pp. 240–244.

13 Groth, C. G., Andersson, A., Bjorken, C., Gunnarsson, R., Hellerstrom, L., Lundgren, G., Petersson, B., Swenne, I., and Ostman, J.: Transplantation of fetal pancreatic microfragments via the portal vein to a diabetic patient. Diabetes *29*(Suppl. 1):80–83, 1980.

14 Najarian, J. S., Sutherland, D. E. R., and Steffes, M. W.: Isolation of human islets of Langerhans for transplantation. Transplant. Proc. *7*:611–13, 1975.

15 Sutherland, D. E. R., Matas, A. J., Steffes, M. W., and Najarian, J. S.: Infant human pancreas: a potential source of islet tissue for transplantation. Diabetes *25*:1123–28, 1976.

16 Mirkovitch, V., and Campiche, M.: Successful intrasplenic autotransplantation of pancreatic tissue in totally pancreatectomized dogs. Transplantation *21*:265–69, 1976.

17 Mosimann, R., Rausis, C., and Mirkovitch, V.: Prevention du diabetes chez le chien pancreatectomise par autotransplantation de tissu pancreatique dans le foie. Helv. Chir. Acta *43*:241–252, 1976.

18 Kretschmer, G. J., Sutherland, D. E. R., Matas, A. J., Cain, T. L., and Najarian, J. S.: Autotransplantation of pancreatic islets without separation of exo and endocrine tissue in totally pancreatectomized dogs. Surgery *82*:74–81, 1977.

19 Kolb, E., Ruchert, R., and Largiader, F.: Intraportal and intrasplenic autotransplantation of pancreatic islets in the dog. Eur. Surg. Res. *9*:149–426, 1977.

20 Kretschmer, G. J., Sutherland, D. E. R., Matas, A. J., Payne, W. D., and Najarian, J. S.: Autotransplantation of pancreatic fragments to the portal vein and spleen of totally pancreatectomized dogs: a comparative evaluation. Ann. Surg. *187*:79–86, 1978.

21 Goetz, F. C., Greenberg, B. Z., Ells, J., and Neinert, C.: A single immunoassay for insulin: application to human and dog plasma. J. Clin. Endocrinol. Metab. *23*:1237–46, 1963.

22 Melani, F., Rubenstein, A. H., Oyer, P. E., and Steiner, D. F.: Identification of proinsulin and C-peptide in human serum by a specific immunoassay. Proc. Natl. Acad. Sci. U.S.A. *67*(1):148–55, 1970.

23 Horowitz, D. L., Rubenstein, A. H., and Katz, A. I.: Quantitation of human pancreatic beta-cell function by immunoassay of C-peptide in urine. Diabetes *26*:30–35, 1977.

24 Herbert, V., Lav., K. S., Gottlieb, C. W., et al.: Coated charcoal immunoassay of insulin. J. Clin. Endocrinol. *25*:1375–84, 1965.

25 Frey, C. F., Child, C. G., and Fry, W.: Pancreatectomy for chronic pancreatitis. Ann. Surg. *184*:403–14, 1976.

26 Braasch, J. W., Vito, L., and Nugent, F. W.: Total pancreatectomy for end stage chronic pancreatitis. Ann. Surg. *188*:317–22, 1978.

27 Warren, K. W.: Surgical management of chronic relapsing pancreatitis. Am. J. Surg. *117*:24–32, 1969.

28 Frey, C. F.: 95% Pancreatectomy. *In* The Pancreas. St. Louis, C. V. Mosby, 1973, pp. 202–29.

29 Matas, A. J., Sutherland, D. E. R., Steffes, M. W., and Najarian, J. S.: Short-term culture of adult pancreatic fragments for purification and transplantation of islets of Langerhans. Surgery *80*:183–91, 1976.

[30] Leonard, R. J., Lazarow, A., McEvoy, R. C., and Hegre, O. D.: Islet cell transplantation. Kidney Int. *6*(Suppl. 1):169–78, 1974.

[31] Jamieson, A. D., Pruitt, K. M., and Caldwell, R. C.: An improved amylase assay. J. Dent. Res. *48*:483. 1969.

[32] Kretschmer, G. J., Sutherland, D. E. R., Matas, A. J., Steffes, M. W., and Najarian, J. S.: The dispersed pancreas: transplantation without islet purification in totally pancreatectomized dogs. Diabetologia *13*:495–502, 1977.

[33] Erlandsen, S. L., Parsons, J. A., Burke, J. P., Redick, J. A., VanOrden, D. E., and VanOrden, L. S.: A modification of the unlabeled antibody enzyme method using heterologous antisera for the light microscopic and ultrastructural localization of insulin, glucagon, and growth hormone. J. Histochem. Cytochem. *23*:666–77, 1975.

[34] Brown, J., Clark, W. R., Molnar, G., and Mullen, Y. S.: Fetal pancreas transplantation for reversal of streptozotocin-induced diabetes in rats. Diabetes *25*:56–64, 1976.

[35] Hogle, H. H., and Reemtsma, K.: Pancreatic autotransplantation following resection. Surgery *83*:359–60, 1978.

[36] Sutherland, D. E. R., Goetz, F. C., and Najarian, J. S.: Clinical segmental pancreas transplantation without duct anastomosis in diabetic renal allograft recipients. Diabetes *29* (Suppl. 1):10–18, 1980.

[37] Cameron, J. L., Mehigan, D. G., Harrington, D. P., and Zuidema, G. D.: Metabolic studies following intrahepatic autotransplantation of pancreatic islet grafts. Surgery. In press, 1979.

[38] Simmons, R. L., Kjellstrand, C. M., and Najarian, J. S.: Kidney technique, complications and results. *In* Transplantation. Philadelphia, Lea and Febiger, 1972, pp. 445–95.

[39] Sutherland, D. E. R., Kretschmer, G. J., Matas, A. J., and Najarian, J. S.: Experience with auto and allotransplantation of pancreatic fragments to the spleen of totally pancreatectomized dogs. Trans. Am. Soc. Artif. Intern. Organs *23*:723–25, 1977.

[40] Kretschmer, G. J., Sutherland, D. E. R., Matas, A. J., and Najarian, J. S.: Preliminary experience with allotransplantation of pancreatic fragments to the spleen of totally pancreatectomized dogs. Transplant. Proc. *11*:537–42, 1977.

Alternatives in Pancreatic Islet Transplantation

Tissue Culture Studies

KEITH REEMTSMA, COLLIN J. WEBER, F. XAVIER PI-SUNYER, ROGER L. LERNER, AND MARK A. HARDY

SUMMARY

Culture of islets isolated from the pancreas of neonatal rats successfully preserved function for 6 days, as indicated by release of insulin into the culture medium and reversal of experimental diabetes by cultured islet isografts. Release of insulin into the culture medium correlated with lowering of fasting blood glucose in the diabetic recipient. Intravenous glucose tolerance was normal in recipients of immediate and 24-h cultured islets but abnormal in recipients of 6-day cultured islets.

Culture of the islets isolated from human pancreases (cadaveric) resulted in islet purification but at the expense of loss of islets, with only 1–5% surviving 1 wk of culture. During 8–10 days in culture, insulin release declined, and histological examination revealed only a few viable islets. Islets isolated from surgical specimens survived the culture conditions as demonstrated by viable cell clumps and insulin secretion. After an 85% pancreatectomy in the patient with chronic pancreatitis, islets were isolated, cultured for 7 days, and then autografted into muscle pockets and the subcutaneous space of the forearm. There was no evidence of function. DIABETES 29 (Suppl. 1): 45–51, 1980.

The last 15 yr have witnessed a remarkable expansion in our understanding of the effects and limitations of pancreas and pancreatic islet transplantation. It is now generally accepted that either whole-organ or isolated islet isografts will reverse hyperglycemia in several experimental models.[1–10] Extensive data exist to support amelioration of diabetic renal morphologic and functional abnormalities by pancreas or islet transplantation.[11–14] Islets have been grafted successfully in a variety of sites, including the peritoneal cavity,[5–9] the portal vein,[6,8,15] the spleen,[16,17] the kidney capsule,[10] and muscle.[18,19] Significant advances have been made in islet isolation and preservation, as witnessed by the data presented in this symposium and in recent articles from several laboratories.[19–28] Preliminary data have been presented attesting to the feasibility and efficacy of segmental pancreatic or islet autografts in selected patients with benign pancreatic disease.[29–33]

The two most serious problems limiting widespread application of islet transplantation in human diabetics are (1) the rapid rejection of pancreatic or islet allografts and xenografts and (2) the low yield of donor islets obtained by presently available techniques of isolation and preservation. A major focus of our laboratory effort in the last several years has been the potential usefulness of tissue culture as a means of isolation and preservation of islets before transplantation, and the results of these experiments are detailed in this report.

MATERIALS AND METHODS

For animal experiments, neonatal Lewis rats were islet donors. Islet recipients (isologous) and concurrently followed controls were adult, streptozotocin-diabetic Lewis rats. An excess of islets (30–35 neonatal donors per recipient) was used in each experiment. Donor islets were transplanted intraperitoneally and intramuscularly. Islet preparation, criteria for grafting in diabetic recipients, maintenance and sampling techniques, hormone assays, and morphologic techniques have been described previously.[9,19,33–35]

Two islet culture techniques have been employed, as outlined in Table 1. Initial studies were done with technique A,[9] modified from the work of Chick[36] and Lambert.[37] Effects of 24-h culture of donor islets before isografting were compared with immediate implantation of islets with regard to reversal of hyperglycemia, glucose tolerance, serum insulin, and islet morphology.

Subsequent studies employed culture technique B,[19,33] modified from that of Hegre.[38] Six-day cultured, neonatal rat islets were isografted intraperitoneally and intramuscularly.

From the Departments of Surgery and Medicine, College of Physicians & Surgeons, Columbia University, New York, New York, and the Section of Endocrinology, Department of Medicine, Cedars-Sinai Medical Center, Los Angeles, California.
Address reprint requests to K. Reemtsma, Department of Surgery, College of Physicians & Surgeons, 630 W. 168th Street, New York, New York 10032.

TABLE 1
Islet culture techniques: specific conditions of techniques A and B

Technique A	
	Mincing
	Collagenase–trypsin–EDTA
	Petri dishes
	Medium 199
	Glucose = 300 mg/dl
	Fetal calf serum
	37°C
Technique B	
	Mincing
	No enzymes
	Grid (Millipore) culture
	95% Oxygen
	Glucose = 300 alternating with 100 mg/dl
	Autologous serum (maternal rodent) or human serum albumin
	Medium–CMRL–1066
	37°C

The insulin content of the culture medium was correlated with reversal of diabetes, and recipients' fasting blood glucose, serum insulin, and glucose tolerance values were compared.

In additional experiments, neonatal rat islet donors were pretreated 24 h before islet culture with Cytoxan (400 mg/kg, intraperitoneally), total-body irradiation (800 rads), antilymphocyte globulin (ALG) (Upjohn, 1.0 mg in 0.1 ml, intraperitoneally), or a combination of these agents. Other cultures were treated by the addition of antilymphocyte globulin to culture medium in concentrations of 1, 2, and 3 mg/ml during 6 days in culture.

Technique A for the isolation and preservation of islets by tissue culture had been developed in more than 100 rodent experiments. We applied this technique initially to studies of six normal cadaveric pancreas specimens from human

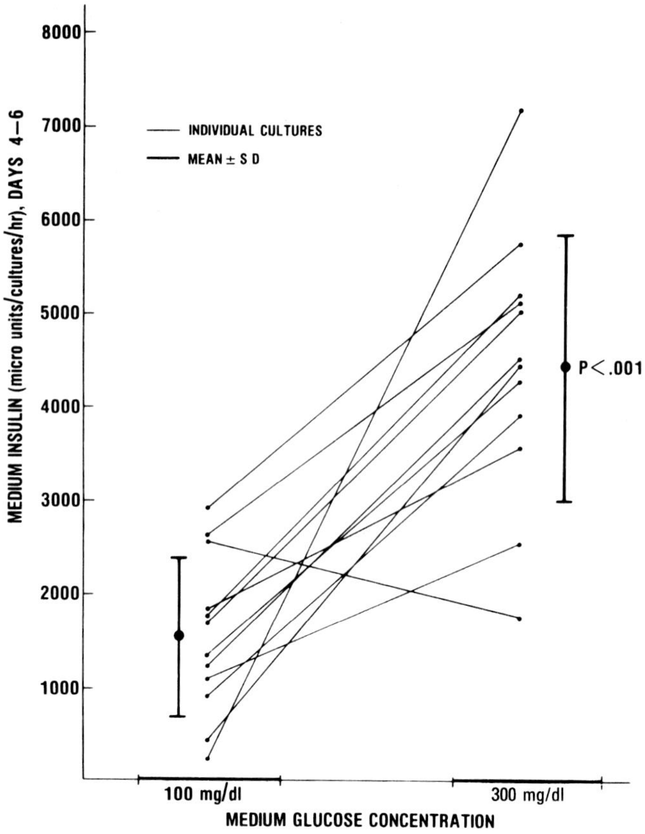

FIGURE 1. Neonatal rat islet cultures: insulin content of medium, days 4–6, with increasing glucose concentration in medium (technique B). Individual and mean ± SD values.

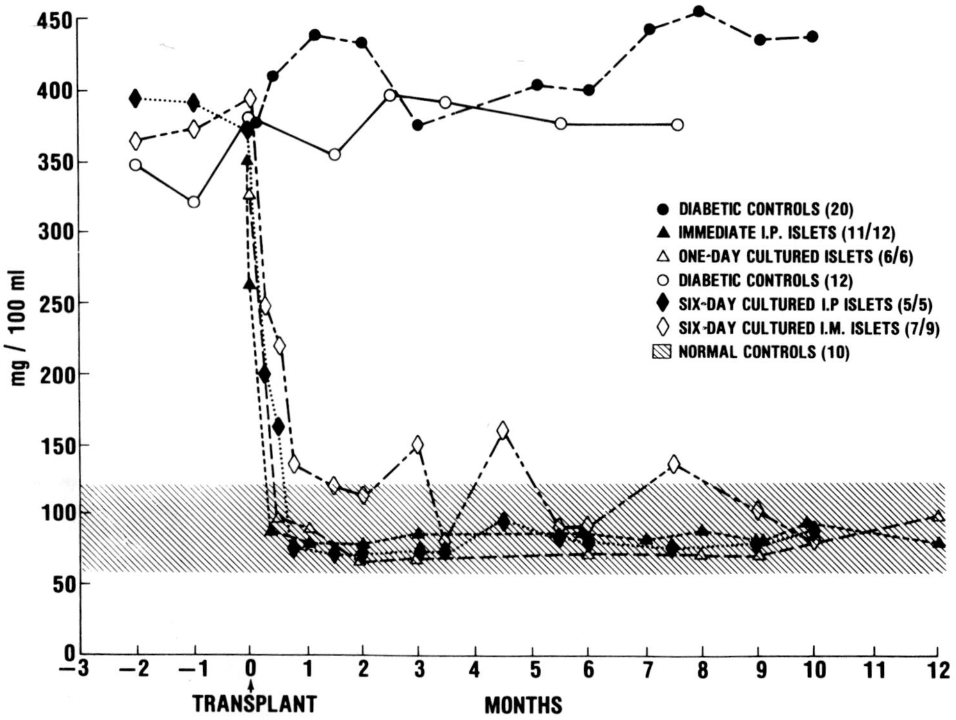

FIGURE 2. Fasting blood glucose over 12 mo in recipients of cultured and immediately implanted neonatal rat islet isografts: mean values.

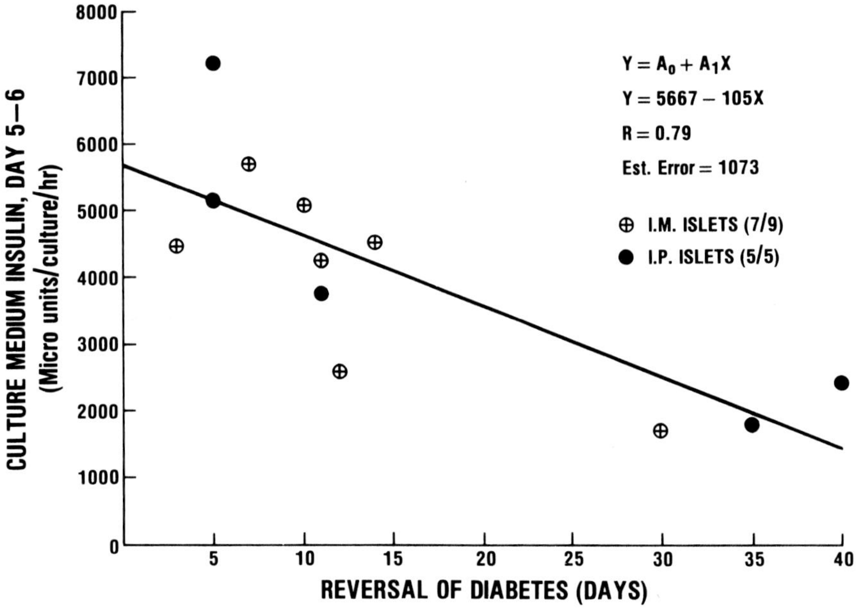

FIGURE 3. Correlation of the insulin content of the culture medium on days 5-6 with time required for reversal of diabetes after intramuscular and intraperitoneal islet isografts. R = correlation coefficient.

donors. Subsequent experience with culture technique B included an additional six pancreas specimens from normal adult human cadavers, two insulinomas, and pancreatic resection specimens from an infant with nesidioblastosis and a patient with severe, relapsing, chronic pancreatitis who underwent an 85% distal pancreatectomy for unremitting pain. A detailed description of the management of this last interesting patient has been published.[19] In brief, the chronic pancreatitis specimen was maintained in culture for 6 days and demonstrated physiologic insulin production, low amylase content, sterility, and histologic viability of islets. The patient recovered satisfactorily from subtotal pancreatectomy but became diabetic. Therefore, after 7 days in vitro, fragments of cultured pancreatic tissue were autografted into muscle pockets and in the subcutaneous space in the nondominant forearm of the patient from which the tissue had been removed. Bilateral antecubital venous samples from before and after the autograft were assayed for glucose, insulin, C-peptide, and glucagon.[19]

RESULTS

Animal studies. Histologically viable neonatal rat islets were identified in tissue culture using both techniques A and B. Increasing the glucose concentration in the medium from 100 mg/dl to 300 mg/dl (days 4–6 in vitro) (technique B) resulted in significantly increased insulin levels in medium ($P < 0.001$) (Figure 1). Amylase and glucagon in medium declined over 6 days of culture.[19]

FIGURE 4. Basal serum insulin levels 8 mo after islet isotransplantation: individual values.

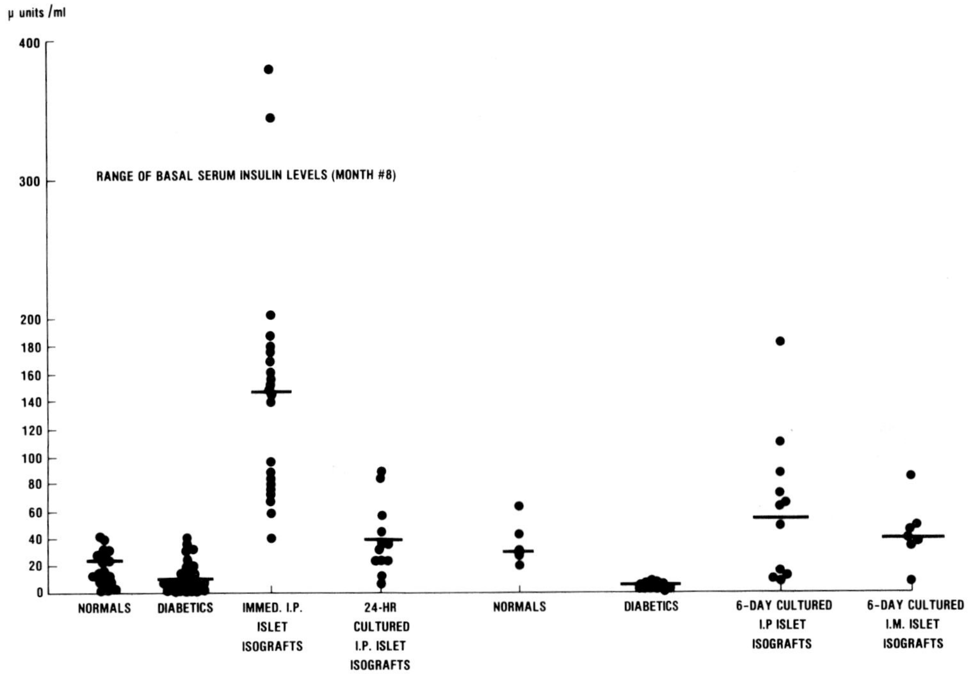

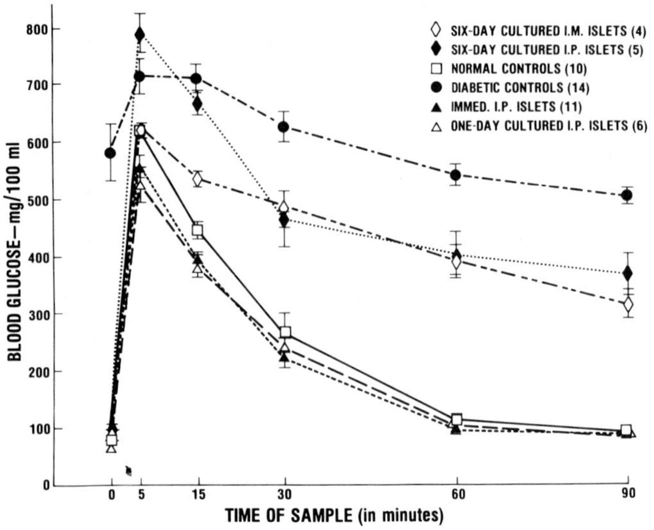

FIGURE 5. Intravenous glucose tolerance in recipients of cultured and immediately isografted neonatal rat islets. Mean ± SD.

Intraperitoneal isografts of islets maintained in culture for 24 h before grafting (6/6) were as effective in reversing experimental diabetes as were immediately implanted islets (11/12) (Figure 2).[9] With 6-day cultured islets isografted intraperitoneally (IP) (5/5) and intramuscularly (IM) (7/9), similar results were obtained (Figure 2).[19]

Reversal of hyperglycemia (fasting blood glucose <130 mg/dl) was inversely correlated with culture-medium insulin values (technique B, IP and IM islets) on days 5 and 6 of culture (Figure 3). Basal serum insulin levels were significantly elevated ($P < 0.001$) in immediate islet recipients (Figure 4) when compared with normal control values. Slight elevation of serum insulin also was observed in recipients of 24-h and 6-day cultured islets. Intravenous glucose tolerance was normal in recipients of immediate and 24-h cultured islets but was abnormal in recipients of 6-day cultured islets (Figure 5).

Islet isografts were readily identified in both intramuscular (Figure 6) and intraperitoneal[34] sites. Accumulation of fat cells and rich vascularity were characteristic findings.

Rat islet cultures from pretreated donors showed uniformly good histologic and functional viability after 6 days in vitro. Similar results were obtained with addition of ALG to culture medium (Figure 7).

Human studies. To date, 16 human pancreatic specimens have been studied (Table 2). In 8- to 10-day cultures of pancreas specimens from normal adult human cadavers, the insulin, glucagon, and amylase levels all declined significantly with time.[22,23] In most instances, amylase and glucagon disappeared from sequential medium samples sooner than did insulin. This was true for both techniques A and B. As shown in Table 2, medium insulin in 7- and 8-day cultures of normal human pancreas using technique A was much greater than when technique B was employed. Con-

FIGURE 6. Neonatal rat islet isograft, biopsied from intramuscular graft site 3 mo after transplantation. Donor islet tissue cultured for 6 days before transplantation. (*Left*) Note adjacent vessel and surrounding fat cells and muscle fibers. (Hematoxylin and eosin, ×160.) (*Right*) Adjacent section, same specimen, same islet. (Aldehyde fuchsin, ×160.)

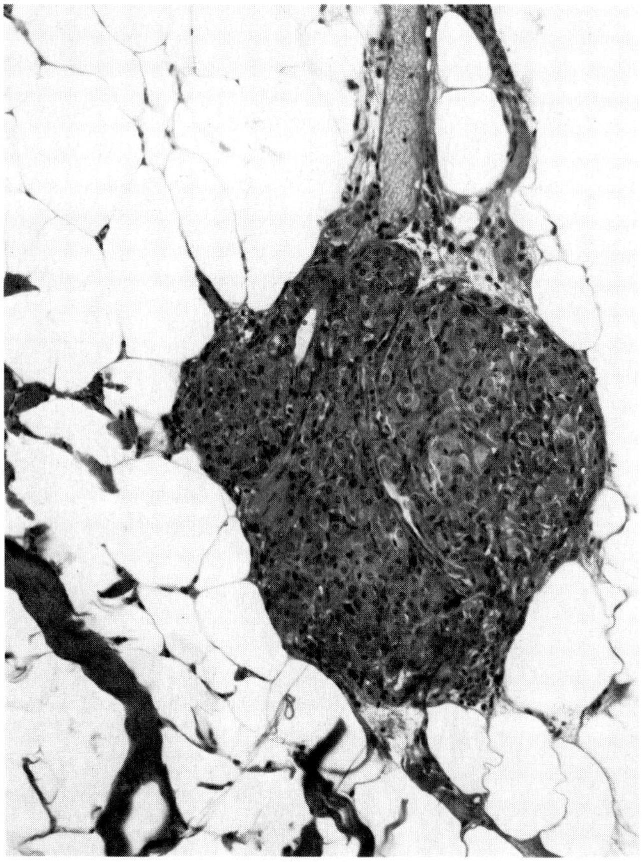

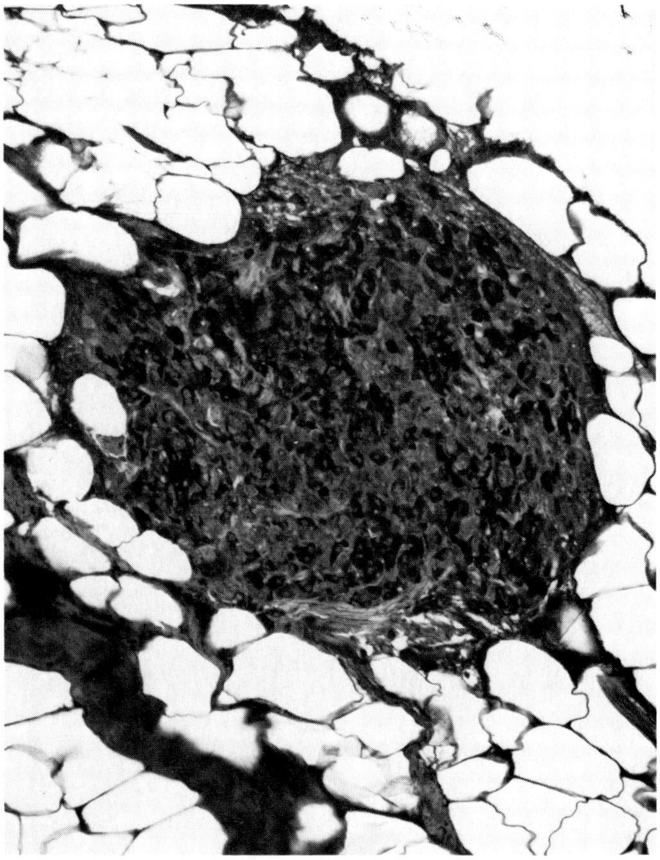

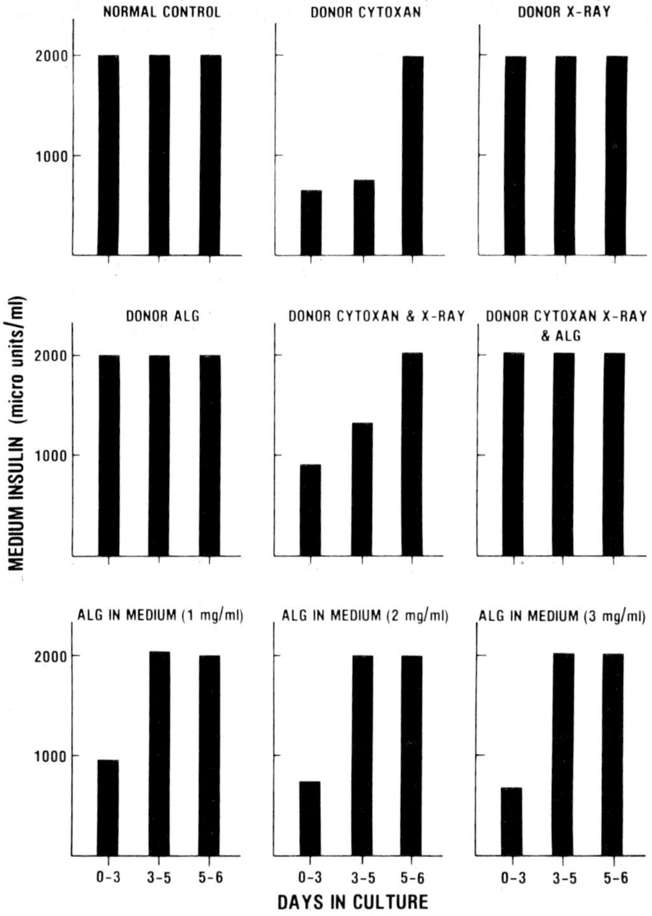

FIGURE 7. Islet donor and islet culture treatment. Insulin in medium, days 0–6 in vitro. Comparison of control and treated islets.

siderable variation in medium insulin levels was noted in cultures done by both techniques, however. Insulin production by abnormal human pancreatic specimens also was variable but was, in general, greater (per gram per day) than that of normal pancreas. Of particular interest was the specimen from a patient with chronic pancreatitis, which produced almost no amylase but significant amounts of insulin throughout 6 days in vitro.[19]

TABLE 2
Insulin content of medium in cultures of human pancreatic specimens

Source and culture technique	Medium insulin (mU/g/day) at days 7–8: No.	Mean ± SD	Range
Technique A (collagenase–trypsin–EDTA, petri dishes, fetal calf serum)			
Normal human pancreas	6	20 ± 13	1.0–37.5
Technique B (mincing, no enzymes, grid, autologous serum)			
Normal human pancreas	6	0.4 ± 0.4	0.06–0.9
Chronic pancreatitis	1	6.7	
Nesidioblastosis	1	13.0	
Insulinoma	2	1.8, 8.9	

Histologic studies of normal human islet cultures at days 8–10 revealed a few viable islets. Characteristic findings were of viable cell clumps, with some aldehyde fuchsin-positive cells, within larger fragments of nonviable tissue (Figure 8).

Cultures of human islet tumors and the chronic pancreatitis specimen showed multiple islets with demonstrable insulin granules,[19,33] corroborating functional data.

In the case of intramuscular autotransplantation of cultured human islets, the graft was well tolerated and glucose tolerance improved after transplantation. Plasma insulin and C-peptide levels were not consistently different in graft arm and nongraft arm venous samples and generally were low. Although the patient has experienced no negative sequelae from the procedure, convincing evidence of graft function is lacking at present.[19,33]

DISCUSSION

The present studies were done to assess the usefulness of tissue culture in the islet transplant effort.

Data obtained from rodent experiments using neonatal donor tissue in excess have been encouraging: sensitivity to glucose was maintained in vitro; insulin levels in medium were predictive of the rapidity of reversal of experimental diabetes; and cultured islets could be transplanted intramuscularly into a graft site, which is a procedure that is appealing for its accessibility and relative patient safety.

Some degree of islet purification compared with acinar tissue can be accomplished by culture but at the expense of islet viability. At present, it must be estimated that only 1–5% of normal human islet tissue will survive 1 wk of culture. Culture affords the opportunity for physiologic, morphologic, and bacteriologic analyses of donor islet tissue before transplantation; and, as Lacy et al.[39] suggested, immunogenicity of donor islets may be altered by a period in tissue culture. Nevertheless, it is at present a laborious technique, rather poorly suited to emergency situations (such as pancreatic resections for trauma) in which islet yield has been low.

Among the alternatives that exist in human islet transplantation, tissue culture may remain as a means for isolation and short-term preservation of donor islet tissue. The storage of islets may eventually be done more efficiently by other means, such as cryopreservation. However, culture techniques will in all probability assume greater importance in immunologic and possibly physiologic alteration of islets. Tissue culture will allow greater flexibility in management of pancreatic disorders in which resectional surgery or islet deficiencies occur.

ACKNOWLEDGMENTS

This work was supported in part by NIH grant AM-19652-01 and by the American Diabetes Association—New York Diabetes Affiliate. The authors gratefully acknowledge the technical assistance of Sandra Rivera, Margaret Freund, Jitka Mucha, and Yim Dam. We thank Frances Langley for preparing the illustrations and Birchard Allen for the photomicrography.

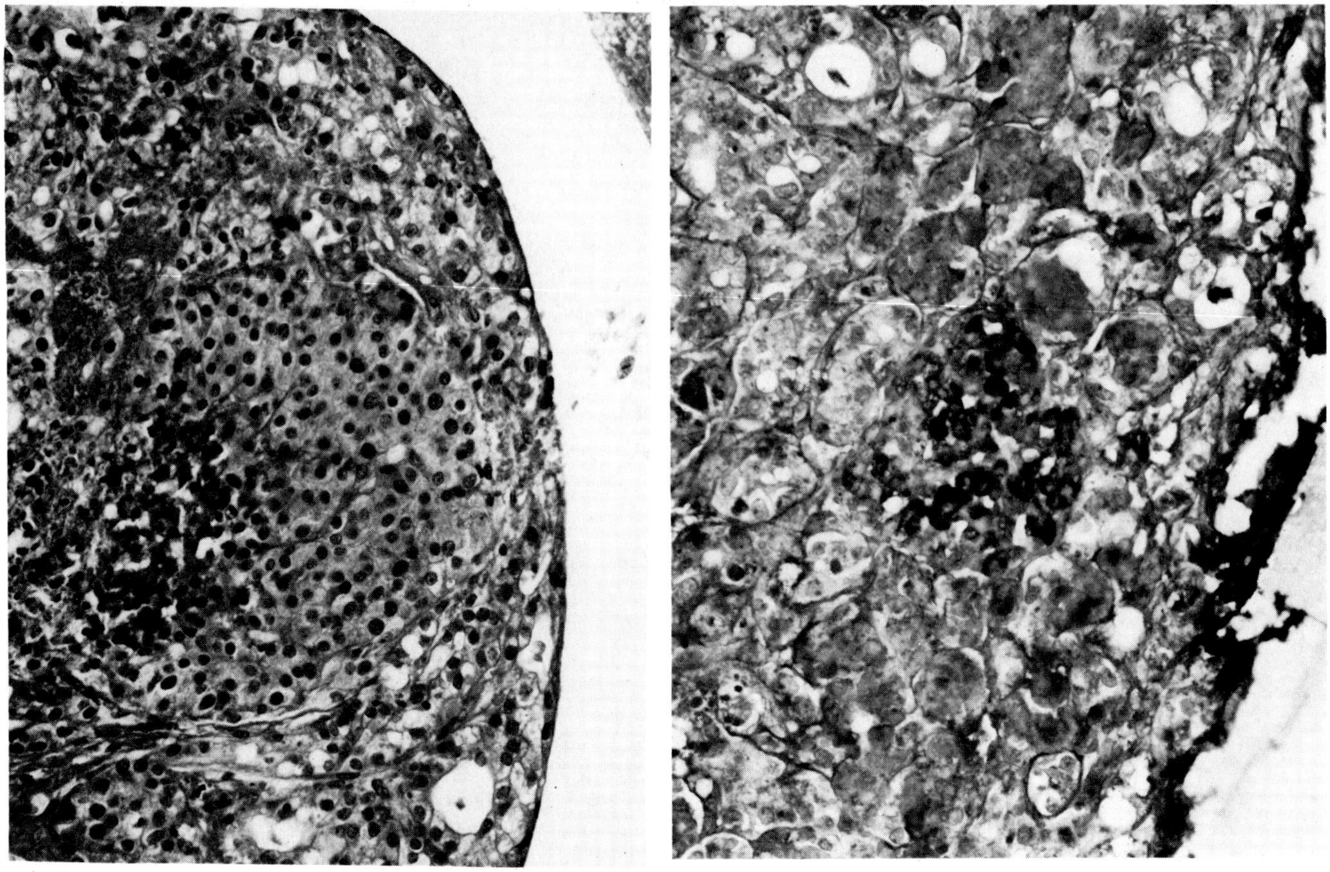

(a) (b)

FIGURE 8. Normal adult, cadaveric human pancreatic islet in tissue culture at 10 days: technique A. (a) Hematoxylin and eosin, ×250. (b) Same islet, adjacent section. (Aldehyde fuchsin, ×400.)

REFERENCES

[1] Lucas, J. F., Jr., Rogers, R. E., and Reemtsma, K.: Homologous pancreatic transplantation in dogs: report of a new technique and studies of endocrine function. Surg. Forum *13*:314–15, 1962.

[2] Reemtsma, K., Lucas, J. F., Jr., Rogers, R. E., Schmidt, F. E., and Davis, F. H., Jr.: Islet cell function of the transplanted canine pancreas. Ann. Surg. *158*:645–54, 1963.

[3] Reemtsma, K., Giraldo, N., Depp, D. A., and Eichwald, E. J.: Islet transplantation. Ann. Surg. *168*:436, 1968.

[4] Ballinger, W. F., and Lacy, P. E.: Transplantation of intact pancreatic islets in rats. Surgery *72*:175–86, 1972.

[5] Leonard, R. J., Lazarow, A., and Hegre, O. D.: Pancreatic islet transplantation in the rat. Diabetes *22*:413–28, 1973.

[6] Barker, C. F.: Transplantation of the islets of Langerhans and the histocompatibility of endocrine tissue. Diabetes *24*:766–75, 1975.

[7] Nozawa, M., Weil, R., III, McIntosh, R., and Reemtsma, K.: Vascularized transplantation of the rat pancreas without duodenum. Transplantation *17*:137–40, 1974.

[8] Kemp, C. B., Knight, M. J., Scharp, D. W., Lacy, P. E., and Ballinger, W. F.: Transplantation of isolated pancreatic islets into the portal vein of diabetic rats. Nature (London) *244*:447, 1973.

[9] Weber, C., Weil, R., III, McIntosh, R., and Reemtsma, K.: Transplantation of pancreatic islets from neonatal to adult rats. Transplantation *19*(5): 442–44, 1975.

[10] Brown, J., Clark, W. R., Makoff, R. K., Weisman, H., Kemp, J. A., and Mullen, Y.: Pancreas transplantation for diabetes mellitus. Ann. Intern. Med. *89*:951–63, 1978.

[11] Weil, R., III, Nozawa, M., Koss, M., Weber, C., Reemtsma, K., and McIntosh, R.: Pancreatic transplantation in diabetic rats: renal function, morphology, ultrastructure and immunohistology. Surgery *78* (2):142–48, 1975.

[12] Mauer, S. M., Steffes, M. W., Sutherland, D. E. R., Najarian, J. S., Michael, A., and Brown, D.: Studies of the rate of regression of the glomerular lesions in diabetic rats treated with pancreatic islet transplantation. Diabetes *24* (3):280–85, 1975.

[13] Weber, C. J., Silva, F. G., Hardy, M. A., Pirani, C. L., and Reemtsma. K.: Effects of islet transplantation on renal function and morphology of short and long-term diabetic rats. Transplant. Proc. *11*:549-56, 1979.

[14] Silva, F. G., Weber, C. J., Pirani, C. L., Hardy, M. A., and Reemtsma, K.: Effects of islet transplantation (Tx) on glomerular basement membrane (GBM) thickness of proteinuria in diabetic Lewis rats. Diabetes *28*:426, 1979.

[15] Kretschmer, G. J., Sutherland, D. E. R., Matas, A. J., Cain, T. L., and Najarian, J. S.: Autotransplantation of pancreatic islets without separation of exocrine and endocrine tissue in totally pancreatectomized dogs. Surgery *82*:74–81, 1977.

[16] Mirkovitch, V., and Campiche, M.: Successful intrasplenic autotransplantation of pancreatic tissue in totally pancreatectomized dogs. Transplantation *21*:265–69, 1976.

[17] Schulak, J., and Reckard, C.: Intrasplenic islet function in the dog following distal splenorenal shunt. Surg. Forum *29*:340, 1978.

[18] Koncz, L., Davidoff, F., DeLellis, R. A., Selby, N., and Zimmerman, C.: Quantitative aspects of the metabolic response to pancreatic islet transplantation in rats with severe ketotic diabetes. Metabolism *25*:147–56, 1976.

[19] Weber, C., Hardy, M. A., Pi-Sunyer, F., Zimmerman, E., and Reemtsma, K.: Tissue culture preservation and intramuscular transplantation of pancreatic islets. Surgery *84*:166–74, 1978.

[20] Andersson, A., Borg, H., Groth, C. G., Gunnarsson, R., Hellerstrom, C., Lundgren, G., Westman, J., and Ostman, J.: Survival of isolated human islets of Langerhans maintained in tissue culture. J. Clin. Invest. *57*:1295–1301, 1976.

[21] Goldman, H., and Colle, E.: Human pancreatic islets in culture: effects of supplementing the medium with homologous and heterologous serum. Science *192*:1014–16, 1976.

[22] Weber, C. J., Hardy, M. A., Lerner, R. L., and Reemtsma, K.: Tissue culture isolation and preservation of human cadaveric pancreatic islets. Surgery *81*:270–73, 1977.

[23] Scharp, D. W., Merrell, R., Feldman, S., Downing, R., Lacy, P., and Ballinger, W.: The use of gyrotation culture for the preservation of isolated islets. Surg. Forum *29*:100, 1978.

[24] Frankel, B., Gylfe, E., Hellman, B., and Idahl, L.: Maintenance of insulin release from pancreatic islets stored in the cold for up to five weeks. J. Clin. Invest. *57*:47–52, 1976.

[25] Kemp, J. A., Mazur, P., Mullen, Y., Miller, R. H., Clark, W., and Brown, J.: Reversal of experimental diabetes by fetal rat pancreas. I. Survival and

function of fetal rat pancreas frozen to −190°C. Transplant. Proc. *9*:325-28, 1977.

[26] Rajotte, R. V., Scharp, D. W., Downing, R., Molnar, G. D., and Ballinger, W. F.: The transplantation of frozen-thawed rat islets transported between centers. Diabetes *28*:377, 1979.

[27] Downing, R., Scharp, D. W., Greider, M., and Ballinger, W. F.: Mass isolation of islets of Langerhans from the dog pancreas. Diabetes *28*:426, 1979.

[28] Ono, J., Lacy, P. E., Michael, H. E. B., and Greider, M. H.: Functional and morphologic status of pancreatic islets cultured at 24°C. Diabetes *28*:427, 1979.

[29] Hogle, H. H., and Reemtsma, K.: Pancreatic autotransplantation following resection. Surgery *84*:359–60, 1978.

[30] Sutherland, D. E. R., Matas, A. J., and Najarian, J. S.: Pancreatic islet cell transplantation. Surg. Clin. North Am. *58*:365–82, 1978.

[31] Najarian, J. S., Sutherland, D. E. R., Matas, A. J., and Goetz, F. C.: Human islet autotransplantation following pancreatectomy. Transplant. Proc. *11*:336–40, 1979.

[32] Traeger, J., Dubernard, J. M., Touraine, J. L., Neyra, P., Malik, M. C., Pelissard, C., and Ruitton, A.: Pancreatic transplantation in man: a new method of pancreas preparation and results on diabetes correction. Transplant. Proc. *11*:331-35, 1979.

[33] Reemtsma, K., Weber, C. J., Pi-Sunyer, F. X., Lerner, R. L., Zimmerman, E., and Hardy, M. A.: Organ culture studies for pancreatic islet transplantation. Transplant. Proc. *11*:1002-10, 1979.

[34] Weber, C., Zatrigi, A., Weil III, R., McIntosh, R., Hardy, M., and Reemtsma, K.: Pancreatic islet isografts, allografts and xenografts: comparison of morphology and function. Surgery *79*:144–51, 1976.

[35] Weber, C. J., Hardy, M. A., Lerner, R. L., Felig, P., and Reemtsma, K.: Hyperinsulinemia and hyperglucagonemia following pancreatic islet transplantation in diabetic rats. Diabetes *25*:944–48, 1976.

[36] Chick, W. L.: Beta cell replication in rat pancreatic monolayer cultures: effects of glucose, tolbutamide, glucocorticoid, growth hormone and glucagon. Diabetes *22*:687–93, 1972.

[37] Lambert, A. E., Blondel, B., Kanazawa, Y., Orci, L., and Renold, A.: Monolayer cell culture of neonatal rat pancreas: light microscopy and evidence for immunoreactive insulin synthesis and release. Endocrinology *90*:239–48, 1972.

[38] Hegre, O. D., Wells, L. J., and Lazarow, A.: Insulin content of fetal rat pancreases grown in organ culture and subsequently transplanted into maternal hosts. Diabetes *21*:193–202, 1972.

[39] Lacy, P. E., Davie, J. M., and Finke, E. H.: Use of in vitro culture (24°C) for prolongation of islet allograft survival. Diabetes *28*:382, 1979.

Evaluating the Benefits of Human Islet Transplantation

FREDERICK C. GOETZ

SUMMARY

For important ethical and practical reasons, present human trials of islet transplantation in diabetes are restricted to subjects already committed to immunosuppression by the need for kidney transplantation. Following the morphology of the transplanted kidney for possible reversal of diabetes-related changes may be the most valuable technique for demonstrating benefit from the restoration of islet function. Amelioration of diabetic vascular disease is the compelling reason for efforts to achieve effective islet transplantation.

DIABETES 29 (Suppl. 1):52–55, 1980.

Why transplant islets? The reflex answer to this question is, of course, "to cure diabetes." But this is not carrying the thought much farther than the mountaineer who says that the reason for climbing Mount Everest is that "it is there."

The matter is simplified somewhat by restricting attention to insulin-requiring, ketosis-prone diabetic patients. Even so, both the metabolic and the vascular components of diabetes require consideration—and both of them are complex.

The purpose of this survey is to present ways to evaluate both the metabolic and vascular benefits of islet transplantation. This is a timely exercise, since much effort is expended attacking the problem, and we should be sure that we can test the benefits of our proposals.

METABOLIC EFFECTS

The demonstration of metabolic benefits is summarized in Table 1. The first two of these goals have already been achieved, although benefit beyond 1 yr remains elusive.

Regarding *hormonal* measurements, beta cell function can now be readily documented by the measurement of insulin in serum and, especially in the early period after transplantation, by measurement of C-peptide in serum and urine.[1] J. Hoiriis-Nielsen has recently provided elegant evidence that the isolated human islet does, indeed, secrete C-peptide in equimolar ratio to insulin,[2] as does the isolated rat islet.[3] For insulin and C-peptide measurements to have full significance, candidates for islet transplantation must have been shown to be devoid of insulin/C-peptide secretion before transplantation.

Glucagon is readily measured in plasma, but no method can distinguish glucagon from the new islets from the recipient's original glucagon source(s). Of main interest will be the question of whether more appropriate glucagon regulation will be seen in the presence of improved beta cell function. To my knowledge, this has not been documented.

Somatostatin and pancreatic polypeptide have not been studied in pancreas transplant recipients, and their significance is at present a matter of conjecture.

Regarding *metabolic substrates,* glucose and ketone metabolism are studied readily, and short-term observations are sensitive indicators of insulin supply. Glycosylated hemoglobin presumably offers an additional way of checking longer-term glucose control. The 24-h pattern of plasma glucose is probably the closest to an ideal indicator of metabolic regulation. Additional substrates and related substances (nitrogen balance, alanine, lactate) are potential subjects for study.[4]

In summary, the tools for demonstration of the major metabolic and hormonal effects of islet transplantation appear to be readily at hand. So far, striking short-term demonstrations of the effectiveness of transplants have been restricted to vascularized transplantation of a single pancreas. All such observations must be qualified by the realization that the patients are required to take corticosteroid permanently.

VASCULAR COMPLICATIONS

Here lies the biggest challenge. In theory, one could demonstrate either slowing of the progress of complications, or reversal, or prevention. End points should be quantitative and precise, and the risks of the observations low.

From the Section of Endocrinology and Metabolism, Department of Medicine, University of Minnesota Hospitals and Medical School, Minneapolis, Minnesota 55455.
Address reprint requests to F. C. Goetz, M.D., Box 93, University Hospitals, Minneapolis, Minnesota 55455.

TABLE 1
Metabolic goals in restoring islet function

Minimum:	Remove the need for injection of insulin
More demanding:	Restore fasting and postmeal plasma glucose levels to normal
Ultimate:	Restore all hormonal and substrate levels to normal

Large vessel disease. Coronary heart disease, arterial disease in the legs, and stroke are serious problems for diabetics; however, they are not specific to diabetes. Clinical methodology for the study of the prevention of coronary disease, in particular, is highly developed (e.g., the Coronary Drug Project).[5] Even in high-risk populations, event rates are relatively low, and, therefore, the number of patients must be large—in the hundreds at least—to make adequate evaluations. The likelihood that islet transplant subjects will be available in such numbers in the near future seems remote.

Retinopathy, nephropathy, neuropathy, and other small vessel changes. These are commonly included under the general term microangiopathy; however, for quantitative observation in controlled studies, each must be considered individually. Ethical considerations, at present, limit the eligibility for pancreas or islet transplantation to those patients already committed to immunosuppression by virtue of a previous kidney transplant and to those for whom immunosuppression is unnecessary (transplantation between identical twins or autotransplantation). For practical purposes then, it is the patient who has already gone to end-stage diabetic nephropathy who is a candidate for pancreas or islet transplantation.[6]

Retinopathy. This offers potentially the best chance for systematic controlled observations. An excellent animal study (by Engerman et al.)[7] indicates that metabolic control in diabetic dogs can retard the development of diabetes-associated retinopathy. Several useful end points are available (visual acuity; morphology on retinal photographs and subjective ophthalmoscopy; vitreous fluorophotometry). Furthermore, most of these have been employed extensively in large clinical trials of other forms of treatment of retinopathy, and there has been extensive experience with the statistics for analyzing data.

Unfortunately, the kidney-transplanted diabetic patient poses severe limitations: experience on our Transplant Service (Table 2) shows that, while almost all such patients already show significant retinopathy at the time of transplant of the kidney, the eye changes are sometimes very advanced and the range of severity is wide. This would make matching of subjects in small groups difficult. Furthermore, after kidney transplantation alone, there is a marked tendency for retinopathy to become inactive (Table 3). Fortunately for these patients—but unfortunately for the purpose at hand—most of the eyes of the kidney-transplant diabetics soon settle into an involutional state in which progression stops but reversal of old scar tissue and ischemic changes is unlikely.[8,9] Photocoagulation treatment is now widely accepted as effective in preventing blindness in eyes with severe proliferative retinopathy.[10,11] It would be unethical to withhold photocoagulation from those eyes with active proliferation.

TABLE 2
Forms of retinopathy present at the time of kidney transplantation in 67 diabetic patients at the University of Minnesota*

Form of retinopathy	Percent of eyes
None	1
Nonproliferative	13
Active proliferative	19
Late proliferative (involutional)	67
All forms	100

* Adapted from Ramsay et al., Am. J. Ophthalmol. *87*:305–10, 1979.[8]

TABLE 3
Persistence of useful vision (better eye > 20/50 corrected acuity) in 70 diabetic patients after kidney transplantation*

Years after kidney transplant	Cumulative percent with useful vision
Baseline	100
0–2	91
2–4	86

* Adapted from Ramsay et al., Am. J. Ophthalmol. *87*:305–10, 1979.[8]

It is also necessary to consider the numbers of subjects required for the likelihood of a statistically significant result. Early figures by Patz[12] suggested that the chances of advanced blindness due to active proliferative retinopathy were about 75% in 2–4 yr. If a treatment such as islet transplantation could reduce this to about 25%, as few as 12–16 treated patients (compared with an equal number of control subjects) would be needed to show that the difference is significant at the conventional level ($P = 0.05$). The much larger experience with over 1700 patients in the Diabetic Retinopathy Study[11] shows a rate of progression in untreated eyes considerably slower than that indicated by Patz's earlier data. This means that the sample size would need to be at least three or four times as large—i.e., 50 or more—for a reasonable chance to demonstrate benefit. For these reasons, retinopathy is not a practical end point for systematic clinical trial under the present circumstances of islet transplantation.

The kidney. The kidney can be studied for changes in morphology and function. Some of the most impressive animal studies of the effects of islet transplantation on kidney function and structure have been carried out on experimentally diabetic rats.[13,14] Some, but not all, of the changes in the human diabetic kidney have a parallel in these animals.

Morphology of the transplanted kidney in the diabetic patient includes regular development of arteriolar hyalinization in 2–4 yr. When both of the glomerular arterioles (afferent and efferent) are involved by this process, the finding is highly characteristic of diabetes.[15,16] A variety of proteins, including albumin and immunoglobulin, can be shown by immunofluorescent staining to be sticking to glomerular and tubular basement membrane.[17] There is moderately severe mesangial thickening as well.

The rat studies suggest that protein adherence and perhaps mesangial thickening might be the changes most likely to reverse after islet transplantation. Arteriolar hyalinosis has not been seen in the rat. The single striking case from Dr. Gliedman's service in Montefiore Hospital,[18] in which a patient receiving simultaneous pancreas and kidney transplants failed to show arteriolar change in the kidney after nearly 4 yr, suggests that this is a preventable lesion.

Kidney function (in contrast to the morphologic changes), as measured by creatinine clearance and serum creatinine level, remains stable for as long as 10 yr after kidney transplantation in diabetics. However, proteinuria by conventional methods has appeared in some subjects after 6–8 yr. It is possible that more sensitive methods of protein measurement applied soon after transplantation might give an additional, useful end point for study. Reversal of proteinuria in diabetic rats has been demonstrated after islet transplantation.[9]

A pertinent question can be raised about the choice of the transplanted kidney for study: if a healthy kidney develops diabetic lesions when transplanted into a diabetic patient, would reversal of those lesions tell us anything about the spontaneous kidney lesions of the typical diabetic patients? In the narrow sense, this is, indeed, an artificial situation, with some features of nephropathy in the transplanted kidney, particularly the accelerated course, distinctly different from spontaneous diabetic glomerulosclerosis. In the broader sense, however, the information should be important and useful. It can be (and is) still argued that glomerulosclerosis is caused by some feature of the diabetic state which is as yet not clearly identified. Reversal of diabetes-related lesions after pancreas or islet transplantation should strengthen the interpretation that it is, indeed, a pancreas- or islet-related effect that causes the kidney damage in the first place (not some extrapancreatic element present in spontaneous diabetes). As in the animal experiments, the simplest interpretation of such a result would seem to be that the morphologic improvement is due to replacement of insulin secretion and resulting improvements in the metabolic state.

Neuropathy. In the kidney-transplanted diabetic patient, muscle function improves steadily after transplant, but the velocity of motor and sensory nerve conduction remains abnormal and stable for years.[20] Short-term animal studies suggest that this abnormality may be reversible by reduction of high blood sugar to normal.[21] Several reports[22,23] indicate that the same may be true in the human being. This is an additional, potentially important end point.

Other vascular lesions. Thickness of the basement membrane of capillaries in the muscle bed has received a great deal of attention as a diabetes-related lesion in humans. Both the methodology and the interpretation of the results and their biological significance are unresolved. Reversal of this lesion in an animal counterpart has not, to my knowledge, been reported. Demonstrations of such reversal in humans seem to have some importance, but less than reversal of kidney or nerve changes. Immunofluorescent studies showing albumin adherence to capillary basement membrane might sharpen the results.[24]

CONTROL SUBJECTS

These should be similar insulin-dependent diabetic subjects, from the same pool of kidney-transplanted diabetic patients in the same transplantation center, taking the same immunosuppressive drugs (corticosteroid and azathioprine). They should differ only in that their diabetes is managed by conventional means rather than by islet transplantation. They should be assigned randomly to the conventionally treated or transplanted groups.

EARLY CASES AND THE PREVENTION OF RETINOPATHY AND OTHER LESIONS

Ultimately it would be highly desirable to test whether early transplantation could effectively prevent the classic severe retinopathy of diabetes. This would require a very certain and low-risk method of transplantation—ideally, one not requiring immunosuppression. Because of the variability of retinopathy, a large number of subjects would be needed, at the very least 50 transplanted and 50 conventionally treated subjects, and they would have to be followed with sensitive methods for 10–20 yr. This sort of trial is far in the future.

FINAL COMMENTS

For many practical and ethical reasons the clinical demonstration of the benefit of pancreas transplantation to diabetic lesions must be studied at present in the patient who has already received a kidney transplant. Because of the advanced problems of these patients, retinopathy cannot be used as an end point. Reversal of lesions in the transplanted kidney and possible reversal of neuropathy and of muscle capillary lesions look like the most promising end points for systematic observation. Observing 10–20 such subjects and an equal number of subjects on standard diabetic treatment could give convincing results in 3–5 yr, especially if reversal of arteriolar hyalinosis in the kidney can be shown.

Why transplant islets?—the question must be faced at last.

Prevention of vascular lesions and their devastating consequences still seems to be the only really compelling reason for efforts to develop effective islet transplantation. Transplantation for metabolic benefits alone will be justified only if a very simple and low-risk method can be developed. This is not yet at hand.

Comments on this position will be welcomed.

REFERENCES

1 Horwitz, D. L., Rubenstein, A. H., and Katz, A. I.: Quantitation of human pancreatic beta-cell function by immunoassay of C-peptide in urine. Diabetes *26*:30–35, 1977.

2 Hoiriis-Nielsen, J.: Discussion. *In* Symposium on the Islet in Juvenile Diabetes. Copenhagen, Steno Memorial Hospital, May 1979.

3 Rubenstein, A. H., Clark, J. L., Melani, F., and Steiner, D. F.: Secretion of proinsulin C-peptide by pancreatic beta cells and its circulation in blood. Nature (London) *224*:697–99, 1969.

4 Noy, G. A., Buckle, A. L. J., and Alberti, K. G. M. M.: Continuous monitoring in vivo of blood glucose, lactate, alanine and 3-hydroxybutyrate. Clin. Chim. Acta. *89*:135–44, 1978.

5 Canner, P. L., Berge, K. G., and Klimt, C. R.: The coronary drug project: design, methods, and baseline results. American Heart Association Monograph No. 38. Circulation *47*:(Suppl. 1) I-1–I-50, 1973.

6 Special Report. Position paper on pancreatic islet and beta cell transplantation in man. Diabetes *23*:987–88, 1974.

7 Engerman, R. L., Bloodworth, J. M. B., and Nelson, S.: Relationship of microvascular disease in diabetes to metabolic control. Diabetes *26*:760–79, 1977.

8 Ramsay, R. C., Knobloch, W. H., Barbosa, J. F., Sutherland, D. E. R., Kjellstrand, C. M., Najarian, J. S., and Goetz, F. C.: The visual status of diabetic patients after renal transplantation. Am. J. Ophthalmol. *87*:305–10, 1979.

9 Ramsay, W. J., Ramsay, R. C., Purple, R. L., and Knobloch, W. H.: Involutional diabetic retinopathy. Am. J. Ophthalmol. *84*:851–858, 1977.

10 Cheng, H.: Multicentre trial of xenonarc photocoagulation in the treatment of diabetic retinopathy. A randomized controlled study. Interim report. Trans. Ophthalmol. Soc. U. K. *95*:351–57, 1975.

[11] The Diabetic Study Research Group: Photocoagulation treatment of proliferative diabetic retinopathy: the second report of Diabetic Retinopathy Study findings. Ophthalmology *85*:82–106, 1978.

[12] Patz, A.: *In* Symposium on the Treatment of Diabetic Retinopathy. Goldberg, M. F., and Fine, S. L., Eds. USPHS Publication No. 1890. Washington, D.C., U. S. Government Printing Office, 1969.

[13] Mauer, S. M., Sutherland, D. E. R., and Steffes, M. W.: Pancreatic islet transplantation. Effects on the glomerular lesions of experimental diabetes in the rat. Diabetes *23*:748–53, 1974.

[14] Lee, S. C., Mauer, S. M., Brown, D. M., Sutherland, D. E. R., Michael, A. F., and Najarian, J. S.: Renal transplantation in diabetes mellitus in rat. J. Exp. Med. *139*:793–98, 1974.

[15] Bell, E. T.: Renal Disease. Philadelphia, Lea and Febiger, 1946, pp. 376–78.

[16] Mauer, S., Barbosa, J., Vernier, R., Kjellstrand, C., Buselmeier, T., Simmons, R., Najarian, J., and Goetz, F.: Development of diabetic vascular lesions in normal kidneys transplanted into patients with diabetes mellitus. N. Engl. J. Med. *295*:916–20, 1976.

[17] Mauer, S., Miller, K., Goetz, F., Barbosa, J., Simmons, R., Najarian, J. S., and Michael, A.: Immunopathology of renal extracellular membranes in kidneys transplanted into patients with diabetes mellitus. Diabetes *25*:709–12, 1976.

[18] Gliedman, M., Tellis, V., Soberman, R., Rifkin, H., and Veith, F.: Long-term effects of pancreatic transplant function in patients with advanced juvenile onset diabetes. Diabetes Care *1*:1–9, 1978.

[19] Mauer, S. M., Brown, D. M., Matas, A. J., and Steffes, M. W.: Effects of pancreatic islet transplantation on the increased urinary albumin excretion rates in intact and uninephrectomized rats with diabetes mellitus. Diabetes *27*:959–64, 1978.

[20] Barbosa, J., Burke, B., Buselmeier, T., Carpenter, A.-M., Goetz, F., Harris, J., Kennedy, W., Kjellstrand, C., Michael, A., Najarian, J. S., and Recker, L.: Neuropathy, retinopathy, and biopsy findings in the transplanted kidney in diabetic patients. Kidney Internatl. *6* (Suppl. 1), S-32–S-36, 1974.

[21] Greene, D. A., De Jesus, P. V., Jr., and Winegrad, A. I.: Effects of insulin and dietary myoinositol on impaired peripheral motor nerve conduction velocity in acute streptozotocin diabetes. J. Clin. Invest. *55*:1326–36, 1975.

[22] Gregersen, G.: Variations in motor conduction velocity produced by acute changes of the metabolic state in diabetic patients. Diabetologia *4*:273–77, 1968.

[23] Graf, R. J., Halter, J. B., Halar, E., and Porte, D., Jr.: Nerve conduction abnormalities in untreated maturity-onset diabetics: relation to levels of fasting plasma glucose and glycosylated hemoglobin. Ann. Intern. Med. *90*:298–302, 1979.

[24] Cohn, R. A., Mauer, S. M., Barbosa, J., and Michael. A. F.: Immunofluorescence studies of skeletal muscle extracellular membranes in diabetes mellitus. Lab. Invest. *39*:13–16, 1978.

Discussion

Sections on Whole-Organ and Islet Transplantation

Discussion on whole-organ pancreas transplantation was directed mainly at the technical aspects of the procedure. The effect of duct ligation on islet cell performance was considered not to be detrimental to endocrine function in segmental pancreas transplants in dog recipients. In open duct grafts drained intraperitoneally, elevations in serum amylase probably reflected absorption of pancreatic enzymes from the peritoneal cavity rather than parenchymal inflammation. In the transplantation models proposed by Sutherland et al., removal of the organ graft after rejection was not considered essential. Participants in whole-organ transplantation protocols were urged to examine graft failures histologically. The supposition that the absence of physiologic function of transplanted tissue was indicative of immune rejection should be supported by histologic evidence of a rejection process. Failure to demonstrate islet cell autoantibodies in recipients of rejected pancreas grafts (Groth) should be confirmed after removal of the transplanted tissue.

Human autografts were acknowledged to provide an appropriate setting for establishing the validity of the various technical procedures employed in islet cell transplants. Compared with whole-organ transplants, transplantation of islet tissue offers the advantage of pooling donor sources. However, the functional efficacy of islet cell preparations in allograft recipients is adversely compromised by both the diabetogenic effect of steroid immunosuppression and the rejection process. These factors may account for the poor results observed with allografted tissue compared with autotransplantation. The potential ability of adult islet cells to replicate after transplantation is supported by preliminary evidence of an increased beta cell mass in mouse recipients (Usadel). Long-term effects of nonpurified and exocrine-contaminated intraportal islet cell preparations require further follow-up.

Perifusion and Culture of Human Fetal Pancreas

JANICE E. MAITLAND, DAVID G. PARRY, AND JOHN R. TURTLE

SUMMARY

Human fetal pancreas has been obtained after the therapeutic termination of pregnancy with prostaglandin F2α. Pancreatic explants were studied in a perifusion system and maintained in organ culture for up to 3 wk. Insulin biosynthesis was stimulated by glucose; however, the incorporation of ^{3}H-L-leucine into proinsulin was surprisingly high (52% after 3 h) vs. insulin (48%), which suggests a possible block in the conversion of proinsulin to insulin. Insulin secretion was stimulated during perifusion with 19.3 mM glucose (1.6× prestimulation level), 1.5 μM glucagon (2.4), 5 mM leucine (2.4), 10 mM arginine (2.7), and 10 mM theophylline (10.0).

Insulin biosynthesis and secretion were maintained in organ culture. After 12 days there was a 3.4-fold increase in insulin secretion in the presence of 22 mM glucose compared with 5.5 mM glucose, and the explant insulin content rose in the presence of high glucose levels by 89%. The acute insulin secretory response to 10 mM theophylline was maintained after culture.

These studies suggest that human fetal pancreas should be considered as a potential source of donor tissue for pancreas transplantation in human diabetes. DIABETES 29 (Suppl. 1):57–63, 1980.

Experimental diabetes mellitus in laboratory animals has been reversed after the transplantation of isolated adult pancreatic islets or neonatal or fetal pancreas.[1–3] In humans, attempts have been made to transplant whole pancreas or isolated islets that have been freshly prepared after collagenase digestion.[4] If it is possible to overcome tissue rejection after the transplantation of insulin-producing tissue in humans, it will be necessary to establish a suitable source of donor tissue before the technique can be applied to the treatment of human diabetes. It has been possible to isolate human pancreatic islets from cadaver donors and to maintain these in tissue culture, but the yields have been low, requiring either cryopreservation or pooling of islets from several donors.[5,6] Neonatal and fetal pancreases have a relatively higher endocrine-to-exocrine ratio and are potentially more suitable for transplantation than adult pancreas.[7,8] Vigorous separation of these two elements has not been necessary for successful transplantation in experimental animals.[9] Furthermore, during culture there has been preferential development of endocrine tissue, with little or no development of exocrine tissue.[10]

Human fetal pancreas obtained after the therapeutic termination of pregnancy could be suitable as donor tissue for transplantation. In the present study, human fetal pancreas was obtained at 14–20 wk gestation after the therapeutic termination of pregnancy with prostaglandin F2α. The tissue synthesized insulin in vitro and responded to a number of stimuli recognized to act as secretagogues in the adult. Pancreatic explants were maintained in organ culture for up to 3 wk, and the properties of this cultured pancreas were examined.

From the Departments of Medicine and Biochemistry, University of Sydney, Sydney NSW, Australia.
Address reprint requests to John R. Turtle, M.D., Department of Medicine, University of Sydney, Sydney NSW 2006, Australia.

MATERIALS AND METHODS

Pancreatic explants. Human fetal pancreas was obtained after the therapeutic termination of pregnancy using the transcervical infusion of prostaglandin F2α (1.5–12 mg by intermittent infusion over 12–36 h). Gestational age was 14–20 wk. Pancreatic tissue was obtained by dissection within 4 h of delivery and frequently within 1 h, but this time did not appear to be critical. The dissected pancreas was placed in tissue-culture medium under sterile conditions, and extraneous material was removed with fine scissors. The cleaned pancreas was placed in fresh medium and sectioned into fragments 1–2 mm^3 in size using razor blades.

Extraction procedure. Hormone content was measured in selected explants after freeze-drying overnight. The dried explants were weighed and then homogenized in a glass microhomogenizer (Calbiochem) with 0.5 ml of an acid-ethanol mixture (18 ml of 10 M HCl per liter of 70% ethanol).[11]

The extraction was permitted to proceed for 24 h at 4°C, after which debris was removed by centrifugation. The supernatant was neutralized, diluted 1:100 with the appropriate buffers for insulin and glucagon assays, and stored at −20°C until the assays were performed. Insulin and glucagon contents are expressed per milligram of freeze-dried pancreas. The diluted acid-ethanol mixture had no effect on the radioimmunoassay for insulin or glucagon at the concentration used for extracted pancreas. Recovery of added crystalline human insulin or crystalline porcine glucagon was 100% using this extraction procedure.

Insulin and glucagon radioimmunoassay. Immunoreactive insulin was determined using the Sorin adaptation of the double-antibody precipitation radioimmunoassay of Hales and Randle.[12] Immunoreactive glucagon was assayed by the method of Faloona and Unger[13] using Unger's pancreatic glucagon-specific antibody 30K. ^{125}I-labeled glucagon was purchased from Nuclear Medical Laboratories and purified porcine pancreatic glucagon was purchased from Novo Industries for use as standard.

Insulin biosynthesis. Pancreatic explants were incubated in 2 ml of Gey and Gey bicarbonate buffer, pH 7.4, containing 50 μCi of ^{3}H-L-leucine (50 Ci/mM, Radiochemical Centre, Amersham), 19 other amino acids (20 μM), 2 or 20 mM glucose, and 10 mg/ml crystalline human serum albumin. The flasks were gassed with 95% oxygen/5% carbon dioxide and were sealed and incubated for 3 h in a shaking incubator at 37°C. At the end of the incubation, the medium was removed and stored at −20°C for radioimmunoassay. The tissue was washed three times with buffer containing leucine before being homogenized in acid-ethanol at room temperature. After precipitation with 10% trichloroacetic acid (TCA), the precipitate was washed three times with 5% TCA and centrifuged 20 min at 2000 × *g*. The resultant pellets were dissolved in 1 M acetic acid.

Fractionation of acid-soluble material containing 1 mg of carrier insulin was performed on a column (1 × 80 cm) of Sephadex G50 (fine) and eluted with 1 M acetic acid. Column eluates were pooled and dried under vacuum. The residue was dissolved in 0.01 M hydrochloric acid, and the pH was adjusted to 8.3 with Tris-glycine buffer and applied to a 10 cm polyacrylamide gel (9% with 0.25% cross-linkage) for electrophoresis. Two-millimeter gel slices were treated with 0.5 ml Soluene 100 (Packard) and counted in a beta spectrometer. Further studies were performed using acid-soluble, TCA-precipitable protein on paper electrophoresis at pH 2 in 20% formic acid, run on Whatman no. 1 paper for 15 h at 5 V/cm. One-centimeter strips were cut and counted in a beta spectrometer.

Perifusion technique. The perifusion apparatus was constructed according to the principles described by Kikuchi et al.[14] The basic perifusion buffer was Krebs-Ringer bicarbonate, pH 7.4, with 25 mM Hepes containing 2 mg/ml crystalline bovine albumin (Calbiochem) and 500 IU/ml Trasylol. The buffer was gassed continuously with 95% oxygen/5% carbon dioxide. Both the buffer reservoir flasks and the perifusion chambers were housed in a 37°C water bath, and buffer was pumped from the flasks to the perifusion chambers by a peristaltic pump at a flow rate of 0.40 ml/min. Buffer changes were effected by a four-way valve, and the time required for a change of medium to reach the collection tube at this flow rate was 5 min. All results have been corrected for this changeover time. A 100-min prestimulation period was performed with 2.8 mM glucose to establish a basal insulin secretion rate, after which a 50-min stimulation period was performed with 19 mM glucose and other secretagogues. A final stimulation period was included with 19 mM glucose plus 10 mM theophylline as a positive insulin-secretory control step to terminate the experiment.

Perifusion fractions were collected at intervals of 5 min on an automatic fraction collector and stored at −20°C until radioimmunoassay. The last five fractions of the prestimulation period (25 min) were used to calculate basal secretion, and a stable basal secretory rate was defined as 1 SD $\leq$ 1 μU of insulin per minute per 10 mg. Five fractions (25 min) were collected during the final stimulatory phase to determine the ability of the tissue to respond to 19 mM glucose plus 10 mM theophylline. Only perifusion profiles exhibiting a stable baseline and a minimum of a fivefold increase over basal insulin release in response to theophylline have been included.

Organ culture. Pancreatic explants were cultured at the liquid gas interface in organ culture dishes (Falcon) on a filter (Nucleopore, 8 μm) supported by a stainless steel grid. Explants were randomly distributed in culture dishes so that each dish contained approximately 10 mg of tissue. All culture media were supplemented with 10% fetal calf serum and 50 μg/ml gentamicin. Cultures incubated for 48 h before perifusion were maintained in TCM199 (5.5 mM glucose) at 37°C in a humidified atmosphere of 95% oxygen/5% carbon dioxide. Long-term cultures (up to 3 wk) were maintained in either TCM199 or RPMI1640 (11 mM glucose), both containing 20 mM Hepes buffer. Incubation was maintained at 37°C in humidified air, and the medium was changed daily. Glucose or amino acids were added as indicated. All culture materials were obtained from Flow Laboratories.

Statistical analysis. Statistical analyses were carried out using Student's *t* test for paired or unpaired data where applicable. Results are expressed as the mean ± SEM.

RESULTS

Insulin and glucagon content of human fetal pancreas. A highly significant correlation was found between gestational age and fetal weight. As reliable estimates of gestational age were not always available, the hormone concentrations of fetal pancreas were related to fetal weight in all experiments. The smallest fetus examined (40 g) had a pancreatic insulin content of 10.5 mU/mg dry weight. The largest (360 g) had an insulin content of 51.6 mU/mg dry weight. Pancreatic insulin concentration showed large variations over the range of fetal weights studied (Figure 1A), and there was no significant correlation between fetal weight and insulin content; however, there was a tendency for the insulin content to rise with increasing fetal weight. The concentration of pancreatic glucagon in relation to fetal weight varied over a wide range in fetal pancreas (Figure 1B). There was no correlation between the insulin and glucagon content. There was a substantial increase in total pancreatic immunoreactive insulin from fetal pancreas weighing approximately 100 mg or more corresponding to a fetal weight of 150 g (Figure 1C).

Insulin biosynthesis. The eluates from the Sephadex gel chromatography showed two peaks (I and II), which had elu-

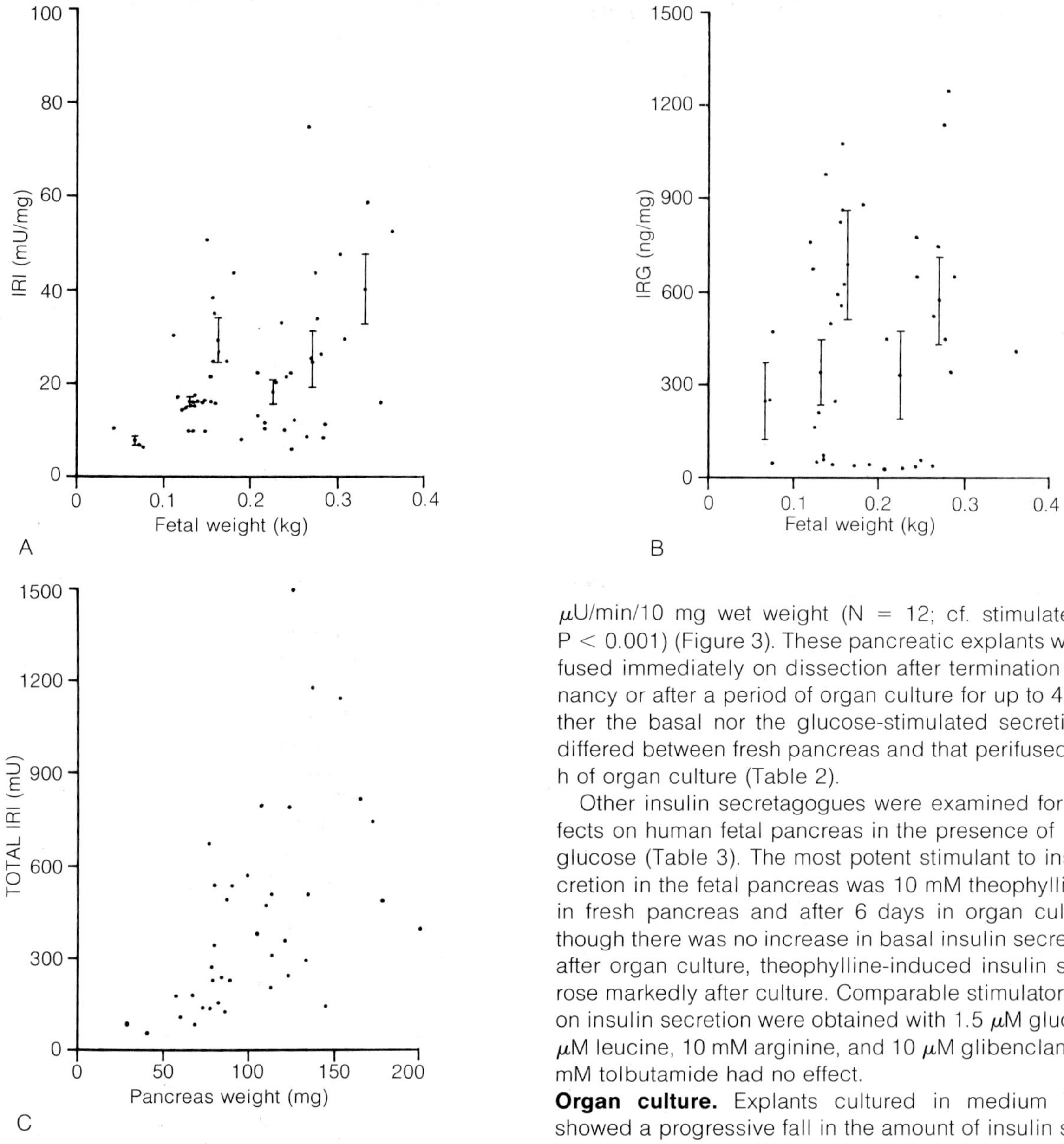

FIGURE 1. Hormone content of human fetal pancreas: (A) Insulin (IRI) content in relation to fetal weight. (b) Glucagon (IRG) content in relation to fetal weight. (C) Total extractable insulin in relation to pancreas weight.

tion properties corresponding to proinsulin and insulin (Figure 2A). These fractions were isolated and dried under vacuum. On polyacrylamide gel electrophoresis, peak I had a proinsulin content of 65% and insulin 35% (Figure 2B), whereas peak II showed 70% insulin and 30% proinsulin (Figure 2C). For both peaks the ^{3}H-L-leucine incorporation into insulin was 48% and into proinsulin, 52%, during the 3-h incubation. The net incorporation of ^{3}H-L-leucine into insulin and proinsulin was increased 2.3-fold during a 3-h incubation with 20 mM glucose compared with 2 mM glucose (Table 1). This incorporation was blocked by cycloheximide.

Insulin secretion. Increasing the glucose concentration of the perifusion buffer from 2.8 to 19.3 mM significantly increased the average rate of insulin secretion from 4.8 to 7.6 μU/min/10 mg wet weight (N = 12; cf. stimulated:basal $P < 0.001$) (Figure 3). These pancreatic explants were perifused immediately on dissection after termination of pregnancy or after a period of organ culture for up to 48 h. Neither the basal nor the glucose-stimulated secretion rates differed between fresh pancreas and that perifused after 48 h of organ culture (Table 2).

Other insulin secretagogues were examined for their effects on human fetal pancreas in the presence of 19.3 mM glucose (Table 3). The most potent stimulant to insulin secretion in the fetal pancreas was 10 mM theophylline, both in fresh pancreas and after 6 days in organ culture. Although there was no increase in basal insulin secretory rate after organ culture, theophylline-induced insulin secretion rose markedly after culture. Comparable stimulatory effects on insulin secretion were obtained with 1.5 μM glucagon, 5 μM leucine, 10 mM arginine, and 10 μM glibenclamide; 1.8 mM tolbutamide had no effect.

Organ culture. Explants cultured in medium TCM199 showed a progressive fall in the amount of insulin secreted into the culture medium over a period of 6 days. An acute insulin response to theophylline or glucose challenge was frequently absent after a week in culture. The use of medium RMPI1640 with 20 mM Hepes decreased the decline in insulin secretion during a 6-day culture (Figure 4). When the medium was supplemented with a sixfold increase in amino acids, insulin secretion into the medium was stabilized over a period of 1 wk (Figure 4). On all occasions, the explants were responsive to an acute stimulus with theophylline, even when the culture period was extended to 3 wk.

The effect of glucose concentration during culture was examined using TCM199 with 20 mM Hepes, supplemented with six times the normal concentration of amino acids, plus either 5.5 mM or 22 mM glucose. At high glucose concentration the insulin secreted during culture in TCM199 (22 mM glucose) was comparable to RPMI1640 (11 mM glucose). Culture in TCM199 (5.5 mM glucose) gave considerably lower insulin secretion than did the other culture conditions. Extraction of the explants after 12 days in culture showed an increase in total insulin content. The total insulin produced

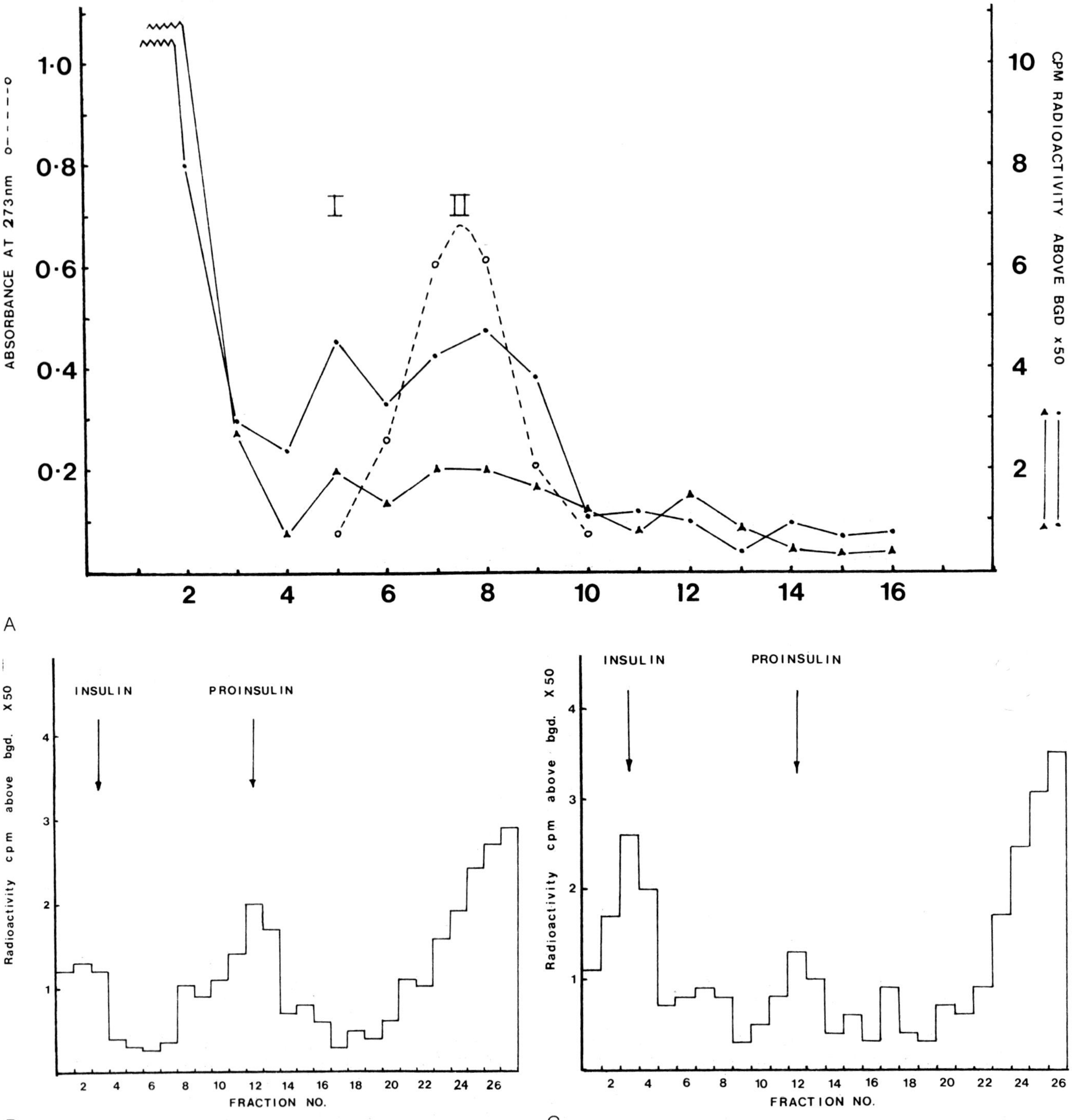

FIGURE 2. Insulin and proinsulin biosynthesis in human fetal pancreas. (A) Sephadex G50 chromatography of an explant extract following a 3-hr incubation with ^{3}H-L-leucine. ●, 20 mM glucose; ▲, 2 mM glucose. (B) Polyacrylamide gel electrophoresis of peak I (from 2A). (C) Polyacrylamide gel electrophoresis of peak II (from 2A).

(medium plus explant) was markedly increased after 12 days in organ culture in the presence of high glucose concentration (Figure 5).

DISCUSSION

Fresh human fetal pancreas explants studied in a perifusion system responded to a glucose challenge with a small but significant increase in insulin secretion. Identical results were obtained for explants maintained in organ culture for up to 48 h. Insulin biosynthesis proceeded rapidly, although the incorporation of ^{3}H-L-leucine into insulin was lower at 3 h, with a corresponding increase in incorporation into proinsulin, than might have been expected from comparable data on adult rat islets or pancreas.[15] Although the incorporation of ^{3}H-L-leucine into proinsulin was marked, no proinsulin could be detected in culture medium or during perifusion when assayed by gel chromatography or specific radioimmunoassay. Contrary to previous reports, these re-

TABLE 1
Glucose-stimulated ^{3}H-L-leucine incorporation into proinsulin and insulin using a human fetal pancreatic slice preparation

	N	^{3}H-L-Leucine uptake* (cpm/μg/3 h)
2 mM Glucose	10	589 ± 169
20 mM Glucose	9	1332 ± 220†
20 mM Glucose + cycloheximide (250 μg/ml)	3	339 ± 39

* Mean ± SEM.
† $P < 0.01$.

sults indicate that the mechanisms involved in glucose-induced insulin secretion as well as synthesis are present in human fetal pancreas,[16,17] although the magnitude of this response is not as great as that obtained by Ballinger and Lacy with isolated human adult islets, which exhibited a fivefold increase in basal insulin secretion in the presence of high glucose.[18] It is of interest, however, that Najarian et al.[19] observed only a 1.7-fold increase in insulin secretion from human islets during perifusion with high glucose. It is probable that significant glucose-induced insulin secretion has been observed in the present study due to the use of a perifusion system to study insulin release with careful monitoring of the viability and secretory competence of the tissue used. Previously negative results had been obtained using modifications of the static incubation procedure of Coore and Randle.[20] Static incubation techniques are adequate for detecting moderate to large changes in insulin release, but they are relatively insensitive to small differences in insulin release from one incubation period to the next, and they are completely insensitive to changes within a single incubation period. Perifusion permits time-dependent changes in insulin release to be followed and small increments above a steady basal secretion rate to be detected. The properties of human fetal pancreas are analogous to those of the rat, in which fetal pancreatic tissue was thought to be unresponsive to glucose;[21] however, perifusion data have shown that this concept is incorrect.[22,23]

During perifusion of adult rat islets the proinsulin-to-insulin ratio may rise to a maximum of 17% after stimulation for 60 min with high glucose.[24] In rat fetal pancreas a delay has been shown for the conversion of proinsulin to insulin.[15] Surprisingly, in the present data, after 3 h, human fetal pancreas showed exceptionally high ^{3}H-L-leucine incorporation into proinsulin and less into insulin (52:48), suggesting a delay in conversion of proinsulin to insulin. In view of the high ^{3}H-L-leucine incorporation into proinsulin in human fetal pancreas, it was considered possible that proinsulin was being preferentially synthesized and released after glucose stimulation and that this was being misinterpreted as insulin release in a cross-reacting insulin radioimmunoassay. However, no proinsulin could be detected during culture or in perifusion during basal, stimulated, or poststimulation theophylline-induced insulin secretion. Certainly proinsulin cannot be considered to be a significant component of the total insulin released from human fetal pancreas in vitro.

In organ culture, there has been no difficulty in maintain-

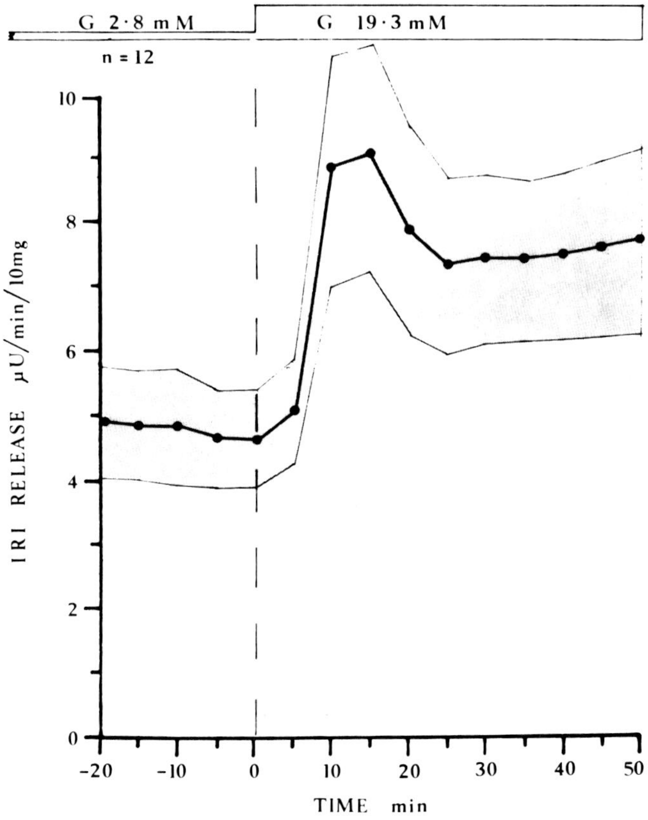

FIGURE 3. Effect of glucose on insulin release from fresh human fetal pancreas explants during perifusion.

TABLE 2
Glucose-stimulated insulin release by human fetal pancreas during perifusion

Condition	N	Insulin release*: Prestimulation— 25 min with 2.8 mM glucose (μU/min/10 mg)	Insulin release*: Stimulation— 50 min with 19.3 mM glucose (μU/min/10 mg)	Ratio (stimulation/ prestimulation)
Fresh explants	5	5.79 ± 1.68	9.44 ± 3.22	1.63†
Explants cultured for 48 h	7	4.1 ± 0.79	6.41 ± 0.67	1.56‡

* Mean ± SEM.
† $P < 0.025$
‡ $P < 0.01$

TABLE 3
Fetal pancreatic insulin secretion during perifusion with insulin secretagogues

Condition	N	Insulin release* Prestimulation, 50 min† (μU/min/10 mg)	Stimulation, 50 min† (μU/min/10 mg)	Ratio (stimulation/ prestimulation)
Tolbutamide, 1.8 mM	4	3.63 ± 0.22	3.54 ± 0.15	0
Glibenclamide, 10 μm	4	3.48 ± 0.14	6.11 ± 0.2	1.8§
Glucagon, 1.5 μm	4	8.33 ± 0.06	12.6 ± 0.3	1.5‡
Leucine, 5 mM	4	8.29 ± 0.3	12.5 ± 0.7	1.5‡
Arginine, 5 mM	4	12.3 ± 0.4	13.9 ± 0.4	1.1
Arginine, 10 mM	3	11.8 ± 0.4	19.9 ± 0.5	1.7§
Theophylline (fresh), 10 mM	5	4.61 ± 0.14	28.8 ± 5.7	6.3§
Theophylline (6 days), 10 mM	3	5.9 ± 0.16	54.2 ± 11.4	9.2§

* Mean ± SEM.
† Glucose 19.3 mM.
‡ $P < 0.01$.
§ $P < 0.001$.

ing viability and response to secretagogues using either medium RPMI1640 or TCM199 supplemented with amino acids. In the presence of high glucose, a steady high rate of insulin secretion was maintained for at least 12 days of culture, and the residual insulin content of the pancreatic explant increased as well by up to 100%. After at least 3 wk, the tissue-insulin response to a theophylline stimulus remained intact.

The net increase in total insulin in response to high glucose indicates that the tissue is potentially capable of responding to the hyperglycemia expected in a diabetic patient after pancreas transplantation. As fetal tissue has a relatively high endocrine content,[8] the difficulties encountered with collagenase digestion of adult pancreas do not occur. Organ culture favors further development of endocrine tissue, while exocrine tissue fails to develop at the same rate.[10] The attenuated response to acute glucose stimulation has not been a problem in the reversal of drug-induced diabetes after transplantation with fetal rat pancreas.[3] It is probable that human fetal pancreas would be suitable as an alternative source of substantial amounts of

FIGURE 4. Insulin release from fetal pancreas explants cultured for 6 days in RPMI1640 (20 mM Hepes) with 10% fetal calf serum. The medium was changed every 24 h. The bars show the effect of amino acid supplementation on insulin release. Results represent the mean ± SEM of duplicate cultures from three fetal pancreases expressed as insulin release per 10 mg pancreas (wet weight).

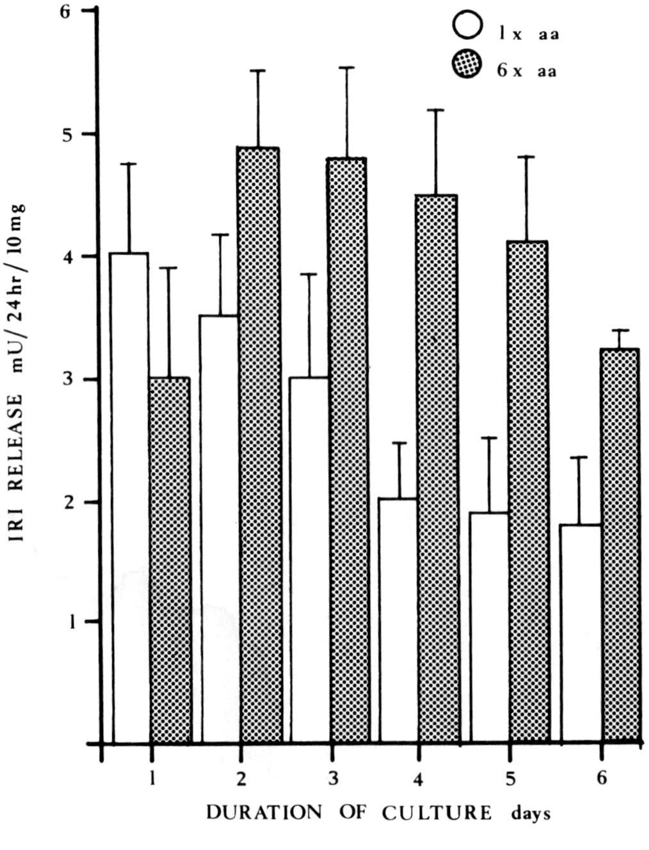

FIGURE 5. Insulin secretion and explant content of insulin following culture of human fetal pancreas for 12 days. All media were buffered with 20 mM Hepes, containing 10% fetal calf serum and a sixfold supplement with amino acids. TCM199 had glucose added to a final concentration of 22 mM. Explants were extracted fresh and after 12 days of culture. Results represent the mean of duplicate cultures from a single fetal pancreas.

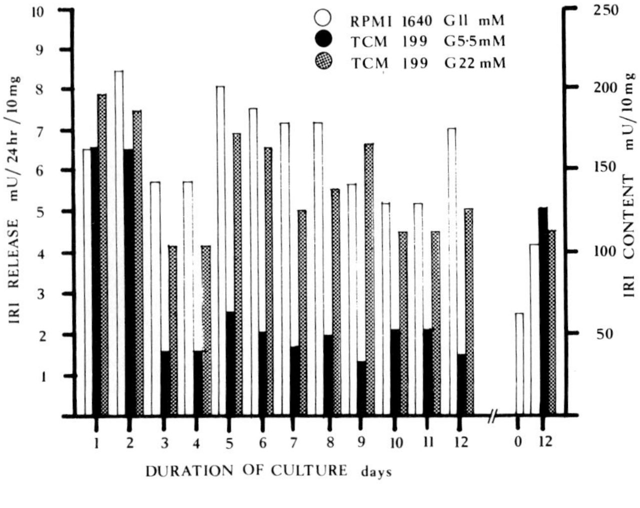

insulin-producing tissue for transplantation. Cryopreservation would not be required, as fetal pancreas remains viable in culture for prolonged periods. While transplantation from a single pancreas may not be sufficient to reverse diabetes, it may provide the basal insulin secretion necessary to convert a highly unstable nonpeptide secretory recipient into a stable diabetic. Furthermore, providing the rejection problems can be overcome, there will be no barrier to transplantation of several fetal pancreases into one recipient diabetic patient.

REFERENCES

[1] Kemp, C. B., Knight, M. J., Scharp, D. W., Ballinger, W. F., and Lacy, P. E.: Effect of transplantation site on the results of pancreatic islet isografts in diabetic rats. Diabetologia 9:486–91, 1973.

[2] Leonard, R. J., Lazarow, A., and Hegre, O. D.: Pancreatic islet transplantation in the rat. Diabetes *22*:413–28, 1973.

[3] Brown, J., Clark, W. R., Molnar, I. G., and Mullen, Y. S.: Fetal pancreas transplantation for reversal of streptozotocin-induced diabetes in rats. Diabetes *25*:56–64, 1976.

[4] Najarian, J. S., Sutherland, D. E. R., Matas, A. J., Steffes, M. W., Simmons, R. L., and Goetz, F. C.: Human islet transplantation: a preliminary report. Transplant. Proc. *9*:233–36, 1977.

[5] Henriksson, C., Claes, G., Gylfe, E., Hellman, B., and Zettergren, L.: Collagenase isolation and ^{45}Ca efflux studies of human islets of Langerhans. Eur. Surg. Res. *10*:343–51, 1978.

[6] Nielsen, J. H., Brundstedt, J., Andersson, A., and Frimodt-Moller, C.: Preservation of beta cell function in adult human pancreatic islets for several months in vitro. Diabetologia *16*:97–100, 1979.

[7] Sutherland, D. E. R., Matas, A. J., Steffes, M. W., and Najarian, J. S.: Infant human pancreas. A potential source of islet tissue for transplantation. Diabetes *25*:1123–28, 1976.

[8] Matas, A. J., Sutherland, D. E. R., Steffes, M. W., and Najarian, J. S.: Insulin and amylase content of human neonatal pancreas. Fed. Proc. *34*:864, 1975.

[9] Hegre, O. D., Schmitt, R. V., and McEvoy, R. C.: Syngeneic transplantation of the fetal rat pancreas IV. Dissociated versus whole organ implantation. Metabolism *28*:157–62, 1979.

[10] Lazarow, A., Wells, L. J., Carpenter, A., Hegre, O. D., Leonard, R., and McEvoy, R. C.: Islet differentiation, organ culture, and transplantation. Diabetes *22*:877–912, 1973.

[11] Andersson, A., Westerman, J., and Hellerstrom, C.: Effects of glucose on the ultrastructure and insulin biosynthesis of isolated mouse pancreatic islets maintained in tissue culture. Diabetologia *10*:743–53, 1974.

[12] Hales, C. N., and Randle, P. J.: Immunoassay of insulin with antibody precipitate. Biochem. J. *88*:137–46, 1973.

[13] Faloona, G. R., and Unger, R. H.: Methods of Hormone Radioimmunoassay. New York, Academic Press, 1974, p. 324.

[14] Kikuchi, M., Rabinovitch, A., Blackard, W. G., and Renold, A. E.: Perifusion of pancreas fragments. A system for the study of dynamic aspects of insulin secretion. Diabetes *23*:550–59, 1974.

[15] Blazquez, E., Lipshaw, L. A., Blazquez, M., and Foa, P. P.: The synthesis and release of insulin in fetal, nursing and young adult rats: studies in vivo and in vitro. Pediatr. Res. *9*:17–25, 1975.

[16] Monteros, A., Driscoll, S. G., and Steinke, J.: Insulin release from isolated human fetal pancreatic islets. Science *168*:111–12, 1970.

[17] Milner, R. D. G., Ashworth, M. A., and Barson, A. J.: Insulin release from human foetal pancreas in response to glucose, leucine and arginine. J. Endocrinol. *52*:497–505, 1972.

[18] Ballinger, W. F., and Lacy, P. E.: Transplantation of intact pancreatic islets in rats. Surgery *72*:175–86, 1972.

[19] Najarian, J. S., Sutherland, D. E. R., and Steffes, M. W.: Isolation of human islets of Langerhans for transplantation. Transplant Proc. *7*:611–13. 1975.

[20] Coore, H. G., and Randle, P. J.: Regulation of insulin secretion studied with pieces of rabbit pancreas incubated in vitro. Biochem. J. *93*:66–78, 1964.

[21] Asplund, K., Westman, S., and Hellerstrom, C.: Glucose stimulation of insulin secretion from the isolated pancreas of foetal and newborn rats. Diabetologia *5*:260–62, 1969.

[22] Asplund, K.: Dynamics of insulin release from the foetal and neonatal rat pancreas. Eur. J. Clin. Invest. *3*:338–44, 1973.

[23] Kervran, A., Guillaume, M., and Jost, A.: The endocrine pancreas of the fetus from diabetic pregnant rat. Diabetologia *15*:387–93, 1978.

[24] Burr, I. M., Stauffacher, W., Balant, L., Renold, A. E., and Grodsky, G.: Dynamic aspects of proinsulin release from perifused rat pancreas. Lancet *2*:882–83, 1969.

Human Fetal Pancreas
Culture and Function in Vitro

A. ÅGREN, A. ANDERSSON, C. BJÖRKÉN, C. G. GROTH, R. GUNNARSSON,
C. HELLERSTRÖM, G. LINDMARK, G. LUNDQVIST, B. PETERSSON, AND I. SWENNE

SUMMARY

Human fetal pancreas, obtained at prostaglandin-induced legal abortions, was maintained in organ culture for 6–14 days in medium TCM 199 (5.5 mM glucose) or RPMI 1640 (11.1 mM glucose) supplemented with 20% calf serum and antibiotics. Light microscopic examination indicated that the cultured explants were composed of fibrous tissue and well-preserved ducts and islets, whereas acinar cells had disappeared. The hormone content (insulin, C-peptide, glucagon, somatostatin) per milligram wet pancreatic weight increased 10–35 times during the culture period.

In static incubations of cultured explants there was a poor insulin response to glucose (16.7 mM). By contrast, insulin release was markedly stimulated in the presence of both glucose (16.7 mM) and theophylline (10 mM). The maximal rate of insulin release in response to glucose plus theophylline was observed after 11 days of culture. When pancreatic explants were incubated in a perifusion system after 7 days in culture, 25% of the fetuses showed a low and monophasic insulin response to glucose alone (15 mM), whereas the remaining ones failed to respond. When perifusions were performed with glucose (15 mM) plus theophylline (5 mM), the insulin response was high in about 25% of the fetuses, intermediate in 40%, and low in 35%. Neither in the static incubations nor in the perifusions was there any clear correlation between the rates of insulin release and the tissue culture medium used.

It is concluded that human fetal B cells may retain viability in organ culture for more than a week. The fetal pancreatic material prepared and stored by this means may be used in attempts to cure human diabetes by transplantation. **DIABETES *29* (Suppl. 1):64–69, 1980.**

From the Departments of Histology, of Obstetrics and Gynecology, and of Clinical Chemistry, University of Uppsala, Uppsala, and the Departments of Surgery and of Internal Medicine, Huddinge Hospital, Huddinge, Sweden. Address reprint requests to Dr. Ambjörn Ågren, Department of Histology, Biomedicum, P. O. Box 571, S-751 23 Uppsala, Sweden.

The most rational and perhaps the only possible way to cure patients suffering from insulin-dependent diabetes mellitus would be the transplantation of pancreatic B cells; however, up to now, attempts to graft the whole, vascularized pancreas have met with limited success, and only three out of more than 75 reported transplants have functioned for more than a year. Likewise, allogeneic transplantation of isolated islets or fragments of adult human pancreas has remained unsuccessful.[1] More promising results have been reported in some recent cases in which autografting of pancreatic fragments was used after pancreatectomy.[2]

An alternative way for transplantation of B cells would be to utilize the fetal endocrine pancreas, which may not only survive but also proliferate after being grafted into the host. Indeed, recent studies indicated that syngeneic transplantation of fetal rat pancreas reversed experimentally induced diabetes in the recipient.[3,4] In addition, there was a rapid growth of B cells in the transplanted tissue which correlated in time with the disappearance of diabetic symptoms in the host.[4] As a first step towards corresponding attempts to cure human diabetes, we report here on studies of the viability of human fetal pancreas obtained at legal abortions. Since fetal pancreatic glands are available only in limited numbers, we have attempted to prolong the survival of the endocrine cells by maintaining the tissue in organ culture. It was hoped that this approach would allow the collection of more viable material in preparation for transplantation and provide a possibility for detailed functional studies before grafting the tissue into the recipient.

MATERIALS AND METHODS

TISSUE PREPARATION

The pancreases from 43 human fetuses obtained at legal abortions were used. The crown-heel length of the fetuses varied between 10 and 38 cm (median length 18 cm). Each abortion was induced by prostaglandin, given either as a single intra-amniotic injection or repeated vaginal administration. Expulsion of the fetus usually occurred within 36 h of prostaglandin induction. Within 1 h, the pancreas was removed aseptically and placed in sterile Hanks' solution. In 19 consecutively collected fetuses, each of the glands was subdivided into three tissue blocks, one of which was used for morphologic studies; the remaining two were quickly blotted and weighed under aseptic conditions on a balance sensitive to 0.1 mg. Of the weighed blocks, the first was extracted for hormone assay (see below) and the remaining one placed in Hanks' solution and chopped into minute fragments (approximately 1 mm^3) which were maintained in culture as described below. In the remaining 24 fetuses the pancreas was immediately processed for tissue culture.

TISSUE CULTURE

The chopped pancreatic tissue was quickly washed in tissue culture medium composed of Parker's solution TCM 199 supplemented with 20% (vol/vol) calf serum, antibiotics (penicillin 100 U/ml, streptomycin 0.1 mg/ml), and glucose to a final concentration of 5.5 mM. In later experiments, TCM 199 was replaced by medium RPMI 1640[5] with a glucose concentration of 11.1 mM. The pieces were explanted into plastic Petri dishes, containing 5 ml of either of the culture media. The dishes were maintained at 37°C in a gas phase of 5% CO_2 in humidified air for a period of 6–14 days (see below). The medium was changed after the first day and subsequently every second day.

HISTOLOGIC EXAMINATION

Pancreatic samples, obtained either from the fresh gland or at the end of the culture period, were fixed in Bouin's solution for 5–24 h and embedded in paraffin. Serial sections 4 μm thick were prepared and stained with a modified aldehyde-fuchsin trichrome method according to Lazarus and Volk.[6] In addition, sections were taken for immunocytochemical localization of insulin. For this purpose, a commercially available batch of anti-bovine-insulin serum raised in guinea pigs (Miles-Yeda Ltd.; Elkhart, Indiana, lot no. GP-5) was used. Horseradish peroxidase-conjugated anti-guinea-pig IgG, also purchased from Miles-Yeda Ltd., was employed as the second antibody. Both antisera were diluted with a phosphate buffer (PBS, pH 7.4, 271 mM) supplemented with NaCl (144 mM), KCl (3 mM), and Triton X-100 (0.3% vol/vol, Packard Instrument, Elmers Grove, Illinois) as described by Hartman et al.[7] Pancreatic sections were hydrated and incubated with insulin antiserum, diluted 1:160 to 1:320, for 24 h at 4°C. They were then rinsed in PBS and treated with peroxidase-conjugated anti-IgG serum, diluted 1:80 to 1:160, for 30 min at room temperature. After rinsing in PBS, immunologically bound peroxidase was histochemically localized by a modification of the method of Graham and Karnovsky[8] using an incubation medium of 0.025 M Tris-HCl buffer, pH 7.6, containing diaminobenzidine-tetrahydrochloride (DAB, 20 mg/ml, Polysciences, Warrington, Pennsylvania, and 0.005% H_2O_2). After incubation for 10 min in this solution, sections were counter-stained with hematoxylin-eosin, dehydrated, and mounted.

To exclude the possibility of unspecific staining, control sections were treated as above, except that either the primary or secondary antibody was omitted. The staining procedure was also applied after adsorption of the primary antibody with either insulin, glucagon, or somatostatin.

HORMONE EXTRACTION

After weighing, the fresh pancreatic fragments were placed in 500 μl of acid ethanol (15 ml of 12 N HCl per liter of 70% ethanol), sonicated for 30 s, and extracted for 18 h at 4°C. The extracts were subsequently frozen and stored at −70°C before estimation of the hormone content by immunoassay (see below).

INSULIN RELEASE

Static incubations. Studies of insulin release into the culture medium began after the initial 12 to 36 h of culture (designated as day 1) and continued every second day up to the 12th day of culture. For this purpose, the culture medium of each dish was exchanged for serum-free TCM 199 supplemented with antibiotics as described above. Incubations of the explants (in this medium) were performed in the culture incubators for three consecutive 4-h periods, during which the glucose concentration was adjusted from 3.3 mM in the first period to 16.7 mM in the second and third periods. In the third period, the medium was also supplemented with 10 mM theophylline. At the end of each 4-h test period, the incubation medium was frozen and stored at −20°C for insulin assay. After the final test period, the explants were resuspended in complete culture medium, and the cultures were continued.

Perifusion. Groups of 25 to 150 uniformly sized pancreatic explants cultured for 7 ± 1 days were placed in a small Millipore chamber and perifused essentially as described by Lacy et al.[9] The perifusion fluid consisted of a bicarbonate medium[10] buffered with 25 mM Hepes and supplemented with 0.5 mg/ml albumin. During the perifusion period, the medium was kept at 37°C and gassed with O_2:CO_2 (95:5). The flow rate was adjusted to 1 ml/min and the glucose concentration maintained at 1.5 mM during the initial stabilizing period of 40 min and then increased to 15 mM for the following 40-min period. During this second period, the medium was also supplemented in some experiments with 5 mM theophylline. In the last 25 min of perifusion, the glucose concentration was lowered to 1.5 mM and theophylline was omitted. Samples of each effluent fraction were frozen for subsequent insulin assay.

HORMONE ASSAY

Insulin was determined according to the method of Heding,[11] using crystalline human insulin as a standard. Glucagon assays[12] were performed using a commercially available kit (Novo A/S, Bagsvaerd, Denmark). Glucagon standards consisted of porcine glucagon, and the antibody was an anti-pig-glucagon rabbit serum K 4023. C-peptide determinations[13] were carried out using synthetic C-peptide as a standard. Antibodies against C-peptide (M 1181, M 1230) were found to have a low cross-reactivity with human proinsulin (Gunnarsson, unpublished data).

Determination of somatostatin was performed using a solid phase technique for separation of free and antibody-bound tracer.[14] The antiserum (R 141) was a generous gift of Dr. Robert P. Elde, University of Minnesota. Synthetic somatostatin and Tyr[1]-somatostatin (Beckman, Geneva, Switzerland) were used for the preparation of standards and labeled somatostatin, respectively.

CALCULATION OF DATA

The results in each experimental group were expressed as the mean ±SEM. When insulin release was measured in static incubations, each experiment represented the average of two to nine observations on pancreatic explants of the same fetus. Statistical significances were evaluated with the aid of Student's *t* test. Results of hormone extractions were calculated as nanograms of hormone per milligram wet weight of extracted pancreas. The values of the insulin release after static incubations were expressed either as nanograms of hormone released per milligram wet weight of the originally explanted pancreatic specimen or as a percentage of the insulin release at 3.3 mM glucose in each experiment. In the perifusion experiments, release of insulin was expressed as a percentage increase of insulin secretion over basal values.

RESULTS

Light microscopic studies were performed on sections of the fresh pancreas from 20 fetuses. In the pancreas of the smaller fetus there was a predominance of loose mesenchymal tissue with only occasional groups of primitive acini. B cells appeared singly or in small groups, whereas, in the older fetuses, these cells formed typical islets (Figure 1a). Each islet was composed of centrally located B cells with a peripheral rim of A_1 and A_2 cells. Morphologic signs of necrosis or extensive tissue damage were absent from all specimens studied.

Examination of pancreatic explants maintained in tissue culture for 6–14 days indicated that marked morphologic changes occurred during the culture period. The explants sometimes attained a spherical shape and often became surrounded by a dense, fibrous capsule. The central core of the explants contained varying amounts of collagen fibers and only rarely did they contain acinar cells. Duct-like structures were common in some explants but absent in others.

FIGURE 1. (a) Aldehyde-fuchsin trichrome-stained pancreatic sections from a human fetus 21 cm in length. A central core of dark (blue-violet) B cells is surrounded by A cells forming a typical "mantle" islet. Acinar cells are seen to the right. (×400.) (b) Section of pancreatic explant from a human fetus 28 cm long, stained for immunocytochemical localization of insulin. Several islets composed of dark (brown) B cells are seen. The explant had been cultured for ten days in RPMI 1640 before being processed for histology. (×250.) (c) Scattered B cells in an explant maintained for 8 days in RPMI 1640. The tissue was obtained from a fetus 31 cm long. Immunocytochemical staining for insulin. (×250.) (d) Higher magnification of FIGURE 1c showing well-preserved B cells scattered in a matrix of fibrous tissue. (×1000.)

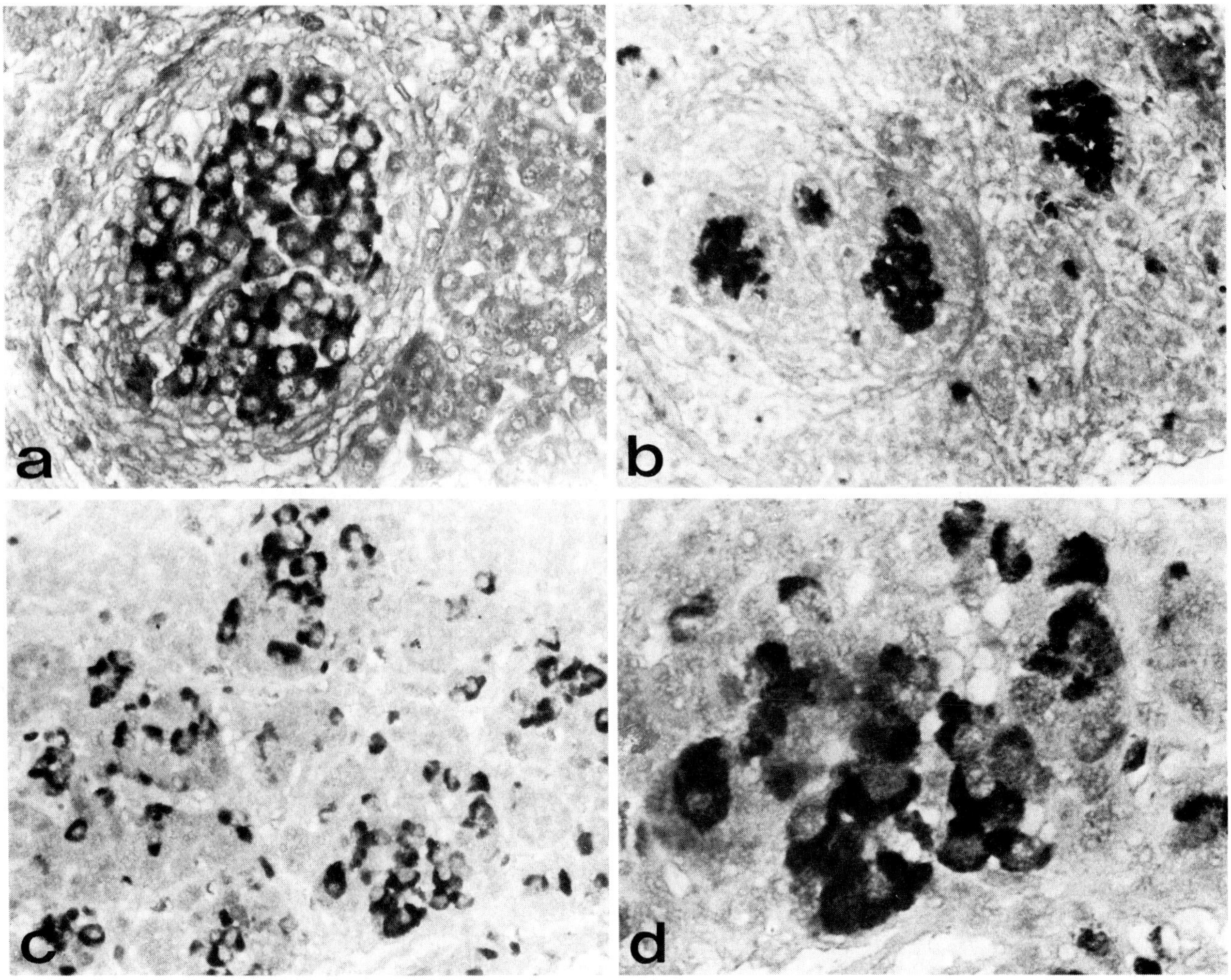

Immunocytochemical staining for insulin demonstrated either heavily stained islets (Figure 1b) or scattered B cells (Figures 1c and d). In some instances the B cells were found intermingled with duct cells. Mostly, however, the B cells formed islets without any apparent direct attachment to the ducts. The morphology of the explants appeared similar, irrespective of whether they had been cultured in TCM 199 or RPMI 1640.

The hormone contents per milligram wet weight of the fresh or cultured pancreas are given in Table 1. It is evident that tissue culture caused a striking increase in the content of the various peptides. Insulin, C-peptide, and glucagon thus increased 11–20 times, whereas the content of somatostatin increased by not less than 35 times after the culture period. A comparison between the content of insulin and that of C-peptide indicated that, on a molar basis, the fresh pancreas contained 1.8 times more C-peptide than insulin, whereas the cultured explants contained 2.7 times more C-peptide.

The insulin release from the fetal pancreatic explants in static incubations is shown in Figure 2a. All data were obtained from explants cultured in TCM 199 and they have been expressed on the basis of the initial wet weight of the explanted tissue, since weighing the tissue in sterile conditions on each culture day was not feasible. It may be seen that glucose alone failed to stimulate insulin release, irrespective of the duration of the culture period ($P > 0.05$). Furthermore, the basal rate of insulin release remained unchanged throughout the observation period. By contrast, addition of 10 mM theophylline in the presence of 16.7 mM glucose evoked a marked insulin response at all the different time points studied. A tendency towards an increased response at the end of the culture period attained statistical significance on culture day 11, when comparisons were made with culture day 1 ($P < 0.005$). When the data were expressed as a percentage of the basal insulin release in each experiment (Figure 2b), there was a slight effect of glucose alone on culture days 1 ($P < 0.01$) and 11 ($P < 0.005$). Again, the effect of glucose plus theophylline on the insulin release was striking, and a significantly enhanced response was seen when a comparison was made between culture days 1 and 11 ($P < 0.005$).

TABLE 1
Hormone contents in acid ethanol extracts of human fetal pancreas obtained either fresh or after culture for 6–14 days in TCM 199*

Immunoreactive peptide	Pancreas	
	Fresh	Cultured
Insulin	104 ± 11 (18)	1460 ± 104 (14)
C-peptide	32 ± 3 (14)	667 ± 92 (15)
Glucagon	5.7 ± 1.0 (15)	63.4 ± 11.6 (10)
Somatostatin	0.8 ± 0.1 (10)	28.6 ± 3.8 (10)

* Values are given as nanograms per milligram wet pancreatic weight for insulin, glucagon, and somatostatin and as picomoles per milligram wet pancreatic weight for C-peptide. Means ± SEM. Number of fetuses (body length 10–24 cm) in parentheses.

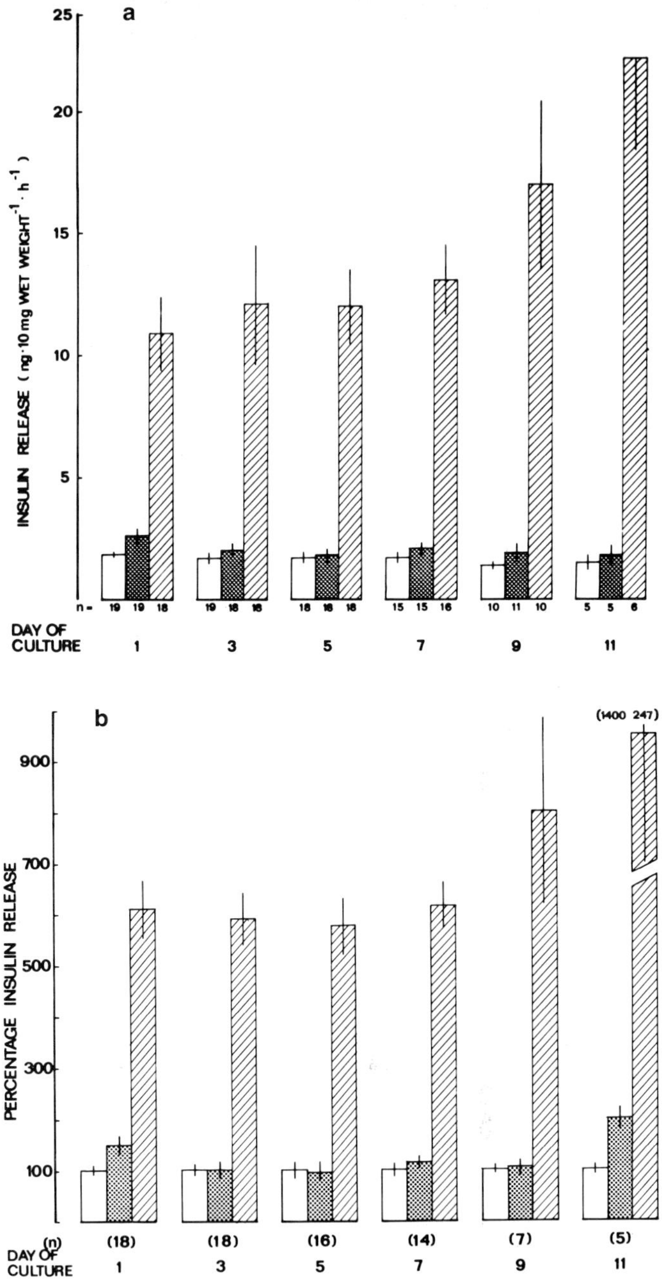

FIGURE 2. (a) Insulin release from fetal pancreatic explants cultured for various times in TCM 199. Static incubations were carried out for 4-h periods in either 3.3 mM glucose (□), 16.7 mM glucose (▩), or 16.7 mM glucose plus 10 mM theophylline (▨). See text for further details. The data (mean ± SEM) have been expressed on the basis of the initial wet weight of the explanted tissue. (b) The same data as in Figure 2a plotted as a percentage of the rate of insulin release at 3.3 mM glucose in each individual experiment. Mean ± SEM.

Tests of islet viability by measurements of insulin release from perifused pancreatic explants were performed after a culture period of 7 days. Out of a total of 22 fetal pancreatic glands, 12 had been maintained in TCM 199 and 10 in RPMI 1640. Since the results obtained in the individual experiments could not for practical reasons be related to islet number, weight, or protein content, the data were grouped according to the pattern of insulin release obtained by plotting, in each experiment, the insulin release as a percentage of the basal value. On this basis, the results of the perifusion experiments could be subdivided into three groups according to criteria given in Figure 3. When perifused with glucose (15 mM) plus theophylline (5 mM), the explants of five cultured pancreases showed a high insulin response; nine showed an intermediate response, and eight a low response. When glucose (15 mM) was used as the only stimulus of insulin release, none of the 15 pancreases (six cultured from TCM 199, nine cultured in RPMI 1640) showed a comparably high response. However, four cultured pancreases responded in an intermediate way and 11 had a response that was either very low or nonexistent. The different culture media used seemed to be equally efficient in maintaining the insulin response to glucose plus theophylline, since three pancreases cultured in TCM 199 and an equal number cultured in RPMI 1640 showed a high rate of release. An intermediate insulin response to glucose alone was observed only in those explants cultured in RPMI 1640.

DISCUSSION

In order to fulfill the aims of the present study, it was necessary to use as simple techniques as possible for tissue preparation so that pancreatic samples arriving in the laboratory at irregular intervals and at any time of the day could be rapidly and efficiently secured for tissue culture. Organ culture of human fetal pancreatic fragments[15,16] appeared ideal for this purpose, since it required a minimal handling of the tissue, yet allowed a series of morphologic and functional studies to be carried out. Initial attempts to apply a collagenase digestion technique for islet isolation[17] were abandoned since, in our hands, the digestion procedure caused a major loss of pancreatic cells and a poor yield of islets. This is at variance with observations in the rat, in which a mild collagenase treatment of the fetal pancreas followed by culture for 1 wk resulted in a selective enrichment of islets.[18]

FIGURE 3. Dynamics of insulin release from fetal pancreatic explants maintained in tissue culture for 7 days. Each curve represents an individual experiment selected as typical for each of three groups of data: (A) high insulin response (○——○), (b) intermediate insulin response (△——△), and (c) low insulin response (■——■). The basal insulin release was expressed as the average of individual measurement performed during the last 10 min of the stabilizing period (−10 to 0 min).

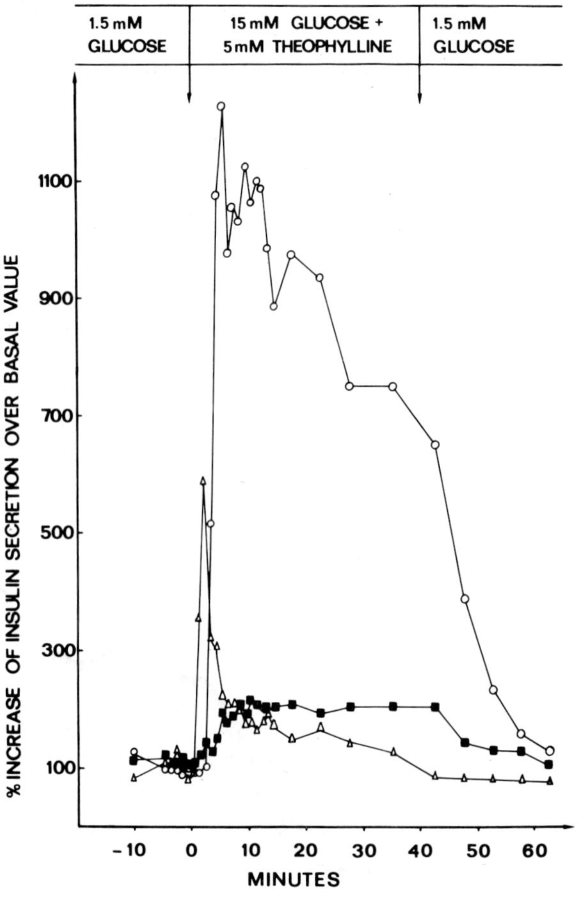

With few exceptions, the fetuses secured for the present studies lacked signs of maceration or autolysis, irrespective of the dosage of prostaglandin or the mode of administration of the drug. The well-preserved structure of the fresh pancreas as seen in the light microscope underlined the impression that the fetal material was useful for the present purpose. Insulin-containing B cells were found at all developmental stages studied, and, in older fetuses, the cells were arranged into typical "mantle" islets. This pattern of development has been described before[19–23] and shows that insulin formation is an early event in the ontogeny of the islets.

Previous studies in the rat indicate a rapid degeneration in vitro of exocrine pancreatic cells which have been maintained either in organ or monolayer culture.[18,24,25] The present observations in the cultured explants corroborate these findings and further suggest that acinar cells were replaced, at least in part, by ducts and/or fibrous tissue. Although this process might have decreased the size of the individual explant, there was still a predominance of nonendocrine cells comprising a potential diffusion barrier to nutrients, hormones, and waste products. Necrotic areas were, however, lacking even in the central parts of the explants, suggesting that the rate of diffusion was compatible with cell survival. In further support of this notion, islets and scattered B cells of normal appearance were present throughout the explants. This, of course, does not exclude that the disappearance of acinar cells was brought about by specific nutritional demands which could not be met by the present culture conditions.

The marked increase in the hormone content per unit wet weight of the cultured explants may reflect the combined effects of several independent processes. Firstly, the loss of acinar tissue may lead to an increase in the proportion of islet cells which becomes manifest as an elevated hormone content of the tissue. Secondly, the lack of blood circulation through the islets may hamper the release of hormones from the islet cells. In support of this we observed a more pronounced immunocytochemical staining for insulin in the cultured islets as compared with that of the fresh pancreas. Furthermore, separate studies indicated the continuous synthesis of both insulin and glucagon for up to 10 days of culture (Andersson and Ågren, unpublished data). Thirdly, a net increase of islet cells through proliferation may occur in culture, but direct evidence of this is still lacking. Irrespective of the precise reason for the enrichment of hormones, it is intriguing that not only the B cells but also the somatostatin- and glucagon-producing cells seemed to retain a capacity for hormone storage throughout the period of tissue culture.

The present observation of a poor insulin release in response to an acute glucose load when fetal explants were studied in either static incubations or in perifusion demonstrates the similarity in this respect between the human pancreas and that of several other species including monkey,[26] rat,[27] and rabbit.[28] Our data also support corresponding observations previously made in the human fetus both in vivo[29] and in vitro.[30] However, the failure to respond to glucose raises immediately the question whether the fetal pancreas is at all suitable for transplantation purposes. Reversal of diabetes after transplantation of fetal pancreas in animal experiments[3,4] indeed suggests that the glucose sensitivity of the B cell becomes manifest soon after grafting into the recipient. In addition, induction of glucose sensitivity in culture has recently been accomplished using fetal rat islets.[18] A poor glucose sensitivity in vitro, therefore, is no reason to refrain from trying the human fetal pancreas for transplantation.

Both the static incubations and the perifusion experiments indicate that insulin was released at a markedly increased rate when the explants were exposed to glucose and theophylline. The observation that the perifused explants could be subdivided into three groups, depending on the temporal pattern and magnitude of the response, demonstrates that the sensitivity of the B cells to glucose plus theophylline varied between different fetuses. We were, however, unable to correlate these different patterns to either fetal age or to the culture medium used. However, the inhomogeneity of the fetal material with regard to age, time of pancreatic ischemia, etc., makes a variability of this kind almost inevitable.

We conclude from the present data that human fetal B cells obtained at prostaglandin abortions may retain viability over a period of more than 1 wk in vitro. The simple organ culture system employed allows the tissue to be rapidly prepared for culture, and it can then be studied as regards sterility, morphology, and hormone release. Preliminary observations suggest that fetal pancreatic material prepared and stored by this means can be used in attempts to cure human diabetes by transplantation.[31]

ACKNOWLEDGMENTS

Financial support from the Swedish Diabetes Association, the Nordisk Insulinfond, Stiftelsen Expressens Prenatalforskningsnämnd, the Medical Faculty of the University of Uppsala, the Swedish Society for Medical Research, the Wiberg Foundation, Allmänna Barnbördsfonden, and the Swedish Medical Research Council (12X-109 and 16X-4527) is gratefully acknowledged.

REFERENCES

1 Najarian, J. S., Sutherland, D. E., Matas, A. J., Steffes, M. W., Simmons, R. L., and Goetz, F. C.: Human islet transplantation: a preliminary report. Transplant. Proc. *9*:233–36, 1977.

2 Sutherland, D. E., Matas, A. J., and Najarian, J. S.: Pancreatic islet cell transplantation. Surg. Clin. North Am. *58*:365–82, 1978.

3 Brown, J., Clark, W., Molnar, G., Kemp, J., Mazur, P., and Mullen, Y. S.: Functional capacity and cryopreservation of foetal rat pancreas in streptozotocin-diabetes. *In* Diabetes. Bajaj, J. S., Ed. Amsterdam, Excerpta Medica, 1977, pp. 535–43.

4 McEvoy, R. C., and Hegre, O. D.: Syngeneic transplantation of fetal rat pancreas. III. Effect of insulin treatment on the growth and differentiation of the pancreatic implants after reversal of diabetes. Diabetes *28*:141–46, 1979.

5 Andersson, A.: Isolated mouse pancreatic islets in culture: effects of serum and different culture media on the insulin production of the islets. Diabetologia *14*:397–404, 1978.

6 Lazarus, S. S., and Volk, B. W.: The Pancreas in Human and Experimental Diabetes. New York, Grune & Stratton, 1962, pp. 261–62.

7 Hartman, B. K., Zide, D., and Udenfriend, S.: The use of dopamine β-hydroxylase as a marker for the central noradrenergic nervous system in the rat brain. Proc. Natl. Acad. Sci. U.S.A. *69*:2722–26, 1972.

8 Graham, R. C., and Karnovsky, M. J.: The early stages of absorptions of injected horseradish peroxidase in the proximal tubules of the mouse kidney: ultrastructural cytochemistry by a new technique. J. Histochem. Cytochem. *14*:291–303, 1966.

9 Lacy, P. E., Walker, M. M., and Fink, C. J.: Perifusion of isolated rat islets in vitro. Participation of the microtubular system in the biphasic release of insulin. Diabetes *21*:987–98, 1972.

10 Krebs, H. A., and Henseleit, K.: Untersuchungen über die Harnstoffbildung im Tierkörper. Hoppe-Seylers Z. Physiol. Chem. *210*:33–66, 1932.

11 Heding, L. G.: Determination of total serum insulin (IRI) in insulin-treated diabetic patients. Diabetologia *8*:260–66, 1972.

12 Heding, L. G.: Radioimmunological determination of pancreatic and gut glucagon in plasma. Diabetologia *7*:10–19, 1971.

13 Heding, L. G.: Radioimmunological determination of human C-peptide in serum. Diabetologia *11*:541–48, 1975.

14 Arimura, A., Lundqvist, G., Rothman J., Chang, R., Fernandez-Durango, R., Elde, R., Coy, D. H., Meyers, C., and Schally, A. V.: Radioimmunoassay of somatostatin. Metabolism *27* (Suppl. 1):1139–44, 1978.

15 Fujimoto, W. Y., and Williams, R. H.: Insulin release from cultured fetal human pancreas. Endocrinology *91*:1133–36, 1972.

16 Leach, F. N., Ashworth, M. S., Barson, A. J., and Milner, R. D. G.: Insulin release from human foetal pancreas in tissue culture. J. Endocrinol. *59*:65–79, 1973.

17 Goldman, H., and Colle, E.: Human pancreatic islets in tissue culture: effects of supplementing the media with homologous and heterologous serum. Science *192*:1014–16, 1976.

18 Hellerström, C., Lewis, N. J., Borg, H., Johnson, R., and Freinkel, N.: Method for large-scale isolation of pancreatic islets by tissue culture of the fetal rat pancreas. Diabetes *28*:769–76, 1979.

19 Ferner, H.: Das Inselsystem des Pankreas. Stuttgart, Georg Thieme Verlag, 1952, pp. 22–48.

20 Björkman, N., Hellerström, C., Hellman, B., and Petersson, B.: The cell types in the endocrine pancreas of the human fetus. Z. Zellforsch. *72*:425–45, 1966.

21 Van Assche, F. A.: The fetal endocrine pancreas. Thesis, University of Leuven, 1970, pp. 1–99.

22 Wellman, K. F., Volk, B. W., and Brancato, P.: Ultrastructure and insulin content of the endocrine pancreas in the human fetus. Lab. Invest. *25*:97–103, 1971.

23 Like, A. A., and Orci, L.: Embryogenesis of the human pancreatic islets: a light and electron microscopic study. Diabetes 21 (Suppl. 2):511–34, 1972.

24 Lazarow, A., Wells, L. J., Carpenter, A. M., Hegre, O. D., Leonard, R. J., and McEvoy, R. C.: Islet differentiation, organ culture, and transplantation. Diabetes *22*:877–912, 1973.

25 Orci, L., Like, A. A., Amherdt, M., Blondel, B., Kanazawa, Y., Marliss, E. B., Lambert, A. E., Wollheim, C. G., and Renold, A. E.: Monolayer cell culture of neonatal rat pancreas. An ultrastructural and biochemical study of functioning endocrine cells. J. Ultrastruct. Res. *43*:270–97, 1973.

26 Chez, R. A., Mintz, D. H., and Epstein, M. F.: Fetal hormonal mechanisms for plasma glucose homeostasis in normal and glucose intolerant pregnancy. *In* Early Diabetes in Early Life. Camerini-Davalos, R. A., and Cole, H. S., Eds. New York, Academic Press, 1975, pp. 141–53.

27 Asplund, K., Westman, S., and Hellerström, C.: Glucose stimulation of insulin secretion from the isolated pancreas of foetal and newborn rats. Diabetologia *5*:260–62, 1969.

28 Milner, R. D. G., Leach, F. N., Ashworth, M. A., Cser, A., and Jack, P. M. B.: Development of pathways of insulin secretion in the rabbit. J. Endocrinol. *64*:349–61, 1975.

29 Grasso, S., Palumbo, G., Messina, A., Mazzarino, C., and Reitano, G.: Human maternal and fetal serum insulin and growth hormone (HGH) response to glucose and leucine. Diabetes *25*:545–49, 1976.

30 Espinosa, M. M. A., Driscoll, S. G., and Steinke, J.: Insulin release from isolated human fetal pancreatic islets. Science *168*:1111–12, 1970.

31 Groth, C. G., Andersson, A., Björkén, C., Gunnarsson, R., Hellerström, C., Lundgren, G., Petersson, B., Swenne, I., and Östman, J.: Transplantation of fetal pancreatic microfragments via the portal vein to a diabetic patient. Diabetes *29* (Suppl. 1):80–83, 1980.

Cryopreservation of Human Fetal Pancreas

JOSIAH BROWN, JOHN A. KEMP, SUSAN HURT, AND WILLIAM R. CLARK

SUMMARY

To determine the optimal conditions for successful cryopreservation of the human fetal pancreas, techniques developed for the rat organ were modified. The parameters studied were the conditions of exposure to the cryopreservation agent dimethyl sulfoxide (DMSO), the rate of cooling and thawing, and the effect of in vitro culture. A total of 33 pancreases, obtained after fetal death due to prostaglandin-induced abortion, was studied. Survival of the pancreas is based on incorporation of ^{3}H-amino acids into protein by pancreas pieces (2 mm^3) during a 4-h incubation compared with nonfrozen control pieces from the same pancreas. Toxicity of DMSO at 37°C was found to be severe after a 4-h exposure. Varying the effects of temperature, time of exposure, and concentrations of DMSO on survival after freeze-thaw revealed that 1.5 M DMSO for 1 h at room temperature was optimal. The cooling rate was 0.22°C/min and thawing was at room temperature. Since these conditions resulted in only 50% survival, a period of culture before exposure to DMSO was added. The optimal duration of culture was 12–16 h. Using this method with addition of culture for 24 h after thawing, survival has varied from 70 to 120% of control. If a functional test for growth and insulin production by the frozen-thawed pancreas is positive, permanent shortage of the human fetal pancreas will be possible. DIABETES *29* (Suppl. 1): 70–73, 1980.

A major consideration in transplantation technology is storage of the donor organ. Because of its small size and, perhaps, other properties unique to fetal tissues, the fetal pancreas lends itself to permanent storage by freezing.[1] Long-term cryopreservation of human fetal pancreases will allow the accumulation of a large bank of donor organs already tissue-typed, thereby improving the HLA compatibility with diabetic recipients. Frozen donor lymphocytes, obtained from the same donor as the fetal pancreas, could be made available for the mixed leukocyte culture reaction with recipient lymphocytes, and time will not be limiting for this test of compatibility. Finally, donor antigens, such as those on liver cells, will be available and might prove useful for the treatment of the recipient before transplantation in order to diminish the rejection reaction.[2,3]

A rat model for reversal of streptozotocin-induced diabetes by transplantation of syngeneic fetal pancreases has been developed.[4,5] A single fetal pancreas will completely reverse diabetes in an adult rat if first placed into a normal rat for 3 wk prior to transfer to the diabetic animal[6] or if the recipient is maintained in a relatively normoglycemic state by treatment with insulin for several weeks after transplantation.[7] Conditions for successful cryopreservation of the fetal rat pancreas[8] include 2 M dimethyl sulfoxide (DMSO) as the cryopreservative and a very slow rate of cooling (0.3°C/min). After freezing under these conditions and storage at −196°C for 9–13 wk, thawed fetal pancreases were transplanted beneath the kidney capsule of normal rats. Vascularization occurred within 2–4 days, and the transplanted organs increased in size. Both beta and alpha cells were observed in the transplanted organ by electron microscopy, and insulin synthesis in the pancreas was demonstrated by radioimmunoassay. The demonstration that a single frozen-thawed fetal pancreas can completely reverse diabetes in an adult rat, equivalent to a nonfrozen organ,[9] suggests that freezing does not appreciably alter the ultimate function of the fetal organ. Additional evidence for the undiminished function of the frozen-thawed fetal rat pancreas is derived from insulin release during perfusion of pancreases removed after 3 wk of growth in normal rats. Both the amount of insulin released and the residual insulin content of frozen-thawed pancreases were the same as from nonfrozen pancreases.[9]

Application of the methods developed for cryopreservation of fetal rat pancreases are being applied to human fetal

From the Department of Medicine, School of Medicine, and the Department of Biology, University of California, Los Angeles, California.
Address reprint requests to Josiah Brown, Department of Medicine, Division of Endocrinology, University of California at Los Angeles, Los Angeles, California 90024.

pancreas and are the subject of this report. It should be emphasized that the test for survival of fetal rat pancreas after freeze-thaw—in vitro incorporation of ^{3}H-amino acids into protein—correlated with function, as judged by insulin content, release, and reversal of diabetes. In judging the survival of human fetal pancreas after freeze-thaw, the criterion is the same—incorporation of amino acids into protein in vitro compared with nonfrozen tissue from the same pancreas.

MATERIALS AND METHODS

Pancreases from 33 human fetuses were obtained after abortion induced by prostaglandins. The mean gestational age was 100 days (range 84–147 days). The exact time of fetal death is unknown; thus, the time of delivery will be used for timing purposes. The interval from delivery to dissection varied from 15–180 min, and the time from dissection to further treatment of the specimens averaged 2.9 h. During this interval, the specimens were in cold phosphate-buffered saline with 15–20% human serum albumin (HSA). Specimens were dissected from surrounding tissues and cut into 2-mm^{3} pieces. Culture medium was Eagle's, containing 5% HSA, glucose 450 mg/dl, and Trasylol 5%. Survival was based on the same method used for fetal rat pancreases, the incorporation of ^{3}H-labeled amino acids into protein during a 4-h incubation.[1] Percent survival is compared with control incubations of randomized pieces of the same fetal pancreas.

RESULTS

In order to determine the toxicity of DMSO for human fetal pancreas pieces, incubations were carried out at 37°C at various concentrations of the cryopreservative (Figure 1). Survival of the tissue was seriously diminished to less than 50% of controls before 4 h in 2.0 M and 1.5 M DMSO and after 4 h in 1 M DMSO. In order to diminish the toxicity of DMSO, pancreas pieces were incubated up to 60 min at various concentrations of DMSO at room temperature and 37°C (Figure 2). The pancreas was then frozen at 0.22°C/min, as described previously,[9] and kept frozen at −196°C for at least 12 h. Survival after freeze-thawing was optimal at 1.5 M DMSO, with equal results when exposed for 60 min at room temperature or 30 min at 37°C. Maximum survival was only about 50% as compared with nonfrozen pieces of the same pancreas.

In order to improve survival of the human fetal pancreas, a period of culture before exposure to DMSO and after thawing was added to the procedure. The results of a varying period of culture before exposure to DMSO in various concentrations followed by freezing and thawing are given in Figure 3. Survival was best if culture lasted longer than 12 h but less than 24 h, followed by exposure to 1.5 M DMSO at room temperature for 60 min.

Using the above technique, survival of human fetal pancreas has varied from 70 to 120% of control. The results of a typical experiment are given in Table 1 and reveal that a period of incubation before and after exposure to DMSO increases ^{3}H-amino acid incorporation in the experiment to 142% of the nonincubated value. Comparison of amino acid incorporation of the frozen-thawed with nonfrozen pancreas reveals no difference (98% of control nonfrozen).

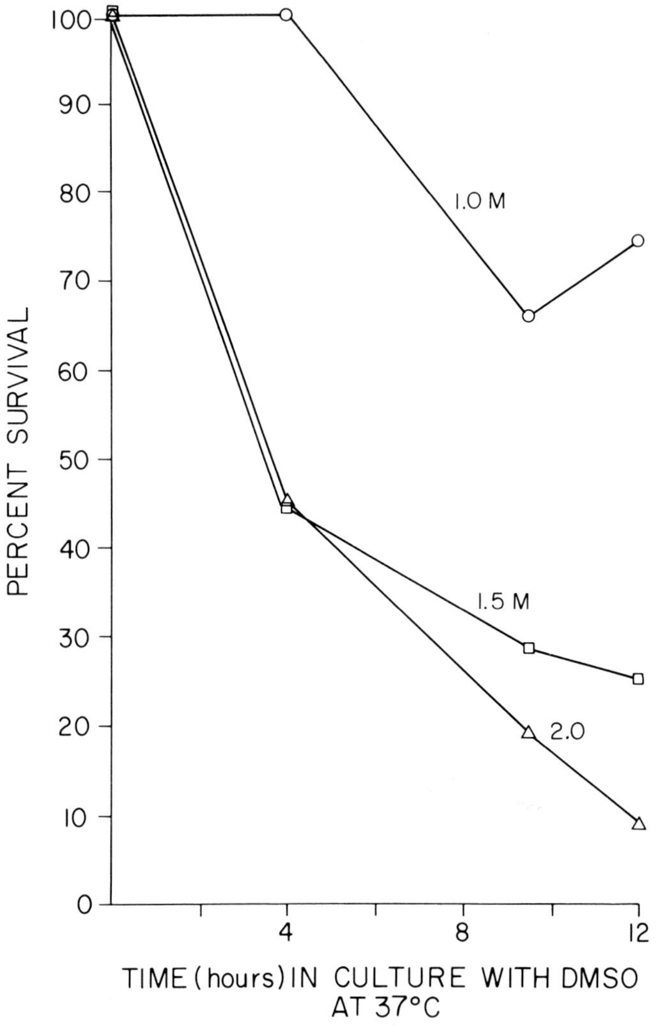

FIGURE 1. Survival of human fetal pancreas segments incubated in various concentrations of dimethyl sulfoxide (DMSO). Survival is determined by ^{3}H-amino acid incorporation into protein expressed as percent of incorporation by random pieces of the same fetal pancreas.

DISCUSSION

Human fetal pancreas fragments have been successfully cryopreserved, as judged by the survival test of incorporation of ^{3}H-amino acids into protein in a 4-h culture. In the rat model there is a close correlation between this test of survival and function after transplantation as determined by growth, insulin synthesis and release during perfusion, and reversal of diabetes. These correlations, combined with the observation that frozen and nonfrozen pancreases after transplantation are indistinguishable ultrastructurally,[10] suggest that changes due to freezing and thawing[11] are reversible. Since the majority of cells in the pancreas are exocrine cells, the survival test (incorporation of amino acids) is essentially a test of exocrine cell survival. However, results obtained in the rat model indicate that endocrine cell's survival and function closely correlate with this test of exocrine cell function after freeze-thaw. We are currently testing the function of frozen-thawed human pancreas fragments by in vitro insulin secretion in response to glucose/theophylline and by transplantation into immunoincompetent or immunosuppressed animal hosts.

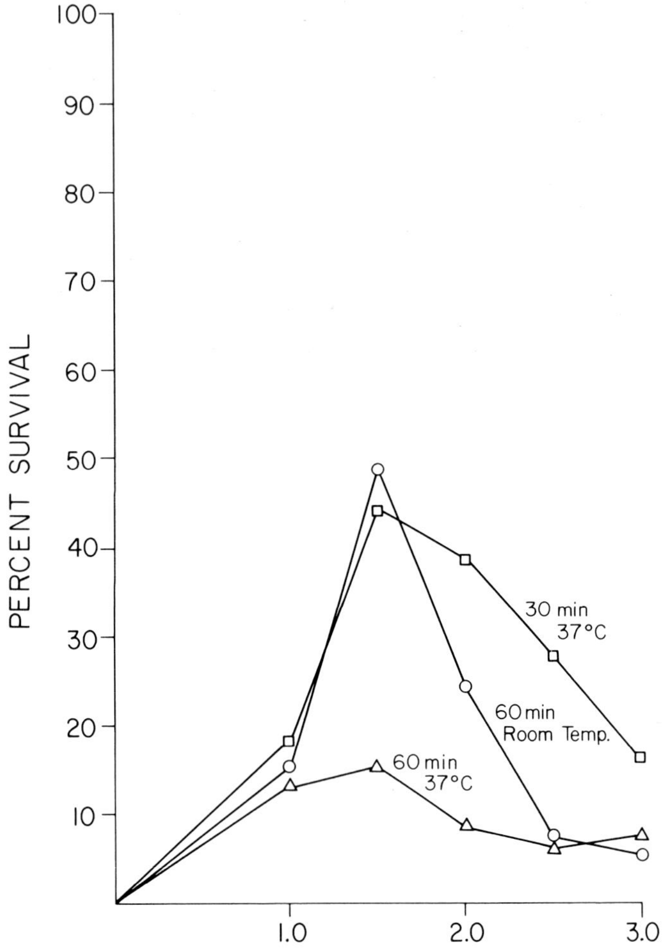

FIGURE 2. Survival of human fetal pancreas segments exposed to DMSO followed by freezing and thawing. Survival is determined by ³H-amino acid incorporation into protein expressed as percent of nonfrozen control by random pieces of the same fetal pancreas.

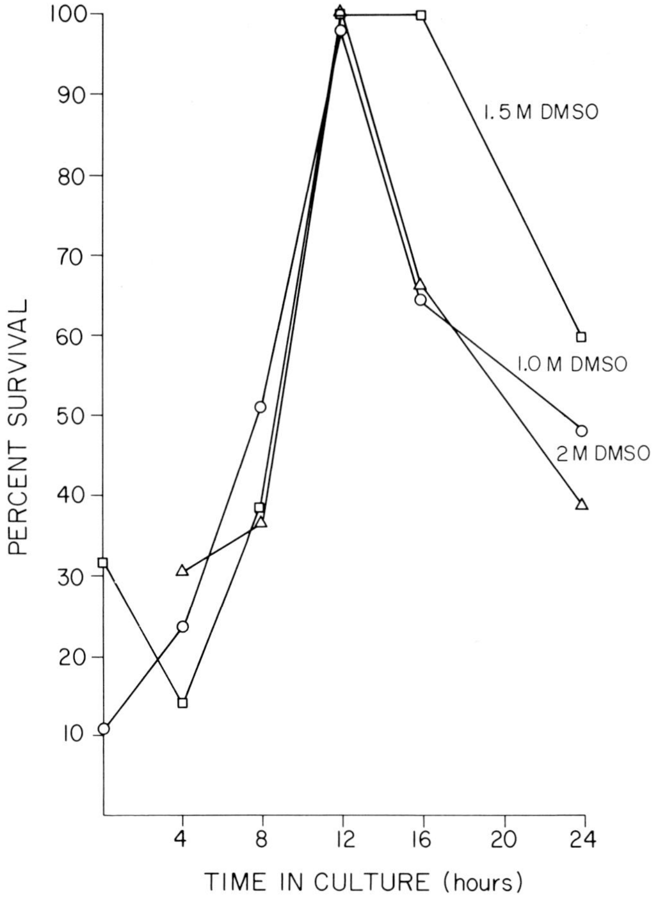

FIGURE 3. Survival of human fetal pancreas segments incubated before exposure to DMSO at various concentrations for 1 h. After freezing and thawing, survival was determined by ³H-amino acid incorporation into protein expressed as percent of nonfrozen control by random pieces of the same fetal pancreas.

In adapting the technical parameters for freezing from the rat model to the human, changes were necessary. The obvious differences between the organs are the larger size and very fibrous nature of the human pancreas. Cutting the human organ into segments of approximately the size of the 17-day rat organ and inclusion of a period of incubation before exposure to DMSO and again after thawing led to survival of 70–120%, which had been achieved in the rat model. The effect of these manipulations on the ultimate total function of the human pancreas may be of great importance. In the rat model system, a single fetal pancreas after a period of growth develops the capacity to completely reverse diabetes in an adult animal, and the frozen-thawed organ also develops this capacity. The results of the experiments presented here suggest that it is possible to successfully cryopreserve human fetal pancreases. Whether the frozen-thawed organ can grow sufficiently to completely reverse diabetes in a diabetic human remains to be determined.

TABLE 1
Effects of preincubation, DMSO, freezing, and postincubation on ³H-amino acid incorporation into protein in vitro by human fetal pancreas

Prefreeze incubation, 19½ h	1.5 M DMSO, 1 h	Freeze	Postfreeze incubation, 24 h	C/Min per μg protein	Percent of control
+	–	–	–	81	
+	+	–	+	115	142
+	+	3× faster	+	0.4	0.3
+	+	+	+	113	98

The advantages of cryopreservation of the human fetal pancreas to the goal of transplantation into diabetic patients are the provision of time. The technique will allow the accumulation and storage of donor organs already tissue-typed for optimal HLA matching with potential recipients, and frozen donor lymphocytes will be available for matching with recipient cells in a mixed leukocyte reaction. Finally, it may be possible to prepare the recipient with such donor antigens as liver cells to diminish the rejection problem.

ACKNOWLEDGMENTS

Secretarial assistance was provided by Pam Meyers and Charlotte Limberg. Financial support was provided by USPHS grants AM17980 and 20827 and by grants from the American Diabetes Association and The Kroc Foundation.

REFERENCES

[1] Mazur, P., Kemp, J. A., and Miller, R. H.: Survival of fetal rat pancreases frozen to −78 and −196°. Proc. Natl. Acad. Sci. U.S.A. *73*:4105–09, 1976.

[2] Pinto, M., Brent, L., and Thomas, A. V.: Specific unresponsiveness to skin allografts in mice. III. Synergistic effect of tissue extracts, *Bordetella pertussis,* and antilymphocytic serum. Transplantation *17*:477–86, 1974.

[3] Brent, L., and Opara, S. C.: Specific unresponsiveness to skin allografts in mice. V. Synergy between donor tissue extract, procarbazine hydrochloride, and antilymphocyte serum in creating a long-lasting unresponsiveness mediated by suppressor T cells. Transplantation *27*:120–26, 1979.

[4] Brown, J., Molnar, I. G., Clark, W., and Mullen, Y.: Control of experimental diabetes mellitus in rats by transplantation of fetal pancreases. Science 184:1377–79, 1974.

[5] Brown, J., Clark, W. R., Molnar, I. G., and Mullen, Y. S.: Fetal pancreas transplantation for reversal of streptozotocin-induced diabetes in rats. Diabetes *25*:56–64, 1976.

[6] Mullen, Y. S., Clark, W. R., Molnar, I. G., and Brown, J.: Complete reversal of experimental diabetes mellitus in rats by a single fetal pancreas. Science *195*:68–70, 1977.

[7] Brown J., Heininger, D., Kuret, J., and Mullen, Y.: Single fetal rat pancreas as a donor organ: capacity for growth and reversal of diabetes. Submitted for publication, 1979.

[8] Kemp, J. A., Mazur, P., Mullen, Y., Miller, R. H., Clark, W., and Brown, J.: Reversal of experimental diabetes by fetal rat pancreas. I. Survival and function of fetal rat pancreas frozen to −196°C. Transplant. Proc. *9*:325–28, 1977.

[9] Kemp, J. A., Mullen, Y., Weissman, H., Heininger, D., Brown, J., and Clark, W. R.: Reversal of diabetes in rats using fetal pancreas stored at −196°C. Transplant. Proc. *26*:260–64, 1978.

[10] Brown, J. (Moderator) et al.: UCLA Conference. Pancreas transplantation for diabetes mellitus. Ann. Intern. Med. *89*:951–56, 1978.

[11] Rajotte, R. V., Steward, H. L., Voss, W. A. G., Shnitka, T. K., and Dossiter, J. B.: Viability studies on frozen-thawed rat islets of Langerhans. Cryobiology *14*:116–20, 1977.

Transplantation of Human Fetal Pancreas

Experience in Thymusaplastic Mice and Rats and in a Diabetic Patient

K. H. USADEL, U. SCHWEDES, G. BASTERT, U. STEINAU, I. KLEMPA, W. FASSBINDER, AND K. SCHÖFFLING

SUMMARY

The aim of the present study was to investigate if thymusaplastic nude mice and rats are favorable as recipients for transplantation of human fetal pancreas. Twenty human fetal pancreases were transplanted subcutaneously to 20 nude mice, and six human fetal pancreases were transplanted to six rats. The xenografts showed histotypical development of islets of Langerhans. Insulin, glucagon, somatostatin, and pancreatic polypeptide immunoreactivities were also seen in very early stages of the transplant development within the monolayered ducts.

With the described "epigastric pouch technique" in rats, we could demonstrate a new in vivo method for selective stimulations and simultaneous blood sampling from tissue-isolated xenografts.

Transplantation of human fetal pancreas to the brachioradial muscle of an insulin-dependent patient in combination with a kidney transplant revealed that rejection crises of the kidney led to necrosis of the pancreas transplant, whereas rejection of the kidney was overcome by steroid pulse therapy. DIABETES 29 (Suppl. 1):74–79, 1980.

In previous reports from this laboratory[1–3] it was shown that subcutaneous isologous transplantation of tissue cell suspensions from fetal rats under the neck skin of adult recipient rats develops to histotypical organs. Pancreas anlage from 14- to 16-day-old rat fetuses have been successfully implanted subcutaneously into the neck of adult rats. Typical pancreatic endocrine tissue, but also exocrine tissue, developed and remained functional for up to 2 yr. By immunohistochemical methods the presence of both insulin- and glucagon-like activity could be demonstrated in the transplanted tissue. Hyperglycemia, induced before transplantation by streptozotocin, was permanently lowered in the examined animals and rose again after removal of the transplant.

The aim of the present study was to investigate if thymusaplastic nude mice and rats are favorable as recipients for transplantation of human fetal pancreas and if there is development of these transplants. Our microsurgical "tissue-isolated transplantation" technique allows new investigations with human tissues under in vivo conditions. Our experience with one clinical case also will be reported.

From the Center for Internal Medicine, Surgery and Gynecology, Johann Wolfgang Goethe University, Frankfurt, Federal Republic of Germany.
Address reprint requests to Prof. K. H. Usadel, Zentrum der Inneren Medizin, Abteilung für Endokrinologie, Theodor Stern-Kai 7, D-6000 Frankfurt a.M., F.R.G.

MATERIAL AND METHODS

ANIMAL RECIPIENTS

Thymusaplastic mutants of mouse (*nu/nu*) and rat (*rnu/rnu*) have previously been described by Pantelouris[4] and Festing et al.[5] The genes governing thymic agenesis and hairlessness proved to be closely linked and inherited as autosomal recessive traits. This defect is linked with a loss of immune-competent T-lymphocytes, resulting in a lack of immune resistance. If nude mice or nude rats are used as recipients, heterologous transplantations can be achieved without any immunosuppressive therapy.[6–13]

nu/nu Mice and rnu/rnu rats. Nude mice of a hybrid strain (NMRI/Balb; initial body weight of approximately 28–30 g; 5–6 wk old) and nude rats (WAG/Rowett; initial body weight of approximately 150–200 g; 10 wk old) served as random-bred recipients.

The animals were protected by means of a laminar flow installation and were maintained under constant environmental conditions (mice at a temperature of 26°C, rats at 22°C; relative humidity 65%; polypropylene cages with sterile bedding). They were offered a special nude mouse and rat diet (Altromin 1414/FRG) and drinking water (mice: 300 mg/L; rats: 600 mg/L oxytetracycline and 500 mg potassium sorbate) ad libitum.

Xenotransplantation in nude mice. The xenografts were sliced into small fragments and immediately transplanted under sterile conditions subcutaneously into the part of the mammary gland which extends into the wall of the thorax.

One mouse was used for each case. Only fresh xenografts were used and transported to the laboratories in a medium (TCM 199, Difco) with 95% air/5% CO_2 water-saturated atmosphere.

Twenty human fetuses (6–23 wk of gestation) were obtained after medically indicated abortions, and the fetal pancreases were prepared and transplanted as described above. Animals were killed between 3 and 17 wk after transplantation. At necropsy, the area of inoculation was inspected macroscopically and microscopically.

FIGURE 1. Epigastric pouch technique in nude rats. (a) Preparation of the epigastric pouch; (b) pedicle immediately after transplantation; (c) plastic pouch.

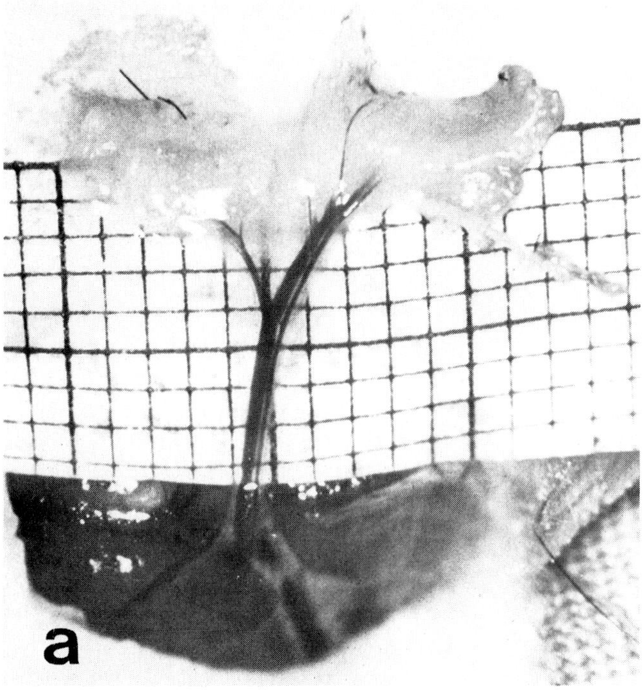

Xenotransplantation in nude rats. After isolation of a 1.5–2.0-cm² patch of dermis and surrounding tissue in the well-vascularized groin region, the vascular pedicle of the patch consisting only of the epigastric artery and vein is carefully dissected up to its origin at the femoral vessels (Figure 1a). The xenografts are implanted into the subcutaneous patch, which is then folded and sutured together (Figure 1b). The pedicle is now inserted into a thin polyethylene pouch where the xenograft can grow separately from the surrounding tissue (Figure 1c). After skin closure above the pouch, the heterotransplanted tissue grows according to its specific growth rate. During the following period, an increase of swelling in the rat's groin can be observed. Sixteen weeks later, an incision in the groin region shows a well-vascularized xenograft covered by the plastic pouch. After preparation of the xenotransplants, the femoral vein can be catheterized proximally and ligated distally from the confluent point of the epigastric vein with the femoral vein. In addition the contralateral femoral vein can be catheterized (Figure 2).

Six human fetal pancreases (12 wk of gestation) were transplanted into six rat pouches.

Histology and immunohistology. For histologic examination, the material was fixed either in Bouin's solution or in formaldehyde immediately after removal of the transplants and was embedded and stained in the usual manner.

Immunohistochemical demonstration of insulin- and glucagon-like activities was performed using a modified immunoperoxidase technique described by Nakane and Pierce[14] and Arnold et al.[15] based on an indirect technique.[16] Antibodies to insulin and glucagon were prepared by immunizing guinea pigs (insulin) and rabbits (glucagon). For the secondary antiserum, peroxidase-conjugated IgG fractions were used (Research Plus Laboratories, Denville, New York). After washing in PBS buffer (pH 7.2), the peroxi-

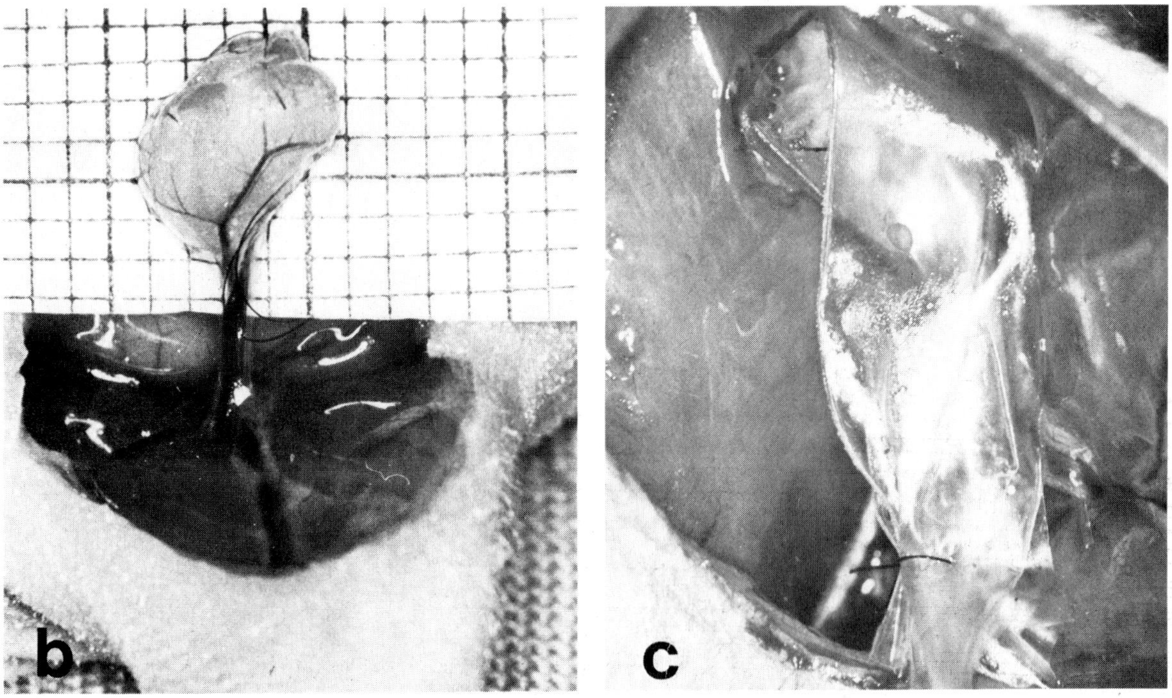

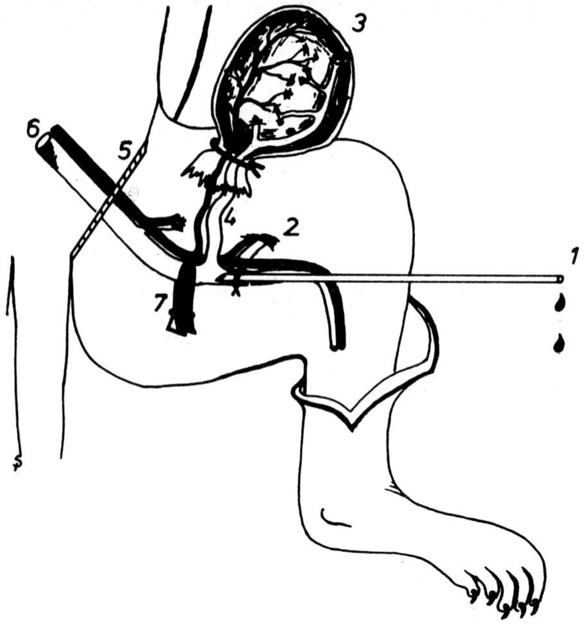

FIGURE 2. Situs of the epigastric pouch in rats. (1) Catheter in "pancreas vein"; (2) profunda femoris artery and vein, closed by tourniquet; (3) plastic pouch; (4) epigastric superficialis artery and vein; (5) ligamentum inguinale; (6) femoral artery and vein; (7) micro clip for blood sampling.

dase reaction was performed according to Graham and Karnovsky.[17] For control reactions, the sections were incubated with buffer solution, normal guinea pig serum or normal rabbit serum, and also with antiserum neutralized with insulin and/or glucagon.

Immunohistochemical reactions for somatostatin and pancreatic polypeptide (PP) immunoreactivity (antibovine PP-serum with 80% cross-reaction to human PP) were performed by Arnold and Creutzfeldt.*

CLINICAL EXPERIENCE

In a 37-yr-old female patient with end-stage renal failure due to insulin-dependent diabetes and severe diabetic retinopathy undergoing kidney transplantation, we additionally transplanted human fetal pancreases (9 and 16 wk of gestation) into the brachioradialis muscle of the right arm. The fresh pancreases were dissected into about 10 pieces, which were inoculated into small pouches prepared in the brachioradialis muscle of the right arm. This method has been used successfully in autologous transplantation of human parathyroid.[18]

RESULTS

Mice. In 15 of the 20 host mice, transplant growth at the implant site occurred (Table 1). The first sign of growth of the transplant could be detected after 21 days. Growth of a heterotransplant from a 10-wk-old human fetal pancreas can be observed at 35 days (Figure 3a) and 77 days (Figure 3b) after transplantation. Some implants have grown up to a size of 6 × 5 × 4 mm at 120 days after transplantation. Microscopy revealed a branched system of small ducts with a monolayered epithelium containing many mitoses and typical islets of Langerhans in older transplants. Numerous buds germinated out of these ducts throughout the experiment.

By immunohistologic examination we found numerous cells containing insulin- (Figures 4a to 4c) or glucgon-like activity (Figure 5b) as well as a few cells containing pancreatic polypeptide- (Figure 5c) or somatostatin-like activity (Figure 5a). These different hormone-producing cells could be detected in all stages of the developing transplant. The number of latter cells was surprisingly high in early stages of the transplant development. The cells were located within the monolayered epithelium of the ducts in early stages of the transplant development. Later, insulin- and glucagon-immunoreactive cells were found concentrated in the buds and islets. B cells were located mainly in the center and A cells in the periphery of the islets of Langerhans.

Pancreases grew when fetuses from 6 to 16 wk of gestation were used for transplantation. The best age of fetal human pancreas for transplantation was 7–12 wk, whereas pancreases older than 16 wk did not grow. In all mice experiments, we never saw histologic signs of transplant rejection.

Rats. In all recipient nude rats, human fetal pancreases developed analogously to the growth in mice. By macroscopic aspect (Figure 6) the "transplant pouch" size reached 6 × 7 × 9 mm 60 days after transplantation and was well-vascularized (Figure 7). There was no difference in histology or immunohistology in comparison to the transplants in mice. There were no difficulties in toleration of the plastic pouch. Preliminary results of catheterizing the pancreas pouch-vein (Figure 2) during glucose tolerance test revealed higher insulin and C-peptide levels in comparison with the contralateral femoral vein. In nude rat recipients, furthermore, we never observed histologic signs of rejection.

Clinical data. In contrast to Sutherland et al.[19] and Dom-

TABLE 1
Data on transplantation of human fetal pancreas to nude mice

Recipient no.	Fetal age (wk)	Necropsy after transplantation (days)	Size of histologically detectable transplants of pancreas
1	6	45	++
2	7	120	+++
3	9	40	+++
4	10	77	+++
5	10	42	+++
6	10	21	++
7	11	28	+++
8	11	21	++
9	12	27	+++
10	12	35	+++
11	12	38	+++
12	15	35	++
13	15	21	+
14	16	31	+
15	16	110	0
16	16	81	+
17	17	110	0
18	21	21	0
19	21	21	0
20	23	21	0

*We are grateful to Prof. R. Arnold and Prof. W. Creutzfeldt (Department of Medicine, Division of Gastroenterology and Metabolism, University of Goettingen, F.R.G.) for their performance of PP and somatostatin reactions.

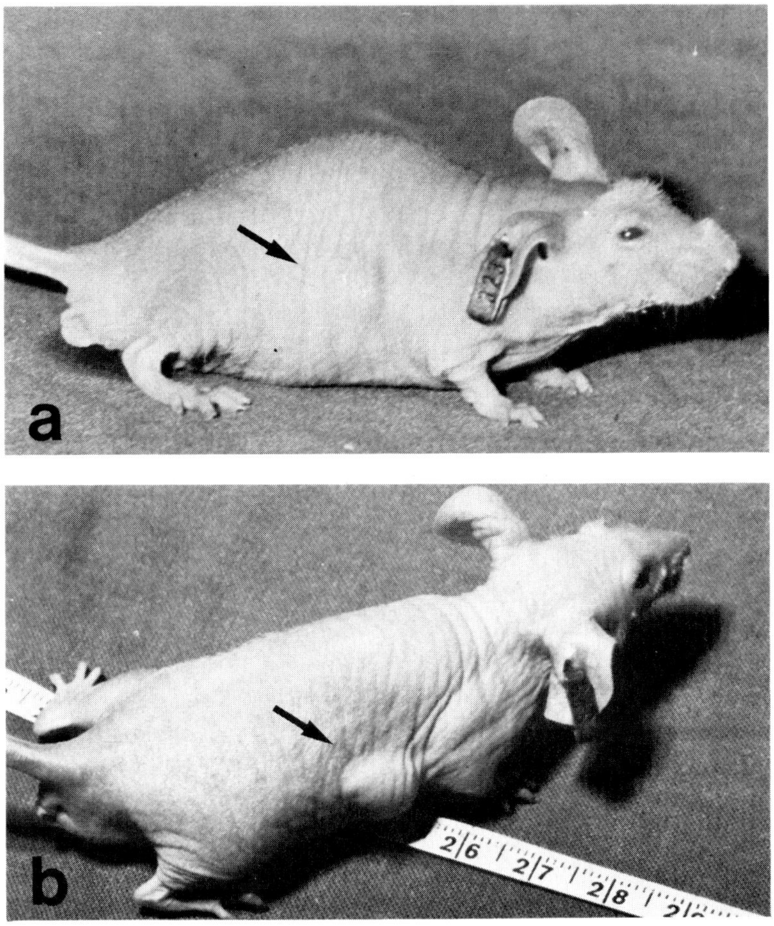

FIGURE 3. Human fetal pancreas transplant (10 wk of gestation) (a) 35 days and (b) 77 days after transplantation in the same host (arrows).

broschke et al.[20] who transplanted autologous isolated islets of Langerhans into the portal vein in patients undergoing total pancreatectomy, we transplanted homologous fetal pancreases into a 37-yr-old, insulin-dependent diabetic woman in 1978. End-stage renal failure, caused by diabetic nephrosclerosis and severe retinopathy, made homologous kidney transplantation necessary after a short (8-wk) period of hemodialysis therapy. Immediately after transplantation, immunosuppressive therapy (100 mg prednisolone and 200 mg azathioprine per day) was begun. On the 6th and 14th postoperative days, respectively, 9- and 16-wk-old human fetal pancreases, resulting from medically indicated abortions, were transplanted. In this early stage of gestation, determinations of ABO blood type and tissue-typing of the fetus are not yet available, but, since the blood group of the recipient was AB, a transplantation seemed worth attempting.

In the fourth and ninth weeks after kidney transplantation, severe rejection crises of the kidney occurred. These were overcome by 16-methyl-prednisolone pulse-therapy. At 12

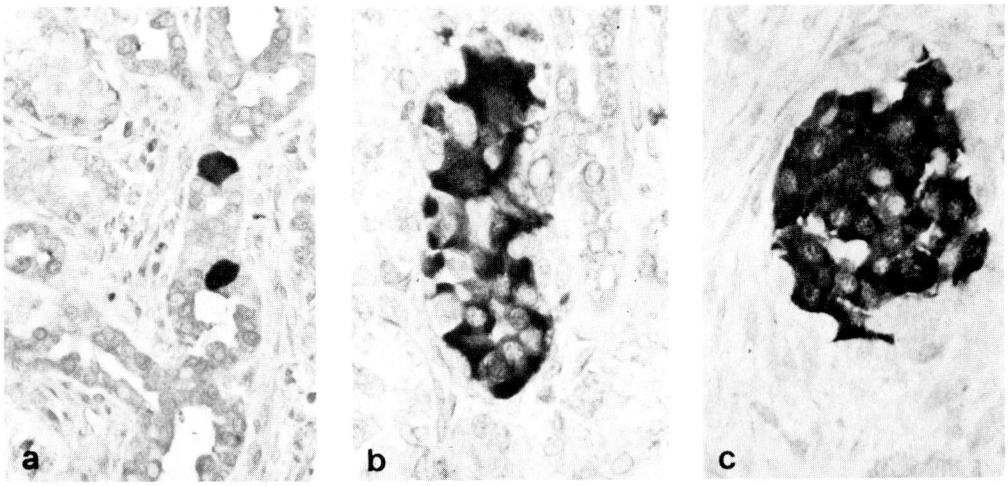

FIGURE 4. Insulin immunoreactivity of human fetal pancreas transplants (10 wk of gestation) to nude mice (a) 21 days, (b) 42 days, and (c) 77 days after transplantation.

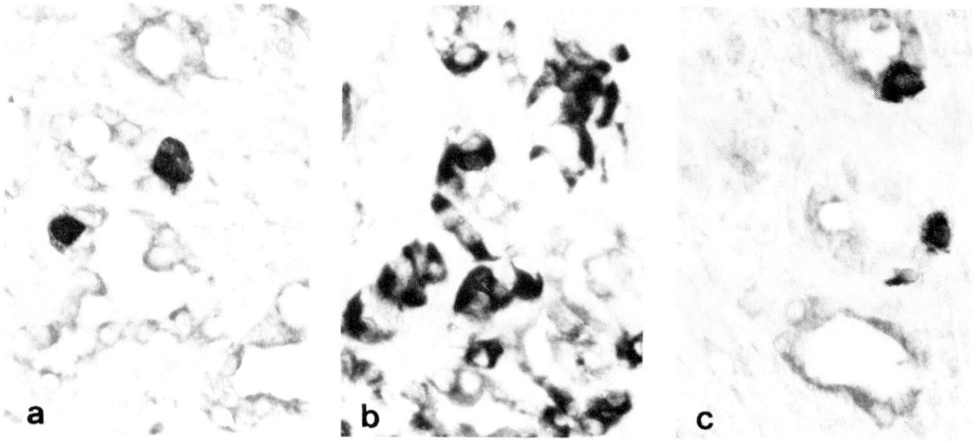

FIGURE 5. Human fetal pancreas transplant (10 wk of gestation) to nude mice 21 days after grafting. (a) Somatostatin, (b) glucagon, and (c) pancreas polypeptide immunoreactivity.

mo after transplantation, the transplanted kidney is still functioning well (creatinine clearance: 58 ml/min).

Before the pancreas transplantation, the patient had no insulin secretion, since there were no measurable serum C-peptide levels using a tolbutamide stimulus. At 10 and at 50 wk after the pancreas transplantation, we repeated the tolbutamide test and again found no C-peptide response in blood samples from the left and right antecubital veins. After pancreas transplantation there was no reduction of the doses of insulin required for treatment of diabetes.

DISCUSSION

Recent emphasis in the field of experimental pancreas transplantation has centered on two methods: (1) isolated islets of adult pancreas of the rat have been isologously transplanted to various locations of the recipient[21–23] and (2) fetal rat pancreas has been used for isologous transplantation to adult recipients.[1,3,24,25] In these experiments, it was shown that isolated adult islets survive after transplantation and that fetal material is able to differentiate to numerous exocrine ducts and to histotypical islets. There is an adequate response in hormone production to stimuli[21,24] when adult as well as fetal materials are used for transplantation.

In the present experiment, it could be demonstrated that human fetal pancreas transplants grow in nude mice and rats and are able to differentiate to a monolayered duct system with buds and numerous histotypical islets of Langerhans. Immunohistochemistry revealed typical A and B cells with insulin- and glucagon-like immunoreactivity as well as D cells with somatostatin and pancreatic polypeptide-like immunoreactivity. It is interesting to point out that all investigated hormone immunoreactivities could already be detected in very early stages of the transplant development within the monolayered epithelium of the ducts. The highest rate of transplant growth was observed when 7- to 12-wk-old pancreases were taken for transplantation, whereas experiments using human fetal pancreases older than 16 wk have not been successful. This indicates that there is a time limit for viability of transplanted pancreatic material. Using the described epigastric-pouching technique in nude rats, we could demonstrate that, in this model, human fetal pancreas develops analogously to that in mouse experiments and that there is an adequate hormone response to tolerance tests. By this new method, selective in vivo tolerance tests of heterotransplants are possible, as we show using human endocrine benign or malignant tissues as grafts.[26–28] Hormone-producing transplant tissue contacts the host only via a single artery and vein.

These results demonstrate that human fetal pancreas has the same chance of development as the rat tissue and that it can be used as a graft in transplantation research. However,

FIGURE 6. Nude rat bearing an epigastric pouch (human fetal pancreas, 12 wk of pregnancy, 60 days after transplantation, arrow).

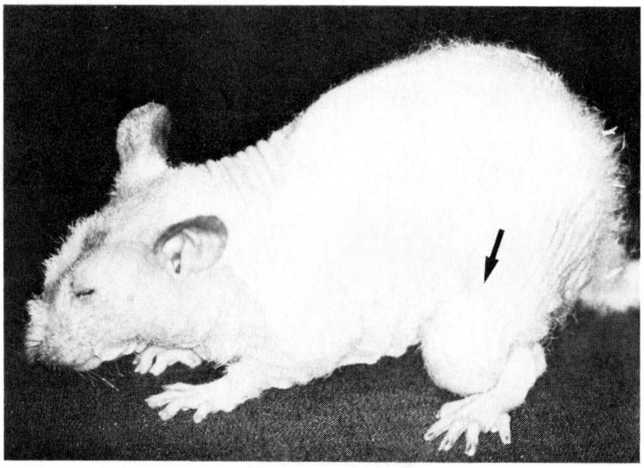

FIGURE 7. The same transplant as in Figure 6 with good vascularization.

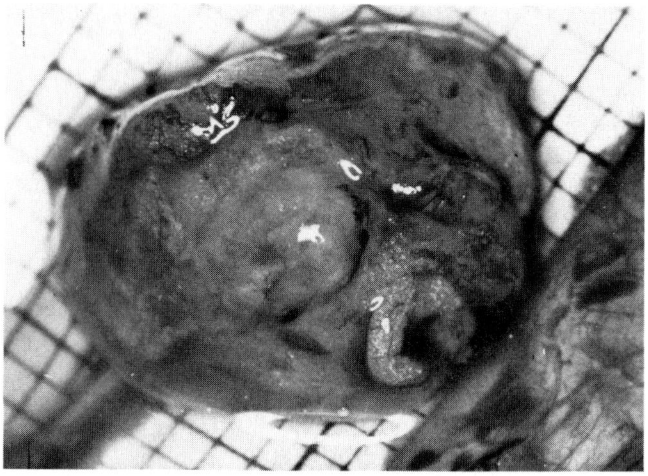

tissue-typing and immunosuppression seem necessary if homologous transplantation is to be useful as therapy in man. As we could show in homologous transplantation experiments in rats, fetal rat pancreas transplants will be rejected by the host on the way to differentiation of the graft. In young, nondifferentiated grafts, rejection is minor.

Summarizing our clinical data, we suggest that the homologous transplants of fetal pancreas did not develop in the patient and that they had no function. This may be attributed to the severe rejection crisis of the kidney transplant during a very early stage of pancreas development, leading to necrosis due to rejection. Further transplantations in the same manner are in progress.

The questions as to what degree in vitro precultivation[29,30] of tissue before transplantation could decrease immunologic problems and to what degree autoantibody graft effects exist in insulin-treated diabetics[31,32] need investigation.

ACKNOWLEDGMENTS

The authors wish to thank I. Obert for her skilled technical assistance and J. Apelbaum for reviewing this manuscript. Dr. H. P. Fortmeyer's technical advice is appreciated. The investigations were supported in part by the Deutsche Forschungsgemeinschaft (Us 8/1 and Schm 177/2).

REFERENCES

[1] Usadel, K. H., Rockert, H., Obert, I., and Schöffling, K.: Entwicklung histiotypischer Organe durch isologe Transplantation von Zellsuspensionen embryonaler Organanlagen bei der Ratte. Klin. Wochenschr. *48*:1417–18, 1970.

[2] Usadel, K. H., Rockert H., Obert, I., and Schöffling, K.: Über die Entwicklung isologer Zellsuspensions-Transplantate aus embryonalen Darm- und Magenanlagen bei der Ratte. Z. Gesamte Exp. Med. *153*:237–49, 1970.

[3] Usadel, K. H., Schwedes, U., Leuschner, U., and Schöffling, K.: Development of isologous transplants of cell suspensions of fetal pancreas in the rat. Acta Endocrinol. Suppl. *184*:97, 1974.

[4] Pantelouris, E. M.: Absence of thymus in a mouse mutant. Nature (London) *217*:370–71, 1968.

[5] Festing, M. F. W., Lovell, D., and Sparrow, S.: The Rowett athymic rat. Symposium: The laboratory rat and biological variation. Cambridge, 1978.

[6] Rygaard, J., and Povlsen, C. O.: Heterotransplantation of a human malignant tumor to "nude" mice. Acta Pathol. Microbiol. Scand. *77*:758–60, 1969.

[7] Povlsen, C. O., Skakkebaek, N. E., Rygaard, J., and Jensen, G.: Heterotransplantation of human foetal organs to the mouse mutant nude. Nature (London) *248*:247–49, 1974.

[8] Giovanella, B. D., Stehlin, J. S., and Williams, L. J., Jr.: Heterotransplantation of human malignant tumors in "nude" thymusless mice. II. Malignant tumors induced by injection of cell cultures derived from human solid tumors. J. Natl. Cancer Inst. *52*:921–27, 1974.

[9] Bastert, G., Althoff, P. H., Usadel, K. H., Fortmeyer, H. P., and Schmidt-Matthiesen, H.: Heterotransplantation of human fetal pituitaries in nude mice. Endocrinology *101*:365–68, 1977.

[10] Bastert, G., Schmidt-Matthiesen, H., Fortmeyer, H. P., Nord, D., Michel, R. T., Gerner, R., and Sturm, R.: Human breast cancer in nu/nu mice. A model for testing in research and clinic. Klin. Wochenschr. *55*:83–84, 1977.

[11] Usadel, K. H., Bastert, G., Schwedes, U., and Fortmeyer, H. P.: Human fetal pancreas transplants in nu/nu mice. Lancet *1*:365, 1977.

[12] Bastert, G., Usadel, K. H., and Althoff, P. H.: Function of human fetal pituitary transplants in nude mice. Acta Endocrinol. Suppl. *215*:13, 1978.

[13] Usadel, K. H., Schwedes, U., Minne, H., Klempa, I., Vlachoyannis, J., Fortmeyer, H. P., and Schöffling, K.: Transplantation of human parathyroid adenoma and carcinoma in nude mice. Acta Endocrinol. Suppl. *215*:55, 1978.

[14] Nakane, P. K., and Pierce, G. B., Jr.: Enzyme-labeled antibodies: preparation and application for the localization of antigens. J. Histochem. Cytochem. *14*:929–31, 1966.

[15] Arnold, R., Deuticke, U., Frerichs, H., and Creutzfeldt, W.: Immunohistologic investigations on human insulinomas. Diabetologia *8*:250–59, 1972.

[16] Weller, T. H., and Coons, A. H.: Fluorescent antibody studies with agents of varicella and herpes zoster propagated in vitro. Proc. Soc. Exp. Biol. Med. *86*:789–94, 1954.

[17] Graham, R. C., Jr., and Karnovsky, M. J.: The early stages of absorption of injected horseradish peroxidase in the proximal tubules of mouse kidney: ultrastructural cytochemistry by a new technique. J. Histochem. Cytochem. *14*:291–302, 1966.

[18] Klempa, J., Steinau, U., Frei, U., Koch, K. M., Usadel, K. H., and Rottger, P.: Morphologische Aspekte der Parathyreoideatransplantation. Chirurg. *49*:704, 1978.

[19] Sutherland, D. E. R., Matas, A. J., and Najarian, J. S.: Pancreatic islet cell transplantation. Surg. Clin. North Am. *58*:365–82, 1978.

[20] Dombroschke, J., Schwemmle, K., Langhoff, G., Laube, H., Bretzel, R. G., and Federlin, K.: Autotransplantation von Langerhansschen Inseln nach totaler Duodenopankreatenktomie bei einem Patienten mit chronischer Pankreatitis. Dtsch. Med. Wochenschr. *103*:1905–10, 1978.

[21] Hegre, O. D., Leonard, R. J., Erlandsen, S. L., McEvoy, R. C., Parsons, J. A., Elde, R. P., and Lazarow, A.: Transplantation of islet tissue in the rat. Acta Endocrinol. (Suppl.) *205*:257–78, 1976.

[22] Kemp, C. B., Knight, M. J., Scharp, D. W., Lacy, P. E., and Ballinger, W. F.: Transplantation of isolated pancreatic islets into the portal vein of diabetic rats. Nature (London) *244*:447, 1973.

[23] Federlin, K., Slijepcevic, M., and Helmke, K.: Islet transplantation in experimental diabetes of the rat. IV. The influence of transplantation site and of histocompatibility on islet function. Horm. Metab. Res. *8*:97–101, 1976.

[24] Brown, J., Clark, W. R., Molnar, I. G., and Mullen, Y. S.: Fetal pancreas transplantation for reversal of streptozotocin-induced diabetes in rats. Diabetes *25*:56–64, 1976.

[25] Mullen, Y. S., Clark, W. R., Molnar, I. G., and Brown, J.: Complete reversal of experimental diabetes mellitus in rats by a single fetal pancreas. Science *195*:68–70, 1977.

[26] Bastert, G., Steinau, U., Eichholz, H., Fortmeyer, H. P., Usadel, K. H., Althoff, P. H., Schwedes, U., Klempa, I., and Schmidt-Matthiesen, H.: Xenografts of human fetal pituitaries in nude rats (epigastric pouching technique). Acta Endocrinol. (Kbh) Suppl. *225*:205, 1979.

[27] Klempa, I., Usadel, K. H., Schwedes, U., Althoff, P. H., Steinau, U., Schneider, M., Bastert, G., Fortmeyer, H. P., and Vecsei, P.: Xenotransplantation of a Conn's tumor in nude rats. Animal experimental model for primary hyperaldosteronism: morphological and functional studies. Acta Endocrinol. (Kbh) Suppl. *225*:339, 1979.

[28] Klempa, I., Steinau, U., Minne, H., Bastert, G., and Usadel, K. H.: Transplantation of human parathyroid tumors in nude mice. An experimental model for hyperparathyroidism. Eur. Surg. Res., 1979. In press.

[29] Lafferty, K. J., Cooley, N. A., Woolnough, J., and Walker, K. Z.: Thyroid allograft immunogenicity is reduced after a period in organ culture. Science *188*:259–61, 1975.

[30] Lacy, P. E., Davie, J. H., and Finke, E. H.: Use of in vitro culture (24°C) for prolongation of islet allograft survival. Diabetes *28* (Suppl.):382, 1979.

[31] Anderson, A.: Islet implantation normalizes hyperglycaemia caused by streptozotocin-induced insulitis. Experiments in mice. Lancet *1*:581, 1979.

[32] Gunnarsson, R., Groth, C. G., Botazzo, G. F., and Lernmark, A.: Islet autoantibodies in human pancreatic transplant recipients. Lancet *1*:926, 1979.

Transplantation of Fetal Pancreatic Microfragments via the Portal Vein to a Diabetic Patient

C. G. GROTH, A. ANDERSSON, C. BJÖRKÉN, R. GUNNARSSON, C. HELLERSTRÖM, G. LUNDGREN, B. PETERSSON, I. SWENNE, AND J. ÖSTMAN

SUMMARY

Human fetal pancreas preserved in culture was used as a donor organ in a 45-yr-old man with diabetes of 14-yr duration complicated by severe retinopathy and nephropathy. Renal failure had been successfully treated by a cadaveric renal transplant 2 yr earlier. Six fetal pancreases, obtained within 30 min of delivery after prostaglandin-induced abortion at 14–20 wk of gestation, were minced and placed in tissue culture for 3 h at the earliest and 15 days at the longest duration. The cultures were harvested 2–3 h before transplantation. Approximately 3 ml of tissue was infused into a right portal vein branch. Azathioprine was continued at 2 mg/kg and prednisolone increased from 10 mg to 100 mg/day on the day of transplantation and gradually reduced to 25 mg/day. Only two doses of antilymphocytic globulin were given because of a severe reaction. During the 40 days since transplantation, insulin requirements have not changed, but C-peptide has appeared in the urine, suggesting function of the transplanted tissue. DIABETES 29 (Suppl. 1):80–83, 1980.

Cure of experimentally induced diabetes mellitus has been achieved in several animal species by transplanting dispersed syngeneic or autologous endocrine pancreatic tissue. In the rodent, success has also been obtained with allogeneic tissue when transplanted into an immunosuppressed host. Hegre and his collaborators suggested the cultured fetal pancreas as a source of pancreatic islet tissue for transplantation,[1–3] and, in 1974, Brown and co-workers reported the cure of streptozotocin diabetes in the rat by transplanting 4–6 syngeneic fetal pancreases.[4,5] Subsequently, these investigators found that complete reversal of experimental diabetes could be achieved with just one fetal pancreas.[6] The cultured fetal pancreas bears several potential advantages:[7,8] (1) it contains a larger proportion of endocrine tissue; (2) the exocrine tissue undergoes atrophy during culture; (3) the fetal tissue possesses a considerable growth potential; and (4) it might be less immunogeneic.

We have recently attempted to transplant cultured fetal human pancreatic microfragments to a diabetic patient via the portal vein. Earlier clinical attempts at transplanting dispersed pancreatic tissue have all involved the use of adult or infant pancreas.[9,10]

From the Departments of Surgery and Medicine, Karolinska Institute, Huddinge Hospital, Stockholm, and the Department of Histology, University of Uppsala, Uppsala, Sweden.
Address reprint requests to Dr. C. G. Groth, Department of Surgery, Huddinge Hospital, 141 86 Huddinge, Sweden.

CASE HISTORY

The recipient was a 45-yr-old man with insulin-dependent diabetes of 14-yr duration. He had developed retinopathy leading to photocoagulation in 1977. Nephropathy resulted in uremia in 1977, and, in April of that year, cadaveric renal transplantation was performed (four HLA-A, -B incompatibilities). Renal function was normalized, and there were no rejection episodes.

METHODS

The fetal graft. The pancreases were procured from fetuses delivered after administration of prostaglandin for legal abortion. The pancreas was harvested within 30 min of delivery and immediately minced into minute fragments (< 1 mm^3) in medium RPMI 1640. One to two hours later, the fragments were suspended for tissue culture in the same medium containing 20% calf serum and antibiotics, as described in detail elsewhere.[11] Six fetal pancreases collected over a 15-day period were used. The size of the fetuses, the estimated time of gestation, and the time the pancreatic tissue was maintained in tissue culture are given in Table 1.

About 3 h before transplantation, small samples of the cultured fragments were taken for morphologic examination and hormone extraction; in addition, samples of the culture medium were saved for bacteriologic control. A subsequent microscopic evaluation of tissue sections submitted to immunocytochemical staining for insulin showed a satisfactory morphologic appearance in all except pancreas no. 2,

TABLE 1
Data on the six human fetal pancreases used for transplantation

Pancreas no.	Size of fetus (cm)	Estimated time of gestation (wk)	Time in tissue culture
1	18	17	15 days
2	30	22	13 days
3	13	14	5 days
4	24	20	24 h
5	22	19	16 h
6	20	18	3 h

which had been cultured for 13 days. Scattered cells or islets staining positive for insulin were seen in all the pancreases (Figure 1). These observations were confirmed by the presence of significant amounts of extractable insulin in each of the glands. All the extracts contained, in addition, immunoreactive glucagon.

The transplantation. The pancreatic explants were harvested from the dishes 2–3 h before transplantation (9 May 1979). When sedimented at 1 × *g* in the culture medium, the total volume of tissue was approximately 3 ml.

After upper midline laparotomy, a catheter was placed in a right portal vein branch via a mesenteric vein. The location of the catheter was checked by radiography, contrast medium being injected into the catheter. A lateral inferior segment of the right liver lobe constituting approximately $^{1}/_{10}$ of the total liver volume was stained (Figure 2). The pancreatic tissue was suspended in 30 ml of normal saline and injected via the catheter over a period of 10 min. There was no change in the portal venous pressure. The pulse rate and the arterial blood pressure were unaffected.

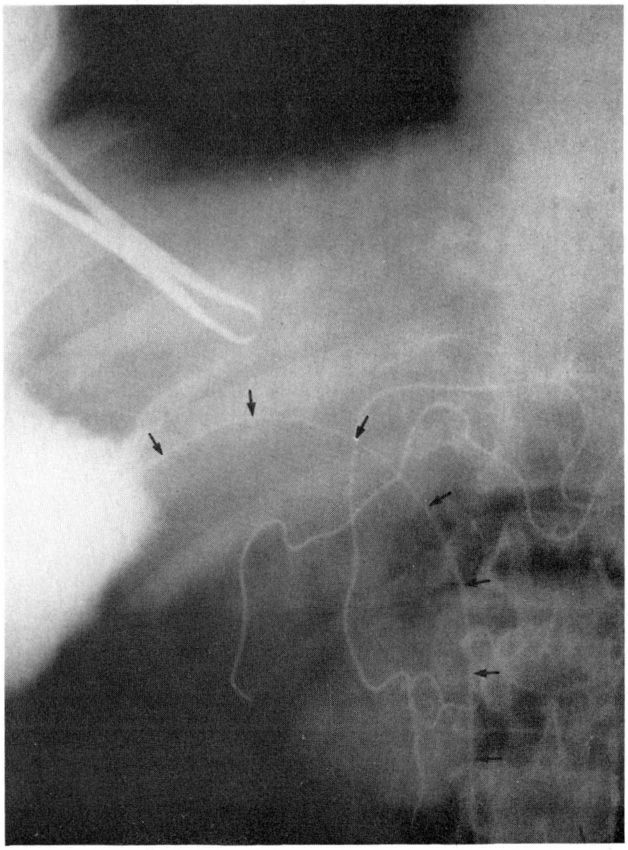

FIGURE 2. Radiograph showing the lateral, inferior segment of the right hepatic lobe (stained) into which the fetal pancreatic fragments were infused. The catheter in the right portal vein branch is also seen (arrows).

Immunosuppression. The patient had been on immunosuppression since the renal transplantation 2 yr earlier. Azathioprine was continued at about 2 mg/kg. On the day of the pancreatic transplantation, the daily prednisolone dose was increased from the previous 10 mg to 100 mg, after which it was gradually reduced to 25 mg. Administration of antithymocyte globulin elicited a severe reaction and had to be abandoned after two doses.

Course after transplantation. During the 40 days since the operation the course has been uneventful. The SGPT rose to 4.59 μkat/L on the day after the infusion, but by day 5 the

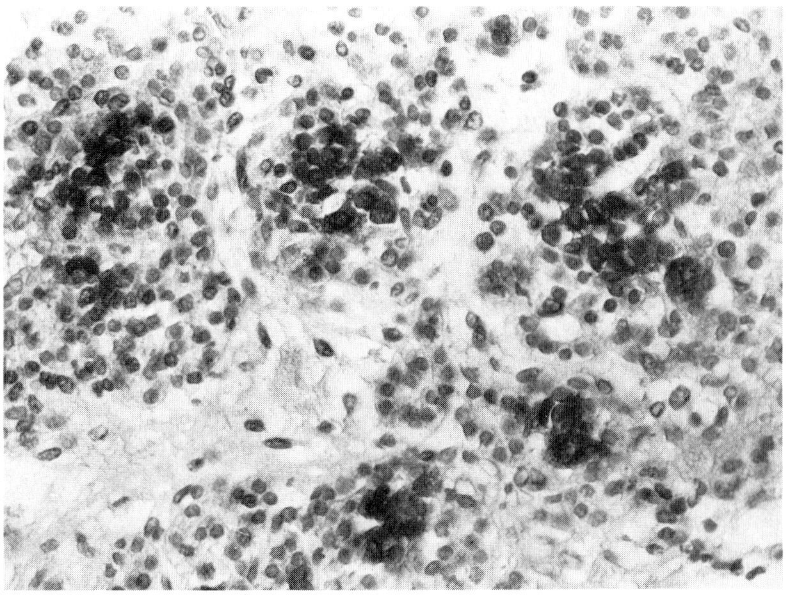

FIGURE 1. Light microscopic view of a fetal pancreatic explant cultured for 24 h before transplantation. Groups of dark-staining B cells containing insulin are scattered throughout the exocrine tissue. Due to the brief period of culture, acinar-like structures can still be recognized. Immunocytochemical staining for insulin[11] (×250).

level had returned to normal (<0.70). A liver scan performed 2 wk after the transplantation disclosed normal conditions not differing from those recorded a few days before the transplantation. There was no increase in serum amylase. Renal function has remained normal.

Before transplantation and during the first postoperative week, no C-peptide[12] was detected in the urine. From day 7 onwards there were, however, small amounts of C-peptide in most of the urine samples, the highest excretion being 820 pmol in 24 h (Figure 3). There seems to be some correlation between urine glucose and C-peptide, suggesting that the transplanted islets respond to a glucose load. The insulin requirement increased somewhat after transplantation, presumably as a result of the increase in the steroid dose (Figure 3). Search for C-peptide in the plasma has been negative throughout.

COMMENTS

The microfragments were transplanted via the portal vein because this has proved to be the most effective route in numerous rodent experiments. To minimize the effects of any liver damage, a small peripheral portal vein branch was used; however, the only untoward effect was a moderate transient rise in the serum transaminases. This feature suggests that the fragments were embolized into the liver as intended; the absence of such a rise would have indicated mere passage of the fragments through the hepatic circulation.

During the short interval since the transplantation was performed there has been no reduction in the patient's insulin requirement; however, no immediate effect on the diabetic state of the grafted endocrine cells could be expected, since the total amount of tissue infused must have been far below that required for a prompt therapeutic action. The appearance of C-peptide in the urine is encouraging, but the concentrations have so far been only a few percent of those recorded for normal subjects at our laboratory (Gunnarsson, unpublished). The transplantation was, however, performed in the hope that growth of the fetal material[6,7,13] would lead to a gradual increase in the insulin production. This would, of course, hinge on there being no rejection. In this respect, the fact that the patient has been immunologically unresponsive to the renal graft is a hopeful sign.

ACKNOWLEDGMENTS

This study was supported by the Swedish Medical Research Council (16X-7527; 12X-109; 12X-2297), the Swedish Diabetes Association, the Edle Johansson Foundation, Nordisk Insulinfond, and Stiftelsen Expressens Prenatalforskningsnämnd.

REFERENCES

1 Hegre, O. D., Wells, L. J., and Lazarow, A.: Response of beta cells to different levels of glucose: fetal pancreases grown in organ culture and subsequently transplanted to maternal hosts. Diabetes *19*:906–15, 1970.

2 Hegre, O. D., Wells, L. J., and Lazarow, A.: Insulin content of fetal rat pancreases grown in organ culture and subsequently transplanted into maternal hosts. Diabetes *21*:193–203, 1972.

3 Hegre, O. D., McEvoy, R. C., Bachelder, V., and Lazarow, A.: Fetal rat pancreas. Differentiation of the islet cell component in vivo and in vitro. Diabetes *22*:577–83, 1973

4 Brown, J., Molnar, I. G., Clark, W., and Mullen, Y.: Control of experimental diabetes mellitus in rats by transplantation of fetal pancreases. Science *184*:1377–79, 1974.

5 Brown, J., Clark, W. R., Molnar, I. G., and Mullen, Y. S.: Fetal pancreas transplantation for reversal of streptozotocin-induced diabetes in rats. Diabetes *25*:56–64, 1976.

6 Mullen, Y. S., Clark, W. R., Molnar, I. G., Kemp, J., and Brown, J.: Complete reversal of experimental diabetes mellitus in rats by a single fetal pancreas. Science *195*:68–70, 1976.

7 Hegre, O. D., Leonard, R. J., Rusin, J. D., and Lazarow, A.: Transplantation of the fetal rat pancreas: quantitative morphological analysis of islet tissue growth. Anat. Rec. *185*:209–21, 1976.

8 Hellerström, C., and Andersson, A.: Isolation, culture and transplantation of human islet tissue. *In* Carbohydrate Metabolism and Its Disorders.

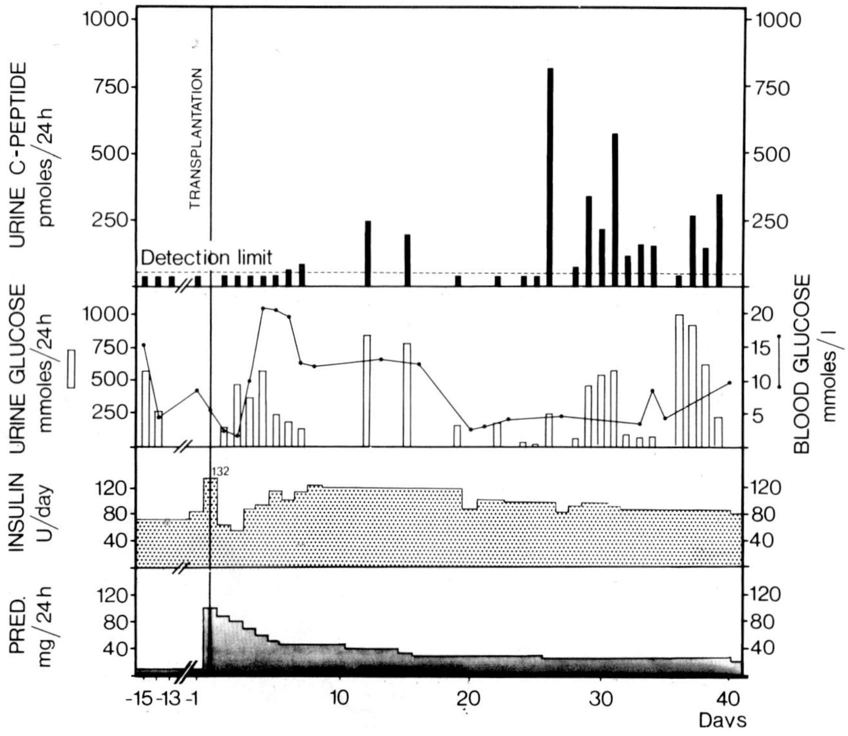

FIGURE 3. Course following intraportal transplantation of fetal pancreatic microfragments (pred. = prednisolone).

Randle, P. J., Steiner, D. F., and Wheelan, W. J., Eds. London, Academic Press, 1979.

[9] Sutherland, D. E. R., Matas, A. J., and Najarian, J. S.: Pancreatic islet cell transplantation. Surg. Clin. North Am. *58*:365–82, 1978.

[10] Sutherland, D. E. R., Matas, A. J., Goetz, F. C., and Najarian, J. S.: Transplantation of dispersed pancreatic islet tissue in humans: autografts and allografts. Diabetes *29* (Suppl. 1):31–44, 1980.

[11] Ågren, A., Andersson, A., Björkén, C., Groth, C. G., Gunnarsson, R., Hellerström, C., Lindmark, G., Lundqvist, G., Petersson, B., and Swenne, I.: Human fetal pancreas: culture and function in vitro. Diabetes *29* (Suppl. 1):64–69, 1980.

[12] Heding, L. G.: Radioimmunological determination of human C-peptide in serum. Diabetologia *11*:541–48, 1975.

[13] McEvoy, R. C., and Hegre, O. D.: Syngeneic transplantation of fetal rat pancreas. III. Effect of insulin treatment on the growth and differentiation of the pancreatic implants after reversal of diabetes. Diabetes *28*:141–46, 1979.

Discussion
Sections on Human Fetal Pancreas

Discussion of the survival of the human fetal pancreas in organ culture and its response to exogenous glucose stimulation was initiated by Hellerström and Turtle and centered on the optimum culture conditions required to achieve functional maturity of the organ. The importance of supplementing the culture media with amino acids was reemphasized by Turtle and may have accounted for the poor insulin response of the fetal explants to exogenous glucose as noted by Hellerström. Comparisons of media supplemented by fetal calf versus human serum are preliminary, although human adult islet cells appear better preserved in homologous serums (Hellerström). The need for a well buffered culture medium was highlighted.

The critical issue of whether the insulin content of the fetal pancreas cultures reflects an increase in number of cells or hormone content per B cell remains unsolved. With regard to functional integrity, pleas were made not to extrapolate the low level in vitro response of fetal pancreas to glucose with the transplant situation, where a period of in vivo maturation may lead to an adequate insulin release. Furthermore, results of theophylline stimulation had a tendency to inflate expectations from cultured tissue and should be taken in context of the physiologic requirement necessary to absolve hyperglycemia.

An important issue requiring further experimentation is the optimum amount of insulin-producing tissue necessary for fetal pancreas or islet cell transplantation in human subjects. From preliminary animal and human research, it is surmised that only a fraction (perhaps 20%) of the original islet cell mass would be adequate to render the diabetic recipient normoglycemic; however, the functional performance of transplanted tissue would depend on a variety of factors, including immunosuppressive agents administered to the recipient (specifically corticosteroids), the nature of the donor tissue (islet cells versus whole organ preparations), site of transplant (intraportal, subcutaneous, or subcapsular beneath the kidney capsule), and possibly histocompatibility match.

Of practical importance was the suggestion that transplantation of islet cell tissue into the forearm may facilitate sampling for functional integrity by drawing blood from the antecubital vein and using the opposite forearm for baseline control values. The measurement of urine C-peptide values in renal transplant recipients receiving pancreas grafts should be interpreted with caution, since renal tissue is the major site of C-peptide metabolism. Furthermore, in kidney recipients, intraportal injection of islets may be preferable to subcapsular transplantation of pancreatic tissue, as the latter graft may be adversely compromised by impaired vascularity and fibrosis of the kidney capsule. The suggestion that only nonresponder kidney-graft recipients be specifically selected as recipients of pancreas transplants was well received. This would require a waiting period after kidney transplantation to establish the responder status of the recipient. Finally, long-term monitoring of transplanted fetal tissue in vivo was emphasized, as animal data has shown that fetal tissue requires a period (weeks to months) of growth before realizing its full functional capacity.

The successful cryopreservation of fetal rat and human pancreases was extended to include similar results for porcine and for neonatal and adult rat islet cells. The importance of a controlled rate of freezing pancreases or islet cells was emphasized. Rates of cooling of approximately 0.25°C/min were considered optimal, with rates greater than 1°C/min adversely compromising isolated islet or whole pancreas survival. However, reports of successful cryopreservation of rat islet cells using an initial rate of cooling of 1.5°/min to a temperature of −35°C followed by 7.5°C/min to −100°C were mentioned. No standardization of thawing rate after cryopreservation was adopted, although room temperature thawing (approximately 7.5°C/min) had been used most frequently by the participants in this discussion. With regard to rat fetal pancreas, room temperature thawing gave better results than 37°C warming. Parenthetically, it was mentioned that allograft rejection with cryopreserved pancreases occurred at a similar rate as nonfrozen controls. The technique of cryopreservation should enable transport of donor organs to histocompatible recipients and allow the temporary storage of islet cells in transplant situations demanding a large number of beta cells.

The histologic survival and growth of xenogeneic human fetal pancreases in immunodeficient nude murine recipients was discussed by Usadel. Pertinent to the work was the comment that, despite normal histologic appearances, grafts transplanted into the subcutaneous or intramuscular sites may be functionally deficient in meeting insulin requirements. Further experimentation is required to confirm this observation. The use of 7–12-wk-old human fetuses posed problems with HLA typing, as histocompatibility antigens were difficult to detect on thymus or liver cells of the fetus before 16 wk of gestational age. Finally, the ability of the nude animal to reject intraperitoneal islet cells highlighted non-T-lymphocyte-mediated mechanisms of immune rejection in such grafts.

Immunologic Problems in Islet Transplantation

CLYDE F. BARKER, ALI NAJI, AND WILLYS K. SILVERS

SUMMARY

Rapid rejection of islet allografts is due to both cellular and antibody mechanisms. Isolated islets transplanted intraportally across a major histocompatibility complex (MHC) barrier in rats are rejected in 3–5 days. However, with MHC identity, the median survival time can be as long as 30.5 days. In mice, isolated islets transplanted between H-2-compatible strains survive no more than 1 wk, only a few days more than with an H-2-incompatible cross. In addition, in certain strains of rats and mice, islet isografts from male donors are rejected by female recipients. Fetal pancreases transplanted beneath the kidney capsule (Lewis to Fisher) are rapidly rejected by 4 days, although long-established grafts of fetal pancreas are not vulnerable to rejection in contrast to adult islets. Minimizing histoincompatibility has been unsuccessful in overcoming rejection because of the universal vulnerability of transplanted islets, and attempts to minimize immunogenicity by use of fetal tissue have not prevented rejection; however, culture of donor tissue may prove helpful in reducing immunogenicity. Transplantation of islet tissue into immunologically privileged sites has not resulted in reliable reversal of diabetes. Immunosuppression by pharmacologic agents such as cyclophosphamide, azathioprine, and corticosteroids was of minor effectiveness, but antilymphocytic serum was quite effective in rodents, even on xenografts when the injections were continued. Immunologic tolerance produced at birth by donor lymphopoietic cells permits later engraftment of isolated donor islets or whole pancreas. However, enhancement by antidonor antibody has not been greatly effective in protecting islets against rejection. The possibility that autoimmunity to islet tissue might interfere with the function of transplanted islets was tested in three types of possible autoimmunity: (1) repeated small doses of streptozotocin, (2) encephalomyocarditis virus, and (3) "BB" rats. In all three cases, transplanted islets were effective in reversing experimental diabetes. **DIABETES 29 (Suppl. 1):86–92, 1980.**

From the Harrison Department of Surgical Research and the Department of Human Genetics, School of Medicine, University of Pennsylvania.

Initial optimism for success of islet allografts was based on the earlier demonstration that some endocrine tissues, such as ovary,[1] when transplanted evoked only a feeble immunologic response as compared with skin grafts, at times even inducing tolerance of subsequent allografts of other tissues from the same donor.[2] It had also been noted that pancreas allografts, when examined histologically after rejection, may possibly display less islet damage than exocrine destruction.[3] Notwithstanding more recent demonstrations that parathyroid[4] and thyroid[5] are other examples of endocrine tissues enjoying some immunologic privilege, initial attempts at transplanting allogeneic isolated islets in rats indicated that these were rejected with profound rapidity, sometimes surviving only 1 or 2 days if transplanted across strong histocompatibility barriers.[6] Indeed, because this anomalously rapid destruction of allografts was difficult to attribute to usual mechanisms of rejection, Matas et al. suggested that it might be caused by technical rather than immunologic factors.[7] Nevertheless, very short-lived functional survival of allografted islets has now been documented by many investigators working with rats,[8] mice,[9] dogs,[10] monkeys,[11] and possibly humans.[12] In contrast, islets transplanted by the same techniques into syngeneic or autologous recipients are able to function indefinitely.

Because strongly histoincompatible islet allografts are so rapidly rejected, Franklin et al. determined the immediate fate of Wistar-Furth (WF) islets when inoculated into the portal vein of MHC (major histocompatibility complex)-incompatible recipients.[13] They found that histologic sections of the livers of the transiently normoglycemic rats had islets of normal appearance after 24 h, but that by 48 h mononuclear cells occurred at the periphery of the islets and by the fourth posttransplant day there was a heavy lymphocytic infiltration accompanied by recurrent hyperglycemia. They concluded that islet destruction was primarily cell mediated, though they noted that some antibody-producing plasma cells also occurred in the cellular infiltrates.

A brisk humoral response has also been observed by us

in rats within a week of their inoculation with allogeneic islets. For examining the possible vulnerability of islets to humoral damage, Naji et al. used Wistar-Furth (WF) rats which had been rendered tolerant of ACI antigens by neonatal inoculation with (WF × ACI) F1 bone marrow cells.[14] When adult, these rats, all of which displayed well-established ACI skin grafts, were rendered diabetic with streptozotocin and then transplanted with allogeneic islets from ACI donors. After 30 days of normoglycemia, they were treated with daily intravenous injections of 1 cm^3 of antiserum raised in WF rats against ACI antigens. Hyperglycemia usually recurred within 1 or 2 days and always by the seventh day. The ACI skin grafts did not suffer acute damage, although in some instances they were chronically rejected after about 30 days, suggesting that the antisera in these rats had abrogated the tolerant (chimeric) state by destroying the neonatally inoculated (WF × ACI) F1 bone marrow cells. The early recurrence of hyperglycemia, however, could only be explained on the basis that the islets were highly sensitive to humoral antibody. Using an identical protocol, Naji and Barker found that parathyroid allografts were not damaged by antibody.[15] Frangipane et al. also demonstrated that transplanted rat islets are easily damaged by antibody.[16] In their experiments, antilymphocyte serum was used to establish intraperitoneally transplanted islets from ACI rat donors in streptozotocin-diabetic mice. The normoglycemic mouse recipients of these islet xenografts were then treated with injections of either mouse anti-rat antibody or an alloantibody raised in WF rats against ACI antigens. In both instances the recurrence of hyperglycemia followed in 1–2 days. The vulnerability to xenoantiserum of rat islets transplanted to immunosuppressed mice was also noted by Delmonico et al.[17] Evidence that islets may be damaged by antibody is also possibly provided by the results of experiments in which attempts to prolong survival of islet allografts by enhancement with antidonor antibody have sometimes been found instead to shorten their survival.[18,19]

The possibility that macrophages are readily attracted to the transplant site has also been suggested as contributing to the rapid destruction of islet allografts, and some evidence that this may be the case is provided by the strikingly prolonged survival reported by Nash and Bell in recipients of rat islet allografts treated with the antimacrophage agents, silica and carrageenan.[20]

ATTEMPTS TO OVERCOME REJECTION

Attempts to avoid rejection of transplanted islets can be grouped into the following categories: (1) minimizing histoincompatibility, (2) minimizing immunogenicity, (3) use of immunologically privileged sites, (4) immunosuppression. Primarily only our own work, published and unpublished, is reviewed here. However, reports of other workers are also mentioned where appropriate, excluding for the most part material to be found elsewhere in this symposium.

Minimizing histoincompatibility. This approach to extending allograft survival has been widely used both experimentally and clinically and has proved particularly effective in the case of some endocrine tissues—e.g., parathyroid,[21] thyroid,[5] and ovary[2]—that may enjoy virtually indefinite survival if donor and recipient are MHC identical. This same principle also holds (though to a considerably lesser extent) for islet tissue. In rats, islets transplanted by portal vein inoculation across an MHC barrier are rejected very rapidly, i.e., WF → ACI 4.8 days,[22] F → ACI 3.7 days,[23] (AS × August)F1 → AS 3.2 days,[24] BN → Lewis 5.5 days,[25] ACI → Lewis 5.2 days.[26] In the more weakly histoincompatible F → L combination, prolongation is not greatly increased (7.8 days),[26] perhaps reflecting the fact that these rats are not truly MHC identical, though both type as $RT1^{l}$.[27] However, in the more closely related, MHC identical DA → ACI (both $RT1^{a}$) combination, median survival was considerably longer, 30.5 days.[28] Similar observations have been made in mice by Frangipane et al. Thus, in this species, H-2-compatible allogeneic islets survive no more than 1 wk, only a few days longer than H-2-incompatible ones.[29] It is somewhat disappointing with regard to the usefulness of this approach and its logical clinical counterpart (that of seeking an optimal histocompatibility match of donor and recipient) that, even when donor and recipient differ only with respect to the comparatively weak H-Y antigen, transplanted islets may be rapidly rejected. Thus, in certain strains of both rats and mice, islet isografts from male donors are rejected by female recipients. In mice, rejection of H-Y-incompatible islets appears to occur only in strains in which females are also capable of rejecting male skin isografts, i.e., C57BL/6 but not C3H/Hej. However, in female C57BL/6 mice, rejection of male islets occurs more rapidly than rejection of skin transplanted across H-Y barrier (<7 days vs. 20–29 days), a finding which provides additional evidence of the unusual vulnerability of transplanted islets.[29]

Minimizing immunogenicity. Several strategies by which donor islets might be presented to recipients in a less immunogenic form are (1) as fetal tissue, (2) after pretransplant culture or other treatment, and (3) as an immediately vascularized graft.

Fetal skin is known to be rejected less rapidly than adult skin (a highly immunogenic tissue). Indeed, in rats and mice, fetal or neonatal skin may not be rejected in situations where adult skin is.[30] Spence et al., therefore, examined the possible advantages of using whole fetal pancreas in rats as a source of allogeneic islets.[31,32] Using the techniques of Brown et al.,[33] he found that syngeneic transplantation of the fetal pancreas under the kidney capsule of diabetic rats resulted in normoglycemia within 20–30 days. However, when Lewis pancreas was transplanted to diabetic Fischer rats, hyperglycemia was never corrected. This result correlated with the histologic finding that destruction of the pancreas by mononuclear infiltration was far advanced within 4 days, so that rejection was complete before the time that normoglycemia occurs after transplantation of syngeneic fetal pancreas. This finding has been confirmed by Brown et al.[34] and by Garvey and Morris.[35]

Despite this disappointing result, we have recently obtained some indirect evidence that fetal pancreas may be preferable to adult isolated islets. This evidence concerns the vulnerability of fetal pancreas and adult islets to adoptive immunity in tolerant recipients. Thus, it was found that, when Fischer rats tolerant of Lewis antigens and cured of their diabetes for 2–6 mo with Lewis fetal pancreas were given normal Fischer lymph node and spleen cells to abrogate tolerance, they did not become hyperglycemic. After an additional 2–6 mo, excision of the transplant confirmed the presence of healthy allogeneic islet tissue and the animals subsequently became hyperglycemic. Apparently, long-established grafts of fetal pancreas do not remain vulnerable to rejection, at least in some instances. Although this finding is in keeping with the general principle that long-standing grafts are more resistant to immune damage than fresh ones, we have consistently found that isolated *adult* allogeneic islets transplanted across the same histocompatibility barrier into tolerant hosts remain fully vulnerable to rejection, being destroyed in about 10 days after abrogation of tolerance. Therefore, it appears that the fetal pancreas may have an immunologic advantage over adult islets, though the demonstration of this requires a complex experimental protocol.

Another method aimed at diminishing immunogenicity is treatment of donor tissue before transplantation. This is not a new idea, and such techniques as perfusion of kidney allografts with RNA, DNA, or Fab fragments have been proposed as possibly altering allografts in some favorable manner.[36] Following the ingenious demonstration by Steinmuller that "passenger leukocytes" trapped within skin grafts and, thus, transplanted along with them were, in themselves, sufficient to sensitize the recipient,[37] attention was given to methods by which various techniques (e.g., perfusion with large volumes of saline or with antilymphocyte serum [ALS]) might remove these cells, conceivably deleting the only component of the graft responsible for immunizing the recipient. These attempts proved unrewarding.[38]

The major impetus for subsequent attempts to attenuate immunogenicity of islets and other tissues was unquestionably provided by Summerlin's reports that, after a period of culture, skin grafts could be grafted to allogeneic mouse or human recipients without provoking rejection.[39] Unfortunately, Summerlin's claims have not been confirmed.[40] Although there were also preliminary reports of successful modulation of islet rejection by this technique,[41] Raaf's careful experiments with cultured thyroid and parathyroid[42] and Hegre's with islet tissue[43] appeared to dispel any likelihood that by employing this technique rejection could be avoided, except possibly in the case of weakly antigenic tissues such as certain tumors.[44] Nevertheless, interest in this approach was recently rekindled by Lafferty's report that thyroid allografts cultured for 21 days or more under conditions of a high O_2 atmosphere could subsequently be transplanted successfully to allogeneic recipients where they enjoyed prolonged survival without rejection.[45] They also presented evidence that the change in immunogenicity occurred on the basis of deletion from the cultured graft of passenger leukocytes, especially macrophages, since these cells could not survive prolonged periods at high oxygen concentrations. Moreover, transplantation of fresh donor leukocytes along with the cultured graft brought about graft destruction. Sollinger et al. reported success with cultured rat thyroid transplanted to xenogeneic mouse hosts.[46] Naji et al. have recently shown that another endocrine tissue (parathyroid) enjoys prolonged survival when transplanted across the strong RT1 barrier in rats (ACI → F) following prolonged (26 days) culture, but only if maintained in an atmosphere of 95% O_2 and 5% CO_2 as compared with the usual 95% air and 5% CO_2.[47] Attempts at maintaining islets for more than a few days at 95% O_2 have been unsuccessful. Barker recently observed that fetal or newborn pancreases of rats and mice also undergo necrosis within 4 or 5 days when exposed to 95% O_2 atmosphere in culture.[48] However, Mandel was able to preserve fetal mouse pancreas for several weeks in vitro and reported that this tissue had prolonged survival when subsequently transplanted into allogeneic hosts.[49] Lacy's recent reports (see his contribution to this symposium) also suggest that by modification of culture conditions isolated islets can be stored long enough to bring about at least small changes in the subsequent survival after transplantation. However, Lacy needed a combination of several manipulations of the donor, such as radiation or pretreatment with silica, both designed to remove passenger leukocytes, as well as ALS treatment of recipients in order to achieve strikingly prolonged survival after transplantation.[50] This may be a further indication that islet tissue is more immunogenic or more vulnerable to rejection than other endocrine tissues, since culturing alone appears to prolong survival of thyroid and parathyroid allografts. Should culturing techniques ultimately prove of clinical usefulness in avoiding rejection, some of the credit will be due to the unfortunate Summerlin.

An older technique of transplanting islet tissue which is likely to be associated with less formidable immunologic problems than isolated islet transplantation is transplantation of the vascularized pancreas. At the time of the initial recognition that allografts of isolated islets in the rat were rejected within a few days, there was little information on survival of whole pancreas allografts in this species, although in large animals, such as the dog, vascularized pancreatic allograft survival was known to be roughly comparable to that of other organs, i.e., 8–12 days.[51] Subsequently, it has been demonstrated by Bitter-Suermann that pancreatic allografts transplanted across major barriers in rats survive about as well as those of kidney or heart (7–12 days).[52] However, Perloff has recently demonstrated that, in Fischer rats, RTI-compatible Lewis pancreases are likely to survive for many weeks,[53] as is also the case for kidney[54] and heart.[55] These findings, in conjunction with the demonstration that isolated islet allografts in several species other than the rat (i.e., dog and pig) are rejected after only a few days, leave little doubt that, in unmodified hosts, isolated islet allografts fare much worse than vascularized whole organs. The demonstration by Naji et al. that established ACI isolated islet allografts in tolerant WF rats are destroyed within 4–8 days if tolerance is abrogated by inoculating the animals with normal WF lymphoid cells clearly indicates that the seemingly increased vulnerability of the isolated islets is not confined to the early posttransplant period when important roles could be played by damage incurred during processing or by ischemia prior to neovascularization.[56] However, the reasons for the anomalously short-lived survival of allogeneic islets remain obscure. Whether or not vascularized allografts of pancreas, like kidney or heart, will consistently have their survival more easily prolonged by immunosuppression, enhancement, or various forms of tolerance than isolated islets remains to be examined by critical experiments employing inbred rats, so that both transplant techniques can be performed and compared under genetically identical conditions. From preliminary results in dogs (and possibly human subjects), however, it appears that the vascularized organ will have the advantage in immunosuppressed as well as in normal hosts.

Immunologically privileged transplant sites. A major theoretical advantage of the isolated islet method of transplantation is that, since such a graft comprises only a small mass, it should be easy to implant anywhere. Not only would this make possible rapid, safe, and relatively painless instillation of islet allografts by simple injection into superficial tissues, but also the use of immunologically advantageous transplant sites might be possible. Early workers in islet transplantation were able to show that fragments of pancreas could be implanted and recovered from the classic privileged sites of the anterior chamber of the eye,[57] hamster cheek pouch,[58] and testicle.[59] In the last site it was also demonstrated by Ferguson and Scothorne that allogeneic islet tissue was protected from immune damage; however, in none of these instances was there convincing evidence that a diabetic status of the pancreas recipient could be altered, although usually only small amounts of islet tissue were transplanted in these experiments. We have found that large numbers of syngeneic islets prepared from up to 20 donors injected intramuscularly, subcutaneously, or into the testicle failed to correct the diabetic state and, in addition, unless separated from acinar tissue with particular care, caused extensive digestion of surrounding tissue through their enzymatic activity. Although successful transplantation of adult islets injected intravenously has been reported,[60] and Weber achieved correction of hyperglycemia by intramuscular implantation of islets isolated from more than 30 neonatal donors,[61] most workers have been able to achieve successful islet transplantation only in the liver, spleen, or peritoneal cavity. Hoping to take advantage of the fetal pancreas' limited enzymatic activity (and thus avoid possible autodigestion of the islet tissue), Spence undertook a systematic study of syngeneic whole fetal pancreas transplanted into superficial tissues that seemed to be promising transplant sites, using a dose of islet tissue (4–12 donors) he had shown to be routinely effective when transplanted under the kidney capsule or into the splenic pulp.[31] He found that, in rats and hamsters, diabetes was not altered by transplantation of fetal pancreas to the intramuscular, subcutaneous, testicular, or cheek pouch sites, and only a few viable islets could ever be identified histologically in these locations. In the case of the intramuscular and subcutaneous grafts, the results were particularly disappointing since there is evidence that both of these sites are immunologically semiprivileged. Naji has shown in the case of parathyroid[21] and Perloff in the case of thyroid[5] that allografts transplanted intramuscularly are rarely rejected when nonmajor (F → L) histoincompatibilities are involved. Billingham recently reported that small allografts of skin transplanted subcutaneously are rejected more slowly than orthotopic ones.[62]

The least favorable implant site in which transplanted islet allograft function has been obtained is the peritoneal cavity, where even very closely histocompatible DA allogeneic islets are rejected in 11.5 days by ACI recipients. In the same donor-recipient combination, intrahepatic islets survive for a median of 30.5 days.[63] Recently we have noted that there is also a strikingly better survival of weakly incompatible (H-Y) islets when transplanted intraportally as compared with intraperitoneally. It could be argued that the intraportal site is a relatively privileged one from the immunologic standpoint, and this viewpoint is supported by the finding of Pfefferman et al. that allogeneic parathyroids implanted directly into the liver (as distinguished from intraportal embolization) enjoy prolonged survival as compared with those transplanted intramuscularly.[64] It could equally well be argued that the peritoneal cavity is an unusually poor transplant site rather than the intraportal one being especially favorable, since an adequate comparison of only these two sites has thus far been carried out. Reckard's demonstration that islets implanted intrasplenically and intraportally are rejected equally rapidly by strongly histoincompatible ACI hosts was claimed by him to show immunologic parity of these two transplant sites.[22] However, to test whether the sites are truly similar will require repetition of these studies with a weakly incompatible donor-recipient combination. Since the spleen is a potentially useful clinical transplant site, it is an encouraging finding that rejection is not unusually abrupt when alien islets are implanted directly into this anatomic component of the immune system.

Another transplant strategy closely related to the immunologically privileged site is the semipermeable chamber. This technique appears to have promise if technological factors and bioincompatibility can be overcome.

Nonspecific immunosuppression. Nonspecific immunosuppressive agents which have been tested in islet allograft systems include pharmacologic agents and antilymphocyte serum. The results with pharmacologic agents have been especially discouraging. Finch and Morris found that (DA × Lewis)F1 islet survival was prolonged in Lewis rats by cyclophosphamide (10 mg/kg/day) only from 4.2 to 6.8 days.[65] Marquet and Heysteck achieved survival with Imuran of up to 25 days in two of five Sprague-Dawley (SD) recipients of WAG/RI5 islets, as compared with a survival of less than 10 days in unmodified hosts.[66] Corticosteroids, another mainstay of pharmacologic clinical immunosuppression, were found to be of no benefit by Nelken et al. in prolonging survival of WF islets in Lewis rats, when used as the sole immunosuppressive agent.[67] Schulack et al. evaluated the potential of high dose, intravenous methylprednisolone to reverse rejection of islets in rats, since this agent is used for this purpose in human renal allograft rejection episodes.[68] He found that it had no beneficial effect in this setting. In dogs, Sutherland et al. actually had the impression[10] that the use of high dose steroids might be detrimental to islet function.

Antilymphocyte serum has been used to prolong the function of islet transplants in rats and mice with substantially greater success than the pharmacologic agents. This is perhaps not surprising, since this agent is known to be particularly effective in extending the survival of other allografts in these species. Reckard et al. made the initial observation that islet allograft survival could be prolonged with ALS, finding that the rejection of intraperitoneal islets from DA donors could be delayed in MHC-compatible ACI recipients from 8.5 to 30.5 days by a 5-day course of treatment.[69] A number of investigators have also lengthened the survival of allogeneic rat islets transplanted across major and minor histocompatibility barriers with ALS.[66,67,70]

Frangipane et al. reported that survival of intraperitoneal isolated islets in mice was extended by ALS therapy, finding that it was effective in both H-2-compatible and-incompatible combinations, but that, in both situations, a brief course of ALS was capable of increasing skin allograft longevity more so than that of islet allografts.[29] An impressive demonstration of the effectiveness of ALS was also provided by us when rat islets were transplanted to diabetic mice being treated with this agent.[71] Indeed, normoglycemia was maintained as long as ALS therapy was continued (30 days) and for approximately an additional 10 days after the agent was discontinued. Few attempts have been made to achieve permanent survival of allotransplanted islets with the use of ALS. However, Gray and Watkins were able to avoid rejection of Lewis islets in all of 10 RTI-compatible Fischer recipients for 227 days by continuing ALS therapy.[72] Ziegler et al. found that, in the more closely related DA → ACI combination, even a short course of ALS was followed by function of islets in two of six recipients for more than 150 days. These long-term islet recipients also accepted ACI skin grafts, indicating that the islets in conjunction with ALS had induced a state of immunologic unresponsiveness.[73]

Further manipulation of the details of regimens of nonspecific immunosuppression in animal islet recipients seems unlikely to generate useful data. Experiments already performed allow us to draw the following conclusions: (1) immunosuppression (especially ALS in rodents) allows significant prolongation of survival of islet allografts and even xenografts; (2) identical immunosuppressive protocols are more effective in prolonging survival of whole organs (kidney, heart) or even of skin allografts than of islets transplanted across the same histocompatibility barriers. Experience with clinical and experimental transplantation of other tissues would lead us to be cautious about expecting that detailed protocols for optimal immunosuppression can be extrapolated from animal experiments to clinical trials in man. Thus, specific immunosuppression protocols for clinical use will probably have to be developed from experience in humans, though general principles learned from laboratory work are applicable.

Specific means of immunosuppression. Enhancement is a specific form of immunologic unresponsiveness which is brought about by administration of donor antigen or antidonor antibody with appropriate timing. Although several groups have reported limited success in extending islet allograft survival by this method (see full discussion by Morris in this symposium), it is clear from Reckard's[74] and Nash's[24] reports that allografts of vascularized whole organs (kidney and heart) are much more responsive than isolated islets to prolongation of survival in this way and that some enhancing protocols may even prejudice islet survival because of their susceptibility to humoral antibody.[19]

Immunologic tolerance is a specific unresponsive state most easily induced in rodents by their inoculation at the time of birth with lymphohematopoietic cells from the donor strain. Several of our experimental protocols have been dependent on this specific form of immunosuppression, which we have shown does allow permanent engraftment of isolated islet or freely grafted whole fetal pancreas allografts.[75] An interesting recent observation by us deserves mention here because of the current interest in the passenger leukocytes as an important, or even the sole, sensitizing influence in islet allografts. In rats, tolerance of subsequent skin allografts can be readily induced only if the neonatally inoculated donor cells are of bone marrow origin. However, if lymph node cells are used instead of bone marrow, a permanent chimeric state ensues and the subjects are tolerant of donor-type lymphoid cells (as shown by mixed lymphocyte cultures). These animals, which almost invariably promptly reject skin allografts of the donor strain, will usually permanently accept vascularized heart allografts of donor type.[76] We have recently found that these "lymph node cell-tolerant" chimeras show no prolongation of survival of donor strain isolated islet allografts. This finding could be explained by several mechanisms, including an islet-specific antigen not present on lymph node cells, but it seems incompatible with the hypothesis that passenger leukocytes are the only sensitizing stimulus present in the islet allograft inoculum, since the recipients are tolerant of these cells.

Further examination of the specific immunosuppressive maneuvers of enhancement and tolerance is warranted, not so much as a preliminary step to clinical application, which seems rather farfetched at present, but to further define the possibly peculiar immunologic properties of islets which are responsible for their anomalously rapid rejection.

POSSIBLE SUSCEPTIBILITY OF TRANSPLANTED ISLETS TO AUTOIMMUNITY

An additional immunologic problem not related to allograft rejection that should be considered in a discussion of islet transplantation is whether insulin-dependent diabetes is based on an autoimmune mechanism, and if so, whether newly transplanted islets would be susceptible to destruction by ongoing or reactivated autoimmunity. Islet transplantation has not been studied in experimental animals in which attempts were made to induce an autoimmune form of the disease by injection of islet tissue in conjunction with Freund's adjuvant. However, it seems unlikely that transplanted islets would succumb to this form of autoimmunity since only histologic changes in the native pancreatic islets and not frank hyperglycemia can be induced in this way. Another animal model of autoimmune diabetes has been examined with regard to the response to islet transplantation. If streptozotocin is administered repeatedly in small doses, hyperglycemia ensues at least partially on the basis of autoimmunity, as evidenced by the suppressive influence of ALS[77] and the finding that diabetes can be induced in secondary hosts by transfer of lymphoid cells.[78] This type of experimental diabetes has recently been shown to respond to treatment by transplanted syngeneic islets without any tendency of recipients to develop recurrent hyperglycemia.[79]

Another type of experimental diabetes is produced by inoculation of mice with encephalomyocarditis virus (EMC). Although actual necrosis of some islet tissue by viral infection occurs, strong suggestion of an autoimmune component is provided by a characteristic mononuclear infiltration of islets[80] and by reports that the disease may be passaged by lymphocytes even after virus can no longer be cultured from tissues.[81] Howard et al.[82] and Naji et al.[83] have shown that the hyperglycemia following EMC infection responds to replacement with syngeneic islets. Howard used a strain of mouse (SWR/J) which usually spontaneously recovers from diabetes within a few weeks, making it necessary for him to carry out islet transplantation very early in the course of the disease, since, later on, normoglycemia on the basis of islet transplant function could not be distinguished from that caused by recovery of native islets. Naji's mice, however, were of a strain (DBA/2) in which some members became permanently hyperglycemic after treatment with virus. Such mice were transplanted only after they had been hyperglycemic for at least 30 days. Transplantation was by insertion of four to eight syngeneic fetal pancreases under the kidney capsule, a technique that is followed by gradual return of normoglycemia over a period of several weeks or months.

After 2–6 mo of normoglycemia, the transplant was excised and the prompt return of hyperglycemia which was observed indicated that previous normoglycemia had been on the basis of the transplanted pancreas. Retransplantation of fetal pancreas to the contralateral kidney capsule was followed by normoglycemia, and, subsequently, excision of the second transplant a month later was again found to result in recurrent hyperglycemia. The entire course of the experiment comprised an 11-mo span, serving to indicate that latent virus was unlikely to damage transplanted pancreas in this experimental model. Taken together, Howard's and Naji's studies constitute strong evidence that neither early or late damage to transplanted pancreas is likely to prevent the beneficial effect of the treatment in virally induced diabetes, despite the fact that this type of diabetes is induced, at least partially, on the basis of autoimmunity.

We have worked with one additional model of diabetes which closely mimics human juvenile-onset diabetes, is of unknown etiology, and seems highly likely to be caused by autoimmunity. About 25% of "BB" rats spontaneously develop diabetes, usually between 60 and 120 days. Characteristic of the syndrome are hypoinsulinemia, ketosis, and severe hyperglycemia.[84] A striking mononuclear infiltration of the pancreatic islets, very similar to that seen in EMC viral diabetes and recent onset human insulin-dependent diabetes, is seen in BB rats if the pancreases are examined at the time of onset of their disease. Naji et al. found that BB rats could be successfully treated with islet transplantation.[83] Since BB rats are outbred, syngeneic donors could not be used. Wistar-Furth ($RT1^{\mu}$) donors were used because serologic typing indicated that BB rats were also $RT1^{\mu}$. Transplanted WF islets were rejected within 7 days in nonimmunosuppressed BB rats, despite relatively close histocompatibility. In ALS-treated BB rats, intraportal transplantation with WF islets resulted in normoglycemia for up to 6 mo, but if immunosuppression was discontinued, hyperglycemia recurred. In 10 long-term recipients of WF islets, histologic examination of the liver demonstrated healthy transplanted islets, while the native pancreatic islets were usually atrophic, indicating that the normoglycemic status of these rats was dependent on the transplanted islets rather than on recovery of the possibly autoimmune insulitis of the BB animals, under the influence of immunosuppression. Nevertheless, in two other long-term ALS-treated transplant recipients, the native pancreatic islets were found to be relatively healthy in appearance, a finding consistent with Like's report that some BB rats can be cured of diabetes with ALS alone.[85]

It appears from the available experimental evidence that transplanted islets can function successfully in animals with several types of probably autoimmune-based diabetes. This argues favorably for the role of transplantation in human diabetes if it proves to be of autoimmune etiology. The finding that immunosuppression alone is useful in treating or preventing some types of experimental diabetes is another intriguing suggestion of the importance of immune mechanisms in this disease.

ACKNOWLEDGMENTS

This work was supported in part by USPHS grants AM19525, CA15822, and AM26007 and by the Thomas McCabe Fund.

REFERENCES

[1] Linder, O. E. A.: Comparisons between survival of grafted skin, ovaries, and tumors in mice across histocompatibility of different strengths. J. Natl. Cancer Inst. *27*:351–73, 1961.

[2] Billingham, R. E., and Parkes, A. S.: Studies on the survival of homografts of skin and ovarian tissue in rats. Proc. R. Soc. B. *143*:550–60, 1955.

[3] Lillehei, R. C., Simmons, R. L., Najarian, J. S., Weil, R., Chida, H., Ruiz, J. O., Kjellstrand, C. V., and Goetz, F. C.: Pancreatico-duodenal allotransplantation, experimental and clinical experience. Ann. Surg. *172*:405–36, 1979.

[4] Russell, P. S., and Gittes, R. F.: Parathyroid transplants in rats: a comparison of their survival times with skin grafts. J. Exp. Med. *109*:571–88, 1959.

[5] Perloff, L. J., Utiger, R. D., Alavi, A., and Barker, C. F.: Thyroid graft: influence of histocompatibility and transplant site on survival. Ann. Surg. *188*:186–96, 1978.

[6] Reckard, C. R., and Barker, C. F.: Transplantation of isolated pancreatic islets across strong and weak histocompatibility barriers. Transplant. Proc. *5*:761–63, 1973.

[7] Matas, A. J., Sutherland, D. E. R., Steffes, M. W., and Najarian, J. S.: Minimal collagenase digestion: Amelioration of diabetes in the rat with transplantation of one dispersed neonatal pancreas. Transplantation *22*:71–73, 1976.

[8] Shulack, J. A., and Reckard, C. R.: Experimental transplantation of pancreatic islet allografts. J. Surg. Res. *25*:562–81, 1978.

[9] Panijananond, P., and Monaco, A. P.: Enhancement of pancreatic islet allograft survival with ALS and donor bone marrow. Surg. Forum *25*:379–81, 1974.

[10] Sutherland, D. E. R., Kretschmer, G. J., Matas, A. J., and Najarian, J. S.: Experience with auto and allotransplantation of pancreatic fragments to the spleen of totally pancreatectomized dogs. Trans. Am. Soc. Artif. Intern. Organs *23*:723–25, 1977.

[11] Scharp, D. W., Murphy, J. J., Newton, W. T., Ballinger, W. F., and Lacy, P. E.: Transplantation of islets of Langerhans in diabetic rhesus monkeys. Surgery *77*:100–05, 1975.

[12] Najarian, J. S., Sutherland, D. E. R., Matas, A. J., Steffes, M. W., and Goetz, F. C.: Human islet transplantation: a preliminary report. Transplant. Proc. *9*:233–36, 1977.

[13] Franklin, W. A., Schulack, J. A., and Reckard, C. R.: The fate of transplanted pancreatic islets in the rat. Am. J. Pathol. *94*:85–95, 1979.

[14] Naji, A., Reckard, C. R., Ziegler, M. M., and Barker, C. F.: Vulnerability of pancreatic islets to immune cells and serum. Surg. Forum *26*:459–61, 1975.

[15] Naji, A., and Barker, C. F.: Differential susceptibility of endocrine tissue to humoral immunity. Surg. Forum *29*:349–51, 1978.

[16] Frangipane, L. G., Poole, T. W., and Barker, C. F.: Vulnerability of allogeneic and xenogeneic islets to alloantisera. Transplant. Proc. *9*:371–73, 1977.

[17] Delmonico, F. L., Chase, C. M., and Russell, P. S.: Transplantation of rat islets of Langerhans into diabetic mice. Transplant. Proc. *9*:367–69, 1977.

[18] Finch, D. R. A., and Morris, P. J.: Passive enhancement of isolated pancreatic islet allografts. Transplantation *22*:508–12, 1976.

[19] Barker, C. F., and Sutherland, D. E. R.: Pancreatic islet cells in management of diabetes. Transplant. Proc. *9*:1257–58, 1977.

[20] Nash, J. R., and Bell, P. R.: Effect of macrophage suppression on the survival of islet allografts. Transplant. Proc. *11*:986–88, 1979.

[21] Naji, A., and Barker, C. F.: The influence of histocompatibility and tranplant site on parathyroid allograft survival. J. Surg. Res. *20*:261–67, 1976.

[22] Reckard, C. R., Franklin, W., and Shulack, J. A.: Intrasplenic vs. intraportal pancreatic islet transplants: quantitative, qualitative and immunological aspects. Trans. Am. Soc. Artif. Intern. Organs *24*:232–34, 1978.

[23] Reckard, C. R.: Personal communication.

[24] Nash, J. R., Peters, M., and Bell, P. R. F.: Comparative survival of pancreatic islets, heart, kidney and skin allografts in rats with and without enhancement. Transplantation *24*:70–73, 1977.

[25] Naji, A., and Barker, C. F.: Unpublished data.

[26] Lacy, P. E., Davie, J. M., and Finke, E. H.: Prolongation of islet allograft survival following in vitro culture (24°C) and a single injection of ALS. Science *204*:312–13, 1979.

[27] Marshak, A., Doherty, P. C., and Wilson, D. B.: The control of specificity of cytotoxic T lymphocytes by the major histocompatibility complex (Ag-B) in system showing no Ag-B restriction. J. Exp. Med. *146*:1773–90, 1977.

[28] Ziegler, M. M., Reckard, C. R., Naji, A., and Barker, C. F.: Extended

function of isolated pancreatic islet isografts and allografts. Transplant. Proc. *7*:743–48, 1975.

[29] Frangipane, L. G., Barker, C. F., and Silvers, W. K.: Importance of weak histocompatibility factors in survival of pancreatic islet transplants. Surg. Forum *28*:294–96, 1977.

[30] Wachtel, S. S., and Silvers, W. K.: The role of passenger leukocytes in the anomalous survival of neonatal skin grafts in mice. J. Exp. Med. *135*:388–404, 1972.

[31] Spence, R. K., Perloff, L. J., and Barker, C. F.: The role of the implant site in rat fetal pancreas transplantation. Trans. Am. Soc. Artif. Intern. Organs *23*:352–57, 1977.

[32] Spence, R. K., Perloff, L. J., and Barker, C. F.: Fetal pancreas in treatment of experimental diabetes in rats. Transplant. Proc. *11*:533–36, 1979.

[33] Brown, J., Molnar, I. G., Clark, W., and Mullen, Y.: Control of experimental diabetes mellitus in rats by transplantation of fetal pancreas. Science *184*:1377–379, 1974.

[34] Brown, J., Clarke, W. R., Makoff, R. K., Weissman, H., Kemp, J. A., and Mullen, Y.: Pancreatic transplantation for diabetes mellitus. Ann. Intern. Med. *89*:951–65, 1978.

[35] Garvey, J. F., and Morris, P. J.: Early rejection of allogeneic fetal rat pancreas. Transplantation *27*:342–44, 1979.

[36] Lemperle, G., Michaelis, W., and Mikatsch, M.: Prolonged survival of kidney allografts after perfusion with RNA or DNA. Transplant. Proc. *3*:477–79, 1971.

[37] Steinmuller, D.: Immunization with skin isografts taken from tolerant mice. Science *158*:127–29, 1967.

[38] Billingham, R. E.: The passenger cell concept in transplantation immunology. Cell. Immunol. *2*:1–12, 1971.

[39] Summerlin, W. T., Broutbar, C., Foanes, R. B., et al.: Acceptance of phenotypically differing cultured skin in man and mice. Transplant. Proc. *5*:707–10, 1973.

[40] Ninnemann, J. L., and Good, R. A.: Allogeneic transplantation of organ cultures without immunosuppression. Transplantation *18*:1–5, 1974.

[41] Boyles, R. R., and Seltzer, H. S.: Reversal of alloxan diabetes in noninbred (allogeneic) rats. Diabetes *24*:420, 1975.

[42] Raaf, J. H., Farr, H. W., and Good, R. A.: Transplantation of fresh and cultured parathyroid glands in the rat. Am. J. Surg. *128*:478–83, 1974.

[43] Hegre, O. D., Leonard, R. J., and Lazarow, A.: Isotransplantation of organ-cultured neonatal pancreas: reversal of alloxan diabetes in the rat. Diabetes *25*:180–89, 1976.

[44] Jacobs, B. B., and Uphodd, D. E.: Immunological modification. Science *185*:582–87, 1974.

[45] Lafferty, K. J., Bootes, A., and Talmage, D. W.: Effect of organ culture on the survival of thyroid allografts in mice. Transplantation *22*:138–49, 1976.

[46] Sollinger, H. W., Burkholder, P. M., and Bach, F. H.: Prolonged survival of xenografts after organ culture. Transplant. Proc. *9*:359–65, 1977.

[47] Naji, A., Silvers, W. K., and Barker, C. F.: Effect of culture in 95% O_2 on the survival of parathyroid allografts. Surg. Forum *30*:109–11, 1979.

[48] Barker, F. G.: Personal communication.

[49] Mandel, T. E.: Organ culture and transplantation of fetal mouse pancreatic islets. Abstracts of the 7th International Congress of the International Transplantation Society, 1978. New York, Grune & Stratton, 1978.

[50] Lacy, P. E., Davie, J. M., Finke, E. H., and Scharp, D. W.: Prolongation of islet allograft survival. Transplantation *27*:171–74 1979.

[51] Zammit, M., Valjee, K. D., and Toledo-Pereyra, L. H.: Comparative study of different pancreas transplantation modalities: islet cell vs. organ pancreas transplantation in pancreatectomized dogs. J. Surg. Res. *26*:308–13, 1979.

[52] Suermann, H. B., and Soderbergh, J. S.: The course of pancreas allografts in rats conditioned by spleen allografts. Transplantation *26*:28–34, 1978.

[53] Perloff, L. J.: Personal communication.

[54] White, E., and Hildemann, W. H.: Allografts in genetically defined rats: differences in survival between kidney and skin. Science *162*:1293–95, 1968.

[55] Barker, C. F., and Billingham, R. E.: Comparison of the fates of Ag-B locus compatible homografts of the skin and heart in inbred rats. Nature (London) *225*:851–52, 1970.

[56] Naji, A., and Barker, C. F.: Relative vulnerability of isolated pancreatic islets, parathyroid, and skin allografts to cellular and humoral immunity. Transplant. Proc. *11*:560–62, 1979.

[57] Browning, H., and Resnick, P.: Homologous and heterologous transplantation of pancreatic tissue in normal and diabetic mice. Yale J. Biol. Med. *24*:141–51, 1951.

[58] House, E. L., Jacobs, M. S., and Pansky, B.: Blood volume, total protein, total cholesterol in normal and diabetic hamsters. Anat. Rec. *144*:25–30, 1962.

[59] Ferguson, J., and Scothorne, R. J.: Extended survival of pancreatic islet allografts in the testes of guinea pigs. J. Anat. *124*:1–8, 1977.

[60] Barker, C. F., and Sutherland, D. E. R.: Pancreatic islet cells in management of diabetes. Transplant. Proc. *9*:1257–58, 1977.

[61] Weber, C. J., Hardy, M. A., Pi-Sunyer, F. X., Zimmerman, E., and Reemtsma, K.: Tissue culture preservation and intramuscular transplantation of pancreatic islets. Surgery *84*:166–74, 1978.

[62] Hamilton, M. S., and Billingham, R. E.: The privileged status of the subcutaneous site for skin allografts in rats. Transplantation *28*:199–202, 1979.

[63] Barker, C. F., Naji, A., Reckard, C. R., and Ziegler, M. M.: The liver as a possible immunologically privileged site for pancreatic islet allografts. Diabetes *24*:418, 1975.

[64] Pfefferman, R., Sakai, A., and Kountz, S. L.: The liver as a privileged site for parathyroid alloimplantation in the rat. Surgery *79*:182–87, 1976.

[65] Finch, D. R. A., and Morris, P. J.: The effect of increasing islet members in survival of pancreatic islet allografts in immunosuppressed diabetic rats. Transplantation *23*:104–06, 1977.

[66] Marquet, R. L., and Heysteck, G. A.: The effect of immunosuppressive treatment on the survival of allogeneic islets of Langerhans in rats. Transplantation *20*:428–31, 1975.

[67] Nelken, D., Morse, S. I., Beyer, M. M., and Friedman, E. A.: Prolonged survival of allotransplanted islet of Langerhans cells in the rat. Transplantation *22*:74–75, 1976.

[68] Shulak, J. A., Franklin, W., and Reckard, C. R.: Morphological and functional changes following intraportal islet allograft rejection: irreversibility with steroid pulse therapy. Surg. Forum *28*:296, 1977.

[69] Reckard, C. R., Ziegler, M. M., and Barker, C. F.: Physiological and immunological consequences of transplanting isolated pancreatic islets. Surgery *74*:91–99, 1973.

[70] Finch, D. R. A., and Morris, P. J.: Failure to demonstrate a synergistic effect between enhancing serum and ALS in recipients of pancreatic islet allografts. Transplantation *23*:386–88, 1977.

[71] Barker, C. F., Frangipane, L. G., and Silvers, W. K.: Islet transplantation in genetically determined diabetes. Ann. Surg. *186*:401–10, 1977.

[72] Gray, B. N., and Watkins, E., Jr.: Prolonged relief from diabetes after syngeneic or allogeneic transplantation of isolated pancreatic islets in rats. Surg. Forum *25*:382–84, 1974.

[73] Ziegler, M. M., Reckard, C. R., and Barker, C. F.: Long-term metabolic and immunological considerations in transplantation of pancreatic islets. J. Surg. Res. *16*:575–81, 1974.

[74] Reckard, C. R., Stuart, F. P., and Schulak, J. A.: Immunologic comparisons of isolated pancreatic islet and whole organ allografts. Transplant. Proc. *11*:563–66, 1979.

[75] Barker, C. F.: Transplantation of the islets of Langerhans and the histocompatibility of endocrine tissue. Diabetes *24*:766–75, 1975.

[76] Barker, C. F., Silvers, W. K., and Lubaroff, D. M.: Lymph node cells: their differential capacity to induce tolerance to heart and skin homografts. Science *172*:1050–52, 1971.

[77] Rossini, A. A., Williams, M. R., and Appel, M. C.: Complete protection from low-dose streptozotocin-induced diabetes in mice. Nature (London) *276*:182–83, 1978.

[78] Buschard, K., and Ruggard, J.: Passive transfer of streptozotocin induced diabetes mellitus with spleen cells. Acta Pathol. Microbiol. Scand. *85*:469–72, 1977.

[79] Andersson, A.: Islet implantation normalises hyperglycemia caused by streptozotocin-induced insulitis. Lancet *1*:581–84, 1979.

[80] Craighead, J. E., Kanich, R. E., and Kessler, J. B.: Lesions of the islets of Langerhans in encephalomyocarditis virus-infected mice with diabetes mellitus-like disease. I. Acute lesions. Am. J. Pathol. *74*:287–300, 1974.

[81] Buschard, K.: Passive transfer of virus-induced diabetes mellitus with spleen cells. Acta Pathol. Microbiol. Scand. *86*:29–32, 1978.

[82] Howard, R. J., Sutherland, D. E. R., and Matas, A. J.: Successful treatment of viral-induced diabetes mellitus by islet transplantation. Surg. Forum *29*:343–44, 1978.

[83] Naji, A., Silvers, W. K., Plotkin, S. A., Dafoe, D., and Barker, C. F.: Successful islet transplantation in spontaneous diabetes. Surgery *86*:218–26, 1979.

[84] Nakhooda, A. F., Like, A. A., Chappel, C. I., Murray, F. T., and Marliss, E. B.: The spontaneously diabetic Wistar rat: metabolic and morphologic studies. Diabetes *26*:100–12, 1977.

[85] Like, A. A., Rossini, A. A., Appel, M. C., Guberski, D. L., and Williams, R. M.: Immune intervention in the spontaneously diabetic bio breeding Worcester rat. Clin. Res. *27*:487, 1979.

Effect of Culture on Islet Rejection

PAUL E. LACY, JOSEPH M. DAVIE, AND EDWARD H. FINKE

SUMMARY

In order to diminish or prevent rejection of transplanted allogeneic islets of Langerhans, in vitro culture was used. After digestion of the rat pancreas and Ficoll separation, islets were handpicked to be free of vascular and ductal tissue. Phenol red in the culture medium imparted a pink color to the islets when observed with a diffuse green light against a black background. Islets cultured at room temperature (24°C) remained functionally and morphologically intact for 1–4 wk. Insulin secretion was 1–3 μU per islet per hour, increasing to 16 μU per islet per hour at 37°C, Culture alone resulted in a modest prolongation of function across a major histocompatibility barrier, Wistar Furth to Lewis (mean survival time, 11.6 ± 1.2 vs. 7.2 ± 0.5 days). However, one injection of antilymphocytic serum (ALS) into 10 recipients at the time of transplantation prolonged survival to greater than 100 days in nine rats. In the combination ACI to Lewis, also a major barrier, the same regimen prolonged function to greater than 100 days in five out of five recipients. Injection of donor peritoneal exudate cells resulted in prompt rejection of islets. These results suggest that culture and ALS either damage or alter passenger leukocytes in the donor tissue, thereby preventing rejection of the islets. DIABETES *29* (Suppl. 1):93–97, 1980.

The use of in vitro culture for the possible prolongation of allograft survival is based upon the concept that passenger leukocytes contaminating the graft are responsible for initiation of immune rejection by the recipient and that these passenger cells could be altered or diminished by in vitro culture of the graft before transplantation. Snell[1] first suggested that donor lymphocytes, carried over in grafts, might play a significant role in invoking immunity. It appears that passenger leukocytes do play a primary role in initiating a local immune reaction against the host within the graft; however, it is not clearly established that passenger leukocytes play a primary role in host-versus-graft reactivity.[2] Lafferty et al.[3] demonstrated that in vitro culture of the thyroid for 26 days in an atmosphere of 95% O_2 before transplantation produced marked prolongation of thyroid allograft survival. The period of time required for in vitro culture could be decreased to 7 days if the donors were pretreated with cyclophosphamide to diminish the lymphoid population[4] or by culturing the thyroid in hyperbaric oxygen.[5] Rejection of the thyroid allografts could be restored by injecting peritoneal exudate cells syngeneic to the donor strain.[6] Kedinger et al.[7] have reported that the survival time of diabetic rats could be prolonged significantly by culturing islets in vitro 4–5 days before transplanting islet allografts directly into the hepatic parenchyma of the liver.

The purpose of this report is to review our studies on prolongation of islet allograft survival across major histocompatibility barriers by procedures that were directed towards elimination or alteration of passenger leukocytes in the islet grafts before transplantation.

From the Department of Pathology, Washington University School of Medicine, St. Louis, Missouri.

EFFECT OF DONOR PRETREATMENT REGIMENS ON ISLET ALLOGRAFT SURVIVAL

We attempted initially to use the in vitro techniques described by Lafferty et al.[3] on isolated adult islets and found that exposure to 95% O_2 resulted in disintegration of the islets after 4–5 days of in vitro culture. In addition, the raft technique of culture used by Lafferty et al.[3] could not be applied to the islets since the individual islets became flattened and disintegrated on the surface of the raft.

Because of these limitations for in vitro culture of the islets, we determined the effect of pretreating donor rats with total body irradiation and intravenous silica to diminish the lymphoid and macrophage population in the islets in conjunction with a brief period of in vitro culture of the islets with rabbit anti-rat lymphocyte serum (ALS) before transplantation.[8] The islets were isolated by the collagenase technique[9,10] and were separated by centrifugation on a Ficoll gradient.[11] In all of the studies reviewed in this report, the isolated islets were transplanted via the portal vein technique,[12] and the recipient Lewis rats were made diabetic by the intravenous injection of streptozotocin (65 mg/kg). Rejection was considered to have occurred in individual recipients when the posttransplant, 24-h urine glucose level was equal to the mean minus one standard deviation of the pretransplant urine glucose level for that particular rat. This procedure made it possible to follow the pattern of rejection as well as to determine the time of rejection.

Unfortunately, none of these donor pretreatment regimens had any effect on prolongation of survival of Ficoll-isolated islets transplanted across either a minor (Fischer [AgB^1] to Lewis [AgB^1]) or a major histocompatibility barrier (WF [AgB^2] to Lewis [AgB^1]). After these discouraging results were obtained, we carried out a careful examination of the tissue present in the islet layer removed from the Ficoll gradient. In this layer we found some islets with attached ductular and vascular tissue, free fragments of vascular and ductular tissue, and, occasionally, small lymph nodes. Since these contaminating structures could be contributing to the immune rejection, the studies were repeated using only islets that were handpicked and free of associated vascular or ductal tissue.

Transplants of handpicked islets across a minor histocompatibility barrier (Fischer to Lewis) after pretreatment of the donors with irradiation and silica in conjunction with in vitro culture of the islets with ALS for 2–3 days before transplantation produced prolongation of the survival time of the transplants.[8] Two of the recipients remained aglycosuric for 90 and 127 days, with rejection still not occurring at 210 and 279 days after transplantation. Pretreatment of the donors alone with irradiation and silica and without in vitro exposure of the islets to ALS did not prolong islet allograft survival.

Since exposure of the islets to ALS appeared to be of importance, we determined the effect of the pretreatment regimen in conjunction with a single injection of ALS into the recipient at the time of transplanting the islets rather than exposing the islets to ALS in vitro.[8] Islet allograft survival across a weak histocompatibility barrier (Fischer to Lewis) was markedly prolonged by either the pretreatment regimen and a single injection of ALS or only a single injection of ALS without donor pretreatment.

These studies were repeated across a major histocompatibility barrier (ACI [AgB^4] to Lewis [AgB^1]). The mean survival time in the control group receiving only freshly isolated islets was 5.2 days. A single injection of ALS into the recipients at the time of transplanting freshly isolated islets produced a slight prolongation of allograft survival, with six of the rats rejecting between 7 and 20 days and one rejecting at 91 days. Pretreatment of the ACI donors with irradiation and silica and a single injection of ALS into the recipients produced a further prolongation of survival, with rejection occurring between 30 and 68 days in four rats; one rat still had a functional transplant at 189 days.[8]

These findings indicated that pretreatment of donor animals with irradiation and silica in conjunction with a single injection of ALS into the recipient would produce prolongation of islet allograft survival across a major histocompatibility barrier; however, the length of survival of the transplant was not comparable to the markedly prolonged survival of thyroid allografts obtained by Lafferty et al.[3]

EFFECT OF IN VITRO CULTURE (24°C) AND ALS (ACI TO LEWIS)

Opelz and Terasaki[13] reported that in vitro maintenance of lymphocytes at a low temperature (22°C) for more than 4 days resulted in a loss of the ability of the lymphocytes to stimulate allogeneic lymphocytes in mixed lymphocyte cultures. Since we were attempting either to diminish or alter the lymphoid elements in the islets before transplantation, we determined whether isolated islets would survive when they were incubated in vitro at room temperature (24°C).

We were surprised to find that the islets remained functionally and morphologically intact after in vitro incubation at 24°C for 1–4 wk.[14] The islets were incubated in tissue culture medium containing glucose (1.5 mg/ml), and the rate of insulin secretion ranged from 1 to 3 μU per islet per hour during the 28-day period of culture at 24°C. When the temperature was increased to 37°C at the end of each of the weekly intervals, the rate of insulin secretion increased to approximately 16 μU per islet per hour and remained stable during a subsequent 7-day period of incubation. This rate of secretion was comparable to control islets, which had been cultured at 37°C for corresponding periods of time.

Since the islets remained morphologically and functionally intact when incubated at 24°C, studies were accomplished to determine the effect of a 7-day period of incubation of ACI (AgB^4) islets at 24°C before transplantation in conjunction with a single injection of ALS into diabetic Lewis (AgB^1) recipients.[15] This pretreatment regimen produced an islet allograft survival of greater than 100 days in all five of the recipients. The mean total weight gain for this group was 100.2 g for the 100-day period. Three of the recipients returned to their individual pretransplant levels between 135 and 150 days after transplantation, whereas the other two recipients still had not rejected their islets at 220 days after transplantation.

EFFECT OF IN VITRO CULTURE (24°C) AND ALS (WF TO LEWIS)

The effect on islet allograft survival of in vitro culture (24°C) for 7 days before transplantation and a single injection of ALS into the recipient was determined across another major histocompatibility barrier (WF [AgB^2] to Lewis [AgB^1]). In 10 recipients receiving islets cultured for 7 days at 24°C and a single injection of ALS, nine had not rejected the allografts at 100 days and one rejected at 12 days.[16,17] Eight of the recipients were aglycosuric throughout the 100-day interval, and one, which remained aglycosuric for 80 days, demonstrated increased urine glucose to 1.75 g/24 h at 100 days. This study confirmed our initial findings and indicated that in vitro culture at 24°C, in conjunction with temporary immunosuppression of the recipient, would produce marked prolongation of islet allograft survival across major histocompatibility barriers.

The effect of only a single injection of ALS on allograft survival of transplants of Wistar Furth islets to Lewis rats was greater than that obtained in our previous investigation using ACI rats as donors. Two recipients receiving only ALS and freshly isolated islets had not rejected the transplant at 100 days.[16,17] The ALS used in these studies was prepared from Wistar Furth lymph node cells. The same lot of ALS was used for the transplantation of ACI and Wistar Furth (WF) islets to Lewis recipients. Thus, it is possible that the ALS may have affected or destroyed passenger leukocytes in WF islets more effectively than passenger leukocytes from the ACI strain.

In vitro incubation of WF islets at 24°C for 7, 14, 21, and 28 days before transplantation without the injection of ALS into diabetic Lewis recipients did not produce a marked prolongation of islet allograft survival.[16,17] Islets incubated for 21 days (24°C) survived slightly longer than control recipients receiving freshly isolated islets (mean survival time, 11.6 ± 1.2 vs. 7.2 ± 0.5 days). These findings indicated that the single injection of ALS into the recipient was required, in conjunction with culture of the islets at 24°C, to obtain marked prolongation of islet allograft survival.

INDUCTION OF REJECTION BY PERITONEAL EXUDATE CELLS

The underlying hypothesis for the experiments on prolonging islet allograft survival by in vitro culture at 24°C and the single injection of ALS was that these procedures were altering or diminishing the passenger leukocyte content of the islet tissue. In order to test this hypothesis, we determined whether the intravenous injection of peritoneal exudate cells (PEC) obtained from the donor strain would induce rejection of established islet allografts.

The two recipients in our initial study[16,17] that had not rejected allografts of ACI islets at 220 days were injected intravenously with 6×10^7 PEC obtained from ACI rats on day 220. Six days after the injection of PEC, rejection was initiated in both animals with a rapid rise in the 24-h urine glucose levels and a precipitous loss of body weight. Similar findings were obtained when Wistar Furth (WF) PEC were injected intravenously into recipients with established WF islet allografts at 219–233 days after transplantation.[17]

These findings indicated that allografts of islets remained immunologically undetected by the recipient until PEC from the donor strain were administered.

REPEATED ISLET TRANSPLANTS AFTER INDUCTION OF REJECTION BY PEC

After induction of rejection of ACI islet allografts by donor PEC[16,17] at 220 days after transplantation, one of these animals was used to determine whether subsequent islet allografts from other strains could be established and whether these allografts could be induced to reject by PEC. A transplant of WF (AgB^2) islets into this animal after in vitro culture (24°C) and ALS in the recipient was successful, and the WF allograft was induced to reject only by Wistar Furth PEC, whereas PEC from ACI rats had no effect on the allograft.[17] A third transplant with islets from the Buffalo strain (AgB^6) was then successfully established after in vitro culture (24°C) and a single injection of ALS. Thus, islet allografts from three different strains of rats (ACI, Wistar Furth, and Buffalo) were successfully established even though rejection of ACI and then WF islets had been induced by PEC syngeneic to the donor strain.

These findings indicated that a remarkable specificity for the PEC was required to induce rejection of the islets and that subsequent islet transplants from different strains could be accomplished, even though rejection of islets from other strains had already been induced in the recipient.

"GREEN-LIGHT" TECHNIQUE FOR ISLET IDENTIFICATION IN VITRO

One of the problems that concerned us was whether small lymph nodes the size of islets would be mistakenly identified and be present even in the handpicked islets used for the transplants. Recently, we have developed a technique that permits the specific identification of islets in vitro.[18] Isolated islets in tissue culture medium containing phenol red have a slightly pinkish color when viewed with ordinary light. This pink color was enhanced by simply viewing the islets under a dissecting microscope with a diffuse green light against a black background. With this lighting arrangement, the islets appear distinctly pink, whereas small lymph nodes, ductal tissue, acinar tissue, and vascular tissue are a bright green. When preparations of handpicked islets were examined with this technique, we found occasional small lymph nodes that had been mistakenly identified as islets. This simple procedure is now used routinely to screen all of the islets before transplantation in order to be certain that small lymph nodes are not included in the transplanted material and that the islets are free of attached acinar, ductal, or vascular tissue.

MECHANISM RESPONSIBLE FOR PROLONGATION OF ISLET ALLOGRAFT SURVIVAL

It would appear that the period of in vitro culture of the islets at 24°C and the administration of ALS to the recipient diminished and/or altered the passenger leukocyte content of the islets below a threshhold level required to initiate rejection. Evidence in favor of this concept is as follows: (1) clean islets, free of associated vascular or ductal tissue, are required for prolongation of islet allograft survival; (2) ALS, prepared against WF lymph node cells, appeared to be more effective in prolonging islet allograft survival of WF islets than of ACI islets when only a single injection of ALS was administered without in vitro culture of the islets; (3) rejection of established allografts of WF islets and ACI islets could be induced by the intravenous injection of PEC lymphocytes and macrophages) that were syngeneic to the donor strain; and (4) the islet cells were apparently not altered since immunologic recognition and rejection of established allografts could be induced by PEC.

Other mechanisms which could play a role in the prolongation of islet allograft survival are the diabetic state of the recipient, the site of implantation of the islets, and the effect of ALS on the recipients. Chemically induced diabetes in mice has been reported to partially suppress the immune system[19–21] and to reduce the nucleated cell content of the thymus and spleen.[22] Obviously the diabetic state did not play a major role in prolonging islet allograft survival, since rejection occurred in control rats regardless of whether the transplants were across a minor or major histocompatibility barrier. In addition, it has also been reported that islet allografts in diabetic rats may be even more susceptible to rejection than other tissues, since islets rejected more rapidly than either skin or heart allografts using the same strain combination.[23,24] Thus, it appears unlikely that the diabetic state played a major role in prolonging islet allograft survival in our investigations; however, a minor effect on suppressing the immune system of the recipients cannot be excluded.

Barker et al.[25] reported a slight increase in the median survival time of islet allografts transplanted across a weak histocompatibility barrier after intraportal transplantation than after intraperitoneal transplantation. When a major histocompatibility barrier was present, the intrahepatic site did not provide prolongation of survival. Since the transplants in our investigations were across major histocompatibility barriers, it appears unlikely that the site of transplantation played a major role in prolonging islet allograft survival; however, a possible synergistic effect of this site on prolonging survival cannot be excluded.

The role of the single injection of ALS in prolonging survival appears to be the destruction of passenger leukocytes in the islet allografts as well as the destruction of passenger leukocytes that may have been altered or damaged after in vitro incubation at 24°C. It is also possible that ALS may have produced a temporary, critical, immunologic window in the recipient, which permitted the establishment of tolerance to the transplanted islet tissue.

FUTURE PROBLEMS

The finding that in vitro incubation of the islets at 24°C and a single injection of ALS into the recipients produces a marked prolongation of islet allograft survival across a major histocompatibility barrier raises several fascinating problems for future investigations. Studies are in progress to attempt to determine whether the T cell, B cell, or macrophage is responsible for the induction of immune rejection of established islet allografts. Once the identity of the stimulator cell or cells has been accomplished, then it will be possible to determine whether the islet cells lack certain loci in the major histocompatibility complex, such as the Ia region.

Techniques are now available for the dispersion and reaggregation of islet cells into small islets,[26,27] making it feasible to determine whether ALS is essential for prolongation of islet allograft survival since these preparations should contain only a few or no passenger leukocyte cells.

It will be of great interest and importance to determine whether the simple procedure used for prolongation of islet allograft survival can be used for prolonging xenograft survival of islets. Sollinger et al.[28] have reported prolongation of thyroid xenografts (rat to mouse) by utilizing the technique described by Lafferty et al.[3]

Studies on different sites of implantation should determine whether the intrahepatic location of the transplants plays a role in the procedures used for prolongation of islet allograft survival.

These studies, in addition to long-term metabolic studies with the optimum method developed for prolongation of islet allograft survival, will be required before islet allografts are attempted as a means of therapy for the diabetic patient.

SUMMARY

This report is a review of our investigations directed toward prolongation of islet allograft survival in the rat. In vitro culture of isolated rat islets at 24°C in conjunction with a single injection of ALS into the recipients produced a 90–100% survival at 100 days after transplantation of islets across major histocompatibility barriers. Rejection of established islet allografts was induced by the intravenous injection of peritoneal exudate cells syngeneic to the donor strain. The simplest explanation for the marked prolongation of islet allograft survival is that the procedure either diminished or altered passenger leukocytes in the islet allografts and that these cells play a primary role in the induction of recognition and rejection of the islet allografts by the recipient. We have discussed other factors that may also be involved in prolongation of the islet allograft survival as well as future problems to be resolved.

ACKNOWLEDGMENTS

This work was supported in part by USPHS grant AM-01226 and by The Kroc Foundation.

REFERENCES

1 Snell, G. D.: The homograft reaction. Annu. Rev. Microbiol. *11*:439–58, 1957.

2 Billingham, R. E.: The passenger cell concept in transplantation immunology. Cell. Immunol. *2*:1–12, 1971.

3 Lafferty, K., Cooley, M. A., Woolnough, J., and Walker, K.: Thyroid allograft immunogenicity is reduced after a period in organ culture. Science *188*:259–61, 1975.

4 Lafferty, K. J., Bootes, A., Killby, V. A., and Burch, W.: Mechanism of thyroid allograft rejection. Aust. J. Exp. Biol. Med. Sci. *54*:573–86, 1976.

5 Talmage, D. W., and Dart, G. A.: Effect of oxygen pressure during culture on survival of mouse thyroid allografts. Science *200*:1066–67, 1978.

6 Talmage, D. W., Dart, G. A., Radovich, J., and Lafferty, K. J.: Activation of transplant immunity: effect of donor leukocytes on thyroid allograft rejection. Science *191*:385–88, 1976.

7 Kedinger, M., Haffen, K., Grenier, J., and Eloy, R.: In vitro culture reduces immunogenicity of pancreatic endocrine islets. Nature (London) *270*:736–38, 1977.

8 Lacy, P. E., Davie, J. M., Finke, E. H., and Scharp, D. W.: Prolongation of islet allograft survival. Transplantation *27*:171–74, 1979.

9 Lacy, P. E., and Kostianovsky, M.: A method for the isolation of intact islets of Langerhans from the rat pancreas. Diabetes *16*:35, 1967.

10 Lacy, P. E., Walker, M. M. and Finke, C. J.: Perifusion of isolated rat islets in vitro. The participation of the microtubular system in the biphasic release of insulin. Diabetes *21*:987–98, 1972.

11 Lindall, A., Steffes, M., and Sorenson, R.: Immunoassayable insulin content of subcellular fractions of rat islets. Endocrinology *85*:218–23, 1969.

12 Kemp, C., Knight, M. J., Scharp, D. W., Ballinger, W. F., and Lacy, P. E.: Effect of transplantation site on results of pancreatic islet isografts in diabetic rats. Diabetologia *9*:486–91, 1973.

13 Opelz, G., and Terasaki, P.: Lymphocyte antigenicity loss with retention of responsiveness. Science 184:464–66, 1974.

14 Ono, J., Lacy, P. E., Michael, H., and Greider, M. H.: Morphologic and functional status of islets maintained 1–4 weeks at 24°C in vitro. Submitted for publication, Am. J. Pathol., 1979.

15 Lacy, P. E., Davie, J. M., and Finke, E. H.: Prolongation of islet allograft survival following in vitro culture (24°C) and a single injection of ALS. Science *204*:312–13, 1979.

16 Lacy, P. E., Davie, J. M., Finke, E. H., and Ono, J.: Prevention of immune rejection of islet allografts by in vitro culture (24°C) and ALS. Diabetes *28* (Program):427, 1979.

17 Lacy, P. E., Davie, J. M., and Finke, E. H.: Induction of rejection of successful allografts of rat islets by donor peritoneal exudate cells. Transplantation *28*:415–20, 1979.

18 Finke, E. H., Lacy, P. E., and Ono, J.: Use of reflected green light for specific in vitro identification of islets following collagenase isolation. Diabetes *28*:612–13, 1979.

19 Ptak, W., Czarnik, Z., and Hanczakowska, M.: Contact sensitivity in alloxan-diabetic mice. Clin. Exp. Immunol. 19(2):319–25, 1975.

20 Mahmoud, A. A. F., Rodman, H. M., Mandel, M. A., and Warrent, K. S.: Induced and spontaneous diabetes mellitus and suppression of cell-mediated immunologic responses: granuloma formation, delayed derman reactivity and allograft rejection. J. Clin. Invest. *57*:362–67, 1976.

21 Nichols, W. K., Spellmann, J. B., Vann, L. L., and Daynes, R. A.: Immune responses of diabetic animals. Diabetologia *16*:51–57, 1979.

22 Nichols, W. K., Spellmann, J. B., and Daynes, R. A.: Immune responses of diabetic animals. Comparison of genetically obese and streptozotocin-diabetic mice. Diabetologia *14*:343–49, 1978.

23 Reckard, C., and Barker, C.: Transplantation of isolated pancreatic islets across strong and weak histocompatibility barriers. Transplant. Proc. *5*:761–63, 1973.

24 Reckard, C. R., Ziegler, M. M., and Barker, C. F.: Physiological and immunological consequences of transplanting isolated pancreatic islets. Surgery *74*:91–99, 1973.

25 Barker, C. F., Naji, A., Reckard, C. R., and Ziegler, M. M.: The liver as an immunologically privileged site for rat pancreatic islet allografts. Diabetes *24*:418, 1975.

[26] Ono, J., Takaki, R., and Fukuma, M.: Preparation of single cells from pancreatic islets of adult rat by the use of Dispase. Endocrinol. Jpn. *24*:265–70, 1977.

[27] Ono, J., Takaki, R., Okuno, H., and Fukuma, M.: Long-term culture of pancreatic islet cells with special reference to the B-cell function. In Vitro, in press, 1979.

[28] Sollinger, H. W., Burkholder, P. M., Rasmus, W. R., and Bach, F. H.: Prolonged survival of xenografts after organ culture. Surgery *81*:74–79, 1977.

Successful Allotransplantation of Mouse Pancreatic Islets to Nonimmunosuppressed Recipients

KERRY M. BOWEN, LINDA ANDRUS, AND KEVIN J. LAFFERTY

SUMMARY

Pancreatic islets from BALB/c (H-2^d) mice are rejected within 14 days of transplantation to the kidney capsule of allogeneic, CBA/H (H-2^k) recipients. Cyclophosphamide pretreatment of the islet donor reduced the intensity of the allograft response, and these islets undergo a more chronic rejection process. Islets from cyclophosphamide-pretreated donors can be cultured in a gas phase of 95% O_2 and 5% CO_2, provided the islets are aggregated into clusters of about 50 islets. After a culture period of 7–12 days, the islet tissue was transplanted to normal allogeneic recipients, where the tissue elicited little or no allograft response over a 3-mo observation period. DIABETES 29 (Suppl. 1):98–104, 1980.

There is now evidence that transplantation antigens on the surface of tissue parenchymal cells are not the major barrier to allotransplantation.[1] It is hematogenous cells carried within the transplanted tissue that play a central role in the induction and expression of allograft reactivity. Stimulator cells that express the S$^+$ phenotype are required for the induction of specific allograft immunity,[2] and the activation of blood cells within the transplant itself can give rise to local inflammatory responses that cause damage to the transplanted tissue.[1]

In the case of mouse thyroid and parathyroid, we have shown that the maintenance of these tissues in organ culture in an atmosphere of 95% O_2 and 5% CO_2 for a period of 3–4 wk before transplantation results in their long-term acceptance by normal allogeneic recipients.[1] The period of organ culture can be considerably shortened if transplant donors are treated with cyclophosphamide before the harvest of tissues for transplantation.[1] The cultured tissue is antigenic and can be rejected if the immune system of the recipient animal is activated with leukocytes of donor origin[3] or an uncultured thyroid of donor origin.[1] Thus, this treatment of tissues before transplantation reduces their immunogenicity for an allogeneic host but does not eliminate their expression of transplantation antigen.

In this paper we describe a procedure that allows mouse pancreatic islet tissue to be cultured in the presence of 95% O_2 for up to 12 days. After this treatment, islet tissue can be successfully transplanted to normal H-2 incompatible recipients where they elicit little or no allograft response over an observation period of up to 3 mo.

From the Department of Immunology, John Curtin Medical Research School, The Australian National University, Canberra City, Australia.

MATERIALS AND METHODS

Experimental animals. Inbred mice of the BALB/c (H-2^d) and CBA/H (H-2^k) strains were used at approximately 8 wk of age. Tissue donors were BALB/c mice and recipients were CBA/H mice of the same sex. Donor pretreatment, where used, consisted of the intraperitoneal injection of cyclophosphamide (Endoxan-Asta, Bristol Laboratories) at a dose rate of 300 mg/kg body weight on days −4 and −2, and tissues were harvested for transplantation on day 0.

Preparation of pancreatic islets. Groups of 8–12 donor animals were anesthetized with ether and killed by cervical dislocation. The following isolation steps were then carried out under sterile conditions. Donor pancreatic tissue was removed, finely diced with scissors, and washed in Hepes-buffered Hank's solution at pH 7.4. The Hepes-buffered Hank's solution was supplemented with bovine serum albumin (0.05%), penicillin (100 U/ml), and streptomycin (100 μg/ml). The minced tissue was allowed to settle at 4° for 4 min, and floating debris was removed with a Pasteur pipette. After three 30-s dicings and subsequent washings, the chopped pancreatic tissue was transferred to a siliconized 15-ml graduated glass centrifuge tube and allowed to settle for an additional 4 min. The volume of chopped tissue was noted, and the tissue was transferred to a siliconized 20-ml glass scintillation vial. Collagenase (Boehringer-Mannheim) was freshly prepared in phosphate-buffered saline (PBS) at a concentration of 10 mg/ml and filtered through a 22-μm Millipore filter. One milliliter of this solution was added to each 1-ml volume of chopped pancreatic tissue, and the volume was made up to 5 ml with Hepes-

Hank's solution. The pancreatic tissue was then digested at 37°C for 17 min in a one-stage procedure, using a water bath with a mechanical shaker oscillating at approximately 200 cycles/min. The digest was then vigorously shaken by hand for approximately 15–20 s to disperse any residual clumps of tissue. The enzymic digestion was slowed down by the addition of 15 ml of chilled Hepes-Hank's solution, and the digest was allowed to settle for 4 min at 4°C. The supernatant liquid was removed, and the washing procedure was repeated two more times. Using a stereomicroscope, individual islets were picked from the digest with the aid of a fine pipette and transferred to a chilled siliconized petri dish. The yield averaged approximately 40 islets per mouse pancreas. At the end of the isolation procedure, RPMI 1640 culture medium, supplemented with 10% heat-inactivated fetal calf serum and antibiotics, was added to the dish.

Organ culture procedure. Groups of approximatley 50 isolated islets were transferred to 35-mm hydrophobic petri dishes (Falcon 1008) containing 2 ml of culture medium. Islets were aggregated by gentle manual oscillation of the dish (Figure 1, left). The islets were then incubated at 37°C in an atmosphere of 95% O_2 and 5% CO_2 for the desired period of time. The culture medium was changed three times a week. At the first and subsequent media changes, sufficient medium was added to just cover the bottom of the culture dishes (approximately 0.75 ml). Individual islets coalesced over a 4–7 day culture period to form tight islet clusters (Figure 1, right) that could be manipulated for transplantation with fine forceps.

Transplantation. Recipient mice were anesthetized with an intraperitoneal injection of Avertin solution.[4] The kidney was exposed through an incision in the left flank, and a single islet cluster was eased into a small pocket under the kidney capsule. In the case of uncultured islets, groups of 50–100 islets were collected in the tip of a siliconized pipette, which was introduced under the kidney capsule where the islets were expelled. The muscle and body wall of the recipient were then closed with autoclips.

Evaluation of transplanted tissue. Tissue transplants were evaluated by histologic examination. At varying times after transplantation, recipient mice were killed by cervical dislocation. The kidney carrying the transplanted islet tissue was fixed in formalin saline, and paraffin sections were stained with hematoxylin and eosin or with aldehyde-fuchsin,[5] which stains the insulin-containing granules of the islet β cells. Tissue sections were examined to determine the degree of islet damage and mononuclear cell infiltration in and around the transplanted tissue.

RESULTS

Transplantation of islets under the kidney capsule of isogeneic recipient mice. Approximately 50 islets from normal or cyclophosphamide-pretreated BALB/c donors were transplanted under the kidney capsule of BALB/c recipients and examined histologically at varying times after transplantation. Islets from both normal and cyclophosphamide-pretreated donors behaved in essentially the same way when transferred to isogeneic recipients. Revascularization of the islets commenced around 4 days after transplantation, and, by 1–2 wk after transplantation, well-vascularized islets lay flat against the kidney parenchyma. When stained with aldehyde-fuchsin, positively stained β cells were seen in the isografted tissue (Figure 2A).

Allograft response to normal islets and islets from cyclophosphamide-treated donors. Groups of 50 islets obtained from normal or cyclophosphamide-pretreated BALB/c donors were transplanted under the kidney capsule of normal CBA recipient mice. Groups of animals were killed 4, 7, and 14 days after transplantation, and the grafted tissue was examined histologically. Table 1 summarizes the results of this study.

There was a violent allograft response to normal islets that began within 4 days of transplantation. By 4 days, the transplant area was lightly to heavily infiltrated by mononuclear cells, including numerous small lymphocytes, lymphoblasts, and macrophages. Polymorphs were occasionally seen around the transplant area. The islets were generally intact at this stage, but some were infiltrated by small pockets of lymphocytes. By day 7, the center of the islets

FIGURE 1. Morphologic appearance of islet clusters (left) at the time of initial cluster formation and (right) after 7 days of organ culture. (×50)

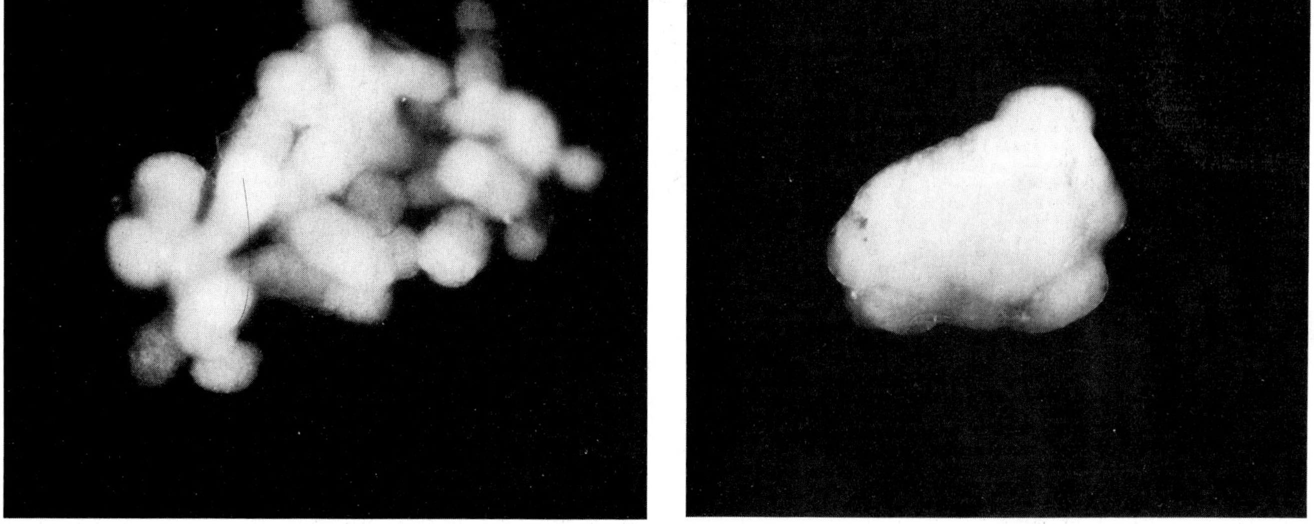

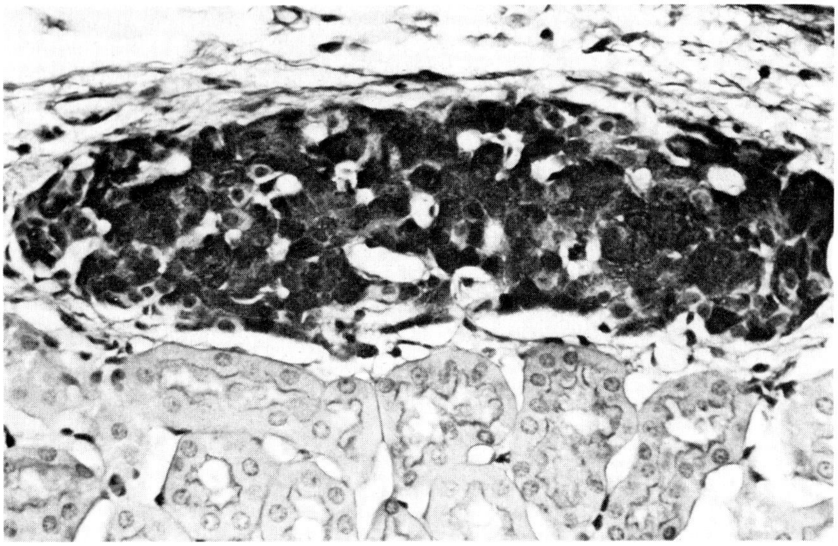

A

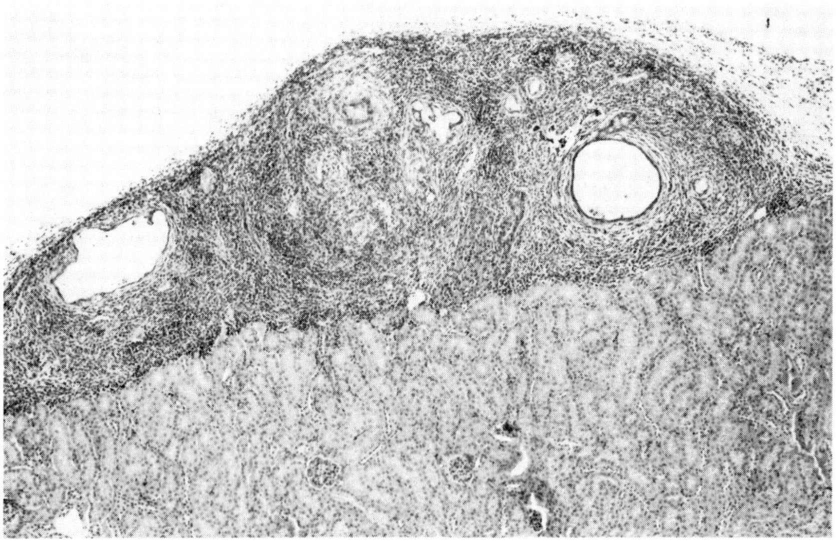

B

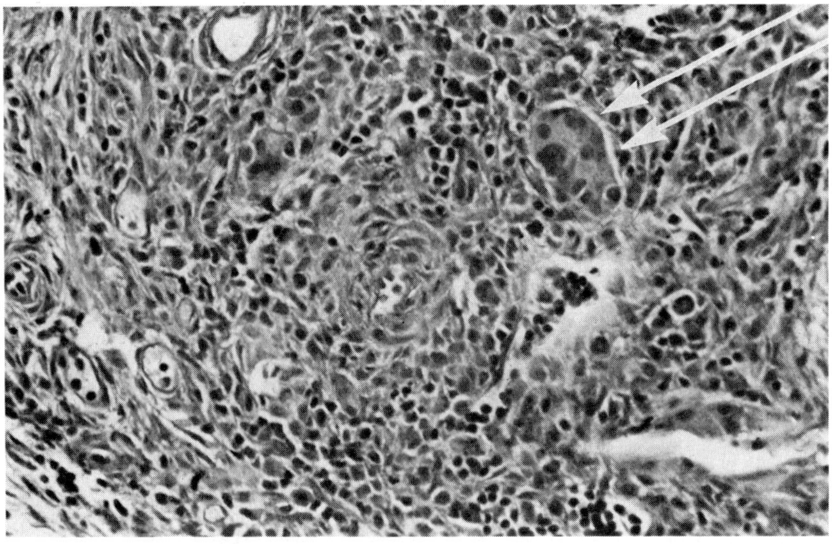

C

FIGURE 2. Host response to transplantation of isogeneic and allogeneic islets under the kidney capsule. (A) BALB/c islets transplanted to BALB/c recipients and examined 3 wk posttransplant. (Aldehyde-fuchsin, ×312.) (B) BALB/c islets transplanted to CBA recipients and examined 2 wk posttransplant. (Hematoxylin and eosin, ×50.) (C) BALB/c islets transplanted to CBA recipients and examined 2 wk posttransplant. Arrows show islet remnants. (Aldehyde-fuchsin, ×312.) (D) BALB/c islets from cyclophosphamide-pretreated donors transplanted to CBA recipients and examined 3 wk posttransplant. (Aldehyde-fuchsin, ×312.)

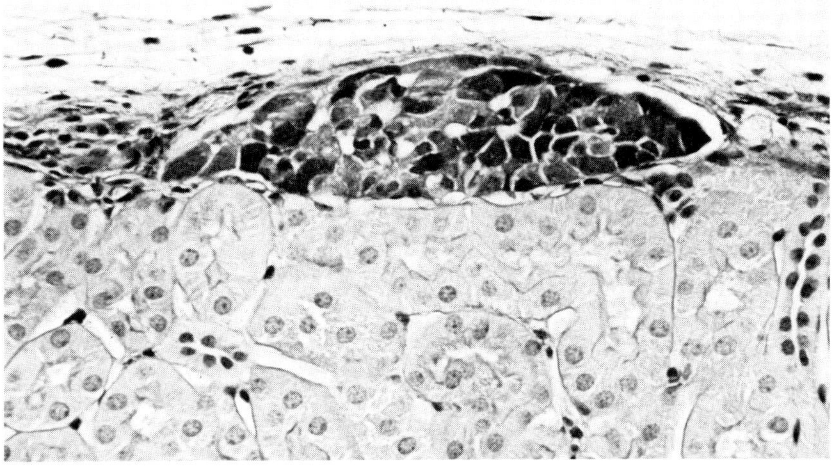

D

TABLE 1
Histologic appearance of islets from normal or cyclophosphamide-treated BALB/c donors * after transplantation to the kidney capsule of CBA recipient mice

Donor pretreatment	Time after transplantation (days)	Histologic score† Mononuclear cell infiltration	Integrity of islets
None	4	+	++++
		+++	+++
		++	++++
		++	+++++
Cyclophosphamide	4	0	+++++
		0	+++++
		+	+++++
		0	+++++
None	7	++	+++
		+++	+++
		++++	+
Cyclophosphamide	7	++	++++
		+	++++
		++	+++++
None	14	++++	+
		++++	+
		++++	+
		++++	+
Cyclophosphamide	14	+	++++
		++++	+
		+	++
		++	++
		++	++++
		++	+++

* BALB/c donors treated with cyclophosphamide (300 mg/kg) on days −4 and −2. Tissue harvested for transplantation on day 0.

† The histologic scores, as determined by histologic appearance, (1) for mononuclear cell infiltration of islets and surrounding tissue: 0, no infiltration; +, light infiltration around transplanted tissue; ++, moderate infiltration around transplant, and a few mononuclear cells within islets; +++, heavy infiltration around graft, and pockets of lymphocytes within islets; ++++, heavy infiltration around transplant, and islets penetrated by many mononuclear cells with severe disruption of islet architecture; and

(2) for integrity of the transplanted islets: +++++, islets completely intact; ++++, outer epithelium disrupted; +++, outer epithelium disrupted and center of islets disorganized; ++, entire islet disorganized; +, islets reduced to remnants.

had become disorganized by infiltrating lymphoid cells, and graft rejection was complete by day 14, when only scattered fragments of islet tissue were seen at the site of transplantation (Figure 2b and c).

Cyclophosphamide pretreatment of the tissue donor before the harvest of tissue for transplantation reduced the intensity of the allograft response. By day 14, there was an obvious response to the grafted tissue; however, some islets were intact and still contained β cells that stained with aldehyde-fuchsin at 21 days posttransplantation (Figure 2d). Islets from cyclophosphamide-pretreated donors generally underwent a more chronic rejection process than islets from untreated donors.

Allograft response to in vitro–cultured islet tissue. Islet clusters, unlike isolated single islets, survive well when cultured in an atmosphere of 95% O_2 and 5% CO_2. The clusters maintain their histologic structure, and aldehyde-fuchsin staining of this tissue showed the presence of β cells in these clusters up to a culture period of 20 days (Figure 3).

When cultured BALB/c islets from cyclophosphamide-treated donors were transplanted under the kidney capsule of CBA mice, little or no allograft response was observed (Table 2). Culture periods of as short as 4 days were effective in conditioning islets for allotransplantation. However, a culture period of around 7 days was generally more convenient because the tight islet clusters produced by 7 days were much easier to manipulate than the somewhat looser aggregates produced after 4 days of culture. In the case of tissue cultured for 7 days, a similar survival pattern was observed, regardless of whether the tissue was obtained from untreated or cyclophosphamide-pretreated donors (Table 2). Fourteen days after transplantation, β cells were obvious in the allografted islet tissue (Figure 4).

By 4 wk after transplantation, the cultured islet tissue was very well vascularized (Figure 5), and only 1 out of 14 allografts showed any sign of islet damage when examined histologically (Table 2). Essentially the same pattern of tissue survival was observed when islets from cyclophosphamide-pretreated donors were cultured for 7–12 days and examined histologically 3 mo after allotransplantation. In this study of five transplanted animals, all transplants were well

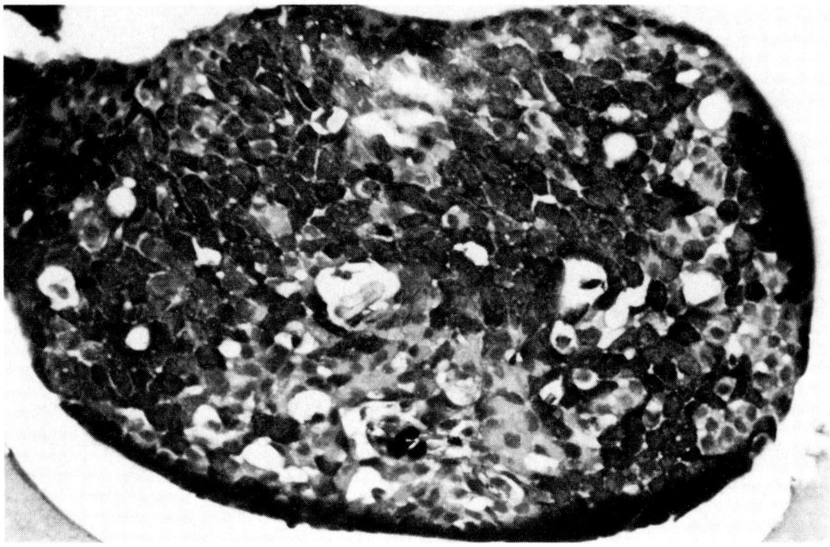

FIGURE 3. Section of islet cluster after 7 days in organ culture, showing presence of darkly stained β cells (aldehyde-fuchsin, ×312).

vascularized when removed from the recipients at 3 mo, and none showed any histologic evidence of an allograft response (Figure 6). Intact β cells were present in the allografted tissue 3 mo after transplantation.

DISCUSSION

Normal pancreatic islets elicit a violent allograft response when transplanted to the kidney capsule of normal allogeneic recipients, and Garvey et al.[6] have reported that it is more difficult to suppress an immune response to transplanted islets than a response to either kidney or skin allografts. However, the data presented in this paper show that the immunogenicity of pancreatic islets can be essentially eliminated by treatment of the islet tissue before transplantation. Our treatment procedures were based on our experience with thyroid allotransplantation, indicating that leukocytes carried within the grafted tissues constitute the major barrier to allotransplantation.[1,3] As was the case with the thyroid, pretreatment of the donor animal with cyclophosphamide does not inhibit the allograft response but results in a somewhat more chronic rejection process. However, when cyclophosphamide pretreatment of the donor was combined with organ culture, little or no immune response to the allografted tissue was detected over a 3-mo observation period. In some transplants, very small pockets of lymphoid cells were seen around the islet tissue 14 days after trans-

TABLE 2
Histologic appearance of cultured islets after transplantation under the kidney capsule of CBA recipient mice

		Histologic score*			
		14 days posttransplantation		28 days posttransplantation	
Donor pretreatment	Culture time (days)	Mononuclear cell infiltration	Integrity of islet tissue	Mononuclear cell infiltration	Integrity of islet tissue
Cyclophosphamide†	4	0	+++++	0	+++++
		0	+++++	0	+++++
		+	+++++	0	+++++
		+	+++++	0	+++++
		+	+++++		
Cyclophosphamide	7	0	+++++	0	+++++
		+	+++++	+	+++++
		0	+++++	+	+++++
		+	+++++	0	+++++
				0	+++++
Cyclophosphamide	12	0	+++++	0	+++++
		0	+++++	0	+++++
		0	+++++	++	++++
		0	+++++	0	+++++
		0	+++++	0	+++++
		+	+++++		
None	7	0	+++++	Not tested	Not tested
		+	+++++		
		0	+++++		
		0	+++++		

* See second footnote to Table 1.
† See first footnote to Table 1.

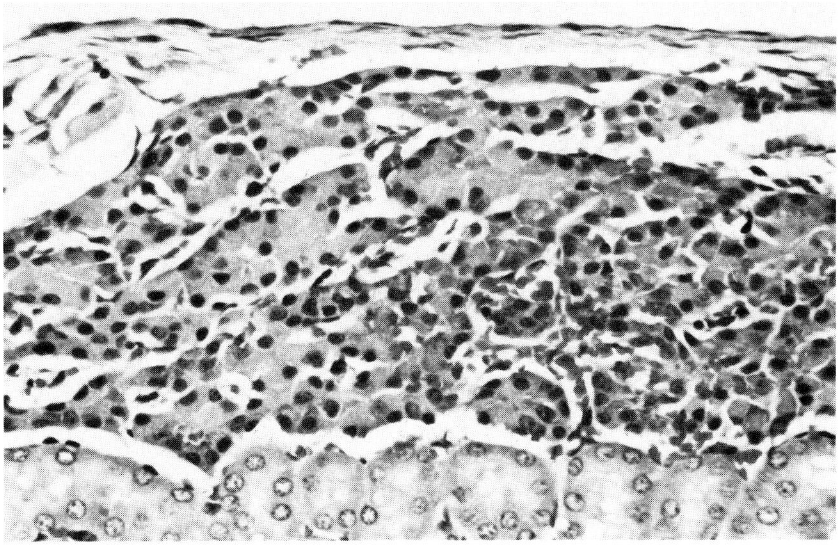

A

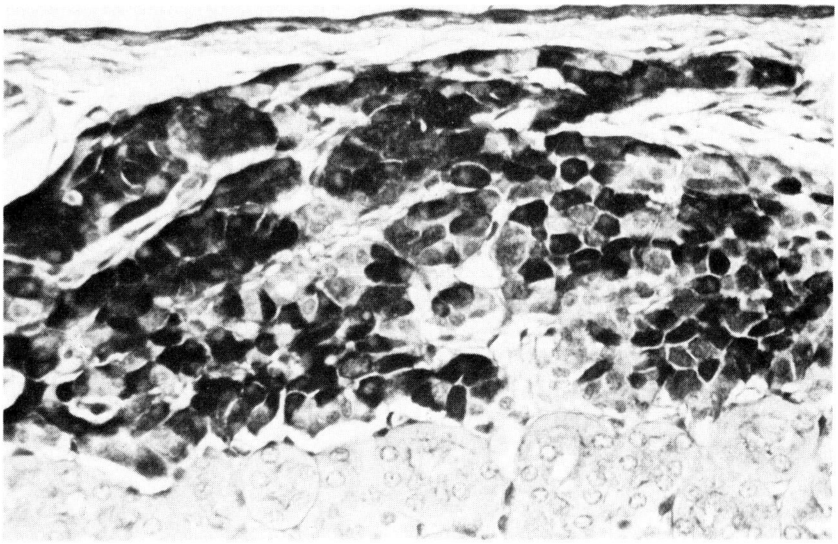

B

FIGURE 4. Host (CBA) response to allograft of islet tissue conditioned by organ culture of BALB/c islet tissue for 7 days before transplantation. Tissue was examined 2 wk after transplantation. (Top) Hematoxylin and eosin, ×312. (Bottom) Aldehyde-fuchsin, ×312.

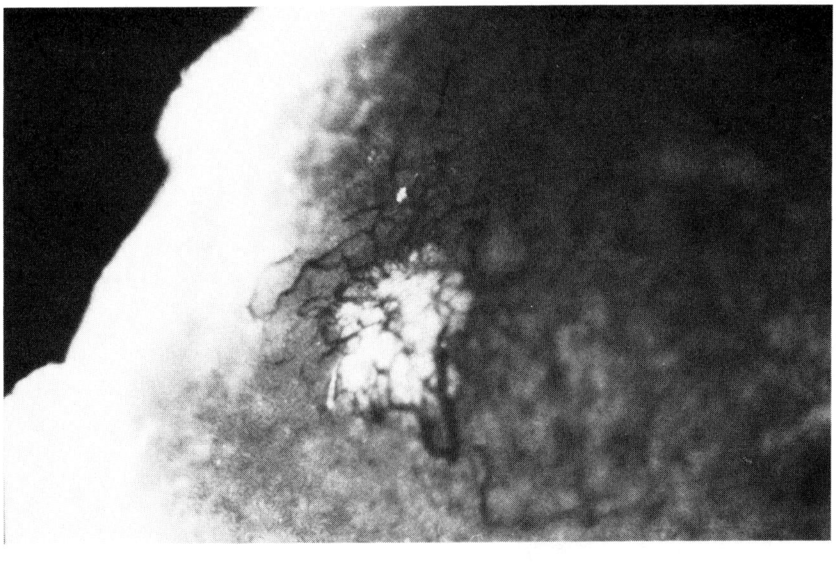

FIGURE 5. Vascular connections to islet tissue (BALB/c) transplanted to the kidney capsule of allogeneic (CBA) recipients 4 wk after transplantation. Islet tissue was conditioned for transplantation by cyclophosphamide treatment of the tissue donor and a 7-day period of organ culture (×50).

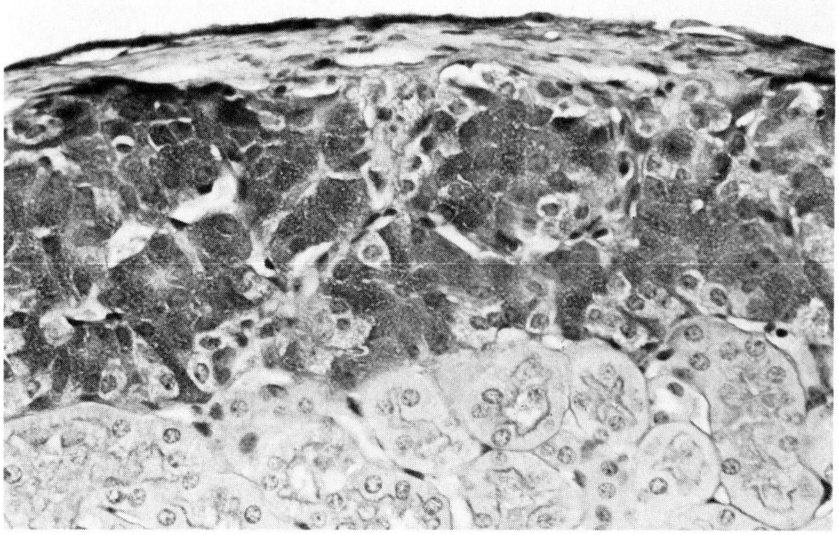

FIGURE 6. Host (CBA) response to allograft of islet tissue conditioned by cyclophosphamide treatment of the islet donors (BALB/c) and a 7-day period of organ culture. Tissue was examined 3 mo posttransplant. (Aldehyde-fuchsin, ×312.)

plantation, but in only 1 out of 38 transplants examined was this reaction extensive enough to cause islet damage. All other allografts had a normal histologic structure and contained obvious β cells when stained with aldehyde-fuchsin. The minor mononuclear cell response to the transplanted tissue appeared to be a transient phenomenon because none of the five allografts examined 3 mo after transplantation showed any trace of an allograft response.

In our previous transplantation studies,[1] tissues were cultured in an atmosphere of 95% O_2 and 5% CO_2 before transplantation. Talmage and Dart[7] reported that the oxygen tension in the gas phase plays an important role in conditioning thyroid tissue for allotransplantation, presumably because of its selective toxicity for blood cells carried within the transplanted tissue. Lacy et al.[8] reported that isolated rat islets degenerate rapidly when cultured in 95% O_2 and 5% CO_2, an effect we have also observed with isolated mouse islets; other attempts to condition islets for allotransplantation have used a gas phase of 5% CO_2 in air.[8–10] In the study reported here, we have shown that, although single islets cannot be cultured in a high oxygen atmosphere, clusters of about 50 islets can be cultured in this way and successfully transplanted to normal allogeneic hosts. Thus, it would appear that oxygen tension in the culture system plays a crucial role in the conditioning of islet tissue for allotransplantation.

In our earlier studies of thyroid allotransplantation[1] we found a synergistic effect of organ culture and cyclophosphamide pretreatment of the donor. In the case of islet tissue, one experimental series showed that organ culture for 7 days was equally effective in conditioning tissue taken from normal or cyclophosphamide-pretreated animals. In the case of the thyroid, organ culture alone for 7 days had little effect on allograft survival. At this stage we are not sure why there is this difference between islets and thyroid; however, it is of considerable practical importance that such a short period of organ culture can have such a dramatic effect on islet allograft survival.

ACKNOWLEDGMENTS

The authors are grateful to Wendy Hughes for technical assistance. This work was supported in part by a grant from the John Claude Kellion Foundation. Kerry Bowen was supported by a NH and MRC Postgraduate Award.

REFERENCES

[1] Lafferty, K. J., and Woolnough, J.: The origin and mechanism of the allograft reaction. Immunol. Rev. *35*:231–62, 1977.

[2] Talmage, D. W., Woolnough, J., Hemmingsen, H., Lopez, L., and Lafferty, K. J.: Activation of cytotoxic T cells by nonstimulating tumor cells and spleen cell factor(s). Proc. Natl. Acad. Sci. U.S.A. *74*:4610–14, 1977.

[3] Talmage, D. W., Dart, G. A., Radovitch, J., and Lafferty, K. J.: Activation of transplant immunity: effect of donor leukocytes on thyroid allograft rejection. Science *191*:385–88, 1976.

[4] Hicken, P., and Krohn, P. L.: The histocompatibility requirements of ovarian grafts in mice. Proc. R. Soc. London B *151*:419–33, 1960.

[5] Bussolati, G., and Bassa, T.: Thiosulfation aldehyde fuchsin (TAF) procedure for the staining of pancreatic β cells. Stain Technol. *49*:313–15, 1974.

[6] Garvey, J. F. W., Morris, P. J., Finch, D. R. A., Millard, P. R., and Poole, M.: Experimental pancreas transplantation. Lancet *1*:971–72, 1979.

[7] Talmage, D. W., and Dart, G. A.: Effect of oxygen pressure during culture on survival of mouse thyroid allografts. Science *200*:1066–67, 1978.

[8] Lacy, P. E., Davie, J. M., and Finke, E. N.: Prolongation of islet allograft survival following in vitro culture (24°C) and a single injection of ALS. Science *204*:312–13, 1979.

[9] Kedinger, M., Haffen, K., Grenier, J., and Elroy, R.: In vitro culture reduces immunogenicity of pancreatic endocrine islets. Nature (London) *270*:736–38, 1977.

[10] Andersson, A., and Buschard, K.: Culture of isolated pancreatic islets: its application for transplantation purposes. Trans. Am. Soc. Artif. Intern. Organs *23*:342–45, 1977.

Effects of Oxygen, Temperature, and Time of Culture on the Survival of Mouse Thyroid and Pancreas Allografts

DAVID W. TALMAGE

SUMMARY

Organ culture of mouse thyroid for 3 wk resulted in survival of allografts. The time in culture has been reduced to 4 days by increasing the oxygen pressure to 1300 mm and to 1 day by culture at 1700 mm and pretreatment of the donor with hydrocortisone. Of 25 BALB/c thyroid grafts cultured for 24 h at 1700 mm O_2 and 37°C, 24 maintained function for 3 wk in C57B1/6 mouse recipients. Culture at room temperature (22–26°C) for 1 day was less effective in preventing rejection, and increasing the oxygen tension was not effective. These culture conditions have been applied to mouse pancreas, and survival of the organ was judged by morphologic and histochemical analysis. Lowering the temperature to 22°C resulted in survival for twice as long as at 37°C. This was true for partial O_2 pressure of 600 mm in which beta cell granulation persisted for 4 days at 22° and only two days at 37°C. At a higher O_2 pressure (1300 mm), beta granulation persisted for 2 days at 22°C and only 1 day at 37°C. Macrophages cultured in 600 mm O_2 survived more than 4 days at 37°C and 30°C, but less than 2 days at 26°C. Since macrophages may play a role in rejection of allografts, culture at 22°C and alteration of O_2 tension may select the desired cell types and enhance allograft survival. **DIABETES *29* (Suppl. 1):105–106, 1980.**

Using the techniques of organ culture and transplantation described by us with Lafferty,[1] we have demonstrated that the time of culture required for mouse thyroid allograft survival can be reduced from more than 3 wk to 4 days by increasing the oxygen pressure during culture from 600 to 1300 mm (reference 2 and experiments 1–4, Table 1). We have thus demonstrated that the major factor in eliminating the immunizing capacity of the thyroid was the oxygen pressure during culture. Since publication of that paper, we have reduced still further the time required for allograft survival by increasing the oxygen pressure to 1700 mm and pretreating the donors with hydrocortisone; 24 out of 25 BALB/c grafts obtained from pretreated donors cultured for only 24 h at this pressure and at 37°C maintained function for 3 wk in C57BL/6 recipients (experiment 5 in Table 1). Compare this with 0 out of 19 functioning grafts cultured for 4 days at 600 mm (experiment 1, Table 1).

When the temperature of culture was reduced to room temperature (22–26°C) and grafts were cultured for 1 day, the percentage of surviving grafts was reduced and further increases in pressure were not effective (experiments 6 and 7). However, when the time of incubation at room temperature was increased to 4 days, a paradoxical result was observed. Fifty percent of the grafts cultured at 600 mm O_2 and 22–26°C survived, but none survived at that pressure if cultured at 37°C or 30°C. (Compare experiments 8 and 10 with experiments 1 and 9.) Grafts cultured at 18° and 26°C survived approximately the same as those cultured at 22°C (data not shown).

DISCUSSION

The data presented in the table show that the time of culture required is a complex function of oxygen pressure and temperature. As indicated in the table, we had already begun to experiment with a lower culture temperature before receiving Dr. Lacy's report.[3] This decision was based on the following rationale: the limiting factor determining the distance oxygen diffuses through tissue is its consumption by that tissue; by lowering the temperature, oxygen consumption should be greatly reduced and, thus, the steady state slope of oxygen tension through the tissue made considerably flatter. Thus, considerably less oxygen might be needed at the surface of the graft to supply an adequate amount to the interior. In addition, oxygen solubility increases as the temperature is reduced.

Since performing the experiments reported in the table we have made another observation which may indicate another reason that lower temperatures are more effective.

From the Webb-Waring Lung Institute and the Departments of Microbiology and Immunology, University of Colorado Medical Center, Denver, Colorado 80262.

TABLE 1
Effects of oxygen, temperature, and time of culture on survival of BALB/c thyroids in C57BL/6 mice.

Exp.	P_{O_2}(mm)	°C	Days	^{125}I uptake*	%
1	600	37	4	0/19	0
2	1000	37	4	4/11	36
3	1300	37	4	8/13	62
4	1300	37	4	15/16†	93
5	1700	37	1	24/25‡	96
6	1700	22–26	1	3/8‡	38
7	2100	22–26	1	3/5	60
8	600	22–26	4	10/20	50
9	600	30	4	0/10	0
10	600	22	4	5/14	36

* A ratio greater than 10 in radioactivity of grafted to ungrafted kidneys 3 wk after transplantation.
† Hydrocortisone added to culture medium.
‡ Hydrocortisone given to donor 24 h before thyroidectomy.

Macrophages cultured in 600 mm O_2 survived more than 4 days at 37°C and 30°C but less than 2 days at 26°C. The critical difference between 26°C and 30°C may be due to the fact that cells can respond adaptively at the higher temperature only. Thus, below 30°C the macrophages may not be able to respond to the high oxygen environment with the production of antioxidant enzymes such as catalase and superoxide dismutase. This is based on the finding of Maccecchini and Burger[4] that 29.5°C is the lowest temperature at which any lymphocyte response to Con A occurs.

In a recent study by Chase et al.[5] we found that histologic evidence of beta cell survival in cultured fetal mouse pancreases persisted approximately twice as long at 22°C as at 37°C. This was true at partial pressures of 1300 and 600 mm O_2. At 1300 mm, beta granulation persisted 1 day at 37°C and 2 days at 22°C. With 600 mm, the survival times were 2 days and 4 days, respectively.

Thus, lowering the temperature increased survival of the endocrine cells and, under some circumstances, reduced the survival of macrophages. For this reason, it is obviously important to determine the optimum temperature for culturing endocrine grafts.

REFERENCES

[1] Lafferty, K. J., Bootes, A., Dart, G., and Talmage, D. W.: Effect of organ culture on the survival of thyroid allografts in mice. Transplantation *22*:138–49, 1976.

[2] Talmage, D. W., and Dart, G. A.: Effect of oxygen pressure during culture on survival of mouse thyroid allografts. Science *200*:1066–67, 1978.

[3] Lacy, P. E., Davie, J. M., and Finke, E. H.: Prolongation of islet allograph survival following in vitro culture (24°C) and a single injection of ALS. Science *204*:312–13, 1979.

[4] Maccecchini, M-L., and Burger, M. M.: Stimulation of lymphocytes by concanavalin A. Temperature-dependent effect of fatty acid replacements. Biochim. Biophys. Acta *469*:33–44, 1977.

[5] Chase, H. P., Ocrant, I., and Talmage, D. W.: The effects of different conditions of organ culture on the survival of the mouse pancreas. Diabetes *28*:990–93, 1979.

Suppression of Rejection of Allogeneic Islet Tissue in the Rat

P. J. MORRIS, D. R. FINCH, J. F. GARVEY, M. D. POOLE, AND P. R. MILLARD

SUMMARY

A variety of immunosuppressive agents was used to prevent rejection of allografts of isolated rat islets of Langerhans injected into the portal vein or spleen, of fetal pancreases placed beneath the kidney capsule, or of vascularized hemipancreases. The agents included antilymphocytic serum (ALS), cyclophosphamide, Cyclosporin A, azathioprine, prednisolone, and donor-specific antiserum. Prolonged tissue culture of fetal pancreas and implantation of xenogeneic neonatal rabbit pancreases in Nucleopore bags were also carried out with the aim of suppressing rejection. In the face of a strong histocompatibility barrier, (DA × Lewis) F1 to Lewis, neither azathioprine nor prednisolone prolonged islet survival, whereas cyclophosphamide and Cyclosporin A prolonged survival by several days. ALS was an effective agent, prolonging islet survival by 26–50 days. Passive enhancement with donor-specific antiserum was modestly effective in DA to Lewis, but much more effective in the heterozygous [(DA × Lewis) F1 to Lewis or DA] combination. Survival of fetal pancreas was most prolonged by ALS, especially (DA × Lewis) F1 to Lewis, with a median survival time of 45 days. In contrast, Cyclosporin A, passive enhancement, and culture for 21 days were ineffective. Cyclosporin A was significantly effective only in prolonging function of the vascularized pancreas for up to 28 days. Nucleopore bags proved ineffective. Pancreatic islet tissue is strongly immunogenic, perhaps because it is not vascularized. A variety of immunosuppressive agents that are effective for other tissues do not protect against rejection of isolated islets or the fetal organ. DIABETES 29 (Suppl. 1): 107–112, 1980.

Although the defects of glucose metabolism in experimental models of diabetes can be corrected in part or in whole by transplantation of pancreatic islets or fetal pancreas, rejection of allogeneic tissue remains a major problem still to be overcome before clinical application of available techniques will be possible. This apparently strong immunogenicity of pancreatic islets or fetal pancreases is in contrast to the behavior of vascularized pancreatic grafts where the immune response to the islet tissue seems less striking. Thus, although transplantation of pancreatic islets or fetal pancreases is an attractive solution to the problem of providing complete and permanent control of diabetes, suppression of the immune response to islet tissue is an obstacle additional to that of provision of sufficient endocrine tissue. In this report, our studies of allogeneic transplantation of pancreatic islet tissue are reviewed. These emphasize the difficulties associated with suppression of the immunologic response to nonvascularized endocrine pancreatic tissue.

From the Nuffield Department of Surgery, Oxford University, John Radcliffe Hospital, Oxford, England.

METHODS AND MATERIALS

ANIMALS

Inbred DA/Ss Wehi (AgB^4, now $RT1^{-avl}$) and Lewis/Ss Wehi (AgB^1, now $RT1^l$) and the (DA × Lewis) F1 hybrid were used in most of our experiments.[1] The DA to Lewis combination represents a very strong histocompatibility barrier and the Lewis to DA a much weaker one, with the (DA × Lewis) F1 to Lewis or to DA models representing weaker immunogenetic combinations than their respective parental donor combinations.[2] Rats weighed between 150 and 250 g.

In some of the xenogeneic transplants of rabbit neonatal pancreas enclosed in a Nucleopore bag, Wistar rats were used as diabetic recipients, whereas Wag rats (AgB^2, $RT1^{\mu}$) were used as recipients in some of the syngeneic intrasplenic transplants.

Fetal pancreases (18-day gestation time) were removed aseptically from Lewis and DA mothers.

INDUCTION OF DIABETES

Diabetes was induced by the single i.v. injection of streptozotocin (Upjohn, Kalamazoo, Michigan) in a dose of 65 mg/kg. Only rats with random blood sugar levels higher than 400 mg/dl (22 mmol/l) and 24-h urine volumes greater than

50 ml, on two estimations at least 1 wk and usually 2 wk after injection, were considered to have established diabetes.

TRANSPLANT MODELS

Adult islets were prepared as described by Ballinger and Lacy.[3] Islets, approximately 600–800 from six donors, were injected either into the portal vein or into the splenic parenchyma, as previously described in detail.[4,5]

Fetal pancreases (6–10) were transplanted under the renal capsule as described by Brown et al.[6] either immediately after removal or after a period in culture for up to 3 wk. The recipients of fetal pancreases were given 1–4 U of Ultralente insulin subcutaneously for 8 days after transplantation to facilitate graft maturation.

Vascularized pancreases were transplanted using the distal half of the pancreas, after splenectomy, with anastomosis of the celiac artery and portal vein to the renal artery and vein, respectively.

DIAGNOSIS OF REJECTION

After transplantation, rats were maintained in metabolic cages, and blood glucose, urinary volume, and body weight were monitored daily. Rejection was defined as the first of two consecutive days in which the blood glucose rose above 200 mg/dl (11 mmol/L) after islet transplantation and above 250 mg/dl (14 mmol/L) after transplantation of the fetal pancreas. The host pancreases were examined histologically in some long-surviving animals for evidence of islet regeneration. In addition, in the intrasplenic and renal subcapsular models, splenectomy or nephrectomy, respectively, was also performed with the same objective.

FETAL PANCREATIC CULTURE

The entire fetal pancreas was placed onto a Millipore raft, pore size 0.45 μm (Millipore SA, Molsheim, France), on a Gelfoam support (Upjohn, Puurs, Belgium) and incubated in a petri dish containing 15 ml medium RPMI 1640 (Flow Laboratories) plus 10% fetal calf serum supplemented with antibiotics in an atmosphere of 95% air and 5% CO_2. Cultures were maintained for up to 3 wk. The final glucose concentration in the medium was 180 mg (10 mmol/L) and the pH 7.2.

XENOGENEIC PANCREAS IN NUCLEOPORE BAGS

Two pancreases from neonatal rabbits were implanted into the peritoneal cavity of diabetic Wistar and DA rats as described by Gates and Lazarus,[7] who collaborated on these experiments. Two Nucleopore bags containing the pancreases of two neonatal rabbits (5–8 days old) were implanted in the peritoneal cavity of streptozotocin-diabetic rats in the following experiments: (1) Wistar male rats, given 85 mg/kg streptozotocin i.v., were implanted at the Wellcome Institute, and their posttransplant serum glucose and urine volumes were monitored in our laboratories; (2) Wistar male rats given 110 mg/kg of streptozotocin at the Wellcome Institute were implanted in our laboratory 1 day later; and (3) our own DA rats, diabetic for at least 2 wk (the diabetic status having been confirmed with two serum glucoses above 25 mmol/L and a urine volume of 50 ml in 24 h), were implanted by Gates and Lazarus in our laboratory and compared with sham-operated diabetic DA rats implanted with only a Nucleopore chamber.

IMMUNOSUPPRESSION

Nonspecific. (1) New Zealand White rabbits were immunized with intraperitoneal injections of 10^8 Lewis and DA thoracic duct lymphocytes as previously described.[8] ALS was given intraperitoneally (i.p.) at days −1, 1, 3, and 5, or i.v. on days 0, 1, 3, and 5.

(2) Cyclophosphamide was given in a dose of 10 mg/kg/day for 14 days. The first dose was given i.v. at the time of transplantation and thereafter intraperitoneally.

(3) Cyclosporin A (Sandoz), a new potent immunosuppressive agent,[9–13] was given orally in olive oil in doses ranging from 5 to 40 mg/kg/day for 14 days.

Specific. DA anti-Lewis or Lewis anti-DA serum was prepared as previously described, using spleen cells with Freund's complete adjuvant.[14] Antisera were administered intravenously into the IVC just before or after the islets were implanted in their recipient site. Doses ranged from 50 μl as a single dose or, alternatively, 2.5 ml over several days, with the first dose being 1 ml followed by subsequent i.v. doses of 0.5 ml.

RESULTS

ISOGENEIC TRANSPLANTS

Intraportal islets. The results are shown in Table 1; 600–800 islets restored normoglycemia within 48 h. Animals remained normoglycemic for at least 12 mo; however, intravenous glucose tolerance tests in these normoglycemic animals were abnormal.

Intrasplenic islets. The results are shown in Table 2; 600–800 islets restored normoglycemia generally within 72 h, but sometimes over a period of several days. Animals remain normoglycemic for at least 12 mo but with abnormal intravenous glucose tolerance tests (IVGTT). Although some islets can be shown to pass into the portal circulation and lodge in the liver, splenectomy immediately makes the rats diabetic once more. Islets from one donor injected into the spleen at weekly intervals were able to restore normoglycemia in all of 10 diabetic animals after 3 wk.

Fetal pancreas. The results are shown in Table 3. All rats became normoglycemic and remained so, but this could take up to 1 mo. In contrast to the intraportal and intrasplenic model, rats given fetal pancreases had normal IVGTT. In some recipients all six pancreases were implanted beneath the capsule of the left kidney. Nephrectomy in five such recipients 40–190 days after transplantation was followed by reversion to the diabetic state. However, nephrectomy in one of these five recipients 230 days after transplantation was not followed by hyperglycemia, showing that regeneration of host islet tissue does occur on occasions.

Culture. Rats receiving fetal pancreases cultured for 21 days became normoglycemic within 21 days, with the exception of one animal that took 43 days (Table 3).

Vascularized pancreas. These animals remained normoglycemic indefinitely. Glucose tolerance tests have been performed and, in two recipients so far studied at 3 mo, the insulin and glucose responses have been similar to normal rats.

ALLOGENEIC TRANSPLANTS

Intraportal islets. No grafts in the DA to Lewis or Lewis to

TABLE 1
Intraportal transplantation of adult islets (600–800) to diabetic DA and Lewis recipients and the effects of ALS, cyclophosphamide, and passive enhancement in preventing rejection

Strain combination	Treatment	No. of rats	Median day of rejection (range)
Lewis → Lewis	Nil	10	>360
DA → DA	Nil	10	>360
DA → Lewis	Nil	5	4 (2–5)
Lewis → DA	Nil	5	4 (4–4)
(DA × L) F_1 → Lewis	Nil	5	4 (4–5)
(DA × L) F_1 → DA	Nil	5	4 (4–6)
ALS			
DA → Lewis	ALS (1 ml, i.p.) days −1,1,3,5	5	26 (22–32)
(DA × L) F_1 → Lewis	"	5	50 (22–>100)
Cyclophosphamide			
(DA × L) F_1 → Lewis	Cyclophosphamide 10 mg/kg/day	5	6 (6–9)
" " (1500–3000 islets)	" "	6	12 (8–>100)
Passive enhancement			
DA → Lewis	500 μl Lewis anti-DA	5	8 (5–11)
(DA × L) F_1 → Lewis	" " "	5	16 (12–>360)
Lewis → DA	500 μl DA anti-Lewis	5	7 (6–8)
(DA × L) F_1 → DA	" "	5	34 (22–>360)

DA combination maintained normoglycemia for more than 6 days, regardless of whether the homozygous parent or the (DA × Lewis) F1 hybrid was used as the donor (Table 1).

Intrasplenic islets. Only the (DA × Lewis) F1 to Lewis combination was tested, but again normoglycemia was not maintained for more than 6 days (Table 2).

Renal subcapsular fetal pancreases. All Lewis and DA recipients of (DA × Lewis) F1 fetal pancreases reverted to the diabetic state by day 10. Subsequent histologic examination at 14 days showed destruction of the graft by a mononuclear cell infiltrate, and, after 1 mo, the only evidence of a graft was a superficial scar (Table 3).

Vascularized pancreas. Lewis recipients rejected DA pancreases within 11 days, and subsequent histologic examination showed a substantial mononuclear and polymorphonuclear infiltrate with evidence of fibrinoid necrosis in the vessels of some grafts (Table 4).

XENOGENEIC

Both DA and Wistar rats were implanted with neonatal rabbit pancreases in Nucleopore bags with several protocols of streptozotocin induction of diabetes, and in only one rat was there a significant and sustained reduction in serum glucose. When this one rat had the bag containing the graft removed, it remained normoglycemic, indicating that the recipient's own pancreas had presumably regenerated some of its islet tissue. Histologic examination of the material within the excised bags revealed no evidence of islet tissue, but there was an extensive fibrotic reaction around the bags.

TABLE 2
Intrasplenic transplantation of adult islets (600–800) and the effect of ALS and Cyclosporin A in preventing rejection

Strain combination	Treatment	No. of rats	Median day of rejection (range)
Lewis to Lewis	Nil	3	>360
WaG to WaG	Nil	6	>360
(DA × L) F_1 → Lewis	Nil	5	5 (5–6)
" "	ALS (1 ml, i.p.), days −1,1,3,5	6	32 (28–38)
DA → Lewis	Olive oil	7	4 (1–6)
"	Cyclosporin A 5 mg/kg/day	4	5 (1–13)
"	" 10 "	5	6 (3–8)
"	" 20 "	6	6 (1–13)
"	" 40 "	6	12 (2–21)

IMMUNOSUPPRESSION: INTRAPORTAL AND INTRASPLENIC ISLETS

Nonspecific. Neither azathioprine (30 mg/kg/day) nor prednisolone (8 mg/kg/day) were able to prolong survival of (DA × Lewis) F1 intraportal islets; rejection occurred within 7 days. Cyclophosphamide (10 mg/kg/day) produced a small but significant prolongation of survival of several days of (DA × Lewis) F1 intraportal islets in Lewis recipients, but if the number of islets transplanted was increased to 1500–3000, obtained from 14–16 donors, then survival was further prolonged, and two out of six animals became long survivors (Table 1).

ALS was an effective immunosuppressive agent in our models. It was able to significantly prolong survival of both DA and (DA×Lewis) F1 intraportal islets in Lewis recipients, the effect being more striking in the (DA×Lewis) F1 to Lewis combination (Table 1). It was equally effective in prolonging survival of (DA × Lewis) F1 intrasplenic islets in Lewis recipients (Table 2). In doses ranging from 5 mg/kg/day up to 40 mg/kg/day, Cyclosporin A produced a very modest but significant prolongation of survival of DA islets given intrasplenically into Lewis recipients (Table 2).

Specific. Both Lewis anti-DA and DA anti-Lewis sera produced small but significant prolongation of survival of intraportal DA and Lewis pancreatic islets, respectively, in a single dose of 500 μl given at the time of transplantation (Table 1). A much larger dose, 2.5 ml of Lewis anti-DA, given over several days produced no prolongation in survival, perhaps due to antibody-mediated damage of the transplanted islets. Passive enhancement was far more impressive when used in the heterozygous (DA × Lewis) F1 to Lewis or DA

TABLE 3
Transplantation of fetal pancreases (6–10) beneath the renal capsule of diabetic rats and the effect of passive enhancement. ALS, Cyclosporin A, and prolonged culture in preventing rejection

Strain combination	Treatment	No. of rats	Median day of rejection (range)
Lewis → Lewis	Nil	9	>150
(DA × L) F_1 → Lewis	"	8	10 (9–10)
(DA × L) F_1 → DA	"	5	10 (9–11)
Passive enhancement			
(DA × Lewis) F_1 → Lewis	Lewis anti-DA (250 μl), days 0,1	6	11 (10–12)
(DA × Lewis) F_1 → DA	DA anti-Lewis (250 μl), days 0,1)	6	9 (9)
ALS			
(DA × Lewis) F_1 → DA	ALS (125 μl, i.v.) days 0,1,3,5	5	9 (9–10)
" "	" 250 μl, "	5	15 (9–15)
" "	" 500 μl, "	5	>100 (11–>100)
(DA × Lewis) F_1 → Lewis	" 500 μl, days 0,1,3,5	4	11 (10–70)
" "	" 750 μl, "	5	45 (18–>100)
Cyclosporin A			
DA → Lewis	Olive oil	7	9 (9–10)
"	CyA 10 mg/kg/day	5	13 (9–14)
"	" 20 "	3	12 (10–13)
"	" 40 "	3	10 (9–15)
Prolonged culture			
Lewis → Lewis	Nil	6	>60 (12–>60)
(DA × Lewis) F_1 → Lewis	Nil	6	11 (10–12)

recipient when, at a dose of 500 μl at the time of transplantation, several animals remained normoglycemic for over a year. Even a dose of 50 μl produced some delay in rejection as did a larger dose of 2.5 ml over several days, in contrast to its use in the recipient of homozygous parental islets, where possible islet damage resulted from the passive administration of antiserum. An increase in the number of (DA × Lewis) F1 islets transplanted, from 600–800 up to 1500–3000, did not result in any increase in the time that DA rats passively enhanced with DA anti-Lewis serum remained normoglycemic, in contrast to immunosuppression with cyclophosphamide described earlier.

Although the combination of passive enhancement and ALS is synergistic in the rat renal allograft model, this did not prove to be so when (DA × Lewis) F1 islets were transplanted intraportally into DA or Lewis recipients. No greater effect of combined therapy was seen with two different protocols of ALS administration than with either ALS or passive enhancement alone.[8]

IMMUNOSUPPRESSION: FETAL PANCREAS

Nonspecific. In both semiallogeneic combinations, ALS was found to be the most immunosuppressive agent. A dose of 500 μl (i.v.) on days 0, 1, 3, and 5 produced long survival of F1 to DA fetal pancreas (three surviving normoglycemic beyond 100 days) and the graft of F1 to Lewis was prolonged to between 28 and 100 days (mean survival time, 45 days). Cyclosporin A, in doses ranging from 5 to 40 mg/kg in olive oil, yielded no significant prolongation (Table 3).

Specific. The use of Lewis anti-DA serum produced no significant prolongation of survival over nonenhanced controls, all the recipients rejecting their grafts and becoming hyperglycemic by day 12. Even in the weakest strain combination (F1 to DA), where as little as 50 μl of antiserum prolongs survival of kidney and adult islet allografts, all recipients became hyperglycemic by day 9, and this period of normoglycemia was shorter than that for nonenhanced control rats. Both these same alloantisera produced extended survival of kidney grafts in the F1 to Lewis and F1 to DA model.

TABLE 4
Transplantation of a vascularized hemipancreas and the effect of Cyclosporin A in preventing rejection

Strain combination	Treatment	No. of rats	Median day of rejection (range)
Lewis → Lewis	Nil	3	>180
DA → Lewis	Nil	4	7 (3–9)
" "	Cyclosporin A 5 mg/kg/day	2	8.5 (8,9)
	" 10 "	2	10.5 (9,12)
	" 20 "	4	24 (19–28)

FETAL PANCREATIC CULTURE

Culture of (DA × Lewis) F1 fetal pancreases for 21 days resulted in a slight prolongation of survival, for rejection had occurred by 12 days in rats receiving cultured pancreases compared with 10 days for those receiving fresh allografts (all recipients received insulin for 8 days after transplantation). Histologic examination of the grafts 9 wk after transplantation showed solid islands of B cells in the cultured isograft but only scar tissue and a few mononuclear cells in the cultured allograft.[15]

VASCULARIZED PANCREAS

Although ineffective in suppressing rejection of adult islets or fetal pancreases, Cyclosporin A was more impressive in this model, survival being prolonged up to 28 days at a dose of 20 mg/kg/day.

DISCUSSION

It is apparent that, although the hyperglycemia of streptozotocin-induced diabetes in the rat can be corrected by the intraportal or intrasplenic transplantation of adult islets or the implantation of fresh or cultured fetal pancreases in syngeneic combinations, once a major histocompatibility barrier is crossed, rejection is rapid. In the strain combinations used in our experiments, no grafts of adult islets survived in nonimmunosuppressed recipients beyond 6 days and fetal pancreases did not survive more than 11 days. It should be remembered that, in the latter instance, insulin is given to the recipient animal for 8 days to facilitate maturation of the fetal pancreases, and rejection probably did occur by day 6–8. Thus, pancreatic islet tissue appers to be as immunogenic as skin, if not more so, although in part the rapid rate of rejection may be attributed to the more sensitive method of detecting rejection of islet tissue, namely, a moderate elevation of blood glucose.

This strong immunogenicity of islet tissue may be due to the nature of the graft, since it is not directly vascularized, as is a renal allograft. Thus, a different immune response to that seen following a vascularized graft may be induced. This is supported by our observation that vascularized hemipancreas grafts are rejected significantly later than isolated islets (4 days vs. 7 days), which is more comparable to the time of rejection of renal allografts in the same strain combination. Furthermore, adult islets were implanted intraportally into the liver or into the splenic parenchyma. The liver is rich in macrophages (Kupfer cells), as is the spleen, and perhaps the induction of an immune response results in such a rapid effector response through the agency of these macrophages. It is relevant that Nash and Bell[16] have shown that suppression of macrophage function by silica pretreatment of the recipient produced extended survival of intraportal islet allografts in the rat. On the other hand, if the abundance of macrophages in the liver and spleen were responsible for the rapid rejection of intraportal and intrasplenic islets, it would be expected that rejection of fetal pancreases beneath the renal capsule would be comparable to skin or kidney. As insulin is given to these animals for 8 days, it is not possible to determine the precise day of rejection, but one suspects it is similar to that of adult intraportal and intrasplenic islets.

There is no information concerning humoral and cellular immune responses after islet transplantation, but this would be relevant, for it has been suggested that islets are more susceptible to humoral antibody,[17] and perhaps an early humoral response results in the rapid rejection of islet tissue. However, it is a little difficult to explain the prolongation of survival of islet tissue produced by the simultaneous administration of enhancing antisera which is donor-specific and cytotoxic if this were the case, for one would have expected to see the onset of accelerated rejection rather than prolonged survival of islet tissue in this situation. Admittedly, large doses of enhancing antisera did not prolong islet survival, which could be interpreted as an effect of antibody-mediated damage. Thus, this question remains unresolved, and for the present the immunogenicity of nonvascularized pancreatic islet tissue is best attributed to sensitivity of the islets to whatever immune response is induced after transplantation, with perhaps macrophage and humoral antibody playing a major role in their rejection.

It is also apparent that suppression of the immune response to pancreatic islet tissue (such that rejection is prevented) is extraordinarily difficult using specific and nonspecific immunosuppressive protocols that are most effective in renal allograft models in the same strain combinations. For example, ALS seems to be the most potent agent, as it was able to prolong the survival of DA intraportal islets in Lewis recipients for 26 days, and no other agent in our hands was capable of delaying rejection for more than a few days in this model. Similar results were achieved by Reckard and Barker.[18] It was also the most effective agent in prolonging the survival of the fetal pancreas, many recipients being normoglycemic beyond 50 days.

Of the other nonspecific immunosuppressive protocols tested, none more forcefully emphasizes the difference between islets and a vascularized allograft than the failure of Cyclosporin A to significantly prolong survival of DA islets in Lewis recipients. In this same strain combination, 10 mg/kg/day of Cyclosporin A given orally for 7 or 14 days completely suppresses rejection of renal allografts, and the recipient rats survive indefinitely.[19] Again demonstrating the difference between vascularized and nonvascularized islet tissue, Cyclosporin A is moderately effective in suppressing rejection of the vascularized hemipancreas in the rat, and it is certainly effective in the dog pancreaticoduodenal allograft model (Calne, personal communication). Cyclophosphamide, another quite potent immunosuppressive agent in the rat renal allograft model,[20] is also relatively ineffective in the pancreatic islet models, although increasing the dose of islets augments its effect. This latter observation also suggests that part of the apparent immunogenicity of islet tissue may be due to the relatively small bulk of functional tissue that is transplanted, which does not provide any functional tissue reserve after damage produced either by ischemia or by the rejection reaction.

Passive enhancement of intraportal islet allografts did prolong survival very moderately in the case of parental donors, but quite strikingly in the case of the F1 hybrid donors. That several animals survived indefinitely after passive enhancement is encouraging, as specific suppression is the ultimate goal of transplant immunologists and would be particularly applicable to islet transplantation, where a relatively safe transplant protocol must be devised before clinical transplantation could be justified in the majority of diabetics. However, this effect was not seen with the fetal pancreas allografts, even in the weak F1 to DA combination. There could be many reasons for this failure of passive enhancement of fetal pancreas: the presence of fetal antigens and the singular vulnerability of the immature islet tissue to donor-specific antibody at an early stage of development are possibilities. So, although fetal pancreas is an ideal donor source for isogeneic transplantation, it is no less immunogenic than adult islet tissue.

Transplantation of Nucleopore bags containing xenogeneic neonatal rabbit pancreases as described by Gates and Lazarus[7] was unsuccessful in our hands in three separate experiments, all of which were performed with the collaboration of those workers. Although attractive in concept, in that chambers might be devised with a pore size sufficient to allow adequate nutrition of the contents and escape of insulin, they are unlikely to prevent escape of antigen with subsequent sensitization of the host. Although the entry of effector cells would be prevented by a relatively large pore size, the use of a chamber with a sufficiently small pore size to prevent the entry of antibody and complement might well compromise the nutrition of the contained islets. Recent models developed by Chick et al.[21] may enable a more precise examination of this concept.

The work of Lafferty,[22,23] showing that mouse allogeneic thyroid tissue cultured for several weeks before transplantation was not rejected, has excited a good deal of interest among those of us working with pancreatic islet transplantation. Unfortunately, in our hands, successful culture of fetal pancreases for up to 21 days resulted in a delay of rejection for only a day or two, although these cultured pancreases were capable of restoring a syngeneic diabetic rat to the normoglycemic state. This failure of prolonged culture to significantly prolong survival of islet tissue may be due to the lack of passenger leukocytes in islet tissue. The thyroid is rich in mononuclear cells, and Lafferty attributes the effects of prolonged culture to the deletion of these passenger leukocytes which play a key role in the induction of the immune response.

Thus, for the present, the immunologic problems of rejection of pancreatic islet tissue, either in the form of isolated islets or fetal pancreases, remain an obstacle of equal magnitude to that of obtaining an adequate amount of functioning islet tissue. Successful clinical application of pancreatic islet transplantation must still seem to be some time away.

ACKNOWLEDGMENTS

This work was supported by the Medical Research Council of the United Kingdom, the Wellcome Trust, and the British Diabetic Association.

REFERENCES

[1] Gill, T. J.: Major histocompatibility complex of the rat. Transplant. Proc. *11*:1174–78, 1979.

[2] Fabre, J. W., and Morris, P. J.: Passive enhancement of homozygous renal allografts in the rat. Transplantation *18*:429–35, 1974.

[3] Ballinger, W. F., and Lacy, P. E.: Transplantation of intact pancreatic islets in rats. Surgery *72*:175–86, 1972.

[4] Finch, D. R. A., and Morris, P. J.: Passive enhancement of isolated pancreatic islet allografts. Transplantation *22*:508–12, 1976.

[5] Finch, D. R. A., Wise, P., and Morris, P. J.: Successful intra-splenic transplantation of syngeneic and allogeneic isolated pancreatic islets. Diabetologia *13*:195–99, 1977.

[6] Brown, J., Clark, W. R., Molnar, I. G., and Mullen, Y. S.: Fetal pancreas transplantation for reversal of streptozotocin-induced diabetes in rats. Diabetes *25*:56–64, 1976.

[7] Gates, R. J., and Lazarus, N. R.: Reversal of streptozotocin-induced diabetes in rats by intraperitoneal implantation of encapsulated neonatal rabbit pancreatic tissue. Lancet *2*:1257–59, 1977.

[8] Finch, D. R., and Morris, P. J.: Failure to demonstrate a synergistic effect between enhancing serum and ALS in recipients of pancreatic islet allografts. Transplantation *23*:386–88, 1977.

[9] Borel, J. F., Feurer, C, Magnee, D, and Stahelin, H.: Effects of new anti-lymphocytic peptide Cyclosporin A in animals. Immunology *32*:1017–25, 1977.

[10] Borel, J. F., Feurer, C., Gubler, H. U., and Stahelin, H.: Biological effects of Cyclosporin A, a new antilymphocytic agent. Agents Actions *6*:468–75, 1976.

[11] Calne, R. Y., White, D. J. G., Rolles, K., Smith, D. P., and Herbertson, B. M.: Prolonged survival of pig orthotopic heart grafts treated with Cyclosporin A. Lancet *1*:1183–85, 1978.

[12] Calne, R. Y.: Pharmacological immunosuppression in clinical organ grafting. Observations on four agents: Cyclosporin A, Asta 5122 (Cytimun), lambda carrageenan and promethazine hydrochloride. Clin. Exp. Immunol. *35*:1–9, 1979

[13] Jamieson, S. W., Burton, N. A., Bieber, C. P., Reitz, B. A., Oyer, P. E., Stinson, E. B., and Shumway, N. E.: Cardiac-allograft survival in primates treated with Cyclosporin A. Lancet *1*:545, 1979.

[14] Fabre, J. W., and Morris, P. J.: Experience with passive enhancement of renal allografts in a (DA × Lewis) F1 to Lewis strain combination. Transplantation *13*:604–09, 1972.

[15] Garvey, J. F. W., Klein, C., Millard, P. R., and Morris, P. J.: Rejection of organ-cultured allogeneic fetal rat pancreas. Surgery, in press, 1979.

[16] Nash, J. R., and Bell, P. R. F.: Effect of macrophage suppression on survival of islet allografts. Transplant. Proc. *11*:986–88, 1979.

[17] Frangipane, L. G., Poole, T. W., Barker, C. F., and Silvers, W. K.: Vulnerability of allogeneic and xenogeneic pancreatic islets to alloantisera. Transplant. Proc. *9*:371–73, 1977.

[18] Reckard, C. F. R., and Barker, C. F.: Transplantation of isolated pancreatic islets across strong and weak histocompatibility barriers. Transplant. Proc. *5*:761–63, 1973.

[19] Homan, W. P., Fabre, J. W., Williams, K. A., Millard, P. R., and Morris, P. J.: Studies on the immunosuppressive properties of Cyclosporin A in rats receiving renal allografts. Transplantation. (In press) 1980.

[20] Winearls, C. G., Fabre, J. W., Millard, P. R., and Morris, P. J.: The combined use of antilymphocyte serum and cyclophosphamide to suppress renal allograft rejection in the rat. Clin. Exp. Immunol. *35*:242–49, 1979.

[21] Chick, W. L., Perna, J. J., Lauris, V., Low, D., Galletti, P. M., Panol, G., Whittemore, A. D., Like, A. A., Colton, C. K., and Lysaght, M. J.: Artificial pancreas using living beta cells: effects on glucose homeostasis in diabetic rats. Science *197*:780–82, 1977.

[22] Lafferty, K. J., Cooley, M. A., Woolnough, J., and Walker, K. Z.: Thyroid allograft immunogenicity is reduced after a period in organ culture. Science *188*:259–61, 1975.

[23] Lafferty, K. J., Bootes, A., Dart, G., and Talmage, D. W.: Effect of organ culture on the survival of thyroid allografts in mice. Transplantation *22*:138–50, 1976.

Specific Immunosuppression for Fetal Pancreas Allografts in Rats

YOKO MULLEN

SUMMARY

This paper is a review of our current work, evaluating the effectiveness of specific immunosuppressive treatment for prolongation of rat fetal pancreas allograft survival. Passively given antidonor antibodies that markedly prolong kidney and heart allograft survival had little effect on allogeneic whole fetal pancreases grafted onto the subcapsular space of the kidney. In contrast, the combination of pretreatment with donor antigen followed by procarbazine hydrochloride (PCH) and antilymphocyte serum (ALS) had a marked effect on fetal pancreas survival. The efficacy of the treatment increased when allograft incompatibility was smaller. Thus, a single injection of both PCH and ALS induced lifelong unresponsiveness to Lewis (LEW) fetal pancreases in 80% of Fischer (F344) recipients across this weak, non-H-1 incompatibility. These allografts were fully functional and completely reversed the host diabetes. Specificity of unresponsiveness was confirmed by prolonged survival of donor-type skin but acute rejection of third-party skin allografts on these recipients. Fetal pancreases surviving more than 300 days in an allogeneic recipient were fully capable of eliciting a rejection reaction in a secondary recipient. When the immunogenetic barrier was greater, stronger immunosuppressive treatment was necessary. In intermediate incompatibility, F344 to LEW, and strong H-1 incompatibility, (LEW × BUF) F1 to LEW, a total of 8–10 injections of PCH and ALS given on alternate days was needed to extend pancreas survivals from 14 days, characteristic of the controls, to 50–70 days with substantial improvement of the host diabetes. Additional approaches for increasing the efficacy of immunosuppressive treatment are discussed. DIABETES *29* (Suppl. 1):113–120, 1980.

In spite of our hope that fetal tissues may be less immunogenic than those of adults, as we found in rat skin allografts,[1] whole pancreases from 17-day-old rat embryos were acutely rejected by allogeneic recipients in all combinations ranging from strong H-1 incompatibility to weak non-H-1 incompatibility.[2] Thus, the most difficult and critical problem in fetal pancreas transplantation remains: how to protect transplants from rejection reaction and how to protect patients from complications associated with nonspecific immunosuppressive treatments often observed in human kidney transplantation. Long-term use of nonspecific immunosuppression based on immunosuppressive drugs, corticosteroids, and antithymocyte globulin, as used in kidney patients, should be avoided in diabetic patients who are already prone to various infections. Instead, specific suppression of host immune reactions to donor antigens, leaving other immune responses intact, is far more desirable. Until specific suppression of the host rejection reaction becomes possible, pancreas transplantation cannot be a practical approach to the treatment of diabetes.

Specific immunotherapy using alloantibodies has been very effective for prolongation of allograft survivals, especially kidney and heart, in experimental animals.[3] Passive enhancement by giving blocking (enhancing) antibodies against donor antigens immediately after transplantation has successfully suppressed rejection reaction against allografts, resulting in long-functioning transplants. The effect of specific immunotherapy can be maximized by combining both antigen pretreatment and passively given antibodies.[4] Although the effectiveness of blocking antibodies is still controversial in human organ transplantation, the longer survivals of kidney allografts in patients who had multiple blood transfusions before the transplantation or those who had multiple pregnancies may be attributable to blocking antibodies.[5] Another approach to specific immunosuppression is induction of specific unresponsiveness to donor antigens. Classic immunologic tolerance induced by donor bone marrow injection during the neonatal state is a state of specific unresponsiveness toward donor antigens, where neither cell-mediated immunity nor antibody response can

From the Dental Research Institute, University of California at Los Angeles, California.

Address reprint requests to Yoko Mullen, Dental Research Institute, School of Dentistry, University of California, Los Angeles, California 90024.

be detected. This permits lifelong acceptance of subsequent tissue transplants from the same donor strain at the adult stage. Many experimental procedures on adult animals which confer a measure of specific unresponsiveness have been reported.[6–9] Some of these treatments may be applicable to and effective in human organ transplantation under certain conditions. Among these procedures, the method developed by Brent and Opara,[6] which used donor antigens, antilymphocyte serum (ALS), and procarbazine hydrochloride (PCH), has a high success rate in the induction of specific unresponsiveness to highly immunologic skin allografts in mice, and a similar treatment may be applicable to human transplantation. Another approach to the induction of specific unresponsiveness is that induced by the total lymphoid irradiation discussed in the paper by Slavin.

The objective of our present study was to evaluate and to improve the effectiveness of various specific immunosuppressive treatments using our rat fetal transplantation model.[10] This paper will review our results to date and discuss possible implications of the application of fetal pancreas transplantation to human diabetics.

MATERIALS AND METHODS

Animals. Adult rats of Buffalo (BUF), Fischer (F344), and Lewis (LEW) inbred strains, 3–5 mo old, were obtained from the Microbiological Associates (Maryland). These rats were used as either pancreas recipients or breeders. Breeding colonies for (LEW × BUF) F1 hybrids, F344, and LEW were set up in our laboratory to provide 17-day-old fetuses as pancreas donors. The gestational age was estimated by daily examination of vaginal smears during the mating period and was further confirmed by careful examination of morphologic features of each fetus.[10] F344 and LEW carry the same $H\text{-}1^{l}/AgB^{1}$ allele but differ at multiple non-H-1 loci. BUF carries the $H\text{-}1^{b}/AgB^{6}$ allele and, thus, is incompatible at the major histocompatibility locus with both F344 and LEW strains. Based upon our previous experience with survival times of kidney[11] and fetal pancreas[2] allografts, fetal pancreas allografts from (LEW × BUF) F1 to LEW served as a model for strong H-1 incompatibility; from F344 to LEW as that for intermediate strength, non-H-1 incompatibility; and from LEW to F344 as that for weak incompatibility.

Induction of diabetes and monitoring of metabolic state. Diabetes was induced by a single injection of streptozotocin (SZ; provided by Upjohn) intravenously. Doses of 65–70 mg/kg of body weight for LEW and of 30–35 mg/kg for F344 induced diabetes with plasma glucose levels of 400–550 mg/dl within a few days. After injection, animals were kept in individual metabolic cages for at least 2 mo after transplantation until normal metabolic states became stable and, thereafter, in individual cages. At monthly intervals rats were placed in metabolic cages for a few days for metabolic studies. Urine volume and glucose excretion were measured daily and plasma glucose was determined weekly from tail blood samples taken between 2:00 and 3:00 p.m. Glucose concentration in blood and urine was measured in duplicate by the glucose oxidase method on a Beckman glucose analyzer. Animals were allowed to eat and drink ad libitum.

Techniques for preparation and transplantation of fetal pancreases. The techniques for dissection and implantation of fetal pancreases are described in detail elsewhere.[10] In short, the entire pancreas, including the ventral portions on the first duodenal loop from 16- and 17-day-old embryos, unless otherwise stated, was dissected from the surrounding tissues and stored in phosphate-buffered saline (PBS) on ice until transplanted. After routine preparation, the recipient kidney was exposed, and a small open space was made between the capsule and surface of the kidney. Three or four fetal pancreases were inserted into this space and spread out evenly on the kidney surface. Each recipient received three to six fetal pancreases from allogeneic donors. Pancreas recipients were treated with daily insulin injection for 10–20 days to control hyperglycemia during the establishment of transplanted fetal pancreases.

Allograft viability. After transplantation, viability of allogeneic fetal pancreases was routinely monitored by the metabolic criteria given above and by occasional visual examination of tissues in situ. Complete reversal of diabetes indicated fully viable, functioning transplants. That was further confirmed by gross observation of the tissue, and such grafts were taken as "fully successful allografts." Partial reversal of diabetes occurred in some recipients in spite of fully grown viable tissues by gross observation. Occasionally diabetes was not improved even with fully viable fetal pancreas allografts. Rejection of allografts was usually indicated by the recurrence of diabetes and was further confirmed by the necrotic change of the tissues. In allografts which did not improve host diabetes, rejection was determined by frequent observation of tissues in situ.

At gross observation, soft but resilient tissues with rich extrinsic and intrinsic vascularization were judged to be fully viable.[2] The intrinsic vascularization appeared as a fine capillary network throughout the transparent tissue. When rejection occurred, the tissue became harder, with turbid whitish-yellow coloration through which the intrinsic vascularization was no longer visible. The extrinsic vascularization remained rich in earlier stages of the rejection reaction but subsequently would disappear. The rejected tissue became necrotic and was often absorbed completely from the grafted site, leaving scar tissue on the kidney surface. The criteria used for viability scoring by gross observation are described in detail elsewhere.[2]

Glucose tolerance test. After overnight fasting, rats were anesthetized with an intraperitoneal injection of 50 mg/kg of methohexital sodium. After the bleeding for the fasting blood glucose level, 0.5 g/kg of 10% glucose solution was injected intravenously through the tail vein, and blood samples were taken from the femoral vein every 10 min for 40 min after glucose injection. Serum glucose concentrations were determined by the glucose oxidase method, and the rate of glucose disappearance (K value) was calculated. Serum from each bleeding was stored at −70° for insulin measurements.

Skin and kidney transplantation techniques. Test skin grafts 1 cm in diameter were placed on the graft bed on the back of the recipients and held in place by three stitches. Recipients were unbandaged on day 10, and graft viability was scored daily thereafter during the first 2 wk and then less frequently if slow rejection was observed to be underway. In one experiment, vascularized and grown fetal pancreases were retransplanted from the primary recipient into the secondary recipient, together with the carrier kidney by the orthotopic kidney transplantation technique.[11] In this experiment, only a right nephrectomy was performed, leaving the left kidney intact.

Immunosuppressive treatment for allograft recipient. The method of rat alloantiserum preparation, fractionation, and titration for blocking antibody treatment was described in detail in our previous paper.[11] In short, antidonor antibodies were prepared in the recipient strain rats by several immunizations with donor spleen cells. IgG-class antibodies were fractionated by ion exchange column chromatography. IgG antibodies from LEW anti-BUF antiserum had antibody titers between 1:64 and 1:512, as measured by the capillary migration hemagglutination test. One milliliter of IgG antibodies (equivalent to the same amount of whole antiserum) was given intravenously to LEW recipients 0, 2, and 4 days after pancreas transplantation from (LEW × BUF) F1 embryos. This treatment protocol prolonged kidney allograft survivals in the same donor-recipient combination for well over 250 days, as we have reported previously.[11]

For treatment with donor tissue extracts, procarbazine hydrochloride, and antilymphocyte serum, tissue extracts were prepared from donor liver by hypotonic destruction of cells according to the method used by Brent and Opara.[6] The prepared semisoluble tissue extracts were adjusted by the addition of PBS to a desired concentration equivalent to a certain wet weight tissue or protein content and adjusted to pH 7.4 by addition of 0.1 N NaOH. Extracts were stored in 1-ml aliquots at −70°C. Antisera against rat lymphocytes were prepared in rabbits by several repeated immunizations with rat thymocytes. Rabbits were bled 7–10 days after the last immunization; serum was separated, heat-activated at 55°C for 30 min, and absorbed with washed rat red blood cells in the ratio of 15:1 overnight at 4°C. These ALS were stored in 1-ml aliquots at −70°C. Each batch of ALS was tested on F344 to LEW skin allografts, and only preparations of ALS that prolonged test skin allograft survival for longer than 20 days when given in 0.5-ml intraperitoneal injections on days 0 and 2 were used for the treatment of fetal pancreas recipients. Procarbazine hydrochloride (provided by Roche Laboratories) was dissolved in PBS in concentration of 39 mg/ml (10% of the LD_{50} per kilogram in 2 ml) just before injection into the peritoneal cavity.

RESULTS

The prolongation of fetal pancreas allograft survival was attempted by two separate methods: (1) passive enhancement by the administration of blocking alloantibodies against donor antigens and (2) the treatment with PCH, ALS, and donor tissue antigens similar to those used in mice to induce long-lasting unresponsiveness to H-2-incompatible skin allografts.[6] The effectiveness of these treatments was tested on fetal pancreas allografts with various histoincompatibilities, since the efficacy of immunosuppressive treatment may vary depending on the intensity of host immune reaction. As we have reported previously,[2,12] a fetal pancreas grafted on each kidney of a normal, nonimmunosuppressed recipient was rejected in 7.5 days in the H-1-incompatible (LEW × BUF) F1 hybrid to LEW strain combination, in 8 days in the F344 to LEW combination differing only at non-H-1 loci, and in 9 days in the reciprocal direction. The differences in times of allograft rejection between three combinations were small but distinctive and reflected the intensity of the host immune reaction, depending on the magnitude of histoincompatibilities. This was demonstrated in kidney allografts where the divergence of host responses was more clearly exhibited, rejection being acute in (LEW × BUF) F1 to LEW, chronic in F344 to LEW, and absent in LEW to F344.[11] Thus, these three combinations were considered to represent allografts with strong, intermediate, and weak immunogenetic disparities.

Passive enhancement fails to prolong fetal pancreas allograft survivals. Specific immunoblocking by alloantibodies against donor antigens was attempted in (LEW × BUF) F1 to LEW fetal pancreas allografts. Five or six pancreases from 17-day-old F1 embryos were grafted into a diabetic LEW recipient which was treated with insulin for 7–10 days after transplantation to control hyperglycemia during maturation of the fetal pancreases. IgG-class antibodies fractionated from high-titer LEW anti-BUF antisera, demonstrated to be the most effective antibodies,[13] were injected intravenously into LEW recipients starting immediately after the transplantation and were followed by an additional injection on days 2 and 4. A total of 3 ml of IgG blocked the host immune reaction very effectively and prolonged kidney allograft survival in this donor-recipient combination. More than 90% of kidney allografts survived for 250–300 days with the passively given antibodies, while the control allografts were rejected within 3 wk. However, the same treatment had little effect on prolongation of fetal pancreas allograft survival. In about 50% of the recipients, F1 fetal pancreases survived 20–35 days without any effect on the diabetes, but allografts in the remaining recipients were rejected within 14 days, similar to the untreated control recipients. The viability of these allografts was judged by gross observation of tissues in situ by repeated laparotomies. Treatment with whole antiserum was less effective than purified IgG antibodies and resulted in the rejection of most allografts within 14 days. A single injection of a small amount (0.5 ml) of blocking antibody at the time of transplantation was also ineffective.

Similarly, blocking antibody treatment was attempted on a small number of diabetic LEW who received F344 fetal pancreases and were treated with LEW anti-F344 antiserum. Again, blocking antibodies had little effect on allograft survivals, and all fetal pancreases were rejected within 17 days, as occurred in the untreated control group, while the same antibody treatment extended F344 kidney allograft survivals from 121 days in the control to longer than 350 days in the treated recipients.

Attempts to induce specific unresponsiveness to fetal pancreas allografts. Among various protocols used to induce unresponsiveness to allografts in adults, the treatment developed by Brent and Opara[6] for mouse skin allografts was evaluated for its effectiveness on fetal pancreas allografts. The original treatment regimen used in mouse skin allografts used one-half of the LD_{50} dose of PCH and 0.5 ml ALS injections on alternate days for 1 wk after transplantation in conjunction with semisoluble donor liver extract injection on −17 days. However, SZ-induced diabetic rats were unable to tolerate such large doses of immunosuppression and died before the treatment was completed. Even one-third of the LD_{50} dose of PCH may be toxic under these conditions. Subsequently, we have found that repeated injections with 10% of the LD_{50} dose of PCH (78 mg/kg) and 0.5 ml ALS diluted in the same volume of PBS could be administered daily for more than a week without severe complication, except for minor weight loss during the treatment, while the leukocyte count in the peripheral blood was depleted to as low as 5,000 cells per microliter, with less than 10% being lymphocytes. Different doses of PCH and ALS were evaluated on fetal pancreas allograft survivals in three conbinations with strong, intermediate, and weak immunogenetic disparities.

Successful induction of specific unresponsiveness to fetal pancreas allografts across weak incompatibility. The combined treatment with donor antigens, PCH, and ALS was very effective for prolongation of LEW fetal pancreas survivals in F344 recipients across weak incompatibilities. Furthermore, few injections of immunosuppressive agents were required for the permanent acceptance of allografts in this combination. Semisoluble LEW antigens extracted from adult liver containing 5–10 mg protein, which was equivalent to about 250–500 mg of wet liver weight, were injected intravenously 16–17 days before the pancreas transplantation. One-third of the LD_{50} dose of PCH (262 mg/kg) was injected into the peritoneal cavity 1 or 2 days before the transplantation, and one or two injections of 0.5 ml ALS were given between the day of transplantation and the third day by the same route. F344 recipients were made diabetic with 30–35 mg/kg of streptozotocin (SZ), transplanted with three to six LEW whole fetal pancreases under the capsule of the kidneys, and given daily insulin for 7–10 days. As shown in Table 1, 12 out of 15 immunosuppressed recipients completely recovered from diabetes within 2 wk and maintained normal metabolism with fully viable transplants for more than 1 yr until the experiment was terminated. In 2 out of the 15 recipients, diabetes reversed completely or partially for a short period but then reverted to the pretransplantation level by 35 and 55 days, respectively. In the remaining recipient the treatment had little effect on suppression of the host immune reaction and all allografts were rejected within 20 days. No difference in the effectiveness of the treatment was observed between male and female F344 recipients.

Metabolic profiles of ten female recipients with successful allografts are depicted in Figure 1. At the time of transplantation, 4 or 5 days after SZ injection, mean values of plasma glucose, urine glucose, and 24-h urine volume of F344 recipients were 392 ± 14 mg/dl (mean ± SEM), 3.7 ± 0.28 g/day, and 40 ± 3 ml/day, respectively. Fourteen days after transplantation, 4 days after the termination of daily insulin treatment, glucose metabolism still remained abnormal, as indicated by plasma glucose (168 ± 18 mg/dl), urine glucose (0.01 ± 0.006 g/day), and urine volume (10 ± 1 ml/day). By 21 days, all three parameters returned to the normal levels (plasma glucose: 138 ± 5 mg/dl; urine glucose: negative; urine volume: 10 ± 1 ml/day), and body weights returned to the pre-SZ injection levels. Thereafter, all recipients had maintained normal metabolism throughout the observation period for more than 12 mo. The control recipients who received the same number of LEW fetal pancreases, but without immunosuppression, reverted to the pretransplantation diabetic state by the end of the third week after transplantation. Fetal pancreases in these control recipients were rejected within 17 days and disappeared from the graft site within 4 wk. Allograft viabilities in the experimental animals were visually examined in situ three or four times during the experimental period to confirm healthy growing tissues. Fully viable fetal pancreases were removed from three recipients in the ex-

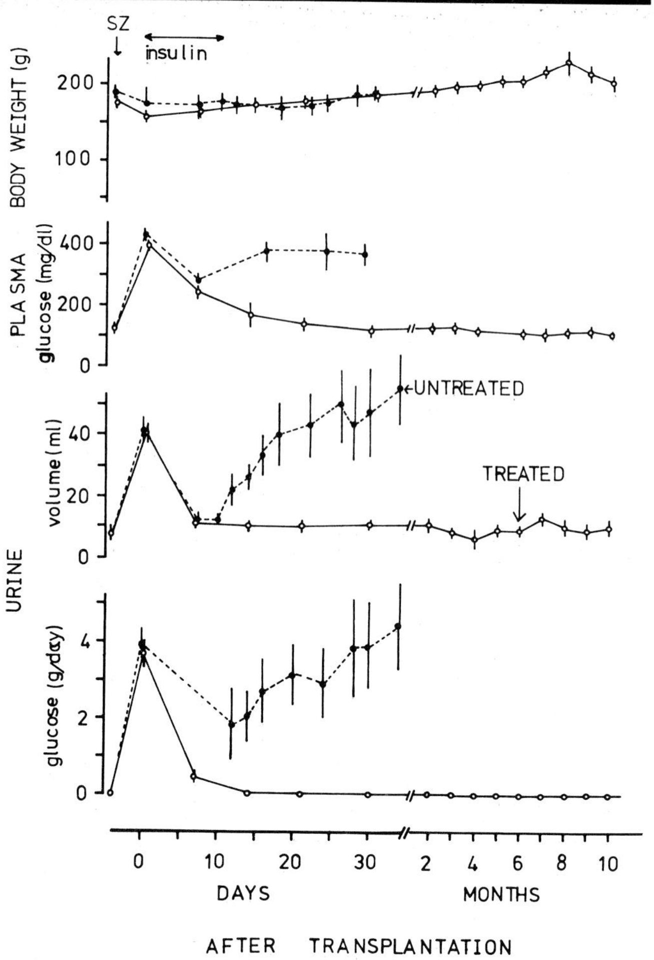

FIGURE 1. Metabolic state in F344 recipients after transplantation of six whole pancreases from 17-day-old LEW embryos. The experimental group contained 10 female recipients that received an i.v. injection of adult LEW liver extracts (equal to 250 mg of wet liver tissue) at −16 days and an i.p. injection of both one-third of the LD_{50} dose of PCH at −1 day and 0.5 ml ALS at 2 days. The control group contained six female recipients transplanted with the same number of LEW fetal pancreases without immunosuppression. Each value represents the mean value of the group and SEM.

TABLE 1
LEW fetal pancreas survival in diabetic F344 recipients treated with donor antigens, PCH, and ALS*

Reversal of diabetes	Allograft survival times	Pancreas survival No.	Pancreas survival %
Complete	>250 days (lifelong)	12	80
Complete	50 days	1	13
Partial	35 days	1	13
None	20 days	1	7

* Adult liver extract equivalent to 250–500 mg wet tissue was given intravenously between 16 and 24 days before transplantation. One-third the amount of the LD_{50} dose of procarbazine hydrochloride (PCH) was injected i.p. 1–2 days before, and one or two injections of 0.5 ml antilymphocyte serum (ALS) was given by the same route 0–3 days after transplantation.

perimental group at 293, 310, and 436 days after transplantation to confirm the functional viability of the allografts. The recurrence of diabetes took place between 3 and 20 days after the removal, when plasma glucose levels reached higher than 200 mg/dl.

Glucose tolerance tests were performed between 280 and 330 days after transplantation on seven diabetes-reversed recipients carrying fully viable allogeneic fetal pancreases. The results are shown in Figure 2. The mean K value for glucose disappearance was 3.3 ± 0.3, which was similar to that obtained in normal, age-matched controls (3.2 ± 0.5). K values became less than 1.0 after the removal of fetal pancreas allografts. Measurements of insulin levels in the test serum samples are currently in progress.

In order to test the host immune state, six recipients carrying fully viable LEW fetal pancreases made possible by successful immunosuppression were grafted with one skin graft from donor LEW and another from third-party ACI-strain rat 340 days after pancreas transplantation. Skin allografts from the pancreas donors (LEW), which were fully viable for more than 50 days, indicated well-established unresponsiveness to donor antigens, while skin allografts from ACI animals were rejected within 2 wk. Thus, suppression of the immune response in these recipients appears to be specific to donor antigens.

Conversely, prolongation of allograft survival might be achieved if the antigenicity of donor tissue is altered. In order to test the possibility of antigenic modulation in transplanted fetal pancreases, LEW fetal pancreases surviving in an allogenic F344 recipient for more than 300 days by the immunosuppressive treatment were retransplanted into a new diabetic F344 recipient together with the carrier kidney. Thus, the only tissue foreign to the new, secondary F344 recipient was that of LEW fetal pancreases. No immunosuppressive treatment was given to the secondary recipient. The metabolic profile of the secondary recipient is depicted in Figure 3. Within 2 days after pancreas-kidney transplantation, plasma glucose and urine volume returned to normal,

FIGURE 2. Intravenous glucose tolerance tests under methohexital sodium anesthesia. Tests were performed between 280 and 330 days after transplantation on seven F344 recipients carrying fully viable LEW fetal pancreases, made possible by successful immunosuppression. The control group contained three normal, age-matched F344. A glucose tolerance test was performed on one recipient twice, once before and again after allograft removal.

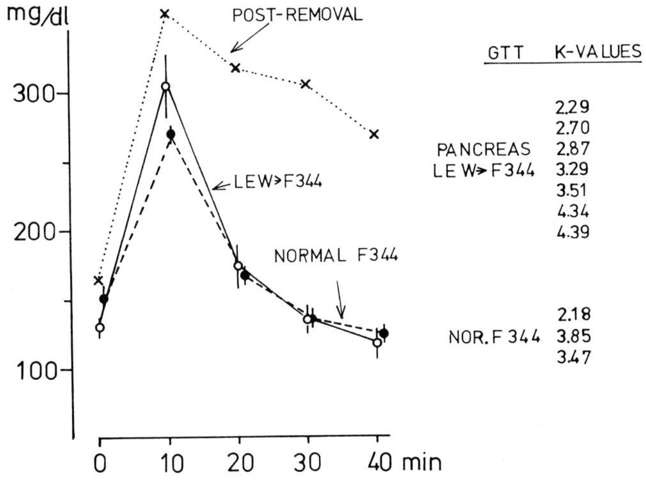

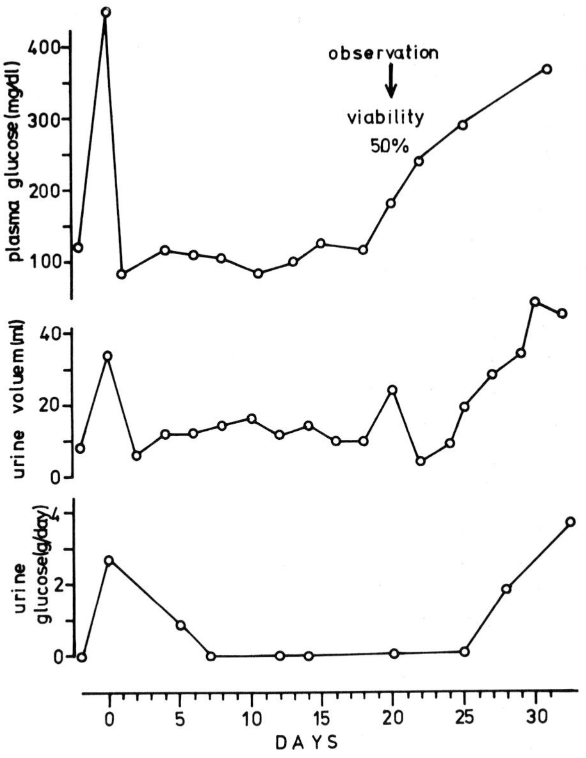

FIGURE 3. Test for antigenic modulation of long-living allogeneic fetal pancreases. Antigenicity of long-surviving LEW fetal pancreases in an F344 recipient who received the immunosuppressive treatment was tested by retransplanting allografts into a diabetic secondary F344 recipient. The glucose metabolism of the secondary recipient returned to normal until 20 days, when rejection started. Viability of grafts was scored as 50% on day 21 and as completely rejected on day 33 by gross observation.

and urine glucose became negative within 1 wk. Normal metabolism continued for about 20 days, and then plasma glucose suddenly rose higher than 150 mg/dl, indicating the onset of rejection. Plasma glucose reached higher than 200 mg/dl by the following day and continued to rise, reaching the pretransplantation level by 30 days after transplantation. Increases in urine volume and urine glucose excretion followed the rise in plasma glucose. Visual examination approximated fetal pancreas viability of 50% on day 21 and complete rejection at 33 days when the tissue was removed for insulin measurement. The removed tissue contained only a trace of insulin. An additional experiment is currently in progress.

Prolongation of fetal pancreas allograft survival across strong and intermediate incompatibilities. The same immunosuppressive regimen which induced lifelong unresponsiveness to LEW fetal pancreases in F344 recipients across a weak immunogenetic disparity was not effective for allografts across stronger incompatibilities. In spite of the treatment, none of the allografts in the F344 to LEW combination, considered as intermediate incompatibility, or in (LEW × BUF) F1 to LEW, a strong incompatibility, survived longer than 2 wk, suggesting the necessity of more intensive immunosuppression. In order to improve the effectiveness of the treatment, several regimens for PCH and ALS administration were tested in these allograft combinations.

Two regimens shown in Table 2 were tested on F344 to LEW allografts. Donor liver extracts containing 10 mg of pro-

TABLE 2
Immunosuppressive treatment for F344 to LEW fetal pancreases

Days	Treatment regimen A	B
−18 to −24	Adult F344 liver extracts (10 mg protein) i.v.	
−10 to −14	SZ (70 mg/kg) i.v.	
−4	PCH	—
−1	PCH	—
0	Transplantation	
	ALS	PCH
1	PCH	ALS
2	ALS	PCH
3	PCH	ALS
4	ALS	PCH
5	PCH	ALS
6	—	PCH
7	—	ALS

PCH: 1/10 of the LD_{50} dose i.p.; ALS: 0.5 ml i.p. SZ, streptozotocin; PCH, procarbazine hydrochloride.

tein (equivalent to 500 mg wet tissue) were injected intravenously between 18 and 24 days before transplantation. Both regimens A and B comprised a total of eight injections of PCH and ALS; however, the distribution of the injections was different. In regimen A, 10% of the LD_{50} dose of PCH injection was started the day of transplantation. After the transplantation, ALS and PCH were given on alternate days until a total of eight injections was reached. As shown in Figure 4, there was essentially no difference in the effectiveness of the two regimens. Both regimens showed clear immunosuppressive effect and markedly prolonged allograft survivals. Seven out of 11 recipients carried fully viable allogeneic fetal pancreases for more than 40 days, which was nearly three times longer than survival time in the untreated control recipients. However, within 70 days all F344 fetal pancreases were rejected.

FIGURE 4. Survival and function of fetal pancreas allografts in the F344 to LEW combination across intermediate incompatibility following the immunosuppressive treatment (Table 2). A total of eight injections of 10% of the LD_{50} dose of PCH and 0.5 ml ALS prolonged allograft survival with complete or partial reversal of host diabetes up to 70 days. ■, reversed; ▧, improved; ▩, no change.

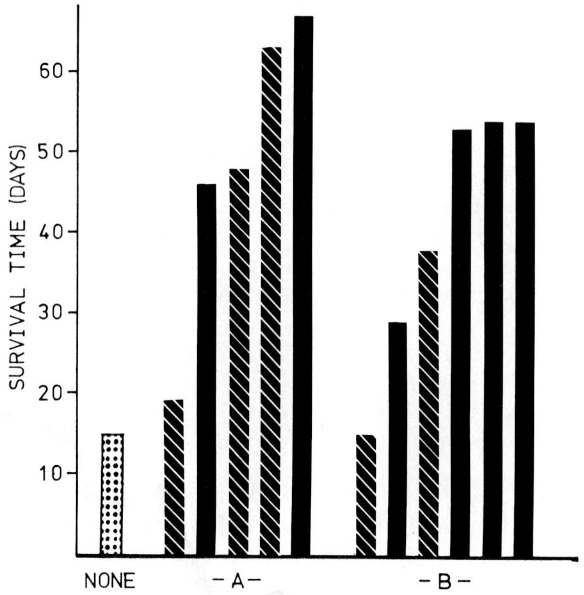

Diabetes was improved in all recipients after transplantation. Total reversal of diabetes was achieved in 6 out of 11 recipients, and significant improvement occurred in the remaining recipients. Rejection was first detected by increased plasma glucose followed by increases in urine glucose and urine volume. Subsequently, all three parameters returned to the pretransplantation diabetic levels.

In the combination across strong H-1 incompatibility, parental BUF liver extract as donor antigens was increased to a dose of 20 mg protein, which was equivalent to about 1 g of wet liver tissue, and was given 17–28 days before transplantation. LEW recipients received five or six (LEW × BUF) F1 hybrid fetal pancreases and were treated by PCH and ALS in three different regimens, as shown in Table 3. Regimens A, B, and C differed in both the number and distribution of injections. In regimen A, PCH injection was started at the time of transplantation and totaled nine injections; in regimen B, one PCH injection was given before transplantation and seven subsequently, and in regimen C, two PCH injections were given before transplantation and eight subsequently. Regimens A and B, which were similar to those applied in the previous F344 to LEW combination, did not have much effect on the prolongation of allograft survival times in the H-1-incompatible F1 hybrid to parental LEW combination (Figure 5). Seven out of 11 recipients rejected allografts within 20 days, and no change in diabetes was observed. In one recipient whose diabetes was substantially improved, rejection occurred 26 days after transplantation. The remaining three recipients whose diabetes was either improved or totally reversed did not reject pancreas allografts for more than 30 days. Interestingly, these long-surviving fetal pancreases in all three recipients were delivered from 15-day-old embryos, although fetal pancreases the same age were rejected within 20 days in one recipient.

In contrast to these results, regimen C, which included more injections, including pretransplantation treatment, showed a marked effect on strong H-1-incompatible F1 fetal

TABLE 3
Immunosuppressive treatment for (LEW × BUF) F1 to LEW fetal pancreases

Days	Treatment regimen A	B	C
−17 to −28	Adult BUF liver extracts (20 mg protein) i.v.		
−14 to −21	SZ (70 mg/kg) i.v.		
−4 to −5	—	PCH	PCH
−1	—	—	PCH
0	Transplantation		
	PCH	PCH	ALS
1	ALS	ALS	PCH
2	PCH	PCH	ALS
3	ALS	ALS	PCH
4	PCH	PCH	ALS
5	ALS	ALS	PCH
6	PCH	PCH	ALS
7	ALS	—	PCH
8	PCH	—	—

PCH: 1/10 of the LD_{50} dose i.p.; ALS: 0.5 ml i.p.

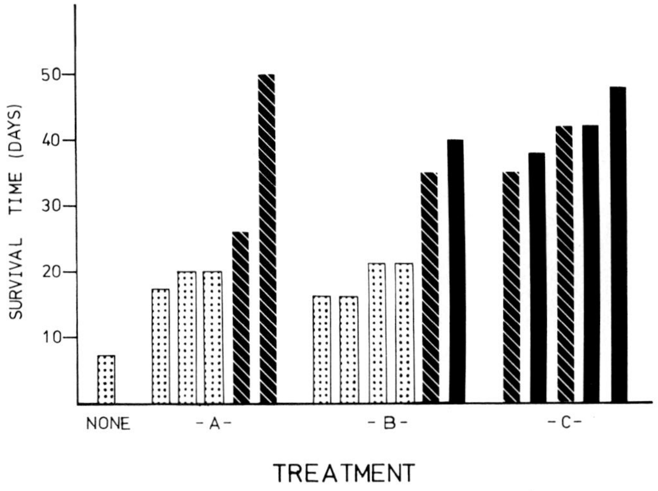

FIGURE 5. Survival and function of fetal pancreas allografts in (LEW × BUF) F1 to LEW combination across strong H-1 incompatibility following the immunosuppressive treatment (Table 3). Only regimen C, which used a total of 10 injections of 10% of the LD_{50} dose of PCH and 0.5 ml ALS starting with two injections before the transplantation, was effective for prolongation of H-1 incompatible allograft survivals up to 50 days. See legend, Figure 4.

pancreas survivals. All allografts in this group survived more than 30 days and improved the host diabetic state. Three recipients returned to normal, but two recipients remained as partial diabetic reversals. Improved metabolism continued until rejection intervened, and all allografts were rejected within 50 days.

DISCUSSION

In spite of the well-established evidence that passively given antidonor antibodies can significantly prolong whole organ (especially kidney and heart) graft survivals, alloantibody treatment for whole fetal pancreas allografts had practically no effect on graft survival. Although some grafts survived for an extended period, the prolongation was limited to 1 mo, and the success rate was low and unpredictable. Finch and Morris[14] have demonstrated prolonged survivals of isolated adult islets with a small dose of alloantiserum but not with larger doses. In our model, however, a small dose had no effect, but the prolonged survival was obtained only by repeated injections of a total of 3 ml of IgG antibodies fractionated from antidonor antiserum which had higher potential than whole antiserum in the passive enhancement of kidney allografts.[11,13] Thus, the amount of antibody used in our experiment was not likely the cause of failure. Indeed, previous results on the effectiveness of alloantibody treatment on isolated adult islet allografts are rather conflicting. Even using a combination treatment protocol of both passive and active enhancement, Reckard et al.[15] have been unable to extend islet allograft survival. Furthermore, islet allografts in the recipients carrying a long-term enhanced kidney from the same donor strain were rejected promptly. Blocking antibody treatment has minimum protection on skin allografts. Skin as well as our fetal pancreases were transplanted without an immediate blood supply. Such grafting conditions may make the efficacy of the blocking antibody minimal as compared with organ transplants which receive an immediate blood supply through vascular connections. The successful immunoblocking with alloantibodies may also require a sufficient amount of antigen released from donor tissue. Although islets injected via the portal vein and lodging in the liver are similar to organ grafts in terms of an immediate blood supply, antigens released from such a small number of cells may not be sufficient for an effective immunoblocking mechanism. Thus, it is not surprising that blocking antibody is effective for the extended survival of adult islets that are transplanted as a whole pancreas with vascular anastomosis. Efficacy of blocking antibodies may not be simply attributable to the immunologic property of the grafted tissue.

On the other hand, host immunosuppression by the combination treatment with donor antigens, PCH, and ALS was very effective for prolongation of fetal pancreas survivals. The efficacy of the treatment increased if allograft incompatibility was weaker. Thus, a single injection of both PCH and ALS produced lifelong unresponsiveness to donor LEW fetal pancreases in F344 recipients across only non-H-1 disparities. These fetal pancreases were not only fully viable in appearance but also functionally capable of reversing diabetes completely for a lifetime. Preliminary examination of histologic sections revealed a mass of healthy beta cells in these long-lived allogeneic fetal pancreases. Functional viability of the long-living fetal pancreases was further confirmed by the recurrence of diabetes after the removal of allografts and by the complete reversal of diabetes in the secondary recipient immediately after transplantation of the long-living allogeneic fetal pancreases together with the kidney of the primary recipient (Figure 3). Immunosuppression induced by this combination treatment appears to be specific to donor antigens, as demonstrated by the markedly extended survival of donor-type skin allografts but the acute rejection of third-party skin in rats carrying pancreas allografts for more than 300 days. Detection of cellular and humoral immune responses directed against donor antigens in these successful allograft recipients is currently being attempted. Fetal pancreases fully functioning for more than 300 days in an allogeneic recipient still carried antigens capable of eliciting an immune response in a new, nonimmunosuppressed recipient. The longer survival time of these fully grown fetal pancreases (about 30 days), as compared with that of the same number of pancreases transplanted directly from 17-day-old embryos (about 2 wk), could be attributed to a larger tissue mass in those fully grown in a diabetic recipient. Fetal antigen involvement in the rejection of these regrafted pancreases is not likely since a rejection reaction against such weak antigens progresses very slowly, if there is any. In addition, we have never observed the rejection of well-established syngeneic fetal pancreases in adult recipients throughout our isograft studies. An experiment to test the involvement of suppressor T lymphocytes in the mechanism of unresponsiveness is now in progress.

When the immunogenetic barrier between donor and recipient was greater, stronger immunosuppressive treatment was necessary. A total of eight injections of PCH and ALS was required for significant prolongation of F344 to LEW allograft survival, while a total of 10 injections starting before transplantation was required for (LEW × BUF) F1 to LEW allografts. However, even with such intense immunosuppression, these allograft survivals were limited to 70 days. Additional treatment to increase the efficacy of host immunosuppression is necessary in order to improve these results.

One approach to this problem may be the use of younger fetal tissues. As shown in the result of F1 hybrid to LEW allografts on regimen A, fetal pancreases from 15-day-old embryos survived significantly longer than those isolated from older embryos, suggesting weaker immunogenicity of these tissues. Expression of various cell surface antigens changes both in quantity and in quality during embryonic development.[16] In the mouse, H-2-linked SD-antigens (H-2K and H-2D) appear on embryonic tissue by day 7 of gestation,[16] while H-2-linked LD-antigens, Ia, are first detected on cells of the 11-day conceptus.[17] Ia expression between days 11 and 16 of gestation is restricted to the liver. After 18 days of gestation, fetal spleen cells but not liver cells become Ia-positive, and their frequency continues to increase after birth. As Ia antigens serve as differential markers of B-lymphocytes, disappearance of Ia antigens from the liver at a certain stage during development may indicate migration of lymphoid cells into other tissues.

If, indeed, pancreatic islets do not express histocompatibility antigens, as indicated in the recent study by Lacy et al.,[18] strong immune reaction directed against the whole fetal pancreas may be elicited by either passenger lymphocytes or by cells other than islets. However, we believe that the role played by donor lymphocytes in induction of rejection reaction against whole fetal pancreases may be small because the long-surviving LEW pancreases in an F344 recipient were still rejected by the secondary F344 recipient in spite of a negligible number of donor-type lymphocytes carried in the transplants. This result indicates that antigens expressed by cells other than islets may be responsible for rejection. Elimination of these cells without disturbing growth and development of the fetal pancreas endocrine tissue is another approach for successful prolongation of allograft survival in rat strain combinations across stronger incompatibilities.

ACKNOWLEDGMENTS

This work was supported by grants from the U.S. Public Health Service (AM 20827 and AM 17980) and from the American Diabetes Association, Southern California Affiliate.

The author wishes to thank Dr. J. Brown for his support and Diane Heininger, Diana Lee, and Yumiko Sugiura for excellent technical assistance.

REFERENCES

[1] Heslop, B. H.: Maturation of histocompatibility antigens and host reactivity in the rat. Transplant. Proc. *1*:560–63, 1969.

[2] Mullen, Y., and Shintaku, P.: Fetal pancreas allografts for reversal of diabetes in rats. 1. Allograft survivals in non-immunosuppressed recipients. Transplantation, in press, 1980.

[3] Carpenter, C. B., d'Apice, A. J. F., and Abbas, A. K.: The role of antibodies in the rejection and enhancement of organ allografts. *In* Advances in Immunology. New York, Academic Press, 1976, pp. 1–65.

[4] Stuart, F. P., Saitoh, T., and Fitch, F. W.: Rejection of renal allografts: specific immunologic suppression. Science *160*:1463–65, 1968.

[5] Opertz, G., and Teraskai, P. I.: Prolongation effect of blood transfusions on kidney graft survival. Transplantation *22*:380–83, 1976.

[6] Brent, L., and Opara, S. C.: Specific unresponsiveness to skin allografts in mice. V. Synergy between donor tissue extract, procarbazine hydrochloride, and antilymphocyte serum in creating a long-lasting unresponsiveness mediated by suppressor T cells. Transplantation *27*:120–25, 1979.

[7] Gowland, G.: Induction of transplantation tolerance in adult animals. Br. Med. Bull. *21*:123, 1965.

[8] Rapaport, F. T., Bachvaroff, R. J., Dicke, K., and Satos, G.: Total-body irradiation and host reconstitution with stored autologous marrow. An experimental model for the induction of allogeneic unresponsiveness in large animals. Transplant. Proc. *11*:1028–31, 1979.

[9] Slavin, S., Strober, S., Fuko, Z., and Kaplan, H. S.: Induction of specific tissue transplantation tolerance using fractionated total lymphoid irradiation in adult mice: long-term survival of allogeneic bone marrow and skin grafts. J. Exp. Med. *146*:34–48, 1977.

[10] Brown, J., Clark, W. R., Molnar, I. G., and Mullen, Y.: Fetal pancreas transplantation for reversal of streptozotocin-induced diabetes in rats. Diabetes *25*:56–64, 1976.

[11] Hildemann, W. H., and Mullen, Y.: The weaker the histocompatibility, the greater the effectiveness of specific immunoblocking antibodies. Transplantation *15*:231–37, 1973.

[12] Brown, J., Clark, W. R., Makoff, R., Weisman, H., Kemp, J. A., and Mullen, Y.: Pancreas transplantation for diabetes mellitus. Ann. Intern. Med. *89*:951–65, 1978.

[13] Mullen, Y., Raison, R., and Hildemann, W. H.: Cytotoxic versus immunoblocking effects of specific alloantibodies. Transplantation *24*:99–105, 1977.

[14] Finch, D. R. A., and Morris, P.: Passive enhancement of isolated pancreatic islet allografts. Transplantation *22*:508–12, 1976.

[15] Reckard, C. R., Stuart, F. P., and Schulak, J. A.: Immunologic comparisons of isolated pancreatic islet and whole-organ allografts. Transplant. Proc. *11*:563–66, 1979.

[16] Pattehy, H., and Edidin, M.: Evidence for the time of appearance of H-2 antigens in mouse development. Transplantation *15*:211–14, 1973.

[17] Delovitch, T. L., Press, J. L., and McDevitt, H. O.: Expression of murine Ia antigens during embryonic development. J. Immunol. *120*:818–24, 1978.

[18] Lacy, P. E., Davie, J. M., and Finke, E. H.: Prolongation of islet allograft survival following in vitro culture (24°C) and a single injection of ALS. Science *204*:312–13, 1979.

Immunosuppression and Organ Transplantation Tolerance Using Total Lymphoid Irradiation

SHIMON SLAVIN, SAMUEL STROBER, ZVI FUKS, AND HENRY S. KAPLAN

SUMMARY

Total lymphoid irradiation (TLI) is a method which delivers irradiation daily in fractionated doses (200 rads) to lymphoid organs while shielding bones, lungs, and the majority of the gastrointestinal tract. TLI is lymphocytopenic in mice, rats, dogs, and humans, and both T cells and B cells are eliminated from the circulation. During the recovery phase in mice, B cells appear before Thy 1.2–bearing T cells, and TL-positive T cells are abundant in the spleen and lymph nodes. These T cells exhibit nonspecific suppressive activity on antibody production and cell-mediated immune responses. TLI permits establishment of specific and long-lasting tolerance to alloantigens. Permanent acceptance of allogeneic bone marrow cells without graft-versus-host disease was achieved in rats and dogs across major histocompatibility barriers. Recipients were tolerant to allografts of skin, hearts, and kidney from animals syngeneic to marrow donors or to organs from the marrow donor. This approach may be suitable for pancreas transplantation in diabetes.
DIABETES *29* (Suppl. 1):121–123, 1980.

The goal of organ transplantation has always been the establishment of tissue-specific transplantation tolerance. Although transplantation tolerance has been successfully induced in neonates from a variety of laboratory animals,[1–3] there has been little success in finding a clinically applicable transplantation tolerance regimen in adult animals. Clinical organ transplantation is based on nonspecific immunosuppression using potent immunosuppressive agents, including cytostatic drugs, antilymphocytic antisera, corticosteroids, and ionizing irradiation on a long-term basis. The available immunosuppressive protocols do not ensure organ engraftment, and infectious, neoplastic, and pharmocologic or radiologic side effects are still far from being satisfactorily controlled. Very limited progress has been achieved during the last few years with new immunosuppressive agents or clinically applicable immunomanipulative regimens.

From the Stanford University School of Medicine, Stanford, California.

The immunosuppressive effects of ionizing irradiation have been noted since the beginning of the century.[4,5] Extensive studies of radiation effects on the immunlogic response have been predominantly concerned with the use of whole body irradiation (WBI) for inducing tolerance to marrow allografts and, to a lesser degree, to kidney allografts. Unfortunately, it was soon found that sublethal WBI was insufficient to prolong the survival of an allograft across major histocompatibility barriers. Higher doses of irradiation proved to be useless due to irreversible bone marrow (BM) aplasia as well as severe gastrointestinal intolerance. More sophisticated approaches included irradiation of the graft site,[6] local irradiation of the allotransplant,[7,8] and extracorporeal irradiation of blood lymphocytes[6–9] and thoracic duct lymphocytes.[6–10] Selective irradiation of lymphocytes was also attempted by injection of lymph-borne radioactive substances into the lymphatic system[8] and by intravascular implantation of a high-energy beta-emitting source.[6,11] None of these approaches is at present in routine clinical use due to unsuccessful attempts in establishing permanent allograft survival, on the one hand, and the technical difficulties in estimating the distribution of the radiation dose in the tissues on the other. Observations on the protective effects of shielding of BM-containing bones[12] and later on hemopoietic cell infusions after exposure of animals to otherwise lethal irradiation doses[13,14] confirmed that the irradiation-induced marrow aplasia could be reversed by infusion of syngeneic or compatible allogeneic hemopoietic cells. The fact that the transplanted hemopoietic cells persisted in the irradiation recipient and replaced the host's immunologic system with donor-type cells enabled the newly conditioned host to accept grafts of other organs from the marrow donor. In the 1960s, a few attempts were made to use the above approach for clinical kidney transplantation.[15] Failures due to the toxic levels of irradiation and the double barrier for successful BM transplantation (establishing engraftment with prevention of graft rejection and the unavoidable graft-versus-host disease) chilled the initial enthusiasm for establishing true transplantation tolerance using organ-donor-type BM transplantation. The interest in the application of a radiotherapeutic approach for immunosuppression and subsequent tolerance induction has recently been revived by introduction of total lymphoid irradiation (TLI). TLI is guided by two major principles: first, the effector lymphocytes in the major lymphoid organs are selectively irradiated by applying radiotherapeutic techniques involving ports of irradiation similar to those used to treat human malignant lymphomas[16]—nonlymphoid organs, such as bones (containing bone marrow), lungs, and the majority of the gastrointestinal tract are thus protected with lead shielding;[17–19] and second, the irradiation is administered in daily fractionated doses of about 200 rads each, achieving a high total cumulative radiation dose (1800–3400 rads). Fractionated irradiation is better tolerated by all animals tested so far, including humans.[16]

The lymphocytopenic effect of TLI has been well established in mice,[17,18] rats,[20] dogs,[19] and humans.[16] After TLI in mice, consisting of 17 daily fractions of 200 rads each, both thymus-derived (T) and bone marrow–derived (B) lymphocytes are eliminated from the circulation. The recovery pattern reveals a generation of B cells before Thy 1.2–bearing T cells, as can be demonstrated by the use of two-stage immunofluorescent techniques and complement-dependent microcytotoxicity assay.[17,18] One remarkable feature is abundance of TL-positive T cells in the spleen as well as in the lymph nodes[20] (Table 1). Spleen and lymph node T cells exhibit nonspecific suppressive activity, as can be demonstrated by inhibition of antibody production in adoptive transfer experiments[21] as well as inhibition of cell-mediated immune responses like the proliferative capacity of the mixed lymphocyte reactivity[22] (Table 1). The most outstanding feature of TLI is the fact that it permits establishment of B-specific and long-lasting tolerant state to alloantigens via establishment of bidirectional tolerance to the donor-type BM allograft.[18,23] Permanent acceptance of allogeneic BM cells without graft-versus-host disease was also achieved without any maintenance immunosuppressive therapy in rats[20] and mongrel dogs[19] across major histocompatibility barriers. Recipients developed specific transplantation tolerance to organ allografts including skin,[17–20] perfused hearts,[20] and kidney allografts (unpublished observations) derived from animals syngeneic to the marrow donors (mice and rats) or the marrow donors themselves (dogs).

Specific suppressor cells could be demonstrated in tolerant mice[22] (Table 1). Tolerance to protein antigens and alloantigens could be transferred adoptively into sublethally irradiated syngeneic recipients, suggesting that suppressor cells played a role in establishing or maintaining the tolerance state following TLI.[21,24]

At present a few centers are involved in adapting the TLI approach for induction of specific transplantation tolerance to BM and organ allografts in large outbred animals, including humans. Based on the experimental model in animals where organ-specific antigens may play a major role in initiating an allograft rejection, it seems reasonable to assume that tolerance to donor-type alloantigens induced by BM cells will enable acceptance of all organs derived from the marrow donor as well. A similar approach may be useful for attempting pancreatic allografts for the treatment of experimental insulin-deficient diabetes, since the potential donors of pancreatic tissues in clinical pancreatic transplantation will be mostly unrelated and, therefore, incompatible cadavers. Lack of engraftment of pancreatic allografts using the available immunosuppressive protocols is still the major barrier to successful application of pancreatic transplantation for the treatment of insulin-deficient diabetic patients, due to the strong antigenicity of pancreatic cells. Diabetic patients are more prone to complications after conventional immunosuppressive regimens, including Imuran and prednisone because of increased susceptibility to infection, on the one hand, and the adverse metabolic side effects of corticosteroids on the other. Therefore, application of an ap-

TABLE 1
Mechanisms of immunosuppression after TLI

Period	Cellular events	Immunologic function	
		Humoral	Cell-mediated
Early radiation effects of TLI 1 mo	No circulating Thy 1.2 cells Low circulating Ig cells	No first response Low second response (IgM, IgG) Memory preserved	No response to PHA, Con A No MLR No allograft rejection Memory preserved
	Low circulating Thy 1.2 cells High TL cells	Low first response (IgM only) Diminished second response (IgM, IgG)	Low PHA response Low/normal Con A response
Early recovery from TLI	High circulating Ig cells Nonspecific suppressor T cells	Thy 1.2–dependent nonspecific suppression	Normal MLR Nonspecific suppression of MLR
	Low circulating Thy 1.2 cells	Low first response (IgM, IgG)	Low PHA response Normal/high Con A response
	High circulating Ig cells	Diminished second response (IgM, IgG)	Normal MLR
Late recovery from TLI	Specific suppressor T cells	In tolerant mice and chimeras:	
		Specific nonresponsiveness to protein antigens	Specific unresponsiveness in MLR and specific transplantation tolerance
		Thy 1.2–dependent antigen specific suppression	Specific suppression of MLR

proach for specific tolerance induction like TLI seems to be particularly suitable for pancreatic transplantation in diabetes mellitus. This approach is now being investigated.

ACKNOWLEDGMENTS

This work was supported by The Kroc Foundation, National Institutes of Health grants AI 15387 and AI 11313, and a Hadassah-Hebrew University Joint Grant. Drs. Slavin's and Fuks's present address is Hadassah University Hospital, Jerusalem, Israel.

REFERENCES

[1] Billingham, R. E., Brent, L., and Medawar, P. B.: Actively acquired tolerance of foreign cells. Nature (London) *172*:603–06, 1953.

[2] Billingham, R. E., and Brent, L.: Acquired tolerance of foreign cells in newborn animals. Proc. R. Soc. London B. *146*:78–89, 1956.

[3] Dorsch, S., and Roser, B.: Recirculating, suppressor T cells in transplantation tolerance. J. Exp. Med. *145*:1144–57, 1977.

[4] Heineke, H.: Uber die Einwirkung der Rontgenstrahlen auf Tiere. Muench. Med. Wochenschr. *50*:2090–92, 1903.

[5] Benjamin, E., and Sluka, E.: Antikorperbildung nach experimenteller schadgung des hematopeostischen Systems durch Rontgenstrahlen. Wien. Klin. Wochenschr. *21*:311–14, 1908.

[6] Hume, D. M., and Wolf, J. S.: Modification of renal homograft rejection by irradiation. Transplantation *5*:1174, 1967.

[7] Cronkite, E. P., Chanana, A. D., and Joel, D. D.: Laisure in Interaction of Radiation and Host Human Defense Mechanisms in Malignancy. Bond, V. P. Hellman, S., Order, S. E., Suit, H. D., and Withers, H. R., Eds. Brookhaven, N.Y., Brookhaven National Laboratory Associated Universities, 1974, pp. 181–206.

[8] Anonymous: *In* Ionizing Radiation: Levels and Effects. New York, United Nations, 1972, pp. 303–78.

[9] Cronkite, E. P., Chanana, A. D., and Schnappauf, H. P.: Extracorporeal irradiation of blood and lymph in animals: its effect on homografts and on lymphoma. N. Engl. J. Med. *272*:456–61, 1965.

[10] Joel, D. D., Chanana, A. D., Cronkite, E. P., and Schiffer, L. M.: Modification of skin allograft immunity by extracorporeal irradiation of lymph. Transplantation *5*:1192, 1967.

[11] Wolf, J. S., and Hume, D. M.: Transplant immunity in animals with lymphocytopenia induced by indwelling beta irradiation. Surg. Forum *16*: 202–04, 1965.

[12] Fabricious-Moeller, J.: Experimental studies of the hemorrhagic diathesis from X-ray sickness. Copenhagen, Levin and Monksgaards Forlag, 1922.

[13] Main, J. M., and Prehn, R. T.: Successful skin homografts after the administration of high dosage X-radiation and homologous bond marrow. J. Natl. Cancer Inst. *15*:1023–29, 1955.

[14] Ford, C. E., Hamerton, J. L., Barnes, D., and Loutit, J. F.: Cytological identification of radiation chimaeras. Nature (London) *177*:452–54, 1956.

[15] Murray, J. E., Merrill, J. P., Dammin, G. J., Dealy, J. B., Jr., Walter, C. W., Brooke, M. S., and Wilson, R. E.: Study on transplantation immunity after total body irradiation: clinical and experimental investigation. Surgery *48*: 272–84, 1960.

[16] Kaplan, H. S.: Hodgkin's disease. Cambridge, Mass., Harvard University Press, 1972, p. 283.

[17] Slavin, S., Strober, S., Fuks, Z., and Kaplan, H. S.: Long-term survival of skin allografts in mice treated with fractionated total lymphoid irradiation. Science *193*:1252, 1976.

[18] Slavin, S., Strober, S., Fuks, Z., and Kaplan, H. S.: Induction of specific tissue transplantation tolerance using fractionated total lymphoid irradiation in adult mice: long-term survival of allogeneic bone marrow and skin grafts. J. Exp. Med. *146*:34–48, 1977.

[19] Slavin, S., Gottlieb, M., Strober, S., Hoppe, R. T., Kaplan, H. S., and Grumet, F. C.: Transplantation of bone marrow in outbred dogs without graft-vs.-host disease using total lymphoid irradiation (TLI). Transplantation *27*:139, 1979.

[20] Strober, S., Gottlieb, M., Slavin, S., Zan-Bar, I., King, D., Hoppe, R. T., Fuks, Z., Grumet, F. C., and Kaplan, H. S.: Allograft tolerance after total lymphoid irradiation (TLI). Immunol. Rev., in press, 1979.

[21] Zan-Bar, I., Slavin, S., and Strober, S.: Induction and mechanism of tolerance to bovine serum albumin in mice given total lymphoid irradiation (TLI). J. Immunol. *121*:1400–04, 1978.

[22] Slavin, S., and Strober, S.: Induction of allograft tolerance after total lymphoid irradiation (TLI): development of suppressor cells of the mixed leukocyte reaction (MLR). Submitted for publication, 1979.

[23] Slavin, S., Fuks, Z., Kaplan, H. S., and Strober, S.: Transplantation of allogeneic bone marrow without graft-vs.-host disease using total lymphoid irradiation (TLI). J. Exp. Med. *147*:963–72, 1978.

[24] Slavin, S., Zan-Bar, I., and Strober, S.: Generation of protein-specific and alloantigen-specific suppressor cells following total lymphoid irradiation in mice. Transplant. Proc. *11*:891–94, 1979.

Discussion

Sections on Rejection and Donor Treatment

The final session of this meeting was introduced by the comprehensive review of the immunologic aspects of pancreatic transplantation by Barker and co-workers. More specifically, the discussion dealt with the influence of in vitro islet cell culture conditions on the ultimate outcome of the allograft survival. Central to the theme of the discussion was the concept of donor-passenger leukocytes (preferably called stimulator cells, SC; Lafferty) and the role of these cells in allograft rejection. In general, culture conditions were designed for optimum islet cell survival and evidence for the concomitant elimination of donor stimulator cells from diminution of rejection. There was uniform agreement that a high oxygen concentration (as opposed to air) was injurious for isolated islet cell cultures and, at the same time, probably cytotoxic for the stimulator cells. In this regard, the evidence presented by Lafferty and co-workers, that clustered islet cells were protected from oxygen toxicity, was considered very encouraging. Observations presented by Morris et al., showing the failure of allogeneic fetal rat islet cells, cultured for 21 days in air, to correct hyperglycemia in vivo, suggested, inter alia, that low tissue oxygen tension may not be adequate for eliminating those cells responsible for the rejection of the islet cell allografts. Parenthetically, fetal rat islets cultured under the same conditions were capable of restoring normoglycemia to syngeneic recipients.

The idiosyncrasies of the culture conditions were further complicated by evidence highlighting the importance of ambient temperature on islet cell growth in vitro.

The influence of physiologic (37°C) versus room temperature (22–24°C) on islet cell growth was compared. With isolated islet cells from newborn or fetal mice (Talmage) or adult rats (Lacy), lower culture temperatures were more protective of the islets in an environment of oxygen than higher (37°C) temperatures. In similar fashion, thyroid allografts, cultured at low (22–24°C) temperatures, show improved survival over those cultures exposed to physiologic temperatures. Although culture in air appeared to result in the best fetal islet survival (Talmage et al.), such conditions were not judged adequate for the elimination of SC. Additional data regarding the effect of culture temperatures on the SC population is awaited.

On an immunologic level, the SC contaminating the islet cell populations were considered more important than parenchymal elements in triggering allograft rejection. Unlike islet or parenchymal cells, donor SC are presumed to stimulate the recipient immune system through the release of soluble mediator(s) (Lafferty et al.). Characteristics of the SC place it among the lymphocyte-macrophage cell lineage. In this regard, the presence of lymphoid tissue interspersed within the pancreatic parenchyma was emphasized. Furthermore, the likelihood that islets may contain integral fixed mononuclear histocytes (similar to the concept of Langerhans cells in the epidermis) was mentioned. The possibility that endothelial (or other) cell types, contaminating islet cell cultures, may trigger a host-immune response by simulating SC or by acting as targets for immune destruction remains to be elucidated. Based on the above discussion, it was concluded that histologically "pure" preparations of islet cells would be most likely to result in an optimum transplant outcome.

Recent reports that mouse islet cells lack surface histocompatibility (H-2) antigens, as determined by immunoferritin staining (E. Parr: J. Exp. Med. *150*:1–9, 1979), raises the future possibility of immune selection of pure islet cell preparations. Whether SC present in fetal transplantation tissue are immunologically mature and contribute to the allograft rejection process remains conjectural at this time. The suggestion was made that islet-cell cell lines (which would theoretically lack SC) be established as a means of elucidating the mechanisms of allograft rejection. Transplantation of such islet cell lines may provide a good model for nonimmune mechanisms of graft rejection. The possibility that stimulatory mediators released from SC may elicit nonspecific inflammatory responses capable of damaging the integrity of the sensitive islet cell elements was raised.

A number of in vivo animal studies was discussed and is relevant to the mechanisms of transplantation rejection and the possible role of SC. Of interest was the pertinent observation by Mullen that viable fetal rat pancreas transplants were still capable of eliciting an immune response when transplanted into a nonimmunosuppressed allogeneic host after 300 days of survival in the original host. One of many possible explanations for this observation was that fixed islet cell histiocytes in the transplanted organ survive despite prolonged in vivo existence in the original host. In contradistinction to the above experiment, Barker reported preliminary findings that, in tolerant rat recipients, allogeneic fetal pancreas grafts were resistant to immune rejection upon restoration of immune competence with host lymphocytes. Further, the same group mentioned that transplant recipients tolerant of allogeneic donor lymph node cells were still capable of rejecting isolated islet cells from the same donor. It was agreed that these apparently discrepant findings highlight the need for further understanding the pathogenesis of pancreas transplantation rejection and the specific role of SC in this immune process.

Numerous methods of suppressing the recipient immune system and prolonging allograft survival were discussed. In general, rejection characterized the transplantation of allogeneic adult islets, fetal pancreas (cultured and noncultured) and vascularized grafts in nonimmunosuppressed rat recipients. Vascularized grafts were considered less prone to the rejection process than isolated islets (Barker). Of the agents used for immunosuppression of the recipient, antilymphocyte serum was the most successful in the rat. Immunologic enhancement by the use of antidonor serum or immunoglobulin failed to produce encouraging results. The use of newer agents, such as Cyclosporin, was found to be beneficial in vascularized grafts and adult islet cell grafts only if continuous immunosuppression was undertaken posttransplantation (Sutherland). Preliminary evidence in dogs suggests that Cyclosporin may be valuable in segmental pancreas transplants. The potential use of total lymphoid irradiation as an immunosuppressive modality in pancreas transplantation awaits further investigation (Slavin). The ability of streptozotocin-treated recipients to regenerate their own islet cells emphasizes the necessity for built-in controls in allograft transplant protocols. Finally, the critical mass of allograft tissue required to permit engraftment and function remains to be established.

Index

Acinar cells, 66
Aldehyde fuchsin staining
of cadaveric human pancreatic islet in tissue culture, 50
of isolated islets, 24
Alloantibodies, specific immunotherapy using, 113-114, 115
Allografts of dispersed islet tissue in humans, 31-44
Allotransplantation of dispersed pancreatic islet tissue to diabetic renal allograft recipients, 39-43
ALS, *see* Antilymphocyte serum
Amylase levels
after islet isotransplantation, 47-49
in open duct grafts, 56
in segmental pancreas transplantation, 11-16
Antilymphocyte globulin, 6
Antilymphocyte serum (ALS)
in immunosuppression for rat fetal pancreas allografts, 114-119
in in vitro culture, 93-96
in islet transplantation, 88-91
in suppression of rejection of rat islet allografts, 109-111
Antithymocyte globulin, 81
Arterial bleeding, potentially fatal, 4
Autografts, human, 56
of dispersed islet tissue, 31-44
Autoimmunity, possible susceptibility of transplanted islets to, 90-91
Azathioprine, 6

Beta cells (B cells, β cells), 102
function, 52
human fetal, 68-69
mass, increased, 56
Bleeding, potentially fatal arterial, 4
Bone marrow aplasia, 121

C-peptide levels
from cultured explants, 67
before and after graft rejection, 7, 8
after intraportal transplantation of fetal pancreatic microfragments, 82, 84
after pancreas transplantation, 12-16
Collagenase digestion islet isolation technique, 20
Corticosteroids in islet allografts, 89
Culture, time of, effect on allograft survival, 105-106
Cyclophosphamide
in islet allografts, 89
in suppression of rejection of rat islet allografts, 108-109, 111
treatment before islet transplantation, 98-104
Cyclosporin A in suppression of rejection of rat islet allografts, 108-111, 125

Diabetes, additional model of, in BB rats, 91
Diabetic patients, pancreas transplantation and, 16-17
Diabetic state, islet allograft survival and, 93
Diabetogeneic effect of steroids, 42, 43
Dimethyl sulfoxide (DMSO), 70-72
Duct anastomosis, clinical segmental pancreas transplantation without, 10-18
Duct ligation
effect on islet cell performance, 56
segmental pancreas transplantation with, 3-9
Ductal distention, 21-28
Ductojejunostomy, 9

Electrolyte solution, balanced, 9
Endocrine-to-exocrine ratio, 57
Enhancement of immunologic unresponsiveness, 90
Enterokinase, 10
Epigastric pouch technique, 75

Fetal pancreas, human, *see* Human fetal pancreas
Ficoll purification islet isolation technique, 20
Fistula, pancreatic, 5-7

Glucagon
antibody staining of isolated islets, 25
immunoreactivity in nude mice, 76, 78
levels in human fetal pancreas, 58-63
levels in islet isotransplantation, 47-48
levels in pancreas transplantation, 13-15
measurements, 52
Glucose
in early experiments in human pancreas transplantation, 1-2
effect plus theophylline on insulin release, 67-68
levels in intraportal transplantation of fetal pancreatic microfragments, 82
levels in islet isotransplantation, 46, 48
levels in pancreas transplantation, 12-16
levels in pancreatectomy, 34-38
levels in rat fetal pancreas allografts, 116
levels in segmental pancreas transplantation, 4
metabolism, 52
-stimulated leucine incorporation into proinsulin, 61

Hematoxylin-eosin staining
of cadaveric human pancreatic islet in tissue culture, 50
of isolated islets, 24
Histocompatability
barriers and islet rejection, 94-96
in pancreatic transplantations, 6
Histoincompatability, minimizing, 98
Human fetal pancreas
advantages, 80
cryopreservation, 70-73, 84-85
culture and function in vitro, 64-69
glucagon levels, 58-59
insulin levels, 58-63
perifusion and culture, 57-63
survival in organ culture, 84
transplantation, 74-79
transplantation via portal vein, 80-83

Immunogenicity, minimizing, 87-88
Immunologic problems in islet transplantation, 86-92
Immunologic unresponsiveness, enchancement of, 90
Immunosuppression
nonspecific, 89-90
in pancreatic transplantations, 6-7
specific, for rat fetal pancreas allografts, 113-120
using total lymphoid irradiation, 121-123
Immunosuppressive therapy, pancreas transplantation and, 17
Immunotherapy, specific, using alloantibodies, 113-114, 115
Imuran in islet allografts, 89
Insulin
antibodies, 8, 9
antibody staining of isolated islets, 25
biosynthesis, 58-59
in early experiments in human pancreas transplantation, 1-2
levels in human fetal pancreas, 58-63
levels in intraportal transplantation of fetal pancreatic microfragments, 82
levels in islet isotransplantation, 47-49
levels in pancreas transplantation, 13-16
levels in pancreatectomy, 34
release, glucose plus theophylline effect on, 67-68
release from human fetal pancreas cultures, 65-69
Irradiation, total lymphoid, *see* Lymphoid irradiation, total
Ischemia, prolonged cold or warm, 42
Islet allotransplantation
intraportal, 42
reasons for failure of, 31
Islet autotransplants
intraportal, 39
after near-total pancreatectomy for chronic pancreatitis, 32-39
Islet cell(s)
antibodies, 8, 9
isolation of viable dog, 19-30
Islet identification in vitro, "green-light" technique for, 93
Islet performance, duct ligation effect on, 56
Islet tissue
auto- and allografts of dispersed, in humans, 31-44
dispersed, 32
dispersed, allotransplantation of, to diabetic renal allograft recipients, 39-43
in rat, suppression of rejection of allogeneic, 107-112
Islet transplantation, 10
donor pretreatment regimens and, 93-94
evaluating benefits of human, 52-55
immunologic problems in, 86-92
immunologically privileged sites for, 89
kidney function and, 53-54
to nonimmunosuppressed recipients, 98-104
peritoneal exudate cells and, 95-96
possible susceptibility to autoimmunity in, 90-91
rejection, attempts to overcome, 87-90
rejection, effect of culture on, 93-97
survival, diabetic state and, 93
tissue culture studies for, *see* Tissue culture studies for islet transplants
Islet yield, estimating, 33
Islets
identification of dog, 23
identification of rat, 23
intraportal, 108, 109
intrasplenic, 108, 109
preparation of, 98-99
problems isolating intact human, 23
pseudoislets, 28-29
storage of, 49

Ketone metabolism, 52
Kidney
function, islet transplantation effects on, 53-54
and pancreas transplantation, simultaneous, 1

Langerhans, islets of, *see* Islet *entries*
Large vessel disease, 53
Leucine incorporation into proinsulin, 61
Leukocytes, passenger, 88, 93, 95-96, 124
Lipase levels after pancreas transplantation, 12, 14
Lymphoid irradiation, total, immunosuppression and organ transplantation tolerance using, 121-123

Methylprednisolone in islet allografts, 89
Microangiopathy, 53

Neoprene, 10
Nephropathy, 53-54
Neuropathy, 54
Nucleopore bags, xenogeneic pancreas in, 108, 109, 111

Oxygen
  atmosphere, high, 98, 104
  effects on allograft survival, 105-106

Pancreas
  fetal, 108-110; *see also* Human fetal pancreas
  human fetal, *see* Human fetal pancreas
  and kidney transplantation, simultaneous, 1
  single-cell preparation from, 26-29
  transplantation of vascularized, 88
  xenogeneic, in Nucleopore bags, 108, 109, 111
Pancreas allografts, oxygen, temperature, and time of culture effects on survival of, 105-106
Pancreas polypeptide immunoreactivity in nude mice, 76, 78
Pancreas transplantation
  diabetic patients and, 16-17
  early experiments in human, 1-2
  immunosuppressive therapy and, 17
  mortality and morbidity, 1
  rejection, 7-8
  segmental, with duct ligation, 3-9
  segmental, without duct anastomosis, 10-18
Pancreatectomy, islet autotransplantation after near-total, 32-39
Pancreatic fistula, 5-7
Pancreatic islet, *see* Islet *entries*
Pancreatic juice, handling of, 9
Pancreatic microfragments, transplanted fetal, 42
Pancreatic polypeptide cells, immunostaining for, 28
Pancreatic transplantation, *see* Pancreas transplantation
Pancreaticoduodenal transplant, 1, 3
Pancreaticojejunostomy, end-to-end, 9
Pancreatin, 34
Pancreatitis, chronic, islet autotransplantation after near-total pancreatectomy for, 32-39
Passenger leukocytes, 88, 93, 95-96, 124
Perifusion technique, 58, 61
Peritoneal exudate cells, islet transplants and, 95-96
Portal vein, transplantation of fetal pancreatic microfragments via, 80-83

Prednisone, 6, 11
Pregnancy, termination of, with prostaglandin F2α, 57, 64-65
Procarbazine hydrochloride (PCH) in immunosuppression for rat fetal pancreas allografts, 114-119
Proinsulin biosynthesis, 60-61
Prostaglandin F2α, termination of pregnancy with, 57, 64-65
Proteinuria, 54
Pseudoislets, 28-29

Renal allograft recipients, diabetic, allotransplantation of dispersed pancreatic islet tissue to, 39-43
Retinopathy, 53, 54
RMPI1640 medium, 59, 62
Roux-en-Y loop, jejunal, 3, 5, 7

Somatostatin
  immunoreactivity in nude mice, 76, 78
  immunostaining for, 28
Steroids, diabetogeneic effect of, 42, 43
Stimulator cells, 124-125

T cells, spleen and lymph node, 122
TCM199 medium, 59, 62
Temperature effects on allograft survival, 105-106
Theophylline, 59, 62
  plus glucose effect on insulin release, 67-68
Thy 1.2-bearing T cells, 122
Thyroid allografts, oxygen, temperature, and time of culture effects on survival of, 105-106
Thyroid tissue, mouse allogeneic, in culture, 112
Tissue culture studies for islet transplants, 45-51
  animal, 47-48
  human, 48-49
Tolerance
  immunologic, 90
  transplantation, using total lymphoid irradiation, 121-123
Transplantation
  of human fetal pancreas, 74-79
  pancreas, *see* Pancreas transplantation
  tolerance using total lymphoid irradiation, 121-123

Uremia, pancreas graft and, 1

Vascular complications in human islet transplantation, 52-54
Vascularized grafts, 125
Vascularized pancreas, transplantation of, 88

Whole body irradiation (WBI), 121

Xenotransplantation
  in nude mice, 74-75, 76, 78-79
  in nude rats, 75-76, 78-79

General Information

COMMITTEE ON SCIENTIFIC PROGRAMS

WILLIAM G. BLACKARD, M.D., *Chairman;* SR. RITAMARY BROWN, R.D., and HAROLD E. LEBOVITZ, M.D., *Vice Chairmen;* EDWARD R. ARQUILLA, M.D., Ph.D., MARTIN J. CONWAY, M.D., WILLIAM DAUGHADAY, M.D., JOHN K. DAVIDSON, MD., Ph.D., WILLIAM C. DUCKWORTH, M.D., SAUL M. GENUTH, M.D., MARILYN P. GILROY, R.D., FREDDA GINSBERG-FELLNER, M.D., ERNEST M. GOLD, M.D., GEROLD M. GRODSKY, Ph.D., DEBBIE SPEEGLE HULL, R.N., M.S.N., LINDA HURWITZ, R.N., ROBERT L. KROC, Ph.D., BILLIE B. LARCH, R.N., RITA M. NEMCHIK, R.N., M.S., J. STUART SOELDNER, M.D., ELIZABETH TANNER, R.N.

REGISTRATION

The Scientific Program is open to members of the medical and allied professions. REGISTRATION FEES: $20.00 for members of the National Professional Section of the American Diabetes Association or The Endocrine Society; $35.00 for nonmembers; $10.00 for residents, interns, and fellows within five years of training following graduation from medical school. Everyone is required to register, and admission is by badge only.

CONTINUING EDUCATION

As an organization accredited for continuing medical education, the American Diabetes Association certifies that this continuing medical education activity meets the criteria for 19 credit hours in category 1 for the Physician's Recognition Award of the American Medical Association. Credit has been applied for with The American Academy of Family Physicians, New York State Nurses Association and The American Dietetic Association.

SCIENTIFIC PROGRAM

Presentation of papers will be ten minutes (with the exception of the Sunday morning, Monday afternoon and Tuesday morning symposia, the Lilly Lecture and the Banting Memorial Lecture), followed by five minutes discussion. All sessions will begin promptly, and speakers have been requested to adhere strictly to the allotted time. Abstracts of papers to be presented at the Sessions begin on page vi and are numbered to correspond with the papers listed through page xxvi.

THE ENDOCRINE SOCIETY

The Sixty-second Annual Meeting of the Endocrine Society will be held Wednesday through Friday, June 18–20, at the Sheraton Washington Hotel, Washington, D.C. Nonmembers of that Society are required to pay a $40.00 registration fee, which includes a copy of the program. However, members of the American Diabetes Association may attend without charge the June 18 (carbohydrate) session upon presentation of their registration badges for the Association's 40th Annual Meeting or their Association membership cards. Copies of The Endocrine Society's program may be purchased at the desk for $10.00 or ordered in advance from the Society's office at 9650 Rockville Pike, Bethesda, Maryland 20014.

PROGRAMS

Distribution of copies of this program without charge is limited to subscribers of *Diabetes* as a Supplement. It is important, therefore, to BRING THIS PROGRAM WITH YOU. Additional copies at the registration desk will cost $5.00 each.

MANUSCRIPTS

The Editors of *Diabetes* and *Diabetes Care* will be pleased to consider for publication papers presented at the Sessions. Manuscripts may be forwarded to the Editorial Office of the Association.

EXHIBITS

The Technical Exhibits will occupy the Washington Room of the Sheraton Washington Hotel. Exhibit dates and hours: Saturday, June 14, 3:00-5:30 p.m., Sunday, June 15, 9:00-5:30 p.m., Monday, June 16, 9:00-5:30 p.m., Tuesday, June 17, 9:00-1:00 p.m.

CASSETTE RECORDINGS

Quality recordings of the Scientific Sessions will be available for purchase. NO tape recorders will be permitted at the Sessions.

APPLICATION FORM FOR SCIENTIFIC SESSIONS
AMERICAN DIABETES ASSOCIATION
40th Annual Meeting

FEE: $20.00—members of the National Professional Section and The Endocrine Society; $35.00—nonmembers; $10.00—Interns, Residents and Fellows. Registration fee must accompany application.

SOCIAL HOUR AND BANQUET: All registrants are invited to attend the Social Hour and Awards Banquet on Saturday evening, June 14, commencing at 6:30 p.m. Dress is informal. Dinner is $26.00 per person.

HOTEL ACCOMMODATIONS: A room reservation card will be sent upon receipt of your registration. If you choose to telephone the Sheraton Washington, you must advise that you are attending the American Diabetes Association meeting to be eligible for our special group rates. The hotel number is (202) 328-2000.

- -

______ I will attend the 40th Annual Meeting of the American Diabetes Association.

______ Professional Member of the American Diabetes Association.

______ Nonmember.

Please reserve:

______ ticket(s) @ $26.00 per person for the Awards Banquet, $ ________

NAME (Please print) ______________________ ADDRESS (Please print) ______________________

NOTE: Please make checks payable to American Diabetes Association, Inc., and return to Harry A. Hansen, American Diabetes Association, 600 Fifth Avenue, New York, New York 10020. Tickets will be held at the Association's Registration Desk.

Schedule of Events

All functions will be held at the Sheraton Washington Hotel

REGISTRATION

Wednesday, June 11—5:00 p.m.-9:00 p.m.	Main Registration Area
Thursday, June 12—8:00 a.m.-5:00 p.m.	Main Registration Area
Friday, June 13—8:00 a.m.-5:00 p.m.	Main Registration Area
Saturday, June 14—8:00 a.m.-9:00 p.m.	Main Registration Area
Sunday, June 15—7:30 a.m.-6:00 p.m.	Main Registration Area
Monday, June 16—8:00 a.m.-5:30 p.m.	Main Registration Area
Tuesday, June 17—8:00 a.m.-4:00 p.m.	Main Registration Area

SOCIAL HOUR AND BANQUET

Saturday, June 14

6:30 p.m.	*Social Hour*	Cotillion Room
7:30 p.m.	*Banquet*	Cotillion Room

SCIENTIFIC SESSIONS

Sunday, June 15

9:00 a.m.-9:15 a.m.	*Opening Remarks*	
	Ronald A. Arky, M.D., President, American Diabetes Association, Inc.	Sheraton Hall
9:15 a.m.-10:45 a.m.	*Open Loop Insulin Delivery*	Sheraton Hall
11:00 a.m.-12:30 p.m.	*Factors in the Development of Diabetic Microangiopathy*	Sheraton Hall
2:00 p.m.-5:00 p.m.	*Complications of Diabetes*	Sheraton Hall
2:00 p.m.-5:00 p.m.	*Hormone Action*	Cotillion Room
2:00 p.m.-3:00 p.m.	*Concepts of Behavioral Change and Compliance*	Maryland Suite
3:00 p.m.-5:00 p.m.	*Behavior and Attitudes Affecting Compliance*	Maryland Suite
5:15 p.m.-5:45 p.m.	*The Lilly Lecture*	Sheraton Hall

Monday, June 16

8:30 a.m.-9:45 a.m.	*Transplantation and Artificial Devices*	Sheraton Hall
8:30 a.m.-9:45 a.m.	*Hormone Secretion I*	Cotillion Room
8:30 a.m.-10:15 a.m.	*Nutritional Management*	Maryland Suite
9:00 a.m.-11:15 a.m.	*Poster Sessions:*	
	Complications of Diabetes	Washington Room
	Hormone Action	Washington Room
	Transplantation and Artificial Devices	Washington Room
	Clinical Physiology	Washington Room
11:30 a.m.-12:30 p.m.	*Banting Lecture*	Sheraton Hall
2:00 p.m.-4:30 p.m.	*Clinical Diabetes*	Sheraton Hall
2:00 p.m.-4:30 p.m.	*Hormone Secretion II*	Cotillion Room
2:00 p.m.-5:00 p.m.	*Methods of Control*	Maryland Suite
3:00 p.m.-5:30 p.m.	*Poster Sessions:*	
	Hormone Secretion	Washington Room
	Health Care Delivery	Washington Room
	Genetics and Immunology	Washington Room

Tuesday, June 17

8:30 a.m.-10:45 a.m.	*Hormone Receptors*	Sheraton Hall
8:30 a.m.-10:45 a.m.	*Clinical Physiology*	Cotillion Room
8:30 a.m.-9:30 a.m.	*Adolescent Concerns*	Maryland Suite
9:30 a.m.-10:30 a.m.	*Legislation and Diabetes*	Maryland Suite
10:00 a.m.-12:30 p.m.	*Poster Sessions:*	
	Clinical Diabetes	Washington Room
	Hormone Receptors	Washington Room
	Metabolism	Washington Room
10:45 a.m.-12:15 p.m.	*Epidemiology and Financial Implications*	Maryland Suite
1:00 p.m.-3:30 p.m.	*Genetics and Immunology*	Sheraton Hall
1:00 p.m.-3:30 p.m.	*Metabolism*	Cotillion Room
1:30 p.m.-3:30 p.m.	*Complications of Diabetes*	Maryland Suite

AWARDS BANQUET
SATURDAY, JUNE 14, 1980
Cotillion Room

Social Hour
6:30 p.m.
Cotillion Room

Banquet
7:30 p.m.
Cotillion Room

Presentation of Awards

Banting Medal	NORBERT FREINKEL, M.D.
Diabetes in Youth	LUTHER B. TRAVIS, M.D.
Outstanding Affiliate Service	NETTI RICHTER
Ames Award	CARELYN P. FYLLING, R.N., M.S.
Pfizer Award	HAROLD RIFKIN, M.D.
Upjohn Award	LEO P. KRALL, M.D.

Other Awards to be Announced

Scientific Program

Membership in the American Diabetes Association is indicated by an asterisk.
Session Co-Chairmen indicated by a double asterisk served as members of the Committee on Scientific Programs.

SUNDAY MORNING, JUNE 15, 9:00 a.m.-12:30 p.m.

Two Consecutive Symposia-Sheraton Hall

9:00-9:15

Opening Remarks
RONALD A. ARKY, M.D.*
President, American Diabetes Association

9:15-10:45

Session I: *Open Loop Insulin Delivery*
J. STUART SOELDNER, M.D.,** *Chairman*

Introductory Remarks
J. STUART SOELDNER, M.D.**
Acting Director, Joslin Research Laboratory, Boston, Massachusetts

A Perspective on Open Loop Insulin Delivery
SAUL M. GENUTH, M.D.*
Director, Saltzman Institute for Clinical Investigation, Mt. Sinai Hospital, Cleveland, Ohio

Practical Application of Open Loop Subcutaneous Insulin Delivery in the Young Diabetic
WILLIAM V. TAMBORLANE, JR., M.D.*
Assistant Professor of Pediatrics, Yale University School of Medicine, New Haven, Connecticut

Long-term Open Loop Insulin Delivery
JOHN A. PARSONS, M.D.
Senior Investigator, National Institute for Medical Research, Mill Hill, London, United Kingdom

Discussion

11:00-12:30

Session II: *Factors in the Development of Diabetic Microangiopathy*
DONALD E. McMILLAN, M.D.,* *Chairman*

Oxygen, Angiogenesis and Diabetic Retinopathy
ARNALL PATZ, M.D.
Chairman, Department of Ophthalmology, The Johns Hopkins Hospital, Baltimore, Maryland

Studies on Diabetic Nephropthy
ALFRED F. MICHAEL, JR., M.D.
Professor of Pediatrics, Department of Pediatrics, Laboratory Medicine and Pathology, University of Minnesota Medical School, Minneapolis, Minnesota

Blood Flow Changes and Blood Vessel Damage in Diabetes
DONALD E. McMILLAN, M.D.*
Director of Diabetes Research, Sansum Medical Research Foundation, Santa Barbara, California

Discussion

Scientific Program

SUNDAY AFTERNOON, JUNE 15

Concurrent Sessions

2:00 p.m.-5:00 p.m.
SHERATON HALL
Session I: *Complications of Diabetes*
KENNETH H. GABBAY, M.D.,* and MARTIN J. CONWAY, M.D.**, *Co-Chairmen*

2:00-2:10 p.m.

1. Progressive Retinopathy with Improved Metabolic Control in Diabetic Dwarfism (Mauriac's Syndrome)
   A. L. DRASH*, D. DANEMAN*, and L. TRAVIS*, Pittsburgh, Pennsylvania and Galveston, Texas

2:15-2:25 p.m.

2. The "Diabetes" of Cystic Fibrosis (CF)
   H. M. RODMAN*, S. WALTMAN, T. KRUPIN, C. KILO, J. R. WILLIAMSON, and L. W. MATTHEWS, Cleveland, Ohio and St. Louis, Missouri

2:30-2:40 p.m.

3. Diabetic Retinopathy: Effects of Pregnancy (P) and Laser Therapy (LT)
   L. J. SINGERMAN, L. M. AIELLO, and H. M. RODMAN*, Cleveland, Ohio and Boston, Massachusetts

2:00 p.m.-5:00 p.m.
COTILLION ROOM
Session II: *Hormone Action*
WILLIAM H. DAUGHADAY, M.D.** and JERROLD M. OLEFSKY, M.D.,* *Co-Chairmen*

2:00-2:10 p.m.

11. Isolation from Rat Adipocytes of a Chemical Mediator for Insulin Activation of Pyruvate Dehydrogenase
    FREDERICK L. KIECHLE, NIRMALA KOTAGAL, DENNIS A. POPP, and LEONARD JARETT*, St. Louis, Missouri

2:15-2:25 p.m.

12. Evidence that a Regulator of Enzyme Activity is Generated by an Insulin-stimulated Proteolytic Reaction at the Plasma Membrane
    JONATHAN R. SEALS, and MICHAEL P. CZECH*, Providence, Rhode Island

2:30-2:40 p.m.

13. Monoclonal Antibodies Against the Rat Adipocyte Intrinsic Membrane Proteins Mimic Insulin Action
    JOANNA BEACHY, Providence, Rhode Island (Introduced by Ora Smith*, New Haven, Connecticut)

2:00 p.m.-3:00 p.m.
MARYLAND SUITE
Symposium
Concepts of Behavioral Change and Compliance
LINDA HURWITZ, R.N.* and T. FRANKLIN WILLIAMS, M.D.*, *Co-Chairmen*

2:00-2:30 p.m.

"Psychological Factors in Health Compliance"
H. L. ROBERT FELDMAN, Ph.D.
Assistant Professor of Health Education, University of Maryland, College Park

2:30-3:00 p.m.

"Educational Principles and Strategies"
DOROTHY DEL BUENO, R.N., Ed.D.
Assistant Dean of Continuing Education, University of Pennsylvania School of Nursing, Philadelphia

2:45-2:55 p.m.

4. Relationship of Vascular Disease to Fasting Plasma Glucose (FPG) and Other Variables in 3583 With Diabetes (DM): A Multinational Study
K. M. WEST*, HARRY KEEN, R. J. JARRETT, J. H. FULLER, ARTHUR TEUSCHER*, A. S. KROLEWSKI, VOLKER SCHLIACK, M. M. S. AHUJA, EISHI MIKI, OSCAR MATEO DE ACOSTA*, VILI GRABAUSKAS, and BERNARD GRAB, Oklahoma City, London, Bern, Warsaw, Berlin GDR, New Delhi, Tokyo, Havana, Phoenix, and Geneva

3:00-3:10 p.m.

5. Reversible Autonomic Nervous System Abnormalities in Juvenile Diabetes, A Pupillographic Study
A. B. HREIDARSSON, Aarhus, Denmark (Introduced by M. W. STEFFES*, Minneapolis, Minnesota.)

3:15-3:45
Intermission

3:45-3:55 p.m.

6. Morphometric Analysis of Autonomic Nerve Fibers in Nondiabetic and Ketonuric Diabetic Chinese Hamsters
A. DIANI*, D. DAVIS, J. FIX, J. SWARTZMAN, and G. GERRITSEN*, Greenville, North Carolina and Kalamazoo, Michigan

2:45-2:55 p.m.

14. Insulin-Stimulated Translocation of Glucose Transport Systems from an Intracellular Pool to the Plasma Membrane in Rat Adipose Cells: Time Course and Reversibility
E. KARNIELI, L. B. SALANS*, and S. W. CUSHMAN*, Bethesda, Maryland

3:00-3:10 p.m.

15. Reconstitution of D-Glucose Transport Activity from Cytoplasmic Membranes: Evidence Against Recruitment of Cytoplasmic Membrane Transporters into the Plasma Membrane as the Major Action of Insulin
CHRISTIN CARTER-SU, Providence, Rhode Island (Introduced by M. F. SHANAHAN*, Madison, Wisconsin)

3:15-3:45
Intermission

3:45-3:55 p.m.

16. Insulin Stimulation of Glycogen Synthase in Human Diploid Fibroblasts
H. HIDAKA, J. LARNER*, and B. V. HOWARD*, Phoenix, Arizona and Charlottesville, Virginia

3:00 p.m.-5:00 p.m.
MARYLAND SUITE
Session III: *Behavior and Attitudes Affecting Compliance*
LINDA A. HURWITZ, R.N.* and T. FRANKLIN WILLIAMS, M.D.*, *Co-Chairmen*

3:00-3:10 p.m.

21. The Effect of Contracting on Patient Compliance
CAROLE MENSING, DEANNE F. BELL, and DURWARD L. BELL, Minneapolis, Minnesota and Austin, Texas

3:15-3:25 p.m.

22. Cognitive and Situational Factors Associated with Diabetic Patient Compliance
S. S. GILBERT, and F. C. PENNINGTON, Ann Arbor, Michigan

3:30-3:40
Intermission

3:45-3:55 p.m.

23. The Relationship of Quality of Life and Quality of Care for a Sample of Diabetic Patients
MARY ETTA C. MILLS, IVAN BAROFSKY, and BEATRICE NORDBERG*, Baltimore, Maryland

Scientific Program

4:00-4:10 p.m.

7. Further Evidence that Streptozotocin-induced Diabetes Accelerates the Catabolism of Recently Synthesized Collagen in Rat Skin
M. SCHNEIR, E. EDLIN-FOLZ, A. HOYRUP, N. RAMAMURTHY, and L. GOLUB, Los Angeles, California

4:15-4:25 p.m.

8. Wound Healing in Spontaneously Diabetic Chinese Hamster: Morphologic and Morphometric Study
E. J. WERINGER*, and E. R. ARQUILLA*, Irvine, California

4:30-4:40 p.m.

9. Increased Catabolism of Glycosylated Low Density Lipoprotein (g-LDL) by Rat Peritoneal Macrophage
H. J. KIM*, and I. V. KURUP, Milwaukee, Wisconsin

4:45-4:55 p.m.

10. Pericyte Necrosis and Muscle Capillary Basement Membrane (CBM) Thickening in Diabetes Mellitus
R. G. TILTON, P. L. HOFFMANN, C. KILO*, and J. R. WILLIAMSON*, St. Louis, Missouri

4:00-4:10 p.m.

17. Calmodulin-Stimulation of Ca^{2+} Transport in Insulin-Sensitive Adipocyte Plasma Membranes
J. M. MCDONALD*, H. A. PERSHADSINGH, and M. LANDT, St. Louis, Missouri

4:15-4:25 p.m.

18. Calmodulin and Inhibitor: Role in Experimental Diabetes and Insulin Action
SOLOMON S. SOLOMON*, MARJORIE PALAZZOLO, JANET MCPHERSON, and AL SMOAKE, Memphis, Tennessee

4:30-4:40 p.m.

19. Elevated Insulin-like Growth Factor II (IGF-II) in Non-islet Tumor Induced Hypoglycemia Detected by a New Specific Radioreceptor Assay
W. H. DAUGHADAY*, B. TRIVEDI, and I. K. MARIZ, St. Louis, Missouri

4:45-4:55 p.m.

20. Functional Correlates of Genetically Defective Receptors for Insulin and Insulin-like Growth Factors in an Infant with Leprechaunism
A. B. KNIGHT, E. E. SCHILLING, J. A. ROMANUS, and M. M. RECHLER, Bethesda, Maryland (Introduced by E. A. H. MCGUIRE*)

4:00-4:10 p.m.

24. Cultural Beliefs Influence Compliance to Therapy for Diabetes Mellitus
CLARISSA S. SCOTT, Miami, Florida (Introduced by JAY S. SKYLER*)

4:15-4:25 p.m.

25. How Diabetic Children Understand Their Illness
ARLENE R. BREWSTER, Detroit, Michigan

4:30-4:40 p.m.

26. Family Characteristics of Diabetic Children: Correlations with Hemoglobin Alc (HbAlc)
B. J. ANDERSON*, W. F. AUSLANDER, and J. P. MILLER, St. Louis, Missouri

4:45-4:55 p.m.

27. Characteristics of "Brittle" Adolescent Diabetics Referred to a University Diabetes Program
D. ORR, M. GOLDEN*, G. MYERS*, and D. MARRERO, Irvine, California

THE LILLY LECTURE

Sheraton Hall—5:15-5:45

Recipient and Lecture topic to be announced.

MONDAY MORNING, JUNE 16

Concurrent Sessions

8:30 a.m.-9:45 a.m.
SHERATON HALL
Session I: *Transplantation and Artificial Devices*
J. STUART SOELDNER, M.D.** and ERROL B. MARLISS, M.D.*, *Co-Chairmen*

8:30-8:40 a.m.

28. Subcutaneous (SC) Open Loop Insulin Delivery: Is a Pump Required?
J. D. NELSON, E. B. MARLISS*, and B. ZINMAN*, Toronto, Canada

8:45-8:55 a.m.

29. Effects of Continuous Subcutaneous Insulin Infusion (CSII) in Non-Insulin-Dependent Diabetes Mellitus (NIDDM) and Insulin-Dependent DM (IDDM)
M. CHAMPION, N. W. RODGER*, and J. DUPRE*, London, Canada

9:00-9:10 a.m.

30. Cellular Stimuli for the Rejection of Islet Allografts
JUNKO ONO, IAN M. ZITRON, PAUL E. LACY*, and JOSEPH M. DAVIE, St. Louis, Missouri

9:15-9:25 a.m.

31. Role of Histocompatibility in Pancreatic Transplantation
G. KYRIAKIDES, A. RABINOVITCH*, L. OLSON, J. MILLER, and D. H. MINTZ*, Miami, Florida

8:30 a.m.-9:45 a.m.
COTILLION ROOM
Session II: *Hormone Secretion I*
RONALD A. ARKY, M.D.* and CHARLES J. GOODNER, M.D.*, *Co-Chairmen*

8:30-8:40 a.m.

33. A Role for Prostaglandin (PG) E in Defective Glucose Potentiation of a Nonglucose Insulin Secretagogue in Diabetics
J. MCRAE, and R. P. ROBERTSON*, Seattle, Washington

8:45-8:55 a.m.

34. Acute Alterations in Prostaglandin Status Fail to Influence Insulin Secretion in Man
R. G. BRODOWS*, Rochester, New York

9:00-9:10 a.m.

35. Somatostatin-like Immunoreactivity (SLI) in Mammalian Plasma
K. A. BOLDT, E. C. LASCHANSKY, C. NIST, D. SIMONOWITZ, J. TABORSKY, and J. W. ENSINCK, Seattle, Washington

9:15-9:25 a.m.

36. Effect of Free Fatty Acids (FFA) on the Gastric and Pancreatic Secretion of Somatostatin-like Immunoreactivity (SLI) in Normal and Alloxan Diabetic Dogs
T. WASADA, A. PIETRI, P. RASKIN*, R. DOBBS*, and R. H. UNGER*, Dallas, Texas

8:30 a.m.-10:15 a.m.
MARYLAND SUITE
Session III: *Nutritional Management*
PATRICIA M. LEAPLEY, R.D.* and HARRY K. DELCHER, M.D.*, *Co-Chairmen*

8:30-8:40 a.m.

38. New Principles of Diet from a Home Glucose Monitoring Program
KATHARINE ALLING, JUDITH BALL, and JOHN R. WILLIAMS, JR.*, Rochester, New York

8:45-8:55 a.m.

39. Assessment of Caloric Intake of Youngsters with Juvenile Diabetes Mellitus (JDM) Compared to Standard Methods of Assessing Caloric Needs
E. KOHLER*, and M. BENZ, Milwaukee, Wisconsin

9:00-9:10 a.m.

40. Dietary Adherence and Metabolic Control with an Unmeasured Diet in Normal Weight Diabetic Patients
C. ABRAIRA*, M. PURICELLI, and A. GALLAGHER, Hines, Illinois

9:15-9:25 a.m.

41. Dietitian Coordinated Diabetes Clinic, Exchange System and Weekly Follow up Visits Decreased Body Weight and Glucose in Obese Individuals
PATRICIA M. LEAPLEY*, Tampa, Florida

Scientific Program

9:30-9:40 a.m.

32. Intrahepatic versus Intrasplenic Pancreatic Islet Transplantation: Effect on Glucose Homeostasis and Hepatic Enzyme Activities
H. SELAWRY*, R. MARGOLIS, and R. T. CURNOW*, Miami, Florida and Charlottesville, Virginia

9:30-9:40 a.m.

37. Immunochemical Studies of Pancreatic Somatostatin
HIDEKI OYAMA, KENNETH GABBAY*, MARIE GREIDER*, and ALAN PERMUTT*, St. Louis, Missouri

9:30-9:40 a.m.

42. Glucose, Insulin and Glucagon Responses to Soya-Fiber Enriched Diet in Obese, Diabetic and Normal Subjects
YORAM KANTER*, ELY ROTENSTERICH, LEA SOLOVEITZIC, BERTA RUBINOVICH, and DAVID BARZILAI, Haifa, Israel

9:45-10:15 a.m.

Introduction of Carelyn P. Fylling, Eden Prairie, Minnesota, the Recipient of the Ames Award

9:00 a.m.-11:15 a.m.
WASHINGTON ROOM
Session IV: *Poster Sessions*

COMPLICATIONS

43. Insulin Treatment of Diabetes Enhances Lysosomal Enzyme Activity and Low Density Lipoprotein (LDL) Degradation by Circulating Mononuclear Cells (MC)
KURT HENZE, and ALAN CHAIT*, Seattle, Washington

44. Salvage of the Inoperable-Ischemic Diabetic Leg with an End-Diastolic Pneumatic Compression Boot - The Circulator Boot-TM
RICHARD S. DILLON*, Philadelphia, Pennsylvania

45. Arterial Glycosaminoglycans in Diabetic Dogs
Dr. O. V. SIREK*, A. SIREK, and E. CUKERMAN, Toronto, Canada

46. Decreased Collagen Extractability in Diabetes: Reversal by B-Aminopropionitrile (BAPN) and D-Penicillamine (D-pen)
J. R. WILLIAMSON*, K. CHANG, J. UITTO, E. A. ROWOLD, G. A. GRANT, and C. KILO*, St. Louis, Missouri

HORMONE ACTION

47. The Relative Roles of Glucose Transport and Metabolism at Varying Glucose Concentrations in Rat Adipocytes
JAMES M. MAY*, Richmond, Virginia

48. Insulin Sensitive Sugar Transport in Rat Adipose Cells: A New Model Based on Substrate Acceleration of Trace 2-deoxyglucose Uptake
JAMES E. FOLEY, ROSEMARY FOLEY, and JORGEN GLIEMANN, Aarhus, Denmark (Introduced by MARIO DiGIROLAMO*, Atlanta, Georgia)

49. *In Vitro* Effects of Tolazamide on Insulin Action
BRUCE MALOFF, and DEAN LOCKWOOD*, Rochester, New York

50. Role of Microtubules in Insulin and Glucagon Stimulation of Amino Acid Uptake by Isolated Rat Hepatocytes
M. PRENTKI, and B. JEANRENAUD*, Geneva, Switzerland

51. Insulin Stimulated Phosphorylation of Ribosomal Protein S6 in Differentiated 3T3-L1 Cells
CHARLES J. SMITH, PETER WEJKSNORA, CHARLES RUBIN, and ORA M. ROSEN*, New York, New York

52. The Effects of Insulin on Cloudman S91 Melanoma Cells
R. A. KAHN, and J. M. PAWELEK, New Haven, Connecticut (Introduced by VIJAY SOMAN*, New Haven, Connecticut)

53. Insulins From Phylogenetically Diverse Species Conserve Growth Promoting Activity in Human Fibroblasts
G. L. KING, and C. R. KAHN*, Bethesda, Maryland

54. Effect of Somatomedin Inhibitors on Insulin-like Action
L. S. PHILLIPS*, and T. D. SCHOLZ, Chicago, Illinois

55. Insulin-like Activity of Bradykinin on Amino Acid Metabolism of the Human Forearm
R. SCHIFMANN, M. WICKLMAYR, I. BOTTGER*, and G. DIETZE, Munich, Federal Republic of Germany

56. Role of Calcium as a Mediator of Hepatic Hormonal Effects
J. R. WILLIAMSON*, E. MURPHY, K. COLL, J. B. HOEK*, and B. E. CORKEY*, Philadelphia, Pennsylvania

57. Role of Ca^{2+} in A-Adrenergic Inactivation of Glycogen Synthase in Rat Hepatocytes and its Inhibition by Insulin
WILLIAM G. STRICKLAND, PETER F. BLACKMORE, and JOHN H. EXTON*, Nashville, Tennessee

Scientific Program

58. Effects of Metabolic Control of Diabetes on Glucagon's Contribution to Epinephrine-induced Hyperglycemia
F. W. KEMMER, H. L. A. LICKLEY*, D. E. GRAY, G. PEREZ*, and M. VRANIC*, Toronto, Ontario, Canada

59. The Effects of Portal versus Peripheral Insulin Administration
W. S. PUTNAM, K. D. ANDERSEN, J. B. HANKS, R. S. JONES, and H. E. LEBOVITZ*, Durham, North Carolina

60. The Effect of Vagotomy on Blood Glucose Changes after Insulin Microinjections into the Hypothalamus
A. J. SZABO*, A. IGUCHI*, and P. D. BURLESON, New York, New York

61. Effect of Insulin (I) Therapy (Rx) on Insulin Resistance (IR) in Type II Diabetic Subjects (D). Evidence for Heterogeneity
H. GINSBERG*, and E. J. RAYFIELD*, New York, New York

62. Characterization of Insulin Resistance in Cultured Human Skin Fibroblasts
M. MARTIN, L. OLANSKY, and S. POHL*, Charlottesville, Virginia

63. Mechanisms of Insulin Resistance in Non-Insulin Dependent Diabetic Subjects (NIDDS)
O. G. KOLTERMAN*, S. GRAY, J. R. INSEL, P. BURNSTEIN*, J. GRIFFIN, and J. M. OLEFSKY*, Denver, Colorado

64. Dual Effect of Epinephrine on Glucose Clearance in Skeletal Muscle
J. L. CHIASSON*, H. SHIKAMA, and J. H. EXTON*, Nashville, Tennessee

65. Relative Importance of the Two Phases of Insulin Release in Glycemic Control
K. STEINER, P. WILLIAMS, S. MOUTON, and A. CHERRINGTON*, Nashville, Tennessee

TRANSPLANTATION AND ARTIFICIAL DEVICES

66. Liposome-Entrapped-Insulin (LEI) Lowers Blood Glucose in Experimental Diabetes
J. ARRIETA, K. ALECK, M. SINHA, C. BROWNSCHIEDLE, J. RIGNEW, L. SHAPIRO, and M. SPERLING*, Los Angeles, California and Cincinnati, Ohio

67. Normalization of Hyperglycemia in Diabetic Rats by Transplantation of Microencapsulated Islets of Langerhans
ANTHONY M. SUN*, FRANK LIM, and PAUL VASINGTON, Toronto, Canada; Richmond, Virginia; and Boston, Massachusetts

68. Effect of Whole Pancreas Transplantation on Glomerular Mesangial Enlargement in Alloxan Diabetic Nephropathy
L. FERNANDEZ-CRUZ, R. H. BELL, S. LEE, H. J. SAYERS*, and M. J. ORLOFF*, San Diego, California

69. Can Treatment of Diabetes with a Portable Insulin Pump Reverse Diabetic Complications?
W. TAMBORLANE*, R. SHERWIN*, M. BERGMAN*, J. EBERSOLE, J. PUKLIN, and P. FELIG*, New Haven, Connecticut

70. Ambulatory Diabetes Management with Pulsed Subcutaneous Insulin (PSI) Using a Portable Pump
JANET SILVERSTEIN, WILLIAM RILEY, and ARLAN ROSENBLOOM*, Gainesville, Florida

71. Five Day Programmed Intraperitoneal Insulin Infusion in Diabetic Man
D. S. SCHADE*, R. P. EATON*, N. M. FRIEDMAN*, and W. SPENCER, Albuquerque, New Mexico

72. Human Pseudo-Islet Formation, Culture and Preservation
D. W. SCHARP*, M. M. FELDMEIER, R. V. RAJOTTE, K. DESCHRYVER, and M. BELL, St. Louis, Missouri

73. Insulin Stimulates DNA Synthesis in B-Cells of Neonatal Rat Pancreas Monolayer Cultures
A. RABINOVITCH*, and D. H. MINTZ*, Miami, Florida

74. In Vivo and In Vitro Evaluation of Insulin Delivery by an Artificial Pancreas using Isolated Islets Perifused with Blood Ultrafiltrate
G. REACH, P. POUSSIER, A. SAUSSE, R. ASSAN, M. ITOH, and J. GERICH*, Rochester, Minnesota and Paris, France

75. Effect of Systemic Venous Drainage and Denervation of the Pancreas on Glucose Tolerance (GT) After Partial Pancreatectomy in Dogs
D. BAUMGARTNER, D. SUTHERLAND*, J. HEIL, J. HUSTAD, and J. NAJARIAN, Minnespolis, Minnesota

CLINICAL PHYSIOLOGY

76. Failure of GIP to Explain the Entero-insular Axis
S. R. BLOOM*, D. L. SARSON, and P. G. KOPELMAN, London, England

77. B-Adrenergic Blockade Inhibits the Hepatic Response to Epinephrine in Diabetic but not in Normal Humans
H. SHAMOON*, Bronx, New York

78. Quantitation of the Factors Controlling Glucose Disposal in Man
RICHARD N. BERGMAN*, LAWRENCE R. PHILLIPS*, and CLAUDIO COBELLI, Los Angeles, California; Chicago, Illinois and Padua, Italy

79. Dietary Prevention of Diabetes in C57BL/Ks (BL/Ks) *db/db* Mice
E. H. LEITER*, and A. B. EISENSTEIN*, Bar Harbor, Maine and Brooklyn, New York

80. Insulin Resistance in Obesity: Differential Effect on Glucose and Amino Acid Disposal
A. R. GLASS, R. BONGIOVANNI, and T. M. BOEHM*, Washington, D.C.

81. Greater Hepatic Insulin (I) Extraction (He_I) during Continuous I Infusion (CII) than Bolus I Injection (BII)
R. V. RAJOTTE*, F. C. RUMPLE, G. D. MOLNAR*, G. CHMURA, and D. M. FAWCETT, Edmonton, Canada

82. Hormone and Insulin Receptor Profiles of Patients Who Did and Did Not Develop Severe Carbohydrate Intolerance During Adaptation to Total Parenteral Nutrition (TPN)
B. M. LIPPE*, S. A. KAPLAN*, S. R. LEVIN*, W. J. BYRNE, C. T. STROBEL, and M. E. AMENT, Los Angeles, California

BANTING MEMORIAL LECTURE

Sheraton Hall — 11:30 a.m.

Ronald A. Arky, M.D.* *Chairman*
NORBERT FREINKEL, M.D.*
"Islet Metabolism and Secretory Performance"

MONDAY AFTERNOON, JUNE 16

Concurrent Sessions

2:00 p.m.-4:30 p.m.
SHERATON HALL
Session I: *Clinical Diabetes*
FREDDA GINSBURG-FELLNER, M.D.**, and DONALD I. BELL, M.D.*, *Co-Chairmen*

2:00-2:10 p.m.

83. C-Peptide Levels and Metabolic Profiles in Diabetes
S. LEICHTER*, Lexington, Kentucky

2:15-2:25 p.m.

84. Effects of Acute Changes in Blood Glucose on Hemoglobin Alc
D. GOLDSTEIN*, S. PETH, J. ENGLAND, R. HESS, and J. DA COSTA, Columbia, Missouri

2:30-2:40 p.m.

85. Evidence of Reversibility of Hemoglobin (Hb) Alc
F. VLACHOKOSTA*, R. KOENIG, G. F. CAHILL, JR.*, and J. S. SOELDNER*, Boston, Massachusetts

2:45-2:55 p.m.

86. LDL/HDL Cholesterol Correlates with Hemoglobin AI and Improves with Insulin Therapy
J. K. SCHMITT, J. R. POOLE, S. B. LEWIS*, and F. FISHER*, Oakland, California and San Francisco, California

2:00 p.m.-4:30 p.m.
COTILLION ROOM
Session II: *Hormone Secretion II*
JOSEPH D. BROWN, M.D.*, and GEROLD M. GRODSKY, Ph.D.*, *Co-Chairmen*

2:00-2:10 p.m.

93. Fasting and Refeeding Control Expression of the Rat Insulin Gene
STEVE GIDDINGS, JOHN CHIRGWIN, and ALAN PERMUTT*, St. Louis, Missouri

2:15-2:25 p.m.

94. The Kinetics of ^{65}Zn and ^{45}Ca Uptake in Granules Isolated from Rat Islets of Langerhans
B. FORMBY, D. FIGLEWICZ, F. SCHMID, A. HODGSON, and G. M. GRODSKY*, San Francisco, California

2:30-2:40 p.m.

95. Use of High Voltage Technique to Determine the Molecular Requirements for Exocytosis in Islet Cells
CAROLINE S. PACE*, Birmingham, Alabama

2:45-2:55 p.m.

96. Role for Calmodulin in Stimulus-secretion Coupling for Insulin Release; Lack of a Role in Exocytosis
YODPHAT KRAUSZ, and GEOFFREY W. G. SHARP*, Boston, Massachusetts

2:00 p.m.-5:00 p.m.
MARYLAND SUITE
Session III: *Methods of Control*
RITA M. NEMCHIK, R.N., M.S.**, and MARTIN J. CONWAY, M.D.**, *Co-Chairmen*

2:00-2:10 p.m.

103. A Rise in Ambient Temperature Accelerates Insulin Absorption from the Injection Site.
V. KOIVISTO, and S. FORTNEY, Helsinki, Finland and New Haven, Connecticut

2:15-2:25 p.m.

104. The Accuracy of Various Methods for Home Glucose Monitoring
N. A. KEANE*, R. S. CLEMENTS, JR.*, K. A. KIRK, and B. R. BOSHELL*, Birmingham, Alabama

2:30-2:40 p.m.

105. Home Monitoring of Blood Glucose by Chemstrip
J. G. SILVESTRI, L. R. ATLES, and L. MILLER*, Los Angeles, California

2:45-2:55 p.m.

106. Reducing Diabetic Ketoacidosis Hospitalizations
LISA PARKER, GAIL GUNTER-HUNT, and MARTHA SPENCER*, Ann Harbor, Michigan

Scientific Program

3:00-3:10 p.m.

87. Hyper-Alpha-Lipoproteinemia (HAL) in Diabetic Children
M. H. BLANC*, R. E. GLEASON*, O. P. GANDA*, and J. S. SOELDNER*, Boston, Massachusetts

3:15-3:25 p.m.

88. Impaired Myocardial Performance in Children with Type I (Insulin-dependent) Diabetes Mellitus
NANCY E. FRIEDMAN, LYNNE L. LEVITSKY*, DEBORAH V. EDIDIN*, DOLORES A. VITULLO, SAMUEL J. LACINA, PIPIT CHIEMMONGKOLTIP, Chicago, Illinois

3:30-3:40 p.m.

89. Insulin Administration Prevents Changes of Myosin Isoenzyme Distribution in the Heart of Diabetic Rats
WOLFGANG H. DILLMANN*, San Diego, California

3:45-3:55 p.m.

90. The Effect of Strict Metabolic Control on Residual B-cell Function. A Control Study
S. MADSBAD, C. BINDER*, T. KRARUP, O. K. FABER, and L. REGEUR, Copenhagen, Denmark

4:00-4:10 p.m.

91. Hypoglycemia may cause Intravascular Coagulation in Juvenile Diabetics
J. HILSTED, J. D. NIELSEN, L. SESTOFT, and J. GORMSEN, Copenhagen, Denmark

3:00-3:10 p.m.

97. Restoration by Ouabain of Glucose-Induced Insulin Release in the Absence of Extracellular Ca.
E. G. SIEGEL, C. B. WOLLHEIM, A. E. RENOLD*, and G. W. G. SHARP, Geneva, Switzerland

3:15-3:25 p.m.

98. Actin Levels in the Islet
J. KELLY, A. E. BOYD, III*, J. BRYAN, and B. R. BRINKLEY, Houston, Texas

3:30-3:40 p.m.

99. Direct Exchange of Nucleotides Between Pancreatic Endocrine Cells
PAOLO MEDA, MYLENE AMHERDT, ALAIN PERRELET, and LELIO ORCI*, Geneva, Switzerland

3:45-3:55 p.m.

100. Modulation of Insulin and Glucagon Secretion by Local Somatostatin Secretion in the Perfused Chicken Pancreas
R. N. HONEY, and G. C. WEIR*, Richmond, Virginia

4:00-4:10 p.m.

101. *In Vitro* Insulin Cycles from the Isolated Canine Pancreas - Possible Control by an Intrinsic Nonadrenergic Nervous System
J. STAGNER, and E. SAMOLS*, Louisville, Kentucky

3:00-3:10 p.m.

107. Control of Diabetes at a Summer Camp: Assessment by Hemoglobin AI and other Measures
D. L. HORWITZ*, E. G. MOORE, D. SHEFTEL, R. STRAUBE, T. UNTERMAN, and M. CHERTACK*, Chicago, Illinois

3:15-3:30
Intermission

3:30-3:40 p.m.

108. Beneficial Effects of Diabetes Teaching: Importance of Self Management by the Patients
VIKTOR JORGENS, PETER BERCHTOLD*, WULF EICKENBUSCH, and EDITH SCHOLZ-THIELEN, Hagen, West Germany

3:45-3:55 p.m.

109. Identifying Patient Responsibilities for Their Care
CHARLES W. GIVEN, BARBARA GIVEN, ROGER BULDAIN, and WILLIAM D. CRANO, East Lansing, Michigan

4:00-4:10 p.m.

110. Differences in Diabetes Care by Hospital-Based Versus Clinic-Based Rural Health Professionals
S. BOATRIGHT*, C. CHANDLER*, and A. RHODES, Lexington, Kentucky

Scientific Program

4:15-4:25 p.m.

92. Effectiveness of Aprotinin (TrasylolR) in Protease-Mediated Insulin (In.) Resistance
G. FREIDENBERG, N. WHITE, S. CATALAND, T. O'DORISIO, J. SOTOS*, and J. SANTIAGO*, Columbus, Ohio and St. Louis, Missouri

4:15-4:25 p.m.

102. The B-Cell Degrades Stored Insulin: A Third Mechanism Controlling Insulin Content
P. A. HALBAN*, and C. B. WOLLHEIM, Geneva, Switzerland

4:15-4:25 p.m.

111. An Out-patient Alternative Program for Regulation of the Insulin-requiring Diabetic Patient
I. J. WHITEHOUSE*, M. S. COX, and D. M. KAHKONEN*, Detroit, Michigan

4:30-4:40 p.m.

112. Perceived Needs of Diabetes Patient Educators
JAMES W. PICHERT, RODNEY A. LORENZ*, ANNE L. TURNER*, and ALAN L. GRABER*, Nashville, Tennessee

4:45-4:55 p.m.

113. Living as a Diabetic
J. GETTINGER*, E. WARREN-BOULTON, G. SPRINGER*, and W. AUSLANDER, St. Louis, Missouri

5:00-7:00 p.m.
Informal Meeting
Allied Health Professionals, Non-Physician
Room to be announced

3:00 p.m.-5:30 p.m.
WASHINGTON ROOM
Session IV: *Poster Sessions*

HORMONE SECRETION

114. Plasma Levels of Somatostatin-Like Immunoreactivity in Healthy Subjects and in Insulin-Dependent Diabetic Patients (IDDM)
G. VALTYSSON, A. I. VINIK*, and S. S. FAJANS*, Ann Arbor, Michigan

115. Decrease of Pancreatic Somatostatin in Neonatal 'Nesidioblastosis'
J. M. POLAK, P. GARIN CHESA, C. M. TIMSON, M. G. BRYANT, and S. R. BLOOM*, London, England

116. Failure of Glucose to Stimulate Insulin Release from Isolated Pure Beta Cells
M. S. BANDISODE*, Augusta, Georgia

117. Isolation, Translation, and Partial Characterization of Messenger RNA Species from Six Human Insulinomas
D. A. HESTER, and H. E. LEBOVITZ*, Durham, North Carolina

118. Transitory Islet Phosphate Depletion: Key Factor in First Phase Stimulated Insulin Release?
ROBERT C. JOHNSON, and NORBERT FREINKEL*, Chicago, Illinois

119. A New *In Vitro* Model to Study Secretion and Biochemistry of Pancreatic Polypeptide (PP)
R. L. GINGERICH*, D. W. SCHARP*, M. H. GREIDER*, E. S. DYE, and K. A. MOUSEL, St. Louis, Missouri

120. Net Changes in Pancreatic Islet Phospholipids During Stimulation by Glucose and cAMP *In Vitro*
R. V. FARESE*, A. M. SABIR, and R. E. LARSON, Tampa, Florida

121. Therapy of Malignant Insulinomas with Monoamine Precursors
J. M. FELDMAN*, C. VERVAERT, C. KLATT, and H. F. SEIGLER, Durham, North Carolina

122. The Effects of Retinoids on Rat Islet Insulin Secretion and Cell Aggregation
B. S. CHERTOW*, N. S. MOSS, B. A. OZUK, J. J. SEWELL, J. C. SHIH, and A. T. WAITE, Huntington, West Virginia

123. Insulin Secretory Defect of Type II Diabetes Reproduced in B cell Deficient Rat Model.
G. C. WEIR*, S. BONNER-WEIR*, E. T. CLORE, and C. J. Z. MACHINSKI, Richmond, Virginia

124. Evidence that the Inhibitory Effect of Vincristine (VCR) on Glucose-Induced Insulin Release is Mediated via Glucose Receptor Mechanisms
J. SHAH*, B. STEVENS, and C. HURKS, Chicago, Illinois

125. Separation of Islet Cell Subpopulations by Fluorescence-activated Cell Sorting
DAVID A. NIELSEN, AKE LERNMARK*, and DONALD F. STEINER*, Chicago, Illinois and Copenhagen, Denmark

126. Ventromedial Hypothalamic (VMH) Lesions Increase Pancreatic Sensitivity to Streptozotocin (STZ) without Obesity
DAVID B. WEST, YUTAKA SEINO, STEPHEN C. WOODS*, and DANIEL PORTE, JR.*, Seattle, Washington and Kyoto, Japan

127. Correlation of Urinary C-peptide with the Integrated Concentration (IC) and Intrinsic Secretion Rate of Insulin (SR-I)
MARY T. MEISTAS, ZVI ZADIK, SIMEON MARGOLIS*, and A. AVINOAM KOWARSKI, Baltimore, Maryland

128. Glucokinase and Glucose-Responsivity of Pancreas
SUVESH CHANDIOK, RHODA MAKOFF, and JOSIAH BROWN*, Los Angeles, California

Scientific Program

129. Mechanism for Chemically Induced Diabetes: Evidence for Oxidant Action and Free Radical Production
ALFRED E. SLONIM*, MELANIE J. SURBER, MARGARET R. CAMERON, and IAN M. BURR*, Nashville, Tennessee

130. Molecular Heterogeneity in Pancreatic Polypeptide
T. PAQUETTE*, and R. GINGERICH*, Seattle, Washington

131. Synchronous Sustained Oscillations of Plasma Epinephrine (E) and Norepinephrine (NE) in M. Mulatta
F. G. HOM*, D. J. KOERKER, C. J. GOODNER*, and J. B. HALTER*, Seattle, Washington

HEALTH CARE DELIVERY

132. Educational Materials for Teaching Children About Diabetes Mellitus at Various Ages
CONNIE KRIEF, CINDY MANLEY, ELAINE KOHLER*, and LINDA HURWITZ*, Milwaukee, Wisconsin

133. Self Management: The Focus on Week Long Diabetes Classes
D. HINNEN*, Wichita, Kansas

134. Microcomputer Utilization in a Diabetes Clinic-Low Cost Data Recording and Monitoring
T. TRUAX, D. LOMATCH, L. ROI, and P. SAVAGE*, Ann Arbor, Michigan

135. Use of the Computer in the Investigation of Diabetes Mellitus
J. R. POOLE, M. M. BLIZIOTES*, T. A. SCHULTZ*, and J. W. JUNG, Oakland, California

136. Effectiveness of a Visual Approach to Diet for Diabetes
JAN ENO*, Toronto, Canada

137. Evaluation of Three Systems for Measuring Blood Glucose
S. L. PIEPHO, H. G. KLOEPFER, and C. SUTHER, Indianapolis, Indiana

138. Utilization of a Self-Care Questionnaire in Patient Assessment
MARGARET A. HOWARD, and LINDA K. STRODTMAN*, Ann Arbor, Michigan

139. Using Guided Design for Teaching Health Professionals How to Plan Patient Education
LINDA K. STRODTMAN*, and CAROL P. BARNETT*, Ann Arbor, Michigan

140. Diabetes by Criteria Mapping with a Weighting of Seriousness of Decision Errors
P. C. DAVIDSON*, E. GREGERSON, and JACK GOODWIN, Morgantown, West Virginia

141. The Prince Edward Island (PEI) Diabetes Control Program - Patterns of Therapy and Cost
M. H. TAN*, and C. WORNELL, Halifax and Charlottetown, Canada

GENETICS AND IMMUNOLOGY

142. Differences in Insulin Antibodies Induced with Varying Antigenic Forms
I. VALDES, R. E. MICHALSKI, R. THOMPSON, and E. R. ARQUILLA*, Irvine, California

143. Two Insulin-like Components in a Family with Hyperproinsulinemia.
D. C. ROBBINS*, H. S. TAGER, M. E. MAKO, K. H. GABBAY*, and A. H. RUBENSTEIN*, Boston, Massachusetts and Chicago, Illinois

144. Mouse Antibody Cytotoxic to Cultured Mouse Beta Cells
M. CHERRY, and E. H. LEITER*, Bar Harbor, Maine

145. Complement-mediated Islet Cell Surface Antibody-induced Block in Insulin Release from Perifused Rat Islet Cells
TAKAHIRO KANATSUNA, AKE LERNMARK*, ARTHUR H. RUBENSTEIN*, and DONALD F. STEINER*, Chicago, Illinois

146. A Genetic Marker in Spontaneously Diabetic Chinese Hamsters
D. W. SAMMONS, L. D. ADAMS, S. L. TOLLAKSEN, and N. G. ANDERSON, Kalamazoo, Michigan and Argonne, Illinois (Introduced by W. E. Dulin*, Kalamazoo, Michigan)

TUESDAY MORNING, JUNE 17

Concurrent Sessions

8:30 a.m.-10:45 a.m.
SHERATON HALL
Session I: *Hormone Receptors*
ROBERT BAR, M.D.* and WILLIAM C. DUCKWORTH, M.D.**, *Co-Chairmen*

8:30-8:40 a.m.

147. Characterization of Specific Growth Hormone Receptors in Isolated Fat Cells
R. SALTMAN, J. GAVIN, III, and W. DAUGHADAY*, St. Louis, Missouri

8:45-8:55 a.m.

148. Tissue Differences in Insulin Receptors: Acute Changes in Insulin Binding with Linearization of Scatchard Plots
J. N. LIVINGSTON*, L. A. POTTICK, and R. T. MOXLEY, Rochester, New York

9:00-9:10 a.m.

149. Removal of an Affinity Regulator from the Insulin Receptor by Lectin Chromatography
J. A. HEDO, L. C. HARRISON*, and J. ROTH*, Bethesda, Maryland

8:30 a.m.-10:45 a.m.
COTILLION ROOM
Session II: *Clinical Physiology*
SAUL M. GENUTH, M.D.** and HARVEY RODMAN, M.D.*, *Co-Chairmen*

8:30-8:40 a.m.

156. Effects of Inhibition of Catecholamine (CA) Release by Clonidine upon Hormone and Substrate Responses to Insulin-Induced Hypoglycemia
S. A. METZ*, and J. B. HALTER*, Seattle, Washington

8:45-8:55 a.m.

157. Plasma Epinephrine Disturbances in Diabetic Subjects during Isometric Exercise
A. B. GUSTAFSON, and R. K. KALKHOFF*, Milwaukee, Wisconsin

9:00-9:10 a.m.

158. The Significance of Cortisol, Glucagon, and HGH for the Development of Ketosis in Insulin Dependent Patients with and without Residual B-Cell Function
C. BINDER*, S. MADSBAD, O. FABER, H. ORSKOV, L. REGEUR, and B. TRONIER, Copenhagen, Denmark

8:30 a.m.-9:30 a.m.
MARYLAND SUITE
Session III: *Adolescent Concerns*
SR. RITAMARY BROWN, R.D.** and J. STUART SOELDNER, M.D.**, *Co-Chairmen*

8:30-8:40 a.m.

165. Adolescent Clinic: A Specialized Treatment Approach
G. GUNTER-HUNT, and L. PARKER, Ann Arbor, Michigan (Introduced by M. SPENCER*)

8:45-8:55 a.m.

166. Diabetes Mellitus in Adolescents: The Relationship between Behavioral, Psychological Variables and Glucose Control
J. SIMONDS, D. GOLDSTEIN*, B. WALKER, and S. RAWLINGS, Columbia, Missouri

9:00-9:10 a.m.

167. Impact of a Recreation Program on Skills, Knowledge and Psychosocial Adjustment in Diabetic Children
DEBORAH V. EDIDIN*, ANNE M. RATH, LYNNE L. LEVITSKY*, CAROL POLLAK, CLARA COEN, JEANETTE WHITE, and EILEEN VENCKUS, Chicago, Illinois

Scientific Program

9:15-9:25 a.m.

150. Insulin-Mimickers Down Regulate the Insulin Receptor: Evidence for a Post Receptor Mechanism
J. F. CARO, and J. M. AMATRUDA*, Rochester, New York

9:30-9:40 a.m.

151. Influence of the Insulin Receptor Compartment on Insulin Clearance
J. PHILIPPE, P. HALBAN*, A. GJINOVCI, and W. DUCKWORTH*, Geneva, Switzerland

9:45-9:55 a.m.

152. Characterization and Significance of Hepatic Receptors for Insulin during Fetal and Neonatal Life
FRANK VINICOR*, and CHARLES CLARK, JR.*, Indianapolis, Indiana

10:00-10:10 a.m.

153. Decreased Spare Hepatic Receptors for Insulin: Possible Importance for Insulin Action
M. B. DAVIDSON*, and H. J. L. FRANK, Los Angeles, California

10:15-10:25 a.m.

154. Insulin Binding and Glucose Transport in Isolated Adipocytes from Obese Patients
T. P. CIARALDI, and J. M. OLEFSKY*, Denver, Colorado

9:15-9:25 a.m.

159. A New Mechanism for the VLDL-TG Removal Defect in Insulin-Deficient Rats
H. BAR-ON, Y-D. I. CHEN, and G. M. REAVEN*, Stanford, California

9:30-9:40 a.m.

160. Insulin-Independent Glucose Disposal During Physiologic Hyperglycemia
S. E. FINEBERG*, S. H. SCHNEIDER*, and D. C. HOWEY*, Indianapolis, Indiana

9:45-9:55 a.m.

161. Diurnal Rhythm of Insulin Sensitivity (IS) in Subjects with Impaired Glucose Tolerance (IGT)
B. SCHULZ, K. P. RATZMANN, G. ALBRECHT, and H. BIBERGEIL, Karlsburg, GDR (Introduced by E. REAVEN*)

10:00-10:10 a.m.

162. Rightward Shift of the Insulin Dose-response Curve for Glucose Disposal in Type II Human Diabetes: Evidence for Decreased Insulin Sensitivity and Impaired Insulin Receptor Function
R. RIZZA*, R. WESTLAND, and L. HALL, Rochester, Minnesota

10:15-10:25 a.m.

163. Long Term Effects of an a-Glucosidase Inhibitor on Catecholamine Levels and Insulin Requirements as Assessed by the Artificial Beta-cell
S. RAPTIS, G. DIMITRIADIS, K. KARAISKOS, J. ROSENTHAL, C. H. R. ZOUPAS, and S. MOULOPOULOS, Athens, Greece and Ulm, Germany (Introduced by C. F. GASTINEAU*, Rochester, Minnesota)

9:15-9:25 a.m.

168. A Therapeutic Paradigm for Discrepant Urine Records
WENDY CITRIN, GEORGE J. ELLIS, III*, and JAY S. SKYLER*, Miami, Florida and Durham, North Carolina

9:30 a.m.-10:30 a.m.
MARYLAND SUITE
Symposium
Legislation and Diabetes
PATRICIA M. LEAPLEY, R.D.*

10:30-10:45
Intermission

10:45 a.m.-12:15 p.m.
MARYLAND SUITE
Session III: *Epidemiology and Financial Implications*
SR. RITAMARY BROWN, R.D.** and J. STUART SOELDNER, M.D.**, *Co-Chairmen*

10:45-10:55 a.m.

169. The Changing Prevalence of Diabetes in the U.S.
M. HARRIS*, and T. DRURY, Bethesda, Maryland

11:00-11:10 a.m.

170. Summary of First Year Results of The First State Registry of Insulin Dependent Diabetes Mellitus
JOY WELLS, JEFFREY ROSEMAN*, and BURIS BOSHELL*, Birmingham, Alabama

10:30-10:40 a.m.

155. Insulin Binding to Erythrocytes and Monocytes from Pima Indians with Various Degrees of Hyperinsulinemia
TOM HUECKSTEADT, FRANK KOSMAKOS*, and DAVE MOTT*, Phoenix, Arizona

10:30-10:40 a.m.

164. Glucose Lowering Effects of Dietary Fiber: Altered Absorption Rather than Metabolism of Carbohydrate
J. WAHREN, O. BJORKMAN, A. JUHLIN-DANNFELT, and P. FELIG*, Stockholm, Sweden and New Haven, Connecticut

11:15-11:25 a.m.

171. The Social and Economic Cost of Diabetes in Kentucky: Final Report
P. H. COLLINS*, A. FISCHER, and C. HERNANDEZ, Lexington, Kentucky

11:30-11:40 a.m.

172. The Social and Economic Costs of Diabetes: An Estimate for 1979
GERALD PLATT, and STEPHEN G. SUDOVAR, Fairfax, Virginia (Introduced by LEONA V. MILLER, M.D.*, Los Angeles, California)

11:45-11:55 a.m.

173. Diabetes and Disability Among Persons Twenty Years and Over
THOMAS F. DRURY, and LOIS LIPSETT*, Hyattsville and Bethesda, Maryland

12:00-12:10 p.m.

174. Ketoacidosis or Coma Mortality in Diabetes
C. A. HERRON, and D. C. MAY, Atlanta, Georgia (Introduced by L. C. DEEB*, Atlanta, Georgia)

TUESDAY MORNING, JUNE 17

10:00 a.m.-12:30 p.m.
WASHINGTON ROOM
Session IV: *Poster Sessions*

CLINICAL DIABETES

176. B-cell Response to Exercise in Diabetic and Non-diabetic Children
L. G. HEDING*, and J. LUDVIGSSON, Denmark and Sweden

177. Increased Hemoglobin Alc (Alc) in Insulin Dependent Diabetics (IDD) During Puberty
D. T. SARGEANT*, J. ACHTENBERG, and J. E. DAVIS, St. Louis, Missouri

178. Longitudinal Growth Studies in Insulin-Dependent Diabetes
J. GUTAI*, E. TSALIKIAN*, and R. LAPORTE, Pittsburgh, Pennsylvania

179. Use of Beta-Cell Function and Insulin Sensitivity in the Classification of Diabetes
J. H. KARAM*, C. W. YOUNG*, A. BURNS, and P. H. FORSHAM*, San Francisco, California

180. The Serum Sugar Responses to Regular Insulin Given Separately and Mixed with NPH Insulin
C. J. BRUHN, E. INGLE, and H. C. KNOWLES*, Cincinnati, Ohio

181. Prediction of Insulin Responsiveness During Therapy with Highly Purified Pork Insulin
J. A. GALLOWAY*, S. E. FINEBERG*, and N. S. FINEBERG, Indianapolis, Indiana

182. Phosphate Therapy in Diabetic Ketoacidosis (DKA)
H. WILSON, S. KEUER, S. LEA, A. E. BOYD, III*, and G. EKNOYAN, Houston, Texas

183. Face-Sparing Partial Lipodystrophy: Clinical Studies of a Large Kindred
RALPH H. STARKEY*, and THOMAS J. CIOTOLA, Danville, Pennsylvania

HORMONE RECEPTORS

184. Evidence that C-peptide Inhibits and Divalent Cations Stimulate Degradation of Insulin by Insulin Protease
GEORGE A. BURGHEN*, RANDOLPH A. MCKENZIE, and TERESA M. HOWARTH, Memphis, Tennessee

185. Models for the Insulin Receptor from Radiation Inactivation Studies
J. T. HARMON, C. R. KAHN*, and M. L. JOHNSON, Bethesda, Maryland and Charlottesville, Virginia

186. Different Reduction States of the Insulin Receptors in Plasma Membranes
J. MASSAGUE, P. F. PILCH, and M. P. CZECH*, Providence, Rhode Island

187. Hormone Receptors on Cultured Cells and Clones Obtained from Islet-cell Tumor
S. J. BHATHENA*, H. OIE, A. GAZDAR, and L. RECANT*, Washington, D.C.

188. Appearance of Insulin Receptor Regulation in Liver Membranes from Zucker Fatty Rats
J. B. CLARK*, and C. M. CLARK, JR.*, Indianapolis, Indiana

189. Effects of Colchicine on Insulin Binding to Isolated Hepatocytes
J. WHITTAKER, V. HAMMOND, and K. G. M. M. ALBERTI*, Newcastle upon Tyne, United Kingdom

190. Insulin Binding to the Blood Brain Barrier: A Direct in vitro Demonstration
H. J. L. FRANK*, and W. M. PARDRIDGE*, Los Angeles, California

191. Acute Downregulation of Monocyte but not Erythrocyte Insulin Receptor Number by Exogenous Insulin in Normal Man
L. MANDARINO, and B. BRICK, Rochester, Minnesota (Introduced by M. HOGAN*)

192. Insulin Binding and Degradation by Livers from Fed and Fasted Rats
SHIGEAKI BABA*, KOICHI YOKONO, YOSHI-MICHI IMAMURA, KOSUI SHII, and HIDEYO SAKAI, Kobe, Japan

193. 'Superinsulins': A Single Amino Acid Substitution at A_8 Causes Increased Receptor Affinity and Biological Activity *in vitro*
M. A. PIRON, P. DE MEYTS*, J. PITTS, J. SIMON, and W. RITTEL, Brussels, Belgium; London, England; Nouzilly, France; and Basel, Switzerland

194. Receptor Linked Degradation of ^{125}I-insulin is Mediated by Internalization in Cultured Human Lymphocytes
E. VAN OBBERGHEN*, J. L. CARPENTIER, P. GORDEN*, and L. ORCI*, Bethesda, Maryland ; and Geneva, Switzerland

METABOLISM

195. Volume, Insulin Binding and Glucose Transport and Oxidation of Adipocytes from Normophagic Rats with Hypothalamic Obesity
J. GOLDMAN*, D. LOCKWOOD, and D. MALCHOFF, Buffalo and Rochester, New York

196. Effects of B-adrenoreceptor Blockade on Insulin- or 2-deoxy-D-glucose-induced Hunger, Thirst and Arginine Vasopressin Secretion in Man
D. A. THOMPSON, U. LILIVIVATHANA*, R. G. CAMPBELL*, S. WELLE, and G. L. ROBERTSON, Rochester, New York

197. Polyol Pathway Activity Increased in Diabetic Cells
J. I. MALONE*, and G. KNOX, Tampa, Florida

198. Insulin Degradation by Hepatocytes in Primary Culture
W. C. DUCKWORTH*, K. R. RUNYAN, R. K. WRIGHT, M. A. HEINEMANN, S. S. SOLOMON*, and P. A. HALBAN, Memphis, Tennessee

199. Defect in Membrane $Na^{+} + K^{+H}$-ATPase in Obese Mouse and Man
M. DELUISE, P. USHER, and J. S. FLIER*, Boston, Massachusetts

200. Physical Training of Zucker Rats Increases Glucose Metabolism in Adipose Cells without Altering Insulin Sensitivity
L. J. WARDZALA, E. D. HORTON, and E. S. HORTON*, Geneva, Switzerland

201. Effects of Acute Insulin Deficiency on Leucine Kinetics in Conscious Dogs
N. N. ABOU-MOURAD*, L. S. JEFFERSON*, S. R. RANNELS, P. E. WILLIAMS, and W. W. LACY*, Nashville, Tennessee and Hershey, Pennsylvania

202. The Effect of Ketone Bodies on Alanine Metabolism in Cultured Rat Skeletal Muscle
ROBERT J. SMITH, and THOMAS T. AOKI*, Boston, Massachusetts

203. Effects of Clofibrate on Alanine Production, Branched Chain Amino Acid Oxidation, and Krebs Cycle Pool Sizes in Isolated Adult Rat Skeletal Muscle Cells
W. M. PARDRIDGE*, L. DUDUCGIAN-VARTAVARIAN, D. CASANELLO-ERTL, M. R. JONES, and J. D. KOPPLE, Los Angeles, California

TUESDAY AFTERNOON, JUNE 17

Concurrent Sessions

1:00 p.m-3:30 p.m.
SHERATON HALL
Session I: *Genetics and Immunology*
ALDO A. ROSSINI, M.D.*, and EDWARD R. ARQUILLA, M.D., Ph.D.**, *Co-Chairmen*

1:00-1:10 p.m.

204. Streptozotocin (SZ)-Induced Insulitis Model in Athymic Mice
ARTHUR A. LIKE*, MICHAEL C. APPEL*, JOHN P. MORDES, and R. MICHAEL WILLIAMS*, Worcester, Massachusetts and Chicago, Illinois

1:15-1:25 p.m.

205. Induction of Diabetes by Streptozotocin is Mediated by T-Cell Functions
SANG-GI PAIK, NORMAN FLEISCHER*, and SEUNG-IL SHIN, New York, New York

1:30-1:40 p.m.

206. Impairment of Cell Mediated Immunity in Chronic Alloxan Diabetic Mice
E. R. ARQUILLA*, R. E. MICHALSKI, and M. D. ROTH, Irvine, California

1:45-1:55 p.m.

207. Immunosuppression in Viral Murine Diabetes
D. DAFOE, A. NAJI, and C. F. BARKER*, Philadelphia, Pennsylvania

1:00 p.m.-3:30 p.m.
COTILLION ROOM
Session II: *Metabolism*
CAROLINE S. PACE, Ph.D.* and HAROLD E. LEBOVITZ, M.D.**, *Co-Chairmen*

1:00-1:10 p.m.

214. Effect of B-hydroxybutyrate on Alanine and Leucine Flux and Leucine N Transfer to Alanine in Man
J. MILES*, and M. HAYMOND*, Rochester, Minnesota

1:15-1:25 p.m.

215. Roles of the Periphery & Liver in the Hypoglycemic Action of Dichloroacetate *In Vivo*
M. P. DIAMOND, W. LACY*, and A. CHERRINGTON*, Nashville, Tennessee

1:30-1:40 p.m.

216. Arachidonic Acid Derivatives (PGE_2 and PGI_2) Produced by Adipocytes Modulate Sympathetic Nervous System Activity.
L. AXELROD*, and L. LEVINE, Boston and Waltham, Massachusetts

1:45-1:55 p.m.

217. Glomerular Prostaglandin Metabolism in Diabetic Rats
D. M. BROWN*, J. M. GERRARD, J. PELLER, G. H. R. RAO, and J. G. WHITE, Minneapolis, Minnesota

1:30 p.m.-3:30 p.m.
MARYLAND SUITE
Session III: *Complications of Diabetes*
FLORENCE R. RUHLAND, R.N.* and HAROLD RIFKIN, M.D.*, *Co-Chairmen*

1:30-1:40 p.m.

224. Regional Localization of Cerebral Edema Associated with Treatment of Diabetic Ketoacidosis
P. A. TORNHEIM, Cincinnati, Ohio (Introduced by KENNETH KREINES*, Cincinnati, Ohio)

1:45-1:55 p.m.

225. Effects of Diabetic Serum and Platelets on Growth of Cultured Vascular Smooth Muscle Cells and Fibroblasts
F. UMEDA, J. P. HALLE, J. ABARCA, S. L. LEUNG, D. J. FRANKS, and P. HAMET*, Montreal, Quebec, Canada

2:00-2:10 p.m.

208. Suppressor Cell Dysfunction in Insulin-Dependent Diabetes
RICHARD S. FAIRCHILD, JOSEPH L. KYNER*, and NABIH I. ABDOU, Kansas City, Kansas

2:15-2:25 p.m.

209. A Prospective Study of Suppressor Cell Activity in Patients with Newly Diagnosed Insulin Dependent Diabetes Mellitus
KARSTEN BUSCHARD, and JORGEN RYGAARD, Copenhagen, Denmark

2:30-2:40 p.m.

210. Rheumatoid Arthritis (RA) in Children with Diabetes
M. RUDOLF, J. DWYER, and M. GENEL*, New Haven, Connecticut

2:45-2:55 p.m.

211. Inherited Autoimmunity versus Coxsackie B4 in Insulin Dependent Diabetes
W. RILEY, N. MACLAREN*, K. RAND, and R. BEJAR, Gainesville, Florida

3:00-3:10 p.m.

212. Islet Cell Antibodies in Gestational Diabetes Mellitus: Prognostic Value
F. GINSBERG-FELLNER*, M. DOBERSEN, E. M. MARK, C. NECHEMIAS*, R. U. HAUSKNECHT, P. RUBINSTEIN and A. L. NOTKINS, New York, New York and Bethesda, Maryland

2:00-2:10 p.m.

218. Pancreatic Immunoreactive Neurotensin (IR-NT) in Obese (ob) and Diabetes (db) Mutant Mice: A Longitudinal Study
M. BERELOWITZ*, C. NAKAWATASE, and L. A. FROHMAN*, Chicago, Illinois

2:15-2:25 p.m.

219. Feeding Alters Hepatic Extraction (HE) of Insulin (I) and Glucagon (Gg)
J. JASPAN*, K. POLONSKY, J. DHORAJIWALA, W. PUGH, and A. MOOSSA, Chicago, Illinois

2:30-2:40 p.m.

220. Possible Role of Defectual Thermogenesis and its Regulation by Insulin in Genetic Obesity
F. ASSIMACOPOULOS-JEANNET, J. SEYDOUX, L. GIRARDIER, and B. JEANRENAUD*, Geneva, Switzerland

2:45-2:55 p.m.

221. Insulin-like and Insulin Antagonistic Effects of Growth Hormone on Glucose Production and Clearance in Man
L. MACGORMAN, and R. RIZZA*, Rochester, Minnesota

3:00-3:10 p.m.

222. Dopaminergic Control of Ketogenesis in Fasting and Diabetic Rats
D. G. JOHNSTON, G. BLESA MALPICA, J. M. BURRIN, H. ORSKOV, and K. G. M. M. ALBERTI*, Newcastle upon Tyne, United Kingdom

2:00-2:10 p.m.

226. Decline in the Cardiovascular Death Rate among Diabetics
M. HARRIS*, Bethesda, Maryland

2:15-2:25 p.m.

227. Incidence of Retinopathy and Cardiovascular Events as a Function of Plasma Glucose
J. R. LISSE, W. C. KNOWLER*, D. J. PETTITT, and P. H. BENNETT*, Phoenix, Arizona

2:30-2:40 p.m.

228. Proliferative Retinopathy with Minimal Visual Symptoms in Insulin-Dependent Diabetes
MARJORIE A. MOSIER*, Irvine, California

2:45-2:55 p.m.

229. Identical Twins and Diabetic Retinopathy
R. D. G. LESLIE, and D. A. PYKE, London, England (Introduced by R. B. GOLDBERG*, Chicago, Illinois)

3:00-3:10 p.m.

230. Improvement in Peripheral Nerve Function in Diabetes After Short-term Treatment with an Artificial Pancreas
M. GOLDEN*, K. NUDLEMAN, G. MYERS*, and A. CHARLES, Irvine, California

Scientific Program

3:15-3:25 p.m.

213. Beta Cell Dysfunction in HLA Identical Siblings of Insulin Dependent Diabetics (IDD)
P. HOLLANDER*, C. ASPLIN, J. HANSEN, and J. P. PALMER*, Seattle, Washington

3:15-3:25 p.m.

223. Effects of Insulin and Glucagon Antisera on the Incorporation of Isotopic Leucine into Myelin Proteins
NORTON SPRITZ*, and BARBARA MARINAN, New York, New York

3:15-3:25 p.m.

231. Prevalence and Associated Findings of Diabetic Foot Ulcer
T. W. KUEBLER, P. BENDICK, J. A. NORTON, JR., O. MARKAND, and F. VINICOR*, Indianapolis, Indiana

Exhibits

Nordisk Insulin — Booth 1

NORDISK INSULIN USA is the American affiliate of the famed NORDISK INSULIN LABORATORIUM, Denmark. We are an independent foundation dedicated to diabetes research, insulin production and treatment of insulin dependent diabetics. NORDISK insulins are of the highest purity and pork species only. These purified pork insulins are now available in the United States.

Shasta Beverages — Booth 2

Auto-Syringe, Inc. — Booth 3

The manufacturer will be displaying its unique line of portable, programmable infusion pumps. In particular, their Model AS*2C will be featured because of its use as an open loop insulin delivery system. The AS*2C can be programmed to deliver any individualized insulin infusion regimen by permitting independent variation of a constant basal rate and pre-prandial boluses.

Hoechst-Roussel Pharmaceuticals — Booths 4-7

Isolab, Inc. — Booth 8

Isolab's innovative products will be displayed and demonstrated. Of especial interest are our Quik-Sep® simplified chromatographic column methodology.

Fast Hemoglobin Test System (for glycohemoglobin levels).

Beckman Instruments — Booth 9

Ames Division, Miles Laboratories, Inc. — Booths 10-12

Sugar Babe Inc. — Booth 13

Libin and Associates — Booth 14

Encyclopaedia Britannica — Booth 15

Batter-Lite Foods Inc. — Booth 16

SweetLite fructose is available in granular form (packets, 8 oz. bulk, 16 oz. bulk, 2 lb canister, 5 lb bulk) powdered (1½ lb. size), liquid (23 oz. or 1 gallon bottle); honey flavored liquid packets.

We carry a line of fructose sweetened cake, cookies, & icing mixes; in addition, we have fructose sweetened drink mixes (lemonade, iced tea, & hot spiced tea), peanut butter, low-cal jams & jellies, and mayonnaise.

Robert J. Brady Company — Booth 17

Pfizer Laboratories — Booth 18

Calorie Control Council — Booth 19

Paddock Laboratories, Inc. — Booth 20

Paddock Laboratories has developed GLUTOSE, a concentrated sugar for treatment of insulin reactions.

GLUTOSE, with its quick open dispenser top, offers the diabetic a quick source of carbohydrate wherever he goes or whatever he does.

GLUTOSE can easily be carried in pocket or purse for immediate use at home, at work, while exercising, vacationing or traveling.

See us at booth #20.

Medical Research Bureau — Booth 21

Lehman Dietetic Confections, Inc. — Booth 22

We manufacture a vast range of chocolates, candies, candy specialties and candy novelties, all sweetened with sorbitol and mannitol. These are available direct from manufacturer, most items not available elsewhere. FREE SAMPLES

Ali Med Inc. — Booth 23

Raven Press — Booth 24

You are invited to stop by Booth #24 where Raven Press will feature an important new title in the field, SECONDARY DIABETES, as well as many other relevant publications in the area of endocrinology.

Coca-Cola, USA — Booth 25

Harvard Apparatus — Booth 26

The exhibit will include the Mill Hill Infuser, a small portable insulin infusion system and other Harvard Apparatus syringe infusion pumps.

Eli Lilly and Company — Booths 27 & 28

National Institute of Arthritis, Metabolism, and Digestive Diseases — Booth 29

Diabetes and the American Pima Indians
Peter H. Bennett, M.D., NIH, Phoenix, AZ
The Pima Indians of Arizona have the world's highest recorded prevalence of diabetes mellitus. Since 1965, NIH has been conducting prospective field studies concerning the distribution of diabetes and its complications in this population. Intensive studies on the various facets of the disease have revealed several interesting results.

AV Scientific Aids — Booth 30

Becton Dickinson Consumer Products — Booths 31-33

The exhibit will feature B-D PLASTIPAK® 1cc. and LO-DOSE® 1/2cc. Insulin Syringes with the MICRO-FINE™ Needle, and B-D Alcohol Swabs as well as current information on the Getting Started™ Program. Brochures will also be available on Proper Injection Technique, Proper Dosage Accuracy and Proper Site Selection and Rotation.

Novo Laboratories, Inc. — Booths 34 & 35

Novo Laboratories, Inc., will be featuring a full line of purified insulins: ACTRAPID® (Purified Pork Insulin Injection); SEMITARD® (Prompt Purified Pork Insulin Zinc Suspension); MONOTARD™ (Purified Pork Insulin Zinc Suspension); LENTARD® (Purified Pork and Beef Insulin Zinc Suspension); ULTRATARD® (Extended Purified Beef Insulin Zinc Suspension).

The Estee Corporation — Booth 36

Special dietary and sugar free foods, including cookies, wafers, mints, gums & bubble gums, puddings and gelatins. Fructose granulated in packets and in bulk, and fructose liquid.

Vision Multimedia Communications — Booth 37

Lido Spa Booth 38

Immunonuclear Corporation Booth 39

Prescription Footwear Association Booth 40

The Upjohn Company Booth 41

Professional representatives of The Upjohn Company are eager to contribute to the success of your meeting. They are here to discuss products of Upjohn research designed to assist you in the practice of your profession. They welcome your inquiries and comments.

Monoject Division Booths 42 & 43

Answering the insulin administration and education needs of patients living with diabetes. Featured items: scale magnifier, travel case, ½cc mini-syringe, insulin injection site selection chart, and up-to-date educational material on diabetes and pregnancy, and insulin administration. Learn how Monoject can help educational programs in your area.

Derata Corporation Booth 44

Fwenz Unlimited Booth 45

FWENZ UNLIMITED presents five charming puppets with voices on casette tape, who offer three programs: "What is Diabetes?", "I Have It And I Hate It!", and "What A Reaction!" PUPPETS TO THE POINT KITS are being used successfully in hospitals, schools, civic groups, ADA Chapters for diabetics, non-diabetics, all ages.

Bio Dynamics/bmc Booths 47 & 48

This exhibit will feature diagnostic systems, including the latest developments in blood and urine glucose testing methods. Featured will be the new Chemstrip bG, a remarkably accurate, 2-minute test for the semiquantitative evaluation of blood glucose levels, and the Stat-Tek System for rapid, quantitative blood glucose determinations.

Bio-Rad Laboratories Booth 49

Bio-Rad's Hemoglobin A_1 Column Test provides a precise and convenient method for measuring glycosylated hemoglobin. Hemoglobin A_1 measurement is not affected by brief or infrequent fluctuations in glucose levels or by external factors at the time of testing, and therefore offers an objective and reliable index of long-term diabetic control.

Alba Foods Booth 50

ALBA FOODS, a division of Weldon Farm Products, Inc., will exhibit ALBA's broad line of nutritious, light-in-calorie sugar free products including ALBA '66 Hot Cocoa Mix, ALBA '77 FIT 'N FROSTY, ALBA SIPPIN' YOGURT Drink Mix, and ALBA Instant Milk products. For more information, contact Alba Foods, 24 West 57th Street, New York, N.Y. 10019

1

Progressive Retinopathy with Improved Metabolic Control in Diabetic Dwarfism (Mauriac's Syndrome)

A.L.DRASH*, D.DANEMAN*, & L. TRAVIS*, Pittsburgh, PA & Galveston, Texas.

We report 4 children (3 boys & 1 girl) aged 11-18½yrs who presented 7-14yrs after the diagnosis of insulin-dependent diabetes. When first seen, all had severe short stature (ht & wt > 3-4 SD below mean for age), 2 had hepatomegaly with abnormal liver enzymes & the older 3 had markedly delayed puberty. They had all been severely underinsulinized & improved control required twice daily insulin injections with large dosage increases. Initial fundoscopy revealed only minimal background changes in the retinal vessels of 3 children. Growth rate improved significantly & hepatomegaly disappeared. Puberty progressed from Tanner stage I to V in less than 1 yr in 2 of the 3 older patients with poor final height. Paradoxically, with improved control retinopathy as assessed by fundoscopy plus fluoroscein angiography &/or fundus photos progressed rapidly in the next 1-9mos with appearance of multiple microaneurysms hemorrhages, exudates & macular edema in all 4 & severe proliferative changes in the older 3. 2 patients required Laser therapy & have had no progression in 2yrs. 1 also developed vitreous changes with blindness in 1 eye. The youngest has stabilized, showing no progression over 1yr.

The reason for these changes remains uncertain but may be related to disturbances in oxygen transport due either to abnormal red cell 2,3 DPG or oxygen-binding capacity associated with high HbA1c levels. These findings suggest that caution is needed when correcting metabolic derangements in patients whose diabetes has been very poorly controlled for a prolonged period.

2

The "Diabetes" of Cystic Fibrosis (CF).

H.M. RODMAN,* S. WALTMAN, T. KRUPIN, L.W. MATTHEWS Cleveland, OH and St. Louis, MO.

With increasing survival 10-15% of CF patients will develop fasting hyperglycemia and glycosuria requiring insulin. Will they also develop the chronic complications of diabetes mellitus? To evaluate this question, fluorescein angiography of the retina, fundus photographs, vitreous fluorophotometry, and electron microscopic measurements of muscle capillary basement membrane thickness (MCBMT) were performed in 25 CF patients (15-36 yrs.). Fajans-Conn criteria were used to classify the patients into: Group 1, normal fasting glucose (FG), normal OGTT; Group 2, normal FG, abnormal OGTT; Group 3, fasting hyperglycemia and glycosuria treated with insulin. Seven percent of Group 3 patients had overt diabetic retinopathy. Ten of 13 Group 3 patients demonstrated breakdown of the blood retinal barrier. Mean vitreous fluorescein concentrations in Group 3, 11.79±3.34 (S.D.) were significantly greater than in Groups 1 and 2, 7.26±1.73 ng/ml ($p<0.0005$). Twenty-one of 25 patients (80%) had increased MCBMT irrespective of carbohydrate tolerance. Mean MCBMT of Group 1 patients was 1065±233A°(S.D.), Group 2, 1280±417A°, and Group 3, 1474±660A°. Mean MCBMT of Group 3 patients was significantly greater than that of Group 1, $p< 0.02$. Conclusions: 1) 7% of CF patients treated with insulin manifested overt diabetic retinopathy; 2) 77% of Group 3 patients had evidence of breakdown of the blood-retinal barrier; 3) 80% of CF subjects had increased MCBMT; 4) Insulin treated hyperglycemia exacerbates the increased MCBMT of CF subjects.

3

Diabetic Retinopathy: Effects of Pregnancy (P) and Laser Therapy (LT).

L.J. SINGERMAN, L.M. AIELLO, H.M. RODMAN,* Cleveland, Ohio and Boston, Mass.

Forty-one diabetic women with no retinopathy or background disease (BR) and 21 with proliferating retinopathy (PDR) were examined with fundus photography prior to P, in each trimester, and 6-12 months postpartum (PP). Eight-five percent of women with no retinopathy or BR progressed to a more advanced stage of BR during P. Seventy percent of these women's BR regressed PP. Five women whose PDR was in remission prior to P had stable retinal vessels and vision during P and PP. Of 10 women treated with LT prior to pregnancy, 7 required no additional treatment during P and PP and maintained good vision. Six other women developed neovascularization of the disc (NVD) during the first trimester. Four of the 6 responded to LT and their PDR remained quiescent during P and PP. Two women developed vitreous hemorrhages in the third trimester. Diabetic women (25) with high risk PDR who had been pregnant in the past were compared to a group with similar lesions but never pregnant in their response to LT. LT was equally effective in reversing retinal lesions and in preserving good vision for both groups of women. Conclusions: 1) BR progresses during P and regresses PP; 2) Women whose PDR is quiescent or who have received LT prior to P can successfully negotiate gestation and the puerperium maintaining good vision; 3) A consideration of pregnancy termination for PDR should be restricted to patients with severe NVD showing progression despite first trimester LT; 4) Prior pregnancy does not impair the effectiveness of LT in preserving good vision.

4

Relationship of Vascular Disease to Fasting Plasma Glucose (FPG) and Other Variables in 3583 With Diabetes (DM): A Multinational Study,

K.M. WEST* HARRY KEEN, R.J. JARRETT, J.H. FULLER, ARTHUR TEUSCHER*, A.S. KROLEWSKI, VOLKER SCHLIACK, M.M.S. AHUJA, EISHI MIKI, OSCAR MATEO DE ACOSTA*, VILI GRABAUSKAS AND BERNARD GRAB, Oklahoma City, London, Bern, Warsaw, Berlin GDR, New Delhi, Tokyo, Havana, Phoenix, and Geneva.

As a subproject of a World Health Organization study, FPG was determined in representative samples of 9 populations (5 races) of diabetics 34-56 years of age. In pooled data, mean FPG was 231 mg/dl in 1204 insulin-takers, 177 in 1697 on oral agents, and 147 in 682 on diet only. FPG was inversely related to age of onset of DM and positively to its duration, to serum cholesterol and triglyceride. A highly significant association was found between FPG and retinopathy. The association of FPG with proteinuria was not so strong but statistically significant. These associations persisted in multivariate analyses that took into account many other variables. After correction for duration, insulin-treated patients had more retinal microaneurysms, hemorrhages, exudates, and neovascularization than those not treated with insulin. Coronary disease was only weakly related to FPG (not statistically significant) but was significantly related to serum cholesterol and even more strongly related to triglyceride. Leg vascular disease was significantly related to FPG and duration of DM. In Oklahoma Indians major Q waves were 3 times as frequent as in Pimas and 5 times more common than in Tokyo. In Warsaw amputation was 3 times as prevalent as in New Delhi and 14 times more frequent than in Tokyo.

5

Reversible Autonomic Nervous System Abnormalities in Juvenile Diabetes, a Pupillographic Study. A.B.HREIDARSSON, Aarhus, Denmark (Introduced by M.W.STEFFES*, Minneapolis, Minn.).

Autonomic nervous function was studied by infrared TV-pupillography in 9 juvenile diabetics, aged 20 to 36 years, with a disease duration from 0 to 3 years, during good (mean blood glucose 140 mg/dl) and poor (mean blood glucose 358 mg/dl) metabolic control. The pupil response to a short pulse of light (25 microlumen) and the pupil size and unrest during continuous illumination (512 microlumen) were measured. During metabolic derangement the 75% redilatation time of the light response was prolonged by 0.64 ± 0.19 sec. (mean change ± SE), 2p=0.012, from 2.26 sec. during good control. Other parameters of the light response i.e. latency time, maximal constriction velocity and response amplitude were unchanged, as was the pupil size in darkness. The relative reduction in pupil size (the degree of miosis) during continuous illumination was decreased by 0.15 ± 0.09, 2p=0.0011, from 0.32 during good control, and the light induced pupillary unrest was decreased by 0.58 ± 0.14 mm^2, 2p=0.0037, from 1.68 mm^2 during good control.Following establishment of good metabolic control the changes returned to normal. It is suggested that the pupillary abnormalities during metabolic derangement are the result of changes within the central autonomic nervous system. The study has thus, for the first time, demonstrated reversible changes in autonomic nervous function, which are related to the diabetic metabolic state and thereby analogous to the previously well established reversible functional changes in the somatic nervous system in early diabetes.

6

Morphometric Analysis of Autonomic Nerve Fibers in Nondiabetic and Ketonuric Diabetic Chinese Hamsters. A. DIANI*, D. DAVIS, J. FIX, J. SWARTZMAN and G. GERRITSEN*, Greenville, N.C. and Kalamazoo, Michigan

Myelinated nerve fibers from the sympathetic trunk (ST) of 8 ketonuric diabetic (KD) Chinese hamsters and 8 age-matched nondiabetics (ND) were quantitatively analyzed to determine frequency distribution. Animals were perfused with Karnovsky's medium and each ST was embedded in plastic. Serial cross-sections were cut at 1μm and randomly selected to eliminate observer bias. Fascicles of ST were photographed and combined into photomontages (875X). A plastic grid with 12 uniform radians was placed over the geometric center of each fascicle. External diameter of all myelinated axons within 2 radians (selected by random number tables) was measured. Composite histograms (diameter vs. frequency) showed population peaks at 4 and 12μm in ND; KD fibers displayed a significant reduction in frequency ($p < .05$) at the same diameters. In contrast to ND, KD fibers showed population densities at 5.5 and 10μm. These findings seemed to suggest that loss of myelin and axon degeneration may be responsible for reduced frequency and diameter of large KD fibers. The distinct KD population at 5.5μm may be the combined result of severe demyelination of large fibers, swelling of small axons and the development of growth cones. In conclusion, these data demonstrate an alteration of white fiber populations suggesting a structural manifestation of autonomic neuropathy in the diabetic Chinese hamster.

Supported by Upjohn & NIH grant AM-21933-02.

7

Further Evidence that Streptozotocin-induced Diabetes Accelerates The Catabolism of Recently Synthesized Collagen in Rat Skin. M. SCHNEIR, E. EDLIN-FOLZ, A. HOYRUP, N. RAMAMURTHY and L. GOLUB, Los Angeles, CA and Stony Brook, N.Y.

We have previously reported (Diabetes 28, 414, 1979) that skins of diabetic rats contain proportionately 3-fold greater amounts of diffusible (^{3}H)hydroxyproline-containing material, 4 hours after (^{3}H)proline injection, compared to that for age-matched control rats. Thus, of the total (^{3}H)hydroxyproline in skin, 27% was diffusible after short-term polytron homogenization in 0.5 N acetic acid compared to 9% for skins from control Non-diabetic rats.

In an effort to test if the above results were caused artifactually during the homogenization process from the degradation of radiolabeled collagen by enzymes present in the diabetic tissues, we co-homogenized skins from control rats that had been injected with (^{3}H)proline with skins from diabetic rats that had not been injected. Rats were 418 g when rendered diabetic by streptozotocin-injection (80 mg/kg body weight). After 20 days, non-diabetic control rats were injected with 1000 μC of (^{3}H) proline and killed 4 hours later. Control and diabetic rats were frozen until skins could be excised and homogenized.

The results show that co-homogenization did not generate more diffusible (^{3}H)hydroxyproline-containing material than obtained by solitary homogenization of skins from non-diabetic rats. This suggests that diffusible (^{3}H)hydroxyproline was present in situ and further supports the proposal that they result from an accelerated catabolism (possibly intracellar) of recently synthesized collagen.

8

Wound healing in spontaneously diabetic Chinese hamster: morphologic and morphometric study. E.J. WERINGER*, Irvine, CA.

Wound healing was examined in normal (N=17) and non-ketotic (N=13) diabetic Chinese hamsters by morphologic (light and electron microscopy) and morphometric (point analysis method of Weibel) methods. Perforating wounds were made in ears of age-matched hamsters and response to injury evaluated in biopsies taken 0, 8 and 16 hrs after injury. Healing in normal hamsters was characterized by vascular proliferation and cellular infiltration. The area within 0.1mm of wound edge (zone I) was heavily infiltrated with polymorphonuclear leukocytes (PMN). The area within 0.2 mm of wound edge, the region between wounded and non-wounded tissue (zone II) contained fibroblasts and capillaries. 8 hrs after injury, wounds of diabetic hamsters revealed less cellular infiltration (fibroblasts, 49.4% of normal (%N); PMN, 47.8%N) and vascular proliferation (46.8%N). At 16 hrs, the %volume occupied by capillaries (86.5%N) and PMN (103.4%N) was not significantly different from normal: fibroblasts, however, (46.5%N) remained depressed. Increased interstitial edema (142.8%N) and vascular degeneration was observed at 8 and 16 hrs after injury in diabetic wounds. At 16 hrs, decreased collagen (54.1%N) was also present. Enhanced edema with reduced vascular proliferation and cellular infiltration, in the early phase of healing, characterize the response of diabetic hamsters to injury. Supported by grants from American Diabetes Association, and Kroc Foundation.

9

Increased Catabolism of Glycosylated Low Density Lipoprotein (g-LDL) by Rat Peritoneal Macrophage. H. J. KIM* and I. V. KURUP, Milwaukee, Wi.

Coronary heart disease in diabetic subjects is frequently associated with high incidence of hypercholesterolemia. However, the association between LDL metabolism and atherogenesis in diabetic man is poorly understood. Persistent hyperglycemia in these patients results in nonenzymatic glycosylation of hemoglobin at N-terminal (HbAlc) or ε-amino group of lysine, due to posttranslational adduction of glucose.

To examine the degree of nonenzymatic glycosylation in LDL in vitro ultracentrifugally purified LDL from nondiabetic subjects was incubated in the presence of [U-^{14}C]-glucose in 15 mM glucose, 0.1M phosphate buffer, PH 7.4 under sterile conditions for 14 days at 37°C. ^{14}C-glucose S.A. and glucose/protein (G/P) ratio in control LDL were increased linearly during this period, while LDL modified with diketene (aLDL-acetoacetylation at lysyl residue) had reduced SA and G/P ratio ($p < 0.01$). The acid hydrolysate of ^{14}C-LDL yielded a product identical with synthetic glycosyl lysine. Since aLDL does not bind to LDL specific receptor in fibroblast but taken up by macrophage, rat peritoneal macrophages were isolated and incubated in Dulbecco's modified Eagle's media (10% serum) for 5 hours with ^{125}I-labelled aLDL, in the presence of various amounts of LDL, gLDL, or aLDL. gLDL competitively inhibited the ^{125}I-aLDL accumulation and degradation as effectively as aLDL. These data suggest that nonenzymatic glycosylation may occur in LDL at ε-amino group of lysine residue and gLDL may be catabolized preferentially by alternate pathway of LDL metabolism.

10

Pericyte Necrosis and Muscle Capillary Basement Membrane (CBM) Thickening in Diabetes Mellitus. R.G. TILTON, P.L. HOFFMANN, C. KILO* AND J.R. WILLIAMSON*. St. Louis, Missouri

These studies were undertaken to determine whether pericyte degeneration analogous to that reported in diabetic retinopathy is associated with muscle CBM thickening. Ultrastructural and morphometric studies including measurement of endothelial area, capillary circumference, percent of capillary circumference covered by pericytes (CCCP), and CBM width (CBMW) were performed on capillaries from 4 muscles (pectoral, abdominal, thigh and calf) obtained at autopsy from 20 diabetics (10 male and 10 female) and 20 age and sex matched nondiabetics. Since pericytes are the only cells completely ensheathed by CBM, accumulations of cell debris within CBM were tabulated as an index of pericyte necrosis.

Percent CCCP, CBMW and pericyte debris increased in the direction of head to foot in both controls and diabetics. The percent CCCP was identical in diabetics and controls, whereas CBMW and pericyte debris were increased (∿2.5 x) in diabetics. Of all the parameters assessed, including duration of diabetes and percent CCCP, only CBM thickening correlated strongly with the presence of pericyte debris ($F=52.4$, $P<0.0001$). These observations suggest that pericyte necrosis occurs more frequently in muscle, as well as in retinal, capillaries of diabetics. In contrast to the retina, regeneration of pericytes in muscle capillaries keeps pace with the increased rate of necrosis to maintain normal numbers of pericytes, i.e., percent CCCP.

Supported in part by USPHS Grant HL 13694 and Kilo Diabetes and Vascular Research Foundation.

11

Isolation from Rat Adipocytes of a Chemical Mediator for Insulin Activation of Pyruvate Dehydrogenase. FREDERICK L. KIECHLE, NIRMALA KOTAGAL, DENNIS A. POPP, and LEONARD JARETT,*St. Louis, Mo.

Adipocytes (Ad) were incubated in the presence (IN) or absence (C) of 100 uUnits/ml of insulin for 10 min. The cells were extracted in boiling 0.2 M acetate buffer, pH 3.8, 0.1 M EDTA and 0.1 mM cysteine. The extract was partially purified by filtration through glass wool and acid washed Norit followed by Sephadex G25 chromatography. Measurement of absorbance at 230 nm revealed a single peak of about MW 1,000-1,500. Total eluate was divided into five fractions which were lyophilized and redissolved in 0.001 M formic acid. Only fraction III (FIII), front of 230 peak, stimulated pyruvate dehydrogenase (PDH) activity in Ad mitochondria. In the presence of ATP FIII from IN caused PDH levels of 17.68±0.18 nmoles/mg/min whereas FIII from C was 10.59±0.19. In the absence of ATP FIII from IN increased PDH to 22.49±1.21 nmoles/mg/min versus 8.66±1.07 for C. NaF, a phosphatase inhibitor, suppressed the stimulation of PDH activity by FIII. Dichloroacetic acid, a kinase inhibitor, had no effect on the stimulation of PDH by FIII in the absence of ATP but stimulated PDH in the presence of ATP and was additive to the FIII effect. Thus insulin stimulates the generation of low MW, acid stable material from Ad which stimulates PDH by activating a calcium sensitive phosphatase. This mechanism is analogous to the one involved in activating the enzyme in the intact cell and involved in insulin activation of PDH in a plasma membrane mitochondrial mixture from Ad. This material appears to be a second messenger for insulin.

12

Evidence that a Regulator of Enzyme Activity is Generated by an Insulin-stimulated Proteolytic Reaction at the Plasma Membrane. JONATHAN R. SEALS and MICHAEL P. CZECH,* Providence, R. I.

Recent studies have shown that insulin (Ins) treatment of a mixture of rat adipocyte plasma membranes (PM) and mitochondria (Mito) stimulates the activity of the Mito enzyme pyruvate dehydrogenase (PDH) (Seals and Jarett, PNAS in press). The PDH regulator is a soluble factor which can be transferred to Mito in the supernatant from which Ins-treated PM have been pelleted by centrifugation. Three lines of evidence suggest that the regulator is a soluble peptide produced by a proteolytic reaction at the PM. First, the peptide nature of the regulator was indicated by the observation that trypsin or chymotrypsin treatment (100 ug/ml, 10 min) of the supernatant from Ins-treated PM removes its stimulatory ability. Second, generation of a PDH stimulator by proteolysis was demonstrated by limited digestion of PM with trypsin (0.01-0.1 ug/ml); the supernatant from these PM stimulated PDH. Third, the involvement of proteolysis in Ins action was demonstrated by pre-treatment of PM with protease inhibitors (ovomucoid or phenylmethylsulfonyl fluoride) or protease substrates (α-N-benzoyl-L-arginine methyl ester or p-tosyl-L-arginine methyl ester) which blocked the ability of PM to respond to Ins. Pre-treatment of PM with esters of lysine, tryosine, or alanine did not interfere with insulin action on PM. These results suggest that an endogenous PM protease with arginine specificity responds to Ins by acting on an endogenous PM substrate to release a soluble peptide which acts as an intracellular enzyme regulator.

13

Monoclonal Antibodies Against the Rat Adipocyte Intrinsic Membrane Proteins Mimic Insulin Action. JOANNA BEACHY, Providence, R.I. (Introduced by Ora Smith*, New Haven, Connecticut).

Antibodies produced in rabbits against rat intrinsic membrane proteins mimic the action of insulin on glucose oxidation in rat adipocytes. (Pillion, D.J. et al, 1979, J. Biol. Chem. 254: 3211-3220). Spleens of SJL mice which had been injected with rat adipocyte intrinsic membrane proteins were fused with 8-azaguanine-resistant, non-secreting mouse myeloma cell line NS-1. The cell medium of the hybrids was tested for its ability to bind to adipocyte plasma membranes and to stimulate the oxidation of glucose to CO_2. Binding of antibodies to the rat adipocyte plasma membrane was assayed by incubating cell medium with plasma membranes followed by further incubation with rat anti-mouse immunoglobulin IgG and ^{125}I protein A. Greater than 50% of the cultures produced immunoglobulins that bound to the plasma membrane of the rat adipocyte while only half of these were biologically active on glucose metabolism. Preincubation of the cell mediums with Staph. aureus and rabbit anti-mouse immunoglobulin IgG to remove mouse immunoglobulin abolished the stimulation of glucose activation. Ten cultures which produced antibodies that stimulated glucose oxidation and/or bound to the plasma membrane were cloned. Two of the clones produce IgG and five produce IgM. The antigenic nature of the proteins is currently under investigation. Thus, in conclusion, monospecific antibodies against the rat adipocyte have been produced which: 1) bind to the fat cell surface and 2) can be divided into two classes- those that mimic insulin action and those that have no biological effect.

14

Insulin-Stimulated Translocation of Glucose Transport Systems from an Intracellular Pool to the Plasma Membrane in Rat Adipose Cells: Time Course and Reversibility. E. KARNIELI, L.B. SALANS,* and S.W. CUSHMAN,* Bethesda, MD.

Insulin(INS) appears to enhance glucose transport in rat epididymal adipose cells by increasing the number of glucose transport systems(GTS) in the plasma membrane(PM). At the same time, INS induces a stoichiometric decrease in the number of GTS in an intracellular pool associated with the microsomes(MIC). The time course and reversibility of these effects of INS on the numbers of GTS, assayed by specific D-glucose-inhibitable ^{3}H-cytochalasin B binding, are compared with the effect of INS on 0.1 mM ^{14}C-3-O-methylglucose (3-O-MG) transport in intact cells. In the basal state, 6.2±1.6(mean±SD) and 64.5±8.9 pmol GTS/mg membrane protein are observed in PM and MIC, respectively, corresponding to a rate of 3-O-MG transport of 0.21±0.14 fmol/cell/min in intact cells. Within 60 sec of exposure to 1000 uU INS/ml, the number of GTS in PM is increased to 22.4±1.3 pmol/mg protein, the number of GTS in MIC is decreased to 46.0±12.0 pmol/mg protein, and the rate of 3-O-MG transport increases to 1.47±0.58 fmol/cell/min. These values represent 65%, 59%, and 60%, respectively, of the maximal effects of INS observed in 5 min. When cells are exposed to INS for 15 min, then to excess anti-INS antibody for 30 min, all values return to the basal levels. These results strongly support the hypothesis that the rapid and reversible glucose transport response to INS in adipose cells is mediated through a translocation of GTS between the intracellular pool and the plasma membrane.

15

Reconstitution Of D-Glucose Transport Activity From Cytoplasmic Membranes: Evidence Against Recruitment Of Cytoplasmic Membrane Transporters Into The Plasma Membrane As The Major Action Of Insulin. CHRISTIN CARTER-SU, Providence, RI (Introduced by M.F.SHANAHAN*, Madison, Wis.)

A cytoplasmic membrane fraction (CM) from rat adipocytes which is less dense than the plasma membrane fraction (PM) was found to contain high levels of cytochalasin B-sensitive D-glucose transport activity when solubilized with 2% cholate and reconstituted with exogenous phospholipids into liposomes. This transporter exhibited the same sugar and inhibitor specificity as the PM glucose transporter but was 3-6 fold higher in activity per mg protein. To determine whether the insulin stimulation of PM glucose transport could be accounted for by recruitment of transporters from the CM to the PM, transport was measured in reconstituted vesicles containing solubilized proteins from CM and PM from both insulin-treated and control adipocytes. Reconstituted PM from insulin-treated adipocytes exhibited 3-10 fold greater transport activity than those from control membranes, while reconstituted CM from control and insulin-treated adipocytes exhibited small and inconsistent differences. Recruitment of transporters from the CM to the PM should not alter the total number of transporters in a combined CM+PM fraction from control and insulin-treated cells. However, hexose transport activity was elevated in the combined preparations derived from insulin-activated compared to control cells. Insulin thus does not stimulate PM transport solely by recruiting transporters. Activation of transporters by insulin must take place.

16

Insulin stimulation of glycogen synthase in human diploid fibroblasts. H. HIDAKA, J. LARNER* and B.V. HOWARD*, Phoenix, AZ and Charlottesville, VA.

We have studied the effect of insulin on glycogen synthase activity in cultured diploid fibroblasts. Physiologic levels of insulin (2×10^{-10}M) increased I activity (the active form of the enzyme) without changing the total activity. Stimulation occurred within 5 min and became maximal in 30 min. Half maximal stimulation of I activity by insulin ($[Ins]_{50}$) was achieved at 3×10^{-9}M (pH 7.4), which corresponds closely with the concentrations of insulin that induce half maximal stimulation of glucose and amino acid uptake in these cells. At lower pH, $[Ins]_{50}$ was increased (10^{-8}M at pH 6.9) and the magnitude of maximal response to insulin was decreased (%I activity increment above unstimulated 34.5±6.8 at pH 7.4 vs 20.7±4.5 at pH 6.9, $p<0.005$). Glucose starvation prior to exposure to insulin increased the magnitude of I activity response to insulin but did not affect $[Ins]_{50}$. Glucose added at the time of insulin addition increased the level of I activity, and the effect of insulin was additive. During in vitro senescence, the total activity declined (634±40 vs 343±37 nmole/mg/hr, $p<0.001$), but $[Ins]_{50}$ was not changed. These data indicate that the regulation of glycogen synthase activity in human diploid fibroblasts is responsive to physiologic levels of insulin. This system appears to be useful to investigate the genetic insulin sensitivity of individuals with various disorders involving insulin resistance.

17

Calmodulin-Stimulation of Ca^{2+} Transport in Insulin-Sensitive Adipocyte Plasma Membranes. J.M. MCDONALD,* H.A. PERSHADSINGH and M. LANDT, St. Louis, Mo.

Adipocyte plasma membranes (PM) have a high affinity (Ca^{2+})-ATPase which is inhibited by direct addition of insulin (Pershadsingh, HA and McDonald, JM, Nature 281:495, 1979). The characteristics of the (Ca^{2+})-ATPase suggested that it was a Ca^{2+} transport enzyme. This study demonstrates Ca^{2+} transport in adipocyte PM which is stimulated by the calcium binding protein, calmodulin. Uptake of $^{45}Ca^{2+}$ was assayed in 200mM sucrose, 2mM $MgCl_2$, 20mM choline chloride, 20mM NaN_3, 10mM Tris-oxalate, 2mM Tris-EGTA, 0-2mM $CaCl_2$ (0-1.7μM ionized Ca^{2+}) and 10mM Tris-PIPES, pH 7.5 at 37°. PM Ca^{2+} transport was distinguished from Ca^{2+} transport in endoplasmic reticulum (ER) on the basis of: 1) sensitivity to KCl, 2) pH optimum and 3) sensitivity to calmodulin. PM transport was insensitive to 20mM KCl, whereas ER transport required KCl for maximal activity (K_m=10mM KCl). The pH optima of PM transport and ER transport were 7.5 and 6.8, respectively. Calmodulin stimulated Ca^{2+} transport by 100-300% and 20-50% in PM prepared with and without EGTA, respectively. ER transport was insensitive to calmodulin. The PM transport system had a K_m of 0.16μM free Ca^{2+} and a Vmax of 3-4 nmol Ca^{2+}/mg/min. Calmodulin stimulation was concentration dependent and saturable with a $K_{0.5}$ of 0.69μg/ml (∼40nM). This calmodulin-sensitive Ca^{2+} transport system appears to be the functional component of the insulin-sensitive (Ca^{2+})-ATPase and may provide an important mechanism whereby insulin regulates intracellular Ca^{2+}.

18

CALMODULIN AND INHIBITOR: ROLE IN EXPERIMENTAL DIABETES AND INSULIN ACTION. Solomon S. Solomon,* Marjorie Palazzolo, Janet McPherson, and Al Smoake; Memphis, Tennessee.

Diabetic ketoacidosis in man is associated with elevation of plasma and tissue levels of cyclic AMP (cAMP) and decrease in cAMP phosphodiesterase (PDE) activity. Calcium dependent regulator or Calmodulin (CM) is a small molecular weight protein essential for full activity of some PDE's. Animals are rendered diabetic by streptozotocin. CM is measured by activation of CM deficient PDE. Animals rendered diabetic by streptozotocin show a 50% decrease in both Vmax of PDE and CM activity in fat ($p < .02$). Insulin restores CM activity to 80% normal ($p < .05$) when administered 24 hours after induction of the diabetes, and 98% control (p = NS) when administered immediately. When preparations from normal and diabetic rat fat and liver are chromatographed on DEAE Sephacel, CM is separated from an inhibitor. Further characterization of CM and inhibitor reveal that the molecular weight of CM is 20,000 and its activity is destroyed by acid hydrolysis; inhibitor isolated from fat has a MW of ≅ 3,500 and appears resistant to acid hydrolysis. Inhibitor competitively inhibits CM activation of cAMP PDE.

Conclusion: Experimental diabetes is associated with a decrease in the activity of cAMP-PDE and CM in rat adipose and liver tissue which is reversed by insulin. A new small molecular weight inhibitor of CM is identified. All of these components appear to play a role in insulin action and diabetes.

19

Elevated Insulin-like Growth Factor II (IGF-II) in Non-islet Tumor Induced Hypoglycemia Detected by a New Specific Radioreceptor Assay. W.H. DAUGHADAY,* B. TRIVEDI, I.K. MARIZ, St. Louis, Mo.

Rat placental membranes contain a separate receptor for IGF-II with an affinity constant of $7 \times 10^{10} M^{-1}$ and a binding capacity of 5.2 pmol/mg of membrane protein. The affinity of IGF-I, MSA and rat somatomedin for this binding site is less than 5% that of IGF-II. Proinsulin, insulin and a variety of hormonal peptides are not bound by this site. Before assay, we have extracted serum with acid ethanol which eliminates binding protein and recovers >90% of added IGF-II. The actual assay was conducted with the same conditions we used for the IGF-I human placental membrane radioreceptor assay. Serum IGF-II in normal subjects between 18 and 69 years of age was 867 ± 42 ng/ml ($\bar{X}$ ± SE, n=25) and for subjects over 70 years was 1056 ± 47 ng/ml (n=25). Cord serum contained 1581 ± 106 ng/ml (n=39). Unlike IGF-I and SmC, IGF-II is little influenced by GH; in pituitary dwarfism, IGF-II concentration was 620 ± 55 ng/ml (n=14) and in acromegaly 869 ± 75 ng/ml (n=22). Five of 6 sera of patients with severe hypoglycemia associated with non-islet cell tumors had elevated serum concentrations of IGF-II (1364, 1802, 2168, 2989, and 3069 ng/ml).

We conclude that not only is there heterogeneity of the structure of insulin-like growth factors but there is heterogeneity in specific receptors and independent regulation of plasma concentrations of IGF-I and II. IGF-II may be the peptide responsible for tumor hypoglycemia in some cases.

20

Functional Correlates of Genetically Defective Receptors for Insulin and Insulin-like Growth Factors in an Infant with Leprechaunism. A.B. KNIGHT, E.E. SCHILLING, J.A. ROMANUS, and M.M. RECHLER, Bethesda, Md. (Introduced by E.A.H. McGUIRE*)

We have reported a profound selective deficit of insulin receptors in fibroblasts cultured from an insulin-resistant infant with leprechaunism (PNAS 76: 5877, 1979). We now examine the effect of this defect on two acute metabolic activities of insulin: glucose incorporation and methylaminoisobutyric acid (AIB) transport. In control fibroblasts, insulin and proinsulin appeared to stimulate both responses via the insulin receptor. The ED_{50} for insulin was ≃5 ng/ml; proinsulin was ≃5% as potent. MSA, an insulin-like growth factor (IGF), stimulated AIB and glucose uptake ≃30 times more potently than its insulin-like potency, presumably via the IGF receptor. In patient's fibroblasts, stimulation of glucose uptake by insulin and MSA was greatly impaired (5-25% of control), whereas stimulation of AIB transport was not affected. Control fibroblasts possess specific IGF receptors. In patient's fibroblasts, specific binding of ^{125}I-IGF I to these receptors was decreased by ≧70%, similar to the reduction in insulin binding to insulin receptors. In conclusion, insulin and IGFs may stimulate glucose and AIB uptake in fibroblasts via insulin or IGF receptors. Both receptors are profoundly impaired in the leprechaun patient's fibroblasts. Stimulation of glucose uptake by insulin and IGFs is impaired but AIB transport is not affected, suggesting functional heterogeneity of receptors. The genetic defect in this patient may alter a component common to insulin and IGF receptors, which may be linked to specific biological functions.

21

The Effect of Contracting on Patient Compliance by CAROLE' MENSING, Minneapolis, Mn., DEANNE F. BELL, and DURWARD L. BELL, Austin, Tx.

From September 1977 through August 1978, 21 registered nurses (specializing in diabetes care and located in various health settings) volunteered to help test health educational concepts and materials. Based on this input, the educational format of a written contract was field tested from September 1978 through August 1979. Nurses and other health professionals participated. A total of 31 clients and their supporters completed contracts and provided written reactions to the contracting process.

It was found that 82% of the clients using contracts were able to meet at least half of their learning objectives, compared with 35% of the noncontract clients. These findings are even more impressive when it is noted that the health educators tended to set more objectives for their patients ehen they formally contracted (4.3 objectives/client) than when conventional teaching techniques were used (3.1 objectives/client).

Thirty-nine percent of the clients using contracts met all learning objectives, as opposed to a 22% compliance rate for those not using contracts. Before contracting, 29% of the clients were very positive toward contracting; afterward 55% were very positive. Initially 32% were neutral or negative; afterwards only 10% fell into this category.

Seventy three percent of the health educators nominated the most effective means of teaching to be "having both patient and supporter complete a contract."

22

Cognitive and Situational Factors Associated with Diabetic Patient Compliance. S.S. GILBERT, F.C. PENNINGTON, Ann Arbor, Michigan.

This study investigated the relationships among factors which have been reported to be associated with patient compliance, especially relationships between these factors and indicators of patient compliance with insulin and dietary regimens. Twenty adult onset insulin managed diabetics were interviewed, and the attending physician for each patient responded to a self-administered questionnaire.

The factors believed to be associated with and influence compliance are the patient's: perceived severity of and susceptibility to complications of diabetes; perceived barriers and benefits to following recommendations; satisfaction with health care provided; health locus of control; and sense of involvement in his/her own management.

Socio-demographic and health background for each of the patients were gathered. These include age, sex, marital status, residential situation, occupation, education, income, age at first diagnosis of diabetes, history of complications, and knowledge of the prescribed regimens.

Indicators of compliance include: patient report of the extent to which he/she follows the dietary and insulin regimens and clinician assessment of the patient's compliance along several criteria.

Results indicate that compliance with dietary instructions is associated with a different set of factors than compliance with insulin-taking instructions.

23

The Relationship of Quality of Life and Quality of Care for a Sample of Diabetic Patients. MARY ETTA C. MILLS, IVAN BAROFSKY, and BEATRICE NORDBERG,* Baltimore, Md.

Twenty-one insulin dependent diabetic patients were studied at the University of Maryland Adult Diabetic Clinic to determine the degree of concordance between a patient's rating of their own status (a quality of life issue) and a provider's rating of the patient's status (a quality of care issue). Both patients and providers rated various aspects of the patient's health status, diet, use of medications (e.g., insulin), self-monitoring knowledgebase and long-term goal setting.

Results indicate that the correlation between a patient's satisfaction with, for example, their diet and a provider's rating of how well a diet was adhered to was low (r=.20) and non-significant. The patient's rating of the impact of their disease on their diet and the provider's rating of how well the diet was kept was also low (r=.10) and non-significant. In contrast, the patient's impact and satisfaction ratings for diet were statistically significant ($r=.48$; $p < .05$). Thus, there appears to be concordance within an individual but not between an individual and the criteria designed to evaluate the care he/she has received.

The implications of this study is that the patient's perceptions of satisfaction and/or impact of disease on quality of life may be minimally related to the quality of care criteria utilized by providers. To what extent patient perceptions are related to the patient's efforts to participate in and control his diabetic condition has yet to be determined.

24

Cultural Beliefs Influence Compliance to Therapy for Diabetes Mellitus. CLARISSA S. SCOTT (Introduced by JAY S. SKYLER*) Miami, Florida.

This study examined the influence on health behavior of culturally-learned beliefs about the safety and effectiveness of particular therapeutic activities. Fifty-eight patients on insulin therapy were interviewed in their homes on two occasions by a medical anthropologist. The majority were low-income, inner-city black Americans. A measure of their insulin bottles was taken each visit and the amount consumed was computed to compare with their verbal statements regarding compliance. All factors of the health belief model were explored; two areas, however, were expanded and dealt with in depth. These were: (a) the patients' culturally-patterned subjective beliefs concerning the efficacy and safety of insulin therapy, diet and weight loss and (b) the use of alternative (folk) therapeutic modalities.

Patients who question the appropriateness of the prescribed diet and the safety of the weight loss plan were significantly less compliant ($p < 0.05$) than those whose beliefs are in accord with their physicians' regarding these two aspects of the diabetes regimen. Patients who use a folk modality and believe it to be equally or more effective than insulin were significantly less compliant ($p < 0.05$) than those who use insulin only.

It is concluded that it is important to sensitively assess cultural beliefs surrounding the treatment of diabetes as an additional predictor of non-compliance.

25

How Diabetic Children Understand Their Illness. ARLENE R. BREWSTER, Detroit, Michigan.

This study investigates the relationship between cognitive development and the childrens understanding of the cause of their illness, intent of medical procedures and role of the medical staff.

Fifty chronically ill, hospitalized children, ages 5 to 12 years, of normal IQ were interviewed (20% juvenile diabetes). Protocol included 5 tasks based on the cognitive theory of Jean Piaget, scored in ascending order of cognitive maturation of responses.

Results indicated correlation coefficient of responses at ($p \leq .01$) among tasks. Analysis of Variance yielded an age related maturation of responses at $p < .01$. There was no significant statistical difference in level of response between high and low affect tasks.

Results demonstrated a predictable sequence of conceptual development of the cause of illness through 3 major stages: 1.) illness is caused by human action; 2.) illness is caused by outside factors, eg., germs; 3.) illness is caused by physical weakness or susceptability. Development of understanding of medical staff intentions followed 3 parallel maturational stages: 1.) procedures viewed as being done to inflict punishment; 2.) correct understanding of the intention, belief that staff's empathy depended on the child expressing pain; 3.) ability of the child to infer both intention and empathy from the medical staff. Specific illness, length of hospitalization did not effect child's level of response.

Children process information about their illness through a predictable maturational cognitive sequence which medical staff must address for comprehension to occur.

26

Family Characteristics of Diabetic Children: Correlations with Hemoglobin A1c (HbA1c). B.J. ANDERSON,* W.F. AUSLANDER, and J.P. MILLER, St. Louis, Mo.

In order to identify specific family parameters related to control in diabetic children, we studied a heterogeneous group of 58 families with children aged 11-19, diabetic more than 1 year. All were participants in a research project at the DRTC at Washington University to collect clinical data on diabetic individuals. Parents and children were interviewed independently, and children were given standardized tests of self-concept (Piers-Harris) and perceived family environment (Moos). HbA1c values were recorded independently and used to measure diabetic control.

Children reporting physical symptoms (slow healing, leg pain, fatigue) had significantly higher HbA1c values. Females ($\bar{X}$=12.5) had significantly higher HbA1c values than males ($\bar{X}$= 10.9), and more females reported negative extra-familial influences on self-management. For parents and children alike, beliefs that the child was in good control and followed the regimen were associated with lower HbA1c values. However, within the same family, parent and child often had discrepant views about family involvement in treatment tasks. Children who believed they were treated the same as siblings and who perceived their family as high on Cohesion (Moos) had lower HbA1c values. Significant positive correlations were also found between family cohesiveness and the child's self-esteem, suggesting a multivariate model in which reports of physical symptoms, beliefs about control and management habits, and family cohesiveness relate to diabetic control.

27

Characteristics of "Brittle" Adolescent Diabetics Referred to a University Diabetes Program. D. ORR, M. GOLDEN,* G. MYERS* and D. MARRERO, Irvine, CA.

Adolescents with insulin dependent diabetes mellitus are often difficult to manage. Widely disparate explanations, from physical-biochemical to emotional, have been proposed. We describe 16 consecutive patients (mean: 16.3 yrs) referred to a University diabetes program for evaluation of diabetic control. Mean duration of diabetes was 5.34 years. Patients referred specifically for "poor control" included 5-recurrent hypoglycemia, 7-recurrent DKA, and 1-both. Expressed concerns for referral were metabolic e.g., receptor abnormalities; not psychologic. Metabolic evaluation, including use of the Biostator(R) in 7 patients, uncovered no unusual insulin requirements. Knowledge of diabetic physiology was adequate. Striking was the high prevalence of psychosocial problems-11/16 had family disruptions and in 8 family dynamics contributed to poor control. Six completed the Offer Self Image Questionnaire for adolescents. Four of 6 indicated maladjustment, ranging from poor impulse control to overt psychopathology. Treatment included education and counseling by multidisciplinary team, an insignificant increase in the mean dosage of insulin (0.94 to 1.03u/kg) with increased flexibility of dosage. 11/16 were referred for psychological counseling (1 inpatient, 3 family, 2 individual, 5 adolescent group treatment). At follow-up 10 patients were improved overall, 4 unchanged, and 2 lost. While education and appropriate insulin therapy are prerequisite to treatment, health professionals must be aware of contribution of psychosocial factors to poor control in adolescents and be prepared to assess and treat these problems.

28

Subcutaneous (SC) open loop insulin delivery: is a pump required? J.D. NELSON, E.B. MARLISS,* and B. ZINMAN,* Toronto, Canada.

SC open loop systems achieve good diabetic control using continuous infusions plus premeal boluses of CZI. To determine the role of the continuous component, we compared glycemias and "free" IRI with 4 boluses (B) alone vs infusion plus boluses (IB) via an indwelling SC catheter. Nine lean IDDM's (mean age 28±3yr) were first studied on the intravenous (IV) closed loop system to determine meal and 24h insulin doses (42± 2U/d). With diet (1677±96kcal) and total insulin constant, IB received continuous (15mU/kg/h) plus boluses 30min premeal. B received only boluses with a bedtime dose of 9x15mU/kg. Fasting glycemia of 108±10mg/dl was obtained prior to each study by overnight IV insulin. All subsequent meal glycemic excursions and IRI were identical in IB and B. Premeal lunch and dinner values were 106±13 and 87±8mg/dl. Peaks post breakfast were 176±11, lunch 134±14 and dinner 119±12mg/dl, and maintained at 99±10mg/dl until 0300h. "Free" IRI showed small excursions from 1.7±0.2 fasting, to peaks of 2.6±0.5ng/ml. However, next morning (0700h), glycemia in B was 240±35 and IRI 0.7±0.2 in contrast to 96±11mg/dl and 1.7±0.5ng/ml ($P < 0.01$) in IB. Pilot studies (n=3) suggest possible correction of overnight hyperglycemia in B by evening Lente. Conclusions: 1) Continuous SC infusion contributes to glycemic control only overnight. 2) Boluses alone (3CZI + 1Lente) via an indwelling SC catheter may be an alternate method of sustaining insulinemia and achieving 24h control. 3) Pumps are not essential for SC delivery systems during the day.

29

Effects of Continuous Subcutaneous Insulin Infusion (CSII) in Non-Insulin-Dependent Diabetes Mellitus (NIDDM) and Insulin-Dependent DM (IDDM) M CHAMPION, NW RODGER,* J DUPRE,* London, Canada

Effects of CSII were compared in NIDDM (n=6, >250 subject-days) and IDDM (n=8, >1600 subject-days). Constant rate insulin infusions were supplemented AC, and meal tolerance was tested with a 75 gm CHO standard mixed meal in diabetic and normal volunteers (n=7). Before treatment with insulin, fasting plasma glucose (PG) was >220 mg/dl in both groups of DM and ketoacidosis was present in IDDM. During optimized conventional depot therapy mean PG AC meals ("basal", mg/dl) was 165±11 in NIDDM and 165±16 in IDDM. The table shows mean PG and free immunoreactive insulin (F-IRI) concentrations before and after meals during CSII, with parameters of the regime.

	NORMAL	IDDM	NIDDM
% Ideal B Wht	101±4	103±4	108±4
PG - AC	90±2	100±5	116±3.9
- PC Peak	151±11	157±17	207±12
F-IRI - AC	7.0±1.1	8.8±1.3	19±2.5
- PC Peak	56±10	30±4.6	48±7.0
CSII Dose U/h	--	0.89±.12	0.85±.22
- AC, U	--	4.4±.55	8.0±.22

CSII resulted in improved control of glycemia in NIDDM as in IDDM. By comparison with basal values on insulin withdrawal in IDDM (F-IRI not detectable) and NIDDM (F-IRI 12±1.3 μU/ml), CSII produced similar increments of F-IRI in both DM groups. Consideration of dose-related increments in F-IRI in NIDDM with CSII suggests that endogenous secretion of insulin may contribute more to basal than PC plasma F-IRI under these conditions.

30

Cellular Stimuli for the Rejection of Islet Allografts. JUNKO ONO, IAN M. ZITRON, PAUL E. LACY*, and JOSEPH M. DAVIE, St. Louis, Mo.

Previous studies in our laboratory have shown that in vitro culture of islets at 24°C for 7 days prior to transplantation and a single injection of ALS into the recipients permits successful transplants of rat islets across major histocompatibility barriers (Sci.204: 312, 1979). Rejection of established islet allografts was induced by injection of peritoneal exudate cells (PEC) syngeneic to the donor strain (Transpl.28: 415, 1979). The cell type(s) responsible for rejection was investigated by using established allografts of WF islets in Lewis recipients. Splenic T cells (double-passed over nylon wool columns), splenic B cells (isolated with anti-Ig immunoabsorbent), or thioglycollate-induced PEC from WF rats were injected I.V., 40-160 days post transplantation. Rejection was monitored by measuring 24 hr. urine glucose, blood glucose and body weight. Recipients of unirradiated T cells or PEC rejected their islet transplants 6-8 days after challenge. Irradiation (1500r) of T or PEC did not abrogate rejection, indicating a proliferation-independent process which we propose to be antigen presentation. As striking as the ability of T and PEC (to induce rejection) was the complete failure of B cells to do so. We interpret our data to indicate that islet allograft rejection is induced by the presentation of antigens which may not be uniformly expressed on leucocyte populations or, alternatively, that B lymphocytes differ from other cell types in their ability to present histocompatibility antigens. (Supported by USPHS AM01226 & Kroc Foundation)

31

Role of Histocompatibility in Pancreatic Transplantation. G. KYRIAKIDES, A. RABINOVITCH,* L. OLSON, J. MILLER, and D.H. MINTZ,* Miami, Florida.

Immunosuppressed mongrel dogs have rejected intraperitoneal segmental vascularized pancreatic allotransplants at 13±4 days (Trans. Proc. 11: 530, 1979). We now studied the role of histocompatibility matching using DLA-typed and MLC-tested pairs of littermate beagles. Recipients were totally pancreatectomized. Four groups (Gr.) were studied: I (n=5) strong MLC reactivity, II (n=5) intermediate MLC reactivity, III (n=5) no MLC reactivity. DLA identical and non-identical dogs were evenly distributed in the three groups. Gr. IV dogs were previously made "tolerant" by total body radiation, autologous marrow implantation, and kidney transplantation from DLA-MLC identical donors without immunosuppression for more than a year before pancreatic transplantation from the same donors was performed. Gr. I-III were immunosuppressed with prednisone and imuran. Gr. IV was not immunosuppressed. Results: Rejection (hyperglycemia) was sudden and unpredictable despite biweekly IVGTT's and serum insulin determinations. Days of normoglycemia: I=8±2, II=15±2, III=60 to >180, and IV >180. Histology at six months showed disappearance of acini and coalescence of islets in III and IV, but with more fibrosis in IV. Conclusions: Pancreatic islets in vascularized grafts may survive indefinitely in the presence of good tissue match, best predicted by MLC testing. Histocompatibility seems to be common enough between kidney and pancreas to allow for long-term survival of both organs transplanted from the same donor (Gr. IV). Steroids may be important in preventing fibrosis of the graft (Gr. III vs. IV).

32

Intrahepatic versus Intrasplenic Pancreatic Islet Transplantation:Effect on Glucose Homeostasis and Hepatic Enzyme Activities. H.SELAWRY*,R.MARGOLIS and R.T.CURNOW*,Miami,FL. and Charlottesville,Va.

Male Wistar-Lewis rats were made diabetic by the intravenous(i.v.)injection of 60 mg/kg streptozotocin.Islets were isolated by a collagenase digestion method.Each of the diabetic rats received either 1 intraportal injection of 1000 islets or 2 successive intrasplenic injections of 1500 islets/implant.Two months after implantation, i.v and oral glucose tolerance tests were done in 4 groups of rats:1) control, 2) diabetic 3)hepatic transplant-improved and 4) splenic transplant-improved.Four months after implantation the livers were excised for enzyme assays.The calculated mean i.v.glucose clearance was 2.57±.15, .58±.04 1.13±.09, and 1.51±.34, in the 4 groups respectively.Intrasplenic rats did not release insulin (IRI) in a physiological manner.Hepatic glycogen synthase in the I form(GS-I) was 17.6±1.1, 6.1±.5, 19.5 ±4.9, and 34.68 ± 5.71 % and GS phosphatase(GS-P) was 3.3 ±.7, .9 ±.4, 1.6 ±.3, and 1.19 ±.09 U/g in the 4 groups respectively.Within group 3 there was a positive correlation between plasma insulin and GS-P(r=.73,$p<.01$).Within group 4 however,there was a negative correlation(r=-.9, $p<.05$) between similar parameters.In conclusion, these data indicate 1)normoglycemia can be achieved with both intrahepatic and intrasplenic transplantation,2) intrasplenic transplants fail to show a normal biphasic IRI response to glucose stimulation, 3)hepatic GS and GS-P are profoundly affected by diabetes and 4) pancreatic islet transplantation variably corrects diabetes-induced changes in hepatic GS & GS-P activities.

33

A Role for Prostaglandin (PG) E in Defective Glucose Potentiation of A Nonglucose Insulin Secretagogue in Diabetics. J. MCRAE, R.P. ROBERTSON*, Seattle, WA.

Diabetics (NIDDM) with fasting hyperglycemia have an impaired ability to recognize glucose signals, manifested by absent acute insulin responses (AIR) to glucose and subnormal glucose potentiation of nonglucose secretagogues. Since prior studies have suggested that PGE may mediate the abnormal AIR to glucose, this study explores whether PGE may also be involved in the abnormal glucose potentiation of nonglucose signals. The effects of a PG synthesis inhibitor, sodium salicylate (SS), on the AIR to arginine (2gIV pulse) in NIDDM and normal subjects were compared. SS (40mg/min IV for 60 min) augmented the AIR (SS=354±46, control=239±36%, $\bar{x}\Delta$2-5'IRI, % basal, n=11, p<.01) in NIDDM but not in normal subjects (SS=384±117; control=326±62%, n=6, p=NS). Conversely, PGE_2 (10mcg/min IV for 30 min) inhibited the AIR in NIDDM (PGE=191±30, control=280±58%, n=7, p<.025) but, again, not in normal subjects (PGE=590±118, control=592±164%, n=5, p=NS), suggesting an increased sensitivity in NIDDM to SS and PGE. The effect of SS on glucose potentiation (GP) of the AIR to arginine was studied by measuring the AIR at two different plasma glucose(G) levels altered by an insulin infusion. GP, expressed by the ratio ΔAIR/Δprestimulus G, was less (p<.005) in NIDDM (1.62±0.67, n=6) than in normals (10.66±2.8, n=4). SS infusion improved GP in NIDDM (4.64±1.74, n=6, p<.05) but not in normals (10.85±4.4, p=NS). These findings suggest a role for endogenous PGE in the defective glucose potentiation of the AIR to nonglucose secretagogues in NIDDM as well as the defective AIR to glucose itself.

34

Acute Alterations in Prostaglandin Status Fail to Influence Insulin Secretion in Man. R.G. BRODOWS* Rochester, New York.

In vitro and in vivo studies on prostaglandins (PG) as regulators of beta cell function often disagree. In vitro, prostaglandins seem to stimulate insulin release. In man, infusion of PGE inhibits the acute insulin response (AIR) to glucose while sodium salicylate, a PG synthesis inhibitor, augments AIR. However, our studies with another PG inhibitor, indomethacin, revealed inhibition of AIR (Clin Res 26:677a, 1978). The present studies were designed to examine AIR to iv glucose pulses before and after (1) increased exogenous (oral PGE_2, 1 mg) and endogenous (iv furosemide, 40 mg) PGs, and (2) decreased endogenous PGs with three PG synthesis inhibitors: aspirin (ASA, 1 g), ibuprofen (IB, 800 & 1600 mg) and sulfinpyrazone (S, 400 mg). The AIR ($\bar{x}\Delta$3-5' IRI) to 5 g iv glucose pulse was unaffected by PGE_2 (35±8 vs 28±6, n=10), furosemide (37±7 vs 36±11, n=9), ASA (24±3 vs 23±5, n=8), S (26±7 vs 24±7, n=5), IB 800 mg (41±14 vs 43±10, n=7) or IB 1600 mg (28±4 vs 29±5, n=8). No drug was associated with changes in basal glucose, insulin or glucagon levels. Glucose disappearance rates were similar before and after PGE_2 (1.28±.2 vs .91±13%/min) and furosemide (.94±.11 vs .83±.13%/min). Thus, acute alterations in PG status in normals did not influence basal or glucose-stimulated insulin release or glucose tolerance. These studies fail to confirm the work of others with iv PGs and PG synthesis inhibitors. Clearly further studies are needed before a consistent theory of PG-beta cell interaction can be developed.

35

Somatostatin-like immunoreactivity (SLI) in Mammalian Plasma. K.A.BOLDT, E.C.LASCHANSKY, C. NIST, D.SIMONOWITZ, G. TABORSKY, J.W.ENSINCK, Seattle, Washington

In unextracted plasma, SLI levels measured by immunoassay requiring ^{125}I-tyr^1 somatostatin (S) as tracer with trasylol plus EDTA to inhibit enzymatic proteolysis have been extremely variable. By means of an antibody recognizing both ^{125}I-tyr^1-S and ^{125}I-tyr^{11}-S analogs, we developed an assay for SLI and an immunoadsorbent of SLI antibody bonded to glass. By the latter technique we found that the ^{125}I-tyr^1 is rapidly cleaved from S by putative amino-peptidases in plasma of several species which, with the exception of the dog, are not blocked by a spectrum of protease inhibitors. Representative mean plasma levels of SLI in the presence of trasylol plus EDTA are given below.

		^{125}I-tyr^1-S	^{125}I-tyr^{11}-S
SLI pg/ml	Human	243	25
	Baboon	361	75
	Rat	> 800	74
	Dog	158	101

Thus, except for the dog, immunoassays with ^{125}I-tyr^1-S in unextracted plasma give spuriously high values which preclude interpretation. In contrast, the use of the ^{125}I-tyr^{11}-S as tracer has permitted a valid assay of SLI in unextracted plasma. In normal and diabetic man, peripheral levels of SLI have been found to oscillate with a periodicity of 4 to 8 minutes. Gradients of SLI across the liver have also been found in man, rat and dog. From the rapid inactivation of ^{125}I-tyr^1-S in plasma at 37° in vitro, it is possible that circulating SLI is in the form of des-Ala-S or des-Ala-Gly-S and may represent the biologically active S.

36

Effect of free fatty acids (FFA) on the gastric and pancreatic secretion of somatostatin-like immunoreactivity (SLI) in normal and alloxan diabetic dogs, T. WASADA, A. PIETRI, P. RASKIN*, R. DOBBS*, and R.H. UNGER*, Dallas, Texas.

A rise in plasma FFA stimulates insulin and suppresses glucagon levels. To determine the influence of FFA levels upon SLI secretion, SLI was measured in 8 normal conscious dogs during changes in plasma FFA concentration produced by infusing triglyceride emulsion (Intralipid®) and heparin. When FFA was raised from 17 ± 2 to 39 ± 3 mg/dl (p<0.001), plasma SLI rose from 145 ± 7 to a peak of 253 ± 44 pg/ml (p<0.05). Neither fat emulsion alone nor heparin alone raised either FFA or SLI levels. Glycerol infusion had no effect on SLI levels. To find the source of the SLI increase induced by FFA, pancreatic and gastric vein plasma of laparotomized dogs was collected during fat-heparin infusion; SLI in the effluent of the pancreas, gastric fundus and antrum increased more than two-fold. To study the response in diabetes, conscious alloxan diabetic dogs were given fat emulsion plus heparin; SLI rose from an elevated basal value of 185 ± 9 to a peak of 310 ± 44 pg/ml (p<0.01). It is concluded that: 1) A rise in FFA levels stimulates SLI secretion in normal and diabetic dogs; and, 2) The SLI rise is derived from the pancreas and stomach. The FFA concentration may be a physiological regulator of SLI secretion and may provide the basis of a stimulatory test of D-cell function.

37

Immunochemical Studies of Pancreatic Somatostatin. HIDEKI OYAMA, KENNETH GABBAY*, MARIE GREIDER*, and ALAN PERMUTT*, HARRY HIRSCH*, St. Louis, MO.

The relationship between pancreatic somatostatin (PS) and tetradecapeptide somatostatin (SRIF) isolated from brain has yet to be determined. Using an antibody to the central portion of SRIF, it was determined that catfish islets contain a large amount of immunoreactive somatostatin (IRS). Two IRS peptides were purified to homogeneity and the sequence of one determined. It contains 8 additional amino acids on the amino terminus of a tetradecapeptide with striking homology to SRIF. Antibodies to this peptide identified specific cells within pancreatic islets by immunoperoxidase staining. A PS radioimmunoassay was developed which measured PS 1000-fold better than SRIF. Using this assay, IRS was measured in extracts of pigeon and rat pancreas. Boiling reduced extractable IRS by 75%. The anti-PS antibody detected 5-10 times more IRS than the SRIF antibody in catfish islets, 5 times more than IRS in rat pancreas but was poorly reactive to pigeon extracts. Displacement curves by rat and pigeon pancreatic extracts were parallel to that with catfish islet extracts. The pancreatic extracts were gel filtered on a Biogel P-60 column. Pigeon pancreatic extracts showed the major IRS coeluting with SRIF, while over 95% of the IRS from rat pancreas migrated as a single peak larger than SRIF, with estimated M_r 3000-4000. In conclusion, purified catfish PS has been used to generate an antibody which has high affinity for fish and rat pancreatic somatostatins. Preliminary observations suggest that the most abundant form of IRS in rat pancreatic extracts is larger than SRIF.

38

New Principles of Diet from a Home Glucose Monitoring Program. KATHARINE ALLING, JUDITH BALL, JOHN R. WILLIAMS, JR.*, Rochester, N.Y.

Achievement of good control of diabetes (which we define as maintaining 90% of blood glucose levels between 50 and 150 mg/dl at any time of day, with none over 200) depends in part upon the patient's understanding of diet. We have over 90 insulin-dependent patients on a home glucose monitoring program whose mastery of control has taught us these basic principles of diet.

Any diet to which a patient will adhere must reflect what the patient wants to eat and can afford. We establish this from a food diary the patient keeps for a week prior to diet counselling. We modify patient desires as little as possible to fit a diabetic diet. Changes of as little as 10 grams of carbohydrate at a meal can alter blood glucose levels by over 100 mg/dl. Since consistent carbohydrate content in meals must be maintained, it is important to allow patients to establish their own quotas. While favored portion sizes vary from one person to another, an individual's portions tend to be consistent. Therefore we never prescribe portions or meal plans.

The patient must understand and be able to compute accurately the carbohydrate content of meals. Both the sources and effects of different carbohydrates, and of proteins and fats, must be understood in order for a patient to plan meals whose effect on blood glucose is consistent.

A patient who understands these fundamentals of diet can learn how variations in dietary intake may be balanced with changes in insulin and/or activity to maintain control as defined above.

39

Assessment of Caloric Intake of Youngsters with Juvenile Diabetes Mellitus (JDM) Compared to Standard Methods of Assessing Caloric Needs. E. KOHLER* and M. BENZ, Milwaukee, WI.

The dietitian established an ADA dietary pattern at a caloric level agreed upon to satisfy the child's appetite for each of 223 JDM youngsters 2-18 years of age through interviews with the child and family. On routine clinic visits this calorie level was continually reassessed by history of intake and revised so that it might reflect actual intake.

Mean energy intake thus estimated was plotted against age in years (yrs) in those children with normal growth, i.e. height and weight following appropriate percentiles, for a total of 583 patient years. Measured as kcal/d, intake for both sexes together was close to Dr. White's rule of thumb (WR = 1000 kcal + 100/yr of age up to 14 yrs for girls and 20 yrs for boys) but > 300 kcal/d below the World Health Organization recommendations (WHO) at all ages and below levels reported from the National Health Survey, 1971-74 (NHS) except at 13-15 yrs of age. In the early yrs, intake of girls and boys separately as kcal/d were close to WR, > 300 kcal/d below WHO and > 200 kcal/d below NHS. However, from 12-16 yrs boys' mean intake was about 200 kcal/d greater than WR and closer to NHS, while girls' over 10 yrs was 100-500 kcal/d less than WR and closer to NHS. Both were still below WHO. The mean intake of both sexes together or separately measured as kcal/kg/d was close to NHS (though lower under 10 yrs of age) and consistently below the intake recommendations of WHO or Nelson's Textbook of Pediatrics.

40

Dietary Adherence and Metabolic Control with an Unmeasured Diet in Normal Weight Diabetic Patients. C. ABRAIRA,* M. PURICELLI and A. GALLAGHER, Hines, IL

Caloric restriction is an unquestioned tenet in the treatment of overweight diabetics. The need for precise caloric prescription in lean adult diabetics has not been tested. In a randomized, single blind prospective study, 50 lean insulin treated patients were assigned to an exchange type fixed composition diet or to an unmeasured diet with sugar restriction and instruction on meal balance. Dietary recalls of 2 days done every 3 months show similar mean caloric intake and composition in both groups over 4 year period. Two thirds of the patients in each group have good adherence to regularity of caloric distribution and day to day consistency. Mean fasting serum glucose and lipids, insulin dosages and reported hypoglycemic reactions are similar in both diets. Body weight remains within normal limits. The degree of fasting blood sugar control in each group is virtually equal, and comparable to that published in other outpatient populations. None of these parameters could be correlated with the regularity of reported intake in either group.

Our earlier pilot study (Am. J. Clin Nutr. 33: May, 1980) suggested that insulin treated lean diabetics spontanously regulate their intake to maintain constant weight in spite of variable glycemia and insulin doses. In addition, the current trial shows no conventionally measurable differences between an exchange type diet and an unmeasured diet in the treatment of these patients.

41

Dietitian Coordinated Diabetes Clinic, Exchange System and Weekly Follow Up Visits Decreased Body Weight and Glucose in Obese Individuals. PATRICIA M. LEAPLEY,* Tampa, Florida.

Obese out patients with elevated blood glucose levels were referred to a dietitian coordinated diabetes clinic for intensive diet therapy. Patients were requested to obtain routine laboratory tests prior to coming to the clinic. They were seen by a physician for a complete history and physical. Individuals then attended an education program taught by the dietitian, nurse, podiatrist and dental hygienist. In addition, the dietitian completed a nutritional assessment prior to giving the patient an individualized meal plan based on the exchange system.

All obese patients were scheduled to be weighed each week by the dietitian. Fasting blood glucose levels were ordered biweekly. Patients then attended a one hour continuing nutrition education program which included behavior modification techniques, menu planning, and other nutrition topics. Patients attended class every week until weight and blood glucose levels were within normal range. Patients returned to the dietitian biweekly and monthly once weight loss was achieved. Intensive and individualized diet therapy was found to be effective in lowering the blood glucose level and weight in obese diabetics.

42

Glucose, Insulin and Glucagon Responses to Soya-Fiber Enriched Diet in Obese, Diabetic and Normal Subjects. YORAM KANTER,* ELY ROTENSTERICH, LEA SOLOVEITZIC, BERTA RUBINOVICH AND DAVID BARZILAI, Haifa, ISRAEL.

We studied the effects of soya-fiber diet (SFD)on the post prandial glucose, insulin and glucagon responses to oral test-meals in 8 obese (OB), 8 non-insulin dependent diabetics (DM) and 8 normal controls (NC).The responses of glucose, insulin and glucagon to standard-test meal were compared to the responses to a 20 Gr soya-fiber enriched test meal given after 3 days. Other biochemical parameters, lipid profiles and hormonal levels were studied. The SFD given during the 3 days between tests, contained 30 cal/kg/day supplemented with 60 Gr of soybean polysacchrides rich material from soybean hulls.

Our findings indicate that SFD not only reduces the levels of glucose (down 24.4% in DM) but may also improve the insulin responses (down 40.8% in OB). No significant changes were noted in glucagon levels.

These results indicate that SFD may be used (as some other dietary-fiber) in the nutritional management of DM and OB patients which seem to benefit from an increase in the soyafiber content in their daily meals.

43

Insulin Treatment of Diabetes Enhances Lysosomal Enzyme Activity and Low Density Lipoprotein (LDL) Degradation by Circulating Mononuclear Cells (MC). KURT HENZE and ALAN CHAIT*, Seattle, WA.

The activity of the lysosomal enzyme acid cholesterol esterase (ACE), which hydrolyzes cholesterol esters (CE), has been shown to be reduced in arterial wall homogenates in experimental diabetes. As a result, CE could accumulate and lead to atherosclerosis. Insulin therapy corrects the impaired ACE activity. Therefore, to determine whether treatment of diabetes in man also is associated with changes in lysosomal activity, lysosomal function was evaluated in freshly isolated circulating MC before and after 1 week of insulin therapy in patients with non-insulin dependent diabetes. ACE increased from .41±.07 to 1.15±.51 nmol/10^6 cells/h (n=5; p<.05) as did the activity of N-acetyl-β-glucosaminidase (NAGA; from 1.91±.29 to 2.7±.22 nmol/10^6 cells/L; n=5; p<.05). Degradation by intact cells of the protein moiety of LDL, the lipoprotein in which most CE is transported, also increased by 25±37%; n=7; p<.05) as a result of insulin therapy. In one non-diabetic subject, infused with insulin and glucose to achieve a euglycemic hyperinsulinemic clamp, lysosomal enzyme activity increased (ACE by 75%, NAGA by 66%) as did LDL degradation by intact MC (+72%) after 4 h of hyperinsulinemia.

Thus, insulin therapy appears to enhance lysosomal enzyme activity in diabetic patients. Impaired cellular catabolism of CE-rich lipoproteins in poorly or uncontrolled diabetics could contribute to CE accumulation in arterial wall cells and play a role in accelerated atherogenesis in the diabetic.

44

Salvage of the Inoperable-Ischemic Diabetic Leg with an End-Diastolic Pneumatic Compression Boot - The Circulator Boot-TM. RICHARD S.DILLON*, Philadelphia, Pennsylvania.

The unique mechanical features of the Circulator Boot (J.Clin Engineering 5:31,1980) and its physiologic operating principles and early clinical results (Angiology, in press) have been published. In this study, 27 consecutive diabetic legs had noninvasive vascular testing both before and after a course of treatment designed to meet their clinical needs. Mean ± SD blood pressure mm Hg (% arm blood pressure) rose from 48.4±42.9 mm Hg (29.4±26.2%) and 65.0±31.2 mm Hg (41.1±19.7%) to 85.6±44.2 mm Hg (67.0±39.8%) and 98.2±40.0 mm Hg (66.3±28.9%) in the dorsalis pedis and posterior tibial arteries respectively. The height of the Doppler pulse tracings increased from 11.3±11.3 and 14.6±13.4 to 23.0±14.0 and 25.8±10.0 mm respectively in the same vessels. Oscillations increased above the ankle from 0.32±0.37 to 1.14±0.62 (normal 1-5). P values varied from <0.02 to <0.001. Of 8 legs with severe claudication, all improved symptomatically and 6 sufficiently to enjoy casual normal life. Of 8 legs with severe rest pain,relief was gained in 7 and no change occurred in 1. Of 10 legs with foot ulcers, 5 healed, 4 improved, and 1 changed little. Of 7 legs with gangrene, 3 healed, 3 stabilized, and one changed little. Minor amputations were successful in 2 patients. 3 patients had major amputations after initial success and loss to followup. Early success was more likely with early aggressive and non-interrupted treatment schedules. Longterm success was increased by close followup and booster treatment as needed.

45

Arterial Glycosaminoglycans in Diabetic Dogs. O.V. SIREK,* A. SIREK, and E. CUKERMAN. Toronto, Canada.

Glycosaminoglycans (GAG) of the arterial wall are subject to hormonal control and the sulphated variety interacts with platelets, binds calcium, fibrinogen and low-density lipoproteins. The GAG composition of a number of large and medium-sized arteries was studied in 10 alloxan-diabetic beagles and compared with 6 normal, age-matched controls. Diabetic animals were maintained on diet and insulin for 100 days. In 6 animals mean fasting plasma sugar concentrations were 150 mg/dl and in the other 4 the fasting values were nearly twice as high. The aortic arch, thoracic and abdominal segments, external iliac, superior mesenteric, renal, common carotid and coronary arteries were analyzed for hyaluronic acid (HA) and for heparan (HS), dermatan (DS) and chondroitin (CS) sulphates. Vascular chemistry was altered in all diabetic animals. Even "well" controlled diabetic dogs displayed significant alterations in that the HA content was reduced in the thoracic aorta and iliac arteries; HS or CS were increased in carotid, iliac and renal arteries. DS, a GAG constituent with a very high affinity for low-density lipoproteins, increased from 1.11 ± 0.04 to 1.34 ± 0.04 mg uronic acid per gm dry, defatted tissue (Mean ± SEM, $p<0.005$) in coronary arteries of all diabetic dogs. Two additional animals, not included in this group, did not become diabetic after alloxanization and showed no abnormalities in arterial GAG content. Early changes in the chemistry of the arterial ground substance seem to provide another clue to the precocious development of atherosclerotic disease in diabetes.

46

Decreased Collagen Extractability in Diabetes: Reversal by β-Aminopropionitrile (βAPN) and D-Penicillamine (D-pen). J.R. WILLIAMSON*, K. CHANG, J. UITTO, E.A. ROWOLD, G.A. GRANT, and C. KILO*. St. Louis, Missouri

Effects of diabetes on collagen crosslink formation and solubility were investigated in granulation tissue collagen induced by polyester fabric implanted subcutaneously in rats at the same time diabetes was produced by injection of streptozotocin. Thus, all of the collagen analyzed was formed in a diabetic milieu. Ten days later the implants were removed; total implant collagen (predominantly type I) and the fraction soluble in 0.5 M acetic acid were determined. Total collagen was the same in diabetic and control implants, however, the acid-soluble fraction in diabetic animals (8.5% ± 1.7 [SD], N=10) was only one half that of controls (17.7% ± 2.8, N=10). The ratio of β to α chains in the acid-soluble fraction was higher in diabetics (0.89) than in controls (0.69). In animals treated with βAPN or D-pen, the acid-soluble fraction of collagen from diabetics equaled that of controls. Blood glucose levels were 111 ± 14 mg/dl in controls and 369 ± 78 mg/dl in diabetics. These observations indicate that both inter- and intra-molecular crosslinks are increased in type I collagen from diabetic rats. Since these crosslinks interfere with degradation of collagen by collagenase, they may contribute to accelerated intimal sclerosis of arteries and to capillary basement membrane thickening in diabetes. Supported in part by USPHS Grant #HL 13694, NIH Research Career Dev. Award 5-K04-AM 0455, and Kilo Diabetes and Vascular Research Foundation.

47

The Relative Roles of Glucose Transport and Metabolism at Varying Glucose Concentrations in Rat Adipocytes. JAMES M. MAY,* Richmond, Va.

Insulin stimulation of adipocyte C-1 glucose metabolism relative to basal rates is optimal (500-800%) at 0.2-1.0 mM medium glucose and falls to 100-200% at physiologic glucose concentrations (5.0 mM-10.0 mM). The role of glucose transport in producing the optimal effect was examined by inhibiting facilitated glucose transport with 50 μM cytochalasin B, and by observing the insulin effect on $[^{14}C]O_2$ production from fructose, the transport of which is not stimulated by insulin. In each case the optimal insulin response was not apparent and 150-200% increments over the entire sugar dose-response range were observed. Conconavalin A and tetramethyl-p-phenylenediamine (TMPD), agents with different sites of action, produced glucose dose-response curves similar to those of insulin also with loss of an optimal response when cytochalasin B or fructose were used. At 5.0-10.0 mM glucose the insulin response was increased to 400% of basal with TMPD, but not with concanavalin A, indicating that metabolism of glucose (increased by TMPD) and not transport was rate-limiting. These studies show that at the sub-physiologic glucose concentrations commonly used in metabolic studies, the optimal responses seen with insulin or insulin-like agents are due to enhanced glucose transport. At physiologic glucose concentrations, however, the relative contribution of glucose transport to metabolism is minimal, bringing into question the importance of insulin-stimulated glucose transport in the normal state.

48

Insulin Sensitive Sugar Transport in Rat Adipose Cells: A New Model Based on Substrate Acceleration of Trace 2-deoxyglucose Uptake. JAMES E. FOLEY, ROSEMARY FOLEY and JØRGEN GLIEMANN, Aarhus, Denmark (introduced by MARIO DiGIROLAMO*,Atlanta, GA.)

In a previous study we have shown that preexposure of adipocytes to glucose (GLU) results in an acceleration of trace 2-deoxyglucose (DG) uptake above those seen in the absence of GLU. This is in contrast to the inhibition seen when GLU and DG are added together. In the present study we have measured trace DG uptake for 1-5 s in the presence of 1-20 mM substrate for 0-60 min. Phosphorylation of DG was not rate limiting during these short pulses. In the presence of insulin, 10 mM GLU had no effect for 5 min and by 30 min the effect was maximal, i.e. a 4-fold higher initial velocity of DG uptake than that seen when DG and GLU were added together. 3.5 mM GLU appears to be a threshold concentration. A smaller effect is seen in the absence of insulin (1.8 fold) using 10 mM GLU and in the presence of insulin (3 fold) using 10 mM mannose. No effect is seen using 10 mM galactose, glyceraldehyde, L-glucose, pyruvate-lactate, fructose and 3-O-methylglucose (3OMG). There is no effect of GLU preexposure on insulin-stimulated 3OMG uptakes. We have previously shown that trace 3OMG is taken up 2 times faster than trace DG even though the ability of the two sugars to inhibit 3OMG transport is the same. These observations suggest that there is an additional partially rate limiting barrier for DG uptake which is not rate limiting for 3OMG and GLU, and that this barrier becomes less rate limiting when aldose-6-phosphates accumulate. We propose that transport is across two independent barriers in series separated by an aqueous pore.

49

In *Vitro* Effects of Tolazamide on Insulin Action
Bruce Maloff and Dean Lockwood*, Rochester, N.Y.

The mechanism(s) by which a sulfonylurea exerts its insulin-like extrapancreatic effects was studied by maintaining rat adipose tissue with tolazamide (TZM, 300 μg/ml) in organ culture for 20-44 h, after which fat cells were isolated by collagenase treatment. Exposure to TZM did not alter the insulin (INS) receptor number or affinity. Basal uptake of 2-deoxyglucose (0.1 mM) was also unaffected by TZM. At each conc. of INS used (10-1000 μU/ml), an additional increase in stimulated glucose uptake of TZM-treated cells was observed (av. incr.; 30.8±2.6%, mean±SEM, $p<.005$). Similar results were found using 3-O-methylglucose. Potentiation was dependent on TZM conc. (3-300 μg/ml), and was not observed with a non-hypoglycemic TZM analog. Glucose conversion to CO_2, total lipids and lactate was determined at 0.1-50 mM glucose. TZM-treatment did not result in a difference in basal metabolism. INS-stimulated metabolism was not potentiated by TZM. Basal utilization at 0.5 mM glucose was 14.3±4.1 nm·10^5cells^{-1}·h^{-1} vs. 18.8±4.2 for the control and TZM-treated cells, respectively; the corresponding values at 1000 μU INS/ml were 43.7±14.8 vs. 44.8±11.7. The difference in TZM action on glucose transport and metabolism may reflect a differential effect of organ culture on the two systems, since under culture conditions the INS responsivity of metabolism was less than that of transport. These studies demonstrate that TZM *in vitro* alters post-receptor INS action without influencing the receptor, and that potentiation of INS-stimulated hexose transport is the major event affected.

50

Role of Microtubules in Insulin and Glucagon Stimulation of Amino Acid Uptake by Isolated Rat Hepatocytes
M. PRENTKI and B. JEANRENAUD*. Geneva, Switzerland

The effect of the microtubule (MT) inhibitor, colchicine, on the action of insulin and glucagon was investigated in isolated hepatocytes from normal fed rats. The action of these hormones on a short term effect (glycogenolysis) and a long term one (α-aminoisobutyric acid, AIB, uptake) was studied. Glucagon-stimulated glucose output or its inhibition by insulin was unaffected by the drug. Within 2 hours of incubation with insulin (0.2-5mU/ml) or glucagon (5.10^{-10}-10^{-7}M), an increase in AIB (0.1mM) uptake was observed. At maximal concentrations, insulin or glucagon stimulated AIB uptake by 2-3 and 4-6 fold, respectively. Colchicine at the low concentration of 5.10^{-7}M did not affect basal uptake of AIB but abolished the stimulatory effect of insulin, and diminished by 40% the stimulatory effect of either glucagon or dibutyryl cAMP. Protein synthesis measured by labeled valine (5mM) incorporation into proteins was unaffected by the drug. The concentration of colchicine (10^{-7}M) required for half-maximal inhibition of amino acid uptake was in the appropriate range for specific MT disruption. Lumicolchicine, the analog that does not bind to tubulin, had no effect.
These data suggest that MT appear to play a role in a long term effect (AIB uptake) of both insulin and glucagon without affecting a short term one (glycogenolysis).

51

Insulin stimulated Phosphorylation of Ribosomal Protein S6 in Differentiated 3T3-L1 Cells.
CHARLES J. SMITH, PETER WEJKSNORA, CHARLES RUBIN and ORA M. ROSEN*. New York, N. Y.

During differentiation the murine preadipocyte cell line 3T3-L1 acquires many of the morphological and biochemical characteristics of mature mammalian adipocytes, including a high concentration of insulin receptors and an insulin-sensitive hexose uptake system. Since many of the acute effects of insulin on fat cell metabolism involve pathways regulated by reversible protein phosphorylation, we incubated 3T3-L1 adipocytes with ^{32}Pi for 50 min and then added insulin [0.1-1nM] for 5-10 min. ^{32}P was incorporated into a 31,000 dalton protein identified as ribosomal protein S6 by sucrose gradient density centrifugation and two-dimensional gel electrophoresis. Incorporation of ^{32}P into this protein was more than 20-fold greater in insulin-treated cells than in control cells. Epidermal growth factor (EGF), antibody to the insulin receptor and a combination of isoproterenol and 1-methyl-3-isobutylxanthine also promoted ^{32}P incorporation into S6 although they were less effective than insulin. Cell-free extracts derived from insulin-treated cells also catalyzed the incorporation of ^{32}P from [γ^{32}P]ATP into ribosomal protein S6. The labeling of S6 *in vitro* mirrored the incorporation of ^{32}P observed in intact cells with respect to the duration and concentrations of insulin required and the efficacy of EGF and cAMP. The magnitude, specificity and sensitivity of S6 phosphorylation may facilitate elucidation of the relationship between insulin action and protein phosphorylation.

52

The Effects of Insulin on Cloudman S91 Melanona Cells
R.A. KAHN and J.M. PAWELEK, New Haven, Ct. (Introduced by VIJAY SOMAN,* New Haven, Ct.)

Insulin is a potent, reversible inhibitor of proliferation in Cloudman S91 mouse melanoma cells. Variants of S91 were isolated which differed from the wild-type (WT) in their response to insulin. Insulin resistant (INS^{res}) variants had the same doubling time independent of the presence of the hormone. One line (INS^{dep}) was found to require insulin for growth. This line was about 15 times more sensitive (half maximal response = 10^{-10}M) to the proliferative effects of insulin than the WT (half-maximal response = $1.5x10^{-9}$M). Revertants of the INS^{dep} line were selected for their ability to proliferate in the absence of insulin. Five out of 5 such revertants were insulin resistant, suggesting that the INS^{dep} line arose as a result of at least two separate mutations. Stimulation of aminoisobutyric acid (AIB) uptake and stimulation of proliferation were not under coordinate control, since AIB uptake was increased equally in the WT cells when proliferation was inhibited and in the INS^{dep} cells when proliferation was stimulated. Binding of ^{125}I-insulin was used to demonstrate the presence of insulin receptors on Cloudman S91 melanoma cells. Both the affinity and specificity of ^{125}I-insulin binding made it likely that binding was to true insulin receptors. The specificity for binding and for the effects on proliferation were the same in both WT and the insulin dependent variant. The two cell lines thus displayed insulin receptors of similar affinity and specificity. Since the effects of insulin on proliferation are opposite in the two cell lines, we propose at least two distinct sites of insulin action, probably located distal to the insulin receptors.

This work was supported by USPHS grant 5 RO1 AM 23032

53

Insulins From Phylogenetically Diverse Species Conserve Growth Promoting Activity in Human Fibroblasts. G.L. KING and C.R. KAHN*, Bethesda, MD.

Insulin's important effects on growth need to be characterized and mapped similarly to the studies on its metabolic effects (e.g. glucose oxidation). Strikingly different orders of potency were obtained when the ability to stimulate a growth response (e.g. thymidine incorporation into nucleic acid of cultured human fibroblasts) from more than 12 different species of animal were compared with their ability to stimulate glucose oxidation in rat adipocytes as a metabolic response. In general, insulin's effect on thymidine incorporation appears to be more conserved among different species than its effect on glucose oxidation. Insulins with high affinities for receptors of metabolic effects (e.g. synthetic human insulin, pork and turkey insulin) have the same relative potency in both assays. Insulin of low receptor binding affinities such as pork proinsulin, casiragua insulin, and bonito insulin show wide divergency between these two effects with an increase of 25-fold for proinsulin, 20-fold for casiragua insulin, and 3 folds for bonito insulins of thymidine incorporation active over that of glucose oxidation. Insulin degradation during these assays were checked and found to be trivial. In conclusion, the data provide, 1)strong evidence that insulin's effect on thymidine incorporation (growth effect) is due to insulin and not an impurity. 2)Support for the postulate that insulin is mediating the growth effect through a different receptor than the receptor for metabolic response. 3)Evidence that the ability of insulin to promote a growth response is more conserved evolutionarily than its ability to stimulate metabolic effects.

54

Effect of somatomedin inhibitors on insulin-like action. L.S. PHILLIPS*, T.D. SCHOLZ, Chicago, IL

Poor growth in diabetes appears due in part to circulating inhibitors which block cartilege stimulation by somatomedins. To determine if the inhibitors have other anti-anabolic effects, we examined their ability to blunt insulin-like action on adipose tissue. Rat epididymal fat pads were exposed to insulin, normal rat serum, or somatomedins (from serum on Sephadrex G-75) with or without added diabetic rat serum, or a somatomedin-inhibiting serum fraction; insulin-like activity was measured by glucose conversion to
1 CO_2. Diabetic rat serum alone lowered glucose utilization 47±8% below buffer (M±SE) but somatomedin inhibitors had no effect. Insulin and somatomedins alone gave parallel dose-response stimulation, while normal rat serum yielded a lower slope. Added diabetic rat serum produced significant decreases in stimulation by insulin (-63±5%) and somatomedins (-66±6%) but less change in stimulation by normal rat serum (-30± 16%). Added somatomedin inhibitors produced small but significant decreases in stimulation by insulin (-21±6%) and normal rat serum (-29±4%) with greater decreases in stimulation by somatomedins (-41±6%). Lineweaver-Burk analysis indicated that inhibition was generally noncompetitive.

Conclusion: Diabetic rats have marked decreases in serum insulin-like activity; somatomedin inhibitors in diabetic rat serum produce noncompetitive decreases in stimulation of adipose tissue by insulin, somatomedins, and normal rat serum. These observations suggest that circulating inhibitory factors may contribute to net tissue catabolism in uncontrolled diabetes.

55

Insulin-Like Activity of Bradykinin on Amino Acid Metabolism of the Human Forearm. R. SCHIFMANN, M. WICKLMAYR, I. BÖTTGER,*and G. DIETZE, Munich, F.R.G.

Since evidence has been accumulated that endogenous kinins might be involved in acceleration of glucose uptake occurring during muscle work and synthetic bradykinin (BK) has been found to exhibit insulin-like activity on carbohydrate metabolism also in resting muscle, it appeared of interest to investigate whether BK also mimics insulin's action on amino acid metabolism in skeletal muscle.

Therefore, balances of oxygen and of 13 amino acids across the human forearm and forearm blood flow (FBF) were determined in normal subjects during the infusion of insulin (250 μUxkg^{-1}xmin^{-1}, n=9), BK (0.2 ngxkg^{-1}xmin^{-1}, n=7) and papaverine (PA) (2 μgxkg^{-1}xmin^{-1}, n=5) into the brachial artery. Uptake of glycine, proline, valine, phenylalanine, leucine, threonine and isoleucine was significantly enhanced during infusion of insulin and the one of glycine, serine, ornithine, valine, leucine, isoleucine and tyrosine during infusion of BK. PA exhibiting an almost identical increase in FBF as BK did not show significant changes in amino acid uptake.

These findings further support the view that endogenous kinins liberated during muscle work may be involved in the work-induced insulin-like effect upon carbohydrate and amino acid metabolism.

56

Role of Calcium as a Mediator of Hepatic Hormonal Effects. J. R. WILLIAMSON*, E. MURPHY, K. COLL, J. B. HOEK*, and B. E. CORKEY*, Phila. Pa. 19104.

It has been postulated that expression of effects induced by binding of a variety of hormones to receptors may be mediated by changes of intracellular Ca^{2+} homeostasis as an alternative to the well documented role of cAMP as second messenger. In order to explore this possibility, methods have been developed using a Ca^{2+}-sensitive electrode or the spectrophotometric Ca^{2+} indicator arsenazo III to determine free Ca^{2+} concentrations in the cytosolic and mitochondrial compartments of isolated hepatocytes and hepatocytes in maintenance culture. The cytosolic free [Ca^{2+}] of normal hepatocytes was about 0.2 μM; it was unaffected by glucagon but was increased up to 3-fold by α-adrenergic stimulation. The time course and dose response relationship of changes of free Ca^{2+} closely matched those of phosphorylase a, and both effects were abolished by α- but not by β- antagonists. Cytosolic free Ca^{2+} increased as a consequence of a stimulation of Ca^{2+} efflux from mitochondria. Rapid cell disruption and centrifugation techniques showed a 25% decrease of the mitochondrial calcium, while mitochondrial free [Ca^{2+}] decreased similarly from normal values of 60 μM. These studies provide support to the concept that cAMP-independent hormonal effects are mediated by increased cytosolic Ca^{2+} and/or decreased mitochondrial Ca^{2+}, thereby affecting the regulation of protein phosphorylations by alterations of calmodulin binding. Studies are in progress to determine the mechanism of stimulation of mitochondrial Ca^{2+} efflux by the $Ca^{2+}/2H^+$ antiporter and the effects of insulin on Ca^{2+} and Mg^{2+} homeostasis.

57

Role of Ca^{2+} in α-Adrenergic Inactivation of Glycogen Synthase in Rat Hepatocytes and its Inhibition by Insulin. WILLIAM G. STRICKLAND, PETER F. BLACKMORE, and JOHN H. EXTON*, Nashville, Tenn.

α-Adrenergic activation of rat liver phosphorylase and inactivation of glycogen synthase (GS) are cAMP-independent phenomena. Much evidence indicates that phosphorylase activation by α-agonists is a Ca^{2+} dependent process (Ca^{2+} being released from mitochondria), but the possible function of Ca^{2+} in GS inactivation by α-agonists has not been defined.

In this study, the role of Ca^{2+} ions in the inactivation of GS and activation of phosphorylase by epinephrine (Epi), vasopressin (Vaso) and the divalent cation ionophore A23187 was examined. Rat liver parenchymal cells were isolated from fed animals and incubated with 30 mM glucose to activate GS. In normal Ca^{2+} containing hepatocytes, Epi, Vaso and A23187 were more potent in inactivating GS than activating phosphorylase. In Ca^{2+} depleted cells (washed and incubated with 1 mM EGTA), the effect of Epi on both enzyme activities was impaired, while the effects of Vaso and A23187 were completely abolished. Insulin (6 nM) was more effective at inhibiting the effects of Epi in Ca^{2+} depleted cells, but was without effect on Vaso and A23187 actions. These findings are consistent with the idea that α-adrenergic inactivation of rat liver GS may be due to the stimulation of a Ca^{2+} dependent protein kinase (possibly phosphorylase b kinase) by Ca^{2+} released from mitochondria into the cytosol.

(Supported in part by NIH grant AM 18660)

58

Effects of Metabolic Control of Diabetes on Glucagon's Contribution to Epinephrine-induced Hyperglycemia. F.W. KEMMER, H.L.A. LICKLEY*, D.E. GRAY, G. PEREZ* and M. VRANIC*. Toronto, Ont., Canada.

Glucagon (IRG) has been shown to mediate to a major degree the effect of epinephrine (E) on glucose production (Ra) in alloxan-diabetic but not in normal dogs. To determine if IRG's contribution to E-induced hyperglycemia depends on the degree of metabolic control, E (0.1 μg/kg-min) was infused with or without somatostatin (ST,0.1 μg/kg-min) in 5 conscious depancreatized dogs. The animals were studied when normoglycemia (basal plasma glucose, 97±5 mg/dl) and hyperglycemia (212±10 mg/dl) were induced by intraportal insulin (220 and 150 μU/kg-min) generating insulin levels of 11±1 and 8±1 μU/ml respectively. Under both metabolic conditions E induced a 150 pg/ml increase in extrapancreatic IRG ($p<0.05$) from 127±43 (normoglycemia) and 166±41 pg/ml (hyperglycemia). ST suppressed IRG below basal. In normoglycemic dogs E induced a sustained increase in Ra from 2.7±0.1 to 6.0±0.2 mg/kg-min ($p<0.01$), which was not diminished by ST. In hyperglycemic dogs basal Ra was 3.2±0.3 and rose to 6.3±0.4 mg/kg-min ($p<0.01$) with E+ST, but with E alone, Ra rose to 8.5±0.2 mg/kg-min ($p<0.01$). Plasma glucose rose by 178±22 mg/dl with E and by 127±17 mg/dl with E+ST ($p<0.01$). In conclusion: E stimulated the release of extrapancreatic IRG in depancreatized dogs. With good metabolic control and constant intraportal insulin levels, E increased Ra independent of IRG as in normal dogs, but with poor metabolic control, IRG contributed greatly to the exaggerated hyperglycemic response to E. Thus, IRG suppression may alleviate diabetic instability of stress but is not effective in countering the actions of E in normoglycemia.

59

The Effects of Portal versus Peripheral Insulin Administration. W.S.PUTNAM, D.K.ANDERSEN, J.B. HANKS, R.S.JONES, and H.E.LEBOVITZ,* Durham, N.C.

The route of insulin(INS) administration is an option in infusion device therapy of diabetes. However, the metabolic consequences of continuous portal(PORT) versus peripheral(PERI) INS infusion are unclear. PERI INS availability and sensitivity as well as hepatic glucose output(Ra) and overall glucose(G) disposal(Rd) were studied in awake normal dogs with chronic PORT venous catheters. 2 mU/kg·min pork INS was given as a primed-continuous infusion for 2.5 hr via either a PERI or PORT vein and produced stable hyperinsulinemia from 15 - 150 min. Fasting euglycemia was held constant by the PERI glucose clamp technique, and averaged 98±7% and 99±2% basal G in PERI(n=5) and PORT(n=4) studies. Ra and Rd were determined from PERI infusion of [3-^{3}H]G, begun 90 min prior to INS infusion.

INS	IRI	Ra (mg/kg·min)			Rd(mg/kg·min)	
ROUTE	μU/ml	BASAL	30-90'	90-150'	30-90'	90-150'
PERI	74±5	4.2±.8	0.2±.4	0.6±.4	9.5±1.4	12.2±2.0
PORT	36±6#	3.4±.2	1.4±.1†	1.3±.3†	5.1±.3†	6.2±.4†

= p<.01, † = p<.05 (PERI vs PORT)

PERI INS infusion caused a 2.5x greater rise in Rd than did PORT INS infusion. Hepatic INS extraction resulted in a 50% reduction of PERI IRI during PORT INS infusion. Ra, however, was not suppressed as greatly by PORT INS infusion, and ranged from 2-7x those levels seen during PERI INS infusion.

We conclude that while INS administration by either route potently suppresses Ra, PERI INS administration causes greater inhibition of Ra, and also necessitates greater G requirements to maintain euglycemia.

60

The Effect of Vagotomy on Blood Glucose Changes after Insulin Microinjections into the Hypothalamus. A.J. SZABO*, A. IGUCHI* and P.D. BURLESON. New York, N.Y.

Rapid decrease in hepatic plasma glucose concentration following stereotaxic microinjections of insulin into the ventromedial hypothalamic nucleus (VMN) suggests that this region functions as a glucoregulator center. To explore the mechanism and efferent pathway of this putative center, subdiaphragmatic vagotomy or sham operation was performed in the experimental rats one day prior to stereotaxic injection of 100 μU insulin in 1 μl saline or 1 μl saline without insulin into the VMN. Hepatic venous blood was collected from a cannula introduced through the jugular vein. Results are shown as changes in mg/dl from the baseline plasma glucose values.

		Baseline	2	5	10	20 min
Vagotomy	Insulin	127.2	+7.5	+3.5	+2.0	+12.7
		±6.1	±2.4	±1.8	±4.1	±6.1
	Saline	125.3	+4.8	+2.6	+4.6	+8.1
		±7.5	±2.6	±3.2	±2.6	±3.8
Sham oper.	Insulin	121.6	-9.3	-11.1	-12.6	-8.0
		±7.0	±2.9	±2.9	±2.5	±4.3
	Saline	117.0	+5.8	+6.3	+5.5	+4.5
		±2.7	±2.7	±3.0	±4.0	±2.1

Significant fall in plasma glucose was observed only in sham operated rats receiving insulin injection into the VMN. Vagotomy effectively blocked this insulin effect. The data suggest that fibres from the vagus nerves carry the efferent impulse from the putative insulin sensitive glucoregulator center.

61

Effect of Insulin (I) Therapy (Rx) on Insulin Resistance (IR) in Type II Diabetic Subjects (D). Evidence for Heterogeneity. H. Ginsberg* and E. J. Rayfield*, New York, N.Y.

In an effort to define the role of I deficiency in the IR of Type II-D, we measured the steady state (SS) plasma (P) glucose (G) during a constant intravenous infusion of I (80 mU/min) and G (6 mg/kg/min) in 13 consecutively recruited Type II-D before and after 6-8 weeks of I-Rx. In 8 subjects, hepatic glucose output (HGO) and PG clearance (CL) were measured by infusion of 3-^{3}H-glucose during SSPG testing.

Retrospectively, we have been able to clearly divide subjects into 2 groups: A (n=9):SSPG>150 mg/dl and B (n=4):SSPG<100 mg/dl. A and B were similar in age (53 vs 46 yrs),%IBW (1.11 vs 1.05) and HbA_{1c} before and after I-Rx. SSPI were the same in A and B during both study periods. However, SSPG was higher in A before I-Rx (347±3.7 vs 201±22.8 mg/dl; p<.01). Although both groups had lower SSPG (increased I sensitivity) after I-Rx, the difference between A and B increased (223±3.9 vs 78±2.5; p<.001). HGO during SSPG testing was greater in A before I-Rx (3.37±0.2 vs 1.89±0.1 mg/kg/min; p<.05) and the difference increased after treatment (3.62±0.4 vs 0.89±0.4; p<.05). A also had lower PG-CL. These studies suggest that the majority of Type II-D have IR that is only partially reversed by I-Rx. The IR is present in both liver and peripheral tissue. However, some Type II-D, may present with IR that is completely corrected by I-Rx. In this study no differences between the two subgroups could be identified prospectively. Thus, these data support metabolic heterogeneity in Type II-D.

62

Characterization of Insulin Resistance in Cultured Human Skin Fibroblasts. M. MARTIN, L. OLANSKY, and S. POHL,* Charlottesville,Va.

We have reported previously that chronic exposure of cultured human skin fibroblasts to insulin induces insulin resistance of α-aminoisobutyric acid (AIB) uptake by decreasing the apparent K_M for insulin (J.Biol.Chem. 254,9976,1979). AIB transport in confluent monolayers with and without chronic insulin exposure was measured as reported previously. Insulin binding was measured directly on confluent monolayers after incubation for 1.25 hr in Hanks balanced salt solution with 20 mM HEPES and 1% BSA,pH 7.4 and 0.1% μCi ^{125}I-insulin with insulin concentrations varying from 10^{-10} to 10^{-7} M. It was found that insulin-induced insulin resistance was not reversed when cells were incubated without insulin for 3 days after the resistance was established. After 24 hrs of incubation with insulin the number of receptors was below the sensitivity of the assay as compared to 3000 receptors/cell for controls. However, the apparent K_M for insulin increased linearly over time up to 48 hrs and did not change significantly thereafter. The apparent K_M for insulin was increased from 3.8 x 10^{-9} to 6.7 x 10^{-9} M when exposed to a chronic concentration of 10^{-9} M, and it continued to increase while cells were exposed to concentrations up to 10^{-6} M. In conclusion, chronic exposure to insulin at concentrations of 10^{-9} M or more produces a decrease in apparent K_M for insulin and this effect occurs over a period of 48 hrs. It is not reversed within 3 days. A decrease in receptors below the sensitivity of the assay occurred within 24 hrs.

63

Mechanisms of Insulin Resistance in Non-Insulin Dependent Diabetic Subjects(NIDDS). O.G. KOLTERMAN*, S. GRAY, J.R. INSEL, P. BURSTEIN*, J. GRIFFIN and J.M. OLEFSKY*, Denver, Colorado.

The insulin(I) resistance in NIDDS could result from decreased I sensitivity (rightward shift in the I-biologic function dose response curve) due to decreased I receptors(R), or decreased I responsiveness (diminished maximal I effect) due to a post-R defect in I action. To evaluate these possibilities, we have measured: 1) I binding to adipocytes, and 2) the dose response relationship between serum I and both overall G disposal and hepatic G production(HGP) in 8 untreated NIDDS (mean FBS 216 mg%) using the euglycemic G clamp technique. IR were decreased by 38% in the NIDDS. Three G clamp studies were performed in each subject at a serum G level of 90 ± 7 mg% with steady state I levels of 342 ± 11, 1054 ± 17, and 10,731 ± 113 μU/ml yielding G disposal rates of 131 ± 16, 138 ± 21, and 157 ± 24 mg/M^2/min in the NIDDS compared to values of 285 ± 19, 353 ± 27, and 369 ± 23 mg/M^2/min for 10 controls. At these steady state I levels, suppression of HGP was 64 ± 9, 84 ± 3, and 90 ± 3% in the NIDDS compared to values of 95 ± 3, 97 ± 2, and 99 ± 2 in controls. Thus, the G disposal dose response curve was shifted to the right with a 59% decrease in maximal G disposal rate, while the dose response curve for HGP suppression was right shifted with normal maximal suppression in NIDDS. In conclusion, the I resistance associated with NIDDS is multifactorial: 1) The defect in G disposal is due to decreased IR and a marked post-R defect in I action, and 2) impaired I mediated suppression of HGP is consistent with decreased IR with no post-R defect in this I action.

64

Dual Effect of Epinephrine on Glucose Clearance in Skeletal Muscle. J.-L. CHIASSON,* H. SHIKAMA, and J.H. EXTON,* Nashville, Tenn.

We have studied the effect of epinephrine on basal and insulin-stimulated glucose clearance in skeletal muscle. Hindlimbs from fed rats weighing 180-220 g were perfused with Krebs' solution containing 33% aged RBC, 4% BSA and 10 mM glucose. Epinephrine and/or insulin were infused for 30 min and glucose uptake was determined at 10 min intervals. Basal glucose clearance in the saline-treated hindlimbs was 0.19 ± 0.01 ml/min/100 g. When muscles were perfused with increasing concentrations of insulin (0.01-10.0 mU/ml) there was a corresponding increase in glucose clearance up to 0.50 ± 0.06 ml/min/100 g. Epinephrine at 10^{-8} and 10^{-7} M also resulted in an increase in glucose clearance to 0.25 ± 0.03 and 0.30 ± 0.02 ml/min/100 g, respectively. These same concentrations of epinephrine, however, suppressed the insulin-stimulated (1 mU/ml) glucose clearance to 0.32 ml/min/100 g. Both the stimulatory and inhibitory effect of epinephrine on glucose clearance were completely reversed by propranolol but were not affected by phentolamine. These data indicate that: 1) epinephrine has a dual effect on glucose clearance, a) a stimulatory effect on basal clearance, and b) an inhibitory effect on the insulin-stimulated clearance; and 2) these two effects are mediated via the beta adrenergic system.

65

Relative Importance of the Two Phases of Insulin Release in Glycemic Control. K. STEINER, P. WILLIAMS, S. MOUTON & A. CHERRINGTON*, Nash., TN

A 4 fold rise in glucagon (G) in the dog causes biphasic insulin(I) release & results in a plasma glucose of 120±3 mg/dl. We studied the relative importance of each phase of release in countering the effects of G on tracer determined glucose production(GP), clearance(Cg) & glycemic control in overnight-fasted conscious dogs. Following a control period in which somatostatin + basal (B) amounts of I & G were given intraportally, G infusion was increased 4 fold in the presence of 1) continued basal I, 2) a square wave increment (1.75B) in I or 3) the latter + an initial 5 min pulse (5B) in I. Glucagon caused a maximum increment in GP of 6.1±0.8 mg/kg-min in the presence of basal I but an increment of only 2.3±0.4mg/kg-min when opposed by a square wave increment in I (avΔ 5μU/ml). Addition of an I pulse (Δ at 5 min of 24μU/ml) lowered the increment in GP to 1.7±0.3mg/kg-min. In the presence of basal I glucagon caused Cg to decline by 0.7± 0.1ml/kg-min. Addition of I caused Cg to rise by an av. of 0.3±0.3 & 0.6±0.2ml/kg-min in groups 2 & 3 respectively. In the absence of extra I release G caused plasma glucose to plateau at 217±15mg/dl. The square wave increment in I reduced the level to 135±12 mg/dl, while addition of the I pulse reduced it to 119±11mg/dl. Our results show that 1) G stimulated GP is extremely sensitive to small changes in I, 2) both phases of I secretion are vital for full glycemic control, but the 2nd phase is dominant, accounting for 80% of regulation, & 3) one third of insulin's antagonism is attributable to restraint of glucose supply & the remainder to enhancement of glucose uptake.

66

Liposome-Entrapped-Insulin (LEI) Lowers Blood Glucose in Experimental Diabetes. J. ARRIETA, K.ALECK,M.SINHA,C.BROWNSCHIEDLE,J.RIGNEW,L.SHAPIRO and M.SPERLING*.Los Angeles,CA & Cincinnati,OH

We investigated the effect of orally administered LEI on blood sugar and plasma insulin concentration in the Spontaneously Diabetic BB Wistar Rat and in alloxan-induced diabetic rabbits.

Negatively charged LEI were prepared using dipalmitoyl phosphatidyl choline, phosphatidic acid and cholesterol in molar ratios of 7:2:1 . Incorporation of insulin within the liposome fraction after Sepharose chromatography ranged from 15 to 23% .All animals received a calculated dose of 5 U/kg ; RIA of Triton X-100 treated LEI yielded values in high agreement with the predicted concentrations. In the rats that responded (n = 9) basal blood glucose was 303 ± 23 mg/dl (mean±SE) falling post LEI to 175 ±28 and 176 ±28 at 1 and 2 hours post LEI (p <0.01 for each). By 4 hours the mean glucose was still lower than basal, but not significantly (244±43). Similarly, in rabbits (n = 6) LEI caused a fall in glucose from 176 ±15 mg/dl to 116±20, 102±23 and 97±20 at 1,2 and 3 hours (p <0.05 for each). In these rabbits plasma insulin rose up to 100 fold of basal.

Some batches of LEI failed to reduce glucose despite apparently adequate preparation, while even with effective batches some animals failed to respond. Oral insulin alone and plain liposomes witout insulin did not affect blood glucose.

The study demonstrates that orally administered LEI can be effective in reducing blood glucose in diabetic animals. Further development of stable effective LEI is necessary before this might be a feasible oral therapy for diabetics.

67

Normalization of Hyperglycemia in Diabetic Rats by Transplantation of Microencapsulated Islets of Langerhans. ANTHONY M. SUN,* FRANK LIM, and PAUL VASINGTON, Toronto, Canada, Richmond, Virginia, and Boston, Massachusetts.

Immunorejection of transplanted islets has made this method of treatment inapplicable for diabetes. Microencapsulation of islets in a polymer membrane which is permeable to glucose and insulin but impermeable to albmumin, antibodies and lymphocytes has been found to give protection against rejection. Histological and electronmicroscopic studies showed that the microencapsulated islets (MI) retained their morphological integrity.

In in vitro experiments, insulin secretion from MI in response to high glucose (300 mg%) was slightly, but not markedly, lower than that from unencapsulated controls (0.48 mU/hr. vs. 0.53 mU/hr). In long-term culture studies the MI remained alive and functional for more than 3 months.

When MI from Wistar rats were injected intraperitoneally into streptozotocin-induced diabetic Wistar Lewis rats, hyperglycemia, polyphagic, polydypsia, and polyuria were all brought within normal limits. Fasting blood glucose decreased from 450-500 mg% before transplantation to 70-80 mg% after. Serum insulin rose from 2-3 μU/ml to 20-30 μU/ml. Further animal experiments are in progress.

68

Effect of Whole Pancreas Transplantation on Glomerular Mesangial Enlargement in Alloxan Diabetic Nephropathy. L. FERNANDEZ-CRUZ, R.H. BELL, S. LEE, H.J. SAYERS,* AND M.J. ORLOFF,* San Diego, Ca.

Serial measurements of the glomerular mesangial area, including nuclear area, were performed over a period of 24 months in 4 groups of inbred male Lewis rats. Group I consisted of 59 normal controls. In Groups II, III and IV, diabetes was induced by the intravenous administration of alloxan (42-44mg/kg). Group II diabetic rats (N=100) were subsequently untreated. Group III diabetic rats (N=91) underwent pancreaticoduodenal transplants 1 wk after diabetes was induced. Group IV diabetic rats (N=118) underwent transplantation of the duct-ligated pancreas. Kidneys were removed monthly from sacrificed animals and stained with periodic-acid-Schiff reagent. Glomerular measurements were made with a camera lucida, and quantitative measurements were done of the mesangial, nuclear, and glomerular areas. Mean results in terms of mesangial area as a percentage of glomerular area were:

Months	Group I	Group II	Group III	Group IV
1- 6	2.56	2.67	2.74	2.78
7-12	3.22†	5.73	3.47†	3.57†
13-18	4.12†	8.42	4.97†	4.77†
19-24	5.58†	10.20	5.61†	6.15†

† = p<.0001 compared to Group II

There were no significant differences at any time between transplanted animals and normal controls. This study demonstrates conclusively that pancreas transplantation early in the course of alloxan diabetes prevents the mesangial enlargement characteristic of diabetic nephropathy.

69

Can Treatment of Diabetes with a Portable Insulin Pump Reverse Diabetic Complications? W. TAMBORLANE,* R. SHERWIN,* M. BERGMAN,* J. EBERSOLE, J. PUKLIN AND P. FELIG*. New Haven, CT.

We have shown that blood glucose can be normalized in juvenile-onset diabetics (JOD) with a portable pump that infuses insulin subcutaneously. To examine whether correction of hyperglycemia reverses diabetic complications, we studied 10 JOD (age 12-29 yrs) given outpatient pump Rx for 3-11 mos. During pump Rx, mean blood glucose (226±20 mg/dl, prepump) fell to 102±6 mg/dl (range 85-120) ($p<0.001$) and HbA_1 (15±1%, prepump) was reduced to normal in all JOD after 8 wk. The effect of pump Rx on sensory nerve conduction is shown in the table. With pump Rx, medial (M) and ulnar (U) action potential latency (LAT, msec) was reduced by 15% and amplitude (AMP, μV) increased by 50-70% (§$p<0.02$). Sural (S) nerve conduction also tended to improve.

LAT:	Prepump	Pump Rx	AMP: Prepump	Pump Rx
M	3.5±.1	3.0±.1§	6.9±.9	11.6±1.3§
U	3.2±.1	2.7±.1§	6.0±1.2	9.0±1.4§
S	3.8±.3	3.4±.5	10.7±1.7	11.4±1.9

In 4 JOD with mild nephropathy (proteinuria without azotemia), pump Rx failed to reduce proteinuria (3.3±1.3 vs 2.2±1.0 g/day, p=NS) or alter creatinine clearance. Furthermore, vitreous hemorrhages occurred 1 and 3 mos. after pump Rx in 2 JOD with proliferative retinopathy. Conclusions: Restoration of normal or near normal blood glucose levels for 3-11 mos. with pump Rx improves sensory nerve conduction in JOD. However, reversal of established microvascular complications was not observed.

70

Ambulatory Diabetes Management with Pulsed Subcutaneous Insulin Using a Portable Pump. JANET SILVERSTEIN, WILLIAM RILEY, ARLAN ROSENBLOOM,* Gainesville, Florida.

A portable pump, programmed to administer intermittent pulses of insulin subcutaneously was used by 8 patients, ages 11 to 26 yrs, for periods of 3 to 11 months. Two boys, 11 and 16 yrs, sought improved growth; 5 young adults desired control to forestall progression of microvascular complications already manifest; a 14-yr-old girl had been incapacitated by unstable diabetes. Maximal control with conventional insulin administration was attempted prior to pump use measured by glycohemoglobin (HgbAl) % and urine and blood sugar levels during 24 hrs and compared to control with pump use. All initially had reduction in 24-hr urine vol (mean 3.3L±0.4SEM-1.4 ±0.2), urine glucose (mean 198gm±81-14±4) and glycemia (mean 258mg/dl±29-135±12). % HgbAl (normal to 9.5%) declined markedly in the 5 who used the pump regularly: 14.4 to 11.4 (5 mos); 12.1 to 9.9 (3.5 mos); 13.8 to 6.8 (3 mos); 16.0 to 10.2 (5 mos); 15.3 to 9.1 (5 mos). Both boys had a doubling of growth pace (5.4 cm/yr-11.4 for 9 mos; 3.3-7.2 for 5 mos). 4 pts continue pump use after 5-11 mos because of improved sense of well-being, weight control and, in one, marked decrease in proteinuria. Cessation of use was because of inconvenience, manipulation with intermittent use, intolerance of normoglycemia or overzealous control attempts with dangerous hypoglycemia. Pump use permits the attainment of levels of control previously not possible, but is extremely demanding for patients and health personnel and must remain an experimental method in carefully selected and monitored patients.

71

Five Day Programmed Intraperitoneal Insulin Infusion in Diabetic Man. D.S. SCHADE*, R.P. EATON*, N.M. FRIEDMAN*, and W. SPENCER, Albuquerque, N.M.

The intraperitoneal (I.P.) route of insulin delivery has the advantage of direct portal vein absorption without venous thrombosis. However, experience with the intraperitoneal route has been limited. Our investigation examined the feasibility of intraperitoneal insulin delivery for 5 continuous days in brittle diabetic man.

Five day I.P. insulin infusion studies were completed in 6 diabetic males characterized by no plasma "C" peptide activity. U-40 insulin was delivered into the peritoneum by an external, portable, 560 gram rotary solenoid peristaltic pump. Acute meal-related bursts of insulin (≃ 15 units) were delivered, separated by a background infusion of ≃ 3/4 units/hour. Plasma glucose concentration was measured every 2 hours throughout the day and night. These results were compared to the glycemic control achieved when each subject was restudied for 5 days receiving subcutaneous (S.C.) insulin injection.

Mean glucose concentration in all 6 diabetics significantly declined from 161 ± 15 mg/dl in the S.C. injection study to 110 ± 6 mg/dl in the I.P. infusion study, $p<0.05$. Instability ("M" value) improved, decreasing from 57 ± 12 in the S.C. study to 14 ± 3 in the I.P. study, $p<0.05$. Hypoglycemic attacks were also reduced with the I.P. route of insulin delivery (S.C.=15; I.P.=6).

These results suggest that prolonged I.P. infusion of insulin may "normalize" plasma glucose concentration in brittle diabetic man. We conclude that I.P. insulin delivery is a potentially feasible route for an implanted insulin delivery device.

72

Human Pseudo-Islet Formation, Culture and Preservation. D.W. SCHARP*, M.M. FELDMEIER, R.V. PAJOTTE, K. DESCHRYVER, M. BELL, St. Louis,MO

We have developed an islet cell isolation technique in the dog producing first pancreatic single cells and then pseudo-islets by selective aggregation from gyrotational tissue culture. This report presents the first human pseudo-islet formation, three week culture, and cryopreservation for one year. We obtained 4 ml of chopped pancreas from a one month old male infant with Nesidioblastosis. Trypsin digestion (100 mg%) produced 5.5 x 10^7 cells with a viability of 77%. 1 x 10^6 cells from each Ficoll layer were placed in 10 ml microfernbach flasks on gyrotational tissue culture for 4 weeks using Media 199 with glutamine, 8.3 mM glucose and 10% calf serum.

Pseudo-islets were solid by four days of culture. Insulin levels in media changes from 10 flasks were 619.3 ± 49.7 uU insulin/ml/24 hr at one day and 233.4 ± 24.3, 300 ± 34.8, 270.7 ± 43.7, and 356.0 ± 51.4 on days 8, 16, 22, and 28 days of culture respectively. In Vitro testing of the pseudo-islets after one week of culture demonstrated no significant increase in insulin secretion in response to glucose challenge but did show a 4 fold increase when theophylline was added thus suggesting a fetal response. Cryopreservation to -196° C using DMSO and a 0.25° C/min freezing rate demonstrated a similar in vitro insulin release in response to glucose and theophylline after 6 and 12 months of cryopreservation. Electron microscopy confirmed the excellent preservation of the pseudo-islets. This preparation of human pseudo-islets may provide a new source of human islet tissue for transplantation.

73

Insulin Stimulates DNA Synthesis in β-Cells of Neonatal Rat Pancreas Monolayer Cultures.
A. RABINOVITCH,* and D.H. MINTZ,* Miami, Florida.

The purpose of this study was to determine whether insulin can directly influence islet β-cell replication. Islet cell monolayer cultures were prepared by trypsin-collagenase digestion of neonatal rat pancreases. DNA synthesis in β-cells was measured by incubating cultures with ^{3}H-dTR and counting labeled nuclei in autoradiographs of aldehyde-thionin stained cells. Addition of insulin (10 μg/ml) to serum-free (SF) medium significantly increased ^{3}H-dTR labeling in β-cells after three days of culture (+76%, $p < 0.001$). The stimulatory effect of insulin on β-cell DNA synthesis was dose-dependent from 0.3 to 30 μg insulin/ml, and the effects were similar in media with 5.6 mM or 16.7 mM glucose. Also, the combination of insulin (10 μg/ml) and the phosphodiesterase inhibitor, IBMX (0.1 mM) in SF, fibroblast-conditioned medium (FCM) stimulated β-cell DNA synthesis to levels significantly greater than in medium supplemented with 10% serum.

Additions to Culture Medium				% of β-Cells Labeled
Serum	Insulin	FCM	IBMX	with ^{3}H-dTR ($\bar{x}$±SEM)
vol.%	10 μg/ml		0.1 mM	
0	-	-	-	4.7 ± 0.3
0	+	-	-	8.0 ± 1.0
0	-	+	-	7.8 ± 0.9
0	+	+	-	11.0 ± 0.5
0	-	+	+	8.1 ± 0.5
0	+	+	+	15.0 ± 0.9
10	-	-	-	9.3 ± 0.9

These results suggest that insulin secreted by β-cells may regulate the growth of its own producer cells.

74

In Vivo and in Vitro Evaluation of Insulin Delivery by an Artificial Pancreas using Isolated Islets Perifused with Blood Ultrafiltrate.
G. Reach, P. Poussier, A. Sausse, R. Assan, M. Itoh, and J. Gerich,* Endocrine Research Unit, Mayo Clinic, Rochester, Minnesota and INSERM U36, Paris, France.

A potentially implantable closed-loop insulin delivery system has been developed and its function evaluated in vitro and in vivo. The device consists of a Millipore chamber containing rat pancreatic islets which are perifused with ultrafiltrate of circulating blood. Use of ultrafiltration instead of diffusion permitted rapid transmission of changes in blood glucose level to the islet compartment (less than 10 min). Insulin release from the device when the glucose concentration of ultrafiltrate of blood from normal rats was increased to 20 mM (73±11 ng/100 islets/24 min) was virtually identical to that observed when the same islets were perifused with 20 mM glucose in Krebs buffer containing 0.3% albumin (69±6 ng/100 islets/24 min, N=4). Connection of the device containing 600 normal rat islets to streptozotocin diabetic rats (N=4) restored appropriate plasma insulin levels in the recipients, decreased their plasma glucose from 411±23 mg/dl to 137±22 mg/dl ($p<0.001$) within 90 min, maintained stable normoglycemia for several hours without overshoot hypoglycemia and rendered subsequent intravenous glucose tolerance tests (0.5 gm/kg) normal. Conclusions: The ability of blood ultrafiltrate to support normal B cell function should permit avoidance of immune rejection with nonsyngenic islet transplantation.

75

Effect of Systemic Venous Drainage and Denervation of the Pancreas on Glucose Tolerance (GT) After Partial Pancreatectomy in Dogs. D. BAUMGARTNER, D. SUTHERLAND*, J. HEIL, J. HUSTAD and J. NAJARIAN Minneapolis, Minnesota

Abnormal GT after segmental pancreas transplantation (Tx) has been attributed to reduced islet mass, systemic rather than portal drainage of pancreatic blood, or denervation of the graft. To study this problem we partially pancreatectomized dogs, leaving only the tail based on the splenic vessels with the duct left open. Group I (n = 23) had no other treatment. Group II (n=4) had a denervation (with skeletonization of the vessels) of the remaining pancreas. Group III (n=8) had the splenic vein anastomosed to the vena cava to establish systemic drainage of the remaining pancreas. Comparison was made to 36 normal (N) dogs. At 2 wks mean ivGTT (.5 gm glucose/kg) K values (%) were: Grp I, -1.2±0.1; Grp II, -1.2±.2; Grp III, -1.2±.2; N, -2.0±0.1 (Grps I, II and III no difference; vs N $p < .001$). Basal insulin levels (μU/ml) were: Grp I, 6±1; Grp II, 5±3; Grp III, 7±2; N, 8±1. Mean insulin levels at 1 min were: Grp I, 32±4; Grp II, 20±4; Grp III, 28±5; N 46±4. Insulin levels from 1 to 30 min were higher in N than in experimental dogs ($p < .05$), but after 60 min were higher in the latter ($p < .02$ at 90 min). Insulin levels in Grp III (systemic drainage) were higher than in Grp I and II from 20 to 180 min ($p < .05$ at 90 min). In oral GTT (.5 gm/kg), glucose and insulin peaks (mg/dl) were not significantly different (glucose at 30 min; Grp I, 155±13; Grp II, 192±17; Grp III, 191 ± 24. Insulin at 30 min: Grp I, 12±2; Grp II, 7±3; Grp III, 13±2). Conclusion: Only reduction of islet mass is an important factor in alteration of GT after pancreatectomy and segmental pancreas Tx. An advantage for either systemic or portal venous drainage or an effect of denervation could not be demonstrated.

76

Failure of GIP to explain the Entero-insular Axis S R BLOOM*, D L SARSON & P G KOPELMAN Royal Postgraduate Medical School, London

GIP is released by oral glucose and is widely held to mediate the entero-insular axis. Fat also releases GIP. Insulin release in normal weight and obese subjects (non-diabetic) was examined using both stimuli against similar blood glucose concentrations. Eleven obese patients (215 ± 5% IBW) and 10 controls (98 ± 3% IBW) were given 100g oral glucose (OG) and one week later 10% glucose IV (IVG) to mimic the blood glucose curve seen after the subjects OGTT Six obese subjects (230% ± 6% IBW) and 6 controls (102 ±4% IBW) also were given 100g fat as unsweetened cream 60 min before IVG, as above. At 60 min glucose concentrations were similar in all tests (obese OG 6.9 ± 0.4 mmol/l IVG 6.6 ± 0.4, normals OG 6.6 ± 0.6, IVG 5.7 ± 0.4, obese IVG after fat 6.8 ± 0.5, normals 5.8 ± 0.3). GIP release after oral stimuli was also closely comparable (obese OG 29.2 ± 2.1 pmol/l, normals 37.6 ± 3.1, obese IVG after fat 37.5 ± 3.7, normals 44.3 ± 3.1). Insulin differed between OG and IVG (obese OG 1152 ± 163 pmol/l, IVG 245 ± 35, $p < 0.001$, normals OG 757 ± 146, IVG 116 ± 18, $p < 0.001$) and between OG and IVG after fat (OG obese 1152 ± 163 pmol/l, normals 757 ± 146; IVG after fat obese 647 ± 119, $p < 0.025$, normals 268 ± 20, $p < 0.01$). Gel chromatography showed 5105 MW GIP release was similar after both stimuli. Thus physiological amounts of GIP after fat, release significantly less insulin than does oral glucose with identical hyperglycaemia, and factors other than GIP must be important in the entero-insular axis.

77

β-Adrenergic Blockade Inhibits the Hepatic Response to Epinephrine in Diabetic But Not in Normal Humans. H. SHAMOON*, Bronx, NY.

Controversy remains as to the relative roles of α-and β-adrenergic receptors in the stimulatory effect of epinephrine (E) on hepatic glucose production (HGP). Therefore, HGP (3-^{3}H-glucose) was measured in 8 normals (NL) and 7 juvenile-onset diabetics (JOD) during a 5h infusion of E alone (1.2 μg/m^2/min) or E + propranolol (P). Plasma E during infusion of E (400 pg/ml) and E+P (800 pg/ml) was comparable in NL and JOD. E alone produced a 5-fold greater rise in plasma glucose in JOD as compared to NL ($P<0.001$) due to a 2-fold greater and more prolonged rise in HGP in JOD. In NL, E caused a transient (<90 min)50% increase in HGP, whereas in JOD HGP rose by 75-100% throughout the 5h infusion. When P was added to E in NL, plasma insulin was unchanged and plasma glucose and HGP rose identically as with E alone. In contrast, P completely abolished the E-induced rise in plasma glucose and HGP in JOD (HGP=2.2±0.2 mg/kg/min basal, 2.1±0.2 mg/kg/min at 5h). To exclude the possibility that an undetected fall in portal insulin accounted for the failure of P to inhibit HGP in NL, insulin (0.15 mU/kg/min) was given with E during P infusion. Despite P and a 75% rise in plasma insulin, E still produced a 50% increase in HGP ($P<0.05$). Conclusions: 1) In JOD, E-induced HGP is exaggerated but totally prevented by β-blockade; 2) in NL, β-blockade, even with simultaneous insulin infusion, does not prevent the E-induced rise in HGP. These data suggest that in JOD, but not in NL, β-adrenergic mechanisms predominate in E-mediated stimulation of HGP.

78

Quantitation of the Factors Controlling Glucose Disposal in Man. RICHARD N. BERGMAN,* LAWRENCE R. PHILLIPS,* and CLAUDIO COBELLI, Los Angeles, CA, Chicago, IL, and Padua, Italy.

We used a new method (Fed. Proc. 39:110,1980) to measure both pancreatic sensitivity to glucose and sensitivity of the periphery to insulin in 19 subjects with varying glucose tolerance (8 normal weight; 11 obese (>140%IBW); K range: 0.5 to 2.4). Mathematical models used to analyze the frequently sampled intravenous glucose tolerance test yield sensitivity of first and second phase insulin secretion to glucose (ϕ_1, ϕ_2) and peripheral insulin sensitivity (S_I). Subjects were bimodally segregated into normal tolerance (K>1.5) and lower tolerance (K<1.5). Parameters for normal weight and tolerance individuals were: ϕ_1=2.3±0.5μU/ml per mg%min, ϕ_2=4.2±0.8μU/ml per mg%min^2, S_I=5.1±1.3 min^{-1} per μU/ml. Normal weight, low tolerance individuals had a 70% decline in ϕ_1 (P<.05) and ϕ_2 secretion (P<.02) with no change in S_I. In contrast, lowered tolerance in obese subjects was due to a 55% decrease in insulin sensitivity (P<.02) despite a paradoxical 7-fold increase in ϕ_1 (P<.002) and normal ϕ_2. Lowered insulin sensitivity was not present in obese subjects with normal tolerance (ϕ_1 was increased (P<.01)). SUMMARY: Lowered glucose tolerance in normal weight individuals is due to diminished sensitivity of insulin secretion to glucose, and due in the obese to peripheral insulin insensitivity uncompensated by increased first-phase insulin secretion. CONCLUSION: This modeling-based non-invasive technique can elucidate the etiology of variable glucose tolerance in man, and may form the basis for physiologically based classification of metabolic disorders. Supp. by Juv. Diab. Fdn.

79

Dietary Prevention of Diabetes in C57BL/Ks (BL/Ks) db/db Mice. E. H. LEITER,* and A. B. EISENSTEIN,* Bar Harbor, Me., and Brooklyn, N.Y.

The gene, diabetes (db), presents in BL/Ks mice as an obesity syndrome accompanied by a severe hyperglycemia and eventual insulinopenia that reflects necrosis of pancreatic B-cells. Drastic restriction of total caloric intake over lifespan has been shown to be the only effective therapy. We have assessed the role of dietary carbohydrate and protein in modulating islet growth, function, and pathological changes. Weanling db/db and normal littermate mice were maintained for 5 mo on isocaloric diets containing either 60% sucrose, 23% casein, 8% corn oil (diet C) or 0% sucrose, 83% casein, 8% corn oil (high protein-no carbohydrate, diet HP). Mutants consumed more diet C than normals, but ate control amounts of diet HP. Mutants fed diet C exhibited 50% mortality between 4-5 mo; survivors exhibited hyperglycemia (> 500 mg/dl). Mutants fed diet HP all remained healthy at 6 mo; although body weight was twice that of normal, mutant ♀s were completely normoglycemic and ♂s were moderately hyperglycemic (ca. 200 mg/dl). Plasma IRG and IRI levels in diet HP-fed mutants were greatly elevated at 6 wk and at 6 mo; pancreatic IRG and IRI contents also increased dramatically as compared to insulinopenic mutants fed diet C. Histology of islets confirmed islet hyperplasia without necrosis in mutants fed diet HP; at 6 mo mutant ♀s on diet HP showed completely regranulated B-cells while in ♂s, only partial regranulation had occurred. These results indicate that dietary protein stimulates islet growth and function in BL/Ks db/db mice without culmination in B-cell necrosis while dietary carbohydrate seems to sensitize B-cells to necrosis.

80

Insulin Resistance in Obesity:Differential Effect on Glucose and Amino Acid Disposal. A.R.GLASS, R. BONGIOVANNI, and T.M.BOEHM*, Washington, D.C.

Obesity is associated with tissue insensitivity to insulin(INS). Since INS mediates cellular uptake of both glucose(GLU) and branched-chain amino acids such as valine(VAL), we examined whether obese subjects showed an equal impairment in disposal of GLU and VAL loads. 17 obese subjects (168±8(SE) % of ideal body weight(IBW)) and 18 control subjects (99±3 %IBW) were given IV bolus injections of 25g GLU or 4g VAL on separate occasions, and plasma GLU, VAL, and INS were measured serially. Plasma levels were fitted to single (GLU) or double (VAL) exponential disappearance curves. There was no difference between obese(OB) and control(CON) subjects in the basal plasma VAL (CON=0.22±0.02 μm/ml; OB=0.25±0.02) or basal plasma GLU (CON=86±3 mg/dl; OB=91±2). OB had higher basal serum INS than CON (15±2 vs 6±1 μU/ml; p<.01) as well as higher incremental INS response to GLU (28±4 vs 11±1 area units; p<.01). Despite this greater INS output, OB had slower rates of GLU disposal (Kg) than CON (0.84±0.06 vs 1.11±0.07 hr^{-1}; p<.01), and in the entire subject group Kg varied inversely with %IBW (r=-0.48, p<.01). In contrast, initial phase VAL disposal rate (α) was faster in OB women than CON women (14±5 vs 6±1 hr^{-1}; p<.05), and in the entire subject group α varied directly with %IBW (r=0.44, p<.01). Second phase VAL disposal rate (β) was similar in OB and CON (CON=0.16±0.04 hr^{-1}; OB=0.12±0.02). There was no correlation between Kg and either α or β. We conclude that moderately obese subjects show a divergence in the degree of impairment of glucose and branched-chain amino acid disposal.

81

Greater Hepatic Insulin (I) Extraction (HE_I) during Continuous I Infusion (CII) than Bolus I Injection (BII). R.V. RAJOTTE*, F.C. RUMPLE, G.D. MOLNAR*, G. CHMURA, D.M. FAWCETT, Edmonton, Canada

Relevant to I infusion for diabetic comas and maintenance of normoglycemia, differences between CII and BII on HE of I and glucose (G) were studied in four normal (N) and six diabetic (D) dogs.

Fasted (24 hrs), anesthetized dogs (N or D: alloxan 50 mg/kg and streptozotocin 35 mg/kg i.v.) received 0.1 unit/kg i.v. porcine I in one minute as BII, or over one hour as CII. BII and CII were in random sequence, each preceded and followed by an hour's saline infusion. Frequent simultaneous blood sampling was from catheters in portal hepatic and hind leg veins and hepatic and femoral arteries. Electromagnetic flow probes on portal vein and hepatic artery gave continuous hepatic blood flow measurements. G analysis was by G oxidase, I as IRI, glucagon as IRG.

CII yielded higher mean HE_I and HE_G. By paired analysis, mean differences between CII and BII were significant:

	HE Insulin CII	HE Insulin BII	HE Glucose CII	HE Glucose BII
	Mean ± SEM%			
N	54.15±4.24	23.35+5.85	-24.95+2.63	-42.07±6.21
D	54.04±3.84	32.17±3.06	-15.14±0.84	-19.32±1.83

Mean Difference % by paired analysis CII vs BII	HE Insulin	HE Glucose
N	33.7 p<0.001	17.12 p<0.005
D	21.9 p<0.001	4.18 p<0.05

CII may be advantageous because of higher and more constant HE_I associated with diminished hepatic G output. Effects of endogenous IRG on HE_I and HE_G are being analysed.

82

Hormone and Insulin Receptor Profiles of Patients Who Did and Did Not Develop Severe Carbohydrate Intolerance During Adaptation to Total Parenteral Nutrition (TPN). B.M. LIPPE*, S.A. KAPLAN*, S.R. LEVIN*, W.J. BYRNE, C.T. STROBEL AND M.E. AMENT. Los Angeles, CA

Mechanisms of adaptation to large doses of IV nutrients were studied in 5 adults receiving a 3.3 L 20% dextrose and AA solution over progressively shorter times in preparation for home TPN. The infusion was over 24hrs in phase (P) 1,17hrs in P-2, and 12hrs in P-3. Four subjects did not have glucosuria but #5 had marked hyperglycemia and glucosuria in P-3. In P-1 glucose (G) was about 100mg/dl with insulin (I) about 60uU/ml. In P-2, G rose slightly at initiation while I rose to a $\overline{M}$ peak of 160uU. In P-3, G rose to a $\overline{M}$ of 190mg and I to 350uU for the 4 tolerant patients. At cessation of the infusion I fell rapidly. Glucagon was somewhat increased (M=220pg/ml); cortisol and growth hormone (GH) were normal. No acute counterregulatory hormonal changes occurred with cessation but no patient became hypoglycemic. Patient #5 was unable to cope with the infusion in P-3, with G reaching 750mg. He developed responses typical of the diabetic state with relative hypoinsulinemia (peak 110uU), hyperglucagonemia (up to 750pg/ml)and increased cortisol and GH. Monocyte insulin binding was increased in P-1, decreased in P-2 and decreased further in P-3 when binding capacity and affinity were very low.

Thus, the capacity for progressive increases in insulin secretion appears responsible for the adaptation to TPN. Downregulation of insulin receptors in P-3 may aggravate the hyperglycemia but could protect against hypoglycemia in the immediate post-infusion state.

83

C-Peptide Levels and Metabolic Profiles in Diabetes. S. LEICHTER*, Lexington, Kentucky.

Important differences may exist in the clinical and metabolic abnormalities among diabetics. We analyzed metabolic parameters of 61 unselected diabetics grouped by fasting serum C-peptide levels, body weight (% IBW), or age as possible determinants of abnormalities. Patients were grouped by C-peptide into: those (n=21) (CP-L) with levels, 0.14 ± 0.04 ng/ml, lower than the normal range for nondiabetic subjects, 0.7-2.5 ng/ml; those (n=31) with levels, 1.48 ± 0.08 ng/ml, within this range (CP-N); and those (n=9), with levels, 3.29 ± 0.21 ng/ml, exceeding this range (CP-H). For all metabolic parameters studied, data for the CP-L group were better than the other groups. HDL-cholesterol levels in the CP-L group, 50.8 ± 2.3 mg/dl, were significantly higher than the levels in the CP-N group, 45.2 ± 2.9 ($p<0.03$), or the CP-H group, 36.2 ± 2.9 ($p<0.001$). Similarly, HDL-cholesterol constituted a higher percent of total cholesterol in the CP-L than CP-N ($p<0.003$) or CP-H groups (p<001). Serum triglyceride and uric acid levels were lower in the CP-L group than the others ($p<0.02$ and 0.005, respectively). Diabetic control was slightly better among the CP-L group than the others ($p<0.05$). Although % IBW and age were greater in the CP-N and CP-H group than CP-L ($p<0.01$ for all comparisons), analyses of this data by % IBW or age did not define groupings of patients with metabolic parameters as distinct as the groups defined by C-peptide. Insulin secretory reserve may itself be a determinant of certain abnormalities in lipid and uric acid metabolism in diabetes. The excellence of diabetic control is not enhanced by residual beta cell function.

84

Effects of acute changes in blood glucose on hemoglobin A1c, D. GOLDSTEIN,* S. PETH, J. ENGLAND, R. HESS and J. DA COSTA, Columbia, Mo.

Recent studies suggest hemoglobin A1c (A1c) is acutely responsive to changes in plasma glucose (GLC) limiting its usefulness as an index of long-term GLC regulation. A1c assayed by column chromatography and GLC were measured in 13 diabetics (D) and 5 controls (C) fasting, 2 and 5h after a standard meal. D but not C showed increases in A1c and GLC at 2h which returned towards baseline by 5h. ΔA1c and ΔGLC 0-2h ($\bar{X}$±SEM); 0.94±.03% and 218 ±12mg/dl. Lability of rapidly formed A1c was studied *in vitro* by measuring A1c in pre- and post-meal blood samples after saline incubations (SAL) of RBC in 0.9%NaCl for 5h at 37°C. A1c decreased in all D and C and for each subject pre- and post-meal A1c's were nearly identical. A1c was then measured pre- and post-SAL in 55D and 7C. A1c decrement was greater in D than C ($\bar{X}$±SEM; 0.91±.07 vs 0.41±.09%, $p<0.001$) and correlated with GLC and pre-SAL A1c (r's=.56 and .58, p's< 0.001). Maximal decrement in %A1c was 2% (decrease in A1c from 14.7 to 12.7%). After dialysis of hemolysates A1c decrease was similar to SAL but unlike SAL increase in A1a+b equaled decrease in A1c. Results suggest A1c exists in 2 chromatographically similar forms, a major portion not affected by short-term ΔGLC and a second form acutely responsive to ΔGLC and represents 10-20% total A1c. These may be identical to stable ketoamine and labile Schiff-base forms of A1c previously described. A1c as measured by column chromatography may reflect recent ΔGLC unless saline incubations of RBC are used.

85

Evidence of Reversibility of Hemoglobin (Hb) AIc. F. VLACHOKOSTA*, R. KOENIG, G.F. CAHILL, JR.*, and J.S. SOELDNER*, Boston, Mass.

Recent studies suggest that glycosylation of Hb is a fast, reversible process. To support this conclusion short (24 hrs) and long term (7 day) in vivo studies were done in diabetic patients controlled by an artificial beta cell (Biostator). Three not well controlled diabetic patients were included in each study.

SHORT TERM STUDY

	Pt A		Pt B		Pt C	
	BG	AIc	BG	AIc	BG	AIc
Time	mg/dl	%	mg/dl	%	mg/dl	%
0	>300	7.9	>350	13.0	>200	10.2
24 hr	100-130	7.1	100-130	12.2	100-130	9.1

LONG TERM STUDY
(7 Day)

	Pt A		Pt B		Pt C	
	BG	AIc	BG	AIc	BG	AIc
Time	mg/dl	Mean±SEM	mg/dl	Mean±SEM	mg/dl	Mean±SEM
0	>300	13.2±.2	>350	11.9±.2	>350	9.9±.2
12 hr	80-120	12.3±.1	80-120	11.2±.1	150-200	9.8±.2
24 hr	80-120	12.4±.2	80-120	11.3±.1	80-130	9.7±.1
48 hr	80-120	11.8±.2	80-120	11.0±.2	80-130	9.2±.1
7-day	80-120	11.1±.1	80-120	10.7±.1	80-130	9.0±.1

Our findings suggest that: 1) A significant fall ($p < 0.001$) of Hb AIc is seen after 12 hrs of euglycemia. 2) The relative lack of change between 48 hrs and 7 days suggest that at 48 hrs only relatively stable Hb AIc is present. In conclusion, glycosylation of Hb is in part a reversible process.

86

LDL/HDL Cholesterol Correlates with Hemoglobin Al and Improves with Insulin Therapy. J.K.SCHMITT, J.R.POOLE, S.B.LEWIS* and F.FISHER*, Oakland, CA. and San Francisco, CA.

Diabetics suffer from increased cardiovascular mortality. Epidemiological studies suggest that the ratio of Low Density Lipoprotein (LDL) to High Density Lipoprotein (HDL) is the most sensitive predictor of cardiovascular risk. In 50 fasting diabetic patients we measured Hemoglobin Al (HBAl), total cholesterol (Chol.) and the LDL and HDL cholesterol subfractions (Chol., LDL and HDL measured in mg/100 ml). Correlation coefficients (r) for HBAl vs. Chol. LDL, HDL, and LDL/HDL follow:

	Chol.	LDL	HDL	LDL/HDL
r	.46	.44	-.28	.54
p	<.001	<.001	<.05	<.001

In 8 fasting, non-ketotic patients HBAl, Chol. LDL, and HDL were measured before and after 2 months of insulin therapy (HBAl measured as percent total HB). Results follow: (Mean ± S.E):

	HBAl	Chol.	LDL	HDL	LDL/HDL
Pre	14.1±1	257±32	149±20	34±7	6.5±1
Post	9.6±.5	181±12	107±9	40±4	3.2±.3
p	<.005	<.05	NS	NS	<.05

Conclusions: 1) There is a good correlation between LDL/HDL and diabetic control in normal weight diabetic patients.
2) With improvement of diabetic control LDL/HDL decreases.

These results would suggest that long term improvement of control of diabetes may decrease cardiovascular mortality.

87

Hyper-Alpha-Lipoproteinemia (HAL) in Diabetic Children. M.H. BLANC*, R.E. GLEASON*, O.P. GANDA*, and J.S. SOELDNER*, Boston, Mass.

Hemoglobin AIc, fasting levels of HDL-cholesterol (C), LDL-C, and triglycerides (TG) were obtained in 75 insulin-dependent diabetic (IDD) boys the day after admission to the Joslin Summer Camp. 15 subjects had HAL (HDL-C ≤ 70 mg/dl, LDL-C ≤ 170 mg/dl), with no history of medication, excessive physical activity or a vegetarian diet.

	HAL	Non-HAL	p
	Mean ± S.D.		
n	15	60	-
Age (yr)	12.1 ± 1.9	12.0 ± 2.2	NS
Duration of diabetes (yr)	4.3 ± 3.3	5.3 ± 3.4	NS
Body Mass Index	18.0 ± 1.8	18.4 ± 2.6	NS
Total C (mg/dl)	193 ± 30	178 ± 35	<.05
LDL-C (mg/dl)	103 ± 29	114 ± 34	NS
HDL-C (mg/dl)	84 ± 11	54 ± 11	<.001
TG (mg/dl)	45 ± 17	51 ± 21	NS
Daily insulin dose: (units/kg)	0.64 ± 0.23	0.81±0.28	<.02
Hb AIc (%)	10.1 ± 2.8	10.0±2.1	NS

Conclusions: 1) The 20% of the IDD with HAL were indistinguishable from the non-HAL with regard to demographic and diabetes related characteristics except daily insulin dose. 2) Subjects with HAL appear to require relatively less insulin. 3) Further studies are needed to characterize the apoproteins in HDL and the plasma free insulin levels. 4) Patients with HAL, despite their diabetes, may be at a lower risk for arteriosclerotic cardiovascular disease.

88

Impaired Myocardial Performance in Children With Type I (Insulin-dependent) Diabetes Mellitus. NANCY E. FRIEDMAN, LYNNE L. LEVITSKY,* DEBORAH V. EDIDIN,* DOLORES A. VITULLO, SAMUEL J. LACINA, PIPIT CHIEMMONGKOLTIP, Chicago, Ill.

Myocardial performance was assessed by M-mode echocardiography in 25 children (ages 6 8/12-16 5/12) with Type I (insulin-dependent) diabetes mellitus of greater than 1 year's duration and in 21 normal children (ages 6 2/12-18 8/12). In order to assess myocardial contractility, ejection fraction and minor axis shortening were obtained from digitized tracings. The mean ejection fraction of the diabetic children was 57.7±1.3% and of controls was 63.8±2.0% ($p<.02$). Mean minor axis shortening in the diabetic children was 25.2±1.1% while in the normals it was 30.8±2.0% ($p<.02$). Nine diabetic children had an ejection fraction more than 1 SD below the mean of the normals and 7 had minor axis shortening more than 1 SD below the mean. Glycohemoglobin levels in children with diabetes (15.8±0.6%, range 10.6-21.7%, normal 5.9-8.7%) correlated with clinical assessment of control ($p<.01$). Age, glycohemoglobin levels, duration of diabetes and clinical assessment of control could not be used to predict myocardial function. We conclude that there is impaired myocardial contractility in some children with insulin-dependent diabetes which is not correlated with duration of diabetes, age, clinical assessment of control or glycohemoglobin levels. The long-term significance of this phenomenon and the effect of improved control remain to be assessed.

89

Insulin Administration Prevents Changes of Myosin Isoenzyme Distribution in the Heart of Diabetic Rats. WOLFGANG H. DILLMANN*, San Diego, CA.

Decreased contractility has been reported in the diabetic heart. The activity of Ca^{++}activated ATPase of purified cardiac myosin ($MCa^{++}ATPase$) is closely correlated to contractility. In addition, it has been shown that ventricular myosin (M) can be separated by pyrophosphate gel electrophoresis into 3 isozymic forms, M-V_1, M-V_2, M-V_3. M-V_1 has the highest mobility and $MCa^{++}ATPase$ (1.3±0.18U), whereas M-V_3 has the lowest mobility and $MCa^{++}ATP$ase (0.12±.02U). M-V_1 and M-V_3 are authentic isoenzymes of M containing a different species of myosin heavy chain. In control (C) rats M-V_1 predominates representing 72%, while M-V_3 constitutes 10% of M. A marked change in isoenzyme distribution occurs in diabetic (D) rats where M-V_3 represents 69% and M-V_1, 12% of M. Due to the predominance of M-V_3 in D, the $MCa^{++}ATPase$ is decreased by 40% from C levels. To investigate the influence of insulin (I) administration on M isoenzyme distribution and $MCa^{++}ATPase$, rats were made D by streptozotocin (65mg/kg BW). Half of the D rats were treated with 2U PCI/day for 4 wks (D+I). When animals were killed, blood sugar was 130±5mg/dl in C rats; 425±71 in D and 183±9 in D+I. Insulin treatment led to a normalization of isoenzyme distribution. In D+I rats, M-V_1 was 70% and M-V_3 10% of total M, vs. 10% M-V_1 and 70% M-V_3 in D rats. In addition, I treatment increased $MCa^{++}ATPase$ from 0.62±0.08µmoles Pi/mg protein/min in D to 1.35±0.25 in D+I. In C, $MCa^{++}ATPase$ was 1.28±0.2µ moles Pi/mg protein/min. Insulin treatment of D rats thus normalizes $MCa^{++}ATPase$ activity by reverting isoenzyme distribution from M-V_3 to M-V_1 predominance.

90

The Effect of Strict Metabolic Control on Residual β-cell Function. A Control Study. S. MADSBAD, C. BINDER*, T. KRARUP, L. Regeur, Copenhagen, Denmark.

The aim was to test whether improvement of metabolic control induces functional regeneration of β-cells in IDDM.

Within 24 hours of diagnosis 15 consecutive patients were randomly allocated to one of two treatment groups: Group A (n=9) treated conventionally (mean BG 11.7±0.5 mmol/l), group B (n=6) treated with 9 daily injections of soluble insulin for 10 days (mean BG 6.4±0.3 mmol/l) and then conventionally. β-cell function was evaluated on day 1,7,14,90, and 180 by means of plasma C-peptide (CP) response to a standard meal.

Average sensitivity of the β-cells to glucose changes in group B was 46 pmol CP/mmol glucose on day 7 and 65 on day 14. This was significantly higher than that of group A (16 and 33 pmol/mmol). CP secretion on day 14 was 18.2±2.6 nmol in group A and 29.0±3.6 nmol in group B ($p<0.05$).

On day 90 both sensitivity and CP secretion had increased further ($p<0.05$) to 43 pmol/mmol and 25.4±4 nmol in group A. Group B exhibited a decline in sensitivity ($p<0.05$) to 30 pmol/mmol and in CP secreted to 24.7±6.6 nmol. On day 180 sensitivity as well as CP secretion had declined in both groups now showing no significant difference.

A similar study of 6 patients with longer duration of disease showed significantly improved β-cell function after one week of group B treatment.

The data show that strict metabolic control leads to functional regeneration of β-cells and further that β-cell function and metabolic control are mutually related.

91

Hypoglycemia may cause intravascular coagulation in juvenile diabetics. J. HILSTED, J.D. NIELSEN, L. SESTOFT*, J. GORMSEN, Copenhagen, Denmark.

Hemostatic parameters were assessed before insulin-induced hypoglycemia and 0, 1 and 2h after discountinuation of insulin infusion in 6 juvenile diabetics, age 32(27-35)ys (mean and range), duration of diabetes 5(0.5-10)ys. The patients were normoglycemic for at least 10h preceeding the study.

Serum glucose levels were 6.5(3.3-10.7)mmol/L before hypoglycemia, 1.7(1.2-2.2)(0h),3.6(2.7-5.3)(1h) and 6.2(3.9-9.7)(2h). Threshold concentrations of ADP required to induce irreversible platelet aggregation was 1.5(1.0-16)µmol/L before hypoglycemia, 0.5(0.25-16)(0h),2.0(1.0-16.0)(1h) and 3.0(1.0-16.0)(2h). Recalcification time in PPP was 132(101-173)sec before hypoglycemia, 97(78-116)(0h),86(59-119)(1h) and 84(64-99)(2h), $p<0.05$. Euglobulin clot lysis time was 136(60-336)min before hypoglycemia, 64(34-110)(0h), 89 (45-141)(1h) and 99(61-138)(2h),$p<0.05$. Platelet counts were 254(168-356) x 10^9/L before hypoglycemia,263(170-400)(0h),226(134-307)(1h) and 213 (103-304)(2h),$p<0.05$. The ethanol gelation test was positive in two patients (1h and 2h).

The enhancement of platelet aggregation followed by a reduction in platelet counts suggests that hypoglycemia causes intravascular platelet aggregation, and the simultaneous acceleration of blood coagulation may lead to intravascular coagulation as indicated by the appearance of a positive ethanol gelation test in two of the patients. The demonstrated abnormalities in hemostasis may play a role in the development of thrombo-embolic complications in juvenile diabetics.

92

Effectiveness of aprotinin (TrasylolR) in Protease-Mediated Insulin (In.) Resistance. G. FREIDENBERG, N. WHITE, S. CATALAND, T. O'DORISIO, J. SOTOS*, J. SANTIAGO*. Cols. OH, St. Louis, Mo.

Five female diabetics, ages 14-27 yrs., developed resistance to subcutaneous (s.c.) In. (2.5-8.5 U/kg/d), as described by Paulsen et al, and had for a period of 2-5 yrs, erratic control, frequent ketoacidosis, and days of hypoglycemia despite no In. administration. Regular pork In. by frequent injections or by s.c. open loop pump resulted in no consistent improvement. Glucocorticoids had no benefit. Control could be easily achieved with constant I.V. In.(0.35-0.9 U/kg/d). Three patients required constant I.V. In. for months. In. antibodies and excess of counterregulatory hormones were excluded. A mixture of Trasylol (Bayer, A.G., F.R.G.), a protease inhibitor, and regular pork In. was given by bolus or pump s.c. Effectiveness was evident from the beginning. With Trasylol, In. levels increased, euglycemia was attained, and ketonuria disappeared.

	prior to Trasylol	during Trasylol	currently
In.(U/kg/d)	4.0 (1.8-6.3)*	1.0 (0.7-1.4)	0.9 (0.6-1.4)
blood glucose (mg%)	323 (117-538)	127 (91-199)	-
glucosuria(gm/d)	(105-308)	(0-65)	0

*mean (range)

Four patients have been well-controlled at home for 3-12 weeks with 2-4 injections daily,and a fifth with a pump (0.6-1.4 U/kg/d), with no adverse effects. The findings support a form of In. resistance resulting from degradation of In. at the injection site and offer the first practical and effective method of management.

93

Fasting and Refeeding Control Expression of the Rat Insulin Gene. STEVE GIDDINGS, JOHN CHIRGWIN, and ALAN PERMUTT*, St. Louis, MO.

Pancreatic insulin content and glucose-stimulated insulin biosynthesis decrease with starvation. β-cells regranulate rapidly with refeeding. To determine whether alterations of preproinsulin mRNA (PPImRNA) could account for these effects, rats were fasted for 4 d and refed for 8, 24, and 48h. Islet mRNA was measured by incorporation of [^{35}S]methionine into protein in an mRNA dependent wheat germ cell-free protein synthesizing system. PPImRNA was estimated by electrophoresis of the translation products. Plasma glucose fell from 6.1±0.5 mM ($\bar{x}$±SE, n=6) to 2.2±0.5 mM and returned to 4.8±0.4 mM with 24h of refeeding. Total islet RNA fell by 50%. Islet mRNA activity was 75±4x10^3 cpm/μg RNA in controls and fell to 25±7x10^3 cpm/μg RNA (p<.001) on fasting. Refeeding for 8h restored translational activity to control values, 80±1 cpm/μg RNA. Refed 24 and 48h values were 150% of controls, 113±1 and 109±3 (p<.001). PPImRNA was 20% of the translational activity in control, 40% in fasted, and 31, 20, and 20% in 8, 24, and 48h refed animals. Fasting decreased PPImRNA by 2/3 even though it was more stable than total message. Only increased rates of PPImRNA synthesis can explain the increase to 150% of control values during refeeding. To assess degradation, fed and 12h fasted rats were given actinomycin D (100 μg/kg). While mRNA synthesis was blocked, fasting still decreased PPImRNA by 50% over a further 10h, indicating increased rates of degradation. These experiments demonstrate that fasting increases the rate of degradation and refeeding increases the rate of synthesis of rat PPImRNA.

94

The Kinetics of ^{65}Zn and ^{45}Ca Uptake in Granules Isolated from Rat Islets of Langerhans. B. FORMBY, D. FIGLEWICZ, F. SCHMID, A. HODGSON, and G.M. GRODSKY,* San Francisco, CA.

Histochemical studies have suggested that B-cell zinc is almost exclusively concentrated in granules, presumably associated with insulin. We found that ^{65}Zn uptake in islets cultured for 24 hr with high or low glucose is a slow process, approaching equilibrium by 24 hr. ^{65}Zn and total endogenous zinc associated with the granular fraction (sucrose gradient) were only 9.5% and 20% of the gradient distribution. ^{65}Zn had not equilibrated with granular endogenous zinc pools by 24 hr. Nevertheless, granular zinc content is sufficient for formation of 2-zinc insulin hexamers. Direct uptake of ^{65}Zn by granules was measured in a 3,000 x g islet supernatant, incubated 20 min at 37°C and pH 7.2. Granules were subsequently isolated on a sucrose gradient. Parallel experiments measuring ^{45}Ca uptake were run as controls. Granular uptake of ^{45}Ca (10 μM) was enhanced 5-fold by 2 mM ATP. ^{65}Zn was taken up in a dose-dependent manner, reaching maximal uptake at a concentration of 5 μM. Uptake was significantly inhibited by 2 mM ATP. ^{65}Zn uptake was also inhibited by the addition of non-hydrolyzable AMP-PNP. ATP-dependent ^{45}Ca uptake was unaffected by Zn, and ^{65}Zn uptake was unaffected by addition of Ca.

In conclusion, these studies show that granules can take up zinc directly by a non-energy-requiring process, whereas ^{45}Ca uptake is energy-dependent. The slow equilibration of ^{65}Zn with granular zinc and the inhibitory effect of ATP on direct ^{65}Zn uptake suggest zinc normally enters granules during their de novo synthesis.

95

Use of a High Voltage Technique to Determine the Molecular Requirements for Exocytosis in Islet Cells CAROLINE S. PACE,* Birmingham, Alabama

Islet cells were subjected to high voltage discharges to render the plasma membrane permeable to small molecular weight substances. Rat islets were subjected to 10 pulses of 2.5 KV/cm (τ = 250 μ sec). Ca^{++} was added to a medium containing EGTA to yield levels of free Ca^{++} from 10^{-8} to 10^{-5} M. Islets preloaded with $^{86}Rb^+$ and then shocked in a medium containing 1 μM Ca^{++} released 92% of the radioisotope within 1 min as compared to a 55% loss from nonshocked islets. Exposure of the islets to ^{14}C-urea and ^{3}H-sucrose at 15 to 20 min after exposure to high voltage discharges indicated that 80% of the intracellular space was occupied by sucrose, whereas sucrose was excluded from nonshocked islet cells. The pores in the plasma membrane resealed between 20 and 30 min after initial formation as indicated by cellular exclusion of sucrose. The [Ca^{++}] yielding half-maximal and maximal secretory responses from shocked islets were 10^{-7} and 10^{-6} M, respectively. The addition of 1 or 5 mM ATP, but not 1 mM glucose, glucose-6-phosphate, phosphoenolpyruvate, or 3-phosphoglycerate augmented the secretory response of shocked islets to 1 μM Ca^{++}. An increase in Mg^{++} from 2 to 10 mM reduced the secretory response to 1 μM Ca^{++} by 63%. Islets, subjected to the high voltage discharges and allowed 30 min to reseal, exhibited a normal secretory response to 16.7 mM glucose. The results indicate that the high voltage technique induces reversible pore formation in β-cells for introduction of ions and solutes into the intracellular environment to determine the factors controlling exocytosis.

96

Role for Calmodulin in Stimulus-secretion Coupling for Insulin Release; Lack of a Role in Exocytosis. YODPHAT KRAUSZ and GEOFFREY W. G. SHARP,* Boston, Ma.

An increase in cytosolic Ca^{++} is an important step in stimulus-secretion coupling. The role of calmodulin (a calcium-dependent regulator protein) in the control of insulin secretion has been examined by the use of trifluoperazine (TFP), a specific inhibitor of the calmodulin-Ca^{++} complex. Rat islets of Langerhans were incubated in KRB buffer for 30 min at pH 7.4 and 37° with various stimulators of insulin release, and in the presence and absence of 100 μM TFP.

TFP inhibited the stimulation of insulin release due to 16.7 mM glucose by 68 ± 4.6%, p<0.001, n=17 (95 ± 12.5 vs. 26 ± 3.9 pg/islet/min). TFP inhibited insulin release induced by D-glyceraldehyde (10 mM) to the same extent, 68 ± 8.8%, p<0.01, n=7. However, insulin release due to 1 mM 3-isobutyl-1-methylxanthine (IBMX) at 2.8 mM glucose was unaffected by TFP (66 ± 4.6 vs. 72 ± 6.2 pg/islet/min, n=7). Release due to the combination of IBMX and 16.7 mM glucose was inhibited by TFP (187 ± 13.9 vs. 151 ± 5.6 pg/islet/min, p<0.05, n=7). However, the increment of insulin release due to IBMX was unaffected, suggesting that only the glucose-stimulated portion of the release was sensitive to TFP. As IBMX is thought to stimulate insulin release by mobilizing intracellular calcium to raise the cytosol Ca^{++} concentration, it is concluded that this mechanism, and exocytosis, is independent of calmodulin. It is also concluded that calmodulin is involved in stimulus-secretion coupling at some point subsequent to the triose steps in glucose metabolism but prior to the elevation of cytosolic Ca^{++}.

97

Restoration by Ouabain of Glucose-Induced Insulin Release in the Absence of Extracellular Ca. E.G.SIEGEL, C.B.WOLLHEIM, A.E.RENOLD* and G. W.G.SHARP, Geneva, Switzerland.

Inhibition of Ca efflux by glucose may contribute to the increase in cytosol Ca^{++} involved in insulin release. Ca extrusion may occur via Na/Ca countertransport driven by the inward Na gradient, in turn maintained by the Na/K pump. Accordingly, inhibition of this pump by 1mM ouabain(O) was compared to effects of glucose(G), 16.7mM. ^{45}Ca efflux and insulin release were measured from perifused rat islets loaded for 2 days with ^{45}Ca. During perifusion at zero Ca, G rapidly inhibited ^{45}Ca efflux, as did O initially, albeit with still more rapid onset. The inhibitory effects of G and O were not additive suggesting that G also affects Na/Ca countertransport. When zero Ca was applied at the time of G-stimulation both phases of insulin were greatly reduced, either as a result of lack of extracellular Ca or of rapid loss of cellular Ca. However, when O was added together with G, or when the Na/K pump was inhibited by removal of K, first phase insulin release was completely restored in the absence of extracellular Ca, and second phase returned to about half-normal. The restoration is probably due to rapid prevention of cellular Ca loss by Na/K pump inhibition. O alone only caused a small, late rise of insulin release. Thus, 1) Glucose may inhibit Ca efflux by interfering with Na/Ca countertransport. 2) Glucose does not need Ca influx to generate first phase, but uses cellular Ca for the first and part of second phase of insulin release.

98

Actin Levels in the Islet. J.KELLY, A.E.BOYD III*, J. BRYAN and B. R. BRINKLEY, Houston, Texas.

We have initiated studies to investigate actin polymerization during insulin secretion. An actin antibody was purified from a patient with chronic hepatitis using an actin affinity column. With indirect immunofluorescence, selective staining of the stress fibers was noted in beta cells grown in monolayer cultures. Treatment of the cultures with cytochalasin B disrupted these actin cables. Actin was measured by the DNAase I assay of Blikstad et al (Cell 15:935,1978) in islets isolated from 10 fed and 10 fasted hamsters. The islets were lysed with 0.5% Triton X-100, homogenized and centrifuged at 12,000g for 10 min. G-actin was measured in the supernatant. The F-actin in the cytoskeleton was measured after depolymerization with 0.75M guanidine-HCl. Actin averaged 1.2% of the total islet protein. Although there were no differences in total actin levels (range 10.5-14.3ng/µg of islet protein) access to food resulted in a 3-fold decrease in the F-actin content. The F-actin values for fasted and fed animals expressed as % of total actin were 17.8±7.0 (SD) vs 6.0±8.0% (p<.005) or 2.2± 1.1ng of actin/µg of total protein vs 0.7±0.9ng/µg protein (p.<005). Ten % polyacrylamide SDS gels of islet cytoskeletons isolated from fasted and fed hamsters revealed a band which comigrated with a rabbit muscle actin standard and was decreased in cytoskeletons from fed animals. Thus the assembly state of actin filaments in islets seem to change depending on the physiologic state of the animal. The decrease in F actin levels in fed animals and the known faciliatory effect of cytochalasin B on insulin secretion suggests a role of actin polymerization in insulin secretion.

99

Direct exchange of nucleotides between pancreatic endocrine cells. PAOLO MEDA, MYLENE AMHERDT, ALAIN PERRELET, and LELIO ORCI,* Geneva, Switzerland.

Intercellular transfer of molecules via specialized regions of the cell membrane, the gap junctions, may play a role in coordinating the secretory activities of the different endocrine cells of the islets of Langerhans. To substantiate this hypothesis, we determined whether endogenous nucleotides were directly exchanged between islet cells in monolayer culture. Islet cells isolated from newborn rats and loaded with ^{3}H-nucleotides after exposure to ^{3}H-uridine (donor cells) were co-cultured with other islet cells devoid of such cytoplasmic labelled molecules (recipient cells). The latter cells were identified by a nuclear labelling following exposure to ^{3}H-thymidine. The transfer of impermeant ^{3}H-nucleotides from donor to recipient cells was assessed by light and electron microscope (EM) autoradiography. The presence of autoradiographic grains over the cytoplasm of recipient cells indicated that ^{3}H-nucleotides had been transferred from donor cells. Such a transfer did not occur via the medium, and took place only between adjacent cells, i.e. cells likely to share gap junctions. EM autoradiography showed that nucleotide exchange occurred between fully differentiated B-cells, and between B- and neighbouring non B-cells. These results show that islet cells are able to directly exchange endogenous nucleotides. The cell-to-cell exchange of molecules to be now defined, may participate to establish a coordinate secretory output of similar and different islet cell types according to needed hormonal balance.

100

Modulation of Insulin and Glucagon Secretion by Local Somatostatin Secretion in the Perfused Chicken Pancreas. R.N. HONEY and G.C. WEIR*. Richmond, Va.

Pancreatic somatostatin has been hypothesized to regulate insulin (I) and glucagon (G) release by local secretion. I and G secretory responses to 8-minute infusions of neutralizing doses of somatostatin sheep antiserum (SSA, Arimura) were measured in the isolated perfused chicken pancreas with duodenum excluded. Effluent concentrations of I and G were measured by radioimmunoassay. In some experiments the perfusate glucose concentration was the normal avian level of 250 mg/dl and in others it was 750 mg/dl.

I effluent concentrations in response to SSA rose rapidly from a baseline average of 5±4 µU/ml to a peak of 32±23 µU/ml at 250 mg/dl glucose. A more pronounced stimulation of I release by SSA was evident at 750 mg/dl glucose. G secretion was promptly stimulated by SSA at 250 mg/dl glucose with the effluent baseline average of 41±14 pg/ml rising to a maximum of 886±87 pg/ml. At 750 mg/dl glucose, G output was rapidly stimulated to the same magnitude by SSA. Control serum did not provoke any change in either I or G release.

These experiments provide direct evidence that endogenous somatostatin secretion continuously suppresses I and G secretion. The effect of SSA on I may be indirect via G. Glucose suppression of G secretion appears to be largely dependent upon local somatostatin secretion.

101

In Vitro Insulin Cycles from the Isolated Canine Pancreas - Possible Control by an Intrinsic Non-adrenergic Nervous System. J. STAGNER and E. SAMOLS*, Louisville, Ky.

Cyclic hormone secretions from the human and monkey pancreas in vivo have recently been confirmed. The liver has been assigned the central role in the production of hormone cycles by pulsatile glucose release. The isolated canine pancreas, perfused in vitro with a constant glucose concentration, demonstrates cyclic insulin secretions similar in period to in vivo cycles. In this in vitro system, the presence of cycles negates the theory of direct hepatic control of cycles and suggests that they may be independent of, but possibly modulated by, the central nervous system. Cycles were disrupted for the duration of infusions of acetylcholine, epinephrine and dopamine by shifting insulin secretion beyond the limits of cycles. Mechanically induced changes in intrapancreatic pressure and flow rate abolished cycles only while being applied. Cycles were not altered by both single and combined infusions of the autonomic blockers propranolol, atropine, dibenzyline, butaclamol and phenothiazines. Initial data from infusions of inhibitors of nerve and ganglionic transmission such as GABA, tetrodotoxin and hexamethonium support the theory of an intrinsic nervous coordinating system. Conclusions: 1) Insulin cycles are not secondary to glucose 2) cycles are not the result of pressure or flow rate changes across the pancreas 3) cycles may be overridden by external nervous modulation 4) cycles may be regulated by an intrinsic nonadrenergic neural system which may serve as a pacemaker and/or communication network to regulate individually secreting islets.

102

The B-Cell Degrades Stored Insulin: A Third Mechanism Controlling Insulin Content. P.A. HALBAN* and C.B. WOLLHEIM, Geneva, Switzerland.

Glucose homeostasis is critically dependent on pancreatic insulin stores.Control of insulin stores is thought to reflect a balance between biosynthesis and release.A third mechanism,intracellular degradation of stored insulin,was studied.Rat pancreatic islets were labelled in culture for 3 days with (^{3}H)leu at 8.3mM glucose (G),followed by a 24h chase.Under all conditions studied,total radioimmunoassayable islet insulin remained unaltered.Radioactive insulin (I*) was measured by immunoprecipitation.I* in islets reached a steady state value of 814±23 dpm/islet during the labelling.A 24h chase at G 8.3mM lowered islet I* to 385±49 dpm/islet,while I* release into the medium was 122±14 dpm/islet. Total I* (islets + medium) was thus reduced from the initial value of 814 dpm/islet to 507.Insulin degradation in the medium was <10% over 24h. Recycling of (^{3}H)leu and reuptake of released insulin were negligible.The loss of 38% of the stored I* therefore occurs by degradation within the B-cell itself.Interestingly,loss of I* from islets due to degradation was greater than the 15% due to release.A 24h chase at G 2.8mM resulted in only 5% I* release and 40% degradation, whilst at G 16.7mM, 47% of stored I* was released and only 8% degraded.The degradation of striking amounts of insulin by the B-cell may be of importance in the regulation of pancreatic insulin content,a mechanism already proposed for other hormone synthesizing cells.

103

A Rise in Ambient Temperature Accelerates Insulin Absorption from the Injection Site. V. KOIVISTO+ and S. FORTNEY, Helsinki, Finland, and New Haven, CT.

Insulin-treated diabetics may experience hypoglycemic symptoms after heat exposure. To examine the mechanism of hypoglycemia after heat exposure, we measured the absorption of 125-I-Actrapid insulin in 6 juvenile diabetics at 35°C, and in 8 patients during and after a sauna at 85°C. Over a 4 hour period at 35°C, insulin disappearance rate was enhanced by 50-60% as compared to room temperature (20°C) ($p<0.01$). The rise in insulin absorption was accompanied by a 25% increase in skin temperature ($p<0.05$) and a 2.3-fold increase in skin blood flow ($p<0.01$). The sauna(25 min. x 2 at 85°C) accelerated insulin absorption by 110% as compared to room temperature ($p<0.01$). At 35°C blood glucose levels tended to be 20 to 25 mg/dl lower than at room temperature, and after sauna, blood glucose was 55 to 60 mg/dl lower than on the control day ($p<0.05$). Furthermore, the fall in blood glucose level after the sauna was proportional to the increase in insulin absorption rate ($r = 0.80$, $p<0.01$).

Conclusions: 1) A rise in ambient temperature augments skin blood flow and insulin absorption, resulting in diminished blood glucose levels. 2) The hypoglycemic effect of the sauna is, at least in part, due to enhanced insulin absorption from the injection site.

104

The Accuracy of Various Methods for Home Glucose Monitoring. N. A. KEANE*, R. S. CLEMENTS, JR.*, and K.A. KIRK, Birmingham, AL.

We evaluated three reagent-strip techniques for the estimation of blood glucose concentration and compared the results with the serum glucose concentration as determined by the ferricyanide technique in 75 samples of blood obtained from patients with diabetes mellitus. Visual inspection of Dextrostix provided a crude estimate of the glucose concentration when the serum glucose concentration was below 250 mg/dl ($r = 0.84$). However, the residual variation with this technique was large (1814.0) and 32% of the determinations were in error by more than 20%. In contrast, when the Dextrostix were quantified with the aid of a reflectance meter, the correlation with the actual serum glucose concentration was excellent ($r = 0.95$), the residual variation was smaller (887.8), and only 11% of the determinations were in error by more than 20%. Similarly, the visual inspection of Chemstrips provided an excellent estimate of the serum glucose concentration ($r = 0.97$), the residual variation was small (629.3), and only 11% of the determinations were in error by more than 20%.

We conclude that both the Dextrostix-reflectance meter technique and the visual inspection of Chemstrips technique are sufficiently accurate to be useful in the estimation of blood glucose concentrations. The latter technique has the advantages that it is slightly more accurate, is technically easier to perform, and is less expensive since it does not require the purchase of a reflectance meter.

105

Home Monitoring of Blood Glucose by Chemstrip. SR. J.G. SILVESTRI, L.R. ATLES, and L. MILLER*, Los Angeles, Calif.

The beneficial effects of home monitoring of blood glucose on: biochemical parameters of diabetes control, on neonatal outcome of infants of diabetic mothers, and on patient self-reliance and compliance have been well-documented (Diabetes Care 3, 57-186, 1980). Patient acceptance has generally been good when professional support and educational programs have been well-planned and executed. One impediment to more widespread use of this technique has been the cost. The two reflectance meters currently on the U.S. market are the Stat-Tek, $650, and the Eyetone, $550. The cost of each blood test using the Eyetone with Dextrostix and controls is $2.00, and with the Stat-Tek and Chemstrip .52¢.

We have evaluated the use of the Chemstrip alone. It is relatively simple to use as no washing is necessary, and its two-color tip facilitates matching with the standard chart. We have found that the measurement of blood glucose with the Chemstrip alone, and with the Chemstrip and Stat-Tek reflectance meter, correlate well with measurements of blood glucose using a laboratory method. The coefficient of correlation between the Chemstrip and Chemstrip with Stat-Tek is .96; the Chemstrip and laboratory .98; and the Stat-Tek and laboratory .99.

It appears that the use of the Chemstrip for home-monitoring of blood glucose is a simple, reliable, and viable alternative to the use of other more expensive methods of monitoring.

106

Reducing Diabetic Ketoacidosis Hospitalizations. LISA PARKER, GAIL GUNTER-HUNT, MARTHA SPENCER*, Ann Arbor, Mi.

The purpose of this study was to break the cycle of repeated hospitalizations associated with diabetic ketoacidosis (DKA). Of 323 IDDM pediatric patients followed in the Michigan Diabetes Research and Training Center (MDRTC), 72 were admitted for DKA in 1979. Sixty-six averaged 1.5 admissions and 5 averaged 15.0 admissions (range 7-25). In the first 9 months of the year, the mean length of stay for these 5 "repeaters" ranged from 4.6 to 11.6 days. The mean time between admissions ranged from 9.7 to 35.5 days.

Various approaches have been tried to alter this pattern. The most successful program involved (1) limitation of activities and visitors, (2) immediate discharge after DKA resolution, (3) team conferences with family members and (4) family counseling. Rewards were given for outpatient treatment, thus eliminating inpatient positive reinforcement.

Three months after this program began, the mean length of stay ranged from 1.5 to 3.8 days ($p < .01$ Wilcoxson Signed Rank) and mean time between admissions ranged from 5.8 to 103.0 days ($p < .01$ Wilcoxson Signed Rank). In addition while no families had previously been in counseling, all are now seeing psychotherapists.

Frequent episodes of DKA may be a result of stressful home situations. Results from this program indicate that these patients respond to a structured inpatient setting and initiation of family counseling. Similar protocols could be implemented in other hospital settings.

107

Control of Diabetes at a Summer Camp: Assessment by Hemoglobin A1 and other Measures. D.L. HORWITZ,* E.G. MOORE, D. SHEFTEL, R. STRAUBE, T. UNTERMAN, AND M. CHERTACK,* Chicago, IL.

This study had three aims: (1) to compare parents' subjective opinions of their child's diabetic control before coming to camp with the opinion of the camp physicians and with hemoglobin A1 (HgA1) determinations; (2) to determine whether control changed at camp, whether 3 weeks of camp was long enough to permit detectable changes in HgA1, and if any changes in HgA1 correlated with other measures of control; (3) to compare 2 chromatographic and one spectrophotometric method of measuring HgA1 in the above studies. 68 children were studied.

75% of parents thought their children were in good or excellent control, while the physicians thought that only 36% of children were this well controlled. Parental opinion of control did not correlate with HgA1, whereas physician control did ($P < .025$). Parents tended to judge control by insulin reactions but not by urine tests, while physicians did the opposite. After 3 weeks of camp, under constant physician supervision, the physicians felt 30 children's control improved, 30 did not change, and 8 became worse. However, change in HgA1 did not correlate with physicians opinion of change in control or with glucosuria at camp. Interestingly, HgA1 rose ($P < .01$) in those children with the most insulin reactions. In the 3 week period, no significant change in mean HgA1 was seen with any method of measurement. No significant differences between any of the methods of HgA1 determination were found.

108

Beneficial effects of diabetes teaching: importance of self management by the patients. VIKTOR JÖRGENS, PETER BERCHTOLD*, WULF EICKENBUSCH and EDITH SCHOLZ-THIELEN, Department of Medicine, Düsseldorf University and General Hospital, Hagen, West Germany.

In order to evaluate the effects of a diabetes teaching program (DTP), insulin-treated patients (P) were re-examined appr. 6 months after hospitalization: 38 P had been subjected to a 15-hour DTP (group A) and 23 P had been discharged from a general hospital without any DTP (group B). The groups did not differ in age, serum-C-Peptide levels and frequency of visits to their physicians. - In group A, 13 P hat continued urine testing (UT) for glucosuria (22 ± 5 times/week) and adaequate self adaptation of insulin dosage (group A1); 12 P had continued UT (19 ± 5 times/week) without self-adaptation of insulin dosages (group A2), and 13 P had discontinued UT (group A3). The P ofgroup B did not practice any UT. The quality of metabolic control on re-examination was:

(means±SD)	A1	A2	A3	B
HbA_I (%)	$8.5 \pm 1.5^{+}$	10.3 ± 1.2	11.9 ± 2.6	10.9 ± 3.0
spontaneous Glucosuria (%)	0.1 ± 0.2	0.3 ± 0.4	$1.6 \pm 1.6^{+}$	1.6 ± 2.5

+ = significantly different from A2 value ($p < 0.05$)

Three P of group B were ketonuric.

The data demonstrate the inefficacy of diabetes treatment without adaequate DTP and the apparent association between the quality of long-term metabolic control and good compliance to the DTP. P practicing self adaptation of their insulin dosage were essentially glucosuria-free and had normal HbA_I-levels.

109

Identifying Patient Responsibilities For Their Care. Charles W. Given, Barbara Given, Roger Buldain, William D. Crano, East Lansing, Michigan.

We have constructed reliable and valid instruments for measuring diabetic patients' knowledge of their disease and therapy; beliefs about the benefits of and barriers to implementing therapy and the effects of diabetes on their social and work roles. A pool of over 200 items was prepared from a review of literature and clinical experience and presented to 154 diagnosed diabetic patients between 21 and 65 years of age who had no evidence of end stage renal disease, no cardiac or cerbral vascular disease and were under treatment at one of five family practice health centers. Standard test scoring procedures were used to select knowledge items with appropriate indices of difficulty. Exploratory and confirmatory factor analyses revealed three scales pertaining to beliefs about the severity of the disease, the benefits of and barriers to compliance with medications and with diet and beliefs about the impact of diabetes upon social role performance and job performance. All scales were determined to be reliable (coefficient alpha $\geq$ .76). These scales were validated using a sample of 100 diabetic patients who responded to interviews and whose medical records were audited to obtain blood sugar levels (outcome measure) clinical severity and indicators of compliance. This work appears to have produced reliable and valid scales suitable for assisting providers to identify patients levels of knowledge and beliefs regarding diabetes and to help patients to become more actively involved in the care of their diabetes.

110

Differences in Diabetes Care by Hospital-Based Versus Clinic-Based Rural Health Professionals. S. Boatright, C. Chandler*, A. Rhodes, Lexington, Kentucky.

We surveyed by record review the performances of nurses and dieticians in 78 diabetic patient records: 34 in rural community hospitals; and 44 in rural county health departments (HDs). Charting behavior, care delivery, and patient instruction differed significantly between these two work situations. Weight changes of these patients were noted in significantly more hospital charts than HD records (χ^2= 9.76, p<0.005), whereas more HD charts noted the type of therapy (χ^2= 8.48, p<0.005). Instruction of patients in 6 areas of diabetes self-care was studied. For all of these areas, more HD patients were taught than hospital patients (p<0.01). Diet counselling was provided more often to patients in HDs than hospitals (χ^2= 15.02, p<0.001), as was foot care instruction (p< 0.001). Diet was reviewed for more patients than other topics at HDs (χ^2= 9.02, p<0.005). In contrast, urine testing methods were taught to hospital patients more often than the other subjects (p<0.05 for all comparisons). Few patients were taught hyperglycemic or hypoglycemic symptoms (<7% of patients), foot care (<18%), or insulin use and administration (<20%) at all of the study sites. We conclude that: 1). care delivery and patient education by allied health professionals may vary with the type of clinical setting; 2). except for instruction on urine testing, patient education is provided less often in rural hospitals than HDs; 3). the majority of patients receiving care at these sites are not adequately taught diabetic self-care.

111

An out-patient alternative program for regulation of the insulin-requiring diabetic patient. I.J. WHITEHOUSE,* M.S. COX and D.M. KAHKONEN,* Detroit, Michigan.

Regulation of diabetes in an outpatient setting is preferred because: 1) the average diabetic patient would rather not be hospitalized; 2) an educational experience can be achieved along with metabolic regulation; 3) the patient's ordinary physical activity can be continued; 4) it is less expensive than inpatient care. For these reasons we are exploring a structured outpatient program for regulation of the insulin-requiring diabetic patient as an alternative to hospitalization.

From 7-1-79 to 2-1-80, we have enrolled 66 patients. Fifty-four have completed a 5-day (35 hours) program which includes a complete physical evaluation, regulation of blood glucose with diet and insulin and initial instruction in the details of diabetic care, as dietary instruction (13 hrs.), insulin instruction (4 hrs.), urine testing, sick day care, exercise, care of the feet and an understanding of hypoglycemia. Pre and post-testing is used. Thirty-six patients used insulin for the first time. Three patients left the program during the week while 9 patients did not begin the program after enrollment. The mean initial BG was 260 mg/dl and the initial total glycosylated hemoglobin averaged 16.0%. Average BG on the 5th day was 149 mg/dl (p<0.001) Only one patient has required hospitalization for an unrelated illness.

We hope third-party carriers perceive the wisdom and success of such programs as they consider fiscal support for diabetes regulation and education in an outpatient setting.

112

Perceived Needs of Diabetes Patient Educators. JAMES W. PICHERT, RODNEY A. LORENZ,* ANNE L. TURNER,* and ALAN L. GRABER,* Nashville, Tenn.

In order to survey local patient education resources and to determine self-perceived needs of practicing patient educators prior to initiating DRTC outreach activities, a modified nominal group approach was employed. Representatives of Middle Tennessee hospitals, visiting nurse agencies, and county health departments were asked to describe and analyze current practices in patient education and to generate a list of needs or obstacles for providing quality educational services. Needs were then rated on the degree to which they were felt to be widespread, personally encountered, and serious.

Twenty-seven needs were listed, 7 of which were considered widespread, personally felt, serious, and worth receiving concerted effort by a majority of participants. These were: a book of patient education resources, community-wide standardization of education practices, better communication between home and hospital care providers, higher administrative priority for in-hospital education services, and continuing education in nutrition, retinopathy, and teaching skills.

The method applied here provided a rapid and inexpensive assessment of available resources and their self-perceived needs; in addition, a cadre of enthusiastic professionals and some services which could be provided by a Diabetes Center were identified.

113

Living as a Diabetic. J. GETTINGER,* E. WARREN-BOULTON, G. SPRINGER,* and W. AUSLANDER, St. Louis, Mo.

The National Commission on Diabetes recommended that knowledge, skills and attitudes of health professionals be improved in order to provide effective diabetic care. Washington University DRTC has responded to this recommendation by conducting continuing education programs for health professionals. Attendees were requested to simulate the lifestyle of a diabetic for four days. To date 93 nurses, 33 dieticians, and 11 other health professionals have participated in this activity.

The goal of the simulation was to improve the quality of patient education by imparting information from a unique perspective - that of a diabetic. During daily staff-guided discussions, participants gained a new appreciation of the complexity of the diabetic regimen, as well as the influence of emotional factors in adherence. Attendees reported that the experience was useful in: 1) acquiring more realistic expectations of patients, 2) identifying the need for flexibility in the regimen, and 3) recognizing the importance of reeducation. This experience was consistently identified as one of the most beneficial components of the course. Evaluations indicate that this is a powerful method of sensitizing health professionals to the daily problems of the insulin-dependent diabetic.

114

Plasma Levels of Somatostatin-Like Immunoreactivity in Healthy Subjects and in Insulin-Dependent Diabetic Patients (IDDM). G. VALTYSSON, A.I. VINIK* AND S.S. FAJANS*, Ann Arbor, MI

An increase in islet somatostatin (SRIF) content has been reported in experimentally-induced insulin deficient diabetes and in IDDM. Concentrations of SRIF in peripheral venous blood have not been reported in IDDM. We have measured plasma somatostatin-like immunoreactivity (SLI) in the basal state and in response to insulin-induced hypoglycemia in 9 healthy nonobese subjects (HS) and in 9 age-, sex-, and weight-matched insulin-treated IDDM (age 20-36 yrs). Healthy subjects received 0.1 units/kg IV; IDDM were given 0.2 units/kg IV. The results were (mean ± SE):

Healthy Subjects:	basal	peak/nadir	Δ from basal
glucose (mg/dl)	91±4	34±2†	58±2
SLI (pg/ml)	232±31	355±23†	122±28
glucagon (pg/ml)	69±5	218±42†	156±36
IDDM patients:			
glucose (mg/dl)	189±26*	48±2†*	140±24*
SLI (pg/ml)	99±16*	214±42†*	115±29
glucagon (pg/ml)	60±11	75±18*	28±12*

*significantly different from healthy subjects
†significantly different from basal

There was an inverse correlation between basal SLI and the $\log_e$ plasma glucose concentrations but none between the change in SLI and the nadir or the change in blood glucose levels. Conclusions: 1) Decreased release of SLI may cause decreased basal SLI in IDDM and may be influenced by insulin treatment. 2) Insulin-induced hypoglycemia results in increases of SLI in peripheral blood in some HS and IDDM, in contrast to an impaired rise in plasma glucagon in IDDM. 3) The impaired glucagon response in IDDM is not due to enhanced SLI release.

115

Decrease of Pancreatic Somatostatin in Neonatal "Nesidioblastosis". J.M. POLAK, P. GARIN CHESA, C.M. TIMSON, M.G. BRYANT and S.R. BLOOM*, RPMS, Hammersmith Hospital, London, U.K.

In addition to the inappropriate insulin release, until recently considered to be the sole or principal cause of severe neonatal hypoglycaemia and "nesidioblastosis", we have recently found a marked decrease of pancreatic somatostatin.

Specimens of pancreas from 8 children with severe hypoglycaemic hyperinsulinaemia and "nesidioblastosis" were examined by immunocytochemistry and radioimmunoassay and compared with age/weight matched controls.

The total endocrine area in the diseased tissue was increased by 22% and consisted mainly of scattered endocrine cells rather than discrete islets. Although the insulin cell area was increased by 20% to 70% in microadenomatous areas, the most dramatic change occured in the somatostatin cell area which, in "nesidioblastosis", was reduced by more than 40% to 0.56±0.07% of background area, controls 1.00±0.12% ($p<0.02$). The normal 2:1 ratio of insulin:somatostatin cells seen in the neonatal period was thus altered to a disproportionately high 5:1 ratio. Similarly the pancreatic content (nmol/g) of insulin and somatostatin in nesidioblastosis was markedly abnormal: insulin: 152±5.6 (controls 37±3) ($p<0.05$): somatostatin: 0.17±0.02 (controls 0.38±0.02) ($p<0.001$). Thus a significant decrease in the content of the insulin inhibitor, somatostatin, is closely involved in the pathogenesis of nesidioblastosis resulting in marked alteration of the normal pancreatic hormone balance.

116

Failure of Glucose to Stimulate Insulin Release from Isolated Pure Beta Cells. M.S. BANDISODE,* Augusta, GA.

In vivo and in vitro studies employing mixed cell preparations have shown glucose to be a major stimulant for insulin release. A technique of isolation of pure beta cells of adult rat pancreas employing collagenase dissociation followed by counterflow sedimentation and gradient centrifugation was developed by me. Light and electronmicroscopy revealed 100% pure preparation with characteristic beta cell morphology. Further characterization was achieved by immunofluorescent staining for insulin, glucagon and somatostatin. Release of insulin was studied by distributing the cells in several flasks and incubating them with different concentrations of glucose, arginine or arginine plus glucose for 15, 30 or 60 min. The cells were separated from the media and the insulin content of the media and acid ethanol extract of the cells was determined by RIA.

Glucose (1, 5, 10 and 20 mM) failed to produce significant insulin release (4.25 to 9.65%). Arginine (1, 5, 10 and 20 mM) produced significant insulin release (14.1, 29.1, 34.9 and 15.05% - 60 min incubation). However, the response to arginine (2.5, 5 and 7.5 mM) plus glucose 5 mM was greater (30.3, 35.3 and 42.1%). In conclusion, glucose does not appear to stimulate insulin release directly from the beta cells. Arginine stimulates insulin release and glucose enhances arginine stimulated insulin release.

117

Isolation, Translation, and Partial Characterization of Messenger RNA Species from Six Human Insulinomas. D.A. HESTER and H.E. LEBOVITZ*, Durham, N.C.

Messenger RNA (mRNA) was isolated by phenol extraction and oligo DT cellulose chromatography from 6 human insulinomas (5 adenomas, 1 carcinoma). The mRNAs increased the incorporation of [^{3}H] leucine into TCA precipitable polypeptides by 2-4 fold in the wheat germ (WG) cell free translation system, and by 4-10 fold in the modified rabbit reticulocyte lysate (RRL) system. The mRNA directed synthetic products were analysed by electrophoresis on 20% polyacrylamide SDS gels: Radiolabelled products of insulinoma mRNAs translated in WG contained a single peak (11,500 dalton) which comprised 21-28% of the total product. Likewise, using the RRL system, the major translation product was an 11,500 dalton (d) protein which accounted for 22-34% of the TCA precipitable products. Immunoprecipitation assay of the translation products, using an anti-porcine insulin antibody, demonstrated, in each, a preproinsulin corresponding to the 11,500 d peak and making up at least 5% of the total polypeptide product. Additional translation products could be identified in the RRL system: A 27,000 d product (7 to 14% of total) made by all 6 preparations; a 45,000 d product made by 4 of the 6 and a 19,000 d product made by 3 of the 6. Thus, human insulinomas contain mRNAs which code for several specific products (detected only by the modified reticulocyte lysate translation system) some of which are constant and some that are variant.

118

Transitory Islet Phosphate Depletion: Key Factor in First Phase Stimulated Insulin Release? ROBERT C. JOHNSON & NORBERT FREINKEL,* Chicago, Ill.

Intracellular disequilibrium during the first phase of ↑ insulin release has not been documented previously even though it might account for the biphasic pattern of B cell stimulus-secretion coupling. We have developed a new technique for simultaneously monitoring phosphate (P_i) influx, efflux and balance during the transitory ↑ efflux which encompasses first phase ↑ insulin (Freinkel et al J Clin Invest 54:1179, 1974). Islets prelabeled with $^{33}P_i$ during basal incubation in KRB containing 0.5 mg/ml glucose were introduced into "cold" KRB overlying dibutyl phthalate in microfuge tubes. Stimulation or maintenance was initiated by introducing more KRB with glucose (to yield 3.0 or 0.5 mg/ml respectively) and $^{32}P_i$. Islets were harvested by centrifugation immediately (t_o) or 8 or 15 min. later (t_8; t_{15} i.e. near the height of first phase or inception of second phase of ↑ insulin release respectively). Net efflux ($\Delta^{33}P_i$), influx ($\Delta^{32}P_i$) and balance of P_i ($\Delta^{33}P_i$-$\Delta^{32}P_i$) were quantified on the basis of dual label counting and known specific activities of the labels. We have found that 3.0 mg/ml glucose effected near-maximal ↑ in efflux by t_8 without disparately affecting influx at that time; by t_{15}, influx was sufficiently greater with 3.0 than with 0.5 mg/ml glucose to nearly rectify the antecedent P_i depletion. Thus, depletion of intracellular P_i and repletion via extracellular sources seem to occur in biphasic fashion and coincident with the end of the first phase and initiation of the second phase of ↑ insulin secretion.

119

A New In Vitro Model To Study Secretion and Biochemistry of Pancreatic Polypeptide (PP). R.L. GINGERICH*, D.W. SCHARP*, M.H. GREIDER*, E.S. DYE, K.A. MOUSEL. St. Louis, Mo.

Secretion and biochemical studies of PP have been hampered by the lack of a suitable in vitro model. Isolated rat islets are not useful since current PP antibodies cross-react minimally with rodent PP. To circumvent this problem, we have developed a method for the formation of canine pseudoislets (PI), islet-like aggregates of pancreatic endocrine cells formed on rotational tissue culture from a trypsin prepared single-cell suspension. By four days of culture, the PIs form into firm, spherical-shaped aggregates containing A-,B-,D- and F-cells plus a few acinar cells. The F-cell is the dominant cell type. A- and B-cells are predominantly located at the periphery, while D-,F- and acinar cells are distributed throughout the PI. Acute stimulation of PIs with carbachol (0.1mM) on day 7 of culture results in a 4-fold increase in PP secretion (from 49.2±7.8 to 235±23.8 pg/PI/90 min). Stimulation values remain significantly elevated and basal levels unchanged through day 21, but by day 28 basal levels are increased and the F cell responds only minimally to stimulation. When studied in a standard perifusion system, carbachol-stimulated PP release is biphasic. PP reaches a peak at 2 min., falls to a nadir at 7 min., then raises during a second phase.

These histologic and functional data show PIs contain viable, healthy F cells. This model makes possible detailed studies of factors and hormonal interactions controlling PP secretion and biosynthesis. (Supp. by NIH AM 25909 and AM 20579.)

120

Net Changes in Pancreatic Phospholipids During Stimulation by Glucose and cAMP In Vitro. R.V. FARESE*, A.M. SABIR and R.E. LARSON, Tampa, FL.

Insulin and zymogens are secreted by exocytosis, and phospholipids (PL) may be involved therein. Pancreatic secretogogues have been shown to enhance Ca++-dependent breakdown of labelled phosphatidylinositol (PI) (Clements et al, JCI 57: 684,1976) and subsequent incorporation of $^{32}PO_4$ into phosphatidic acid (PA), PI and other derivatives of CDP∼diacylglycerol (Freinkel et al, Eur J Biochem 59:245,1975). However, it is uncertain to what extent these isotopic experiments reflect net changes in tissue PL concentrations. To evaluate the latter, we incubated relatively large amounts of rat pancreatic tissue (prepared by collagenase digestion) in Krebs-Ringer Bicarbonate buffer containing 0.5 g albumin and 60 (low) or 500 (high) mg glucose/dl. PL were extracted, purified by TLC, and quantified by P measurement. After 60 min preincubation in low glucose, incubation in low glucose, incubation for 30 min in high glucose cause PI to decrease 26% from 17.96 to 13.30 nmol/mg protein. This decrease in PI was accompanied by a 56% increase in PA from 2.03 to 3.16, and a 44% increase in phosphatidylglycerol (PG) from 6.75 to 9.70 nmol/mg protein. Polyphosphoinositides did not change with glucose stimulation, nor did phosphatidylcholine. cAMP (5mM), another secretogogue, induced similar changes in PL.

Conclusions: (a) pancreatic secretogogues cause relatively large changes in net levels of PI, PA and PG; (b) the decrease in PI following stimulation is accompanied by a comparable increase in PA + PG; (c) any or all of these PL changes may be important in secretion of insulin and zymogens.

121

Therapy of Malignant Insulinomas With Monoamine Precursors. J. M. FELDMAN*, C. VERVAERT, C. KLATT and H. F. SEIGLER, Durham, NC.

The hyperinsulinemia and hypoglycemia produced by malignant insulinomas is a difficult therapeutic problem. The non-polar monoamine precursors 5-hydroxytryptophan (5-HTP), L-3,4-dihydroxyphenylalanine (L-DOPA) and DL-threo-dihydroxyphenyserine are readily taken up by normal hamster pancreatic islets and are converted intracellularly to serotonin, dopamine (DA) and norepinephrine (NE). These intracellular monoamines then inhibit glucose-stimulated insulin secretion. In the present study we determined if the monoamine precursors could modify the severe hypoglycemia of hamsters bearing a rapidly-growing transplantable insulinoma. One hour after receiving the respective precursor there was a 9, 16, and 54-fold increase in the concentration of serotonin, DA or NE in the insulinomas. 24-hours after the administration of the respective precursors there were the following changes in plasma glucose in the respective groups: 5-HTP, 37 to 91 mg/dl; L-DOPA 29 to 68 mg/dl; and DOPS 40 to 102 mg/dl. In general the increase in plasma glucose was associated with a decrease in plasma insulin. To determine if this therapeutic approach could modify the rapidly fatal outcome of the tumor-bearing hamsters, they received saline, or DOPS or pargyline plus DOPS every two days. The survival of the groups (M±SEM) were: saline 8.4 ± 1.1 days; DOPS 17.9 ± 3.5 days; and pargyline plus DOPS 23.3 ± 4.8 days. The present study suggests that increasing the monoamine content of malignant insulinomas may favorably modify the course of these devastating tumors.

122

The Effects of Retinoids on Rat Islet Insulin Secretion and Cell Aggregation. B. S. CHERTOW,* N. S. MOSS, B. A. OZUK, J. J. SEWELL, J.C. SHIH, and A.T. WAITE, Huntington, West Virginia.

To elucidate subcellular mechanisms of insulin release, the effects of retinoids on intercellular membrane adhesiveness and aggregation of dispersed islet cells were related to effects on biphasic insulin release from perifused isolated rat islets. Adult rat islets were dispersed using trypsin in low concentrations. A suspension of 10^6 islet cells was incubated for 60 min in Hanks balanced salt solution at pH 7.35. The number of free cells and number of clumps after 60 min of incubation were counted in control and treated suspensions.

10^{-6}M all-trans retinoic acid (RA) and 13 cis RA significantly increased the number of free cells clumping at 60 min of incubation to 133% and 130% of control (C), respectively and increased the number of clumps to 169% and 200% of C, respectively. 10^{-5}M and 10^{-4}M 13-cis RA caused all cells to aggregate into one large clump and as a result, free cells were not available for counting. At 10^{-4}M, 13-cis RA, significantly increased glucose (16.7 mM)-induced second phase insulin release to 170% of C. 10^{-6}M RA stimulated second phase release but not significantly.

In conclusion, all-trans and 13-cis RA increased aggregation of dispersed islets cells. At high concentrations, 13-cis RA stimulates insulin release. At high concentrations of 13-cis RA, a marked increase in intercellular membrane adhesiveness may facilitate beta cell-to-cell communications and, in turn, insulin release.

123

Insulin Secretory Defect of Type II Diabetes Reproduced in B Cell Deficient Rat Model. G.C.WEIR* S. BONNER-WEIR*, E.T. CLORE, and C.J.ZMACHINSKI, Richmond, Va.

Studies in Type II diabetes have revealed a minimal insulin response to a glucose pulse, but preservation of the response to arginine and isoproterenol. A rat model has been developed with similarities to Type II diabetes. Two day old neonatal rats are injected with streptozotocin (90 mg/kg) which is followed two days later by hyperglycemia (275-400 mg/dl, fed), and by age 10 days glucose normalizes, but at 6 wks, hyperglycemia develops which at 8 wks is noted to be more severe in males (247±26) than females (187±6). There is an accompanying 35% reduction of a B cell number, as determined by counting immunocytochemically stained cells.

Islet secretion of hyperglycemic male rats, age 10 weeks, was evaluated by isolated pancreas perfusion. With perfusate glucose at 140 mg/dl insulin secretion was higher in control (C) than in streptozotocin (SZ) rats (102±50 vs 16±6 μU/ml). When perfusate glucose was increased to 400 mg/dl there was a marked peak insulin output in C (875±336) with almost no response by SZ (29±19). In response to arginine 10 mM the peak C response was 836±299 and the peak SZ response was 381±114. Insulin responses to isoproterenol are also preserved. Thus a reduction of B cell number leads to hyperglycemia and a severe functional defect in glucose-stimulated insulin secretion, whereas arginine and isoproterenol-stimulated secretion is partially preserved. This functional impairment may be secondary to chronic exposure of B cells to an unnatural level of hyperglycemia.

124

Evidence That the Inhibitory Effect of Vincristine (VCR) on Glucose-Induced Insulin Release is Mediated via Glucose Receptor Mechanisms. J. SHAH,* B. STEVENS, and C. HURKS, Chicago, Il.

We have recently shown that, 1) in the intact rat at 60 min after VCR (0.15mg/kg, iv) glucose-induced insulin release and glucose disappearance rate (K_G) were impaired in the absence of any morphological alteration of the beta cell microtubular structures; 2) even though VCR inhibited glucose-induced insulin release, it had no effect on arginine-induced insulin release. The present study further evaluated the mechanism of inhibition of VCR on glucose-induced insulin release. Glucose (500 mg/kg) was infused over one min into fasting rats with indwelling vascular catheters. Five min later VCR (0.15mg/kg, iv) or vehicle (control) was injected. Sixty min after VCR or vehicle treatment, insulin release in response to a 150 mg, iv glucose pulse was examined. Baseline, as well as in response to the glucose pulse, serum glucose and insulin levels were similar at all time intervals in the VCR-treated and the control rats. Similarly, mean K_G of 2.9 $\pm$ 0.1 in the VCR-treated rats was not significantly different from that of 2.8 $\pm$ 0.2 observed in the control rats. Therefore, in the intact rat, prior exposure to elevated glucose levels protected the beta cell from the inhibitory effect of VCR on glucose-induced insulin release. These findings, along with our previous observations, strongly suggest that *in vivo* the effect of VCR on glucose-induced insulin release is mediated via alteration of the beta cell glucose receptor rather than microtubular structures.

125

Separation of Islet Cell Subpopulations by Fluorescence-activated Cell Sorting. DAVID A. NIELSEN, ÅKE LERNMARK*, DONALD F. STEINER*, Chicago, IL. and Copenhagen, Denmark.

Isolated rat pancreatic islets dissociated into single cell suspensions (0.5-1.5 x 10^6 cells per experiment), were analyzed and sorted in a Fluorescence-activated Cell Sorter (FACS III, Becton Dickinson, Calif, USA). By forward-angle light scattering analysis the islet cells were contained within a broad peak distinctly separated from particles of low scatter intensity. Fluorescein diacetate staining demonstrated that 90% of the total viable cells were contained in the islet cell peak and that, within this peak, 75% of the cells were viable. The presence of alpha, beta, and D cells in this peak was confirmed by electron microscopy. Immunoassays of 3-75 x 10^3 cells sorted from different regions of the scatter distribution revealed an overlapping distribution of endocrine cells. The glucagon-containing cells were concentrated towards the left side of the islet cell peak; insulin-containing cells were abundant in the middle and right slope, while somatostatin-containing cells were confined to the far right slope. Sodium dodecyl sulfate slab gel electrophoresis and autoradiography of islet cells (20-40 x 10^3 cells), sorted from various regions of the peak, and labeled with ^{35}S-methionine, showed that cells from the far left slope contained mainly 18Kd proglucagon and its 13Kd and 10Kd conversion intermediates (Patzelt, et al., Nature 282, 260, 1979), while 12.5Kd prosomatostatin (PNAS, In press) was greatly enriched in cells from the far right side of the peak. These results demonstrate that viable, single cell islet subpopulations enriched in different cell types can be routinely obtained by this method. Supported by grants AM 13914 and AM 20595.

126

Ventromedial Hypothalamic (VMH) Lesions Increase Pancreatic Sensitivity to Streptozotocin (STZ) Without Obesity. DAVID B. WEST, YUTAKA SEINO, STEPHEN C. WOODS,* and DANIEL PORTE, JR.*, Seattle, Wa and Kyoto, Japan.

It has been suggested that obese animals are more sensitive to the diabetogenic action of STZ when the drug is given on a body weight basis. To determine if this change of sensitivity is due to obesity per se or to some difference of effective dosage, VMH-lesioned rats were tested for sensitivity to STZ prior to the development of obesity STZ was administered intravenously to weight-matched rats 48 hr following bilateral lesions of the VMH or sham surgery. Fifty-eight percent (19/33) of the VMH-lesioned rats receiving 50 mg/kg STZ died of hyperglycemia within 6 wk whereas none of the sham-operated animals died. Slightly smaller doses (30 and 35 mg/kg STZ) yielded comparable results (57% mortality for the lesioned rats) and a higher dose (65 mg/kg) killed 100% of the lesioned rats within 6 wk. Surviving lesioned rats were comparably hyperglycemic to the sham-operated rats. Since the lesioned rats had not gained more weight than their controls by the time of the STZ administration, the increased sensitivity must be attributed to the lesion and not to the development of obesity. This suggests that islet cell function may be an important parameter of sensitivity to islet destruction. Parasympathetic activation of the islet following the lesion is suggested as mediating the response.

127

Correlation of Urinary C-peptide with the Integrated Concentration (IC) and Intrinsic Secretion Rate of Insulin (SR-I). MARY T. MEISTAS, ZVI ZADIK, SIMEON MARGOLIS*, and A. AVINOAM KOWARSKI, Baltimore, MD.

A practical method for determining the daily SR-I would be quite useful, especially if applicable to diabetic patients. As a first step in the development of such a method, we used the 24 hour IC of plasma insulin in 16 normal, nonobese subjects to calculate the SR-I and correlate it with the daily urinary excretion of C-peptide.

The average IC of insulin was 0.35 $\pm$ 0.14 ng/ml. The SR-I is equal to the product of the IC and the total body metabolic clearance rate, which was estimated by using a previously reported value (850 $\pm$ 140 ml/min/m^2). The average calculated SR-I of the 16 subjects was 18.5 $\pm$ 8 U/24 hours. The daily excretion of C-peptide was 33.5 $\pm$ 10.8 µg/gm creatinine. The correlation between the SR-I and the 24 hour urinary C-peptide was statistically significant ($r = 0.88$, $p < 0.001$).

Because of the administration of exogenous insulin and interference with the immunoassay of insulin by insulin antibodies, this method cannot be used to measure the SR-I in insulin-treated diabetics. However, our finding that 24 hour urinary C-peptide correlated with SR-I in normal individuals suggests that measurement of urinary C-peptide may allow estimation of the SR-I in diabetic patients. Determination of the IC and SR of C-peptide may also prove useful for this purpose.

128

Glucokinase and Glucose-Responsivity of Pancreas. Suvesh Chandiok, Rhoda Makoff, Josiah Brown*. Los Angeles, California

Glucose must be metabolized by the β cell to elicit glucose mediated insulin release. This mechanism is not present in the fetus. A high Km glucose phosphorylating enzyme glucokinase is ideally suited for this function. Appearance of glucokinase in the pancreas of fetal and neonatal rats was measured as NADPH production using a sensitive spectrofluorometer. Fetal pancreases were transplanted into normals and diabetics; function evaluated in-vitro by perfusion studies.

RAT PANCREAS (u moles NADP reduced/mg protein/min)	TOTAL	HEXOKINASE	GLUCOKINASE
18-19 day fetal	0.372	0.333	-
19-20 day fetal	0.215	0.243	-
21 day fetal	0.684	0.684	-
Newborn (<12 hrs)	0.410	0.256	0.154
1 day neonatal	0.376	0.242	0.134
2 days neonatal	0.528	0.242	0.286
7 days neonatal	0.662	0.312	0.350
26 days neonatal	0.510	0.200	0.310
Fetal pancreas transplanted (a) normal adult rats	0.330	0.215	0.115
(b) diabetic adult rats (cured)	0.462	0.027	0.435

Conclusions: (a) glucokinase is not detectable in fetal pancreas (b) the appearance of glucokinase in rat pancreases correlates with the appearance of glucose responsivity as shown by other workers (c) glucokinase in transplanted pancreas correlates with insulin release during perfusion and transplant function in reversing diabetes. Thus, glucokinase may be a mediator of glucose induced insulin release.

129

Mechanism for Chemically Induced Diabetes: Evidence for Oxidant Action and Free Radical Production. ALFRED E. SLONIM,* MELANIE J. SURBER, MARGARET R. CAMERON AND IAN M. BURR,* Nashville,Tn.

Previously it was noted that the chemical diabetogenic agents, streptozotocin (Sz) and alloxan(AL) both induce a change in the redox state of RBC's and islets (fall in reduced glutathione (GSH) to oxidized glutathione (GSSG) ratio.)

Free radical production in vitro was assessed by malondialdehyde (MDA) formation. AL, (0.01 mM to 10 mM) induced a dose dependent increase in MDA in rat liver microsomes. 1 mM AL induced a 4-fold rise in MDA. Sz failed to demonstrate increased MDA production from liver microsomes. However, both Sz and AL induced a dose-dependent increase in MDA production from rat pancreatic microsomes. 10 mM Sz of AL increased MDA 3-fold.

Vitamin E (200 u/d for 2 days IM) given to male Wistar rats, prior to either Sz (45 mg/Kg IV) or AL (95 mg/Kg IV), protected against diabetes. Rats on Vitamin E and selenium (Vit E+Se) deficient diet were more susceptible to Sz (45 mg/KgIV) which induced rapid severe diabetes with 100% mortality within 72 hours. This was shown to be due to diabetes, as insulin administration (2 u NPH/d) started 24 hrs. after Sz, prevented this lethal effect. A lower concentration of Sz(25 mg/Kg IV) caused glucose intolerance in Vit E+Se deficient rats, but not in control animals.

Conclusion: 1) In vitro studies demonstrate that Sz and AL act as oxidants. 2)Both Sz and AL induce free radical production in pancreatic microsomes, yet only AL has this effect on liver microsomes. 3) Antioxidant Vit E protects against Sz or Al induced diabetes, while diabetogenic effect of Sz is enhanced in the antioxidant depleted state.

130

Molecular Heterogeneity in Pancreatic Polypeptide T. PAQUETTE and R. GINGERICH* Seattle, Wa. and St. Louis, Mo.*

Cultures of canine pancreatic F-cells were analyzed for different molecular forms of pancreatic polypeptide (PP). Cultures were extracted in 8 M urea 2% sodium dodecylsulfate (SDS) 4% mercaptoethanol or in 6 M guanidine hydrochloride 4% mercaptoethanol. Extracts were then subjected to electrophoresis in 17% acrylamide SDS gels or to molecular seive chromatography on columns of BioGel P-100. Gels were sliced, eluted, and immunoassayed with either rabbit or guinea pig anti PP antibodies; column fractions were diluted and immunoassayed. Most of the immunoactivity migrated and eluted from the gel or column in the position a porcine PP (4200 molecular weight) standard but 1-5% of the immunoactivity was found at respective migration and elution positions corresponding to 7500 molecular weight. This larger molecular weight immunoactivity could be a biosynthetic precursor to PP. PP sized material eluted from the SDS gel was further analyzed by isoelectric focusing (IEF) in BioLyte 3/10 ampholyte. Cultures biosynthetically labeled with ^3H leucine were extracted and subjected to SDS electrophoresis, elution, IEF and elution. We found several peaks of immunoactivity in IEF gel slice eluates. One peak corresponded in isoelectric point to pPP standard but surprisingly the major peak of radioactivity was associated with a peak of immunoactivity with an isoelectric point two pH units below pPP itself. These results raise the question whether PP is the only endocrine product of the pancreatic F-cell.

131

Synchronous Sustained Oscillations of Plasma Epinephrine (E) and Norepinephrine (NE) in M. mulatta. F.G. HOM*, D.J. KOERKER, C.J. GOODNER* and J.B. HALTER*, Seattle, WA.

We have reported that plasma insulin, glucagon, glucose and C-peptide exhibit synchronous oscillations, with periods averaging 9 minutes, in the fasting rhesus. Glucose and C-peptide oscillate in phase while glucagon oscillates out of phase with insulin.

Six time studies for insulin, E and NE were performed to determine if plasma catechols might oscillate in synchrony with insulin. Plasma E and NE were both shown to oscillate with a period of approximately 9 minutes, the same as for insulin. The mean E level was 326 $\pm$ 47 (SE) pg/ml with the amplitude/2 of the oscillations averaging 29 $\pm$ 4%. For NE the mean plasma level was 390 $\pm$ 70 pg/ml with the amplitude/2 averaging 24 $\pm$ 5%. Plasma insulin in these studies averaged 50 $\pm$ 12 uU/ml with the amplitude/2 being 43 $\pm$ 1%. By cross-correlation with insulin, the peaks of plasma E and NE trailed the peak of insulin by 6 minutes, in synchrony with plasma glucagon. In conclusion, plasma E and NE oscillate every 9 minutes in fasted rhesus, in phase with glucagon and out of phase with insulin. As previous studies have shown no effect by sympathetic nervous system blocking agents upon insulin oscillations; and insulin oscillations have been observed in non-innervated perfused pancreas preparations, the oscillating plasma catecholamines are not part of a CNS oscillator which is in turn, driving insulin oscillations. Rather, the sympathetic nervous system and aderenal medulla probably couple in synchrony with the oscillating levels of insulin and glucagon for control of metabolic fuels. The site and mechanism of coupling remains to be determined.

132

Educational Materials for Teaching Children About Diabetes Mellitus at Various Ages. CONNIE KRIEF, CINDY MANLEY, ELAINE KOHLER,* and LINDA HURWITZ,* Milwaukee, WI.

Inexpensive materials have been developed for the education of the diabetic child. Children in kindergarten and early grades begin with coloring, cutting and pasting of the steps in urine testing, insulin injection and sugar digestion and metabolism. They learn about diabetes in puppet shows and games like "fish" with diabetes related words.

For children in older grades percent of sugar in urine has been graphically demonstrated, the symptoms of too little and too much sugar listed and drawn. Individualized patterns of insulin action, caloric intake and expenditure are drawn on diagrams of the child's usual day's activity to show how metabolic balance may be achieved. The importance of exercise for fitness as well as self care for metabolic balance is emphasized in questionnaires and handouts. Concepts of sugar metabolism are explained simply including storage and release by hormones, effects of growth and stress. Games are played like hidden word and crossword puzzles with terms relating to diabetes.

High school youngsters progress from problem solving, balance of caloric output and intake and insulin dosage adjustment, to more long range concerns like budgetting for diabetic care, evaluation of health care resources, recognition of complications and how diabetes affects career goals and family life. Quizzes have been devised appropriate to the age level. These materials are used in the framework of a coordinated grade appropriate curriculum.

133

Self Management: The Focus on Week Long Diabetes Classes. D. HINNEN* Wichita, Kansas

The premise for diabetes education classes at UKSM-W is to teach patients self management skills in order that they might attain the ultimate goal of maintaining normoglycemia 75-85% of the time. A 34 hr. family seminar is taught by 4 faculty with 7 additional faculty represented by video tape presentations. Guidelines for insulin & calorie adjustment by the patient are clearly delineated & reinforced through the education process. Literature in patient manuals, slide presentations, role playing, & discussions demonstrate common self adjustments made in diabetes regimens. These guidelines serve as protocol for the health care team when assisting the patient & family with urine record & blood sugar evaluations on subsequent follow-up visits. The responsibility for adjusting calories with changes in exercise, growth & illness on a day to day basis is left primarily to the patient & family after completing the education class. METS levels, urine or blood sugars along with height & weight records may be utilized as patient guidelines for calorie adjustments during exercise. Similarly specific information is provided for individuals making insulin adjustments. Better control can be achieved with few insulin reaction by education of the patient & family in self management skills than by rigid control at long distance by the health care team. Rehospitalization rate of 3% suggests that the well educated family with diabetes with little alteration in life styles can maintain control of the diabetes with infrequent rehospitalization.

134

Microcomputer Utilization in a Diabetes Clinic - Low Cost Data Recording and Monitoring. T. TRUAX, D. LOMATCH, L. ROI and P. SAVAGE*, Ann Arbor, Mi.

Incomplete recording of data available to health care providers in an outpatient clinic makes monitoring of patient care difficult. A microcomputer-based data recording and management system has been developed which enables medical staff to directly and rapidly enter and retrieve medical data on a microcomputer video screen (cathode ray tube). The use of the computer to control data entry on a formated screen allows utilization by medical staff with minimal training and no previous computer experience. Location of the computer in the clinic and direct use by health professionals allows immediate checking for errors in data entry and computer generated requests for additional information. Data are evaluated on entry for unusual values and for compliance with predetermined standards of care. When out of range entries are detected, the computer immediately alerts the health care provider. The provider can request a video display of diagnostic information, criteria of care and patient management strategies ("help screens").

The microcomputer stores patient data and "help screens" locally using floppy disks. Data are also transmitted via telephone to a large computer where they are maintained using a relational data base management system, a form of storage which facilitates retrieval and linkage of data sets. Development of profiles of provider performance and statistical analysis of group data are possible on the main computer. This "distributed processing system" has the advantages of both a low cost, dedicated microcomputer and the processing power and storage capacity of a large computer.

135

Use of the Computer in the Investigation of Diabetes Mellitus. J.R. POOLE, M.M. BLIZIOTES,* T.A. SCHULTZ,* J.W. JUNG, Oakland, California.

The systematic management and study of a chronic disease afflicting a large patient population such as diabetes mellitus requires the ability to store, retrieve, and analyse clinical data obtained over many years.

In our diabetes clinic all history, physical, and laboratory data is entered into a computer. At each clinic visit the physician reviews a computer printout of the patient's recent history. In addition, serial diabetes-related data including hemoglobin A_1, blood glucose, lipids and mode of therapy is summarized in chronological order.

The computer provides the option for retrieving selected pieces of data (such as hemoglobin A_1 and lipid profile) from an individual patient file or from any number of files in the entire patient population.

Linear regression analysis can be applied to any combination of 30 diabetes-related laboratory values and the data points plotted by the computer.

Statistical analysis of selected data from hundreds of patients can therefore be obtained in seconds.

Conclusion: A computerized data base provides a valuable tool for the management and investigation of chronic multifaceted diseases such as diabetes mellitus.

136

Effectiveness of a Visual Approach to Diet for Diabetes. Jan Eno*, Toronto, Canada.

The Canadian Diabetes Association Task Force which included one dietitian from each Province developed a colour-coded poster illustrating individual foods. A prototype in English was tested nationally, as a teaching aid. The sample of 593 was divided into readers (R) and non-readers (NR); 68.4% (376) of the R and 20.9% (9) of the NR could correctly plan an example meal using the poster; this difference being significant at $p<0.001$. Similarly Indians (I) and non-Indians (NI) were compared and were not found to be significantly different. The meal planning concepts which needed explanation most frequently for NR were: 1) That foods within a group are interchangeable, and 2) That numbers in the eating plan mean number of food portions from corresponding groups. Significantly fewer ($p<0.001$) R needed explanation of these concepts. Difficulty with the interchangeability concept did not vary significantly when I and NI were compared. The poster was an effective aid in learning about diet, but it did not stand alone. As expected, the NR had greater difficulty planning their meals using the poster suggesting that: 1) Words on the poster aided understanding, and 2) NR need more intensive teaching than R.

137

Evaluation of Three Systems for Measuring Blood Glucose. S.L. PIEPHO, H.G. KLOEPFER, C. SUTHER, Indianapolis, IN.

Three systems applicable for use by patients in monitoring blood glucose were evaluated. Studies were conducted at 5 sites. Systems evaluated were Bio-Dynamics/bmc StatTek and ChemStrip bG and Ames Eyetone. All systems utilize reagent impregnated strips. StatTek and Eyetone use reflectance meters for quantitation. ChemStrip bG is a visually read strip. A minimum of 200 patient samples was analyzed at each site by these 3 methods. Each sample was also analyzed by a routine laboratory method: Beckman glucose analyzer at sites 2, 4, and 5, YSI glucose analyzer at site 1 and the AutoAnalyzer Hoffman-ferricyanide method at site 3. All work was performed by trained laboratory personnel. A summary of the results obtained is shown below:

	Site 1	Site 2	Site 3	Site 4	Site 5
Eyetone					
Range	0-350	0-350	0-350	0-350	0-350
r2	0.868	0.988	0.986	0.955	0.925
$\bar{x}$ Ref.	107.6	149.4	125.0	109.6	115.2
$\bar{x}$ Eyetone	119.6	145.5	118.7	102.9	113.5
StatTek					
Range	0.350	0-350	0-350	0-350	0-350
r2	0.942	0.989	0.983	0.906	0.904
$\bar{x}$ Ref.	107.6	149-4	125.0	109.6	119.0
$\bar{x}$ StatTek	104.7	146.1	124.0	101.8	110.2
ChemStrip bG					
Range	0.800	0.800	0.800	0.800	0-800
r2	0.930	0.957	0.986	0.867	0.886
$\bar{x}$ Ref.	177.8	166.3	179.9	121.5	126.1
$\bar{x}$ Chemstrip bG	160.5	164.5	177.6	108.8	111.6

It is concluded that all three methods give reliable results and are suitable for patient use.

138

Utilization of a Self-Care Questionnaire in Patient Assessment. MARGARET A. HOWARD and LINDA K. STRODTMAN*, Ann Arbor, Mi.

The self-report method of obtaining data from patients has been underutilized by health professionals. The reasons are varied but one suspects that self-report has been discounted as being unreliable.

The adult Diabetes Center Unit has been using a patient self-care questionnaire. It is completed by the patient prior to or on admission to the unit. It asks for demographic data and diabetes self-care information. It also asks the patient to rate their understanding about diabetes and how it affects their work/school, sports, hobbies, sexual relations, traveling and budget.

To date 231 questionnaires have been analyzed (71 IDDM-mean age 32 yrs., duration 13.7 yrs. and 160 NIDDM-mean age 54 yrs., duration 10.8 yrs.). Fifty-eight subjects who had rated their understanding had also taken a 38 item knowledge pretest. Their rating of understanding correlated with their test scores (TS):Good=TS of 71% $\pm$ 13, Fair=TS of 64% $\pm$ 18, Poor=TS of 52% $\pm$ 20($p \leq .02$). There was no significant difference between the IDDM and NIDDM patients in their degree to which DM affected their activities of daily living. If DM affected the IDDM's work/school it also affected their other activities($p<.01$). For the NIDDM patients if work was affected only hobbies, travel and sports correlated($p.<.01$).

Besides finding out what the person knows about their self-care the questionnaire has given much information as to how the person feels about having DM. Since objective data has shown to correlate with patient self-report this assessment tool should be more widely used by health professionals.

139

Using Guided Design for Teaching Health Professionals How to Plan Patient Education. LINDA K. STRODTMAN* and CAROL P. BARNETT*, Ann Arbor, Mi.

Traditional methods of teaching health professionals how to plan patient education have usually focused on specific details of delivery such as group versus individual instruction or the type of media. Little consideration has been given to teaching the process of developing written educational plans.

Guided Design, a decision-making model, was selected to teach patient care planning. Guided Design is an educational strategy developed by Wales and Stager to educate engineering students. The model simultaneously accomplishes several goals, it 1) teaches subject content using step-by-step feedback, 2) facilitates the development of decision-making skills, 3) permits the application of content to real-world problems and 4) provides an organized group experience in which participants can practice interaction skills. The project uses a case presentation in which step-by-step feedback is given to teams of 5-8 professionals as they make decisions in planning care for a patient with diabetes mellitus.

Nearly 250 health professionals (dietitians, nurses, physicians, and social workers) have participated in an one and one-half hour workshop using this project. The workshop is part of a two day symposium on diabetes.

The response of the participants to this approach has been positive. The workshop evaluations have been rated good to excellent and the most frequent benefit identified by the participants has been the "team experience".

140

Diabetes by Criteria Mapping with a Weighting of Seriousness of Decision Errors. P.C. DAVIDSON, E. GREGERSON, and JACK GOODWIN, Morgantown, WV

An audit of the management of diabetes in a metropolitan university hospital revealed that 7% of patients with diabetes were optimally managed and 36% were unsatisfactorily managed by criteria agreed upon in advance. Ninety-six consecutive medical records of persons with a discharge diagnosis of diabetes, glucose >140 mg/dl fasting or >300 mg/dl random, on insulin, or on oral hypoglycemic agents were audited by a branching logic system of quality assessment known as criteria mapping. Twelve possible decision errors were present on the criteria map. Ninety-nine such errors occurred per 100 diabetic patients. Each error was weighted as to the probability that a clinical problem would arise from the error (p). The most serious stops were discharging patients with ketosis not on insulin (1%, p 0.9) or discharging the patient in a hyperosmolar state (7%, p 0.7). The more prevalent problems included treating a patient without any dietary restrictions (15%, p 0.6) and not assessing or supplementing the patient's knowledge of diabetes (13%, p 0.6). These latter items had the highest probability times incidence score. Other high scores included missing overt cases of diabetes, discharging patients with blood sugars >300 without evidence of physician awareness, and dropping hypoglycemic agents without assessing effect. This information has been useful in implementing measures to provide improved diabetic management. A repeat audit one year later is in progress. An area wide audit is underway.

141

The Prince Edward Island (PEI) Diabetes Control Program - Patterns of Therapy and Cost. M. H. TAN,* and C. WORNELL, Halifax and Charlottetown, Canada.

The PEI Diabetes Control Program provides insulin, oral agents and urine testing materials free of charge to diabetics who register annually with the Department of Health. Since 1964 it has served as an informal registry of diabetics in PEI whose population is 122,000. It also offers free diabetes education to patients.

To determine the patterns of therapy of diabetes, the diabetics were classified according to their treatment. In 1978 there were 2047 diabetics. Of these 20% were on diet alone, 48% on oral agents and 32% on insulin. In 1979 there were 2306 diabetics. The % in each treatment category were 23%, 43% and 34% respectively.

To determine the cost of providing free medications to diabetics, the total cost was analysed. In 1978 the cost of running the program was $137,326. Of this 34% was spent for education, 14% for urine testing materials, 11% for oral agents and 41% for insulin. When expressed as cost per diabetic per year the cost analysis showed: education=$23.06, urine testing materials=$9.38, oral agents=$14.87 and insulin=$84.50. In 1979 the figures were $22.50, $7.94, $12.60 and $93.14 respectively. The oral agents and urine testing materials are dispended directly by the provincial pharmacy. Bulk purchasing of drugs by generic name, no dispensing fee and provision of 3 month supplies contribute to the low cost of providing oral agents and urine testing materials.

142

Differences in Insulin Antibodies Induced with Varying Antigenic Forms. I. VALDES, R. E. MICHALSKI, R. THOMPSON, and E. R. ARQUILLA*, Irvine, Ca.

Insulin antisera contain at least two major populations of antibodies: those operative in the radioimmune assay (ABr), the others operative in the immune hemolysis assay (ABh) (Arquilla, et al., Diabetes 25, 1976). ABr interact with B-chain determinants while ABh interact with A-chain determinants. Hartley Mongrel guinea pigs were immunized with either monocomponent (MC) insulin, Zn-crystalline insulin, Ni-crystalline insulin, or fibrillar insulin. Each antigen preparation was from a single lot of MC bovine insulin prepared in our laboratory. The antiserum obtained from each guinea pig was titrated in both radioimmune assay and immune hemolysis assay to determine the respective levels of ABr and ABh. Antisera raised against Zn and Ni insulin had significantly higher ABh titers (2670 $\pm$ 511 and 3593 $\pm$ 1062, respectively) than antisera raised against MC and fibrillar insulin (1266 $\pm$ 318 and 910 $\pm$ 290, respectively). When either Zn or Ni insulin is the antigen, more antibodies directed toward A-chain determinants are produced. Animals immunized with MC insulin produced the antisera with the highest ABr titers (24,000 and 16,500). When Zn or Ni insulin is the antigen, antisera with high levels of antibodies directed toward A-chain determinants are produced. Immunizing with MC insulin is best for obtaining antisera with high levels of antibodies directed toward the B-chain determinants, which can be used to establish very sensitive radioimmune assays for insulin. Supported by grants from USPHS #AM13441-12 and the KROC Foundation.

143

Two Insulin-like Components in a Family with Hyperproinsulinemia. D. C. ROBBINS, H. S. TAGER, M. E. MAKO, K. H. GABBAY* and A. H. RUBENSTEIN,* Boston, Massachusetts and Chicago, Illinois.

Proinsulin-like material (PLM) from a hyperproinsulinemic family is relatively resistant to normal conversion and tryptic cleavage (PNAS 76: 2881-2885, 1979). About 10% of the serum immunoreactive insulin (IRI) in these subjects is 6000 MW material (ILM), which may be the products of both normal and defective precursors. ILM was obtained by affinity chromatography and purified by gel filtration. On 15% polyacrylamide gel electrophoresis (PAGE), the ILM separated into 2 bands at both pH 4.5 and 8.7. One band co-migrated with normal human insulin, diluted in parallel to human insulin standards in radioimmunoassay (RIA) and had normal biological activity in stimulating 2-deoxyglucose uptake in rat adipocytes. The second band migrated further than insulin at pH 8.7 but less than insulin at pH 4.5, suggesting the loss of a basic amino acid. Its electrophoretic mobilities and resistance to carboxypeptidase-B, however, indicated that the component is not desoctapeptide insulin. Furthermore, the material lacked biological activity and dilutions were not parallel to human insulin standards in RIA. Conclusion: Abnormal structure of the proinsulin molecule may cause aberrant cleavage(s) and the production of this unusual ILM. The presence of a biologically active ILM that co-migrates on PAGE with normal insulin suggests the expression of a co-dominant, normal insulin gene in this family.

144

Mouse Antibody Cytotoxic to Cultured Mouse Beta Cells. M. CHERRY and E. H. LEITER,* Bar Harbor.

Islets of Langerhans were isolated from CBA/J mice affected with Exocrine Pancreatic Insufficiency syndrome. Three allogeneic strains [A/J, C57BL/6J, and C57BL/KsJ (BL/Ks)] were given multiple injections of homogenized islets plus adjuvant. Only the pooled serum from the BL/Ks mice produced significant anti-CBA antibody (titering at 1/160 in the chromium release cytotoxicity test using CBA/J lymph node cells as targets). Extensive cytolysis in 14-day cultures of CBA/J islet cells was observed within 4 hr after introduction of immune serum (1%), but only in the presence of rabbit serum (5%, agarose absorbed) as a complement source. This cytolysis, which was not effected by BL/Ks normal serum, was accompanied by acute IRI and IRG release, as well as efflux of chromium-51 from pre-labeled islet cells. Ultrastructural survey showed degenerate beta cells, but normal appearing alpha cells. The appearance of distended profiles of rough endoplasmic reticulum that often contained intracisternal type A retrovirus budding into them was the major feature distinguishing antiserum-treated from control beta cells. The combined effect of a hyperglycemic milieu, effected by high medium glucose, and complement-mediated immune cytolysis produced degenerative changes similar to those seen in adult BL/Ks db/db beta cells in situ. The antiserum has a general specificity in that CBA thymus cell absorption effectively eliminates cytotoxicity to CBA/J islet cells. However, its specificity does not seem to be H-2K, since an anti-H-2K^k antibody cytotoxic to lymphocytes did not produce islet cell cytolysis at a 1% concentration.

145

Complement-mediated Islet Cell Surface Antibody -induced Block in Insulin Release from Perifused Rat Islet Cells. TAKAHIRO KANATSUNA, AKE LERNMARK*, DONALD F. STEINER*, Chicago, IL.

Antibodies reactive with the cell surface of rat pancreatic islet cells were raised in rabbits. An islet specific antiserum was obtained after extensive absorption to both spleen cells and hepatocytes. To investigate the effect of surface antibodies on the dynamics of insulin release a system allowing perifusion of single cells was developed. Suspensions of dispersed islet cells were prepared by mechanical treatment of collagenase-isolated rat pancreatic islets in Ca^{2+}-free medium. The dispersed islet cells representing about 60% single cells were mixed with 1 ml small polyacrylamide beads in two perifusion-chambers run in parallel. The dynamics of insulin release in response to glucose was biphasic (5mmol/l glucose 373±149 and 30 mmol/l glucose 1301±166 ng insulin released per 5×10^5 cells and 60 min). Addition of the anti-rat islet cell surface antibodies did not affect the release of insulin. However, 10% (v/v) guinea-pig serum as a source of complement added to cells previously exposed to islet cell surface antibodies resulted in an inability of the β-cells to release insulin in response to 30 mmol/l D-glucose.

A cytotoxic effect of islet cell surface antibodies and complement was also indicated by a marked release of ^{51}Cr-radioactivity (normal rabbit serum 1.3% and rat islet cell antiserum 28.1% of total cell radioactivity in 10 min) from rat islets prelabelled with $Na_2\,{}^{51}CrO_4$ before perifusion.

It is concluded that β-cells exposed to islet cell surface antibodies and complement are unable to release insulin in response to glucose.

146

A Genetic Marker in Spontaneously Diabetic Chinese Hamsters. D.W. SAMMONS and L.D. ADAMS, Kalamazoo, MI; S.L. TOLLAKSEN and N.G. ANDERSON, Argonne, IL (Introduced by W.E. Dulin*, Kalamazoo, MI)

The Upjohn colony of highly inbred nondiabetic and diabetic Chinese hamsters is being used to systematically search for genetic markers for diabetes. With two-dimensional gel electrophoresis, which allows charge and size discrimination of hundreds of protein gene products, we examined patterns of liver protein gene products from animals of 6 diabetic and 3 nondiabetic sublines. Within an inbred subline the patterns were nearly identical, whereas between sublines there were consistent pattern differences. One difference characteristic of all diabetic sublines was an aberrant protein whose position was unexpected and was shifted from that observed for the same gene product in the nondiabetic sublines. This variant protein did not result from a post-translational modification associated with high blood glucose levels because it occurred in young animals before the onset of hyperglycemia. In addition to being present in all highly inbred diabetics, the aberrant protein seemed to segregate with diabetic offspring in a hybrid subline (ZM) that had originated from a cross between a diabetic (Z) and a nondiabetic (M) subline. While additional experimental crosses will be required to prove conclusively the association between diabetes and this protein, its segregation with diabetes in the ZM subline and its presence in all established diabetic sublines suggest that this variant protein is a genetic marker for diabetes. (Supported in part by U.S. DOE under contract number W31-109-ENG-38.)

147

Characterization of Specific Growth Hormone Receptors in Isolated Fat Cells. R. SALTMAN, J. GAVIN, III, and W. DAUGHADAY,* St. Louis, Mo.

The isolated adipocyte has served as a useful model for the study of correlations between hormone receptor binding and activation of hormone-sensitive biologic responses. In studying the mechanisms through which various agents influence insulin sensitivity, we have further investigated the interaction of GH with fat cells. We now describe a specific receptor for GH in isolated rat fat cells. Binding of ^{125}I-hGH is rapid, reversible, shows time and temperature dependence with maximum specific binding at 37°C in 30-40 min. In contrast to other hormone receptors in these cells, there is a striking pH dependence with 3 to 4-fold greater specific binding occurring at pH 4.85 than at pH 7.4. Ca^{++} and Mg^{++} conc. over a 10-fold range have no effect on binding. Tracer degradation is less than 15% over 90 min at 37°. ^{125}I-hGH binding is inhibited by as little as 0.5 ng/ml of hGH. No inhibition is observed with insulin, glucagon, TSH, or hPRL at conc. up to 1 µg/ml. This receptor does not discriminate between mGH, rGH, bGH and pGH. At low pH, Scatchard analysis reveals curvilinear plots compatible with heterogeneous receptors or site-site interactions. Binding sites are approx. 60×10^3/ cell under these conditions. At pH 7.4, Scatchard plots are linear with $K_a \sim 10^{11}\ M^{-1}$ and 15×10^3 sites/cell. This striking effect of pH change on receptor binding is under further study.

Specific GH receptors in these cells facilitate the study of regulation of insulin and GH receptors in metabolic settings where opposite biologic effects may be observed.

148

Tissue Differences in Insulin Receptors: Acute Changes in Insulin Binding with Linearization of Scatchard Plots. J.N. LIVINGSTON*, L.A. POTTICK, and R.T. MOXLEY. Rochester, NY.

Wheat germ agglutinin (WGA) markedly enhances insulin binding(IB) and insulin (I) sensitivity of rat adipocytes (Am. J. Physiol.,in press). Further studies of WGA effect on IB (^{125}I-insulin, 5×10^{-10}M) were conducted using membranes from rat adipocytes (AM), rat liver (LM), human placenta (PM) and intact human monocytes. WGA stimulated IB in AM and LM by 480±30% and 260±15% above control (100%) respectively, whereas enhancement for PM was 140±8% and monocytes did not respond. Maximum stimulation required 1 µg/ml WGA for AM, and 5 µg/ml for LM and PM. WGA caused a decrease in I dissociation; this effect was greatest with AM followed by LM then PM. Results from Scatchard analysis of IB in the presence (+) and absence (-) of WGA were:

Prep.	Kd($\times 10^{-10}$M) High Aff. (-)	High Aff. (+)	Low Aff. (-)	Low Aff. (+)	R_o Value (pg.I/30 µg prot.) (-)	(+)
AM	8.0	2.5	42	absent	780	280
LM	7.0	5.5	51	absent	620	260
PM	6.0	5.0	70	46	90	76

WGA treatment of AM and LM linearizes the curvilinear Scatchard plots to one high affinity component while reducing the maximum binding capacity (R_o). In contrast, both affinity components were retained by PM and R_o was reduced by only 15%. These results indicate differences in receptor structure and/or its membrane environment in these different tissues. The acute and reversible nature of WGA effects make the lectin a useful probe to study changes in IB affinity.

149

Removal of an Affinity Regulator From the Insulin Receptor by Lectin Chromatography. J. A. HEDO, L. C. HARRISON*, and J. ROTH*. Bethesda, MD.

The insulin receptor is a glycoprotein, and its interaction with lectins alters its binding properties. We here demonstrate a permanent increase in the affinity of the solubilized insulin receptor after lectin chromatography. When membranes from human placenta and IM-9 lymphocytes were solubilized in Triton X-100 and filtered through agarose columns containing immobilized lectins, insulin binding activity was retained by concanavalin A, lentil, pea, ricin I and II, and wheat germ. After desorption with sugars, the insulin binding capacity (R_o) of the receptor was increased by up to 50-fold. In addition, there was a clear increase in the affinity of the receptor as evidenced by: 1) a decrease in the concentration of unlabeled insulin causing half maximal reduction of ^{125}I-insulin binding (from 11 to 4 ng/ml), and 2) an increase in Bound/Free ^{125}I-insulin (tracer binding) greater than the increase in binding capacity (saturation binding). The binding properties of the insulin receptor not retained by six other lectins (Bandeiraea Simplicifolia, gorse seed, horse gram, peanut, Sophora Japonica and soybean) were unaltered. The increase in receptor affinity mimics that observed after irradiation of the receptor and in certain in vivo situations, e.g. acromegaly, obesity after 72 hr fast, normal subjects 5 hrs after glucose. Our findings suggest the existence of a regulator of the insulin receptor that normally inhibits the affinity of the binding site and which is separated from it by chromatography on lectins.

150

Insulin-Mimickers Down Regulate the Insulin Receptor: Evidence for a Post Receptor Mechanism. J.F. CARO and J.M. AMATRUDA, Rochester NY.

The mechanism(s) by which insulin(Ins) regulates its receptor(Rec) is uncertain. It has been postulated that this effect is mediated through the Rec itself by complex degradative processes requiring protein synthesis. We have evaluated down regulation of the Ins Rec in primary cultures of rat hepatocytes with Ins,10^{-7}M, Ins Rec antibodies (Science 200:1283,1978) and the Ins mimickers H_2O_2 (0.3 mM),Vit K_5 (0.3 mM), spermine (0.3 mM) and wheat germ agglutinin (10 µg/ml). While having no acute effects on Ins binding, all decrease Ins binding after 18 hours of culture to approximately 50% of control. Analyses of binding indicate a decrease in the number of receptors without a change in the apparent affinity (high affinity Kd ∿ 1.0×10^{-9}M). Down regulation is not observed if cells are cultured with cyclohexamide,0.1 mM. These agents have no effect on glucagon binding or cell viability. The biological activity of the Ins mimickers is equal to Ins as shown by their ability to stimulate lipid synthesis.

In summary, Ins and agents with "insulin-like" activity specifically down regulate the Ins Rec. This phenomenon is unrelated to Rec occupancy since Vit K_5,H_2O_2 and spermine, which act distal to the Ins Rec, have similar effects. These studies demonstrate that the regulation of the Ins Rec is a complex intracellular biological response to Ins and may explain why in some cases Ins resistance is not related to changes in Ins Rec number.

151

Influence of the Insulin Receptor Compartment on Insulin Clearance. J. PHILIPPE, P. HALBAN*, A. GJINOVCI and W. DUCKWORTH* Geneva, Switzerland

Cells from streptozotocin (strep.) diabetic rats display increased insulin receptor binding. Since it has been suggested that insulin receptors may trap up to 75% of extrapancreatic insulin, we have studied the influence of the insulin receptor compartment on plasma insulin clearance in normal and strep. diabetic rats. Diabetics were studied 8 days after injection of 50mg/kg strep. (plasma insulin lowered by 50%, plasma glucose: 500-600mg/dl). (^{3}H)insulin (I*) was injected intravenously (3.5µCi,14.5mU/100g) and blood drawn from a jugular catheter at set times up to 60min. Plasma samples were chromatographed to separate intact I* from degradation products. The rate of I* clearance from plasma was increased by 70% in diabetics. Increased extracellular space did not fully account for this change. I* in urine was negligible. In order to displace I* from insulin receptors, 10U unlabelled insulin were injected 6min after the I* injection. This approach permits evaluation of the insulin receptor compartment. I* clearance following the unlabelled insulin injection was decreased by 46% in diabetics and by only 27% in normals. This difference was due to the increased I* displacement in diabetics compared to controls, indicating a larger receptor compartment in strep. diabetic rats. Changes in the receptor compartment thus affect insulin clearance, a finding of potential interest when considering plasma insulin clearance in man.

152

Characterization and Significance of Hepatic Receptors for Insulin during Fetal and Neonatal Life. FRANK VINICOR* and CHARLES CLARK, JR.*, Indianapolis, IN.

During late gestation, fetal tissues a) are especially sensitive to insulin(I); and b) store fuels and experience rapid growth. To determine the role of the I receptor in these processes, we have examined I binding in partially purified rat liver membranes during the perinatal(PN) period. Compared to adult(A), membranes from 21 day fetal(21dF), 1 day(1dN) and 7 day neonatal (7dN) rats bound 98, 84 and 50% more insulin, respectively: A - 76± 6(fmol/mg, mean±SEM); 21dF-150± 15(p<0.001 vs.A); 1dN-139±15 (p<0.01 vs.A); 7dN-114± 8 (p<0.01 vs.A). By 10 postnatal days, I binding was comparable to A. Only 14% of insulin was degraded by 1dN liver membranes compared to 66% with A hepatic tissues (p<0.01). Even when I degradation by A liver membranes was inhibited by incubation at 4°C however, PN membranes still bound 30% more insulin. In both A and PN liver membranes, comparable negative cooperativity was present: 40 fold dilution-51%(1dN) and 44%(A) dissociation of I; 40 fold dilution + excess I-70%(1dN) and 62%(A) dissociation. Scatchard and average affinity profile analyses of I binding revealed both increased receptor affinity (K_e) and greater I receptor concentration in PN liver membranes. These studies suggest that increased I binding by PN hepatic membranes a) is due to greater I receptor affinity and concentration, and diminished I degradation; and b) contributes to heightened tissue sensitivity to I which insures storage of fuel and growth of the organism.

153

Decreased Spare Hepatic Receptors for Insulin: Possible Importance for Insulin Action. M.B. DAVIDSON*, and H.J.L. FRANK, Los Angeles, Ca.

Approximately 5% and 20% of receptors in fat and muscle respectively need to be occupied for maximal insulin action. The presence of spare receptors in liver has not been evaluated because of the lack of a suitable bioassay. We have developed an assay for insulin action in rat hepatocytes by measuring ^{14}C-glucose incorporation into glycogen at 37°C for 1 hour. This pathway is sensitive to physiological insulin concentrations with an effect detectable at 1 ng/ml, a ½ maximal effect noted at 3 ng/ml and a maximal effect (doubling of basal incorporation) between 10 and 20 ng/ml. Insulin binding at equilibrium was measured at both 20°C and 37°C. Comparison of insulin binding and action on the same cells revealed that maximal action occurred when only 35% of the receptors were occupied whether binding was measured at 20°C (n=8) or at 37°C (n=5). Thus, 65% of hepatic insulin receptors are "spare". Scatchard analysis of the curvilinear plots of 7 paired binding studies at the 2 temperatures revealed no differences in either high or low affinity constants but significant increases ($p < .02$ or better) in both binding capacities at 20°C compared to 37°C. Conclusions: 1) Hepatic insulin action is not maximal until 35% of receptors are occupied compared to maximal effects at 5% occupancy in fat and 20% occupancy in muscle; 2) The lower % of spare receptors in the liver may allow a continued response at high portal vein insulin levels at which peripheral tissues would have ceased to respond; 3) Binding temperatures affect capacities but not affinities or % of spare receptors.

154

Insulin Binding and Glucose Transport in Isolated Adipocytes from Obese Patients. T.P. CIARALDI and J.M. OLEFSKY*, Denver, Colorado.

To study cellular mechanisms of insulin(I) resistance in human obesity and the relationships between I binding and glucose transport(GT), initial rates of 3-O-methyl glucose (50 μM) uptake and I binding to adipocytes were measured in 9 obese and 11 control subjects. I receptors(R) were decreased by 42% in adipocytes from the obese patients. I led to a dose dependent 2-fold increase in GT from 1.03 to 2.14 pmoles/2 X 10^5 cells/10 sec with a 1/2 maximally effective I level of 0.55 ng/ml in cells from normals. In 2 mildly hyperinsulinemic obese patients (fasting I = 27 μU/ml) I increased GT from 1.01 to 2.23 with a 1/2 maximal I level of 1.1 ng/ml, indicating a rightward shift in the dose response curve with no change in maximal GT rates, consistent with a decrease in IR. These patients also exhibited normal maximal in vivo rates of G disposal during G clamp studies. In 9, more severely obese, hyperinsulinemic patients (fasting I = 58 μU/ml) I increased GT from 0.30 to 0.89 with a 1/2 maximal I level of 1 ng/ml, indicating a rightward shift in the curve plus a marked decrease in basal and maximal GT rates, consistent with both a decrease in IR and a post-R defect in the GT system. These patients also exhibited decreased (45%) maximal in vivo rates of G disposal during G clamp studies. In conclusion: 1) In mildly hyperinsulinemic obese patients cellular I resistance is due to decreased IR whereas it is due to decreased IR plus a post-R defect in the GT system in more severely hyperinsulinemic obese patients. 2) These in vitro data correlate well to in vivo studies of I action on overall G disposal.

155

Insulin Binding to Erythrocytes and Monocytes from Pima Indians with Various Degrees of Hyperinsulinemia. TOM HUECKSTEADT, FRANK KOSMAKOS,* AND DAVE MOTT,* Phoenix, AZ.

Pima Indians have marked insulin resistance. To determine the role of the insulin receptor in this resistance, Pima receptors were characterized and examined under various degrees of hyperinsulinemia. The interaction of insulin with the RBC insulin receptor was normal in specificity, reversibility, and time-, temperature-, and pH-dependence of binding. Receptor number and affinity were determined using both monocytes and RBC from 17 subjects with various degrees of hyperinsulinemia (10-61 μU/ml). Fasting insulins were not significantly correlated with high or low affinity receptor numbers on Pima RBC. However, RBC receptor affinity did decrease with increasing insulin levels ($r=0.68$, $p<0.004$). The concurrent monocyte studies were similar to those of the RBC in that a correlation between high or low affinity receptor number and fasting insulins was not detected. In contrast to the RBC, monocyte receptor affinity did not change with fasting insulin levels. When either high or low affinity receptor number or receptor affinity was compared between RBC and monotyes of the same subject, a significant correlation was not observed. These results with Pima cells suggest: 1) the insulin receptor is normal by a variety of binding criteria; 2) the monocytes and red cells are not comparable systems for monitoring receptor status; and 3) the mechanisms for insulin mediated regulation of insulin binding to RBC is via altered receptor affinity, while receptor regulation was not observed in monocytes.

156

Effects of Inhibition of Catecholamine (CA) Release by Clonidine upon Hormone and Substrate Responses to Insulin-Induced Hypoglycemia. S.A. METZ* and J.B. HALTER*, Seattle, WA.

The role of CA in the counterregulation of hypoglycemia is poorly defined. We previously reported that clonidine (CLON) reduced basal norepinephrine (NE) but not basal epinephrine (EPI) levels in normal male subjects. To determine whether CLON reduces stimulated EPI and NE release and whether such effects modify responses to insulin-induced hypoglycemia (IH), CLON (0.5mg p.o.) was administered to 6 subjects 90min. prior to induction of hypoglycemia with insulin (0.05 U/kg IV). Despite a hypoglycemic nadir of 44±5mg/dl ($\bar{x}$±SEM), no increase of NE or EPI occurred during CLON. However, the glucose (GLU) nadir during CLON was slightly (9±3mg/dl; $p<.05$) less deep than during control studies. Therefore additional studies were performed using a higher insulin dose (0.06-0.075 U/kg) in subjects receiving CLON. Identical GLU nadirs (saline=34±3; CLON=35±2mg/dl) and rates of fall of GLU were now achieved. CLON still reduced CA response (0-60 min. area) by 83% ($p<.02$), with both EPI and NE being diminished, but did not alter the magnitude of the glucagon (IRG) response (control=2066±378; CLON=1587±414 pg/ml·hr; p=NS). Nevertheless, the early GLU recovery rate (ΔGLU 0-15 min. after each subject's own GLU nadir) was blunted compared to control studies (saline=1.75±0.27; CLON=0.96±0.29mg/dl/min, $p<.05$). We conclude that CLON markedly inhibits the CA but not the IRG rise during IH. Thus increments in CA are not required for the IRG response to hypoglycemia. Selective inhibition of CA secretion leads to a transient inhibition of the GLU homeostatic response.

157

Plasma Epinephrine Disturbances in Diabetic Subjects during Isometric Exercise. A. B. GUSTAFSON and R. K. KALKHOFF*, Milwaukee, Wi.

Little is known about the metabolic effects of isometric exercise on diabetic subjects. Ten healthy, insulin-dependent diabetic patients (IDD) were matched in age, weight and sex to 10 control adults (C). Blood samples were obtained and mean blood pressure (MBP) and heart rate (HR) were measured in an a.m. basal state after 30 min of absolute bedrest and sequentially during 10 min of upright posture, 5 min of handgrip at 30% of maximum voluntary contraction, and after 15 min of rest while still upright. In C and IDD groups, respectively, basal plasma norepinephrine (NE: 180 ± 22 vs. 169 ± 27 pg/ml), epinephrine (E: 24 ± 4 vs. 33 ± 8 pg/ml) as well as glucagon (GON), HR and MBP did not differ. Fasting plasma glucose concentrations were 81 ± 2 and 165 ± 30 mg/dl (a.m. insulin withheld). Measured parameters excepting glucose rose during standing, reached peak values during handgrip and fell partially toward baseline at rest. No differences in MBP nor excursions of plasma NE or GON in the two groups were observed. However, plasma E in IDD subjects exceeded C values 1.5 to 2.5-fold during each period as did HR during standing and recovery ($p < 0.05$). Mean plasma glucose increments in IDD were 21 and 41 mg/dl above baseline during grip and recovery as contrasted to 3-4 mg/dl increments in C.

We conclude that plasma E disturbances exist in this IDD group during standing and isometric exercise. This is physiologically linked to exaggerated increments of heart rate and plasma glucose concentrations during these periods.

158

The Significance of Cortisol, Glucagon, and HGH for the Development of Ketosis in Insulin Dependent Patients with and without Residual β-cell Function. C. BINDER*, S. MADSBAD, O. FABER, H. ØRSKOV, L. REGEUR, B. TRONIER, Copenhagen, Denmark.

The response of cortisol, HGH, and glucagon was studied postabsorptively during 12 hours of insulin deprivation and continued fasting in 8 insulin dependent patients with (group A) and in 7 without residual β-cell function (group B). Study design and metabolic responses have been published recently (Brit.Med.J. 2:1257-59,1979).

Mean plasma cortisol showed normal morning values followed by a normal diurnal decline for 2 hours. Then it increased significantly in group B at a time when blood glucose as the only metabolite had deviated from that of group A. Final levels were significantly correlated with final concentration of glucose ($R=0.64$, $P<0.02$), 3-OH-butyrate ($R=0.68$, $P<0.02$), and NEFA ($R=0.73$, $P<0.01$).

Mean plasma HGH was significantly higher in group B (16.1±1.8 ng/ml) compared to group A (8.3±0.9 ng/ml) in which it was only slightly above normal. Glucagon rose similarly in both groups from 88±6 to 120±10 pg/ml. There was no correlation between changes or final concentrations of HGH and glucagon to changes or final concentrations of any metabolite measured: glucose, 3-OH-butyrate, NEFA, glycerol, lactate, and alanine.

Mean and final concentrations of cortisol, HGH, and glucagon were not correlated with each other, and in group A they were not correlated with mean C-peptide concentration.

The results point to cortisol as a key hormone rather than glucagon in the development of ketosis in insulin dependent patients deprived of insulin.

159

A New Mechanism for the VLDL-TG Removal Defect in Insulin Deficient Rats. H. BAR-ON, Y-D.I. CHEN and G.M. REAVEN*. Stanford, Ca.

Hypertriglyceridemia in insulin-deficient rats is secondary to decreased removal of very low density lipoprotein (VLDL)-triglyceride (TG) from plasma, and recent evidence suggests that this defect is not due entirely to reduced tissue lipoprotein lipase activity. In this study we have attempted to define other mechanisms that might be responsible for this phenomenon. Endogenously labeled (^{3}H-glycerol) VLDL-TG was prepared in control (C) and streptozotocin-induced diabetic (D) rats, and its half-time of disappearance ($t_{1/2}$) determined following its injection into normal recipient rats. Recipient rats received between 1.4-1.8 ml of plasma containing prelabeled VLDL-TG. In each experiment the amount of total injected TG obtained either from diabetic or control rats was kept constant. Mean (± SEM) $t_{1/2}$ (in minutes) of VLDL-TG removal was significantly prolonged (8.6±0.9 vs 4.7±0.3, $p<0.0001$) following the injection into normal recipients of plasma from D (=10) as compared to C ($n=9$) rats, and this abnormality persisted following exhaustive dialysis. However, the differences in $t_{1/2}$ disappeared when prelabeled VLDL-TG from D and C was isolated and injected into normal recipients in the absence of the d>1.006 infranate. Thus, the defect in removal of VLDL-TG from D rats could be due to either an abnormal VLDL-TG (which is repaired by plasma cofactors present in recipient rats) or to inhibitors of VLDL-TG removal present in D plasma. In either case, it is suggested that these changes contribute to the hypertriglyceridemia of insulin deficiency.

160

Insulin-Independent Glucose Disposal During Physiologic Hyperglycemia. S.E. FINEBERG*, S.H. SCHNEIDER*, and D.C. HOWEY*. Indianapolis, IN.

Glucose disposal during physiologic hyperglycemia remains normal over a wide range of insulin concentrations. Increased glucose disposal in normal individuals may be independent of changes in insulin. We have tested this hypothesis by induction of local hyperglycemia during dose-ranging and dose-response studies in forearms of normal individuals. During 11 studies, forearm arterial glucose concentrations were increased from 20 to 200 mg/dl for 1 hour. Glucose uptake was markedly enhanced by hyperglycemia alone and was directly related to glucose increment (GI). The range of deep (D, muscle) and superficial (S, fat and skin) glucose uptake during baseline was .45-2.05 and .02-.40 uMole·100 ml tissue^{-1}·min^{-1} and depending on GI, increased to 2.06-9.27 and .29-2.67 uMole·100^{-1} ml·min^{-1}, both $p<.001$ when paired with baseline. The slope of GI vs glucose uptake was linear, $r=.76$, $p<.02$. This relationship was confirmed in 9 studies in which there were GI of 17, 30 and 63 mg/dl: GI vs arteriovenous differences of glucose across D, $r=.89$, $p<.005$ and S, $r=.92$, $p<.001$. An increase in forearm insulin concentrations (350 uU/ml) in the presence of hyperglycemia shut off lipolysis in S and promoted K+ uptake in D and S; but insulin had no additional effects upon glucose disposal. We conclude that in normal man glucose disposal during physiologic hyperglycemia is largely independent of changing insulin concentrations. This suggests that comparative studies between normal and diabetic individuals must take glucose concentrations into account.

161

Diurnal Rhythm of Insulin Sensitivity (IS) in Subjects with Impaired Glucose Tolerance (IGT). B. SCHULZ, K.P. RATZMANN, G. ALBRECHT and H. BIBERGEIL, Karlsburg, GDR (Intr. by E. REAVEN*).

Although diurnal variations in carbohydrate tolerance (CT) have been previously described, it is not known if there are also diurnal variations in IS. Furthermore, if such variations do exist, can they be seen in subjects with both normal and IGT? To answer these questions, five nonobese subjects with IGT and five controls were connected to a glucose controlled insulin infusion system (BIOSTATOR) for at least 27 hr. This technique involved a static plus dynamic control for insulin infusion. Glucose was infused at a fixed rate of 2 mg/kg/min. The amount of insulin needed to keep glycemia at a concentration of 80 mg/dl was used as an index of IS. During the whole period of investigation subjects were at bed rest and did not receive any food.

Despite the continuous glucose infusion, the C-peptide levels did not change in either group. The mean amount of insulin necessary to metabolize 1 g of glucose was 219 mU and 83 mU in subjects with IGT and controls, respectively ($p<0.01$). Both groups demonstrated regular oscillation of insulin requirement throughout the study. The highest IS was observed between 2PM and 6 PM and the lowest between 11PM and 4 AM. A circadia rhythm was found by autocorrelation. The periods had a mean duration of 20 and 25 hr (p=N.S.) in subjects with IGT and controls, respectively.

In conclusion, diurnal variations in IS do occur. Although mean IS is reduced in subjects with IGT, the diurnal variation was seen in both groups. Thus, diurnal variations in IS are independent of degree of CT.

162

Rightward Shift of the Insulin Dose-response Curve for Glucose Disposal in Type II Human Diabetes: Evidence for Decreased Insulin Sensitivity and Impaired Insulin Receptor Function. R.Rizza,* R. Westland, and L. Hall, Endocrine Research Unit, Mayo Clinic, Rochester, Minnesota.

To assess insulin action in type II diabetes, insulin dose-response curves for glucose disposal were determined in nonobest type II diabetics (fasting plasma glucose 145±16 mg/dl) and in age-weight and sex matched nondiabetic controls using sequential insulin infusions and the glucose clamp technique. Plasma glucose was maintained at 95±2 mg/dl in both groups (C.V=4.8±0.4%). Steady-state glucose infusion rates (SSGIR, mg/kg/min) required to maintain euglycemia were used to quantify responses to insulin. Infusion of insulin at 0.5, 1.0, 2.0 and 5.0 mU/kg/min, each for 2 hrs, increased plasma insulin to 51±3, 105±12, 250±27 and 758±94 μU/ml in diabetics and to 52±3, 96±6, 231±12, and 719±46, in controls and resulted in SSGIRs of 2.9±0.4, 6.7±0.5, 9.0±0.8 and 10.5±0.8 in diabetics and 4.7±0.5, 7.9±0.3, 9.6±0.4 and 10.7±0.3 in controls. Plasma insulin concentrations required for half-maximal effect (Km) in diabetics (81±4 μU/ml) were greater than those in controls (59±3 μU/ml, $p<0.01$) but maximal responses to insulin were comparable in both groups. Km's correlated with both monocyte and RBC insulin binding (r=.67 and .75, $p<0.05$) and iv glucose tolerance (r=.67, $p<0.05$). Conclusion: Rightward shift of the insulin dose-response curve for glucose disposal with a normal maximal response to insulin indicates decreased insulin sensitivity in type II diabetes. Associated changes in monocyte and RBC insulin binding suggest insulin receptor dysfunction may be responsible.

163

Long Term Effects of an α-Glucosidase Inhibitor on Catecholamine Levels and Insulin Requirements as Assessed by the Artificial Beta-cell. S.RAPTIS, G.DIMITRIADIS, K.KARAISKOS, J.ROSENTHAL, CHR.ZOUPAS and S.MOULOPOULOS Athens,Greece; Ulm, Germany (Introduced by G.F.GASTINEAU*,Rochester Minn).

The α-Glucosidase inhibitor (Bay-g-5421) was studied in 10 male juvenile type diabetics (age 20-38 years) who exhibited no measurable C-Peptide levels. All patients were kept on a constant diet and treated with Bay 200mg/tid p.o. for periods of up to 6 months.Before and at 1,2 and 6 months under Bay the participants were connected for 48 hours to the artificial beta-cell(Biostator GCIIS). Before treatment insulin requirements were 70±11 units/24h, at 1 month 38±12 and almost unchanged at 6 months (42±8). Postprandial blood glucose increments before treatment were 53±9 mg%, 33±11 and 65±17 (after breakfast, lunch and dinner), the corresponding values at 1 month of Bay were 32±8,15±4 and 16±5 and at 6 months 28±11, 12±6 and 19±8. Catecholamine levels decreased from 122±16pg/ml to 94±32 for epinephrine and from 353±48pg/ml to 290±60 for norepinephrine (mean values during multiple daily determinations) at 1 month with no important changes up to 6 months.

We concluded that Bay induces smoothening of the blood glucose curve together with an insulin sparing effect which is accompanied by lower catecholamine levels. Conceivably, this compound can be used as adjunct therapy in insulin dependent diabetics. (Supported by grants from Social Ministry Athens, Greece and the Alexander S. Onassis Foundation Vaduz, Liechtenstein).

164

Glucose Lowering Effects of Dietary Fiber: Altered Absorption Rather than Metabolism of Carbohydrate. J. WAHREN, O. BJORKMAN, A. JUHLIN-DANNFELT, and P. FELIG*. Stockholm, Sweden, and New Haven, Ct.

Dietary fiber reduces postprandial hyperglycemia and lowers insulin requirements in diabetics. The mechanism of these actions has not however, been determined. In the present study the effects of dietary fiber on insulin sensitivity and secretion and on disposal of glucose by splanchnic versus peripheral tissues were examined using the glucose clamp technic and hepatic vein catheterization. In 10 normal subjects plasma glucose was acutely raised and maintained at 125 mg/dl above fasting (by a variable glucose infusion) for 3 hrs. After 1 hr 5 of the subjects ingested 10 gm guar gum (fiber). The rise in plasma insulin after fiber was no greater than in the control study (60-80 μU/ml). Total glucose metabolized (an index of total body insulin sensitivity) was the same with and without fiber (12.4±2.7 vs 12.8±3.0 mg/kg/min). Splanchnic glucose uptake was also the same with and without fiber (1.6±0.3 vs 1.8±0.1 mg/kg/min). In a second series of studies, the effect of fiber on carbohydrate absorption was determined by administering orally 25 gm xylose with and without 10 gm guar. Blood xylose levels 1-3 hrs after fiber were 25-40% lower than after oral xylose alone ($P<0.05$-0.01). Conclusions: 1) Dietary fiber fails to increase insulin secretion, total body insulin sensitivity or hepatic uptake of glucose. 2) Dietary fiber decreases and/or delays carbohydrate absorption. The glucose lowering effect of dietary fiber is thus a consequence of changes in carbohydrate absorption rather than metabolism.

165

Adolescent Clinic: A Specialized Treatment Approach. G. GUNTER-HUNT and L. PARKER, Ann Arbor, Mi., (Introduced by M. SPENCER*).

Diabetes treatment programs are often difficult for adolescents struggling with developmental issues such as independence and self-identity. These issues are manifested by feelings such as ambivalence, rebelliousness and self-assertion. Resulting treatment problems (e.g. noncompliance) alerted our team to the need for a specialized approach - an adolescent clinic.

The clinic offers a group experience for teens led by the nurse clinician and for parents led by the social worker. Adolescent input regarding education and discussion topics was obtained through the use of a mailout questionnaire (N=40). Guided by the results of this survey, topics such as birth control/pregnancy, heredity, long-term complications, exercise and alcohol/drugs have been scheduled for adolescent breakfast sessions. The less structured parent rap sessions have generally focused on topics such as adolescent rebellion and noncompliance. Clinic meets monthly with patients attending at their regularly scheduled appointments. As of January 1980, 18 sessions have been held where 50 adolescents and their parents have attended. Twenty-three have returned more than once.

Development of the program involved assessing patient interest and needs, eliciting staff support and obtaining staff time commitments. Preliminary feedback from parents and adolescents indicates that the program is responsive to their needs. A formal program evaluation is in progress. It is anticipated that this program could serve as a prototype for other health providers working with adolescent populations.

166

Diabetes Mellitus in Adolescents: The Relationship between Behavioral, Psychological Variables and Glucose Control. J. SIMONDS, D. GOLDSTEIN*, B. WALKER, S. RAWLINGS, Columbia, Missouri.

We are investigating the relationship between glucose control as reflected by Hemoglobin A1c (HbA1c) and psychological variables such as locus of control, self image, personality traits and behavioral factors in a group of 50 insulin dependent diabetic (at least 5 years duration) adolescents. HbA1c values are compared with data obtained from standardized questionnaires and self report questionnaires that assess feelings, self care versus parental care, compliance, behavioral adjustment and perception of environmental reactions. There are 6 parent and 5 subject questionnaires set up on a Likert type scale that requires a response from 0 to 6 (i.e. never to always) in relationship to the previous 2 month period. Total scores are summed for each questionnaire. Initially a test-retest reliability study of the 11 self report questionnaires was completed on 27 diabetic subjects 11 years to 18 years of age. At the time of clinic visits mothers and subjects were asked to report on the frequency of feelings and behaviors during the previous 2 months. Two weeks later each subject and parent completed the same questionnaires. Correlation coefficients for the 11 questionnaires ranged from .58 to .86 with 10 questionnaires having acceptable limits of reliability (i.e. above .70).

Thus far 7 subjects have completed this project. Results indicate that better glucose control, as estimated by HbA1c, correlated positively with the degree of parental supervision and negatively with the degree of adolescent self care.

167

Impact of a Recreation Program on Skills, Knowledge and Psychosocial Adjustment in Diabetic Children. DEBORAH V. EDIDIN,* ANNE M. RATH, LYNNE L. LEVITSKY,* CAROL POLLAK, CLARA COEN, JEANETTE WHITE, and EILEEN VENCKUS, Chicago, Ill.

Thirteen preadolescent diabetic children (ages 8-12 years) participated in a 6 month twice-monthly recreational/educational program. Diabetes knowledge, self-care skills, regimen adherence, attitude, self-esteem, anxiety and control were evaluated pre- and post-program. Initial positive attitude toward diabetes (questionnaire) correlated with older age at onset (9.8 ± 0.8 vs 5.3 ± 1.3 yrs, $p<.02$), recent diagnosis (1.8 ± 0.5 vs 5.8 ± 1.4 yrs, $p<.02$), and female sex (0/5 boys vs 6/8 girls). Nine children had increased anxiety (Castaneda et al. anxiety scale), and 7 had low self-esteem (modified Kaplan self-esteem scale). Ten (5/5 boys) exhibited magical thinking about the cause or course of their disease unrelated to age, duration or knowledge and skills assessment. Nine children (5/5 boys) felt isolated pre-, and only 5 did post-program (questionnaire). Knowledge and skill scores (questionnaire, demonstration) increased post-program ($p<.005$, knowledge, $p<.01$ skills) but adherence scores did not. Glycohemoglobin fell in 10/12 children (N.S.). The program was associated with improvement in knowledge and skills, as well as amelioration of feelings of isolation. However, neither adherence nor control improved significantly. Age-inappropriate magical thinking may influence the effect of diabetes education in the preadolescent child.

168

A Therapeutic Paradigm for Discrepant Urine Records. WENDY CITRIN, GEORGE J. ELLIS, III,* and JAY S. SKYLER,* Miami, Florida and Durham, North Carolina.

The use of glycosylated hemoglobin determinations as an objective parameter for the assessment of diabetic control has permitted the identification of a new category of patients -- those in whom there is marked discrepancy between control as determined by glycosylated hemoglobin and control as reflected in urine glucose records. Assuming erroneous testing techniques and altered renal threshold are excluded, the discrepancy may be accounted for on the basis of several mechanisms. We have developed a diagnostic/therapeutic classification of patients with discrepant urine records, based on the presumed underlying reason for discrepant results. Reasons for discrepant results include: (1) seeking of perfection; (2) denial; (3) seeking of approval; (4) expression of resentment or anger; (5) avoidance of punishment; (6) avoidance of confrontation; (7) avoidance of depression; (8) guilt (e.g. following dietary indiscretions). Using this scheme and a non-judgemental therapeutic approach that seeks patient input in defining causes and outcome, it is possible to develop a long-term plan that promotes truthfulness, lessens discrepancy between urine testing and other control parameters, and thereby improves not only the utility of urine testing as a monitoring procedure, but hopefully also improves patient self-concept.

169

The Changing Prevalence of Diabetes in the U.S.
T. Drury and M. Harris*, Bethesda, MD.

Data from U.S. National Health Surveys, complemented by community-based studies, are used to document a 6-fold increase in the prevalence of diabetes between 1936 and 1978. Age/sex/race-specific rates illustrate that each demographic group has experienced increases in prevalence. These changes can be ascribed to increases in the incidence of new cases and the duration of prevalent cases, both of which can be sorted into a number of subcomponents. Increases in incidence rates for age groups above 55 years are approximately 2-fold greater than for younger groups. Trends in severity at the time of diagnosis indicate that milder, asymptomatic cases, emerging from a reservoir of approximately 4 million undiagnosed diabetics, may constitute the bulk of newly discovered diabetes. Social factors such as intensive screening for diabetes, Medicare legislation, and improvements in the technology for glucose measurement confound what may be real etiologic increases, such as those associated with increasing obesity of the U.S. population. Changes in the mean duration of diabetes and declines in mortality due to diabetes, particularly cardiovascular mortality since 1968, contribute to the increased prevalence of this disease in the U.S.

170

Summary of First Year Results of The First State Registry of Insulin Dependent Diabetes Mellitus.
JOY WELLS, JEFFREY ROSEMAN*, and BURIS BOSHELL*, Birmingham, Al.

In November, 1978, Alabama became the first state to make Insulin Dependent Diabetes Mellitus (IDDM) a reportable disease. All reported cases are included in the Alabama Juvenile Onset Diabetes Registry. This presentation will be a summary of the first full year of the Registry.

In 1979, 200 cases of IDDM were reported. The approximate equal sex distribution (48% male, 52% female) is similar to those reported on clinic samples and population samples from other countries. Since 30.4% of the individuals below 30 years of age in Alabama are black, the racial distribution (73% white, 27% black) suggests that the incidence of IDDM in blacks is not much lower than whites as has been suggested by others. This difference may reflect bias in ascertainment. In general the age of onset distributions for males and females are consistent with what has been reported by others with peak incidence in the 7-15 age group. The peak month of onset was October and the month with the fewest reported cases was June.

We feel that this number of reported cases represents under-reporting. In the summer of 1979 a telephone survey of a 10% random sample of Alabama physicians (n=354) was conducted. The survey revealed that the majority of physicians were unaware that IDDM was reportable. Efforts are underway to determine the validity and reliability of the Registry. These will be discussed.
(Supported by grants from the Appalachian Regional Commission (ARC-78-156 AL6350-78-I-302-0613) and the Diabetes Trust Fund.)

171

The Social and Economic Cost of Diabetes in Kentucky: Final Report.
P. H. COLLINS*, A. FISCHER, C. HERNANDEZ, Lexington, Kentucky.

We compiled data on the mortality, morbidity and economic loss attributable to diabetes in Kentucky. Such data was attributed to diabetes whenever: diabetes was listed as the primary diagnosis (Dx); diabetes was a secondary Dx for a complication, as diabetic nephropathy, not expected to occur among nondiabetic populations; the data represented the increment in occurrence of a diabetic complication over the expected occurrences in nondiabetic populations. In 1978, the death rate due to diabetes as a primary Dx was 17.7/100,000 people; the overall death rate among diabetic Kentuckians was 42.7/100,000; the death rate directly attributable to diabetes plus its complications was 30.3/100,000. Diabetes was the leading cause of hospital admission, by disease. Admissions directly attributable to diabetes accounted for 2.7% of 324,364 hospital admissions examined, and diabetics, admitted for any reason, accounted for 5.23% of all admissions. Diabetes was the primary diagnosis in 27.5-33.2% of cases and diabetic complications were the primary diagnosis in 23.6%. Almost half of the admissions due to complications were due to heart disease, without acute infarction. Hyperglycemic or hypoglycemic emergencies accounted for 2.7-3.4% of admissions due to diabetes. Direct medical costs attributable to diabetes were estimated at $88,384,981-$134,174,670/year. The average diabetic hospital stay, costing $1037-1248, was more expensive than nondiabetics stay ($p<0.01$). We conclude that diabetes is a more serious cause of social and economic loss than previously supposed.

172

The Social and Economic Costs of Diabetes: An Estimate for 1979.
GERALD PLATT, PH.D. and STEPHEN G. SUDOVAR, Fairfax, VA (Introduced by LEONA V. MILLER, M.D.,* Los Angeles, CA).

This study estimates the magnitude and associated costs of diabetes in the U.S. during 1979, and estimates the proportions attributable to insulin-dependency.

It has been estimated that there were 8.3 million diabetics in the U.S. during 1979.

This prevalence figure has been shown to be biased toward elderly, toward females, and toward non-whites. Further, it has been shown that 14.6 percent of the above prevalence figures represent new cases ("incidence") during 1979.

A breakdown of the 8.3 million prevalence estimate in terms of treatment regime reveals that 1.9 million are insulin-dependent, 2.9 million are non-insulin oral-dependent, 1.6 million are diet-only dependent, and approximately 1.8 million have undiagnosed diabetes.

The study shows that the 8.3 million diabetics generated a total cost of $15.4 billion in 1979. The "average" diabetic generated costs of $1,845.32 during 1979, about two-thirds (65.8%) of which were indirect and almost half (48.3%) of which were the result of lost workdays.

The 1.9 million diabetics who were insulin-dependent during 1979 have been separately analyzed in terms of the $4.5 billion costs they generated.

On a per-capita (or per-patient) basis, the total costs are 21 percent higher for an insulin-dependent diabetic than for an "average" diabetic.

173

Diabetes and Disability Among Persons Twenty Years of Age and Older. THOMAS F. DRURY and LOIS LIPSETT,* Hyattsville, Md. and Bethesda, Md.

It has long been recognized that the Health Interview Survey of the National Center for Health Statistics is an important source of information on the prevalence and impact of known diabetes. Only recently, however, has the secondary analytic potential of this national household survey for diabetes epidemiology and health care policy issues been recognized and utilized. During the last two years collaborative efforts between staff members of the Division of Health Interview Statistics within the National Center for Health Statistics and of the National Diabetes Information Clearinghouse within the National Institute of Arthritis, Digestive and Metabolic Diseases have led to the identification and construction of data sets which make possible on the basis of available data a far more comprehensive description of the health and medical care aspects of known diabetes than has hitherto been possible from this data source. The proposed paper will present highlights from preliminary analyses of several of these data sets which shed important light on disability among persons twenty years of age and older with diabetes by making possible comparisons between diabetics and nondiabetics on a variety of short-term and long-term disability indicators with selected demographic characteristics controlled.

174

Ketoacidosis or Coma Mortality in Diabetes. C.A. HERRON, D.C. MAY, (Introduced by L.C. DEEB,*) Atlanta, Georgia

Ketoacidosis and coma are diabetic complications considered to be preventable. Their occurrence in specific populations may reflect adequacy of care. In cause-of-death reporting, diabetes with mention of acidosis or coma (DKA) is differentiated, as ICDA code #250.0, from diabetes without such mention, ICDA #250.9, permitting analysis of deaths due to these complications through standard mortality data.

Deaths from DKA as underlying cause on NCHS mortality tapes for 1968-72 were analyzed by age, race, and sex for both cause-specific death rates and for proportional mortality ratios relative to all diabetes deaths (ICDA 250.0 + 250.9). Mean annual age-specific death rates for DKA ranged from 0.11/100,000 in persons aged <10 yrs. to 15.2/100,000 in those aged $\geq$80 yrs. Rates were generally higher in females than males, consistent with differences in diabetes prevalence. By race, however, rates for adults among other-than-whites (OTW) exceeded those in whites beyond expected from disease prevalence alone. Among diabetes deaths in adult age groups the relative risk by race (OTW:white) of DKA being causal ranged from 1.6 to 1.9.

County-and race-specific DKA death rates and proportional ratios tended to correlate directly with proportions of families with incomes below poverty and inversely with median income levels, with the racial difference persisting at all income levels. This association with economic indicators suggests that these mortality measurements may indeed indicate adequacy of health care delivery to diabetic persons.

175

Insulin Action, Insulin Binding, and Aging. R.A. DE FRONZO*. New Haven, Ct.

Previous studies employing the hyperglycemic and insulin clamp techniques have demonstrated an age-related decline in glucose metabolism which is primarily due to the presence of insulin resistance. In the present study we have quantitated tissue sensitivity to insulin employing the insulin clamp technique in 23 young (23±1 yr) and 17 old (63±2) normal weight (obesity index = 95-113%) subjects. Plasma insulin is raised by ~100 μU/ml and plasma glucose is held constant at basal levels. Under these steady state conditions of euglycemia all of the infused glucose is taken up by cells and provides a measure of insulin-mediated glucose metabolism (M). M was reduced by 30% in old (5.30±0.33 mg/kg·min) compared to young (7.61±0.29) subjects, p<0.001. Total ^{125}I-insulin specific binding to circulating monocytes was also reduced by a similar percentage in old (6.6±0.3%) vs young (9.1±0.2%), p<0.001. Both M (r=-0.620, p<0.001) and insulin binding (r=-0.656, p<0.001) were inversely correlated with age. A very strong positive correlation (r=-0.729, p<0.001) was observed between insulin binding and M. In both young and old groups insulin binding was inversely correlated to the fasting plasma insulin conc, p<0.001. Conclusions: (1) tissue sensitivity to insulin declines with age; (2) insulin binding also decreases with age and is highly correlated with the age-related decline in insulin-mediated glucose metabolism. These results suggest that a decrease in the number of insulin receptors on target tissues may contribute, in part, to the tissue insensitivity to insulin that occurs with advancing age.

176

B-cell Response to Exercise in Diabetic and Non-diabetic Children. L.G.HEDING* and J.LUDVIGSSON, Denmark and Sweden.

20 non-diabetic and 11-insulin dependent diabetic (IDD) children underwent short time exercise followed by a 10 minute rest. Glucose, IRI, C-peptide and proinsulin were determined prior to and at the end of exercise, and again after 10 minutes' rest.

In the non-diabetic children significant decreases were observed in IRI, C-peptide and proinsulin during exercise. After 10 minutes' rest, glucose as well as the three B-cell secretory products increased significantly. The change in glucose was significantly (p<0.001) correlated to the change in IRI. During the rest period IRI rose more the C-peptide. In some patients IRI even rose without simultaneous rise in C-peptide indicating a release of tissue bound IRI.

The group of IDD children did not show any significant changes in glucose and total IRI, while the endogenous insulin, as measured by C-peptide, did show a fall during exercise. The same was found for proinsulin. No increase in endogenous secretion was observed during the rest period, probably due to suppression of the B-cell by hyperinsulinism.

177

Increased Hemoglobin Alc(Alc) in Insulin Dependent Diabetics(IDD) During Puberty. D.T. SARGEANT*, J. ACHTENBERG, J.E. DAVIS St. Louis, Mo.

Among diabetic children, adolescence is associated with increased insulin requirements and difficulties in attaining optimal glucose control. To determine the effect of puberty on Alc, we analyzed 3 years of data on 188 children with IDD for more than 2 years.

In 90 males mean ±SE Alc rose progressively between Tanner Stages(TS) I and III (from 10.8±.3 to 13.0±.5) and then declined at TS IV to V (13.0±.4, 11.8±.5). The increase in Alc between TS I-III ($p<0.001$) occurred despite an increase in total daily insulin dose(0.76±.02 to 1.04±.07 U/kg, $P<.001$). In 98 females Alc rose progressively from TS I to TS IV (11.0±.4, 12.6±.5, 13.4±.5, 14.1±.4). In females mean insulin dose ranged from 0.9 to 1.1 U/kg and was unrelated to TS. Physician awareness of Alc helped identify patients in poor glucose control but did not lead to a reduction in follow-up Alc's, since subsequent values increased in 63% and decreased in only 36% of follow-up visits.

Thus, among children diabetic for more than 2 years, mean glucose control deteriorates significantly during puberty even when accompanied by a significant increase in insulin doses. The cause of high Alc's during puberty is unknown but an element of relative resistance to insulin is suggested since, after age 19, lower Alc's were found with lower insulin doses. Moreover, knowing a patient's Alc may not of itself result in improved control in a clinical practice in which insulin is given twice daily and changes in insulin dose and hypoglycemia are infrequent.

178

Longitudinal Growth Studies in Insulin-Dependent Diabetes. J. GUTAI*, E. TSALIKIAN* & R. LAPORTE. Pittsburgh, PA.

The data on the linear growth was evaluated on 519 girls and 544 boys with insulin dependent diabetes mellitus followed in the pediatric diabetes clinic 1965-1976. We did not consider the duration of disease in the analysis of growth pattern. The median height & the fifth percentile of diabetic boys & girls was compared to that of normal children at the same age. (Figs)

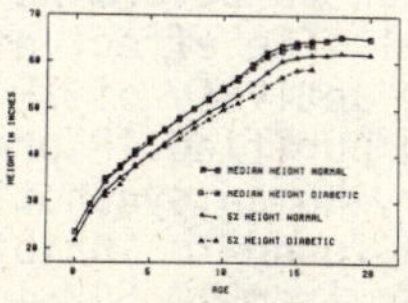

GIRLS

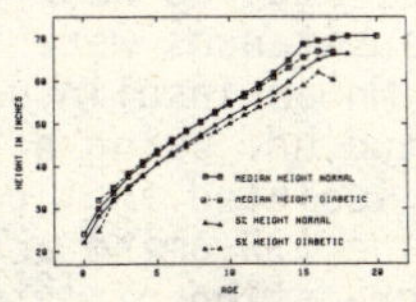

BOYS

The median height of diabetic children began to differ from that of normals at age 10 & was lower throughout the pubertal years. The greatest difference in median height of female diabetics compared to median height of normals was 2.5cms at 14yrs while that of male diabetics was 6.0cms at 16yrs. Beginning at age 7yrs, the fifth percentile height of diabetic children was also lower than normal children. The greatest difference in the fifth percentile height of diabetic boys compared to a normal population was 10cms and occurred at age 15 while the difference of diabetic girls was 8.5cms and occurred at 14yrs. Since the height differences are most marked during the pubertal yrs we therefore speculate that the delayed onset of puberty may be a factor responsible for the height difference during yrs 10-16.

179

Use of Beta-Cell Function and Insulin Sensitivity in the Classification of Diabetes. J.H. KARAM,* C.W. YOUNG,* A. BURNS, and P.H. FORSHAM,* San Francisco, CA.

A currently recommended classification of diabetes mellitus carefully defines Type I as insulin-dependent (IDDM) on the basis of proneness to ketosis, severe insulinopenia, islet-cell antibodies and HLA linkage. Less well categorized is non-ketotic diabetes, which includes the obese and nonobese as subgroups of Type II, non-insulin-dependent diabetes (NIDDM). To further characterize NIDDM, we assessed islet-cell secretory capacity after overnight fasting in 14 normals and 28 diabetics with 50 g oral glucose combined with 30 g arginine i.v. over 30 min and terminated with an i.v. bolus of 0.5 g tolbutamide and 0.5 mg glucagon. C-peptide levels (ng/ml; Mean±SEM), peaking 5 min after the final injection, were 15.7±1.4 in 14 normals, < 2 in 11 IDDM, 5.3±1 in 10 nonobese NIDDM, and 17.4±3.3 in 7 obese NIDDM, despite comparable fasting hyperglycemia (>140 mg/dl) in all diabetic subclasses. Only IDDM showed no fall in free fatty acids and a supranormal plasma glucagon rise to arginine.

Concurrent studies with an insulin tolerance test (N=7) previously standardized in diabetics, and a euglycemic clamp measuring glucose disposal during constant insulin infusion (N=8), showed normal insulin responsiveness in nonobese diabetics and insensitivity in obese NIDDM.

These findings of deficient beta-cell capacity in nonobese NIDDM suggest that their functional disorder is much closer to Type I (IDDM) than to that of their insulin-resistant obese cohorts of Type II, and grouping them with the latter may be physiologically unsound.

180

The Serum Sugar Responses to Regular Insulin Given Separately and Mixed with NPH Insulin. C. J. BRUHN, E. INGLE, H. C. KNOWLES*, Cincinnati, Ohio.

There is great current interest in achieving precise control of Type I diabetes. Regular insulin is mixed with intermediate action insulin to obtain added effect, but it is uncertain if the time of response of the regular is altered. Six newly diagnosed insulin requiring diabetics received morning mixtures of NPH and regular insulins in ratio of 2 to 1. After initial stabilization the insulins were given on alternate days as mixed and separate injection, 3 days each. Serum sugar and insulin were measured fasting and hourly from 8 AM to 8 PM. Regression curves were calculated from 10 AM to 4 PM since the trend was downward except for a small postprandial rise.

$$\text{Mixed } \hat{Y} = 420 - 18.5\,X$$

$$\text{Separate } \hat{Y} = 346 - 12.2\,X$$

Within each person the common slope was more negative in the mixed group. By covariance analyses with pooled common regressions the slope of the mixed group curve was significantly negatively greater than that of the separate injections ($P<0.02$). The summed insulin increment levels (9 AM to 4 PM) above fasting were 228 and 235µ respectively in mixed and separate groups and not significantly different.

The estimated decrease in sugar in the mixed group was 235 to 124 mg/dl and in the separate group 224 to 151 mg/dl. The reasons for the greater rate of fall in the mixed group are unclear. It is not possible to evaluate the insulin levels for rate of absorption because of the presence of some endogenous insulin.

181

Prediction of Insulin Responsiveness During Therapy with Highly Purified Pork Insulin. J. A. GALLOWAY,* S. E. FINEBERG,* and N. S. FINEBERG. Indianapolis, Ind.

When patients are switched from unchromatographed beef or mixed beef-pork (BP) insulins to the purified pork insulins (PI), a marked and lasting reduction in dose has been reported. From a group of 212 patients with IDDM switched after 3 mos. from BP "single peak" insulin to PI, 38 normal weight patients with completely comparable clinical characteristics were categorized with respect to their insulin responsiveness (IR) to PI. Ten individuals had decreased IR (G1), 11 had no change (G2), and 17 had increased IR (G3).

Prior to the change, % initial binding of radioactive beef insulin exceeded that for pork in all groups. Total serum insulin concentrations as well as antibody capacity in G3 exceeded that in G1+2: 1.45±.30 vs .86±.20 mU/ml ($p < .05$); G3, beef 11.72±2.71 U/L vs 6.32±1.78 U/L in G1+2 ($p < .05$). Antibody capacity for beef and pork insulin was highly correlated in all groups.

When IR was decreased or remained unchanged after the switch, it was stable for 4 months. In G3 increased IR was evident after 2 months and disappeared after 4 months of therapy. Total insulin concentrations and antibody binding capacity were highest in patients with increased IR. Also, differentiation with regard to pork and beef binding did not predict IR. Finally, the increased IR with PI was transient.

The change from "single peak" BP to PI is shown in this study to have little long range impact on IR.

182

Phosphate Therapy in Diabetic Ketoacidosis (DKA) H. WILSON, S. KEUER, S. LEA, A. E. BOYD III* and G. EKNOYAN, Houston, Texas.

Phosphate depletion occurs during DKA, but the therapeutic efficacy or dosage of PO_4 for its replacement has not been defined. This prospective randomized study compares 3 groups of patients: Group I, 14 subjects, received no PO_4; Group II, 17 subjects, received 15mM (475 mg) PO_4 at 4th hr of therapy; Group III, 10 subjects, received 3 doses of 15mM PO_4 at the 2nd, 6th and 10th hr of therapy. PO_4 was given as the sodium salt. All patients were treated with a standard protocol of intravenous insulin (0.1U/kg/hr), fluids and potassium chloride. All 3 groups were similar in age, sex, admission glucose and pH. The mean ± SD of the serum phosphate (mg/dl) in the 3 groups was

Time (hr)	0	4	8	16
Group I	5.1±2.3	3.9±1.6	2.1±0.8	1.8±0.6
Group II	4.9±2.3	3.7±2.0	2.8±0.8*	2.4±0.8
Group III	4.9±1.8	4.7±2.4	2.9±1.3*	2.6±1.7*

*denotes significant difference from Group I

Serum calcium at 24 hrs, duration of DKA and insulin dosage was similar in all three groups with no evidence of hemolysis, cardiomyopathy, or liver dysfunction. On admission and throughout therapy, creatinine phosphokinase was elevated in 2 Group I, 4 Group II and 3 in Group III patients. Aldolase was elevated in one patient of each group. These results indicate: 1) 3 doses of 15mM PO_4 are adequate to maintain normal serum PO_4 and does not induce hypocalcemia; 2) phosphate replacement does not reduce the duration of DKA or the dose of insulin and 3) evidence for muscle injury is often present on admission with DKA and was not altered by the PO_4.

183

Face-Sparing Partial Lipodystrophy: Clinical Studies of a Large Kindred. RALPH H. STARKEY* and THOMAS J. CIOTOLA, Danville, PA.

The syndrome of face-sparing partial lipodystrophy (F-SPL) is a rare form of lipoatrophic diabetes with dominant transmission in which detailed family studies have not been performed. We have studied 25 and gathered historical information on an additional 40 members of a large affected kindred spanning five generations; included is the first male ever studied (second reported) with the full syndrome.

The frequency of the various parts of the syndrome was:

	Examined (n=25)	By History (n=40)	Total (n=65)
Lipoatrophy (LA)	6	4	10
Diabetes (DM)	10	12	22
Acanthosis Nigricans (AN)	4	?	4(+?)
Hyperlipidemia (HL)	10	?	10(+?)

None of the patients were previously recognized as having LA and 6/10 with glucose intolerance were asymptomatic and not known diabetics. All six patients with LA had insulin-resistant DM, four had AN, and five had HL. The four examined non-lipoatrophic diabetics did not have insulin resistance. One man had the full syndrome and four had parts: diabetes and/or HL. HLA typing (loci A, B, and C) failed to reveal an association between any parts of the syndrome and the tested loci.

Conclusions: F-SPL is probably more frequent than previously believed, the clinical picture is variable, men may be affected (usually only DM and/or HL), and no relation with HLA loci is apparent.

184

Evidence that C-peptide Inhibits and Divalent Cations Stimulate Degradation of Insulin by Insulin Protease. GEORGE A. BURGHEN*, RANDOLPH A. MCKENZIE and TERESA M. HOWARTH, Memphis, TN.

Insulin protease (IP) is thought to be the major enzyme responsible for the intracellular degradation of insulin. A very potent competitive inhibitor of IP was isolated from rat liver and found to have a mol. wt. of about 3500. Because of the simularity in mol. wt. of IP-inhibitor and C-peptide, studies were undertaken to determine if these substances were identical. The effect of Ca, Mg and Mn on insulin degrading activity of IP was also studied. Using a 700-fold purified IP preparation isolated from rat liver, human synthetic C-peptide (35 amino acids) was found to inhibit the degradation of ^{125}I-insulin from 10-50% in a linear fashion at concentrations of C-peptide ranging from 0.2-5.0 ng/ml. At a concentration of 10 ng/ml C-peptide produced 73% inhibition of insulin degradation. Kinetic studies revealed that C-peptide is a competitive inhibitor for IP with a K_i of 13 ng/ml. Partially purified rat liver IP-inhibitor contained only a small amount of C-peptide as measured by radioimmunoassay compared to the large percentage of insulin degrading inhibitory activity.

EDTA and EGTA in a concentration of 1mM produced approximately 50% inhibition of the enzyme, whereas Ca, Mg, and Mn stimulated insulin degrading activity.

It appears from these data that both C-peptide and IP-inhibitor are potent competitive inhibitors of IP and may be important in the regulation of insulin degradation. In addition, divalent cations may also play a role.

185

Models for the Insulin Receptor From Radiation Inactivation Studies. J.T. HARMON, C.R. KAHN*, & M.L. JOHNSON, Bethesda, Md, & Charlottesville, VA.

We have previously shown that high energy ionizing radiation can be used to determine the molecular weight of the insulin receptor in situ in rat liver membranes. When the log of the fraction of specific insulin binding was plotted versus radiation dose, complex results were observed. Binding increased 2-3 fold reaching a maximum at 12 Mrad and then decreased at higher doses of radiation. Similar results have been observed with adipocyte membranes, IM-9 lymphocyte membranes and Triton X-100 solubilized rat liver membranes. From equilibrium studies, it was concluded that the increase in binding at low radiation doses was due to an increase in the binding affinity. The total number of receptors decreased at all radiation doses. These data were used to test several proposed models for the insulin receptor: a model in which the binding component is associated with a high molecular weight affinity-modulating component; a polymer model in which the binding components are able to form reversibly multimeric complexes; an isomerization model in which a conformational change occurs upon insulin binding causing a change in the affinity of the insulin sites; and a multisite model in which there are binding components of differing affinities. Computer analysis of the results of radiation inactivation studies are most consistent with a model in which there is a separate affinity-modulator associated with the insulin receptor. Upon binding insulin there is a dissociation of the binding and modulating components. Whether the modulator is the insulin-effector system remains to be determined.

186

Different Reduction States of the Insulin Receptor in Plasma Membranes. J. MASSAGUE, P.F.PILCH, and M.P.CZECH*. Providence, R.I.

Rat liver, adipocyte and heart muscle plasma membrane insulin receptors crosslinked to receptor-bound ^{125}I-insulin by disuccinimidyl (DS)derivatives (DSsuberate, DSadipate, DSsuccinate) can be detected in gels following SDS-polyacrylamide gel electrophoresis (SDS-PAGE). After SDS-PAGE in the absence of dithiothreitol (DTT), three major radioactive bands (Mr 290,000, 320,000, and 350,000) appeared in the gels,whereas a single major band (Mr 125,000) appeared after SDS-PAGE in the presence of 50 mM DTT. All three bands derived from SDS-PAGE without DTT migrated as Mr 125,000 when they were subjected to second dimentional SDS-PAGE with DTT.

Two additional bands (Mr 200,000 and Mr 160,000) were observed after SDS-PAGE of pure liver plasma membrane in the absence of DTT. After second dimentional SDS-PAGE with 50 mM DTT, both bands migrated as Mr 125,000. These two bands were generated in adipocyte and heart muscle plasma membranes if DTT was present at low concentration (0.5 mM to 1.5 mM) during SDS-PAGE. This suggests that the insulin receptor exists in several disulfide-linked forms containing two or more different-sized subunits, and that insulin binds to a Mr 125,000 subunit. The results also suggest that partially reduced forms of the insulin receptor are present in liver plasma membrane.

187

Hormone Receptors on cultured cells and clones obtained from Islet-cell tumor. S. J. BHATHENA,* H. OIE, A. GAZDAR, L. RECANT,* Washington, D.C.

Rat islet-cell tumor produced by Chick, was passaged in culture. The cells secreted/24 hrs. predominantly insulin (I) (3000 uU/10^7 cells), some somatostatin (S), (1.0 ng/10^7 cells) and glucagon (G) (400 pg/10^7 cells). Hormone (H) secretions were responsive to secretagogues such as glucose, arginine, theophylline, and elevated K^+ and Ca^{++}. Specific receptors (R) for I, G and S were demonstrated in these parent cells N=15). Maximum specific binding (B) during 1 hr. incubation at 20° C. for $2x10^6$ cells was 5.3% for I, 2.1% for G and 1.5% for S. B for all 3 H was linear with cell number and was maximal at 1 hr. Bound I and S were dissociable and "down-regulation" of B was seen with increased H concentration. The cells were cloned and examined for H binding. Predominantly I secreting clones (I-cl) (2.5 to 15 mU/10^7 cells) bound 5.0% I, 0.82% G and 1.45% S (N=15) compared with predominantly S secreting clones (S-cl) (0.5-5.0 ng/10^7 cells) which bound 9.2% I, 1.1% G and 2.9% S (N=6).

Scatchard analyses and affinity plots were carried out on parent cells and subclones of I-cl and S-cl. Subclones of S-cl showed the highest number of R for I and S, while R numbers were similar in parent and subclones of I-cl. A greater affinity for G and S was found in I-cl.

The existence of specific R for all 3 H on parent cells and their clones supports the likelihood that all 3 H may interact to regulate alpha, beta and delta cells.

188

Appearance of Insulin Receptor Regulation in Liver Membranes from Zucker Fatty Rats. J.B. CLARK*, and C.M. CLARK, JR.*, Indianapolis, IN.

Zucker fatty rats (F) are obese, normoglycemic animals with marked hyperinsulinemia. Whereas one would expect very low numbers of insulin receptors on liver plasma membranes (LPM) of F, varying results have been previously reported. We herein report that the presence or absence of down regulation in this model is a function of age. LPM were isolated from F and their lean littermates (L) at ages 2.5, 5 and 12 mos. Purification of the LPM was identical in all groups. The plasma insulin concentrations (I) in uU/ml and the limiting values of Bound/Free (B/F) determined in displacement studies of F with 125-I insulin are summarized below (the numbers of animals is in parentheses):

Age:	2.5 mos.	5 mos.	12 mos.
I	750 ± 271 (7)	1522 ± 225 (4)	396 ± 75 (9)
B/F	0.86±0.18 (3)	0.17±0.05 (3)	0.41±0.06 (4)

I and B/F remained constant in the L animals (I = 42 ± 5 and B/F = 0.85 ± 0.4). Affinity values from 125-I insulin displacement curves were similar in all age groups. The B/F of the LPM from the youngest F group did not differ from that of L in spite of hyperinsulinemia. Down regulation is evident in the LPM of the older F groups ($p < 0.001$, 5 mos, $p < 0.01$, 12 mos. as compared to L). We conclude that down regulation does occur in the LPM of F by at least 5 mos. Whether liver insulin receptor regulation in F requires very high I or some added factor associated with age remains to be determined. The studies also suggest that F may be a model for studies on the regulation of the insulin receptor.

189

Effects of Colchicine on Insulin Binding to Isolated Hepatocytes. J WHITTAKER, V HAMMOND and K G M M ALBERTI*, Newcastle upon Tyne, U.K.

Since insulin is internalised by adsorptive pinocytosis, plasma membrane receptors must be continually replaced to maintain steady state binding in the presence of insulin. As plasma membrane proteins are replaced through the fusion of secretory vesicles with the membrane during exocytosis, the integrity of the microtubule system may be essential for normal turn-over of insulin receptors. The effects of colchicine on insulin binding to isolated rat hepatocytes have therefore been examined.

Competitive binding studies with unlabelled insulin in concentrations of $6x10^{-11}M$ to $10^{-7}M$ were performed in the presence or absence of 10^{-5} M colchicine at 37°C. No significant differences were observed. This was independent of the duration of pre incubation with colchicine. To accelerate internalisation cells were incubated for 1 or 2 hrs. with $10^{-8}M$ insulin at 37°C. When steady state tracer binding with $3x10^{-10}M$ ^{125}I-insulin was measured in colchicine treated cells, binding was reduced by 40-70% after 1 hr. with no further change at 2 hrs. There was no change in control cells. This effect was not found at 20°C, a temperature at which the rate of adsorptive pinocytosis is low. After trypsinisation to destroy insulin receptors, there was no recovery of binding in colchicine treated cells whereas control cells recovered at 8-12% of initial binding/hr. Colchicine($10^{-5}M$) had no effect on protein or glyco-protein synthesis.

We conclude that colchicine probably blocks receptor turn-over by effects on the secretory mechanism of the hepatocyte.

190

Insulin Binding to the Blood Brain Barrier: A Direct in vitro Demonstration. H.J.L. FRANK* and W.M. PARDRIDGE,* Los Angeles, Ca.

Recent in vivo autoradiographic studies by van Houten and Posner (1979) have suggested that circulating insulin may bind to the brain capillary wall, i.e., the blood-brain barrier (BBB). In the present studies, the putative BBB insulin receptor was examined directly by measuring I^{125}-insulin binding to capillaries isolated from fresh bovine cerebral cortex. The microvessels, prepared by gentle homogenization and trapping on nylon mesh, were greater than 95% viable based on trypan blue exclusion. I^{125}-insulin binding to these isolated capillaries was rapid, specific, and reversible. Maximum specific binding of 23% per mg protein was reached by 45 min., with ½ max. binding achieved by ∿5 min. I^{125}-insulin was not displaced by excess thyrotropin, prolactin, or growth hormone, and only minimally displaced by proinsulin. A 50% displacement of I^{125}-insulin by unlabeled insulin occurred at approximately 0.9 nM. Conclusions: These studies confirm the presence of a specific insulin receptor at the BBB. Although insulin does not cross the BBB (Goodner and Berrie, 1977), the operation of the BBB insulin receptor provides a mechanism by which blood-borne insulin may influence brain cell metabolism. The isolated cerebral capillary may provide a suitable preparation for future investigations of the possible chemical signals generated by insulin binding to the BBB.

191

Acute Downregulation of Monocyte but not Erythrocyte Insulin Receptor Number by Exogenous Insulin in Normal Man. L. Mandarino and B. Brick (Introduced by M. Hogan*), Endocrine Research Unit, Mayo Clinic, Rochester, Minnesota.

Prolonged exposure to insulin in vitro decreases the number of insulin receptors on hepatocytes and lymphocytes. To date, in man acute alterations in plasma insulin have been associated with changes in insulin receptor affinity but not receptor number. Therefore, to determine whether acute increases in plasma insulin to levels observed in insulin resistant states could decrease insulin receptor number in man, 8 normal overnight fasted human subjects were infused with insulin at different rates (0.2-5.0 mU/kg/min) for up to 8 hrs while euglycemia was maintained by the glucose clamp technique. Monocytes (MC) and erythrocyte (RBC) insulin binding was determined before and after insulin infusions by conventional methods. Under all conditions, specific insulin binding to RBCs was not affected. However, under conditions in which plasma insulin had been increased to approximately 600 μU/ml, insulin binding to MC decreased 40% from 15.8±1.3 to 9.6±1.1% per 10^7MC, p<0.001. This was due to a decrease in receptor number (22,106±3710 vs 15,016±2284, p<0.05) since average empty site affinity did not change (5.34± 0.66 x 10^8M^{-1} vs 5.25±1.10 x 10^8M^{-1}). Conclusions: Acute increases in plasma insulin to levels observed in insulin resistant states can decrease MC but not RBC insulin receptor number within 8 hrs in man. RBC insulin receptors appear to be regulated differently than MC insulin receptors and may not be an appropriate model to study acute changes in insulin receptor function.

192

Insulin Binding and Degradation by Livers from Fed and Fasted Rats. SHIGEAKI BABA*, KOICHI YOKONO, YOSHIMICHI IMAMURA, KOSUI SHII, and HIDEYO SAKAI, Kobe,

Insulin specific binding(IB) to isolated liver plasma membranes was time and temperature dependent with a slower but higher binding achieved at a lower temperature(4°C). In contrast, IB decreased at higher temperatures(24°C, 37°C) in proportion to the increase of insulin degradation(ID) by membranes. Unlabeled insulin competed with ^{125}I-insulin for binding to membranes with half-maximal inhibition of binding being observed with less than 2ng/ml. Liver membranes of 72 hrs-fasted rats bound two times as much insulin as did membranes of fed rats. Scatchard analysis showed that the enhancement of IB in fasted rats was due to a increase of insulin receptor concentrations in the membrane. ID activity by membranes, which was 10% of the soluble fraction, showed no significant difference between fed and fasted group. On the other hand, ID activity in the soluble fraction was significantly lower than fed rats in fasted ones (p<0.02). Quantitative analysis of ID in this fraction revealed a similar Km for both groups (1.8 to 2.5x10^{-7} M), whereas maximal velocities in fasted rats was significantly lower than fed rats (p<0.02). Antiserum to insulin-degrading enzyme purified from pig skeletal muscle inhibited ID activity not only in the soluble fraction (34±7 vs 79±3%control, p<0.001) but also in plasma membranes (49±7 vs 81±6 %control, p<0.01) as compared with normal rabbit serum. Furthermore, IB significantly increased in the presence of antiserum (121±9%control, p<0.05). These data suggest that, as in the muscle, insulin levels are regulated by intracellular enzyme(s) including insulin-degrading enzyme rather than ID system of plasma membranes in the liver.

193

"Superinsulins" : a Single Amino Acid Substitution at A_8 Causes Increased Receptor Affinity and Biological Activity *in vitro*.

M.A. PIRON, P. DE MEYTS*, J. PITTS, J. SIMON and W. RITTEL; Brussels, Belgium; London, England; Nouzilly, France; and Basel, Switzerland.

Chicken and turkey insulins have affinities for the insulin receptor and biological activities *in vitro* that are 2-3 times higher than do porcine, bovine or human insulins. Among the six residues changed in the bird insulins, the A_8 His (Ala in bovine, Thr in human and porcine insulins) lies just outside the putative receptor-binding region of the insulin molecule. It was speculated that the changes at A_8 may result in stabilizing interactions with receptor residues (Pullen *et al*.Nature, 259,369,1976). We demonstrate this in studies of the bird insulins and totally synthetic insulins having the sequence of human insulin except for the substitution of His, Lys or Phe in the A_8 position. All five insulins were more potent biologically than porcine (A_8 His = 2-2.6, A_8 Phe and A_8 Lys = 1-2 times more). Similar increased potencies were found in competition of the unlabeled analogues with ^{125}I-porcine insulin for binding, and in direct binding studies of the labeled analogues. Slightly increased initial rates of association and decreased dissociation rates concurred with the increased affinity of all analogues, except for A_8-Phe insulin, which had the same off-rate as porcine insulin. All analogues were fully "negatively cooperative" except for A_8-Phe, which had a slightly impaired cooperativity. These data show that a single substitution during evolution can markedly affect the ability of insulin to bind to its receptor.

194

Receptor Linked Degradation of ^{125}I-insulin is Mediated by Internalization in Cultured Human Lymphocytes. E. VAN OBBERGHEN*, J.-L. CARPENTIER, P. GORDEN*, and L. ORCI*. Bethesda, MD, USA; and Geneva, Switzerland.

Using quantitative EM autoradiography we have shown in IM-9 lymphocytes that ^{125}I-insulin is internalized in a time- and temperature dependent fashion. In the present study we examine by EM autoradiography and gel chromatography the fate of ^{125}I-insulin in IM-9 cells. When cells are incubated at 37°C with ^{125}I-insulin and the cell associated radioactivity is studied at the end of each incubation period from 15 to 180 min, the radioactivity dissociates from the cells to the same level. However, with increasing association time there is a small but progressive increase in the fraction of degraded radioactivity dissociating from the cells (% intact insulin = 95 and 64% after 15 and 180 min of association, respectively) and remaining associated with the cells (% intact insulin = 91 and 77% after 15 and 180 min of association, respectively). By EM autoradiography an increasing proportion of radioactive grains is internalized with increasing incubation time. After 120 min of association, a further modest increment in the proportion of internalized grains associated with lysosome-like structures is observed with increasing dissociation times.

We conclude that in the IM-9 cells (i) a portion of receptor bound insulin is internalized and preferentially associated with lysosome-like structures, (ii) the amount of ^{125}I-insulin degraded is quantitatively similar to the proportion of the ligand internalized.

195

Volume, Insulin Binding and Glucose Transport and Oxidation of Adipocytes from Normophagic Rats with Hypothalamic Obesity. J. GOLDMAN*, D. LOCKWOOD and D. MALCHOFF. Buffalo and Rochester, New York.

Isolated adipocytes were obtained from male Sprague-Dawley rats 2 weeks after placement of ventromedial hypothalamic lesions. Control rats received sham lesions. Adipocyte volume and triglyceride content were markedly increased in lesioned rats (6.0±0.5 vs 3.6±0.4 nanoliters TG/cell). At insulin concentrations of 0.25, 1.0 and 5.0 x 10^{-9}M, specific insulin binding was not significantly different comparing intact adipocytes from lesioned and control rats, although non-specific binding was nearly twice normal in lesioned rats. Basal 2-deoxyglucose uptake per 10^5 cells was 110 picomoles in lesioned rats and 19 picomoles in control rats. Insulin stimulated uptakes were 920 vs 516 picomoles respectively. Basal glucose oxidation per 10^5 cells was 1272 picomoles in lesioned rats and 409 in controls. Insulin stimulated values were 8813 picomoles and 4244 respectively.

Conclusions are 1) hypothalamic obesity without hyperphagia is characterized by adipocyte enlargement, 2) basal and insulin stimulated glucose transport and oxidation are greatly increased in adipocytes of rats with such obesity, and 3) in the face of increased circulating insulin levels, there is no decrease in insulin binding to adipocytes of these rats.

196

Effects of B-adrenoreceptor Blockade on Insulin- or 2-deoxy-D-glucose-induced Hunger,Thirst and Arginine Vasopressin Secretion in Man. D.A. THOMPSON,U.LILIVIVATHANA*,R.G.CAMPBELL*,S.WELLE, and G.L.ROBERTSON, Rochester, N.Y.

We have previously shown that glucoprivation induced by 2 deoxy-D-glucose(2DG)intravenous infusion(50 mg/kg/20 min)increases hunger and thirst ratings on a linear scale and food and water intake in overnight fasted normal subjects (Sci.198:1065,1977). To determine whether B-adrenoreceptor stimulation modulates arginine vasopressin(AVP)secretion,thirst and hunger during 2DG-or insulin(0.15 units/kg)-induced glucoprivation,propanolol(3 mg/3 min.followed by 80μg/min)or saline were infused continuously before and after 2DG and insulin injections in eight male volunteers.Peak responses to 2DG and insulin infusions with and without propranolol:

Condition	Hunger mm	Food kcal	Thirst mm	Water ml	AVP pg/ml	PRA ng/ml/hr
NS-2DG	66	680	27	649	5.3	3.66
Prop-2DG	67	553	21	830	7.1	0.62
NS-NS	15	--	9	87	1.9	0.53
NS-Insul	47	--	27	261	4.0	1.70
Prop-Insul	22	--	23	323	4.4	0.84

Glucoprivation increased hunger and thirst ratings and AVP and PRA levels significantly while B-adrenoreceptor blockade suppressed only the PRA response to glucoprivation. Epinephrine levels increased significantly during glucoprivation. Mean arterial pressure,plasma sodium and osmolality changes following 2DG were not sufficient to increase thirst and AVP levels.Thus hunger,thirst and AVP response to glucoprivation are not mediated by B-adrenoreceptor stimulation, hyptotension or changes in PRA and osmolality.

197

Polyol Pathway Activity Increased In Diabetic Cells. G. Knox, J.I. Malone*, Tampa, Florida

Sorbitol has been shown to accumulate in the human red cell in response to the surrounding glucose concentration. The kinetics of glucose to sorbitol conversion plus the blockade produced by an aldose reductase inhibitor suggest that red cell sorbitol concentration reflects polyol pathway activity. Heparinized blood was collected from 136 insulin dependent diabetics (IDD) and 47 non diabetics (ND) after an 8 hour fast. The plasma and red cells were separated by centrifugation. Glucose and sorbitol were measured using glucose oxidose and sorbitol dehydrogenase respectively. The mean sorbitol/glucose ratio for IDD (21.0 ± 9.9) was significantly greater ($p < .005$) than the mean ND level (13.1 ± 7.9). Washed red cells from both IDD and ND groups were resuspended in Krebs bicarbonate buffer pH 7.4 and incubated in replicate in 3 different glucose concentrations for 3 hours at 37°C. Incubated red cells from diabetics had significantly greater ($p < .005$) mean sorbitol/glucose ratios when compared to red cells from ND.

Media	Sorbitol as mean ± SD		
Glucose	100 mg/dl	300 mg/dl	500 mg/dl
ND	26.5 ±11.0(11)	12.9 ±4.8(11)	12.9±6.5(11)
IDD	46.7 ±17.0(9)	31.5 ±10.9(9)	26.7±8.4(10)

In vivo and *in vitro* sorbitol accumulation in the red cell suggests that some factor in addition to ambient glucose concentration alters polyol pathway activity and increases intracellular sorbitol accumulation in the cells of people with spontaneous diabetes.

198

Insulin Degradation by Hepatocytes in Primary Culture. W.C. DUCKWORTH,*, K.R. RUNYAN, R.K. WRIGHT, M.A. HEINEMANN, S.S. SOLOMON,* Memphis, TN.

Receptor-bound insulin is internalized and proteolytically degraded. The exact mechanism of the degradative step is not known. Degradation of ^{125}I-insulin was studied in isolated rat liver cells which had been maintained 48 h in primary culture as attached monolayers. Conversion of ^{125} I-insulin to TCA-soluble products was linear over 4 h at 37° and was dependent on cell concentration. No degradative activity was detected in media which had been exposed to cells. Studies with [phe^{B1}-^{3}H] insulin showed that when the extract from cells was chromatographed on Sephadex G-50, the amount of radioactivity eluting with intact insulin decreased with time while labeled substances appeared in the void volume and salt peak. Degradation of ^{125}I-insulin was reduced to 20% of control values by N-ethylmaleimide (NEM), Kunitz pancreatic trypsin inhibitor (KPTI), and bacitracin. No significant inhibition of insulin degradation was seen with sodium azide, phenylmethylsulfonyl fluoride (PMSF) TPCK, NH_4Cl, chloroquine, or procaine. The effect of these inhibitors on purified insulin protease was also examined. NEM, KPTI, and bacitracin inhibited the purified enzyme while PMSF, TPCK, NH_4Cl, chloroquine, and procaine had no effect.

These data suggest that insulin degradation in hepatocytes is not sensitive to classical lysosomal inhibitors but is sensitive to agents known to inhibit the enzyme insulin protease.

199

Defect in Membrane Na^+ + K^+-ATPase in Obese Mouse and Man. M. DELUISE, P. USHER and J.S. FLIER*, Boston, Mass.

Evidence suggests that obesity may be associated with impaired cellular thermogenesis, a fundamental process linked to the membrane sodium pump, the Na^+ + K^+-ATPase. In support of this thesis, the activity and concentration of this enzyme is known to be reduced in liver and muscle of the obese-diabetic (ob/ob) mouse. We have used three separate probes of this enzyme to further characterize its status in the ob/ob mouse, and demonstrate for the first time a related defect in human obesity. The rate of Na^+ + K^+-ATPase dependent ATP hydrolysis is reduced in homogenates of liver (by 70%) and heart (by 20%) of 7-16 week old obese mice when compared to thin littermates. In contrast, the same animals show no reduction of ATPase mediated transport of ^{86}Rb when intact pieces of liver, heart, and whole erythrocytes are used, suggesting an altered relationship between enzyme units and enzyme activity in the obese animal. In a group of 16 obese patients (>150% of ideal body weight) the number of Na^+ + K^+-ATPase units on circulating RBC's as measured by ^{3}H-ouabain binding is reduced when compared to controls (0.632 ± 0.028 vs. 0.545 ± 0.034 picomoles bound/10^9 cells). Enzyme activity as measured by ouabain inhibitable ^{86}Rb uptake is also reduced in obese vs. control RBC's (103.2 ± 2.4 vs. 94.6 ± 4.4 nanomoles/10^9 cells/hr). It is concluded that abnormalities of the membrane Na^+ + K^+-ATPase are present in both ob/ob mice and a heterogenous group of obese humans. Further studies of this defect could provide important clues into a fundamental defect in obesity.

200

Physical Training of Zucker Rats Increases Glucose Metabolism in Adipose Cells Without Altering Insulin Sensitivity. L.J. WARDZALA, E.D. HORTON, and E.S. HORTON*. Geneva, Switzerland.

To determine if physical training effects glucose metabolism and insulin sensitivity in isolated adipose cells(AC) of the Zucker rat, 4-5 week-old control and obese animals were trained for 6 wks on a treadmill (2h/d, 5d/wk, 0.7mph, 8%grade). 48 hrs after the last exercise, total AC 1-^{14}C-glucose metabolism (0.56mM) was measured, ± varying insulin concentrations. Untrained obese rats had higher basal and insulin-stimulated glucose metabolism than controls, with a rightward shift of the insulin dose-response (decreased sensitivity). Cell size was greater in obese than in lean and not changed by training. Training resulted in 2-3-fold increases in basal and insulin-stimulated glucose metabolism in AC of controls. Similar but smaller increases were observed in trained obese rats.

Glucose Metabolism (fmol/cell/h) in AC

	Lean		Obese	
	Untrained	Trained	Untrained	Trained
BASAL	125±8	300± 5	375±10	430± 5
INS.(MAX)	250±6	675±15	870±10	1350±20

Training of lean and obese rats did not result in shifts of insulin-dose response curves (no change in sensitivity). Conclusions: 1) physical training increases the capacity of AC to metabolize glucose without changing the sensitivity to insulin; 2) the effects observed are probably distal to the insulin-receptor complex and may involve increased transport of and/or changes in intracellular metabolism of glucose.

201

Effects of Acute Insulin Deficiency on Leucine Kinetics in Conscious Dogs: N.N. ABOU-MOURAD,* L. S. JEFFERSON,* S.R. RANNELS, P.E. WILLIAMS, and W.W. LACY,* Nashville, Tn. and Hershey, Pa.

With acute or chronic insulin deficiency, plasma leucine (leu) rises. While many in vitro studies have shown an effect of insulin on protein turnover, no in vivo data are available to indicate whether increased inflow or decreased removal predominate in changing plasma leu on withdrawal of insulin. We measured the effect of acute insulin withdrawal on the rate of appearance (Ra) and disappearance (Rd) of plasma leu, utilizing a constant infusion of 4,5 3-H leucine. Two groups of overnight fasted dogs were utilized. One saline infused group (n=5) served as control. In the other group (n=4) a selective insulin deficiency was produced by the infusion of somatostatin (0.8μg/kg/min) and intraportal replacement of glucagon (0.65ng/kg/min).

In the control dogs constant leu specific activity (SA) was attained by 120 min and both SA and leu (125 ± 10μmol/L) remained constant for 300 min., with Ra and Rd being equal (3.2 ± 0.03μmol/kg/min). With insulin withdrawal, plasma leu increased from 125 ± 3 to 200 ± 6 μmol/L. Ra did not rise, while Rd fell by 10% in 2 hrs. After 3 hrs of insulin deprivation, Rd returned to normal, but since leu level increased by 60%, clearance fell by 36% and persisted.

In conclusion, acute insulin deficiency results in a rise in plasma leu by inducing a decrease in Rd and not by a change in Ra. The data are consistent with a physiologic role of basal insulin in determining net protein synthesis.

202

The Effect of Ketone Bodies on Alanine Metabolism in Cultured Rat Skeletal Muscle. ROBERT J. SMITH and THOMAS T. AOKI*, Boston, Massachusetts

We have studied the effects of ketone bodies on alanine synthesis and release by rat skeletal muscle myotubes (L6) in long term culture in order to determine the role of hyperketonemia during adaptation to starvation. On incubation in Eagle's minimal essential medium supplemented with 10% dialyzed bovine serum, L6 myotubes form and release alanine at a rate of 32.3 nmol/h/mg cell protein. When ketone bodies are added to the medium (β-hydroxybutyrate 5.1mM, acetoacetate 1.7mM) and cultures are studied over the subsequent 48 hours, alanine release is decreased by 26%. The intracellular alanine concentration remains constant at 17mM, consistent with a decrease in net alanine synthesis in response to ketone bodies. The intracellular pyruvate concentration increases by 24%, suggesting that ketone bodies do not alter alanine release by limiting supplies of pyruvate. When medium glutamine (6.5mM) is the principle source of amino groups, ketone bodies do not affect alanine formation and release. When branched chain amino acids (4.0mM) are the principle sources of amino groups, however, ketone bodies decrease alanine release by 24%. We conclude that alanine formation and release in cultured rat skeletal myotubes are decreased by ketone bodies. In contrast to reported findings with short term in vitro studies of muscle tissue, ketone bodies do not appear to limit glycolysis, but selectively interfere with alanine formation from branched chain amino acids. This mechanism may underly the decline in alanine release from skeletal muscle following trauma or starvation.

203

Effects of Clofibrate on Alanine Production, Branched Chain Amino Acid Oxidation, and Krebs Cycle Pool Sizes in Isolated Adult Rat Skeletal Muscle Cells. W.M. PARDRIDGE*, L. DUDUCGIAN-VARTAVARIAN, D. CASANELLO-ERTL, M.R. JONES AND J.D. KOPPLE, Los Angeles, Ca.

The branched chain amino acids (leucine, isoleucine, valine) are believed to be important donors of carbon both to the Krebs cycle and for the synthesis of alanine in skeletal muscle. Recent studies have shown that clofibric acid, a drug which causes myopathy in man, selectively inhibits the oxidation of ^{14}C-branched chain amino acids in both the diaphragm and the L_6 myogenic line (Clin.Res. 28:52A, 1980). Therefore, the present studies were designed to investigate the effects of clofibrate on alanine production and on Krebs cycle metabolites in isolated skeletal muscle cells obtained from adult rats and grown in primary tissue culture. Under conditions in which glucose or lactate were not utilized, the rate of metabolism of the branched chain amino acids increased 4-fold, concomitant with the net production of pyruvate, alanine, and citrate. A 2 mM concentration of clofibrate resulted in a 76% inhibition of branched chain amino acid utilization, a marked decrease in the production of alanine and citrate, a 50% decrease in pool size of malate, citrate and α-ketoglutarate, but no change in cell ATP. Conclusions: The utilization of branched chain amino acids as the primary carbon source in skeletal muscle cells results in the net production of alanine and citrate, and these processes are blocked by acute clofibrate treatment.

204

Streptozotocin (SZ)-Induced Insulitis Model in Athymic Mice: ALDO A. ROSSINI*, ARTHUR A. LIKE*, MICHAEL C. APPEL*, JOHN P. MORDES and R. MICHAEL WILLIAMS*. Worcester, MA and Chicago, IL.

The multi-dose SZ-induced model of diabetes in CD-1 mice features: 1) delayed onset hyperglycemia, 2) destructive insulitis, and 3) induction of type C virus within surviving beta cells. Previous experiments suggest that cell-mediated autoimmune destruction of beta cells causes the diabetic syndrome. To study the role of thymus-dependent T-cells in the etiology of the syndrome, two strains of nude mice were used. Nude is a mutant allele on chromosome 11 of mice. Homozygous (Nu/Nu) animals are hairless, lack a normal thymus, and manifest severe reduction in T-cell numbers. The Nu mutation exists on both BALB/c and SWR/J inbred strains. Normal BALB/c, BALB Nu/+ and BALB Nu/Nu mice are all resistant to both single and multi-dose SZ. Normal SWR mice given single or multiple injections of SZ evidence hyperglycemia comparable to that previously observed in CD-1 mice. SWR Nu/+ mice given five daily I.P. injections of SZ (35 mg/kg BW) developed delayed hyperglycemia (P.G. 331±18 mg%, N=20) on the 10th day following the first injection. SWR Nu/Nu littermates treated identically remained normoglycemic throughout the experiment (P.G. 165±6 mg%, N=28). On the 12th day animals were sacrificed for pancreatic histology. Insulitis was found in SWR Nu/+ but not in Nu/Nu mice. These data suggest that insulitis and delayed onset hyperglycemia in the multi-dose SZ model are mediated through thymus derived T-lymphocytes.

205

Induction of Diabetes by Streptozotocin Is Mediated by T-Cell Functions. SANG-GI PAIK, NORMAN FLEISCHER* and SEUNG-IL SHIN, New York, NY.

To examine the role of autoimmune processes in the etiology of experimental diabetes, we investigated the development of insulin-dependent hyperglycemia in streptozotocin(SZ)-treated athymic nude (nu/nu) mice and their phenotypically normal heterozygous (+/nu) littermates of BALB/c origin.

Injection of a single high dose of SZ (200 mg/kg) rapidly led to severe and persistent hyperglycemia in both +/nu and nu/nu mice (>500 mg plasma glucose/dl). In contrast, injection of 5 daily doses of 40 mg SZ/kg resulted in diabetes in 100 % of +/nu mice but very rarely in nu/nu mice. To prove directly that this resistance to multiple low doses of SZ was due to the defect in thymic functions, nude mice were transplanted with neonatal thymus from +/nu mice and later tested for inducibility of diabetes with low dose injections of SZ (5 X 40 mg/kg/day). Only those nude mice in which the thymus graft had resulted in successful T-cell reconstitution, as shown by the production of antibodies against sheep RBC, developed diabetes. Furthermore, splenic T-cells isolated from diabetic +/nu mice, induced with multiple low doses of SZ, caused significant impairment of glucose tolerance when injected into naive nu/nu mice. Our results demonstrate that the development of diabetes in mice treated with repeated low doses of the beta cell toxin requires host T-cell functions, and support the view that this type of experimental diabetes may be mediated by autoimmune mechanisms, presumably involving T-cells sensitized against beta cell-associated self-antigens.

206

Impairment of Cell Mediated Immunity in Chronic Alloxan Diabetic Mice. E.R. ARQUILLA*, R.E. MICHALSKI, and M.D. ROTH, Irvine, California.

We have demonstrated that the delayed hypersensitivity (DH) response of sensitized chronic diabetic mice to 2,4 dinitrofluorobenzine (DNFB) was attenuated (20%) compared to the response observed in sensitized normal mice (Barg, et al, Diabetes 27, 1978). The DH response was passively transferred to normal nonsensitized recipients with either normal or diabetic sensitized spleen cells. In either case, the DH response was of equal magnitude. The DH response could not be transferred to nonsensitized diabetic recipients with either normal or diabetic sensitized spleen cells. Consequently, the diabetic nonsensitized mice cannot host the passive transfer of DH. Insulin treatment of chronic diabetic mice improves the attenuated DH response to approximately 50 to 60% of normal. Normal mice made insulinopenic with antisera have an impaired DH response (40% of normal). Spleen hypertrophy following DNFB challenge demonstrable in normal sensitized mice is absent in diabetic sensitized mice. Normal sensitized mice treated with insulin antisera do not have spleen hypertrophy but diabetic sensitized mice treated with insulin have a very marked hypertrophy of the spleen following DNFB challenge. These observations are presented as evidence that there is significant impairment of the cellular immune response in the chronic alloxan diabetic mouse which is related to the persistent insulinopenia. This impairment is qualitatively demonstrable following challenge and significantly attenuated in the primary DH response. Supported by grants from the Juvenile Diabetes and KROC Foundations.

207

Immunosuppression in Viral Murine Diabetes D.DAFOE, A.NAJI, C.F. BARKER*, PHILA. PA

In virally induced diabetes the importance of an autoimmune phase reinforcing betatropic infection is controversial. Reports that the murine disease can be passaged by lymphocytes from infected animals have not been confirmed. The influence of immunosuppression was studied since if autoimmunity were responsible for islet destruction this should be protective, but if infection itself is responsible, immunosuppression might emphasize damage. Prior to inoculation of SWR/J mice with EMC virus they were treated with the following agents: antilymphocyte serum (ALS), silica (an anti-macrophage agent), anti-θ serum (cytotoxic specifically for T lymphocytes). Cyclophosphamide (CY) was used in a dose which selectively depletes suppressor cells but not cytotoxic T cells. Normal SWR/J mice had a mean plasma glucose of 173 $\pm$ 36 mg/dl. Those treated with only EMC virus were hyperglycemic 5 days later (389$\pm$ 138). Protection from diabetes was conferred by ALS (144 $\pm$ 45; $p < .001$), by silica plus anti-θ (138 $\pm$ 53; $p < .001$) and to a marginal degree by silica alone (305 $\pm$ 138); but not by CY (347 $\pm$ 199). However, CY treated mice failed to make the usual rapid recovery (glucose 296 $\pm$ 112 after 4 weeks vs. 197 $\pm$ 26 for mice treated with virus alone) arguing that suppressor cells are important in the recovery phase. The findings support the importance of autoimmunity in viral diabetes.

208

Suppressor Cell Dysfunction in Insulin-Dependent Diabetes. RICHARD S. FAIRCHILD, JOSEPH L. KYNER*, and NABIH I. ABDOU, Kansas City, Ks.

Insulin-dependent diabetes (IDD) is in part an immune-mediated disorder. Because of the association of certain autoimmune diseases with suppressor cell (SC) dysfunction, non-specific and specific in vitro SC activity was evaluated in 11 patients with IDD, 4 with non-IDD, and 11 normal controls. Non-specific SC function was evaluated by measuring pokeweed mitogen stimulated B cell IgG biosynthesis in concanavalin A SC-activated (experimental) and nonactivated (control) cultures. Antigen specific SC function was evaluated by SC activation with 100μg guinea pig islet cell homogenate (experimental culture) or splenic cell homogenate (control culture) for 24 hr. Experimental and control cultures were washed and co-cultured with fresh cells stimulated with 1.0μg islet cell homogenate. Coculture cell proliferation rates were measured by ^{3}H-thymidine incorporation. SC activity was scored by dividing the values obtained for experimental cultures by those for control cultures. IDD non-specific SC function was less efficient than controls; IDD group 1.42±0.66 and control group 0.61±0.08 ($p<0.02$). Specific SC activity was 1.15±0.23 for IDD, 0.77±0.05 for non-IDD and 0.79±0.33 for controls; the difference between the IDD and other 2 groups was statistically significant ($p<0.02$). The two IDD patients tested with disease duration >5 years had no evidence of specific SC dysfunction. In conclusion, IDD is associated with SC dysfunction, not noted in hyperglycemic non-IDD, which may be an early transient event and could play a key role in the induction of the disease.

209

A Prospective Study of Suppressor Cell Activity in Patients with Newly Diagnosed Insulin Dependent Diabetes Mellitus. KARSTEN BUSCHARD and JØRGEN RYGAARD, Copenhagen, Denmark.

The aim was to investigate prospectively the suppressor cell activity (SCA) in patients with newly diagnosed insulin dependent diabetes mellitus (IDDM).

SCA of patients peripheral blood lymphocytes was tested after 48 hours preincubation with concanavalin A. Suppression (S) was measured as the ability of the lymphocytes to inhibit ^{3}H-thymidine incorporation in concanavalin A stimulated normal donor lymphocytes. Suppressor index (SI) expresses the S-value of a patient in relation to the S-values of simultaneously investigated healthy control persons (normal SI being 1.00).

Seventeen diabetics were investigated 5 ± 1 (SEM) days after their diagnosis. The mean S-value ± SEM was 23 ± 6 and the mean SI-value was 0.58 ± 0.15. The SI-values were correlated to the patients' β-cell function expressed by C-peptide measurements ($p<0.02$). The patients were re-tested 5 ± 1 months later and the mean S-value was then 44 ± 4 and the mean SI-value 1.25 ± 0.14. It is concluded that SCA is significantly depressed in patients with IDDM at time of diagnosis ($p_S<0.05$, $p_{SI}<0.01$).

As several studies have demonstrated the importance of autoreactive lymphocytes in diabetogenesis, it is suggested that an impaired SCA, causing a decreased inhibition of lymphocytes, may be implicated in the pathogenesis of IDDM.

210

Rheumatoid Arthritis (RA) In Children With Diabetes M. RUDOLF, J. DWYER and M. GENEL*, New Haven, CT

Type I diabetes mellitus (DM-I) is frequently associated with the thyrogastric cluster of autoimmune diseases, but not with the lupus cluster. We have identified 6 children (4F, 2M) with diabetes >5 yrs duration and RA. Four also have thyroiditis and/or other autoimmune disorders.

Immunological studies revealed significant ANA titres in 5, strongly positive rheumatoid factor (RF) in 2 and mitochondrial antibodies (MA) in 2. Positive organ specific antibodies (OSA) were found in 5: thyroid microsomal (TMA) in 4, thyroglobulin (TGA) in 3, parietal cell (PCA) in 2 and adrenal (AA) in 1. No patient had antibodies to islet cells (measured by Dr. N. Maclaren) reticulum cells or smooth muscle. Coomb's tests, C3 and DNA binding were normal. Five had HLA alleles at risk for DM-I (B8,15,18, DRw3,4) and for RA (B27, DRw3,4,8).

	F1	F2	F3	F4	M1	M2
JRA	⟵	polyarticular		⟶	pauciarticular	
RF	+ + +	-	+ +	-	-	-
ANA	+ +	+	+ +	+ + +	-	+
Misc	↓C4		↓IgA	↓C4/MA		MA
OSA	TGA	TMA	TM/TGA AA	TMA PCA		TM/TGA PCA
HLA	B8,15 DRw4	B27 DRw3,4		B18 DRw3	B27 DRw3,8	B8 DRw3,4

Although the presence of OSA and these HLA antigens in DM-I is not unusual, our children also exhibit clinical and serological features of the lupus cluster. This association has not heretofore been recognized. Our children may represent a unique subgroup of DM-I in whom more generalized immunological dysfunction occurs.

211

Inherited Autoimmuniuty versus Coxsackie B4 in Insulin Dependent Diabetes. W. RILEY, N. MACLAREN,* K. RAND and R BEJAR, Gainesville, Florida.

Autommunity has been increasingly implicated in the pathogenesis of insulin dependent diabetes mellitus (IDDM); however, interest in a viral etiology has been reawakened by isolation of Coxsackie B4 which induced diabetes in mice, from a patient with recently diagnosed IDDM (Yoon et al. 1979). 26 probands with recent (20<2weeks) onset of IDDM and their families were studied for neutralizing titers to Coxsackie B4 (McLaughlin strain). The probands with IDDM and family members had similar titers. Islet cell antibodies (ICA) were found in 68% of the patients, but in none of the other household members. We also found no ICA in another 10 patients recovering from Coxsackie B infections (meningitis, pericarditis). In a large study of family members of IDDM probands, the following autoantibodies were found:

Relatives	n	ICA	(THYROID) TMA	(GASTRIC) PCA
Mothers	155	7(4.5%)	36(23%)	17(11%)
Fathers	31	0	4(13%)	2(6%)
Siblings	36	0	2(5.5%)	0
IDDM	404	146(36%)	80(20%)	34(8.5%)

These data indicated a strong familial predisposition for organ specific autoimmunity. Our findings that ICA was absent in patients convalescing from proven Coxsackie illnesses, that antibodies to Coxsackie were similar in the household contacts and the probands at the time of diagnosis and that transient ICA was not seen among relatives of probands at the time of diagnosis do not support an acute viral illness (Coxsackie B4) as a frequent etiology of IDDM.

212

Islet Cell Antibodies in Gestational Diabetes Mellitus: Prognostic Value. F.GINSBERG-FELLNER*, M.DOBERSEN, E.M.MARK, C.NECHEMIAS*,R.U.HAUSKNECHT P. RUBINSTEIN and A.L.NOTKINS, New York,N.Y. and Bethesda, Md.

Previous studies have indicated that 35-50% of gestational diabetic women develop overt diabetes mellitus within ten years following pregnancy. As the presence of islet cell antibodies (ICAs) in non-insulin dependent adult diabetics has already been shown to portend the future need for insulin therapy, it was hypothesized that such studies in gestational diabetics might allow a similar prediction. Accordingly, 47 recently diagnosed Class A diabetic women, ages 18 to 41 years (mean age 27 years) and 23 Class A diabetic women participating in a longitudinal study that started in 1969 were investigated. 15/47 (32%) of the present gestational diabetics demonstrated ICAs on serial serum specimens obtained during the second and third trimesters of pregnancy. The presence of ICAs did not correlate with hemoglobin A1C levels or birth weights of their infants. However, 11/15 ICA positive women had HLA DRW3 or DRW4. 11/23 (48%) of the older group of gestational diabetics (mean age during pregnancy 26 years, mean present age 35 years) were similarly found to have ICAs in stored serum specimens. Of this group, 8 (73%), are presently insulin-dependent for a mean duration of 3.2 years. Furthermore, only 1/12 (8%) ICA negative women is currently receiving oral antidiabetic therapy.

The data suggest that the presence of ICAs in pregnancy may enable prediction of which gestational diabetic women will develop true insulin-dependent diabetes mellitus in the future.

213

Beta Cell Dysfunction In HLA Identical Siblings of Insulin Dependent Diabetics (IDD) P.HOLLANDER, C. ASPLIN, J. HANSEN and J.P.PALMER*, Seattle,Wa.*

HLA typing allows identification of non-diabetic individuals most likely to have inherited the susceptibility gene for IDD, i.e. HLA identical siblings of young IDD (S-IDD). We have investigated 8 non-diabetic SIDD (age 14-27) for subclinical abnormalities of beta cell secretion and/or carbohydrate metabolism. An oral glucose tolerance test (OGTT) (100g), an intravenous glucose tolerance test (IVGTT)(25g), and an intravenous arginine stimulation test (5g) were performed. During the OGTT, S-IDD when compared to 8 non-diabetic controls (ND) showed an exaggerated peak glucose level ($\bar{X}\pm SE$, 156.83±10.18 vs 119.4±6.95 mg/dl $p<.05$) and decreased disposal of glucose, (S-IDD glucose area=286.71±16.75 mg/dl/3 hours vs ND=119.66±33.21 mg/dl/3 hours, $p<.03$). Acute insulin response (AIR) to the IVGTT (insulin area 0-10 min post glucose), was elevated in the S-IDD, 94.24±9.69 uU/ml.10' compared to ND, 52.13± 5.83 uU/ml.10' ($p<.005$). When individual AIR of the S-IDD were compared to the ND with the use of confidence limits, six out of eight were significantly elevated, $p<.01$. The two S-IDD with normal AIR also had normal insulin and glucose values on their OGTT, but were not separable from the 6 abnormal S-IDD by HLA type. The AIR to arginine showed no difference between the two groups. Conclusion: 3/4 of the S-IDD evaluated exhibited abnormalities in insulin secretion and/or carbohydrate metabolism. Inheritance of the susceptibility gene may result in mild subclinical abnormalities of beta cell function and/or glucose metabolism before the onset of overt IDD.

214

Effect of β-hydroxybutyrate on alanine and leucine flux and leucine N transfer to alanine in man. J. MILES* and M. HAYMOND*, Endocrine Research Unit, Mayo Clinic, Rochester, MN.

Infusion of β-hydroxybutyrate (βOHB) in man decreases plasma alanine (ala) in the absence of changes in plasma insulin (I), suggesting that ketone bodies may decrease proteolysis during fasting. If this were true, infusion of βOHB should decrease ala and leucine (leu) production (Ra) and diminish transfer of leu nitrogen (N) to ala. To test this hypothesis, 6 normal postabsorptive volunteers were infused with D-βOHB (15 μmol/kg-min) for 3 hrs. Rates of leu and ala Ra, disappearance (Rd) and clearance (MCR) were determined using the stable isotopes [6,6,6-$^2H_3$] leu and [2, 3,3,3-$^2H_4$] ala. Rates of leu N conversion to ala were assessed with [^{15}N]leu. Arterialized-venous samples were analyzed by GC/MS. During infusion of D-βOHB plasma total ketone body concentration increased from 0.2 mM to a stable plateau of 2.3 mM. Plasma ala decreased from 250 μM to 221 μM by 3 hr ($p < 0.05$). Ala Ra increased from 5.3 ± .3 μmol/kg-min to 7.8 ± 0.6 μmol/kg-min by hr 3; ala MCR increased from 22 ± 2 to 35 ± 3 ml/kg-min by 3 hr ($p< 0.02$). Plasma I and leu Ra, Rd and MCR did not change, but the rate of transfer of leu N to ala increased from 0.66 ± .08 to 1.40 ± 0.20 μmol/kg-min and the % of leu N incorporated into ala increased from 26 ± 3 to 45 ± 5% ($p < 0.02$). Plasma pyruvate doubled ($p < 0.05$). Conclusion: infusion of βOHB in man increased ala Ra, transfer of leu N to ala and ala MCR, without altering leu turnover. These results suggest that ketone bodies do not decrease proteolysis and that changes in the plasma ala may be due to increased pyruvate availability.

215

Roles of the Periphery & Liver in the Hypoglycemic action of dichloroacetate in vivo. M.P. DIAMOND, W. LACY* & A. CHERRINGTON*, Nash., TN

Examination of the effects of dichloroacetate (DCA) in vivo has been complicated by the fact that the compound can alter the secretion rate of insulin. We previously failed to detect any effect of DCA on glucose production (GP) or clearance (Cg) in fasted dogs possibly because the direct effects of DCA were offset by the consequences of the fall in plasma insulin. To test this hypothesis DCA was infused (0.4 mg/kg-min) for 5h into a group of 48h fasted conscious dogs whose insulin (I) & glucagon (G) levels were clamped at basal values by peripheral infusion of somatostatin & intraportal replacement of I (300 μU/kg-min) & G (1 ng/kg-min). Metabolite balances across the liver were measured using an A-V difference technique, glucose and alanine turnovers were determined using tracer techniques & gluconeogenesis was assessed by following conversion of gluconeogenic precursors into glucose. In the presence of fixed concentrations of I (13 μU/ml) & G (166pg/ml) DCA caused the arterial levels of alanine & lactate to fall by 84±1 and 52±13% respectively, decreased their hepatic uptake by 65±3 & 54±10% respectively & reduced their conversion to glucose by 64±8%. Coincident with these changes GP fell by 19±9%, Cg increased by 55±16%, and the plama glucose level fell (107 ±10 to 56±6 mg/dl). These data demonstrate in 48h fasted dogs that 1) 2/3 of DCA's hypoglycemic action is attributable to an effect on peripheral glucose uptake while 1/3 is attributable to a curtailment of glucose supply & 2) in vivo, small DCA induced changes in I (Δ5μU/ml) can mask the direct effects of DCA on GP & Cg.

216

Arachidonic Acid Derivatives (PGE_2 and PGI_2) Produced by Adipocytes Modulate Sympathetic Nervous System Activity. L. AXELROD* and L. LEVINE, Boston, MA and Waltham, MA

We studied the production rate (PR) of arachidonic acid (AA) derivatives by isolated rat adipocytes, using radioimmunoassay. During norepinephrine (NE)-induced lipolysis, there was a significant increase in PR of prostaglandin E_2 (PGE_2), prostacyclin (PGI_2, measured as 6-keto-$PGF_{1\alpha}$) and $PGF_{2\alpha}$. Indomethacin (INDO) inhibited the PR of PGI_2 and $PGF_{2\alpha}$, but did not prevent a 3½ fold increase in the PR of PGE_2. Insulin (10,50,100 μU/ml) significantly inhibited the NE-induced increment in PR of PGE_2 (and $PGF_{2\alpha}$) but not of PGI_2.

The endogenous NE-induced PR of PGI_2 by adipocytes, calculated from the PR of PGI_2 observed in our studies (2.2 ng/10^6cells/2 hrs) and from the number of fat cells in the normal organism, was 1.46 ng/kg/min for rats, 4.46 ng/kg/min for men and 11.86 ng/kg/min for women, comparable to the exogenous PGI_2 infusion rate that alters platelet aggregation (5 ng/kg/min) and blood pressure (20 ng/kg/min) in man. PGI_2 failed to modify lipolysis.

We conclude that AA derivatives produced by adipocytes modulate sympathetic nervous system activity: (1) PGE_2 is a negative feedback modulator of lipolysis. During NE-induced lipolysis, PGE_2 inhibits lipolysis; during inhibition of lipolysis by insulin, the decrease in PGE_2 PR offsets the antilipolytic effect of insulin. Previous objections to this concept based on failure of INDO to enhance lipolysis are not valid, since INDO does not inhibit PGE_2 PR. (2) The PR of PGI_2 by adipocytes is sufficient to modify platelet aggregation and blood pressure.

217

Glomerular Prostaglandin Metabolism in Diabetic Rats. D.M. BROWN*, J.M. GERRARD, J. PELLER, G.H. R. RAO, J.G. WHITE, Minneapolis, Minnesota.

Prostaglandins (PG) regulate smooth muscle and vascular responsiveness. Increased synthesis of thromboxane (TxB_2), a potent vasoconstrictor, has been found by platelets from diabetic (D) rats whereas synthesis of prostacyclin (6-Keto-$PGF_{1\alpha}$) (PGI_2) by aortas is decreased. Since several hemodynamic and mesangial functions are altered by diabetes and since the glomerulus is known to be capable of synthesizing several PG metabolites, the metabolism of the PG precursor arachidonic acid (AA) was studied using glomeruli isolated from rats diabetic for 1.5 and 6 months as compared with age-matched controls (C). Results are expressed as % of AA for each metabolite. Other metabolites included: $PGF_{2\alpha}$, PGE_2, PGD_2, 12-hydroxy-5,8,10,14-eicosatetraenoic acid (HETE) and 12-hydroxy-5,8,10 heptadecatrienoic acid (HHT).

PG metabolite	% Arachidonic Acid 1.5 mos. D	1.5 mos. C	6 mos. D	6 mos. C
TxB_2	5.74	0.71	6.77	2.73
PGI_2	0.32	0.21	0.37	0.41
$PGF_{2\alpha}$	0.87	1.07	1.30	0.99
PGE_2	4.46	1.83	2.95	1.83
PGD_2	0.64	0.62	0.66	0.49
HETE	3.31	2.11	4.66	3.39
HHT	4.38	1.53	2.84	2.38

Diabetic glomeruli synthesize increased PG metabolites in both cyclooxygenase and lipooxygenase pathways, increased amounts of the potent vasoconstrictor TxB_2 and increased amounts of PGE_2 and of HETE. Altered PG synthesis is postulated to contribute to the pathophysiology of functional abnormalities of glomeruli in diabetis mellitus.

218

Pancreatic Immunoreactive Neurotensin (IR-NT) in Obese (ob) and Diabetes (db) Mutant Mice: A Longitudinal Study. M. BERELOWITZ,* C. NAKAWATASE, and L.A. FROHMAN,* Chicago, IL.

Neurotensin, a hypothalamic peptide with potent hyperglycemic effects, stimulates glucagon and inhibits insulin release. IR-NT has recently been demonstrated in normal pancreas with an increased content reported in streptozotocin-diabetic rats. We have measured pancreatic IR-NT in relation to metabolic status during development of obese and diabetes syndromes in mutant C57BL mice. Female 6J and KsJ mice with ob/ob or db/db genes and littermate controls were killed at age 6-24 wk and 2N acetic acid extracts of pancreas assayed for IR-NT by a specific RIA. The obese syndrome in ob/ob and db/db 6J mice resulted in progressive weight gain, moderate hyperglycemia and marked hyperinsulinemia from 6 wk. Pancreatic IR-NT was similar at all ages in obese and control mice. A progressive fall in IR-NT occurred with increasing age in 6J ob/ob mice and controls from ± 750 pg/g at 6 wk to ± 200 pg/g at 24 wk ($p < 0.001$) but was not seen in 6J db/db mice or controls. The diabetes syndrome in db/db and ob/ob KsJ mice resulted in a similar metabolic state until 9-10 wk when increasing hyperglycemia followed falling serum insulin levels. Pancreatic IR-NT was markedly elevated from 10 wk in KsJ db/db and ob/ob mice compared to controls ($p<0.001$). In all groups a fall in IR-NT occurred from 6-24 wk. The results indicate that mouse pancreas IR-NT levels are similar to those in rats and fall progressively with age. Pancreatic IR-NT is increased in insulinopenic diabetes but is unaffected by obesity with insulin resistance, suggesting a role for the peptide in diabetes.

219

Feeding Alters Hepatic Extraction (HE) of Insulin (I) and Glucagon (Gg). J. JASPAN,* K. POLONSKY, J. DHORAJIWALA, W. PUGH, A. MOOSSA. Chicago, Ill.

The effect of glucose (G) and protein (prot.) on HE of I and Gg was studied in 6 conscious dogs by sampling from catheters placed 21 days before in portal vein (PV), femoral artery and hepatic (hep.) vein. Hep. plasma flow was measured by cardiogreen. Simultaneous samples were drawn from each vessel before and every 30 min. after 25 gm. G (n=3) or 60 gm. prot. (n=3) given orally. I (μu/ml) and Gg (pg/ml) levels and hep. G output (HGO) (mg/kg/min) were measured. Results of G feeding were analyzed in three, 120 min. periods based upon changes in HGO.

	BASELINE	0-120'	120-240'	240-360'
PV I	38±3	108±25	42±5	29±2
PV Gg	174±10	105±12	161±21	189±9
HE(I)%	33.5±12.3	58.9±11.4	49±0.4	25.5±5.9
HE(Gg)%	22.6±2.6	8.3±6.1	12.3±4.3	17.9±5.1
HGO	2.7±0.3	-0.6±0.3	1.6±0.7	2.8±0.4

After G, HE(I) doubled. This temporary increase in HE(I) coincided with the period of hep. G uptake, while suppressed Gg levels were associated with reduced HE(Gg), which returned to basal by 4-6 hr. In the first 120 min. after prot., the 50% increase in PV I was associated with hep. G uptake but no significant change in HE(I). In this period PV Gg doubled but HE Gg fell from 33±0.9% to 23±3%. Over the next 4 hr. HGO was restored and although PV Gg remained elevated, HE Gg returned to basal (34±2%). Conclusions: 1) Changes in HE of I and Gg induced by feeding are correlated with changes in hep. G handling. 2) The changing HE of I and Gg after meals makes peripheral levels a poor reflection of PV levels and hep. hormone delivery. 3) Nutrient-mediated changes in HE of I and Gg may influence nutrient disposal.

220

Possible Role of Defectual Thermogenesis and its Regulation by Insulin in Genetic Obesity
F. ASSIMACOPOULOS-JEANNET, J. SEYDOUX, L. GIRARDIER, and B. JEANRENAUD*, Geneva, Switz.

Obese hyperinsulinemic rodents have impaired thermogenesis when exposed to temperatures lower than neutrality. Brown adipose tissue (BAT) from lean and obese (ob/ob) mice was studied in vitro. Three indices of metabolic activity (referred to as "metabolism") were measured: NAD (P) redox state during electrical nerve stimulation or norepinephrine addition, glycerol and heat output during norepinephrine stimulation. BAT from fed obese mice (IRI: 46±7ng/ml) showed no change in BAT "metabolism" in response to nerve or noradrenaline stimulation, while lean mice responded by a marked increase in BAT "metabolism" under these same conditions. Three days of fasting (IRI: 3.0±0.1) and to a greater extent cold adaptation at 5°C (IRI:19±4) resulted in a partial recovery in the response to nerve stimulation and norepinephrine-induced heat production in BAT from ob/ob mice. These data suggest that: 1) although the main effector of BAT "metabolism" is the sympathetic nervous system, its response may partly be modulated by chronic changes in hyperinsulinemia; 2) decreased BAT thermogenesis of the obese mice may contribute to greater metabolic efficiency, hence to obesity per se.

221

Insulin-like and Insulin Antagonistic Effects of Growth Hormone on Glucose Production and Clearance in Man. L. MacGorman and R. Rizza,* Endocrine Research Unit, Mayo Clinic, Rochester, Minnesota.

To determine the effect of physiologic increments in plasma growth hormone (GH) on human glucose homeostasis, six normal subjects were infused with HGH (100 ng/kg/min) for 6 hrs along with somatostatin (100 μg/hr, to suppress endogenous insulin, glucagon, and GH secretion) and sufficient insulin (100 μU/kg/min) to maintain plasma insulin constant; during the final 2 hrs, glucose (2 mg/kg/min) was infused. On another occasion (control studies), saline was infused instead of HGH. Glucose production (mg/kg/min) and clearance (ml/kg/min) were determined isotopically using $3H^3$-glucose. Infusion of HGH, which increased plasma GH to 30-40 ng/ml, resulted in a greater decrease in plasma glucose than that observed in control studies (60±2 vs 67±1 mg/dl respectively, $p<0.05$). This was due to both greater suppression of glucose production (1.13±0.07 vs 1.21±0.03, $p<0.05$) and stimulation of glucose clearance (2.7±0.1 vs 2.4±0.1, $p<0.05$) during GH infusion. Subsequently when glucose was infused, GH caused greater hyperglycemia (133±4 mg/dl) than that observed in control studies (104±6 mg/dl, $p<0.01$) due to impaired suppression of endogenous glucose production (0.4±0.04 vs 0.19±0.14, $p<0.01$) and greater suppression of glucose clearance (1.6±0.1 vs 2.1±0.1, $p<0.01$). Conclusions: Physiologic increments in plasma GH have an early transient insulin-like effect and a late persistent insulin antagonistic action on glucose production and glucose clearance in man. Thus, growth hormone-induced insulin insulin resistance may involve hepatic as well as peripheral glucose metabolism.

222

Dopaminergic Control of Ketogenesis in Fasting and Diabetic Rats. D.G. JOHNSTON, G. BLESA MALPICA, J.M. BURRIN, H. ØRSKOV and K.G.M.M. ALBERTI,* Newcastle upon Tyne, U.K.

The role of dopamine in the ketonaemia of starvation and diabetic ketoacidosis was investigated. Normal male Wistar rats receiving the specific dopamine antagonists, metoclopramide 4mg/kg/24h (n=12) or domperidone 4mg/kg/24h (n=6) were compared with placebo (n=12) during a 48h fast. In addition, metoclopramide 4mg/kg/24h (n=6) or placebo (n=6) were administered to insulin-deprived streptozotocin (120mg/kg) diabetic animals during a 48h fast. Metoclopramide decreased blood ketone body concentrations at 24h and 48h in fasted normal rats (2.28±0.66 mmol/l metoclopramide; 3.43±0.72 mmol/l placebo; $p<0.01$). Plasma NEFA, blood glucose, serum insulin and plasma glucagon levels were unaltered by metoclopramide. A similar decrease in blood ketone body concentrations (30.6% decrease compared with placebo at 24h, $p<0.02$; 30% at 48h, $p<0.05$) was obtained with domperidone. In insulin deprived fasted diabetics, metoclopramide caused a 34% decrease in ketone body concentrations at 24h ($p<0.05$), but this difference had disappeared at 48h. Blood glucose was similar in metoclopramide and placebo-treated rats at 24h and 48h. Dopamine blockade thus decreased the ketonaemic response to starvation in normals and the early hyper-ketonaemia of insulin-deprivation in diabetic animals. This action was independent of lipolysis or changes in circulating hormone levels, suggesting a role for dopamine in production of the ketonaemia.

223

Effects of Insulin and Glucagon Antisera on the Incorporation of Isotopic Leucine into Myelin Proteins.
NORTON SPRITZ* and BARBARA MARINAN
New York, New York

We have shown previously that, in an in vitro system, incorporation of amino acid precursors into sciatic nerve myelin proteins is generally diminshed in experimental diabetes in the rat, but incorporation into a protein of 10,500 daltons (B protein) is not decreased and in some instances, increased. Insulin, when added at high concentrations (10^{-7} M) to nerves of normal animals, increased incorporation generally, but not in the B protein. Glucagon in contrast, enhanced incorporation into B protein. In order to establish, further, the role of these hormones in modulating metabolic activity of this protein, we utilized insulin antiserum and found that it reproduces, in vitro, the effects of diabetes. In 7 studies, incorporation into higher molecular weight myelin proteins and total incorporation into proteins was diminshed by greater than 50% when compared to the effect of non-immune serum (NIS); but incorporation into B protein was unaffected or slightly enhanced. In contrast, in 6 studies utilizing glucagon antiserum (compared to NIS) incorporation into B protein diminshed by an average of 28%. We thus provide further evidence that the altered pattern of amino acid incorporation in myelin proteins in experimental diabetes relates to the high glucagon, low insulin state that characterizes that model; and that the Schwann cell which probably synthesizes myelin is modulated by these hormones.

224

Regional Localization of Cerebral Edema Associated with Treatment of Diabetic Ketoacidosis, P. A. TORNHEIM, Cincinnati, Oh. (Introduced by KENNETH KREINES*, Cincinnati, Oh.)

Occasionally, diabetic patients suffer lethal cerebral edema following agressive therapy with fluids and insulin. In order to localize this form of edema, streptozotocin-diabetic rats selected for plasma ketosis were treated by constant intravenous infusion with saline and regular insulin. At the end of 2 and 5 hours of therapy, rats were sacrificed and tested for density of cerebral cortex, corpus callosum, thalamus, caudate-putamen, and medulla, using an organic density gradient. Density data from treated rats were compared with those from normal control animals to determine change in brain water content.

Animals sacrificed after 2 hours of therapy demonstrated increase in brain water content that was similar in magnitude for all regions tested and was less than the 5% change considered clinically significant. After 5 hours of therapy, there was further increase in water content of cortex, with a tissue volume for treated animals that was 6.5% higher than control values. For white matter, there was also continued increase in water content, less than that seen for cortex. Other regions tested showed values after 5 hours of therapy similar to those seen after 2 hours.

These findings suggest that the cerebral edema associated with treatment for diabetic ketoacidosis accumulates preferentially in the cerebral cortex. Increase in water content of white matter suggests, but does not document, an interstitial component to this form of cerebral edema. This study was supported by NIH Grant HL 22106.

225

Effects of Diabetic Serum and Platelets on Growth of Cultured Vascular Smooth Muscle Cells and Fibroblasts. F. UMEDA, J.P. HALLE, J. ABARCA, SL. LEUNG, D.J. FRANKS, and P. HAMET*. CLINICAL RESEARCH INSTITUTE OF MONTREAL, QUEBEC, CANADA
Platelets and platelet derived factors appear to play a major role in the pathogenesis of atherosclerosis. The effects of serum and platelet extract (PE) containing platelet growth factor (PGF) obtained from 5 male insulin-dependent, diabetics (IDDM) on the growth rate of rat SMC, mouse 3T3, and WI-38 cells were studied and compared with 6 age-matched control subjects. Growth rate was determined by incorporation of ^{3}H thymidine into DNA. Diabetic plasma derived serum (PDS) was significantly less effective in supporting growth of SMC, 3T3 and WI-38 than control. In contrast, whole blood serum (WBS) from diabetics was more growth supportive to 3T3 and WI-38 than control WBS. Little difference was observed in SMC. A similar effect of WBS on the growth of SMC and 3T3 were observed in experimental diabetes (insulin-treated streptozotocin induced diabetic rats and spontaneously diabetic rats). Furthermore, the growth promoting activity of PE from diabetics was greater in all cultured cells studied. These results suggest abnormal activities of plasma and platelet derived growth factors are present in human and experimental IDDM and may be involved in the development of vascular disease. Heterologous as well as homologous cell culture models may be useful systems for evaluating the development and severity of vascular complications in diabetes. Supported by NIH 1RO1 AM21299 and Canadian Heart Foundation.

226

Decline in the Cardiovascular Death Rate among Diabetics. M. HARRIS,* Bethesda, MD

The 1973-75 Health Interview Surveys of the NCHS show that 600,000 new cases of diabetes (DM) were diagnosed in each of those years while the prevalence of DM increased by 300,000 cases annually. The difference can be attributed to the annual number of deaths of diabetics. However, during this period US mortality statistics allocated only 37,000 deaths annually to DM as the underlying cause (UC) of death. Data From Rochester, Minn., and Pennsylvania substantiate the assertion that DM is coded as the UC in only about 10% of DM deaths. This gross underestimation indicates that DM mortality analyses based on national data are of limited value. Improvements can be made by analyzing DM as UC and as contributing cause(CC) of death. To assess the complexity of deaths among DMs, Iowa multiple cause of death data are analyzed to determine which conditions are associated with death due to DM and for which conditions DM is considered a CC of death. Declines from 1972-77 in DM deaths where cardiovascular (CV) diseases were or were not present on the death certificate are analyzed to show that DMs with CV diseases have experienced a 2-fold greater decline in death rate than DMs without these conditions. In contrast, decline in the CV death rate where DM was present as a CC was the same as when DM was absent, indicating no increased mortality due to DM among persons who die of CV diseases.

227

Incidence of Retinopathy and Cardiovascular Events as a Function of Plasma Glucose. J.R. LISSE, W.C. KNOWLER*, D.J. PETTITT, P.H. BENNETT*, Phoenix, Az.

590 Pima Indians, at least 25 years old, with normal EKG's and retinae, had plasma glucose concentrations (PG) determined two hours after 75 gms of oral carbohydrate at an initial exam. Six year incidence rates of retinopathy, defined as microaneurysms, hemorrhages, or neovascularization; and EKG changes, defined by U.S. Pooling Project Study criteria, were stratified by the PG.

In 131 autopsies the presence of atherosclerotic cardiovascular disease (ASCVD), including old myocardial infarction (MI), sudden death, and death due to stroke or MI, was determined. Prevalence rates of ASCVD at death were stratified by the subjects' most recent PG.

Retinopathy incidence increased steadily with PG, from 1.5% in people with PG <130 mg/dl to 48% with PG $\geq$500 mg/dl ($p<.0001$). In contrast, EKG changes and ASCVD at death showed little relationship with PG.

Thus PG was a strong risk factor for the development of retinopathy (microvascular disease), but not for ASCVD (macrovascular disease).

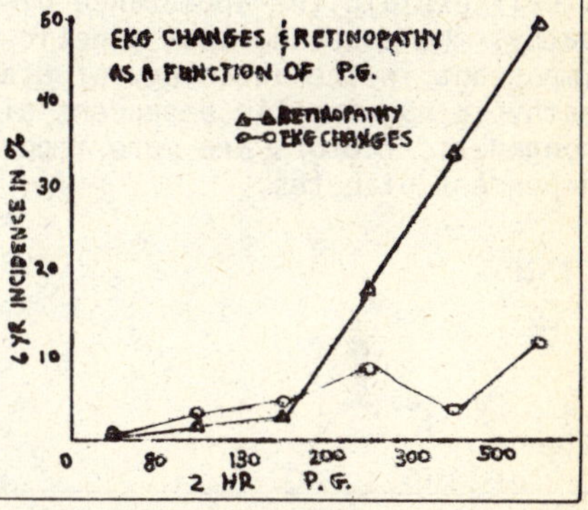

228

Proliferative Retinopathy with Minimal Visual Symptoms in Insulin-Dependent Diabetes

MARJORIE A. MOSIER*, Irvine, Calif.

The potential for rapid development of retinopathy in the young, insulin-dependent diabetic is not generally appreciated. There is, consequently, inadequate utilization of available therapeutic measures which are effective in the early stages of proliferative retinopathy. The purpose of this report is to emphasize the occurrence of, and potential for, rapid loss of vision in the young, insulin-dependent diabetic.

We studied ten insulin-dependent diabetic subjects under the age of 40 with duration of diabetes from 15 to 23 years. All demonstrated a pattern of rapid development of retinovascular proliferation with few or late symptoms. Retinal changes which threatened or ultimately destroyed vision developed while good visual acuity was maintained. Fifty per cent of these had advanced beyond the stage at which treatment is most beneficial when first examined. We conclude that the "silent" progression of this blinding disorder permits it to escape detection and therapeutic intervention prior to a stage of advanced damage. Early and regular ophthalmic assessment of the young, insulin-dependent diabetic is essential for the prevention of blindness.

229

Identical Twins and Diabetic Retinopathy. R.D.G. LESLIE and D. A. PYKE, Kings College Hospital, London, England (Introduced by R. B. Goldberg,* Chicago, IL.)

The prevalence and features of diabetic retinopathy have been examined in 68 pairs of concordant identical twins--31 with insulin dependent diabetes. Optic fundi were examined after pupillary dilatation and when retinopathy was classified as nil, background or proliferative changes 35 of the 37 non insulin dependent diabetic pairs were in the same category ($p < 0.001$). However, there was no tendency for insulin dependent diabetic pairs to fall into the same category and even when we consider the duration of diabetes a striking difference for retinopathy was observed in 5 pairs of twins. There was no significant difference for retinopathy between 31 concordant and 27 discordant insulin dependent diabetic twin pairs. Diabetic retinopathy was not observed in 52 unaffected cotwins of diabetics suggesting a genetic predisposition to diabetes does not of itself explain the appearance of diabetic retinopathy. We conclude that genetic factors may be important in the aetiology of diabetic retinopathy in non insulin dependent diabetes but that nongenetic factors are more important in insulin dependent diabetes.

230

Improvement in Peripheral Nerve Function in Diabetes After Short-term Treatment with an Artificial Pancreas. M. GOLDEN,* K. NUDLEMAN, G. MYERS,* and A. CHARLES, Irvine, CA.

In patients with diabetes mellitus, motor nerve function correlates with degree of hyperglycemia, while sensory nerve function may not. To determine the effect of short-term excellent diabetic control on peripheral nerve function (PNF), 6 young($\bar{x}$ 19.5 yrs) insulin-dependent diabetic patients were studied before and after 48 hours of treatment with the Biostator(R). Patients had clinical and/or electrophysiologic(E.P.) evidence of peripheral neuropathy. Motor nerve conduction velocity(MNCV), terminal latencies, sensory nerve conduction velocity(SNCV), amplitude, and duration of the evoked response were measured in upper and lower limbs under temperature control. Diabetic and non-diabetic controls were also studied at 48 hour intervals to define non-treatment related variation. Diabetics had significantly decreased function in all measurements(e.g.mean median nerve SNCV controls 53.8 $\pm$ 1.5m/sec vs. diabetics 43.4$\pm$3.5, $p<.05$). No sigficant differences were seen in non-diabetic controls or non-Biostator treated diabetics when studied at 48 hour intervals. 48 hours of Biostator control improved motor(e.g.peroneal MNCV 43.4$\pm$4.2m/sec before and 47.4$\pm$3.8 after, $p<.01$) and sensory E.P. functions. In this small group, patients with the most clinical neuropathy tended to have the largest improvements. No symptomatic changes occurred. This suggests that short-term optimal control of hyperglycemia may improve E.P. PNF in insulin-dependent diabetics. A relationship to long-term clinical improvement remains to be demonstrated. Further studies are in progress.

231

Prevalence and Associated Findings of Diabetic Foot Ulcer. T.W. KUEBLER, P. BENDICK, J.A. NORTON, JR., O. MARKAND, F. VINICOR* Indianapolis, IN.

A cross-sectional sample of 300 adult diabetics contained 13 patients with foot ulcers (4.3%). Diabetics with foot ulcers (FU) had a significantly higher mean fasting plasma glucose (fpg) than those with no foot ulcers (NFU): FU mean fpg = 305; NFU mean fpg = 240, P =.05. Whereas the mean duration of diabetes was 13.1 years in FU and 10.1 yrs in NFU this difference was not significant (P>.05). The motor nerve conduction velocity in the median nerve was 30.7 (M./sec.) in FU and 40.9 in NFU (P=.02) and in the common peroneal nerve was 35.4 in FU and 41.1 in NFU (P=.05). The sensory nerve conduction velocity in the median nerve was 38.2 in FU and 44.6 in NFU (P>.05). The percentage of FU with prior amputations was 42.9% and 1.6% in NFU (P=.002). A doppler ultrasound examination was performed to assess occlusive arterial disease and no significant differences were found. Clinically, neither claw foot deformity, sole callus, nor dorsal toe callus were more frequent in FU than in NFU; however, 50% of FU and 27.7% of NFU had bunions.

Thus, FU were present in 4.3% of our patients in association with higher plasma glucose, prior amputations, and decreased motor conduction velocity. Doppler ultrasound examinations were not significantly different between the two groups. These data suggest a neuropathic etiology of the ulcers.

CLINICAL DIABETES

232

Adult Respiratory Distress Syndrome (ARDS) in Diabetic Coma
Robert Matz*, Bronx, New York

In a 15 month period 3 patients who presented in diabetic coma (ketoacidotic and hyperosmolar) developed an adult respiratory distress syndrome (ARDS). Ages ranged from 23-68; none were infected; all had clear lung fields on physical and x-ray examination on admission; two were hypotensive; all were treated with crystalloids, colloid (one), and insulin. Clinical ARDS did not become evident until 8 - 18 hours after admission although all had an arterial pO_2 between 52-60 mm Hg on admission.

Thus all 3 patients had hypoxemia on admission which became an overt ARDS. No cause was evident except uncontrolled diabetes. All received positive end expiratory pressure (PEEP) ventilation and oxygen. The sole survivor required 20 cm PEEP and a 95% F_{IO_2}.

Conclusion: ARDS maybe a manifestation of diabetic coma. A low arterial pO_2 in the absence of infiltrates, infection, pulmonary embolus or abnormal pulmonary physical findings should lead one to anticipate the development of an ARDS in the comatose diabetic.

233

Do Diabetics Need Pneumococcus Vaccine?
JAMES M. MOSS, Alexandria, Virginia

It is generally accepted that patients with diabetes have decreased resistance to infection and therefore should be protected by better hygiene, improved sanitation, increased immunization and prophylactic antibiotics. This belief is based upon studies performed on untreated patients and does not apply to properly controlled diabetics. However, diabetes is listed as an indication for the use of the new polyvalent pneumococcus vaccine. Pneumococcus pneumonia was present in only 0.8% in 6765 admissions of diabetic patients to the Los Angeles County Hospital. A survey of twenty-four physicians with more than a half million patient-years of experience in treating diabetes gave an incidence of pneumococcus pneumonia that was less than one in twenty thousand patient-years of diabetes. Pneumococcus pneumonia is not a significant risk in patients with diabetes. Diabetes is not a valid indication for the use of pneumococcus vaccine.

234

Interrelations of Feto-Placental Maturation, Maternal Glycemic Indices, and Birth Weight.
W. LUQMAN, W. MOORE, C. SAUNDERS, R. KULWIN, M. SMITH, and B. FARISS*, Tacoma, Wa.

It has been suggested that a glucose tolerance test performed prior to 24 weeks gestation could not exclude gestational diabetes in the high risk population. We examined, retrospectively, the relationship between indices of maternal glycemia and (1) gestational age at the time of testing (mean ± SD 31.31±4.08) and (2) gestational age at onset of labor and delivery (mean ± SD=40.06 ± 1.074) in 52 subjects at risk for glucose intolerance tested after 24 weeks of gestation. All pregnancies terminated in spontaneous labor at 40 ± 2 weeks of the calculated gestation. They were selected because of fasting serum glucose (FBS<110 mg%, 2-hour post-testing serum glucose {2 hrPP} <140 mg%, and lack of medical complications. These findings were tested by linear regression and partial correlation applied to the principle of random occurrence within the high risk population studied.

Birth weight correlated with maternal indices of obesity (r=0.316, p=0.02). FBS correlated with birth weight if the contribution of obesity was allowed for (partial correlation r=0.273, p=<0.03). The 2 hrPP/FBS ratio correlated positively with the gestational age at the time of testing (r=0.279, p=0.03) but negatively with gestational age at onset of labor (r=-0.381, p=0.003).

Obesity is a recognized risk for glucose intolerance. It is possible that the macrosomia reported with obesity is mediated via precipitation of glucose intolerance due to counter-regulatory mechanisms beyond 31 weeks of gestation.

235

A Revised Classification and Modified Treatment for Pregnant Diabetics. D.R. HOLLINGSWORTH*, L. COUSINS and S.S.C. YEN, La Jolla, Ca

Pregnant Type I (insulin deficient) and Type II (non insulin deficient) diabetics differ metabolically and require therapeutic reassessment. We studied 6 Type I and 6 Type II patients by measuring plasma glucose (PG) excursions throughout the 24 hr. metabolic clock at 25 and 35 wks. gestation. Insulin dosage was monitored each week by evaluating 24 hr. quantitative fractional urine glucose loss and serial PG throughout the day. All infants were assessed for morbidity.

We found Type II women significantly (P< 0.001) more obese, more insulin resistant (mean pregnancy insulin dose ↑ 94% vs 33% in Type I) and free from hypoglycemia and ketosis. Type I diabetics had wider 24 hr. PG excursions, significant, but usually unrecognized daytime and nocturnal hypoglycemia (PG < 40 mg/dl) and occasional ketonuria. Twenty-four hr. fractional urinary glucose loss precisely mirrored 24 hr. PG excursions and was more useful in adjusting insulin requirements than frequent random PG values. Insulin resistant Type II patients responded poorly to usual split doses of intermediate and regular insulin, but did well on 3 daily doses of regular insulin given before meals. Infant morbidity was higher in "mild" Type II diabetics whose infants had significant polycythemia (P< 0.001 despite similar birth weights 3475 gm. vs 3493 gm., P=NS) and 2 congenital heart lesions. We concluded (1) Pregnancy accentuates metabolic differences between Type I and Type II diabetics; (2) Pregnancy in Type I and Type II diabetics requires management reappraisal; and (3) Infant morbidity is higher in "mild" Type II diabetics.

236

The Time Course of Elevation of Glycohemoglobins in Diabetic Rhesus Monkeys. W. MUELLER, I.Y. ROSENBLUM,* and B. BILLHYMER, Holloman AFB, N.M.

A chronic insulin-dependent diabetic state, characterized by permanent hyperglycemia, glucosuria and ketonuria, was chemically induced in 7 young adult rhesus monkeys (Macaca mulatta). Hemoglobin A_{1c} (Hb A_{1c}) and total glycosylated hemoglobin (Hb A_1) fractions, determined by the method of high pressure liquid chromatography, were measured prior to and at monthly intervals for 3 months following diabetes induction. Hb A_1 was significantly elevated at the 1st (9.9 ± 0.7%), 2nd (13.2 ± 0.4%) and 3rd (13.5 ± 1.1%) monthly intervals compared to baseline (7.1 ± 0.6%). Hb A_{1c}, which was absent in baseline bloods, was detected in 3 of 7 animals at 1 month (4.8 ± 1.5%), in 5 of 6 animals at 2 months (5.7 ± 1.1%) and in 3 of 4 animals at 3 months (5.5 ± 0.4%). Comparison of glycohemoglobin levels to the average daily fasting blood glucose values (FBG) calculated for the corresponding monthly intervals revealed: (1) both Hb A_1 and A_{1c} elevations occur within 1 month (one erythrocyte life span) of the establishment of severe hyperglycemia (435 ± 26 mg/dl 1st month FBG vs. 62 ± 1 mg/dl baseline); and (2) both Hb A_1 and A_{1c} levels plateau at the 2nd and 3rd months despite a decreased severity of hyperglycemia (336 ± 26 mg/dl FBG and 273 ± 19 mg/dl FBG, respectively). Although the rhesus monkey apparently lacks the Hb A_{1c} fraction under normoglycemic conditions, the relationship between Hb A_{1c} or Hb A_1 elevation and long term glycemic control appears to mimic observations in diabetic humans.

237

Glucose Intolerance In The Chimpanzee. I. Y. ROSENBLUM,* Holloman AFB, N.M. 88330

The examination of carbohydrate management in selected adult chimpanzees (Pan troglodytes) has revealed significant glucose intolerance in 4 animals. Based on results of intravenous glucose tolerance tests these animals displayed the following changes compared to nondiabetic controls: (1) abnormally low glucose disappearance rates (0.87 ± 0.05 vs. 2.67 ± 0.37 %/min.) (2) inappropriately low serum levels of immunoreactive insulin (IRI) and C-peptide (CPR); (3) elevated serum levels of immunoreactive glucagon (IRG) and (4) mild-to-moderate glucosuria and proteinuria. Tolbutamide challenges, conducted in 2 of the chimpanzees to further characterize the nature of the glucose intolerant states, failed to elicit significant increases in serum IRI levels. As a group, the glucose intolerant chimpanzees had elevated levels of serum triglycerides (318 ± 68 mg/dl vs. 190 ± 14 mg/dl for controls) and serum total lipids (508 ± 68 mg/dl vs. 350 ± 54 mg/dl for controls), but not of serum cholesterol (262 ± 25 mg/dl vs. 229 ± 13 mg/dl for controls. Histologic examination of pancreatic tissue from one of the glucose intolerant animals demonstrated the presence of both normal-appearing and hypercellular islets. Use of a modified Gomori's aldehyde-fuchsin staining method demonstrated the presence of islets that were completely or predominately depleted of beta cells. The blood chemistry data together with the histologic findings suggest the occurrence of noninsulin-dependent diabetes mellitus similar in characteristics to the human adult-onset type diabetic disorder.

238

Xylitol-a potential Sweetener for Diabetics

W.Hassinger,G.Sauer,U.Cordes,J.Beyer,K.H.Baessler Mainz,Germany

Xylitol has been discussed as a potential sweetener in diabetic diet.To study insulin requirement and blood glucose when xylitol is given as part of diabetes diet a standard diabetes diet was compared with diets containing in breakfast either 30 gm sucrose or 30 gm xylitol isocalorically exchanging 30 gm starch in 14 insulin dependent diabetics.Insulin requirement and blood glucose was determined continuosly by a glucose controlled insulin infusion system.Mean amplitude of glycemic excursions(MAGE)after sucrose shows large fluctuations of blood glucose compared to MAGE after starch or xylitol(tab.) Food induced insulin requirement(FIIR)was significantly higher after sucrose compared intraindividually to starch,but there was no difference after xylitol compared to starch.Insulin requirementafter xylitol was less than after starch during second hour(tab.).After 4th hour there was no difference in blood glucose or insulin consumption.Single dose of 30 gm xylitol exchanged against starch could be used as sweetener in diabetic diet regardless to insulin application.

Tab.		MAGE (2h)	FIIR 30	60	120 min.
sucrose	m	59	5,91	5,40	3,68
	s	29,9	2,57	2,67	2,64
starch	m	32	2,15	3,23	3,65
	s	11,9	1,98	1,22	2,56
xylitol	m	33	2,58	2,42	1,85
	s	18,3	1,47	1,81	1,41

239

C-Peptide Response in the Infected Patient: K. THALER, V. KAMDAR*, A. BESSMAN*, Downey, Calif.

Insulin requirements during stress are known to increase in diabetic patients(DP). There are data implicating catabolic hormones (epinephrine, glucagon,etc.)in humans. Depressed insulin secretion in septic animals has been reported. Data about insulin secretion in adult onset DPare lacking.

Baseline and 1 mgm. iv.glucagon stimulated serum C-peptide(CP) and glucose levels were measured in 10 adult onset DP and 5 non-diabetic (ND) patients. In the first study each patient had clinical and laboratory evidence of infection; in the second study each had recovered.

Glucose levels(GL) rose in all patients following glucagon. GL were significantly higher in the DP but were not different in the two test situations in either DP or ND subjects.

C-peptide levels (ng./ml.)after Glucagon

Time	Diabetic Infec.	Diabetic Non-Infec.	p	Non-Diabetic Infec.	Non-Diabetic Non-Infec.	p
0	3.1+0.17	5.0+0.68	<.01	2.8+0.19	2.8+0.39	NS
5	3.6±0.12	5.8±0.72	<.05	4.6±0.18	4.8±0.69	NS
10	3.5±0.17	5.6±0.69	<.05	4.7±0.17	5.2±0.51	NS
15	3.5±0.18	5.5±0.68	<.01	4.5±0.25	4.9±0.59	NS
	p value	0:peak=NS		p value	0:peak=<.05	

In the infected compared to the non-infected adult onset DP, baseline insulin secretion is suppressed. In the ND, glucagon evoked a 70% (infected) and 85% (non-infected) increase in CP levels. However in the DP, glucagon evoked only slight increases in CP levels. Although the differences are not statistically significant, ND patients had a smaller % rise in glucagon stimulated CP levels when infected.

240

Glycosilated Haemoglobin(HbA1)in Insulin-Dependent Diabetics(IDD)after 4 Months of Self-Monitoring of Blood Glucose(BG).U. RAGGI,P. MICOSSI*,G. VIBERTI,A. GRECHI,M. NEGRATI,B. GARIMBERTI,M. BEVILACQUA,and G. NORBIATO.Milan, Italy

Sixtythree IDD were instructed for home self-monitoring of BG(Dextrostix)and urinary glucose (UG,Clinitest)and to modify accordingly insulin therapy,diet and physical exercise,and allowed to choose between 2 protocols.Thirtythree IDD chose the self-monitoring of BG(glycaemic profiles every 15 days + extra BG in case of symptoms)and UG 3 times a day(Group 1).Thirty chose self-monitoring of UG alone(Group 2).Before entering the study no difference was found between the 2 groups in the % of body weight variation,mean and fasting BG and UG,HbA1 and insulin daily dosage.Only 12 out of 33 in group 1 and 21 out of 30 in group 2 followed the program for at least 4 months.HbA1 and mean UG were reduced in group 1 (respectively $p<.02$ and $p<.001$)after 4 months, whereas no difference was found in group 2.The self-performed BG and UG highly correlated with HbA1(respectively $r=.64, p<.001$and $r=.57, p<.001$).

In conclusion,with the same educational program only self-monitoring of BG induced a significant reduction of HbA1 and UG.However the adherence to the program in group 1 was much lower suggesting that only highly motivated patients can follow it.

241

The Use of Intramuscular Injection of Regular Insulin in Treating Diabetes. JOHN R. WILLIAMS, JR*, D. DEILE, A. MATTIS, K. ALLING, Rochester, N.Y.

Statistically significant differences in blood insulin levels and in blood glucose levels between intramuscular (i.m.) and subcutaneous (s.c.) injections of insulin in both normal and diabetic patients are demonstrated. The inconsistencies of action between s.c. and i.m. injections previously reported in the literature are explained.

Use of i.m. regular insulin has helped us to maintain good control in over 90 insulin-dependent diabetic patients. We have defined good control as maintaining 90% of the day's blood glucose levels between 50 and 150 mg/dl at any time of day, with none over 200. These patients can live the life-style of their choice as regards diet and activity with a single daily dose of intermediate-acting insulin s.c. and an occasional dose of regular insulin i.m.

I.M. regular is of value in allowing a patient to eat a normal breakfast 30 minutes after injection without loss of glycemic control. It enables the patient to eat additional carbohydrate as desired, or to lower an unusual elevation of blood glucose. The amounts of regular insulin used i.m. for any of these purposes is small in comparison to its use s.c.: 3 to 4 units will enable most patients to eat 25 grams of extra carbohydrate without a rise in blood glucose, or to lower an elevated level shortly after eating. Even smaller amounts must be used if the patient has not recently eaten, particularly at bed time.

242

Nerve Conduction Velocity in Diabetes.MAUNG H. AUNG,and ARYE LEV-RAN*,La Jolla,California.

To investigate the influence of hyperglycemia and diabetic con'rol on objective parameters of diabetic neuropathy,we studied conduction velocity in median and peroneal nerves as well as sensory median and sural latencies in 110 diabetics (57 insulin-dependent and 53 non-insulin dependent).In the non-insulin-dependent patients the glycemia was calculated as the mean of fasting and 2h postprandial plasma glucose; in insulin-dependent diabetics glycemia was calculated as the mean of fasting,3h after breakfast and 3h after lunch plasma glucose values.Glycohemoglobin was determined as an indicator of long-term diabetes control.Both sensory and motor nerve latencies tended to correlate with the control of diabetes,but none reached the significance level.Mean glycemia and glycohemoglobin did correlate significantly with median and peroneal conduction velocities in both groups of patients (correlation coefficients from -0.277 to -0.414, $P<0.05$).In all 10 patients followed up dynamically,the changes in the diabetic control correlated with the corresponding changes in sural nerve latencies.The parameters studied did not correlate with age,sex,duration or type of diabetes or the presence of other diabetic complications. These data support the view that diabetic neuropathy depends,at least in part,on diabetic control.

243

Control of Diabetes is Correlated with a Measure of In Vivo Platelet Activation.ARYE LEV-RAN*,GWEN REISS,and MARK H.GINSBERG, La Jolla,California.

Diabetics are at increased risk for the development of vascular disease and diabetic platelets are reported to be "hyperactive" in vitro. In order to evaluate the relationship between a measure of in vivo platelet activation and various manifestations of diabetes mellitus,we have determined the plasma levels of a platelet specific antigen,platelet factor 4 (PF 4),in 50 diabetics. In a normal population the plasma PF 4 level was 2-20 ng/ml (mean 7.6 ng/ml). Elevated plasma PF 4 ($>$ 20 ng/ml) was observed in 24 diabetics.Plasma PF 4 levels were significantly correlated with the mean daily plasma glucose ($r=+0.503$, $P<0.001$) and glycohemoglobin ($r=+0.642$, $P<0.001$). Elevated plasma PF 4 levels were not correlated with age,duration of diabetes,its insulin-dependence or use of oral drugs,obesity, neuropathy,nephropathy,retinopathy,hypertension, history of arteriosclerotic heart disease, plasma cholesterol or triglycerides.These data indicate potential relationship between in vivo platelet activation and diabetic control.Since platelets may contribute to vascular disease, these data also suggest a potential pathogenetic link between control of diabetes and the progression of vessel disease.

244

Effect of Metoprolol (M) and Propranolol (P) on Oral Glucose Tolerance Test (OGTT) and Insulin-Induced Hypoglycaemia (IIH) in Hypertensive Diabetic Patients. P. MICOSSI*, G. POLLAVINI, U. RAGGI, S. CORALLO, M.C. LIBRENTI, L. ZANABONI, P. BEGGI, M. BEVILACQUA, G. NORBIATO, and A. FASOLI, Milan, Italy.

Glucose tolerance, insulin (IRI) and glucagon (IRG) production were studied in 2 groups of 8 hypertensive diabetic patients (8 on diet; 8 on glibenclamide) while IIH was performed in a third group of insulin dependent diabetics. After 1 week wash-out period (placebo), patients were given P 160 mg/die and M 200 mg/die, each one for 4 weeks, according to a cross-over design. In neither group difference was observed between the 2 drugs on blood pressure and heart rate reduction as well as plasma glucose levels during OGTT. In G treated patients only P and not M reduced IRI production (30 min : $p < .01$; 60 min : $p < .05$) while in patients on diet no difference was observed because of the larger insulin storage showed by these patients ($p < .02$). In this group of patients P and not M reduced IRG production. In patients treated with oral hypoglycaemic drug P and M were not able to reduce IRG secretion already inhibited by G. In the third group, symptoms of IIH (tachicardia and sweating) were masked by P and not by M.

In conclusion only P reduces IRI secretion during OGTT without any modification of glucose tolerance; it also reduces IRI and IRG production and inhibits symptoms related to IIH. M does not show the above mentioned effects. The cardioselective M seems to be more suitable in the treatment of arterial hypertension in diabetic patients.

245

Accelerated Lipogenesis and Adipose Cell Proliferation in Culture as Factor(s) in Human Obesity and Maturity Onset Diabetes Mellitus. I.WAHEED, W.J.POZNANSKI*, Ottawa, Canada.

Previous studies in this laboratory have shown that cultured adipose cells obtained from some obese subjects proliferate faster than those from non obese donors or exhibit accelerated lipogenesis which correlates with the degree of obesity. The purpose of this study was to determine whether this abnormal and possibly inherent behaviour in fat cells occurs as a single or as a combined phenomenon and whether it coexists with hyperglycemia.

Adipose cells(pre-and adipocytes)from obese and non-obese donors were cultured through six passages.Rate of proliferation and rate of lipogenesis were determined using ^{14}C glucose, ^{3}H-Oleic Acid or ^{3}H-Triolein as substrate. Cells from 25 obese subjects showed both accelerated growth rate{0.24±0.04 vs. 0.14±0.05(p<.05)no. of generations per day} and increased lipogenesis:

	CPM x 10^3 per mg Protein		
	^{14}C-glucose	^{3}H-Oleic Acid	^{3}H-Triolein
Normal	5.0 ± 0.1	10 ± 2.0	7.8 ± 0.5
Obese	10.5 ± 2.7	15 ± 1.3	13.2 ± 1.0

Cells from 8 other obese subjects showed similar increase in lipogenesis without acceleration of cell replication. Cells from six subjects showed normal rate of lipogenesis and cell replication.Hyperglycemia was found only in the first obese group, which showed both increased proliferation and lipogenesis.

246

Enhancement of the Hyperglycemic Effect of Gliburate(G) in Maturity Onset Diabetes(MOD) by Concommittant Administration of Enteric-Coated Aspirin(ECA).Evidence for an Extra-Pancreatic Mechanism of Action.POZNANSKI,W.J.*,KUWAYTI,K. Ottawa, Canada.

We have demonstrated previously that short periods of a combined therapy using sulphonureas and ECA produced greater hypoglycemic effects in MOD than therapy involving a single agent.

The present study endeavours to elucidate the mechanism of action of those drugs in MOD when used in combination over a prolonged period (8 weeks).

Ten MOD patients of normal weight and on isocaloric diet were treated with either ECA(2 gm/day) or G(20 mg/day) alone or in combination.Each agent when given alone reduced significantly both fasting and post-prandial blood glucose(BG)(14% and 16% respectively). It also increased serum insulin levels by 18% and 19% respectively.

When both agents were given simultaneously, further reduction of BG(mean:40% from baseline) and enhancement of insulin release (38%) were obtained (p<.001 compared to single agent).

Each agent produced a significant decrease of HbA1 (p<.05). The combination reduced it further (p<0.001).

Statistical analysis of the data suggests additive effect rather than synergism of action. However,magnitude of change in insulin-glucose ratios(22%) could not explain the hypoglycemic effect by an enhancement of insulin production alone, rather it suggests an action of salicylate on peripheral glucose utilization.

247

Myocardial Infarction: the value of HbA_1 as an epidemiological and diagnostic marker for diabetes mellitus. N.G. SOLER*, D. MAHAM, G. MOTL, S. FRANK, Springfield, Illinois.

Hyperglycemia is a risk factor for myocardial infarction (MI) but stress hyperglycemia makes diagnosis of diabetes difficult immediately after the acute episode. We have tested the hypothesis that glycosylated hemoglobin (HbA_1), an integral measurement of glycemia in the weeks before the infarct, can be more useful in this acute situation. Follow-up studies have also been carried out to investigate the value and reproducibility of the HbA_1 recorded during stress.

200 consecutive patients were admitted to an intensive care unit with suspected MI. 33 patients who were known diabetics are not considered further and of the remaining 167 patients 99 had a confirmed MI. Plasma glucose on admission was higher in patients with MI (p<0.005) and showed a poor correlation with HbA_1 (r=0.22) whereas plasma glucose and HbA_1 were strongly correlated (r=0.67) in patients without MI. Among patients with and without MI 54% and 37% respectively had a fasting plasma glucose (FPG) >115 mg% but only 12% of each group of patients had a HbA_1 above normal (>8.5%).

48 patients with an initial FPG >115 mg% were followed up three months later. The follow-up FPG was significantly lower in patients with and without MI but HbA_1 did not change significantly in either group. The original HbA_1 had a good correlation with follow-up FPG (r=0.56) and follow-up HbA_1 (r=0.49).

Conclusion: HbA_1 is a valuable epidemiological marker and diagnostic index for diabetes mellitus after acute MI.

248

Effect of Glucomannan(Konjac Mannan) on Carbohydrate and Lipid Metabolism in Diabetics. KUNIHIRO DOI,* MASAAKI MATSUURA, AKIRA KAWARA, MASAHIKO TAKEDA, KEIKO SUMINOE, RINZO UENOYAMA, KAZUNORI NISHIKAWA, Kobe, Japan

In recent years, dietary fibres have been successfuly used to treat diabetes. We have therefore investigated the influence of glucomannan(GM, prepared from the tubers of Amorphophallus, Konjac) on glucose and lipid metabolism of diabetics, and the effect of GM on glucose tolerance compared with guar gum.

During 50g oral glucose tolerance test(OGTT), the peaks of blood glucose and serum insulin concentrations were slightly reduced by addition of 2.6g GM in both 5 healthy men and 10 diabetics, however significantly reduced by 3.9g GM in 8 healthy men($p<0.05$). In addition of 2.6g or 3.9g guar gum the OGTT showed slightly improvement in 8 healthy men, but there were not statistically significant. Plasma glucagon levels were unchanged in both fibres.

When 14 non-insulin dependent diabetics had their metabolic diets supplemented with 7.8g GM daily for 90 days, their mean serum cholesterol at the 20 day fell by 11.2%($p<0.1$) and their mean fasting blood glucose fell by 29%($p<0.025$, for 30 days), and insulin or hypoglycemic agents were reduced in doses.

Serum total bile acids levels were reduced during the EGG tolerance test with the additional of 3.9g GM and the composition of the bile salt pool was markedly altered.

We concluded that GM might be usefull for the treatment of diabetics as well as guar gum.

249

Direct Measurement of Plasma Proinsulin in Chemical Diabetics and Maturity Onset Diabetics, YOSHIMICHI IMAMURA, KOICHI YOKONO, HIDEYO SAKAI, and KOSUI SHII, Kobe, Japan

There is little information about the proinsulin levels in diabetics. We have developed a direct measurement of proinsulin in human plasma by the use of insulin-degrading enzyme(IDE) which purified from pig skeletal muscle. After plasma was incubated with IDE, the remaining proinsulin was assayed by the double antibody radioimmunoassay. Plasma levels of proinsulin, insulin and C-peptide during 50g glucose tolerance test were studied in 22 patients with maturity-onset diabetics and 10 with chemical diabetes, and compared to those in 13 normal subjects. Fasting levels of proinsulin in maturity-onset diabetics, chemical diabetics and normal subjects were 0.56 ± 0.04, 0.44 ± 0.03 and 0.24 ± 0.02ng/ml(mean$\pm$SE), respectively. Proinsulin levels after glucose loading in maturity-onset diabetics and chemical diabetics were significantly higher than those in normal subjects. Chemical diabetics had greater responses of proinsulin, insulin and C-peptide to compare with maturity-onset diabetics. In maturity-onset diabetics, proinsulin responses to oral glucose were low, whereas fasting levels of proinsulin were high. In addition, more lower responses of proinsulin, insulin and C-peptide were seen in older maturity-onset diabetics. These finding suggest that the hypersecretion of proinsulin in chemical diabetes may due to the inability of processing mechanism in secretary granules, and that the increased proinsulin in maturity-onset diabetes may be secondary to beta cell exhaustion.

250

Temperature Dependence of the Chromatographic Assay of Hemoglobin A_1 and Application to Clinical Evaluation of Diabetic Control. M.JOHNSON, G.DOBREA, R. BENDEZU and R.WIELAND*, Dept. of Medicine, St. Luke's Hospital, Cleveland, Ohio

We investigated the temperature dependence of the cation-exchange chromatographic properties of hemoglobin A_1 (HbA_1) using the "Fast Hemoglobins Test System" from Isolab, Inc., Akron, Ohio in a temperature controlled chamber. Six samples, two each from the "normal" range (5-8.5%), "transitional" range (8.5-12.0%) and "uncontrolled diabetic" range (12-20%) described by Isolab were assayed. Assay temperatures were 20°C, 22°C, 24°C, 26°C and 28°C. For each 2°C increment, mean assay results increased .8%, 1.1% and 1.6% for each sample range. Therefore the temperature dependence is partially a function of HbA_1 concentration. The controlled temperature reduced assay variation to less than 5%. The assay, when applied to screening HbA_1 levels in 77 diabetics revealed 26% of the patients in the "normal" range, 43% in the "transitional" range, and 31% in the "uncontrolled diabetic" range. When divided on the basis of therapy patient distribution becomes:

Therapy group	n	Normal	Transitional	Uncontrol.
Diet Controlled	15	27%	53%	20%
Oral Agents	14	29%	29%	42%
Insulin Requir.	48	25%	44%	31%

Measurements of HbA_1 levels of 7 patients with ketoacidosis revealed elevated levels in 6. This confirms the presence of a period of uncontrolled diabetes preceding the acute ketoacidosis.

251

Time Course of Action of NPH Insulin in Children with Insulin-Dependent Diabetes Mellitus (IDDM). RICHARD D. KAYNE, MICHAEL S. KAPPY*, AND LESLIE P. PLOTNICK*, Baltimore, MD,

Although individual reactions to intermediate acting insulins (e.g., NPH) are presumed to be different (A,B,&C reactors, Hallas-Moller, Diabetes 5:7, 1956), a study of this phenomenon in children is lacking.

The integrated concentration of plasma glucose was measured every 30 min for 24 hrs by continuous blood withdrawal. Nine subjects, ages 10-19 years, all of whom had IDDM for at least 3 years, were studied. They received their usual morning dose of NPH insulin alone. All injections were given subcutaneously in the abdomen and all subjects were on appropriate ADA diets. The time course of action of the NPH insulin was determined by the ratio of the mean nighttime plasma glucose concentration (midnight to 6 am) to the mean plasma glucose concentration for the entire 24 hour period. In 7 of the subjects, the ratio was close to 1 (0.84 ± 0.12, mean $\pm$ SD) corresponding to B reactors, whereas the remaining 2 subjects had ratios of 1.28 and 0.35, corresponding to A and C reactors respectively. This demonstrates that the variability of the time course of NPH action is also seen in the pediatric age group.

252

Low I.V. Intermitent Doses of Insulin as a Routine Treatment in Acute Diabetic Hyperglycemia. RICARDO QUIBRERA and MANUEL NAVA, San Luis Potosí, S.L.P., México.

The efficacy of low insulin doses in the treatment of diabetic coma has been demostrated. We established this method in a general hospital as "a routine" in acute hyperglycemic complications, five years ago (1975-79). 116 patients have been admitted: 74(63.7%) females and 42 (36.3%) males. The diagnosis was: ketoacidosis (K.A.) in 60(51.7%), severe hyperglycemia (S.H.) without coma or acidosis in 47(40.6%) and hyperosmolar coma (H.C.) in 9(7.7%). All patients received I.V. cristaline insulin, five units every hour. The fluid replacement was conventional. Insulin was stopped when the blood glucose was around 150 mg/dl;total insulin used was in K.A.: 51.9 U., in H.C.: 72.2 U. and 30.8 U. for S.H., time from beging treatment to normoglycemia was in average of 10.39 h. for K.A., 14.42 h. for H.C. and 6.19 h. for S.H. 4 patients had hypoglycemia. We did not observed hypokalemia. This method is simple, it does not require continous infusion pump or albumin, we recommend it in the emergency wards of general hospitals.

253

Seven Day Fast for Plasma Glucose Control Increases Proteinuria of Plasma Origin M. NAGULESPARAN*, E. V. FLOCK*, A. L. KENNEDY, P.H. BENNETT*, Phoenix, AZ.

To determine if plasma glucose (PG) control would improve proteinuria, urinary proteins of plasma origin were measured in Type II diabetics during control of PG by fasting, followed by caloric restriction. Eighteen subjects were on a 300 g carbohydrate weight-maintaining diet for at least three days before 24-hr urine collections and OGTT. Five subjects had normal glucose tolerance [FPG<115 mg/dl and 2 hr<140], 5 impaired glucose tolerance [IGT] [FPG<140 and 2 hr 140-200] and 8 were diabetic [2 hr>200]. All were fasted for 7 days and 24-hr urines were collected on days 1, 3, 5 & 7. The subjects were then fed a hypocaloric diet for 2 weeks, and 24-hr urines were collected twice a week. Proteins were measured in unconcentrated urine with antisera to whole human serum using the laser nephelometer. Urinary albumin was measured using a specific antibody to human albumin. During the fast PG decreased from 169±32 mg/dl to 82±10 mg/dl in the diabetics. The urinary proteins fell on the first day of fast in most subjects, and then increased, reaching maximal levels by the 7th day. In the diabetics, prefast protein excretion was 16-93 mg/24 hr (range) and increased to 20-289 mg/24 hr on day 7. The increases were moderate in IGT and even smaller in normal subjects. On refeeding the proteinuria decreased rapidly to prefast levels in all. Similar changes were found in urinary albumin. In conclusion, control of PG by fasting produced an increase instead of a decrease in proteinuria.

254

Multiple Insulin Injections Vs. Portable Insulin Delivery Systems (IDS) in Unstable Diabetics. LOIS MENTH, EDWARD SZALAPSKI, RICHARD SIMMONS, DAVID SUTHERLAND*, JOHN EATON, ROBERT BONNER*, JOHN NAJARIAN*, and JOSE BARBOSA*.

We have compared a regimen of multiple daily insulin injections (Rx A) with the IDS (Auto-Syringe and Mill Hill) (Rx B) in brittle diabetics. In 3 of the 5 patients Rx A was used before and after Rx B. The patients were monitored by home blood glucoses, 24 hr. urine glucose and glucosylated hemoglobin (HgAl). Results for the Auto-Syringe are shown.

	Rx A(#5)	Rx B(#5)	p
Days	1110	541	
FBG†	209±5‡	148±7	<.001
NFBG††	210±20	151±4	<.02
HgAl	11.4±1.2	8.1±1.3	NS

†fasting glucose, ‡nonfasting glucose, ††mg/dl, Mean±SEM.

24 hr. urine glucose showed significant improvement; the daily maximal BG excursions did not. One of the patients deteriorated after stopping the IDS; the other 2 did not. Factors others than the IDS may have played a role in the improvement of these patients. The results obtained with the British IDS were identical. We conclude that the use of the IDS in brittle diabetics in an ambulatory setting seems to result in levels of control better than those achieved with multiple injections but do not normalize control (AM20742, Ames Co., Eli Lilly Co.).

255

Post-Prednisone Urinary C-peptide--A Simple Test of Human Beta Cell Reserve. B. J. HOOGWERF, F.C. GOETZ*. Minneapolis, Minnesota

As a simple test of human beta cell reserve we measured urinary C-peptide (UCP) before and after oral prednisone (PR) in 11 healthy subjects on controlled diet and activity for 2 consecutive days. Serial urine collections for C-peptide were obtained in 4 and 12 hr. specimens. All subjects had morning serum C-peptides (SCP) and plasma glucoses (PG), and 3 subjects had PG and SCP drawn between 1600 and 2000. On Day 2 each subject was given PR 20 mg. p.o. at 0800 and 1600.

There was a consistent rise in UCP 8 to 12 hr. after the first dose of PR (Table 1), and a concomitant rise in PG and SCP on Day 2 compared to the baseline day (Table 2). FPG was unchanged, but SCP was elevated over baseline values 24 hr. after the first dose of PR.

TABLE 1 - UCP (pmol/min)

Time	Day 1	Day 2
0800-1200	17.4±7.0	20.7±11.0
1200-1600	19.9±10.4	25.4±15.4
1600-2000	25.3±12.9	38.2±18.8
2000-0800	10.5±5.8	22.8±10.2°°

Values = Mean ± S.D.

TABLE 2 - PG (mg/dl) / SCP (ng/ml)

	PG (mg/dl)		SCP (ng/ml)		
Time	Day 1	Day 2	Day 1	Day 2	Day 3
0800	88±9	89±14	2.8±0.3	3.0±0.7	3.9±1.2°
1600	86±8	113±16°	3.5±0.6	4.6±1.7	
2000	86±8	142±7°°°	4.8±1.4	5.7±1.1	

P values by paired t test °<.05, °°<.01, °°°<.001

We conclude 1)PR caused an increase in PG and insulin secretion as measured by SCP and UCP, 2) PR effect on glucose metabolism is apparent by 8 hr. and largely gone by 24 hr., 3)UCP reflects SCP and is a useful tool to measure beta cell reserve.

256

Serum Insulin Levels in the Management of Insulin Dependent Diabetes. J.I. MALONE*, G. HOUGH and A.W. ROOT, Tampa, Florida.

The quantity of insulin administered to insulin dependent children (IDC) is based on empiric data (U/kg) and indirect criteria, i.e. urine and blood glucose concentrations. Measurement of therapuetic insulin levels is limited by interfering antibodies. Blood was collected from 133 IDC (insulin treated > 1 yr.) 24 hrs. after receiving a single s.c. dose of NPH or Lente insulin. Plasma C-peptide and insulin were measured by RIA after treatment with polyethylene glycol. Plasma glucose was measured with glucose oxidase. Hemoglobin Al_c (HbAlc) was quantitated by HPLC. None of the children had measurable C-peptide. IDC (98/147) had measurable insulin levels (MI) while 28/100 NPH and 21/47 Lente treated IDC had no MI. IDC (30) had acetone in their urine at the time of blood collection. No MI was found in 18 of the 30. Those with MI had 3.9 ± 1.8 μU/ml of free insulin FI. Those with no MI as a group had PG 298 ± 94 mg/dl, $HbAl_c$ 12.2 ± 2.8%; those with FI between 1 and 10 μU/ml had PG 238 ± 85, $HbAl_c$ 12.4 ± 3.6%; those with FI > 10 μU/ml had PG 200 ± 102, $HbAl_c$ 9.1 ± 2.6. The mean insulin dose for the 3 groups were (0.6 ± 0.18 U/kg, 0.67±0.21 U/kg, 0.92 ± 0.4 U/kg). The SD for each group indicates that some individuals with high insulin doses had no MI and some with low insulin doses had MI. Higher FI was found following BID insulin administration, but 12/20 had FI < 10 μU/ml and 5 had no MI. FI > 10 μU/ml is associated with a greater degree of control in IDC. The measurement of FI can provide information useful to improve control in IDC.

257

Correlation of Parameters of Urine Testing Procedure. D.W. GUTHRIE*, D. HINNEN* Wichita, Ks.

Urine testing is not considered by many to be a useful device in guiding the control of D.M. Until continuous glucose monitoring is common in clinical settings the urine test is a useful guide for a day to day management of the disease. Previous studies by us have shown that pre-meal & bedtime samples for first & second voided specimen contain the same amount of glucose 72% of the time & 1st voided have more glucose in the urine than the second voided specimen 23% of the time. The mean volume of urine in the first & second voided samples against the percentage amount of glucose & in relation to fluid intake have been determined & will be discussed. Also, urine glucose has been thought to change if urine has been left standing for a period of time. 25 refrigerated & non-refrigerated urine specimens were tested 4 to 6 hrs. after initial determination to see if or how much the urine glucose was altered.

Again, in order to find if urine testings for people with know renal thresholds is a useful guide of diabetes control, 100 urine samples were tested in a double blind study using ketodiastix & 2 drop clinitest method. It was found that urine glucose by ketodiastix reading was not only depressed by ketones but also by urine glucose greater than 5%. Other parameters of urine tests to be reported are comparison with A_1CHb, age & duration of disease.

258

Clinical Use Of Closed Loop Artificial Beta Cell R.A. GUTHRIE*, B.P. CHILDS*, Wichita, Kansas.

We have performed 645.5 hrs. of control & an additional 167 hrs. of monitoring by the use of the Biostator glucose monitor-controller, the production model of the closed loop artificial beta cell being tested for Life Science Instruments & the Food & Drug Administration. We have performed clinical trials of the Biostator in a community hospital setting over the last nine months. We have controlled 3 patients for 42 hrs. during labor & delivery & bilateral tubal ligations; 1 pt. for 33½ hrs., for open heart surgery, 202.5 hrs. for major & minor surgery, including eye surgery, caesarean section, GI surgery, dental extractions, etc., & 7 pts. for 139.5 hrs. for treatment of diabetic ketoacidosis. We have also completed 16 pts. for 394 hrs. monitoring & controlling (M&C) in pregnant women & pts. with management problems for reregulation for tighter control of the D.M. Such M&C has identified some interesting absorption patterns for shor & intermediate acting isulins. These patterns will be discussed. Data for monitoring & control will be reported in each of the clinical settings of our experience.

259

Free Insulin Assay in Evaluating Patients with Severe "Insulin Resistance". N. WHITE*, D. SARGEANT*, L. RIGG*, St. Louis, Mo.

Massive insulin requirements are sometimes due to excessive degradation of injected insulin. Measurement of free insulin concentrations(FI) in plasma was used to study diabetics with "insulin resistance" and to select appropriate treatment.

In 10 non-resistant diabetics treated with intravenous(IV) or subcutaneous(SC) insulin, basal and post prandial FI concentrations required to achieve euglycemia were 27±7 and 98±55 uU/ml (mean ± SD). Four "insulin resistant" patients (more than 4 U/kg/day) with normal or low insulin antibody titers were studied. Two women requiring over 4 U/kg/day SC had low FI levels but responded dramatically to .5 - .9 U/kg/day of insulin IV. They had "insulin resistance" only with SC insulin and responded to SC injection of insulin mixed with a protease inhibitor, aprotinin. A boy given 30 U/kg/day SC and 2.5 U/kg/day IV had low FI levels. Aprotinin given IV (100,000 KIU/hr) reduced closed loop IV insulin requirements by 46% but had no effect when mixed with insulin and given SC. He had massive clearance of insulin injected IV and SC. An obese woman in month 8 of pregnancy required SC 4.7 and IV 3.5 U/kg/day and had markedly elevated FI (274±165 uU/ml). She was thus truly insulin resistant.

A low FI with massive insulin requirements helps identify patients with excessive insulin degradation and distinguishes them from those truly "resistant". Once identified, some of the former may respond to IV insulin or to inhibition of insulinase activity with aprotinin, especially when insulin degradation occurs primarily SC.

260

Comparative Characteristics of the Diabetic and General Population. R.G.HISS, B.M.BROCK, F.C. PENNINGTON, D.M. McCLARAN, Ann Arbor, Michigan

During the investigation of public health issues which followed the polybrominated biphenyl (PBB) accident in Michigan in 1973, two surveys of the Michigan population were done to determine health beliefs and numerous health practices. The surveys were constructed to represent a true cross section of the state of Michigan, with attention to the details of randomization, sampling and high response rate. Survey I included a randomly selected adult from 3,088 households; 1,300 children, one from each household which had children, were additionally surveyed. Survey II recorded responses from one adult in 3,200 households, similarly chosen.

The response to the question, "Were you ever told you were diabetic?" was 4.7% of adults in Survey I, 1.1% of children, and 4.0% of Survey II. Data are available from these surveys to determine the difference of this diabetic subset from the total population with respect to the following (partial listing of total of 258 items available): age, race, sex, hypertension, heart and kidney disease, cancer, stroke, physical restrictions, hospitalization rate, frequency of clinic visits, concern for health, perception of health compared to others, smoking and drinking habits, income, education and employment.

This study used good survey technique and statistical design, and avoids some of the bias present in analyses of clinic populations. It should be a complement to the National Ambulatory Care Study (HANES), which did not assess most of the items reported here.

261

Total Glycosylated Hemoglobin (HgbAl) in Childhood Diabetes Management. ARLAN L. ROSENBLOOM,* JANET H. SILVERSTEIN, KATHRYN GAITANIS, Gainesville, Florida.

240 insulin dependent patients age 1-26 yrs. had 660 determinations of HgbAl during an 18 month period, using rapid microcolumn separation (Isolab, normal 5.0 - 9.5%). Levels correlated significantly ($p<.0001$) with concommitant plasma glucose concentration. Means of most recent tests for each pt. increased significantly with duration of diabetes up to 3 yrs with no difference thereafter (<1 yr, 13.0% $\pm$ .6 SEM; 1-3 yrs, 14.3 $\pm$ .4; 3-5 yrs, 15.6 $\pm$ .5; 5-7 yrs, 15.4 $\pm$ .5; 7-9 yrs, 15.1 $\pm$ .5; 9+ yrs, 15.2 $\pm$ .4; n = 31 -56/gp). Control estimate based on hospitalizations, school/work record, symptoms and urine tests in clinic and from home records correlated well with HgbAl means: good n=34, 11.4 $\pm$ .5; fairly good n=78, 14.3 $\pm$ .3; fair n=101, 16.0 $\pm$ .2; poor n=27, 17.0 $\pm$ .4 for most recent evaluation and good n=75, 12.0 $\pm$ .3; fairly good n=246, 14.5 $\pm$ .2; fair n=252, 16.5 $\pm$ .2; poor n=87, 18.5 $\pm$ .3 for all 660 specimens. There were no differences related to presence or severity of limited joint mobility nor correlation with growth pace (height age change/chronologic age change) over the previous 6-12 mos. Normal levels were seen with short diabetes duration, management with portable pump infusion of insulin for 4-11 months in 4 pts, and "overcontrol" with hypoglycemia in 3 pts. Discrepancies between individual control estimates, despite statistical correlation, and longitudinal data support the view of HgbAl as an objective serial measure of control of great help to patient and physician.

262

Continuous Subcutaneous Insulin Infusion (CSI) Reduces the Exercise-Induced Hypoglycemia and Albuminuria in Juvenile Onset Diabetics (JOD). VEIKKO A. KOIVISTO,* NIILO-PEKKA HUTTUNEN, and ESKO A. NIKKILÄ, Helsinki, and Oulu, Finland.

JOD treated with daily insulin injections are characterized by a rapid fall in blood glucose (BG) and an excessive albuminuria during exercise. To examine the effect of CSI on BG and albuminuria during exercise, we studied 8 JOD (age 22 - 40 yrs) who performed a 40 min ergometer exercise (intensity 120 W) during conventional insulin Rx and after 1 wk of CSI with a portable infusion pump. During CSI, mean daily BG (184 $\pm$ 13 mg/dl pre-pump, measured at 2 - 4 hr intervals) fell to 111 $\pm$ 13 mg/dl ($p < 0.005$) and glycosuria (54 $\pm$ 14 g/day pre-pump) fell to 4 $\pm$ 1 g/day ($p < 0.05$). The exercise-induced fall in BG (148 $\pm$ 29 mg/dl pre-pump) was reduced to 30 $\pm$ 8 mg/dl during CSI ($p < 0.005$). The exercise-induced albuminuria (measured by RIA) was 3.9 $\pm$ 1.1 µg/min during conventional Rx and fell to 0.8 $\pm$ 0.9 µg/min during CSI ($p < 0.02$). The heart rate response to exercise was comparable both during conventional and pump Rx (136 $\pm$ 3 vs 138 $\pm$ 2 beats/min, respectively).

Conclusions: 1) While the metabolic control is improved, the risk for exercise-induced hypoglycemia is reduced by CSI. 2) A decrease in exercise-induced albuminuria during CSI indicates that a good metabolic control can reverse the altered glomerular permeability in JOD and may delay the development of diabetic nephropathy.

263

Lack of Correlation Between Plasma and Urine Glucose in Diabetes, LAWRENCE MORRIS,* JIM MCGEE, and ABBAS KITABCHI,* Memphis, Tn.

Semi-quantitative urine glucose measurements on spot urine specimens have found widespread acceptance by patients and physicians alike in the monitoring of diabetic control. Implicit in the concept of urine glucose testing is an assumption that plasma glucose levels are reflected by the concentration of glucose in the urine. There have never been any studies to validate the use of the glucose concentration of spot urine specimens as a reflection of plasma glucose in an outpatient setting with adult diabetics.

To determine whether spot urine specimens measured semi-quantitatively (or quantitatively) for glucose provide an accurate reflection of prevailing plasma glucose, we compared 390 second-voided urines to simultaneous plasma glucose from 246 adult diabetics routinely visiting a city hospital outpatient department. In spite of fair general correlation of quantitative urine glucose to plasma glucose, when urine glucose measurements were stratified into the corresponding urine scale readings of the semi-quantitative urine testing agents (viz. Neg., Trace, 1+, etc.), there was considerable false negative error (up to 60% for Negative and up to 90% for Trace urine glucose). Urine glucose readings of 3+ and 4+, however, did correlate well with plasma glucose greater than 200 mg/dl. Because of this considerable false negative error we feel that, except for detection of marked hyperglycemia, the use of spot urine glucose measurements (regardless of the method), in the clinical assessment and management of diabetic patients is inappropriate.

264

Plasma Angiotensin II and Blood Pressure in Diabetes Mellitus. P. SULLIVAN,* B. FERRISS, M. CROWLEY, D. O'SULLIVAN,* and H. GONGRYPP. Cork Regional Hospital, Cork, Ireland.

Plasma angiotensin II (A2) and blood pressure (BP) were studied in 101 patients attending a diabetic clinic and 65 age and sex matched normal controls. No patient had evidence of ketoacidosis or fluid depletion. Blood was taken for A2, sodium (Na^+), creatinine (Cr), packed cell volume (PCV) and glucose (Glu). A2 was measured by radioimmunoassay. Diabetics were grouped as follows a) all together (Gp1), b) those without complications (Gp2), c) those with neuropathy (Gp3). BP, Cr and Glu were significantly higher in all diabetic groups compared to controls. A2 in Gp1 and Gp2 was similar to control values. However, A2 in Gp3 was significantly lower than in Gp2 ($p<0.003$). BP was inversely correlated with A2 in all diabetic groups (Gp1-$p<0.002$, Gp2-$p<0.03$, Gp3-$p<0.04$), and these relationships were independent of age and all other variables studied. On the other hand, in normals BP correlated positively with A2 ($p<0.007$) and also with Glu ($p<0.04$). Na^+ and PCV were inversely related to Glu in all diabetic groups suggesting an expansion of blood volume associated with hyperglycaemia. These findings indicate that a raised blood volume may contribute to hypertension in diabetes and would also explain the inverse relationship between A2 and BP in this condition, as opposed to normal controls in whom blood pressure appears, at least in part, to be A2 dependent.

265

The prevalence of diabetes mellitus (DM) in Melanesians and Polynesians in New Caledonia. P.ZIMMET*, D.CANTELOUBE, G.LeGONIDEC, P.COUZIGOU, M.PEGHINI, P.BENNETT*, and T.KUBERSKI, Melbourne, Australia; Noumea, New Caledonia; and Phoenix, Arizona.

With modernization of lifestyle, there has been a dramatic rise in prevalence of DM in Polynesians and Micronesians. However, in Melanesians, information about DM prevalence, and the effect of modernization is sparse. This study investigated the prevalence of DM in the Melanesian population of mainland New Caledonia and Melanesians and Polynesians of Ouvea, Loyalty Islands.

Prevalence rates for impaired glucose tolerance (IGT) and DM are summarized in the table (population $\geq$20 years):

	No.	IGT	DM
Mainland - Melanesians	172	5.8%	1.7%
Ouvea - Melanesians	533	5.1%	3.2%
- Polynesians	401	8.5%	6.5%

These groups maintain a similar lifestyle (diet and activity patterns) and no major differences in degree of obesity and mean age exist. Therefore, given similar environmental influences, these differences in DM prevalence are the result of a difference in susceptibility to the disease. This variability in susceptibility is possibly due to genetic factors.

Supported by NIH grant 1 RO1 AM25446-01

266

Value of Glycosylated Hemoglobin in the Diagnosis of Diabetes Mellitus. E. TAMAGNA* and D. KUMAR*, Los Angeles, Ca.

In several reports, levels of HbA_{1c} are considered useful in establishing the diagnosis of diabetes mellitus. Therefore, we evaluated the relationship of oral glucose tolerance tests to HbA_1% in 34 subjects. HbA_1 correlated with FPG (r.85), peak glucose (r.70) and area under the glucose curve (r.76) for the entire group. HbA_1 ranged from 8.3 to 15.4% in the overt diabetics and from 5.7 to 9.5% in the other subjects, who had normal (N), non-diagnostic (Non-Dx), or impaired GTT (IGT). The relationships of HbA_1 and GTT results were:

HbA_1%	No. of subjects				
Range	Tot	DM	IGT	Non-Dx	N
5.7-7.7	17	0	2	4	11
7.8-10	11	4	1	3	3
>10	6	6	0	0	0

Conclusion: HbA_1 concentrations greater than 10% may be used to confirm the diagnosis of overt diabetes mellitus, while values in the normal range may exclude this diagnosis. HbA_1 concentrations between 7.7 and 10% are nonconclusive, and GTT may be required for further evaluation.

267

Treatment of Hypertensive Diabetic Patients with Prazosin. DARLENE MOORE, ALICE M. POPE, FLONA J. TODD, ROBERT J. ROSENQUIST* and LOREN G. LIPSON*, Los Angeles, Calif.

Impotence is a severe problem in diabetic men. It is often caused by neurovascular complications of diabetes mellitus, but it may be psychogenic. In the hypertensive diabetic patient, however, there may be another important cause of impotence - that of a side effect of the antihypertensive medication which is used.

We have observed 5 Type II diabetic patients (age 51 $\pm$ 5 years, duration of diabetes 11.6 $\pm$ 3 years) who had essential hypertension for 5.4 $\pm$ 1.2 years. They complained of sexual dysfunction for a mean duration of 24 $\pm$ 12 months, while on antihypertensive therapy with methyldopa or clonidine. When these patients were then treated with prazosin (Minipress), all 5 patients had subjective improvement in sexual function within 3 to 6 months, and also had better compliance in taking their antihypertensive medication.

From these preliminary data it appears that prazosin should be considered in the treatment of the hypertensive male diabetic patient who requires more than phiazide therapy.

Diabetic Control in Pancreatectomized Patients. D. BAJORUNAS*, G. CHAVENT, H. KELLER, J. FORTNER, New York, New York.

On a 1-8 week program of home glucose (G) monitoring, diabetic control was assessed in 8 pancreatectomized patients (pts). A high calorie (27-62 cal/kg), 3 meal, 4 snack diet limited in sucrose, maintained pts' weights at 90-114%(mean 95.5%) of ideal body weight. Preprandial and one hour postprandial fingerstick G were obtained. Despite intensive pt education and good compliance, euglycemia was not achieved. On split insulin doses of 0.32-1.2 u/kg, Hb A_{1c} levels ranged from 9.8-14.9% and random 24 hour urinary G from 1.8-76.5 gm.

PT	MEAN G RANGE	MAXIMUM G EXCURSION°	MEAN FASTING G	%POSTPRANDIAL G 60-180 mg/dl
1	217±9†	199±9†	126±7†	40
2	127±19	126±20	95±19	43
3	165±12	152±11	200±17	45
4	243±9	215±9	121±8	31
5	169±11	125±19	146±10	56
6	235±15	203±14	89±7	23
7+	230±24	198±20	202±24	17
8#	130±13	120±13	230±19	4

In 5 pts.G<50mg/dl comprised 3.2-18% of total G values. We conclude: 1)Significant G instability does occur in diabetics lacking pancreatic glucagon. 2)Home G monitoring permits detection of frequent, often asymptomatic hypoglycemia. 3) Whether euglycemia can be achieved without intolerable hypoglycemia in these pts is not at present clear.

†-Mean±SEM +-concurrent illness #-noncompliant
°-largest unidirectional change in consecutive G

Hyperglycemic Coma Following Suprasellar Surgery. GARY FREIDENBERG, EDWARD KOSNIK, and JUAN SOTOS.* Columbus, Ohio.

Within the past 8 months three patients developed diabetes insipidus following suprasellar surgery. Fluids containing 5% dextrose were given to replace urine output plus insensible water loss. Dexamethasone 4-10 mg every 6 hours was administered. Between 1 and 3 days postoperatively, two of the patients had seizures and respiratory arrest. All had life threatening nonketotic hyperosmolar coma, with serum osmolalities between 351 and 381 mOsm/kg and serum glucoses of 667 to 1240 mg%. Hourly rates of intravenous glucose administration exceeded known maximum tolerable limits of exogenous glucose utilization (3.4-14.2 mg/kg/min). In one of the patients extreme hyperinsulinemia was found together with a low tolerance to exogenous glucose (2.6-3.0 mg/kg/min), suggesting, in addition, some degree of insulin resistance. The serum growth hormone was 1.0 ng/ml, insulin 950 μU/ml, and ADH 31.9 mU/ml when the serum glucose was 490 mg%. Subcutaneous and intravenous pitressin were both ineffective in controlling the osmotic diuresis despite negative free water clearance. The polyuria and hyperglycemia resolved quickly upon diminishing the glucose input and exogenous insulin did not seem to be necessary.

This unknown hyperglycemic complication probably has gone undetected and likely occurs more frequently in less severe forms. Prevention should be possible by using pitressin to control the diabetes insipidus and maintaining infused glucose rates below 3.0 mg/kg/min, which is equivalent to approximately 5.2 L/M^2/d of a 2.5% dextrose solution.

Improvement of Lipid Status in Diabetic Boys: The 1971 and 1979 Joslin Camp Lipid Levels. O.P. GANDA*, M.H. BLANC*, R.E. GLEASON*, Boston, Mass.

Since 1972 our young diabetic patients have been advised to use a diet low in cholesterol and with a high fraction of unsaturated fat. Mean fasting cholesterol (Chol) and triglyceride (TG) levels at admission to the Camp in 1971 (Kaufmann et al, Diabetes 24:672, 1975) and in 1979 were compared.

	Mean ± S.D. 1971	1979	P
n	122	79	-
Age (yrs)	12.5 ± 1.6	12.5 ± 4.7	NS
Duration of DM (yrs)	5.2 ± 3.3	5.2 ± 3.6	NS
Weight (kg)	43.1 ± 9.4	41.6 ±11.4	NS
Chol mg/dl	224 ± 62	180 ± 36	<.001
TG mg/dl	71 ± 39	50 ± 20	<.001

In 1971, 20% of the boys demonstrated a hyperlipoproteinemia (Type II=12, Type IV=13) vs 7.6% (Type II=6) in 1979.

Conclusions:

1) The serum lipid status has improved in diabetic boys since the introduction of a diet with low cholesterol and an increased fraction unsaturated fat. 2) Prevalence of Type IV hyperlipoproteinemia has dropped dramatically. 3) A decrease in arteriosclerotic cardiovascular disease in juvenile onset diabetics may be expceted but prospective studies are needed to confirm this possibility.

Arginine-stimulated Fall in Free Fatty Acids (FFA) as an Index of Insulin Reserve in Diabetics. J.K. SCHMITT, N.V. BOHANNON, J.H. KARAM,* and P.H. FORSHAM,* San Francisco, CA.

To investigate whether FFA response to arginine reflects insulin reserve, we measured plasma C-peptide (CPR), glucagon (IRG), glucose and FFA responses to i.v. arginine (250 mg/kg over 30 min) in 16 nonobese insulinopenic diabetics and 8 normals and correlated these with the CPR response. There was no detectable rise in CPR in 8 diabetics (CPR-), as compared with a mean peak of 3.28±0.3 ng/ml in 8 diabetics (CPR+) and 4.48±0.19 in normals (P<0.01).

(min)	FFA (mM/L) 0	30	45
a) CPR-	.878±.08	.816±.05	.879±.04
b) CPR+	.756±.04	.591±.05	.554±.04
c) Normals	.659±.05	.429±.03	.413±.02
P a vs b	NS	< 0.02	< 0.001
P a vs c	< 0.05	< 0.001	< 0.001
P b vs c	NS	< 0.02	< 0.02

After arginine, diabetics showed a higher plasma glucose (P<0.005) and higher plasma IRG rise (P<0.05) than normals. Linear regression coefficient for CPR rise vs FFA fall (0 - 45 min) was 0.8 (P<0.001).

CPR- patients showed no sustained fall in FFA during arginine, followed by a rebound at 45 min to basal levels--a phenomenon also present in one pancreatectomized patient who was totally devoid of CPR. CPR+ patients showed a continuous fall in FFA after discontinuation of arginine.

The fall in FFA during arginine infusion affords a simple, sensitive index of insulin reserve.

272

Value of Specific Food Testing for Assessing Insulin Resistance. JOHN E. POTTS* and MELVIN S. LANG, Walla Walla, WA

The amount and frequency of ingestion of specific foods may improve or impair GT by means not yet elucidated. Of many foods tested over a two year period, corn was chosen for a comparison to glucose in the GTT. Fasting and 1 hour blood glucose and insulin assays were performed as a measure of tolerance. One hundred gm of glucose and 50 gm of CHO as whole kernel corn was given as the respective test dose.

Fifty-five subjects received both tests at appropriate intervals. Twenty-two obese subjects were divided into 2 groups of 11 each, gr 1, 1 hr G on GTT ⩽159; gr 2, 1 hr GTT⩾160. Group 2, as expected, showed G 201> than gr 1, G 106. Insulin resistance demonstrated in gr 2, 152, vs gr 1, 74. The non-obese gr 3 revealed intermediate, GTT 1 hr glucose 152, I, 66; corn test 1 hr G 123, I 32.

		GTT 1 hr		Corn 1 hr	
	ob. ind.	Gmg/dl	μU/ml	Gmg/dl	μU/ml
1 hr<159 gr 1	1. 3	106	74	102	38
1 hr⩾160 gr 2	1. 4	201	152	141	42
	p<	0. 01	0. 05	0. 01	n. s.

Thirty-four % of total subjects on GTT showed G 1 hr⩽160; in 27% of subjects 1 hr G> for 50 gm corn than 100 gm glucose; 15% of total subjects 1 hr insulin levels were corn> than glucose. Other foods show similar results for individual patients. Omission of corn and other foods causing elevated 1 hr levels of G and I improved glucose metabolism.

273

Measurement of Glycosylated Hemoglobin: Comparison of Colorimetric and Ion-Exchange Resin Chromatography Methods. J. DA COSTA, R. HESS, J. ENGLAND, and S. PETH, Columbia, Mo. (Introduced by T.W. BURNS*, Columbia, Mo.)

The level of glycosylated hemoglobin (GHb) is thought to reflect long-term blood glucose regulation. Most widely used methods for quantitating GHb employ ion-exchange chromatography (IEC). A colorimetric assy for GHb based upon 2-thiobarbituric acid (TBA) color formation has been developed and studies show high degree of correlation between GHb by IEC and TBA color. In those studies actual GHb by IEC often showed large differences from that predicted by TBA color (up to 6% GHb) raising questions about the relationship between both methods. We previously found GHb measured by IEC exists in stable and labile forms possibly identical to ketoamine and Schiff-base forms of GHb previously described. The labile form is acutely responsive to changes in blood glucose. Saline incubation (SAL) of RBC (0.9%NaCl, 37°, 5h) removes labile form. The relationship between GHb measured by TBA color formation and IEC with and without prior SAL of RBC was studied. TBA color was not affected by SAL suggesting stable GHb forms. Relationship between predicted GHb by TBA color and actual GHb by IEC was determined by linear regression in 40 diabetics and controls. Correlation coefficients between TBA color and GHb were similar with and without saline incubations (r's=.964 and .968). Difference between predicted GHb from TBA color and actual GHb by IEC were ($\bar{X}$±SEM): SAL, .32±.01%(range=.06-.8%); nonSAL .85±.09%(range=.1-1.96%). GHb by TBA predicts GHb by IEC accurately after SAL of RBC. GHb by TBA and IEC may reflect same pathophysiological process.

274

Outpatient Management of the Pregnant Diabetic Using an Open Loop Portable Insulin Infusion Pump. DONALD R. COUSTAN*, MARY C. RUDOLPH, and MYRON GENEL*, New Haven, Conn.

Aggressive management with home glucose monitoring has enabled normalization of glucose metabolism in pregnant insulin-requiring diabetics, with improvement of pregnancy outcomes. Some pregnant diabetics can't successfully be controlled despite multiple insulin injections. Our previous success in normalizing carbohydrate metabolism in adolescent diabetics using a portable insulin infusion pump on an outpatient basis (Tamberlane et al, NEJM, 300:573, 1979), prompted us to apply this technique to pregnant diabetics.

Four Class C through FR diabetics have been studied; all were difficult to control prior to initiation of pump therapy, despite frequent glucose monitoring and multiple dose insulin regimens. One subject has delivered at term, after 54 days on the pump, a 2900 gm baby with a normal glucose disappearance curve (K_t=0.625, nl 0.8 ± 0.23) in the first 6 hours of life. The 2 weeks prior to pump therapy are compared with the 2 weeks prior to delivery. Mean plasma glucose fell from 148.2 mg/dl to 108.9 mg/dl. Hb $A1_{A-C}$ fell from 9.2% to 6.5% (IsoLab Kit, normal 5.0 to 8.0%). Hypoglycemia (blood glucose < 45 mg/dl) fell from 7.3% of values to 2.6%; severe hyperglycemia (>150 mg/dl) fell from 36.5% to 11.8%. The other subjects have shown similar improvement in glucose metabolism, but have not yet delivered.

Pregnancy is an especially appropriate time for outpatient use of the insulin pump; it is a finite period of time when good metabolic control is important.

275

Abnormal EEGs in Diabetic Ketoacidosis (DKA):Lack of Correlation with B-Hydroxybutyrate (BOH) and Alanine (A) Levels. E. TSALIKIAN*, D.J. BECKER *, P.K. CRUMRINE, G.M. VALERIANO, Pittsburgh, PA.

Abnormal EEGs in long standing diabetes mellitus were previously attributed to hypoglycemia. EEG changes during episodes of diabetic ketoacidosis have not been reported. We performed serial EEGs at 1,12,24 hrs. & 5 days after initiation of treatment for DKA on 28 patients aged 11/12-16 yrs 22 patients were in ketoacidosis, 6 patients in ketosis only. Abnormal EEGs were found in 20 of the 28 patients on admission. The EEG changes at 1 hr., classified in 5 stages in order of increasing severity, were correlated with the serum glucose (G) & osmolarity (OSM)(p:<.01 &<.001 respectively) but not with the bicarbonate (Bi), BOH & alanine levels or the clinical presentation. The mean ± SD are tabulated:

EEG (1 hr)	G mg/dl	OSM mOsm/L	Bi meq/L	BOH mM	Alanine μ M
Stage V	1447±731	394±41	13.5±6	8.2	85
" IV	625±254	323±18	10.4±5	7.6±3.4	162±56
" III	525±217	323±14	10.2±6	9.5±2.3	189±74
" II	507±184	309±16	13 ±6	7.1±3.6	134±41
" I	423±232	301±10	17 ±4	4.1±1.8	142±51

EEG changes persisted in 5 of 11 children on day 5 despite clinical recovery in all & normal BOH levels in 3. BOH levels were elevated (.62±.2mM) in all children with normal EEGs at 5 days. Alanine levels remained low (192±110μM). 5 of the 6 previously abnormal EEGs repeated 2-5 mos. later remained abnormal. The severity and persistence of EEG changes appears unrelated to the degree of metabolic events such as ketosis, acidosis or the severity of the clinical presentation & recovery.

276

Glucosylated Serum Protein, Serum Glucose and Glycosylated Hemoglobin in Diabetes. A.L. KENNEDY, T. MEHL, T.J. MERIMEE*, Gainesville, Florida.

Non-enzymatically glucosulated serum protein (G.P.) was measured in 100 diabetic and 86 non-diabetic patients by a thiobarbituric acid technique, using 5-hydroxymethylfurfuraldehyde (HMF) as a standard. We found that spurious elevation of G.P. levels was produced by the addition of glucose (up to 350 mg per 100 ml) to nondiabetic sera immediately before assay, so all serum samples in this study, obtained after an overnight fast, were dialyzed against N saline before assay.

Mean ± SEM G.P. in the diabetics was 0.72 ± 0.03 nmol HMF per mg protein compared to 0.33 ± 0.015 in controls ($p<0.001$). A positive correlation was found, in the diabetics, between fasting serum glucose and G.P. levels, $r=0.37$, $p<0.01$. In 38 diabetics with Type II diabetes, the correlation between serum glucose and G.P. was much stronger than in the 62 with Type I diabetes - r values 0.69 and 0.29 respectively. G.P. levels correlated also with glycosylated hemoglobin levels in 77 diabetics ($r=0.54$).

Treatment of 4 poorly controlled diabetics by continuous subcutaneous insulin infusion resulted in a 38% (0.83 to 0.51) mean fall in G.P. within a week compared to a 6% (15.3 to 14.3% HbA_1) mean fall in glycosylated hemoglobin.

These results confirm that glucosylation of serum proteins is enhanced in the diabetic state and suggest that such glucosylation reflects glycemia over a shorter period than does glycosylated hemoglobin.

277

Factors Associated with the Early Remission of Insulin dependent Diabetes. A Prospective Study. P.VAGUE*, B.VIALETTES J.P.MOULIN, E. ALTOMARE, V. LASSMANN, M.J. SIMONIN. Marseille FRANCE.

Thirty diabetics less than 35 years old and needing insulin for initial keto acidosis or O.H.A. failure were randomly assigned to two treatment groups. Blood glucose was normalized with an artificial pancreas in one, with carefully adapted multiple SC insulin injections in the other. Frequency of remission (no insulin, urine tests negative, all B.G. values lower than 7.8mM/l) was 8/15 and 10/15 respectively, higher than in a matched retrospective study (8/30) with less careful control. Remission lasted for 3 to more than 24 months.

The 18 patients with remission did not differ from the 12 others by age, R.B.W. HbA1c and basal or stimulative C peptide levels at admission. But apparent duration of diabetes was shorter, HLA B18 more frequent (5/8 versus 0/11) B7 less frequent (1/18 versus 4/11) while B8 was equally distributed.

Three months after the end of remission degree of control and insulin dose compared favourably with the non remission group.

Early and optimal treatment promotes occurence of remission but factors related to the patient and/or his disease are equally involved.

278

Automated Spectrophotometric Assay for Glycosylated Hemoglobin. EDWIN G. MOORE, STEPHEN D. STROUPE, and LAWRENCE J. BLECKA, North Chicago, Illinois

We have developed a method for assaying glycosylated hemoglobin which is based on the functional and spectrophotometric properties of hemoglobin. The method does not involve ion exchange resins or column chromatography. Instead, the method is based upon the position of glycosylation on HbA_1, functional changes of hemoglobin induced by inositol hexaphosphate (IHP) and spectrophotometric changes in hemoglobin associated with the functional changes.

Our data support the position of glycosylation in HbA_1 at the N-termini of the β chains. Since this position forms part of the binding site for diphosphoglyceric acid (DPG), the binding of DPG and DPG-analogues, such as inositol hexaphosphate is sterically prohibited. Hence, IHP induced functional and spectrophotometric changes are inhibited in glycosylated hemoglobin, but are measurable in non-glycosylated hemoglobin.

The assay based on this method is rapid and easily automatable. In addition, it retains specificity for hemoglobin which is glycosylated only at the N-termini of the β chains (HbA_1). Interferences from other hemoglobin variants are also reduced. Fetal hemoglobin (HbF) is the only common variant which is known to interfere.

Data will be presented to support the validity of this methodology.

279

The Spectrum of Secondary Diabetes. STEPHEN PODOLSKY,* Boston, Massachusetts.

Recent research suggests that diabetes mellitus is a heterogeneous group of diseases rather than a single disease. This situation is much like that which prevailed in the field of hypertension 25 years ago, before it was realized that there are a large number of relatively uncommon forms of secondary hypertension with specific etiologies, in addition to essential hypertension.

The term "Secondary Diabetes" has been used to indicate diabetes mellitus (or sustained inappropriate hyperglycemia) induced by a specific cause. There is a growing and widespread medical literature on secondary diabetes, which sometimes may be reversible. Chronic calcifying pancreatitis is one type which appears to be increasing throughout the world. Chronic pancreatitis may have different etiologies (alcohol abuse, gallstones, possibly cassava ingestion in the tropics), although the ensuing clinical diabetes is often quite similar. Viral infections of the pancreas, autoimmunity, pancreatectomy, pancreatic carcinoma, hemochromatosis, nonpancreatic endocrine diseases, therapeutic agents and pesticides, and severe electrolyte disturbances, may all be underlying causes of diabetes. While many of these conditions are rare, together they make up a surprising percentage of clinical diabetes.

In a sense, even obesity may be considered a cause of secondary diabetes in the non-insulin-dependent person. A crucial question that remains to be determined is whether specific etiologies such as the above induce diabetes in everyone affected, or only in those already having a genetically programmed decreased insulin reserve.

CLINICAL PHYSIOLOGY

280

Effect of different Temperatures and local Massage on the Absorption of s.c. injected Insulin (scI). P.BERCHTOLD*, H.J. CÜPPERS, V.JÖRGENS, M.BERGER* Düsseldorf, W.-Germany

We recently demonstrated that absorption of scI can be altered by muscular exercise or by the addition of aprotinin. This study was performed to assess the effects of alterations of the local and the systemic temperature and local massage of the injection site on the absorption of exogenous insulin. Ten U of Actrapid Insulin were injected in the leg of fasting healthy volunteers. Veinous blood was drawn at repeatet time intervals up to 300 min post injection (pi). Under all experimental conditions blood glucose fell to 40-50 mg/dl 60 to 90 min pi and serum C-peptide decreased as expected. In resting subjects at room temperature serum IRI rose from $8 \pm .4$ to a plateau of 17 ± 1.6 μU/ml which lasted up to 150 min pi. Then IRI gradually fell to 11 ± 1 μU/ml at 300 min pi. The pi rise of IRI was significantly decreased by a cold bath of 22°C, but accelerated and increased during the first hour pi by a 42°C - bath or by putting a hot water bottle on the injection site. Massage of the injection site increased IRI to 18 ± 1.4 μU/ml at 10 min pi and IRI remained significantly elevated over control values from 10 to 50 min pi. A sauna bath had no effect on the absorption of scI. These data demonstrate the variability of the insulin absorption process. The clinical significance of increasing and accelerating the early insulin peak by alteration of the temperature or local massage remains to be elucidated.

281

Isoproterenol-Stimulated C-Peptide and Insulin Secretion in Diabetic and Nonobese Normal Subjects : Decreased Hepatic Extraction of Endogenous Insulin in Diabetes. H. SANDO, Y. S. LEE, Y. IWAMOTO, M. IKEUCHI, and K. KOSAKA, Tokyo, Japan (Introduced by WILFRED Y. FUJIMOTO*, Seattle, WA.)

Following intravenous injection of 2 μg isoproterenol, peripheral plasma insulin and C-peptide concentrations were measured in 16 nonobese normal subjects and 53 maturity-onset diabetic subjects. Basal insulin and C-peptide levels ($P < 0.005$), and insulin increments following isoproterenol ($P < 0.025$) were high in obese diabetic subjects, compared to the nonobese normal subjects. However, C-peptide increments were not significantly higher in obese diabetics than in the nonobese normals.

Hepatic insulin extraction was measured by comparing the ratios of insulin increment to C-peptide increment after isoproterenol injection (ΔIRI/ΔCPR). Mean ΔIRI/ΔCPR (molar ratio) was higher in both diet-treated (0.82 ± 0.10, mean$\pm$SE, $P < 0.005$, and 0.84 ± 0.17, $P < 0.005$, in the nonobese and obese subjects, respectively) and sulfonylurea-treated (0.74 ± 0.08, $P < 0.01$, and 0.75 ± 0.07, $P < 0.005$, in the nonobese and obese subjects, respectively) groups, compared to the normal group (0.48 ± 0.05). No significant differences in the ratios were noted between nonobese and obese diabetics, or diet and sulfonylurea therapy. Age, sex, duration of disease, familial predisposition to diabetes, fasting blood glucose level, and diabetic retinopathy did not influence the ratios.

These studies indicate that hepatic insulin extraction decreases in nonobese and obese diabetic subjects.

282

What constitutes Immuno-Reactive Insulin (I.R.I.) in Normals ? D.R. OWENS*, SANDRA RAINBOW, L.G. HEDING, Cardiff, Wales.

Metabolic day profiles-glucose, CPR (C-peptide), I.R.I., Pro-In (Proinsulin) In (Insulin) - were determined in 2 groups of 5 normal subjects given (i) isocaloric (Normal) meals on 2 separate days (ii) identical test meals/day, sampling half-hourly. Correlation coefficients with glucose: CPR 0.39; I.R.I. 0.65; Pro-In 0.25; Insulin 0.62.

Fasting Pro-In as % of I.R.I. (μU/μU was 10-20% increasing to 40-50% 2-3 hours after breakfast, the equivalent mean molar ratios (pmol/pmol) being 0.5 increasing to 3.6. Pro-In: CPR ratio double over this period. Subsequent pre and post-meal values reflected the differing Pro-In and In half-lives. Pro-In's contribution to I.R.I. especially preprandially being much higher and varying according to meal frequency. Therefore In not I.R.I. should be used to assess β cell response thus avoiding contribution by non-converted Pro-In to I.R.I.

283

Increased Glucose Utilization with Triglyceride Feeding: Studies in Normal and Insulin Dependent Diabetics(IDDs). J. TILLINGHAST, S. CATALAND, J.V. SANTIAGO*, St. Louis, Mo. and Columbus, Ohio.

Studies were conducted to compare the role of enteric factors as enhancers of glucose utilization(M). Using a closed loop system (Biostator, GCIIS, Miles Labs) plasma glucose was clamped at 216 mg/dl for 1 hr and then maintained for 2 hrs after giving 100 ml Lipomul orally(TF) in 8 normal and 5 lean IDDs. M was calculated as the amount of glucose required to maintain the hyperglycemic clamp. In IDDs insulin was given at 40 mU/m^2/min for 3 hrs. Gastric inhibitory polypeptide(GIP) and plasma free insulin(I) were measured every 15 minutes.

In normals not given TF, I rose progressively every hour (52±8, 68±12, 115±16 uU/ml) while M remained constant (7.4±1.5, 7.6±2.5, 8.0±1.5 mg/kg/min) and GIP did not change. TF caused a 106-188% increase in I and M (196±40 and 238±60 uU/ml and 15.8±4.0 and 22±3.9 mg/kg/min) after 1 and 2 hours, respectively. The timing and magnitude of the change in I and M was variable and correlated poorly with GIP responses. The increase in M due to TF was abolished by prior infusion of insulin at high rates (400 mU/m^2/min). In IDDs I was fixed at 65-70 uU/ml for 3 hrs. M was 4.5±.7 and increased to 6.1±.6 and 6.4±.5 mg/kg/min 1 and 2 hrs after TF, increases of 36 and 42%. GIP responses to TF in IDDs were twice controls

In normals the increase in M after TF is due mostly to increased I, can be eliminated with hyperinsulinemia, and cannot be accounted for by GIP alone. In IDDs the deficient M response after TF is not due to deficient GIP release.

284

Rise in Plasma Glucose with Exercise During Maintenance of Strict Normoglycemia in Diabetics. M. MARTIN, R. BERGENSTAL, B. LAGRANGE, P. BLIX and D. ROBBINS, Burlington, Vt. and Chicago, Ill.

The metabolic response to exercise in diabetics may vary depending on their control, site of insulin injection, or in relation to meals. The effect of 30 minutes vigorous stationary bicycle exercise (pulse ~150/min) in 5 male type I diabetics (D) and 5 normal controls (N) was examined 18 hrs after their last meal and insulin injection. D initially had higher plasma glucose (PG) (203±34 mg/dl) and free fatty acids (FFA) (0.86±.06 mM) than N (91±2 mg/dl and 0.52±.03 mM respectively). D were then given intravenous insulin (68±25 μU/Kg/min) to achieve euglycemia and maintained at this level (82±4 mg/dl) for 4 hours prior to exercise during continued insulin infusion. At the onset of exercise there was no difference between the D and N in PG (79±6 v. 85±10 mg/dl), free insulin (9.2±2.1 v. 10.4±1.9 μU/ml), serum lactate (1.2±.2 v. 1.3±.1 meq/l), glucagon (77±12 v. 91±9 pg/ml) and FFA concentrations (1.0±.14 v .88±.18 mM). During and 30 minutes after exercise, however, D sustained an elevation in PG (Δ 13±3 mg/dl, p<.01), while there was no change in N. This increment in PG could not be accounted for by changes in free insulin, C-peptide or plasma lactate concentrations. FFA concentrations were also unchanged. The D had a larger mean increment in plasma glucagon than N during exercise (28 v. 11 pg/ml), but the difference was not significant (p<.3). Conclusion: Vigorous exercise in euglycemic insulin dependent diabetics, in contrast to normals is accompanied by an elevation in PG that persists for 30 mins.

285

Influence of Sodium (Na) on the Oral Glucose (G) Tolerance Test. E. FERRANNINI, S. BEVILACQUA, E. BARRETT,* New Haven, CT.

It is well known from in vitro studies that active intestinal absorption of G is closely coupled to Na absorption. Studies in vivo using perfused intestinal segments have also demonstrated enhancement of G transport by Na. However, the overall glycemic response to Na addition has not been assessed. In the present study, we therefore examined the influence of Na on the plasma G response to a standard oral G tolerance test. We administered equimolar solutions of G (780 mM, Glucola^R), containing either 77 mM NaCl or 145 mM mannitol, to 10 normal subjects on two successive days. Plasma G and insulin levels and G disappearance rates (measured with ^{3}H-glucose) were determined basally and at 15 min intervals for 210 min following G ingestion. When Na was substituted for mannitol in the drink, plasma G levels were significantly (p<0.01) higher at 60, 75, 90 and 105 min post-feeding. The mean plasma G increment above basal with Na (37±8 mg/dl) was ∿25% greater (p<0.005) than with mannitol (30±7). The mean plasma insulin response was slightly, though not significantly, greater with Na. The higher plasma G levels observed with Na addition could not be explained by differences in the rate of G disappearance, which was similar in the Na (1202±101 mg/kg over 210 min) and mannitol (1109±150) studies.

Conclusion: The addition of Na enhances the rate of absorption of an oral G load. Thus, standard G tolerance testing, performed with Na-free drinks, may overestimate the tolerance to salt-containing carbohydrate meals.

286

Decreased Glucosuria in Non-Insulin Dependent Diabetics Following Fasting Via Decreased Glucose Production. F.L. GREENWAY,* D. HEBER, R. RUBY,* and R.T. CHLEBOWSKI. Torrance, California.

The observation that obese non-insulin dependent diabetics (NIDD) decrease their glucosuria for up to two weeks following a 3-day fast prompted us to investigate the mechanism of this phenomenon. Six NIDD patients were admitted to our CRC and placed on an 1800 cal/m^2 ADA diet for 5 days, fasted for 3 days, and then placed back on 1800 cal/m^2 for 7 days. Blood glucose (G) and insulin levels (I) were determined on days 4, 8, 14 and G and I were determined after an OGTT on days 5, 9, and 15. 24 hr. urine samples were collected on days 1 to 15 for glucose, creatinine and sodium. In these patients, mean glucose excretion decreased from 162±36 gm/24 hrs on days 1 to 5 to 86±34 gm/24 hrs on days 10 to 14 (p<0.05). GFR, urinary Na, blood glucose and insulin, and responses to OGTT were unchanged despite decreased glucosuria. Renal glucose threshold, glucose utilization and glucose production were studied in one patient. Renal threshold and glucose utilization rate determined by IV GTT were unchanged on day 4 vs. day 14 despite a decrease in glucosuria from 69.4 to 46.1 gm/24 hrs. Glucose production rate determined by ^{3}H-glucose infusion was decreased from 3.2 mg/kg/min on day 4 to 2.1 mg/kg/min on day 14. We conclude that decreased glucose production occurs following a three-day fast in NIDD patients and accounts for a significant decrease in glucosuria at a time when renal threshold, glucose utilization, and blood insulin and glucose levels have returned to pre-fasting diets.

287

Heterogeneity of Glucose Metabolism in Non-Insulin Dependent Diabetes Mellitus (NIDDM). E.D. BRANSOME*, T.A. HUFF*, R.A. HICKS AND L.B. HENDRY, Augusta, Georgia.

Postabsorptive hyperglycemia can be attributed to impaired glucose uptake, and/or an inappropriately high rate of glucogenesis. We subjected normals and diabetics to constant i.v. infusions of 3-^{13}C-L-alanine (5 mg/min) and $^{2}H_{5}$-α-D-glucose (2 mg/min) until an approximate steady state level of enrichment of plasma glucose and alanine was achieved (3 hrs). After chemical derivativization the ratios of $^{13}C:^{12}C$ and $^{2}H:^{1}H$ in plasma glucose were measured by selected ion monitoring with a gas chromatograph-mass spectrometer. Endogenous glucose production, glucose from alanine and glucose uptake were calculated. We found that the efficiency of glucose uptake was impaired in all diabetics but were surprised to find that this measurement did not correlate with the extent of hyperglycemia within a heterogenous group of NIDDM. The rate of glucose production was below normal in subjects with glucose intolerance (FBS <110 mg/dl), approximately normal in some moderate diabetics and elevated in others.

Averages	Blood Sugar mg%	Glucose Production mg/kg/min	Glucose Uptake %
Normal	80	2.1	5.7
Glucose Intolerance	93	1.6	4.1
Moderate A	150	2.3	3.8
Moderate B	191	3.5	4.2

The results of studies after several months of treatment with an oral sulfonylurea suggest that these agents may not be effective in diabetics with elevated rates of glucogenesis.

288

Effectiveness of Insulin Therapy on Altered Renal Transport of Magnesium in Experimental Diabetes. BETH HOSKINS*, Jackson, MS.

The uptake of magnesium-28 by kidney cortex slices from normal rats and from rats with streptozotocin (STZ)- or alloxan (ALX)-induced diabetes was studied. The results of these studies are summarized as follows:

Magnesium uptake expressed as slice-to-medium (S/M) ratios (cpm/g ÷ cpm/ml) was increased significantly after one week and was doubled after 3 weeks of ALX-induced diabetes. STZ-induced diabetes produced less effect on magnesium uptake, S/M ratios being significantly increased over controls after 3 weeks' duration of diabetes.

Early insulin therapy (initiated 72 hours after injections of ALX or STZ) reversed the effect of diabetes on magnesium transport, S/M ratios being equal to those of controls after 3 weeks of therapy. Late insulin therapy (initiated after 4 weeks of diabetes) was ineffective in restoring S/M ratios to normal in either group of diabetic animals during 3 weeks of continuous therapy.

The alterations in magnesium transport occurred prior to any evidence of nephropathy (e.g., BUN levels were normal and there was no proteinuria).

Since insulin therapy was given such that control of blood glucose was not established, the data indicate that promptness of therapy is more important than maintenance of normoglycemia in the prevention of early disturbances in renal function.

COMPLICATIONS OF DIABETES

289

Renal Functions in Spontaneously Diabetic Chinese Hamsters with Different Profiles of Plasma and Renal Glycohydrolases. A.Y. CHANG*, Kalamazoo, MI.

Increased activity of plasma N-acetyl-β-D-glucosaminidase (NAG) has been observed in diabetic human patients and animal models. Decreased activities of NAG, α-D-mannosidase (MAN), and β-D-galactosidase (GAL) were also found in the kidneys of various diabetic animals. It has been speculated that these degradative enzymes may play important roles in the development of diabetic complications. In a colony of Chinese hamsters, two highly inbred sublines, AC and XA, produced diabetic animals with distinctly different profiles of plasma and renal glycohydrolases. Although animals from AC and XA sublines had higher levels of plasma MAN and GAL than those from the nondiabetic subline M, the AC's showed subnormal activity of plasma NAG whereas the XA's had excessive level of plasma NAG. Statistically significant differences in renal MAN and GAL activities were evident among animals of these three sublines in the following order: M>AC>XA. The AC's also had depressed renal NAG level but the XA's and M's showed similar activities of renal NAG. Polyuria and excessive urinary MAN, GAL, and NAG (U/day) were found in both AC's and XA's with no apparent difference between these two diabetic sublines. Creatinine clearance rate and plasma and urinary creatinine levels were not significantly different between the nondiabetic M's and the diabetic AC's or XA's or between the AC's and XA's. Thus the significance of abnormal plasma and renal glycohydrolase levels in the development of diabetic nephropathy remains uncertain.

290

New Aspects of Bladder Disturbance in Diabetes Mellitus and Their Management, ZAFAR KHAN, GERALD J. FRIEDMAN,* New York.

Bladder pressure studies, urethral sphincter studies, and evoked potentials of the sacral spinal cord were performed in a group of patients with diabetes mellitus.

Using new, sophisticated, methods it was shown that the diabetics had bladder distention with loss of proprio-ceptive sensation, while maintaining their ability to contract; indicating the absence of a motor deficit.

The urethral sphincter studies demonstrated a normal "coordinated" relaxation during bladder contraction in the majority of diabetics. However, a small group demonstrated "uncoordinated" sphincter contraction during bladder contraction, precipitating poor urinary flow or urinary retention.

The evoked potential studies were abnormal only in those diabetics with clinical evidence of neuropathy.

The studies demonstrate that sensory, and not motor loss is the major underlying problem in the diabetic patient with urinary tract dysfunction. The treatment of choice will be presented and discussed.

291

Subclinical Thyroiditis and Lipid Levels of the Insulin Treated Diabetic Patients. SIDIKA KASIM,* WILL G. RYAN,* Downey, CA, & Chicago, IL.

The increased prevalence of Anti-thyroid antibodies (ATA) has been reported in diabetic patients (DP). In the general population subclinical thyroiditis (presence of ATA) is reported to be an atherogenic risk factor possibly by altering cholesterol metabolism. We founded ATA in 17% (44/264) of insulin treated DP. The prevalence of ATA was 7.8% (6/76) in black, 11.1% (8/72) in Mexican, 26.6% (29/109) in caucasian patients. $HgbA_1C$, T4, T3 resin uptake (T3R), free thyroxin index (FTI) and TSH levels (TableI) and lipid levels (Table II) in age and sex matched ATA positive and ATA negative insulin treated DP are listed (Mean ±SD).

Table I	No.	Age	$HgbA_1C$ %	T4 mcg/dl	T3R %	FTI	TSH mcIU/ml
ATA (-)	14	57.8 ±13	13.1 ±2.4	8.2 ±1.8	31.3 ±4.3	2.49 ±.36	6.3 ±1.8
ATA (+)	14	56.2 ±13	12.5 ±2.6	7.2 ±1.1	30.0 ±3.0	2.19 ±.38	7.2 ±3.2
		N.S	N.S	p<.1	N.S	p<.05	N.S

Table II	No.	Triglyceride mg/100ml	Total Cholesterol mg/100ml	HDL-Cholesterol mg/100ml
ATA (-)	14	221±164	237±53	41.7±13.8
ATA (+)	14	264±168	246±58	35.0 ±9.1
		N.S	N.S	p<0.1

The DP with subclinical thyroiditis showed a significantly lower FTI. HDL-Cholesterol levels in this group were also lower. ATA positivity may be a risk factor for atherogenesis in DP.

292

Infants of Diabetic Mothers (IDM): The Effect of Maternally Administered Dexamethasone on Fetal Rat Lung: Phospholipid Synthesis. M.Y. TSAI, M. W. JOSEPHSON and D.M. BROWN*, Minneapolis, MN.

IDM are at greater risk than normal infants in developing respiratory distress syndrome (RDS). The mechanism of this increased risk is not well understood. RDS in premature infants of non-diabetic pregnancies can be prevented by maternal administration of glucocorticoids which enhances the production of fetal pulmonary surfactant. However the efficacy of this mode of therapy in IDM is not known. In the present investigation, we studied surfactant synthesis in fetal lungs of streptozotocin diabetic rats. Fetuses of 19 day gestational age were employed and the effect of dexamethasone was studied by maternal administration on days 16, 17 and 18 of gestation. Phosphatidylcholine (PC) synthesis was assessed by incubation of lung slices with ^{14}C-palmitate or ^{3}H-choline. Incorporation of ^{14}C-palmitate into total phosphatidyl choline (TPC) was moderately increased (16%), while incorporation into disaturated phosphatidylcholine (DSPC) was not different between the diabetic and control groups. Incorporation of ^{3}H-choline into TPC and SPC was higher (18% and 40% respectively) in diabetic than the control group. Maternal dexamethasone treatment significantly increased choline incorporation into TPC (65%) and DSPC (87%) in the control group. In contrast, this treatment had no effect on the incorporation of choline into either TPC or DSPC in IDM. The results suggest IDM are not deficient in PC synthesis, although glucocorticoid stimulation of phospholipids synthesis is inhibited. Further studies are required to determine the usefulness of dexamethasone therapy for prevention of RDS in IDM.

293

Comparison of Results of Sympathectomy in Diabetics and Non-Diabetics with Respect to Protection from Amputation or Further Surgery. M.J. DaVALLE, T.S. RILES, N. GROVER-JOHNSON,* F.G. BAUMANN, A.M. IMPARATO, New York, NY.

The efficacy of lumbar sympathectomy in the treatment of lower extremity ischemia has been debated for five decades. Some patients with threatened limb loss appear to be spared limb amputation after sympathectomy. Nevertheless, predicting which patients will benefit from sympathectomy remains difficult. The results of 93 lumbar sympathectomies performed over a 5 year period on 54 diabetic and 39 non-diabetic patients were compared in terms of subsequent amputations or required further surgery using life table analysis methods. Significant differences in amputation or required further surgery rates in favor of non-diabetics were noted at 5 years and most shorter 6 month intervals. A possible explanation for this finding in terms of the prior spontaneous denervation of diabetic blood vessels is suggested. The results demonstrate that better predictive indices for lumbar sympathectomy are needed.

294

Quantitative Ultrastructural Evidence of 'Autosympathectomy' Causing Denervation in Epineurial Blood Vessels of the Diabetic Lower Limb. N. GROVER-JOHNSON,* F.G. BAUMANN, A.M. IMPARATO, T.S. RILES, New York, NY.

Quantitative ultrastructural methods were used to compare innervation of arterioles from the sural nerve of 6 diabetic and 6 non-diabetic non-sympathectomized patients obtained after amputation for end-stage peripheral vascular disease. Results showed: a) average nerve-muscle distance was 8.20 µm in diabetics and only 4.63 in non-diabetics ($p<.05$). b) in non-diabetics 88.9% of axons were found within a functionally effective distance of the media (within 7 µm); in diabetics only 42.7% of axons were within this distance ($p<.001$). c) average number of axons less than 7 µm from the media was 70 in diabetics and 313 in non-diabetics ($p<.01$). Furthermore, when 6 sympathectomized diabetics were compared with the 6 non-sympathectomized diabetics there was no statistically significant difference between the diabetic groups in average nerve-muscle distance, proportion of axons found less than 7 µm from the media, or average number of axons less than 7 µm from the media. Thus, diabetic epineurial arterioles of the lower limb are significantly denervated and sympathectomy does not result in significant additional denervation.

295

The Effects of Diabetes and Insulin Therapy on the Contractile and Relaxing Activity of an Isolated Blood Vessel Preparation. R. HILMAN, A. DARBY AND *M. A. PFAFFMAN, Jackson, MS.

Contractures induced by 10^{-4}M phenylephrine (PE) or 70 mM KCl and their relaxation by 10^{-2}M theophylline (Theo) were observed in aortae isolated from untreated and insulin-treated streptozotocin-diabetic rats for 12 weeks after the induction of diabetes. Diabetes consistently caused an average decrease of 40% in the PE and K-induced contractures. Treatment of diabetic animals with 2.0-3.5 U NPH insulin/day partially prevented diabetes-induced decreases in the PE contractures while completely preventing them in the K-contractures. Relaxation of the PE-contractures, which were more susceptible to Theo than were the K-contractures in control tissues, was not affected by either untreated or insulin-treated diabetes until 12 weeks after the induction of diabetes. While insulin therapy did not reverse diabetes-induced decreases in the Theo-induced relaxation of the PE contractures, it did prevent the diabetes-induced increases in the relaxation of the K-contractures which were observed after 4 weeks. The results indicate that while the mechanisms involved in mediating the PE and K-contractures are inhibited by diabetes, insulin is more effective in preventing the effects of diabetes on the K-contractures and their relaxation than on the induction and relaxation of the PE contractures. (Supported by BRSG Grant 5 S07 RR05386 and a grant from the AHA-Mississippi Affiliate.)

296

Does Untreated and Insulin-Treated Diabetes Affect the Cardiovascular System of the Rat? *M. A. PFAFFMAN, R. HILMAN AND A. DARBY, Jackson, MS.

The effects of untreated and insulin-treated streptozotocin-induced diabetes was observed on the heart rate, blood pressure and isolated blood vessels of male Wistar rats for a period of 12 weeks. The heart rate, which decreased 20% within 6 days after the 2nd intraperitoneal injection of streptozotocin (65 mg/kg), remained depressed throughout the 12 week observation period in the untreated diabetic rats. Within 4 days after institution of treatment with NPH insulin (1 U/day subcutaneously) the heart rates of the treated diabetic rats returned to control values. A decrease in blood pressure was observed in the untreated diabetic rats 6 weeks after the induction of diabetes while there was no difference between blood pressures in the control and insulin-treated animals. The maximal KCl (70 mM) and phenylephrine (PE-10^{-4}M) contractile responses in aortae isolated from untreated diabetic rats were 57 and 48%, respectively, of those from control animals, while those of tissues from insulin-treated rats did not differ from controls. Diabetes increased theophylline (Theo-10^{-2}M)-induced relaxation of the K-contracture but decreased relaxation of the PE-contracture. Insulin-treatment prevented the effects of diabetes on relaxation of the K but not the PE-contracture. These results indicate that insulin-treatment will reverse diabetes-induced decreases in the heart rate and will prevent the observed diabetes-induced decreases in the blood pressure and vascular contractile responses. (Supported by BRSG Grant 5 S07 RR05386 & AHA-MS Affil. Grant.)

297

Treatment of Retinal Neovascularization after Panretinal Photocoagulation. GERALD D. ROGELL,* Rockville, Md.

Panretinal photocoagulation (PRP) is an effective means of eradicating neovascularization in proliferative diabetic retinopathy. Sometimes, however, new vessels recur or progress after PRP. How should these eyes be treated?

Since early 1978, the author has treated such cases with additional PRP therapy. These cases were reviewed, and the results are presented. Fifteen such eyes were identified, with an average followup of 24 months from first laser treatment.

In all cases, progression of proliferative retinopathy was successfully halted. Good vision was retained in all cases, with 14 of the 15 eyes currently seeing 20/40 or better. Only one significant vitreous hemorrhage was seen; it cleared rapidly. No eyes became legally blind. Fundus appearance is currently stable in all eyes.

These results demonstrate that further PRP treatment is effective in controlling neovascularization which has progressed or recurred after initial PRP.

298

Study of Methods for Clinical Trials in Diabetic Polyneuropathy. D.A. GREENE*, M.J. BROWN, S.N. BRAUNSTEIN*, S.S. SCHWARTZ*, and A.I. WINEGRAD*, Philadelphia, Pa.

Diabetic polyneuropathy is assoc. with p. nerve lesions that are only partially reversible; uniform severity in nerves of the arms and legs is not documented. The electrophysiological tests (EPTs) used in clinical trials (mostly in arms) provide composite values with disproportionate contributions from large fibers, but are often the primary basis for assessing responses. Nine chronic insulin-requiring diabetics, age 21-59, with symptomatic polyneuropathy were selected for the absence of complicating illness and other forms or causes of neuropathy. Sural SNCV and sensory amplitude (SAmp) were uniformly abnormal as were median and ulnar MNCV, but there was a striking variation in the distribution of abnormal median, radial, and ulnar SNCV and SAmp both between and within pts. unrelated to the extent of s. deficits in the arms. Diet and insulin were adjusted on CRC adm. and at weekly intervals; multivitamins and either a placebo or myoinositol (av 2 g/day) were adm. in hopes of obtaining a range of responses. Symptoms and s. deficits and a battery of EPTs were assessed at 0,2,4, and 6 mos. Four pts. had sig. improvement in both symptoms and s. deficits in the legs but without improvement in sural SNCV or SAmp or in peroneal MNCV. The same pts. had improvement in symptoms and s. deficits in the arms but with only isolated instances of improvement in initially abnormal EPTs in the ulnar, median, and radial nerves, which lacked a consistent pattern. Clinical improvement probably reflects improved function of restricted components of a chronically diseased p. nervous system.

299

Differential Sensitivity of Normal and Diabetic Isolated Rat Hearts to Calcium. D.R. BIELEFELD and B.R. BOSHELL* Birmingham, Alabama

The effect of Ca^{2+} on the function of isolated perfused hearts obtained from normal and diabetic rats was determined. Rats injected with 40 mg/kg of streptozotocin developed a plasma glucose level of 400-600 mg% and were maintained without treatment for 2 to 3 months before sacrifice. The working heart preparation with an afterload of 100 cm H_2O and a left ventricular filling pressure of 10 cm H_2O was used. The glucose concentration in the perfusate was 11 mM. The influence of 0 to 4.5 mM Ca^{2+} on left ventricular pressure yielded a half-maximal response at 0.6 mM and 1.0 mM Ca^{2+} in control and diabetic hearts, respectively. Initiation of aortic output (a.o.) was obtained with 0.7 mM Ca^{2+} in normal hearts whereas in diabetic hearts a.o. was obtained with 1.0 mM Ca^{2+}. Maximum a.o. was achieved in both preparations at 2.5 mM Ca^{2+}. A decrease in $[Ca^{2+}]$ increased the coronary flow (c.f.) in diabetic hearts in spite of a decrease in a.o., whereas both c.f. and a.o. decreased in normal hearts. Epinephrine (10 nM) and insulin (10 nM) augmented the Ca^{2+} sensitivity of the normal and diabetic hearts; however, the influence of insulin on the diabetic heart was transient. The results indicate that chronic untreated diabetes leads to an impairment in cardiac performance associated with Ca^{2+} sensitivity. This suggests that there may be a diabetes related defect in the regulation of a crucial Ca^{2+} sensitive reaction in myocardial tissue.

300

Rest Electrocardiographic Patterns (REP) in Diabetics without Evidence of Ischemic Heart Disease (IHD). MOSHE Y. FLUGELMAN, YORAM KANTER,* EDWARD G. ABINADER and DAVID BARZILAI, Haifa, ISRAEL.

We have studied the REP of 42 diabetics without evidence of IHD. All were under 50 years of age, with normal levels of blood pressure and weight. All had normal lipid profiles and smoked less than 10 cigarettes per day. There was no evidence of IHD by history or physical examination, no evidence or retinopathy or nephropathy and with no Q's or bundle branch blocks on ECG.

A double-standard double-speed 12 leads REP was studied, and QT as RR intervals were measured. The QT was corrected by the Bazzet formula $QTc=QT/\sqrt{RR}$.

In 31 subjects, abnormal REP as ST elevations, junctional depressions, T wave invertions or prolonged QT intervals were noted.

In 24 (57.1%) subjects we have found repolarization changes, mainly at the inferior and lateral walls. In 15 (35.7%) subjects the QTc was above 0.425 and the QT was prolonged. The mean QT interval for all the 42 subjects was 0.420.

These results show the presence of an abnormal REP in diabetics without evidence of IHD. These REP changes might be related to the diabetic heart per se, as a part of "Diabetic Cardiopathy" which might preceed any ischemic changes of IHD.

301

Sorbitol Dehydrogenase and Aldose Reductase Activity in Normal and Diabetic Rat Brain, S.E. OROSZ, S.F. TOWNSEND, P.A. TORNHEIM, and C.M. BROWNSCHEIDLE, Cincinnati, Ohio (Introduced by KENNETH KREINES*, Cinti., Ohio)

During hyperglycemia, cerebral accumulations of sorbitol and/or fructose may predispose the CNS to cerebral edema associated with the treatment of diabetic ketoacidosis. Presumably, these osmotically active particles accumulate as the result of an increased metabolism of glucose through the polyol pathway. In the present investigation, the brains of normal and diabetic rats were examined histochemically to determine the precise location of the enzymes of the polyol pathway in the CNS and whether there is a change in activity of these enzymes in diabetes.

Adult male rats were sacrificed 2 and 10 weeks following injection with streptozotocin (75 mg/kg I.P.) or vehicle. Sections of cortex, corpus striatum, thalamus, medulla, and cervical spinal cord were analyzed for sorbitol dehydrogenase (SDH) and aldose reductase (AR)(Johnson '65,'67).

SDH and AR activities were demonstrated in control groups in choroidal epithelium, ependymal cells and outer leptomeninges throughout the CNS. Activity could not be detected intraneuronally in any of the regions examined. Diabetics showed activity in the same cell types as the vehicles. Comparison between diabetics and vehicle groups did not demonstrate any alterations in activity for SDH and AR.

The extraneuronal location of these enzymes and the absence of any detectable change in activity between diabetics and vehicles fails to support the polyol theory as an explanation for acute cerebral edema. Study supported NIH-HL-22106

302

Induction of Suction Blisters in Diabetic and Normal Skin. J.E. BERNSTEIN, C. YUNG, M. MEDENICA and K. SOLTANI, Chicago, IL. (Introduced by J.B. JASPAN*, Chicago, IL.)

Diabetes mellitus is associated with a characteristic rare bullous eruption, as well as with a more common but less specific increased susceptibility to friction blisters. In order to investigate whether fragility of the dermo-epidermal junction (DEJ) is the cause of such easy blistering in diabetics, we evaluated the mechanical force necessary to induce suction blisters in insulin-dependent diabetic and normal subjects. Our suction apparatus utilized a 0.10 HP vacuum pump, a manometer, and 36 cm polyvinyl tubing attached to a glass mouth 1 cm in diameter. Suction was applied to normal flexor forearm skin of diabetic and sex-and age-matched normal volunteers at a pressure of 200 mm Hg until an incipient blister was formed, and the time required to produce such a blister recorded. The mean suction blister threshold for diabetics was 36 minutes, while that for the normal volunteers was 64 minutes, a highly significant difference ($P < .01$). The suction blister threshold decreased with age in both groups. Histologic examination of suction blisters from normal and diabetic skin revealed separation at the DEJ level. These results suggest that an intrinsic defect at the DEJ in insulin-dependent diabetics renders their skin more susceptible to blister formation.

303

Growth regulation of fibroblasts from primary and secondary diabetics by the metabolic control of diabetes.T.KOSCHINSKY*,C. BÜNTING,F.A.GRIES. Düsseldorf,F.R.Germany

The contribution of genetic and metabolic factors to the increased growth of fibroblasts(F) from diabetics, which has been related to the increased angiopathic risk, is unknown. Therefore, F were cultured from 6 primary diabetics (PD) with poor and from 1 PD with good metabolic longterm control (age: 10-40 yrs., duration of diabetes: 1-7 yrs.), from 4 secondary diabetics (SD) (9-24 months after total pancreatectomy, no family history of diabetes,age: 41-45 yrs.) with poor metabolic control and from 5 age matched healthy controls. Growth of F in DME+10% diabetic or normal human serum was measured til confluency.

F growth from SD increased with normal serum by 30-70% as compared to normal F and matched the growth increase of F from PD with poor metabolic control. In contrast, F growth from 1 PD with good metabolic control matched normal F. Diabetic sera from poorly controlled diabetics increased growth in all F-lines by 25-50% as compared to normal sera without changing the group specific growth differences.

This suggests a major regulatory effect of the metabolic long term control of diabetes on changes of growth capacity of F. As far as this model operates in the vascular wall, selection of cells with a high susceptibility to growth stimulation by metabolic factors present in poorly controlled diabetics may occur. This would provide an additional rational for optimal metabolic longterm control of diabetes.

304

Diabetic Angiopathy of Lower Extremities. A. GILFER, M. FEIGIN*, Chicago, IL.

There had been examined more than 1000 diabetic (D) patients. Out of this there were 112 cases (11.2%) with diabetic angiopathy of the lower extremities (DALE), including 41 cases (4.1%) with diabetic gangrene and 16 cases (1.6%) with diabetic osteoarthropathy.

To clear up earlier disorders of the periferal circulation in lower extremities plethysomograms were taken from the big toes and simultaneously speed spreading of the pulse wave (SSRW) of LE arteries was determined.

Feet skin t° on the same patient big toes and skin was determined. Restoration of this t° was measured after taking down the tight from the femur. Analysis of given result in different age categories led to the conclusion that functional disturbance in small vessels precedes some compacting changes of the walls of large vessels.

Given changes in skin t° , plethysomogram decreasing without changes in oscillogram and SSPW we can consider that micro-angiopathy predominates. Straight dependence of the perifernal circulation disturbance from degree of diabetes severity and lingering was marked.

The problem of patient treatment with a different manifestation of diabetic angiopathy LE would be discussed in the report.

305

DIABETES AND MICCARDIAL INFARCTICN. MARK FEIGIN* CHICAGO, ILLINOIS.

WITH A PURPOSE OF RESEARCH SOME PECULIARITYS OF CURRENT MIOCARDIAL INFARCTION IN DIABETIC PATIENTS WE MADE SOME COMPARISON OF THE EXPONENTS OF MIOCARDIAL INFARCTION IN DIABETIC (D) PATIENTS -137 CASES AND NON-DIABETIC (ND) PATIENTS WITH INFARCT-IN 1448 CASES.

68,6% D HAD LARGE INFARCTION,11,6% OF THIS AMOUNT HAD ANEURISM. AMONG ND LARGE INFARCTION WAS DIAGNOSED IN 57,7%,ANEURISM-IN6,3%. ANGINA PECTORIS WAS PRECEDED BY INFARCTION IN 73% CASES BY D AND IN 62% BY ND.

MORTALITY WAS IN 36,5% BY D AND IN 30,3% BY ND. IN BOTH GROUPS MORTALITY AMONG WOMENS WAS HIGHER THEN AMONG MENS. REPEATED INFARCTION WAS NOTED IN 27%CASES BY D AND 21%BY ND.

IN THE 40-49 AGE GROUP INFARCTICN BY ND AMONG MEN WAS IN75,6%, AMONG WOMEN-IN 24,4%.

INFARCTION BY D AMONG MEN WAS IN 61,5% AND AMONG WOMEN IN 38,5%.

IN THE 50-59 AGE GROUP INFARCTION BY ND WAS IN 63,5% AMONG MEN AND IN 36,5% AMONG WOMEN. BY D IN 50,7% AMONG MEN AND IN 49,3% AMONG WOMEN.

OBVIOUSLY AMONG D QUANTITY OF WOMEN WITH INFARCTION SERIOSLY INCRESED, ESPESSIALY IN THE SECOND AGE GROUP.

GIVEN RESEARCH ALLOWED TO CONCLUDE THAT CURRENT OF MIOCARDIAL INFARCTICN BY D IS MORE OPPRESSIVE THAN BY ND AND TO MARC SOME PECULIARITIES IN THE CLINICAL PICTURE OF MIOCARDIAL INFARCTION BY D.

WE DIDN'T NOTE A STRAIGHT DEPENDENCE BETWEEN THE DEGREE AND LINGERING OF DIABETES AND ORIGIN OF MIOCARDIAL INFARCTICN.

306

The Relationship of Plasma Renin Activity (PRA) Urinary Aldosterone (Aldo) and Sodium Excretion in Juvenile Insulin Dependent Diabetics. SONGJA PANG, MARIA I. NEW*, SHARON E. OBERFIELD, and LENORE S. LEVINE* New York, New York

Since abnormalities of the renin-angiotensin-aldosterone system have been reported in adult patients with complications of diabetes mellitus, we have studied this system in 42 ambulatory patients (18 male, 24 female) with insulin-dependent juvenile diabetes (age range: 3 $^{7}/_{12}$ - 23 years). The duration of diabetic disease was 1 month to 19 years with a mean of 7.5 years. All the patients were normotensive and in good health without severe hyperglycemia or ketoacidosis, although the degree of glycosuria varied. Creatinine clearances were within the normal range in all patients. Two patients had proteinuria (500 mg/day) and 3 patients had early mild diabetic retinopathy. No patients had diabetic neuropathy. Ambulatory plasma renin activity (ng/ml/hr) and urinary aldo excretion ($\mu g/m^2$/day) were appropriate for sodium excretion in all diabetic patients compared to those of normal children. The renin-aldosterone system in the patients with proteinuria or retinopathy was normal. This study demonstrates that in the baseline ambulatory state, the renin-aldosterone system in non-complicated juvenile diabetics was essentially normal, similar to the findings in adult patients with non-complicated diabetes mellitus.

307

Myocardial Mitochondria in Depancreatized Dogs. M.D. WIDER, A.J. WHITTY, E.A. ELFONT and R.A. BOTA Sinai Hosp. of Detroit, Detroit, Mi.

Male mongrel dogs were depancreatized under pentobarbital anesthesia and maintained on daily injections of Ultralente insulin sufficient to keep blood glucose under 175 mg/dl. They were fed a high protein diet with pancreatic enzyme supplements and none of the animals lost weight during the study. The dogs were sacrificed after 1 to 7 weeks and the heart removed rapidly and placed in ice cold saline. Mitochondria from the left ventricular wall were isolated by rate zonal centrifugation using an iso-osmotic Ficoll gradient. The subendocardial layer showed a single, slowly migrating peak with none of the rapidly migrating mitochondria which normally comprise 65% of the subendocardial population. Histologic examination by light (LM) and electron (EM) microscopy revealed no evidence of inflamation or vascular disease. There were, however, extensive subendocardial inclusion bodies and an increase in collagen bundles and strands. EM studies showed mitochondria that were more electron lucent than normal and resembling those seen in ischemic myocardium. There was no evidence of microtubular alterations however, nor any change in the Z and I bands that are seen in ischemia. These morphologic changes in the mitochondria could reflect functional alterations caused by the diabetic changes in metabolism even though the animals were kept under reasonable control.

308

Prostacycline Stimulation of cAMP Accumulation in Diabetic Platelets. JOHN COMSTOCK*, Houston, TX.

Previous studies in diabetic subjects have shown increased platelet aggregation _in vitro_ which is thought to be important in the development of vascular disease. Although the bio-regulation of platelet function is not precisely understood, increased levels of cAMP prevent platelet aggregation probably by inhibiting prostaglandin (PG) synthesis. Prostacyclin (PGI_2), a potent inhibitor of aggregation acts by stimulating platelet adenylate cyclase. The effect of PGI_2 on [^{3}H]cAMP accumulation from the precursor [^{3}H]adenine was measured in platelet-rich plasma from 10 male diabetics (D) and 7 matched controls (C). Results are reported as percent conversion of the total platelet [^{3}H]adenosine nucleotide pool to [^{3}H]cAMP (% cAMP). The time course of [^{3}H]cAMP accumulation showed 2 peaks at 2 and 60 min. Effects of 0.25 µM PGI_2 (rate-limiting) were determined:

	% cAMP			
Time (min)	0	1	30	
C	.17±.01	2.03±.32	2.84±.58	$\bar{X}$ ±SEM
D	.10±.01	2.80±.80	3.79±.68	
	(NS)	(NS)	(NS)	

Responses to increasing [PGI_2] (10^{-8} to 10^{-6}M) were measured at 1 and 30 min:

Model Form: $ln(\frac{C-y}{y})=\alpha-\beta \cdot ln\ [PGI_2]$.

y=% cAMP; C=extent of % cAMP increase: 4.9 at 1 min, 6.5 at 30 min. for both D and C (NS); β= rate constant:~1.0 for C and D (NS); α=intercept: ~5.0 for C and D (NS). Prostacyclin stimulated cAMP accumulation is normal in diabetic platelets, eliminating the hypothesis that reduced negative control of PG synthesis is responsible for increased aggregation.

309

Lack of Plasma Glucagon (GL) Response to Insulin (I) Hypoglycemia in Experimental Diabetic Rats. D.G. PATEL*, T.D. MAHER*, B. ANDALORO, L. ROTH and E. BERNSTEIN. Auburn-Syracuse, NY.

It has been previously reported that diabetics with autonomic neuropathy do not secrete GL during insulin-hypoglycemia (ITT). Streptozotocin (STZ, 65 mg/kg) was injected i.v. to a group of rats (D) while weight matched control rats (C) were injected i.v. with citrate buffer. Three weeks after induction of diabetes oral glucose tolerance test was performed and plasma glucose (G) concentrations were estimated. Fasting G in C and D was 74.13 ± 7.1 and 212.0 ± 138.4 mg% respectively. Sixty minutes after oral glucose load G values increased to 102.6 ± 43.0 mg% in C and 267.6 ± 39.1 mg% in D. G and GL were measured at intervals during I (0.5U/kg i.p.) induced hypoglycemia. Fasting GL in C and D was 87.6 ± 29.4 and 341.2 ± 181.3 pg/ml respectively. During ITT the G nadir was approximately 30 mg% in both groups. GL levels during hypoglycemia were 242.5 ± 98.4 pg/ml in C and 141.2 ± 75.9 pg/ml in D. Seventy-two hours following ITT the animals were sacrificed and whole brain dopamine (DP) and Serotonin (5HT) were assayed by liquid chromatography. DP levels in D were (1.31 ± 0.09 µg/g, significantly lower than in C (2.13 ± 0.68 µg/g, p<0.01). However, 5HT values were similar in both C (1.20 ± 0.40 µg/g and D (1.30 ± 0.09 µg/g).

The results demonstrate a positive correlation of DP depletion in the central nervous system and lack of GL response to ITT. The STZ diabetic animal may be suitable for studying the biochemical aspects of diabetic neuropathy.

310

Sensitive Methods for Evaluating Autonomic Nervous System Dysfunction in Diabetes Mellitus. M.A. PFEIFER,* J. BRODSKY AND D. COOK, Seattle, WA.

Autonomic neuropathy (AN) is a major complication of diabetes. Therefore, methods that quantitate sympathetic nervous system (SNS) and parasympathetic nervous system (PNS) function in man were evaluated. Dark adapted pupil diameter (light intensity of 1 foot candle[FC] for 15 min) and responses to dark stimulation (decrease from 65 FC to 1 FC for 10 sec) were measured by a pupillometer. Compared to 19 aged-matched normals (N), 21 diabetics subjects (D) had decreased dark adaptation (5.56±0.21mm, $\bar{x}$±SEM vs. 6.27±0.29, $p<.05$) and dark responses (Δ= +0.94±0.11 vs. Δ= +1.36±0.12, $p<.01$). Since impaired dark adaptation persisted in D during PNS blockade with 1% tropicamide (D: 6.54±0.22, vs. N:7.58±0.43, $p<.02$), the impaired pupil dilation is due to decreased SNS activity.

PNS activity was assessed by measuring heart rate (HR) and the variability of RR intervals (RR-VAR) 30 min after 10mg of IV propranolol during supine deep inspiration (5/min) for 5 min. D had a greater HR (63±2 vs. 53±1 beats/min, $p<.001$) and decreased RR-VAR (42±13 vs. 82±11 msec, $p<.02$) compared to N. In N, coordination of SNS and PNS activity was indicated by the relationship between dark adapted pupil size and both HR (n=.81, $p<.001$) and RR-VAR ($r=.62$, $p<.03$). In contrast, these measures of SNS and PNS function were not related in D. D without clinical AN also had a decrease in dark response (Δ= +0.90±.17, n=9, $p<.025$) and an increase in HR (62±4, n=8, $p<.03$). Thus, these measurements are sensitive, quantitative methods which may be used to detect early AN in patients with diabetes.

311

Age of Onset Distribution and Prevalence of Complications From A Retrospective Record Review of 5341 Diabetics. KAREN ANDREWS, JEFFREY ROSEMAN*, and KATHARINE KIRK Birmingham, AL

The Diabetes Hospital and Outpatient Clinic of the University of Alabama in Birmingham began seeing patients in 1972. As a first step in the development of a diabetes research database, a retrospective review of all diabetics was begun in 1978. The sample, which consisted of 5341 diabetics on whom information was available, was 70% White and 30% Black; 62% female and 38% male.

Analysis of the age of onset distributions revealed the following results. In insulin dependent diabetics with an age of onset less than or equal to 25, two major peaks were noted at ages 6-7 and10-12. In the latter peak, the male mode was one year later than the female mode in both races. There was a suggestion of a peak in Black males at an age of onset less than 2. In diabetics with onset greater than 25, the peak age of onset was in the 45-55 age group.

Analysis of the prevalence of various complications was performed. There was no difference in prevalence of retinopathy between those with onset before 30 and after 30 years of age when duration was controlled. Even controlling for duration, nephropathy was significantly increased in the younger age group and neuropathy was significantly increased in the older age group. Controlling for duration and age of onset, diabetics who required insulin for control had significantly increased prevalence of retinopathy and neuropathy. There was no significant difference in nephropathy. (Supported by grants from the Appalachian Regional Commission and Diabetes Trust Fund.)

312

Possible Hormonal Effects on the Linear Decline of Renal Function in Diabetic Nephropathy. JOHN A. LINFOOT*, JEANETTE S. NAKAGAWA, and PETER A. LINFOOT, Berkeley, California.

The factors which influence the rate of progression of diabetic renal disease (DRD) are not known. A study on the effects of alpha particle pituitary irradiation (APPI) on 48 adult (AOD) and 119 juvenile insulin dependent (JID) diabetic patients with proliferative retinopathy (PDR) was initiated in 1958. Data indicated an apparent improved survival when compared to other groups with PDR and/or DRD. Using constant proteinuria as the criteria for DRD, three groups of patients were defined: <1, 1-4, >4 gm of protein per 24 hours. All groups showed a slower decline in glomerular filtration rate, measured by endogenous creatinine clearance; and the observed differences were significantly less than predicted by Mogensen, i.e., ~1 ml/min/mo. To further assess deterioration of renal function, the reciprocal of serum creatinine (μmol/l) was analyzed in each of the three groups. Although there is great variability between diabetics, the decline in renal function in any given diabetic is linear after the serum creatinine reaches 200 μmol/l (2.3 mg/dl). We found that the rate of development of moderately advanced or severe renal failure was significantly reduced in our patients in spite of PDR and renal angiopathy, and correlated with improved survival. Conclusions: 1) DRD was not the leading cause of death in 167 AOD and JID diabetics with PDR treated with APPI. 2) The apparent slowed progression of DRD after APPI suggests an hormonal role in diabetic angiopathy.

313

Relationship of Hypertension to other Cardiovascular Risk Factors and Atherosclerosis: A Multivariate Analysis in Diabetics with and without Peripheral Vascular Disease. H.U. JANKA*, E. STANDL, H. MEHNERT*, Munich, W. Germany

Much evidence suggests that diabetics have a higher prevalence of hypertension than non-diabetics, but its role as contributor to the excess prevalence of atherosclerosis among diabetics is still under debate.

In a study of 623 non-selected diabetic outpatients hypertension ($\geqslant$ 160/95 mmHg) was found to be the most frequent cardiovascular risk factor (50.4 %). In order to define the relationship of elevated blood pressure values to other risk factors and to peripheral vascular disease (PVD) an univariate and multivariate analysis of variance (SSPS- MANOVA computerized program) was performed.

Systolic hypertension was associated significantly with serum cholesterol ($p< 0.02$) and serum triglycerides ($p< 0.03$), even after adjustment for age and overweight. In contrast, diastolic hypertension was only significantly correlated to duration of diabetes ($p< 0.05$).

PVD was significantly associated with systolic blood pressure values ($p< 0.0005$) which in turn correlated with serum cholesterol in these patients ($p< 0.05$).

While the cause of these interrelationships has to be determined our results indicate that hypertension in diabetics is generally associated with elevated blood lipids. Since, especially, patients with PVD exhibited this risk constellation a pathogenetic role is suggested.

314

Renal Glomerular Studies in Bio Breeding/Worcester (BB/W) Diabetic Rats. A.A. LIKE*, M.C.APPEL*, and S. ERICSON, Worcester, Mass.

The Bio Breeding/Worcester (BB/W) rat is a model of spontaneous, non-obese, ketosis prone, insulin deficient diabetes mellitus (Diabetes 26, 100, 1977), characterized by genetic susceptibility and a probable autoimmune pathogenesis (Science 206, 1423, 1979). Bacterial and viral agents are not involved in the syndrome's etiology (Diabetes 28, 27, 1979). To examine the BB/W rat as a model of diabetic renal disease, normal (N=7), glucose intolerant (GI=9) and diabetic (D=6) animals were housed in metabolic cages. Plasma glucose (PG), 24 hour urine volume (UV) and urinary glucose (UG) were quantitated for 4 months and correlated with renal glomerular morphology at sacrifice. Mean PG, (mg/dl) UV (ml) and UG (mg) of N and GI rats were indistinguishable. (N: PG=98.3, UV=10.2, UG= 3.6) (GI: PG=94.8, UV=9.1, UG=3.4). D rats segregated into well controlled (DWC=3) and poorly controlled (DPC=3) on the basis of PG, UV and UG. (DWC: PG=238.6, UV=15.5, UG=952). (DPC: PG=572, UV=76.9, UG=6685). Immune fluorescence studies of N & GI renal glomeruli (RG) were indistinguishable. Both revealed 1/2-1+ and 1-3+ deposits of IgG and IgM. DWC and DPC RG revealed similar IgM deposits (3+): IgG deposits were more severe in DPC (3-4+) than DWC (1-2+). N, GI, DWC and DPC were indistinguishable on the basis of glomerular C3, and fibrinogen was absent. The data suggest that the BB/W rat is a valid model of diabetic renal disease and that RG IgG deposits mirror diabetic severity.

315

Platelet Aggregation in Yucatan Miniature Swine which Differ in Glucose Tolerance. NELSON WESTMORELAND and R.W. PHILLIPS* Ft. Collins, Colo.

We have developed lines of miniature swine which differ greatly in their ability to remove an I.V. injected bolus of glucose from their circulation. The low glucose tolerance (LGT) swine have a reduced insulin level in the peripheral circulation in response to the glucose. Platelets from these LGT animals show greater maximal aggregation and delayed disaggregation when compared with platelets from animals with high glucose tolerance (HGT). The platelets from the LGT pigs are less sensitive to inhibition of aggregation by citrate.

Maximal aggregation and disaggregation slopes at various concentrations of ADP were measured on platelet rich plasma (PRP) isolated from blood which had been mixed with citrate at three concentrations. PRP was prepared from 5 LGT and 5 HGT swine. At the high citrate level (1ml cit. to 9ml blood), platelets from both lines of animals had maximal aggregation inhibited to the 40-50% range. At the lowest citrate concentration (.5ml cit. to 9.5ml blood), they both aggregated equally well in the 80-90% range. At the intermediate concentration (.75ml cit. to 9.25ml blood), platelets from the LGT animals had a higher max. aggregation (p .005). Disaggregation slopes were greater for the aggregates formed from platelets from the LGT animals (p .025 for low cit.; p .05 for intermediate).

Similar response data have been seen in platlets from glucose intolerant humans.

Supported by the Kroc Foundation. Instnument loaned by Sandy Simons of Sienco, Inc.

316

Relationship Between Diabetic Control and Degenerative Complications. Rene N. Charles*, Port-au-Prince, Haiti.

Two groups of Diabetes were studied to evaluate the incidence of diabetic complications in relation to glycemic control.

Group I comprises 700 patients (mean age 53 years) treated in other clinics and poorly controlled; with mean blood glucose of 200 mg over several years (mean 7 years).

Retinopathy increases from 8% in patients with known duration of diabetes of less than 5 years to 75% in patients with Diabetes of more than 15 years; Nephropathy from 4 to 25%; Neuropathy from 8 to 50%; Atherosclerosis from 20 to 50%.

Failure to oral hypoglycemic agents reached 53%-Diet was not well observed.

Group II comprises 1500 patients (mean age 55 years) followed in our clinic from the onset of their disease. Mean blood glucose is 140 mg.

Retinopathy increases from 4 to 35% after 15 years; Nephropathy from 2 to 12.5%; Neuropathy from 5 to 25%; Atherosclerosis from 4 to 25%. Thirty per cent of patients were controlled with Diet only. There were 16% failure to oral agents.

The incidence of complications increases with duration of Diabetes Mellitus and is also related to poor glycemic control.

317

Early Diabetic Retinopathy in Young Patients with Insulin Dependent Diabetes Mellitus (IDDM) Detected by Green Monochromatic Light Photography. E. TOPPER, Y. YASSUR, R. SIEGAL, I. BEN SIRA, Z. LARON*, and M. KARP*, Tel Aviv, Israel.

Monochromatic light photography (MLP) with green light (540 and 570 nm) was found to be much superior to white light (color) photography and as reliable as fluorescein angiography, in detecting early changes of diabetic retinopathy.

Early diabetic microangiopathy (MA) was found by this photographic technique to be quite common in young patients with IDDM treated in our clinic. It existed in 54 out of 124 (44%) patients aged 3 - 34 years with diabetes duration of half - 19 years. Of these it was found in 20 out of 61 patients (30%) with diabetes duration of less than 5 years, and in 35 out of 94 patients (37%) who were below the age of 20 years. It is noteworthy that the incidence of MA in our patient population is lower than that reported by other groups.

MLP is a reliable non-invasive diagnostic technique that may be used routinely for screening of IDDM populations.

318

Platelet Adhesion in Experimental Diabetes Mellitus. R.J. CUNNINGHAM*, B.H. BROUHARD and L.B. TRAVIS*, Galveston, Texas.

Platelet adhesion and aggregation have been implicated as important steps in the pathogenesis of diabetic vascular disease. Previous studies have indicated that platelets obtained from patients with Diabetes (DM) are more sensitive than platelets from non-diabetics to a variety of stimuli which induce platelet aggregation; platelet adhesiveness is also increased in diabetics, particularly in those with evidence of vascular disease. The present study examined the effects of DM and insulin therapy(I) on adhesion of platelets to collagen coated glass. Alloxan (100 mg/kg) was given IV to a group New Zealand white rabbits; blood glucoses were tested 48 hours later and found to be >300 mg/dl. Four rabbits were treated with daily insulin (2.5 units NPH IM/day), six were not treated. Fourteen days later, the animals were exsanguinated, blood collected using acid citrate dextrose as the anticoagulant and platelets were isolated and washed. Platelets were incubated with ^{51}Cr and adhesion to collagen coated glass was measured.

Platelets obtained from the rabbit with DM adhered less (30,341 ± 4951 platelets/mm^2) than those obtained from normal rabbits (49,437 ± 5231). Platelets from the DM rabbits treated with I were more adherent than normals (58,795 ± 5584). The differences are statistically significant at the $p < 0.01$ level. These results indicate that insulin treatment markedly increases the platelet adhesiveness in the insulin-deficient diabetic rabbit. Hyperinsulinemia as well as hyperglycemia may have significant effects on platelet adhesion and may be an important factor in the development of vascular disease.

GENETICS & IMMUNOLOGY

319

HLA DRW_3, DRW_4 and Islet Cell Antibodies (ICA) in Insulin Dependent Diabetes Mellitus (IDDM) in Israel. M. KARP*, C. BRAUTBAR, S. ASSA, Z. LARON*, R. ZAMIR, I. COHEN, C. LEVENE and T. COHEN, Tel Aviv and Jerusalem, Israel.

The association between HLA antigens and IDDM is not uniform over populations. Also the relationship between ICA and the development of IDDM in genetically susceptible individuals is not clear. 72 randomly selected IDDM patients (41 Ashkenazi; 31 non-Ashkenazi) and 7 multiplex families with more than one IDDM patient were studied. The Ashkenazi patients showed an increase in B8 frequency - 32% (RR=4.3; P=0.09 vs. Ashkenazi control). Non-Ashkenazis showed low B8 frequency - 6% (P=NS vs. non-Ashkenazi controls). Both groups showed an increase in DRW_3 (Ashkenazi: 44% vs. 18%. RR=3.6; P=0.006. Non-Ashkenazi: 71% vs. 10%; RR=17.8; $P<2x10^{-6}$) and in DRW_4 (Ashkenazi 83% vs. 46%; RR=5.0; P=0.0009; non-Ashkenazi: 78% vs. 26%; RR=10.2; $P<3x10^{-5}$). Seven families with 20 affected and 23 healthy children were studied. Of the 13 non proband affected sibs 8 (62%) shared both haplotypes and 3 (23%) one haplotype with the proband. Of the 23 healthy sibs 8 (35%) shared the same haplotype as the proband (x^2=7.25; P<0.01). ICA were found in 2 of the patients and none in the healthy sibs and their parents, whereas 14/15 of newly diagnosed IDDM patients had positive ICA. It is concluded that DRW_3 and DRW_4 are predisposing to IDDM with an increase in B8 only in Ashkenazis. ICA might not serve as a diabetes marker in healthy sibs of multiplex families with an IDDM proband.

320

Two subsets of Insulin Dependent Diabetes (IDD): Differentiation by Immune Responses C.M. ASPLIN, P. HOLLANDER, R. PECORARO, J. HANSEN, J. CROSSLEY, M. COONEY, J. BRODSKY, R. WARD, and J.P. PALMER, Seattle, Wa.*

To identify subsets of IDD, we have measured antibodies (AB) to insulin (I), pancreatic polypeptide (PP), glucagon (G) and somatostatin (SRIF) cross sectionally in 90 randomly selected I treated diabetics and in addition have also determined histocompatability antigens (HLA), islet cell antibody (ICA) titer and AB titer to Coxsackie (Cox) B3, B4, B5 prospectively in newly diagnosed IDD. All 90 I treated diabetics had AB-I, 42 had AB-PP, 9 had AB-G and none AB-SRIF. There was no relationship of AB-I and/or AB-PP with any clinical characteristic, including glycosylated hemoglobin concentration, except AB-PP negative patients had a shorter mean duration of I therapy (5.5 vs 14.3 years; p<.01) and presented more often with glycosuria than ketoacidosis (p<.01). 37 children were studied prospectively for 1 year or longer after starting I therapy, 26 at exactly one year. AB-PP was detected in 49%. 7 of the 26 IDD had a low AB-I response, were also AB-PP negative (p<.01) and were non-HLA B8 (p<.05). The AB-PP status was not related to HLA, ICA, Cox B5 or mode of onset of IDD, but 11 IDD classified as hyporesponders to Cox B3/4 tended (p<.01) to be AB-PP negative. Conclusions: (A) AB-I, AB-PP and AB-G have no beneficial or detrimental clinical effects when evaluated cross sectionally (B) we have identified 2 subsets of IDD characterized by (1) low AB-I, absent AB-PP and non-HLA-B8 (2) low AB-PP and low AB-Cox B3/4.

321

Gene Dosage and Susceptibility to Insulin-Dependent Diabetes. RICHARD S. SPIELMAN, LESTER BAKER,* and CHESTER ZMIJEWSKI, Philadelphia, Pa.

Most studies of shared HLA haplotypes among sib pairs with insulin-dependent diabetes (IDDM) have focused on only two extreme possibilities for the mode of inheritance of susceptibility: dominant or recessive. The analyses have been controversial, and contradictory conclusions have been reached from the same data. We have analyzed the HLA data on affected sibs, allowing for the possibility that although heterozygotes for a susceptibility allele are susceptible, a second "dose" of the allele confers increased susceptibility (penetrance). The analysis incorporates data on recurrence in relatives, and allows for recombination between HLA and the susceptibility locus, S.

With either our own data on 31 IDDM sib pairs or a sample of 164 assembled by pooling with published data, the maximum likelihood estimate of the two-dose penetrance is 71%, of the one-dose, 6.5%. The hypothesis of differential penetrance according to gene dosage provides a significantly better explanation than either simple dominant or simple recessive inheritance.

Estimates of the recombination fraction between HLA and S are very sensitive to the proportion of affected sib pairs sharing neither HLA haplotype, which varies considerably among the samples pooled. With the pooled data the recombination fraction is estimated as 3%, but in view of the strong associations with particular HLA alleles seen in population data, this should probably be considered an upper limit.

322

The HLA D Region Of Chromosome 6 In Diabetes Mellitus. JOSE BARBOSA*, FRITZ H. BACH, University of Minnesota, Minneapolis, Minnesota.

We have studied patients with insulin dependent diabetes (IDD) and maturity onset hyperglycemia of the young (MOHY) using homozygous typing cells (Dw), serology (DRw), and primed lymphocyte testing (PLT).

Antigens	Cont. (400)	IDD Mult. (#17)‡		IDD Rand.‡(#38)	
	%	%	RR††	%	RR††
Dw2	18	0†	.1	0(?1)†	.06
Dw3	15	44†	5	39†	4
Dw4	12	56†	8	50†	7
Dw3/4	2	19†	11	13†	7

‡Probands of selected multiplex and random families; ††Relative Risk; †$p < .02$.

Similar results obtained for DRw antigens and the risk was also increased for DRw 4/4. PLT cells prepared against the DRw2-Dw2 haplotype and Dw2 alone were used to test 9 IDD patients, 4 of whom were B7+ (in linkage disequilibrium with Dw2). None of the diabetic cells gave strong restimulation, or expressed serologically as DRw2. PLT with T cell clones prepared against Dw2 is underway. No heterogeneity of the RR's was found for age at onset or family history. MOHY patients had normal frequencies of all D antigens. The most striking finding is the apparent absence of Dw2(DRw2) in IDD; this may reflect a genetic protective factor or the dysmetabolism of IDD. (AM20729, NO1-HD-82846)

323

Detection of Soluble Immune Complexes in Patients with Diabetes Mellitus (D.M.) G. VIRELLA, H. WOHLTMANN*, J. SAGEL, MARIA F. LOPES-VIRELLA, M. KILPATRICK, and J. COLWELL*, Charleston, S.C.

A series of 154 diabetic patients has been studied for the presence of soluble immune complexes (IC) using five different screening techniques. The percentage of positive results was maximal (68%) using a technique specific for insulin-anti-insulin IC. Free anti-insulin antibodies were detected exclusively in insulin-treated D.M.; insulin-anti-insulin IC were found in patients with free anti-insulin antibodies, but also in two patients that had no record of previous insulin administration. The agreement between methods was not perfect, ranging from a minimum of 41% to a maximum of 69%. To express numerically the overall degree of positivity in individual patients, we calculated IC scores by giving a value of 0 to a negative result, 1 to a borderline result, and 2 to a positive score. The added up score was then divided by the theoretical maximum score (no. of tests x 2), a score of 1 meaning across the board positivity and 0 meaning across the board negativity. With this approach, the percentage of patients with high rates of positivity (scores higher than 0.66) is 19%. No significant correlations were seen between IC scores and duration of disease, type of diabetes, insulin dosage, and indexes of metabolic control, but significant correlations were found between IC scores and abnormal proteinuria ($p < 0.001$) and clinical evidence of microangiopathy ($p < 0.005$). (Supported by the Kroc Foundation, the S.C. state appropriation for Research, and VA Institutional Research Funds).

324

Isolation and Characterization of Soluble Insulin-Anti-Insulin Immune Complexes Formed In Vitro and In Vivo in Sera from Patients with Diabetes Mellitus, J.M. KILPATRICK, and G. VIRELLA, Charleston, S.C. (Introduced by * J. Colwell).

The formation of insulin anti-insulin IC in vitro was studied by adding ^{125}I-insulin to the sera of patients with anti-insulin Ab; insulin co-precipitated with proteins with 5% polyethylene glycol, was eluted in the high-molecular-weight fractions when the precipitated material was fractionated by gel filtration, and remained bound at neutral pH when these fractions were submitted to affinity chromatography on protein A-Sepharose. When the bound immune complexes were recovered by acid elution and immediately filtered through a Sephadex G-50 column equilibrated with the same acid buffer, free antigen (^{125}I-insulin) and antibody were recovered. This antibody, after neutralization, showed binding capacity when remixed with radioiodinated insulin. This protocol was applied to a serum that gave positive results in several screening methods for soluble IC. Insulin was detected by radioimmunoassay in the high-molecular-weight fractions separated from the 5% polyethylene glycol precipitate and in the fractions retained by Protein A. Anti-insulin antibodies were recovered after acid gel filtration in Sephadex G-50. Negative results were obtained with a serum with no soluble IC. These results prove that soluble IC can be formed easily in sera containing anti-insulin antibodies and can be recovered from sera of diabetic patients containing native IC. (Supported by The Kroc Foundation and by the state of South Carolina Appropriation for Research).

325

Frequency of Lewis Negative Blood Group Not Increased in Insulin-Dependent Diabetes. LESTER BAKER,* RICHARD S. SPIELMAN, HAROLD A. WURZEL, and CHESTER M. ZMIJEWSKI, Philadelphia, Pa.

It has been reported (Diabetologia 15:33, 1978) that the Lewis negative red blood cell phenotype (Le a-b-) is significantly more frequent in diabetics, regardless of insulin dependence, than in controls. We have tried to confirm this finding by typing the red cells of 22 unrelated Caucasian insulin-dependent diabetics, 13 of whom have a parent, sib, or offspring affected with IDDM. The distribution of phenotypes found is: Le (a+b-) - 6; Le (a-b+) - 15; Le (a-b-) - 1. The frequencies of the three phenotypes are 27%, 68%, and 5% respectively and do not differ significantly between diabetics with and without affected first degree relatives. These proportions are in excellent agreement with results from a large control sample (Amer. J. Phys. Anthrop. 9: 115, 1951) where the phenotype frequencies were found to be 22%, 72%, and 6% respectively. In various Caucasian control series, the frequency of Le (a-b-) has ranged from 6% to 18%. Thus our findings provide no evidence for an increased frequency of Le (a-b-) in IDDM.

326

Metabolic Features Associated with Specific HLA Types(B8, B15, B18)and Sharing of Haplotypes with a Diabetic Sibling. TJ ORCHARD, BS RABIN, DK WAGENER, M SALAS, M BANKS, AL DRASH.Pittsburgh PA.

Siblings, irrespective of how many HLA haplotypes they share with a diabetic brother or sister, showed similar glucose tolerances after a standard oral glucose load(1.75 gm/kg body weight 75 grams maximum)in a study of relatives of insulin dependent diabetics. However, the peak insulin value increased($p<0.05$)with the number of haplotypes shared(61.4 uU/ml no shared haplotypes n=24, 68.8 uU/ml one shared haplotype n=42 and 74.3 uU/ml both haplotypes shared n=17). The insulin ratio 15 min.: peak(15:PKI)decreased with the number of shared haplotypes as did the 3 hour insulin: glucose area ratio. There was a suggestion of reduced growth hormone and glucagon suppression during the OGTT and delayed growth hormone peaks in those siblings sharing both haplotypes with their diabetic sibling. Unlike other workers, however, we found no difference in fasting glucose and insulin values according to the number of shared haplotypes. HLA B15 positive relatives(parents & siblings n=25)had higher glucose levels during an OGTT(3 hr area=116)than B15 negative relatives(n=198 3 hr area=86.2 $p<0.05$). B8 positive relatives had lower growth hormone peaks than B8 negative relatives($p<0.05$)whilst B18 positive relatives had lower glucagon levels throughout the oral glucose tolerance test. Analysis for confounding variables is in progress. Overall, of 266 relatives tested, 13(9 males & 3<16 yrs) had "impaired glucose tolerance"(IGT) & both 2(both males)"diabetes"(NIH Criteria). Early results suggest that IGT was associated with a decreased 15:PKI ratio and delayed insulin peaks.

327

Interferon Effect on Encephalomyocarditis Virus Infection of Cultured Mouse Pancreatic Beta Cells. G. WILSON, S. BELLOMO, P. BONAZINGA AND J. CRAIGHEAD, Burlington, Vt. (Introduced by E. DANFORTH*, Burlington, Vt.)

The M variant of encephalomyocarditis virus (EMC) produces beta cell necrosis and insulitis associated with a diabetes-like disease in some strains of mice; other strains are relatively resistant to the diabetogenic effect of this virus, although insular lesions occur. The basis for the unique beta cell tropism of the M variant and the basis for the difference between mouse strains remains to be determined.

The interferon system is the earliest-appearing of the known host defenses and is believed to be central to the control of many viral infections. This study was undertaken to investigate the role of interferon in modulating beta cell injury induced by the M variant of EMC *in vitro*. Initial work revealed that the M variant is a potent inducer of interferon in mouse fibroblast cells compared to other nondiabetogenic strains of EMC. Interferon was added to monolayer beta cell cultures 24 hours before infection and changes in the insulin release and virus production were determined periodically to assess its effect. These experiments showed that beta cell damage and virus replication are delayed, but not prevented, in cultures derived from both diabetes-prone CD-1 and resistant C57BL/6 mice. Thus, interferon *in vivo* might act in concert with other host defense mechanisms to influence susceptibility or resistance of beta cells to viral infection.

Supported by NIH grant #PHS R01 20790.

HEALTH CARE DELIVERY

328

Dietitians' Practices and Problems. J. WYLIE*, R. MAZZE, S. ROSEN, New York, N.Y.

One hundred and forty dietitians/nutritionists were surveyed to determine: (1) diabetic patient assessment practices, (2) desired changes in practice and, (3) obstacles to change. A self-administered protocol consisting of 20 variables was used.

Forty-five percent of the respondents indicated that they did not assess the patient's knowledge of breakdown of macronutrients. One-fourth did not include evaluation of the patient's understanding of the pathophysiology of diabetes. In contrast, more than 95% of the respondents assessed dietary and weight history, attitude toward diet, and physical activity.

Greater than 50% of the dietitians indicated that they were dissatisfied with their current practice because of need for more complete patient assessment and counseling, lack of patient education material and need to organize patient groups. The obstacles to resolving these problems were identified as: (1) lack of staff (62%), (2) lack of funding (43%), (3) inability to obtain third party payments for counseling (32%), and, (4) lack of both nursing and dietary department support (23%). Further analysis revealed that 75% of those surveyed worked within hospital or nursing home dietary departments in which they indicated nutrition counseling was only a small portion of their overall patient care responsibility.

On the basis of this pilot study as well as three years training experience in a Diabetes Research and Training Center, we conclude that the systemic defects in hospital-based nutritional services resulting in compartmentalized care may contribute to inadequate health care of the diabetic.

329

Relationship Between Personality Characteristics, Demographic Data, and the Physiological Control of Adult Insulin-Dependent Diabetics. *JANICE JENKINS and CONNIE WEBB, Opelika, Al.

Several reports have suggested the relationship between personality traits and demographic data of diabetics. The purpose of this study was to identify personality characteristics of adult insulin-dependent diabetics who were in good plasma glucose control (GPGC= PG averaged 200mg% or less for the preceeding 12 months; no more than 10% $<$50mg% and no more than 10% $>$250mg%) and those in poor plasma glucose control (PPGC= PG averaged 200mg% or more for preceeding 12 months, and/or more than 10% $\leq$50mg%, and/or more than 10% $\geq$250mg%).

Forty adult insulin-dependent diabetics who were outpatients (17 in GPGC and 23 in PPGC) were given Jackson's Personality Research Form which measured 20 personality characteristics. The two groups differed statistically only in Abasement, $p < .05$. No statistical differences were found comparing quantitative variables (age, educational level, duration of diabetes, insulin dosage, and number of insulin injections/day) and qualitative variables (marital and employment status, sex, race, and complications of diabetes).

In conclusion, personality characteristics, qualitative, and quantitative variables were not shown to have statistical significance in relation to the degree of physiological control of adult insulin-dependent diabetic outpatients.

330

Specialty Variability in the use of Oral Hypoglycemic Agents (OHA) in a 340-Bed Community Hospital. STEPHEN E. DIPPE* and BARRY BARNES, Scottsdale, Arizona.

During a 5-month period, July-November 1977, 166 patients (pts.) with diabetes were identified through a medical records search. Diabetes was the primary diagnosis in 56 pts. and a secondary diagnosis in 110 pts. Insulin was used to treat 50% of the pts., OHA 16%, diet or no treatment the remainder. Family Practitioners (FP) cared for 56% of all diabetes, Internal Medicine (IM) 40% and surgeons 13%. One case was treated with insulin by a pediatrician. FP used OHA in 20% of their pts. compared to 24% for surgeons and 9% for IM.

A pharmacy records search was also completed during the same period. A total of 49 pts. received OHA (24-chlorpropamide, 12-tolazamide, 9-tolbutamide, 4-acetohexamide). The diagnosis of diabetes was never recorded at discharge for 17 (35%) pts. who received OHA, led by surgeons with 7/15 (45%) pts. followed by FP 7/22 (32%) pts. and IM 3/12 (24%) pts.

There was considerable difference in the choice of OHA with 12/15 (80%) surgical pts. receiving chlorpropamide as compared to only 8/22 (35%) for FP pts. and 4/12 (34%) for IM pts. FP prescribed 75% of the tolazamide.

In conclusion, surgeons used OHA more frequently than either FP or IM. The preferred OHA by surgeons was chlorpropamide. Also, 17 pts. received OHA for diabetes but were discharged without the diagnosis of diabetes. Diabetes is frequently not recorded at discharge even though treatment is given.

331

The Prevalence of Diabetes in Kentucky. S. LEICHTER*, C. HERNANDEZ, A FISCHER, P.H. COLLINS*, Lexington, Kentucky

We studied the prevalence rates (PR) of active, diagnosed cases of diabetes (ADM) and "borderline" diabetes (BDM) among 34,126 people, or 1% of the Kentucky population, in 7 counties. Prevalence rates of ADM were 2.08 cases/100 people $<$ 17 years of age, and 19.33 cases/1000 people, 17-45 years of age. Analysis of reported national prevalence data and this Kentucky data disclosed an exponential increase in prevalence by age ($r= 0.99$, $p<0.01$). A linear correlation was noted between the rate of increase in prevalences in Kentucky between the two age groups (AG) studied and the $\log_e$ [unemployment rates X 100] for the populations of these counties ($r=0.8737$, $p<0.025$). Therefore, the Kentucky PRs among specific AGs were estimated from linear plots of $\log_e$ [PR] versus AG and may be predicted by the formula:

$$\log_e [PR] = \frac{\log_e [\text{unemployment rate} \times 100] + 0.957}{31.57}(AG) - 0.62$$

Using this formula and the raw data, the prevalence of active cases of ADM was 150,721 or 4.4% of the population. BDM was estimated to affect 83,324 persons, or 2.4% of the population. PR in rural areas was up to 3 fold higher than urban areas. In total, both forms of diabetes afflicted 6.8% of the population. We conclude that: 1). the prevalence of diabetes in certain rural areas of Kentucky is extremely high; 2). the prevalence is related in part to unemployment rates; 3). unemployment rates may be a "marker" for other, causal socioeconomic factors, not understood clearly, at present.

332

Perceived Benefits of Interaction Among Diabetics in a Hospital Based Education Program. S. SARVER and M. HOWARD, Ann Arbor, Mi. (Introduced by C. BARNETT*).

A discharge evaluation was administered to 73 Michigan Diabetes Research and Training Center (MDRTC) patients over 7 months to gather information on what patients perceived as benefits of their hospital experience. The questionnaire contained 9 items rated on a 4-point scale and 4 open-ended statements. Rated items included improvement in knowledge, satisfaction with care, strengthened coping abilities and need for length of hospitalization. The open-ended statments required written information about the best and worst aspects of the program. The health care team was reported to be a "best experience" by 39% of the respondents. 21% felt that the classes were most valuable and 20% responded that sharing ideas and experiences about diabetes with other patients was most beneficial.

Traditionally, patient education is planned and delivered through classes, individual contact with care givers and use of audiovisual and printed materials. The members of the health team are recognized as the people sharing information with the patient and family, thereby providing care. Education and care are usually not thought of as being delivered by other patients. Group interaction may be an overlooked benefit in most clinical settings.

333

Perception of Health Status & Use of Health Care Among Adult Diabetics, J.J. KRONENFELD, M.G. ORY, R. STERMAN, Birmingham, Alabama.

153 diabetics who were receiving care at the Diabetes Hospital Outpt. Clinic at the Univ. of Al. in Birmingham from Oct. 1978 to Jan. 1979 were interviewed in their home to obtain information about perceptions of their health status & their health care use. The majority of the pts. (91.5%) were adult onset diabetics & 62% of these were currently insulin dependent. 2/3 of the pts. had been diagnosed at least 3 years. This group of diabetics is relatively old (median age = 53.5), predominantly female (69%), and heavily black (62%). Education levels are fairly low (40% have not graduated from high school) and the median income is $6500 a year.

This group of pts. had a number of other chronic health problems beyond diabetes. Only 9% reported no other health problems while the mean for the sample was 2.8 health problems. Similarly, the mean number of disability days was 43 & over 25% had 30 or more disability days. When asked to evaluate their own health status, 54% described it as fair or poor. As expected, these pts. visit the physician regularly on an outpt. basis (mean number of physician visits per year = 6,S.D.=4). Despite the presence of other chronic problems, 86% of their outpt. visits are related to diabetes. Pts. with more chronic conditions or more disability days use more health care in general, although a lower proportion of their outpt. care is diabetes related. Blacks use more health care than whites & a slightly higher proportion of their health care is diabetes related, partially because whites in this study have more chronic conditions than do blacks.

334

Limited Usefulness of Urine Glucose Testing in Diabetes Mellitus. MAVIS VERRONNEAU, R. J. GARDINER,* and H. ALEYASSINE,* Montreal, Canada.

We evaluated the usefulness of urine glucose testing by monitoring the levels of fasting plasma glucose (FPG), glycosylated hemoglobin (GHb) and urine glucose in more than 600 adult ambulatory diabetic patients. The percentage of GHb was measured by both cation exchange column chromatography and gel electrophoresis. Plasma and single-voided urine specimens, collected before breakfast, were tested on the Beckman glucose analyzer using a glucose oxidase reagent. Simultaneous urine glucose testing was also carried out with the use of Clinitest and Labstix. The results have shown that in more than two-thirds of the patients the presence of glucose in urine was undectable (less than 100 mg%) by Labstix and Clinitest methods. This finding was also confirmed by the glucose analyzer. However, in 70% of these patients with "negative" glycosuria, GHb and FPG values were above the normal range. Elevated GHb and FPG were also observed in all subjects with "positive" glycosuria, with the exception of 4 patients. Thus, the overall analysis of the results revealed that only one-third of the diabetic subjects showed evidence of glycosuria, while in 80% of the patients elevated FPG and GHb levels were present.

It is concluded that with the ready availability of FPG and GHb tests in the outpatient diabetic clinics, the routine glucose testing of urine should be abandoned since in the majority of the patients the absence of glycosuria tends to create the false assurance of satisfactory blood glucose control.

335

An Analysis of All Recognized Cases of Maternal Diabetes in South Carolina, 1978. L.C. DEEB,* Atlanta, Georgia, C.W. GOLLMAR, and F.C. WHEELER, Columbia, South Carolina

Charts of all women and their infants discharged from S.C. hospitals in 1978 with a diagnosis of delivery and diabetes (DM) were reviewed.

DM occurs in 4.7/1000 births; white and black rates are 4.4 and 5.2; insulin treated DM rates are 2.1 in whites and 2.3 in blacks. Age-specific rates in whites increased from 1/1000, ages 15-19, to 12.3, ages 35-44; and in blacks increased from 1.4, ages 15-19, to 24, ages 35-44. Rates of DM and ITDM in urban and rural areas are comparable; and are similar to those found by the national collaborative perinatal study.

Perinatal DM mortality rates (PMR) are 56/1000 for whites and 85 for blacks as compared to 19 in all whites and 31.5 in all blacks. ITDM PMR are 103 in whites and 145 in blacks. All 16 DM perinatal deaths were stillbirths. There were no neonatal deaths. Fourteen of these were in ITDM.

Obstetricians provide primary care in 96% of DM cases. 61% of ITDM and 29% of those treated on diet alone were delivered by caesarean section. Congenital anomalies were noted prior to discharge in 6.7% of DM births. None were fatal. Glucose was measured in 44% of the infants in hypoglycemia (<30) was found in 45%.

This study provides a statewide population-based description of recognized maternal diabetes and its care and outcomes.

HEALTH EDUCATION

336

Effect of Camping Experience on Diabetic Youngsters' Attitudes Toward Diet. MARION J. FRANZ, Minneapolis, Mn.

Attitudes toward dietary management of diabetes were surveyed in 125 youngsters before, shortly after, and six months after each spent one week at a camp for diabetic children. Parents also were surveyed after six months.

Of the 125 campers, 109 (87%) said they had a meal plan (diet) for use at home, while 16 (13%) replied they did not. 85% use the exchange system for meal planning.

The following conclusions were drawn:

1. Campers feel diet is important: 32% rated diet extremely important before camp, compared with 46% after camp ($p > 01$).
2. 81% said they understood their diet well before camp, compared with 89% after ($p > .02$). Also 58% said they understood diet better after camp.
3. 83% of the campers said they usually or always followed their diets. Parents agreed.
4. 69% of the campers did not find following a meal plan difficult, and 77% said their plans were ok or flexible. 81% did not perceive diet as a family problem. Parents agreed.
5. 72% reported dietitians as primary providers of instruction; 27% relied on a doctor. When the dietitian was the instructor, 34% felt diet was extremely important and 43% understood diets well; with physician instructors, corresponding figures were 27 and 21%. ($p > .05$).
6. Campers believe diet is more important and understand meal planning better when diets are reviewed every three months instead of at intervals of one year or longer.

337

The Development of a Statewide Model Outpatient Diabetes Education Program. ROBERT M. ANDERSON, ROBERT W. GENTHNER, and MARIA ALOGNA.*

In early 1978 the Diabetes Control Project (DCP) a joint project of Medical Care Development, Inc. and the State of Maine Department of Human Services, surveyed Maine's acute care hospitals and found only four comprehensive outpatient diabetes education programs.

During 1979 the DCP formed a task force of diabetes educators which reviewed local and national diabetes outpatient education programs. Most programs that were studied focused on skills and knowledge and lacked a coordinated approach to addressing the psychosocial aspects of having diabetes. The DCP and the Task Force designed a model outpatient diabetes education program that utilized a counseling approach for influencing behavior. The program has a comprehensive format for providing diabetics and their families with knowledge and skills and also has a systematic approach for assessing and influencing attitudes. The program contains individual assessment, one-to-one and group classes, and follow-up visits.

The nursing and dietary program instructors needed substantial training in knowledge of diabetes, one-to-one interviewing, and classroom teaching skills. Therefore, the DCP developed and presented a week-long teaching skills workshop which was attended by 23 nurses and 14 dieticians. The workshop was staffed by a diabetes nurse specialist, a psychologist and an educator.

The program is being implemented in over 25 sites throughout Maine (serving 80% of the diabetic population)and is being systematically evaluated using a revised version of Leona Miller's Assessment Questionnaire.

338

CONTINUITY OF CARE IN AN OBSTETRIC/DIABETIC PROGRAM Suren, J.V.*, Holland, N., Papatheodorou, N.H. Los Angeles, CA. The Obstetrics (OB) & Diabetes (D) Programs of UCLA Med. Cr. combined efforts to form the OB/D Program. It's purpose is to provide continuity of care, patient (pt) participation in care delivery, optimal psychological support to the pregnant diabetic pt. To promote continuity, the OB nurse specialist follows the pt. in the clinic(cl), through hospitalizations &delivery. The D. Program team(nurse specialist & social worker) does the same with the addition that once referred to the D. Cl., they have ongoing contact with the pt. there also. Using the ADA AADE Guidelines for education of Diabetics, team approach, & concept of Alliance, the OB/D Program developed 1. a standard care plan, 2.checklist for education & counceling documentation & 3.audit criteria. The three documents include Survival Level D. knowledge & skills, an attitude assessment about the pregnancy & the overlay of D., & a detailed itemization of cost, risks, & inconvenience compared to a noncomplicated pregnancy. The checklist is retained in the chart as an information vehicle for both in pt. & cl. staff. Unique aspects of the program are 1. utilization of pts. as teachers about D. selfcare, pregnancy information, preparationfor procedures, & to give psychological support.2.pts continue self care in hospital & in clinic 3.pts see the same care providers both in & out of hospital 4. the cl. is conducive to active exchange & offers emotional support 5. although hospitalized, the pt can still attend cl.for this prupose.
Besides profiding quality care, the pts.need for psychological support are of equal importance in the OB/D Program. Details to be discussed.

339

INTERDISCIPLINARY MANAGEMENT OF TEMPORARY DIABETES IN LEUKEMIC CHILDREN. Suren, J.V., Wiley, F.M., Papatheodorou, N.H. Los Angeles, Ca. L-Asparaginase (L-Asp) & Prednisone, drugs used in the induction phase of Acute Lymphocytic Leukemia (A.L.L.), may cause secondary, temporary diabetes mellitus (D.M.) When D.M. occurs, the child's & family's focus is usually on the life threatening malignancy, not on the inconvenience nor implications of the transient D.M. In light of this, the oncology & D.M. Nurse Specialists, & the D.M. Social Worker of the UCLA Med. Ctr. collaborated to develop an approach & education program specific to the needs of these children & their families. The treatment of the A.L.L. starts within days of diagnosis; if D.M. occurs, it usually ensues within 2 wks. The cancer chemotherapy invariably causes severe neutropenia. The consequent increased susceptability to infections necessitates careful control of the blood glucose levels with insulin therapy. When the L-Asp & Prednisone are discontinued as the child achieves remission, the D.M. promptly recedes. The educational perspective is on maintaining reasonable blood glucose with the least inconvenience. The usual juvenile D.M. teaching manuals are inappropriate because tight control for possible prevention of long range complications has no relevance with transient D.M. Only the Survival Level of the ADA/AADE Guidelines for Education of Diabetics is taught. Frequent phone monitoring of the D.M. is necessary: as it recedes, the insulin requirements decrease. In most cases, the family emotionally concentrates on the life threatening A.L.L., & does not have the concerns that preoccupy families with the usual juvenile D.M. Discussion will focus on these unique needs and strategies for their management.

340

The Organization and Operation of a Summer Camp for Children with Diabetes Mellitus. MARCIA FRANK* and ROBERT M. EHRLICH,* Toronto, Ontario, Canada.

The Diabetes Association of Ontario (DAO) has been operating a camp for children with diabetes mellitus (DM) for 15 years. Initially a 2 week period was available using facilities and personnel of another camp. This was found to be unsatisfactory. For 9 years at a camp site purchased by the DAO 80 children aged 8-15, in 4, 2 week periods have enjoyed an active program including waterfront activities, canoe tripping, camp craft, and land sports. Medical and dietary supervision is blended into the camp program. Urine glucose is tested 3x per day. Each morning a physician reviews the previous days tests and prescribes insulin. Two physicians, 3 nurses and 3 dieticians are present during each camp period. The health center is equipped to deal with diabetic emergencies. Careful attention to routines allows early detection and treatment of medical problems. In the pre-camp period counsellors are trained to understand DM and deal with hypoglycemia. 50% of the counsellors are former campers. The camp is operated by a lay group from the DAO with help from medical and dietary personnel. Financing is through camp fees, proceeds of an annual lottery, provincial grants and donations. Our experience will be valuable to groups interested in starting a camp for children with DM.

341

Response to Recruitment: Fear of Long Term Complications. G. Lauger, A. Miraglio and F.K. Thorp,* Chicago, IL

Studies have shown that the fear component of the Health Belief Model increases compliance to appointment-keeping and a variety of therapeutic regimens. Fear of long term complications from diabetes can be used as a method to change health behaviors, but the effect of such an approach on personal adjustment and long range compliance is unknown. Two levels of fear were used in letters sent to parents and children with insulin-dependent diabetes being recruited for a patient education study in the pediatric clinic facility of the University of Chicago Diabetes Training and Research Center. Although identical in most respects, one of the two letters mentioned specific, unsuspected complications resulting from diabetes and was written with an urgent tone. Effects of the fear component on the willingness to make and keep the clinic visits will be described. Significant background variables will be related to the theoretical construct for patient behavior.

342

Diabetes Mellitus: Importance and Impact of Education During Adolescence. J.W. STEPHENS*, R. KHARDORI, and L. BURKE, Portland, Oregon.

Diabetes mellitus with its inception during the childhood can pose certain frustrating problems both to the family and physician alike. The real problems arise when older children resent their parental supervision and authority. At this point it becomes imperative on part of the treating physician to evaluate the understanding and knowledge of his patient before the care can be entrusted to him without any direct parental supervision. Recent studies have repeatedly emphasized the role of education of diabetic patients and our experience also suggests that well informed patient is less likely to get into acute crisis situations. The role of teaching younger diabetic population does not, however, seem to be always emphasized.

We had an opportunity to study a group of 47 juvenile onset diabetics aged 14-16 years and it was surprising to find how poorly informed some of these youngsters were, and entrusting their care entirely to themselves would have resulted in a major catastrophy. Majority of these kids had not been through any teaching/education program. These kids were completely proficient in measuring insulin and administering it. Apparantly these two parameters alone had been taken in to the consideration by the health professionals providing the health care as sufficient to let their patients assume a full charge. Our interaction with this group before and after formal teaching showed that these youngsters were quite capable of learning the basic aspects of diabetes and that it is important to educate them for good care.

343

Anxiety Response During Clinical Trials Related To The Use Of The Artificial Pancreas.
B. P. CHILDS*, D. W. GUTHRIE*, R. BARNETT, Wichita Kansas

During the clinical field testing for the FDA & Life Science Instruments, Miles Laboratories Inc., of the Biostator continuous glucose Monitor-Controller, it was noted that various patients expressed alterations of anxiety response. This anxiety state appeared to be relieved through the question-answer process. The patient population included children, over the age of ten, & adults with diabetes mellitus. The artificial pancreas was used on adults during labor, delivery, & surgery; & on adults & children to reverse ketoacidosis & to aid in regulation of blood glucose during a 24-hour ± period. This particular study included 20 subjects. Ten subjects were given minimal information & were not subjected to questions by others. The other ten subjects were given optimal information & were present whild others had their questions answered. Spielberger's STATE-trait anxiety inventory was administered on first contact with the patient & was repeated prior to actual attachment of the Biostator. At the end of the control period a knowledge test was administered. Those individuals receiving optimal amounts of information were found to be less anxious than those receiving minimal information.

It was also noted through observation that professionals anxiety decreased as more information was provided & questions answered.

344

Calorie Point System. J.FRIFSEN* Wichita,Kansas

Education in nutrition,through the use of the calorie point system, promotes independence. Then hours of applied nutrition education is included in our 34 hour diabetes education program. The concept of the calorie point system is that 75 calories equal one point. Individuality and flexibility are the basic premises for this method of meal planning. Nutrient education is strongly emphasized with presentations on iron, calcium, vitamins, protein, carbohydrate and fat.

Primary responsibility for nutrient assessment, recording, self-adjustment of calorie level with growth, illness and exercise, are shifted to the patient. The dietitian acts as a consultant in meal-planning and supports the patient with continuing education under the auspices of a physician.

For the person with diabetes, well-educated in timing, portions, and distribution of food intake, the calorie point system can offer flexibility that is important in lifestyles of today. Many of our 600 patients have opted to change from other diet plans to calorie points to meet their need for flexibility in meal planning and continue to stay in optimal control of their diabetes.

345

Determination of Priorities for Community Educational Interventions. J.A.SOCHALSKI, M.L. BOUTAUGH, R.G.HISS, B.G.HELMS, Ann Arbor, MI

A stated aim of the Michigan Diabetes Research and Training Center (M-DRTC) is to identify the educational needs of health professionals providing care to diabetics in Michigan communities. To accomplish this task, information about the current practice behaviors of diabetes care providers was compared to a profile of desired practice behaviors. The data about current practices was collected through a series of interviews with 185 diabetics, family members, and a variety of professionals involved in diabetes care. These interview data were summarized and compiled into statements of need.

A Profile of Ideal Psychosocial Adjustment was also developed, enumerating all desired behaviors in diabetes care. These behaviors were rated by a cross section of health professionals in M-DRTC according to the perceived importance and changeability of each. Those behaviors which had been rated as both important and changeable were compiled and then compared with the list of stated needs generated from the community interviews. A list of "gaps" between current practice behaviors and desired ones were identified. The gaps fell into three categories: professional education, patient education, and health-care delivery issues. Several implications for health professionals were suggested, such as directives for professional education programs, ideas for patient education curriculum development, and an impetus to examine and stimulate development of an interdisciplinary approach to diabetes care.

346

Genesis of a Symposium on Diabetes: A Model of Integrating DRTC Educational Resources. R. KNOPF*, D. MCCLAREN, P. BARR and G. HESS, Ann Arbor, Mi.

The Michigan Diabetes Research and Training Center (MDRTC) has conducted five 2 day Symposia on Diabetes in Michigan communities. The two major purposes of the symposia were to provide a review and update on diabetes topics for health professionals and to link educational resources of the MDRTC to the practice problems of the communities.

The development of these symposia required the collaboration and integration of the resources of three MDRTC core facilities: the Diabetes Center Unit (DCU), Educational Development and Evaluation (EDEV) and Continuing Education and Outreach (CEDO). The DCU is an inpatient/outpatient resource which conducts clinical research, trains health professionals and teaches patients. The DCU developed the symposia content and provided medical expertise as well as the speakers. EDEV designed and developed instructional materials and evaluation instruments. CEDO established communication with community health professionals, performed an initial needs assessments, and executed the logistics of the symposia.

The collaborative efforts among members of the 3 cores permitted clearly defined roles and responsibilities, open communication and cooperation, and responsiveness to course participants. The collaboration developed in this process is being strengthened and has become the basis of several new program initiatives.

A Compliance Score for Diet Histories of Children with Diabetes Mellitus.
A. Miragio, G. Lauger and F.K. Thorp,* Chicago, IL

The analysis and quantifying of food records for diet histories has value in patient assessment, patient education, clinical evaluation and research. At the Pediatrics Nutrition Clinic of the University of Chicago Diabetes Training and Research Center, a method of quantifying and scoring food records was developed for patients with insulin-dependent diabetes mellitus. The method addresses the problems of the distribution of carbohydrates and the total daily intake of carbohydrate, fat and protein.

The method was tested and revised with patient records in the out-patient facility. Validation of the relative weights assigned to the foods was done with in-patients. The concurrent measures were urine sugar tests, plasma glucose and glycosylated hemoglobin levels, dietary records, and direct observation of consumed food. The method was determined to be accurate, valid, and easy to master. The supporting data, a description of the method, and its value in a variety of settings will be presented.

HORMONE ACTION

348

Dietary Management Guidelines for Celiac Diabetes Mellitus. BETTY WEDMAN, Hinsdale, IL.

Four celiac diabetes cases are profiled: 3 female, 1 male; ages 25 to 45 years. Case 1 was diagnosed diabetic when fasting blood sugar showed elevated glucose as contributing factor to recurring vaginal infections. This patient was instructed on traditional diabetic meal plan including milk and wheat products. Continued reduction in carbohydrate level of meal plan was needed to reduce fasting blood glucose to less than 180mg/100ml. Omiting wheat and diary products resulted in significant blood glucose drop and marked reduction in insulin requirements. Case 2 is diabetic male suffering from severe diarrhea which led to small intestinal biopsy. Patient's poor dietery compliance to regime limited blood glucose control. Case 3 is known celiac patient with elevated fasting blood glucose on routine physical following patient complaint of weight loss. Case 4 is celiac patient with increasing hypoglycemic symptoms. Carbohydrate intolerance and low insulin levels noted on semi annual glucose tolerance - insulin assay testing. Diet modifications were adapted to food exchanges. Insulin therapy adjustments and blood glucose decline correlated to dietary adherence. Patient education modalities for diet instructions are outlined.

349

SOME PROPERITES OF A MONOMERIC INSULIN FROM THE PORCUPINE (HYSTRIX CRISTATA)
R. Horuk, T. L. Blundell, London, England; N. R. Lazurus, R. W. J. Neville, D. Stone, Kent, England and A. Wollmer, Aachen, Germany.
Introduced by P. H. Sönksen,* London, England.

This communication reports on the primary structure and unusual properties of a hystricomorph insulin, that of the porcupine (Hystrix cristata). The insulin differs at only 7 amino acid residues from the primary structure of bovine insulin but these substitutions have quite pronounced effects on the aggregation, conformation, and biological properties of the hormone.

On the basis of data from zinc binding experiments, it is suggested that porcupine insulin is incapable of forming zinc insulin hexamers. CD (circular dichroism) studies of the hormone provide further evidence for its inability to self associate and also reveal conformational changes in the three dimensional structure of the molecule. Since all the residues implicated in the formation of dimers and hexamers in bovine insulin are conserved in porcupine insulin its failure to self associate is ascribed to the structural changes in its tertiary structure. These are thought to arise mainly from the substitution B_{22} Arg to Asp, in the primary structure of porcupine insulin, which destroys the B_{22}-A_{21} ion pair implicated in the stabilisation of the tertiary structure of bovine insulin.

Examination of the biological properties of porcupine insulin reveal a discrepancy between receptor binding, 25% and biological activity, 4%, of the hormone previously only shown by hagfish insulin.

350

Insulin Production Rate and Splanchnic Glucose Exchange in Not Insulin Dependent Diabetics. W.WALDHÄUSL*, P.BRATUSCH-MARRAIN, S.GASIC, A.KORN, and P.NOWOTNY, Wien, Austria.

Insulin production rate (IPR) and splanchnic glucose exchange were studied in obese not insulin dependent diabetics (NIDDM, n=20) both in the postabsorptive state and after glucose ingestion (25 g and 100 g). IPR was calculated from splanchnic C-peptide output as reported previously for healthy subjects (Diabetologia 17, 221-227, 1979). The hepatic venous catheter technique was employed.

The obtained data demonstrate in obese diabetics a basal IPR of 33±2 mU/min ($\bar{x}$±SEM) being twofold above normal values ($p < 0.0005$). Following an oral glucose load IPR rose to 7±1.3 U/150 min after ingestion of 25 g, and to 9.9±1.7 U/150 min following 100 g of glucose, which was not different from that reported in healthy controls.

Splanchnic glucose output (SGO) was 133±9 mg/min in NIDDM in the basal state (normal 125±7 mg/min). It rose to 5.1±2.4 g/150 min after 25 g of oral glucose and to 30.6±6.3 g/150 min following 100 g of glucose (ns. vs. normal). Contrary to our findings in normals no relation was found after an oral glucose load between splanchnic glucose retention (SGR: amount of ingested glucose - SGO above basal) and IPR. Surprisingly, three patients displayed an inappropriately high SGR in spite of a low IPR, whereas two had a low SGR associated with an elevated or normal IPR.

We conclude that obese not insulin dependent diabetics may represent a heterogenous group which displays either 1. normal IPR, SGR and peripheral insulin resistance, or 2. elevated or normal IPR, impaired SGR and possibly hepatic insulin resistance.

351

Hyperinsulinism in the Dog: The Metabolic and Hormonal Consequences of Chronic Exogenous Insulin Infusion. A.M. ALBISSER, A. BAHORIC, Y. GORIYA. TORONTO, CANADA.

Glycemic normalization by infused insulin in diabetes is frequently accompanied by hyperinsulinism. To explore the consequences of this state we studied a group of 3 dogs initially as normoinsulinemic (NI) controls and then used a portable pump to establish hyperinsulinemia (HI) after 21 to 56d during which time the insulin infusion rate was escalated to 12mU/min. Diet was constant as was body weight (12.8±0.7kg).

After 5 to 29d of HI the animals were subjected to repeated OGTTs (1g/kg). Comparing NI to HI, we found fasting blood glucose fell from 94±1 to 56±10mg/dl ($p < 0.005$) but rose to similar values at 30min. At 2h it was 40±3mg/dl, significantly lower than fasting in both groups ($p < 0.04$). IRI rose from 10±1 to 29±4uU/ml, was always higher ($p < 0.03$), and the 30min peak was delayed to 108±18min. Fasting IRG rose from 75±5 to 108±18pg/ml ($p < 0.03$), remained constant in NI but fell in HI to 79±12 at 1h and rose to 143±28 at 3h. Lactate levels were not different but pyruvate and alanine levels were lower at all times. FFA and 3-hydroxybutyrate levels were lower and dropped transiently during OGTT.

CONCLUSIONS: exogenous hyperinsulinemia produces chronic asymptomatic hypoglycemia, hyperglucagonemia and atypical insulin secretion with consistent alterations in other fuel substrates in response to oral glucose in the dog.

352

Effect of Insulin on Sodium and Potassium Balance in Normal and Electrolytes-Depleted Dogs. ARTUR CZYŻYK*, MARIANNA BAK, EWA SZCZEPANSKA-SADOWSKA, JANUSZ KRZYMIEN and STANISŁAW KOZŁOWSKI, Warsaw, Poland.

Severe depletion of electrolytes (ED) may occur in uncontrolled diabetes. The purpose of this study was to compare the effect of therapeutic doses of insulin (0.05U/kg/h i.v. in 4% glucose) on plasma concentration (P_{Na} and P_K) and renal excretion ($U_{Na}V$ and U_K) of sodium and potassium in normal (N) and ED dogs. ED was produced by repeated i.v. infusions of 20% mannitol decreasing extracellular sodium content by 13.0±2.7%. In N dogs infusion of insulin transiently increased P_{Na} by 3.1±0.9 mEq/l (n=10, $P < 0.01$) and $U_{Na}V$ by 48.9±17.4 µEq/min ($P < 0.05$), decreased P_K by 0.9±0.1 mEq/l ($P < 0.001$) and U_KV by 13.6±5.4 µEq/min ($P < 0.05$). Resting values of P_{Na}, P_K, $U_{Na}V$ and U_KV were lower in ED than in N dogs. In ED dogs infusion of insulin caused a prolonged elevation of P_{Na} with a peak increase by 4.2±0.8 mEq/l (n=9, $P < 0.001$) a slight decrease in $U_{Na}V$ and no changes in U_KV. P_K decreased by 0.5±0.1 mEq/l. This decrement was markedly lower than in N dogs ($\bar{d}$=0.40±0.14 mEq/l, $P < 0.001$). The results indicate that the effect of insulin on sodium and potassium balance may depend on total body stores of electrolytes.

353

Failure of Gastric Inhibitory Polypeptide (GIP) to Exert Insulin-like Activity on Glucose Metabolism in the Adipocyte. D.L. SEVERSON and S.A. ROSS*, Calgary, Alberta, Canada.

GIP is now recognized as the key insulinotropic hormone released from the small intestine following the ingestion of food resulting in an augmentation of insulin levels and an increased rate of disposal of glucose. GIP has also been demonstrated to increase lipoprotein lipase activity in isolated adipocytes, to inhibit glucagon-induced lipolysis and reduce glucagon-stimulated cyclic AMP levels in the adipocyte. These findings suggest that GIP may have peripheral insulin-like action. Therefore, the effect of GIP, insulin, and GIP plus insulin on rates of glucose oxidation in isolated adipocytes was determined. Adipocytes were obtained from male Sprague Dawley rats and incubated in Krebs-Ringer buffer with U-C^{14}-glucose. The degree of stimulation of glucose oxidation was assessed by the production of $^{14}CO_2$ in the presence of insulin, (varying concentrations from 0-4 ng/ml), with 1 µg/ml of GIP alone, and with GIP added to each of the tested insulin concentrations. Glucose oxidation reached a maximum of 30-fold stimulation with increasing concentrations of added insulin. GIP alone added to the incubation media did not stimulate glucose oxidation and the addition of insulin plus GIP to the incubation medium did not increase the stimulation of glucose oxidation above that already observed with insulin alone. Thus GIP appears to have no influence on glucose metabolism in the isolated adipocyte and its anabolic effects in the adipocyte appear to be confined to fat metabolism only.

354

Do Ocytocin and Insulin Share a Common Post-receptor Mechanism in Rat Adipocytes? DOUGLAS B. MUCHMORE AND CHRISTOPH DE HAËN, Seattle, WA. (Introduced by ALAN CHAIT‡ Seattle, WA)

Like insulin, ocytocin is known to preferentially stimulate glucose-C1-oxidation over glucose-C6-oxidation (EC_{50} around 10^{-9}M), incorporation of glucose into lipids and incorporation of amino acids into proteins, but does so to a lesser extent than insulin. In contrast to insulin, ocytocin reportedly failed to accelerate 2-deoxyglucose uptake or glucose incorporation into glycogen. Since ocytocin and insulin do not compete for binding sites, ocytocin promised a means for separating hexose transport stimulation from other post-receptor events mediated by insulin. However, we now report that ocytocin (5×10^{-7}M) does stimulate 2-deoxyglucose uptake by 60% (cf 500% for insulin) and 3-*O*-methylglucose uptake by 30% (cf 60% for insulin). Low doses of insulin (2.5×10^{-10}M) and maximal doses of ocytocin (5×10^{-7}M) showed additive effects on glucose transport and oxidation as well as intracellular H_2O_2 production. At a slightly higher dose of insulin (2.5×10^{-9}M) the effects were intermediate between those of maximal doses of insulin and ocytocin alone, and at maximal doses of insulin (5×10^{-8}M), insulin dominated. This behavior is characteristic of competition by hormones for a common mechanism. In further support, inhibition of oxidative phosphorylation affected insulin and ocytocin stimulation in the same manner. Like insulin, ocytocin also inhibited β-adrenergically stimulated lipolysis. These findings suggest that while insulin and ocytocin act through separate receptors, they share a common post-receptor mechanism, and differ primarily in intrinsic activity.

355

Plasma Insulin and Glucose Uptake by Muscle in Eviscerated Obese (Zucker) Rats. ORA L. K. SMITH,* New Haven, CT.

Evisceration was used to isolate the peripheral tissues of congenitally fat rats, so that the effects of obesity on insulin stimulated glucose uptake by the intact skeletal muscles could be measured. Evisceration, including functional hepatectomy and nephrectomy, was performed on 11-14 week old female fa/fa fatty or lean Zucker rats. Then glucose uptake was compared by measurement of the rate of disappearance of glucose from the plasma after a single iv load of 50% glucose. It was found that supramaximal doses of up to 1000 mU of regular insulin iv failed to restore uptake in fa/fa preparations to levels found in lean littermates (102 and 147 mg/100 g/h respectively). Additionally, levels of plasma insulin were manipulated over the physiological range by iv infusion. Results showed 1) the level required for maximal stimulation of glucose uptake was raised from 40 in lean to 170 μU/ml in fa/fa preparations. 2) Obesity also suppressed the rate of disappearance of glucose to about 65% of lean (from 39.5 ± 1.80 to 25.8 ± 0.62 mg/100 g/h, $p < 0.0005$) at the lowest concentrations of insulin (lean = 13.4 ± 2.4, fa/fa = 22.2 ± 3.1 μU/ml). Conclusion: The shift in dose response curve suggests there are abnormalities in the insulin receptors, but the findings also indicate that post receptor defects in carbohydrate disposal by muscle can play a major role in the production of insulin resistance in animal models of obesity.

356

Calcitonin lowers circulating levels of both glucagon and glucose in juvenile type diabetics (JOD). ACHIM STARKE, ELMAR KECK, ERNST CHANTELAU, MICHAEL BERGER+ and HORST ZIMMERMANN, Department of Medicine, University of Düsseldorf, West Germany.

Previously, we have shown in normal volunteers that Ca^{++}-infusions inhibit the arginine- and the hypoglycaemia-induced stimulation of glucagon (IRG) -secretion. In this study, the effects of Ca^{++} and calcitonin (CT) were investigated in JOD. In 14 JOD 3 experimental protocols were used: (1) control infusions of saline, (2) infusions of 15 mg Ca^{++} per kg body weight over 2 h, (3) infusions of 4.5 IU salmon calcitonin per kg b.wt. over 2 h. Blood samples were drawn at intervals up to 300 min after the onset of the infusions from a contralateral antecubital vein. Basal IRG (assayed using the antibody 30K) was elevated in JOD (109± 65 pg/ml; normal range 57±15 pg/ml). Plasma calcium rose from 2.2±0.2 to 3.2±0.3 mmol/l during Ca^{++}-infusions and remained constant during saline infusions and fell slightly from 2.15±0.1 to 2.0± 0.1 mmol/l during CT-infusions.

During saline infusions blood glucose (BG) rose slightly (by +9±12% of basal levels), IRG, CT, and C-peptide remained unchanged. Ca^{++}-infusions induced a fall of BG (-23±9%, $p<0.001$) and IRG (-26± 15%, $p<0.001$), CT rose to levels twice normal and C-peptide levels decreased slightly. CT-infusions induced a fall of BG (-26±8%, $p<0.001$) and IRG (-23±6%, $p<0.001$), whereas serum-C-peptide levels remained unchanged.

Conclusion: an increase of circulating CT levels, induced by Ca^{++} infusions or by exogenous CT depress circulating IRG and glucose levels in JOD.

357

Interaction of Cholecystokinin and Glucose on Insulin Secretion from the Perfused Rat Pancreas. MAKOTO OTSUKI, CHOITSU SAKAMOTO, ATSUSHI OHKI, HOSAI YUU. Kobe, Japan.

IRI-releasing effect previously attributed to CCK has been shown to be due to contaminating GIP present in impure preparation of CCK. The present study was undertaken to reinvestigate the effect of CCK and synthetic caerulein (Cn) on IRI release and to demonstrate the interaction of CCK and glucose concentrations on IRI release with paying attention to pancreatic exocrine secretions. The experiments were performed on the isolated and perfused pancreas of Wistar strain male rats weighing about 250 g. CCK and Cn produced a dose-related increase in IRI and exocrine pancreatic secretions in the presence of 50, 100 and 150 mg/dl glucose. The maximally effective doses for the effects on exocrine (CCK: 0.5-10 mU/ml, Cn; 0.05-1 ng/ml) and endocrine (CCK>50 mU/ml, Cn>10 ng/ml) pancreas were quite different in the hypoglycemic state (50 mg/dl). On the other hand, even submaximal dose of CCK (0.1 mU/ml) and Cn (0.01 ng/ml) for the effects on exocrine pancreas could also stimulate IRI release in the presence of 100 and 150 mg/dl glucose. Based on the effects on exocrine responses, these doses were considered to be within the physiological range. The effectiveness of CCK and Cn as insulinotropic agents increased with increasing glucose concentrations. Moreover, pre-perfusion of CCK and Cn led to a significant enhancement of IRI response to a subsequent glucose stimulation.

CONCLUSION: Physiological doses of CCK stimulate IRI release directly and augment IRI response to glucose stimuation. Thus, CCK should be considered as a possible member of the incretin family.

358

Phosphodiesterase activity in human adipose tissue: Findings in starvation and diabetes mellitus. P. ENGFELDT, P. ARNER, and J. ÖSTMAN*, Huddinge, Sweden.

Using Pöchs method the cyclic AMP phosphodiesterase activities (PDE) were essentially determined in segments of adipose tissue, since isolation of fat cells by collagenase procedure results in erroneously low Vmax. The PDE (low and high Km) was like peak level of cyclic AMP (at 10 min.) and rate of glycerol release (2h) correlated to the mean size of the incubated fat cells. In subcutaneous adipose tissue removed from the gluteal and abdominal regions of 10 obese patients submitted to therapeutic fasting for one week, the Vmax of PDE was markedly decreased. The decrease was significantly related to the increase in cyclic AMP level. Similar changes were seen in isolated fat cells. In 7 patients with newly discovered diabetes mellitus adequate treatment was associated with decreased rate of lipolysis and increased PDE in subcutaneous adipose tissue.

The findings suggest that changes in PDE is one major factor in regulating the rate of lipolysis in human adipose tissue.

359

Isolation from Rat Adipocyte Plasma Membrane of a Factor Which Simulates Activation of Pyruvate Dehydrogenase by Insulin. NIRMALA KOTAGAL, FREDERICK L. KIECHLE, DENNIS A. POPP, and LEONARD JARETT,* St. Louis, Mo.

Insulin added to an adipocyte (Ad) plasma membrane (PM) mitochondrial mixture stimulates pyruvate dehydrogenase (PDH) by activation of the phosphatase. A factor from insulin treated Ad and muscle mimics insulin action in the in vitro system. A similar factor (F) now has been isolated from the Ad PM. PM were spun in a microfuge for 40 seconds. A F in the supernatant stimulated PDH in both Ad and hepatic mitochondria. NaF, a phosphatase inhibitor, suppressed this increase in PDH activity. Dichloroacetic acid (DCA), a PDH kinase inhibitor, had no effect on the F's activity in the absence of ATP, but stimulated PDH in the presence of ATP and was additive to the F effect. The F was partially purified by Sephadex G25 chromatography of the supernatant. Absorbance at 230 nm revealed one peak at about MW 1,000-1,500. The eluate was divided into five fractions. The peak was divided into two fractions; fIII and fIV. Only fIV stimulated Ad mitochondrial PDH; by 7.17 ± 0.72 nmole/mg/min in the presence of ATP and by 8.27 ± 0.47 nmole/mg/min in the absence of ATP. NaF and DCA exerted the same effects on fIV's activity as they did on the F in the supernatant. The F isolated from Ad PM is similar to the factor isolated from insulin treated Ad and muscle. These factors have properties suggesting that they function as a second messenger for the rapid intracellular effects of insulin.

360

Comparison of Methods for the Assessment of Insulin resistance. M.S. GREENFIELD*, L. DOBERNE, F. KRAEMER, T. TOBEY, and G.M. REAVEN*.Stanford,Ca

We have quantified insulin resistance by determining steady state plasma glucose (SSPG) and insulin (SSPI) responses during a continuous infusion of epinephrine (Epi), propranolol (Prop), insulin and glucose. Epi and Prop inhibit endogenous insulin release, SSPI levels are similar in all subjects, and SSPG levels provide a direct estimate of insulin sensitivity. The "euglycemic clamp" technique estimates insulin sensitivity by determining the amount of glucose metabolizes (M) in order to maintain euglycemia during a period of exogenous hyperinsulinemia. Although a more complicated procedure, this latter approach avoids the need to infuse Epi and Prop. In order to see if the two techniques provide similar data, we have quantified insulin sensitivity in 25 patients with varying degrees of glucose tolerance. Both methods clearly demonstrated that there was a high degree of correlation between the magnitude of the plasma glucose response to oral glucose and insulin resistance as estimated by either M ($r = 0.56$, $p<0.001$) or SSPG ($r = 0.66$, $p<0.001$). In addition, there was a strong degree of correlation between the two methods ($r = 0.86$, $p<0.001$). Thus, in spite of theoretical questions concerning the use of Epi and Prop, estimates of insulin resistance provided by the simpler SSPG method closely approximate those achieved with the more complicated "euglycemic clamp". Both methods indicated that patients with glucose intolerance have lost normal insulin sensitivity, and that the magnitude of their insulin resistance correlates with the severity of their diabetes.

361

Effects of pH on Hexose Uptake by BHK Fibroblasts V.R. LAVIS*, R. DAVENPORT, and E.R. WEIDMAN*, Houston, Texas

We have previously shown that accumulation of products of glycolysis leads to H^+-mediated inhibition of hexose uptake, when quiescent fibroblasts are cultured in the presence of insulin and 25mM glucose. We now report further studies of the effect of pH on hexose uptake. Culture medium contained 5mM glucose, and was buffered with 15mM HEPES. Hexose uptake was assessed as the initial rate of entry of either [^{3}H]-2-deoxyglucose (2DG) or the nonphosphorylated sugar, [^{3}H]-3-O-methylglucose (3OMG). Basal uptake of both hexoses varied linearly with medium pH over the range 6.5 to 8.0, as did glucose utilization. At pH 6.8, the insulin dose-response curve for stimulation of 2DG uptake was shifted to the right compared to pH 7.7. Insulin stimulation of 3OMG uptake was independent of pH, over the range 6.5 to 8.0. After a shift of medium pH from 6.8 to 7.7 or vice versa, 2DG uptake changed to its new rate gradually, over 4 hrs. Conclusions: Extracellular H^+ ion regulates both glucose transport and phosphorylation, and modulates insulin action on phosphorylation. The slow time course of pH-induced changes in hexose uptake suggests the involvement of biosynthetic and/or degradative processes. These phenomena may play a role in the "insulin resistance" of diabetic ketoacidosis.

362

Improvement of the Insulin Sensitivity in "Brittle" Diabetes After Prolonged Euglycemia Achieved by the Artificial Beta Cell. MARSHALL K. GROSSMAN, ALAN N. ELIAS* and LUBOMIR J. VALENTA*, Irvine, California.

An insulin sensitivity test (IST) has been developed using the artificial beta cell (ABC). Gradually increasing amounts of dextrose such as 100, 200, 300 and 400 mg/min (D100-D400) are infused while euglycemia is maintained by insulin infusion via ABC. The insulin consumption rate (ICR) is then a measure of peripheral insulin sensitivity. In normal euglycemic controls the ICR was <30 at D100, <50 at D200, <70 at D300,and <100 mU/min insulin at D400. Two poorly controlled diabetics were studied. Their initial fasting blood glucose was in the range of 300-600 mg/dl. The blood glucose was maintained for 48 hrs in the range of 100-140 mg/dl by ABC. IST was performed at the beginning and at the end of the 48-hr period. Initially maximum ICR of 920 mU/min failed to maintain euglycemia at D50-D100. Following 24 hrs of euglycemia one of the patients still showed marked insulin resistance, ICR at D100 being 465 mU/min. After 48 hrs of euglycemia the insulin sensitivity in both patients markedly improved so that it was 47 & 175 mU/min respectively at D100, 73 & 181 at D200, 81 & 185 at D300, 103 & 192 at D400. It is concluded that IST using the artificial beta cell is a useful clinical test of peripheral insulin sensitivity. Two poorly controlled diabetics studied demonstrated marked insulin resistance which could be corrected to near normal by prolonged euglycemia. Poor control of diabetes thus can be due, at least in part, to reversible insulin resistance.

363

ß-Endorphin and Leucin-Enkephalin Levels during Stimulation with Glucose and Arginine in the Isolated Perfused Rat Pancreas. G.SACHSE, H.LAUBE, J.SVEDBERG, TH. BREIDENBACH, H.TESCHEMACHER, Giessen, FRG (Introduced by B.WILLMS+, Bad Lauterberg)

Endorphins have been reported to enhance the release of insulin and glucagon in the isolated perfused dog pancreas.By other investigators a supression of insulin by enkephalin was observed.To establish a further involvement of endorphins and enkephalins in the regulation of islet secretion the following studies were carried out in the isolated perfused rat pancreas as described by Sussman et al.without any adjacent organ such as stomach or spleen.The stimulating substances(glucose 5.5 mMol/min.,arginine 25 mMol/min.)were infused for different periods into the cannulated aorta.ß-endorphin,leucin-enkephalin,insulin,and glucagon were measured by radioimmunassay.During stimulation with glucose there was no change in ß-endorphin and leucin-enkephalin levels,during stimulation with arginine,however,there was a significant increase of ß-endorphin levels,and a significant decrease of leucin-enkephalin levels.($p < 0.001$)
These results suggest that ß-endorphin, leucin-enkephalin,and related substances may provide an important and different link between endocrine secretion and metabolism.

364

Role of Glucagon in Insulin-Induced Natriuresis in the Chicken. L.K. NIEMAN, B.R. RENNICK, P.J. DAVIS,* F.B. DAVIS, F.B. CERRA and L. EDWARDS, Buffalo, NY.

Recent observations from this laboratory have defined natriuretic effects of both insulin (I) and glucagon (G) administration in the Sperber model (unanesthetized, intact chicken). Unilateral renal venous infusion of porcine I (120 U/hr) or of chicken I (0.7 U/hr) caused a bilateral 3-4-fold rise ($p < 0.001$) in urinary Na excretion ($U_{Na}V$) and no change in $U_K V$ or blood sugar content. Because these results excluded a direct renal effect of I on $U_{Na}V$ and because G also increased $U_{Na}V$ without influencing $U_K V$, we studied the possibility that the I effect on $U_{Na}V$ was mediated by endogenous G release. Porcine I was infused in the Sperber model, as above, and serum immunoreactive G was measured by RIA with the 30-K antibody. Serum G rose 3-fold ($p < 0.005$) in concert with porcine I infusion and onset of Na diuresis. Infusion of chicken I caused a 10-fold increase in serum G.

The natriuretic effect of I in the chicken contrasts with the anti-natriuretic action of I in mammals. G is natriuretic in both chicken and mammals and the present study indicates that I-induced natriuresis in the Sperber model depends upon I enhancement of endogenous G release.

365

Insulin Stimulates Protein Phosphorylation in Cultured Skeletal Muscle Cells. MICHAEL A. BUSH*, Los Angeles, Ca.

Insulin has been shown to stimulate protein phosphorylation in intact liver and fat cells. If this is an important general mechanism for insulin's action, it should be possible to demonstrate it in insulin's third important target tissue, muscle. Studies in muscle, however, have been hampered by the lack of a suitable isolated cell preparation. We have used the L_6 cultured skeletal muscle cell line for such studies. After growth for 10-14 days in Dulbecco's modified Eagle's medium with 10% fetal calf serum, cells were incubated for 2 hrs. in Krebs-Ringers-Hepes buffer with 100uCi/ml of $^{32}P_i$ and then exposed to insulin. After the incubation they were prepared for SDS polyacrylamide gel electrophoresis, autoradiographs were made, and ^{32}P incorporation estimated by quantitative densitometry.

Insulin stimulated the phosphorylation of only a single muscle cell peptide, that of MW 29,000. This stimulation, 100% over control, was seen at 5 min., was maximal at 20 min. and returned to baseline by 60 min. Half-maximal stimulation was seen with 1mU/ml, which is similar to the amount of insulin required to stimulate ^{14}C-glucose incorporation into glycogen in these cells. The 29K MW peptide was located in the 105,000g pellet which is consistent with either a plasma membrane or microsomal site for this protein.

Summary: Insulin stimulates the phosphorylation of a single peptide in cultured skeletal muscle cells. Thus, insulin-stimulated protein phosphorylation has been shown in all major target tissues for this hormone, and probably represents a crucial mechanism for insulin action.

Hormone-stimulated Phosphorylation of Citrate Cleavage Enzyme. M. ALEXANDER, J. PALMER, E. KOWALOFF and J. AVRUCH.* Boston, MA

In isolated rat hepatocytes, the phosphorylation of citrate cleavage enzyme (CCE) is increased by both insulin and glucagon. We have attempted to define the mechanism of hormone-stimulated phosphorylation of CCE.

CCE purified from ^{32}P-labelled hepatocytes, in the presence of NaF+EDTA, has a ^{32}P content identical to that immunoprecipitated (IP) directly from unfractionated cytosol, indicating complete recovery of ^{32}P through purification. The phosphate content of this enzyme is 1 mole P/500,000g Lowry protein (=1 mole CCE). Insulin (1 mU/ml) induces a 100-200% increase in the ^{32}P content of IP-CCE, whereas glucagon (10^{-8}M) gives a 50% increase. With both hormones, 90% of the initial ^{32}P content is recovered after purification. The phosphate on purified CCE in all cases is entirely acid-stable and localized to a 57 K dalton tryptic fragment, clearly distinguishing it from the acid-labile phosphoenzyme intermediate, which migrates with a 68 K tryptic fragment.

CCE isolated from unstimulated hepatocytes is a substrate for the catalytic subunit of the cAMP-dependent protein kinase. Up to 4 moles of ^{32}P is incorporated/mole CCE. Tryptic digests of ^{32}P CCE phosphorylated by catalytic subunit in vitro exhibit ^{32}P peptides indistinguishable from those observed in tryptic digests of ^{32}P CCE purified from glucagon-treated ^{32}P hepatocytes.

We conclude that glucagon-stimulated phosphorylation of CCE is mediated by the cAMP-dependent protein kinase. Insulin-stimulated phosphorylation is mediated by an as yet unidentified protein kinase.

367

Role of Glucagon in Increasing Precursor Incorporation into Glomerular RNA in Streptozotocin (STZ) Diabetes. F.DUMLER, K.K.VENKATACHALAM, P.CORTES, J.GOLDMAN* and N.W.LEVIN, Detroit, Michigan.

We have shown previously that ^{3}H-orotate incorporation (^{3}Hinc) into glomerular RNA (expressed as % dpm infused incorporated into RNA/mg DNA) is increased in early STZ diabetes (control:0.15% vs diabetic:0.32%) and that hyperglucagonemia may be a major factor in causing this increase (Kidney Int. 16:790; 1979). In the present study we have attempted to separate more clearly the effects of hyperglucagonemia, hypo-insulinemia and hyperglycemia on the increased ^{3}Hinc. Glomeruli were separated from 10-20 pooled rat renal cortices, 48hr after STZ injection, after a 2hr intravenous infusion of ^{3}H-orotate. Three groups of diabetic rats were studied: untreated (D), insulin (.5 u/day) treated (D+I) and insulin (.5 u/day) + glucagon (.86 ug/day) treated (D+I+G). Insulin and glucagon were given as continuous intravenous infusions for 38hr starting 10hrs after STZ. Results are given as mean $\pm$ SEM.

	Plasma Glucose (mg/dl)	Plasma Insulin (uU/ml)	Plasma Glucagon (pg/ml)	% ^{3}Hinc → RNA
D	430 $\pm$ 10	27 $\pm$ 4	280 $\pm$ 33	0.196
D+I	459 $\pm$ 4	51 $\pm$ 5	166 $\pm$ 12	0.172
D+I+G	426 $\pm$ 10	57 $\pm$ 3	290 $\pm$ 37	0.278

^{3}Hinc into glomerular RNA varied directly with plasma glucagon and independently of plasma glucose and insulin levels. These results further support a dominant role for hyperglucagonemia in the altered glomerular RNA metabolism and possibly in the renal hypertrophy of early experimental diabetes.

Characterization of a 25-Hydroxy-1-hydroxylase Assay From Porcine Kidneys to Study Hormone Action. E. MARTIN SPENCER and DAUNA MARSHALL, San Francisco, CA (Introduced by C. Young, San Francisco, CA.)

Clinical reports suggest that diabetics are at risk for osteopenia. In diabetic rats we have found low 1-hydroxylase (1-OHase) activity and others have reported low plasma 1,25-$(OH)_2D_3$ levels. To establish whether insulin or a secondary factor affects 1-OHase activity we have developed a mammalian assay.

Homogenates of porcine cortex (10%) were prepared from a 30 kg pig raised on a normal Ca and P diet. 3 mls in 0.25 M sucrose, 15 mM Tris-acetate, 2.0 mM $MgCl_2$ and 5 mM sodium succinate at pH 7.4 were incubated for 30 min at 37 C with 545 pmol of ^{3}H-25-OH-D_3 (s.a. 0.72 Ci/mmol.) Homogenates were extracted by the method of Bligh and Dyer and chromatographed on Sephadex LH-20 to quantitate ^{3}H-1,25-$(OH)_2D_3$ produced.

Control samples converted approximately 20% of the label to ^{3}H-1,25-$(OH)_2D_3$ and produced 8.2 pmol/min/g. K_m and V_{max} were 0.9 10^{-7} and 12.05 pmol/min/gm. Ca (2.4 mM) decreased 1-OHase activity to 20% of control while insulin (1.2 ug), PRL (5 ug), GH (5 ug) and db-cAMP had no stimulatory effect. Preliminary results suggest that renal slices produce 1,25-$(OH)_2D_3$ and may be superior for testing polypeptide hormone actions.

Summary: A mammalian 1-OHase assay has been developed to test hormone actions.

369

Mechanism of Decreased Glucose Transport Response to Insulin in Enlarged Adipose Cells of Obese Rats: Depletion of the Insulin-Responsive Intracellular Pool of Transport Systems. P.J. HISSIN, E. KARNIELI, and L.B. SALANS,* Bethesda, MD.

Increasing epididymal adipose cell size in the aging, obese rat is accompanied by an increasing basal, but unchanging insulin(INS)-stimulated, rate of glucose transport(GT)/cell. Further, INS appears to stimulate GT in small cells through a translocation of glucose transport systems(GTSYS) from an intracellular pool associated with the microsomes(MIC) to the plasma membrane(PM), as assayed by specific D-glucose-inhibitable ^{3}H-cytochalasin B binding. The relative distribution of GTSYS between MIC and PM in small and large cells, prepared from 180 and 800 g rats, respectively, is examined following their incubation in the absence or presence of 1000 uU INS/ml. In the basal state, small cells contain an estimated total number of 2.21$\pm$0.04(mean$\pm$SD) X 10^6 GTSYS/cell, of which roughly 95% and 5%, respectively, are associated with MIC and PM. While large cells contain no more than a 2-fold greater total number of GTSYS/cell, those in MIC and PM represent roughly 30% and 70%, respectively, values similar to those observed in small cells following INS stimulation. INS stimulation of large cells has little effect on either the total number of GTSYS/cell or their distribution. These results suggest that adipose cellular enlargement is accompanied primarily by a marked redistribution of GTSYS from MIC to PM, thereby increasing the basal rate of GT/cell and greatly diminishing the stimulation of GT by INS through a depletion of the intracellular pool from which GTSYS are translocated to PM in response to INS.

370

Evidence for a Post-Receptor Defect as the Cause of Insulin Resistance in Lipoatrophic Diabetes. JONATHAN R. INSEL, and ORVILLE G. KOLTERMAN*, Denver, Colorado.

Lipoatrophic diabetes(LD) is characterized by either generalized or partial loss of adipose tissue and insulin(I)-resistant diabetes. 3 LD patients - 1 generalized and 2 partial - with evidence of I-resistant diabetes with fasting hyperinsulinemia (38 μU/ml) and fasting hyperglycemia (175 mg%) were studied. The mechanism of the I resistance was evaluated by measuring: 1) I binding(IB) to erythrocytes and monocytes, and 2) the dose response relationship between serum I and both overall glucose(G) disposal and hepatic glucose production(HGP) using the G clamp technique. The 3 patients demonstrated normal IB to erythrocytes, 7.5 ± .8% vs 6.4 ± .6% (controls), and monocytes, 4.2 ± .9% vs 4.2 ± .2% (controls). The patients underwent 3 separate G clamp studies where serum G was maintained at euglycemic levels (90 ± 5 mg%) while I was infused at rates of 120 $mU/M^2/min$, 240 $mU/M^2/min$ or 1200 $mU/M^2/min$ giving steady state serum I levels of 281 ± 10, 624 ± 72, and 8303 ± 1022 μU/ml, respectively. The G disposal(D) rate(R) during the 3 studies was 104 ± 11, 124 ± 9, and 134 ± 13 $mg/M^2/min$ compared to values of 269 ± 16, 319 ± 19, and 368 ± 27 $mg/M^2/min$ for controls. Although I inhibited HGP by 90-100% during all 3 infusions in patients with LD and in controls, the basal HGP in LD was 2.5 times that of controls. In conclusion, 1) patients with LD exhibited decreased G disposal rates at submaximal and maximal I levels in the absence of a change in IB, consistent with a post-receptor defect in peripheral G utilization, and 2) I had a normal ability to inhibit HGP.

371

Insulin Resistance (IR) in Uremia: Evidence for Receptor and Postreceptor Defects. D. SMITH, New Haven, Ct (Introduced by N. MARIEB, New Haven,Ct)

Tissue sensitivity to insulin (I), quantitated with the I clamp technique (plasma I=110±5 μU/ml), was reduced by 54% in 17 uremic subjects (3.8±0.2 vs 7.2±0.5 mg/kg·min). The observed IR could result from impaired I binding (IB) or a postreceptor defect. To distinguish between these possibilities we measured IB to monocytes in 8 uremic subjects. Total ^{125}I-Insulin binding was reduced by 32% in uremics (5.4±0.6%) vs controls (8.0±0.3%), p<0.001 To further examine the contribution of decreased IB to the IR, we constructed dose response curves relating in vivo I-mediated glucose (G) metabolism to plasma I. Since I action is associated with IB to a small percentage (∿ 10 %) of available receptors, with a receptor defect normalization of the I response would be expected if a sufficiently high I conc is attained; in contrast with a postreceptor defect decreased insulin response would be expected at all I conc. Plasma I was raised by 100, 500, 1000 μU/ml while maintaining plasma G constant at basal levels. Under these steady state conditions the amount of G metabolized (M) equals the G infusion rate and is a measure of tissue sensitivity to I. At all three I plateaus M was significantly reduced (p<0.01) in uremics (3.4±0.3 vs 7.2±0.5; 5.9±0.2 vs 9.9±0.5; 7.0±0.5 vs 10.9±0.5 mg/kg·min). These data represent a rightward shift in the dose response curve relating plasma I to M and a failure to normalize I-mediated G metabolism even at maximally effective plasma I. These results are the predicted consequence of a postreceptor defect in I action. Conclusion: both decreased IB & impaired postreceptor events contribute to IR in uremia.

372

Does Insulin Hyperpolarize Rat Skeletal Muscle by Stimulating an Electrogenic Pump? ELLEN M. ROGUS* AND KENNETH ZIERLER, Baltimore, Maryland.

The mechanism by which insulin hyperpolarizes skeletal muscle has not been agreed upon. On the one hand, it is postulated that the hyperpolarization results from decreased passive permeability to Na^+ and K^+. On the other, it is claimed that insulin stimulates an electrogenic Na-K pump. The latter claim is based on findings that ouabain, at 10^{-3} or 10^{-4} M, prevents or abolishes insulin-induced hyperpolarization. However, it is not certain that ouabain at such high concentrations acts solely to inhibit the pump and has no adverse effects on passive membrane properties. To reduce that possibility, experiments were done using concentrations of ouabain sufficiently low to have negligible effect on resting membrane potential, but sufficiently high to block hyperpolarization by 10^{-6} M isoproterenol, which hyperpolarization is generally attributed to stimulation of an electrogenic pump in skeletal muscle. Results were: 10^{-6} M isoproterenol hyperpolarized rat caudofemoralis in the absence of ouabain but not when 10^{-5} M ouabain was added simultaneously or subsequently. Insulin, 100 mU/ml, hyperpolarized even when added simultaneously with 10^{-4} M ouabain. This hyperpolarization was not significantly different from that produced by insulin alone. It is concluded that insulin-induced hyperpolarization is not due to stimulation of an electrogenic pump in rat skeletal muscle since it is not abolished by ouabain at a concentration ten times higher than that required to block isoproterenol-induced hyperpolarization.

373

Dissociation of Insulin's Effects on Cell Metabolism and on Subcellular Calcium Transport. D.M. MALCHOFF and D.E. BRUNS (Introduced by P.E. DONALD*) Charlottesville, Va.

Redistribution of subcellular calcium has been proposed to mediate insulin's effects. The azide (N_3)-insensitive calcium uptake systems found in a variety of cells appear capable of altering the subcellular distribution of calcium. However, reports of insulin's effects on these systems are contradictory: the N_3-insensitive calcium pump of adipocytes was increased by insulin while that of hepatocytes was decreased.

To further study this question, confluent 3T3-L1 cells were grown with insulin (10 μg/ml) to promote adipocyte differentiation; insulin was removed from the medium 2-5 days prior to study. Calcium uptake by membrane vesicles in the 600g supernatant of the cell homogenate was assessed using $^{45}Ca^{2+}$ and rapid millipore filtration. The assay was done at 37°C and in an isotonic buffer, pH 6.8, containing 5 mM $MgCl_2$ and ATP, 10 mM N_3 and 10 mM oxalate. Calcium uptake was ATP-dependent and stimulated by oxalate. It had a K_m of 4 μM Ca^{2+} and a V_{max} of 6.4 nmol Ca^{2+}/mg protein/min. Treatment of cells with insulin (I mU/ml) for 10-90 min induced progressive and signficant 2-14 fold increases in cell accumulation of (^{3}H)-D-glucose and incorporation of ^{3}H into lipid. In contrast, insulin had no effects on the N_3-insensitive or N_3-sensitive calcium transport systems or on passive calcium binding to membranes. These results suggest that an acute stable effect of insulin on intracellular calcium pumps is not an essential step in the mechanism of insulin's action on 3T3-L1 adipocytes.

Regulation of Glycogen Metabolism by Glucagon and Glucose. R.H. POINTER,* S.J. ROSE, and J. AVRUCH,* Boston, Ma.

The relative contribution of glucagon to the physiological control of hepatic glycogen metabolism by glucose was studied in isolated rat hepatocytes. Glucagon (10^{-10} to 10^{-6} M) added in the absence of glucose caused a rapid increase in phosphorylase A activity. Glycogen synthase activity measured in the absence of glucose-6-phosphate (glycogen synthase I) was low initially and was not further altered by glucagon. Total glycogen synthase activity (glycogen synthase D) was not altered when measured at saturating concentrations of glucose-6-phosphate.

Glucose administration in the absence of glucagon led to a rapid fall in phosphorylase A activity followed after a short lag by a slower rise in glycogen synthase I activity. (Glycogen synthase D activity was unaltered.) When glucagon was added along with glucose the fall in phosphorylase A activity was blunted and delayed and the subsequent rise in synthase I activity was substantially inhibited.

These studies suggest that the control of hepatic glycogen metabolism by glucagon is superimposed on a fundamental control exerted by glucose and its metabolites.

376

Initial Lag-phase in the Action of Insulin on Glucagon Stimulated cAMP-levels in Hepatocytes. H.U. HÄRING, B. KRAUS*, D. BROCKS, C. SCHUDT, W. KEMMLER, Munich, Germany

Kinetic studies in fat cells have shown that the insulin signal from the receptor to the glucose transport and cAMP-system is transmitted with a delay of 40-50 sec. Modifications of this characteristic coupling time by several means proved to be a suitable way to characterize the postreceptor signal transfer. To establish an analogous kinetic model in liver cells we studied the early time-courses of the insulin effect on glucagon stimulated cAMP-levels in freshly isolated and cultured rat hepatocytes. Basal cAMP-levels were 6.7 ± 0.9 pmol/10^6 in freshly prepared cells. In these cells glucagon in a submaximally effective concentration of 5 nM stimulates cAMP within 20 sec by 180 ± 16 %, a maximal effect of 330 ± 36 % is reached within 2 min and maintained for > 10 min. Insulin (100 μU/ml) had no effect on basal cAMP and simultaneously given with glucagon it didn't affect the initial rise of cAMP up to 20 sec, while a reduction of the cAMP levels was significant at later time points (at 2 min 200 ± 14 % over basal value). Addition of insulin 4 min after glucagon lowered cAMP-levels after a lag-period of 30-60 sec significantly. The kinetics of the insulin effect were analogous in both types of cell preparation. Simultaneous I^{125}-insulin binding studies suggest, that the delay in the transfer of the insulin signal is caused on the postreceptor level.

375

Insulin Stimulated Protein Synthesis Diminishes Gluconeogenesis. SAMUEL P. BESSMAN and CHANDRA MOHAN, L.A., CA. (Intro. by V. Kamdar*, L.A., CA.)

The effect of insulin on gluconeogenesis from ^{14}C-alanine, ^{14}C-glycerol and ^{14}C-acetate was studied in diabetic rabbits by measurement of both pool size and total activity of alanine, glucose, lactate and protein pools. Insulin (0.2 U/Kg/hr) caused an immediate net drop in the alanine, lactate, pyruvate and glucose pool sizes. Tracer carbon was shunted from glucose to protein during insulin administration concurrent with the fall in plasma levels of 3-carbon compounds measured. Insulin caused total activity of the glucose pool to decrease more than pool size. The decrease in pool size was about half the decrease in delivery of radioactivity from amino acid pool. 94% of the total radioactivity administered was recovered in muscle and plasma components and as expired CO_2. 38.5% of the carbon lost from the glucose pool was incorporated into muscle and plasma protein, 34.6% was expired as CO_2 and 7.3% was incorporated into muscle glycogen. This suggests that the major carbon flow is directed away from glucose towards protein synthesis by insulin. Experiments with ^{14}C-acetate which can be incorporated into glucose through the activity of PC-PEPCK show that although its incorporation into protein is increased significantly by insulin its incorporation into glucose is unaffected. These results are consistent with the conclusion that insulin "inhibits" gluconeogenesis primarily by stimulating resynthesis of amino acids into protein before they are converted to glucose.

377

Insulin Enhances Low Density Lipoprotein Catabolism In Vivo. ALAN CHAIT*, DONALD G. MILLER and EDWIN L. BIERMAN*, Seattle, WA.

Low density lipoprotein (LDL) is catabolized in vitro by a specific cell surface receptor mediated pathway. Insulin enhances the degradation of LDL by increasing the number of LDL receptors on cultured cells. Since LDL degradation in vivo also is believed to be largely receptor mediated, the effect of endogenous hyperinsulinemia on LDL catabolism was evaluated. Five patients were studied prior to and following commencement of total parenteral nutrition (TPN), started for a variety of indications. Plasma insulin levels rose from 15±10 to 174±52 uU/ml during TPN ($p < .005$). These marked increases in circulating insulin levels were associated with enhanced LDL degradation (measured as the urine/plasma ratio of injected ^{125}I-LDL) in 4 of the 5 subjects. TPN was associated with a reduction in plasma cholesterol levels in all subjects (146±56 to 110±60 mg/dl; $p<.05$) accounted for by a reduction in both LDL (74±32 to 49±18 mg/dl) and high density lipoprotein (HDL) cholesterol (38±11 to 21±6 mg/dl). The fall in HDL-cholesterol was not related to the increase in plasma triglycerides (123±43 to 269±212 mg/dl) observed. To test whether these changes in lipoprotein transport were due to insulin or some other effect of TPN, a single non-TPN requiring subject was infused with exogenous insulin (and glucose to maintain euglycemia). Plasma insulin levels increased more than 10-fold during the infusion and LDL removal rate increased from 0.28/day to 0.55/day. Thus, insulin appears to regulate LDL (and HDL) catabolism in vivo, presumably by enhancing receptor mediated degradation of these lipoproteins.

HORMONE RECEPTORS

379

Demonstration of Insulin Receptors in the Rat Fetus *in vivo*. F.R. SODOYEZ-GOFFAUX, J.C. SODOYEZ*, Y.M. THIRY-MORIS and C.J. DE VOS, Liege, Belgium.

[^{125}I] Monoiodoinsulin (^{125}I-Ins) was injected into the vitelline vein of 17, 19 and 21 day-old fetuses *in utero*. The liver, kidneys and heart concentrated ^{125}I-Ins, the highest specific activity (S.A.) being found in the liver. Carcass, placenta and lungs had a low S.A. except for the lungs of the 17 day-old fetuses. Concomitant injection of excess unlabeled insulin (Ins) inhibited the uptake of ^{125}I-Ins by the liver (saturable) but not by the kidney (non saturable). Radioautographs of the liver demonstrated silver grains mainly on the membranes of the hepatocytes and not on the hematopoietic cells following ^{125}I-Ins alone and in the vascular compartment following ^{125}I-Ins + unlabeled Ins. In the kidneys, silver grains were selectively localized in the proximal tubules.

When ^{125}I-Ins and unlabeled Ins were injected sequentially, the S.A. of the liver briskly decreased whereas plasma intact ^{125}I-Ins increased. Liver binding however was not fully reversible, possibly because of internalization of the label as suggested by radioautographs. Insulin induced increments of plasma ^{125}I-Ins conc. measured after stepwise increasing the delay between ^{125}I-Ins and Ins injection allowed to evaluate that the half life of ^{125}I-Ins in the receptor compartment was 6 min.

In the 3 age groups tested, the liver binding capacity (pmoles/g liver) was already in the same range as in adult rats, interestingly at a time of well documented marked hyperinsulinemia.

378

Rapid Reversal of Decreased Erythrocyte Insulin Binding Following Delivery in Normal and Diabetic Pregancy. M.D. HARRIS, D.R. HOLLINGSWORTH*, L. COUSINS, P.F. KRAUS and S.S.C. YEN, La Jolla, Ca.

Pregnancy is associated with resistance to insulin, but the mechanism(s) governing this phenomenon is unclear. This study was designed to examine one possible mechanism, i.e. the insulin binding characteristics by erythrocytes. Measurements were made in normal nonpregnant women and in pregnant women with and without Type II (non insulin deficient) diabetes. Each pregnant subject was studied during late gestation (35-40 wk.) and again at 6, 12 and 24 hours postpartum. The RBC insulin binding assay was similar to that of Gambhir and yielded a mean maximum specific binding in the nonpregnant controls of 9.4 ± 1.4% (N=12). During late pregnancy, maximum specific binding was signficantly reduced in normal women (N=6, 7.0 ± 0.8%, $P < 0.01$) and in 5 Type II diabetics (5.6 ± 0.8%, $P < 0.01$). In both groups this change reflected a decrease in receptor concentration. A modest increase in insulin binding was observed at 12 hr. postpartum ($P > 0.05$). By 24 hours postpartum, binding had returned to the normal nonpregnancy range in both normal and diabetic subjects. The increase in binding following delivery resulted from an increase in binding affinity rather than a change in concentration of receptor sites.

These findings suggest that the insulin resistance observed during pregnancy is at least in part reflected by a decrease in RBC binding. The rapid reversal in binding as well as the increase in receptor affinity may reflect the disappearance of diabetogenic hormones following delivery.

380

Carbohydrate Metabolism and Insulin Receptor Response in Humans with Acute Viral Infection. J. H. ANDERSON, JR.* and G. MERRILL, Frederick, Md.

The effect of acute illness produced by sandfly fever virus (SFV) on insulin secretion, carbohydrate metabolism and insulin receptor physiology was evaluated in 3 males who granted fully informed consent to oral glucose (1.75 g/kg) tolerance tests (OGTT) and insulin receptor studies both prior to SFV inoculation and at onset of fever. Fasting glucose (106 ± 4 mg/dl) was elevated ($P < 0.01$) above control (93 ± 4 mg/dl) at onset of fever, but prior to changes in dietary carbohydrate intake. Fasting immunoreactive insulin (IRI) values were also increased (22 ± 4 μU/ml compared to 12 ± 2 μU/ml, $P < 0.05$). Glucose values during OGTT were elevated at all points compared to preinoculation controls and failed to return to fasting by 120 min. Insulin response was elevated (50-130%, $P < 0.05$) at each time point. Increased insulin:glucose ratios during illness suggest insulin resistance as an explanation for the carbohydrate intolerance. Insulin receptor studies on peripheral mononuclear cells demonstrated a 7.5-30% decrease in binding at onset of illness, compared to preinoculation values. The decreased binding was associated with a 25-75% loss of insulin receptors during infection ($P < 0.05$). Receptor affinity remained the same in 2 volunteers, but was markedly increased in one. In conclusion, the onset of mild viral illness in man is associated with hyperinsulinism, glucose intolerance, insulin resistance and decreased binding of insulin to peripheral mononuclear leukocytes, attributed to decreased receptor numbers.

381

Identification of Insulin Receptor Subunits by Antireceptor Antibody in Gel Electrophoresis. M. KASUGA*, E. VAN OBBERGHEN*, L. C. HARRISON*, and K. YAMADA. Bethesda, Maryland.

Insulin binding proteins have been identified in SDS-PAGE by other investigators using crosslinking of ^{125}I-insulin to cell membranes. In this study we investigated insulin receptors of lymphocyte membranes. ^{125}I-insulin was crosslinked to membranes by disuccinimidyl suberate. SDS-PAGE of this preparation revealed a single ^{125}I-labeled band with MW 130K. The same band was observed when the crosslinked preparation was solubilized, immunoprecipitated with antireceptor antibody, and subjected to SDS-PAGE. Monovalent ^{125}I-Fab fragments (MW 50K) prepared from antireceptor antibodies were crosslinked to membranes as above. SDS-PAGE of these preparations revealed 2 bands at 180K and 230K. Neither band was observed when ^{125}I-Fab fragments were crosslinked to membranes in the presence of an excess unlabeled insulin or Fab fragments. Partially purified insulin receptors were subjected to SDS-PAGE and subsequent incubation with ^{125}I-antireceptor antibodies revealed a band at MW 63K. We conclude: 1) Crosslinking of ^{125}I-insulin to its receptor in lymphocyte membranes followed by SDS-PAGE reveals a 130K complex which is precipitated by antireceptor IgG; 2) The 180 and 230K bands seen after crosslinking of ^{125}I-monovalent antireceptor antibody may represent complexes of the 130K component with one and two (50K) Fab fragments. 3) Failure to detect the 130K component by binding of ^{125}I-antireceptor antibodies to gels after electrophoresis of the partially purified receptor may be due to loss of its immunoreactivity after exposure to SDS.

382

Analysis of Cooperativity in Insulin Binding to Rat Adipocytes and Human Erythrocytes. H.J. GOREN, J.S. BECK, A. RESCIGNO, Calgary, Canada (Introduced by P.M. CROCKFORD,* Edmonton, Canada).

A method of analysis of ligand-receptor binding based on a model where rate constants (association and dissociation) and equilibrium constant are dependent upon occupancy of receptors has been developed. The analysis leads to 3 kinds of experiments: 1) equilibrium measurements which permit quantitative determinations of a dissociation equilibrium parameter as a function of receptor occupancy, 2) measurements prior to equilibrium which yield the same information, and 3) measurements prior to equilibrium which reveal quantitatively the dependence of both association and dissociation rate parameters, separately, on occupancy. This new procedure for analyzing ligand-receptor binding has been applied to insulin-receptor systems (rat epididymal fat cell and human erythrocyte). Adipocytes have decreasing affinity for insulin with increasing occupancy - 50% decrease from 1% to 100% occupancy. In the red blood cell, below 1% occupancy affinity for insulin remains unchanged; above 1% occupancy the equilibrium dissociation constant increases sharply (at 10% 4-fold and at 50% occupancy 25-fold). Presently, data for fat cells indicate that both the association and dissociation rate constants for insulin binding decrease with receptor occupancy, the former decreasing more than the latter. The method will be compared with previously described analyses of ligand-receptor binding studies and the data will be discussed with reference to insulin binding to the IM-9 lymphocyte. (Supported by the Canadian Diabetes Association.)

383

Lipoatrophic Diabetic Plasma Inhibits Insulin Receptor Regulation In-Vitro. D.M. MOTT* and H. KATZEFF, Phoenix, AZ.

Plasma from a 32 yr old male with congenital lipoatrophic diabetes (LD) with documented severe insulin resistance has been studied for its effects on insulin mediated down regulation (DR) of fibroblast insulin receptors. Percent DR was calculated from the amount of insulin binding/cell following a 16 hour, 37°C incubation of normal diploid fibroblast monolayers in medium with 20% plasma or 0.1% bovine serum albumin (BSA) and varied insulin concentrations. Maximum DR using LD plasma was significantly reduced compared to the mean obtained using plasma from 4 normal subjects (37±6% vs 60±5%, $p<0.001$). When compared to normal plasma over a range of insulin concentrations, LD plasma caused a significant reduction in DR at 2.5 ($p<0.002$), 10.0 ($p<0.001$) and 100 ($p<0.008$) ng/ml insulin. The concentration of insulin required for ½ maximum DR was increased for the LD (2.0±0.1 for normals vs 8.0±0.8 ng/ml for LD). 20% plasma from normals or LD had no effect on maximum specific insulin binding/cell when compared to preincubation of cells with 0.1% BSA. Normal plasma had no significant effect on DR when compared with BSA over the range of insulin concentrations studied. LD plasma did not differ from normals when tested for insulin degradation and did not contain antibodies against insulin or the insulin receptor. We conclude that 1) insulin mediated DR of insulin receptors can be used to detect plasma factors which may contribute to insulin resistance; 2) LD plasma contains factor(s) which alter the sensitivity and magnitude of insulin mediated DR.

384

Human Erythrocyte Insulin Binding Decreases as an Exponential Function of Cell Age. ROBERT F. DONS, LAURENCE M. CORASH, and PHILLIP GORDEN*. Bethesda, Maryland.

The insulin receptor of mononuclear cells has been used to reflect the ambient state of insulin receptors in target tissues. Recently, red cells have been used in the same manner. Human red cells were fractionated according to age to determine whether there is heterogeneity in the specific binding of ^{125}I-insulin [I] to different red cell age-variants. Mean cell age (MCA) was determined from the cumulative distribution frequency of the cells in an isotonic (290 mOsm/kg) density gradient, and confirmed by assay for pyruvate kinase, an age-dependent enzyme. [I]-binding to red cells was found to decrease exponentially as a function of their MCA in 6 subjects when expressed either individually or as grouped data. [I]-binding to a red cell preparation containing 31% reticulocytes from a glucose-6-phosphate dehydrogenase deficient patient was 37.5% / 4.5 x 10^9 cells. This value was in good agreement with that predicted by extrapolation of the linear relationship of log % [I]-binding versus MCA determined for normals. [I]-binding to leukocyte-free whole blood (60 days MCA) was 7.2 ± 2% while that to the oldest red cells was < 1% as estimated by extrapolation of the normal curves. We conclude: (1) [I]-binding to human erythrocytes does occur in a heterogeneous fashion related to cell age, and (2) since the [I]-binding to younger red cells is several fold greater than that to older red cells, it is possible that only younger cells respond to factors that regulate insulin receptors.

385

Diabetogenic Action of L-Asparaginase: Decreased Insulin Receptors. MASASHI KOBAYASHI,* HIROSHI MAEGAWA, MAKOTO IWASAKI, YUKIO SHIGETA. Ohtsu, JAPAN.

L-asparaginase (LA) is a potent antitumor agent and is known to be diabetogenic because it decreases insulin (I) secretion. However, hyperinsulinemia with hyperglycemia is seen in some of the patients treated with LA. To clarify another diabetogenic action of LA, i.e. I resistance, rats were injected with 40,000 U/kg of LA i.v. and I binding (B) to isolated adipocytes from these rats was examined. IB decreased at 6 hrs after LA injection to 72 % and at 24 hrs further decreased to 52 % of control at a trace concentration of I. At 48 hrs it recovered to 78 % and by 2 weeks IB completely recovered. This decreased IB was totally accounted for by decreased number of I receptor (R). I action in these cells with 50 % decreased I R was tested by 2-deoxyglucose transport study, and the I dose response curve was shifted to right, which is a concequence of decreased number of IR. Direct incubation of adipocytes or placenta membrane with LA for up to 6 hrs at 37°C did not affect IB. Plasma concentration of asparagine in these rats was 42 ± 6 nmole/ml before injection, 0 nmole/ml at 6 hrs after injection, 4 ± 1 nmole/ml at 24 hrs after injection and 29 ± 11 nmole/ml 48 hrs after injection. Plasma I concetration was not significantly elevated in these rats whereas plasma glucose was minimaly elevated.

Conclusion: LA decreased IR on rat adipocytes and consequently affect I action in glucose transport. Decreased IR was not a direct action of LA but probably due to decreased concentration of asparagine which may be necessary for IR synthesis.

386

The Effect of Medium Glucose Concentration on Insulin Binding in Cultured Chinese Hamster Kidney Epithelial Cells. B.M. WYSE and A.Y. CHANG*, Kalamazoo, MI.

Binding of insulin to cultured epithelial-like Chinese hamster kidney cells showed typical characteristics of insulin-receptor interaction, e.g., specificity and negative cooperativity. Optimal binding occurred at pH 8 and 2½ hours of incubation at room temperature. The effect of glucose concentration in culture medium on insulin binding was studied in two substrains derived from an established cell strain by growing (10 or more passages) in media containing 100 mg/dl (L) and 400 mg/dl (H) glucose, respectively. Insulin binding was greater in H (11.9±0.7 μU/10^8 cells) than in L (6.6±0.5 μU/10^8 cells). This difference, however, could be reversed by growing substrain H in 100 mg/dl glucose. After 4 more passages in media containing either 400 mg/dl or 100 mg/dl glucose, insulin binding in substrain H decreased from 12.3 μU/10^8 cells to 9.5 μU/10^8 cells. These data suggest that the ability of cultured cells to bind insulin may be increased by prolonged exposure of the cells to elevated levels of glucose.

387

***In Vitro* Insulin Induced Alterations of Insulin Receptor Affinity in the Turkey Erythrocyte.** FRANK KOSMAKOS,* Phoenix, AZ.

In vivo or in vitro exposure of cells to insulin results in a loss in the number of insulin receptors. Previous studies with IM-9 lymphocytes have shown that insulin induced loss in receptor number is mediated via the insulin receptor and requires at least one step beyond binding. Since the turkey erythrocyte has an insulin receptor that is identical to other characterized insulin receptor systems and lacks active macromolecular synthetic processes, it was used to investigate the mechanism by which insulin mediates receptor loss. Preincubation of turkey erythrocytes with insulin for 18 hr at 30° produced a marked increase in ^{125}I-insulin binding. This increase was due entirely to an increase in receptor affinity with no apparent change in receptor number. The effect of insulin was specific and mediated through the insulin receptor, since either insulin or proinsulin could increase receptor affinity, with the increase predicted by each hormones affinity for the insulin receptor. Further, the increase in affinity was dependent on the concentration of insulin in the preincubation medium. The increase was manifest by 8 hr of exposure to insulin and reached a plateau by 20 hr. Removal of insulin from medium reversed the effect so that by 10 hr, insulin binding was restored to the level observed in cells not exposed to hormone. The ability of insulin to induce alterations in recptor affinity in avian erythrocyte provides a simple cellular model to examine the different mechanisms by which exposure to insulin can alter the total level of insulin binding.

388

Chemical Properties of Insulin Receptors of Rat Islets of Langerhans. Hermann P.T. Ammon* and Eugen J. Verspohl, Tuebingen, F.R.G.

100 Collagenase isolated islets were preincubated in KRB-albumin buffer without and with trypsin, neuraminidase, phospholipase A_2, p-chloromercuribenzoate, Ellman's reagent, carbodiimid and tetranitromethan for 30 min. In the presence of increasing concentrations of exogenous insulin, specific binding of [^{125}I]insulin to islets and glucose-induced insulin secretion (RIA) were measured.

Trypsin and neuraminidase decreased the amount of insulin receptors, in addition trypsin decreased the receptor affinity; this was associated with a decrease of the inhibitory effect of exogenous insulin on insulin secretion. Phospholipase A_2 and the sulfhydryl reagents neither changed binding of insulin nor its effect on insulin secretion. Carbodiimid (carboxyl-reagent) diminished the amount of receptors, tetranitromethan (reacting with sulfhydryl-, tyrosyl- and tryptophan-groups) strongly decreased affinity and amount of insulin receptors.

Conclusion. Binding of insulin to insulin receptors of the pancreatic islets depends on protein structure, carboxyl-, tyrosin- and/or tryptophan-groups; it does not depend on phospholipids and sulfhydryl-groups. With respect to phospholipase A_2 and trypsin insulin receptors of pancreatic islets are different from those of other tissues.

389

Insulin Receptor Number Increased by Glucocorticoid Stimulation of Protein Synthesis in Cultured Human Lymphocytes. D. R. BORREBACH and D. B. JARRETT, Pittsburgh, PA (Introduced by SIGRID HAGG,* Pittsburgh, PA).

Glucocorticoid hormones increase insulin binding to cultured human lymphocytes (line IM-9). This effect, which is specific for cortisol and dexamethasone, is both time and concentration dependent reaching a maximum of 30% after a 14 hour incubation with 10μg/100 mls cortisol. The increase is due to an increase in receptor number (60,000 to 78,000 sites/cell) and the average affinity profile shows no change in K_e or K_f. Cortisol does not increase labeled growth hormone binding to its receptors on these same cells. Using glucose free culture media, the cortisol effect is not inhibited, with viability >90% (trypan blue exclusion). Receptor recovery following down regulation with insulin (10^{-7} M for 6 hours) is accelerated in the presence of cortisol (10μg/100 mls) with receptor number being greater than spontaneous recovery at all time points studied. The cortisol effect is unrelated to cell growth as judged by cell number and ^{14}C-thymidine incorporation. Also, preventing mitosis with 0.5μg/ml N-desacetyl-N-methylocolchicine (Colcemid®) is without effect upon the cortisol stimulated increase in receptor number. The cortisol effect can be blocked by both cycloheximide (5μg/ml) and actinomycin D (1μg/ml). Cortisol is also without effect upon ^{3}H-uridine incorporation which suggests that the stimulation of insulin receptor is due to a direct action of cortisol on protein synthesis.

390

A Possible Regulatory Role of Amino Acids on Insulin Receptors. RICHARD A. GALBRAITH, CURTIS WISE, and MARIA G. BUSE*, Charleston, S. C.

The adaptation of insulin receptors to the metabolic milieu is poorly understood. Possible regulation by amino acids (AA) was studied in erythroblastic leukemic (EBL) cells, which grow rapidly and have copious insulin receptors (22,300/cell). EBL cells were passaged in rat pups and isolated from the liver. Cells (1-3 X 10^6/ml) were incubated at 37°C in primary culture for 1 hr with 1 or 5 X physiologic serum AA, then washed twice in binding buffer at 4°C and assayed for specific insulin binding at 37°C for 5 min (at equilibrium). Cells incubated in 5 X AA bound 53% more insulin than those in 1 X AA (n = 7, $p < 0.05$). Direct addition of AA to the insulin binding assay did not affect binding. Incubation with cycloheximide (1 μg/ml) did not affect maximum binding with 1 X AA but reduced binding with 5 X AA (cyclohex. 6.7 ± 0.26 vs control 8.67 ± 0.54; $p < 0.05$). Incubation with insulin (100 mU/ml) decreased subsequent insulin binding to 41% of control values in 1 X AA and to 37% in 5 X AA ($p < 0.01$). Parallel incubations with ^{125}I-albumin showed 0.063% trapping, insufficient to account for the down-regulation observed. Conclusions: 1) In EBL cells, AA conc. modulates maximum specific insulin binding. The effect is not directly on binding and seems to require protein synthesis. 2) EBL cells exhibit insulin induced down-regulation within 1 hr. 3) High ambient AA may be required in rapidly growing cells as structural components to maintain fast insulin receptor synthesis; alternatively, one or more specific AA may exert a regulatory influence on receptor homeostasis.

391

Receptor Depletion in Ketoacidosis Prone Diabetes Mellitus: Response to Tolbutamide Therapy. R. GALAGAN, R.P. EATON,* E. KAUFMAN and R. ALLEN, Albuquerque, New Mexico

The mechanism commonly held responsible for severe insulin resistance is neutralization of insulin by antibodies, however, many cases of insulin resistance are not explained by this hypothesis. Oral sulfonylurea agents have been demonstrated to reverse insulin resistance but their mode of action has not been established. We studied erythrocyte receptor binding of insulin, insulin antibody binding, endogenous insulin secretion (assessed by C-peptide levels) and the effects of Tolbutamide therapy in two patients with recurrent diabetic ketoacidosis secondary to severe insulin resistance.

On admission, the patient's erythrocyte receptor binding of insulin was abnormally low owing to a reduction of insulin receptor concentration. (Table) Following Tolbutamide therapy, ketoacidosis corrected and diabetic control improved. On remeasurement, erythrocyte receptor binding of insulin had normalized with a substantial increase in insulin receptor concentration. Insulin antibody titers did not change with treatment and C-peptide levels surprisingly decreased.

Patients	Specific (^{125}I) Insulin Bound *	Receptor Concentration: In 4.5x10^9 Red Blood Cells (ng/ml)	Receptor Concentration: Binding Sites/Cell
E.T. Before Tolbutamide	3.78 ± 1.7%	0.9	20
E.T. On Tolbutamide	7.5 ± 1.6%	3.0	68
J.M. Before Tolbutamide	4.25 ± 0.8%	0.9	20
J.M. On Tolbutamide	9.0 ± 0.8%	6.3	142
Normal Men (N-11)	6.25 ± 1.8%	3.0	69

*0.1 ng/ml (^{125}I) insulin per 4.5x10^9 RBC/ml

These results suggest that diabetic ketoacidosis and severe insulin resistance may result from a reduction in cellular insulin binding. Tolbutamide may ameliorate severe insulin resistance by restoring cellular insulin receptor concentration.

392

Insulin Binding to Pancreatic Beta Cells. C. BRADLEY, J. YOON, J. ARCHER, J. SANUSI, L. CARTER, H. JAMES, and P. CARSON. Washington, D.C. (Introduced by J. T. Williams,* Washington, D.C.)

The effect of insulin in regulating its own secretion has not been clearly defined. To demonstrate the interaction of insulin with the beta cell (B.C.), a modification of the insulin radioreceptor assay was used to demonstrate specific insulin receptors in monolayered cultured mouse cells. Incubation of 3.2 x 10^5 B.C./ml., at pH 6, 7, 7.6, and 8 resulted in specific insulin binding of 9.2%, 11.9%, 13.2%, and 7.2%, respectively. Thus the optimal pH was 7.6. Studies on the effect of varying temperature (4°, 15°, 30°) and time (30 min. to 24 hrs.) showed optimum for these parameters to be 15°C and 3.5 hrs.. With an increase of B.C. from 0.8 x 10^5/ml. to 3.2 x 10^5/ml., the specific insulin binding increased from 1.0% to 12.8%. To study the effect of insulin binding on insulin secretion, flourescein-labelled anti-insulin antibody stains and selected electron micrographs were used to determine the number of B.C. containing immunoreactive insulin (IRI) granules in monolayers cultured with and without exogenous insulin (EI), and in high (HG), 300mgs%, and low (LG), 100mgs%, glucose media. After 5 days of culture with no EI, 1.2% of those B.C. in HG media and 29% of those in LG media contained IRI granules. When cultured an additional 4 days with EI, IRI granules were present in 7% of the B.C. grown in HG and in 20% of those in LG. These studies demonstrate that insulin does bind specifically to its own secretory organ, and under varying conditions may stimulate or inhibit its own secretion.

393

Decreased ^{125}I Insulin Binding By Human Red Blood Cell After Administration of Dexamethasone or Prednisone. KEIGO YASUDA and ABBAS KITABCHI,* Memphis, Tn.

Hypercortisolism in experimental animals has produced variable results in regard to the insulin binding in target tissues depending on the type of steroid used to induce hypercortisolism. Very few studies have been conducted in man. Recent investigation using prednisone in man demonstrated an increase rather than a decrease in binding of ^{125}I insulin to monocytes. We have investigated the effect of overnight 1 mg. dexamethasone administration on ^{125}I insulin binding to red blood cells in nine normal lean subjects. Various kinetic and binding characteristics were studied including the average affinity profile ($\bar{K}e$: 10^{-7} M^{-1}), receptor numbers, and dissociation curves. Dexamethasone significantly decreased ^{125}I binding in all subjects (9.6% control vs. 6.7%, $p < 0.01$) with significant change in $\bar{K}e$ (0.93 vs. 0.62, $p < 0.01$) but without change in receptor numbers. Overnight administration of prednisone (10 mg. every 6 hours for one day) also reduced ^{125}I insulin binding to red blood cells with similar results to those of dexamethasone. No changes in dissociation curves, nonspecific insulin binding, insulin degradation or number of reticulocytes were noted.

These data suggest that acute hypercortisolism induced by dexamethasone or prednisone in man reduces ^{125}I insulin binding to red blood cells. This reduction is due to decreased affinity rather than a decrease in number of insulin receptors.

394

Regional Differences in Binding of Insulin to Human Adipocytes: Relation to Insulin Effects. ULF SMITH* and MARIO DiGIROLAMO*, Göteborg, Sweden and Atlanta, Georgia.

The relationship of insulin binding to human adipocytes (A) with insulin effects is still undetermined. It was observed previously that subcutaneous adipose tissue from the femoral region was markedly less responsive to the antilipolytic effect of insulin than tissue from the abdominal region.

To clarify this relationship, the binding of ^{125}I-insulin to isolated A from biopsies of femoral and abdominal adipose tissue was compared in 9 subjects (7 males, 2 females) varying in age from 52 to 70 years and in relative body weight from 96 to 125% of desirable. Femoral A (mean cell weight = .538 µg. lipid) were on average 28% larger than abdominal A (.387 µg. lipid). Specific insulin binding, expressed on a per cell basis, was similar in both regions at insulin concentrations varying from 2 to 24 ng./ml.; at higher insulin concentrations (44 ng./ml.), femoral A tended to bind greater amounts of insulin than abdominal cells. When expressed per unit of A surface area, binding of insulin was not significantly different in the two regions.

The results show that binding of insulin to two different adipose regions from the same subjects cannot explain the marked difference found in the antilipolytic effect of insulin. Thus, regional differences in the capacity of the adipocytes to respond to insulin must be attributed to a postreceptor alteration rather than to a receptor abnormality.

395

Insulin Receptors in Cultured Retinal Pericytes. S.M. LUCAS*, D. PARKER, S. KHILNANI, R. FRANK, Detroit, Michigan.

Although abnormalities of insulin homeostasis are associated with microvascular disease, little is known about the interaction of insulin with microvessel cells. Selective loss of the capillary intramural pericytes is an early feature of diabetic retinopathy. We have cultured pure cell lines of bovine retinal pericytes and characterized the specific binding of insulin to these cells. Pericytes were isolated from retinal microvessels by the use of sieves and centrifugation. The cells were incubated in supplemented Hams F12 medium with 20% fetal calf serum at 37°C in a humidified incubator in an atmosphere of 95% air 5% O_2. At 4°C binding of porcine I^{125} insulin reached equilibrium at 5 hours. A sharp pH optimum at pH 7.8 was observed. Binding was specific in that glucagon prolactin and growth hormone did not compete (10^{-6}M) whereas native porcine insulin produced a dose related inhibitory response. Curvilinear Scatchard plots suggested either two classes of binding sites or one class of negatively cooperative sites. Specific binding was decreased by preincubation with 10^{-6}M insulin. Thus, these binding sites have the characteristics of physiologic insulin receptors. This system of cultured retinal pericytes provides a unique in vitro model for the study of the action of insulin in modulating the metabolic activities of a specific cell type which may play a major role in the pathogenesis of the microvascular complications of diabetic retinopathy.

396

The Erythrocyte (E) Insulin Receptor (IR) of Sheep: Presence in the Fetus (F) and Absence in the Adult (A). M. SINHA, N. VELAYO, S. VOINA, S. GANGULI, Intro. by M. McCARROLL, Cincinnati, OH

Developmental loss of E glucose transport with postnatal maturation has been reported in some mammals including sheep. To assess whether this loss is related to postnatal changes in the characteristics of EIR, we compared EIR in the F or A sheep to A humans. EIR was characterized with respect to binding of mono-iodinated ^{125}I-insulin ($\sim 3.5 \times 10^9$cells/ml) in the presence or absence of unlabeled ligand and by Scatchard analysis to determine binding sites and their affinities. In 7 healthy human males, specific binding was 7.1 ± 0.7%(mean±SE) while non-specific binding did not exceed 1.5%. Scatchard plots were curvilinear; for high affinity (HA) Ka was $1.8 \pm 0.2 \times 10^9$M with 4.8 ± 0.3 sites/cell while low affinity (LA) Ka was $1.2 \pm 0.2 \times 10^8$M with 44.4 ± 3.6 sites/cell. In 5 sheep fetuses between 124 and 140D gestation(Term=150D) specific binding was 3.8 ± 0.5; Scatchard plots were also curvilinear yielding HA Ka of $2.0 \pm 0.2 \times 10^9$M and 2.4 ± 0.6 sites/cell and LA Ka of $1.9 \pm 0.4 \times 10^8$M with 12.5 ± 3.0 sites/cell. Thus, though, quantitatively less than A human, F sheep EIR exhibit similar characteristics. In marked contrast to both A human and F sheep, A sheep(n=11) were completely devoid of ^{125}I-insulin binding or measurable EIR even when assays were run in parallel to F sheep E. These findings held true for pregnant or virgin sheep or rams. We conclude that the EIR disappears postnatally in the sheep. We propose that the maturational loss of EIR may be related to loss of E glucose transport; both phenomena may represent postnatal adaptation to a major change in nutrient sources.

397

Ontogenesis of Insulin (I) and Glucagon (G) Receptors and Adenylate Cyclase (AC) in Rabbit Fetal Liver Plasma Membrane (FLPM). S. GANGULI, S. VOINA N. VELAYO, U. DEVASKAR, M. SPERLING*, Cinti, OH.

We investigated the maturation of I and G receptors as well as hormone sensitive AC. (c-AMP production) in FLPM between 25D and 30D gestation (Term=31D). Fetal livers (4 to 8) from each pregnancy (n=11) were pooled to prepare FLPM. 50ug of FLPM protein was used in all subsequent assays. There was a rapid and significant increase in I binding (2.7 vs 13.8%) and total I binding capacity (12.5 vs 37.5×10^{-11}M/L) between 25D and 27-30D gestation. However, Ka for high affinity sites (HA) (4 vs 5×10^{8}) and low affinity sites (LA) (1 vs 2×10^{8}) were not different at any gestational time. Similarly, G binding was 5.2% at 25D, 8% at 27-29D and 15% at 30D. Corresponding total binding capacities were 3, 11, and 24x 10^{-11}M/L. For HA, Ka (1.8, 1.7, 1.4×10^{9}M) and binding capacity (3, 2.8, 4.4×10^{-11}M/L) were not different. LA were not detected prior to 27D, scatchard plots being linear at 25D but curvilinear thereafter, increasing progressively (8 vs 21 $\times 10^{-11}$M/L). Ka for the LA (3.25 vs 3.8×10^{8}M) were not significantly different. G (10^{-9}-10^{6}M) failed to stimulate AC at any gestational age with or without GTP in the generating medium. In contrast PGE (10^{-7}-10^{-4}) produced a dose response curve for c-AMP production in all groups; responses with 10^{-5}M (306±41pm/mg/10min) or 10^{-4}M (397±63) were significantly higher than the basal value (191±20). Conclusion - (1) I and G receptors increase with a sharp rise occuring late in gestation. (2) G receptor maturation involves both number and affinity. (3) Hormone sensitive AC developes independently of the G receptors.

HORMONE SECRETION

398

A Comparison of C-Peptide Secretion in Obese Versus Non-Obese Maturity Onset Diabetic (MOD) Patients Controlled by Diet Alone. E NICKOLOFF, HM DREW, M HINNENKAMP, J ZARRIELLO, M RENDELL* Baltimore, Maryland

Two groups of MOD patients were successfully treated by caloric restriction. The obese group consisted of 14 patients. After dietary success, mean fasting plasma glucose (FPG) in this group was 113±10 mg/dl (Mean±2S.E.). Mean 4 PM glucose (4 PM G) was 107±10 mg/dl. Average weight reduction was 8±3% and mean final relative weight (FRW) was 1.41±0.06. A standard 5 hour GTT with concurrent C-peptide measurement was performed in these patients. Mean summed glucose values (ΣG) was 1041±160 mg/dl. Mean summed C-peptide values (ΣC) was 7.9±1.8 pM/ml.

The non-obese group consisted of 7 patients. The average weight reduction was 11±4% and FRW was 1.04±0.02. FPG was 103±10 mg/dl, 4 PM G was 108±14 mg/dl. ΣG in this group was 1080±128 mg/dl. ΣC was 7.2±2.8 pM/ml. None of these parameters differed statistically from the values in the obese group.

10 normal volunteers at ideal body weight underwent a similar GTT with C-peptide sampling. In this group, FPG was 81±3 mg/dl. ΣG was 669±64 mg/dl and ΣC 6.1±0.9 pM/ml, Both FPG and ΣG differed statistically from those of the two diabetic groups, but the differences in ΣC were not statistically significant.

It is concluded that, in MOD patients successfully treated by diet alone, the degree of body weight excess within 50% of ideal body weight does not significantly influence the parameters of insulin secretion. In diet controllable MOD patients, endogenous insulin secretion is normal.

399

C-Peptide Secretion in Previously Ketonuric Maturity Onset Diabetic (MOD) Patients Successfully Treated by Diet Alone. M RENDELL,* J ZARRIELLO, HM DREW, E NICKOLOFF, Baltimore, Md

Seven MOD patients presented with severe hyperglycemia and ketonuria. Six had positive serum ketones. Three had accompanying acidosis. In only one case was a precipitating factor (periodontal disease) identified. In each case, insulin was initially administered. In all cases, it was eventually possible to withdraw insulin and control hyperglycemia by diet alone. The average (Mean±2S.E.) weeks. Mean fasting plasma glucose (FPG) was 110±13 mg/dl. Mean 4 PM glucose was 98 ±8 mg/dl. Average weight reduction at time of control was 7±2%. Mean final relative weight was 1.27±0.18.

In each case, a standard 5 hour GTT (100 gm glucose) with concurrent C-peptide measurement was performed. Mean summed glucose (ΣG) was 894±190 mg/dl. Mean summed C-peptide (ΣC) was 6.8±2.5 pM/ml. Mean ratio of ΣG to ΣC was 153±48.

By comparison, in a group of 10 normal volunteers, ΣG was 669±64mg/dl, ΣC 6.1±0.9pM/ml, and ΣG/ΣC 116±22. Only ΣG was statistically significantly different from the ketonuric MOD group.

The presence of ketonuria in MOD does not exclude the possibility of eventual dietary control. Complete reversal of hyperglycemia is possible with restoration of normal insulin secretion as well as sensitivity to endogenous insulin.

400

Insulin Secretion by Cultured Islet Cells is Enhanced by Amino Acids. A.EISENSTEIN* I. STRACK, J. NEBBIA, Brooklyn, N.Y.

Pancreatic islet cells secrete insulin (I) when grown in standard tissue culture media. Since these media were not developed for islet cells they may lack factors that affect cell survival and function. To ascertain whether the amino acid content of Eagle's MEM is optimal, islet cells obtained by enzymatic digestion of rat pancreases were placed in tissue culture. On culture day 6, cells were maintained in MEM (5.5mM glucose) for 24 h. On day 7, cells were placed in high glucose MEM (16.5mM) or in high glucose MEM supplemented with 2-fold and 4-fold increases of amino acid (AA) content or by adding leucine or lysine (3.43mM). Media were removed after 4 h and fresh media of the same composition were added and incubation continued for an additional 20 h.

Percent Increase of Insulin Secretion Induced by High Glucose

	MEM	MEM + 2xAA	MEM + 4xAA	MEM + Leucine	MEM + Lysine
4 hrs	587±35	775±88	1176±133	950±95	649±19
20 "	231±30	245±28	282±40	337±43	241±25

Two-fold and 4-fold increases of AA in MEM and addition of leucine caused substantial but transient enhancement of glucose induced I secretion. These findings indicate that composition of tissue culture media is an important factor affecting function of cultured islet cells.

401

Calcium and Insulin-Hypersecretion by Islets from Zucker "Fatty" Rats. A. R. PANSINI and E. L. TOLMAN,* Pearl River, New York 10965.

The influence of obesity on the involvement of calcium (Ca^{++}) in the insulin secretory response to glucose was studied using islets of Langerhans isolated from Zucker "fatty" rats and their lean counterparts.

Islets from "fatty" rats secreted 1.5 to 3 times as much insulin as did the lean rat islets over a glucose concentration range of 0 to 27.7 mM. Maximum rates of secretion occurred at 11.1 mM glucose for both "fatty" rat islets (70-90 μU/islet/25 min.) and lean rat islets (50-60 μU/islet/25 min.). Over the same glucose concentration range, Ca^{++} accumulation was greater in islets from the "fatty" rats than from the others and the maximum rates of uptake (90 pg/islet/25 min. for "fatty" rat islets and 40 pg/islet/25 min. for lean rat islets) were attained in both at about 8.3 mM glucose. Both insulin secretion and Ca^{++} uptake rates were 2 to 3-fold greater for islets from "fatty" rats than those from the lean animals over an extracellular Ca^{++} concentration range up to 5 mEq/L. Maximum rates for both were achieved at 2 mEq Ca^{++}/L in "fatty" rat and lean rat islets. Thus, for islets isolated from Zucker "fatty" rats insulin hypersecretion in response to both glucose and extracellular Ca^{++} is associated with enhanced Ca^{++} accumulation.

402

Cultured Islet Cell Systems for the Study of Alloxan (A) Cytotoxicity and Islet Cell Regeneration. KENNETH C. GORRAY and WILFRED Y. FUJIMOTO,* Seattle, WA.

Previous investigators have explored the mechanism of A toxicity for islet B cells using short term incubations of islet preparations treated with A *in vitro*. Our studies have evaluated the long-term effects of A treatment *in vitro* on islet cell function utilizing 3 different systems of cultured islet cells: newborn rat pancreatic monolayers (NRP) and dispersed islet cell cultures of adult rat (ARI) and guinea pig (AGPI). Cultures were treated with different doses of A for 5 min and rates of insulin release (IR) were followed for one week after A treatment. IR (expressed as % of buffer-treated control) by cultures at the end of this period are shown below:

NRP		ARI		AGPI	
A (mM)	IR	A (mM)	IR	A (mM)	IR
0.2	96.72	1	45.11	1	107.32
1	73.64	2	7.75	2	60.37
2	28.72	5	3.64	5	30.19
10	7.27	40	2.60	40	3.23
20	1.64	60	1.50	60	5.09

Glucagon release, as a measure of specificity of the drug for B cells, was unaltered even at the highest doses of A in these systems.

Conclusions: 1) Long-term effects of A in these systems appear to be B-cell specific. 2) ARI and NRP respond similarly to A. 3) AGPI cells are somewhat A-resistant but this resistance can be overcome by using high doses of A. 4) The results for AGPI cells cannot explain the cycle of B cell degeneration followed by regeneration which we have observed after high dose A treatment of GPs *in vivo*.

403

Diurnal Episodic Pattern of Insulin Secretion in the Dog. W.P. VANHELDER, A. SIREK, O.V. SIREK,* K.H. NORWICH, Z. POLICOVA and T. VANHELDER. Toronto, Canada.

Sampling portal blood every 15 minutes by means of indwelling cannulae, we have found evidence that basal insulin secretion in non-anesthetized dogs takes place in 6-7 major secretory episodes over a 24-h period. Reproducible patterns were obtained in four experiments conducted on three normal animals. When frequency of peaks was plotted against the log of insulin concentration, a normal distribution was obtained (lognormal distribution). The means and variances were similar in the three animals: N(3.55, 0.51), N(2.69, 0.81) and N(2.72, 0.88). Low levels of insulin (10-25 μU/ml) alternated with peaks which were occasionally higher than 200 μU/ml. The average duration of a peak was 30 minutes and was independent of ambient glucose levels. The surges observed in the portal circulation seemed to be unrelated to oscillations known to take place in peripheral (posthepatic) insulin concentrations. Surgical hypophysectomy produced inconsistent changes in the pattern of basal insulin secretion of four dogs. The data are in keeping with the notion that the insulin peaks are not solely governed by the hypophysis, implicitly by growth hormone surges, but also by spontaneous repetitive discharges along neuronal pathways functionally related to insulin secretion.

404

The Precise Stimulus by Monosaccharides to Gastric Inhibitory Polypeptide (GIP) Secretion from the Canine Intestine. S.A. ROSS*, Calgary, Alta.

GIP is an enteric hormone released following the ingestion of glucose or galactose. It is not known whether GIP secretion is elicited by the presence of carbohydrate on the cell surface or whether intracellular metabolism of the carbohydrate is required before GIP is released. To examine the precise stimulus to GIP secretion, dogs were surgically prepared with a chronic duodenal fistula and GIP secretion measured after infusion of glucose, 2-deoxy-D-glucose or 3-0-methylglucose into the fistula. 2-deoxyglucose is phosphorylated by the same process as D-glucose but undergoes no further metabolism; 3-0-methylglucose is transported on the D-glucose carrier but no further metabolism takes place within the cell. After overnight fast, 10 gm. of each substrate was infused on separate occasions into the duodenal fistula over a 15 minute period. Immunoreactive GIP (IRGIP) was measured over a 2 hour period. Following the infusion of D-glucose (N=6), the total hormone production was 2.5 $\pm$ .1 ng/ml.min. The infusion of 2-deoxyglucose (N=5) resulted in a smaller but significant release of IRGIP, mean hormone secretion 1.0 $\pm$ .08 ng/ml.min. Following the infusion of 3-0-methylglucose (N=4) there was a small nonsignificant IRGIP rise over the test period. These data would indicate that the presence of glucose at the mucosal cell is not a sufficient stimulus for the release of GIP and that initial metabolism of the carbohydrate within the GIP secreting cell is required before the stimulus to GIP secretion is evoked.

405

Interplay between K^+ conductance, membrane potential and Ca^{2+} influx in islet cells. A. HERCHUELZ, N. THONNART et W.J. MALAISSE*. Brussels, Belgium.

The release of insulin evoked by glucose coincides with changes in K^+ conductance, membrane potential and Ca^{2+} flux in or out the pancreatic B-cell. The interplay between these variables was investigated. Raising the extracellular K^+ concentration from 5 to 20 mM increased ^{45}Ca net uptake, ^{45}Ca fractional outflow rate (FOR) and insulin release from isolated islets. In the absence of extracellular Ca^{2+}, 20 mM K^+ failed to affect ^{45}Ca FOR, while glucose provoked a sustained decrease in ^{45}Ca FOR, whether at 5 or 20 mM K^+. Tetraethylammonium (TEA), a specific blocker of K^+ conductance, reduced ^{86}Rb FOR to the same extent as glucose 4.4 mM. In the absence of glucose, TEA failed to affect ^{45}Ca FOR, ^{45}Ca uptake and insulin release from isolated islets. TEA lowered the threshold concentration of glucose required to stimulate Ca^{2+} influx and insulin release and increased the cationic and secretory responses to intermediate glucose concentrations. In the presence or absence of TEA, the effect of glucose to stimulate ^{45}Ca efflux required the presence of extracellular Ca^{2+}. These findings support the view that glucose, by decreasing K^+ conductance and hence causing B-cell depolarization, provokes the gating of voltage-sensitive Ca^{2+} channels, leading to stimulated Ca^{2+} influx. However, the inhibitory effect of the sugar upon Ca^{2+} outflow appears unrelated to changes in K^+ conductance and membrane potential.

406

Important Role of Glucose in Regulating Pancreatic Somatostatin Secretion. S. SEINO, H. SAKURAI*, Y. SEINO*, K. TANIGAWA, K. TSUDA, H. KUZUYA, and H. IMURA, Kyoto, Japan.

Since the D cells are closely located to the A and B cells within the pancreatic islet, glucose known to affect insulin and glucagon release possibly plays an important role in regulating somatostatin (IRS) secretion. To test this, effects of glucose alone and glucose together with arginine on IRS secretion were studied using the isolated perfused rat pancreas. After equilibration period, glucose concentration was increased progressively at 15 min intervals from 0 to 16.7mM and then lowered to 4.4mM. Basal IRS levels were 21$\pm$6 pg/ml (mean $\pm$SE) in the absence of glucose. No significant increase in IRS levels was observed when glucose concentration was raised to 4.4mM. IRS secretion, however, was slightly increased at 8.8mM glucose and markedly increased at 16.7mM glucose. Total IRS increments above basal level ($\Sigma\Delta$IRS) were 57$\pm$27 pg/ml and 385$\pm$101 pg/ml during the stimulation of 8.8mM and 16.7mM glucose, respectively. In different series of experiment, following the equilibration period, arginine stimulus (19mM, 15min) was applied in the presence of varying glucose concentrations. IRS response to arginine expressed as $\Sigma\Delta$IRS was not evident in the absence of glucose, but 135$\pm$31 pg/ml and 442$\pm$36 pg/ml in the presence of 4.4mM and 11mM glucose, respectively. Thus, arginine enhanced IRS secretion in proportion to glucose concentration.

These results lead us to conclude that glucose directly stimulates IRS secretion and potentiates arginine-induced IRS secretion.

407

Effect of tolbutamide on Na^+-K^+-Mg^{++}-ATPase in fish islet (Brockmann body) and rat liver <u>in vitro</u>. S.KAWAZU*,M.IKEUCHI, H.SANDO,M,KIKUCHI, Y.KANAZAWA* and K.KOSAKA,TOKYO,JAPAN

We attempted to study the effect of tolbutamide on Na^+-K^+-Mg^{++} ATPase activity <u>in vitro</u>, comparing with those of other insulin secretagogues (glucose,L-arginine, X537A, A23187 etc.), using the tissue homogenates or membrane fractions from fish islet and rat liver. ATPase activity in the presence of Na^+,K^+,Mg^{++} (140:14:5 mM) and EDTA(0.5 mM), which was inhibited about 80% with ouabain (1 mM),was dose dependently depressed with tolbutamide (0-5000 µg/ml), but not with glucose (0-16.7 mM). $CaCl_2$ (10 mM) and X537A (100 µM) strongly inhibited the activity of Na^+-K^+-Mg^{++} ATPase, but A23187 (20 µM) did not. These effects on ATPase in fish islet and rat liver were not largely different. Tolbutamide is reported to potentiate ^{45}Ca uptake in islets of Langerhans, probably through the ionophoretic system of plasma membranes without entering into the cell. In conclusion, tolbutamide acts also on the energy-dependent cation movement across cell membranes, either directly or indirectly, to some extent mimicking X537A.

408

Reduced A Cell and Increased D Cell Responsiveness in Spontaneously Diabetic BB/W Rats with Absolute Insulin Deficiency. G. BODEN,* C. BARKER, A. NAJI and F. MATSCHINSKY,* Philadelphia, PA.

Non-obese BB/W rats spontaneously develop destructive inflammation of the pancreatic islets. This results in insulin dependent diabetes which closely resembles the early stages of human insulin dependent diabetes. There are presently no detailed data on the effects of this form of islitis on the secretory function of the major hormone producing islet cells. Using the isolated perfused pancreas technique, we have studied the release of immunoreactive glucagon (IRG), insulin (IRI) and somatostatin (SLI) in 4 diabetic and in 3 non-diabetic BB/W rats after stimulation with amino acids (AA, 15 mM) and after AA + glucose (G, 10 mM). No IRI release was detectable in diabetic rats after AA or AA + G. The IRG response to AA was reduced in diabetics to 25% of controls (7.2±3.6 ng vs. 27.6±8.1 ng per 25 min., $p < 0.05$) and G failed to exert the physiological suppression of AA stimulated IRG release (AA vs. AA + G = 7.2±3.6 ng vs. 6.4±2.6 ng per 25 min., $p > 0.05$). The SLI response to AA + G was markedly enhanced in diabetics as compared to controls (36.1±7.1 ng vs. 7.9±1.2 ng per 25 min., $p < 0.05$). The absolute insulin deficiency is consistent with the clinical picture and published morphological data. The low *in vitro* response of the A cells to AA is surprising, yet the hyperglucagonemia observed *in vivo* could be due to glucose resistance of these cells. The hyperresponsiveness of D cells to glucose resembles data obtained by our team in 5 day starved rats. Its etiology and significance remain uncertain.

409

Index of B-cell Response: A measure of the Severity of Diabetes? A. HADJI-GEORGOPOULOS, D. MEHIGAN, P. BROE, J. CAMERON, and A.A. KOWARSKI (Introduced by S. MARGOLIS*), Baltimore, MD.

Insulin resistance in obese subjects affects their glucose tolerance (GT); therefore measuring GT does not adequately reflect the severity of their diabetes. An index based on insulin secretion may be more appropriate. The relation of GT and B-cell response to glucose and secretin was studied in 6 control dogs and in 10 with pancreatic autotransplants in the spleen. GT was measured by the glucose assimilation rate (Kg = min^{-1} x 100). The transplanted animals had varying degrees of glucose intolerance with Kg values 0.1-0.9 vs 0.9-1.7 in the controls. Peripheral blood glucose levels and portal integrated insulin concentrations were measured continuously. After a baseline period, an i.v. bolus of a 50% glucose solution (0.15 g/kg) was administered, followed by an i.v. bolus of secretin (0.1 U/kg) 2 h later. The fasting blood glucose level (FBG) was used to separate the transplanted animals into 6 mild diabetics (FBG<140 mg/dl) and 4 moderate diabetics (FBG>140 mg/dl). We measured the percent change in insulin during the initial 5 min after glucose (IGR) and secretin (IGS). We also calculated an index of B-cell response (IBR): IBR=IGR+IGS. In the controls Kg values correlated with both the IBR (r=0.976) and IGR (r=0.871); and similarly in the mildly diabetic dogs (IBR: r=0.896; r=0.933). However, in the moderately diabetic dogs the IBR was better correlated with the Kg values (r=0.793) than the IGR (r=0.538). Conclusion: the IBR might be useful in assessing the severity of moderate diabetes in obese subjects.

410

Studies on the Glycoprotein Components of β-cell Plasma Membranes from Rat Insulinoma. N.A.PANJWANI, W.L.CHICK,* and R.G.SPIRO,* Boston, Ma.

Carbohydrates of the β-cell surface, by acting as receptors or antigens, may play a role in many processes that affect the metabolism of this cell. Plasma membranes were isolated by density gradient centrifugations from insulinomas previously shown to consist of well-differentiated β-cells (yield: 68 mg membrane/100 g tumor). Total carbohydrate of the membranes was 8 mg/100 mg peptide and it was present as galactose, mannose, glucose, fucose, xylose, glucosamine (GlcN), galactosamine (GalN) and sialic acid (SA). After delipidation the membranes retained 74% of their carbohydrate and were shown to contain at least 5 glycoprotein components (apparent M.W.= 50 to 140K) by polyacrylamide gel electrophoresis. With a chloroform-methanol extraction procedure a glycoprotein fraction (GP) was obtained which primarily contained two of the components (M.W.= 100 and 140K). The total saccharide of this fraction was 20 mg/100 mg peptide and was present as galactose, mannose, fucose, GlcN, GalN and SA in molar ratios of 0.9:1.0:0.1:2.1:0.7:1.7 respectively. GP reacted strongly with wheat germ agglutinin (WGA) by precipitin reaction and 85% of ^{3}H-labeled GP was retained on WGA-Sepharose column permitting further purification. After treatment with neuraminidase GP reaction with WGA was abolished but interaction with peanut lectin became evident; this suggested the occurrence of chains with a sialic acid-galactose-N-acetylgalactosamine sequence.

The plasma membrane glycoproteins being characterized in this study may contribute to an understanding of cell surface reactions which regulate islet function.

411

Exponential Loss of β-cell Function and Islet Mass is Asynchronal with Hyperglycemia after Low Doses of Streptozotocin. VAGN BONNEVIE-NIELSEN, Copenhagen, Denmark. Introduced by M.W. STEFFES.

Mice (C 57 Bl/KsJ) were given streptozotocin (40 mg/kg) in 5 daily i.p.-injections. Non-fasting hyperglycemia was present on experimental day 7, whereas an increase in fasting blood glucose was not detectable until day 12.

At day 6, 8, 12 and 15 insulin release in response to glucose was determined by perfusion of the isolated mouse pancreas. *In situ* perfusion of each pancreas with dithizone was shown to stain the pancreatic islets specifically allowing a morphometric quantitation of the total islet area as well as islet number. Progressively with time the streptozotocin treatment resulted in a decreased release of insulin in response to 30 mmol/l glucose, affecting both the initial and the secondary phase. Consequently, the total amount of released insulin decreased being 21% of the controls on day 6, 12% on day 8, 5% on day 12 and 3% on day 15. In parallel both islet area ($p < 0.02$) and number ($p < 0.01$) were markedly reduced in good correlation with the loss in functional capacity of the gland. Light microscopy of the perfused glands showed inflammation of the islets on each experimental day.

The results indicate that fasting hyperglycemia after low doses of streptozotocin does not appear until the functional capacity and islet mass is reduced to 5-6% of the controls. In addition, a major impairment of the β-cell function is present before non-fasting hyperglycemia develops.

412

HPLC Preparation of High Specific Activity I^{125}-Labels of Insulin, Proinsulin and Other Polypeptide Hormones. BRUCE H. FRANK (Introduced by RONALD E. CHANCE*) Indianapolis, Indiana

We have investigated the use of HPLC to isolate high specific activity and specifically labelled I^{125} tracers of beef and pork insulins and proinsulins as well as other polypeptide hormones. Iodination was usually done by the Lactoperoxidase method. The specific radiolabel of interest was then isolated directly from the reaction mixture using a reverse-phase C_{18} HPLC system. This isolation procedure was quite rapid (less than 1 hour) and was specific in terms of the tracer isolated. With beef insulin for example, the I^{125} Insulin isolated was labelled on the A14-tyrosine. In addition, the same HPLC procedures were used to isolate the monoiodo-labels (I^{125} in each case on the A14-tyrosine) of pork insulin, and beef and pork proinsulins. We have also applied the same methodology to the rapid isolation of specific radiolabels of bovine pancreatic polypeptide, insulin A and B chain derivatives, and glucagon. All of these radiolabelled proteins have been quite stable. Moreover, because of their specific nature and high specific activity, these radiolabels have yielded greater sensitivity and more accuracy in radioimmuno- and radioreceptor assays than conventionally prepared and purified radiolabels of these same peptides.

413

Effect of Variations in Islet Size and Shape on Glucose-stimulated Insulin Secretion. EVE REAVEN*, GERALD GOLD and WILMER WALKER, Stanford, Ca.

Although it is known that collagenase-isolated islets of Langerhans vary in size and shape, it has not been clear what impact the size of an islet or its geometry has on its function. The present study considers the effect of islet size and shape on in vitro glucose-stimulated insulin secretion. Eight experiments were carried out. Islets were obtained from young (200-300 gram) rats and rapidly sorted into three size categories before incubation with 16.7 mM glucose (45 incubation vials; 20 islets/vial). Following incubation, the diameters of each islet (900 in all) were measured and values for surface area and volume, assuming various spheroidal or ellipsoidal shapes, were calculated for each islet. These various figures were correlated with the measured insulin secretion values from the same islets and a regression curve was generated for each different islet shape. The results indicate that insulin secretory rates increase directly as a function of islet size (r = 0.78; standard error of estimate = 0.71). Identical correlation coefficients were observed whatever shape was considered, whether islet area or islet volume was considered, or whether first or second order curves were calculated for each shape. Thus, within the range tested, the larger an islet is the more insulin it secretes (regardless of its shape) and studies utilizing isolated islets should be normalized for this factor. Measurements of islet diameter provide an easy and accurate solution to this problem.

414

Prostaglandins (PGs) and glucagon release : effect of phospholipase A_2 and indomethacin on isolated islets. Alfred S. LUYCKX* and Pierre J. LEFEBVRE*, Liège, Belgium.

Previous results from our Laboratory suggest that endogenous PGs stimulate glucagon secretion. We now report the influence of bee venom phospholipase A_2 (PhA, which increases arachidonate availability from membrane phospholipids) on glucagon release (GR) from isolated guinea-pig islets incubated *in vitro*.

Under control conditions (GEY and GEY buffer ; albumin 2 g/l ; glucose 1.7 mM/l), GR averaged 64 ± 4 pg/islet/90 min *i.e.* 1.5 ± 0.2 % of the islet glucagon content (IGC). GR was significantly increased in the presence of various concentrations of PhA ranging from 0.1 to 2.5 µg/ml. Expressed in % of IGC, glucagon release reached 4.5 ± 0.9 in the presence of 2.5 µg/ml PhA ($p < 0.005$ *versus* control conditions). This stimulatory effect was reduced by 67 % when the islets were preincubated and incubated in the presence of 100 µmol/l indomethacin (INDO). Using two successive 45 min incubation periods with 0.1 µg/ml PhA, we found that the stimulatory effect decreased with time and was totally blocked by INDO during the second incubation period. These results support the view that endogenous PGs indeed modulate glucagon release.

415

Suppressive Role of Prostaglandins on Insulin and Glucagon Secretion in Superfused Pancreatic Monolayer Cell Cultures. J.T. BRAATEN*, Y. SIDDIQUI, and C. ANDREADIS, Ottawa, Ontario.

The role of prostaglandins (PGs) in the regulation of insulin (IRI)and glucagon(IRG)secretion is controversial. To evaluate this question a superfusion system with monolayer cell cultures of neonatal rat pancreatic islets consisting mainly of purified endocrine cells, was used. The cultures were superfused continuously with tissue culture medium 199 (glucose 5.6mM). The IRI and IRG were measured in the superfusate collected every 10 min. At time 0 the precursor of PG-2 series, Linoleic acid(LA)3.6 µM; $PGF_{2\alpha}$ 2.8 µM or the PG synthetase inhibitor acetyl salicylic acid (ASA) 0.1 mM was added. The maximum effect of these substances on the hormone secretion was found at 30→40 min:

	IRG pg/min/culture		IRI ng/min/culture	
	-10→0	30→40min.	-10→0	30→40min.
LA	267±68	52±17*	12.2±1.9	8.9±1.5*
$PGF_{2\alpha}$	104±11	55± 3†	11.4±1.0	6.7±1.1†
ASA	153±25	265±43Φ	5.1±1.1	11.1±2.1Φ

* p<.04; † p<.01; Φ p<.003 N=6 Mean SEM

The obtained data indicate that both insulin and glucagon secretion were significantly suppressed by exposure to a precursor of PG and to $PGF_{2\alpha}$. On the contrary, the inhibition of endogenous PG synthesis by ASA resulted in a stimulation of insulin and glucagon secretion.

This study suggests that prostaglandins play a suppressive role in the regulation of insulin and glucagon secretion at a secretory dependent step common to both alpha and the beta cell.
(Supported by M.R.C. and C.D.A.).

Effect of Myo-inositol on Cell Division, Insulin Synthesis and Insulin Secretion in Cultured Rat Pancreatic Islets.

R.S. CLEMENTS, JR.* and C.S. PACE,* Birmingham, Al.

Although myo-inositol (MI) is recognized as an essential growth factor for most mammalian cells in culture, a requirement for exogenous MI has not been documented for cultured pancreatic islets. We cultured batches of adult rat islets for 6 days in CMRL-1066 medium containing 11 mM D-glucose and varying concentrations of MI. After the culture period, the incorporation of ^{3}H-thymidine into DNA and ^{3}H-leucine into proinsulin and insulin were measured as were the islet insulin content and capacity to secrete insulin in response to 16.7 mM D-glucose. As shown below, with the exception of DNA synthesis, a progressive increase was observed in all dimensions analyzed as the medium MI content was increased. DNA synthesis was maximal at 20 ug/ml MI. We conclude that cell division, insulin synthesis and the ability to secrete insulin in response to glucose may be critically dependent upon the MI concentration to which cultured islets are exposed in vitro.

Dimension Analyzed	Myo-inositol Content of Culture Medium (ug/ml) 0	20	40
DNA synthesis (dpm/islet/3 hrs)	60.7 ±4.6	256.2 ± 41.8*	53.0 ± 19.4
Proinsulin synthesis (dpm/islet/3 hrs)	2885 ±301	4527 ± 976	6903 ± 403*
Insulin synthesis (dpm/islet/3 hrs)	1982 ±181	2214 ± 500	4756 ± 277*
Insulin content (mU/islet)	0.49 ±0.19	1.05 ±0.08	1.60 ± 0.12*
Insulin secretion (%Δ vs. 5.5 mM glucose)	-14.2 ±23.9	+84.9 ± 23.7*	+229.5 ± 0.12*

*p versus absence of myo-inositol in the medium < 0.01

418

Effect of Repeated Injections of Islet Activating Protein (IAP) in Spontaneously Diabetic Animals.

TAKAYOSHI TOYOTA*, MASAEI KAKIZAKI, YOSHIO GOTO, MOTOYUKI YAJIMA, TAKESHI OKAMOTO, Sendai, Japan.

IAP extracted from B. pertussis culture medium has been shown to potentiate the acute phase insulin release to glucose in animals. A single injection lowers blood glucose for up to 30 days.

This study examined in 2 types of spontaneously diabetic animals - the Wistar rat and the Shionogi mouse, the effect of repeated intraperitoneal (i.p.) injections of IAP (1 mcg/Kg) on oral glucose tolerance (2 gm/kg glucose).

Seven Wistar rats received 8 i.p. injections of IAP over a period of 300 days. Pre-treatment ΣOGTT-glucose values were similar in this group and in 7 untreated control rats (1000 mg/dl). Post-treatment values were unchanged in the control group, but significantly lowered (p<0.01) in the IAP treated group (720 mg/dl).

The Shionogi mouse develops insulitis at 60 days resulting in diabetes and death in ketoacidosis by approx. 140 days. IAP was administered i.p. at 30, 72 and 120 days to 6 mice. Compared to control mice IAP significantly lowered the glucose response by increasing insulin release in response to the oral glucose load at days 30 and 72 only.

No anaphylactic reactions to IAP were observed.

417

Insulin Secretion: Effect of Simultaneous Parasympathetic and Sympathetic Neural Inputs. L. ARTHUR CAMPFIELD* and FRANCOISE J. SMITH, Los Angeles, CA.

Sympathetic (S) and parasympathetic (P) neural inputs can modify glucose induced insulin secretion (IS). We investigated the effects of both simultaneous and consecutive application of S and P inputs at an intermediate glucose (G) concentration, 10 mM. IS was determined by statically incubating 10 isolated rat islets in KRB with neurotransmitter for 30 to 60 min. Exposure of islets to NE or ACH resulted in dose-dependent inhibition or enhancement of IS, respectively. Near maximal concentrations were selected to assess the interaction of S and P inputs on IS: 30 μM ACH (A) and 0.3 μM NE (N). A significantly increased IS by 78 ± 10%, while N significantly inhibited IS by 38 ± 4%. When islets were simultaneously exposed to N + A, IS was inhibited by 39 ± 4% (n=7) and was not different than N alone. Thus, under these conditions, S was dominant. Consecutive incubations with A followed by N + A resulted in similar inhibitions of IS by N + A. However, consecutive incubation with N followed by N + A resulted in IS as follows: N: -33 ± 1%; N + A: -12 ± 6%. Thus, N completely inhibited A enhanced IS, while A partially overcame N inhibition of IS. Therefore, at 10 mM G, P enhances IS, S inhibits IS and S + P can also inhibit IS. The degree of inhibition of IS by S + P was dependent on the order of input application. We conclude that the effects of neural inputs on IS are a complex function of both the magnitudes and order of application of S and P inputs in addition to the local glucose concentration. (Supported by USPHS AM 23111, NSF PCM-78-006644)

419

Immunoreactive Gastric Inhibitory Polypeptide in a Glucagonoma. DAVID G. JOHNSON,* HUGO V. VILLAR, PHILLIP H. SMITH,* and JOHN C. BROWN, Tucson, Az.

Immunoreactive gastric inhibitory polypeptide (GIP) has been identified by immunoperoxidase histochemistry in A-cells of several mammalian species and a few human glucagonomas. We removed a 4 x 2.5 x 2 cm glucagonoma from a 47 year old woman with mild diabetes mellitus. Preoperative plasma glucagon was 2009 pg/ml. Fractionation on a Biogel P-30 column revealed peaks of both higher molecular weight and 3500 dalton glucagon. Pieces of the tumor were fixed immediately for subsequent immunohistochemical identification of immunoreactive glucagon, insulin, somatostatin, pancreatic polypeptide, and GIP. Although the tumor cells appeared homogeneous by conventional staining, scattered single cells stained for glucagon and GIP. No cells stained for insulin, somatostatin, or pancreatic polypeptide. A 0.5 N acetic acid extract of tumor tissue contained 18 μg of glucagon and 94 ng of GIP per g fresh tissue. Fractionation of tumor extract on a Biogel P-30 column revealed that immunoreactive glucagon was present mainly in the 3500 dalton peak. Immunoreactive GIP was detected in three peaks that did not co-elute with glucagon. Neither of the two GIP peaks that represented molecular species larger than glucagon eluted in the same fractions as the large molecular weight glucagon found in preoperative plasma. These results suggest that glucagonoma cells make a GIP-like polypeptide that is different from both normal glucagon and the high molecular weight glucagon released into plasma.

420

Enhancement of Epinephrine-stimulated Glucagon Secretion by Tolbutamide. BARBARA PETRACK,* ANDREW J.CZERNIK and JUSTIN ANSELL, Ardsley, N.Y.

The effects of tolbutamide (T) on glucagon and insulin secretion from the isolated, perfused rat pancreas were examined under a variety of experimental conditions. At 50 μM, T stimulated insulin release under basal conditions (80 mg% glucose in perfusate) and potentiated the release of insulin by 20 mM arginine. T inhibited arginine-induced glucagon secretion. These effects of T were rapid in onset and readily reversible upon removal of the drug from the perfusate. To test whether the suppression of glucagon was a direct effect on the α-cell or an indirect result of T-stimulated insulin release, conditions were devised to eliminate endogenous insulin secretion. Epinephrine (270 nM) was used to stimulate glucagon secretion in pancreases isolated from rats which were acutely pretreated with streptozotocin (75 mg/kg i.v.) Under these conditions, no insulin secretion was detected, but surprisingly, T markedly potentiated the epinephrine-stimulated release of glucagon. Using pancreas preparations from untreated rats, this effect of T on glucagon secretion was much less pronounced. Glyburide (G) was also tested in similar experiments. The effect of 20 nM G on epinephrine-stimulated glucagon secretion in acutely streptozotocin-treated rats was small compared to T, and G appeared to have a prolonged duration of action under conditions of basal and arginine perfusion.

If these findings extend to the clinical situation, enhancement of epinephrine-induced glucagon secretion by T might be detrimental to diabetics, especially under conditions of stress or exercise, when catecholamine levels are elevated.

421

Selective Impairment of Beta-cell Responses by Ethionine-induced Pancreatitis in Rats. KATHLEEN VERMITSKY and F.X. PI-SUNYER,* New York, N.Y.

We previously found that secretin (0.1 U/ml) fails to increase insulin secretion by perfused rat pancreases in which pancreatitis was induced by 2 weeks of 0.5% DL-ethionine feeding (E). Secretin does stimulate insulin release by pancreases isolated from food-restricted controls (C) to 218% of basal. To further investigate this impairment of islet function in pancreatitis, we perfused E and C pancreases with 5.5 mM glucose and: 1) 1.5 μM vasoactive intestinal peptide (VIP) which is structurally similar to secretin; 2) 0.05 μM somatotropin release inhibiting factor (SRIF) which, like secretin, is effective in preparations of intact pancreases but may not be in those with disrupted islet-acinar relationships; 3) 0.5 μM isoproterenol which has been postulated to bind to the same islet receptor as secretin.

VIP increased insulin and glucagon secretion by both E and C pancreases. SRIF inhibited arginine-stimulated insulin and glucagon release by E and C pancreases. In contrast, isoproterenol failed to stimulate insulin secretion from E pancreases, whereas the response of C pancreases was 211% of basal. These findings suggest that ethionine-induced pancreatitis selectively damages a receptor or effector common to secretin and isoproterenol, thereby supporting the hypothesis that these agents act upon the same islet receptor.

422

Effects of Calcium, Magnesium and Potassium on Pancreatic D-cell Function in Vitro. L. Mandarino, M. Itoh, W. Blanchard, and J. Gerich,* Endocrine Research Unit, Mayo Clinic, Rochester, Minnesota.

Extracellular calcium (Ca^{++}), magnesium (Mg^{++}), and potassium (K^+) modulate insulin (IRI) and glucagon secretion but the effect of these cations on somatostatin (IRS) release has not been determined. Therefore, the effect of selective deficiency of these cations and their dose-response relationship with both IRS and IRI release from cat pancreases perfused in vitro were investigated. To minimize intraislet variables, supraphysiologic concentrations of exogenous glucagon (0.05 μM) were used to stimulate hormone secretion. Glucagon in the presence of Ca^{++} (2.1 mM), Mg^{++} (1.2 mM) and K^+ (4.4 mM) stimulated biphasic release of IRS and IRI. Omission of Ca^{++} or Mg^+ from perfusate decreased both basal and stimulated IRS release; omission of K^+ increased basal but decreased stimulated IRS release. Omission of K^+ or Ca^{++} decreased basal and stimulated IRS release; omission of Mg^{++} increased basal but not stimulated IRI release. When Ca^{++} (2.1-16.8 mM) was added to perfusate, IRS and IRI secretion increased with different dose-responsive kinetics; IRI, but not IRS, release was inhibited at 16.8 mM Ca^{++}. Addition of K^+ (1.1-17.6 mM) enhanced both IRS and IRI secretion; large spikes of IRS and IRI release occurred at 8.7 and 17.6 mM K^+ probably due to depolarization. Addition of Mg^{++} (0.6-7.2 mM) decreased both IRS and IRI secretion with no apparent dose-response relationship. Conclusions: Extracellular Ca^{++} and K^+ are essential for both IRS and IRI release but appear to modulate islet B- and D-cell function differently whereas Mg^{++} depresses both B- and D-cell function similarly.

423

Sympathetic Nerve Stimulation Suppresses Secretion Rates of Somatostatin and Insulin: Differing Effects of Adrenergic Blockade. MARK W. ROY, M. SUE JONES, and RALPH E. MILLER*., Lexington, Ky.

Pancreata of mongrel puppies (3-6 kg) were isolated (including exclusion of the duodenum) in situ and perfused in a nonrecirculating system with oxygenated Krebs-Ringer bicarbonate buffer. Bilateral 3 min. splanchnic nerve stimulation (stim., 5 Hz, 20 V, 1 msec) or 3 min. norepinephrine (NE) infusion (10μg/ml) were tested for effect on the pancreatic immunoreactive somatostatin secretion rate (SSR), immunoreactive insulin secretion rate (ISR), and perfusion pressure in control experiments (no blockade) and during infusion of phentolamine (PN, 10μg/kg.·min) or propranalol (PR, 2μg/kg.·min). Results are in the Table. (↑ = increase, p<.05; ↓ = decrease, p<.05; – = no change).

Blocker	Dogs	SSR		ISR		Perfusion Pressure	
		Stim	NE	Stim	NE	Stim	NE
None	10	↓	↓	↓	↓	↑	↑
PN	3	↓	↓	↑	↑	–	↑
PR	3	↓	↓	↓	↓	↑	↑

Since phentolamine infusion reverses the effect of sympathetic nerve stimulation or norepinephrine infusion on the secretion rate of insulin but not somatostatin, we conclude that the adrenoceptors regulating the output of these hormones are different.

Dept. of Pharmacology, University of Kentucky Medical Center, Lexington, Ky. Supported by NIH grant # AM17082 and the Isabell Kircher Fund.

424

.timulus Effects on Membrane Potential [E_m] and Intracellular Ca Activity (a_{Ca}) during Secretion J. O'Doherty and R.J. Stark and W. McD. Armstrong (introduced by S. Wentworth*) Indianapolis, IN

It is proposed that the initial membrane receptor-secretion regulator interaction causes changes in E_m that result from translocation of Na, K, and Cl ions and alters a_{Ca} to activate an effector system controlling excytosis. The fly salivary gland has emerged as a model system for examining secretory control. In this epithelial system, Serotonin (5-HT)-induced changes in E_m and a_{Ca} are conc. dependent. Cells stimulated with 10^{-8}M 5-HT produced a 5 mV hyperpolarization in E_m and when impaled with a Ca selective electrode produced spontaneous oscillations in the Ca-potential (E_{Ca}). These oscillatory deflections had a mean amplitude of 9.8 $\pm$ 0.6 mV and resulted from a short phasic 2-3 fold increase in aC_a. Higher conc. of 5-HT (10^{-7}M) resulted in depolarization of both E_m (14 $\pm$ 1.3 mV) and E_{Ca} (64 $\pm$ 2.1 mV). A dramatic increase in a_{Ca} was observed that was directly related to the stimulus duration. Prolonged stimulation with 10^{-7}M 5-HT (5-10 min.) increased a_{Ca} to (2.5 $\pm$ 0.3) x 10^{-4}M with a loss of the spontaneous buffering of a_{Ca} observed with 10^{-8}M 5-HT. Recovery of the original E_{Ca} depended solely on how quickly 5-HT was washed away with the normal saline soln. These results suggest that stimulation of secretory cells with higher than physiological concs. of hormone could interfere with the normal a_{Ca} regulation and lead to misinterpretation of the mechanism of stimulus-secretion coupling. (Supported by American Diabetes Assoc. and USPHS AM 26246, AM 12715, and HL 23332.

425

Analytical Fractionation of B-Cells. AUSTIN C. MIRCHEFF, LOREN G. LIPSON*, MICHAEL J. BUSH, AEREE YOON and JOHN J. BARISH, Los Angeles, Cal.

As the first stage in identifying factors which control the release of insulin, we are devising methods for analytical fractionation of B-cells and, in particular, for the simultaneous isolation of plasma membranes and secretory granules. Preparations of islets(at least 80% B-cells) were homogenized in an isotonic sorbitol buffer containing 40% ficoll and 0.3 mM $MgCl_2$. Total particulate fractions were applied to linear gradients of 5 to 35% ficoll containing 5% sorbitol and 0.5 mM EDTA and centrifuged at 60,000 rpm for 90 min. 50% of the potassium-stimulated phosphatase (K-PNPPase), a plasma membrane marker, was resolved into a symmetrical peak centered at 10% ficoll. Peak alkaline phosphatase, believed associated with plasma membranes, overlapped the high density portion of K-PNPPase. Adenylate cyclase overlapped the lower density portion of the K-PNPPase peak. It was enriched 4 fold over the homogenate. Less than 10% of the insulin remained in the sample layer, suggesting that the secretory granules were intact. Insulin showed a plateau in the higher density region of the gradient with a specific content 4 fold over the homogenate and suggests that the granules are contaminated to only a minor extent by other subcellular components.

The resolution of our fractionation procedure is now sufficient that we expect to be able to distinguish plasma membrane-associated and granule membrane-associated substrates for protein phosphorylation.

426

Neural Control of Pancreatic Somatostatin Release. GERALD J. TABORSKY, JR.,* THOMAS L. PAQUETTE, and JOHN W. ENSINCK,* Seattle, WA.

To test the hypothesis that pancreatic D-cells are under neural control, we first examined the effect of a systemic infusion of a beta-adrenergic agonist on somatostatin (SLI) output from the in situ dog pancreas. Isoproterenol (ISO, 2 μg/min x 60 min, IV) increased both insulin (IRI) ($\bar{x}\Delta$ = +3,675 $\pm$ 1153 mU/min, $p<0.01$) and SLI output ($\bar{x}\Delta$ = +201 $\pm$ 74 pg/min, $p<0.025$, n = 10). To provide direct neural input to the pancreatic D-cells, we next electrically stimulated the pancreatic nerves (8 Hz, 1 msec pulses, 10 mAmp) for 5 minutes. Norepinephrine (NE), but not epinephrine (EPI), increased consistently in pancreatic vein plasma (ΔNE= +372 $\pm$ 94 pg/ml, $p<0.01$; ΔEPI = +27 $\pm$ 15 pg/ml, p = NS) confirming localized sympathetic stimulation. Both IRI and SLI output decreased (ΔIRI= -1,045 $\pm$ 342 mU/min, $p<0.01$; ΔSLI= -179 $\pm$ 64 pg/min, $p<0.025$, n = 8). This inhibition of SLI was apparently not due to a generalized decrease of pancreatic hormone output for both glucagon (IRG) and pancreatic polypeptide (PP) remained unchanged during nerve stimulation. Summary: 1) Systemic ISO infusion increases both pancreatic SLI and IRI output. 2) Local nerve stimulation decreases both SLI and IRI output with no significant effect on IRG or PP output. Conclusion: 1) Pancreatic somatostatin is under neural control. 2) Beta adrenergic stimulation increases somatostatin release, whereas alpha adrenergic and/or cholinergic stimulation may decrease pancreatic somatostatin secretion.

427

Hyperglycemia During Adrenergic Stimulation Compensates for Impaired Insulin Release. J. BEARD*, D. PORTE, JR.,* Seattle, WA.

Glucose regulates pancreatic islet function by stimulating insulin (IRI) secretion and by enhancing (potentiating) the acute insulin response (AIR) to non-glucose stimuli. Epinephrine (EPI) inhibits the insulin response to glucose, but does EPI affect glucose potentiation? To examine this question, we measured AIR ($\bar{x}$ ΔIRI, 2-5') to 5 gm IV arginine (ARG) in normal subjects during saline (SAL) infusion and, on separate days, EPI infusions: 15 ng/kg/min (LO-EPI) and 80 ng/kg/min (HI-EPI). AIR during HI-EPI did not differ from AIR during SAL (59 $\pm$ 7 μU/ml vs 64 $\pm$ 18, $\bar{x}$ $\pm$ SEM; n = 5, p = NS). However, HI-EPI infusion raised prestimulus glucose (PG) levels above those observed during SAL (187 $\pm$ 6 mg/dl vs 99 $\pm$ 4, n = 5, $p < .001$). Therefore, variable glucose infusions were used to obtain three stepwise-increasing PG levels on each study day, with each subject's levels on the SAL day matched to his levels on the EPI days. At matched PG levels ranging from 142 to 251 mg/dl, HI-EPI inhibited AIR by 77 $\pm$ 5% compared to AIR during SAL (n = 6, $p < .001$). With PG matched, LO-EPI produced a smaller inhibition of AIR (39 $\pm$ 8%, n = 10, $p < .001$). To quantify EPI's effect on glucose potentiation, the change in AIR accompanying a given increment of PG was expressed as a slope: ΔAIR/ΔPG. These glucose potentiation slopes were inversely related to log plasma EPI (r = -.83, n = 10, $p < .002$). Thus, the potentiating effect of PG elevation on AIR to ARG declines as EPI concentration increases. We conclude that arginine-stimulated insulin secretion during EPI infusion can appear normal only because the induced hyperglycemia compensates for EPI's inhibitory effect on glucose potentiation.

428

Piroglíride-Induced Alteration of Beta Cell Responsiveness. Walter S. Zawalich*, Victoria A. Weill, Franz M. Matschinsky*, Philadelphia, PA.

Piroglíride (McNeil 3495) is an effective potentiator of glucose (G)-induced insulin release (IR) and glucose usage (GU). Experiments were conducted to further characterize its effects on collagenase isolated islets. IR was determined during islet perifusion and GU by the rate of T_2O formation from 5-T-G. In the presence of 5.5 mM G, Piroglíride (P) potentiated insulin release at 10μM and above. Maximal potentiation (350%) was noted with 100μM P. Higher concentrations reduced the secretory response. GU was accelerated by P in a dose dependent manner. However concentrations above 100μM, reduced GU. Comprehensive studies with different G concentrations and 100μM P demonstrated that the compound shifted the dose-response curve for both IR and GU to the left, reducing the K_m for both responses while not effecting the maximal response.

In the absence of G, 100μM piroglíride has no effect on IR. This contrasts with 500μM tolbutamide which causes a spike of IR under this condition. Omission of calcium from the perifusion medium abolished P effects on glucose-induced IR, while the addition of atropine (500μM) had no effect of P-potentiated IR. P(100μM) potentiated the insulin secretory response to 7mM α-ketoisocaproate and 15 mM N-acetylglucosamine.

P, or a derivative, may prove to be important not only as a probe for elucidating the processes which govern islet cell responsiveness, but also in the therapy of non-insulin dependent diabetes.

429

Insulin Release in the Diabetic Chinese Hamster Pancreas: Why an Excess Response to Theophylline? B.J. FRANKEL,* A. HELDT, and G.M. GRODSKY,* San Francisco, CA.

Pancreases from adult Chinese hamsters (male & female) from 1 normal and 3 diabetic (insulin-deficient type) sublines inbred 15 or more generations were perfused in vitro with: (1) glucose 5.5 mM + arginine 20 mM (gluc+arg); (2) theophylline 10 mM (theoph); or (3) KCl 18.3 mM (K); n = 5 to 8 in each group; total = 150. Mean fed plasma glucose = 97±2 and 321±9 mg/dl, respectively.

The diabetics showed subnormal insulin release to gluc+arg (-66%; P<<.001) and to K (-47%; P<<.001), but excessive responses to theoph (+97%; P<.001). One diabetic subline consistently showed excess glucagon responses to all stimuli (P<.005 - .05). In certain diabetic sublines, females showed less insulin release than males in response to gluc+arg and K, while, in normals, females showed more insulin release than males to gluc+arg. Sex differences are unexplained.

Because diabetic pancreases show excess insulin responses to theoph, their subnormal insulin responses to gluc+arg and K cannot be due solely to their decreased pancreatic insulin content (-78%; P<<<.001).

Siegel et al. (Biochem. J. 180:233,1979) showed gluc+IBMX-induced insulin release but little ^{45}Ca efflux in diabetic hamster islets. One possibility is that the diabetic hamster B cell may have a defect in its Ca metabolism such that Ca stores are glucose-inaccessible but cAMP-accessible. Diabetics' insensitivity to K indicates a defect distal to any defect(s) in the recognition or metabolism of glucose and arginine.

430

Differential Effects of K^+ on Glucagon Secretion in a Cultured Islet-cell Tumor and its Clones. S. SMITH, S. BHATHENA,* H. OIE, A.GAZDAR, S. WILKINS and L. RECANT,* Washington, D.C.

In the isolated rat pancreas perfusion under arginine-glucose stimulation, we have shown that elevated $[K^+]$ decreased glucagon (IRG) secretion and increased insulin (IRI) secretion. We now report that decreased $[K^+]$ has the reverse effect on these hormones, and that when period to period K^+-induced changes in IRG secretion are plotted against corresponding changes in IRI secretion, a significant negative correlation is obtained (p<.001; 13 perfusions). This suggests a possible intra-islet regulation of hormone secretion. While insulin seems a likely mediator for such regulation, further experiments using diabetic pancreas, glucose-free media, or insulin clamp methods show persistence of IRG responses to K^+ without measureable changes in IRI release.

We investigated these mechanisms further using a cultured islet-cell tumor line secreting mostly IRI, with appreciable somatostatin (SRIF) and small amounts of IRG. Clones secreting predominantly IRI or SRIF were also studied. The parent cell line showed the same response to K^+ as the pancreas perfusion; however, most clones showed increased IRG secretion in response to elevated $[K^+]$. No correlations could be made between changes in IRG secretion and corresponding changes in either SRIF or IRI. These data suggest that elevated $[K^+]$ may have a direct stimulatory action on islet cells, and that islet architectural organization, perhaps maintained to some extent in the parent cell line, may be required for elevated $[K^+]$ to inhibit IRG release.

431

Sensitivity of Insulin (I) Secretion to Feedback Inhibition by Hyperinsulinemia (HI) is Impaired in Diabetes. O FABER, E FERRANNINI, J WAHREN, R DeFRONZO, New Haven, CT, Stockholm, Sweden, Copenhagen, Denmark.

The ability of I to inhibit its own secretion has been the subject of much controversy. In the present study we have examined the effect of physiologic HI on endogenous I secretion, using C-peptide (CP). In 15 normal subjects a steady state plateau of HI was created while plasma glucose (G) was held constant at basal levels by a variable G infusion. I was infused at three rates (0.25-0.5, 1.0, or 5-10 mU/kg·min) and resulted in steady state plasma I of 43±4, 97±9, and 828±210 μU/ml. Fasting CP, 0.29±0.02 pmol/ml, fell significantly in all subjects by 60 min to 0.20±0.2 (p<0.01) and declined further to 0.14±0.03 (p<0.001) at 120 min. The decline in CP was similar in all three I infusion groups and was unrelated to the steady state plasma I. Fasting CP (0.34±0.03 pmol/ml) in 8 normal maturity-onset diabetic (MOD) with fasting hyperglycemia (168±4 mg%) was similar to controls. When I was infused at 1 mU/kg·min (plasma I=119±5 μU/ml), the decline in CP was markedly blunted. No decrease was observed at 60 min and by 120 min CP had declined to only 0.28±0.03 pmol/ml (p<0.001 vs controls). Conclusions: (1) basal I secretion is inhibited by small physiologic increments in plasma I independent of changes in plasma G, (2) supraphysiologic elevations in plasma I do not further decrease I secretion above that with mild HI, (3) the ability of HI to inhibit endogenous I secretion is impaired in MOD. This attenuated suppressive effect of HI on I secretion may result from a stimulatory action of hyperglycemia.

432

Transitory Inhibition by Morphine Sulfate of Glucose-Stimulated Insulin Release From Rat Pancreatic Islets. STEVEN W. RYDER, Bronx, N.Y. (Introduced by ROSALYN S. YALOW* Bronx, N.Y.)

Numerous metabolic and endocrine effects of opiate compounds have been described, including effects on pancreatic insulin release. We investigated the influence of morphine sulfate (MS) on glucose stimulated insulin (Ins) release from rat pancreatic islets (PI). PI were isolated by collagenase digestion from 200-250g male Sprague-Dawley rats fed ad libitum. Four sets of PI were initially superfused for 50 min with buffered 1.7 mM glucose then superfused for an additional 50 min with buffered 5.5 mM glucose, 2 sets with (+) and 2 without (-) MS ($5x10^{-5}$M). Aliquots of superfusion effluent were collected and radioimmunoassayed for Ins (rat Ins standards). During control period Ins in effluents averaged 1.44±12 ng/min/30 islets. Ins in effluents during experimental periods are shown in Table:

Time	Insulin (ng/min/30 islets) (Mean ± SEM, N=2) (-) MS	(+) MS
at 6 min	3.70 ± .69	2.93 ± .48 (NS)
18-22	3.50 ± .30	1.55 ± .09 (p<.05)
46-50	3.18 ± .38	3.68 ± .04 (NS)

These results demonstrate that MS inhibits glucose-stimulated Ins release only transiently from isolated rat PI and are consistent with prior observations using this superfusion system (Ryder et al, Horm Metab Res, in press) of a transient inhibitory effect of MS on glucose plus arginine-stimulated insulin release from rat pancreatic islets.

434

Microtubular-Microfilamentous System's Role in Development of Glucose-Induced Insulin Release. RONALD S. HILL & WILLIAM B. RHOTEN*, Urbana, IL.

The role of microtubules (MT) & microfilaments (MF) in the onset & maturation of glucose-induced insulin secretion in the rat β cell (day 17 of gestation, D17G, to 6 days postnatally, D6PN) was examined in a perifusion system. D6PN β cells showed a rapid onset of release (early phase: 2-12 min post-stimulus) followed by sustained release (late phase: 15-45 min). This reflects maturation to the adult pattern from a glucose refractory state at D17G. Vinblastine (VB) inhibited the maximal secretory rate (peak) and/or the total amount released (tot) in response to 3.5 mg/ml glucose at D6PN, D21G & D20G. Cytochalasin B (CB) increased secretion in response to high glucose. The arginine-induced response at D17G was not detectably altered by VB or CB.

Effect of VB(20μM) & CB(10μg/ml): % Δ controls

AGE	VINBLASTINE early PHASE peak	VINBLASTINE early PHASE tot	VINBLASTINE late peak	VINBLASTINE late tot	CYTOCHALASIN B early PHASE peak	CYTOCHALASIN B early PHASE tot	CYTOCHALASIN B late peak	CYTOCHALASIN B late tot
D6PN	77λ	79	46λ	49†	230	208	126	137
D21G	79λ	77λ	64†	70	213λ	188λ	183	163
D20G	71†	67§	67†	63†	211†	191λ	179λ	190λ
D17G	108	88	43	54	91	107	86	65

λ,p < .05; †,p < .005; §,p < .002

Since agents that modify MT or MF altered the D20G secretory dynamics, the subsequent maturation to a fully biphasic pattern is probably not dependent upon the MT-MF system. However, the onset of glucose responsiveness of the fetal β cell may be correlated with development of some aspect of the MT-MF system. Aided by a grant from the American Diabetes Association-Downstate Illinois Affiliate and the C. J. Diffenderger Fund.

433

Glucose Modulation of Insulin and Somatostatin Release from the Isolated Perfused Rat Pancreas. D.V. LINDELL, R.L. SORENSON*, and R.P. ELDE, Minneapolis, MN.

Glucose stimulation of somatostatin (SS) has been previously reported. However, the extent of this response and its characteristics have largely gone unnoted. The objective of this study was to characterize the SS response to glucose and its possible contribution to glucose stimulated insulin release.

Perfusion of pancreata at a sustatined 300 mg/dl glucose concentration resulted in a 10 fold increase of SS (198±20 pg/ml) over basal 50 mg/dl (18±2 pg/ml) whereas insulin increased 25 fold (.47±.12 ng/ml to 12.8± 1.7 ng/ml). Stimulation was sustained over the 20 minute 300 mg/dl treatment period and rapidly declined to basal release during 50 mg/dl perfusion. The response of both hormones was biphasic, with the first phase response of SS slightly, but consistently, delayed with respect to that of insulin.

The effect of a glucose gradient on the release of insulin and SS was also tested. As the glucose concentration in the perfusate increased linearly from 50 mg/dl to 300 mg/dl over a 40 minute period, insulin and SS were released in parallel, with a slight lag in the initial SS response. The first detectable release greater than basal level occurred at 88.5±1.8 mg/dl glucose for insulin and 97.5±4.5 mg/dl for SS.

When exogenous SS was perfused along with the glucose gradient the insulin response at 10^{-9}M SS was identical to controls except that basal release was depressed. In addition to inhibiting basal release, SS at 10^{-8} and 10^{-7} M delayed the insulin response to glucose (to 103 mg/dl at 10^{-8}M; to 153 mg/dl at 10^{-7}M), and suppressed insulin release throughout the duration of the gradient. The K_I was estimated to be $3.4X10^{-8}$M SS. When SS antisera was perfused with the gradient, no significant difference from the controls was observed.

In spite of the marked 10 fold stimulation of SS release in response to glucose, the estimated intra-islet concentration of SS ($1X10^{-9}$M) is not sufficiently great to modulate glucose stimulated insulin release in the isolated perfused rat pancreas.

435

Portal Vein Insulin Response of Low Glucose Tolerant Yucatan Miniature Swine to Common Secretogogues. RONALD S. SPANGLER and ROBERT W. PHILLIPS; Ft. Collins, Colorado

Low glucose tolerant miniature swine (low K) exhibited an impaired portal vein insulin response to an intravenous glucose tolerance test (IVGTT) when compared to that of control animals (6.74 ± 1.25 ng vs. 37.75 ± 4.70 ng; p<.001). The portal vein insulin response to infusions of arginine, leucine and isoproterenol were examined. A significant difference was noted in the insulin response to a 30-minute infusion of arginine (.5 g/kg) between low K and control animals (8.09 ± 2.22 ng vs. 17.22 ± 2.99 ng; p<.05). An equivalent response was seen to a .2 g/kg leucine infusion (16.59 ± 2.93 ng vs. 32.00 ± 10.93 ng). Both groups exhibited a similar response to a 90-minute infusion of isoproterenol (.05 ug/kg·min.) when the average of the 20-, 25- and 30-minute values were compared (4.34 ± 1.35 ng/vs. 5.00 ± 2.53 ng). A second IVGTT was performed at the 30-minute time point during the course of the isoproterenol infusion. A significant difference between the two groups was again evident, with the low K group exhibiting an insulin response of 13.90 ± 12.81 ng and the control group a response of 69.70 ± 22.12 ng (p<.05). These data indicate that porcine islets respond via different mechanisms to the secretogogues tested. The secretory defects noted in the low K group are similar to those seen in some human diabetics. (Supported by the Kroc Foundation).

METABOLISM

437

Alanine Turnover in Normal and Diabetic Dogs. F. FERY and E.O. BALASSE*, Brussels, Belgium.

The metabolism of two major gluconeogenic amino acids, alanine (ALA) and glutamine (GLN), was studied in 6 control dogs and in 10 depancreatized diabetic dogs deprived of insulin for 24-48 h. In the latter group, glucose and ketone concentrations averaged respectively 368 ± 25 mg/dl (mean ± SEM) and 3.24 ± 0.84 μmols/ml. The rate of production of ALA was estimated using a primed constant infusion of U-^{14}C-ALA or 2,3-^{3}H-ALA.

In diabetic dogs, the mean concentration (0.65 ± 0.19 μmols/ml) and rate of production (20.8 ± 5.4 μmols/kg.min) of ALA exceeded but not significantly those observed in normals (0.35 ± 0.08 μmols/ml and 9.23 ± 0.70 μmols/kg.min). Plasma ALA correlated positively with its rate of production ($r = 0.94$; $p < 0.001$) over the wide range of concentrations observed in the normal and diabetic animals. In this latter group, both ALA production and ALA concentration correlated positively with glucose levels ($r = 0.65$; $p < 0.05$ and $r = 0.73$; $p = 0.01$) but were unrelated to ketone-body levels. GLN concentrations were similar in the 2 groups.

In conclusion : 1) Diabetes in dogs has variable effects on plasma ALA concentration which occasionally reaches very high levels. 2) The concentration of ALA is mostly dependent on its rate of production rather than being regulated at its (presumably hepatic) site of uptake. 3) The degree of hyperglycemia is positively correlated to the concentration and the rate of production of ALA.

436

Immunocytochemical Localization of Glycerol-3-phosphate Dehydrogenase to Pancreatic Alpha Cells. D.A. GAPP*, Clinton, NY (introduced by I.Y. ZEYTIN, Amherst, NH)

L-glycerol-3-phosphate dehydrogenase (GPDH) catalyzes the conversion of dihydroxyacetone phosphate into glycerol-3-phosphate. Antiserum to the adult isozyme form of mouse GPDH has been used for the peroxidase-antiperoxidase localization of the enzyme in sections of Bouin's-fixed pancreatic tissue obtained from normal and diabetic C57BL/Ks and C57BL/6 mice. Using adjacent sections stained for GPDH or for insulin, glucagon, somatostatin, or pancreatic polypeptide, GPDH was localized to the A cells of the islets with no demonstrable activity in other islet or in exocrine cells. Adsorption of GPDH antiserum with excess GPDH, but not excess glucagon, eliminated the staining completely. There appeared to be no significant differences in staining intensity or cellular distribution of the enzyme between the two strains of mice, nor did the presence of the diabetes gene alter the apparent A cell content of GPDH during various stages of diabetes. Present findings demonstrate an enzyme marker which is apparently unique to A cells among the islet cells, and which may provide new insights to A cell as well as islet metabolic processes.

Supported in part by NIH Grant AM05750.

438

HbAI and Glucose Control in Diabetics. FAUSTO SANTEUSANIO, GEREMIA BOLLI*, MARIA GIULIA CARTECHINI, PIETRO COMPAGNUCCI, PAOLO BRUNETTI, Perugia, Italy.

To investigate the relationship between glucose control and HbAI, we measured fasting and postlunch plasma glucose (FPG, PLPG) and total glycosylated fractions of Hb (HbAI, by high performance liquid chromatography) in 15 untreated JOD subjects (GI), in 32 diabetics with poor control (GII), in 67 subjects with abnormal OGTT, but normal FPG (GIII) and in 40 with normal OGTT (normals, N). At the 1st visit HbAI (mean±SEM) was: GI 14.1±0.5%, GII 12.6±0.6%, GIII 7.7±0.09%, N 6.4±0.08% ($p<.05$ between groups). All GI and 10 GII diabetics were given a careful insulin treatment. The other GII diabetics received oral agents and/or ipocaloric diet only. FPG, PLPG, HbAI were determined weekly until 90 days after start of treatment. HbAI decreased significantly earlier in diabetics on insulin as compared to those on oral agents or diet. All considered groups showed the same nadir of HbAI decrease on day 60 (8.8±0.9%). HbAI correlated with FPG, PLPG on admission ($r=0.81$, $r=0.78$) and later during therapy with FPG, PLPG of the previous 2-4 wks in GI and GII. Significant correlations were found between HbAI and OGTT response in all subjects with normal FPG (groups N+GIII).

Conclusions: HbAI reflects closely different degrees of glucose tolerance not only in clinically overt diabetics, but also in subjects with normal FPG, but abnormal OGTT. Moreover, as HbAI determination during therapy is strictly related to PG changes, it represents also an important proof of a really improved glycemic control of the previous 2-4 weeks.

439

Do HbAI Rapid Changes Occur in Diabetics? PAOLO BRUNETTI, PIETRO COMPAGNUCCI, MARIA G. CARTECHINI, GEREMIA BOLLI*, FAUSTO SANTEUSANIO*, Perugia, Italy.

To answer the question we planned 3 protocols. Total glycosylated fractions of Hb (HbAI) were determined by high performance liquid chromatography at +18°C. First: 6 diabetics, whose HbAI was stable for 2 weeks ($13.7 \pm 0.2\%$, mean$\pm$SEM), were connected to a Biostator for 3 days. Mean blood glucose (MBG) decreased from 16 to 7 mM/1 after 4h treatment. HbAI changed slightly after 1 and 2 days ($13.5 \pm 0.2\%$; $12.9 \pm 0.3\%$, p=ns), but decreased significantly after 3 days ($12.6 \pm 0.3\%$; $p < 0.05$). Second: 24h after insulin withdrawal in 5 JOD subjects in good glycemic control and steady-state HbAI ($8.8 \pm 0.4\%$), HbAI increased up to $9.2 \pm 0.4\%$ ($p < 0.01$), while MBG rose from 8.1 ± 0.3 to 16.3 ± 1.4 mM/1. HbAI reversed to basal values after RBC incubation in vitro in glucose-free saline (GFS) at +37°C for 6h. Third: RBC from 5 nondiabetics (fasting BG 4.7 ± 0.1 mM/1) were incubated for 6h (+37 °C) at 14; 22; 100 mM/1 glucose. HbAI rose from $6.5 \pm 0.2\%$ to $7.5 \pm 0.2\%$; $8.3 \pm 0.2\%$; $13.8 \pm 0.3\%$, reversing to basal values in GFS.

Conclusions: a rapid and marked glycosylation of Hb occurs in vitro at 100 mM/1 glucose, i.e. at glucose molarity (GM) which never realizes in vivo. The rapid HbAI increase in vitro is much more lower at lower GM (14 and 22 mM/1), which are usually observed in poorly controlled diabetics. Deglycosylation in GFS occurs in RBC incubated both at high and low GM.

Our results in vivo approximate those obtained in vitro and suggest that rapid HbAI changes really occur in insulin-requiring diabetics, but their clinical relevance is very limited.

440

Physiological role of glutamine as a fuel for pancreatic islet cells. W.J. MALAISSE*, A. SENER and J. CHRISTOPHE. Brussels, Belgium.

Oxygen uptake occurs at a sustained rate (8.1 ± 0.7 pmol/min per islet) in isolated rat islets deprived of exogenous nutrients. The nature of the endogenous fuels utilized by the islets is not known. L-glutamine (10 mM) increased O_2 consumption by 0.7 ± 0.1 pmol/min per islet, a value lower than the rate of $^{14}CO_2$ production from L-[U-^{14}C]glutamine, i.e. 3.4 ± 0.3 pmol/min per islet. At a physiological concentration (1.0 mM), L-glutamine oxidation averaged 71 ± 6 % of that found at 10 mM. In the presence of L-glutamine 10 mM, the production of metabolic end-products increased above basal value (pmol/120 min per islet) by 633 ± 33 for NH_4^+, 305 ± 26 for glutamate, 14 ± 3 for γ-aminobutyrate and 14 ± 6 for lactate, the calculated rate of glutamate utilization (157 ± 19) being close to the antimycin A-sensitive rate of L-[G-^{3}H]-glutamine conversion to ^3H_2O (162 ± 26). Although minimizing the fall in ATP content and ATP/ADP ratio found in nutrient-deprived islets, L-glutamine (10 mM) suppressed $^{14}CO_2$ output from islets prelabelled with [U-^{14}C]palmitate to a level comparable to that found in the presence of antimycin A (10 µM). The metabolic fate and effect of L-glutamine were little affected by the presence of glucose in the incubation medium. Glutamine failed to provoke any sustained increase in NAD(P)H content or insulin release in islets deprived of other exogenous nutrients. It is concluded that under physiological conditions, L-glutamine represents one of the major nutrients for pancreatic endocrine cells.

441

Effect of Alloxan on Cell Glucose Metabolism. F. ISHIBASHI AND B.V. HOWARD*, Phoenix, AZ.

The influence of alloxan (A) on uptake and metabolism of glucose (G) in mammalian cells has been studied using cultured human diploid fibroblasts. When cell monolayers were exposed to [U-^{14}C]-G, the presence of A (0.31-1.87mM) resulted initially in dose-dependent stimulation (maximum $151 \pm 2.7\%$ of non-A control) of total cell G incorporation. This stimulation was observed within 2 min and began to decline after 6 min. Thereafter A inhibited [U-^{14}C]-G incorporation (minimum $50 \pm 4.5\%$ of non-A control). When hexose transport was examined directly using G analogues, A neither stimulated nor inhibited the time course of 3-O-methyl-D-glucose or 2-deoxy-D-glucose uptake. When distribution of incorporated [U-^{14}C]-G was examined chromatographically, 11% was incorporated into glycogen, 20% into G-6-PO_4, 31% into lactate in the medium, 32% into nucleotides and 3% into CO_2. Under these conditions, changes induced by A were primarily an initial stimulation and subsequent inhibition of nucleotides and CO_2, and initial inhibition and subsequent stimulation of lactate. Alloxanic acid (0.62-1.87 mM), a decomposition product of A, did not affect G incorporation in fibroblasts. In addition, prior exposure to A (0.62-1.87 mM) for 6 minutes did not influence trypan blue exclusion, nor impair [^{3}H]-leucine incorporation into TCA precipitable material. These results suggest that A may directly influence cell G metabolism beyond the level of phosphorylation, possibly at the pentose phosphate shunt. These effects of A on G metabolism in fibroblasts may be related to the A-stimulation and subsequent inhibition of G-induced insulin release in pancreatic islets.

442

2-Tetradecylglycidic Acid (McN-3802). An Inhibitor of Mitochondrial Carnitine Palmitoyltransferase <u>In Vivo</u>. G.F. TUTWILER, M.T. RYZLAK and J. JOSEPH, Fort Washington, PA.

2-Tetradecylglycidic acid (McN-3802) is an oral hypoglycemic agent which has been reported to inhibit long chain but not short chain fatty acid oxidation in isolated rat hepatocytes, muscle preparations and liver mitochondria. <u>In vitro</u>, the site of this effect was the irreversible inhibition of mitochondrial carnitine acyltransferase with evidence indicating that the actual inhibitor was the CoA ester of McN-3802. McN-3802 also inhibited this enzyme <u>in vivo</u>. Doses of McN-3802 (1-10 mg/kg, p.o.) which lowered blood glucose and ketones of fasted rats markedly inhibited (84-99%) the ability of rat liver mitochondria to convert palmitoyl-CoA and ^{3}[H]CH_3-L-carnitine into palmitoyl-[^{3}H]CH_3-L-carnitine. Fatty acyl-CoA synthetase was not inhibited. Only the enzyme designated carnitine palmitoyl transferase I (CPT I), which was released from mitochondria by freeze-thawing and which catalyzes the production of palmitoyl carnitine outside the mitochondrial permeability barrier for acyl-CoA, was inhibited. CPT I was much less inhibited 36 hours after a single dose of McN-3802. Interestingly, even though McN-3802 failed to lower the blood glucose of <u>ad libitum</u> fed or pair-fed rats, CPT I was still inhibited. However, compared to the fasted state, inhibition was somewhat less (67-85%). One possible explanation for this lesser effect might be the enhanced rate of esterification of acyl-CoA derivatives in the fed state. Preliminary evidence suggests that McN-3802 can be esterified into lipids <u>in vivo</u> and thus in the fed state may be less available to CPT I.

443

Pharmacokinetics and antidiabetic effects of glipizide: Acute/long-term studies in maturity-onset diabetes mellitus. J. ÖSTMAN*, I. CHRISTENSON, B. JANSSON and L. WEINER. Huddinge, Sweden.

In 13 patients with maturity-onset diabetes mellitus that had not responded to diet alone the serum concentration of glipizide, blood glucose concentration (B-G), and serum immunoreactive insulin (S-IRI) were monitored hourly over 12 h after administration of a placebo, and an initial dose of glipizide (5 mg p.o.) and long-term treatment with glipizide in doses, which produced a fasting B-G of 8 mmol/l. The drug was administered as a single or a 3-part dose. The immediate effects of the glipizide on the B-G, S-IRI and S-IRI/B-G ratio lasted 9, 4.5 and 6.5 h respectively. The apparent half life of glipizide was 4.1 h, the distribution volume 0.123 l/kg and the plasma clearance 0.0023 l/kg h. The kinetics of glipizide, given as a long-term treatment (mean dose 10.4 mg, range 7.5-20 mg), on the B-G, S-IRI and S-IRI/B-G ratio lasted for up to 12 h. The mean B-G for 12 h was lower after the single than after the 3-part dose regime (7 and 8.7 mmol/l). In part, the prolonged antidiabetic effect of glipizide is explained by a serum concentration within the therapeutic range over a great part of the day.

444

Effect of Physiologic Levels of Glucagon on Ketone body Production and Utilization Rates in Normal Man. U. KELLER*, G.E. SONNENBERG, and W. STAUFFACHER, Basel, Switzerland.

Glucagon has been reported to be ketogenic in insulin-deficient diabetic man. To determine the effect of various levels of glucagon on ketone body (k.b.) turnover rates with basal insulin maintained, somatostatin (SRIF) was infused for 120 min without or in combination with 2 replacement doses of glucagon while insulin was replaced by i.v.infusion at 150 μU/kg/min. K.b.turnover rates were determined using primed-constant infusions of 3-^{14}C-acetoacetate and a previously validated pool model in 14 hrs fasted normal subjects.

SRIF alone induced a 120±32 % increase in k.b.production and a 30±3 % decrease in k.b.clearance. Replacement of insulin (level: 11±2 μU/ml) during SRIF (n=6) without glucagon (glucagon level 89±16 pg/ml) resulted in no change of the basal k.b.production rate (5.6± 0.8 μmol/kg/min) and of the basal k.b.clearance (16± 1 ml/kg/min). The addition of glucagon at 2 and 4 ng/kg/min (resulting in glucagon levels of 340± 45 and 799±104 pg/ml, n=6 each dose) did not affect k.b.production and clearance while plasma insulin was maintained at 12±1 and 12.5±1 μU/ml, respectively. Concentrations of acetoacetate, βOHB and acetone were also unchanged. FFA levels increased during SRIF infusion alone by 78± 20% and were readily restrained by insulin replacement. Neither dose of glucagon affected the FFA levels.

Thus, glucagon at 3 different physiologic levels was unable to alter total k.b.production and utilization rates in the presence of insulin.

445

Inhibition of Hepatic Gluconeogenesis By (+)-Octanoycarnitine. S.A. BLUMENTHAL*, Syracuse, New York.

In studies with perfused livers of fasted rats, 0.5 mM palmitate (P) (complexed with defatted albumin in a 1:1 molar ratio) significantly increased glucose formation from 5 mM lactate (16.22->23.69 μmol/gm wet wt liver/h, p<0.01). Hence, "physiologic" concentrations of albumin-bound long-chain fatty acids stimulate gluconeogenesis even when the supply of reducing equivalents is not limiting. In subsequent studies, the technique of Berry (J. Cell Biol. 43:506, 1969) was used to isolate hepatocytes from 150-200 gm male Sprague-Dawley rats fasted for 48 hours. Hepatocytes were incubated for 30 minute periods in media containing 5 mM pyruvate as gluconeogenic substrate. Control rates of glucose and total ketoacid production averaged 0.8 μmol and 0.7 μmol/mg DNA/30 min respectively. Addition of P to the medium caused a 2.4-fold increase in glucose production (p<.05), a 2.8-fold increase in ketoacid production (p<.001), and a 2.4-fold increase in the β-hydroxybutyrate: acetoacetate ratio (0.34->0.80, p<.05). Stimulation of gluconeogenesis and ketogenesis by P was completely suppressed by the further addition of 0.5 mM (+)-octanoylcarnitine (OC), an inhibitor of fatty acid oxidation. Preliminary data indicate that OC alone may reduce conversion of pyruvate to glucose.

Conclusion: Selective blockade of P oxidation by OC also blocks P-induced hepatic gluconeogenesis in fasted rats. Thus, OC and its congeners may lower plasma glucose levels in diabetic animals.

446

Site of Enhanced Insulin Sensitivity in Year Old Rats Adapted to Hypergravitational Force. C.E. MONDON*, C. DOLKAS AND J. OYAMA. Stanford and Moffett Field, Ca.

Although normal fasted rats exhibit a relative glucose intolerance and hyperinsulinemia with increase in age, older rats exposed to hypergravity by continuous centrifugation at 4.1 g show significantly lower plasma insulin levels after oral glucose than age or weight-matched control rats. To assess insulin sensitivity of specific organs, glucose uptake by perfused hindlimb muscle (M) and liver (L) from year old fasted hypergravic (H) rats was compared with perfused organs from 10 week old weight-matched control (C) rats. Hindlimb M received a continuous infusion of glucose (102 nmol/min/g muscle) in the absence and presence of low perfusate insulin levels (35 μU/ml) and glucose uptake was assessed as a metabolic clearance (k). Hepatic glucose uptake was measured at perfusate insulin levels of 40 μU/ml after prior elevation of perfusate glucose to 16 mM. The results show that k was 24% faster in HM than CM in the absence of insulin (10.6 ±.4 vs 8.1 ±.6 μl/min/g muscle) and was more than 2-fold faster at low perfusate insulin levels (23.0 ±3.0 vs 9.5 ±1.4). Conversely, glucose uptake by L from H rats was significantly less (p<.001) than L from C rats (10.3 ±2.2 vs 27.8 ±2.8 μmol/g). These findings suggest that greater insulin sensitivity in older hypergravic rats following glucose loading entails an alteration in glucose disposal with skeletal muscle showing increased responsiveness to insulin-induced glucose uptake accompanied by decreased removal of glucose by the liver.

447

A Humoral Satiety Factor After Intestinal Bypass Surgery. R.L. ATKINSON* and E.L. BRENT, Charlottesville, Va.

Weight loss after intestinal bypass is due predominantly to a decrease in food intake, the mechanism for which is unknown. In 2 experiments, we tested the hypothesis that bypass produces a humoral satiety factor. Two groups of 3 Sprague-Dawley rats had end-to-side jejunoileal bypass or sham bypass surgery. After 14 days, the rats were anesthetized with ether and exsanguinated by aortic puncture. The heparinized plasma was injected intraperitoneally into 18-hour-fasted recipient rats and food intake measured at 1, 5 and 10 hours after injection. After 1 hr., recipient rats receiving bypass plasma ate 29% less chow than recipients receiving sham bypass plasma. At 5 and 10 hr., food intake was reduced by 17% and 10% respectively. Another group of 22 rats (mean wt. 538 gm.) were weight-matched into 2 groups and underwent bypass or sham bypass surgery, respectively. The rats were anesthetized and exsanguinated 2 weeks after surgery. The heparinized plasma was infused via an indwelling femoral vein catheter into 22 18-hour-food-deprived recipient rats (mean wt. 477 gm.) over a 30 min. period. Food was offered immediately after the infusion. After 1 hr., rats receiving bypass plasma ate 25% more than rats receiving bypass plasma. After 10 hr., sham bypass plasma recipients again ate 25% more than bypass plasma recipients (p<.01). Summary: Food intake is decreased at 1, 5 and 10 hr. in recipient rats infused with bypass plasma as compared to rats receiving sham bypass plasma by intraperitoneal or intravenous injection. Conclusion: Bypass plasma contains a humoral factor which inhibits food intake.

448

Low Protein, High Carbohydrate Diet Prevents Development of Hyperglycemia in dbdb Mice. P.DONALD* and S.POHL*, Charlottesville, Va.

We have studied the role of dietary protein level in mice genetically predisposed to obesity and diabetes. Six-week old dbdb mice, weighing 33 g, were fed ad libitum isocaloric diets containing 2, 5, 10, and 15 or 25% lactalbumin protein for 10 weeks. Each diet contained 10% fat and the rest of the energy as carbohydrate from starches and sucrose. Mean body weight and plasma glucose (glu) values at 4 and 10 weeks, and immunoreactive insulin (IRI) at 10 weeks, for the 2%, 5% and 15% protein-fed groups are shown below:

Weeks		2% Protein	5% Protein	15% Protein
4	wt(g)	37.3±1.1	37.3±0.9	41.2±1.2
	glu(mg%)	150±16	554±95	561±120
10	wt	43.5±1.5	32.8±0.7	38.1±1.4
	glu	186±35	1108±273	942±80
	IRI(μU/ml)	22.7±9.0	19.9±5.2	18.7±5.6

Values are means ± standard error, n=4-6

All 5 groups were hyperinsulinemic compared to chow-fed nondiabetic mice (9μU/ml). At 6.5 weeks the 2-10% protein-fed groups had gained an average of 5-6 and the 15% and 25% protein-fed groups had gained 9.6 and 10.5 g, respectively. Thereafter, the 2% protein-fed groups continued to gain and became quite obese with very fatty livers at sacrifice, while the other 4 groups lost weight steadily throughout the remainder of the study. In conclusion, the 2% protein diet prevented hyperglycemia but not obesity in the dbdb mice.

449

Influence of Inorganic Chromium (III) on Circulating Lipids, Glucose, and Insulin. REBECCA RIALES, Parkersburg, WV, and MARGARET J. ALBRINK,* Morgantown, WV.

A double-blind 12-wk study of 23 normal males ages 31 to 60 was conducted to investigate the effects of Cr(III), 200 mcg/d, 5 d/wk, or placebo (water, W), on lipoprotein metabolism, as reflected in fasting levels of serum HDL-cholesterol (HDL-C), LDL-cholesterol, total cholesterol, triglycerides, and phospholipids. Half had glucose tolerance tests with measurement of plasma glucose and insulin fasting and at 30, 60, and 90 min following a 75-g glucose load. Blood was collected at 0, 6, and 12 wk.

Between 0 and 12 wk mean weight decreased in the Cr group (185 to 183 lb, $P \simeq 0.02$), but remained unchanged in the control group (190 lb).

HDL-C was the only lipid which changed significantly. In the Cr group it rose between 0 and 12 wk from 35 to 39 mg/dl ($P \simeq 0.05$), but it remained unchanged in the control group (34 mg/dl).

Summation of the values at four times for glucose (sigma-glu) and insulin (sigma-ins) revealed decreases in each parameter in the Cr group at 6 wk which were partially lost at 12 wk (a: P< 0.005: b: P< 0.20, compared to baseline).

	Cr0	Cr6	Cr12	W0	W6	W12
sigma-glu	541	470[a]	522	535	490	506
sigma-ins	260	230[b]	241	294	312	272

Cr may influence HDL through effect on glucose tolerance.

450

Renal Ornithine Decarboxylase (ODC) Activity in Streptozotocin Diabetic (SD) Rats: Regulation by Age and Sexual Maturity. J. H. LEVINE*, A. B. LEAMING, AND D. A. SENS, Charleston, S. C.

The activity of ODC, the rate-limiting enzyme in polyamine biosynthesis, is altered by diabetes in several tissues. The pathogenesis of diabetic nephropathy remains unknown. Since renal disease is extremely rare prepubertally, we have compared the effects of SD on renal ODC activity in sexually immature and mature male and female rats. All rats received either 120 mg/kg streptozotocin or vehicle i.p. after an 18h fast. They were fed ad lib and decapitated on the second or third day of diabetes. ODC activity is expressed in units (nanomoles $^{14}CO_2$/g kidney/30 min.)

SD in mature male rats (150-200 g) caused an increase in renal ODC activity from 36.2±2.2 (M±SEM; n = 4-6 rats) to 70.5±4.0 U. In contrast, SD in immature male rats (50 g) produced a decrease in ODC activity from 50.9±4.2 to 13.7±1.0 U. Similar patterns were observed with female rats of the same sizes. Castration 1 wk prior to SD in mature male rats did not prevent the two-fold increase in enzyme activity. Immature male and female rats were treated with 100 ug testosterone (T)/day for 1 wk before SD. In both sexes T treatment alone did not stimulate renal ODC activity. T-treated diabetic rats showed a two-fold increase in renal ODC activity rather than the decrease seen in untreated rats. Conclusion: The effect of SD on renal ODC activity is age but not sex dependent. The renal ODC response to SD is not dependent on testicular activity. Androgen treatment of sexually immature rats converts the diabetic kidney enzyme response to an adult pattern.

451

Acute Hypernatremia Induces Hypoglycemia in Young Mice: Possible Mechanisms of Action. JEAN H. THURSTON,* RICHARD E. HAUHART and JOHN A. DIRGO, St. Louis, MO.

Deaths have occurred in healthy individuals following the use of hypertonic saline as an emetic, for therapeutic abortion, and following the accidental substitution of salt for sugar in infant formulas. Stimulated by the pathophysiology of this disaster, we developed a model of acute salt poisoning in normal nursing 17 to 23-day-old mice. Animals received 1 M NaCl, 30 ml/kg s.c. followed by another 30 ml/kg i.p. (total dose 60 mEq/kg of Na^+); controls received 0.9% NaCl. Other littermates received an equal volume of 2 M urea. Salt loading increased plasma [Na^+] from 141 ± 1 mEq/l (mean ± SE) (N=13) to 199 ± 2 mEq/l (N=24); urea lowered plasma [Na^+] to 125 ± 1 mEq/l (N=14) (P vs control <0.001 in each case). Acute hypernatremia caused a progressive lowering of plasma glucose concentration. At 60 min plasma glucose was reduced 66%, 3.56 ± 0.41 mM (N=24) vs 10.31 ± 0.42 mM (N=13) in controls, P <0.001. At this time there were severe neurologic deficits. Hypernatremia-induced hypoglycemia was not due to increased insulin secretion. In 10 controls plasma insulin was 0.35 ± 0.10 ng/ml; in each of 9 salt-loaded mice plasma insulin was <0.2 ng/ml. Nor was it due to hyperosmolality per se - equiosmolar urea had no effect on plasma glucose levels. Furthermore, urea-injected animals did not exhibit neurologic dysfunction. The possibility of Na^+-induced stimulation of glucose uptake and glucose metabolism in muscle in vivo is under investigation.

The data raise the important question of reduced blood (and brain) glucose levels in acute hypernatremia in man.

452

Effects of "Caloric Clamping" in Rats on Metabolite Levels in vivo and on Ketogenesis in Isolated Hepatocytes. W.F. WOODSIDE and A. HAYEK (Introduced by E. KAUFMAN*), Albuquerque, N.M.

We have developed a new technic called "caloric clamping" (CC) to study metabolic events in rats at various levels of caloric balance. Freely-moving, conscious rats with chronic stomach cannulas were connected to an apparatus and infused for 22 hrs. with varying amounts of glucose from 6.25 to 0 Kcal/(kg)$^{.75}$/hr (KKh). Blood glucose (G), ketones (K), and fatty acids (FA) changed slightly with 6.25-1.25 KKh, but from 1.25-0 KKh, G decreased (dec.) and K and FA increased (inc.) linearly from 5.6, 0.2, and 0.2 to 4.2, 0.9 and 0.5 mM, respectively. Liver glycogen dec. linearly with decreasing caloric infusion (CI). Ketogenesis was assessed in hepatocytes incubated with 1 mM oleate (OL) and in other cells prepared with 40 mM G to preserve glycogen and incubated with 1 mM OL plus 20 mM G. Rates with OL alone inc. linearly with decreasing CI until a maximum was reached with 2.5-1.25 KKh. With OL and G, rates inc. linearly with decreasing CI to 0 KKh, and were lower than that obtained with OL alone at each level of CI. Optimal ketogenic response to glucagon in vitro with OL alone was obtained with cells from rats infused with 5 KKh whereas with OL plus G, optimal response was obtained with cells from rats infused with 2.5 KKh. In both cases, 10^{-9}M glucagon maximally stimulated rates by 80-100%; conc. for half-maximal stimulation was 2×10^{-10}M. CC provides a systematic method for defining optimal conditions for investigation of hormonal regulation of hepatic ketogenesis in vitro.

453

Chronic Intravenous (iv) Infusion of Glucose Reduces Food Intake of Baboons. STEPHEN C. WOODS,* LESLIE J. STEIN, and L. DAVID McKAY, Seattle, Wa.

It has previously not been possible to demonstrate acute satiety by the elevation of circulating nutrients. We have recently suggested that insulin may be a long-term regulator of appetite in the baboon, thus implying that iv nutrients, via their insulin stimulatory capacity, should be effective regulators of appetite in long-term infusion experiments.

To test this, adult male baboons were chaired in sound-attenuating chambers. They had access to a nutritionally complete liquid diet for 7 hr/day. Two venous catheters enabled simultaneous infusion and sampling. After a 2-wk baseline period when only saline was infused and food intake was stable, glucose was added to the infusate to provide 25 or 50% of each baboon's average daily caloric intake spread over 24 hr. This caused a significant reduction of food intake (-21 and -36% over 2 wk for the two infusion rates, respectively). However, the decrease of food intake was not usually apparent for several days and grew larger over days. By 3 wk, the animals still were not compensating fully. Plasma immunoreactive insulin (IRI) levels taken from fasted animals in the morning averaged 65 μU/ml during the baseline period. The two infusions raised them by 28 and 45% respectively. There was a significant inverse correlation between IRI output (calculated from IRI samples taken every 20 min over the day) and food intake over the subsequent 3 days. These results are consistent with the hypothesis that insulin levels feed back to the central nervous system to influence appetite on a long-term basis.

454

Metabolic Influences on Susceptibility of C57BL/6 (ob/ob) Mice to Encephalomyocarditis Viral Diabetes. B.J. D'ANDREA, J.E. CRAIGHEAD and G.L. WILSON, Burlington, Vt. (Introduced by E.A. SIMS,* Burlington, Vt.)

The M variant of EMC virus causes an insulin-dependent diabetes in certain inbred strains of mice. Other strains appear more resistant to the diabetogenic effect of this virus. Previous studies in our laboratory suggest the involvement of undefined metabolic factors in the variable response of mice to infection. We hypothesized that metabolic stimulation of the beta cell, resulting from spontaneous obesity, might alter resistance to EMC-induced diabetes. C57BL/6 mice were used because homozygous normal (+/+) mice are relatively resistant to EMC-induced hyperglycemia. In addition, the homozygous ob/ob genotype on the C57BL/6 background causes hypertrophy and hyperplasia of beta cells during the expression of obesity. C57BL/6-ob/ob adult, male mice were infected with EMC M virus (100 PFU/mouse), and matched, lean colony-mates (ob/+ and +/+) were treated similarly. Blood glucose levels of infected obese mice were higher than those of uninfected obese controls 3-5 days after exposure to EMC. Light microscopic evaluation of pancreatic tissue revealed varying degrees of inflammation and islet cell cytolysis in both lean and obese animals, but the most severe changes were observed in the obese group. Thus, in vivo metabolic effects on the beta cell appear to increase the susceptibility of C57BL/6 mice to viral infection associated with enhanced insular damage and diabetic symptoms.

Supported by NIH grant #PHS R01 20790.

455

Changes of Glucose Tolerance in Obese Patients Following Prolonged Starvation. LUBOMIR J.VALENTA and ALAN N. ELIAS*, Irvine, California

Nine female obese patients, average weight 102 ± 42 kg, range 85 to 202 kg, were subjected to a 3-week fasting regimen with daily intake of cca 70 kcal. The average weight loss was 10.2 ± 2.9 kg, range 5 to 15 kg. Standard oral glucose tolerance test (GTT) was performed at the beginning (Control) and the end of the prolonged fast. Serum glucose, immunoreactive insulin (IRI), C-peptide (C-p), cortisol and growth hormone were measured on each blood sample. The values given in the Table are: fasting (F), maximum increase (Δ max), 2 hour postprandial (2PP) and 4 hour PP (4PP). Post Fast, hyperglycemia persisted during the late phase of GTT. Fasting IRI was lower than on Control GTT, but maximum IRI and C-p response to glucose load remained the same. Compared to Control, IRI and C-p were markedly elevated during the late phase of Post Fast GTT. This apparent insulin resistance was in contradiction with known increase in sensitivity to exogenous insulin in obesity following prolonged fast which was also demonstrated in the present study by using a peripheral insulin sensitivity test and ^{125}I-insulin binding to the patients' erythrocytes. It is suggested that it was due to the secretion of insulin of low biologic activity, possibly proinsulin.

	Serum glucose (mg/100 ml)			
	F	Δ max	2PP	4PP
Control	100 ± 8	182 ± 33	122 ± 30	57 ± 19
Post Fast	93 ± 12	210 ± 54	192 ± 64	144 ± 34

	Serum IRI (μU/ml)				Serum C-peptide (ng/ml)			
	F	Δ max	2PP	4PP	F	Δ max	2PP	4PP
Control	14 ± 9	85 ± 22	63 ± 40	13 ± 5	2.9 ±.8	7.8 ± .8	5.4 ± 1	3 ± 1
Post Fast	4 ± 3	78 ± 27	66 ± 26	50 ± 31	2.6 ±.9	7.8 ±1.8	7.6 ± 2	6 ± 2

456

Quantitation of Non-Enzymatic Glucosylation of Platelet Membrane Glycoproteins in Diabetic Patients and Normal Controls. B.C.O'MALLEY*, G. SWANK and R.K. KELLER, Tampa, FL.

The basic cause of the platelet hypersensitivity found in diabetes has not yet been established. Platelet membrane glycoproteins are thought to be the surface receptors of several agents which induce adhesion and/or aggregation, such as ADP, thrombin, collagen, etc. Increased non-enzymatic glucosylation of several proteins (including those of the red cell membrane) has been demonstrated in diabetes but those of the platelet membrane have not yet been studied. Although the platelet itself has a relatively short half-life, exposure of the megakaryocyte to hyperglycemia might result in excessive glucosylation of platelet membranes with possible subsequent alterations in function.

Serum and membranes from both RBCs and platelets were prepared from whole blood collected from diabetic patients and normal controls. Each fraction was assayed for glucosylated proteins using 5-hydroxymethylfurfural as standard (Fluckinger and Winterhalter, FEBS Letts 71:356, 1976). All values were calculated on a per mg protein basis (BioRad assay). In addition, Hb was isolated from RBCs and percent HbA_{1c} determined by HPLC.

The data obtained indicate a significant elevation in percent HbA_{1c} and glucosylation of serum and RBC membrane proteins from blood of diabetic patients, in confirmation of the work of others. Preliminary results have failed to demonstrate a significant increase in glucosylation of platelet membrane glycoproteins from diabetic patients.

457

Extreme Hyperlipidemia in Mild Diabetes: Defect in Feedback Regulation of Plasma Very Low Density Lipoprotein Synthesis. A. KISSEBAH,* R. MURRAY,* N. VYDELINGUM,* and C. HUSSEY, Milwaukee, Wi.

Extreme hypertriglyceridemia leading to recurrent abdominal pain and progressive angina might occur in nonketotic mild diabetes. To unravel mechanisms underlying the lipid disorder, we examined 1) 2 diabetic patients with extreme hypertriglyceridemia (EHTG) studied before and after reduction of plasma triglycerides (TG) by repeated plasma exchange (PE), 2) 8 diabetic patients with moderate hypertriglyceridemia (MHTG), and 3) 13 normal subjects (NS). VLDL-TG, β and CII apoproteins and extrahepatic lipoprotein lipase (LPL) were analyzed. Plasma VLDL was labeled in the β and TG moieties with I^{131} and C^{14}-palmitate, respectively, and synthetic rates (SR) were determined from radioactivity decay curves. The results were as follows:

	NS	MHTG	EHTG (PE)			
VLDL	Range	Range	Pre	Post	Pre	Post
TGmg%	46-18	210-340	2188	213	1860	314
TG/β	8-13	9-13	37	11	26	12
CII/TG†	11-18	9-14	4	14	5	12
TG SR‡	226-453	630-868	1120	1380	980	1160
β SR‡	9-26	25-42	32	63	34	58
LPL††	28-40	22-38	11	46	9	42

† = x10^3. ‡ = mg/kg/hr. †† = μeq FFA/ml/hr.

The extreme hypertriglyceridemia of mild diabetes results from overproduction of triglyceride enriched VLDL. The rebound increase in VLDL secretion after PE suggests a defect in feedback regulation of VLDL synthesis. Saturation of the removal system leads to hyperchylomicronemia. The apparent deficiency of LPL and its activator protein, CII, might be secondary events.

458

Effects of dietary induced phosphorus depletion on cardiac composition. HUEY G. MCDANIEL,* WILMER W. NICHOLS and THOMAS J. FULLER, Birmingham, Ala. and Gainesville, Fla.

Hypophosphatemia is a complication of therapy of diabetic ketoacidosis. Recent animal and human studies suggest that hypophosphatemia and/or phosphorus depletion (PD) has a deleterious effect on cardiac function. The mechanism(s) for both the noted decrease in resting myocardial performance as well as the decrease in myocardial reserve are poorly understood. In order to investigate this the effects of 5 weeks of dietary induced PD on cardiac high energy phosphates and glycogen (G) was studied in 6 control and 5 P-depleted dogs:

Results:	Control	PD
Serum Pi(mg/dl)	4.9 ± 0.7	1.1± 0.4 @@
Cardiac Pi(umol/g)	10.8 ± 1.2	6.9± 1.3 @
ATP(umol/g)	5.0 ± 0.6	4.4± 0.8
ADP(umol/g)	0.73± 0.15	.45± 0.1 @
AMP(umol/g)	0.12± 0.02	.05± 0.01@
Creatine Phosphate (umol/g)	2.5 ± 0.4	2.2± 0.4
Glycogen(mg/g)	4.0 ± 0.3	5.3± 0.5 @

Conclusion: Dietary induced PD severely decreases cardiac ADP and AMP while ATP and creatine phosphate are maintained. Glycogen content is significantly increased.

Data: Mean ± Standard error, @ p<0.05, @@ p<0.01.

459

Free and esterified cholesterol (CH) levels in plasma of acutely diabetic rats (eviscerated with functional liver), J.C. PENHOS*, M. MONTALBERT-SMITH and E.R. RAMEY*, Washington, D.C.

We used an eviscerated rat model with a functional liver and kidneys in which the pancreas could be left *in situ* or removed (acute diabetes). In this last condition a significant elevation above normal of plasma CH (free and esterified) was observed. When the liver circulation was occluded (evisceration with non-functional liver), the plasma esterified CH level decreased, but total CH was unchanged. With a functional liver plus nephrectomy the levels of esterified CH were the same as those seen with the kidneys *in situ*. Complete restoration of plasma CH patterns to control values was seen only when the pancreas, liver and kidneys were all functioning in the eviscerated normoglycemic rats. These data indicate that in this model the G.I. tract per se does not make a significant contribution to plasma CH and that the critical determinants of plasma CH levels appear to be the liver and the endocrine pancreas.

460

Insulin Responsiveness of Glucose Metabolism in Rat Fat Cells: Variations among three depots. S. K.FRIED, M.LAVAU, and F.X.PI-SUNYER.* New York,NY.

Most studies of fat cell (FC) metabolism and insulin responsiveness are conducted on FCs from the epididymal(E) depot. This study was initiated to determine whether these results apply to FCs from other sites. FCs from the E, retroperitoneal (R), and dorsal subcutaneous(S) depots of 150g male Wistar rats had similar cell sizes. Basal(B) (1-^{14}C)glucose(G) oxidation and conversion to fatty acids(FA) were lower in S than R and E FCs, while glyceride-glycerol(GG) synthesis was similar. The rates of G oxidation and FA synthesis with 2.8 nM insulin were both decreased by 80% in S vs E FCs. Incorporation of G into GG was similar in all FCs. The insulin concentration that gave 50% of maximal response of G metabolism was similar in each FC type. Activities of acetyl CoA carboxylase, fatty acid synthetase(FAS), citrate cleavage and malic enzymes, and glucose-6-phosphate and 6-phosphogluconate dehydrogenases were reduced by 70% in S and 25% in R vs E FCs, paralleling the rates of FA synthesis. Furthermore, activity of FAS was highly correlated(r=.97) with I-stimulated G metabolism in all FCs. B and maximally I-stimulated ^{14}C-2-deoxyglucose uptake was depressed by 30% in S vs E and R FCs, but % stimulation and sensitivity to submaximal I were unaffected. The decreased response of G metabolism to I in S FCs is therefore not due to decreased I effect on G transport and/or phosphorylation.

In conclusion, S FCs exhibit an impaired response to I in terms of G oxidation and FA synthesis compared to E and R FCs which is not a function of cell size and is probably due to lower lipogenic enzyme activities.

461

Diabetogenic Effects of Episodic Growth Hormone Secretion in Normal Man. K. Mackes, K. Greene, J. King, and T.Rambis (Introduced by M. Haymond*), Endocrine Research Unit, Mayo Clinic, Rochester, MN

The present studies were undertaken to assess the effects on glucose homeostasis in normal man of episodic growth hormone secretion producing increments in plasma growth hormone (HGH) within the physiologic range. For this purpose, growth hormone secretion was induced concomitant with meal ingestion (breakfast, snack, lunch, snack, dinner) by subcutaneous administration of subemetic doses of apomorphine (0.36 mg) in 10 normal subjects. Plasma glucose, insulin, growth hormone and glucagon were determined at 15-30 min intervals throughout the day. Following apomorphine administration, plasma HGH increased to peak levels of 6-12 ng/ml during each meal. Postprandial plasma glucose levels increased progressively throughout the day compared to those observed in control studies when meals were consumed without apomorphine administration ($p<0.001$). This occurred despite postprandial plasma insulin responses which were increased 50-100% ($p<0.01$), indicating insulin resistance had been induced. Plasma glucagon responses were unaffected. These effects of apomorphine appeared to be specifically due to its stimulation of HGH secretion since episodic infusion of exogenous HGH (100 ng/kg/min for 30 min) in the same subjects during ingestion of meals (N=5), which resulted in peak plasma HGH levels of 8-20 ng/ml completely reproduced the effects seen with apomorphine administration. Conclusions: Episodic GH secretion increasing plasma GH to levels within the physiologic range can cause insulin resistance and deterioration of glucose tolerance in normal man.

462

Studies on Glucose Uptake in Isolated Porcine Adipose Tissue cells. J. SCHRAGE, P. LANGLEY, and T. BURNS* Columbia, Missouri.

Of several species we have studied, porcine adipose tissue is unique in the striking degree of potentiation of lipolytic peptide substances caused by theophylline (Th). Th alone, and in the presence of isoproterenol (Is), also decreased glucose uptake.

The present studies were done to gain more information on the regulation of glucose utilization in porcine adipose tissue. Porcine adipocytes were prepared from subcutaneous adipose tissue and incubated with lipolytic substances, insulin, and Th. Percent incorporation of total available carbon label from ^{14}C(U)-glucose was determined.

ACTH (0.1 U/ml), TSH (0.1 U/ml), and Is (10^{-5}M) decreased carbon label incorporation into triglyceride. Insulin (100 μU/ml or 320 μU/ml) returned incorporation to control levels when incubated with ACTH or Is:

Addition	None	ACTH	TSH	Is
None	1.61±0.056*	0.99±0.18	0.83±0.20	0.75±0.08
Insulin	2.06±0.210	1.58±0.08	1.21±0.28	1.59±0.16
P-value	.10	0.025	0.50	0.005

*% label incorporation, mean and S.E.M.

Th (3.2 mM/ml) reduced carbon label incorporation alone and in the presence of lipolytic substances:

Addition	None	ACTH	TSH	Is
None	1.69	1.37	1.42	0.98
Th	0.71	0.56	0.47	0.36

*mean % label incorporation

Several lipolytic substances reduce glucose conversion to triglyceride as measured by percent incorporation of labeled carbon from ^{14}C(U)-glucose. Insulin diminishes and Th enhances this effect.

463

In Vitro Glycosylation of Hemoglobin (Hb). D. DANEMAN,* N. SCHANE & D. BECKER,* Pittsburgh, Pa.

To study the rate & reversibility of Hb glycosylation, we incubated intact & hemolysed RBCs from normal (N) & diabetic (IDD) subjects in glucose (G) solutions of increasing concentrations (0-2000 mg%) for 4-48h at 21°C. Before incubation the RBCs were washed in saline to remove any G present. Postincubation ½ of each intact RBC specimen was rewashed to remove G to <10mg%. HbA1 was measured by column chromatography at 22-24°C. The table shows the mean %HbA1 after incubation for 4 & 48h compared to that in whole blood as baseline (B) ($\overline{X} \pm$ SEM glucose in N adults & IDD children=83.6 ± 6 & 293 ± 44 mg% respectively).

	B	4h incubation (n10each)				48h (n5each)	
G		0	150	500	2000	500	2000
N							
URBC	5.8	*5.4	*6.3	*7.3	*11.5	*8.9	*14.7
WRBC	5.7	5.3†	5.6†	6.0†	*7.5†	*7.6†	*10.4†
IDD							
URBC	13	12.7	13.2	*14.3	*18.7	--	*19.4
WRBC	12.3	12.3	12.7	13.1†	*14.3†	--	*16.1†

* p <0.01 from baseline † p <0.01 from URBC
URBC = unwashed RBCs WRBC = washed RBCs

There were no significant differences between 24 & 48h incubations or between hemolysed & intact unwashed RBCs. The maximum HbA1 achieved was 21.7% (?saturation of glycosylation). We suggest that (1) a small, significant component of glycosylation is rapid & reversed or arrested by washing RBCs, (2) intact RBC membranes are not essential for glycosylation. These HbA1 changes, although only ≤1% in G range of most IDD, may be important in ongoing assessment of control. To standardize techniques we advise washing specimens soon after venipuncture.

464

Marked Decrease in Insulin Requirements in Diabetics During Labor and Delivery. DONNA YOUNGER,* FREDERICKA VLACHOKOSTA,* JOHN KITZMILLER,* LOUIS VIGNATI,* THOMAS AOKI,* Boston, Massachusetts

A glucose controlled insulin infusion system (GCIIS) was used to monitor the blood glucose and insulin requirements in 2 groups of well controlled, insulin-dependent diabetic pregnant women. Group A: 4 patients, 1 class-C and 3 class-D (White's classification) were monitored 8-10 hrs before C-section and 4 hrs postpartum. Group B: 5 patients, 3 class-B, 1 class-C and 1 class-D were monitored during oxytocin-induced labor and 4 hrs postpartum. All patients received regular insulin before supper the night before C-section or induction of labor, and a snack at 9pm, and were NPO after midnight. On the day of C-section or labor and delivery all patients received D5W-125 cc/hr and were euglycemic on insulin feedback (GCIIS).

RESULTS	GROUP	MEAN BLOOD GLUCOSE BEFORE DEL. (±SEM)	INS.REQ. (mU)	CORD GLUCOSE (MEAN±SEM)
	A	78 ± 3	2.066	64 ± 4
	B	75 ± 4	Zero	88 ± 5

Only one infant developed hypoglycemia in the first 3 days of life. We concluded that well controlled insulin dependent diabetic pregnant women require almost no insulin on the day of delivery. This may be due to: 1. Normal or increased sensitivity of various tissues to insulin. 2. Utilization of glucose by the fetus. 3. Increased glucose utilization related to the "exercise of labor". 4. Decrease in caloric intake. Well controlled blood glucose before and during the intrapartum period might prevent neonatal hypoglycemia.

465

Lipoprotein Disorders in Obese Moderately Well-Controlled Diabetics. R. B. GOLDBERG,* and A. H. RUBENSTEIN.* Chicago, Illinois

Although lipoprotein disorders are common in diabetics, their relationship to the clinical status of these patients is not clear. We report here the serum triglyceride (Trig), cholesterol (Chol), HDL-cholesterol (HDL-Ch) and apolipoprotein (apo) A-I, A-II and B levels in 62 diabetics, divided into (25) normal weight (NWtI) and (22) obese (ObI) insulin treated, and (15) non-insulin treated (NonI, 119% of IBW) groups, and in 48 controls (C). Diabetic control as judged by HbA1 was similar in the 3 groups (12.1±0.6%, 13.2±1% and 11.3±0.8%, respectively). Results in mg/dl;

	Trig	Chol	HDL-Ch	A-I	A-II	B
NWtI	96±16	176±9	56±2	118±3	24±2	90±5
ObI	169±25†	208±8†	47±3†	116±3	23±1	117±6§
NonI	159±23†	205±11ʃ	44±4†	106±5†	22±2	112±9ʃ
C	59±4§	169±4	55±2	121±3	26±1	75±3†

(ʃp<0.05, †p<0.02, §p<0.001, compared with NWtI).

Females had higher HDL-Ch and apo A-I in each group. Despite similar diabetic control, HDL-Ch but not apo A-I was lower in ObI than in NWtI and (C), suggesting that HDL composition may be altered in ObI. Both HDL-Ch and apo A-I were decreased in NonI. There was an inverse correlation between HDL-Ch and Trig (r = - 0.56, p<0.001) but not between HDL-Ch and HbA1 or degree of obesity. Conclusion: non-obese, moderately well-controlled diabetics have minimally altered lipoprotein profiles, whereas obese subjects matched for diabetic control have significantly altered lipoprotein levels. These findings may have relevance to the development of atherosclerosis in these diabetic subgroups.

466

The Hepatic Glucose (G) and Amino Acid Response to Oral Amino Acids (AA) in Dogs. E BARRETT*, J TEPLER, R JACOB, R HENDLER, R GUSBERG, New Haven, Ct

Studies in man have demonstrated an important role for the splanchnic bed in the disposal of AA from ingested protein. We examined the individual roles of the liver (L) and extrahepatic splanchnic (EHS) tissues in the G and AA response to oral AA in 7 dogs with chronic portal, hepatic venous and arterial catheters. Blood levels of AA, plasma G, insulin (I) and glucagon (Gg) levels and rates of G disappearance (^{3}H-glucose) were determined postabsorptively and for 3 h following the ingestion of 0.7 g/kg of an AA mixture. Basally, L released G at a rate of 2.8±0.2 mg/min·kg and removed alanine at a rate of 3.9±0.4 μM/min·kg, while EHS consumed G at a rate of 0.7±0.1 and released alanine at a rate of 1.2±0.8. After feeding, portal plasma I and Gg peaked at 79±24 μU/ml and 383±203 pg/ml. Over 3 h, EHS alanine output exceeded the oral alanine load by 40% and alanine removal by L was 3-fold greater than the amount contained in the load. For 4 other glucogenic AA (ϕala, ser, gly, pro), all of the load appeared in the portal vein and was extracted by L. EHS tissues utilized 215±21 mg/kg·3 h of G, a 48% (p<.05) increase above basal, and L released 650±66 mg/kg·3 h of G, 27% (p<.025) more than basal. Total G disappearance (686±114 mg/kg) slightly exceeded G appearance (671±110) thus accounting for the small but significant (p<.02) fall in arterial plasma G (98 ±3 to 93±4 mg/dl). Conclusions: a) EHS tissues extract G and produce alanine in the fasting and fed state; b) following AA ingestion, L removes glucogenic AA very effectively. If converted to G, these AA can contribute to the observed G output.

467

Trifluorperazine Inhibition of Glucose Stimulated Insulin Release. R. KARL and H. RASMUSSEN, Chicago IL and New Haven, CT (introduced by Eli Ipp*)

Trifluorperazine (TFP, Stellazine) has been shown to bind to calcium dependent regulator protein (CDR) and inhibit its activation of adenylate cyclase and phosphodiesterase. We have studied the effect of TFP on glucose (G) stimulated insulin release and islet cyclic AMP(cAMP) levels. Collagenase isolated rat islets were first perifused with 2.75mM G ± TFP (1-20μM) and then switched to 27.5mM G ± TFP. Marked inhibition of glucose stimulated release was noted at 10μM TFP. (see Table A) Islets were quick frozen and extracted for radioimmunoassay of cAMP two minutes after switching from 2.75mM G ± 10μM TFP to 2.75mM G ± 10μM TFP or 27.5mM G ± 10μM TFP. (see Table B) These results show that 27.5mM G increased cAMP levels two fold above controls and that TFP did not affect cAMP levels in control (2.75mM G) or glucose stimulated (27.5mM G) islets.

TABLE A - Insulin Release in Response to 27.5mM G

TFP	0μM	1μM	5μM	10μM	20μM
insulin(μU/ min/100 islets	109±13 (n=6)	70±8 (n=4)	64±2 (n=4)	22±2 (n=4)	18±2 (n=4)

TABLE B - cAMP Levels 2 Minutes After Exposure To:

	2.75mM G	2.75mM G 10μM TFP	27.5mM G	27.5mM G 10μM TFP
cAMP(fmoles/ islet):	1.83±.22	1.48±.23	3.66±.82	2.79±.50

These data are consistent with the hypothesis that a CDR protein is intimately involved in insulin release and that elevated cAMP levels per se are not sufficient to cause insulin secretion.

468

Effect of Energy Source on Protein and Glucose Metabolism During Dietary Therapy of Adolescents, W.H. Dietz and R.R. Wolfe*, Boston, Mass.

We have studied the interrelationship of protein and glucose metabolism in 7 obese adolescents consuming 1.5 gm meat protein/kg $IBW/_d$ and either 1 gm glucose/kg $IBW/_d$ (P+CHO) or an isocaloric quantity of fat (P+F). IBW was determined by measuring total body water with H_2O^{18}. Each dietary period lasted 21 days; periods were separated by 1 month of weight maintenance.

Nitrogen losses (by N-balance) were significantly larger during P+F. The mean basal rate of glucose production (R_a), measured by means of a primed, constant infusion of U-^{13}C-glucose, was 1.92 ± .36 mg/kg·min and was similar prior to each dietary period. Expressed on the basis of IBW, R_a was comparable to that observed in young adult males. R_a was significantly lower (75% baseline) at the end of each dietary period. R_a during P+F did not differ significantly from R_a during P+CHO. Suppressibility of hepatic glucose production, measured during the infusion of 1 mg unlabelled glucose/kg·min, was equal to the rate of administration.

When 24 hour glucose production was calculated from R_a and corrected for CHO intake, the improved balance observed with CHO could not be explained simply by an equimolar substitution of exogenous glucose for endogenous production.

*Supported by grants from the American Diabetes Association and the Weight Watchers Foundation.

469

Modulation of the Blood Glucose Levels by the Putative Insulin Sensitive CNS Glucoregulator Following Alimentary Glucose Loads. A. IGUCHI*, P.D. BURLESON and A.J. SZABO*, New York, N.Y.

To investigate the possible role of the putative insulin sensitive CNS glucoregulator on alimentary hyperglycemia, glucose,1 gm/kg,was introduced into the stomach of overnight fasted anesthetized rats. Immediately thereafter insulin, 100 μU in 1 μl saline, or 1 μl saline was injected through a stereotaxic needle into the VMN or LHA. Blood samples were obtained from a hepatic venous cannula introduced through the jugular vein. Plasma glucose values for rats injected into the VMN are expressed as mg/dl increases from the baseline.

	Baseline	2	5	10	20	30 min
Saline	85.4 ±3.0	10.7 ±3.5	19.1 ±2.1	43.9 ±4.5	69.7 ±7.2	85.0 ±7.2
Insulin	90.5 ±5.6	3.6 ±1.4	9.3 ±1.0	28.6 ±3.5	47.2 ±4.2	41.3 ±8.3
		$p<0.05$	$p<0.01$	$p<0.05$	$p<0.05$	$p<0.05$

The data show significantly lower plasma glucose levels in rats receiving insulin injections into the VMN than in saline injected controls. However, rats injected with insulin into the LHA showed identical glucose tolerance curves to those injected with saline into the same area. Plasma immunoreactive insulin increased after glucose administration in all four groups of rats. Though the mechanism of these changes requires further elucidation (altered absorption, blood flow or metabolism), it is evident, that insulin injection into the VMN significantly lowers blood glucose levels after intragastric glucose loads.

470

Competition between Glutamate and Palmitoyl-CoA as Substrate for Cardiac Mitochondria from Normal and Diabetic Rats. STEVE W. PUCKETT and WILLIAM J. REDDY*, Birmingham, Alabama.

Fatty acids and glucose are the major fuels for cardiac metabolism. In the diabetic animal the contribution of fatty acids to cardiac metabolism increases, and the contribution of glucose decreases. Glucose utilization is dependent on the removal of cytoplasmically generated reducing equivalents by the malate-aspartate shuttle. Previous work from this laboratory has demonstrated that glutamate translocase is a rate-limiting step in the malate-aspartate shuttle, and glutamate translocase activity is regulated by insulin. The present study was carried out to investigate the relationship between glutamate and palmitoyl-CoA metabolism by heart mitochondria and the effect of diabetes. Palmitoyl-CoA competitively inhibited the oxidation of [1-^{14}C]glutamate to $^{14}CO_2$ by mitochondria from either normal or diabetic rats, with apparent Ki values of 22.7 μM and 16.7 μM palmitoyl-CoA, respectively. Glutamate was demonstrated to inhibit $^{14}CO_2$ evolution from [1-^{14}C]palmitoyl-CoA in mitochondria from normal and diabetic rats with apparent Ki values of 1.6 mM and 4.9 mM glutamate, respectively. In the diabetic rats as compared to the normal rats, palmitoyl-CoA resulted in a greater inhibition of glutamate oxidation and glutamate had a smaller effect of palmitoyl-CoA oxidation as demonstrated by the differences in the apparent Ki values. It is suggested that the increased fatty acid oxidation of diabetic hearts is in part a consequence of decreased glutamate translocase activity.

471

Skeletal Muscle Metabolism in Diabetics with Peripheral Vascular Disease: Studies on the Lower Limb during Rest and Exercise. E.STANDL, H.U.JANKA*, H. MEHNERT*, Munich, W.-Germany

Calf muscle metabolism was investigated in 9 insulin-dependent diabetics with peripheral vascular disease (PVD) and 6 nondiabetics with PVD during rest, a submaximal workload for 10 min and the postexercise period (sampling of venous blood via a catheter from the popliteal vein; determination of muscle blood flow by recording the local clearance of ^{133}Xenon).

After insulin withdrawal there was - similar to diabetics without PVD - a net muscle efflux of glucose, even during exercise, in most of the diabetics with occlusive vascular disease, whereas in the nondiabetics with PVD glucose was consistently taken up by muscle. In the diabetics with PVD the release of free fatty acids and glycerol was increased, the percental uptake of ketone bodies diminished and the production of lactate significantly reduced (lactate release after 10 min of exercise: diabetic 40.31 ± 13.18 µmol/100 g x min; nondiabetics 81.15 ± 19.93; $\bar{x}$ ± SEM). Muscle blood flow was comparable in both groups.

These results indicate that production of lactate is dependent not only on ischemia and site of obliteration but also on diminished glycolysis during insulin deficiency.

472

Endogenous Glucose Production in Pregnant Insulin Dependent Diabetic Women During the Third Trimester. R.M. Cowett, C.B. Kahn*, J.B. Susa, C. Cha, W. Oh, B. Giletti and R. Schwartz*, Providence, RI

The effect of insulin dependent diabetes on glucose homeostasis in pregnant women has not been evaluated systematically. Therefore, glucose kinetic studies have been performed at the end of the third trimester using D(U-^{13}C) glucose with the prime constant infusion technique to define endogenous glucose production (EGP). Pregnant non-diabetic women of comparable gestation served as controls. All subjects were studied after an overnight fast (before a.m. insulin) and received 0.9% saline during the study. Plasma glucose, glucagon, beta hydroxybutyrate (β-OH B), human chorionic somatomammotropin (HCS), amino acid profiles, Hb A_{Ic} and glucose 13/12$_C$ ratio were measured during the steady state. EGP rates were derived.

M±SD		PLASMA			EGP
		Glucose	Glucagon	β-OH B	
	(n)	mg/dl	pg/ml	mM	mg/kg/min
Normal	(6)	75±3	359±234	0.27±0.10	1.9±0.3
Ins. Dep.	(7)	72±15	183±222	0.17±0.08	2.5±1.7

Hb A_{Ic} was 5.7±0.3 vs 7.3±2.3% (control vs diabetic). There were no differences in means between the two groups for the parameters listed or for HCS and amino acid profiles. However, Hb A_{Ic} values in the diabetics (5.4-12.0%) indicated variable prior metabolic control. Two subjects with normal Hb A_{Ic} had normal EGP, while five subjects with elevated Hb A_{Ic} had inconsistent EGP, i.e. low to high values. Despite normal plasma glucose, glucagon and β-OH B, compatible with adequate insulin therapy at the time of study, EGP was unpredictable in the diabetic.

473

Role of H_2-receptors in Gastrogenic Hyperglycemia and Hyperinsulinemia. V.SCHUSDZIARRA*, D.ROUILLER, and R.H.UNGER*, Dallas, Tx. and Ulm, West-Germany

Recent studies have suggested that gastric factors other than gastrin may stimulate islet cell function. The present study was designed to examine the role of histamine H_2-receptors in this gastro-insular axis. In anesthetized dogs with a bisected pylorus and a gastric fistula 250 ml 20% liver extract (LE) at pH7 or pH2 was instilled intragastrically. LE pH2 (N=7) elicited a significant rise in inferior vena cava plasma insulin by 15 uU/ml, glucagon by 100 pg/ml and glucose by 25 mg%, while after LE pH7 (N=7) only glucagon rose significantly. During the infusion of cimetidine, a specific histamine H_2-receptor antagonist, at a rate of 1 mg/kg/h starting 45 min before the instillation of the meal LE pH2 (N=6) elicited a significant rise in inferior vena cava plasma insulin by 10 uU/ml, glucagon by 90 pg/ml and glucose by 17 mg%. This was not significantly different from the controls. In response to LE pH7 (N=5) glucagon rose significantly by 70 pg/ml and insulin by 14 uU/ml whereas glucose levels did not change. The present data demonstrate that during the gastric phase the effect of a meal at low pH upon islet cell function and glucose homeostasis is not altered during the infusion of cimetidine whereas in response to a neutral meal insulin release is stimulated in the presence of H_2-receptor antagonists suggesting that H_2-receptors participate in the regulation of postprandial insulin release during the gastric phase of a meal in dogs.

474

Effect of Acute Treatment with Insulin on Hepatic Lipase in Diabetic Rats. M. BLIZIOTES*, J. ANSON, J. COYLE, S. LEWIS*, Oakland, CA.

We evaluated the acute effects of insulin in restoring the level of hepatic lipase (HL) in isolated, perfused livers of streptozotocin-diabetic rats. Perfusions were performed in fasted male Sprague-Dawley rats; venous collections were made at one minute intervals after an intra-arterial bolus of 10 units (u) of heparin. HL activity was assayed in the cell-free perfusate and expressed as u/gm of tissue (1 u = 1 nmol FFA/ml/h). Peak HL activity (PA) was found 1 min after heparin bolus in all experiments. PA in normal animals (NL) was 2536±96 u/gm (mean±S.E.). Untreated animals (DM) had significantly lower PA (653±94 u/gm, p<.001 vs. NL). In another experiment, diabetic animals were given a pre-infusion of either 1000 µU/ml of insulin (I) or saline for 30 min, and then treated with 10 u of heparin. PA in I-treated rats was no different from control (1120±240 u/gm vs. 1038±209, p=NS). Another group of diabetic rats was pretreated with 1 u of I i.p. 4 hours prior to perfusion. Mean blood glucoses before treatment with I were higher than those 4 hours after I (369±7 mg/dl vs. 59±34, p<.001). PA in I-treated rats was not different from DM (1074±426 vs. 653±94, p=NS). Conclusions: 1) insulinopenic diabetes is associated with a reduced level of heparin-releasable hepatic lipase, 2) acute administration of insulin to diabetic rats does not reverse the deficiency in hepatic lipase, and 3) restoration of hepatic lipase in insulinopenic diabetes may require prolonged priming with insulin.

475

Ketone and alanine turnover rates in health, diabetes, obesity and starvation. S.E.H. HALL, Ottawa, Ontario. (Introduced by G.HETENYI*, Ottawa, Ont.)

In diabetic patients the degree of hypoalaninemia is inversely related to the blood ketone concentration. Experiments have been designed to measure the turnover rates(RT) and metabolic clearance rates(MCR) of alanine and the ketone bodies, acetoacetate(AcAc) and β-hydroxybutyrate, simultaneously over a wide range of ketone concentration. So far experiments have been carried out in 5 newly diagnosed, insulin requiring diabetic patients, 5 obese patients before and after 1-2 wk starvation and 3 normal subjects before and after a high protein diet(HP). All subjects were infused IV for 4h with ^{3}H-2-3 alanine and ^{14}C-3-Na AcAc. RT was calculated from the ratio of the rate of infusion (dpm/min): specific activity (dpm/mmol) plateau.

Blood ketone concentration rose in both normal (HP) and obese starved subjects whereas alanine concentration fell. RT alanine (μmol $min^{-1}kg^{-1}$) fell from 2.0±0.5 to 1.7±0.5 in the obese and from 2.6 ±0.2 to 1.3±0.05 in normal subjects. Basal alanine MCR(ml/min) was normal in diabetic patients 704± 61. In all obese subjects alanine MCR rose after starvation(869±49 to 1117±165). In normal subjects on HP it fell from 681±124 to 505±90. RT_{AcAc} (μmol $min^{-1}kg^{-1}$) was higher in diabetic patients 4.86± 1.1 and obese 2.5±0.5 than normals 1.0±0.3. Starvation caused a 3 fold increase in RT_{AcAc} but AcAc MCR fell from 2839.9±330 to 1066±246.5. In diabetic patients MCR AcAc was lower 1436±156 than normal 2669±88. Thus in diabetes MCR AcAc is lower for a given ketone concentration than in health, obesity or starvation. Starvation is associated with an increase in alanine MCR which is not seen in diabetes. Supported by the MRC (Canada).

476

Effect of Age on Glucose Metabolism and Insulin Response of Cultured Hepatocytes. N. KALANT,* and N. FUKUSHIMA, Montreal, Que.

To determine the effect of maturation on hepatic carbohydrate metabolism we have studied glucose utilization in primary cultures of hepatocytes obtained from rats of increasing age. Cells were cultured in medium L-15 (which contains 5mM galactose) supplemented with 8mM glucose and 20% fetal bovine serum. When maintained for more than 24 hours, the medium was changed daily. Cells from 2-week rats, prior to weaning, showed net utilization of galactose and net production of glucose during the first day in culture. As donor age increased to 6 weeks galactose utilization fell to approximately 30% of that at 2 weeks and remained at that level subsequently; glucose utilization increased to reach a plateau at 8 weeks. A similar pattern of decreasing galactose utilization and increasing glucose utilization was seen with hepatocytes cultured up to 6 days. Insulin binding was identical in cultures from 3-week and 8-week rats but the rate of degradation rose with age of donor and age in culture. In the standard medium insulin had no effect on glucose utilization or glucose incorporation into glycogen. Dexamethasone (10^{-8} M) added to cultures from 3-week rats decreased insulin binding but stimulated glucose incorporation into glycogen by >300%; in cultures from 8-week rats glycogen synthesis was stimulated only 50-70%. It is concluded that: (1) age changes in hexose utilization in vivo are paralleled by changes with age in culture; (2) age changes in glucose utilization and responsiveness to insulin are independent of the level of insulin binding.

477

Dichloroacetate: Inhibition of Rat Liver HMG-CoA Reductase, PETER W. STACPOOLE,* Nashville, Tn.

Dichloroacetate (DCA) reduces serum cholesterol (C) in patients with Fredrickson types IV, IIB or homozygous IIA. To investigate the mechanism of C reduction, the effect of DCA on rat liver microsomal HMG-CoA reductase activity (RA) was studied in normocholesterolemic, reverse light-cycled animals.

Oral DCA (50 or 100mg/kg) administration for 4 days inhibited RA 50% (p=.003) without significantly affecting serum C. In isolated rat hepatocytes incubated for 1 hr with DCA, inhibition of RA was observed at 0.1 (33%) and 1.0 (45%; p=.02) mM DCA. Higher doses resulted in decreased cell viability. Glyoxalate and oxalate, hepatic metabolites of DCA, also markedly reduced RA in isolated cells at 1mM concentrations.

Conclusions: 1) DCA (and/or its metabolites) inhibits rat liver HMG-CoA reductase activity in vivo and in vitro; 2) Reduction of serum C in man may thus be due, at least in part, to inhibition of the rate-limiting enzyme in C biosynthesis.

478

Diabetes Decreases Net Whole Body Cholesterol Synthesis in the Rat. NANCY L. YOUNG, JOSEPH KRASOVSKY, and CHRISTOPHER SAUDEK,* New York, NY

We found earlier that hydroxymethylglutaryl-Co A reductase activity in hypercholesterolemic diabetic rats is low in liver but as a result of hyperphagia is high in small intestine. The effect of diabetes on whole body cholesterol synthesis was studied directly with ^3H_2O incorporation. Male rats on chow ad lib were injected iv. with 45 mCi ^3H_2O at mid dark. Whole body ^{3}H-cholesterol was isolated by digitonin precipitation & thin layer chromatography. In controls plasma water specific activity was constant from ¼ to 4 hr after injection; ^{3}H-cholesterol was 0 at 0 hr and increased linearly to 4hr. Six diabetics and 6 controls were studied 8 days after injection of streptozotocin at 65 mg/kg or of buffer and 4 hr after injection of ^3H_2O. It was assumed that 22 stable H atoms of cholesterol come from H_2O. Data are means ± SEM.

Experiment		Diabetic	Control	
I	plasma insulin	29 ± 5	81 ± 12	μU/ml
	glucose	522 ± 25	167 ± 4	mg/dl
	cholesterol	90 ± 10	50 ± 1	mg/dl
II	body weight day 0	309 ± 4	301 ± 8	gm
	day 8	310 ± 6	338 ± 11	gm
	plasma water	144 ± 3	141 ± 5	μCi/ml
	^{3}H-cholesterol	313 ± 18	405 ± 22	nCi/rat
	cholesterol synthesis	82 ± 6	100 ± 5	mg/(kg·day)

There was a signifigant decrease ($P < 0.05$) in net cholesterol synthesis with diabetes. This may result from increased intake of cholesterol from 24 to 49 mg/(kg·day) with hyperphagia, from failure to gain weight, from conversion of more ^{3}H-cholesterol to bile acids, or from direct effects of lower insulin on hepatic cholesterol synthesis.

479

Effects of Glucagon and Insulin on the Synthesis of L-carnitine by Cultured Human Skin Fibroblasts. J.F. ORAM, Seattle, WA. (Introduced by E.L. BIERMAN,* Seattle, WA.).

Cultured human skin fibroblasts synthesize L-carnitine when incubated with carnitine-deficient medium as evident by an increase in the L-carnitine content of both the medium and the cell. The synthesis of carnitine depends on the availability of L-lysine in the medium. The addition of either L-lysine or γ-aminobutyrate to lysine-free growth medium resulted in a dose-related increase in the amount of carnitine produced by the cell. Addition of high concentrations of glucagon (100 ng/ml) to the medium (plus lysine) increased carnitine production several-fold. A small increase (15-30%) was also evident in the presence of physiological concentrations of glucagon (1.0 ng/ml). Addition of 100 to 10,000 uU/ml insulin to the medium had no apparent effect on carnitine synthesis either in the presence or absence of glucagon. These results suggest that peripheral cells have the ability to synthesize carnitine and that the synthetic process is under hormonal regulation.

TRANSPLANTATION

480

Effects of Dichloroacetate on Amino Acids in Diabetic Dogs. R. PARK, W. J. LEACH and A. I. ARIEFF,* San Francisco, Ca.

Dichloroacetate (DCA) may be useful in the treatment of diabetes and certain disorders of lactate (Lac) metabolism by enhancing the oxidation of glucose derived substrates in extrahepatic tissues such as skeletal muscle (Musc), thereby decreasing the normal release of substrates such as Lac, pyruvate, and alanine (Ala) which are used for hepatic gluconeogenesis. To further explore the effects of DCA, we studied the effects of a 4 h infusion, 300 mgm/kg/h, on blood levels of Lac and 24 amino acids (AA) and their arteriovenous differences across hind limb Musc and extrahepatic splanchnic bed (gut). In diabetic dogs, glutamine (Gln) and Ala together accounted for most of the AA found in arterial plasma and for most of AA released from Musc. Gut utilized large quantities of Gln, and produced significant amounts of Ala, glutamate, citrulline, and proline. DCA treatment lowered blood levels of the gluconeogenic substrates Lac and Ala to 35% and 32% of control, respectively. The DCA effect on Ala was mediated by an 87% decrease in Musc release ($p < 0.01$); whereas gut release was not affected. DCA treatment appeared to increase gut utilization of Gln since there was increased release of the degradation products of Gln (glutamate, citrulline, and proline) from gut tissue ($p < 0.02$).

Conclusions: DCA 1) lowers blood glucose in diabetic dogs in part by decreasing the release of gluconeogenic substrates from extrahepatic sites; 2) appears to enhance the gut utilization of Gln; and 3) may be useful in the treatment of diabetes and lactic acidosis.

481

Observations on survival of Rat-Pancreas Cultures differently Frozen-Thawed. V.ESPOSITO, V.MEZZOGIORNO, G.MELLUSO, M.PAPA*, G.P.PAPACCIO. Naples - Italy

We have determined the effects of four different cooling programs on cultured pancreas survival. Rat pancreas fragments were cultured in SRI-8 modified and added up with pilocarpine 40mg% and aprotininum[∞] 6.8ml% to purify endocrine pancre as from exocrine digestive enzymes. The purified islets were placed in 10% dimethyl-sulfoxide and kept at 4C/45min in 2-methylbutan bath, then cooled in liquid nitrogen according to the following programs: 1) rapid cooling (500C/min); 2) cooling at a constant rate of 0.6C/min to -7C, plateau/20 min, then cooling at rate of 2.4C/min to -196C; 3) cooling rate of 0.12C/min to -40C and cooling rate of 9C/min to -196C; 4) cooling rate of 0.25/min to -80C and cooling rate of 3C/min to -196C.

All samples were rapidly (37C) and slowly (room-temperature) thawed.

Islet purification was tested by measuring insulin/amylase ratio every hour. The functional recovery of the frozen-thawed pancreas was assessed by in vitro stimulation with glucose and glucose-tolbutamide. The islets cooled slowly enough to allow them to come into equilibrium with external ice, and room-temperature thawed, showed on morphological and biochemical examination an high survival rate and suggest their useful application to reverse experimental diabetes. [∞](Trasylol)

482

Transplantation of Cultured Rat Pancreas into the Spleen. V.ESPOSITO, V. MEZZOGIORNO, G.MELLUSO, M. PAPA* Naples-Italy

The spleen seems to be bettor than other sites for endocrine pancreas allograft, because in case of rejection it can be easily removed without vital damage for the recipient. A short-time pancreas culture (4h) in SRI-8 modified and added up with pilocarpine 40mg% and aprotininum (Trasylol) 6.8ml% before transplantation allows to achieve a high amount of islets purified from exocrine enzymes. Therefore the implant with islets from a single donor reduces the immunological consequences due to the allograft from several donors.

Sprague-Dawley rats received pancreas from Wistar. They had been immunosuppressed with ALS two doses (8ml/Kg) gived on days -1 and +1 and with corticosteroides (5mg/Kg).

Between the 2nd and 6th day after trasplantation 75% of recipients showed normal Glicemic Levels (GL), normal urine volume weight gain and Insulin Serum Levels (ISL) were 22± 2.4 µU/ml and are presently aglycosuric at 50/60 days. Whereas in diabetic controls high GL and ISL 6.0±1.5 µU/ml occurred. The recipients not immunosuppressed died in high rate.

Some animals are regularly sacrified for histological and histochemical B cells studies. The results suggest a successful use of cultured pancreas and spleen as grafting site in clinical practice.

483

The Effect of Exogenous Human Growth Hormone (hGH) on Blood Glucose Concentrations and Insulin Requirements During Closed Loop (Biostator ®-GCIIS) Control of Diabetes Mellitus. G. BRIGHT, T. MELTON, A. ROGOL, W. CLARKE*, Charlottesville, Va.

The effects of continuous intravenous hGH at two different rates [1µg/kg/hr(L) or 2µg/kg/hr(H)] on blood glucose concentrations and insulin requirements were compared in 5 insulin-requiring diabetic subjects whose blood glucose concentrations were controlled with a closed loop insulin delivery system. Each individual served as his own control (saline infusion) and was studied on 3 separate days for periods of 8 to 10 hours. Diet, physical activity and Biostator control algorithms were identical on each study day while the order of the studies was randomized.

	"BASAL" hGH MEAN ng/ml±SEM	GLUCOSE MEAN mg/dl±SEM	INSULIN MEAN Units/Study
C	3.0 ± 0.7	141 ± 10	44.1 ± 6
L †	7.1 ± 0.8	142 ± 21	45.9 ± 9
H ††	9.8 ± 0.8	138 ± 10	45.1 ± 6

†p<0.01 ††p<0.025

Although mean basal hGH concentrations (average hGH concentration excluding transient physiologic rises) were significantly different on each of the study days, mean blood glucose concentrations and mean insulin required to maintain blood glucose concentrations remained unchanged. These studies indicate that short term sustained elevations in mean hGH similar to those reported in poorly controlled diabetic subjects, do not necessitate increased insulin delivery in subjects whose blood glucose concentrations are being controlled with a closed loop insulin delivery system.

484

The Management of Diabetes Mellitus in a Pregnant Diabetic Using a Portable Insulin Infusion Pump. ERIC A. ORZECK*, Houston, Tx.

A twenty-four-year-old woman with a ten-year history of insulin-dependent diabetes (White's Class C) was started on constant subcutaneous insulin infusion (CSII) via a portable pump (Auto-Syringe TM) during the last ten weeks of pregnancy. Her mean prepump plasma glucose level was 117.5 mg/dl with a standard deviation of 67.0 mg/dl. After initiation of CSII her mean plasma glucose level fell to 91.8 mg/dl with a standard deviation of 35.3 mg/dl. This represented a significant tightening of control in this patient, which is further reflected in her plasma glucose levels for the thirty days prior to delivery, as with only four exceptions, two-hour post-prandial plasma glucose levels under 125 mg/dl were maintained. Basal insulin allowances and preprandial bolus doses were calculated with adjustments made as necessary to accommodate the changing insulin requirements imposed by pregnancy. Glycosylated hemoglobin (HbA_{1c}) fell from 12.7% to 9.1% after 10 weeks of CSII (4.2%-9.1% normal range). A healthy male infant (Apgar 8 at one minute, 9 at five minutes) weighing 3.8 kg. was delivered at term. The child's plasma glucose level remained above 45 mg/dl, and no problems with hypocalcemia or hyperbilirubinemia were encountered.

485

L-Asparaginase Diabetes in Rabbits: Effect of Single vs. Multiple L-Asparaginase Dose Regimen. ROBERT L. LAVINE* AND DEBORAH M. DICINTIO, Philadelphia, Pa.

We have demonstrated that a single intravenous dose of 10,000 I.U. E. coli L-asparaginase (A)/kg b.w. induces an insulin resistant, hyperinsulinemic diabetic syndrome in male NZW rabbits. Since this observation was different from the effect observed in patients and animals receiving multiple doses of A, male NZW rabbits were injected I.V. with 1000 I.U. E. coli A/kg b.w. daily for 10 days to observe any differences in the diabetic syndrome induced by a multiple dose regimen as compared to the single dose regimen. All animals were weighed and blood for serum glucose (G) and insulin (IRI) was obtained prior to the injection of A and on the 11th day after 10 daily doses of A. Control animals (C) were injected with an amount of mannitol equivalent to that in the A dose and were followed in the same manner.

	Δ wgt.	G (mgm/dl)		IRI (pgm/ml)	
	Day 11	Day 0	Day 11	Day 0	Day 11
A	-0.47±0.16(5)	108±7(8)	377±42(5)	109±4(8)	66±12(5)
C	+0.26±0.02(5)	107±6(5)	108±4(5)	107±3(5)	106±1(4)

mean ± S.D. (#)

Regular insulin (0.1 U/kg b.w. I.V.) caused a significant decline in glucose levels (40%) in the diabetic animals. These results demonstrate that multiple doses of A induce a hypoinsulinemic insulin sensitive diabetic syndrome while a single I.V. dose, similar in quantity to the multiple dose regimen, induces a hyperinsulinemic insulin resistant diabetic syndrome in male NZW rabbits.

486

Skin Conductance and Heart Rate as Indicators of Hypoglycemia. N.M. FRIEDMAN*, R.P. EATON*, D.S. SCHADE*, J.G. DAVIS, Albuquerque, NM.

Nocturnal hypoglycemia is the principal complication of insulin therapy in diabetic man. We examined the feasibility of monitoring changes in skin conductance (SC) and heart rate (HR) as indicators of hypoglycemia for use in a patient alarm system.

Normoglycemic characterization of SC and HR was determined in five subjects using an automated portable recording system. During 63 cumulative hours, the mean SC was 8 ± 3 μmho/cm^2 and the mean HR was 73 ± 3 beats/min.

A total of 7 hypoglycemic insulin reactions were monitored with a mean glucose nadir of 54 ± 7 mg/dl. The simultaneous changes in SC and HR were (mean ± SEM).

	Δ from baseline	Duration (min)	Significance
SC μmho/cm^2	11 ± 3	26 ± 7	$p<0.05$
HR beats/min	25 ± 9	18 ± 3	$p<0.05$

Thirteen additional events occurred with comparable changes in SC and HR during the day in response to non-hypoglycemic stimuli. No events that fit our criteria were observed during the 22 hours of sleep monitoring.

These results suggest that significant changes in SC and HR are characteristic of hypoglycemia in man. Specificity and sensitivity may be sufficient to identify nocturnal hypoglycemic events. We conclude that an alarm system monitoring SC and HR as indicators of nocturnal hypoglycemia is feasible.

487

Normalization of Blood Glucose through Pregnancy, Labor and Delivery. L. JOVANOVIC, P. ALLEN, C.M. PETERSON, New York, N.Y.

A program to normalize maternal blood glucose (BG) throughout pregnancy has been developed with the use of a home glucose monitoring system during pregnancy and an artifical B cell Biostator during labor and delivery.

Over the past three years, 48 insulin dependent diabetic women (White Class B=10, C=10, D=8, R=3, F=1, G=16) have completed the program. All 48 began the program in their 12th week or less of gestation. On entry into the program all 48 were not in "control" (mean BG=219±83 mg/dl, hemoglobin A_{1c} (HbA_{1c}) 10±2%, MAGE 150±64 mg/dl). After one week, BG normalized (mean 86±8 mg/dl, MAGE 43±6 mg/dl) and after 6 weeks HbA_{1c} normalized to 4.1±1.4%. Insulin requirements rose from .7 to.8 u/kg/day at 32±2 weeks. Insulin requirement at term was 1.0 u/kg/day but with decreasing overnight requirement. Caloric requirement was 30 kcal/kg and mean weight gain during pregnancy was 11 kg.

Normalization was maintained during labor and delivery utilizing a Biostator. Despite the fact that the last subcutaneously administered insulin was given 8 hours prior to induction, no insulin was required for the duration of labor (group mean 7±3 hours), whereas the glucose infused over the same period to maintain BG at 74±4 mg/dl was 2.55 ±0.20 mg/kg/min. The incidence of macrosomnia, hypoglycemia, hyperbilrubinimia, hypocalcemia, erythemia, respiratory distress and major congenital anormalies was 0%. No infant or maternal morbidity was encountered in the pre-, peri- or post-partum period.

488

Prevention of Glomerular Basement Membrane Thickening by Whole Pancreas Transplantation in Alloxan Diabetes. M.J.ORLOFF,* R.H. BELL, L. FERNANDEZ-CRUZ, S. LEE, and H.J. SAYERS,* San Diego, Ca.

Serial thickness measurements of the glomerular basement membrane were performed over a 24-month period in inbred male Lewis rats. Group I consisted of 44 normal controls. In Groups II, III and IV, diabetes was induced by intravenous alloxan (42-44 mg/kg). Group II rats (51 diabetic controls) were subsequently untreated. Group III animals (N=72) underwent pancreaticoduodenal transplants 1 week after alloxan injection. Group IV rats (N=68) underwent transplantation of the duct-ligated pancreas. The glomerular capillary basement membrane was measured in sacrificed animals monthly in each group by a quantitative morphometric technique. Results were as follows:

BASEMENT MEMBRANE THICKNESS (Å)

Age (mos)	Group I	Group II	Group III	Group IV
1- 6	2256±102	2257±296	2292± 90	2364± 83
7-12	2927± 96†	3842±115	2992± 90†	2842± 84†
13-18	3352± 78†	4418±162	3529±100†	3451± 64†
19-24	3687±276†	5033±171	3458±295†	3982±118†

† = p<.001 compared to Group II

There were no significant differences at any time between transplanted animals and normal controls. This study demonstrates conclusively that whole pancreas transplantation early in the course of experimental diabetes completely prevents the basement membrane thickening associated with diabetic nephropathy.

489

Portal Vein Insulin Placement via Cutaneous Bowel Loop Wall Injection. E. DENNIS MURPHY*, KURT A. BUZARD, EDWARD F. SCANLON, Evanston, Illinois

In diabetes, intermittent subcutaneous insulin administration poorly mimics the non-diabetic state as judged by blood glucose control. Constant subcutaneous insulin administration has been shown in several recent studies to more closely reproduce blood glucose and selected metabolic parameters.

We have chosen to imitate another aspect of non-diabetic insulin secretion, that of portal venous system placement of insulin. To do this we have established cutaneous isolated small bowel loops with intact mesenteric blood supply in surgically diabetic dogs. Insulin was then injected into the bowel loop wall, providing access for the first long term studies of the effects of portal venous system insulin administration.

Our experience to date with bowel loop insulin injection will be reviewed. We obtained Iodine-131 labeled insulin kinetic data, short term experiments were also conducted over a few hours time comparing blood glucose after bowel loop versus subcutaneous insulin injection with a meal. Long term, two week management periods have shown continued control of blood sugar with bowel loop insulin injections. Finally we present data comparing the results of continuous pump insulin infusion via bowel loop versus subcutaneous routes with pre-programmed post-prandial waveforms.

490

Central Venous Insulin Delivery for Prolonged Glycemic Normalization in Ambulatory Adolescent Diabetics. K. PERLMAN, R.M. EHRLICH*, R.M. FILLER, and A.M. ALBISSER*, Toronto, Canada.

With informed consent from both subjects and parents, five non obese uncomplicated Type 1 diabetics (aged 14-17y) were studied in hospital for 14-23d with open-loop intravascular insulin infusion (IVI). Activity was otherwise not restricted. The usual diabetic diet was of constant caloric content and was provided as three meals at 0900, 1200 and 1700h. Under local anaesthesia a silicone rubber indwelling catheter was placed in a branch of an external jugular vein, advanced to the superior vena cava and tunnelled subcutaneously to exit in the supramammary region where it was connected to the miniature, portable pumping system (Diabetes Care 3(2), 1980). The pattern of insulin infusion involved a basal rate which was augmented 4-5X, 10-15' after the beginning of a meal. 90-120' later it was reduced back to basal over the next 120-180' in a two step fashion. Mean fasting plasma glucose before IVI was 315 ± 56 and dropped to 84 ± 6mg/dl on IVI. This was accompanied by normal meal excursions (mean a.c. glucose 80 ± 8mg/dl, with a mean glucose rise of 33 ± 6mg/dl at 44 ± 4 minutes). Plasma C-peptide was detectable in only one subject 0.08pmol/ml (normal fasting 0.41 ± 0.12). Mean urine glucose was 52 before and 1.3g/d during IVI. Serum cholesterol and triglycerides dropped from 248 ± 45 and 422 ± 123mg/dl to 154 ± 13 and 155 ± 13mg/dl respectively. Initial mean HbA was 14.6% and declined to 9.7% with IVI (Normals:6.5-8.5%). All indices of control showed improvement with $p < 0.05$. There were no catheter related complications. The system was well accepted by all subjects. We conclude that in ambulatory adolescent diabetics continuous open-loop IV insulin infusion by central vein is feasible for the prolonged normalization of glycemia and other indices of control.

491

Long-Term Insulin Pump Rx of Diabetes: Effect on Insulin and Fuel Metabolism. M. BERGMAN,* W. TAMBORLANE,* V. SOMAN,* R. HENDLER* and R. SHERWIN,* New Haven, CT.

Normalization of blood glucose by peripheral (rather than portal) insulin (I) infusion may result in hyperinsulinemia. The latter would be potentially harmful if it caused abnormal reductions in amino acids (AA), lipids and a fall in I binding. We therefore measured fasting and post-meal free I, plasma AA and lipids and I binding to RBCs in 10 JOD on outpatient I pump Rx for 3-11 months (FBS 81±8, 2h post-meal 130±13 mg/dl). Fasting free I levels in JOD on pump Rx (29±5 uU/ml) were moderately elevated as compared to normal controls (16±2 uU/ml, $p<0.05$). Nevertheless, fasting plasma branched chain AA (361±27 uM), cholesterol (158±9 mg/dl) and triglycerides (68±8 mg/dl) were all comparable to control values (p=NS). With the pre-meal I dose, peak free I levels were similar to those obtained in normals consuming identical meals. Beyond 2-3 h, free I remained increased in JOD, but returned to baseline in normals. Despite elevations in free I, post-meal increments in branched chain AA (125±26 uM) were similar to control values (118±20, p=NS). I binding to RBCs was not suppressed by I pump Rx and, in fact, tended to be higher as compared to values in normal subjects (10±1% vs 8±1%, p=NS). Conclusion: Despite altered free I profiles, long-term subcutaneous I pump Rx in JOD results in normal AA and lipid concentrations and does not reduce I binding. These data suggest that long-term I pump Rx corrects hyperglycemia without inducing the metabolic consequences of hyperinsulinemia.

492

Effect of In Vitro Culture on Pancreatic Islet Allotransplantation. W.J.TZE, J.TAI, Vancouver, British Columbia. (Introduced by A.R.CAIRNS*, Vancouver, British Columbia)

Prolongation of islet allograft survival across major histocompatibility barrier has been achieved by in vitro culture in conjunction with ALS in the recipient rat. This study reports (i) the survival time of Lewis(AgB^1) islets cultured at 26°C, 32°C and 37°C and atmosphere of 5% CO_2 in air or 5% CO_2 in 95% O_2 for 7 days and subsequently transplanted intraportally into streptozotocin-induced diabetic ACI(AgB^4) recipient rats, (ii) the daily anti-Le antibody level in the recipients with C'dependent cytotoxicity test and (iii) the vulnerability of islets to immunorejection tested by IV administration of 10^7 Le spleen cells to the host. With islets cultured at 26°C, prolonged graft survival of 14 to over 120 days were found. Islet allografts cultured at 32°C or 37°C were rejected around 5 days similar to fresh islet allograft. Islets cultured in O_2 rich atmosphere also achieved prolonged allosurvival. The peak anti-Le titers achieved by cultured islets was less than 1:3 which was significantly lower than 1:80 found in recipients of fresh islets. The ACI recipient rats with over 120 days of functioning Le islet allograft reverted back to diabetic state 2 days following the IV administration of Le spleen cells. These data indicate that (i) islet cultured at 26°C for 7 days without host immunosuppression prolonged allograft survival, (ii) significantly lower Ab titers in ACI recipients of cultured islets, (iii) no correlation between Ab titers and graft survival time and (iv) islet allograft with prolonged survival was still susceptible to host immunorejection.

493

A Pocket Sized Directly Readable Insulin Delivery System. D. WHITNEY, E.C. LAYNE, L.J. THOMAS, A.N. BESSMAN*, J. GAUME and S.P. BESSMAN, Los Angeles and Downey, CA.

The piezoelectric pump system previously used continuously for months transcutaneously in dogs, has been designed to be worn externally and to deliver insulin at controllable rates. The unit consists of a special case, rechargeable battery and directly readable refillable reservoir containing 3.5 ml. The reservoir consists of a spiral of thin plastic tubing. The volume delivered can be read by the wearer by the position of the meniscus referred to a calibration chart. The smallest readable change is about 1.2 µl. The system can pump a bolus from every 0.5 to every 10 minutes.

Four different pumps have been tested in human volunteers for 8 hours to check the volume delivery of an inert substance. Each volunteer wore the unit attached to his belt with the needle inserted subcutaneously in the abdominal wall. Each was totally ambulatory. The volume delivered was read by the wearer at hourly intervals and was checked in the laboratory after each test. The average bolus delivered in 7 tests in volunteers was 0.71 µl and in laboratory was 0.66 µl. There is no significant difference (paired t test) between the volume delivered at no back pressure (laboratory) and subcutaneously. Apparently the subcutaneous tissue pressure is negligible in relation to the 150-175 mm. Hg. pressure capability of the system. The system functions reliably in an in vivo setting for the 8 hour period tested.

494

Islet Cell Antibodies Appearing at Rejection of a Fetal Pancreatic Graft in a Diabetic Patient. R. GUNNARSSON*, H. ZUHLKE, Z. FREEDMAN, G.F. BOTTAZZO, A. ANDERSSON, C. HELLERSTRÖM*, C.G. GROTH, Huddinge, Sweden.

A 45-year old male diabetic, on maintenance immunosuppression following a successful cadaveric renal transplantation two years previously for end-stage nephropathy, received an intraportal injection of fetal pancreatic microfragments. This tissue had been harvested from 6 fetuses, and maintained in culture for periods up to 14 days.

One month after the pancreatic transplantation, small amounts of C-peptide appeared in the urine. Its level then increased over a 3-month period to reach a maximum of about 5 per cent of normal. Within the following week, C-peptide excretion ceased abruptly. Simultaneously, islet cell surface antibodies (ICSAb) appeared in the patient's serum. The amount seemed to rise during the following month, and then to decline. A search for islet cell cytoplasmic antibodies was negative. The patient required the administration of insulin throughout.

The cessation of graft function may have been due to allograft rejection, the rise in ICSAb then being a secondary phenomenon. However, since there is evidence that autoimmune processes are involved in the pathogenesis of insulin-dependent diabetes mellitus, it may be speculated that the transplantation caused recurrence of autoimmunity against islet tissue, this resulting in graft destruction.

OTHER

495

Peripheral Hyperinsulinism, a Prerequisit for Good Metabolic Control under Feedback Regulated Insulininfusion. W. KEMMLER, B. KRAUS*, K. GERBITZ, M. HAUNER, K. PIWERNETZ, K.D. HEPP, R. RENNER, Munich, Germany

Hyperinsulinism, a possible causal factor for the development of macroangiopathy is usually observed under conventional s.c. insulin therapy. It is thus far unclear which insulin levels are needed under feed back regulated i.v. therapy. Ten diabetics of type I (TI) and 4 of type II (TII) were treated with a glucose regulated insulin infusion by a minipump. The infusion rates were set according to especially developed algorithms. Two identical meals were administered at 8 and 11^{45} a.m. Every 30 min free insulin (FI), bound insulin and C-peptid were measured under s.c. and i.v. therapy. Five healthy subjects served as controls (C). The glucose levels under i.v. therapy were almost normalized in TI and TII and significantly improved as compared to those under s.c. therapy. The mean FI levels were under i.v. infusion: TI 68±21.7 μU/ml (s.c. therapy 74.4±14 μU/ml) TII 77.5±10.9 μU/ml, C 42.1±7.9 μU/ml. The FI levels between the meals and the postprandial insulin peaks in TI and TII were almost double as high as in C. The infusion rate necessary after the meal at 8 a.m. was significantly higher than after the meal at 11^{45} a.m. (ratio 1.6:1) resulting however in identical FI levels. The FI were not correlated with the infusion rates, the C-peptide or the bound insulin. These results indicate that also under feedback regulated i.v. therapy hyperinsulinism is necessary for good metabolic control. The higher need of insulin in the morning is possibly caused by differences in insulin metabolism rather than in the insulin sensitivity.

496

Psychosocial Profile of Adult Diabetics. R. MAZZE*, J. MURPHY, D. ENGSTROM, S. ROSEN, NEW YORK, N.Y.

Three self-administered protocols were developed to evaluate adult diabetic patients for (1) depression, (2) anxiety, and (3) problems of adjustment (comprised of seven areas: medical, job, social, personal, psychological, marital and sexual) to determine whether they differ significantly from a comparable non-diabetic sample.

A random sample (N=25) was drawn from the 125 enrolled diabetic patients at a city hospital diabetes clinic (CDC). A second sample (N=28) was drawn from the 300 diabetic patients at a voluntary hospital diabetes clinic (VDC). A sex and age matched non-diabetic group (N=25) also completed the three protocols. Subjects in each group ranged in age from 24 to 64 and consisted of 40% males and 60% females.

The Student's t Test was used to determine whether a significant difference existed between the non-diabetic group (ND) and each of the samples (CDC and VDC). A significant difference between ND and CDC ($p<.05$) and ND and VDC ($p<.005$) was found for the protocol on problems of adjustment. Closer analysis revealed that perceived medical status ($p<.02$ for CDC and VDC) and job related problems ($p<.005$ for CDC and VDC) were the principal contributing factors which explained the difference between the non-diabetic and the diabetic groups. In contrast, this study showed no significant difference between the non-diabetic and the diabetic groups for depression and anxiety. All groups scored at the lower end of the two scales.

One implication of the pilot study is that adult diabetics may be coping far better than we suspected with the psychological aspects of diabetes.

497

Glucose- and Caerulein-induced Insulin Release from Rat Insulinomas. TSUTOMU KAZUMI, CHOITSU SAKAMOTO ATSUSHI OHKI, GEN YOSHINO, MAKOTO OTSUKI, SHIGEAKI BABA* Kobe, Japan

Effect of glucose(G) and caerulein(Cn) on insulin (IRI) release were studied in the isolated perfused rat pancreas bearing insulinomas induced by streptozotocin and nicotinamide(Cancer Res. 38:2144, 1978. Endocrinology 103:154;, 1978). Perfusion without recirculation(JCI. 63:478 , 1979) for 50 min (10-20 min interval) was done before and after removal of the tumors or sham-operation. Results are expressed as the integrated IRI output(ng/10 min) calculated on the basis of the experiments.

		before	after
G, 50 mg/dl	Insulinoma:	324 ± 76[1]	87 ± 20[1]
	Control :	8 ± 1	8 ± 2
G, 150 mg/dl	Insulinoma:	2162 ± 718[1]	257 ± 74[1]
	Control :	285 ± 27	862 ± 75
Cn, 0.1 ng/ml	Insulinoma:	3198 ± 826[1]	256 ± 70[1]
+G, 150 mg/dl	Control :	824 ± 85	925 ± 123
G, 50 mg/dl	Insulinoma:	1095 ± 226[1]	103 ± 24[1]
	Control :	78 ± 7	98 ± 12

Mean ± SEM of 6 - 10 experiments.

[1]: $p<0.005$ or less vs. respective controls.

G- and Cn-induced changes in IRI secretion from tumor-bearing pancreases were elevated in magnitide but were similar in pattern between the two groups. IRI contents of the tumors averaged 13.4 ± 1.8mg/g wet weight and 92 ± 2% of the total IRI migrated in the insulin region on gel filtration.

The study shows that rat insulinoma B cells, like normal pancreatic B cells, can store and secrete insulin, and suggest that pancreatic B cell function is suppressed by a large amount of insulin released from insulinomas.

498

The Effect of Fenfluramine on Glucose Homeostasis in Lipodystrophy. T.WILSON, T. MELTON, W. CLARKE*, Charlottesville, Va.

Diabetes associated with lipodystrophy (L) is characterized by insulin resistance. Fenfluramine (F), a cogener of dextro-amphetamine, has been shown to reduce fasting glucose concentrations and improve glucose tolerance in some patients with L. We evaluated the effect of F on glucose homeostasis (G.H.) independent of its effect on appetite in 3 patients with L over a 3 - 12 month period. Patient A has total acquired L and chemical diabetes while patients B & C are siblings with total congenital L and overt diabetes. Studies included HbA_1, 5 hour oral glucose tolerance test (OGTT) and continuous blood glucose monitoring or control with a closed loop insulin delivery system (Biostator ® - GC11S) prior to and during F therapy. OGTT results are expressed as the sum of individual glucose values, while the continuous glucose concentrations over a 16 hour period are expressed as mean ± S.E.

Pt.	F mg/day	HbA_1 %	OGTT Σ mg/dl	16 hr Glucose mg/dl±SE	Insulin Infused units/16 hr
A	0	6.8	1028	108±1	-
	120	7.5	923	95±1	-
B	0	13.9	2317	166±1	-
	60	10.5	902	101±1	-
C	0	16.1	3994	192±4	97
	100	17.2	3769	198±1	132

While F appeared to improve G.H. in B and to have a small effect in A, it did not improve G.H. in C whose diabetes was more severe. Thus, the beneficial effect of F on G.H. in L is not uniform and appears to be limited to those individuals with mild to moderate impairments in G.H.

499

Coronary Vascular and Myocardial Responses to Hypoxia in Diabetic Newborn Lambs. JOHN C. LEE*, JOHN C. WERNER and S. EVANS DOWNING, NEW HAVEN,CT.

The purpose of this investigation was to examine changes in cardiac performance and coronary reactivity during hypoxia in diabetic lambs. Diabetic mellitus (DM) was produced in 6 animals, 4-11 days of age, by giving alloxan monohydrate, 150 mg/kg, 24 hours prior to study. These lambs were compared with 7 controls (C). Measurement of LV dp/dt max, LVEDP, coronary sinus flow (CF) and myocardial oxygen extraction (O_2EXT) were made using a hemodynamically controlled preparation described previously (AJP 244: 1381, 1973). The average arterial glucose concentration in C and DM lambs was 86.7 (± 10.7SE) and 532.8 (±117.2SE) mg%, respectively. Parasympathetic and β-adrenergic blockades were produced in each lamb by giving atropine (1mg) and practolol (4mg/kg), respectively. Hypoxia was produced by addition of N_2 to the respirator. As the PO_2 fell from ~ 100 mmHg to ~25 mmHg, CF and O_2 EXT increased progressively in both C and DM lambs. The responses of the two groups were quantitatively identical. Phentolamine (2mg/kg) reduced coronary vascular resistance in DM but not in C lambs. During hypoxia, LV dp/dt increased significantly in both groups while LVEDP was unchanged. These findings indicate that diabetic lambs have more alpha-adrenergic tone in the coronary vessels, but the coronary vascular and myocardial contractility responses to hypoxia were not altered by the acute diabetic state.

500

Dynamic Time Course Studies of the Diabetic "BB" Wistar Rat. G.S. TANNENBAUM, E.COLLE, and T.A. SEEMAYER (Intro. by M.M.BELMONTE*) Montreal,Canada

The development of diabetes was studied in 37 male "BB" Wistar rats. Successive 6-hr plasma glucose (G), insulin (IRI) and growth hormone (GH) profiles were obtained from unanesthetized,freely-behaving chronically cannulated rats at various times prior to and after onset. During the prediabetic stage (2-18 days prior to onset) normal basal plasma G (138±2 mg/dl), IRI (1.2±0.6 ng/ml) and GH secretory episodes were found. Glucose tolerance (2 gm/kg iv) was normal up to 10 days before onset. Plasma G levels were significantly elevated (284.5±5 mg/dl) during feeding 2 days prior to onset with inappropriately low, but measurable, plasma IRI (2.02±.06 ng/ml). Following detection, there was marked elevation of G (484±5 mg/dl) and decrease of IRI (0.38±.01 ng/ml). GH secretory episodes were normal early but decreased when weight loss occurred. Pancreatic IRI concentrations were severely depressed 1-2 days post detection (1.46±.27 vs 61.4±18.3 ng/mg wet weight in control littermates). Pancreatic glucagon concentrations were normal (3.65±.55 ng/mg vs 2.05±.48 ng/mg in littermates) in the early stage, but significantly depleted in the terminal stage (0.79±.12 ng/mg). Light and electron microscopy of the early stage showed lymphocytic infiltration of islets, hyperplasia of beta cell endoplasmic reticulum, and evidence of beta cell injury and necrosis with sparing of alpha cells. Islets from end stage diabetics were reduced in number with rare beta cells and no lymphocytes. Thus, this model mimics human diabetes in that hormonal profiles are normal until 2-3 days prior to overt disease at a time when pancreatic pathology is well established

501

Risk Factors for Ten-Year Mortality in Adult-Onset Diabetes. B. HAWKINS, C. MEINERT, H. KNOWLES*, F. GOETZ*. Baltimore, Maryland

Laboratory definition of non-ketotic diabetes remains difficult and depends in part on evidence that hyperglycemia is a risk factor for vascular disease. Multiple regression procedures have been used with data from the University Group Diabetes Program (UGDP) to identify characteristics which are related to mortality. The analyses include results from 600 patients who were originally assigned to the placebo, insulin-standard, and insulin-variable treatment groups. Mild to more severe, non-insulin dependent diabetics with a baseline SUM GTT (the sum of the fasting, 1-, 2-, and 3-hour blood glucose levels) between 500 and 1500 mg/dl were enrolled in the study. Patients studied were under follow-up for a minimum of 10 years.

Twenty-four different baseline characteristics were used in the analyses including age at entry, sex, race, various cardiovascular risk factors, and the blood glucose levels. The characteristics with the highest predictive value, other than age, were cardiovascular risk factors including absence of arterial pulses in the lower extremities, digitalis use, and heart rate. Neither the SUM GTT nor any of the four baseline blood glucose values had any significant predictive value. The analyses suggest that mild glucose intolerance is associated with the same mortality as more severe hyperglycemia.

502

Polyploidy in Islets of Normal and Diabetic Humans. F.J. SWARTZ*, M.N. POHL, and P.H.B. CARSTENS, Louisville, Ky.

This pilot study was initiated to determine if the increased polyploidization of pancreatic B-cells in diabetic mice, previously reported from this laboratory, is also characteristic of human diabetes.

Nuclei of H & E stained islet cells were traced by camera lucida and their volumes determined by semiautomatic particle size analysis. Previous studies have confirmed that, in mouse and human islets, nuclear volume is a reliable index of polyploidy. Five insulin independent, and three insulin dependent human diabetics, and their age and sex matched controls, were studied.

The major findings were: (1) Percentages of polyploid nuclei in insulin independent diabetic islets were elevated significantly over controls in four out of five cases. The one exception was an 85 year old male who was diagnosed as a diabetic only two months prior to death. (2) Of the three insulin dependent diabetics, one, whose islets appeared otherwise normal, had a significantly greater percentage of polyploid nuclei than the controls; the other two, whose islets were markedly hyalinized, exhibited percentages of polyploid nuclei within normal ranges. Percent polyploidy in the entire group of diabetics was significantly elevated over the controls.

The implications of increased percentages of polyploid nuclei in diabetic islets, and the interpretation of these results relative to previous studies on genetically diabetic mice, will be discussed. (Supported by Grant PHS-AM 21120)

503

Differential Development of the Exocrine and Endocrine Pancreas of the Mouse Neonate. B.A. DORE, W.M. GROGAN, G.E. MADGE, and S.R. WEBB,* Richmond, Va.

Neonate mice provide the optimum source for islet isolation using the collagenase digestion technique. We examined newborn, 5, 10, 15, 20, 30, and 120 day old SWR/J mice to define pancreas development and determine why there exists a critical period beyond which acceptable quantities of islets are difficult to isolate.

We examined pancreas weight, DNA, amylase, insulin and then cells by histology and DNA flow cytometry. From birth to day 5 body weight increased more rapidly than pancreas weight, but after day 10 the pattern was reversed. Exocrine and endocrine pancreas development proceeds continuously but at different rates, resulting in a biphasic pattern. The first phase was dominated by proliferation and growth of endocrine cells from birth to day 10. Phase 2 was dominated by exocrine development and was not pronounced until after day 15. DNA content of diploid cells was 7.9 pg/cell. Increase in cell number, determined by DNA analysis and flow cytometry, correlated well with the biphasic pattern. Histology confirmed these observations. Most islets obtained adult form by 15 days and massive exocrine proliferation occured at 20 days. The optimum age for islet isolation was that period after primary endocrine development and differentiation into their adult form and before the second, or exocrine, phase of development -- that would be days 10 to 15 of neonatal development. (Supported by NIH grant AM21730.)

504

Cell Cycle Analysis of the Mouse Pancreas during Neonatal Development. S.R. WEBB,* B.A. DORE, and W.M. GROGAN, Richmond, Va.

A variety of approaches have been used to examine changes in prancreas cells during development. Most have relied heavily on some form of light microscopic technique. We examined pancreas development of the mouse by DNA flow cytometric analysis. This permitted more precise statistical characterization of cell number and the proportion of cells in each phase of the cell cycle, as well as polyploidy.

Pancreases from newborn, 5, 10, 15, 20, 30, and 120 day old SWR/J mice were disrupted and the nuclei stained with propidium iodine. Nuclei were subjected to flow microflurometric DNA analysis using a Coulter TPS-1 cell analyzer. Total pancreatic DNA was also determined by diphenylamine analysis. Through day 15 of neonatal development most pancreas cells were in G_0-G_1 phase (diploid) with only 4.5-7.5% in S phase (DNA synthesis) and 2.0-4.2% in G_2-M phase (tertaploid, before cell division). Begining at day 20 the proportion of G_0-G_1 cells decreased through day 120 to 60% as both S and G_2-M phase cells increased. Polyploidy was not detected until day 20 when 3.3% were polyploid. The number increased to 3.8% by day 30 and 9.5% by day 120. Octaploidy was never seen. The newborn pancreas has 4.1×10^6 cells, the number increased to 74×10^6 by day 120. Two periods of rapid increase in cell number occured, the first between birth and day 5, the second between days 15 and 20. These correlate well with primary endocrine and exocrine cell proliferation respectively. (Supported by NIH grant AM 21730.)

505

Corticosterone Enhances the Survival and/or Growth of the Delta Cells in Cultured Fetal Rat Islets. ROBERT C. MCEVOY,* New York, NY.

Fetal rat islets were cultured using the method of Hellerstrom, et al. (Diabetes 28:769, 1979). After one day in culture, half of the plates were continued in control medium and half were grown in medium with corticosterone (CS), 0.1 ug/ml. Media were changed daily and culture was continued for a total of 8 days. The hormone contents of the media were determined daily. The hormone contents of the tissue were also determined at the time of plating and after 1 and 8 days in vitro. Islets were fixed on Day 8 and the cells containing each of the hormones were identified by immunocytochemistry. Based on hormone content, about 14% of the A and B cells were plated and about 7% remained attached on Day 1. Only 8% of the D cells survived dissociation and 4% were attached on Day 1. CS supplementation resulted in 3-fold greater SRIF content in the medium. The insulin and glucagon contents of the CS media were slightly reduced. On Day 8, there was no difference in the insulin content of the cultured tissue regardless of media. The glucagon and SRIF contents of the tissue grown on CS medium were greater (1.8 and 3.1-fold, respectively) than tissue grown on control medium. D cells were rare in the control islets (0.4%), but were more numerous in islets grown on CS medium (2.2%). Preliminary study of the secretion of these cultured islets suggests that the islets grown on CS medium have a reduced insulin secretory response to 22 mM glucose. Supported by NIH grants HD-00285 and AM-25257 and a grant from the JDF.

506

Experience with a Diabetic Registry. J. ACHTENBERG, A. DREXLER*, St. Louis, Mo.

The Diabetic Registry of the Washington University DRTC was established in 1975 to 1) provide a controlled, documented database from which to select patients for detailed study, 2) provide data for prospective longitudinal study of the natural history of DM, 3) improve patient care.

Patients are hospitalized 3-5 days annually (adults) or biannually (children) for complete medical exam and routine lab plus HLA typing, fluorescein angiography and fluorophotometry, studies of skeletal development and density, muscle capillary basement membrane thickness, and glycosylated hemoglobins. A flexible computer program permits inclusion of data reflecting evolving research trends to the pre-existing core of the database.

1000 admissions of 500 patients are on file, 1/3 of whom have been followed for 3 or more years. Mean age-at-onset is 20, 70% onset before age 30. Mean disease duration is 9 years, 5% duration 25 years or more. 92% are insulin treated. Complications: Retinopathy, 40%; Neuropathy, 52%; Cataracts, 13%; Nephropathy, 39%; Coronary Artery Disease, 5%; Peripheral Vascular Disease, 9%; Hyperlipoproteinemia, 34%.

Accumulation and maturation of the database has generated increasing interest in Diabetes research across many disciplines. Users represent at least 9 medical school departments, behavioral scientists, and those outside the University. In 1979 alone, at least 30 articles abstracts or book chapters have been published using data from the Registry.

507

Pathology of Alloxan Diabetic Dog Endocrine Stomach and Pancreas. W. ALLEN SHANNON, JR. and RICHARD E. DOBBS,* Dallas, TX.

Pathological changes in alloxan diabetes are important in understanding pathophysiology of models and the relations to human diabetes.

Alloxan diabetic dogs were sacrificed at 4 mo. to 7 yrs. Splenic pancreas and oxyntic mucosa were processed for electron microscopy and indirect immunofluorescence for glucagon (A-cells) or somatostatin (D-cells).

In the stomach, increased numbers of A-cells and D-cells/mm^2 were observed, up to 45% and 61%, respectively. EM indicated increased A-like and ECL cells in addition. Hypersecretion was notable in D-cells. In the islets, in addition to complete or partial destruction of B-cells, numerous A, D and ECL cells were present. Many A-cells exhibited secretion often appearing to be of a holocrine type. Numerous cytolysosomes were also present possibly in response to increased cell activity. Islet capillary endothelium lacked fenestrae except adjacent to typical B-cells (base line insulin). The endothelium and basal lamina also tended to be thicker. Some remaining B-cells, especially in the 7 yr. dog, expressed hypersecretion.

Increased extrapancreatic endocrine cells indicate a functional relationship to the chronic loss of B-cells and possible dysfunction of islet A and D-cells. Islet A-cell phenomena may result from secretory response to lack of normal vascular permeability. The pathophysiology may be associated at least in part with these phenomena, especially the absence of capillary endothelium fenestrae, a basic structural defect. Support: VA and ADA, N. Tx. Affl.

508

Plasma Osmolality in Normal and Diabetic Dogs Following Glucose Infusion. Elsa Janle-Swain*, Steven R. Ash, James M. Carter, H.D. Jackson, and Ronald Barile, W. Lafayette, IN 47907.

Equations such as $\pi = 0.0556$ Glucose + 0.357 BUN + 1.75 Na + 10.1 (Edelman, J.S., et al. J. Clin. Invest. 37 1236, 1958) have been developed to relate osmolality to major plasma constituents in heterogeneous groups of fasting patients. We tested the ability of this equation to predict prospective variations in osmolality in normal and diabetic dogs during a baseline period and after IV infusions of 1 gm/kg of glucose.

If glucose changes could be reliably predicted from osmolality changes, an osmolality sensor might be used instead of a glucose sensor in an artificial pancreas.

After glucose infusion, plasma osmolality rose significantly in diabetics ($p < 0.05$) but not in normals. In normal dogs the correlation between glucose and osmolality was low ($r = 0.29$) because there is a wide range of osmolalities in the normal glucose range. In diabetic dogs, the correlation was higher ($r = 0.59$).

Variations in other plasma solutes would also cause variations in plasma osmolality. Therefore Na, K, BUN and protein were also measured. In diabetics, Na was lower than in normals and BUN was higher, but none of these solutes showed any significant changes after glucose infusion in either normal or diabetic dogs.

An osmole gap between measured and calculated osmolalities was found in both normal and diabetic dogs, but the osmole gap in diabetic dogs (20 mOs/kg) was significantly greater than in normal dogs ($p < 0.05$).

509

Virus Induced Abnormalities in Insulin Release in Perifused Hamster Islets. E.J. RAYFIELD,* Y. SETO, S.B. WALSH, New York, NY.

We previously demonstrated a sustained diminution in glucose (G) stimulated insulin release (IR) and abnormal glucose tolerance of shorter duration in golden hamsters following inoculation with the TC-83 vaccine strain of Venezuelan Encephalitis Virus (VEV). To understand better the mechanisms of this defect in IR, we studied IR in response to several test agents in isolated perifused islets from control and 24 day post VEV infected hamsters. IR data were expressed as μU insulin/minute/50 islets normalized/μg DNA and total IR for each test agent during a 30 minute perifusion period from control (C) and VEV infected (INF) islets. Following perifusion of basal G (3mM), high G (20mM) resulted in a 45% decrease of IR in INF islets compared to C islets ($p < 0.001$) similar to in vivo findings. 15mM arginine in combination with 17mM glucose resulted in a 32% decrease in IR in INF islets ($p < 0.02$). IR following 1mM tolbutamide (T) stimulation was similar in C and INF islets and T + 20mM G completely corrected the diminished IR present with 20mM G alone. 10mM theophylline + 20mM glucose also corrected the decrease in IR noted with 20mM G alone. Further, 1mM dibutyryl cAMP in combination with 20mM G resulted in similar IR in C and INF islets (76 vs 74 μU insulin/30 min/50 islets/μg DNA respectively). These data suggest that VEV induces a defect in glucose as well as arginine stimulated IR from hamster beta cells. However, IR responses to dibutyryl cAMP and phosphodiesterase inhibitors in the high glucose experiments are consistent with normal beta cell function distal to the cAMP system.

510

Effect of Alloxan on Non-Islet B-Cells in the Guinea Pig Pancreas. DENIS G. BASKIN, KENNETH C. GORRAY, Seattle, WA (Introduced by MICHAEL A. PFEIFER*, Seattle, WA).

Guinea pigs recover from the diabetogenic effects of alloxan but the mechanism of resistance is not known. We therefore evaluated morphological changes in the B-cell population of the guinea pig pancreas by light microscopic immunocytochemistry following alloxan treatment. Guinea pigs were injected (i.v.) with 200 mg/kg alloxan in citrate buffer; controls received only buffer. At 24 hr intervals up to 120 hrs after alloxan injection, the pancreas was collected from 3 alloxan and 3 control guinea pigs and fixed in Bouin's. Sections from three pieces of pancreas per animal were analyzed by morphometric techniques after immunoperoxidase staining for insulin. The results showed that by 72 hrs the alloxan treated guinea pigs had significantly more small, non-islet cell clusters (1-4 cells) which stained for insulin in comparison to controls ($162 \pm 8.1\%$, $p < .01$). This suggests that the number of non-islet B-cells increased in response to alloxan treatment. Further, compared to controls the volume of B-cell cytoplasm relative to pancreatic volume was also elevated at 72 hrs after alloxan treatment ($p < .05$), and the ranked staining intensity of B-cells was significantly higher ($p < .025$) at 96 hr. These results indicate that insulin-producing cells hypertrophy after alloxan treatment. We conclude that recovery from alloxan could in part be due to the temporary production of insulin by non-islet B-cells. This hypothesis suggests that compensatory production of insulin by non-islet cells could reduce the effects of some pancreatic insults which may lead to diabetes.

511

Testicular Pathology in the Spontaneously Diabetic BB Wistar Rat. J.R. WRIGHT, A.J.YATES, H.M. SHARMA, P. THIBERT, C. SHIM, D.A. SENHAUSER. Columbus, OH (Introduced by M. TZAGOURNIS*, Columbus, OH).

Testicular histology, mass, and testicular/body mass ratios were studied in 63BB Wistar(BBW) diabetic(d), 12BBW nondiabetic(nd), and 17 stanard Wistar(W) rats. Moderate or severe testicular atrophy was observed histologically in 32% of BBWd, 25% of BBWnd, and 0% of W rats. Atrophy in BBWd was bilateral in 17 of 20 cases and was characterized by partial or total loss of the germinal epithelium in the seminiferous tubules and an apparent preponderance of Sertoli cells. Several atrophic testes had tubules with multinucleate giant cells in the lumens. Leydig cells appeared normal. Many normal testes in BBW were hypocellular or aspermatic. One BBWd had subacute orchitis; another had a granuloma.

Mean testicular masses were: BBWd with atrophy ($\bar{c}$).62gm., BBWd without atrophy($\bar{s}$)1.34gm., BBWnd $\bar{c}$ .64gm., BBWnd$\bar{s}$ .95gm., and W$\bar{s}$ 1.57gm. Mean testicular mass/body mass ratios for BBWd$\bar{c}$, BBWd$\bar{s}$, and W$\bar{s}$ were 0.00196, 0.00453, and 0.00493 respectively. Analysis of variance for the latter values revealed that BBWd$\bar{c}$ differ significantly ($p<.001$) from either BBWd$\bar{s}$ or W$\bar{s}$. No difference was apparent between BBWd$\bar{s}$ and W$\bar{s}$. Age differences were corrected by analysis of covariance. Following age adjustment, testicular masses for the 2 groups still differed significantly ($p<.01$). Atrophy may be responsible for the lower breeding success observed in BBW rats. (Supported by Dept. of Pathology, College of Medicine, and Graduate School, Ohio State University; the Upjohn Company)

512

The degu: A New Model of Spontaneous Diabetes. GERALD S. SPEAR* and DAVID K. BORAKER, Irvine, Ca. and Burlington, Vt.

The degu, a S. American Hystricomorph, is a new model of diabetes reported by others without further detail to have cataracts and islet amyloid, and to have crystalline cytoplasmic bodies in α cells increasing as diabetes progressed, virus-like particles 20 nm diameter in cytoplasm and ER of exocrine cells and to manifest apparent horizontal transmission of diabetes to guinea pigs.

The present studies demonstrate that the diabetes is a non-obese model sometimes characterized by hyperlipidemia and ketoacidosis, in the latter setting the islets sometimes exhibiting cytolysis in the absence of inflammation. Typical herpes viruses are present in the nucleus and cytoplasm of presumed pancreatic acinar cells, in both normal and diabetic animals. Such viral infested cells are uncommon and generally unaccompanied by inflammation. Similar cells more commonly are present and are more numerous in salivary glands of both normal and diabetic animals. The salivary gland always is infested when the pancreas is infested. Virus is not evident in other organs. Islet amyloid is uncommon, is seen both in normal and diabetic animals, and both in the presence and absence of virus. The cytoplasmic crystalline inclusions are not more evident in diabetic animals than in controls.

513

Glucose Intolerance in Athymic Nude Mice: A New Animal Model for Spontaneous Diabetes Mellitus. ADINA ZEIDLER*, CLARA TOSCO, DINESH KUMAR*, SURAJA RASHEED, and JOHN PARKER, Los Angeles, Ca.

Athymic nude mice BALB/C (nu/nu) have been described as having abnormal gonadal and adrenal changes. In an attempt to evaluate the endocrine pancreas which has not been previously investigated in nude mice, we studied fasting plasma glucose (FPG) in 1, 8 and 12 week old nude mice and controls BALB/C (C). Nude mice at 1 week (n=12) had normal FPG which was similar to C (96±11 vs 91±7 mg/dl). Eight and 12 week old nude mice had a higher FPG (187±5 and 204±2 mg/dl) as compared to C (140±7 and 161±7 mg/dl). Fasting IRI levels were lower in 8 week old nude mice compared to C (3.7±1.1 vs 22.7±2.7 uU/ml, p<.05). Glucose tolerance test using 2 mg/gm of BW 20% dextrose I.P. in 8 week nude mice was different in 6 of 8 animals studied:

Time (min)	Plasma Glucose (mg/dl) C (n=6)	nude (n=6)
0	139±7	187±5
30	194±6	337±7*
60	191±6	310±9*
120	130±5	313±9*
180	139±5	283±7*

*p<.05

Blood and organ cultures were negative for bacterial and C-viral growth.

Conclusions: 1) Athymic nude mice present spontaneous hyperglycemia, abnormal glucose tolerance and decreased IRI. 2) Those abnormalities may indicate overt diabetes and may possibly relate to the immune deficient state of this animal model.

514

Influence of Age and Sex on Susceptibility to Streptozotocin Diabetes. JOHN P. MORDES and ALDO A. ROSSINI*. Worcester, MA.

A single injection of streptozotocin (SZ) at a dose of 50 mg/kg body weight classically produces diabetes in adult rats. We investigated the effect of age and sex on this phenomenon. Either citrate buffer or SZ in doses of 40,60,80 or 100 mg/kg was injected intraperitoneally into male and female albino rats 1, 2, 3, 4, 5, 10 and 26 weeks of age. At least 5 animals of each sex were injected at all ages and dosage levels. Seventy-two hours after injection animals were sacrificed. Serum glucose was measured and the pancreata were fixed in Bouin's solution. Diabetes was defined as a blood sugar > 3 standard deviations above the mean for buffer injected controls. From one to four weeks of age only SZ 100 mg/kg regularly produced diabetes. Animals of both sexes were resistant to smaller doses of SZ. By 5 weeks of age SZ 80 mg/kg produced diabetes in 86% of males but only 27% females. At 10 and 26 weeks of age essentially all animals became diabetic at a dose of 40 mg/kg. Histologic study of the pancreata of animals given SZ 80 mg/kg showed some degree of islet destruction at all ages, but increased destruction with increasing age. Greatest numbers of surviving beta cells were seen in preweaning animals. These data suggest that susceptibility to the diabetogenic effect of SZ is age dependent. Preadolescent animals are most resistant to SZ. Females may also be more resistant than males at 5 weeks of age. The basis of these effects is unknown, but may be sex-hormone dependent.

515

Purification and Properties of 5'-Nucleotidase from Normal and Streptozotocin Diabetic Rat Liver Plasma Membranes. V. CHANDRAMOULI and JAMES R. CARTER, JR.*, Cleveland, Ohio.

5'-Nucleotidase was purified from isolated liver plasma membranes by solubilization in Lubrol Px followed by affinity chromatographic separation on con A-polyacrylic hydrazide agarose and 5'-AMP sepharose 4B. Specific activity of the enzyme from the normal was 3500 μmol Pi/h/mg and for the diabetic 3200 μmol Pi/h/mg. Physical properties of membrane bound and purified enzymes showed interesting differences. Km's of purified enzymes from normal and diabetic livers were 39 μM and 36 μM while membrane bound enzyme had Km's of 43 μM and 40 μM respectively. Purified enzyme also hydrolysed 5'-UMP, 5'-GMP, 5'-TMP and 5'-CMP. Maximum activities were 82, 38, 22 and 70% of that for 5'-AMP for the normal and 100, 49, 30 and 87% for the diabetic. Membrane enzyme from normals hydrolysed 5'-UMP, 5'-TMP and 5'-CMP 116, 50 and 93% of that of 5'-AMP and 95, 39 and 78% from diabetic. Low concentrations of con A and higher concentrations of RCAI, WGA and LCA inhibited the purified enzymes. Purified normal enzyme activity was inhibited more than the diabetic enzyme by lectins, but this was not so for the membrane bound enzymes. Both purified and membrane diabetic enzyme were more resistant to heat denaturation than normal. Arrhenius plot of temperature effects showed no differences. Activation energies were 10565 cal/mole and 11157 cal/mole. These changes in purified enzyme properties as compared with membrane bound enzyme suggest differences in structural composition. (Supported by NIH and a grant from Cleveland Diabetes Association.)

516

Long Term Effect of Streptozotocin in Inbred Lewis Rats. J.TAI, W.J. TZE, S.KROEGER and J.E.DIMMICK, Vancouver, British Columbia. (Introduced by A.R.CAIRNS* Vancouver, British Columbia)

Long term effect of streptozotocin (SZ) has been examined in 43 inbred male Lewis rats. SZ at 50mg/kg body weight (BW) was administered intravenously and the animal was weighed and examined at 10 to 14 day intervals. Determination of fasting blood glucose and insulin; daily urine output; urine for glucose,ketone and protein; and IV glucose tolerance test were performed. Four trends in weight changes were observed. (i) continued weight loss; (ii) relatively constant weight; (iii)&(iv) spontaneous increase in weight after a period of weight loss before and after 12 months respectively. Groups (i)&(ii) were characterized by continued hyperglycemia of over 400 mg/dl and marked polyuria of 116±13ml/24hr. Groups (iii)&(iv) demonstrated initial high blood glucose with dramatic reduction to normal or hypoglycemic levels concomitant with significant increases in BW and changes in mean insulin level from 15μU/ml to 27 μU/ml. Normal glucose disappearance rates (K = 3.4±0.7) was also observed. Kidney tumor and liver cysts were found in 64% of the animals while pancreatic tumour was present in 5%. Segmental glomerulosclerosis was more frequent in (i)&(ii). The tumor tissue resembled benign renal adenoma. Pancreatic sections showed an increase in number of islets in (iii)&(iv). Cataract increased in a linear fashion from 19% to 83% over 10 months. The finding of spontaneous reversal of diabetic state in one third of SZ treated rats after 6-18 months following diabetic induction queries the suitability of using this diabetic animal model for long-term studies.

Sequential events in the development of diabetes mellitus associated with islet amyloid.

CHARLES F. HOWARD JR.*, Beaverton, Oregon

Diabetes mellitus spontaneously develops in *Macaca nigra* owing to a lesion in the islets of Langerhans. The sequence of which appears first --cellular aberrations or deposition of islet amyloid--has now been established.

Four groups of monkeys were identified: nondiabetic (ND), incipient diabetic (ID), borderline diabetic (BD), and diabetic (D). Significant

	Amyloid (%)	IRG (pg/ml)	$\Delta I/\Delta G$	K (%)	Glucose (mg/dl)	Insulin (μU/ml)
ND	0-trace	663	1.5	2.7	64	33
ID	0-trace	1622	0.6	2.6	71	29
BD	5-50	2807	0.3	1.7	92	20
D	25-80	364	0.2	0.9	132	19

changes first occurred in ID monkeys: increased immunoreactive glucagon (IRG) and decreased insulin response per glucose change ($\Delta I/\Delta G$) by 15 min in IV-GTT. K values (% glucose clearance/min in IV-GTT), glucose and insulin altered significantly only in the later stages of diabetes.

Pancreatic sections (biopsy and autopsy) were examined by light and electron microscopy. More than 85% of the ND and 70% of the ID monkeys had no visible amyloid and the rest had only a trace; BD and D monkeys had significantly greater concentrations.

Conclusions: islet secretory cell metabolic aberrations occur before amyloid appears; hormonal and pathologic changes allow recognition of developing diabetes in monkeys long before clinical detection. Diabetes in *Macaca nigra* appears similar to that in many aging human beings.

Index

Authors of all abstracts printed in this Supplement are listed alphabetically, along with the number(s) of the abstract(s). Membership in the American Diabetes Association is indicated by an asterisk.

A

Abarca Jorge, 225
Abdou Nabih I., 208
Abinader Edward G., 300
Abou-Mourad N.N.,* 201
Abraira C.,* 40
Achtenberg J., 177, 506
Adams L. D., 146
Ahuja M. M. S., 4
Aiello Lloyd M., 3
Alberti K. G. M. M.,* 189, 222
Albisser A. M.,* 351, 490
Albrecht G., 161
Albrink Margaret J.,* 449
Aleck Kirck A., 66
Alexander M., 366
Aleyassine H.,* 334
Allen P., 487
Allen Richard, 391
Alling Katharine, 38, 241
Alogna Maria,* 337
Altomare E., 277
Amatruda J. M., 150
Ament M. E., 82
Amherdt Mylene, 99
Ammon Hermann P. T.,* 388
Andaloro B., 309
Andersen D. K., 59
Anderson B. J., 26
Anderson J. H., Jr.,* 380
Anderson N. G., 146
Anderson Robert M., 337
Andersson A., 494
Andreadis C., 415
Andrews Karen, 311
Ansell Justin, 420
Anson J. R., 474
Aoki Thomas T.,* 202, 464
Appel Michael C.,* 204, 314
Archer Juanita A., 392
Arieff A. I.,* 480
Armstrong W. McD., 424
Arner P., 358
Arquilla E. R.,* 142, 206
Arrieta Jose F., 66
Ash Steven R., 508
Asplin C. M., 213, 320
Assa S., 319
Assan R., 74
Assimacopoulos-Jeannet F., 220
Atkinson R. L.,* 447
Atles L. R., 105
Aung Maung H., 242
Auslander W. F., 26, 113
Avruch J.,* 366, 374
Axelrod L.,* 216

B

Baba Shigeaki,* 192, 497
Bach Fritz, 322
Bahoric A., 351
Bajorunas Daiva,* 268
Bak Marianna, 352
Baker Lester,* 321, 325
Balasse E. O.,* 437
Ball Judith, 38
Bandisode M. S.,* 116
Banks Melanie, 326
Barbosa Jose,* 254, 322
Barile Ronald, 508
Barish John, 425
Barker Clyde F.,* 207, 408
Barnes Barry, 330
Barnett C.,* 309, 332
Barnett Carol,* 139
Barnett R., 343
Barofsky Ivan, 23
Bar-On H., 159
Barr P., 346
Barrett Eugene,* 285, 466
Barzilai David, 42, 300
Baskin Denis G., 510
Bässler Karl H., 238
Baumann F. G., 293, 294
Baumgartner D., 75
Beachy Joanna, 13
Beard J.,* 427
Beck J. S., 382
Becker D.,* 275, 463
Beggi Paola, 244
Bejar R., 211
Bell Deanne F., 21
Bell Durward L., 21
Bell Martin, 72
Bell R. H., 68, 488
Bellomo S., 327
Belmonte M. M.,* 500
Bendezu Rafael, 250
Bendick P., 231
Bennett P., 265
Bennett Peter H.,* 227, 253
Ben Sira I., 317
Benz M., 39
Berchtold Peter,* 108, 280
Berelowitz M.,* 218
Bergenstal R., 284
Berger Michael,* 356
Berger M.,* 280
Bergman M.,* 69, 491
Bergman Richard N.,* 78
Bernstein E., 309
Bernstein Joel E., 302
Bessman Alice N.,* 239, 493
Bessman Samuel P., 375, 493
Bevilacqua Maurizio, 244
Bevilacqua Stefano, 285
Be Vilacque M., 240
Beyer Jürgen, 238
Bhathena Sam J.,* 187, 430
Bibergeil H., 161
Bielefeld David R., 299
Bierman E. L.,* 377, 479
Billhymer B., 236
Binder Christian,* 90, 158
Bjorkman Ola, 164
Blackmore Peter F., 57
Blanc M. H.,* 87, 269
Blanchard W., 422
Blecka Lawrence J., 278
Blix P., 284
Bliziotes M. M.,* 135, 474
Bloom S. R.,* 76, 115
Blumenthal Stanley A.,* 445
Blundell T. L., 349
Boatright Shelly,* 110
Boden G.,* 408
Boehm T. M.,* 80
Bohannon N. V., 271
Boldt Kenneth A., 35
Bolli Geremia,* 438, 439
Bonazinga P., 327
Bongiovanni R., 80

Bonner Robert,* 254
Bonner-Weir S.,* 123
Bonnevie-Nielsen Vagn, 411
Boraker David K., 512
Borrebach Donald R., 389
Boshell Buris R.,* 170, 299
Bota R. A., 307
Bottazzo G. F., 494
Böttger I.,* 55
Boutaugh Michele Louise, 345
Boyd A. E. III,* 98, 182
Braaten J. T.,* 415
Bradley Carole J., 392
Bransome Edwin D., Jr.,* 287
Bratusch-Marrain Paul, 350
Braunstein S. N.,* 298
Brautbar C., 319
Breidenbach Th., 363
Brent E. L., 447
Brewster Arlene R., 25
Brick B., 191
Bright George Matthew, 483
Brinkley B. R., 98
Brock Bruce M., 260
Brocks D., 376
Brodows Robert G.,* 34
Brodsky J., 320
Brodsky Joel, 310
Broe P., 409
Brouhard B. H., 318
Brown David M.,* 217, 292
Brown John C., 419
Brown Josiah,* 128
Brown M. J., 298
Brownschiedle Carol M., 66, 301
Bruhn Charles J., 180
Brunetti Paolo, 438, 439
Bruns D. E., 373
Bryan J., 98
Bryant M. G., 115
Buldain Roger, 109
Bunnag Srichitra C., 161
Bünting Christina E., 303
Burghen George A.,* 184
Burke Elizabeth, 342
Burleson Paul D., 60, 469
Burns A., 179
Burns Thomas W.,* 273, 462
Burr Ian M.,* 129
Burrin J. M., 222
Burstein P.,* 63
Buschard Karsten, 209
Buse Maria G.,* 390
Bush Michael A.,* 365,
Bush Michael J., 425
Buzard Kurt A., 489
Byrne W. J., 82

C

Cahill George F., Jr.,* 85
Cairns A. R.,* 492, 516
Cameron J., 409
Cameron Margaret R., 129
Campbell R. G.,* 196
Campfield L. Arthur,* 417
Canteloube D., 265
Caro J. F., 150
Carpentier Jean-Louis, 194
Carson Phyllis, 392
Carstens P. H. B., 502
Cartechini Maria Giulia, 438, 439
Carter James M., 508
Carter James R., Jr.,* 515
Carter Laurenda, 392
Carter-Su Christin, 15
Casanello-Ertl D., 203
Cataland S., 92, 283
Cerra F. B., 364
Cha Chung-Ja, 472
Chait Alan,* 43, 354, 377
Champion Malcolm C., 29
Chance Ronald E.,* 412
Chandiok Suvesh, 128
Chandler Cynthia,* 110
Chandramouli V., 515
Chang A. Y.,* 289, 386
Chang K., 46
Chantelau Ernst, 356
Charles A., 230
Charles Rene N., 316
Chavent Georgia, 268
Chen Y-D. I., 159
Cherrington A.,* 65, 215
Cherry Marianna, 144
Chertack M. M.,* 107, 502
Chertow B. S.,* 122
Chesa Pilar Garin, 115
Chiasson J.-L.,* 64
Chick W. L.,* 410
Chiemmongkoltip Pipit, 88
Childs B. P.,* 258, 343
Chirgwin John, 93
Chlebowski R. T., 286
Chmura G., 81
Christenson I., 443
Christophe J., 440
Ciaraldi T. P., 154
Ciotola Thomas J., 183
Citrin Wendy, 168
Clark Charles M., Jr.,* 152, 188
Clark Julia B.,* 188
Clarke W.,* 498
Clarke William L.,* 483
Clements R. S., Jr.,* 104, 416
Clore E. T., 123
Cobelli Claudio, 78
Coen Clara, 167
Cohen I., 319
Cohen T., 319
Coll K., 56
Colle E., 500
Collins Peggy,* 171, 331
Colwell John A.,* 323, 324
Compagnucci Pietro, 438, 439
Comstock John P.,* 308
Cook Daniel L., 310
Cooney M., 320
Corallo Sandro, 244
Corash Laurence M., 384
Cordes Uwe, 238
Corkey B. E.,* 56
Cortes P., 367
Cousins L., 235, 378
Coustan Donald,* 274
Couzigou P., 265
Cowett Richard M., 472
Cox Mary S., 111
Coyle J. J., 474
Craighead J. E., 327, 454
Crano William D., 109
Crockford Peter M., 382
Crossley J., 320
Crowley M., 264
Crumrine P., 275
Cukerman E., 45
Cunningham R. J.,* 318
Cuppers H. J., 280
Curnow R. T.,* 32
Cushman S. W.,* 14
Czech Michael P.,* 12, 186
Czernik Andrew J., 420
Czyzyk Artur,* 352

D

Da Costa Jose, 84, 273
Dafoe Don, 207
D'Andrea B. J., 454
Daneman D.,* 1, 463
Danforth E.,* 327
Darby A., 295, 296
Daughaday W. H.,* 19, 147
Da Valle M. J., 293
Davenport R., 361
Davidson Mayer B.,* 153
Davidson P. C., 140
Davie Joseph M., 30, 31
Davis D., 6
Davis F. B., 364
Davis J. E., 177
Davis J. G., 486
Davis P. J.,* 364
Deeb L. C.,* 174, 335
DeFronzo Ralph A.,* 431
De Haën Christoph, 354
Deile D., 241
DeLuise Mario, 199
De Meyts P.,* 193
Deschryver K., 72
Devaskar U., 397
De Vos C. J., 379
Dhorajiwala J., 219
Diamond M. P., 215
Diani A.,* 6

DiCintio Deborah M., 485
Dietz William H., 468
Dietze G., 55
DiGirolamo Mario,* 48, 394
Dillmann Wolfgang H.,* 89
Dillon Richard S.,* 44
Dimitriadis G., 163
Dimmick J. E., 516
Dippé Stephen E.,* 330
Dirgo John A., 451
Dobbs Richard E.,* 36, 507
Doberne L., 360
Dobersen M., 212
Dobrea George M., 250
Doi Kunihiro,* 248, 249
Dolkas C., 446
Donald P. E.,* 373, 448
Dons Robert F., 384
Dore B. A., 503, 504
Downing S. E., 499
Drash Allan L.,* 1, 326
Drew Helen Mikesell, 398, 399
Drexler A.,* 506
Drury Thomas F., 169, 173
Duckworth W. C.,* 151, 198
Duducgian-Vartavarian L., 203
Dulin W. E.,* 146
Dumler F., 367
Dupre John,* 29
Dwyer J., 210
Dye E. S., 119

E

Eaton John, 254
Eaton R. Phillip,* 71, 391, 486
Ebersole J., 69
Edidin Deborah V.,* 88, 167
Edlin-Folz E., 7
Edwards L., 364
Ehrlich R. M.,* 490
Ehrlich Robert,* 340
Eickenbusch Wulf, 108
Eisenstein Albert B.,* 79, 400
Eknoyan G., 182
Elde R. P., 433
Elfont E. A., 307
Elias Alan N.,* 362, 455
Ellis George J.,* 168
Engfeldt P., 358
England Jack D., Jr., 84, 273
Engstrom D., 496
Eno Jan, 136
Ensinck John W.,* 35, 426
Ericson Sandra, 314
Esposito V., 481, 482
Exton John H.,* 57, 64

F

Faber Ole K., 158, 431
Fairchild Richard S., 208
Fajans S. S.,* 114
Farese R. V.,* 120
Fariss B., 234
Fasoli Angelo, 244
Fawcett D. M., 81
Feigin Mark, 304, 305
Feldman J. M.,* 121
Feldmeier M., 72
Felig Philip,* 69, 164
Fernandez-Cruz L., 68, 488
Ferrannini Eleuterio, 285, 431
Ferriss B., 264
Fery F., 437
Figlewicz D., 94
Filler R. M., 490
Fineberg N. S., 181
Fineberg S. E.,* 160, 181
Fischer Angela, 171, 331
Fisher F.,* 86
Fix J., 6
Fleischer Norman,* 205
Flier Jeffrey S.,* 199
Flock Eunice V.,* 253
Flugelman Moshe Y., 300
Foley James E., 48
Foley Rosemary, 48
Formby B., 94
Forsham P. H.,* 179, 271
Fortner Joseph G., 268
Fortney Suzanne M., 103
Frank Bruce H., 412
Frank Harrison J. L., 153, 190
Frank Marcia,* 340
Frank Robert N., 395
Frank S., 247
Frankel B. J.,* 429
Franks Douglas J., 225
Franz Marion J.,* 336
Freedman Z., 494
Freidenberg Gary, 92, 270
Freinkel Norbert,* 118
Fried S. K., 460
Friedman Gerald J.,* 290
Friedman Nancy E., 88
Friedman N. M.,* 71, 486
Friesen J.,* 344
Frohman L. A.,* 218
Fujimoto Wilfred,* 281, 402
Fukushima N., 476
Fuller J. H., 4
Fuller Thomas J., 458

G

Gabbay Kenneth,* 37, 143
Gaitanis K., 261
Galagan Robert, 391
Galbraith Richard A., 390
Gallagher A., 40
Galloway John A.,* 181
Ganda O. P.,* 37, 269
Ganguli S., 396, 397
Gapp David A., 436
Gardiner R. J.,* 334
Garimberti B., 240
Gasic Slobodan, 350
Gastineau C. F.,* 163
Gaume J., 493
Gavin J., III, 147
Gazdar Adi F., 187, 430
Genel Myron,* 210, 274
Genthner Robert, 337
Gerbitz K., 495
Gerich J.,* 74, 422
Gerrard Jonathan M., 217
Gerritsen G.,* 6
Gettinger J.,* 113
Giddings Steve, 93
Gilbert S. S., 22
Giletti Bruno, 472
Gilfer A., 304
Gingerich R. L.,* 119, 130
Ginsberg Henry,* 61
Ginsberg Mark, 243
Ginsberg-Fellner F.,* 84
Girardier L., 220
Given Barbara, 109
Given Charles W., 109
Gjinovci A., 151
Glass A. R., 80
Gleason R. E.,* 87, 269
Gliemann Jørgen, 48
Goetz Frederick C.,* 255, 501
Gold Gerald, 413
Goldberg R. B.,* 229, 465
Golden M.,* 27, 230
Goldman J.,* 195, 367
Goldstein David E.,* 84, 166
Gollmar C. W., 335
Golub L., 7
Gongrypp H., 264
Goodner Charles J.,* 131
Goodwin Jack, 140
Gorden Phillip,* 194, 384
Goren H. J., 382
Goriya Y., 351
Gormsen J., 91
Gorray Kenneth C., 402, 510
Goto Yoshio, 418
Grab Bernard, 4
Grabauskas Vili, 4
Graber Alan L.,* 112
Grammes Charles F.,* 183
Grant G. A., 46
Gray D. E., 58
Gray S., 63
Grechi A., 240
Greene D. A.,* 298
Greene K., 461
Greenfield M. S.,* 360
Greenway F. L.,* 286

Gregerson Estelle, 140
Greider Marie H.,* 37, 119
Gries F. Arnold, 303
Griffin J., 63
Grodsky G. M.,* 94, 429
Grogan W. M., 503, 504
Grossman Marshall K., 362
Groth C. G., 494
Grover-Johnson N.,* 293, 294
Gunnerson Rolf,* 494
Gunter-Hunt Gail, 106, 165
Gusberg Richard, 466
Gustafson A. B., 157
Gutai J.,* 178
Guthrie D. W.,* 257, 343
Guthrie R. A.,* 258

H

Hadji-Georgopoulos A., 409
Hagg S., 389
Halban P. A.,* 102, 151
Hall L., 162
Hall Susan E. H., 475
Halle Jean Pierre, 225
Halter Jeffrey B.,* 131, 156
Hamet Pavel,* 225
Hammond V., 189
Hanks J. B., 59
Hansen J., 213, 320
Häring H. U., 376
Harmon Joan T., 185
Harris, M. D., 378
Harris Maureen I.,* 169, 226
Harrison Len C.,* 149, 381
Hassinger Wieland, 238
Hauhart Richard E., 451
Hauner H., 495
Hausknecht R. U., 212
Hawkins Barbara, 501
Hayek A., 452
Haymond M.,* 214, 461
Heber D.,* 286
Heding Lise G.,* 176, 282
Hedo José A., 149
Heil J., 75
Heinemann M. A., 198
Heldt A., 429
Hellerström C.,* 494
Helms Brenda G., 345
Hendler Rosa,* 466, 491
Hendry Lawrence B., 287
Henze Kurt, 43
Hepp K. D., 495
Herberg L., 238
Herchuelz A., 405
Hernandez Carlos, 171, 331
Herron C. A., 174
Hess G., 346
Hess Randall L., 84, 273
Hester D. A., 117
Hetenyi G., Jr.,* 475
Hicks R. Anthony, 287
Hidaka H., 16
Hill Ronald S., 434
Hilman R., 295, 296
Hilsted Jannik, 91
Hinnen D.,* 133, 257
Hinnenkamp Marilyn, 398
Hirsch Harry, 37
Hiss Roland G., 260, 345
Hissin P. J., 369
Hodgson A., 94
Hoek J. B.,* 56
Hoffmann P. L., 10
Hogan M.,* 191
Holland N., 338
Hollander P.,* 213, 320
Hollingsworth D. R.,* 235, 378
Hom Frederick G.,* 131
Honey R. N., 100
Hoogwerf Byron J., 255
Horton E. D., 200
Horton E. S.,* 200
Horuk R., 349
Horwitz D. L.,* 107
Hoskins Beth,* 288
Hough Gerald, 256
Howard Barbara V.,* 16, 441
Howard Charles F., Jr.,* 517
Howard Margaret A., 138, 332
Howarth Teresa M., 184
Howey D. C.,* 160
Hoyrup A., 7
Hreidarsson A. B., 5
Hueckstead Tom, 155
Huff Thomas A.,* 287
Hurks C., 124
Hurwitz Linda,* 132
Hussey C., 457
Hustad J., 75
Huttunen Niilo-Pekka, 262

I

Iguchi Akihisa,* 60, 469
Ikeuchi Masatoshi, 281, 407
Imamura Yoshimichi, 192, 249
Imparato A. M., 293, 294
Imura Hiroo, 406
Ingle Elizabeth, 180
Insel Jonathan R., 63, 370
Ipp Eli,* 467
Ishibashi Fukashi, 441
Itoh M., 74, 422
Iwamoto Yasuhiko, 281
Iwasaki Makoto, 385

J

Jackson H. D., 508
Jacob Ralph, 466
James H., 392
Janka H. U.,* 313, 471
Janle-Swain Elsa,* 508
Jansson B., 443
Jarett Leonard,* 11, 359
Jarrett David B., 389
Jarrett R. J., 4
Jaspan Jonathan B.,* 219, 302
Jeanrenaud B.,* 50, 220
Jefferson L. S.,* 201
Jenkins J.,* 329
Johnson David G.,* 419
Johnson M. L., 185
Johnson Mark W., 250
Johnson Robert C., 118
Johnston D. G., 222
Jones M. R., 203
Jones M. Sue, 423
Jones R. S., 59
Jörgens Viktor, 108, 280
Joseph J., 442
Josephson Mark W., 292
Jovanovic L., 487
Juhlin-Dannfelt A., 164
Jung J. W., 135

K

Kahkonen Dorothy M.,* 111
Kahn Charles B.,* 472
Kahn C. Ronald,* 53, 185
Kahn Richard A., 52
Kakizaki Masaei, 418
Kalant N.,* 476
Kalkhoff R. K.,* 157
Kamdar Vikram,* 239, 375
Kanatsuna Takahiro, 145
Kanazawa Y.,* 407
Kanter Yoram,* 42, 300
Kaplan S. A.,* 82
Kappy Michael S.,* 251
Karaiskos K., 163
Karam J. H.,* 179, 271
Karl Richard C., 467
Karnieli E., 14, 369
Karp M.,* 317, 319
Kasim Sidika,* 291
Kasuga Masato,* 381
Katzeff Harvey, 383
Kaufman Ellen,* 391, 452
Kawara Akira, 248
Kawazu Shoji,* 407
Kayne Richard D., 251
Kazumi Tsutomu, 497
Keane N. A.,* 104
Keck Elmar, 356
Keen Harry, 4
Keller Helen, 268
Keller R. K., 456
Keller Ulrich,* 444
Kelly J., 98

Kemmer F. W., 58
Kemmler W., 376, 495
Kennedy A. Laurence, 276
Kennedy Annette L., 253
Keuer S., 182
Khan Zafar, 290
Khardori Romesh, 342
Khilnani S., 395
Kiechle Frederick L., 11, 359
Kikuchi M., 407
Kilo C.,* 46, 192
Kilpatrick J. M., 323, 324
Kim H. J.,* 9
King George L., 53
King J., 461
Kirk Katharine, 311
Kirk K. A., 104
Kissebah A.,* 457
Kitabchi Abbas E.,* 263, 393
Kitzmiller John,* 464
Klatt C., 121
Kloepfer H. G., 137
Knight A. B., 20
Knopf R.,* 346
Knowler William C.,* 227
Knowles Harvey C., Jr.,* 180, 501
Knox Gail F., 197
Kobayashi Masashi,* 385
Koenig Ronald, 85
Koerker Donna J., 131
Kohler Elaine,* 39, 132
Koivisto Veikko A.,* 103, 262
Kopelman P. G., 76
Kolterman Orville G.,* 63, 370
Kopple J. D., 203
Korn Adrienne, 350
Kosaka K., 281, 407
Koschinsky Theodor, 303
Kosmakos Frank C., 155, 387
Kosnik Edward, 270
Kotagal Nirmala, 11, 359
Kowaloff E., 366
Kowarski A. Avinoam, 127, 409
Kozlowski Stanislaw, 352
Knight A. B., 384
Kraemer F., 360
Krarup Thure, 90
Krasovsky Joseph, 478
Kraus B.,* 376, 495
Kraus P. F., 378
Krausz Yodphat, 96
Kreines Kenneth,* 224, 301
Krief Connie, 132
Kroeger S., 516
Krolewski A. S., 4
Kronenfeld Jennie J., 333
Krupin T., 2
Krzymien Janusz, 352
Kuberski T., 265
Kuebler T. W., 231
Kulwin R., 234
Kumar Dinesh,* 266, 513
Kurup I. V., 9
Kuwayti K., 246
Kuzuya Hideshi, 406
Kyner Joseph L.,* 208
Kyriakides George, 31

L

Lacina Samuel J., 88
Lacy Paul,* 30
Lacy W. W.,* 201, 215
La Grange B., 284
Landt M., 17
Lang Melvin S., 272
Langley Paul E., 462
Laporte R., 178
Larner J.,* 16
Laron Z.,* 317, 319
Larson R. E., 120
Laschansky Ellen C., 35
Lassmann V., 277
Laube H., 363
Lauger G., 341, 347
Lavau M., 460
Lavine Robert L.,* 485
Lavis V. R.,* 361
Layne E. C., 493
Lazurus N. R., 349
Lea S., 182
Leach W. J., 480
Leaming A. B., 450
Leapley Patricia M.,* 41
Lebovitz H. E.,* 59, 177
Lee John C.,* 499
Lee S., 68, 488
Lee Ying Shih, 281
Lefebvre Pierre J., 414
LeGonidec G., 265
Leichter Steven,* 83, 331
Leiter Edward H.,* 79, 144
Lernmark Åke,* 125, 145
Leslie R. D. G., 229
Leung Hélène, 225
Levene C., 22
Levin N. W., 367
Levin S. R.,* 82
Levine J. H.,* 450
Levine L., 216
Levine Lenore S.,* 306
Levitsky Lynne L.,* 88, 167
Lev-Ran Arye,* 242, 243
Lewis S. B.,* 86, 474
Librenti Maria C., 244
Lickley H. L. A.,* 58
Like Arthur A.,* 204, 314
Lilivivathana U.,* 196
Lim Frank, 67
Lindell D. V., 433
Linfoot John A.,* 312
Linfoot Peter A., 312
Lippe B. M.,* 82
Lipsett Lois, 173
Lipson Loren G.,* 267, 425
Lisse Jeffrey R., 227
Livingston J. N.,* 148
Lockwood Dean,* 49, 195
Lomatch D., 134
Lopes-Virella Maria F. L., 323
Lorenz Rodney A.,* 112
Lucas Stephenie M.,* 395
Ludvigsson Johnny, 176
Luqman W., 234
Luyckx Alfred S., 414

M

MacGorman L., 221
Mackes K., 461
Maclaren Noel,* 211
Madge G. E., 503
Madsbad Sten, 90, 158
Maegawa Hiroshi, 385
Maham D., 247
Maher T. D.,* 309
Mako M. E.,* 143, 284
Makoff Rhoda, 128
Malaisse W. J.,* 405, 440
Malchoff D., 195
Malchoff, D. M., 373
Maloff Bruce, 49
Malone John I.,* 197, 256
Malpica G. Blesa, 222
Mandarino L., 191, 422
Manley Cindy, 132
Margolis R. N., 32
Margolis Simeon,* 127, 409
Marieb N.,* 371
Marinan Barbara, 223
Mariz I. K., 19
Mark E. M., 212
Markand O., 231
Marliss E. B., 28
Marrero D., 27
Marshall Dauna, 368
Martin M. J., 284
Martin Marsha S., 62
Massague Joan, 186
Mateo De Acosta Oscar,* 4
Matschinsky Franz M.,* 408, 428
Matsuura Masaaki, 248
Matthews LeRoy W., 2
Mattis A., 241
Matz Robert,* 232
May D. C., 174
May James M.,* 47
Mazze R., 328, 496
McCarroll A. M.,* 396
McClaran Diane M., 260, 346
McDaniel Huey G.,* 458
McDonald J. M.,* 17

McEvoy Robert C.,* 505
McGee Jim, 263
McGuire E. A. H.,* 20
McKay L. David, 453
McKenzie Randolph A., 184
McPherson J., 18
McRae J. R., 33
Meda Paolo, 99
Medenica Maria, 302
Mehigan D., 409
Mehl Thomas, 276
Mehnert H.,* 313, 471
Meinert Curtis L., 501
Meistas Mary T., 127
Melluso G., 481, 482
Melton Terry W., 483, 498
Mensing Carole', 21
Menth Lois, 254
Merimee Thomas J.,* 276
Merrill G., 380
Metz S. A.,* 156
Mezzogiorno V., 481, 482
Michalski R. E., 142, 206
Micossi Piero,* 240, 244
Miki Eishi, 4
Miles J.,* 214
Miller Donald, 377
Miller Joshua, 31
Miller J. P., 26
Miller Leona V.,* 105, 172
Miller Ralph E.,* 423
Mills Mary Etta C., 23
Mintz Daniel H.,* 31, 73
Miraglio Angela, 341, 347
Mircheff Austin C., 425
Mohan Chandra, 375
Molnar G. D.,* 81
Mondon C. E.,* 446
Montalbert-Smith M., 459
Moore Darlene, 267
Moore E. G., 107
Moore Edwin G., 278
Moore W., 234
Moossa A., 219
Mordes John P., 204, 514
Morita Saidrio, 357
Morris Lawrence,* 263
Mosier Marjorie A.,* 228
Moss James M.,* 233
Moss N. S., 122
Motl G., 247
Mott David M.,* 155, 383
Moulin J. P., 277
Moulopoulos S., 163
Mousel K. A., 119
Mouton S., 65
Moxley R. T., 148
Muchmore Douglas B., 354
Mueller W., 236
Murphy E., 56
Murphy E. Dennis, 489
Murphy J., 496
Murray R.,* 457
Myers G.,* 27, 230

N

Nagulesparan Murugasu,* 253
Najarian John,* 75, 254
Naji Ali, 207, 408
Nakagawa Jeanette S., 312
Nakawatase C., 218
Nava Manuel, 252
Nebbia Judy, 400
Nechemias C.,* 212
Negrati M., 240
Nelson J. D., 28
Neville R. W. J., 349
New Maria I.,* 306
Nichols Wilmer W., 458
Nickoloff Eileen, 398, 399
Nielsen David A., 125
Nielsen J. D., 91
Nieman L. K., 364
Nikkilä Esko A., 262
Nishikawa Kazunori, 248
Nist Claudine, 35
Norbiato Guido, 240, 244
Nordberg Beatrice, 23
Norton J. A., Jr., 231
Norwich K. H., 403
Notkins A. L., 212
Nowotny Peter, 350
Nudleman K., 230

O

Oberfield Sharon E., 306
O'Doherty J., 424
O'Dorisio T., 92
Oh William, 472
Ohki Atsushi, 357, 497
Oie Herbert K., 187, 430
Okamoto Takeshi, 418
Olansky Leann, 62
Olefsky J. M.,* 63, 154
Olson Les, 31
O'Malley B. C.,* 456
Ono Junko, 31
Oram Jack, 479
Orchard Trevor J., 326
Orci Lelio,* 99, 194
Orloff M. J.,* 68, 488
Orosz Susan E., 301
Orr D., 27
Ørskov Hans, 158, 222
Ory Marcia G., 333
Orzeck Eric A.,* 484
Ostman Jan,* 358, 443
O'Sullivan D.,* 264
Otsuki Makoto, 357, 497
Owens D. R., 282
Oyama Hideki, 37
Oyama J., 446
Ozuk B. A., 122

P

Pace Caroline,* 95, 416
Paik Sang-gi, 205
Palazzolo M., 18
Palmer J., 366
Palmer J. P.,* 213, 320
Pang Songja, 306
Panjwani N. A., 410
Pansini A. R., 401
Papa M.,* 481, 482
Papaccio G., 481
Papatheodorou Noreen, 338, 339
Paquette Thomas L., 130, 426
Pardridge William M.,* 190, 203
Park R., 480
Parker D., 395
Parker John W., 513
Parker L., 165
Parker Lisa, 106
Patel D. G.,* 309
Pawelek John M., 52
Pecoraro R., 320
Peghini M., 265
Peller Janet, 217
Penhos J. C.,* 459
Pennington Floyd C., 22, 260
Perez G.,* 58
Perlman K., 490
Permutt Alan,* 37, 93
Perrelet Alain, 99
Pershadsingh H. A., 17
Peterson Charles,* 137
Peterson C. M.,* 487
Peth Steven B., 84, 273
Petrack Barbara,* 420
Pettitt David J., 227
Pfaffman M. A.,* 295, 296
Pfeifer Michael A.,* 310, 510
Philippe J., 151
Phillips Lawrence R., 78
Phillips Lawrence S.,* 54
Phillips Robert W.,* 315, 435
Pichert James W., 112
Piepho S. L., 137
Pietri Angel, 36
Pilch Paul F., 186
Piron M. A., 193
Pi-Sunyer F. Xavier,* 421, 460
Pitts J., 193
Piwernetz K., 495
Platt Gerald, 172
Plotnick Leslie P.,* 251
Podolsky Stephen,* 279
Pohl Donald P., 448
Pohl M. N., 502

Pohl S.,* 448
Pohl Stephen L.,* 62
Pointer R. H.,* 374
Polak Julia M., 115
Policova Z., 403
Pollak Carol, 167
Pollavini Giorgio, 244
Polonsky K., 219
Poole J. R., 86, 135
Pope Alice M., 267
Popp Dennis A., 11, 359
Porte Daniel, Jr.,* 126, 427
Pottick L. A., 148
Potts John E.,* 272
Poussier P., 74
Poznanski W. J.,* 245, 246
Prentki M., 50
Puckett Steve W., 470
Pugh W., 219
Puklin J., 69
Puricelli M., 40
Putnam W. S., 59
Pyke D. A., 229

Q

Quibrera Ricardo,* 252

R

Rabin Bruce S., 326
Rabinovitch Alexander,* 31, 73
Raggi Umberto, 240, 244
Rainbow Sandra, 282
Rajotte R. V.,* 72, 81
Ramamurthy N., 7
Rambis T., 461
Ramey E. R.,* 459
Rand K., 211
Rannels S. R., 201
Rao Gundu H. R., 217
Raptis S., 163
Rasheed Suraja, 513
Raskin Philip,* 36
Rasmussen Howard, 467
Rath Anne M., 167
Ratzmann K. P., 161
Rawlings S., 166
Rayfield Elliot J.,* 61, 509
Reach G., 74
Reaven Eve P.,* 161, 413
Reaven G. M.,* 159, 360
Recant Lillian,* 187, 430
Rechler M. M., 20
Reddy William J.,* 470
Regeur Lisbeth, 90, 158
Reiss Gwenn, 243
Rendell Marc,* 398, 399
Renner R., 495
Rennick B. R., 364
Renold A. E.,* 97
Rescigno A., 382
Rhodes Anne, 110
Rhoten William B.,* 434
Riales Rebecca, 449
Rigg L.,* 259
Rignew Jeanette L., 66
Riles T. S., 293, 294
Riley William, 70, 211
Rittel W., 193
Rizza R.,* 162, 221
Robbins D. C., 143, 284
Robertson G. L., 196
Robertson R. P.,* 33
Rodger N. Wilson,* 29
Rodman Harvey M.,* 2, 3
Rogell Gerald D.,* 297
Rogol Alan, 483
Rogus Ellen M.,* 372
Roi L., 134
Romanus J. A., 20
Root Allen W., 256
Rose S. J., 374
Roseman Jeffrey,* 170, 311
Rosen Ora M.,* 51
Rosen S., 328, 496
Rosen Sam, 51
Rosenbloom Arlan L.,* 70, 261
Rosenblum I. Y.,* 236, 237
Rosenquist Robert J.,* 267
Rosenthal J., 163
Ross Stuart A.,* 353, 404
Rossini Aldo A.,* 204, 514
Rotensterich Ely, 42
Roth Jesse,* 149
Roth L., 309
Roth M. D., 206
Rouiller D., 473
Rowold E. A., 46
Roy Mark W., 423
Rubenstein A. H.,* 143, 465
Rubin Charles, 51
Rubinovich Berta, 42
Rubinstein P., 212
Ruby R.,* 286
Rudolph Mary C., 274
Rudolf M., 210
Rumple F. C., 81
Runyan K. R., 198
Ryan Will G.,* 291
Ryder Steven W., 432
Rygaard Jorgen, 209
Ryzlak M. T., 442

S

Sabir A. M., 120
Sachse G., 363
Sagel J., 323
Sakai Hideyo, 192, 249
Sakamoto Choitsu, 357, 497
Sakurai Hideo,* 406
Salans L. B.,* 14, 369
Salas M., 326
Saltman R., 147
Sammons D. W., 146
Samols E.,* 101
Sando H., 281, 407
Santeusanio Fausto, 438, 439
Santiago J. V.,* 92, 283
Sanusi Jemi, 392
Sargeant D. T.,* 177, 259
Sarson D. L., 76
Sarver Sue, 332
Saudek Christopher,* 478
Sauer Gottfried, 238
Saunders C., 234
Sausse A., 74
Savage P. J.,* 134
Sayers H. J.,* 68, 488
Scanlon Edward F., 489
Schade D. S.,* 71, 486
Schane N., 463
Scharp D. W.,* 72, 119
Schifmann R., 55
Schilling E. E., 20
Schliack Volker, 4
Schlichtkrull Jørgen,* 209
Schmid F., 94
Schmitt J. K., 86, 271
Schneider S. H.,* 160
Schneir M., 7
Scholz T. D., 54
Scholz-Thielen Edith, 108
Schrage Jon Paul, 462
Schudt C., 376
Schultz T. A.,* 135
Schulz B., 161
Schusdziarra V.,* 473
Schwartz Robert,* 472
Schwartz S. S.,* 298
Scott Clarrisa S., 24
Seals Jonathan R., 12
Seemayer T. A., 500
Seigler H. F., 121
Seino Susumu, 406
Seino Yutaka,* 126, 406
Selawry H. P.,* 32, 165
Sener A., 440
Senhauser Donald A., 511
Sens D. A., 450
Sestoft L.,* 91
Seto Y., 509
Severson D. L., 353
Sewell J. J., 122
Seydoux J., 220
Shah J. H.,* 124
Shamoon Harry,* 77
Shanahan M. F.,* 15
Shannon W. Allen, Jr., 507
Shapiro Larry, 66
Sharma Hari M., 511
Sharp Geoffrey W. G.,* 96, 97

Sheftel D., 107
Sherwin R.,* 69, 491
Shigeta Yukio, 385
Shih J. C., 122
Shii Kosui, 192, 249
Shikama H., 64
Shim Chull, 511
Shin Seung-il, 205
Siddiqui Y, 415
Siegal R., 317
Siegel E. G., 97
Silverstein Janet H., 70, 261
Silvestri J. G., Sr., 105
Simmons Richard, 254
Simon J., 193
Simonds John F., 166
Simonin M. J., 277
Simonowitz David A., 35
Sims E. A.,* 454
Singerman Lawerence J., 3
Sinha Madhur A., 66, 396
Sirek A., 45, 403
Sirek O. V.,* 45, 403
Skyler Jay S.,* 24, 168
Slonim Alfred W.,* 129
Smith Charles J., 51
Smith Douglas, 371
Smith Francoise J., 417
Smith M., 234
Smith Ora L. K.,* 13, 355
Smith Phillip H., 419
Smith Robert J., 202
Smith Stewart S., 430
Smith Ulf,* 394
Smoake A., 18
Sochalski Julie A., 345
Sodoyez J. C.,* 379
Sodoyez-Goffaux F. R., 379
Soeldner J. Stuart,* 85, 87
Soler N. G.,* 247
Solomon Solomon S.,* 18, 198
Soloveitzic Lea, 42
Soltani Keyoumars, 302
Soman Vijay,* 52, 491
Sönksen P. H.,* 349
Sonnenberg Gabriele E., 444
Sorenson R. L.,* 433
Sotos Juan,* 92, 270
Spangler Ronald S., 435
Spear Gerald S.,* 512
Spencer E. Martin, 368
Spencer M.,* 165
Spencer Martha,* 106
Spencer W., 71
Sperling Mark A.,* 66, 397
Spielman Richard S., 321, 325
Spiro R. G.,* 410
Springer G.,* 113
Spritz Norton,* 223
Stacpoole Peter W.,* 477
Stagner J., 101
Standl E., 313, 471
Stark R. J., 424
Starke Achim, 356
Starkey Ralph H.,* 183
Stauffacher Werner,* 444
Steffes M. W.,* 5, 411
Stein Leslie J., 453
Steiner Donald F.,* 125, 145
Steiner K., 65
Stephens John W.,* 342
Sterman Robert, 333
Stevens B., 124
Stone D., 349
Strack Inge, 400
Straube R., 107
Strickland William G., 57
Strobel C. T., 82
Strodtman Linda K.,* 138, 139
Stroupe Stephen D., 278
Sullivan P.,* 264
Suminoe Keiko, 248
Sun Anthony M.,* 67
Sunovar Stephen G., 172
Surber Melanie J., 129
Suren J. V.,* 338, 339
Susa John B., 472
Suther C., 137
Sutherland David,* 75, 254
Svedberg J., 363
Swank G., 456
Swartz F. J., 502
Swartzman J., 6
Szabo Andrew J.,* 60, 469
Szalapski Edward, 254
Szczepanska-Sadowska Ewa, 352

T

Taborsky Gerald J., Jr., 35, 426
Tager H. S., 143
Tai J., 492, 516
Takeda Masahiko, 248
Tamagna E.,* 266
Tamborlane W.,* 69, 401
Tan M. H.,* 141
Tanigawa Keiichiro, 406
Tannenbaum G. S., 500
Tepler Jeff, 466
Teschemacher H., 363
Teuscher Arthur,* 4
Thaler Kenneth, 239
Thibert Pierre, 511
Thiry-Moris Y. M., 379
Thomas L. J., 493
Thompson, D. A., 196
Thompson R., 142
Thonnart N., 405
Thorp Frank K.,* 341, 347
Thurston Jean H.,* 451
Tillinghast J., 283
Tilton R. G., 10
Timson C. M., 115
Tobey T., 360
Todd Flona J., 267
Tollaksen S. L., 146
Tolman E. L.,* 401
Topper E., 317
Tornheim Patricia A., 224, 301
Tosco Clara, 513
Townsend Samuel F., 301
Toyota Takayoshi,* 418
Travis L. B.,* 1, 318
Trivedi B., 19
Tronier Bente, 158
Truax T., 134
Tsai Michael Y., 292
Tsalikian E.,* 178, 275
Tsuda Kinsuke, 406
Turner Anne L., 112
Tutwiler G. F.,* 442
Tzagournis Manuel,* 511
Tze W. J., 492, 516

U

Uenoyama Rinzo, 248
Uitto J., 46
Umeda Fumio, 225
Unger Roger H.,* 36, 473
Unterman T., 107
Usher Patricia, 193

V

Vague P.,* 277
Valdes I., 142
Valenta Lubomir J.,* 362, 455
Valeriano G., 275
Valtysson G., 114
Vanhelder T., 403
Vanhelder W. P., 403
Van Obberghen Emmanuel,* 194, 381
Vasington Paul, 67
Velayo N., 396, 397
Venckus Eileen, 167
Venkatachalam K. K., 367
Vermitsky Kathleen, 421
Verronneau Mavis, 334
Verspohl Eugen J., 388
Vervaert C., 121
Vialettes B., 277
Viberti G., 240
Vignati Louis,* 464
Villar Hugo V., 419
Vinicor Frank,* 152, 231
Vinik A. I.,* 114
Virella G., 323, 324
Vitullo Dolores A., 88
Vlachokosta Fredericka,* 85, 464
Voina S., 396, 397
Vranic M.,* 58
Vydelingum N.,* 457

W

Wagener Diane K., 326
Waheed I., 245
Wahren John, 164, 431
Waite A. T., 122
Waldhäusl Werner K.,* 350
Walker Beth, 166
Walker Wilmer, 413
Walsh S. B., 509
Waltman Stephen, 2
Ward R., 320
Wardzala L. J., 200
Warren-Boulton E., 113
Wasada Taro, 36
Webb C., 329
Webb S. R.,* 503, 504
Wedman Betty, 348
Weidman E. R.,* 361
Weill Victoria A., 428
Weiner L., 443
Weir Gordon C.,* 100, 123
Wejksnora Peter, 51
Welle S., 196
Wells Joy, 170
Wentworth S.,* 424
Weringer Elora J.,* 8
Werner John C., 499
West David B., 126
West K. M.,* 4
Westland R., 162
Westmoreland Nelson, 315
Wheeler F. C., 335
White James G., 217
White Jeannette, 167
White N.,* 259
White N., 92
Whitehouse Fred, 25
Whitehouse Iris J.,* 111
Whitney D., 493
Whittaker J., 189
Whitty A. J., 307
Wicklmayr M., 55
Wider M. D., 307
Wieland Ralph G.,* 250
Wiley F. M., 339
Wilkins Samuel D., 430
Williams John R., Jr.,* 38, 241
Williams J. T., 392
Williams P., 65
Williams P. E., 201
Williams R. Michael,* 204
Williamson John R.,* 56, 192
Williamson Joseph R.,* 10, 46
Willms B.,* 363
Wilson G., 327
Wilson G. L., 454
Wilson H., 182
Wilson Thomas, 498
Windsor Richard A., 333
Winegrad A. I.,* 298
Wise Curtis, 390
Wohltmann H., 323
Wolfe Robert R.,* 468
Wollheim C. B., 97, 102
Wollmer A., 349
Woods Stephen C.,* 126, 453
Woodside W. F., 452
Wornell C., 141
Wright James R., Jr., 511
Wright R. K., 198
Wurzel Harold A., 325
Wylie J.,* 328
Wyse B. M., 386

Y

Yajima Motoyuki, 418
Yalow Rosalyn S.,* 432
Yamada K., 381
Yassur Y., 317
Yasuda Keigo, 393
Yates Allan J., 511
Yen S. S. C., 235, 378
Yokono Koichi, 192, 249
Yoon Aeree, 425
Yoon Ji-Won, 392
Yoshino Gen, 497
Young C.,* 368
Young C. W.,* 179
Young Nancy L., 478
Younger Donna M.,* 464
Yung Cheuk Wo, 302
Yuu Hosai, 357

Z

Zadik Zvi, 127
Zamir R., 319
Zanaboni Laura, 244
Zarriello Joan, 398, 399
Zawalich Walter S.,* 428
Zeidler Adina,* 513
Zeytin I. Y., 436
Zierler Kenneth, 372
Zimmermann Horst, 356
Zimmet P., 265
Zinman Bernard,* 28
Zitron I. M., 30
Zmachinski C. J., 123
Zmijewski Chester M., 321, 325
Zoupas Chr., 163
Zuhlke H., 494

Notes